Language Intervention Strategies in Aphasia and Related Neurogenic Communication Disorders

FIFTH EDITION

Language Intervention Strategies in Aphasia and Related Neurogenic Communication Disorders

FIFTH EDITION

Editor

Roberta Chapey, Ed.D.

Professor
Department of Speech Communication Arts and Sciences
Brooklyn College
The City University of New York
Brooklyn, New York

Wolters Kluwer | Lippincott Williams & Wilkins
Health
Philadelphia · Baltimore · New York · London
Buenos Aires · Hong Kong · Sydney · Tokyo

Editor: Peter Sabatini
Managing Editor: Lisa Koepenick / Kevin C. Dietz
Marketing Manager: Allison Noplock
Compositor: Aptara, Inc.
Printer: RRD-Willard

First Edition, 1981
Second Edition, 1986
Third Edition, 1994
Fourth Edition, 2001

Library of Congress Cataloging-in-Publication Data

Language intervention strategies in aphasia and related neurogenic
communication disorders / editor, Roberta Chapey. — 5th ed.
    p. ; cm.
 Includes bibliographical references and indexes.
  ISBN-13: 978-0-7817-6981-5 (hardcover)
  ISBN-10: 0-7817-6981-7 (hardcover)
 1. Aphasia—Treatment. 2. Language disorders—Treatment. I. Chapey,
Roberta.
  [DNLM: 1. Aphasia—therapy. 2. Language Disorders—therapy. 3.
Language Therapy—methods. 4. Speech Disorders—therapy. WL 340.5
L2872 2008]
  RC425.L37 2008
  616.85'5206—dc22

                                                          2007038506

To purchase additional copies of this book, call our customer service department at **(800) 638-3030** or fax
orders to **(301) 824-7390**. International customers should call **(301) 714-2324**.

To the memory of my dad,
Robert (Bob) Chapey,
for his boundless generosity, kindness, love,
understanding, tolerance, support, humanness,
and humor—and for his truly brilliant strategies
for living. He was a super parent.

R.C.

Preface

Welcome to the fifth edition of *Language Intervention Strategies in Aphasia and Related Neurogenic Communication Disorders*. The first edition of this book was published in 1981, the second in 1986, the third in 1994, and the fourth in 2001. All four editions grew out of the realization that the discussion of aphasia therapy had become a major theme in clinical aphasiology literature but that the specification of numerous types or strategies of intervention was of fairly recent origin.

All five texts grew out of the belief that there continues to be a substantial number of approaches applicable to the remediation of language-disordered adults that should be brought together and shared. The five texts are also grounded in the realization that a variety of different therapeutic principles and approaches need to be articulated, assembled, applied, and critiqued in order to strengthen the quality of future work in our field.

The major purpose of the fifth edition is to bring together significant thoughts on intervention and to stimulate further developments in the remediation of adults with aphasia. It should be noted that some of the models presented in this text still need to be supported by controlled studies and long-term clinical application.

Each edition of this text is increasingly informed by the view that language is cognitively based (Chapey, 2008) and socially constructed by participants communicating with someone, about something, for some reason; and that judgments of competence/incompetence involve evaluations about issues such as role, context, intent, timing, volume, movements, intonation, gender, age, taste, group membership, etc. (Bloom and Lahey, 1988; Kovarsky, Duchan, and Maxwell, 1999). In addition, the **dual goals of communication**—that of **transaction** or the exchange of information and that of **interaction** or the fulfillment of social needs (such as affiliation with other people, assertion of individuality, demonstration of competence, gaining and maintaining membership in social circles, etc. (Simmons-Mackie, 2008) are increasingly reflected in the texts.

Further, the texts increasingly reflect the fact that we have a responsibility to individuals with aphasia and their significant others to foster their membership in a communicating society and their participation in personally relevant activities (Simmons-Mackie, 2008). The texts also emphasize the belief that **two of the most important factors in positive human health** for all individuals are living a life of purpose and quality connection to others.

The fifth edition contains 36 chapters organized into five sections. **Section I** covers basic considerations such as definitions of aphasia and stroke, incidence of stroke, the neural basis of language disorders, medical aspects of stroke, and the assessment of language disorders in adults.

Section II contains five chapters on principles of language intervention such as research methods appropriate to our field, treatment recovery, prognosis, and clinical effectiveness, teams and partnerships in clinical practice, as well as treatment of bilingual and bicultrurally diverse individuals. A number of issues related to service delivery are discussed.

Section III contains five chapters on psychosocial and functional approaches to intervention—models that focus on improving ability to perform communication activities of daily living. Such approaches consider the impact of aphasia on the well-being of the individual, their family, and the environment.

Section IV, the largest section, covers 'Traditional Approaches to Language Intervention.' It is divided into four units containing seven stimulation approaches, four cognitive neuropsycological and four neurolinguistic approaches, and three 'specialized' interventions.

Section V provides suggestions for remediation of disorders that frequently accompany aphasia or are related to or confused with aphasia; namely, traumatic brain injury, right hemisphere damage, dementia, apraxia, and dysarthria.

The chapters can be read in any order. In addition, all the chapters do not need to be read at one time. For example, when I teach our graduate course in adult aphasia, I typically use about 12 to 15 chapters as a core, and then refer to other chapters as they come up in class discussions, presentations or term papers, and/or when students ask questions about a specific individual that they are observing or working with in clinical practicum. I use the remaining chapters to give additional options, depth, and resources for actual work with individuals affected by aphasia.

Language Intervention Strategies in Aphasia and Related Neurogenic Communication Disorders—Fifth Edition can be used in classes for advanced undergraduate and graduate students in speech language pathology. Clinical aphasiologists who are no longer formal students, but who desire to keep abreast of new ideas in their field will also find the material of interest. Further, the material will be valuable to students and professionals in nursing, medicine, and other health-related disciplines.

Roberta Chapey,
Ed.D. Professor

References

Bloom, L., and Lahey, M. (1988), *Language Disorders and Language Development*. New York: Macmillan.

Chapey, R. (2008). Cognitive Stimulation: Stimulation of Recognition/Comprehension, Memory, Convergent Thinking, Divergent and Evaluative Thinking. In R. Chapey (Ed.)., *Language Intervention Strategies in Aphasia and Related Neurogenic Communication Disorders*—Fifth Ed. Baltimore, MD.: Lippincot Williams and Wilkins.

Kovarsky, D., Duchan, J. and Maxwell, M. (1999). *Constructing (In) Competence. Disabling Evaluations in Clinical and Social Interaction*. Mahwah, NJ: Lawrence Erlbaum.

Simmons-Mackie, N. (2008). Social approaches to aphasia intervention. In R. Chapey (Ed.)., *Language Intervention Strategies in Aphasia and Related Neurogenic Communication Disorders*—Fifth Ed. Baltimore, MD.: Lippincott Williams and Wilkins.

Acknowledgments

To those who have contributed to my personal life and professional career, past and present, I express my deep appreciation. I am also grateful to the authors and publishers who granted me permission to quote from their works.

Many concerned and dedicated people have helped bring this textbook to fruition. Sincere appreciation is extended to each. Special thanks are extended to Argye E. (Beth) Hillis for her professionalism and enthusiasm in organizing the section on cognitive neuropsychology. As editor, I would especially like to thank each contributor for helping to make this text a kaleidoscope of enriching and rewarding experiences for me as well as for each of our patients. I am deeply appreciative of their caring and support and for many "one and only moments" of connection.

I am also thankful to the staff of Lippincott Williams & Wilkins for their dedication to making this a first rate text and for facilitating so many relentless details of this project. For the tireless support and help, I thank Peter Sabatini, Acquisitions Editor; Lisa Koepenick, Managing Editor; and Susan Katz, Vice President, Health Professions.

Contributors

Donna L. Bandur, MCISc
Profession Leader
Speech-Language Pathology
London Health Sciences Centre
London, Ontario, Canada

Kathryn A. Bayles, PhD
Professor-Emerita
Department of Speech, Language and Hearing Sciences
The University of Arizona

Pelagie M. Beeson, PhD, CCC-SLP
Associate Professor
Department of Speech, Language, and Hearing Sciences
Department of Neurology
The University of Arizona
Tucson, Arizona

Rita Sloan Berndt, PhD
Professor
Department of Neurology
University of Maryland School of Medicine
Baltimore, Maryland

Margaret Lehman Blake, PhD
Assistant Professor
Department of Communication Sciences and Disorders
University of Houston
Houston, Texas

Roberta Chapey, EdD
Professor
Department of Speech Communication Arts and Sciences
Brooklyn College
City University of New York
Brooklyn, New York

Leora R. Cherney, PhD, BC-ANCDS
Associate Professor
Physical Medicine and Rehabilitation
Northwestern University, Feinberg School of Medicine
Clinical Research Scientist
Center for Aphasia Research
Rehabilitation Institute of Chicago
Chicago, Illinois

Carl A. Coelho, PhD
Professor and Head
Communication Sciences
University of Connecticut
Storrs, Connecticut

Hanna Damasio, MD
Dana Dornsife Professor of Neuroscience and
Director, Dana & David Dornsife Cognitive Neuroscience
    Imaging Center,
University of Southern California
Los Angeles

Judith F. Duchan, PhD, CCC
Professor
Department of Communicative Disorders
    and Sciences
State University of New York at Buffalo
Buffalo, New York

Joseph R. Duffy, PhD
Professor
Consultant and Head
Division of Speech Pathology
Department of Neurology
Mayo Clinic College of Medicing
Rochester, Minnesota

Roberta J. Elman, PhD, CCC-SLP, BC-ANCDS
President/Founder
Aphasia Center of California
Oakland, California

Timothy J. Feeney, PhD
School of Community Supports
Project Director
NYS Neurobehavioral Resource Project
New York, New York

Linda J. Garcia, PhD
Associate Professor and Chair
Audiology and Speech-Language Pathology
    Program
University of Ottawa
Ottawa, Ontario, Canada

April Gibbs Scott, MS, CCC-SLP
PhD Student
Department of Communication Science and
    Disorders
University of Pittsburgh
Pittsburgh, Pennsylvania

Lee Ann C. Golper, PhD
Associate Professor
Department of Hearing and Speech Sciences
Vanderbilt University
Nashville, Tennessee

Brooke Hallowell, PhD
Director
School of Hearing, Speech and Language Sciences
Associate Dean
College of Health and Human Services
Ohio University
Athens, Ohio

Maya L. Henry, MS, CCC-SLP
Department of Speech, Language, and Hearing
    Sciences
University of Arizona, Tucson, AZ

Argye Elizabeth Hillis, MD, MA
Professor of Neurology, Physical Medicine and
    Rehabilitation, and Cognitive Science
Executive Vice Chair, Department of Neurology
Director, Neurology Residency Program
Co-Director, Cerebrovascular Division
Johns Hopkins University School of Medicine
Baltimore, Maryland

Tammy Hopper, PhD
Assistant Professor
Department of Speech Pathology and Audiology
University of Alberta
Edmonton, Alberta, Canada

Karen Hux, PhD
Associate Professor
Special Education and Communication Disorders
University of Nebraska at Lincoln
Lincoln, Nebraska

Aura Kagan, PhD, Reg CASLPO, S-LP (C)
Program, Research, and Education Director
The Aphasia Institute
Toronto, Ontario, Canada

Richard C. Katz, PhD
Chair
Audiology and Speech Pathology Department
Carl T. Hayden VA Medical Center
Phoenix, Arizona
Adjunct Professor
Department of Speech and Hearing Science
Arizona State University
Tempe, Arizona

Kevin P. Kearns, PhD
Professor and Director
Communication Sciences and Disorders
Massachusetts General Hospital Institute of Health
    Professions
Boston, Massachusetts

Rosemary B. Lubinski, EdD
Professor
Department of Communication Disorders and Sciences
University of Buffalo
Buffalo, New York

Jon G. Lyon, PhD, CCC-SLP
Director
Living with Aphasia, Inc
Mazomanie, Wisconsin

Robert C. Marshall, PhD
Professor
Rehabilitation Sciences
University of Kentucky
Lexington, Kentucky

Malcolm R. McNeil, PhD
Distinguished Service Professor and Chair
Department of Communication Science
    and Disorders
University of Pittsburgh
Research Scientist
Speech Motor, Aphasia, Cognition Laboratory
    (SMAC)
VA Pittsburgh Healthcare System
Pittsburgh, Pennsylvania

E. Jeffrey Metter, MD
Medical Officer
Clinical Research Branch
National Institute On Aging
National Institutes of Health
Gerontology Research Center
Baltimore, Maryland

Charlotte C. Mitchum, MS, CCC-SLP
Research Associate
Department of Neurology
University of Maryland School of Medicine
Baltimore, Maryland

Anthony G. Mlcoch, PhD
Speech-Language Pathologist
Audiology and Speech Pathology Service
Hines Veterans Affairs Hospital
Hines, Illinois
and
Adjunct Professor of Neurology
Speech Pathology and Audiology
Stricht School of Medicine, Loyola University

Shirley Morganstein, MA, CCC-SLP
Partner
Speaking of Aphasia, LLC
Montclair, New Jersey

Penelope S. Myers, PhD
Speech Pathologist
Rochester, Minnesota

Stephen E. Nadeau, MD
Professor
Department of Neurology
University of Florida College of Medicine
Staff Neurologist
Geriatric Research, Education and Clinic
Malcolm Randall VA Medical Center
Gainesville, Florida

Melissa Newhart, BS
Research Assistant
Stroke and Cognitive Disorders Laboratory

Janet P. Pattersion, PhD
Associate Professor
Department of Communicative Sciences and Disorders
California State University East Bay
Hayward, California
Research Associate
Center for Aphasia and Related Diseases
VA Northern California
Martinez, California

Richard K. Peach, PhD
Professor
Otolaryngology, Neurological Sciences and
    Communication Disorders and Sciences
Rush University Medical Center
Chicago, Illinois

Bruce Earl Porch, PhD
Associate Professor
Speech and Hearing Sciences and Neurology
University of New Mexico
Albuquerque, New Mexico

Anastasia M. Raymer, PhD
Professor
Department of Early Childhood, Speech Pathology and
    Special Education
Old Dominion University
Norfolk, Virginia

Patricia M. Roberts, PhD
Associate Professor
Department of Health Sciences
University of Ottawa
Ottawa, Ontario, Canada

Randall R. Robey, PhD
Director
Communication Disorders Program
University of Virginia
Charlottesville, Virginia

John C. Rosenbek, PhD
Professor and Chair
Department of Communicative Disorders
University of Florida
Gainesville FL

Leslie J. Gonzalez Rothi, PhD
Professor
Department of Neurology
University of Florida
Program Director and Career Research
    Scientist
Brain Rehabilitation Research Center
Malcolm Randall VA Medical Center
Gainesville, Florida

Victoria L. Scharp, MS, CCC-SLP
PhD Student
Department of Communication Science and
    Disorders
University of Pittsburgh
Pittsburgh, Pennsylvania

Cynthia M. Shewan, PhD, CCC
Director, Research and Scientific Affairs
    Department
American Academy of Orthopaedic
    Surgeons
Rosemont, Illinois

Linda I. Shuster, PhD, CCC/SLP
Associate Professor
Department of Speech Pathology and Audiology
West Virginia University

Nina Simmons-Mackie, PhD
Professor and Scholar in Residence
Department of Communication Sciences and Disorders
Southeastern Louisiana University
Hammond, Louisiana

Michele Page Sinotte, MS, CCC-SLP
Communication Sciences Department
University of Connecticut
Storrs, Connecticut 06269-1085

Marilyn Certner Smith, MA, CCC-SLP
Partner
Speaking of Aphasia, LLC

Robert W. Sparks, MSc
Chief, Speech Pathology/Audiology (retired)
Veterans Affairs Medical Center
Boston, Massachusetts

Shirley F. Szekeres, PhD
Dean of Health and Human Services
Professor
Speech and Language Pathology
Nazareth College
Rochester, New York

Cynthia K. Thompson, PhD
Professor
Department of Communication Sciences and Disorders, and Neurology
Northwestern University
Evanston, Illinois

Connie A. Tompkins, PhD
Professor
Department of Communication Science and Disorders
University of Pittsburgh
Pittsburgh, Pennsylvania

Mark Ylvisaker, PhD
Professor
Department of Communication Sciences and Disorders
College of Saint Rose
Albany, New York

Sarah Wallace, MA, CCC-SLP
Doctoral Student
Special Education and Communication Disorders
University of Nebraska at Lincoln
Lincoln, Nebraska
Speech-Language Pathologist
Quality Living, Inc
Omaha, Nebraska

Julie L. Wambaugh, PhD, CCC/SLP
Associate Professor
Deptartment of Communication Sciences and Disorders
University of Utah
Researcher
VA Salt Lake City Healthcare System
Salt Lake City, UT, USA

Kristy S.E. Weissling, SLPD, CCC-SLP
Lecturer
Department of Special Education and Communication Disorders
University of Nebraska at Lincoln
Lincoln, Nebraska

Contents

Section I. **BASIC CONSIDERATIONS** 1

1 Introduction to Language Intervention
Strategies in Adult Aphasia 3
Brooke Hallowell and Roberta Chapey

2 Neural Basis of Language Disorders 20
Hanna Damasio

3 Medical Aspects of Stroke Rehabilitation 42
Anthony G. Mlcoch and E. Jeffrey Metter

4 Assessment of Language Disorders in Adults 64
Janet P. Patterson and Roberta Chapey

APPENDIX 4.1 Pre-interview or Referral
Form for Collecting Family and Medical
History and Status Information 153

APPENDIX 4.2 Examples of Auditory
Retention and Comprehension Tasks 158

APPENDIX 4.3 Various Tasks Used to Assess
Auditory Comprehension of Syntax 160

Section II. **PRINCIPLES OF LANGUAGE INTERVENTION** 161

5 Research Principles for the Clinician 163
Connie A. Tompkins, April Gibbs Scott, and Victoria L. Scharp

6 Aphasia Treatment: Recovery, Prognosis,
and Clinical Effectiveness 186
Leora R. Cherney and Randall R. Robey

7 Delivering Language Intervention Services to
Adults with Neurogenic Communication
Disorders 203
Brooke Hallowell and Roberta Chapey

8 Teams and Partnerships in Aphasia Intervention .. 229
Lee Ann C. Golper

9 Issues in Assessment and Treatment for
Bilingual and Culturally Diverse Patients 245
Patricia M. Roberts

APPENDIX 9.1 Addresses for Ordering Tests ... 275

Section III. **PSYCHOSOCIAL/FUNCTIONAL APPROACHES TO
INTERVENTION: FOCUS ON IMPROVING ABILITY TO
PERFORM COMMUNICATION ACTIVITIES OF DAILY
LIVING** 277

10 Life-Participation Approach to Aphasia:
A Statement of Values for the Future 279
Roberta Chapey, Judith F. Duchan, Roberta J.
Elman, Linda J. Garcia, Aura Kagan,
Jon G. Lyon, and Nina Simmons-Mackie

11 Social Approaches to Aphasia Intervention 290
Nina Simmons-Mackie

APPENDIX 11.1 Examples of Strategies for
Communication-Partners of People with Aphasia ... 318

APPENDIX 11.2 Advocacy Strategies for
Supporting Participation of the Person
with Aphasia 318

12 Environmental Approach to Adult Aphasia 319
Rosemary Lubinski

13 Focusing on the Consequences of Aphasia:
Helping Individuals Get What They Need 349
Linda J. Garcia

APPENDIX 13.1 Interview Guidelines for
Looking at Functioning 374

14 Group Therapy for Aphasia: Theoretical and
Practical Considerations 376
Kevin P. Kearns and Roberta J. Elman

Section IV. **TRADITIONAL APPROACHES TO LANGUAGE
INTERVENTION** 401

A. **STIMULATION APPROACHES**

15 Schuell's Stimulation Approach to Rehabilitation ... 403
Carl A. Coelho, Michele P. Sinotte, and Joseph R. Duffy

16 Thematic Language-Stimulation Therapy 450
Shirley Morganstein and Marilyn Certner-Smith

APPENDIX 16.1 Thematic Language
Stimulation (TLS) Unit on Books with
Instructions for Creating TLS Units 461

17 Cognitive Stimulation: Stimulation of Recognition/
    Comprehension, Memory, and Convergent,
    Divergent, and Evaluative Thinking 469
    Roberta Chapey

18 Early Management of Wernicke's Aphasia:
    A Context-Based Approach 507
    Robert C. Marshall

19 Rehabilitation of Subcortical Aphasia 530
    Stephen E. Nadeau and Leslie J. Gonzalez Rothi

20 Primary Progressive Aphasia and Apraxia of
    Speech 543
    Joseph R. Duffy and Malcolm R. McNeil

    APPENDIX 20.1 Information Resources 564

21 Global Aphasia: Indentification and Management . . 565
    Richard K. Peach

B. COGNITIVE NEUROPSYCHOLOGICAL APPROACHES TO
    TREATMENT OF LANGUAGE DISORDERS

22 Cognitive Neuropsychological Approaches to
    Treatment of Language Disorders:
    Introduction 595
    Argye E. Hillis and Melissa Newhart

    APPENDIX 22.1 Selected Interdisciplinary
    Centers for Aphasia Research and
    Rehabilitation 605

    APPENDIX 22.2 Glossary 606

23 Impairments of Word Comprehension and
    Production 607
    Anastasia M. Raymer and Leslie J. Gonzalez Rothi

    APPENDIX 23.1 Stimuli from the Florida
    Semantics Battery 630

    APPENDIX 23.2 Glossary 631

24 Comprehension and Production of
    Sentences 632
    Charlotte C. Mitchum and Rita Sloan Berndt

25 Comprehension and Production of Written
    Words 654
    Pelagie M. Beeson and Maya L. Henry

    APPENDIX 25.1 Johns Hopkins University
    Dyslexia and Dysgraphia Batteries 678

    APPENDIX 25.2 Rank Order of Phoneme
    Occurrences in Word Corpus and the Common
    Associated Graphemic Representations 687

    APPENDIX 25.3 Glossary 688

C. COGNITIVE NEUROLINGUISTIC APPROACHES TO
    THE TREATMENT OF LANGUAGE DISORDERS

26 Language Rehabilitation from a Neural
    Perspective 689
    Stephen E. Nadeau, Leslie J. Gonzalez Rothi, and
    Jay Rosenbek

27 Treatment of Syntactic and Morphologic
    Deficits in Agrammatic Aphasia: Treatment
    of Underlying Forms 735
    Cynthia K. Thompson

    APPENDIX 27.1 Treatment Protocols 754

28 Language-Oriented Treatment: A Psycholinguistic
    Approach to Aphasia 756
    Donna L. Bandur and Cynthia M. Shewan

    APPENDIX 28.1 Language-Oriented
    Treatment Goals Form 798

    APPENDIX 28.2 Language-Oriented
    Treatment Data Record Form 799

29 Treatment of Aphasia Subsequent to the Porch
    Index of Communicative Ability (PICA) 800
    Bruce E. Porch

D. SPECIALIZED INTERVENTIONS FOR PATIENTS
    WITH APHASIA

30 Communication-Based Interventions: Augmented
    and Alternative Communication for People
    with Aphasia 814
    Karen Hux, Kristy Weissling, and Sarah Wallace

31 Melodic Intonation Therapy 837
    Robert W. Sparks

32 Computer Applications in Aphasia Treatment 852
    Richard C. Katz

    APPENDIX 32.1 Clinical Examples 874

    APPENDIX 32.2 Sources for Software and
    Other Relevant Technology 875

    APPENDIX 32.3 Web Sites of Interest 876

Section V. **THERAPY FOR ASSOCIATED NEUROPATHOLOGIES OF SPEECH- AND LANGUAGE-RELATED FUNCTIONS** 877

33 Communication Disorders Associated with Traumatic Brain Injury 879
Mark Ylvisaker, Shirley F. Szekeres, and Timothy Feeney

APPENDIX 33.1 Aspects of Cognition 955

APPENDIX 33.2 Conventional Versus Functional Approaches to Intervention after Brain Injury: Communication, Behavior, and Cognition 956

APPENDIX 33.3 Examples of Compensatory Strategies for Individuals with Cognitive Impairments 958

APPENDIX 33.4 Rationale for Collaborative Relationships with Everyday People 960

APPENDIX 33.5 Communication-Partner Competencies for Supporting and Improving Cognition in Individuals with Cognitive Impairment 961

34 Communication Disorders Associated with Right-Hemisphere Damage 963
Penelope S. Myers and Margaret Lehman Blake

35 Management of Neurogenic Communication Disorders Associated with Dementia 988
Tammy Hopper and Kathryn A. Bayles

36 The Nature and Management of Neuromotor Speech Disorders Accompanying Aphasia 1009
Julie Wambaugh and Linda Shuster

APPENDIX 36.1 Consonant-Production Probe 1035

APPENDIX 36.2 Example of Lists of Balanced Multisyllabic Words 1036

APPENDIX 36.3 Examples of Sentence-Completion Items 1037

APPENDIX 36.4 Metronome and Hand-tapping Treatment 1039

APPENDIX 36.5 Eight-Step Continuum 1040

APPENDIX 36.6 Original Sound-Production Treatment Hierarchy 1040

APPENDIX 36.7 Modified Sound-Production Treatment 1041

APPENDIX 36.8 Modified Response Elaboration Training 1042

Author Index 1043

Subject Index 1073

Section I

Basic Considerations

Chapter 1

Introduction to Language Intervention Strategies in Adult Aphasia

Brooke Hallowell and
Roberta Chapey

OBJECTIVES

The objectives of this chapter are to present a concise and comprehensive definition of aphasia, consider appropriate ways to refer to individuals with aphasia, explore conceptual frameworks for study and clinical practice in aphasia, review key etiologic and epidemiological factors related to aphasia, highlight the interdisciplinary nature of aphasiology, present a rationale for language intervention for adults with neurogenic communication disorders, and address future trends in aphasiology.

The present text grew out of a desire to bring researchers and practitioners together in adult neurogenic communication disorders to present an accurate and coherent picture of current practice in language assessment and intervention and to make it available in useful form. Foremost is the desire to coalesce significant thoughts on language intervention, while stimulating further study concerning the effectiveness of the approaches presented.

Before proceeding with the discussion of specific intervention strategies, we will consider several general issues that are relevant to clinical aphasiology. In this chapter we consider a brief definition of aphasia; ways to refer to people with aphasia; frameworks for conceptualizing aphasia; etiology and epidemiology; the interdisciplinary nature of aphasia; the importance of appreciating the life-changing effects of aphasia; a rationale for intervention; and future trends in aphasiology.

APHASIA BRIEFLY DEFINED

The study of aphasia is complex because of the variable manifestations of aphasia, the heterogeneity of its underlying neurologicsubstrates, and the sophistication required to understand the mechanisms behind its associated symptomatology. Therefore, there are many ways of conceptualizing it. However, students and professionals interested in exploring the world of neurogenic communication disorders often need to be able to articulate a clear and concise definition of aphasia. Such a definition might be **"aphasia" is an acquired communication disorder caused by brain damage, characterized by an impairment of language modalities: speaking, listening, reading, and writing; it is not the result of a sensory or motor deficit, a general intellectual deficit, confusion, or a psychiatric disorder** (e.g., Brookshire, 1992; Darley, 1982; Goodglass, 1993).

What is critical to an adequate definition is the mention of four primary facts: it is neurogenic; it is acquired; it affects language; and it excludes general sensory and mental deficits.

1. **Aphasia is neurogenic.** Aphasia always results from some form of damage to the brain. The specific structures affected vary among cases, as do the means by which the damage may occur. Still, the underlying cause of aphasia is always neurologic. Aphasia is most often caused by stroke, but may also arise from head trauma, surgical removal of brain tissue, growth of brain tumors, or infections.
2. **Aphasia is acquired.** Aphasia is not characterized as a developmental disorder; an individual is not born with it. Rather, it is characterized by the partial or complete loss of language function in a person who had previously developed some language ability. It is important to note that most people with aphasia retain many linguistic abilities; many experience problems of reduced efficiency of formulation and/or production, reduced access to linguistic information still stored in the brain, and reduced retention of new linguistic information, not necessarily a complete lack of ability in any given area of language processing.

   The term "childhood aphasia" refers to an acquired language problem in children; it is not, by definition, applicable to children who never had language abilities to lose. (Childhood aphasia is not discussed in this text.) It should be noted, though, that children who have suffered neurologic incidents such as gunshot wounds, surgical removal of tumors, or even stroke, may develop a true form of "aphasia" if those incidents cause them to lose communication abilities they had gained earlier in life.

3. **Aphasia involves language problems.** Aphasia is often described as symbolic processing disorders, a multimodal problem of formulation and interpretation of linguistic symbols. In defining aphasia it is important to recognize that any or all modalities of symbolic communication may be affected: speaking, listening, reading, writing, and receptive and expressive use of sign language. Most cases involve at least some impairment in all language modalities.

4. **Aphasia is not a problem of sensation, motor function, or intellect.** Aphasia excludes general sensory and mental deficits. By definition, aphasia does not involve a problem of sight, touch, smell, hearing, or taste. Although aphasia may be *accompanied* by any number of other deficits in perceptual acuity, its definition excludes such deficits. Further, aphasia is not a result of general intellectual deterioration, mental slowing, or psychiatric disturbance. Aphasia is also not due to motor impairment. The exclusionary characteristics of the definition of aphasia are especially critical in the differential diagnosis of a wide array of neurogenic language, speech, cognitive, motor, and perceptual disorders.

A NOTE ON REFERRING TO PEOPLE WITH APHASIA

Before progressing with further study of aphasia and its management, it is important to note that the term "aphasic" is not a noun but an adjective, just as are most of the words we use to describe disabilities. While one might defend the stylistic use of the adjectival form as a label for a person who has aphasia ("an aphasic"), such labeling may convey a lack of respect for, and sensitivity toward, individuals who have aphasia (Brookshire, 2007).

Indeed, the World Health Organization (WHO) has launched worldwide efforts to modify the ways in which we refer to persons with disabilities, as discussed later in this and other chapters. The WHO classification emphasizes that disablement is not considered an attribute of an individual, but rather the complex interactions of conditions involving a person in the context of his or her social environment (WHO, 2001). Health-care professionals and researchers throughout the world are following suit by deemphasizing the reference to individuals according to medically based diagnostic categories, focusing instead on

their holistic functional concerns and what might be done to address them (Hallowell. 2007).

While, occasionally, the term "aphasic" may be used to refer to an "individual with aphasia" in the writings of diverse authors, there is a widespread movement among health care professionals to heighten sensitivity to individuals served by choosing terminology that does not objectify and label people primarily through their impairments or disabilities. Readers are encouraged to join this movement, and to help sensitize others to the importance of using person-first language. Guidelines for writing and talking about persons with aphasia and related disorders are summarized in Table 1–1.

CONCEPTUAL FRAMEWORKS OF APHASIA

Although it is simple to define the term "aphasia," there are a number of in-depth definitions or frameworks for studying the nature of aphasia. An understanding of basic differences among ways of conceptualizing aphasia is essential to developing a solid theoretical framework of one's own.

Propositional Language Framework

According to Hughling Jackson, aphasia is an impairment in one's ability to make propositions, or to convey the intent of an utterance (Jackson, 1878). In referring to the "propositional" aspects of language, Jackson emphasizes the intellectual, volitional, and rational aspects of language that involve the use of linguistic symbols for the communication of highly specific and appropriate ideas and relationships. In a proposition, both the words and the manner in which they are related to one another are important. Jackson contrasts propositional aspects of language with subpropositional aspects, which he characterizes as inferior, automatic, highly learned responses (Goodglass & Wingfield, 1997; Head, 1915; Jackson, 1878).

Within this framework, a person with aphasia is seen as having difficulty communicating specific meaning and integrating words into particular contexts to express specific ideas and relationships. Patients may know words, but may habitually use them incorrectly, and often fail at embedding words in a variety of sentence forms. Jackson noted that even when propositional language is impaired, many patients retain automatic language. For example, even with severe propositional deficits, an individual may be able to name the days of the week, complete sentences such as "The grass is _____," or produce highly learned responses such as "Hi. How are you?"

According to proponents of the framework, an individual with aphasia has an impairment in the use of spontaneous language to communicate *specific meaning*. The more propositional language required in a particular communication context, the more difficulty the patient has communicating.

TABLE 1–1

Guidelines for Writing and Talking about Persons with Aphasia and Related Disorders

Recognize the importance of currency and context in referring to individuals with disabilities.	There are always variances in the terms that particular consumers or readers prefer, and it is essential to stay current regarding changes in accepted terminology as well as to be sensitive to preferences for referents within a given communicative context.
Consider reference to "disabilities".	Although the very term "disability" may be considered offensive to some (with its inherent focus on a lack of ability), it is currently generally preferred over the term "handicap" in reference to persons with physical, cognitive, and/or psychological challenges or "disabilities".
Avoid using condition labels as nouns.	Many words conveying information about specific disabilities exist in both noun and adjectival forms, yet should primarily be used only as adjectives, or even better, modified into nouns corresponding to conditions. For example, it is not appropriate to call an individual with aphasia "an aphasic".[1] Likewise, it is not appropriate to call an individual with paraplegia "a paraplegic," or to call persons with disabilities "the disabled".
Use person-first language.	Person-first language helps emphasize the importance of the individuals mentioned rather than their disabilities. Although the term "an aphasic individual" would be preferred to the use of "an aphasic", such labeling still conveys a disability-focused identity. It is more appropriate, for example, to refer to a "person with anomia" or an "individual with dementia," than to an "anomic person" or a "demented individual".
Consider use of the term "individual" or "person" rather than "patient".	Consistent with the aim of focusing on individuals and their broad life contexts, rather than on people being treated in a medical context, use of the word "person" or "individual" is generally preferable to use of the term "patient". In some contexts, such as in academic texts and articles, when people with and without language disorders are being discussed, use of the term "patient" may help to provide clarity of referents and to simplify explanations. In some contexts, the term "client" or "consumer" may be preferred to "patient" when referring to a person who is receiving professional services.
Avoid language of victimization.	Do not use language suggesting that clients are "victims" or people who "suffer" from various forms of disability. For example, say, "the client had a stroke" rather than "the client is a stroke victim." Say, "She uses a wheelchair," rather than "she is confined to a wheelchair." Say "her leg was amputated . . . " instead of, "the client suffered an amputation of the leg".
Avoid words with negative connotations.	Words that evoke derogatory connotations should be avoided in every context. These include such words and phrases as affliction, crazy, crippled, defective, deformed, dumb, insane, invalid, lame, maimed, mute, retard, and withered.
Encourage others in appropriate language use.	By modeling appropriate language in writing about persons with disabilities, including those with language disorders, students, clinicians and researchers take an important step in helping others to improve in this area. It is vital to help others learn to implement guidelines such as these directly through course work and other educational experiences. Likewise, polite and constructive corrections of others using inaccurate language helps encourage more positive communication as well as more enabling positive societal attitudes, widening the arena for empowering persons with disabilities.

[1]Brookshire, R.H. (2007). *An introduction to neurogenic communications disorders.* St. Louis: Mosby – Year Book.
(Adapted from Hallowell, in press).

Assessment involves an analysis of the patient's ability to use spontaneous speech to express specific ideas. Intervention focuses on stimulation of the patient's ability to use propositional language.

Concrete-Abstract Framework

Goldstein and Scheerer (1948) observed that having an "abstract attitude" implies an ability to react to things in a conceptual manner. This attitude is necessary to isolate properties that are common to several objects, and for the formulation of concepts as opposed to sensory impressions of individual objects. It is also used to comprehend relationships between objects and events in the world. An abstract attitude gives the individual the power to inhibit actions or reactions and to use past experiences. These experiences help the individual organize perceptual rules and therefore to create and continue interactions with other people. Language that reflects an abstract attitude is propositional language. In contrast, the individual in the concrete attitude passively responds to reality and is bound to the immediate experience of objects and situations. Concrete language consists of speech automations, emotional utterances, sounds, words, and series of words (Goldstein & Scheerer, 1948).

In general, impairment in abstract attitude is reflected in propositional language. If one cannot abstract, one cannot symbolize or embed symbols in appropriate contexts. An individual who is impaired in abstract attitude, then, is unable to consider things that are possibilities rather than actualities, to keep in mind simultaneously various aspects of a situation, to react to two stimuli that do not belong intrinsically together, to inhibit reactions, and to ideationally isolate parts of a whole.

Goldstein and Scheerer (1948) developed a number of tests of ability to assume the abstract attitude. These tests include object-sorting tasks involving form, color, and combined color and form sorting. When observing sorting test results, one may ask: Is the sort concrete (perceptual) or abstract (conceptual)? Can the individual verbally account for the type of sort presented by the examiner (abstract)? The intervention implications of this framework would be to stimulate the patient to comprehend and produce language that is increasingly more abstract.

Thought Process Framework

Wepman (1972a) suggested that aphasia may be a thought process disorder in which impairment of semantic expression is the result of an impairment of thought processes that "serve as the catalyst for verbal expression" (p. 207). He noted that patients with aphasia frequently substitute words that are associated with words they are attempting to produce, and that the remainder of the individual's communicative effort appears to relate to the approximated rather than the intended word. An inaccurate verbal formulation may lead to interference with thought processes, as there is a drive to establish consonance between the thought process and the actual utterance. For example, if a patient is trying to say "circle" and instead utters "square," the concept of circle may be modified to be consistent with the utterance, and the patient may begin to think of a circle as a square.

Individuals who cannot retrieve the most appropriate lexical symbol for a context are impaired in their ability to communicate a number and variety of specific propositional ideas. When the continued efforts relate to the approximated rather than the intended word, spontaneous language becomes even more impaired.

Within a framework in which aphasia is seen primarily as a disorder of thought process, assessment involves determining whether individuals can follow a train of thought in their communication or spontaneous language, and whether they can expand on topics and ideas. For Wepman (1972b, 1976), the first stage of therapy is thought-centered or content-centered discussion in which patients are stimulated to attend to their thoughts and remain on topic. During the second stage of therapy, patients are encouraged to elaborate on various topics.

Unidimensional Framework

A unidimensional view of aphasia relates language behaviors to a single common denominator. The expressive and receptive, as well as the semantic and syntactic components of language are considered to be inseparable. This view suggests that damage to the language mechanism results in general language impairment in which there is an effect on all aspects of language. Aphasiologists who subscribe to this framework do not promote the use of Broca's-Wernicke's, fluent-nonfluent, sensory-motor, receptive-expressive, or input-output dichotomies in aphasia.

One of the most popular and in-depth unidimensional theories, proposed by Schuell and her colleagues (Schuell, Jenkins, & Jimenez-Pabon, 1964), regards aphasia as a general language impairment that crosses all language modalities: speaking, listening, reading, and writing. These authors noted that the behaviors impaired in aphasia involve integrations that cannot be attributed merely to organization of motor responses or to events in outgoing pathways; rather, they involve use of an ability that is dependent on higher-level integrations.

According to proponents of this framework, aphasia is not modality-specific. Rather, it involves the inability to access or retrieve words and rules of an acquired language for communication (Schuell et al., 1964). The person with aphasia has lost functional spontaneous language, or the ability to use connected language units to communicate according to the established conventions of the language.

Schuell's concept of the cause of this general language breakdown reflects a broad and dynamic view of the language process.

The assessment implications of the unidimensional framework involve an analysis of the patient's ability to comprehend and produce language within all four modalities, and in contexts ranging from single words to spontaneous discourse. Schuell's test, the Minnesota Test for Differential Diagnosis of Aphasia (MTDDA) (Schuell, 1973) is based on this model (see Chapters 4 and 17).

The intervention applications are similarly unidimensional and multimodal. Treatment focus is on stimulation: the use of strong, controlled, and intensive auditory activation of the impaired symbol system to maximize patient reorganization of language. The clinician manipulates and controls specific dimensions of stimuli to make complex events happen in the brain, thus aiding the patient in making maximal responses (see Chapter 17).

Microgenetic View

Several authors challenge the notion that language production can be explained by an array of cortical speech centers and connecting pathways that convey memories and images from one processing center to another. Brown (1972, 1977, 1979) proposes a conceptual framework in which language processing is conceived as an event that emerges over different levels of the brain corresponding to different levels of evolutionary development, not across specific cortical areas. Phylogenetically older limbic mechanisms are thought to mediate early stages in cognition and linguistic representation, while the more recently evolved left lateralized neocortex (encompassing Broca's and Wernicke's areas) mediates the final stages in cognition and linguistic processing. Having evolved from common limbic structures, the anterior and posterior language zones are considered to be fundamentally united. Language is considered to be processed simultaneously by complementary systems in the anterior and posterior part of the brain, rather than sequentially from one component to the next. The function of cerebral pathways is considered to be the coordination of different regions of the brain rather than the mere conveyance of information between regions.

According to this view, varying forms of aphasia correspond to lesions of brain structures that have emerged at varying stages of evolution. A lesion in one of the language areas of the brain gives rise to the relative prominence of an earlier stage of language processing. Thus, the symptoms of aphasia serve to magnify the processing events that, in normal language, would be mediated by the lesioned area. Adherents to this framework envision treatment as facilitating the transition from one stage to the next in the microgenetic sequence.

Multidimensional Frameworks

Proponents of a multidimensional framework conceptualize aphasia as having multiple forms, each corresponding to a different underlying site of lesion and having a characteristic list of hallmark features. For individuals who hold a multidimensional view of aphasia, assessment involves determining what symptomatology is present and subsequently classifying a patient in one category or another. Some conceptualize aphasia dichotomously, for example, as Broca's versus Wernicke's, fluent versus nonfluent, semantic versus syntactic, or anterior versus posterior. Usually, such dichotomies are associated with the cerebral localization of the lesions that result in aphasia. The Boston Diagnostic Aphasia Examination (BDAE) (Goodglass, Kaplan, & Baressi, 2001), the Western Aphasia Battery (Kertesz, 1982; Kertesz & Poole, 1974), and the Language Modalities Test for Aphasia (Wepman & Jones, 1961) reflect such classification systems. Intervention, according to this framework, is oriented toward specific deficits. That is, the clinician attempts to rehabilitate a specific language modality (such as speaking) or behavior (such as confrontation naming or phonemic production) that is found to be impaired (c.f., Cubelli, Foresti, & Consolini, 1988).

Classification of Multidimensional Types of Aphasia

For the sake of simplicity and presentation of basic terminology, one may consider the basic subtypes of aphasia across different multidimensional classification schemes to fall into the categories of "fluent," "nonfluent," and "other" aphasias. The reader should be aware, though, that the terms fluent and nonfluent are not highly descriptive terms in and of themselves. It is important to specify what is meant by the use of these terms when describing the language of any individual patient. An individual may appear to be nonfluent for any of a variety of reasons, or according to any of a large array of measures. Generally, persons with aphasia are considered fluent if they are able to speak in spontaneous conversation without abnormal pauses, abundant nonmeaningful filler phrases, or long periods of silence. Nonfluent patients tend to have a reduced rate of speech and to express less communicative content per unit of time than normal speakers do. Of course, patients who are completely nonverbal are nonfluent. Damasio (1998) presents an excellent synopsis of the various categorical terms used throughout the history of the study of aphasia. A more thorough discussion of the classification of aphasia according to neuroanatomic substrates is presented in the next chapter.

Fluent Aphasias

There are three basic types of fluent aphasia: conduction aphasia, Wernicke's aphasia, and transcortical sensory aphasia.

Wernicke's Aphasia. The critical features of Wernicke's aphasia are impaired auditory and reading comprehension and fluently articulated but paraphasic speech (Goodglass et al., 2001) in which syntactic structure is relatively preserved. In many cases, patients with Wernicke's aphasia present with logorrhea, or press of speech, characterized by excessive verbal production. Paraphasias are most often in the form of sound transpositions and word substitutions (Goodglass, Quadfasel, & Timberlake, 1964). Patients with Wernicke's aphasia experience naming difficulty that is severe in relation to their fluent spontaneous speech (Goodglass et al., 1964). Neologisms are frequent. Those who produce frequent neologistic expressions are often unintelligible and are sometimes referred to as having "jargon aphasia" (Wepman & Jones, 1961). Patients with Wernicke's aphasia also have difficulty reading, writing, and repeating words (Damasio, 1998). They often demonstrate a lack of awareness of their deficits, especially compared to patients with other types of aphasia. Some authors and many clinicians use the term "receptive aphasia" to refer to the disability of patients with Wernicke's aphasia because of their primary deficit in the area of linguistic comprehension. Likewise, because lesions that lead to this form of aphasia tend to be located in the temporal lobe, Wernicke's aphasia represents a classic form of "posterior" aphasia.

Conduction Aphasia. The speech of persons with conduction aphasia is fluent, although generally less abundant than the speech of those with Wernicke's aphasia (Damasio, 1998). A hallmark feature is impaired repetition of words and sentences relative to fluency in spontaneous speech, which is often normal or near normal. Auditory comprehension is also relatively spared (Goodglass et al., 2001). Most patients "repeat words with phonemic paraphasias, but often they will omit or substitute words, and they may fail to repeat anything at all if function words rather than nouns are requested" (Damasio, 1998, p. 35). Literal paraphasias repeatedly interfere with speech.

Transcortical Sensory Aphasia (TSA). Individuals with TSA have fluent, well-articulated speech with frequent paraphasias and neologisms (Goodglass et al., 2001). Global paraphasias occur more frequently than phonemic paraphasias (Damasio, 1998). A key feature that differentiates TSA from conduction aphasia is intact repetition ability. Auditory comprehension is generally poor. Confrontation naming is impaired, and the patient may offer an irrelevant response or echo the words of the examiner (Goodglass et al., 2001).

Nonfluent Aphasias

There are three basic types of nonfluent aphasia: Broca's, transcortical motor, and global aphasia.

Broca's Aphasia. Broca's aphasia is the most classic form of nonfluent aphasia. It is often considered the "opposite" of Wernicke's aphasia (Damasio, 1998, p. 35). The essential characteristics of Broca's aphasia include awkward articulation, restricted vocabulary, agrammatism, and relatively intact auditory and reading comprehension (Goodglass et al., 2001). Typically, writing is at least as severely impaired as speech. Persons with Broca's aphasia are usually aware of their communicative deficits, and are more prone to depression and sometimes catastrophic reactions than are patients with other forms of aphasia. Some authors and clinicians use the term "expressive aphasia" to refer to the disability of patients with Broca's aphasia because of their primary deficit in the area of language formulation and production. Likewise, because lesions that lead to this form of aphasia tend to be located in the frontal lobe, Broca's aphasia represents a classic form of "anterior" aphasia.

Transcortical Motor Aphasia (TMA). In patients with TMA, repetition is intact relative to "otherwise limited speech" (Goodglass et al., 2001). Such patients exhibit phonemic and global paraphasias, syntactic errors, perseveration, and difficulty imitating and organizing responses in conversation (Damasio, 1998; Goodglass et al., 2001). Confrontation naming is usually preserved, but auditory comprehension is impaired.

Global Aphasia. Global aphasia is a disorder of language characterized by impaired linguistic comprehension and expression. It is often considered a combination of both Wernicke's and Broca's aphasia. Patients with global aphasia tend to produce few utterances and have a highly restricted lexicon. They have little or no understanding in any modality and little or no ability to communicate effectively (Wepman & Jones, 1961).

Other Forms of Aphasia

Anomic Aphasia. Anomic aphasia is a form of aphasia characterized primarily by significant word retrieval problems (Damasio, 1998; Goodglass, 1993; Goodglass & Wingfield, 1997). It is differentiated from the symptom of anomia, or dysnomia, which is typical in most forms of aphasia. Speech is generally fluent except for the hesitancies and pauses associated with word- finding deficits. Grammar is generally intact.

Primary Progressive Aphasia. Primary progressive aphasia is a type of aphasia that has an insidious rather than an acute onset. The term "primary" refers to the fact that deficits in language are the primary symptoms noted, with cognitive skills remaining intact relative to linguistic skills. The term "progressive" refers to the fact that the condition is degenerative, with communication skills worsening over time. The underlying etiology for progressive aphasia may be any of a number of degenerative diseases affecting the brain. Many patients with this form of aphasia eventually present with significant cognitive deficits as part of a syndrome of dementia (Ceccaldi, Soubrouillard, Poncet, & Lecours, 1996; Damasio, 1998).

Alexia and Agraphia. Alexia, a deficit in reading ability, occurs in most forms of aphasia, especially in those forms involving significant auditory comprehension deficits, such as Wernicke's aphasia or TSA. Consequently, it is infrequently considered a form of aphasia in and of itself. There are some rare patients, though, who present with deficits in reading that are markedly more severe than other communicative deficits, such as auditory comprehension and speech. Such forms of alexia may occur with or without agraphia, a deficit in writing ability. Forms of aphasia involving alexia with and without agraphia are described in formidable detail by Damasio and Damasio (1983), Goodglass (1993), and Geschwind (1965).

Exceptions to Multidimensional Aphasia Subtypes

Numerous systems for the multidimensional categorization of aphasia have been proposed. Further, most textbooks addressing aphasia offer creative means of categorizing the various subtypes of aphasia based on derivations of previous authors' suggestions. Acknowledging the diversity in diagnostic criteria and nomenclature used throughout the history of the study of aphasia, Damasio (1998) refers to the task of classifying the subtypes of aphasia as a "necessary evil" (p. 32). Most aphasiologists might agree with Damasio that "attempting to review the classification systems of aphasia is probably foolhardy" (p. 32). Most clinical aphasiologists attest to the fact that it is common to meet patients with forms of aphasia that do not fit neatly into any one category described according to a known multidimensional classification scheme (c.f., Caplan & Chertkow, 1989). Even an individual with a form of aphasia that fits a particular classification at one point in time may demonstrate a different form of aphasia as his or her condition evolves. Patients with right or bilateral cerebral dominance for language functions, subcortical lesions, degenerative conditions, traumatic brain injury, and multiple or unknown sites of lesion often present further challenges to the classification of aphasia subtypes, as explored in other chapters of this book. Still, it is essential that those studying aphasia and working with people who have aphasia understand traditional multidimensional models of classification. Such an understanding helps ensure improved communication among clinicians and researchers, improve the validity and reliability of diagnostic reporting, clarify theoretic differences in how experts differ in their ways of conceptualizing aphasia, and highlight the similarities and distinctions between one's idealized concept of any subtype of aphasia compared to the actual manifestations of aphasia in an individual patient.

Psycholinguistic/Problem Solving/Information Processing Framework

Psycholinguistic approaches to language recognize its three integrated and interrelated components: cognition, language, and communication (Muma, 1978), as well as the integration of language content, form, and use (Bloom & Lahey, 1978). **Content** involves meaning. **Language** refers to the structures of language or the rule-based systems of phonology, morphology, syntax, and semantics. **Communication** involves the use, purpose, or function that a particular utterance or gesture serves at any one time and its contextual realization. **Cognition** involves the acquisition of knowledge of the world, and the continued processing of this knowledge. Cognition refers to all of the mental processes by which information is transformed, reduced, elaborated, stored, recovered, and used (Neisser, 1967). Cognition can be operationally defined as the mental operations in the Guilford (1967) Structure-of-Intellect Model, namely, recognition/understanding; memory; and convergent, divergent, and evaluative thinking (see Chapter 17).

In a psycholinguistic framework, aphasia may be defined as an acquired impairment in language content, form, and use and the cognitive processes that underlie language, such as memory and thinking (convergent, divergent, and evaluative thinking). The impairment may be manifested in listening, speaking, reading, writing, and sign language, although not necessarily to the same degree in each.

Aphasia may be seen as an impairment in problem solving and information processing. Problem-solving and information processing both involve the use of all five cognitive operations (recognition/understanding; memory; and convergent, divergent and, evaluative thinking); the four types of content (figural, symbolic, semantic [content, form, and use], and behavioral [use/pragmatics]; and the five products or associations [units, classes, relations, systems, and transformations] of the Guilford (1967) model (see Chapter 17). The specific components that are used depend upon the problem presented and/or the information being processed.

Within this model, assessment of individuals with aphasia centers on an analysis of the cognitive, linguistic, and communicative strengths and weaknesses of each individual. Intervention focuses on the stimulation of these abilities, but especially on the stimulation of the cognitive processes underlying language comprehension and production (see Chapter 17).

Body Structure and Function, Activity, and Participation Framework

The WHO has launched a worldwide effort to redefine functioning and disability in an effort to heighten awareness of its holistic components and the complex interaction of conditions within each individual and in the environment that affects each individual's functioning. An earlier classification scheme proposed by the WHO, the International Classification of Impairments, Disabilities and Handicaps (ICIDH) employed the general terms "impairment," "disability," and "handicap," while a more recent scheme, the ICIDH-2, employed the terms "impairment," "activity," and "participation," to refer to the various contextual aspects of disabling conditions one might experience. The two primary levels within the most recent WHO International Classification of Functioning, Disability and Health (ICF) are (1) body structure and function and (2) activity and participation (WHO, 2001).

For individuals with aphasia, **body structure and function** refers to impairments of brain and brain functions. **Activity limitations** primarily involve the four language modalities: speaking, listening, reading, and writing as well as tasks necessary for daily living, such as conversing with the nurse or family member, writing a check, making a phone call, reading a paper or menu, and so forth. These modalities have been the traditional focus of assessment and intervention in aphasia. During the past 20 years, such tasks have increasingly been the focus of care.

The constructs of **activities and participation** capture the notion of engagement in daily life and realizing immediate and long-term real-life goals. This might include playing golf, shopping for clothes, getting a job, going on vacation, participating in clubs and organizations, and so forth. We may discuss limitations of "activities" in a similar way to our use of the term **disability.** We may discuss limitations of "participation" in a similar way to our use of the term **handicap.** For people with aphasia, these constructs represent the ability to use language in context. **Environment** is another key construct in the ICF. It includes the assistive technology, relationships with and support from others, support services, policies and regulations, physical environmental factors, and the attitudes of individuals with aphasia and their significant others.

The WHO classification schemes provide a framework for moving away from the classic biomedical model and take into consideration the organic and the complex functional consequences of disease. Viewing aphasia in this framework helps us consider social exclusion and inclusion as fundamental to the context in which people with aphasia communicate and engage in daily life activities. People with aphasia are not seen as solely responsible for the social consequences of their aphasia. The framework highlights the dynamic interaction of important variables such as social support, risk factors, causes, genetics, capabilities, environmental factors, and life habits of social participation in examining health, handicap, and disability. For example, consistent and dependable support from friends and family will likely decrease the impact of impairment; a depressed, uninvolved spouse may increase it. All individuals in the environment—and the environment itself—impact functioning and participation in

life (see Chapter 10). Therefore, assessment and treatment focus not just on the restoration of language functions, but also on individual communication of wants and needs and the social and environmental supports that might contribute to full participation. Assessment and treatment target all major areas in the classification scheme from day one.

This framework also helps clinicians and researchers focus on the core features of health and well-being. It encourages us to focus on seeing aphasia as a contextualized life-affecting condition requiring resources and compensatory and adaptive services for full life participation (Parr, Byng, & Gilpin, 1997). Health, well-being, and quality of life are considered essential to understanding aphasia and in helping those affected by it. Vitally related to a focus on life participation is the Life Participation Approach to Aphasia (LPAA Project Group, 2000) (see Chapter 10).

ETIOLOGY AND EPIDEMIOLOGY OF STROKE AND APHASIA

Stroke

Stroke, or cerebrovascular accident (CVA), is the most prevalent cause of aphasia. A stroke occurs when blood flow to an area of the brain is interrupted by the blockage of a blood vessel or artery, or by the rupturing of an artery. Blood carries essential nutrients, especially glucose and oxygen, to brain cells. Since brain cells do not have the capacity to store these nutrients, they are in need of constant blood supply. Even brief periods of interruption in blood supply to the brain can have lasting devastating effects on brain tissue (see Chapters 2 and 3).

Stroke is the third leading cause of death in the United States and the most common cause of adult disability (American Heart Association, 2006). In the United States alone, approximately 700,000 individuals experience a stroke each year (Centers for Disease Control and Prevention, Division for Heart Disease and Stroke Prevention, 2006). According to Zivin and Choi (1991), roughly 30 percent of those who have a stroke die, and "20 to 30 percent become severely and permanently disabled" (p. 56). For at least 40 percent of those who survive, stroke is a seriously disabling disease. Many survivors have lasting problems with movement and motor control of the body, perceptual deficits, cognitive problems, and swallowing disorders, as well as problems of speech and language.

There are several types of stroke. Chapters 2 and 3 contain a discussion of the most common forms of stroke leading to aphasia, namely thrombotic, embolic, and hemorrhagic strokes.

Incidence of Aphasia

Statistics regarding the incidence of aphasia and of the various subtypes of aphasia are variable, owing to subject sampling and description methods (c.f., Scarpa, Colombo, Sorgato, & DeRenzi, 1987). Marquardsen (1969) estimates that approximately one-third of patients who survive the first week of stroke have aphasia. Pedersen, Jorgensen, Nakayama, Raaschou, & Olsen (1995) report incidences as high as 40% in patients evaluated within the first three days of stroke. Scarpa et al. (1987) estimate that about 55% of patients with strokes affecting the left hemisphere have aphasia when examined 15 to 30 days after a stroke. Approximately 80,000 Americans develop aphasia each year, and about one million people in the United States—about one in 300 people—currently have aphasia (National Institute for Deafness and Other Communication Disorders, 2006).

Risk Factors for Stroke and Aphasia

Diagnoses of hypertension, heart disease, diabetes, and high cholesterol are factors that increase an individual's likelihood of experiencing stroke and aphasia, as are lifestyle factors of smoking, stress, inactivity, excessive consumption of alcohol, and dietary intake high in cholesterol, fat and sodium (NIDCD, 2006; Silvestrelli et al., 2006).

Although some studies have reported gender differences in the incidence of aphasia and in the location of associated lesions (Kertesz & Sheppard, 1981; Kimura, 1980; McGlone, 1980; Wyller, 1999), other researchers have discounted such findings (Hier et al., 1994; Pedersen et al., 1995; Scarpa et al., 1987). The prevalence of stroke is higher among men up to the age of approximately 80 years, after which it becomes higher in women. Women are, on average, six years older than men when they experience a first stroke (Roquer, Rodríguez-Campello, & Gomis, 2003). A majority of studies indicate that the case-fatality rate is higher in female than in male stroke patients; there is also some evidence, albeit relatively weak, indicating a better functional outcome in men (Roquer et al., 2003). Gender differences in risk factor profile and treatment response appear to be weak.

Handedness does not appear to be significantly associated with stroke incidence or severity (Pedersen et al., 1995). Given the low incidence of left- compared to right-handed individuals, the heterogeneity of left-handed people in terms of cerebral dominance for language, and also the fact that researchers commonly exclude left-handed individuals from aphasia studies, data are lacking as to the etiologic and epidemiologic associations between handedness and aphasia.

While advancing age is consistently associated with stroke (Stegmayr, Asplund, & Wester, 1994), reports of the influence of age on the incidence of aphasia within stroke patient populations have not been substantiated in studies employing controlled sampling and subject description methods (Habib, Ali-Cherif, Poncet, & Salamon, 1987; Miceli, Caltagirone, Gainotti, Masullo, Silveri, & Villa, 1981). Although the risk of acquiring aphasia increases with age, it is important to note that age has not been causally linked to aphasia.

Data from the 42-year-long Framingham Study conducted by the National Institutes of Health (Willich, 1987) suggest that strokes are twice as likely to occur between 6:00 a.m. and noon than at any other time of the day and that more than half (especially hemorrhagic strokes) occur on Mondays. Other studies have confirmed this finding, attributing it to the fact that those times correspond to periods when the body's supply and demand for oxygen is at its greatest level of imbalance—that is, when there is an increase in oxygen requirements simultaneous with reduced levels of blood flow (Flack & Yunis, 1997).

Racial, Ethnic, and Cultural Factors Influencing Incidence of Stroke and Aphasia

Many researchers report an influence of racial and ethnic origins on the incidence of stroke and aphasia. Stroke mortality is generally reported to be substantially higher in African American and Hispanic populations than in Caucasians (Gaines, 1997; Hoyert, Heron, Murphy, & Kung, 2006; Sacco et al., 1998). Discrepancies among reports on the relationship of race and ethnicity to stroke and aphasia may be attributable to sampling methods and to the sophistication and accuracy of diagnostic methods (c.f., Gillum, 1994, 1995). Most of the racial differences in the incidence of stroke and aphasia may be accounted for by differences in cultural influences on such lifestyle factors as diet, exercise, smoking, and access to health care services (Kuller, 1995). Persons of lower socioeconomic status also have higher risk factors for stroke, further influencing epidemiologic studies of stroke and aphasia (Centers for Disease Control and Prevention, 2006; Feigin, 2005; Feigin et al., 2006).

The role of race, ethnicity, socioeconomic status, and culture have important implications not only for the incidence of aphasia, but also for its diagnosis and treatment. It is for this reason that an entire chapter of this book and several components of other chapters are devoted to multicultural issues pertinent to intervention in adult aphasia.

Geographic location appears to play an important role in the prevalence and incidence rates of stroke and aphasia. For example, the southeastern region of the United States has been labeled by many as the "Stroke Belt" because of higher stroke mortality rates than other geographic areas, even when researchers account for age, gender, and race. Regional differences appear to be primarily influenced by the levels of risk factors such as high blood pressure, obesity, poor diet, and smoking, not on the physical properties of the areas involved (Casper et al., 1995; Centers for Disease Control and Prevention, 2006; Gaines, 1997).

Prevention

Data pertaining to risk factors enable researchers, clinicians, and laypersons to better reduce the likelihood of any individual experiencing the life-altering consequences of stroke and aphasia. A summary of strategies to prevent stroke at the individual level is provided in Table 1–2. Of course, public health programs to support health and wellness and access to health care are critical factors in prevention, as well as in recovery through medical and rehabilitative treatment following stroke (Centers for Disease Control and Prevention, Division for Heart Disease and Stroke Prevention, 2006). Recognizing the tremendous cost-saving advantages of preventing stroke, many health insurance companies have launched programs to promote wellness and help reduce consumers' risk of stroke (Thomas, 1997). Key lifestyle changes to reduce the risk of stroke and aphasia include dietary modification (e.g., reduced cholesterol and sodium intake, increased dietary fiber, vitamin therapy, moderation of consumption of caffeine and alcohol, and weight reduction in overweight patients), increased physical activity, smoking cessation, and stress reduction (He & Whelton, 1997; Gottlieb, 2006; Khaw, 1996; Labarthe, Biggers, Goff, & Houston, 2005; Shinton, 1997).

TABLE 1–2

Summary of Strategies to Prevent Stroke

- If you are overweight, lose weight. Maintain proper weight.
- Lower intake of salt or maintain low salt intake.
- Eat fruits and vegetables daily.
- Take in sufficient amounts of potassium.
- Keep cholesterol intake low.
- Maintain a low-fat diet.
- Engage in no more than moderate alcohol consumption.
- Be physically active. Exercise regularly. Engage in regular resistance training.
- Drink several glasses of water daily.
- Develop and nurture a calm, relaxed, optimistic, and even-tempered attitude.
- Get a flu shot.
- If you smoke, quit.
- Reduce exposure to second-hand smoke.
- Seek medical treatment for disorders that increase risk of stroke, including diabetes, atrial fibrillation, sickle cell disease, carotid artery disease, and heart failure.
- Seek medical advice. A doctor may recommend andarterectomy, aspirin or other blood-thinning therapy, medicines that help lower blood pressure, or alternatives to drugs known to raise blood pressure.
- Know the warning signs of stroke; seek medical attention as soon as symptoms occur.

Numerous pharmacologic treatments reduce the risk of stroke by helping to control hypertension and blood lipids (Centers for Disease Control and Prevention, 1999). In light of the increased risk of stroke in the early morning hours and on Mondays, scheduling of stressful tasks at times other than these is advised, as is the careful timing of the daily administration of antihypertensive medications (Flack & Yunis, 1997; Metoki, 2006).

Many preventive health programs focus on the core features of positive human health, well-being and quality of life, namely, leading a life of purpose, quality connection to others, positive self-regard, and a sense of mastery and accomplishment (Kahneman, Diener, & Schwarz, 1999). Active intervention programs focusing on these factors is especially important for patients and their significant others to prevent further illness such as additional strokes in individuals with aphasia (see section "Impairment, Activities, Participation in Life") and disease in their significant others.

Etiologies Other Than Stroke

Much of the empirical literature on aphasia is based on the study of patients who acquired aphasia because of a cerebrovascular accident. There are two good reasons for this. First, the majority of patients who have a clear and definite diagnosis of aphasia have had a stroke. Second, because stroke patients tend to have well-defined, localizable focal lesions, the etiologies associated with their manifestations of aphasia can be documented in research reports and controlled for in experimental paradigms, making such patients attractive research participants. Still, it is important to acknowledge that many other etiologies may be associated with aphasia. For example, patients who have experienced traumatic brain injury, brain surgery, infections, tumors, degenerative conditions, or exposure to neurotoxic agents may present with aphasia. The diffuse brain damage and frequently ill-defined sites of lesion associated with such etiologies preclude a large volume of controlled research pertaining specifically to aphasia in these complex populations. It is nonetheless important to recognize and treat patients who have aphasia regardless of the underlying cause. The Centers for Disease Control and Prevention, Division for Heart Disease and Prevention (2006) report that approximately 1.4 million adults per year in the United States experience a traumatic brain injury, far exceeding the number who have strokes. Approximately 43,800 new cases of brain and central nervous system tumors are diagnosed annually in the United States (Central Brain Tumor Registry of the United States, 2005). Millions more are diagnosed each year with other neurologic disorders affecting language abilities (e.g., dementia, Parkinson's disease, multiple sclerosis).

While the nature of aphasia is not always best studied with non-stroke populations, there is a growing body of treatment research pertaining to such populations. This book includes several chapters that address issues especially relevant to intervention with patients with traumatic brain injury and varied forms of dementia. Additionally, much of what has been learned about the treatment of aphasia in stroke patients may be applied to the treatment of acquired neurogenic communication problems in other patient populations.

Other Acquired Neurogenic Disorders

The study of aphasia is vitally related to the study of other acquired neurogenic communication disorders. Clinical aphasiologists are ideally trained in the diagnosis and treatment of a host of neurogenic conditions and have a solid understanding of their underlying neuropathologies. Academic knowledge and clinical expertise in the areas of dementia and other cognitive disorders, right-brain damage, traumatic brain injury, motor-speech disorders, confusional states, dysphagia, and normal aging are essential to excellence in clinical aphasiology. Also essential is competence in interdisciplinary research and clinical collaboration, given that individuals who experience any acquired neurogenic communication disorder are likely to also experience multiple additional concomitant disorders and medical conditions.

Aging and Communication

The past three decades have brought an increasing interest in age-related changes in adults. Toward this end, numerous professionals have measured cognition, perception, sensation, mobility, communication, and other neurologic and psychological systems in an attempt to identify key variables that may or may not change with age. Although an increase in incidence with age is reported for many diseases and other problems affecting the cardiovascular, pulmonary, gastrointestinal, genitourinary, hematologic, musculoskeletal, metabolic, and endocrine systems (Abrams & Berko, 1990), some research has focused on positive changes and functioning in the elderly. The "myth . . . that to be old is to be sick, sexless and senile" (Frady, Gerdau, Lennon, Sherman, & Singer, 1985) is being countered by many vigorous and independent aging adults. In fact, gradual improvement has been seen in the overall health of elderly people (Manton, Stallard, & Corder, 1998; National Academy on an Aging Society and Merck Institute of Aging and Health, 2004; Philip, 2004). The majority of those who are over 85 are continuing to care for themselves (Elias, 1992; U.S. General Accounting Office, 2002).

Studies suggesting relationships between age and health or cognitive factors are often confounded by concomitant problems faced by elderly individuals. For example, those who perform poorly on mental ability tests may have other problems, such as depression, amnesia, dementia, vitamin deficiencies, or alcoholism. Additionally, they may be hindered by medications, including sedatives and/or nonsteroidal anti-inflammatory drugs, or by environmental insults such as pollution and stress.

New neuroimaging and behavioral methods, as well as evolving technology for the molecular study of the nervous system, have allowed researchers to conclude that, despite the loss of neurons with aging, the brain undergoes continuous adaptation as it ages. Evidence of neurobiologic changes that may come with age can be derived from animal research, which suggests that elderly animals are as capable of growing new connections between brain cells as are younger animals (van Praag, Shubert, Zhao, & Gage, 2005; Wu, Zou, Rajan, & Cline, 1999). This also appears to be true in humans (Abrous, Koehl, & Le Moal, 2005; Eriksson et al., 1998; Jin et al., 2006; Saurwein-Teissl, Schonitzer, & Grubeck-Loebenstein, 1998). Mesulam (1987) claims that age-related changes may underlie "wisdom," suggesting that the progressive death of neurons and the sprouting of new connections may actually be healthy and a sign of maturity in the most positive sense.

INTERDISCIPLINARY APPROACHES TO APHASIOLOGY

The study of aphasia and related neurogenic communication disorders is inherently interdisciplinary (see Chapter 8). Although clinical practice in intervention for patients with aphasia requires specific training, certification, and/or licensure in much of the world, the study of aphasia does not fall within the bounds of any single discipline. Disciplines that help understand the nature of neurogenic communication disorders and provide the most effective intervention include speech-language pathology, audiology, neuroscience, cognitive science, biology, engineering, physics, psychology, pharmacology, linguistics, communication, social work, counseling, anthropology, sociology, multiculturalism, mathematics, rehabilitation, physiatry, neurology, gerontology, physical therapy, occupational therapy, music therapy, and health care administration. This list is far from exhaustive. It is interesting to note that many of the disciplines just mentioned are also hybrid ones, drawing from basic science, theory, and practice in a variety of content areas. Thus, the student or professional who is truly committed to the study of aphasia must also be committed to lifelong learning across disciplinary boundaries.

LIFE-CHANGING EFFECTS OF APHASIA

Within a matter of minutes, the lives of individuals who have aphasia change completely. They may feel that they are prisoners in their own minds. Many, through the effects of neurologic impairments, may feel that they are prisoners in their own bodies as well. Some want to move and walk but cannot; many have much to say but are significantly limited in their ability to express themselves. Persons who were employed prior to acquiring aphasia may be unable to maintain employment, leading not only to financial stress but also to feelings of isolation, frustration, and worthlessness. Some people with aphasia are lonely and desperate. Others tolerate the condition remarkably well.

Despite worldwide efforts to improve the ways that individuals with disabilities are treated and regarded, negative attitudes toward and discomfort with persons with communicative and physical disabilities remain. Individuals with stroke and aphasia are susceptible to attitudinal barriers, lack of important information, loss of companionship with loved ones, marginal social status, rejection, distrust, stigmatization, and loss of esteem (Boone & Zraik, 1991; Croteau & LeDorze, 2006; Love, 1981; Murphy, 2006; Post & Leith, 1983).

Patients' significant others are usually dramatically affected by the onset of aphasia in a friend, colleague, or loved one. The onset of acquired aphasia, so life-changing in practically every dimension of daily living, inspires many to appreciate just how central communicative ability is to being and feeling human.

Language: The Human Essence

The need for socialization is the core of human existence, and the ability to communicate with others is the essence of that socialization. Language is basic to what Chomsky (1972) calls the "human essence." More than any other attribute, language distinguishes humans from other animals. It is the most basic characteristic of the intellect and the very means through which the mind matures and develops. Language enables individuals to describe and clarify their thoughts for themselves and others.

Human experience and interaction are welded to language. According to Goodman (1971), the ability to share experience through language is a means of homeostasis that enables human beings to maintain and/or restore an equilibrium in which they can survive. Goodman also observes that language is the basis of personality, revealing our innate being and our psychic ties with the world.

Language is also the essence of maturity, which is defined as an ability to relate warmly to and intimately with others — with their goals, aspirations, and hopes. It involves a "fitting in," carrying one's share of personal and social responsibility, and conveying one's seasoned intelligence. Thus, definitions of maturity involve and revolve around the ability to use language effectively.

Insofar as persons with aphasia are impaired in their ability to use language, they are impaired in their human essence. Part of the personality often appears lost, and the ability to maintain interpersonal relationships, to convey wants and needs, and to be a mature self-reliant, self-actualized person is impaired.

There is tremendous variability in how aphasia affects an individual's sense of self and social ability. The effects may be disproportionate to the degree of neurologic impairment. Even mild deficits may be traumatizing to persons who closely identify with their active roles as communicators. Others with severe neurologic impairments and language deficits tolerate the effects of their condition with remarkable serenity.

EVIDENCE-BASED PRACTICE

Evidence-based practice is a construct receiving increasing attention from researchers, clinicians, patients, and health insurance companies, as well as agencies that rate quality of care in a wide array of health care contexts. As with many other health-related disciplines, the frequency of use of the term in the neurogenic communication disorders literature has expanded dramatically over the past decade. It refers to the skilled use of empirical support to make diagnostic and intervention decisions (c.f., Sackett, Rosenberg, Gray, Hayes, & Richardson, 1996; Sackett, Straus, Richardson, Rosenberg, & Haynes, 2000). The concept of using evidence to inform practice is not a new one. However, it has become a growing focal point due to: the expansion of our knowledge base; the increased accessibility of data and other information via recent advances in print- and web-based publishing; the growing demand for accountability from consumers, employers and insurance companies; and the continuous quality improvement- and outcomes-focused programs in which we engage as clinicians to ensure that we provide the best services we can. The "evidence" we use to inform our clinical decisions may come in the form of expert opinion, or from research involving a variety of methods, including case studies, randomized clinical studies, and randomized controlled clinical trials (c.f., Frattali & Worral, 2001; Robey, 1998; Robey & Schultz, 1998). The way we incorporate the evidence is ideally influenced by our careful consideration of the methodologic quality and validity of specific research studies, our own clinical judgment about the relevance and importance of research findings to a specific patient, the values of the patient, the feasibility of applying research findings in a given intervention context, and our own and others' expert opinion (c.f., Woolf, Grol, Hutchinson, Eccles, & Grimshaw, 1999).

The Academy of Neurologic Communication Disorders and Sciences (ANCDS) has developed evidence-based practice guidelines founded on careful literature reviews and analysis by teams of clinical researchers in specialty areas within neurogenic communication disorders. Examples of guidelines published to date include those on cognitive-communicative disorders resulting from traumatic brain injury (Turkstra, Ylvisaker, Coelho, Kennedy, Sohlberg, & Avery, 2005). ANCDS writing groups are now developing guidelines for additional areas, including aphasia and dementia. The American Speech-Language-Hearing Association (ASHA) has supported the development of evidence-based clinical practice guidelines based on reviews of the research literature in several areas of clinical practice, and has recently initiated the National Center for Evidence-Based Practice in Communication Disorders. Information about related initiatives is updated regularly online (ASHA, 2007).

As clinicians we require a basic knowledge of the processes used to engage in and document evidence-based clinical practice. We must also keep abreast of the literature regarding which assessment and therapeutic techniques are effective with specific types of patients and under what conditions. It is critical that we continuously find, document, and evaluate our practices and test whether our therapeutic techniques are effective.

RATIONALE FOR LANGUAGE INTERVENTION IN APHASIA

A rationale for language intervention in persons who have aphasia is based on the belief that language is vital to one's human essence and that treatment can affect a change in a patient's communicative performance. Aphasia is not considered by most to be a disorder that can be cured. Still, skilled intervention enables many individuals to be able to comprehend and produce language and to communicate more effectively. Through intervention, aphasiologists attempt to heighten each patient's potential to function maximally within his or her environment, to facilitate meaningful relationships, and to restore self-esteem, dignity, and independence (Wepman, 1972a).

It is unfortunate that many posttrauma and poststroke patients with good potential for rehabilitation are left untreated. Many individuals have the capacity to communicate more effectively and yet are not enabled to do so (Wepman, 1972a). Quality health care means going beyond the provision of basic physical care and meeting the holistic needs of patients with high standards and dignity. Individuals should be granted the right to be treated by qualified clinicians providing the best techniques known. Not to allow persons to communicate to the best of their ability is to deprive them of their own human essence.

FUTURE TRENDS

The explosion of new knowledge and new technology is leading scientists to a progressively greater understanding of the brain's biology. Molecular answers are now increasingly available for questions we have addressed only indirectly. New and evolving imaging methods provide promise for richer information about the nature of neurogenic disorders in adults, and about their treatment. New approaches to pharmacologic intervention are producing promising preliminary results related to facilitation of cerebrovascular recovery following stroke or brain injury, as well as cognitive improvement through neurotrophic factors. Biologic interventions hold promise for stimulating or repairing injured brain areas. The future may also bring tissue transplantation, perhaps using stem cells, and electronic prostheses, perhaps using cortical electrode grids to facilitate function (Wineburgh & Small, 2004). Emerging technology will continue to expand our alternatives as aphasiologists for assessment and treatment.

Research in all the areas related to the study of aphasia will continue to illuminate our understanding of neurogenic communication disorders. Many of these research areas are explored further in this book. It is important that aphasiologists continue to learn about how the brain organizes language and to reflect on how this kind of knowledge can affect the growth and development of new approaches to treatment. The more we know about how intervention changes brain function, the more effective we can make our intervention approaches. The accelerated emphasis on evidence-based practice within our profession and the emergence of additional collaborative efforts among researchers and clinicians to enhance the evidence base in our discipline bode well for improved efficacy, efficiency, outcomes, accountability, and quality in our services.

Demographic characteristics of patient populations will continue to stimulate new development in adult language intervention. Increased life expectancies and the progressive aging of the world's population will continue to influence the nature of the patients served by clinical aphasiologists, as will the growth of multilingual and multicultural populations. Other important influences will include the increased incidence of certain relevant etiologic and associated risk factors such as obesity, hepatitis, and HIV and AIDS (ASHA, 1989a; Centers for Disease Control and Prevention, 2006; Larsen, 1998; Flower & Sooy, 1987).

RATIONALE FOR THIS TEXT

The primary purpose of the present text is the presentation of various models of intervention for adult patients with aphasia and for patients with related disorders. Such models can provide a framework with which to focus therapy, to generate intervention tasks, and to analyze empirically the efficiency of rehabilitation efforts. Some of these strategies have appeared in part or in whole in previous literature; others have not. It should be recognized, however, that it is not the purpose of this text to assess any of the models or to resolve the inconsistencies in these approaches. These functions are better performed in appropriate professional journals.

It is hoped that this text will provoke theoretic speculation and that those chapters that are rich conceptually will prompt the collection of further data and generate the production of new approaches. The readings are organized into sections to help shape the reader's perspective on the field. However, the sections of the book—and its chapters—may be used in any order.

▶ *Acknowledgment*—This work was supported in part by grant DC00153-01A1 from the National Institute on Deafness and Other Communication Disorders. Thanks to Meggan Moore for editorial assistance.

KEY POINTS

1. There are four essential features to a definition of aphasia.
2. The term "aphasic" is an adjective, not a noun.
3. Varied theoretic frameworks influence the way one conceptualizes aphasia and therefore may influence the diagnosis and treatment of aphasia.
4. Multiple etiological factors are associated with aphasia, the most common of which is stroke.
5. Traditional classification schemes help to elucidate various manifestations of aphasia, but are often limited in terms of characterizing the conditions of individual patients.
6. The study of aphasia is interdisciplinary.
7. A solid rationale for language intervention in adult aphasia is based on the notion that language is essential to one's human essence and that treatment can affect a change in a patient's communicative competence.

ACTIVITIES FOR REFLECTION AND DISCUSSION

1. Write your own definition of the term "aphasia," employing each of the four components mentioned for an ideal definition. Compare your definition with those of your colleagues. How might the way one conceptualizes aphasia influence one's choice of words in defining aphasia?
2. Create an interactive exercise for students and clinicians to practice the use of appropriate terms to refer to individuals with a variety of neurogenic language disorders.

3. Review the means of reducing stroke risk in Table 1–2. Considering yourself a role model for an individual at risk of stroke (and repeat strokes), what specific steps would be important for you to undertake to demonstrate a lower stroke risk in your own life style? Develop a personal action plan for reducing your own stroke risk.
4. A background in basic terminology used in the study of communication disorders is assumed by the authors of this book. Reviewing terminology as presented in other texts may be helpful. Define in your own words the following terms used to describe the symptoms associated with aphasia:
   - agraphia
   - alexia
   - anomia
   - catastrophic reaction
   - logorrhea
   - neologism
   - paraphasia (including the terms literal, phonemic, semantic, verbal, and global paraphasia)
   - perseveration
   - press of speech
   - transposition

   Note that some authors use the prefix *dys*- rather than *a*- for many of these terms, referring, for example, to dysnomia, dyslexia, dysgraphia, and even dysphasia rather than using the corresponding terms anomia, alexia, agraphia, and aphasia. What is the literal semantic distinction between terms beginning with *dys*- as compared to *a*-? The choice of prefixes in the usage of such terms among aphasiologists appears to be a function of stylistic convention more than a function of the literal significance of the prefixes in question.
5. Explain why many patients with "fluent" aphasia are also considered to have "receptive" aphasia.
6. Describe the hallmark features of each of the classic subtypes of aphasia described: Wernicke's aphasia, transcortical motor aphasia, conduction aphasia, Broca's aphasia, global aphasia, transcortical sensory aphasia, anomic aphasia, alexia, and primary progressive aphasia. As you read the upcoming chapter, it will be helpful to continue to reflect on how these hallmark symptoms are associated with the underlying neuropathologies of aphasia. As you consider diagnostic issues in aphasia as discussed further in this text, it will be helpful to consider further how the way in which one conceptualizes aphasia is relevant to the diagnostic process.
7. How might the way you conceptualize the nature of aphasia, and classify its subtypes, influence your own assessment of an individual with aphasia? How might it influence treatment?

References

Abrams, W., & Berko, R. (1990). *The Merck manual of geriatrics.* Rahway, NJ: Merck, Sharp & Dohme Research Laboratories.

Abrous, D. N., Koehl, M., & Le Moal, M. (2005). Adult neurogenesis: From precursors to network and physiology. *Physiology Review, 85,* 523–569.

America Speech-Language-Hearing Association (2007). *Evidence-based practice.* Retrieved September 28, 2007, from http://www. asha.org/members/ebp/default.

American Heart Association. (2006). *Heart disease and stroke statistics: 2006 Update.* Dallas: American Heart Association.

Bloom, L., & Lahey, M. (1978). *Language development and language disorders.* New York: Wiley.

Boone, R. R., & Zraik, R. I. (1991). Spouse attitudes toward the person with aphasia. *Journal of Speech and Hearing Research, 34,* 123–128.

Brookshire, R. H. (2007). *An introduction to neurogenic communications disorders.* St. Louis: Mosby-Year Book.

Brown, J. W. (1972). *Aphasia, apraxia and agnosia: Clinical and theoretical aspects.* Springfield, IL: Charles C Thomas.

Brown, J. W. (1977). *Mind, brain and consciousness.* New York: Academic Press.

Brown, J. W. (1979). Language representation in the brain. In H. Steklis & M. Raleigh (Eds.), *Neurobiology of social communication in primates.* New York: Academic Press.

Caplan, D., & Chertkow, H. (1989). Neurolinguistics. In D. P. Kuehn, M. L. Lemme, & J. M. Baumgartner (Eds.), *Neural bases of speech, hearing, and language* (292–302). Austin, TX: Pro-Ed.

Casper, M. L., Wing, S., Anda, R. F., Knowles M., & Polland R. A. (1995). The shifting stroke belt: Changes in the geographic pattern of stroke mortality in the United States, 1962 to 1988. *Stroke, 26*(5), 755–760.

Ceccaldi, M., Soubrouillard, C., Poncet, M., & Lecours, A. R. (1996). A case reported by Serieux: The first description of a "primary progressive word deafness"? In C. Code, C. W. Wallesch, Y. Joanette, & A. Roch (Eds.), *Classic cases in neuropsychology* (pp. 45–52). East Sussex, UK: Psychology Press.

Centers for Disease Control and Prevention. (1999, August). Achievements in public health, 1900–1999. *Morbidity and Mortality Weekly Report, 48*(30), 1283–1286.

Centers for Disease Control and Prevention (2006). Epidemiology of HIV/AIDS-United States, 1981–2005. *Morbidity and Mortality Weekly Report, 55*(21), 589–592.

Centers for Disease Control and Prevention, Division for Heart Disease and Stroke Prevention. (2006). *Fact sheets and at-a-glance reports.* Retrieved October 10, 2006, from http://www.cdc.gov/dhdsp/library/fs_stroke.htm.

Central Brain Tumor Registry of the United States. (2005–2006). *Fact sheet.* Retrieved October 10, 2006, from http://www.cbtrus.org/factsheet/factsheet.html.

Chomsky, N. (1972). *Language and mind.* New York: Harcourt, Brace & World.

Croteau, C., & LeDorze, G. (2006). Overprotection, "speaking for," and conversational participation: A study of couples with aphasia. *Aphasiology, 20*(10–04), 327–336.

Cubelli, R., Foresti, A., & Consolini, T. (1988). Reeducation strategies in conduction aphasia. *Journal of Communication Disorders, 21,* 239–249.

Damasio, A. (1998). Signs of aphasia. In M. T. Sarno (Ed.), *Acquired aphasia* (25–41). New York: Academic Press.

Damasio, A., & Damasio, H. (1983). The anatomic basis of pure alexia. *Neurology, 33,* 1573–1583.

Darley, F. L. (1982). *Aphasia.* Philadelphia: W.B. Saunders.

Elias, S. (1992). What is independence? *Generations, 16*(1), 49–52.

Eriksson, P. S., Perfilieva E., Bjork-Eriksson T., Alborn A. M., Nordborg C., Peterson D. A., et al. (1998). Neurogenesis in the adult human hippocampus. *Nature Medicine, 4*(11), 1313–1317.

Feigin, V. L. (2005). Stroke epidemiology in the developing world. *Lancet, 365*(9478), 2160–2161.

Feigin, V., Carter, K., Hackett, M., Barber, A. P., McNaughton, H., Dyall, L., et al. (2006). Ethnic disparities in incidence of stroke subtypes: Auckland Regional Community Stroke Study. *Lancet, Neurology, 5*(2), 130–139.

Flack, J. M., & Yunis, C. (1997). Therapeutic implications of the epidemiology and timing of myocardial infarction and other cardiovascular diseases. *Journal of Human Hypertension, 11,* 23–28.

Flower, W., & Sooy, D. (1987). AIDS: An introduction for speech-language pathologists and audiologists. *ASHA, 29,* 25–30.

Frady, M., Gerdau, R., Lennon, T., Sherman, W., & Singer, S. (1985, December 28). *Growing old in America.* ABC News Close-Up.

Frattali, C., & Worral, L. E. (2001). Evidence-based practice: Applying science to the art of clinical care. *Journal of Medical Speech-Language Pathology, 9,* ix-xiv.

Gaines, K. (1997). Regional and ethnic differences in stroke in the southeastern United States population. *Ethnicity and Disease, 7,* 150–264.

Geschwind, N. (1965). Disconnexion syndromes in animals and man. *Brain, 88,* 237–294, 585–644.

Gillum, R. F. (1994). Epidemiology of stroke in Native Americans. *Stroke, 26*(3), 514–521.

Gillum, R. F. (1995). Epidemiology of stroke in Hispanic Americans. *Stroke, 26*(9), 1707–1712.

Goldstein, K., & Scheerer, M. (1948). Abstract and concrete behavior in experimental study with special tests. *Psychological Monograph, 53,* 2.

Goodglass, H. (1993). *Understanding aphasia.* San Diego: Academic Press.

Goodglass, H., Kaplan, E. & Baressi, B. (2001). *The Assessment of aphasia and related disorders* (3rd ed.). Philadelphia: Lea & Febiger.

Goodglass, H., Quadfasel, F., & Timberlake, W. (1964). Phrase length and type and severity of aphasia. *Cortex, 1,* 133–153.

Goodglass, H., & Wingfield, A. (1997). Anatomical and theoretical considerations in anomia. In H. Goodglass & A. Wingfield (Eds.), *Anomia: neuroanatomical and cognitive correlates* (pp. 20–29). San Diego: Academic Press.

Goodman, P. (1971). *Speaking and language: Defense of poetry.* New York: Random House.

Gottlieb, S. H. (2006). Stroke. Feared but preventable. *Diabetes Forecast, 59*(9), 39–41.

Guilford, J. P. (1967). *The nature of human intelligence.* New York: McGraw-Hill.

Habib, M., Ali-Cherif, A., Poncet, M., & Salamon, G. (1987). Age-related changes in aphasia type and stroke location. *Brain and Language, 31*(2), 245–251.

Hallowell, B. (2007). Using NSF-sponsored projects to enrich students' written communication skills. In J. Enderle & B. Hallowell (Eds.), *2006 Annual review of engineering design projects to aid persons with disabilities.* Mansfield Center, CT: Creative Learning Press/National Science Foundation.

He, J., & Whelton, P. K. (1997). Epidemiology and prevention of hypertension. *Medical Clinics of North America, 81*(5), 1077–1097.

Head, H. (1915). Hughlings Jackson on aphasia and kindred affections of speech. *Brain, 38,* 1–27.

Hier, D. B., Yoon, W. B., Mohr, J. P., Price, T. R., & Wolf, P. A. (1994). Gender and aphasia in the stroke data bank. *Brain and Language, 47,* 155–167.

Hoyert, D. L., Heron, M. P., Murphy, S. L., & Kung, H. (2006). Deaths: Final data for 2003. *National Vital Statistics Reports, 54* (13), 1–20. Hyattsville, MD: National Center for Health Statistics.

Jackson, H. H. (1878). On affectations of speech from disease of the brain. *Brain, 1,* 304–330.

Jin, K., Wang, X., Xie, L., Mao, X. O., Zhu, W., Wang, Y., et al. (2006). Evidence for stroke-induced neurogenesis in the human brain. *Proceedings of the National Academy of Sciences of the United States of America, 103*(35), 13198–13202.

Kahneman, D., Diener, E., & Schwarz, N. (1999). *Well-being.* New York: Russell Sage Foundation.

Kertesz, A. (1982). *Western aphasia battery.* New York: Grune & Stratton.

Kertesz, A., & Poole, E. (1974). The aphasia quotient: The taxonomic approach to the measurement of aphasic disability. *Canadian Journal of Neurological Science, 1,* 7–16.

Kertesz, A., & Sheppard, A. (1981). The epidemiology of aphasic and cognitive impairment in stroke: Age, sex, aphasia type and laterality differences. *Brain, 104,* 117–128.

Khaw, K. (1996). Epidemiology of stroke. *Journal of Neurology, Neurosurgery, and Psychiatry, 61,* 333–338.

Kimura, D. (1980). Sex differences in intrahemispheric organization of speech. *Behavioral and Brain Sciences, 3,* 240–241.

Kuller, L. H. (1995). Stroke and diabetes. In National Diabetes Data Group (Eds.), *Diabetes in America.* (2nd ed., pp. 449–456). Bethesda, MD: National Institutes of Health.

Labarthe, D. R., Biggers, A., Goff, D. C., & Houston, M. (2005) Translating a plan into action: A public health action plan to prevent heart disease and stroke. *American Journal of Preventive Medicine, 29*(1), 146–151.

Larsen, C. (1998). *HIV-1 and communication disorders: What speech and hearing professionals need to know.* San Diego: Singular.

Love, R. J. (1981). The forgotten minority: The communicatively disabled. *ASHA, 23,* 485–490.

LPAA Project Group (in alphabetical order: Roberta Chapey, Judith F. Duchan, Roberta J. Elman, Linda J. Garcia, Aura Kagan, Jon Lyon, & Nina Simmons-Mackie) (February, 2000). Life participation approach to aphasia: A statement of values for the future. *The ASHA Leader, 5,* 3.

Manton, K. G., Stallard, E., & Corder, L. S. (1998). The dynamics of dimensions of age-related disability 1982 to 1994 in the U.S. elderly population. *Journals of Gerontology: Series A: Biological Sciences and Medical Sciences, 53A*(1), B59–B70.

Marquardsen, J. (1969). The natural history of acute cerebrovascular disease: A retrospective study of 769 patients. *Acta Neurologica Scandinavica, 45* (supplement 38).

McGlone, J. (1980). Sex difference in human brain asymmetry: A critical survey. *Behavioral and Brain Sciences, 3,* 215–263.

Mesulam, M. M. (1987). Involutional and developmental implications of age-related neuronal changes: In search of an engram for wisdom. *Neurobiology of Aging, 8*(6), 581–583.

Metoki, H. (2006). Prognostic significance of night-time, early morning, and daytime blood pressures on the risk of cerebrovascular and cardiovascular mortality: The Ohasama Study. *Journal of Hypertension, 24*(9), 1841.

Miceli, G., Caltagirone, C., Gainotti, G., Masullo, C., Silveri, M. C., & Villa, G. (1981). Influence of age, sex, literacy and pathologic lesion on incidence, severity and type of aphasia. *Acta Neurologica Scandinavica, 64*(5), 370–382.

Muma, J. (1978). *Language handbook: Concepts, assessment and intervention.* Englewood Cliffs, NJ: Prentice-Hall.

Murphy, J. (2006). Perceptions of communication between people with communication disability and general practice staff. *Health Expectations, 9,* 49–59.

National Academy on an Aging Society and Merck Institute of Aging and Health (2004). *The state of aging and health in America.* Retrieved December 4, 2006, from http://www.agingsociety. org/agingsociety/publications/state/index.html.

National Institute for Deafness and Other Communication Disorders. (2006). *Aphasia.* Retrieved December 4, 2006, from http://www.nidcd.nih.gov/health/voice/aphasia.asp.

Neisser, U. (1967). *Cognitive psychology.* New York: Appleton-Century Crofts.

Parr, S., Byng, S., & Gilpin, S. (1997). *Talking about aphasia.* Buckingham, UK: Open University Press.

Pedersen, P. M., Jorgensen, H. S., Nakayama, H., Raaschou, H. O., & Olsen, T. S. (1995). Aphasia in acute stroke: Incidence, determinants, and recovery. *Annals of Neurology, 38*(4), 659–666.

Philip, I. (2004). *Better health in old age.* United Kingdom: Department of Health.

Post, J., & Leith, W. (1983). I'd rather tell a story than be one. *ASHA, 25,* 23–26.

Robey, R. (1998). A meta-analysis of clinical outcomes in the treatment of aphasia. *Journal of Speech, Language, and Hearing Research, 41,* 172–187.

Robey, R. R., & Schultz, M. C. (1998). A model for conducting clinical outcome research: An adaptation of the standard protocol for use in aphasiology. *Aphasiology, 12,* 787–810.

Roquer, J., Rodríguez-Campello, A., & Gomis, M. (2003). Sex differences in first-ever acute stroke. *Stroke, 34,* 1841.

Sacco, R. L., Boden-Albala, B., Gan, R., Chen, X., Kargman., D. E., Shea, S., et al. (1998, Feb). Stroke incidence among white, black, and Hispanic residents of an urban community: The Northern Manhattan Stroke Study. *American Journal of Epidemiology, 147*(3), 259–268.

Sackett, D. L., Rosenberg, W. M. C., Gray, J. A. M., Hayes, R. B., & Richardson, W. S. (1996). Evidence based medicine: What it is and what it isn't. *British Medical Journal, 312,* 71–72.

Sackett, D. L., Straus, S. E., Richardson, W. S., Rosenberg, W., & Haynes, R. B. (2000). *Evidence-based medicine: How to practice and teach EBM.* London: Churchill Livingstone.

Saurwein-Teissl, M., Schonitzer, D., & Grubeck-Loebenstein, B. (1998). Dendritic cell responsiveness to stimulation with influenza vaccine is unimpaired in old age. *Experimental Gerontology, 33*(6), 625–631.

Scarpa, M., Colombo, P., Sorgato, P., & DeRenzi, E. (1987). The incidence of aphasia and global aphasia in left brain-damaged patients. *Cortex, 23,* 331–336.

Schuell, H. (revised by J. Sefer) (1973). *Differential diagnosis of aphasia with the Minnesota Test.* Minneapolis, MN: University of Minnesota Press.

Schuell, H., Jenkins, J. J., & Jiminez-Pabon, E. (1964). *Aphasia in adults.* New York: Harper Medical Division.

Shinton, R. (1997). Lifelong exposures and the potential for stroke prevention: The contribution of cigarette smoking, exercise, and body fat. *Journal of Epidemiology and Community Health, 51*(2), 138–143.

Silvestrelli, G., Paciaroni, M., Caso, V., Milia, P., Palmerini, F., Venti, M., et al (2006). Risk factors and stroke subtypes: results of five consecutive years of the perugia stroke registry. *Clinical & Experimental Hypertension, 28*(3/4), 279–286.

Sohlberg, M., Avery, J., Kennedy, M. R. T., Coelho, C., Ylvisaker, M., Turkstra, L., et al. (2003). Practice guidelines for direct attention training. *Journal of Medical Speech-Language Pathology, 11,* 3, xix–xxxix.

Stegmayr, B., Asplund, K., & Wester, P. O. (1994). Trends in incidence, case-fatality rate, and severity of stroke in northern Sweden. *Stroke, 25*(9), 1738–1745.

Thomas, T. N. (1997). The medical economics of stroke. *Drugs, 54*(3), 51–58.

Turkstra, L., Ylvisaker, M., Coelho, C., Kennedy, M. R. T., Sohlberg, M. M., & Avery, J. (2005). Practice guidelines for standardized assessment for persons with traumatic brain injury. *Journal of Medical Speech-Language Pathology, 13*(2), ix–xviii.

U.S. General Accounting Office (2002). *Aging baby boom generation will increase demand and burden on Federal and state budgets.* Report GAO-02-544Y. Washington, D.C.: U.S. General Accounting Office.

van Praag, H., Shubert, T., Zhao, C., & Gage, F. H. (2005). Exercise enhances learning and hippocampal neurogenesis in aged mice. *Journal of Neuroscience, 25,* 8680–8685.

Wepman, J. (1972a). Aphasia therapy: A new look. *Journal of Speech and Hearing Disorders, 37,* 203–214.

Wepman, J. (1972b). Aphasia therapy: Some relative comments and some purely personal prejudices. In M. Sarno (Ed.), *Aphasia: Selected readings.* New York: Appleton-Century-Crofts.

Wepman, J. (1976). Aphasia: Language without thought or thought without language. *ASHA, 18,* 131–136.

Wepman, J., & Jones, L. (1961). *Studies in aphasia: An approach to testing: The Language Modalities Test for Aphasia.* Chicago: Education-Industry Service.

Willich, S. N., Levy, D., Rocco M. B., Tofler, G. H., Stone, P. H., & Muller, J. E. (1987, Oct.). Circadian variation in the incidence of sudden cardiac death in the Framingham Heart Study population. *American Journal of Cardiology, 60*(10), 801–806.

Wineburgh, L., & Small, S. (2004). Aphasia treatment at the crossroads: A biological perspective. *The ASHA Leader, 9*(8), 6–7, 18–19.

Woolf, S. H., Grol, R., Hutchinson, A., Eccles, M., & Grimshaw, J. (1999). Potential benefits, limitations, and harms of clinical guidelines. *British Medical Journal, 318,* 527–530.

World Health Organization (2001). *ICF: International Classification of Functioning, Disability, and Health.* Geneva, Switzerland: Author.

Wu, G. Y., Zou, D. J., Rajan, I., & Cline, H. (1999). Dendritic dynamics in vivo change during neuronal maturation. *Journal of Neuroscience, 19*(11), 4472–4483.

Wyller, T. B. (1999). Stroke and gender. *Journal of Gender-Specific Medicine, 2*(3), 41–45.

Yusuf, H. R., Giles, W. H, Croft, J. B., Anda, R. F., & Casper, M. L. (1998). Impact of risk factor profiles on determining cardiovascular disease risk. *Preventive Medicine, 27*(1), 1–9.

Zivin, J., & Choi, D. (1991, July). Stroke therapy. *Scientific American, 265*(1), 56–63.

Chapter 2

Neural Basis of Language Disorders

Hanna Damasio

OBJECTIVES

This chapter considers the neural basis of abnormal language processing and is based on the study of pathologic neuroanatomy in patients with aphasia due to focal brain damage. Aphasia refers to a compromise in the process of comprehending language, formulating language, or both, which occurs in a language-competent and intellectually competent individual. Specifically, aphasia is a breakdown in a two-way translation process that establishes the relation between thought and language. As a consequence, individuals with aphasia have an inability to translate, with reasonable fidelity, a nonverbal set of images (thoughts) into linguistic symbols and grammatical relationships (or they have the inverse problem, translating a received language message into thought).

Aphasia is a defect in language processing and not a defect of perception or movement or thought. Deafness, even when due to central processes, precludes comprehension of language through the auditory channel but not through the visual channel. Incoordination of speech movements causes dysarthria but not a linguistic breakdown of speech output. A thought disorder such as schizophrenia does not cause aphasia but rather produces a correct linguistic translation of a deranged thought process. As discussed in other chapters of this text, aphasia can compromise varied aspects of language processing (e.g., syntax, the lexicon, the phonemic and morphemic morphology of a word). In each individual patient several or even all of these aspects can be compromised, but the emphasis of the defect can also fall on one particular aspect only.

Aphasia is not the exclusive province of auditory-based languages. Languages based on visuomotor communication, such as American Sign Language (ASL), can also be compromised following focal brain damage, along similar symptom clusters (Bellugi, Poizner, & Klima, 1983).

Most often aphasia is the result of cerebrovascular disease leading to stroke, but it can also appear following head injury, cerebral tumors, and degenerative diseases such as Alzheimer's or Pick's. The constellation of defects does not really depend on the underlying pathologic process but rather on the specific brain region that becomes affected. The differences one might witness between aphasias caused by some of these pathologic processes, or others, have more to do with the way the process affects the underlying brain tissue than with a specific effect on the language dysfunction. (For example, see Anderson, Damasio, & Tranel, 1988, 1990; Damasio, 1987a.)

Most aphasic syndromes are seen in disease processes affecting the left hemisphere given that the vast majority of individuals share a left-hemisphere language dominance, even when they are left-handed. However, in some instances, some left-handers develop aphasia after lesions of the right hemisphere (or may fail to show aphasia after lesions in language areas of the left hemisphere), possibly because both hemispheres are more involved in language processing than is standard. Even more rarely, we can witness either the presence of aphasia with a right-hemisphere lesion in a right-handed person, or conversely, the absence of aphasia with a typical left-hemisphere insult also in a right-handed subject. These cases are known as "crossed aphasia" and "crossed non-aphasia," respectively.

HISTORICAL OVERVIEW

The history of aphasia and the history of neuroscience share the same starting point: neuroscience began with the description, in 1861, of a patient who had lost the ability to communicate through the spoken word because of damage to the left frontal operculum. The original description was outlined by Paul Broca (1861), and it formed the basis for what was later coined Broca's aphasia, a severe disruption of language output which far exceeded a difficulty in language comprehension. About a decade later Carl Wernicke was to describe another seminal patient with aphasia (Wernicke, 1874, 1886). The cause was another lesion of the left hemisphere but this time in the posterior temporal region rather than in the frontal lobe. So began what was later termed Wernicke's aphasia, in which the deficit in language comprehension far exceeded the disruption of language output. It did not take long to transform these observations of specific language deficits, which occurred after circumscribed areas of left-hemisphere damage, into generalizations about the neural basis of language. The idea that the left hemisphere was the site of human spoken language became accepted. With it came the idea that there were brain "centers" responsible for this function—an anterior center responsible for the production of language located in the frontal operculum or Broca's area and a posterior center responsible for language comprehension, located in the posterior half of the superior temporal gyrus or Wernicke's area. Further studies of patients with differently placed lesions and slight variations of the presenting deficits helped cement the traditional view, which mapped language-related brain areas to Broca's and Wernicke's areas, and their anatomic connection through a unidirectional fiber tract, the arcuate fasciculus, which carried speech signals from Wernicke's area to Broca's area. This cartoon of the key set of structures necessary to receive and produce language still pervades most textbooks and monographs on the subject, and even some modern texts on cognitive science and linguistics continue to use this phrenologic picture of the language brain despite their otherwise non-phrenologic models of the processes of thought and language. In the meantime, however, much has occurred in the history of aphasia. This includes a major backlash against localizationism that occurred along with the advent of behaviorisms in psychology, an approach that led to the opposite point of view—namely, that nothing but the whole brain was responsible for cognition. During the heyday of this approach, virtually all and any part of the brain was seen as equipotential, and language processes were no longer localized. The other initial historical development occurred when Norman Geschwind, working in the mid-1960s, struck a healthy balance between the excesses of phrenology and those of behavioristic theories. With his landmark articles on disconnection syndromes (Geschwind, 1965) he placed the classical observations on the anatomy of aphasia in a new functional perspective. He also went further in the anatomic explanations he provided for some of the previously described aphasic syndromes and enlarged the original set of language-related areas to include the left supramarginal gyrus and the left angular gyrus, both located in the inferior sector of the parietal lobe (see also Geschwind, 1971). At about the same time, detailed evaluation of aphasic patients was beginning to be performed with measurement tools that considered the linguistic and cognitive aspects of language processing. Modern test batteries and classifications of the aphasias started in earnest in the 1960s.

Over the years numerous other aphasia classifications have appeared, all having their origin in the difficulties encountered by previous classifications in the accommodation to the unavoidable variability in the presentation of patients with aphasia. I will not discuss the several available classification systems of aphasia, or their respective advantages and disadvantages. This topic is covered in other chapters in this book. In general, I will follow the separation of aphasic syndromes associated with the Boston and Iowa schools (Benton & Hamsher, 1978; Goodglass & Kaplan, 1982).

The availability of MR imaging and more recently 3-D reconstruction of the human brain has empowered the human lesion method and made way for a new wave of cognitive experiments. (For more on the lesion method see Damasio, 2000; Damasio & Damasio, 1989.) The results of these studies have shown that language processing is not "centered" on Broca and Wernicke's areas, but rather on systems composed of many neural sites working in close cooperation. Two of these sites include Broca's and Wernicke's areas. Language processing will, for instance, engage several regions of left temporal and prefrontal/premotor cortices in the left hemisphere, which lie outside the classical language areas (Damasio, 1990; Damasio, Damasio, Tranel, & Brandt, 1990; Damasio & Tranel, 1993; Goodglass, Wingfield, Hyde, & Theurkauf, 1986). It has also been shown that structures in the left basal ganglia, thalamus, and supplementary motor areas are engaged in language production (Damasio, Damasio, Rizzo, Varney, & Gersh, 1982; Graff-Radford, Damasio, Yamada, Eslinger, & Damasio, 1985; Graff-Radford, Schelper, Ilinsky, & Damasio, 1985; Naeser, Alexander, Helm-Estabrooks, Levine, Laughlin, and Geschwind, 1982).

The literature on language processing in normal subjects has grown immensely in recent years due to the availability of functional magnetic resonance (fMR), as well as, earlier on, developments such as positron emission tomography (PET) and several aspects of electrophysiology. Functional studies do address language processing and its neural underpinnings, but do so mostly on the basis of normal language in normal subjects. Given that this chapter is meant to address the neural basis of language disorders, I will not review the extensive literature on functional studies in normal language processing, but will rather concentrate on the "aphasias."

ANATOMICAL OVERVIEW
Sulci, Gyri and Cytoarchitectonic Fields

To understand the neural underpinnings of the aphasias, we must begin with an understanding of normal brain anatomy.

Knowledge of neuroanatomy has been gathered over the years mostly through the study of brains at the autopsy table, although today it is possible to study macroscopic anatomy at the computer screen, thanks to the technique of magnetic resonance (MR) imaging and to programs that manipulate MRI information and allow for 3-dimensional (3-D) reconstruction of brain tissue viewed at the computer screen. The brain anatomy reviewed in this chapter is based on normal brains, that is, brains of normal individuals without any neurologic or psychiatric disease. The brains I use have been reconstructed in 3-D from thin MR slices (1.5-mm thick). The slices are contiguous, T1-weighted, and obtained in the coronal direction. A collection of about 124 such coronal slices is stripped of scalp, meninges, blood vessels, cerebellum, and brainstem, and reconstructed in 3-D on the computer screen (of silicon graphics workstation, personal computers, or Apple workstations) using Brainvox (Damasio & Frank, 1992; Frank, Damaio, & Grabowski, 1997). Brainvox

is a family of programs developed to analyze normal and lesioned brains at the computer screen. It allows us to identify and color code sulci, gyri, lesions, or any structure on the 3-D rendered volume, on the original coronal slices, or on any slice obtained by slicing through the 3-D volume. Any such markings are immediately available on any 2-D view intersecting the marked structure and on the 3-D reconstructed brain. The 3-D reconstructed brain can be viewed in any direction, can be split into smaller regions, and can be measured volumetrically. Surface and linear measurements can also be obtained.

Figure 2–1 shows the left hemisphere of such a reconstructed normal brain seen from the lateral and mesial views. Some major sulci that divide the hemispheres into their basic constituents, the lobes and the gyri, are marked. (See also Damasio, 2005; Duvernoy, 1991; Ono, Kubik, & Abernathey, 1990; among others, for more anatomic information.) On the lateral surface the most prominent sulcus is

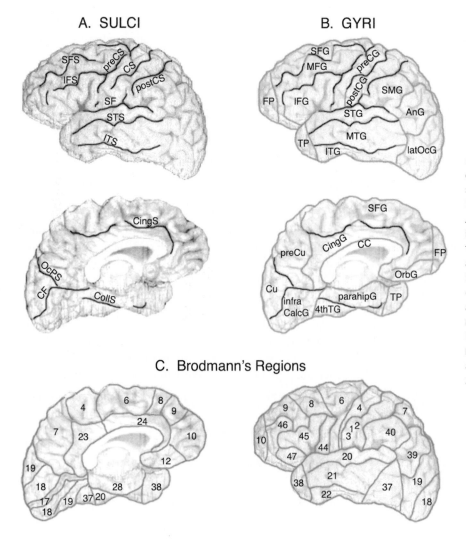

Figure 2–1. A. Lateral and mesial views of the left hemisphere of a brain reconstructed in 3-D from thin MRI slices using Brainvox. The major sulci are identified. Abbreviations are as mentioned in the text. **B.** The same lateral and mesial views of the left hemisphere, with the different gyri and their sulcal limits as seen in **A** (dark lines). The light gray lines show the remainder of the gyri limits (some are sulci, others are arbitrary lines). **C.** The same lateral and mesial views seen in **A** and **B**, here with Brodmann's cytoarchitectonic fields marked. (For more details on sulcal, gyral and cytoarchitectonic fields see Damasio, 2005.)

the sylvian fissure (SF), a mostly horizontal sulcus running anteroposteriorly. The SF separates the temporal lobe, below, from the frontal and parietal lobes, above. The posterior end of the SF usually shows an asymmetric course when the right and left hemispheres are compared (Damasio, 2005). It tends to be longer and lower on the left, and shorter and turning upward on the right. The other prominent sulcus, usually continuous, on the lateral surface of the hemispheres is the central sulcus (CS). It runs from the interhemispheric fissure (the separation between the two hemispheres) above, toward the SF, below, taking a posteroanterior course. It may or may not reach the sylvian fissure proper. This sulcus separates the frontal lobe, in front, from the parietal lobe (behind). Parallel to the central sulcus are two other sulci, which are more often than not subdivided into more than one segment. They are, anteriorly, the pre-central sulcus (preCS), and posteriorly, the post-central sulcus (postCS). Together with the central sulcus they define the pre-central and post-central gyri (preCG, postCG), respectively, the most posterior sector of the frontal lobe, often designated as the motor cortex (where the primary motor cortex or Brodmann's field 4 can be found), and the most anterior sector of the parietal lobe, the sensory cortex (where primary sensory cortices or Brodmann's fields 3, 1, and 2 are seen). Very often we speak of these two gyri as the "sensorimotor" cortices. There are two other prominent sulci to consider in the dorsolateral surface of the frontal lobe, namely the superior frontal sulcus (SFS) and the inferior frontal sulcus (IFS). Both run anteroposteriorly from the pre-central sulcus toward the polar region of the frontal lobe, usually stopping before reaching the pole. In relation to "language," the inferior frontal sulcus is probably the more important of the two, given that it forms the superior limit of the inferior frontal gyrus (IFG), in which we find the frontal operculum. The inferior frontal gyrus comprises distinct subdivisions corresponding to Brodmann's fields 44, 45, and 47. The combination of field 44 and 45 on the left is traditionally called Broca's area. Between the inferior frontal sulcus and the superior frontal sulcus lies the middle frontal gyrus (MFG) occupied by Brodmann's fields 46, 9, 8, and 6. The superior frontal sulcus constitutes the lateral and inferior limit of the superior frontal gyrus (SFG), which continues into the mesial surface of the hemisphere. On this dorsolateral aspect of the gyrus we find Brodmann's fields 9, 8, and 6. The most anterior sector of the frontal lobe, the polar region just in front of the three horizontal frontal gyri just described, also known as the frontal pole, is occupied by Brodmann's field 10.

In the temporal lobe there is one consistent sulcus, more or less parallel to the sylvian fissure, the superior temporal sulcus (STS). Together with the sylvian fissure it delineates the superior temporal gyrus (STG), which corresponds to Brodmann's field 22. Another sulcus, also parallel, can be seen on the lateral surface, the inferior temporal sulcus

(ITS). This sulcus is constituted, more often than not, by several small segments and can be difficult to recognize. It creates the separation between the middle temporal gyrus (MTG) containing Brodmann's field 21, above, and the inferior temporal gyrus (ITG) containing Brodmann's field 20, below. The posterior sector of both these gyri contain Brodmann's field 37, which continues into the inferomesial surface of the temporal lobe.

The parietal lobe is also subdivided by a prominent anteroposteriorly running sulcus, the intraparietal sulcus (IPS), starting at the post-central sulcus and going in the direction of the occipital lobe. This sulcus is more easily seen when looking at the brain from above (Fig. 2–2), and it separates the inferior parietal lobule (IPL), containing Brodmann's field 40 and 39, from the superior parietal lobule (SPL), containing Brodmann's field 5 and 7. The inferior parietal lobule is itself subdivided into two major gyri, namely the supramarginal gyrus (SMG), anteriorly (Brodmann's area 40), sitting on top of the sylvian fissure and around its posterior end, and the angular gyrus (AnG), or Brodmann's field 39, sitting behind and below the former, around the posterior end of the superior temporal sulcus.

No sulcal demarcation exists between the parietal, temporal, and occipital lobes on the lateral surface of the hemispheres.

On the mesial surface of the hemispheres, several major sulci are to be considered. One is the cingulate sulcus (CingS), continuous or subdivided into several segments, more or less parallel to the contour of the corpus callosum (CC). The corpus callosum is the midline white-matter structure containing the fibers connecting the cortices of the two hemispheres. Together with the pericallosal sulcus, directly around the corpus callosum, it creates the limit of the cingulate gyrus (CingG), containing prominently Brodmann's fields 23 and 24, plus several other regions buried within the sulcus itself. At its posterior end, the cingulate sulcus turns upward in what is known as the ascending branch of the cingulate sulcus.

In the mesial aspect of the temporal lobe there is one consistent sulcus, parallel to the long axis of the temporal lobe, the collateral sulcus (ColluS), which separates the fifth or parahippocampal gyrus (parahipG), containing Brodmann's field 28, from the inferotemporal region, the name often given to the temporal cortices between the collateral sulcus and the superior temporal sulcus described earlier (see also Fig. 2–2 for a better view of this sulcus). This inferotemporal region also includes the inferior temporal gyrus (ITG) and the fourth temporal gyrus (4thTG), containing both Brodmann's fields 20 and 37.

Mesially, the parietal lobe, the sector behind the ascending branch of the cingulate sulcus, is clearly separated from the occipital lobe by a sulcus running superoinferiorly and slightly posteroanteriorly, the occipitoparietal sulcus (OPS). The parietal region in front of this sulcus is also known as the precuneus (preCu) or Brodmann's field 7.

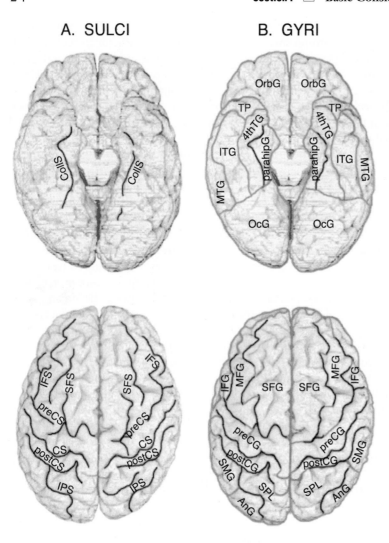

A. SULCI   B. GYRI

Figure 2–2. **A.** The inferior and superior views of the brain with markings of the most important sulci seen in those views. **B.** The same views as in **A**, here with identification of the gyri. It is important to note that these views show a very large surface of brain, something that viewing only the lateral and mesial aspects, as in Figure 2–1, may not be evident.

No distinct sulcus separates the occipital from the temporal lobe. However, in the mesial aspect of the occipital lobe itself there is a distinct and consistent sulcus, running anteroposteriorly—the calcarine fissure (CF)—whose two lips contain the primary visual cortex or Brodmann's field 17. The calcarine fissure separates the mesial aspect of the occipital lobe into two sectors: the supracalcarine region (sCR), or cuneus (CU), containing Brodmann's fields 18 and 19, and the infracalcarine region (iCR), also containing Brodmann's fields 18 and 19.

Typically, the occipitoparietal sulcus and the calcarine sulcus join just behind the posterior end of the corpus callosum, which is also known as the splenium. The cortex between the splenium and the juncture of the occipitoparietal and calcarine sulci is usually referred to as the "retrosplenial" area, which contains several different cytoarchitectonic areas.

Most of the cerebral cortex is actually not readily visible in any of the views we have been dealing with but rather are hidden within the hemispheric sulci, something that can be more easily appreciated if we look at coronal cuts throughout the hemispheres (Fig. 2–3). Furthermore, two surfaces of cortex are completely hidden from view when we look only at lateral, mesial, inferior, or superior views. These are the insula (In) and the Heschl's gyrus (HG), the latter also known as primary auditory cortex containing Brodmann's fields 41 and 42 (Fig. 2–3). Heschl's gyrus occupies the superior surface of the superior temporal gyrus. This structure divides the superior temporal gyrus into two distinct segments, one anterior and one posterior to it, both containing Brodmann's field 22. The posterior sector is also known as the planum temporale, which typically shows a marked asymmetry between the right and the left hemispheres, being usually larger on the left, where it constitutes the major portion of the classical Wernicke's area. The insula is also completely hidden. It can be found by opening up the sylvian fissure, separating the temporal lobe from the frontoparietal operculum. (See Damasio, 2005, for images depicting all these hidden structures.)

Figure 2–3. Two coronal cuts through the same brain seen in Figures 2–1 and 2–2, and whose left hemisphere is depicted on the right. The lines on the 3-D-reconstructed hemisphere represent the placement of the cuts seen on the left. Note that most of the cortical rim is actually not on the visible surface of the hemisphere but rather buried within the sulci. The ventricles appear as clearly delineated black structures. The subcortical gray areas, as well as the insula, can easily be identified in these cuts. Abbreviations are those used in the text. (The coronal slices are presented according to the radiologic convention, with the right hemisphere on the left and the left hemisphere on the right. This convention is respected in all illustrations. Brain slices are always presented from anterior to posterior or from the most inferior view to the most superior view.)

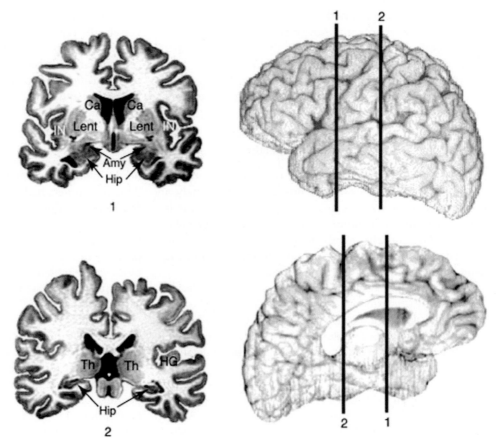

Figure 2–4. 3-D reconstruction of the brain of a patient with stroke. Acutely the patient had Broca's aphasia and mild right-arm and facial paresis as a result of an infarction in a middle branch of the MCA (pre-central artery). Recovery was fairly quick. In the chronic epoch there were no motor defects and language had improved remarkably. The lesion occupies the anterior half (lower two-thirds) of the pre-central gyrus, not damaging the motor cortex in the central sulcus (arrows) in the left hemisphere. The lesion also damages the posterior sector of the inferior frontal gyrus (the pars opercularis of the frontal operculum). It does not damage insula or basal ganglia, which can be seen to be intact in the coronal slices. In summary, it is a lesion that partially damages premotor cortices 6 and 44, but leaves most of Broca's area intact.

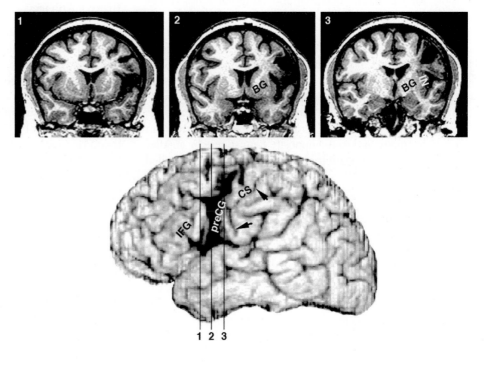

We should also refer briefly to some of the more important subcortical gray matter structures (Fig. 2–3). Within the temporal lobe, in the depth of the parahippocampal gyrus, we find the hippocampus proper (Hip) and the amygdala (Amy). Within the frontal lobe we find the basal ganglia (BG) with its separate constituents, the caudate nucleus and the lenticular nucleus.

Vascular Supply of the Cerebral Hemispheres

Before we begin our discussion about the neurologic underpinnings of the aphasias, we need one more aside, namely, a very brief overview of the brain's vascular supply. This is important as the most common cause of aphasia is a vascular lesion, and because the vascular lesions causing aphasia have allowed us to use the lesion method efficiently to find the neural underpinnings of language disorders.

The brain's vascular supply comes from the internal carotid artery (the external carotid giving blood supply to the extracranial tissues). (See also Day, 1987; Damasio, 1987b; Lazorthes, Gouaze, & Salamon, 1976; Szilda, Bouvier, Hori, & Petrov, 1977; and Waddington, 1974 , for more detail of the vascular supply of the brain.)

The blood supply for each hemisphere comes mostly from the internal carotid artery (ICA), which is subdivided into two major branches: the anterior cerebral artery (ACA) mesially, and the middle cerebral artery (MCA) laterally. The ACA supplies most of the mesial and orbital sectors of the frontal lobe and the mesial sector of the parietal lobe. The MCA provides the blood supply for most of the inferior and lateral sectors of the temporal lobe, and the lateral sector of the frontal, parietal, and occipital lobes. The blood supply for the mesial occipital and temporal lobes comes from the posterior cerebral artery (PCA), a branch of the basilar artery.

The mesial aspect of the most anterior sector of the temporal lobe gets its blood supply from the anterior choroidal artery (antChA), a branch of the internal carotid artery before the internal carotid subdivides into middle and anterior cerebral arteries. The three main vascular territories mentioned, the ACA, MCA, and PCA, are interconnected in each hemisphere and to the opposite hemisphere by smaller vessels, the communicating arteries, forming what is called the circle of Willis.

The area at the edges of each of the three main territories receives capillaries from the three arterial territories as they meet. This "horseshoe" region occupies a sector on the superior frontal gyrus, the superior parietal lobule and the angular gyrus, and the posterolateral aspect of the occipital lobe, continuing on the inferior surface of the temporal lobe toward the temporal pole. It is normally designated as the watershed area. It is important to have an idea about this region for two specific reasons. First, because of its dual blood supply, this region is more resistant to infarction.

Second, because its supply is achieved by terminal, thinner vessels, the region is more vulnerable to severe decreases in arterial blood pressure. In such events, as, for example, in cases of cardiac arrest, this is one of the regions that suffers the most intense deprivation of oxygen. In a stroke caused by a severe and sustained drop in blood pressure, these areas may be compromised. When this happens in the left hemisphere the consequence can be an aphasia of the transcortical type.

Another region is supplied by terminal arteries, but does not have dual blood supply: the region of the basal ganglia. This region gets its blood supply from multiple, thin, and fragile perforating vessels that leave the stem of the middle cerebral artery at almost right angles. This configuration makes them very vulnerable to sudden decreases in blood pressure in the main supplying vessel as well as to arterial blockage by emboli. Damage in these territories in the left hemisphere may lead to infarcts in the basal ganglia causing "atypical aphasias."

Because the blood supply to the brain is carried out by small vessels that penetrate the hemispheres through the cortex in the direction of the underlying white matter, an obstruction of any of the major supply vessels tends to create an area of infarct that is broader on the surface than in the depth. It is the reason for the well-known and traditional description of the image of a stroke as a wedge-shaped form with the base turned toward the cortex.

NEUROANATOMICAL CORRELATES OF THE APHASIAS

Classic Aphasias

Broca's Aphasia

Broca's description of the language impairment seen in his patient Leborgne suggests that the condition was worse than what we associate today with a typical Broca's aphasia. The speech output was so sparse that it was largely confined to the word "tant," and comprehension of spoken language was also severely compromised (Broca, 1861). In modern terms, the disorder that began the history of aphasiology and whose lesion became associated with Broca's aphasia, would probably be described as a global aphasia. Usually, Broca's aphasia is characterized by sparse agrammatical discourse, but not by complete absence of speech.

Even today, there are still unresolved issues about the anatomical underpinnings of Broca's aphasia. For instance, in 1978 Mohr and collaborators pointed out that infarctions confined to the inferior frontal gyrus cause only a brief period of mutism, which resolves into effortful speech but generally does not cause significant linguistic deficits (Mohr, Pessin, Finkelstein, Funkenstein, Duncan, & Davis, 1978). They claimed that such lesions do not cause a Broca's aphasia in the proper sense. The same investigators suggested

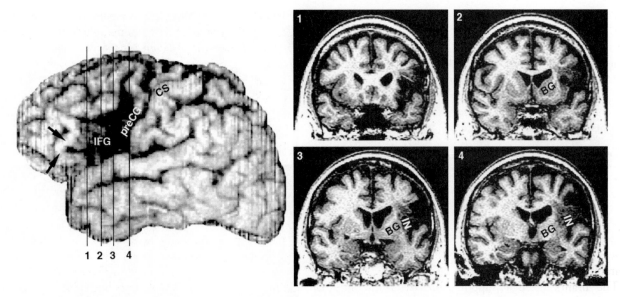

Figure 2–5. 3-D reconstruction of the brain of a patient who acutely also had Broca's aphasia together with facial and arm paresis as a result of an infarction in the territories of the anterior and middle branches of the MCA (pre-frontal and pre-central arteries). Compared to the image in Figure 2–4 the damage is larger anteriorly. This patient also recovered but was left with mild weakness in the right arm and with language deficits that were still classified as a mild Broca's aphasia. The lesion occupies the inferior third of the entire pre-central gyrus, involving the central sulcus region in the left hemisphere (Brodmann's fields 6 and 4). It also involves the posterior two-thirds of the inferior frontal gyrus corresponding to the entire frontal operculum (pars opercularis and triangularis and even part of pars orbitalis); all of Broca's area is involved (fields 44, 45, and part of 47). It is only the outer rim of the inferior frontal gyrus that is spared (arrows). The lesion also extends further into the underlying white matter than in the previous case (Fig. 2-4). It damages insula but does not damage the basal ganglia (see the two lower coronal cuts on the right).

that the lesion necessary to produce the more severe language disturbance usually classified as Broca's aphasia is far larger, requiring the involvement of all of the frontal operculum and of the insula. In our experience, chronic and long-lasting language deficits conforming to the characteristics of a Broca's aphasia in the chronic epoch do indeed require damage of a sizable area of the frontal operculum and surrounding tissue. However, in the acute epoch of the condition, a small and circumscribed infarct of the frontal operculum can also produce a nonfluent language deficit with all the characteristics of a typical Broca's aphasia (Fig. 2–4). Similar findings have been described by Tonkonogy and Goodglass (1981). These authors pointed out that a small lesion involving the frontal operculum had caused linguistic deficits in the acute epoch, although the deficits were not long-lasting. In the same study, the authors showed that an equally small lesion placed in an immediately posterior position, in the rolandic operculum, did not cause any phonemic, lexical, or syntactical processing difficulties, but rather dysarthric and dysprosodic speech output (see also Schiff, Alexander, Naeser, & Galaburda, 1983).

When language deficits are classified as a Broca's aphasia in the acute phase and when they persist for months, it is usually the case that damage in a large sector of the inferior frontal gyrus is found, as seen in Figure 2–5, for example. (See also Alexander, Naeser, & Palumbo., 1990, and Naeser & Hayward, 1978.) In other cases, the infarct may be in the territory of most of the anterior branches of the MCA and will have damaged not just the cortex of the frontal operculum (Brodmann's fields 44 and 45), but also have extended into the underlying white matter and involved the insula and the basal ganglia, as well as the inferior sector of the pre-central gyrus. Other such chronic Broca's aphasias will have started as a global aphasia in the acute period. (See also the section on Global Aphasia, below, and Fig. 2–9.)

Wernicke's Aphasia

There has never been the same degree of controversy in relation to the symptom complex or to the anatomical correlate of the prototypical fluent aphasia: Wernicke's aphasia. Wernicke's original description of the language impairment and of its underlying brain damage (Wernicke, 1886) is consonant with contemporary investigations (Damasio, 1981, 1987a; Kertesz, 1979; Kertesz, Harlock, & Coates, 1979; Kertesz, Lau, & Polk, 1993; Knopman, Selnes,

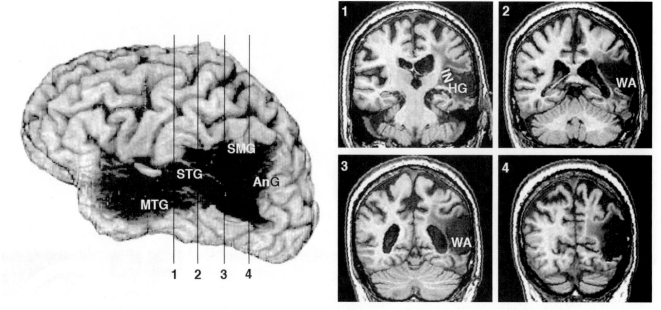

Figure 2–6. 3-D reconstruction of the brain of a patient who acutely presented with Wernicke's aphasia and right hemianopsia as a result of an infarction in the territory of the temporal branches of the MCA. The visual field persisted in the chronic epoch as did the aphasia. The lesion involves most of the dorsolateral aspect of the left temporal lobe. The superior and middle temporal gyri are completely occupied by damaged tissue (Brodmann's fields 22, 21, and part of 37), as well as the inferior sector of the supramarginal gyrus (field 40), and the anterior sector of the angular gyrus (field 39). The damage extends deep into the underlying white matter, destroying the posterior segment of the insula and reaching the ventricle in the posterior cuts (see coronal slices 2 and 3). Cortical areas that are destroyed beyond the insula include the primary auditory cortices in the transverse gyrus of Heschl (fields 41 and 42) and all of the surrounding superior temporal gyrus (field 22), which in the posterior portion forms Wernicke's area (also seen in the coronal slices on the right).

Niccum, & Rubens, 1984; Mazzocchi & Vignolo, 1979; Naeser & Hayward, 1978; and Selnes et al., 1983; 1984; 1985, among others). A typical case of Wernicke's aphasia due to an infarct of the temporal arteries is depicted in Figure 2–6. The lesion is seen in the posterior sector of the superior temporal gyrus (Brodmann's field 22). This region is the core of Wernicke's area. The lesion also extends into the posterior region of the middle and inferior temporal gyri (part of Brodmann's fields 37, 20, and 21), and into part of the inferior parietal lobule, destroying the lower sector of the supramarginal and the angular gyri (Brodmann's fields 40 and 39). In such cases, recovery is limited and a severe fluent aphasia may persist for months. A noticeable aphasia may persist for years.

Conduction Aphasia

When damage is limited to the supramarginal gyrus (Brodmann's field 40) the result is a fluent aphasia, distinct from Wernicke's aphasia, known as "conduction aphasia." The fundamental clinical characteristic of conduction aphasia is a severe inability to repeat verbatim a heard sentence. In severe cases, even single words are not repeated. This repetition deficit is disproportionately severe in comparison to the ability to produce spontaneous speech or to understand speech. (See Benson, Sheremata, Bouchard, Segarra, Price, & Geschwind, 1973; Geschwind, 1965; Konorski, Kozniewska, & Stepien, 1961; Liepmann & Pappenheim, 1914, for the early descriptions of the syndrome and its underlying brain damage, and Damasio & Damasio, 1980; Kertesz et al., 1979; Naeser & Hayward, 1978; Rubens & Selnes, 1986, among others, for later descriptions.)

Typical cases of conduction aphasia are often caused by damage to the supramarginal gyrus (see Fig. 2–7 for an example). This is the case of a patient who, at age 33, suffered an intracerebral hemorrhage to the left parietal lobe that lead to the diagnosis of an intracerebral arteriovenous malformation (AVM). To excise the entire malformation, the neurosurgeon had to remove the entire supramarginal gyrus, while being able to spare the entire superior temporal gyrus. After surgery this patient presented with a

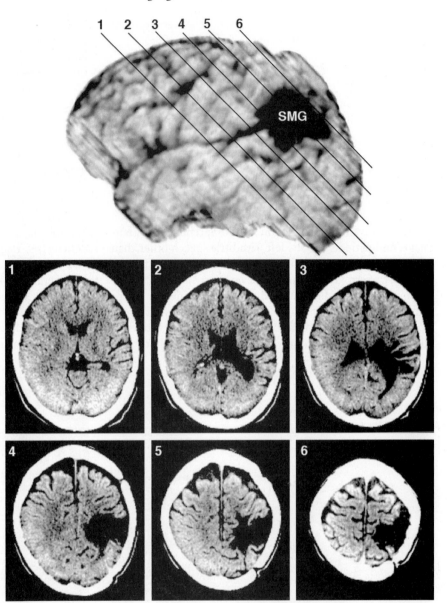

Figure 2–7. 3-D reconstruction (in this instance from a thin-cut CT scan) of the brain of a patient with conduction aphasia resulting from an arteriovenous malformation that ruptured and bled. The condition required the subsequent surgical removal of most of the supramarginal gyrus. In the chronic epoch this patient continues to display a mild conduction aphasia. The lesion involves the supramarginal gyrus (Brodmann's field 40). Wernicke's area is mostly intact.

typical conduction aphasia. She was unable to repeat even short sentences, for example, "Take this home." As is typical of conduction aphasia, comprehension of the sentences to be repeated was preserved. For example, asked to repeat "The orchestra played and the audience applauded," verbatim, the patient failed entirely. Yet, when asked about the meaning of the sentence she paraphrased it as "There was music and they liked it, they clapped." Even today, almost 20 years after the onset of her aphasia, this patient has difficulty in repeating sentences longer than three or four words, although her other acute deficits, for example, her naming impairment, have improved remarkably.

Damage to the cortex of the supramarginal gyrus and to its underlying white matter compromises the arcuate fasciculus,

the pathway that connects posterior and anterior language areas as first described by Dejerine (1906). Geschwind (1965) proposed that the inability to repeat was a result of damage to the pathway and although the essence of this explanation may well be correct for some cases of conduction aphasia, it may not be adequate for all. It is certainly the case that conduction aphasia can result from somewhat different lesion patterns. In 1980 we described patients with lesions in left auditory cortex and insula, without involvement of supramarginal gyrus, who presented with a typical conduction aphasia (Damasio & Damasio, 1980). Rubens and Selnes (1986) also described a similar presentation with exclusively left insular damage. Interestingly, the arcuate fasciculus seems not to course exclusively in the depth of the supramarginal gyrus as described by Dejerine but may instead be a large sheath of white matter whose lower segment courses under the insula (Galaburda & Pandya, 1983).

Global Aphasia

While occlusion of some of the anterior branches of the middle cerebral artery causes a nonfluent Broca's type of aphasia, and occlusion of posterior temporal and parietal branches causes a fluent, Wernicke's type of aphasia, occlusion of the middle cerebral artery itself, prior to its branching, causes extensive damage to frontal, parietal, and temporal regions, and results in a more severe language deficit known as "global aphasia." As the description indicates, the ensuing deficits involve both production and comprehension of language, and patients may be left with little speech other than for stereotyped and automated words and stock sentences. This sort of stroke also causes a severe restriction of movement in the right side of the body, a right hemiplegia. A typical image of the brain lesion of such a patient is shown in Figure 2–8. The signs of global aphasia—namely, little language output, severe comprehension deficits in both oral

and written form, inability to repeat, and inability to write— may appear in association with more restricted lesions. A large left frontal-lobe lesion, involving not only Broca's area but extending into other frontal gyri, the pre- and post-central gyri, the supramarginal gyrus, the insula, and the basal ganglia, sparing the temporal lobe altogether, may present as a severe global aphasia. Such an "acute" global aphasia may resolve into a less severe albeit remarkable language deficit and be eventually classified as a severe Broca's aphasia (see Fig. 2–9 for an example).

One other anatomical presentation of global aphasia deserves mention. The severe and pervasive linguistic deficit of global aphasia, which is usually accompanied by a right hemiplegia, may, on occasion, present without any motor deficits (see Legatt, Rubin, Kaplan, Healton, & Brust, 1987, and Tranel, Biller, Damasio, Adams, & Cornell, 1987). Such a presentation is the consequence of two separate lesions due, for instance, to multiple emboli causing infarctions in both anterior and posterior branches of the middle cerebral artery. In other words, instead of a blockage of the main trunk of the artery, at the level of the stem, resulting in one

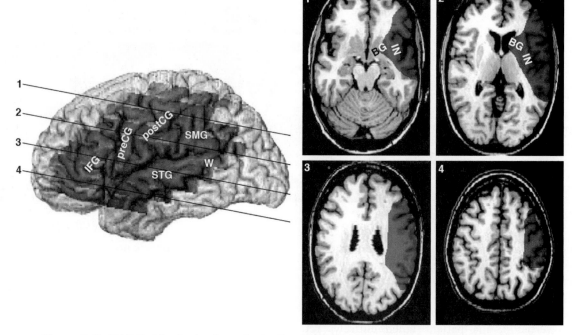

Figure 2–8. MAP-3 of the brain of a patient with a large left MCA infarct resulting in severe global aphasia and right hemiparesis. (MAP-3 is a technique that allows the 3-D visualization of lesions of individual subjects in a common normal target brain. For details about the technique see Damasio, 2000, 2005, and Frank et al., 1997). The lesion involves most of the frontal-lobe structures in the territory of the anterior branches of the MCA, including the inferior frontal gyrus with Broca's area (Brodmann's fields 44, 45, and 47), most of the sensorimotor cortices in the pre-central and post-central gyri (fields 6, and 4, and 3, 1, and 2), and the supramarginal gyrus (field 40), as well as all of the superior temporal gyrus (fields 22, 41, and42), including Wernicke's area (W). The insula and the basal ganglia, as well as the white matter in the frontal and parietal lobes, are also damaged.

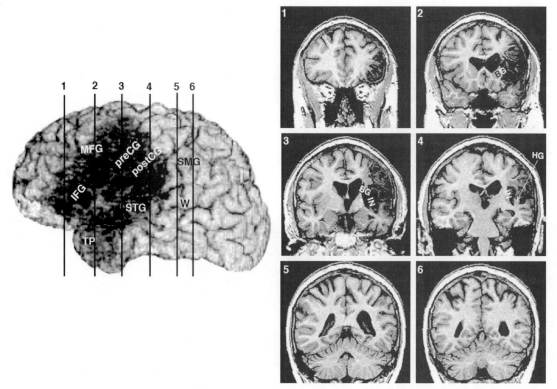

Figure 2–9. 3-D reconstruction of the brain of a patient with a large infarct in the territory of the anterior frontal branches of the left MCA as well as the anterior-temporal branches. This patient also presented acutely with a right hemiparesis and global aphasia. In the chronic epoch, however, language had improved enough to have the aphasia reclassified as a severe Broca's aphasia. The infarct involves prefrontal cortices in both the inferior and part of the middle-frontal gyri (Brodmann's fields 45, 47, and part of 46 and 9), premotor regions in the same gyri (Brodmann's fields 44 and 6), sensorimotor regions in the pre- and post-central gyri (Brodmann's fields 4, 3, 1, and 2), the anterior sector of the superior temporal gyrus (Brodmann's field 22), and the dorsolateral sector of the temporal pole (Brodmann's field 38). The insula is equally damaged and the infarct extends deep into the subcortical structures, damaging the basal ganglia (caudate and putamen), as seen in the coronal cuts on the right. The important feature to note is that the primary auditory cortex (Brodmann's fields 41 and 42) in Heschl's gyrus is only partially damaged (see cut 4) and that both Wernicke's area (posterior Brodmann's field 22) and the supramarginal gyrus (Brodmann's field 40) are spared, as can be seen in the two cuts in the bottom row and in the 3-D-reconstructed hemisphere on the left.

large lesion, more peripheral blockages occur and thus result in more than one lesion. As described in Tranel et al. (1987), there may be an area of infarct in the left prefrontal/premotor cortices, and then another in the left posterior temporal-parietal region, sparing the sensorimotor cortices in between (Fig. 2–10). As is to be expected from the lesion placement, patients with this form of global aphasia recover faster and better than do those with classic global aphasia.

Transcortical Aphasias

The transcortical aphasias are characterized by normal word and sentence repetition. Transcortical sensory aphasia is diagnosed when a patient presents with fluent paraphasic speech and with poor auditory comprehension but with intact word and sentence repetition. There is a practical value in recognizing this type of aphasia as separate from Wernicke's aphasia because it indicates to the clinician that both the primary auditory cortices (Brodmann's fields 41 and 42 in the transverse gyrus of Heschl) and the posterior sector of the superior temporal gyrus (Wernicke's area proper) are spared. In transcortical sensory aphasia, the damage is posterior and inferior to the above-mentioned regions. It may involve the angular gyrus (Brodmann's field 39) and the posterior sector of the middle temporal gyrus (Brodmann's field 37).

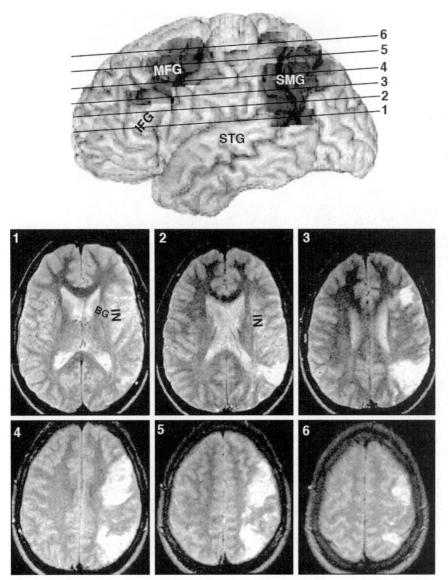

Figure 2–10. T2-weighted MR image and MAP-3 of the brain of another patient who acutely presented with global aphasia, but this time without hemiparesis. This patient improved rapidly and was eventually left with only a mild language deficit. Note the two separate areas of infarction in the left hemisphere: the more anterior lesion is in the territory of the anterior branches of the MCA, damaging the superior sector of the frontal operculum in the inferior frontal gyrus (Brodmann's field 45), and the posterior sector of the middle frontal gyrus (field 6); the more posterior lesion is in the territory of the posterior branches of the MCA, damaging the supramarginal gyrus (field 40) and probably a portion of the posterior sector of the superior temporal gyrus (field 22). The sensorimotor cortices in the pre- and post-central gyri, the insula, and the basal ganglia are intact, as is most of the frontal operculum and most of Wernicke's area (which, however, is not completely spared).

On occasion the lesions may extend into the lateral aspect of the occipital lobe (Brodmann's fields 19 and 18) or into more anterior sectors of the middle temporal gyrus (Brodmann's field 21) See Alexander, Hiltbronner, & Fischer, 1989b; Damasio, 1981, 1987a; Freedman, Alexander, & Naeser, 1984; and Kertesz et al., 1979, among others.) In some instances, this same type of aphasia can be detected with exclusively subcortical lesions underlying the cortical regions mentioned above, as described in Damasio (1987a). See Figure 2–11 for an example of a transcortical sensory aphasia.

When patients present with a nonfluent language deficit and preserved repetition, we talk about a transcortical motor aphasia. The location of the lesions responsible for this type of aphasia is less consistent than for the transcor-

tical sensory type. We may find transcortical motor aphasia in patients with small subcortical lesions located immediately anterior to the frontal horn of the left lateral ventricle, a part of the so-called anterior watershed area (Fig. 2–12). We also may find transcortical motor aphasia with lesions in the left frontal lobe involving prefrontal and premotor cortices (Brodmann's fields 10, 9, 46, 8, and 6, respectively).

Isolation of the Speech Areas

The combinations of the lesions described for transcortical motor aphasia with those responsible for transcortical sensory aphasia may result in an extensive lesion that isolates the "speech area." Patients with such lesions have a

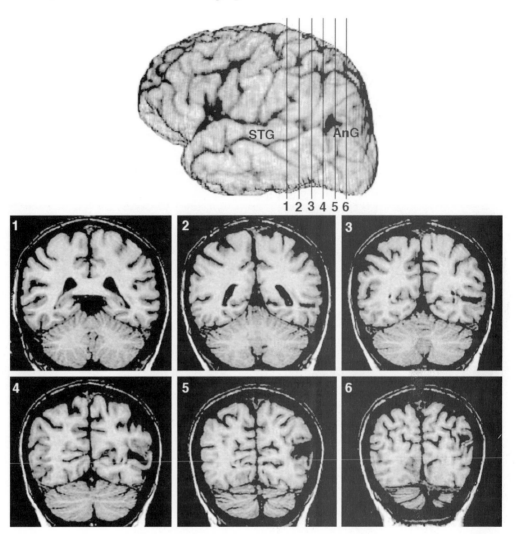

Figure 2–11. 3-D reconstruction of the brain of a patient who presented with a fluent aphasia but intact repetition. This is a typical presentation of transcortical sensory aphasia. The cause of the syndrome was an acute intracerebral hemorrhage in the left hemisphere. In the chronic epoch, after resolution of the hemorrhage, we see an area of encephalomalacia in the left angular gyrus (Brodmann's field 39) and underlying white matter but no damage to the posterior sector of the superior temporal gyrus. There is also evidence of some enlargement in the anterior sector of the sylvian fissure, possibly due to atrophy in the frontal gyri. However, no brain-tissue damage can be detected in these regions.

severe dual deficit in language comprehension and intentional language formulation, associated with a remarkably preserved capacity for aural repetition of even long sentences, devoid of any proper comprehension of sentence meaning. The repetition is achieved with so much ease that it is best described as echolalia, the immediate and rather accurate repetition of any verbal material received auditorily. When asked a question the patient may actually repeat the question verbatim instead of providing an answer. Geschwind described one of these rare cases, which was due to severe carbon monoxide poisoning (Geschwind, Quadfaset, & Segarra, 1968). The underlying pathology was a watershed infarction nearly occupying the totality of the watershed region between the anterior and middle cerebral arteries and the posterior and middle cerebral arteries.

Crossed Aphasia

As mentioned earlier, the diagnosis of crossed aphasia applies when a fully right-handed subject has a lesion in the right hemisphere and becomes aphasic as a consequence of that lesion (Fig. 2–13). The incidence of such cases is low (Alexander, Fischette, & Fischer, 1989a; Castro-Caldas, Confraria, & Poppe, 1987). The same sort of individuals may fail to develop aphasia following lesions located in "language-related" areas of the left hemisphere, a situation known as "crossed non-aphasia" (Fig. 2–14).

Atypical Aphasias

With the advent of the modern neuroimaging techniques, beginning with early CT scans in 1972 and then with MRI

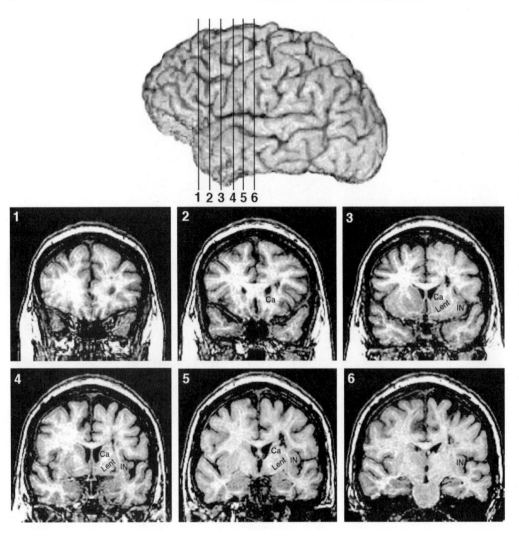

Figure 2–12. 3-D reconstruction of the brain of a patient who suffered a relatively small infarct in the left hemisphere, in the region of the anterior watershed territory. The external surface of the brain is intact, including all of the cortical mantle in Broca's and Wernicke's areas. The area of damage can only be seen in the coronal slices as an area of decreased signal in the white matter just anterior to the frontal horn of the left ventricle (see the first coronal cut). It extends posteriorly lateral to the lateral ventricle. It does not damage the caudate nucleus or the insula. This patient showed the typical presentation of transcortical motor aphasia.

scans since the early 1980s, it became possible to identify the neural underpinnings of some aphasic presentations that were classified as "atypical". The atypicality was usually the result of a mixture of features of nonfluent and fluent aphasias that produced a blend quite distinctive from the severe and all-encompassing deficits of a global aphasia.

In the early 1980s several authors provided anatomical evidence for the connection between such a mixture of symptoms and infarcts in the basal ganglia. More specifically, the infarcts were located in the left hemisphere, in the head of the caudate nucleus, and in the putamen (Aran, Rose, Rekate, & Whiteaker, 1983; Brunner, Kornhuber, Seemiuller, Suger, & Wallesch, 1982; Damasio et al., 1982; Damasio, Eslinger, & Adams, 1984; Fromm, Holland, Swindell, & Reinmuth, 1985; Naeser et al., 1982). No aphasia at all is seen when the damage occurs in the right hemisphere. The vascular territory affected here

was that of the striate arteries, a set of small terminal arteries arising from the stem of the middle cerebral artery. When infarcts are placed more laterally, involving only the lateral aspect of the putamen and the external and extreme capsules, and even the anterior insula, no aphasia is observed although the patient may show dysarthria and dysprosodia.

The early reports, based on relatively low-resolution scans of the 1970s, raised the possibility that there might be undetected damage in cortical regions. In a postmortem study, however, Barat and colleagues demonstrated that there was no damage outside the basal ganglia (Barat, Mazaux, Bioulac, Giroire, Vital, & Arne, 1981). Under the microscope, no area of abnormality could be seen in the cortical language areas. Modern, high-resolution MR scans confirm that this syndrome does occur as a result of damage to the left basal ganglia without involvement of the cortical language regions (Fig. 2–15).

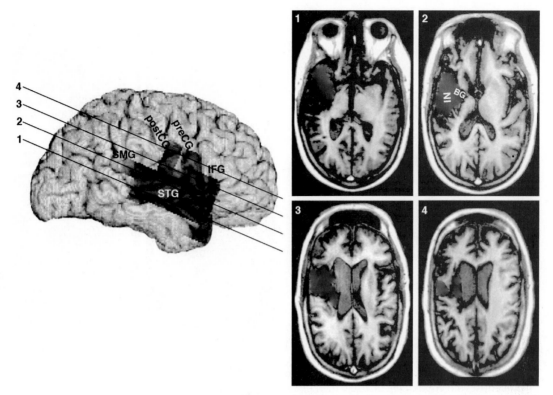

Figure 2–13. T1-weighted MR image and MAP-3 of a right-handed patient with an infarct in the territory of the right anterior branches of the MCA (pre-frontal, pre-central, and central) and the territory of the anterior and middle temporal arteries. He presented with a left hemiparesis, visual neglect, anosognosia, visuospatial deficits, and severe atypical aphasia—a typical presentation for a "crossed aphasia." There is damage to the right hemisphere in the frontal operculum of the inferior frontal gyrus (part of Brodmann's fields 44, 45, and 47), the sensorimotor cortices in the lower tier of the pre- and post-central gyri (fields 6 and 4, and 3, 1, and 2), the inferior sector of the supramarginal gyrus (field 40), most of the anterior sectors of the superior temporal gyrus (field 22), the auditory cortices in Heschl's gyrus (fields 41 and 42), as well as extension into insula and deep structures such as the basal ganglia. There is no sign of damage in the left hemisphere.

The occurrence of aphasia with damage in the left thalamus has been noted with vascular lesions (Alexander & Loverme, 1980; Cappa & Vignolo, 1979; McFarling Rothi, & Heilman, 1982; Mohr, Wafters, & Duncan, 1975), and with thalamic tumors (Arseni, 1958; Cheek & Taveras, 1966). The modern neuroimaging techniques have helped establish a precise anatomical basis for these aphasias (Archer, Ilinsky, Goldfader, & Smith, 1981; Cohen, Gelfer, & Sweet, 1980; Graff-Radford & Damasio, 1984; Graff-Radford, Damasio, et al., 1985; Graff-Radford, Schelper, et al., 1985). Lesions in the anterior nuclei of the left thalamus, involving mostly the lateroventral and anteroventral nuclei were related to aphasias of the transcortical type (Fig. 2–16). Lesions of the left thalamus that spare the anterior nuclei, and lesions of the right thalamus, result in sensory and motor deficits but not in aphasia.

Anomic Aphasia

Difficulty in producing the words that denote concrete entities presented visually, the most typical situation of "confrontation naming," is often present in most types of aphasia. On occasion, however, such a deficit is disproportionate in relation to other language deficits, or can even occur in isolation, something that was noted as early as 1898 by Pities (Pitres, 1898). In such situations, it may be reasonable to use the label "anomic aphasia" or "amnesic aphasia."

In 1986 Goodglass called attention to the fact that a dissociation between the production of words denoting actions and those denoting concrete entities could be found in patients with both nonfluent and fluent aphasia, respectively (Goodglass et al., 1986; see also Daniele, Giustolisi, Silveri, Colosimo, & Gainotti, 1994). In 1984 Warrington and Shallice had called attention to the presentation of different

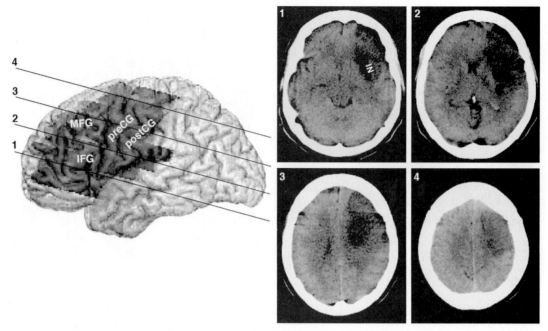

Figure 2–14. CT scan and MAP-3 of the brain of a right-handed patient with a very large left MCA infarct followed by a partial frontotemporal brain resection. Neither the infarct nor the subsequent surgery resulted in aphasia; there was only mild dysarthria. The patient, however, did present severe impairment of visual memory, visuoconstructional abilities, and some degree of anosognosia. These symptoms are suggestive of a lesion in the nondominant hemisphere, suggesting reversed language dominance in this right-handed subject. We would talk about a "crossed non-aphasia."

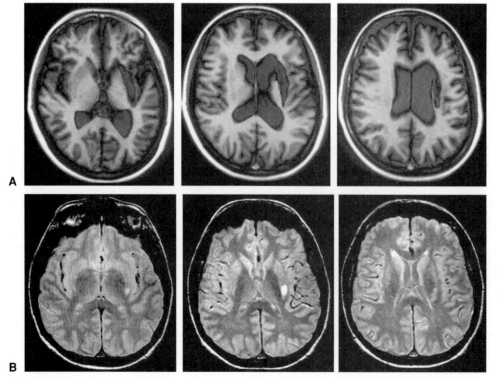

Figure 2–15. A. T1-weighted MR image of a patient who presented acutely with a left basal ganglionic hemorrhage and an atypical aphasia. This scan, obtained in the chronic epoch, shows a lesion in the head of the caudate nucleus and the putamen, as well as the internal capsule. However, there is no damage to cortical regions in the frontal operculum, nor to posterior temporal cortices. **B.** T2-weighted MR image of a patient who presented acutely with dysarthria, but no aphasia, as a result of a ventriculostriatal infarct affecting the posterior sector of the putamen. Most of the putamen is, however, spared, as is the caudate nucleus.

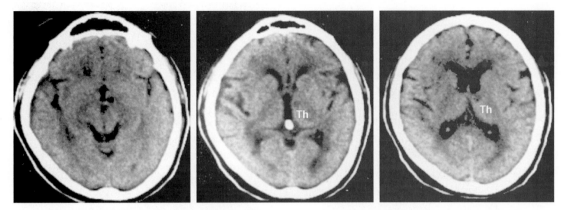

Figure 2–16. CT scan of a patient who presented acutely with an atypical aphasia due to an infarct of the anterior thalamic arteries. There is a low-density lesion in the anteromesial region of the left thalamus.

patients with category-specific semantic impairments (Hart, Berndt, & Caramazza, 1985; Hillis & Caramazza, 1991; Semenza & Zettin, 1989; Silveri & Gainotti, 1988; Warrington & McCarthy, 1994; Warrington & Shallice, 1984).

The possible anatomical underpinnings for such category-specific word retrieval deficits only began to be elucidated over the past decade. Today there is ample evidence that the inferotemporal cortex of the left cerebral hemisphere can be segregated into distinct areas whose damage causes category-specific word retrieval defects for visually presented concrete entities (Caramazza & Hillis, 1991; Damasio et al., 1990; Damasio & Tranel, 1993; Damasio, Grabowski, Tranel, Hichwa, & Damasio, 1996; Hillis & Caramazza, 1991; Miozzo, Soardi, & Cappa; 1994; Perani, Cappa, Bettinardi, Bressi, Gorno-Tempini, Matarrese, & Fazio, 1995; Tranel, Damasio, & Damasio, 1997; Tranel, Logan, Frank, & Damasio, 1997). Convergent findings have come through functional studies of nonlesioned brains (Buchel et al., 1998; Bunn et al., 1998; Damasio et al., 1996; Frith, Friston, Liddle, & Frackowiak, 1991; Martin et al., 1996; Mazoyer et al., 1993; Nobre et al., 1994; Ojemann, 1983; 1991; Petersen et al., 1988; Schlaghecken, 1998).

Work from our laboratory has shown that lesions located exclusively in the left temporal pole can cause deficits in the retrieval of proper names for unique persons, in the presence of normal recognition of those persons (Damasio et al., 1996; Damasio, Tranel, Grabowski, Adolphs, & Damasio, 2004). Such deficits are not seen with lesions in the temporal pole of the nondominant hemisphere although damage to the right temporal pole may result in a deficient recognition of unique persons (Tranel, Logan, et al., 1997). (See Damasio et al., 1996; 2004, and Tranel, Logan, et al., 1997, for details of the testing procedures required to separate the processes of recognition and name retrieval.) When the lesion extends into the left anterior sector of the inferior temporal lobe, in addition to damaging the temporal pole, the deficit encom-

passes not only the retrieval of words denoting unique persons but also those of nonunique animals. If the lesion spares the temporal pole but damages the anterior sector of the IT region, the deficit may be limited to the retrieval of words denoting animals alone. Again, recognition is not affected (in order for recognition of animals to be affected, the lesions must involve the mesial occipitotemporal cortices, especially those in the right hemisphere). When the retrieval of words denoting nonunique manipulable tools is the predominant feature of a naming deficit, the lesion usually involves the left posterior IT region at the level of the lateral occipitotemporal junction. See Figure 2–17 for a summary of lesions producing category-specific deficits.

We should consider here another group of patients who often present with pure naming deficits in the early stages of disease, the so-called "progressive aphasias." The term refers to subjects who show a progressive impairment in language performance, usually starting with a deficit in unique name retrieval, later proceeding to encompass deficits in the retrieval of words denoting nonunique entities, and finally encompassing more typical features of aphasia. The underlying damage is usually found in the left temporal lobe in the form of atrophy. The atrophy usually starts in the polar region and gradually comes to involve more of the temporal region, especially in IT regions. Many of these patients have a progressive degenerative disease, for example, a variant of Pick's disease. On occasion, the disease may affect first the frontal lobe, with particular atrophy in the inferior frontal gyrus. In such cases, the presenting signs are those of difficulty retrieving words denoting actions and words denoting relationship of entities.

Mutism

Mutism is a condition that is not strictly an aphasia but is often taken as such. For instance, patients with akinetic mutism do not have abnormal language: they simply do not

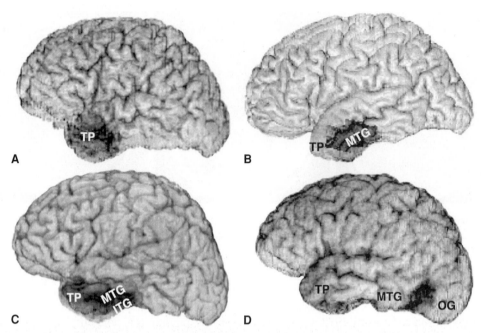

Figure 2–17. 3-D reconstruction (**A, C, D**) and MAP-3 (**B**) of the brains of four different patients with anomia. **A.** A subject with left temporal lobectomy who after surgery was left with severe impairment of naming of unique persons whom the patient could, however, recognize. The excised area was limited to the temporopolar region (Brodmann's field 38). **B.** A subject with a resection of an arteriovenous malformation in the anterior sector of the left temporal lobe. After surgery there was a lesion in the anterior sector of the middle and inferior temporal gyri (fields 21 and 20) without extensive damage to the temporal pole. This subject showed a deficit in retrieval of words denoting living entities such as animals, which he could, however, recognize. There were no other aphasic symptoms, nor were there deficits in the retrieval of unique names. **C.** A subject with left temporal lobectomy, more extensive than the one depicted in **A.** In this case the excision included the temporopolar region (field 38) as well as the most anterior sector of the middle and inferior temporal gyri (fields 21 and 20). This subject not only showed impairment in retrieving the name of unique persons he still recognized, but also showed deficits in retrieving words denoting animals. Once again there were no other language deficits. The damage in this patient could be described as a sum of the damage seen in **A** and **B. D.** A subject with a lesion in the posterior sector of the left middle and inferior temporal gyri and the anterior sector of the occipital gyri (Brodmann's fields 37 and 19). This subject showed deficits in the retrieval of words denoting manipulable tools, in the setting of some further cognitive deficits that would characterize her as having a transcortical sensory aphasia. (For more details about lesions causing naming deficits see Damasio et al. 2004.)

communicate in any form or fashion. They do not speak spontaneously; they do not speak when spoken to; and they fail to show any intention to communicate with the interlocutor. This attitude is in sharp contrast with that of the patients discussed so far. A hallmark of patients with aphasia is the intent to communicate albeit with incorrectly found language. Akinetic mute patients are usually immobile, in body and speech. Akinetic mutism occurs with lesions of the anterior cingulate gyrus, either bilateral or unilateral, usually as a result of infarcts of the anterior branches of the anterior cerebral artery. Rupture of an anterior communicating aneurysm can produce vascular spasm in both anterior cerebral arteries and also cause such infarcts. The patients may remain akinetic and mute for weeks or months and eventually recover without language deficits. Predictably, the recovery is speedier with unilateral infarcts. See Figure 2–18 for an example of such a lesion. When the lesion occurs only in the supplementary motor area (mesial section of Brodmann's field 6), the condition is restricted to mutism, with only minor akinesia. During the recovery of the latter sort of patient, the condition may resemble a transcortical motor aphasia.

▶ *Acknowledgment*—This work was supported by NIH Program Project Grant P01NS19632.

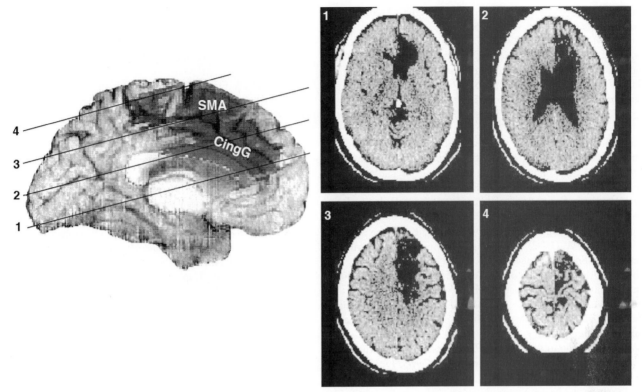

Figure 2–18. CT scan and MAP-3 (mesial view of the left hemisphere) of a patient who suffered the rupture of an anterior communicating aneurysm and had, as a result, an infarct in the territory of the middle branches of the ACA (internal-frontal and paracentral arteries). The patient presented suddenly with what was thought to be right hemiplegia and mutism. The infarcted region occupies the anterior cingulate gyrus (Brodmann's field 24 and part of field 23), and the mesial aspect of the superior frontal gyrus, including the supplementary motor area (field 6) and part of the mesial motor region (field 4). It was soon recognized that in fact there were some motor deficits in the right leg but that there were no motor deficits in the right arm. The patient was simply akinetic. The patient improved over a period of a few weeks and began using sparse, non-aphasic language that in time became completely normal.

KEY POINTS

1. The anatomical descriptions of classic Broca's and Wernicke's aphasias have stood the test of time. The location of the lesions that can produce those aphasias is, in essence, the same that was proposed originally.
2. The notion of "language centers" derived from those early anatomical studies did not prevail. All aspects of language performance depend on the concerted functioning of multi-component systems. The deficits caused by a lesion in a specific location correspond to the removal of the contribution of a particular anatomical component toward the overall function of the system.
3. The traditional Broca's and Wernicke's "language areas" are not sufficient to explain all that goes on in language production and comprehension. Many other areas must be added to the list if we are to explain normal language processing and account for the language deficits due to focal brain lesions.

References

Alexander, M. P., Fischette, M. R., & Fischer, R. S. (1989a). Crossed aphasia can be mirror image or anomalous. *Brain, 112*, 953–973.

Alexander, M. P., Hiltbronner, B., & Fischer, R. (1989b). The distributed anatomy of transcortical sensory aphasia. *Archives of Neurology, 46*, 885–892.

Alexander, M. P., & Loverme, S. R., Jr. (1980). Aphasia after left hemispheric intracerebral hemorrhage. *Neurology, 30*, 1193–1202.

Alexander, M. P., Naeser, M. A., & Palumbo, C. (1990). Broca's area aphasia. *Neurology, 40*, 353–362.

Anderson, S. W., Damasio, H., & Tranel, D. (1988). The use of tumor and stroke patients in neuropsychological research: A methodological critique. *Clinical and Experimental Neurpsychology, 10*, 32.

Anderson, S. W., Damasio, H., & Tranel, D. (1990). Neuropsychological impairments associated with lesions caused by tumor or stroke. *Archives of Neurology, 47*, 397–405.

Aran, D. M., Rose, D. F., Rekate, H. L., & Whiteaker, A. (1983). Acquired capsular/striatal aphasia in childhood. *Archives of Neurology, 40*, 614–617.

Archer, C. R., Ilinsky, I. A., Goldfader, P. R., & Smith, K. R. (1981). Aphasia in thalamic stroke: CT stereotactic localization. I. *Computer Assisted Tomography, 5*, 427–432.

Arseni, C. (1958). Tumors of the basal ganglia. *Archives of Neurology and Psychiatry, 80*, 18–26.

Barat, M., Mazaux, J. M., Bioulac, B., Giroire, J. M., Vital, C., & Arne, L. (1981). Troubles du langage de type aphasique et lesions putamino-caudees. *Revista de Neurologica (Paris), 137*, 343–356.

Bellugi, V., Poizner, H., & Klima, E. S. (1983). Sign language aphasia. *Human Neurobiology, 2*, 155–170.

Benson, D. F., Sheremata, W. A., Bouchard, R., Segarra, J. M., Price, D. L., & Geschwind, N. (1973). Conduction aphasia: A clinicopathological study. *Archives of Neurology (Chicago), 28*, 339–346.

Benton, A. L., & Hamsher, K. (1978). *Multilingual aphasia examination.* Iowa City: Benton Laboratory of Neuropsychology.

Broca, P. (1861). Remarques sur le siege de la faculte de langage articule, suivie d'une observation d'aphemie (perte de la parole). *Bulletin de La Societe Anatomie, 36*, 330–357.

Brunner, R. J., Kornhuber, H. H., Seemiuller, E., Suger, G., & Wallesch, C. W. (1982). Basal ganglia participation in language pathology. *Brain and Language, 16*, 281–299.

Buchel, C., Price, C., & Friston, K.: A multimodal language region in the ventral visual pathway. *Nature, 394*, 272–277, 1998.

Bunn, E. M., Tyler, L. K., & Moss, H. E.: Category-specific semanticdeficits: The role of familiarity and property type reexamined. *Neuropsychology, 12*, 367–379, 1998.

Cappa, S. F., & Vignolo, L. A. (1979). "Transcortical" features of aphasia following left thalamic hemorrhage. *Cortex, 15*, 121–130.

Caramazza, A., & Hillis, A. (1991). Lexical organization of nouns and verbs in the brain. *Nature, 349*, 788–790.

Castro-Caldas, A., Confraria, A., & Poppe, P. (1987). Nonverbal disturbances in crossed aphasia. *Aphasiology, 1*, 403–413.

Cheek, W. R., & Taveras, J. (1966). Thalamic tumors. *Journal of Neurosurgery, 24*, 505–513.

Cohen, J. A., Gelfer, C. E., & Sweet, R. D. (1980). Thalamic infarction producing aphasia. *Mount Sinai Journal of Medicine (NY), 47*, 398–404.

Damasio, A., Damasio, H., Rizzo, M., Varney, N., & Gersh, F. (1982). Aphasia with nonhemorrhagic lesions in the basal ganglia and internal capsule. *Archives of Neurology, 39*, 15–20.

Damasio, A. R. (1990). Category-related recognition defects as a clue to the neural substrates of knowledge. *Trends in Neuroscience, 13*, 95–98.

Damasio, A. R., Damasio, H., Tranel, D., & Brandt, J. P. (1990). Neural regionalization of knowledge access. *Symposia on Quantitative Biology, 55*, 1039–1947. New York: Cold Spring Harbor Laboratory Press.

Damasio, A. R., & Tranel, D. (1993). Nouns and verbs are retrieved with differently distributed neural systems. *Proceedings of the National Academy Of Sciences USA, 90*, 4957–4960.

Damasio, H. (1981). Cerebral localization of the aphasias. In M. T. Sarno (Ed.), *Acquired aphasia.* New York: Academic Press.

Damasio, H. (1987a). Anatomical and neuroimaging contributions to the study of aphasia. In H. Goodglass (Ed.), *Handbook of neuropsychology: Vol. I. Language.* Amsterdam: Elsevier.

Damasio, H. (1987b). Vascular territories defined by computer tomography. In J. H. Wood (Ed.), *Cerebral blood flow: Physiologic and clinical aspects* (pp. 324–332). New York: McGraw-Hill.

Damasio, H. (2000). The lesion method in cognitive neuroscience. In J. Grafman (Ed.), *Handbook of neuropsychology, Vol. 1.* Amsterdam: Elsevier.

Damasio, H. (2005). *Human brain anatomy in computerized images* (2nd ed.). New York: Oxford University Press.

Damasio, H., & Damasio, A. (1989). *Lesion analysis in neuropsychology.* New York: Oxford University Press.

Damasio, H., & Damasio, A. R. (1980). The anatomical basis of conduction aphasia. *Brain, 103*, 337–350.

Damasio, H., Eslinger, P., & Adams, H. P. (1984). Aphasia following basal ganglia lesions: New evidence. *Seminars in Neurology, 4*, 151–161.

Damasio, H., & Frank, R. (1992). Three-dimensional in vivo mapping of brain lesions in humans. *Archives of Neurology, 49*, 137–143.

Damasio, H., Grabowski, T. J., Tranel, D., Hichwa, R. D., & Damasio, A. (1996). A neural basis for lexical retrieval. *Nature, 380*, 499–505.

Damasio, H., Tranel, D., Grabowski, T., Adolphs, R., & Damasio, A. (2004). Neural systems behind word and concept retrieval. *Cognition, 92*, 179–229.

Daniele, A., Giustolisi, L., Silveri, M. C., Colosimo, C., & Gainotti, G. (1994). Evidence for a possible neuroanatomical basis for lexical processing of nouns and verbs. *Neuropsychologia, 32*, 1325–1341.

Day, A. L. (1987). Arterial distributions and variants. In J. H. Wood (Ed.), *Cerebral blood flow: Physiologic and clinical aspects* (pp. 19–36). New York: McGraw-Hill.

Dejerine, J. (1906). L'aphasie sensorielle et 1'aphasie motrice. *Presse Medicale, 14*, 437–439, 453–457. From Dejerine, J. (1901). *Anatomie des centres nerveux.* Paris: Reuff.

Dejerine, J., & Marie, P. (1971). Society of Neurology of Paris, Meeting of June 11, 1908: Discussion on aphasia. *Revue Neurologique, 16*, 1–611. In M. F. Cole & M. Cole (Eds.), *Pierre Marie's papers on speech disorders.* New York: Hafner.

Duvernoy, H. (1991). *The human brain: Surface, three-dimensional sectional anatomy and MRI.* Vienna: Springer-Verlag.

Frank, R J., Damasio, H., & Grabowski, T. J. (1997). Brainvox: an inter-active, multimodal, visualization and analysis system for neuroanatomical imaging. *Neuroimage, 5*, 13–30.

Freedman, M., Alexander, I. M. P., & Naeser, M. A. (1984). Anatomic basis of transcortical motor aphasia. *Neurology, 34*, 409–417.

Frith, C. D., Friston, K. J., Liddle, P. F., & Frackowiak, R. S. J. (1991). A PET study of word finding. *Neuropsychologia, 29*, 1137–1148.

Fromm, D., Holland, A. L., Swindell, C. S., & Reinmuth, O. M. (1985). Various consequences of subcortical stroke. *Archives of Neurology, 42*, 943–950.

Galaburda, A. M., & Pandya, D. N. (1983). The intrinsic architectonic and connectional organization of the superior temporal region of the rhesus monkey. *Journal of Comprehensive Neurology, 221*, 169–184.

Geschwind, N. (1965). Disconnexion syndromes in animals and man. *Brain, 88*, 237–294.

Geschwind, N. (1971). Aphasia. *New England Journal of Medicine, 284*, 654–656.

Geschwind, N., Quadfaset, F. A., & Segarra, J. M. (1968). Isolation of the speech area. *Neuropsychologia, 6*, 327–340.

Goodglass, H., & Kaplan, E. (1982). *The Assessment of aphasia and related disorders.* Philadelphia: Lea & Febiger.

Goodglass, H., Wingfield, A., Hyde, M. R., & Theurkauf, J. (1986). Category specific dissociations in naming and recognition by aphasic patients. *Cortex, 22*, 87–102.

Graff-Radford, N., & Damasio, A. (1984). Disturbances of speech and language associated with thalamic dysfunction. *Seminars in Neurology, 4*, 162–168.

Graff-Radford, N., Damasio, H., Yamada, T., Eslinger, P., & Damasio, A. (1985). Nonhemorrhagic thalamic infarctions: Clinical, neurophysiological and electrophysiological findings in four anatomical groups defined by CT. *Brain, 108*, 485–516.

Graff-Radford, N., Schelper, R. L., Ilinsky, I., & Damasio, H. (1985). Computed tomography and post mortem study of a nonhemorrhagic thalamic infarction. *Archives of Neurology (Chicago), 42,* 761–763.

Hart, J., Berndt, R. S., & Caramazza, A. (1985). Category-specific naming deficit following cerebral infarction. *Nature, 316,* 439–440.

Hillis, A. E., & Caramazza, A. (1991). Category-specific naming and comprehension impairment: A double dissociation. *Brain, 114,* 2081–2094.

Kertesz, A. (1979). *Aphasia and associated disorders.* New York: Grune & Stratton.

Kertesz, A., Harlock, W., & Coates, R. (1979). Computer tomographic localization, lesion size, and prognosia in aphasia and nonverbal impairment. *Brain and Language, 8,* 34–50.

Kertesz, A., Lau, W. K., & Polk, M. (1993). The structural determinants of recovery in Wernicke's aphasia. *Brain and Language, 44,* 153–164.

Knopman, D. S., Seines, O. A., Niccum, N., & Rubens, A. B. (1984). Recovery of naming in aphasia: Relationship to fluency, comprehension and CT findings. *Neurology, 34,* 1461–1470.

Konorski, J., Kozniewska, H., & Stepien, L. (1961). Analysis of symptoms and cerebral localization of audio-verbal aphasia. *Proceedings of the VIIth International Congress on Neurology, 2,* 234–235.

Lazorthes, G., Gouaze, A., & Salamon, G. (1976). *Vascularisation et circulation de i'encephale.* Paris: Masson.

Legatt, A. D., Rubin, A. J., Kaplan, L. R., Healton, E. B., & Brust, J. C. (1987). Global aphasia without hemiparesis. *Neurology, 37,* 201–205.

Liepmann, H., & Pappenheim, M. (1914). Uber einem fall von sogenannter leitungsaphasie mit anatomischem befund. Zentralblatt der Neuroanatomie und Psychiatrie, 27, 111.

Mazzocchi, F., & Vignolo, L. A. (1979). Localization of lesions of aphasia: Clinical CT scan correlations in stroke patients. *Cortex, 15,* 627–654.

Martin, A., Wiggs, C. L., Ungerleider, L. G., & Haxby, J. V. (1996). Neural correlates of category-specific knowledge. *Nature, 379:*649–652.

Mazoyer, B. M., Tzourio, N., Frak, V., Syrota, A., Murayama, N., Levrier, O., Salamon, G., Dehaene, S., Cohen, L., & Mehler, J.: The cortical representation of speech. *J. Cog. Neurosci., 5,* 467–479, 1993.

McFarling, D., Rothi, L. J., & Heilman, K. M. (1982). Transcortical aphasia from ischemic infarcts of the thalamus. *Journal of Neurology, Neurosurgery, and Psychiatry, 45,* 107–112.

Miozzo, A., Soardi, S., & Cappa, S. E. (1994). Pure anomia with spared action naming due to a left temporal lesion. *Neuropsychologia, 32,* 1101–1109.

Mohr, J. P., Pessin, M. S., Finkelstein, S., Funkenstein, H. H., Duncan, G.. W., & Davis, K. R. (1978). Broca's aphasia: Pathologic and clinical. *Neurology, 28,* 311–324.

Mohr, J. P., Wafters, W. C., & Duncan, G. W. (1975). Thalamic hemorrhage and aphasia. *Brain and Language, 2,* 3–17.

Naeser, M. A., Alexander, M. P., Helm-Estabrooks, N., Levine, H. L., Laughlin, S. A., & Geschwind, N. (1982). Aphasia with predominantly subcortical lesion sites. *Archives of Neurology, 39,* 2–14.

Naeser, M. A., & Hayward, R. W. (1978). Lesion localization in aphasia with cranial computed tomography and the Boston Diagnostic Aphasia Exam. *Neurology, 28,* 545–551.

Nobre, A. C., Allison, T. & McCarthy, G. (1994). Word recognition in the human inferior temporal lobe. *Nature, 372:*260–263.

Ojemann, G. A.: Brain organization for language from the perspective of electrical stimulation mapping. *Behav. Brain Sci., 189,* 230, 1983.

Ojemann, G. A. (1991). Cortical organization of language. *Journal of Neuroscience,* 11:2281–2287.

Ono, M., Kubik, S., & Abernathey, C. D. (1990). *Atlas of the cerebral sulci.* Stuttgart: George Thieme Verlag.

Perani, D., Cappa, S. F., Bettinardi, V., Bressi, S., Gorno-Tempini, M., Matarrese, M., & Fazio, F. (1995). Different neural systems for the recognition of animals and man-made tools. *Neurology Report, 6,* 1637–1641.

Petersen, S. E., Fox, P. T., Posner, M. I., Mintun, M., Raichle, M. E.: Positron emission tomographic studies of the cortical anatomy of single-word processing. *Nature, 331,* 585–589, 1988.

Pitres, A. (1898). L'aphasic amnesique et ses varietes cliniques. *Frog. Med., 28,* 17–23.

Rubens, A., & Selnes, O. (1986). Aphasia with insular cortex infarction. *Proceedings of the Academy of Aphasia Meeting,* Nashville, TN.

Schiff, H. B., Alexander, M. P., Naeser, M. A., & Galaburda, A. M. (1983). Aphemia: Clinical-anatomic correlations. *Archives of Neurology, 40,* 720–727.

Schlaghecken, F.: On processing BEASTS and BIRDS: An events-related potential study on the representation of taxonomic structure. *Brain & Lang., 64,* 53–82, 1998.

Selnes, O. A., Knopman, D. S., Niccum, N., & Rubens, A. B. (1985). The critical role of Wernicke's area in sentence repetition. *Archives of Neurology, 17,* 549–557.

Selnes, O. A., Knopman, D. S., Niccum, N., Rubens, A. B., & Larson, D. (1983). Computed tomographic scan correlates of auditory comprehension deficits in aphasia: A prospective recovery study. *Archives of Neurology, 13,* 558–566.

Selnes, O. A., Niccum, N., Knopman, D. S., & Rubens, A.B. (1984). Recovery of single word comprehension: CT scan correlates. *Brain and Language, 21,* 72–84.

Semenza, C., & Zettin, M. (1989). Evidence from aphasia for the role of proper names as pure referring expressions. *Nature, 342,* 678–679.

Silveri, M. C., & Gainotti, G. B. (1988). Interaction between vision and language in category specific semantic access impairment. *Cognitive Neuropsychology, 5,* 677–709.

Szilda, G., Bouvier, G., Hori, T., & Petrov, V. (1977). *Angiography of the human brain cortex.* Berlin: Springer-Verlag.

Tonkonogy, J., & Goodglass, H. (1981). Language function, foot of the third frontal gyrus, and rolandic operculum. *Archives of Neurology, 38,* 486–490.

Tranel, D., Biller, J., Damasio, H., Adams, H., & Cornell, S. (1987). Global aphasia without hemiparesis. *Archives of Neurology, 44,* 304–308.

Tranel, D., Damasio, D., & Damasio, A. R. (1997). On the neurology of naming. In H. Goodglass & A. Wingfield (Eds.), *Anomia: Neuroanatomical and cognitive correlates* (pp. 67–92). New York: Academic Press.

Tranel, D., Logan, C. G., Frank, R. J., & Damasio, A. R. (1997). Explaining category-related effects in the retrieval of conceptual and lexical knowledge for concrete entities: Operationalization and analysis of factors. *Neuropsychologia, 35,* 1329–1339.

Waddington, M. M. (1974). *Atlas of cerebral angiography with anatomic correlation.* Boston: Little, Brown & Co.

Warrington, E. K., & McCarthy, R. A. (1994). Multiple meaning systems in the brain: A case for visual semantics. *Neuropsychologia, 32,* 1465–1473.

Warrington, E. K., & Shallice, T. (1984). Category specific semantic impairments. *Brain, 107,* 829–853.

Wernicke, C. (1874). *Der aphasische symptomen-komplex.* Breslau: Cohn & Weigert.

Wernicke, C. (1886). Einige neuere arbeiten fiber aphasie. *Fortschritte der Medizen 4,* 377–463.

Chapter 3

Medical Aspects of Stroke Rehabilitation

Anthony G. Mlcoch and
E. Jeffrey Metter

OBJECTIVES

Stroke is a leading cause of death and disability. Each year, it is estimated that nearly 731,000 individuals will suffer from the sequelae of stroke, including death, paralysis, sensory loss, mental status changes, and speech and language disturbances (Broderick et al., 1998). By definition stroke is a "... sudden and severe attack ... " implying that the signs of stroke occur abruptly with little warning and are usually persistent (Dorland's Illustrated Medical Dictionary, 1994). The etiology of stroke is vascular in origin and is due to an interruption of blood flow to various brain regions or to bleeding within the brain or spinal cord. The term "cerebrovascular accident" (CVA) is used synonymously with the term "stroke" to denote this vascular etiology. Keeping in mind the sudden onset, the persistent nature, and the vascular origins, the World Health Organization (1989) defines stroke as a series of "... rapidly developing clinical signs of focal (or global) disturbance of cerebral function, with symptoms lasting 24 hours or longer or leading to death with no apparent cause other than of vascular origin."

It is important for the health-care professional to know the warning signs of stroke, how strokes are manifested, diagnosed, and treated for several reasons. First, the nurse, physical therapist, occupational therapist, or speech pathologist may be the first to recognize that a stroke is occurring. As will be reviewed in this chapter, early detection of the signs of stroke are critically important since acute treatment may minimize the effects that a stroke will have on the individual. Second, these professionals will be working with others or within a dedicated team of stroke professionals. A command of the stroke vernacular is necessary to communicate effectively with these professionals and to develop and participate in a plan of treatment for the stroke victim. Lastly, the health-care professional will be responsible for counseling the patient and his or her family, providing information pertaining to the prognosis, treatment, and outcome of stroke. An understanding of the pathogenesis, diagnostic procedures, and the purpose of various treatments is obviously needed.

The purpose of this chapter is to provide the information outlined above. It will review the risk factors (epidemiology), the etiology and diagnosis of stroke including the major neuroimaging procedures, and the current acute and chronic stroke treatments. In addition, future research directions for treatments and their effect on stroke recovery will be reviewed.

EPIDEMIOLOGY

Stroke ranks third behind heart disease and cancer as cause of death in the United States. Approximately 158,000 deaths occur per year in the United States, which is 1 in every 15 deaths (Thom et al., 2006). The annual incidence is approximately 2 per 1,000, with about 1.7 per 1000 being first events, while the prevalence rates are between 4 and 8 per 1000 (Thom et al., 2006). These numbers imply that for 2003 approximately 2.4 million individuals were living after suffering from a stroke, with 700,000 individuals having suffered from a stroke, and about 20% having died related to the stroke. The event rates are higher for men and African Americans. The overall cost of stroke is estimated at 58 billion dollars for 2006. Costs will continue to rise as more individuals survive a stroke, as can be seen with the increase prevalence of noninstitutionalized stroke suviviors, which has risen from 1.5 million in the early 1970s to 2.4 million in the early 1990s (Thom et al., 2006).

The incidence of stroke increases exponentially with age and is primarily a disorder of the elderly. For example, for white females the incidence rate increases from 0.8 per 1000 women for 45 to 54 year olds to 16.5 per 1000 women at ages greater than 85 years (Thom et al., 2006). About 1 in 4 men and 1 in 5 women aged 45 will have a stroke if they live to an age of 85 (Bonita, 1992).

Epidemiologic studies (see Whisnant, 1983) demonstrated that the annual incidence of strokes declined from the 1950s through the 1970s. However, from 1980 the rates have been increasing. For example, in Rochester, Minnesota, the incidence of stroke increased from 1980 to 1984 (Broderick, Phillips, Whisnant, O'Fallon, & Bergstralh, 1989) and from 1985 to 1989 (Brown, Whisnant, Sicks, O'Fallon, & Wiebers, 1996). The increases are likely due to improved diagnostic methods caused by the introduction of CT scanning and better identification of hemorrhagic strokes (Mayo, Goldberg, Leve, Danys, & Bitensky, 1991). More recently, the stroke death rate has been declining and went down by 18.5% from 1993 to 2003 (Thom et al., 2006).

Preventive measures may contribute to lowering the incidence of major disability and mortality as well. Table 3–1 lists factors that have been associated with increased risk for stroke. Many of these factors can be altered by life style changes, proper counseling, and earlier recognition of changes in patient health status. Improved recognition and treatment of such factors have helped to reduce the incidence of stroke. As an example, the improved treatment of hypertension by lowering blood pressure has been shown to decrease the incidence of stroke and myocardial infarctions (Veteran's Administration Cooperative Study Group on Antihypertensive Agents, 1970; SHEP Cooperative Research Group, 1991). The recognition of transient ischemic attacks (described below) can also forewarn of impending disaster and appropriate referral becomes critical. Improved recognition and treatment of such factors have helped to reduce the incidence of stroke.

Stroke-related mortality results from the stroke itself and from other vascular diseases, particularly coronary artery disease and associated heart attacks. Early mortality varies between 17% and 34% during the first month post stroke (Bonita, 1992), with 7.3% mortality for ischemic and 33.1% for hemorrhagic stroke observed in the Atherosclerotic Risk in Communities (ARIC) Cohorts (Rosamond, 1999). The most significant factors associated with early mortality have been alteration in consciousness, which implies a greater and more extensive stroke, and increasing age (Truscott, Kretschmann, Toole, & Pajak, 1974). Myocardial infarction, congestive heart failure, and hypertension have been correlated with early mortality in some studies (Ford & Katz, 1966). Late mortality occurs after the initial hospitalization and is much higher than for the general age-adjusted population.

The scope of the problem becomes more clear when examining what becomes of stroke survivors. In the Framingham Heart Study Cohort, 43% of elderly stroke survivors had moderate to severe disabilities that were more prevalent in the oldest individuals (Kelly-Hayes, et al., 2003). Marquardsen (1969), in an extensive review of the literature, noted that of unselected stroke survivors, 1% to 25% were able to return to work, 50% to 75% were able to walk unaided and discharged home, and 20% to 30% required continued institutionalization. Held (1975) notes, "the percentage of patients who can resume their capability to earn wages is lower than in virtually all other handicaps, physical or intellectual." From these observations it is apparent that stroke can have a devastating effect on the patient and the entire family.

STROKE ETIOLOGY

The most common cause of stroke-like illnesses are related to vascular disease. A partial differential diagnosis for stroke is shown in Table 3–2. The two main mechanisms are related to either loss of blood circulation to parts of the brain through thrombosis with infarction or to hemorrhage of blood into or surrounding the brain. Both mechanisms result in rapid disruption of the ability of neurons to function properly, and if severe and persistent, to the death of neuronal tissue. Resulting symptoms depend on the area of the brain damaged, and the effect that the damaged region has on the remainder of the brain.

The circulation to the brain arises from two pairs of arteries: the internal carotids and the vertebrals. The carotid arteries course in the anterior aspects of the neck and divide into an external and internal branch. The internal carotid artery proceeds to enter the cranium and supply much of the forebrain. The internal carotid artery bifurcates into the anterior and middle cerebral arteries, which supply the cerebral hemispheres over the anterior and much of the lateral surfaces of the cerebral hemisphere (Williams, 1995; Parent, 1996).

The vertebral artery is the first branch of the subclavian artery and proceeds into the cranium through the foramen

---

TABLE 3–1

Risk Factors Associated with Ischemic and Hemorrhagic Stroke

Hypertension
Hypercholesterolemia
Cigarette smoking
Cardiac disease
Diabetes mellitus
Alcohol
Obesity
Homocysteinemia
Sickle cell disease
Male sex
African-American race
Hyperviscosity
Lack of physical activity
Transient ischemic attacks

TABLE 3–2

Partial Differential Diagnosis for Stroke

Vascular Pathology
　Hemorrhage
　　Intracranial hemorrhage
　　Subarachnoid hemorrhage
　　　Aneurysm
　　　Arteriovenous malformation
　　Subdural hematoma
　　Epidural hematoma
　Infarction
　　Thrombotic
　　Embolism
Etiology
　Hypertension
　Atherosclerosis
　Heart disease
　Rheumatic valvular disease
　Atrial fibrillation
　Prosthetic valve
　Infectious endocarditis
Infectious
Trauma
Drugs
　Anticoagulants
　Antiplatelets
　Heparin
Arterial dissection
Cocaine
Congenital absence or atresia of artery
Radiation fibrosis
Trauma
Vasculitis
HIV
Fibromuscular hyperplasia
Moyamoya disease
Hypertensive encephalopathy
Sickle cell disease

magnum. The two vertebral arteries unite to form the basilar artery. The basilar artery continues along the midline of the pons. At the upward end of the pons, the artery divides into two posterior cerebral arteries, which proceed posteriorly to the inferior medial surfaces of the hemispheres to the occipital lobes. The artery supplies blood to those regions including the brain stem, inferior and medial aspects of the hemispheres, and the occipital area.

At the base of the brain, interconnections occur between the carotid and vertebral arteries, forming a circular passage that allows for mixing of blood from the anterior and posterior circulations. This interconnection is called the circle of Willis. Collateral circulation, which refers to the ability of blood from separate brain arteries to redistribute to other brain areas, is extensive, including the circle of Willis, connections between the external and internal carotids, between the left and right anterior cerebral arteries via the anterior communicating artery, and connections between the three cerebral artery systems. Collateral circulation is particularly important when the principle artery to a region becomes compromised. If collateral circulation is adequate, no brain damage may occur. This is accounted for by the ability of collateral arteries to take over and supply an adequate blood supply to the affected internal carotid (Gillilan, 1980).

Ischemic Strokes

Ischemic strokes occur with the complete or partial occlusion of arteries. When blood flow to a region falls below a critical level needed to maintain cellular function and to remove accumulating toxic waste (e.g., lactic acid), cells begin to die and an infarct develops with necrosis and loss of tissue bulk (Plum & Posner, 1980; Raichle, 1983). Typically, in ischemic regions, there will be an inner zone of infarction with a surrounding zone of ischemia called the penumbra (Schlaug et al., 1999). The goals of treatment are to prevent the infarction by early intervention and to protect the ischemic zone by preventing the infarct from getting larger and thus limit functional disability.

The most common causes of ischemic strokes are thrombotic and/or embolic occlusion of the artery related to atherosclerosis. Atherosclerosis is a proliferation of the smooth muscle cells in the intima of the arterial wall with an expansion and deposition of lipid within the associated connective tissue (Ross & Glomset, 1973; Ross, 1980). Atheroma deposition within the arterial wall results in narrowing or stenosis of the artery. If the stenosis reaches a critical level, usually considered greater than about 70%, changes occur in distal blood flow. As stenosis increases and flow becomes stagnate, the likelihood of thrombosis within the artery increases. A second change results from injury to the friable and easily damaged atherosclerotic lesion, with the development of an ulcer. The blood system responds to the ulcer as it would to any other injury within the arterial wall with the laying down of fibrin material, platelet adhesion, and trapping of blood cells. This deposition is called a "thrombus." It can either occlude the blood vessel, which is called a thrombosis, or break apart and be released into the bloodstream as an embolus, which can occlude a distal artery. Embolism can result from thrombus formed for any reason, not just from ulcerated arterial lesions. Other sites of embolic material include the atria of the heart, with embolus formation in relationship to the presence of atrial fibrillation, and the left ventricle of the heart when the chamber has been significantly damaged by a myocardial infarction. These two mechanisms—thrombosis and embolus—are the principle causes of ischemic strokes. The clinical picture with ischemic stroke, as with any neurologic disorder, depends on

TABLE 3–3

Focal Neurologic Findings in Stroke

Middle cerebral artery distribution
    Hemiplegia/hemiparesis
    Hemisensory loss
    Homonymous hemianopsia
    Perceptual dysfunction
    Aphasia
Anterior cerebral artery distribution
    Hemiparesis, legs more than arms
    Hemisensory loss, legs more than arms
    Mutism
    Decreased spontaneity
    Bradyphrenia
    Apraxia
    Abulia
    Akinetic mutism
Posterior cerebral artery distribution
    Coma
    Hemiplegia
    Ataxia
    Tremor
    Hemiballismus
    Sensory loss
    Intractable pain
    Vision loss (uni or bilateral hemianopsia)
    Prosopagnosia
Vertebral-basilar artery distribution
    Paresis
    Sensory loss
    Cranial nerve
    Ataxia
    Diplopia
    Dysarthria
    Vertigo
    Coma

the regions of the brain damaged and the involved artery (Table 3–3).

Hemorrhagic Strokes

A hemorrhagic stroke results from the rupture of a blood vessel within the intracranium. The hemorrhage can occur within three different spaces: the parenchyma of the brain, the subarachnoid space, or the subdural space. The most frequent type of hemorrhage that would result in consultation with a speech-language pathologist would be an intraparenchymal hemorrhage. Such hemorrhages occur secondary to rupture of a small artery within the brain, or occasionally by bleeding from a complex of abnormally formed blood vessels, called an arteriovenous malforma-tion. Intracerebral hemorrhage causes symptomatology by mass displacement of brain tissue, increased pressure in adjacent and distal brain regions, and tissue destruction at the site of bleeding. Current imaging techniques allow for the identification of even small hemorrhages, which have a good prognosis.

Clinical features are relatively distinct depending on type and location of the hemorrhage. The onset frequently occurs during activity or exertion. The patient has the sudden onset of a severe headache, with rapid development of alteration of consciousness. Neurologic symptoms are similar to corresponding strokes resulting from infarctions (Table 3–3).

Transient Ischemic Attacks

Transient ischemic attacks (TIA) are particularly important for the speech-language pathologist to understand because an individual who has such an attack is at a high risk of having a stroke. In fact, there is a 10% to 20% chance of having a stroke within one year, and a 30% to 60% chance of having one in five years. Half of the strokes occur within 24 to 48 hours after the TIA (Albers et al., 2002).

Because of the high risk associated with TIA, it is important to understand clearly what does and does not constitute an attack. A TIA is a brief focal cerebral event in which the symptoms develop rapidly. The duration of an attack ranges from 2 to 30 minutes, to as long as 24 hours, while most are less than 2 to 3 hours in duration. The patient may have two or more such attacks over a variable period of time (Joint Committee for Stroke Facilities, 1974). During a TIA, part of the brain has temporarily become ischemic, resulting in the clinical symptoms. With resolution of the ischemia, the symptoms disappear. Recently, an emphasis has been put on the fact that the vast majority of TIAs resolve in less than an hour (Albers et al., 2002). This focus on the short-term transient nature of TIAs is important as the use of thrombolytic therapy for ischemic stroke is most successful within 3 hours of onset. The ability to separate the two related conditions maximizes the therapeutic potential of the treatment.

Carotid territory TIAs show one or more of the following (Joint Committee, 1974): (1) Hemiparesis—muscular weakness or clumsiness of an arm and/or leg on one side of the body; (2) hemisensory changes; (3) transient aphasia; (4) amaurosis fugax—transient loss of vision in one eye; and/or (5) homonymous hemianopsia—transient loss of vision with an inability to see one side of the visual field.

Vertebrobasilar TIAs show a different combination of symptoms determined by the structures that receive the blood flow from this arterial complex. Symptoms include one or more of the following: (1) motor dysfunction involving one or more extremities; (2) sensory changes involving one or more extremities, usually including the face; (3) visual loss, both total or partial; (4) gait or posture instability with ataxia, imbalance, or unsteadiness but not vertigo; and/or (5) double vision (diplopia), swallowing problems (dysphagia), dysarthria, or vertigo occurring in combination with the above.

The following are not considered as TIAs since each of the symptoms commonly occur and are not associated with stroke: (1) altered conscious or faints; (2) dizziness; (3) amnesia alone; (4) confusion alone; (5) seizure activity; (6) progression of motor or sensory symptoms; (7) vertigo alone; (8) diplopia alone; (9) dysphagia alone; (10) dysarthria alone; or (11) symptoms associated with migraine, such as scintillating scotomata (Joint Committee, 1974).

Diagnosis of TIAs is based on the transient clinical presentation, the absence of other explanations for the event, and the absence of evidence for ischemia on CT or MRI. MRI with diffusion-weighted images is the most sensitive in demonstrating the presence of small subtle infarctions that could be missed by CT.

Treatment for TIAs is successful at decreasing the risk of impending strokes. It attempts to prevent the formation of thrombus and the release of emboli. Two major approaches are being used (Sacco et al., 2006). The surgical approach is to remove the atheromatous material from within the carotid artery (i.e., endarterectomy). Recent cooperative studies have shown that carotid endarterectomies are beneficial to patients with recent hemispheric or retinal transient ischemic attacks (Barnett et al., 1991; Mayberg, et al., 1991; European Carotid Trialists' Collaborative Group, 1991). Patients with stenosis greater than 70% of the vessel lumen to their symptomatic carotid artery were less likely to incur a stroke after undergoing an endarterectomy than if they had received only antiplatelet treatment (e.g., aspirin). Patients with stenoses in the 50% to 69% range showed less consistent benefits (Barnett et al., 1998). However, there is a risk from the arteriogram required to define the anatomy of the blood vessels, and from the surgical procedure itself (Whisnant, Sandok, & Sundt, 1983). Endarterectomy seems warranted only when overall morbidity and mortality from the angiogram and surgical procedure are less than 5% (Sundt, Sandok, & Whisnant, 1975). Under the right circumstances, carotid endarterectomy can lead to a greater reduction of stroke risk than medical treatment (Sacco et al., 2006).

The second treatment approach is medical and consists of preventing thrombus formation. The main medical treatment has been antiplatelet agents such as aspirin. Aspirin decreases the stickiness of platelets so that they will not adhere to the atheromatous lesions. A number of studies have shown that the use of aspirin lowers the risk of subsequent TIA, strokes, and death, particularly in males (Fields, Lemak, Frankoski, & Hardy, 1977; Canadian Cooperative Study Group, 1978; Antiplatelet Trialists Collaboration, 1994). At present, the optimal dose of aspirin has not been determined and no dose has been shown to be definitely most efficacious (Dalen, 2006). The low risk of complications other than gastrointestinal symptoms make this an appealing treatment.

Other antiplatelet medications may prove to be more beneficial either alone or in combination with aspirin, while having less risk of hemorrhage (Lutsep, 2006; Leonardi-Bee et al., 2005). It is unclear whether using these other medications is superior to aspirin, but frequently a combination with aspirin may give some further reduction in risk.

Other recommendations for stroke prevention address many current public-health policies for improved cardiovascular health. Hypertension, diabetes mellitus, lipid abnormalities, obesity, cigarette smoking, and inadequate physical activity are associated with increased risk for stroke. Each of these can be addressed to lower the risk for vascular events including stroke (Sacco et al., 2006).

In subjects with atrial fibrillation, rapidly irregular beating of the heart not associated with rheumatic heart disease, anticoagulation has been found to be a better treatment than antiplatelet therapy (Koudstaal, 2006). Anticoagulants prevent the formation of the thrombus, thus preventing the release of emboli, and can reduce the risk of subsequent stroke by almost 70%. The risk of anticoagulants is bleeding, and this can be a high risk. In using these medications, bleeding parameters of the blood, primarily the prothrombin time, need to be followed carefully and adjusted. In general, the physician attempts to keep the value at 2.0 to 3.0 International Normalized Ratio (INR) for atrial fibrillation, which minimizes the bleeding risk (Sacco et al., 2006). In general, treatments for TIAs can reduce the risk of subsequent strokes by 20% to 40%.

Other Causes

A large number of other disorders can result in stroke-like syndromes (Table 3–2). Such illnesses include brain tumors, chronic subdural hematomas, infections of the brain, multiple sclerosis, residual of head trauma, and so on. At times clinical clues suggest that what appears to be a stroke may be something else. Recognition of such differences in clinical course suggest that something is occurring other than a "simple stroke." The key is that over time the patient is not showing normal recovery, but rather is becoming worse. This can appear as slowly increasing weakness, seizures, increasing confusion, aphasia, or the development of new signs or symptoms that were not noted previously.

DIAGNOSIS

A diagnosis is made based on a history, physical examination, and diagnostic studies. The history is the most important part of the evaluation. Without adequate information, the physician typically does not know what to look for. The purpose of the physical examination is to confirm the history.

In making a neurologic diagnosis, answers are needed to several key questions. The first question is whether the problem is based on a nervous system dysfunction. For example, a patient being seen because of a sudden episode of loss of consciousness lasting two to three minutes, could have had a seizure which is of neurologic origin, or a syncopal episode (faint), which is usually not neurologic but more likely of cardiovascular origin. The second question asks where in the nervous system does the dysfunction occur? Can the clinical picture be explained by a single or multiple lesion. The third question is what is the etiology of the lesion. The answer to these three questions dictates the nature and extent of intervention.

DIAGNOSTIC STUDIES

The role of diagnostic studies in stroke patients is to help identify the location, etiology, and pathophysiology of the problem. Stroke is associated with disease in a number of other body organs and caused by other medical conditions.

Laboratory Evaluation

A variety of non-atherosclerotic causes of stroke syndromes can occur (Table 3–2). Routine tests are usually done to define hematologic, connective tissue, and inflammatory disorders. Typically blood studies include counts of the red and white blood cells. A screening panel is done that examines blood electrolytes (sodium, potassium, chloride, bicarbonate, and calcium), glucose level, and liver and kidney function. Other blood tests include syphilis serology, as well as screening tests for connective tissue diseases. Routine studies also include an electrocardiogram to evaluate the heart. Additional cardiac studies are frequently done, including 24-hour ambulatory monitoring of the heart and transthoracic or transesophageal echocardiography. These tests are done because of their low cost, safety, and high return of information that may not be available from other sources.

Noninvasive Carotid Studies

Since carotid endarterectomy has become an appropriate therapy for non-hemorrhagic strokes related to atherosclerotic disease, techniques are needed to evaluate the extent of disease at the carotid bifurcation. The ideal would be to have a procedure that would be 100% accurate in detecting the extent of disease, and would carry no risk. The accepted procedure to evaluate this area is cerebral angiography, but this carries a definite risk. Other tests have been developed that can evaluate the carotid bifurcation and intracranial arterial structure with 80% to 90% accuracy and far less risk, with 3% to 5% false-positives in experienced laboratories.

Ultrasound approaches are used to study the carotid bifurcation. The first is based on the doppler effect, that is, a sound source that moves towards you has a higher pitch than if it is standing still, and a lower pitch if it is moving away from you (Evans, McDicken, Skidmore, & Woodcock, 1989). Doppler imaging registers echoes of ultrasound waves in relation to the velocity of blood flow. It presents an image of the vessel lumen and in particular the blood column. The second approach uses B-scan mode ultrasonography, which registers echoes related to variations in the acoustical carrying properties of tissues. It images the vessel wall instantaneously as a real-time image.

Doppler techniques have been applied to the study of intracranial arteries. The procedures allow for the estimation of whether intracranial arterial stenosis, aneurysm, or arteriovenous malformations are present. The procedure is valuable in assisting the physician in understanding the blood-flow dynamics in patients with complex cerebrovascular problems (Asslid, 1992).

Cerebral Angiography

Cerebral angiography represents the "gold standard" for determining the nature and extent of the vascular abnormality in cerebral blood vessels. Angiography is particularly necessary when considerations are being made to do a surgical procedure, or when clinical diagnosis is uncertain. Typically, the procedure is carried out by placing a small-bore tube into the femoral artery in the groin and passing it up the artery to the aortic arch and into the appropriate arteries, including both carotid arteries and a vertebral artery. When in place, contrast medium is forced through the tube and into the arterial circulation, while x-ray pictures are taken in rapid sequence over a 10- to 20-second period. Pictures are taken in several planes, resulting in three-dimensional reconstruction of the arteries. In the hands of a good angiographer, the risk is typically less than 1% morbidity and mortality. The major risk from this procedure is the development of a stroke during or shortly after the procedure.

Magnetic resonance angiography has been developed; it takes advantage of the power of magnetic resonance imaging (MRI) (see below) and has become the most common approach for studying the cerebral arteries. This technique offers the advantage of imaging carotid and intracerebral circulation without the use of injected contrast media (Ruggieri, Masayk, & Ross, 1991).

Brain Imaging

The techniques examined so far have studied what occurs within the blood vessel. An important issue for the physician is the kind and extent of the brain damage that has occurred.

This can be studied by several imaging technologies. Two types of neuroimaging methods have emerged that enable the physician to obtain three-dimensional images of the central nervous system; those that measure the transmission of energy through tissue such as computed transmission tomography, and those producing images from natural or introduced energy sources, which include magnetic resonance imaging, positron emission tomography, and single photon emission tomography.

Transmission tomography examines differential tissue absorption of externally administered energy and includes standard radiography and computer tomography (CT). In standard radiography, the brain is irradiated by x-ray. The x-rays that are unabsorbed or transmitted through the brain are recorded by sensitive film or a video image device (fluoroscopy). This provides a planar or two-dimensional image that has excellent spacial but poor contrast resolution (i.e., the ability to distinguish white matter from gray matter). CT obtains three-dimensional images of the brain by measuring the amount of transmitted radiation using multiple detectors placed around the head. The amount of transmitted radiation at each integral point (pixel) is then calculated using a dedicated computer. A three-dimensional image of the brain is constructed using this information.

CT studies brain structure, pathology, and anatomy. Contrast between structures depends on the amount of x-ray absorbed and the thickness, density, and atomic number of the structures. For example, bone, which contains a high concentration of calcium, absorbs x-ray much more readily than other tissues, and is clearly delineated by both conventional radiography and CT. Distinctive structures within the brain are more difficult to see because specific gravity differences between adjacent structures are small. CT is capable of differentiating tissues with small absorption differences. With standard x-ray, resolution is basically continuous, while with CT it is dependent on pixel size, since each pixel represents an average value of transmitted radiation within its borders (Oldendorf, 1981; Ketonen, 1997). CT is commonly used when a patient first presents with an acute event, and is being considered for immediate treatment to identify an intracerebral hemorrhage or other potential causes for a stroke-like presentation (Moonis & Fisher, 2001; Bonaffini, Altieri, Rocca, & Di Piero, 2002).

Emission tomography produces images utilizing data from internal energy sources. Such sources include magnetic, radionuclides injected intravenously, intraarterially, or by inhalation, and the electrophysiologic characteristics of the brain. Emission techniques include MRI, positron emission tomography (PET), and single photon emission computed tomography (SPECT).

MRI does not use radioactive substances but examines the response of selected elements in response to a large magnetic field. Current techniques are primarily concerned with the study of proton distribution—water. The resolution of MRI is on the order of CT, but has better contrast in distinguishing gray from white matter. The technique is particularly useful in studying the posterior fossa, where CT has difficulty.

MRI utilizes a very different set of physical properties, taking advantage of the behavior of nuclei as small dipoles or very weak magnets. Under normal circumstances, the axes of the nuclei point in random directions. In a strong magnetic field, the nuclei line up so that their dipoles are either parallel or antiparallel with the field. The nuclei can flip back and forth between the parallel and antiparallel positions, which requires energy absorption and the emission of a radiowave. MRI uses this property, by applying a radiofrequency wave, to the fixed magnetic field, encouraging nuclei to flip back and forth (resonate) between parallel and antiparallel positions and measuring the radiowaves emitted in the process (Bradley, 1982).

Each element in a magnetic field resonates at specific frequencies, making the physical properties of the fields specific to a given element. Hydrogen is most commonly scanned because of its excellent resonating ability and abundance in tissue as a component of water and all organic molecules. Two measures usually studied are magnetic relaxation times "T1" and "T2," and are dependent on nuclear density and environment. T1 is the "thermal relation" or "spin-lattice" reaction time and represents the time for the nuclei to become aligned and magnetized when placed in a magnetic field. T1 depends on the physical properties of the sample, for example, liquids are held together by looser forces than are solids, and will become magnetized more quickly than solids, and will have a shorter T1.

T2 is the "spin-spin" or "transverse" relaxation time. Nuclei tend to spin much as a top does. As a top spins it points perpendicular to the ground when under stable conditions. If a second energy source is applied (as by touching it with a finger), it begins to wobble. The wobble represents a torque, which describes a second axis of rotation for the top. Nuclei in a strong magnetic field when pulsed by a radiofrequency wave behave in a similar manner. T2 is a measure of how well and how long this wobble is maintained, following the radiofrequency pulse. For solids, T2 is very short, because of the fixed rigid structure of the molecules, while it is long for liquids (Bradley, 1982).

In ischemic strokes, MRI is more sensitive than CT. Recent techniques have added new methods to the standard T1 and T2 imaging. A diffusion-weighted image (DWI) applies two gradients across the radiofrequency pulse that leads to an image with hyperintensity in an ischemic region due to the accumulation of intracellular water early in the process. DWI can be useful in differentiating stroke subtypes, extent of the damage, and appropriateness for specific acute therapy (Moonis & Fisher, 2001; Bonaffini et al., 2002), but it is not necessarily better than other approaches (Hand et al., 2006). Perfusion weighted images show changes in ischemic regions outside the area of primary infarction. When PWI is used with DWI, PWI abnormalities outside those shown by DWI represent the penumbra, which is brain tissue potentially salvageable (Schlaug et al., 1999). MRI can be useful with acute brain attacks in making the decision for thrombolytic therapy. The limitation is that the decision for therapy has to be made quickly, which typically precludes time for MRI, and favors the use of CT.

MRI can be used to study blood flow. Such applications are being used to study how the brain responds to specific tasks.

PET and SPECT are two tomographic techniques based on the technology of detecting gamma-ray emissions from intravenous injected radioisotopes. PET and SPECT are designed to measure functional changes such as regional cerebral blood flow (rCBF), metabolism, and neurotransmitters. These methods are distinguished by the type of radiopharmaceuticals and equipment each employs. The half-lives of these isotopes are usually short, necessitating the availability of a cyclotron, which adds considerable expense to the procedure. These isotopes are also unique since the annihilation of their electrons produces two gamma photons that discharge at 180 degrees from each other. Detection of both photons is made by a gamma camera with a series of parallel gamma-ray detectors. Using a dedicated computer, the site at which the dual photons were emitted is located with excellent accuracy.

SPECT also employs isotopes that are injected intravenously. At present only two SPECT radioisotopes are approved by the Federal Food and Drug Administration for clinical use: N-isopropyl-p-iodoamphetamine (IMP) and 99mTc hexamethylpropylene amine oxide (HMPAO). These radiotracers have relatively long half-lives and do not require an on-site cyclotron. They are either made from kits or are shipped directly from the manufacturer. They also differ from those isotopes used by PET in that they emit one gamma photon. The site at which the photon was emitted is located by using a collimator, which is a lead shield with a series of holes cut into it. The collimator is mounted on the head of the gamma camera. Spatial resolution is less than the other imaging methods.

SPECT has not been used extensively in the diagnosis of stroke. The reason is that while SPECT detects focal and diffuse changes of cerebral blood flow (CBF), it is insensitive to the specific etiology, such as discerning whether the observed behavioral changes are ischemic, neoplastic, or metabolic. At best the physician requests a SPECT scan in those cases where the CT and MRI are negative and the patient exhibits mental status changes that are stroke-like. In these cases SPECT might be helpful in determining whether these changes are secondary to a progressive dementia or to neuropsychiatric disease (Talbot, Lloyd, Snowden, Neary, & Testa, 1998).

Brain Imaging in the Study of Aphasia

X-ray Computed Tomography

CT has been a powerful tool in correlating brain structural abnormalities with speech and language pathology. Within the past 10 to 15 years, CT has been supplanted by MRI serving the same role. However, CT studies were the first to describe the relationship between lesion site and type of aphasia (Hayward, Naeser, & Zatz, 1977; Naeser & Hayward, 1978; Kertesz, Harlock, & Coates, 1979; Mazzocchi & Vignolo, 1979; Noel, Bain, Collard, & Huvelle, 1980). Specific lesions have resulted in specific aphasia syndromes in a manner consistent with classical descriptions. The pre-rolandic/post-rolandic separation of nonfluent and fluent aphasias seems well supported by CT (Naeser & Hayward, 1978; Kertesz et al., 1979). A number of cases do not fit within the model (Mazzocchi & Vignolo, 1979; Metter, Wasterlain, Kuhl, Hanson, & Phelps, 1981). For example, investigations using CT have demonstrated that the location of brain lesions can be predicted from aphasia type with reasonable accuracy; however, the reverse does not appear to be true (Noel et al., 1980). In general, larger lesions result in poorer outcome and more severe aphasia than do small single lesions (Kertesz et al., 1979; Yarnell, Monroe, & Sobel, 1976). Lesion localization independent of size may also be critical for recovery, as noted by the poor prognosis of patients with lesions involving the posterior superior temporal and infrasylvian supramarginal regions, which are associated with poor comprehension (Selnes, Knopman, Niccum, Rubens, & Larson, 1983). Some large lesions are less devastating than very critically placed smaller lesions. The value of knowing the site of brain lesions in predicting the recovery potential of patients with aphasia has been demonstrated (Selnes et al., 1983). Such information may be of value in planning language therapy for aphasic patients. Patients without lesions in specific areas may benefit from early intensive therapy to facilitate recovery.

CT has been particularly valuable in the identification of subcortical lesions and their correlation to language disturbance. Subcortical infarctions of the dominant hemisphere with basal ganglia involvement have resulted in aphasia that is characterized by word-finding difficulties, phonemic paraphasia, intact repetition, and rapid recovery (Brunner, Kornhuber, Seemuller, Suger, & Wallesch, 1982). A specific type of "thalamic speech" has also been recognized that characterizes the aphasia associated with thalamic CT lesions, with paucity of spontaneous speech, hypophonia, anomia, perseveration, and neologisms with intact comprehension and word repetition (Alexander & LoVerme, 1980).

Positron Emission Computed Tomography

Glucose is the main substrate used by the brain to produce the energy required for it to function. Normal brain function is dependent on the availability and utilization of glucose. Flourodeoxyglucose (FDG) positron emission tomography (PET) studies have demonstrated decreased cerebral glucose metabolism (hypometabolism) in the brains of stroke patients that extends beyond the zone of infarction as determined by CT (Kuhl, et al., 1980; Metter et al., 1981; Metter et al., 1985). Similar changes remote from the site of infarction have been found in many stroke cases (Kuhl et al., 1980; Metter et al., 1981; Lenzi, Frackowiak, & Jones, 1981; Baron et al., 1981; Martin & Raichle, 1983; Metter et al., 1987). Distant regions of hypometabolism suggest that the function in undamaged tissue may be aberrant, and might account for some aspects of the aphasic language disturbance and in the recovery process (Metter, Jackson, Kempler, & Hanson, 1992). Furthermore, functional activation studies in aphasia have shown changing brain organization with increasing activity in the right hemisphere (Muller et al., 1999; Heiss, Kessler, Thiel, Ghaemi, & Karbe, 1999; Cappa & Vallar, 1992).

Studies that examine brain regional blood flow and metabolism demonstrate that focal brain regions have clear effects on other parts of the brain. Such observations appear to allow for more unifying concepts regarding the development of aphasia following stroke. For example, it has been found that essentially all patients with aphasia studied by FDG PET demonstrated metabolic abnormalities in the left temporoparietal regions independent of where the structural lesion causing the aphasia is located (Metter et al., 1990). Furthermore, differences between Wernicke's, Broca's, and conduction aphasias were found to differ on the extent of metabolic abnormalities in the prefrontal cortex, a part of the brain not believed to be directly responsible for most aphasias (Metter et al., 1989). The data also suggested that language function may not be attributable only to the structural lesion, but rather to what occurs in other brain areas when the perisylvian region (which functions as a unit involved with language function) is structurally damaged.

Studying brain metabolism has also demonstrated aspects of the role of subcortical brain structures in aphasia (Metter, 1992). Differences in the location of subcortical structural damage are associated with differences in the location changes in overlying cortex. For most middle cerebral artery distribution strokes, the presence of subcortical extension of the infarct will be associated with frontal lobe hypometabolism. These metabolic changes and the associated subcortical structural changes are associated with the expressive aspects of the aphasia (Metter, Riege, Hanson, Phelps, & Kuhl, 1988).

Single Photon Emission Computed Tomography

Like PET, single photon emission computed tomography (SPECT) often detects areas of reduced cerebral blood flow larger than and remote from the ischemic lesion identified on CT and MRI. These areas include subcortical infarcts resulting in cortical hypoperfusion, and cortical frontoparietal infarcts resulting in contralateral cerebellar diaschisis (Bogousslavsky, Miklossy, & Regli, 1988; Vallar et al., 1988; Megens, van Loon, Goffin, & Gybels, 1992; Okuda, Tanaka, Tachibana, Kawabata, & Sugita, 1994; Halkar, Sisterhen, Ammons, Galt, & Alazraki, 1997; Abe, Ukita, Yorifu, &Yanagihara, 1997). The behavior associated with this phenomenon (i.e., ataxia and aphasia) often resolves as perfusion returns to the remote region (Vallar et al., 1988; Megens et al., 1992). In addition to the distant effects associated with cerebral infarction, the size of the cerebral blood-flow defect is inversely correlated with stroke recovery (Lee, Hillman, & Holman, 1984; Defer, Moretti, & Cesaro, 1987; Bushnell et al., 1989; Giulibei, Lenzi, & Dipiero, 1990; Limburg, Royen, Hijdra, & Verbeeten, 1990; Gupta et al., 1991). That is, the larger the defect the less likely the patient will exhibit good recovery. Using SPECT, Yamaguchi, Meyer, Sakai, & Yamamoto (1980) showed that poor recovery from aphasia was associated with failure of increased cerebral blood flow in the frontotemporal regions in both cerebral hemispheres in response to counting, conversational speech, and listening to music. Similarly Knopman, Rubens, & Selnes (1983) and Cardebat et al. (1994) found that good recovery from aphasia was associated with increases of cerebral blood flow in the right inferior frontal region and the right middle temporal cortex, respectively, in response to a listening task. Good recovery appeared to be associated with reduced but not absent cerebral blood flow activity in the language region in the left cerebral hemisphere early following the stroke and with improvement in flow with recovery. The language regions remained hypoperfused during recovery in patients with poor language recovery (Tikofsky et al., 1985; Mlcoch, Bushnell, Gupta, & Milo, 1994).

Functional MRI (fMRI)

MRI offers an opportunity to study brain activity, as estimated by regional changes in blood flow, during the performance of specific activities, thus examining how brain regions are selectively responding to specific tasks. Currently, fMRI represents the most dynamic approach to understanding the impact of brain damage on language function in health and with aphasia, and during recovery from stroke (Wise 2003; Price & Crinion, 2005). Recent work suggests a sequential but complex response by the brain to aphasia resulting from an ischemic stroke. One study (Saur et al., 2006) suggests a sequential response by the brain to an ischemic stroke in a select group of aphasic subjects. During the acute phase immediately following the onset of the stroke, little activity is found in noninfarcted left hemisphere language areas. This is followed subacutely by increased activity in the left and activation of homologous regions in the right hemispheres. In the chronic phase, a shift occurs back towards the left hemisphere. Others have noted persistent changes in the response in the right hemisphere to both speech production and to comprehension tasks (Price & Crinion, 2005). The reorganization with increasing activity in the contralateral hemisphere leads to an alternate strategy for language processing and communication. The new strategies can result in improved communication and language. The resulting improvements in language likely reflect the extent of damage and functional loss in the dominant language areas, and the ability of both the dominant and nondominant hemispheres to adapt.

TREATMENT

The treatment of a patient who has developed a stroke can be divided into two parts. The initial or acute therapy is directed to the preservation of life and to preventing expansion of the disability associated with the stroke. The second part or, chronic therapy, is directed towards rehabilitation with the reestablishment of as normal a life style as possible.

Acute Therapy

With ischemic strokes a region of infarction is surrounded by a zone whose tissue can either recover or progress to infarction. This zone is called the "ischemic penumbra" and extensive efforts have been made to develop methods to protect and improve blood flow to this region during the early stages of stroke. These include the use of vasodilators to increase cerebral blood flow and to increase arterial pressure in an attempt to force blood into the zone, and the use of corticosteriods, drugs aimed at reducing the swelling of the brain associated with the acute stage of stroke. Unfortunately, none of these neuroprotective methods have proved to be beneficial and until recently the medical treatment of acute ischemic stroke has been limited to the preservation of life.

In 1995 the National Institute of Neurological Disorders and Stroke Study Group (NINDS) reported a double-blind study to determine the efficacy of recombinant tissue plasminogen activator (t-PA) for the treatment of acute ischemic stroke. t-PA is a drug delivered intravenenously and is essentially a "clot buster" in that it breaks the embolism apart, allowing blood flow to return to the deprived region of the brain. The NINDS found that patients who had received t-PA within 3 hours of onset of stroke symptoms demonstrated significantly better recovery at 3 months post-onset. As compared with a placebo control group, patients treated with t-PA were at least 30% more likely to have minimal or no disability at three months poststroke onset. The one negative result was that at 36 hours after onset there was a higher incidence of symptomatic intracerebral hemorrhage in the t-PA group (6.4% vs. 0.6%). However mortality was lower for the t-PA group at three months (17% vs. 21%).

Based on the findings of the NINDS study, t-PA received formal Food and Drug Administration approval in 1996 for the treatment of patients with acute ischemic stroke. To be eligible for this drug, the patient must have had the onset of symptoms of an ischemic stroke within 3 hours of taking the drug; had a CT scan showing no evidence of intracranial hemorrhage; had not had another stroke or serious head trauma within the preceding 3 months; had not undergone major surgery within 14 days; had no history of subarachnoid or intracranial hemorrhage; showed no evidence of significant hypertension; did not have a history of gastrointestinal or urinary tract hemorrhage within 21 days; and were not taking anticoagulants. Since approval t-PA has been shown to be an effective treatment of ischemic stroke in community hospitals as well large medical centers (Chui et al., 1998; Grand et al., 1998). However, since FDA approval t-PA has been substantially underused (Bambauer, Johnson, Bambauer, & Zivin, 2006), for three primary reasons. First, the population as a whole has not been educated as to the signs and symptoms of stroke and the importance of getting to the hospital immediately when they occur. Second, owing to the relatively high incidence of intracerebral bleeding, physicians have been reluctant to provide t-PA due to possible liability. Third, the t-PA procedure has not been adequately reimbursed. Hopefully, with better education of the population, physicians, and third-party payers, t-PA will be better utilized in the future.

For those patients who do not meet the above stringent criteria and cannot take t-PA, treatment is dependent on identifying the etiology, or where the stroke-producing emboli is formed; primarily from the internal carotid artery or the heart. Treatment of the former is by either removing the thrombus from the artery by a surgical procedure called a "carotid endarterectomy," or by providing antiplatelets such as aspirin. CEA has been shown to significantly reduce the chances of having a second stroke (North American Symptomatic Carotid Endarterectomy Trial Collaborators, 1991a, 1991b; Mayberg et al., 1991; Haynes et al., 1994; Gasecki et al., 1994; Moore et al., 1995). The relative risk of having a second symptomatic stroke within 3 years is reduced as much as 50% after undergoing a CEA when compared to medically treated patients (ECSTC, 1991). On the other hand, if the etiology is cardiogenic, anticoagulants such as heparin and warfarin (coumadin) are given to prevent further embolization. Evidence suggests that such treatment reduces overall morbidity and mortality (Easton & Sherman, 1977; Ezekowitz & Levine, 1999).

Chronic Therapy

Chronic therapy begins as soon as the patient is medically stable. The goals of treatment are rehabilitative at this stage and are generally aimed at teaching or providing the means whereby the patient can walk, communicate, and carry out activities of daily living (ADLs). Initially, this might be as simple as preventing contractures and decubiti (breakdowns and ulcerations of the skin) from forming, especially in seriously disabled patients. This entails passive ranging of a hemiparetic arm and/or leg and rotating the patient in his or her bed routinely. Another goal is to provide stimulation by either talking to the patient or having him or her actively participate in their ADLs and gradually getting the patient into a lounging or wheelchair for progressively longer periods each day. Early mobilization is advocated whenever possible (U.S. Department of Health and Human Services, 1995). This will help the patient actively participate in a rehabilitative program by preventing her or him from becoming deconditioned.

Formal rehabilitation entails the disciplines of physiatry; nursing; social services; psychology; and physical, occupational, speech-language, and vocational therapy. Rehabilitation programs can be conducted in a number of settings. There is evidence that patients do better in a dedicated stroke unit. Stroke care can be provided in a rehabilitation unit, nursing facility, outpatient clinic, or in the home. At present, recommendations are that rehabilitation units should be used for patients with multiple disabilities and those who can tolerate at least 3 hours of physical activity each day (U.S. Department of Health & Human Services, 1995; Duncan et al., 2005).

The goals and techniques utilized by each type of therapy are beyond the scope of this chapter. The extent and intensity of rehabilitation is still unclear (Kwakkel, Wagenaar, Koelman, Lankhorse, & Koetsier, 1997). Furthermore, the time of recovery varies. For example, continued improvement in language performance can be observed for many years following the onset of aphasia (Hanson, Metter, & Riege, 1989). An American Heart Association panel has stated that there are six major areas of focus in stroke rehabilitation: (1) dealing with co-morbid illnesses and complications; (2) maximizing independence; (3) maximizing psychosocial coping for both patient and family; (4) promotion of societal reintegration; (5) improving quality of life; and (6) preventing recurrent vascular events (Gresham et al., 1997; U.S. Department of Health & Human Services, 1995). However, it is important to note which factors affect overall stroke rehabilitation or outcome.

The severity of the neurologic impairment has been shown to have the most effect on the outcome of stroke recovery (Lorenze, DeRosa, & Keenan, 1958; Gersten, Ager, Anderson, & Cenkovich, 1970). Patients demonstrating severe to profound neurologic impairment and/or hemiplegia (vs. hemiparesis) tend to stay longer in the hospital and become less functional (Harvey et al., 1998). Degree of communication deficit also plays a role in the stroke recovery. Patients with global aphasia or hemineglect tend to respond poorly to rehabilitative efforts aimed at teaching ADLs and improving mobility (Paolucci et al., 1998).

Patients with these deficits are likely to be less independent than those with other types of aphasia (with better comprehension of spoken language) or without sensory neglect (the ability to attend to events in the left or right hemispace) (Paolucci et al., 1996). Lastly, the effects of psychiatric disorders such as depression and apathy may also have a negative effect on stroke recovery. Surprisingly, poststroke depression has not been found to be consistently correlated with outcome or length of stay on a rehabilitative unit (Eastwood, Rifat, Nobbs, & Ruderman, 1989; Sinyor et al., 1986). Stroke patients with depression are not less functionally competent but tend to have less active life styles than patients without depression (Clark & Smith, 1998). In contrast, patients demonstrating an "apathy syndrome" or "negative symptom complex" tend to stay longer in rehabilitation and are less functionally competent and independent at the end of treatment (Galynker et al., 1997; Clark & Smith, 1998). This type of patient is indifferent to the surrounding environment. He or she expresses no concerns about the effect of the stroke has on others, often explaining lack of motivation as being tired. He or she shows little or no ambition and makes feeble efforts at achieving independence. These patients respond poorly to rehabilitation regardless of their degree of physical disability (Dombovy, Sandok, & Basford, 1986; Schmel'kov, 1982). However, the clinician should not assume that this behavior is purposeful. It is often the sequela of brain damage such as "abulia" (lack of willfulness) associated with frontal lobe disease or "anasognosia" (lack of awareness of disability) resulting from right cerebral hemisphere or left temporal lobe damage.

RESTORATIVE NEUROLOGY

For many years it was believed that the brain was a static organ, hard-wired after puberty and immutable. Subsequently, brain damage resulted in a loss of function, and recovery from brain damage, such as from a stroke, was a result of a reorganizational process within the brain. In the past 20 to 30 years this concept has undergone a radical change. We now know that the brain is capable of and does produce new cells that have the ability to take over the function of damaged brain regions and that after a stroke the remaining neurons are capable under certain circumstances to either partially or completely take over the lost function. The term used to refer to the brain's ability to undergo structural and functional modifications is *brain plasticity* or *neuroplasticity*. These modifications happen as a result of neurologic injury and/or external stimulation (i.e., behavioral management such as the stimulation provided in speech and language therapy). These changes occur at all levels including the cortex, the subcortex—the level at which neurons network and communicate—the cellular, and the biochemical. What precipitates these changes has been of particular interest to researchers as well as to clinicians who treat stroke victims.

Specifically, research has concentrated on what can be done to enhance the brain's ability to learn after a brain injury, thus enhancing recovery. The term used to describe those treatments that modify or enhance brain plasticity is *restorative neurology* (Druback, Makely, & Dodd, 2004).

In the past 10 to 15 years researchers have concentrated on three methods to potentiate the brain: electrical cortical stimulation, transcortical magnetic stimulation, and neuropharmaceutical stimulation. While much of the work has been done with animal models, human translation studies have begun to emerge.

Electrical cortical stimulation (ECS) is a method by which subthreshold electrical impulses are applied to target cortical areas. "Subthreshold" refers to a level of brain stimulation that does not result in a motor or cognitive action such as stimulating the hand area of the motor cortex, resulting in the movement of that appendage. The thrust of the research has been to determine whether the application of ECS concurrently with rehabilitative therapy results in better recovery of function. That is, whether undamaged cortical regions can be enhanced or positively potentiated by subthreshold electrical stimulation.

Atkins-Mair and Jones (2003) studied both the behavioral and dendritic effects of combining ECS with motor-skill training in rats with induced motor cortex infarcts. In this study rats were trained on a skilled forelimb-reaching task and then underwent an operation that induced ischemic lesions to the sensorimotor cortex. Ten to 14 days later electrodes were implanted in the perilesional cortex. The rats then began 10 days of rehabilitative training at which time they either received 50-Hz (subthreshold) stimulation, 250-Hz stimulation, or no stimulation. Of the three groups, the subthreshold group demonstrated a significantly greater rate of improvement of forelimb movement. In addition, they showed a greater density of dendritic processes in the perilesional cortex, indicating that the structural cortical changes were associated with the positive potentiation of the brain.

In a similar study, Klein et al. (2003) investigated whether ECS with rehabilitative training enlarges the cortical region responsible for forelimb movement after focal ischemic infarct. To answer this question, cortical maps were made after rats underwent 2 weeks of a food-pellet task. An infarct to the forelimb cortical region was then induced and cortical electrodes were placed around the lesion. As might be expected the cortical region surrounding the infarcted area that represented forelimb movement was larger for rats receiving ECS than those found in rats receiving no stimulation during postinfarct training. Teskey, Flynn, Goertzen, Monfils, & Young (2003) in a nearly identical investigation found that rats receiving stimulation during retraining had larger polysynaptic potentials. They conjectured that training with ECS most likely results in "strengthened synaptic

efficacy," which in turn involves long-term cortical potentiation associated with learning.

ECS combined with motor training has also been studied in nonhuman primates. Plautz et al. (2003) found that monkeys receiving hand-movement training with subthreshold ECS 3.5 to 5 months after incurring an induced infarct to the motor hand cortical region demonstrated a significant improvement in addition to having a larger peri-infarct region representing the hand. Importantly, this study showed that poststroke interventions are not limited to the period immediately after the brain insult but can be successful after the period associated with spontaneous recovery.

ECS has been also studied on a limited basis with human subjects. Brown, Lutsep, Cramer, & Weinand (2003) presented a case report of a 65-year-old patient who had a right spastic hemiparesis secondary to a subcortical infarct . The infarct occurred 19 months prior to undergoing a combination of subthreshold epidural (electrodes placed on the dura above the cortical region of interest) motor ECS and occupational therapy for 3 weeks. Before treatment the patient was unable to flex or extend his fingers; after treatment he could pick up a pencil, print letters, and pick up ball bearings. Cramer et al. (2005) employed the same protocol on 13 patients with infarcts to the brain stem, cortex, subcortex, and subcortical/cortical regions. The strokes had occurred 9 to 68 months before receiving 3 weeks of physical therapy combined with epidural ECS to the motor cortex. In comparison to a sham group those patients who received ECS showed significant improvement of arm motion. Brown, Lutsep, Weinand, & Cramer (2006) used a protocol identical to that used by Cramer et al. (2005). In this study patients were limited to those who had cortical and/or subcortical strokes that resulted in upper extremity paresis. Like that found in the previous study, patients in the active treatment group improved significantly better than patients receiving rehabilitation treatment only. These studies tend to show that regardless of the infarcted region ECS of the motor cortex will enhance arm recovery even after the period of spontaneous recovery has ended.

Although more extensive large sample studies are needed, several observations were made with the above investigations. First, the combination of ECS and rehabilitative therapy appears to enhance recovery from stroke . Second, the behavioral changes induced by ECS appear to be correlated with changes in cortical representation as well as structural cortical changes (i.e., increased dendritic density). In turn this most likely represents the long-term potentiation of the brain. Last, ECS and epidural ECS appear to be well-tolerated and safe.

To date no studies have looked at the combination of ECS (cortical or epidural) and language treatment for patients with aphasia. However, as of this writing a project is ongoing at the Rehabilitation Institute of Chicago and the University of Chicago, looking at the effectiveness and safety in combining epidural ECS and aphasia therapy. It is called the "Northstar project." In this investigation subthreshold epidural ECS is applied to the language region in the left cerebral hemisphere while the patient receives language treatment, 3 hours a day, 5 days a week, for 6 weeks. We anticipate the results from this study in the near future.

Transcranial magnetic stimulation (TMS) is another method that has been shown to be an effective way of potentiating as well as depotentiating the brain. TMS entails placing a figure-eight coil on the scalp and delivering a magnetic pulse to the underlying brain region. Slow pulses (1 Hz) reduce excitability of the region while rapid pulses (>3Hz) increase the excitability or potentiates the brain region of interest (Pascual-Leone et al., 1998; Hoffman & Cavus, 2002; Fraser et al., 2002). One area of TMS research has been to identify those intact cortical regions that may contribute to stroke recovery.

To determine whether the intact (undamaged) motor cortex has a role in recovery, Werhahn, Conforta, Kadon, Hallet, & Cohen (2003) applied TMS to the motor cortex of the intact and damaged cerebral hemispheres of chronic stroke patients with a paretic hand. In normal subjects, stimulating the motor cortex on one side of the brain results in abnormal motor performance in the contralateral hand and arm, but not by the ipsilateral hand and arm. When TMS was applied to the stroke patients, the stimulation of the intact cortex was associated with delayed reaction times of the contralateral nonparetic hand and not the paretic hand, while TMS to the damaged hemisphere resulted in delayed reaction times to the paretic hand and not the nonparetic hand. The pattern of response was similar in the healthy and the subjects with stroke. The investigators concluded that recovery of motor function was primarily due to the reorganization of the intact motor cortex of the damaged cerebral hemisphere.

Fridman et al. (2004) also found that the intact motor cortex of the affected hemisphere was capable of reorganizing impaired movement. TMS was applied to the primary motor cortex, dorsal premotor cortex, and ventral premotor cortex of the affected and intact cerebral hemispheres. TMS applied to the dorsal premotor cortex of the damaged hemisphere resulted in delays in the reaction times of the paretic hand.

In a treatment study, Takeuchi, Chuma, Matsuo, Watanabe, & Ikoma (2005) applied slow TMS (1 Hz) to the contralesional brain to determine whether deactivating this region would result in better motor improvement for patients with stroke. Using a double-blind method, they found that those patients receiving slow TMS to the contralateral region had a greater pinch acceleration than patients receiving sham TMS. This suggests that the contralesional region of the intact hemisphere actually inhibits rather than promotes recovery.

TMS has also been used to study the clinical recovery from aphasia. Specifically, it has been used to determine the relative importance of the right cerebral hemisphere of patients with aphasia. In a unique investigation, Naeser et al. (2005) administered slow TMS to the right Broca's area for 10 days in four patients with aphasia who were 5 to 11 years post-onset of a left middle cerebral artery stroke. As a group these patients were able to name significantly more pictured objects and at significantly reduced reaction times. This improvement was maintained for 2 months for one patient and 8 months for three patients. These researchers interpreted their results to indicate that activation patterns seen in the intact right cerebral hemisphere are "maladaptive." That is, activation or hyperexcitability of regions on the intact right cerebral hemisphere often seen in PET and fMRI poststroke studies may interfere rather than promote aphasia recovery (such as that found in the use of slow TMS and hemiparetic recovery). In a study combining PET with fast TMS (4 Hz) Winhuisen et al. (2005) found that of 11 patients with aphasia, three demonstrated PET activation of the left inferior frontal gyrus (IFG), while the remaining eight patients showed activation of the IFG in both hemispheres. When fast TMS was applied to each of these regions, stimulation of the right IFG resulted in increased reaction times on a semantic task for five patients, while six patients showed a similar response when TMS was applied to the left IFG. However, lower verbal scores were associated without the right-sided TMS effect, indicating that while the right IFG may be important for language function in some patients, its compensatory value is more limited. That is, the left IFG may be better suited to assist language recovery.

In conclusion, more stroke recovery and treatment studies involving TMS are needed, especially studies that are double-blinded and employ a large patient sample size. However, the above investigations demonstrate several important trends that deserve further study, including the identification of cortical regions affecting recovery, those that inhibit recovery and thereby might be a maladaptive response of the brain to damage, and those that enhance recovery indicating that these regions are more predisposed to assisting recovery. In the future TMS may be an important adjunct to language treatment of stroke patients with aphasia. As we found with ECS, TMS may enhance recovery from aphasia, not as a monotherapy but in combination with language therapy.

The effects of pharmaceuticals on stroke recovery had also been studied. Much of this research has stemmed from the stroke patient's need for drugs for the treatment of complications that may compromise his or her health and overall recovery. These include seizures, hyperanxiety, depression, and hypertension. Many of these drugs have been shown to impede recovery in laboratory animals and the motor recovery of patients with stroke (Table 3–4)

TABLE 3-4

Common Drugs and Their Effect on Stroke Recovery in Laboratory Animals and Human Beings

Neurotransmitter Action	Clinical Use	Effects	
		Animal	Human
Norepinephrine agonists			
Amphetamine	Stimulant	+	+
Methylphenidate (Ritalin)	Stimulant	+	+
Norepinephrine antagonists			
Prazosin	Antihypertensive	−	ID
Clonidine	Antihypertensive	−	ID
Propranolol	Antihypertensive	NE	NE
Dopamine agonists			
Bromocriptine	Stimulant	ND	ID
Apomorphine	Stimulant	+	ND
Dopamine antagonists			
Halperidol (Haldol)	Tranquilizer	−	ID
Spiroperidol	Tranquilizer	−	ND
GABA agonists			
Diazepam	Anxiolytic	−	ID
Phenytoin (Dilantin)	Anti-seizure	−	ID
Phenobarbital	Anti-seizure	−	ID
Carbamazepine (Tegretol)	Anti-seizure	NE	ID
Serotonin (5-HT) agonists			
Trazodone	Antidepressant	−	+
Desipramine	Antidepressant	+	ND
Fluoxitine	Antidepressant	NE	+
Amitriptyline (Elavil)	Antidepressant	NE	NE
Nortriptyline (Pamelor)	Antidepressant	ND	NE

Key: + positive effect; NE = negative effect; ID = insufficient data; ND = no data.

(Goldstein, Matchar, Morganlander, & Davis, 1990; Goldstein, 1995; also see Goldstein, 1997, 1998a, 1998b for a review).

Essentially these retrospective studies have shown that patients taking commonly prescribed drugs, including the antihypertensives clonidine and prazosin, dopamine-receptor antagonists, anxiolytics, and the antiseizure agent phenytoin, tend to demonstrate significantly poorer motor recovery and were less independent in their performance of ADLs. However, the major drawback to these retrospective studies is that it is difficult to determine whether the negative effect was due to the drugs or the disorders treated by the drugs (e.g., depression, anxiety, etc.). A double-blind prospective investigation of a specific drug or class of drugs is needed to determine their effect on stroke recovery.

Pharmacologic agents that specifically act on the central nervous system have been studied as to whether they enhance stroke recovery. These agents can be classified according to whether they increase production or retard metabolism (agonists), or impede production or enhance the metabolism (antagonists) of specific neurotransmitters such as norepinephrine (NE), gamma-aminobutyric-acid (GABA), serotonin (5-HT), and dopamine (DA). Of these only the effects of NE and DA agonists have been extensively studied in both animals and human beings after brain injury.

Norepinephrine is produced within the pons and the lateral tegmental areas of the midbrain and is projected to all areas of the cerebral cortex, and to specific thalamic and subthalamic nuclei. It acts on the sympathetic nervous system in that it prepares the brain to cope with stressful situations and is associated with wakefulness and alertness. A reduction of NE has been found in rat and cat brain stems after cerebral infarction (Cohen, Waltz, & Jacobson, 1975). Based on the assumption that motor deficits secondary to cerebral injury might be reversed by increasing the production of NE, several investigations have looked at the effect that amphetamine, a powerful NE agonist, has on the motor recovery in laboratory animals (Feeney, Gonzalez, & Law, 1982; Boyeson & Feeney, 1984; Hovda & Feeney, 1984). The common finding of these studies is that amphetamine tends to accelerate the motor recovery in rats and cats after cerebral injury is induced and that the improvement is enduring. Also common to these studies is that improvement only occurred when amphetamine was given in conjunction with motor training. Amphetamine treatment alone did not accelerate recovery, indicating that this psychostimulant is a "performance-enhancing" drug.

Similar findings have been found in human beings. Crisostomo, Duncan, Propst, Dawson, & Davis (1988) showed that patients with stroke who took amphetamine with physical therapy demonstrated a rate of improvement 40% greater than patients who received physical therapy and a placebo. Walker-Batson, Smith, Curtis, Unwin, & Greenlee (1995) also showed that this accelerated recovery continues after the patient stops taking amphetamine and well past the period of spontaneous recovery. Hemiplegic patients who received 10 mg of amphetamine every fourth day for 10 sessions paired with physical therapy demonstrated continued accelerated motor recovery up to 12 months after the onset of stroke. Methylphenidate (Ritalin), another NE agonist, has also been shown to have a positive effect on stroke recovery (Grade, Redford, Chrotowski, Toussaint, & Blackwell, 1998). Patients with acute stroke receiving this drug exhibited significant improvements in mood, ability to carry out ADLs, and motor functioning. In addition the effects of combining motor training with amphetamine has also been shown to result in motor plasticity (i.e., the recruitment of brain tissue surrounding the infarcted region) (Tegenthoff, Cornelius, Pleger, Malin, & Schwenkries, 2004).

Combining amphetamine with language treatment of patients with aphasia has also been studied in open-labeled and double-blind placebo-controlled studies. Using a similar experimental paradigm, Walker-Batson and her colleagues (1991, 1992) studied six patients within 30 days of their strokes. Each was given 10 to 15 mg of amphetamine followed by a 1-hour session of intensive speech and language therapy every fourth day for 10 sessions. The Porch Index of Communicative Ability (PICA) was administered 3 days prior to initiation of treatment, 1 week after the treatment was terminated, then again at 3 months post-stroke onset. Comparisons of their 3-month PICA overall scores and their 6-month predicted overall PICA scores were

made. Of the six patients, four had achieved over 94% of their projected 6-month score at the end of the d-amphetamine and language therapy sessions. At 3- months post-onset, five of the six patients with aphasia demonstrated over 100% of their 6-month predicted score. Using a nearly identical treatment paradigm but this time in a double-bind placebo-controlled study, Walker-Batson et al. (2001) demonstrated again that combining amphetamine with language treatment accelerates aphasia recovery. Twenty-one patients with acute onset of aphasia were randomly assigned to either receive a 10-mg dose of dextroamphetamine or a placebo, combined with language therapy. One week after the 10 sessions of combined treatment, the amphetamine group demonstrated significantly greater language improvement. At 6 months the differences between the groups continued to increase but were found to be insignificant. Regardless, the two studies show that amphetamine can be a powerful adjunct to aphasia therapy. However, large sample, controlled studies, addressing the safety, the amount of dosage, and the dosing schedule, are needed before this psychostimulant can be prescribed as a "standard of care" for stroke patients with aphasia.

The neurotransmitter dopamine (DA) is produced in the substantia nigra and the ventral segmental regions and projected to the caudate nucleus, putamen, globus pallidus, and mesial frontal cortex. Dopaminergic agents such as Sinemet and bromocriptine have been used for many years to improve the initiation and ease of movement of patients with Parkinson's disease. Other uses include the treatment of akinetic mutism (Echiverri, Tatum, Merens, & Coker, 1988) and apathy due to bilateral thalamic strokes (Catsman-Berrevoets & Harskamp, 1988).

The effect of bromocriptine on stroke recovery from aphasia has been studied. Early studies were promising, indicating that this drug may improve the speech fluency of patients with nonfluent aphasia secondary to stroke (Albert, Bachman, Morgan, & Helm-Estabrook, 1988; Bachman & Morgan, 1988; Gupta & Mlcoch, 1992; MacLennan, Nicholas, Morley, & Brookshire, 1991; Sabe, Leiguarda, & Starkstein, 1992; Gold, VanDam, & Silman, 2000; Raymer et al., 2001). However, the data from these studies were generally episodal, employing a single-subject test-retest design without adequate experimental controls, such as including a placebo condition and blinding the patient and the examiner.

Four group double-blind, placebo-controlled investigations have been since undertaken (Gupta, Mlcoch, Scolaro, & Moritz, 1995; Sabe, Salverezza, Cuerva, Leiguarda, & Starkstein, 1995; Bragoni et al., 2000; Ashtry, Janghorbani, Chitsaz, Reisi, & Bahrami, 2006). The studies by Gupta and her colleagues (1991, 1992, 1995) and Sabe et al. recruited patients with chronic, nonfluent aphasia. In each study the patients took a daily dose (15 mg and 60 mg, respectively) of bromocriptine and after a wash-out period were placed on placebo tablets. Language skills were measured before and after each phase (drug and placebo trials). Regardless of the dosage given in each study, bromocriptine had no effect on the patient's ability to speak fluently, to name objects, to write, and to understand spoken and printed language when compared to the placebo condition. Bromocriptine did not prove to be an effective treatment of chronic nonfluent aphasia. The third study, conducted by Bragoni et al. (2000) was different in that each patient was given a 60-mg dose of bromocriptine combined with aphasia therapy, though information pertaining to the type and intensity of treatment was not given. Of the eleven patients, six dropped out due to secondary side effects. The remaining five patients showed significant language improvement. High doses of bromocriptine were not found to be a reasonable treatment due to significant side effects. The last study by Ashtry et al. (2006) employed 38 patients with acute nonfluent aphasia who were randomly assigned to either a group receiving a 10-mg dose of bromocriptine or a placebo. At 4 months no difference was seen between the groups' verbal fluency, gesture to command, naming, or overall global language score, though each group had significantly improved from baseline.

Interestingly, the question of whether bromocriptine (or DA agonists in general) may be performance-enhancing drugs, like amphetamine, was not tested. Three studies used patients with chronic nonfluent aphasia while one used patients with acute-onset of aphasia in which drug administration was not tightly coupled with language therapy. In fact, three of the four studies did not provide language treatment to their patients. To date there has been no investigation of whether bromocriptine is performance-enhancing drug in either laboratory animals or human beings. Obviously a study of this type is needed.

FUTURE TRENDS

Since the fourth edition of this book was printed in 2000, some things have changed but much is unchanged in the diagnosis and treatment of stroke. For the most part, stroke remains a neurologic disease of prevention. The physician's responsibility is to identify those risk factors associated with stroke and to eliminate or minimize their potential effects by educating patients regarding the risks and associated diseases. Areas that need to be considered by the health-care provider include recommendations for implementing life style changes that can reduce the associated risks, by management of established diseases, and by treating the patient surgically (i.e., carotid endarterectomy) and/or pharmaceutically (i.e., antiplatelet, antihypertensive, and anticoagulation therapy) as needed based on the specific needs of the individual patient.

In the past 15 years much effort has been directed at reducing the extent of functional brain damage resulting from stroke. In an attempt to save the tissue surrounding the infarct (i.e., ischemic penumbra) many potential neuro-protective agents have been studied. Unfortunately, except for t-PA, none have been found to be effective in stopping the cascade of events resulting in brain-cell death. As reviewed, t-PA has the potential to reduce the degree of brain damage by quickly returning blood flow to the affected region. This will hopefully enhance the stroke patient's overall recovery.

The future of stroke treatment lies in how we view the brain. In the past we considered the brain as a "static organ," one that is "hard-wired" and changes little after puberty. We now understand that the brain is a "dynamic structure," one that is constantly changing as the environment requires and is continually adding new cells that may have the power to enhance the cognitive skills of the individual. It is this view that has lead researchers to the implantation of fetal brain-stem cells into the brains of patients with Parkinson's disease as well as adult brain-stem cells created by specialized tumors into patients with stroke. In addition, as was reviewed in the last section of this chapter, many new therapies are on the horizon that have the potential to enhance the brain's ability to learn, thereby increasing the effectiveness of stroke treatments such as language therapy. The importance of speech–language pathologists will lie in their ability to select the appropriate treatments. While the preliminary results (published and unpublished) from this research are mixed and in their infancy, it may potentally lead to an effective treatment of brain disorders, including stroke, within the near future.

KEY POINTS

1. Stroke is a neurologic disorder manifested by sudden changes in the patient's sensory, motor, cognitive, and/or speech and language skills.
2. Stroke is a neurologic disease of prevention and depends on eliminating or minimizing those risk factors associated with cerebrovascular disease.
3. Strokes are secondary to vascular disease including embolic, thrombotic, and hemorrhagic etiology.
4. Patients with transient ischemic attacks are at a high risk of having a major stroke within 5 years.
5. The initial examination of the patient with stroke should include procedures designed to identify where the vascular etiology emanates. These include noninvasive and invasive cerebral angiography and echocardiography.
6. Acute treatment is directed toward the preservation of life and limiting the area of cerebral infarction,

thereby preventing the expansion of disability associated with stroke.

7. Chronic therapy begins as soon as the patient with stroke is medically stable and is directed at his or her rehabilitation.
8. Commonly prescribed drugs can have a detrimental effect on stroke recovery.
9. The brain is a "dynamic structure" that is constantly adapting and adding new cells that may have the ability to enhance the cognitive skills of the individual.
10. In the future, electrical cortical, transcranial magnetic, and pharmaceutical stimulation of the brain may be used as adjuncts to behavioral stroke treatments, thereby enhancing the effectiveness of these therapies.

References

Abe, K., Ukita, N., Yorifuji, S., & Yanagihara, T. (1997). Crossed cerebellar diaschisis in chronic Broca's aphasia. *Neuroradiology*, *39*, 624–626.

Albers, G. W., Caplan, L. R., Easton, J. D., Fayad, P. B., Mohr, J. P., Saver, J. L., et al. (2002). Transient ischemic attack—Proposal for a new definition. *New England Journal of Medicine*, *347*, 1713–1716.

Albert, M. L., Bachman, D. L., Morgan, A., & Helm-Estabrook, N. (1988). Pharmacotherapy for aphasia. *Neurology*, *38*, 877–879.

Alexander, M., & LoVerme, S. R. (1980). Aphasia after left hemispheric intracerebral hemorrhage. *Neurology*, *30*, 1193–1202.

American Heart Association (1992). *Heart and stroke facts*. Dallas, American Heart Association.

Antiplatelet Trialists Collaboration (1994). Collaborative overview of randomized trials of antiplatelet therapy. Prevention of death, myocardial infarction and stroke by prolonged antiplatelet therapy in various categories of patients. *British Medical Journal*, *308*, 81–106.

Ashtry, F., Janghorbani, M., Chitsaz, A., Reisi, A., & Bahrami, A. (2006). A randomized, double-blind trial of bromocriptine efficacy after stroke. *Neurology*, *66*, 914–916.

Asslid, R. (1992). *Transcranial Doppler sonography*. New York: Springer-Verlag.

Atkins-Mair, D. L., & Jones, J. A. (2003). Cortical electrical stimulation combined with rehabilitative training: Enhanced functional recovery and dendritic plasticity following focal ischemia in rats. *Neurological Research*, *25*, 780–788.

Bachman, D. L., & Morgan, A. (1988). The role of pharmacotherapy in the treatment of aphasia: Preliminary results. *Aphasiology*, *2*, 225–228.

Bambauer, K. Z., Johnson, S. C., Bambauer, D. E., & Zivin, J. A. (2006) Reasons why few patients with acute stroke receive tissue plasminogen activator. *Archives of Neurology*, *63*, 661–664.

Barnett, H. J. M., Taylor, D. W., Haynes, R. B., Sackett, D. L., Peerless, S. J., & Ferguson, G. G. (1991). Beneficial effect of carotid endarterectomy in symptomatic patients with high-grade carotid stenosis. *New England Journal of Medicine*, *325*, 445–453.

Barnett H. J., Taylor, D. W., Eliasziw, M., Fox A. J., Ferguson, G. G., Haynes, R. B., Rankin, R. N., Claqett, G. P., Hachinski, V. C., Sackett, D. L., Thorpe, K. E., Heldrum, H. E., Spence, J. D. (1998). Benefit of cartoid endarterectomy in patients with symptomatic moderate or severe stenosis. North American symptomatic cartoid endarterectomy trial collaborators. *New England Journal of Medicine 339*, 1415–1425.

Baron, J. C., Bousser, M. G., Comar, D., Duquesnoy, N., Sastre, J., & Castaigne, P. (1981). Crossed cerebellar diaschisis: A remote functional depression secondary to supratentorial infarction in man. *Journal of Cerebral Blood Flow Metabolism*, *1*(Suppl 1), S500–S501.

Bogousslavsky, J., Miklossy, J., & Regli, F. (1988). Subcortical neglect: Neuropsychological correlations with anterior choroidal artery territory infarction. *Annals of Neurology*, *23*, 448–452.

Bonaffini, N., Altieri, M., Rocca, A., & Di Piero, V. (2002). Functional neuroimaging in acute stroke. *Clinical and Experimental Hypertension*, *24*, 6476–657.

Bonita, R. (1992). Epidemiology of stroke. *Lancet*, *339*, 342–344.

Boyeson, M. G., & Feeney, D. (1984). The role of norepinephrine in recovery from brain injury. *Society of Neuroscience Abstracts*, *10*, 638.

Bradley, W. G. (1982). *NMR tomography*. Diasonic Interactive Education Program. Diasonics, Militas, CA.

Bragoni, M., Altieri, M., DiPiero, V., Padovani, A., Mostardini, C., & Lenzi, G. L. (2000). Bromocriptine and speech therapy in non-fluent chronic aphasia after stroke. *Neurological Science 21*, 19–22.

Broderick, J., Brott, T., Kathari, R., Miller, R., Khoury, J., Pancoli, A., et al. (1998). The Greater Cincinnati/Northern Kentucky Stroke Study: Preliminary first-ever and total incidence rates of strokes among blacks. *Stroke*, *29*, 415–421.

Broderick, J. P., Phillips, S. J., Whisnant, J. P., O'Fallon, W. M., & Bergstralh, E. J. (1989). Incidence rates of stroke in the eighties: The end of the decline in stroke. *Stroke*, *20*, 577–582.

Brown, J. A., Lutsep, H., Cramer, S. C., & Weinand, M. (2003). Motro cortex stimulation for enhancement of recovery after stroke: Case report. *Neurological Research*, *25*, 815–818.

Brown, J. A., Lutsep, H. L., Weinand, M., & Cramer, S. C. (2006). Motor stimulation for enhancement of recovery from stroke: A prospective, multicenter safety study. *Neurosurgery*, *58*, 1–8.

Brown R. D., Whisnant J. P., Sicks J. D., O'Fallon W. M., & Wiebers D. O. (1996). Stroke incidence, prevalence, and survival: Secular trends in Rochester, Minnesota, through 1989. *Stroke*, *27*, 373–380.

Brunner, R. J., Kornhuber, H. H., Seemuller, E., Suger, G., & Wallesch, C. W. (1982). Basal ganglia participation in language pathology. *Brain and Language*, *16*, 281–299.

Bushnell, D. L., Gupta, S., Mlcoch, A. G., & Barnes, E. (1989) Prediction of language and neurologic recovery after cerebral infarction with SPECT imaging using N-isopropyl-p-(I123) iodoamphetamine. *Archives of Neurology*, *46*, 665–669.

Canadian Cooperative Study Group. (1978). A randomized trial of asp sulfinpyrazone in threatened stroke. *New England Journal of Medicine*, *299*, 53–59.

Cappa S. F., & Vallar G. (1992). The role of the left and right hemispheres in recovery from aphasia. *Aphasiology, 6,* 359–372.

Cardebat, D., Demonet, J. F., Celsis, P., Puel, M., Vaillord, G., & Marc-Vergnes, J. P. (1994). Right temporal compensatory mechanism in a deep dysphasic patient: A case report with activation study by SPECT. *Neuropsychologia, 32,* 97–103.

Catsman-Berrevoets, C. E., & Harskamp, F. V. (1988). Compulsive pre-sleep behavior and apathy due to bilateral thalamic stroke. *Neurology, 38,* 647–649.

Chui, D., Krieger, D., Villar-Cordova, C., Kasner, S. E., Morgenstern, L. B., Brantina, P. L., et al. (1998). Intravenous tissue plasminogen activator for acute ischemic stroke: Feasibility, safety, and efficacy in the first year of clinical practice. *Stroke, 29,* 18–22.

Clark, M. S., & Smith, D. S. (1998). The effects of depression and abnormal illness behavior on outcome following rehabilitation from stroke. *Clinical Rehabilitation, 12,* 73–80.

Cohen, M. P., Waltz, A. G., & Jacobson, R. L. (1975). Catecholamine content of cerebral tissue after occlusion or manipulation of the middle cerebral artery in cats. *Journal of Neurosurgery, 43,* 32–36.

Cramer, S. C., Bensen, R. R., Himes, B. S., Burra, V. C., Janowsky, J. S., Weinand, M. E., et al. (2005). Use of functional MRI to guide decisions in a clinical stroke trial. *Stroke, 36,* e50–e52.

Crisostomo, E. A., Duncan, P. W., Propst, M. A., Dawson, D. V., & Davis, J. N. (1988). Evidence that amphetamine with physical therapy promotes recovery of motor function in stroke patients. *Annals of Neurology, 23,* 94–97.

Dalen, J. E. (2006). Aspirin to prevent heart attack and stroke: What's the right dose? *American Journal of Medicine, 119,* 198–202.

Defer, G., Moretti, J. L., & Cesaro P. (1987). Early and delayed SPECT using N-isopropyl-p-iodoamphetamine iodine 123 in cerebral ischemia: A prognostic index for clinical recovery. *Archives of Neurology, 44,* 715–718.

Dombovy, M. L., & Bach-y-Rita, P. (1988). Clinical observations on recovery from stroke. *Advances in Neurology, 47,* 265–276.

Dorland's Illustrated Medical Dictionary, 26th Edition. Saunders, Philadelphia, 1994.

Druback, D. A., Makely, M., & Dodd, M. L. (2004). Central nervous system plasticity: A new dimension in the car of neurologically impaired patients. *Mayo Clinic Proceedings, 79,* 796–800.

Dumbovy, M. L., Sandok, B. A., & Basford, J. R. (1986). Rehabilitation for stroke: A review. *Stroke, 17,* 363–369.

Duncan, P. W., Zorowitz, R., Bates, B., Choi, J. Y., Glasberg, J. J., Graham, G. D., et al. (2005). Management of adult stroke rehabilitation care: A clinical practice guideline. *Stroke, 36,* e100–e143.

Easton, J. D., & Sherman, D. G. (1977). Stroke and mortality rate in carotid endarterectomy: 228 consecutive operations. *Stroke, 8,* 565–568.

Eastwood, M. R., Rifat, S. L., Nobbs, H., & Ruderman, J. (1989). Mood disorders following CVA. *British Journal of Psychiatry, 154,* 195–200.

Echiverri, H. C., Tatum, W. O., Merens, T. A., & Coker, S. B. (1988). Akinetic mutism: Pharmacologic probe of dopminergic mesencephalofrontal activating system. *Pediatric Neurology, 4,* 228–230.

ECSTC (1991). MRC European carotid surgery trial: Interim results for symptomatic patients with severe (70–90%) or with (0–29%) carotid stenosis. *Lancet, 337,* 1235–1243.

European Carotid Trialists' Collaborative Group MRC /European Carotid Surgery Trial. (1991). Interim results for symptomatic patients with severe (70–99%) or with mild (0–29%) carotid stenosis. *Lancet, 1,* 1235–1245.

Evans D. H., McDicken W. N., Skidmore R., & Woodcock J. P. (1989). *Doppler ultrasound physics, instrumentation, and clinical applications.* Chichester: John Wiley & Sons.

Ezekowitz, M. D., & Levine, J. A. (1999). Preventing strokes in patients with atrial fibrillation. *JAMA, 281,* 1830–1835.

Feeney, D., Gonzales, J., & Law, W. (1982). Amphetamine, haloperidol and experience interact to affect rate of recovery after motor cortex injury. *Science, 217,* 855–857.

Feeney, D., & Hovda, D. A. (1983). Amphetamine and apomorphine restore tactile placing after motor cortex injury in the cat. *Psychopharmacology, 79,* 67–71.

Feigenson, J. S., McCarthy, M. L., Meese, P. D., Feigenson, W. D., Greenberg, S. D., Rubin, E., et al. (1977). Stroke rehabilitation. I. Factors predicting outcome and length of stay-an overview. *New York State Journal of Medicine, 77,* 1426–1434.

Fields, W. S., Lemak, N. A., Frankoski, R. F., & Hardy, R. J. (1977). Controlled trial of aspirin in cerebral ischemia. *Stroke, 8,* 301–315.

Ford, A. B., & Katz, S. (1966). Prognosis after strokes. *Medicine (Baltimore), 45,* 223–246.

Fraser, C., Power, M., Hamdy, S., Rothwell, J., Hobday, D., Hollander, I., et al. (2002). Driving plasticity in adult motor cortex is associated with improved motor function after brain injury. *Neuron, 34,* 831–840.

Fridman, E. A., Hanakowa, T., Chung, M., Hummel, F., Leiguarda, R. C., & Cohen, L. G. (2004). Reorganization of the human ipsilateral premotor cortex after stroke. *Brain, 127,* 747–758.

Galynker, I., Prikhojan, A., Phllips, E., Facsenseanu, M., Ieronimo, C., & Rosenthal, R. (1997). Negative symptoms in stroke patients and length of hospital stay. *Journal of Nervous and Mental Disease, 185,* 616–621.

Gasecki, A. P., Ferguson, G. G., Eliasziw, M., Cagett, G. P., Fox, A. J., Hachinski, V., et al. (1994). Early endarterectomy for severe carotid artery stenosis after a nondisabling stroke: Results from the North American Symptomatic Carotid Endarterectomy Trial. *Journal of Vascular Surgery,* 288–295.

Gersten, J. W., Ager, C., Anderson, K., & Cenkovich, F. (1970). Relation of muscle strength and range of motion to activities of daily living. *Archives of Physical Medicine and Rehabilitation, 51,* 137–142.

Gillilan, L. A. (1980). Anatomy of the blood supply to the brain and spinal cord. In Cerebrovascular Survey Report for Joint Council Subcommittee on Cerebrovascular Disease National Institute of Neurological and Communicative Disorders and Stroke and National Heart and Lung Institute.

Giubilei, F., Lenzi, G. L., & Dipiero, V. (1990). Predictive value of brain perfusion single photon emission computed tomography in acute ischemic stroke. *Stroke, 21,* 895–900.

Gold, M., VanDam, A., & Sillman, E. R. (2000). An open-label trial of bromocriptine in nonfluent aphasia: A qualitative analysis of word storage and retrieval. *Brain and Language, 74,* 141–156.

Goldstein, L. B. (1995). Common drugs may influence motor recovery after stroke. *Neurology, 45,* 865–871.

Goldstein, L. B. (1997). Influence of common drugs and related factors on stroke outcome. *Current Opinion in Neurology, 10,* 52–57.

Goldstein, L. B. (1998a). *Restorative neurology: Advances in pharmacotherapy for recovery after stroke.* Armonk, NY: Futura.

Goldstein, L. B. (1998b). Potential effects of common drugs on stroke recovery. *Archives of Neurology, 55,* 454–456.

Goldstein, L. B., Matchar, D. B., Morganlander, J. C., & Davis, J. N. (1990). The influence of drugs on the recovery of sensorimotor function after stroke. *Journal of Neurological Rehabilitation, 4,* 137–144.

Grade, C., Redford, B., Chrotowski, J., Toussaint, L., & Blackwell, B. (1998). Methlphenidate in early poststroke recovery: A double-blind placebo controlled study. *Archives of Physical and Medical Rehabilitation, 79,* 1047–1050.

Grand, M., Stenzel, C., Schmullins, S., Rudolf, J., Neveling, M., Lechleuthner, A., et al. (1998). Early intravenous thrombolysis for acute stroke in a community-based approach. *Stroke, 29,* 1544–1549.

Gresham G. E., Alexander D., Bishop D. S., Giuliani C., Goldberg G., Holland A., et al. (1997). Rehabilitation. *Stroke, 28,* 1522–1526.

Gupta, S., Bushnell, D., Mlcoch, A. G., Eastman, G., Barnes, W. E., & Fisher, S. G. (1991). Utility of late N-isopropyl-p-(I 123)-iodoamphetamine brain distribution in the predictive recovery/outcome following cerebral infarction. *Stroke, 22,* 1512–1518.

Gupta, S. R., & Mlcoch, A. G. (1992). Bromocriptine treatment of nonfluent aphasia. *Archives of Physical and Medical Rehabilitation, 73,* 373–376.

Gupta, S. R., Mlcoch, A. G., Scolaro, C., & Moritz, T. (1995). Bromocriptine treatment of nonfluent aphasia. *Neurology, 45,* 2170–2173.

Halkar, R. K., Sisterhen, C., Ammons, J., Galt, J. R., & Alazraki, N. P. (1997). Tc-99m ECD SPECT imaging in aphasia caused by subcortical infarct. *Clinical Nuclear Medicine, 22,* 850–851.

Hand, P. J., Wardlaw, J. M., Rivers, C. S., Armitage, P. A., Bastin, M. E., Lindley, R. I., et al. (2006). MR diffusion-weighted imaging and outcome prediction after ischemic stroke. *Neurology, 66,* 1159–1163.

Hanson, W. R., Metter, E. J., & Riege, W. H. (1989). The course of chronic aphasia. *Aphasiology, 3,* 19–29.

Harvey, R. L., Roth, E. J., Heinemann, A. W., Lovell, L. L., McGuire, J. R., & Diaz, S. (1998). Stroke rehabilitation: Clinical predictors of resource utilization. *Archives of Physical and Medical Rehabilitation, 79,* 1349–1355.

Haynes, R. B., Taylor, D. W., Sackett, D. L., Thorpe, K., Ferguson, G. G., & Barnett, H. J. (1994). Prevention of functional impairment by endarterectomy for symptomatic high-grade carotid stenosis. *Journal of the American Medical Association, 271,* 1256–1259.

Hayward, R. W., Naeser, M. A., & Zatz, L. M. (1977). Cranial computed tomography in aphasia. *Radiology, 123,* 653–660.

Heiss W. D., Kessler J., Thiel A., Ghaemi M., & Karbe H. (1999). Differential capacity of left and right hemispheric areas for compensation of poststroke aphasia. *Annals of Neurology, 45,* 430–438.

Held, J. P. (1975). The natural history of stroke. In S. Licht (ed.), *Stroke and its rehabilitation.* Baltimore: 1975.

Henry, J. M., Barnett, D., Taylor, W., Eliasziw, M., Fox, A. J., Ferguson, G. C., et al. for the North American Symptomatic Carotid Endarterectomy Trial Collaborators (1998). Benefit of carotid endarterectomy in patients with symptomatic moderate or severe stenosis. *New England Journal of Medicine, 339,* 1415–1425.

Hoffman, R. E., & Cavus, I. (2002). Slow transcranial magnetic stimulation, long term potentiation, and brain hyperexcitability disorders. *American Journal of Psychiatry, 161,* 928.

Hovda, D. A., & Feeney, D. (1984). Amphetamine and experience promotes recovery of locomotor function after unilateral frontal cortex injury in the cat. *Brain Research, 298,* 358–361.

Joint Committee for Stroke Facilities. (1974). XI. Transient focal cerebral ischemia: Epidemiological and clinical aspects. *Stroke, 5,* 276–287.

Kelly-Hayes, M., Beiser, A., Kase, C. S., Scaramucci, A., D'Agostino R. B., & Wolf, P. A. (2003). The influence of gender and age on disability following ischemic stroke: The Framingham Study. *Journal of Stroke and Cerebrovascular Disease, 12,* 119–126.

Kertesz, A., Harlock, W., & Coates, R. (1979). Computer tomographic localization, lesion size and prognosis in aphasia and nonverbal impairment. *Brain and Language, 8,* 34–50.

Ketonen L. (1997). Computerized tomography in clinical neurology. In R. J. Joynt & R. C. Griggs (Ed.), *Clinical Neurology.* Philadelphia: Lippincott Williams & Wilkins.

Klein, J. A., Bruneau, R., Vandenberg, P., MacDonald, E., Mulrooney, R., & Pocock, D. (2003). Motor cortex stimulation enhances motor recovery and reduces infarct dysfunction following ischemic insult. *Neurological Research, 25,* 789–793.

Knopman, D. S., Rubens, A. B., & Selnes, O. (1983). Right hemisphere participation in recovery from aphasia: Evidence from xenon-133 inhalation rCBF studies. *Journal of Cerebral Blood Flow Metabolism, 3*(Suppl 1), S250–S251.

Koudstaal, S. R. (2006). Anticoagulants versus antiplatelet therapy for preventing stroke in patients with nonrheumatic atrial fibrillation and a history of stroke or transient ischemic attack. *Cochrane Library, Issue 2.*

Kuhl, D. E., Phelps, M. E., Kowell, A. P., Metter, E. J., Selin, C., & Winter, J. (1980). Effects of stroke on local cerebral metabolism and perfusion: Mapping by emission computed tomography of 18FDG and 13NH3. *Annals of Neurology, 8,* 47–60.

Kwakkel, G., Wagenaar, R. C., Koelman, T. W., Lankhorst, G. J., Koetsier, J. C. (1997). Effects of intensity of rehabilitation after stroke a research synthesis. *Stroke, 28,* 1550–1556.

Lee, R. G., Hillman, T. C., & Holman, B. L. (1984). Predictive value of perfusion defect size using N-isopropyl-(I-123)-p-iodoamphetamine emission tomography in acute stroke. *Journal of Neurosurgery, 61,* 449–452.

Lenzi, G. L., Frackowiak, R. S., & Jones, T. (1981). Regional cerebral blood flow (rCBF), oxygen utilization (CMRO2) and oxygen extraction ratio (OER) in acute hemispheric stroke.

Journal of Cerebral Blood Flow Metabolism, 1(Suppl 1), S504–S505.

Leonardi-Bee, J., Bath, P. M. W., Bousser M., Davalos, A., Diener H., Guiraud-Chaumeil, B., et al. (2005). Dipyridamole for preventing recurrent ischemic stroke and other vascular events: A meta-analysis of individual patient data from randomized controlled trials. *Stroke, 36*, 162–168.

Limburg, M., Royen, E. A., Hijdra, A., & Verbeeten, B. (1991). RCBF-SPECT in brain infarction: When does it predict outcome? *Journal of Nuclear Medicine, 32*, 382–387.

Lorenze, E. J., DeRosa, A. J., & Keenan, E. L. (1958) Ambulation problems in hemiplegia. *Archives of Physical Medicine and Rehabilitation, 39*, 366–370.

Lutsep, H. L. (2006). MATCH results: Implications for the internist. *American Journal of Medicine, 119*, 526.e1–526.e7.

MacLennan, D. L., Nicholas, L. E., Morley, G. K., & Brookshire, R. H. (1991). The effects of bromocriptine on speech and language function in a with transcortical motor aphasia. In T. E. Prescott (Ed.), *Clinical aphasiology*, Vol. 20 (pp. 145–156). Boston: College Hill.

Marquardsen, J. (1969). The natural history of acute cerebrovascular disease. *Acta Neurologica Scandinavica, 45* (suppl 38), 1–192.

Martin, W. R. W., & Raichle, M. E. (1983). Cerebellar blood flow and metabolism in cerebral hemisphere infarction. *Annals of Neurology, 14*, 168–176.

Mayberg, M. R., Wilson, S. E., Yatsu, F., Weiss, D. G., Messina, L., & Colling, C. (1991). Carotid endarterectomy and prevention of cerebral ischemia in symptomatic carotid stenosis. *Journal of the American Medical Association, 266*, 3289–3294.

Mayo, N.E. Goldberg, M. S., Leve, A. R., Danys, I., & Korner-Bitensky, N. (1991). Changing rates of stroke in the province of Quebec, Canada. *Stroke, 22*, 590–595.

Mazzocchi, F., & Vignolo, L. A. (1979). Localization of lesions in aphasia: Clinical-CT scan correlation in stroke patients. *Cortex, 15*, 627–653.

Megens, J., van Loon, J. Goffin, J., & Gybels, J. (1992). Subcortical aphasia from a thalamic abscess. *Journal of Neurology and Neurosurgery, 55*, 319–321.

Metter, E. J. (1992). Role of subcortical structures in aphasia: Evidence from resting cerebral glucose metabolism. In G. Vallar, S. F. Cappa, & C. W. Walesch (Eds.), *Neuropsychological disorders associated with subcortical lesions* (pp. 478–500). New York: Oxford University Press.

Metter, E. J., & Hanson, W. R. (1985). Brain imaging as related to speech and language. In J. Darby (Ed.), *Speech evaluation in neurology* (pp. 123–160). New York: Grune and Stratton.

Metter, E. J., Hanson, W. R., Jackson, C. A., Kempler, D., Van Lancker, D., & Mazziotta, J. C. (1990) Temporoparietal cortex in aphasia, evidence from positron emission tomography. *Archives of Neurology, 47*, 1235–1238.

Metter, E. J., Jackson C. A., Kempler D., & Hanson W. R. (1992). Temporoparietal cortex and the recovery of language comprehension in aphasia. *Aphasiology, 6*, 349–358.

Metter, E. J., Kempler, D. Jackson, C., Hanson, W. R., Mazziotta, J. C., & Phelps, M. E. (1989). Cerebral glucose metabolism in Wernicke's, Broca's, and conduction aphasias. *Archives of Neurology, 46*, 27–34.

Metter, E. J., Kempler, D., Jackson, C. A., Hanson, W. R., Riege, W. H., & Camras, L. R. (1987). Cerebral glucose metabolism in chronic aphasia. *Neurology, 37*, 1599–1606.

Metter, E. J., Mazziotta, J. C., Itabashi, H. H., Mankovich, N. J., Phelps, M. E., & Kuhl, D. E. (1985). Comparison of x-ray CT, glucose metabolism and postmortem data in a patient with multiple infarctions. *Neurology, 35*, 1695–1701.

Metter, E.J., Riege, W. H., Hanson, W. R., Phelps, M. E., & Kuhl, D. E. (1988). Evidence for a caudate role in aphasia from FDG positron computed tomography. *Aphasiology, 2*, 33–43.

Metter, E. J., Wasterlain, C. G., Kuhl, D. E., Hanson, W. R., & Phelps, M. E. (1981) 18FDG positron emission computed tomography in a study of aphasia. *Annals of Neurology, 10*, 173–183.

Mlcoch, A. G., Bushnell, D. L., Gupta, S., & Milo, T. J. (1994). Speech fluency in aphasia: Regional cerebral blood flow correlates of recovery using Single photon emission computed tomography. *Journal of Neuroimaging, 4*, 6–10.

Moonis, M., & Fisher, M. (2001). Imaging of acute stroke. *Cerebrovascular Diseases, 11*, 143–150.

Moore, W. S., Barnett, H. J., Beebe, H. G., Bernstein, E. F., Brener, B. J., Brott, T., et al. (1995). A multidiscipline consensus statement for the Ad Hoc Committee, American Heart Association. *Stroke, 26*, 188–201.

Muller R. A., Tothermel R. D., Behen M. E., Muzik O., Chakraborty P. K., & Chugani H. T. (1999). Language organization in patients with early and late left-hemispheric lesion: A PET study. *Neuropsychologia, 37*, 545–557.

Naeser, M. A., & Hayward, R. W. (1978). Lesion localization in aphasia with cranial computed tomography and the Boston Diagnostic Aphasia Exam. *Neurology, 28*, 545–551.

Naeser, M. A., & Helm-Esterbrooks, N. (1985). CT scan lesion localization and response to melodic intonation therapy with nonfluent aphasia cases. *Cortex, 21*, 203–223.

Naeser, M. A., Martin, P. I., Nicholas, M., Baker, E. H., Seeking, H., Kobayashi, M., et al. (2005). Improved picture naming in chronic aphasia after TMS to part of the right Broca's area: An open-protocol. *Brain and Language, 93*, 95–105.

National Institute of Neurological Disorders and Stroke Study Group (1995). Tissue plasminogen activator for the acute ischemic stroke. *New England Journal of Medicine, 333*, 1581–1587.

Noel, G., Bain, H., Collard, M., & Huvelle, R. (1980). Clinicopathological correlations in aphasiology by means of computerized axial tomography: Interest of using printout and prospective considerations. *Neuropsychobiology, 6*, 190–200.

North American Symptomatic Carotid Endarterectomy Trial Collaborators (1991a). Beneficial effect of carotid endarterectomy in symptomatic patients with high-grade carotid stenosis. *New England Journal of Medicine, 325*, 445–453.

North American Symptomatic Carotid Endarterectomy Trial Collaborators (1991b). North American Symptomatic carotid endarterectomy trial. Methods, patient characteristics, and progress. *Stroke, 22*, 11–20.

Okuda, B., Tanaka, H., Tachibana, H., Kawabata, K., & Sugita, M. (1994). Cerebral blood flow in subcortical global aphasia. Perisylvian cortical hypoperfusion as a crucial role. *Stroke, 25*, 1495–1499.

Oldendorf, W. H. (1981). Nuclear medicine in clinical neurology: An update. *Annals of Neurology, 10,* 207–213.

Paolucci, S., Antonucci, G., Gialloret, L. E., Traballes, M., Lubich, S., Pratesi, L., et al. (1996). Predicting stroke inpatient rehabilitation outcome: The prominent role of neuropsychological disorders. *European Neurology, 36,* 385–390.

Paolucci, S., Antonucci, G., Pratesi, L., Traballesi, M., Lubich, S., & Grasso, M. G. (1998). Functional outcome in stroke inpatient rehabilitation: predicting no, low, and high response patients. *Cerebrovascular Diseases, 8,* 228–234.

Parent A. (1996). *Carpenter's Human Neuroanatomy,* 9th ed. Baltimore: Williams & Williams.

Pascual-Leone, A., Tormos, J. M., Keenan, J., Tarazona, F., Canete, C., & Cataldo, M. D. (1998). Study of modulation of human cortical excitability with transcranial magnetic stimulation. *Journal of Clinical Neurophysiology, 15,* 333–343.

Plautz, E. J., Narbay, S., Frost, S. B., Friel, K. M., Dancause, N., Zoubina, E. V., et al. (2003). Post-infarct cortical plasticity and behavioral recovery using concurrent cortical stimulation and rehabilitation. *Neurological Research, 8,* 801–810.

Plum, F., & Posner, J. B. (1980). *The diagnosis of stupor and coma,* (3rd ed.). Philadelphia: Davis.

Porch, B. (1982). *The Porch index of communicative abilities.* Palo Alto, CA: Consulting Psychologists Press.

Price, C. J., & Crinion, J. (2005). The latest on functional imaging studies of aphasic stroke. *Current Opinion in Neurology, 18,* 429–434.

Raichle, M. E. (1983). The pathophysiology of brain ischemia. *Annals of Neurology, 13,* 2–10.

Raymer, A. M., Bandy, D., Adair, J. C., Schwartz, R. L., Williamson, D. J., Gonzalez-Rothi, L. J., et al. (2001). Effects of bromocriptine in a patient with crossed nonfluent aphasia: Case report. *Archives of Physical Medicine and Rehabilitation, 82,* 139–144.

Rosamond, W. D., Folson, A. R., Chambless, L. E., Wang, C., McGovern, P. G., Howard, G., et al. (1999). Stroke incidence and survival among middle-aged adults: 9-year follow-up of the Atherosclerosis Risk in Communities (ARIC) Cohort. *Stroke, 30,* 736–743.

Ross, R. (1980). Atherosclerosis. In *Cerebrovascular Survey Report for Joint Council Subcommittee on Cerebrovascular Disease National Institute of Neurological and Communicative Disorders and Stroke and National Heart and Lung Institute.*

Ross, R., & Glomset, J. A. (1973). Atherosclerosis and the arterial smooth muscle cell. *Science, 180,* 1332–1339.

Ruggieri, P. M., Masayk, T. J., & Ross, J. S. (1991). Magnetic resonance angiography: Cerebrovascular applications. *Current Concepts of Cerebrovascular Disease and Stroke. 26,* 29–36.

Sabe, L., Leiguarda, R., & Starkstein, S. E. (1992). An open-label trial of bromocriptine in nonfluent aphasia. *Neurology, 42,* 1637–1638.

Sabe, L., Salverezza, F., Cuerva, A. G., Leiguarda, R., & Starkstein, S. (1995). A randomized double-blind, placebo-controlled study of bromocriptine in nonfluent aphasia. *Neurology, 45,* 2272–2274.

Sacco, R. L., Adams, R., Albers, G., Alberts, M. J., Benavente, O., Furie, K., et al. (2006). Guidelines for prevention of stroke in patients with ischemic stroke or transient ischemic attack: A statement for healthcare professionals from the American Heart Association/American Stroke Association Council on Stroke: Co-sponsored by the Council on Cardiovascular Radiology and Intervention: The American Academy of Neurology affirms the value of this guideline. *Stroke, 37,* 577–617.

Saur, D., Lange R., Baumgaertner, A., Schraknepper, V., Willmes, K., Rijntjes, M., et al. (2006). Dynamics of language reorganization after stroke. *Brain, 129,* 1371–1384.

Schlaug, G., Benfield, A., Baird, A. E., Siewert, B., Lövblad, K. O., Parker, R. A., et al. (1999). The ischemic penumbra: Operationally defined by diffusion and perfusion MRI. *Neurology, 22,* 1528–1537.

Schmel'kov, V. N. (1982). Restoration of motor function in stroke patients: Peculiarities relating to damage of the right or left hemisphere. *Neuroscience and Behavioral Psychology, 12,* 96–100.

Selnes, O. A., Knopman, D. S., Niccums, N., Rubens, A. B., & Larson, D. (1983). Computed tomographic scan correlates of auditory comprehension deficits in aphasia: A prospective recovery study. *Annals of Neurology, 5,* 558–566.

SHEP Cooperative Research Group (1991). Prevention of stroke by antihypertensive drug treatment in older persons with isolated systolic hypertension—Final results of the systolic hypertension in the elderly program (SHEP). *Journal of the American Medical Association, 265,* 3255–3264.

Sherman, D. G., Goldman, L., Whiting, R. B., Jurgensen, K., Kaste, M., & Easton, D. (1984). Thromboembolism in patients with atrial fibrillation. *Archives of Neurology, 41,* 708–710.

Sinyor, D., Amato, P., Kaloupek, D. G., Becker, R., Goldenberg, M., & Coopersmith, H. (1986). Post-stroke depression: Relationship to functional impairment, coping strategies, and rehabilitative outcome. *Stroke, 17,* 1102–1107.

Sundt, T. M., Sandok, B. A., & Whisnant, J. P. (1975). Carotid endarterectomy: Complications and preoperative assessment of risk. *Mayo Clinic Proceedings, 50,* 301–306.

Takeuchi, N., Chuma, T., Matsuo, Y., Watanabe, I., & Ikoma, K. (2005). Repetative transcortical magnetic stimulation of contralesional primary motor cortex improves hand function in stroke. *Stroke, 36,* 2681–2690.

Talbot, P. R., Lloyd, J. J., Snowden, J. S., Neary, D., & Testa, H. J. (1998). A clinical role for 99m Tc-HMPAO SPECT in the investigation of dementia? *Journal of Neurosurgery and Psychiatry, 64,* 306–313.

Tegenthoff, M., Cornelius, B., Pleger, B., Malin., J. P., & Schwenkries, P. (2004). Amphetamine enhances training-induced motor cortex plasticity. *Acta Neurology Scandinavica, 109,* 330–336.

Teskey, G. C., Flynn, C. D., Goertzen, C. D., Monfils, M. H., & Young, N. A. (2003). Cortical stimulation improves skilled forelimb use following a focal ischemic infarct in the rat. *Neurological Research, 8,* 794–800.

Thom, T., Haase, N., Rosamond, W., Howard, V. J., Rumsfield, J., Manilio, T., et al. (2006). Heart disease and stroke-2006 update. *Circulation, 105,* 1–69.

Tikofsky, R. S., Collier, B. D., Hellman, R. S., Sapena, V. K., Zielonka, J. S., Krohn, L., et al. (1985). *Cerebral blood flow patterns determined by SPECT I-123 iodoamphetamine (IMP) imaging and WAB AQs in chronic aphasia: A preliminary report.* Poster presented at the Academy of Aphasia, Nashville, Tennessee.

Truscott, B. L., Kretschmann, C. M., Toole, J. F., & Pajak, T. F. (1974). Early rehabilitative care in community hospitals: Effect on quality of survivorship following a stroke. *Stroke, 5,* 623–629.

U.S. Department of Health and Human Services (1995). *Clinical practice guidelines, number 16, post-stroke rehabilitation.* Rockville, MD: Public Health Service, AHCPR Publication 95-0662.

Vallar, G., Perani, D., Cappa, S., Messa, C., Lenzi, G. L., & Fazio, F., (1988). Recovery from aphasia and neglect after subcortical stroke: Neuropsychological and cerebral perfusion study. *Journal of Neurological and Neurosurgical Psychiatry, 51,*1269–1276.

Veteran's Administration Cooperative Study Group on Antihypertensive Agents. (1967). Effect of treatment on morbidity in hypertension. I. Results in patients with diastolic blood pressure averaging 115 through 129 mm Hg. *Journal of the American Medical Association, 202,* 116–122.

Veteran's Administration Cooperative Study Group on Antihypertensive Agents. (1970). Effect of treatment on morbidity in hypertension. II. Results in patients with diastolic blood pressure averaging 90 through 114 mm Hg. *Journal of the American Medical Association, 213,* 1143–1152.

Walker-Batson, D., Curtis, S., Natajan, R., Ford, J., Dronkers, N., Salmoron, E., et al. (2001). A double-blind, placebo-controlled study of the use of amphetamine in the treatment of aphasia. *Stroke, 32,* 2093–2098.

Walker-Batson, D., Devous, M. D., Curtis, S. S., Unwin, H., & Greenlee, R. G. (1991). Response to amphetamine to facilitate recovery from aphasia subsequent to stroke. In T.E. Prescott (Ed.), *Clinical aphasiology, Vol. 20.* Boston: College Hill.

Walker-Batson, D., Smith, P., Curtis, S., Unwin, H., & Greenlee, R. (1995). Amphetamine paired with physical therapy accelerates motor recovery after stroke: Further evidence. *Stroke, 26,* 2254–2259.

Walker-Batson, D., Unwin, H., Curtis, S., Allen, E., Wood, M., & Smith, P. (1992). Use of amphetamine in the treatment of aphasia. *Restorative Neurology and Neurosciences, 4,* 47–50.

Werhahn, K. J., Conforta, A. B., Kadon, N., Hallett, M., & Cohen, L. G. (2003). Contribution of the ipsilateral motor cortex to recovery after chronic stroke, *54,* 464–472.

Whisnant, J. P. (1983). The role of the neurologist in the decline of stroke. *Annals of Neurology, 14,* 1–7.

Whisnant, J. P., Sandok, B. A., & Sundt, T. M. (1983). Carotid endarterectomy for unilateral carotid system transient cerebral ischemia. *Mayo Clinic Proceedings, 58,* 171–175.

Williams, P. L. (Ed) (1995). *Gray's anatomy.* Edinburgh: Churchill Livingstone.

Winhuisen, L., Theil, A., Schumackher, B., Kessler, J., Rudolf, J., Haupt, W. F., et al. (2005). Role of the contralateral inferior frontal gyrus in recovery of language function in poststroke aphasia: A combined repetitive transcranial magnetic stimulation and positron emission tomographic study. *Stroke, 36,* 1759–1763.

Wise, R. J. S. (2003). Language systems in normal and aphasic human subjects: Functional imaging studies and inferences from animal studies. *British Medical Bulletin, 65,* 95–119.

World Health Organization (1989). Stroke 1989: Recommendations on stroke prevention, diagnosis, and therapy: Report of the WHO task force and other cerebrovascular disorders. *Stroke, 20,* 1407–1431.

Yamaguchi, F., Meyer, J. S., Sakai, F., & Yamamoto, M., (1980). Case reports of three dysphasic patients to illustrate rCBF responses during behavioral activation. *Brain and Language, 9,* 145–148.

Yarnell, P., Monroe, P., Sobel, L. (1976). Aphasic outcome in stroke: A clinical neuroradiological correlation. *Stroke, 7.*

Chapter 4

Assessment of Language Disorders in Adults

Janet P. Patterson and
Roberta Chapey

OBJECTIVES

As a result of reading this chapter, reviewing the key points, and completing the learning activities, the reader will be able to:

1. Describe the dynamic process of assessment of adults with neurogenic communication disorders, considering the three interrelated components of cognitive abilities, linguistic skills, and pragmatic behavior.
2. Identify several instruments and procedures that assess an individual's communication abilities and deficits within the World Health Organization's International Classification of Functioning, Disability and Health.
3. State the theoretic foundation and practical application of several models of assessment of language and communication abilities, such as a cognitive neuropsychological model, a psycholinguistic model, or a functional communication model.
4. Identify standardized and nonstandardized assessment instruments and procedures that can be used during the differential diagnosis of persons with neurogenic communication disorders, such as aphasia, dementia, a motor speech disorder, and right hemisphere communication disorder.
5. Describe several instruments and procedures that can be used to assess an individual's functional communication abilities through structured testing and an observational profile.
6. Identify several variables, such as biographic variables, medical variables, or environmental variables, that influence assessment decisions and contribute to prognostic statements.

7. Define quality of life (QOL) as a concept; identify several measures to assess QOL in persons with neurogenic communication disorders, and describe how QOL contributes to the assessment process.

LANGUAGE

Language has three highly interrelated and integrated components: cognitive, linguistic, and pragmatic (Muma, 1978) (Fig. 4–1). The **cognitive** component refers to the manner in which individuals acquire knowledge about the world and in which they continue to process this knowledge. It refers to all of the processes by which sensory input is transformed, reduced, elaborated, stored, recovered, and used (Neisser, 1967). Through the use of cognitive processes we achieve knowledge and command of our world; that is, we process information and use it to influence people and events in our environment. High-level cognitive processing activities such as planning and organizing are governed by the executive function system (Hillis, 2005). According to Chapey (1986) these processes can be defined operationally within the five mental operations in the Guilford (1967) Structure of Intellect (SOI) model: recognition/understanding/comprehension (attention/perception), memory, convergent thinking, divergent thinking, and evaluative thinking.

The **linguistic** component refers to language form and content. Language **form** consists of three rule systems that dictate the structure of an utterance in order to convey meaning: phonology, morphology, and syntax. Language **content**, or semantics, is the meaning, topic, or subject matter involved in an utterance (Plante & Beeson, 2004).

The **pragmatic** component refers to the system of rules and knowledge that guides the use of language in social settings (Bates, 1976). It includes knowledge of how to converse with, and what to say to, different partners in different contexts, and how to initiate, maintain, and terminate discourse events such as conversation and narrative (Craig, 1983). It also refers to the use, function, or purpose that a particular utterance serves. For example, the same form and

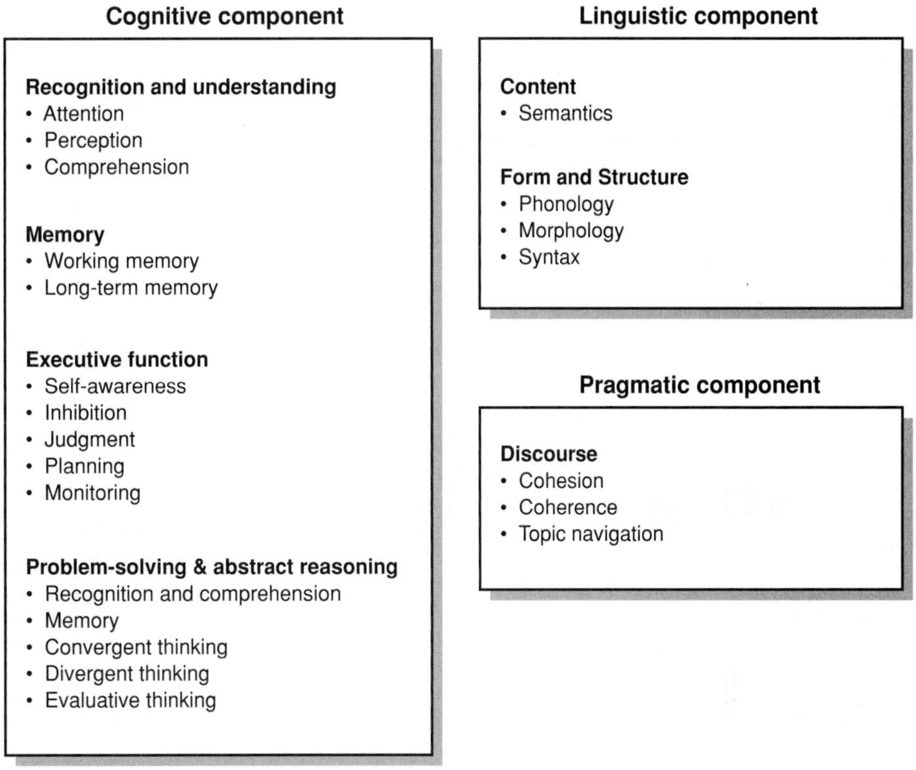

Cognitive component

Recognition and understanding
- Attention
- Perception
- Comprehension

Memory
- Working memory
- Long-term memory

Executive function
- Self-awareness
- Inhibition
- Judgment
- Planning
- Monitoring

Problem-solving & abstract reasoning
- Recognition and comprehension
- Memory
- Convergent thinking
- Divergent thinking
- Evaluative thinking

Linguistic component

Content
- Semantics

Form and Structure
- Phonology
- Morphology
- Syntax

Pragmatic component

Discourse
- Cohesion
- Coherence
- Topic navigation

Figure 4–1. Modified from Murray & Chapey, 2001; Chapey 1994; Muma, 1978.

content, "It is cold in this room" can be used to report an observation or to indirectly request an action to turn up the thermostat.

Within this model of language, **adult aphasia** is defined as an acquired impairment in language production, comprehension, or cognitive processes that underlie language. Aphasia is secondary to brain damage and most frequently caused by stroke (LaPointe, 2005). It is characterized by a reduction or impairment in the ability to access language form or structure, language content or meaning, language use or function, and the cognitive processes that underlie and interact with language such as attention, memory, and thinking (Murray & Chapey, 2001). Aphasia is a multi-modality disorder, since it may affect listening, speaking, reading, writing, and gesturing, although not necessarily to the same degree.

Aphasia does not refer to single modality deficits including perceptual impairments such as agnosia, or motor impairments such as apraxia of speech or a dysarthria. **Agnosia** refers to an inability to imitate, copy, or recognize the significance of incoming sensory information in the absence of sensory deficit in the affected sensory modality (Bauer, 2006). For example, in auditory agnosia an individual would be unable to recognize an incoming auditory signal as the word "table" even though the auditory sensation is intact. **Apraxia of speech** is a motoric impairment that disrupts central motor planning and consequently, voluntary

positioning of the speech musculature and sequencing of muscular movements. This disruption is in the absence of impairment in muscular control (Duffy, 2005; Darley, Aronson, & Brown, 1975). **Dysarthria** is a group of motor speech deficits caused by impaired strength, speed, or coordination of the speech musculature (Duffy, 2005; Darley et al., 1975). Agnosia, apraxia of speech, and dysarthria can co-occur in an individual with aphasia. Therefore, an important part of assessment involves determining which, if any, of these disorders exist and subsequently defining the nature and extent of each particular disorder and its interaction with the aphasia.

Body Functions and Structures, Activities, and Participation in Life

Aphasia can also be defined within the context of the World Health Organization's International Classification of Functioning, Disability and Health (International Classification of Functioning, Disability and Health: ICF, 2001; Towards a Common Language for Functioning, Disability and Health, 2002). The model classifies an individual's functioning and disability as they are associated with health conditions. **Functioning** refers to body functions and activities and participation in life events; **disability** refers to impairments, activity limitations, and participation restrictions that prevent an individual from participating fully in

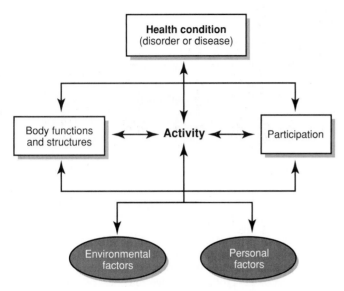

Figure 4–2. World Health Organization International Classification of Functioning Disability and Health (ICF, 2001)

his or desired life activities. This classification system proposes four levels, namely, (1) health condition (disorder or disease), (2) body functions and structures, (3) activity, and (4) participation. Figure 4–2 shows the WHO ICF model and illustrates the interrelatedness of the levels of the model as well as the environmental and personal factors that influence an individual's state.

One purpose of this model is to heighten awareness of the holistic components of functioning and participation in life activities, and the very complex interaction of conditions between an individual and his or her environment that affects functioning. That is, the WHO model takes into consideration both the organic and the functional consequences of the health condition. Fougeyrollas et al. (1997) expanded on this definition and attempted to show the dynamic interaction of important variables such as organic systems and capabilities, environmental factors, and life habits of social participation that contribute to functioning in what they termed the "Handicap Creation Process." Included in an assessment of aphasia should be examination of the aspects of an individual's life that may overtly or unintentionally lead to creating a handicapping situation and preventing full participation in life.

For individuals with aphasia, body functions and structures refer to impairments of brain and brain functions. Activity limitations primarily involve the four language modalities of speaking, listening, reading, and writing, as well as tasks necessary for daily living such as conversing with a heath-care provider or family member, writing a check, making a phone call, or reading a paper or a menu. Traditionally, the four language modalities, at the levels of impairment and activity limitations, have been the focus of

assessment and intervention in aphasia. In recent years, however, functional tasks have increasingly become the focus of diagnosis. This focus includes participation in daily life and the realization of immediate and long-term real-life goals (Chapey et al., 2001) such as playing golf, shopping for clothes, getting a job, volunteering, or participating in clubs and organizations. The effect of aphasia on an individual's pursuit and enjoyment of these activities is the concern of classifications such as ICF and the Handicap Creation Process.

The literature on aphasia and life participation supports the notion that the core features of positive human health or well-being involve leading a life of purpose, quality connection to others (zest for life comes from such interactions), positive self-regard, and mastery (Byng & Duchan, 2005; Kahneman, Diner, & Schwartz, 1999; Ryff & Singer, 1998). Subsequent to the loss of language due to stroke, all of these areas may be affected not only for the person with aphasia but also for significant individuals in that person's environment. This, in turn, has an impact on the health, well-being, and quality of life for the person with aphasia, as the relationship between an individual with aphasia and his or her family and friends is interactive with each influencing the other.

Further, without a reason or a cause to communicate there is no practical need for communication. Therefore, within this definition of aphasia as related to body functions and structures, activity, and participation, assessment and treatment must target all three areas from the outset and focus on a reason for the individual to communicate as much as on communication skills and ability to repair faulty communication. A result of using classifications such as these is an increased focus on the social and physical environmental factors that contribute to full participation in life (Chapey et al., 2001; Elman, 2005).

Assessment Defined

Assessment is an organized, goal-directed evaluation of the interrelated, integrated components of communication: cognitive, linguistic, and pragmatic. It also includes evaluation of an individual's quality of life, communicative interactions within the family or social unit, and role in the larger unit of society. An evaluation is carried out to determine a patient's language strengths and weaknesses and the degree to which language strengths can be fortified and language weaknesses modified (Chapey, 1994; Lahey, 1988; Murray & Chapey, 2001; Murray & Clark, 2006). Ideally, evaluation explores "the nature of the language impairment and indicate(s) what aspects of language performance are more appropriate for treatment" (Byng et al., 1990, p. 67). This type of in-depth assessment may seem contrary to current health-care philosophy, which underscores frugality and efficiency (Holland & Hinckley, 2002). However, it is essential that clinicians advocate for the best-quality services for their patients, which includes requesting sufficient time and funding to complete a sensitive, valid, and reliable assessment from which to develop the most appropriate treatment goals and procedures. A thorough, specific, and detailed assessment is essential if one is to see patterns of a patient's communicative and cognitive behavior, describe the complexity of the behavior, and develop a hierarchy of therapeutic goals that are appropriate for the individual with a neurogenic communication disorder and his or her family. That is, there should be a strong connection between a clinician's definition of language and communication, the description of a patient's language and communication abilities, and the goals that are established for treatment (Chapey, 1994; Murray & Chapey, 2001). Indeed, as Brookshire (2003) states, clinicians "must work to ensure that gains in economy and efficiency do not come at the expense of their patients' impairments and do not compromise their ability to provide the most efficacious treatment for those impairments" (p. 206).

Assessment Goals

Assessment of communicative and cognitive abilities in a person with a neurogenic communication disorder is multifaceted and involves the person with aphasia as well as his or her family or caregiver. The purposes are: (1) to describe language behavior in terms of both strengths and weaknesses; (2) to identify existing problems; (3) to determine intervention goals; and (4) to define factors that facilitate the comprehension, production, and use of language (Chapey, 1994; Murray & Chapey, 2001). Within these general goals, specific assessment goals vary according to factors such as the stage of the disorder (i.e., acute or chronic), the setting in which the assessment occurs (i.e., a hospital, residential facility, outpatient facility, or patient's home), the severity of the communication disorder, and concomitant physical, emotional, or psychosocial disorders that may be present. Consideration should be given to identifying a patient's current communicative environment and needs, the modality of communication (i.e., verbal speech, gesture, writing, or another augmentative or alternative communication method (Buzolich, 1995; Garrett & Lasker, 2005) and any factors that may interfere with communication. Specific goals are divided into etiologic goals, cognitive/linguistic/pragmatic/life goals, and treatment goals (Table 4–1) (Chapey, 1986, 1994; Murray & Chapey, 2001).

Hallmarks of a Quality Assessment

The nature of the language or communication deficit in the patient with aphasia dictates the need to perform a high-quality and thorough assessment. Some of the characteristics that typify a quality evaluation include the following. (1) A current knowledge of significant characteristics and

---

TABLE 4–1

Specific Goals of Assessment

Etiologic Goals
1. Determine the presence or absence of aphasia.
2. Identify and definition of complicating conditions that have precipitated or are maintaining the communication deficit to determine whether they can be eliminated, reduced, or changed.

Cognitive, Linguistic, Pragmatic, or Life Goals
(For each of the following goals, behaviors are analyzed to specify the nature and extent of the strengths and weaknesses in that particular behavior.)
3. Cognitive abilities.
4. The ability to comprehend language content.
5. The ability to comprehend language form.
6. The ability to produce language content.
7. The ability to produce language form.
8. Pragmatic abilities.
9. Quality of life with aphasia.

Treatment Goals
10. Determination of candidacy for and prognosis in treatment.
11. Specification and prioritization of treatment goals.

---

patterns of the patient's language impairment, as well as restrictions to personal activities and participation in life based both on first-hand experiences with patients with aphasia as well as a dedicated review of the aphasia language and disability literature. (2) A collection of comprehensive and detailed language samples of a patient performing tasks at varying levels of difficulty. (3) Repeated observation of communicative behavior, abstraction of behavior patterns, and formulation of hypotheses to account for the language and communicative deficit. (4) A quantitative and qualitative description of performance to generate information regarding the course, extent, and scope of treatment. (5) Respect for each and every individual patient, including a patient's history and accomplishments as well as his or her future contributions to the family unit and to society.

THE ASSESSMENT PROCESS

Assessment in aphasia and related neurogenic communication disorders involves three interrelated components: **data collection, hypothesis formation, and hypothesis testing** (Chapey, 1994; Murray & Chapey, 2001; Whitworth, Webster, & Howard, 2005). **Data collection** is the process of obtaining information that is linked directly or indirectly to the language strengths and weaknesses of the patient

(Lahey, 1988). Information should be obtained from the individual with aphasia, family members, caregivers, and other persons within the individual's social network (Blackstone & Berg, 2003). **Hypothesis formation** involves categorizing the data or forming taxonomies based on regularities in the data or similarities observed in the collected information. Furthermore, it requires interpreting the data and making decisions regarding the presence of aphasia, candidacy for treatment, prognosis and appropriate treatment goals. **Hypothesis testing** is the third component germane to the assessment process, involving the ongoing assessment and analysis of target behaviors, treatment goals, procedures, and patient progress (Lahey, 1988; Whitworth et al., 2005).

Data Collection

The data collected during the assessment process are based upon reported observations of a patient's language and communication abilities as well as on direct observation of the individual during language tasks and communicative interaction (Lahey, 1988).

Reported Observations

Reported observations are those data gathered from persons who have assessed the patient or who are familiar with the patient's current communicative abilities and communicative, vocational, or social history. These observations may be collected via interviews and written correspondence as well as in a review of the patient's pertinent medical records. For example, the clinician may interview professional workers or review the written reports of physicians, nurses, nursing assistants, occupational therapists, physical therapists, neuropsychologists, and social workers who have already assessed or treated the patient. When possible, the patient's perceptions of his or her current language and communication strengths and weaknesses should also be explored. Likewise, family members, friends, and/or members of the community who live with or who have frequent contact with the patient can provide valuable information concerning the patient's current language skills, activities, and participation in life. These friends and relatives may be asked to keep a diary or log, or to complete checklists or rating scales that relate their perception of the patient's language abilities. For example, a spouse might compile a diary of how her husband typically makes his needs and wants known in different contexts or with different communication partners throughout the day.

One tool for gathering such information is the Communicative Effectiveness Index (Lomas et al., 1989). This index requires a respondent to rate the patient's current performance in communication skills in specific daily communicative situations, using a continuum from "not at all able" to "as able as before the stroke" (Table 4–2). The

---

TABLE 4–2

The Sixteen Items of the Communicative Effectiveness Index (CETI)[a]

Please rate _____'s performance for that particular communication situation.
1. Getting somebody's attention.
2. Getting involved in group conversations that are about him or her.
3. Giving yes and no answers appropriately.
4. Communicating his or her emotions.
5. Indicating that he or she understands what is being said to him or her.
6. Having coffee-time visits and conversations with friends and neighbors (around the bedside or at home).
7. Having a one-to-one conversation with you.
8. Saying the name of someone whose face is in front of him or her.
9. Communicating physical problems such as aches and pains.
10. Having a spontaneous conversation (e.g., starting the conversation and/or changing the subject).
11. Responding to or communicating anything (including yes and no) without words.
12. Starting a conversation with people who are not close family.
13. Understanding writing.
14. Being part of a conversation when it is fast and a number of people are involved.
15. Participating in a conversation with strangers.
16. Describing or discussing something in-depth.

(From Lomas J., Pickard, L., Bester, S., Elbard, H., Finlayson, A., & Zoghaib, C. (1989). The Communicative Effectiveness Index: Development and psychometric evaluation of a functional communication measure for adult aphasia. *Journal of Speech and Hearing Disorders, 54*, 113–124.)

---

respondent places a mark on a 100- mm line for each item. Comparison of multiple response opportunities across time can be used to examine changes in perception about an individual's communicative abilities.

Social Network Theory provides another means of gathering information about the communication needs and abilities of an individual and his or her communication partners (Blackstone & Berg, 2003). In Social Network Theory an individual is at the center of a series of concentric circles, each of which represents a communication partner. The partners in the circles nearest to the center have the closet relationship to the patient (Fig. 4–3). The partners in the outside circles represent communication partners who are unfamiliar with the patient but who may have a specific role in communicative interactions (e.g., transportation workers or wait staff at a restaurant). Using an interview procedure, the clinician discovers the communication needs of the interaction between the individual and these partners.

Activity 1: Circles of communication partners

Directions: Please fill out your circle of communication partners.
1. Who is in your 1st, 2nd, 3rd, 4th, 5th circle?
2. Write initials/role of each person on the appropriate circle.
   For circle 5, write categories.
3. Raise your hand when you are finished.

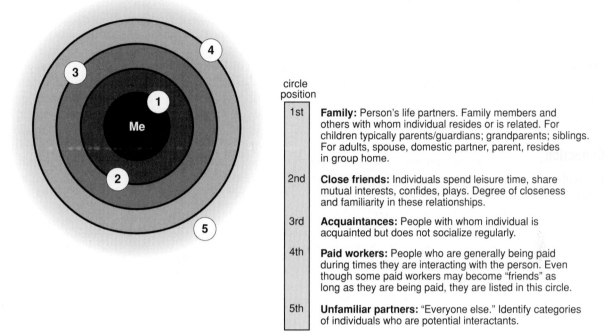

Figure 4–3. Blackstone, S., & Berg, M. (2003). Social Networks: A Communication Inventory for Individuals with Complex Communication Needs and Their Communication Partners. Monterey CA: Augmentative Communication, Inc. *Reprinted with Permission.*

Time, reliability and validity may present barriers to reported observations. For example, if an individual does not quickly and easily interact with a clinician, and the time allotted for observation is short, the data collected in the observation may be insufficient to allow the clinician to draw reliable conclusions about a patient's behavior. While acknowledging the importance of reported observations, professionals and paraprofessionals working in medical settings may not have the time to complete lengthy interviews or questionnaires. Holland and Hinckley (2002) discuss the importance to the diagnostic process of the information gathered from reported observations and describe several methods of gathering this information, such as conversational analysis and streamlined functional communication checklists. This information is particularly important for diagnosis of pragmatic functioning. Boles and Bombard (1998) provide suggestions for accomplishing conversational analysis that is efficient yet generates sufficient data for diagnosis.

Direct Observations

During direct observation, the clinician observes the patient, preferably over several sessions. Repeated observa-

tions are important to maximize the patient's ability to respond and to minimize fatigue, stress, and possible failure. Multiple samples are also essential because qualitative and quantitative aspects of the language abilities of patients with aphasia vary across different communication contexts, contents, tasks, and partners (Murray & Chapey, 2001). In addition, the communicative success of a person with aphasia may also vary despite identical communication conditions (Boyle, Coelho, & Kimbarow, 1991), since "an inconsistent response is one of the most striking results produced by a lesion of the cerebral cortex" (Head, 1920). Therefore the clinician should elicit language in several contexts, such as unstructured, moderately structured, and highly structured contexts, and appraise the effect of sampling methodology on the language elicited (Davidson, Worrall, & Hickson, 2003; Lahey, 1988; Murray & Chapey, 2001; Murray & Clark, 2006).

Unstructured Observation

In unstructured observation, the clinician describes the patient's cognitive, linguistic, and pragmatic behaviors in a natural setting when there is a minimum of control or interference. The setting should be familiar to the client and provide the opportunity for the individual to interact verbally with others. For example, a clinician working in a home-health setting may spend part of a session early in the treatment program observing the spontaneous communicative interactions among the patient and spouse or other family members during a meal. In this observation the clinician may be able to identify maladaptive behavior strategies (e.g., a spouse who pretends to understand the aphasia jargon produced by his or her partner) that lead to communicative interference or breakdown. The clinician may also observe positive strategies (e.g. an individual with aphasia who requests repetitions, or a spouse who accompanies his or her speech with gesture) that the patient or spouse currently use to facilitate communication interaction (Kagan et al., 2004; LeDorze & Brassard, 1995). In a medical setting a clinician might observe how the patient communicates with the reception area staff, again observing maladaptive or facilitative strategies used by both the staff and the patient.

Moderately Structured Observation

At times, the clinician may take a moderately active role in structuring observations and use predetermined questions or tasks to observe comprehension of and to elicit production of spontaneous communicative interaction (speech and language) (Croteau et al., 2004). For example, a client may be asked to retell a story, describe pictures, or answer direct requests, such as, "How do you change a tire?" or "How do you make scrambled eggs?" The clinician and patient may also role play specific situations such as (a) ordering in a restaurant and paying the bill, (b) relating the date and time of a doctor's appointment, or (c) answering the telephone and relaying a message (Chapey, 1994; Murray & Chapey, 2001). When possible, descriptive, narrative, procedural, and conversational types of discourse should be elicited since several studies have documented that type of discourse may significantly affect quantitative and qualitative aspects of a patient's language (Armstrong, 2000; Cherney, Shadden, & Coelho, 1998; Li et al., 1996; Penn, 1999; Shadden et al., 1991). The use of moderately structured observations allows the clinician to collect and observe a larger and more varied sample of communicative behavior than otherwise might be possible in an unstructured observation. In addition, this observation style fosters exploration of specific aspects of spontaneous language production and comprehension that may not have emerged during an unstructured observation (Chapey, 1994; Holland & Hinckley, 2002; Lahey, 1988; Murray & Chapey, 2001).

Highly Structured Observation

The language and communication assessment also includes highly structured observations based on results of bedside and screening assessment tools, comprehensive aphasia batteries, and/or tests of specific language functions. The American Speech-Language-Hearing Association publishes a list of speech-language assessments that can be accessed by ASHA members (Directory of Speech-Language Pathology Assessment Instruments, 2006).

Screening Tests. Screening tests provide an efficient means to determine the presence or absence of aphasia and to develop ideas for further assessment and initial treatment procedures (Al-Khawaja, Wade, & Collin, 1996; Salter et al., 2006). However, since they are short in length and sample a limited amount of language and communicative behavior, they do not provide a detailed description of the patient's language ability. Screening tests are most useful in three situations: in the early post-acute stages of recovery when patients may be too ill to complete a lengthy aphasia evaluation; in certain clinical settings where the length of stay in the facility is brief; or when the cost containment necessitates fast clinical information without extensive testing.

Spreen and Risser (2003) describe three screening procedures relevant to aphasia diagnosis: the bedside clinical examination, published screening instruments, and standardized tests that are limited to a specific aspect of language function. **Bedside tests** are rooted in classic neurology evaluation where interaction between the patient and examiner provides diagnostic data, and ranges from unstructured conversations to structured task sets (Spreen & Risser, 2003). Spreen and Risser (2003), Davis (2000), and Brookshire (2003) agree that an experienced clinician is able to make maximal use of patient responses and obtain a satisfactory aphasia screening under almost any set of clinical circumstances. Brookshire (2003) cautions however, that "...an unsystematic approach may lead the examiner to miss important signs, and may invalidate comparisons of the patient's performance with that of other patients or with the same patient on subsequent visits." (p. 165).

There are several frequently used aphasia **screening instruments** (Table 4–3), such as the Aphasia Language Performance Scales (Keenan & Brassell, 1975). This instrument consists of four scales (i.e., Listening, Talking, Reading, and Writing), each of which has 10 items of increasing difficulty. The screening requires minimal administration and scoring time and is suitable for patients regardless of aphasia severity or type. A Spanish version is also currently available. The Frenchay Aphasia Screening Test (Enderby & Crow, 1996; Enderby, Wood, & Wade, 2006; Enderby et al., 1987) was designed for use by individuals who are not trained speech-language pathologists, to screen for language disturbances in persons with aphasia. There are four sections to this test (i.e., Comprehension, Expression, Reading, and Writing). The test is short and easy to administer, and provides excellent value (Salter et al., 2006). Nkase-Thompson et al. (2005) introduced the Mississippi Aphasia Screening Test (MAST) as a screening

TABLE 4–3

Screening or Bedside Tests of Aphasia

Instrument	Source
Acute Aphasia Screening Protocol (AASP)	Crary et al. (1989)
Aphasia Language Performance Scales (ALPS)	Keenan & Brassell (1975)
Bedside Evaluation Screening Test, 2nd ed. (BEST-2)	Fitch-West & Sands (1998)
Frenchay Aphasia Screening Test, 2nd ed.	Enderby et al. (2006); Enderby & Crow (1996)
Reitan-Indiana Aphasia Screening Test	Reitan (1991)
ScreeLing	Doesborgh et al. (2003)
Sheffield Screening Test for Acquired Language Disorders	Syder et al. (1993)
Sklar Aphasia Scale (SAS)	Sklar (1983)
The Aphasia Screening Test (AST)	Whurr (1996)
Quick Assessment for Aphasia	Tanner & Culbertson (1999)

test designed to detect changes in language abilities over time. It was developed by a team of neuropsychologists, physiatrists, and speech-language pathologists, and has nine subtests designed to measure receptive and expressive language abilities. The Multimodal Communication Screening Task for Persons with Aphasia (Garrett & Lasker, 2005) is a cognitive-linguistic and behavioral assessment protocol for communicators with aphasia who may benefit from Augmentative or Alternative Communication Systems (AAC). This tool consists of eight tasks presented in picture format and designed to communicate a specific message. Responses are rated for accuracy in conveying the message, number of cues provided, number of attempts, and the examiners rating of message adequacy. Scores are summarized to determine whether the patient is an independent or partner-dependent communicator.

Shortened versions of several comprehensive tests of aphasia are also available to be used for screening purposes. These include the Minnesota Test for Differential Diagnosis of Aphasia (Powell, Bailey, & Clark, 1980) and the Porch Index of Communicative Ability (PICA; DiSimoni, Keith, & Darley, 1980). DiSimoni, Keith, and Darley report that shortened PICA scores accurately predict full PICA scores. However, Holtzapple and colleagues (1989) suggest using the shortened version of the PICA with caution as it may not always provide the same results. The third edition of the Boston Diagnostic Aphasia Examination (Goodglass, Kaplan, & Baressi, 2001) contains a short form that is valid for a constrained assessment session. The WAB-E (Kertesz, 2006) also contains a shortened version meant to be administered at the bedside.

Tests for specific aspects of language functioning have also been shortened to serve as screening tools. For example, The Token Test (Spellacy & Spreen, 1969) and the Boston Naming Test (Fastenau, Denburg, & Mauer, 1998) both have short forms. The reliability and validity of the shortened versions, as compared to the original tests, have been demonstrated and these tests should prove useful as screening instruments.

Several scales exist to screen, very briefly, for aphasia and other physical and neuropsychological sequelae that may accompany stroke (NIH Stroke Scales, 2003; Stroke Scales, 2006). These scales are primarily intended for use by physicians at the first sign of stroke in an individual. Some include only one or two items to assess speech, language, and mental status (i.e., Miami Emergency Neurologic Deficit (MEND) Prehospital Checklist (Miami Emergency Neurologic Deficit (MEND) Prehospital Checklist, 2001)), while others have several items to examine speech and language (NIH Stroke Scale, 2003).

Comprehensive Aphasia Tests. In many instances clinicians rely on comprehensive aphasia batteries to provide the major portion of their highly structured observations. These tests are designed to obtain a diverse sampling of performance at different levels of task difficulty (Spreen & Risser, 2003) and to evaluate language input and output modalities along a continuum of complexity (Brookshire, 2003). Many comprehensive aphasia batteries are available, each of which differs in terminology, internal organization, and the number of modalities tested, and each is associated with particular administration and interpretation of strengths and weaknesses (Lezak, Howieson, & Loring, 2004). Five tests that are commonly used in North America are the Minnesota Test for the Differential Diagnosis of Aphasia (MTDDA; Schuell, 1965), the Boston Diagnostic Aphasia Examination (BDAE; Goodglass et al., 2001), the Western Aphasia Battery (WAB; Kertesz, 1982; 2006), the Aphasia Diagnostic Profiles (ADP; Helm-Estabrooks, 1992), and the Porch Index of Communicative Ability (PICA; Porch, 1967, 1981).

One of the oldest and most comprehensive test batteries for aphasia is the MTDDA (Schuell, 1965). It consists of

46 subtests that are designed to assess a patient's strengths and weaknesses in speaking, listening, reading, and writing. A plus/minus scoring is used for most subtests. In addition, a severity rating scale from 0 to 6 can be used to quantify performance in the four assessed language modalities. The test provides a classification system based on Schuell's view that aphasia is a unidimensional, multi-modality impairment. This system categorizes an individual's performance according to whether the patient presents with aphasia alone, or whether he or she presents with aphasia plus sensory and/or motor deficits. For example, a patient may have a diagnosis of simple aphasia, aphasia with sensorimotor involvement, or aphasia with visual impairment. The test manual provides guidelines for the prediction of recovery based on Schuell's extensive clinical experience.

The third edition of the BDAE-3 (Goodglass et al., 2001) provides a comprehensive exploration of a range of communicative abilities. The results of the BDAE are used to classify patient's language profiles into one of the localization-based classifications of aphasia: Broca's, Wernicke's, anomic, conduction, transcortical motor, transcortical sensory, and global aphasia syndromes. The BDAE contains 34 subtests that assess conversational and narrative speech, auditory comprehension, oral expression, repetition, reading, and writing. The test provides for detailed scoring of conversational and narrative speech using a five-level aphasia severity rating scale, and several seven-point rating scales that comprise a profile of speech characteristics: melodic line, phrase length, articulatory agility, grammatical form, paraphasia in running speech, repetition, word-finding, and auditory comprehension. Raw scores on the subtests vary from a plus/minus scoring procedure, to rating scales, to frequency counts. These scores are converted to percentiles and registered on the Subject Summary Profile. The pattern of scores can be compared to examplar profiles to help determine aphasia classification. The BDAE-3 consists of an Extended Standard Form for in-depth study of aphasia symptoms, including grammar and syntax, and a Short Form that takes only 30 to 45 minutes to complete. The Boston Naming Test and the Visuospatial Quantitative Battery are included as part of the BDAE-3. They are designed to assess visual confrontation naming (BNT) and visuospatial skills sensitive to parietal-lobe lesion. New to this edition is a videotape in which the authors demonstrate assessment and scoring procedures with individuals with aphasia.

Like the BDAE-3, the WAB (and WAB-Enhanced (WAB-E)) (Kertesz, 1982; 2006) is designed to diagnose localization-based aphasic syndromes. However, unlike the BDAE, the WAB identifies syndromes on the basis of specific test scores, and provides summary scores that allow documentation of progress. The oral language abilities portion of the WAB contains 10 subtests that assess spontaneous speech (i.e., content and fluency), auditory comprehension, repetition, and naming. The seven subtests of visual language and the other subtest portions examine reading, writing, praxis, and construction abilities. Three summary scores can be calculated from WAB performances: (a) an Aphasia Quotient (AQ), which is derived from performance on the oral language subtests; (b) a Language Quotient (LQ), which is derived from performance on all language subtests (i.e., oral language abilities subtests as well as reading and writing subtests) (Shewan & Kertesz, 1984), and (c) a Cortical Quotient (CQ), which is derived from performance on all subtests.

The WAB-E (Kertesz, 2006) contains 32 tasks within eight subtests, and measures spontaneous speech (content and fluency), auditory comprehension, repetition, and naming, as well as reading and writing. Supplemental tests measure drawing, calculation, block design, and praxis. In addition, two new supplemental tasks (reading and writing of irregular words and nonwords) were included to aid in distinguishing between surface, deep, and visual dyslexia. The WAB-E provides six criterion quotient scores: Aphasia Quotient, Cortical Quotient, Auditory Comprehension Quotient, Oral Expression Quotient, Reading Quotient, and Writing Quotient. The WAB-E has revised administration instructions for each subtest and expanded scoring guidelines, and can be purchased with or without the manipulatives required for administration. In addition, the test battery contains a Bedside WAB-E that can be administered in approximately 15 minutes to assess briefly a patient's level of functioning.

The ADP (Helm-Estabrooks, 1992) provides for documentation of the nature and severity of aphasia, the communicative value of a patient's responses, and information concerning the general social-emotional status of a patient. The test contains nine subtests that assess speaking, listening, reading, writing, and gesture modalities (the reading and writing portions are short and therefore may require follow-up testing in some patients with aphasia). The ADP is designed to emphasize conversational interaction with the patient. The scoring methods vary across subtests, from a four-point scale and plus/minus scoring, to calculation of the number of correct information units and phrase length for verbal fluency tasks. Subtest raw scores are converted to standard scores and percentiles and used to create composite scores for five profiles: Aphasia Classification Profile, Aphasia Severity Profile, Alternative Communication Profile, Error Profile, and Behavioral Profile. Like the WAB, subtest and summary standard scores are used to determine aphasia type in terms of the Boston classification of aphasia. In addition to these nonfluent and fluent types of aphasia classifications, the ADP includes a borderline fluent aphasia type. Clinicians can also plot confidence ranges (i.e., standard error of measurement intervals) for each subtest and summary standard scores that can be used to determine patient progress over time.

The PICA (Porch, 1967; 1981) is a standardized test designed to provide a reliable measure of deficit severity and

TABLE 4–4

Multidimensional Scoring System of the Porch Index of Communicative Ability

Score	Level	Description
16	Complex	Accurate, responsive, complex, immediate, elaborative response to test item
15	Complete	Accurate, responsive, complete, immediate response to test item
14	Distorted	Accurate, responsive, complete response to test item, but with reduced facility of production
13	Complete-delayed	Accurate, responsive, complete response to test item that is significantly slow or delayed
12	Incomplete	Accurate, responsive response to test item that is lacking in completeness
11	Incomplete-delayed	Accurate, responsive, incomplete response to test item that is significantly slowed or delayed
10	Corrected	Accurate response to test item self-correcting a previous error without request or after a prolonged delay
9	Repetition	Accurate response to test item after a repetition of the instructions by request or after a prolonged delay
8	Cued	Accurate response to test item stimulated by a cue, additional information, or another test item
7	Related	Inaccurate response to test item that is clearly related to or suggestive of an accurate response
6	Error	Inaccurate response to test item
5	Intelligible	Intelligible response that is not associated with the test item; for example, perseverative or automatic responses or an expressed indication of inability to respond
4	Unintelligible	Unintelligible or incomprehensible response that can be differentiated from other responses
3	Minimal	Unintelligible response that cannot be differentiated from other responses
2	Attention	Patient attends to test item but gives no response
1	No response	Patient exhibits no awareness of test item

(From Porch, B. (1971). Multidimensional scoring in aphasia testing. *Journal of Speech and Hearing Research, 14,* 776–792.)

recovery progress. It contains 18 subtests that assess verbal, gestural, and graphic modalities through the use of 10 common objects. It does not, however, contain any tasks that assess spontaneous production of connected speech in discourse tasks. Performance on items in each subtest is scored using an elaborate 16-point multidimensional scoring system that encodes five dimensions of behavior: completeness, accuracy, promptness, responsiveness, and efficiency (see Table 4-4). The numbers assigned to a patient's responses are averaged to provide individual subtest scores, overall performance scores, and scores for each of six modalities: pantomime, reading, auditory, visual, writing, and copying. In the 1981 revision, Porch added diacritical markings to the scoring system to provide a greater degree of specific and sensitive response characterization. For example, an intelligible response that was rated a 5 would be augmented by a diacritical "p" if it was a preservative response. The PICA scoring system is highly informative; however, it requires a recommended 40 hours of formal training for skillful use (Martin, 1977; McNeil, Prescott, & Chang, 1975).

The batteries described above are among the most frequently used by clinicians. In addition, several other comprehensive aphasia tests are available. The Comprehensive Aphasia Test (CAT; Swinburn, Porter, & Howard, 2004) contains a cognitive screen, language battery, and disability questionnaire, and can be used to assess performance across a range of tasks. The Neurosensory Center Comprehensive Examination for Aphasia (Spreen & Benton, 1977; Spreen & Strauss, 1998) assesses language comprehension, language production, reading, and writing in 20 subtests. Examining for Aphasia (Eisenson, 1994) assesses oral and written receptive and expressive language functions, agnosia (visual, auditory, and tactile), and simple mathematic skills.

For patients whose first language is not English or who do not speak English, aphasia batteries are available in other languages (Kennedy & Chiou, 2005), such as the Aachen Aphasia Test (Huber, Poeck, &, Willmes, 1984; Huber et al., 1983; Kusunoki, 1985; Miller, Willmes, & DeBleser, 2000). Aphasia batteries originally written in English have been translated to other languages; two examples are the BDAE (Laine et al., 1993; Mazaux & Orgogozo, 1981) and the WAB (Sugishita, 1988). In addition, a few aphasia batteries such as the Multilingual Aphasia Examination (Benton et al., 1994; Rey & Benton, 1991), and the Bilingual Aphasia Tests (Paradis & Libben, 1987; 1993) assess various language abilities of patients who are bilingual or multilingual. These tests provide different language versions (e.g., Spanish, Arabic, Chinese, Swedish) that appear functionally and culturally equivalent in content and not simply direct translations of stimulus items from one version to the next.

Two other comprehensive batteries, the Boston Assessment of Severe Aphasia (BASA: Helm-Estabrooks et al., 1989) and the Assessment of Communication Effectiveness in Severe Aphasia (Cunningham et al., 1995) have been developed for patients with severe language problems. Because these batteries are designed to measure the language abilities of patients who are severely aphasic, their test procedures differ from those of traditional aphasia tests. For example, the BASA probes for spared language abilities across a variety of tasks and modalities including auditory, visual, and gestural expression and comprehension, as well as visuospatial and praxis tasks. The scoring system on this measure includes the identification of affect and perseveration, as well as partial verbal and gestural responses. Consequently, clinicians can acquire more explicit information regarding the communication strengths and weaknesses of their patients who have severe aphasia than can typically be obtained using one of the traditional aphasia batteries.

Tests of Specific Language Functions. Clinicians may need to supplement or substitute comprehensive aphasia batteries with tests of specific language functions to allow more in-depth quantification and/or qualification of abilities in a specific language modality than can be obtained from a general assessment battery, or to include a greater range of item difficulty. This testing may be particularly important when a person with aphasia scores at either a basal (very low) or ceiling (very high) level on an aphasia battery. In either of these cases little information is obtained with respect to areas of relative strength or weakness in a patient's communicative abilities. Such information is valuable for treatment diagnosis as well as treatment planning. Table 4–5 contains a list of some of the tests available for measuring auditory comprehension, verbal expression, reading comprehension, writing, and gestural abilities of patients with aphasia.

For many of these tests, normative data are provided in the test manual so that the performance of a person with aphasia may be compared with those of brain-damaged or non-brain-damaged peers. For other tests, clinicians must look to the empirical literature to find the appropriate normative data. For example, several studies have been conducted to extend the normative sample of the Boston Naming Test (Goodglass et al., 2001) to individuals who (a) live in institutionalized or community settings (Neils et al., 1995), (b) represent a wide age range (Henderson et al., 1998; Tombaugh & Hubley, 1997; Welch et al., 1996), and (c) represent diverse educational, racial, and socioeconomic backgrounds (Henderson et al., 1998; Kohnert, Hernandez, & Bates, 1998; Neils et al., 1995; Tombaugh & Hubley, 1997). Likewise, expanded normative data for verbal fluency tests such as the Controlled Oral Word Association Test (Benton et al., 1994) and the Thurstone Word Fluency Test (Thurstone & Thurstone, 1962) are also available in the research literature (Heaton, Grant, & Matthews, 1992; Ivnik et al., 1996; Kempler et al., 1998). Further expansion of norms for many published language tests is needed since

the demographic characteristics of the population of individuals with aphasia who live in North America is slowly changing over time (Neils-Strunjas, 1998).

Nonstandard Observation

Nonstandardized observations are useful in diagnosing the presence and severity of aphasia. Indeed, some tests of aphasia and some measures of specific language function rely primarily on nonstandard observations. These observations can be moderately or highly structured and typically do not have published norms (Lahey, 1988). They may be cited as tasks in empirical research studies or in doctoral dissertations or master's theses. These tasks can easily be adopted for assessment purposes and often lend valuable insight into the language, communication, or cognitive abilities and impairments of individuals with aphasia.

One example of a nonstandard observation is the Shewan Spontaneous Language Analysis (Shewan, 1988a, 1988b). The SSLA is a comprehensive and in-depth method for analyzing samples of spontaneous connected speech in picture description tasks. The SSLA contains several scoring dimensions, such as time of utterances, melody, and error analysis. Another example is divergent semantic naming tasks (Chapey, 1983; Murray & Chapey, 2001). For example, a clinician might ask a client to "Name as many objects as you can that can be folded," or "Name as many objects as you can that will break if they are dropped," or "Name as many ways as you can think of to use a hammer." The client's responses can be scored on several dimensions: fluency (the number of responses), flexibility (the variety of responses), originality, or elaboration. These tasks, while useful in diagnosis, do not have published norms for comparison.

Luria (Christensen, 1975) approached aphasia diagnosis through nonstandard observation across a variety of modalities and functions. He developed a series of bedside tasks, and recorded and rated a patient's responses according to level of performance. For example, the functions of reading and writing were examined through analysis of responses on letter identification and production tasks, reading words, reading phrases, and copying simple and complex forms. Performance pattern was related to site of lesion. Christensen (1975) formalized the tasks for use in clinical settings.

Qualitative assessment approaches the assessment process from a discovery perspective, using authentic, functional, and descriptive measures (Tetnowski & Franklin, 2003). Tetnowski and Franklin reviewed several principles of qualitative analysis: collect holistic data, focus on data in authentic settings, engage in a rich description of the communication phenomenon, approach assessment with an open stance to data collection, and collect data from the perspective of the individual being evaluated. Damico and colleagues (1999) illustrated these principles in qualitative analysis of communication skills in persons with aphasia.

TABLE 4–5

Tests of Specific Language Functions That May Be Used to Augment or Replace Comprehensive Aphasia Batteries

Language Function	Instrument	Source
Auditory comprehension	Auditory Comprehension Test for Sentences	Shewan (1979)
	Functional Auditory Comprehension Task	LaPointe & Horner (1978)
	Discourse Comprehension Test	Brookshire & Nicholas (1997)
	Peabody Picture Vocabulary Test-3	Dunn & Dunn (1997)
	Psycholinguistic Assessments of Language Processing in Aphasia	Kay et al. (1992)
	Pyramids and Palm Trees	Howard & Patterson (1992)
	Revised Token Test	McNeil & Prescott (1978)
	Test for Reception of Grammar – 2nd Version	Bishop (2003)
	Test for Reception of Grammar - Electronic	Bishop (2005)
	Test of Adolescent and Adult Language	Hammill et al. (1994)
Naming	Action Naming Test	Obler & Albert (1979)
	An Object and Action Naming Test	Druks & Masterson (2000)
	Boston Naming Test	Goodglass et al. (2001)
	Comprehensive Assessment of Spoken Language	Woolfolk (1999)
	Comprehensive Receptive and Expressive Vocabulary Test-Adult – 2nd Version	Wallace & Hammill (2002)
	Controlled Oral Word Association Test	Benton et al. (1994); Ruff et al. (1996)
	Florida Semantics Battery	Raymer et al. (1990)
	Object Naming Test	Newcombe et al. (1971)
	Psycholinguistic Assessments of Language Processing in Aphasia	Kay et al. (1992)
	Test of Adolescent/Adult Word-Finding	German (1990)
	The Naming Test	Williams (2000)
	The Word Test-Adolescent	Bowers et al. (2005)
Syntax	Northwestern Syntax Screening Test	Lee (1971)
	Shewan Spontaneous Language Analysis	Shewan (1988a, 1988b)
	Test of Adolescent and Adult Language	Hammill et al. (1994)
	The Reporter's Test	DeRenzi & Ferrari (1978)
	The SOAP (A Test of Syntactic Complexity)	Love & Oster (2003)
Reading comprehension	American NART	Grober & Sliwinski (1991)
	Gates-MacGinitie Reading Tests – 4th ed.	MacGinitie et al. (2000)
	Gray Oral Reading Tests - 3	Wiederholt & Bryant (2002)
	Johns Hopkins University Dyslexia Battery	Goodman & Caramazza (1986b)
	National Adult Reading Test	Nelson & Willison (1991)
	North American Adult Reading Test	Blair & Spreen (1989)
	Peabody Individual Achievement Test -Revised	Markwardt (1998)
	Psycholinguistic Assessments of Language Processing in Aphasia	Kay et al. (1992)
	Reading Comprehension Battery for Aphasia-2	LaPointe & Horner (1998)
	Reading subset of the Kaufman Functional Academic Skills Test (K-FAST)	Kaufman & Kaufman (1994)
	Test of Adolescent and Adult Language	Hammill et al. (1994)
	Test of Reading Comprehension-3	Brown et al. (1995)
	Wechsler Test of Adult Reading	Wechsler (2001)
	Wide Range Achievement Test-3	Wilkinson (1993)
Writing	Johns Hopkins University Dysgraphia Battery	Goodman & Caramazza (1986a)
	Psycholinguistic Assessments of Language Processing in Aphasia	Kay et al. (1992)
	Test of Adolescent and Adult Language	Hammill et al. (1994)
	Test of Written Language-3	Hammill & Larson (1996)
	Thurstone Word Fluency Test	Thurstone & Thurstone (1962)
	Wide Range Achievement Test-3	Wilkinson (1993)

TABLE 4–5

Tests of Specific Language Functions That May Be Used to Augment or Replace Comprehensive Aphasia Batteries (*continued*)

Language Function	Instrument	Source
	Writing Process Test	Warden & Hutchinson (1993)
	Written Language Assessment	Grill & Kirwin (1989)
Gesture	Florida Apraxia Screening Test – Revised (FAST-R)	Rothi, Raymer et al. (1997)
	Florida Action Recall Test (FLART)	Schwartz et al. (2000)
	Pantomime Recognition Test	Benton et al. (1993)
	Test of Apraxia	van Heutgen et al. (1999)
	Test of Oral and Limb Apraxia	Helm-Estabrooks (1991)
	15 item battery of movement to imitation	Haaland & Flaherty (1984)

Nonstandardized observation must be reliable to be of greatest value in a clinical setting (Cordes, 1994; Tetnowski & Franklin, 2003). Cordes described the theoretic foundation for observation and four common methods of measuring reliability: correlation based on classical test theory, interjudge percent agreement calculations, analysis of data from more than one observer, and generalizability theory, which is a method of estimating reliability from sources of error. Regardless of the method selected for measuring reliability in nonstandardized observation, the success of the measurement depends largely on the careful description of the behavior to be observed and the assurance that results were not influenced by error, which is inherent in human judgment (Dollaghan & Campbell, 1992).

Psychometric Considerations

Clinicians should be knowledgeable about the basic psychometric properties of aphasia batteries or tests used to assess an individual with a neurogenic or cognitive communication disorder. Specifically, each test or procedure used should be evaluated in terms of its validity, reliability, and standardization (Carmines & Zeller, 1979). In addition, when selecting a test clinicians should also consider the social and ethical consequences of using the test in terms of costs and benefits as well as possible side effects as a result of using the test, and consequences that might arise as a result of using the data from the test. Messick (1980) labeled the consideration of psychometric properties of a test as the **evidential bias** of test interpretation, and consideration of social and ethical consequences as the **consequential bias**. Skenes and McCauley (1985) reviewed nine tests for use with persons with aphasia and found several to be lacking in one or more categories of psychometric factors. Clinicians are cautioned to carefully review test manuals prior to administration to be assured that the test selected is psychometrically rigorous and addresses the goals of the evaluation (McCauley & Swisher, 1984).

Validity

Three categories of validity are important in language sciences: content, construct, and criterion-related validity. Each of the categories has several subtypes of validity that allow a fine-grained analysis of a test procedure (Messick, 1980). **Content validity** involves determining whether the test contains items that adequately represent the full domain of behaviors that should be measured. In aphasia assessment a test should contain language and communication behaviors that are perceived as being theoretically and functionally germane for successful communication (Carmines & Zeller, 1979; Spreen & Risser, 2003). A fine-grained analysis of content validity might include examination of the range and diversity of the content. **Construct validity** refers to determination of the extent to which a test relates to other measures of the same construct. In the case of aphasia assessment those constructs would be aphasia characteristics or language abilities. Spreen and Risser (2003) suggest that few aphasia tests have known validity; thus, to demonstrate construct validity test administrators may use factor-analytic statistical techniques. These techniques demonstrate whether test items contribute to one or more major factors that represent language or communication function. **Criterion-related validity** refers to the hypothesis about the relationship between a test and the criterion to which it is to be compared (Messick, 1980). In aphasia assessment, criterion validity refers to the accuracy with which a test can determine whether or not a patient meets the criterion for a diagnosis of aphasia. Concurrent and predictive validity are two types of criterion-related validity. Aphasia tests with good concurrent validity should be able to discriminate between the presence or absence of aphasia in an individual. Ideally an aphasia test should be able to discriminate not only between individuals with aphasia and non-brain-damaged individuals, but also between individuals with aphasia and other neurogenic communication disorders, such as right hemisphere disorder or dementia (Spreen & Risser, 2003; Strauss, Sherman, & Spreen, 2006). A test with good predictive validity should be suitable for measurement of change over time. A single aphasia test may not be appropriate for both concurrent and predictive validity purposes.

Unfortunately, aphasia batteries have been questioned on the basis of all forms of validity. Spreen and Risser (2003), and Strauss, Sherman, and Spreen (2006) note that although an aphasia test may have strong criterion-related validity, analysis often does not indicate whether trivial test items are responsible for discriminating performance of individuals with aphasia from non-brain-damaged individuals. The content and construct validity of some aphasia tests are also suspect because they include no clear operational definition of what is being assessed and/or fail to stipulate the specific model of language on which test construction was based (Byng et al., 1990; Chapey, 1986; 1994; David, 1990; David & Skilbeck, 1984; Kay et al., 1990; Martin, 1977; Murray & Chapey, 2001; Weniger, 1990). For example, the conceptual schemata underlying aphasia tests have often ignored the complexity factor in language (Chapey, 1986; 1994; Murray & Chapey, 2001). Tests have not reflected the fact that the communication of meaning is the essence of language (Goodman, 1971), and results do not supply enough information about the content, context, intent, structure, relevance, and meaningfulness of utterances (Chapey, 1994). Furthermore, most aphasia batteries do not provide a description of the patient's language impairment in relation to recently advanced cognitive neuropsychologic models of language (Ellis & Young, 1988; Hillis, 2002a; Patterson, Coltheart, & Marshall, 1985; Raymer & Rothi, 2000) and consequently fail to yield information concerning the nature of the underlying disorder. As Byng et al. (1990) suggest, "most standardized tests neither clarify what is wrong with the patient, nor specify what treatment should be provided" (p. 67). Lastly, many tasks in aphasia batteries assess composite abilities or more than one linguistic and/or cognitive ability at a time. For example, instructing a patient to "Put the pen on top of the book, then give it to me" (WAB item) engages linguistic processing abilities as well as attention, memory, initiation, and limb praxis abilities. Because linguistic and cognitive skills are both composite abilities and because they are highly interrelated processes, testing one particular aspect of language (e.g., confrontation written naming) without directly or indirectly involving associated processes (e.g., visuoperception or graphomotor constructional abilities) involves at best sophisticated clinical skill and acumen to provide an accurate diagnosis.

Reliability

Reliability refers to the consistency, stability, and accuracy of a test's sores during repeated administration under similar testing conditions (Anastasi & Urbani, 1996; Murray & Chapey,

2001). Spreen and Risser (2003) suggest that three types of reliability are most relevant for aphasia tests: the **internal consistency of the test, test-retest stability,** and **interrater reliability.** Aphasia test manuals should report correlation coefficients of at least 0.80 for these measures of reliability. The standard error of measurement for the test should also be reported. Although measuring any phenomenon is always associated with some degree of chance error, a test should contain detailed administration and scoring instructions as well as examples of correct and incorrect responses in order to minimize intra- and inter-examiner measurement error that can affect test reliability as well as validity.

Because of the extensive physiologic changes that typically occur during the early, acute phases of recovery, the reliability of aphasia tests can be poor (Murray & Chapey, 2001). To improve reliability, Spreen and Risser (2003) suggest that ". . . reliability is best demonstrated with normal, healthy subjects, since the measurement error in patient populations and the likelihood of change in performance due to changes in the patient's condition are high." Many aphasia tests demonstrate reliability using patients who have chronic aphasia rather than patients with acute aphasia, because language and communication deficits related to aphasia are considered to be stable. Considering only time post-onset of aphasia, these individuals are likely to show less variability and thus better reliability than individuals with acute aphasia. Clinicians should carefully examine the standardization sample on which reliability data are reported and examine the reliability of both overall test scores and individual scores (Cordes, 1994; Meline, 2005).

Standardization

Test administration procedures should be standardized (Cronbach, 1990; Spreen & Risser, 2003) to minimize measurement error and to allow valid and reliable comparison of patient performance to published norms. Standardization procedures reflect both test structure and administration instructions. The test structure should allow for minor variations in administration that routinely occur (i.e., variations related to individual clinical settings) but indicate deviations that may result in incorrect interpretation of test results. Test administration and scoring instructions must be clearly stated. Three areas where clarity of administration and scoring instructions are particularly important are (a) clarifying the range of scoring options left to the judgment of the clinician (i.e., use of an equivalent vocabulary term); (b) determining whether repetition of instruction is permitted; and (c) limiting stimulus and response format to that specified in the test (i.e., not allowing extra time for a response, or giving cues to elicit a response). Permitting variations in procedures may provide valuable diagnostic information; however, they render comparison to standardization norms inappropriate (Spreen & Risser, 2003).

To establish norms for comparison, standardized tests are administered to a large number of individuals who represent a cross-section of the population to whom the test will be administered in clinical practice. In addition, many test authors revise their tests in an attempt to improve sampling procedures and to expand normative data to a greater variety of reference groups (e.g., increased age range, or improved minority representation in the normative sample). When selecting a test for use with individuals with aphasia, clinicians are advised to examine carefully the characteristics of the standardization sample (i.e., age, education, time post-onset), the details of administration instructions, the parameters of scoring principles, reliability and validity data, and information about test revision (Jackson & Tompkins, 1991; Strauss, Spreen, & Hunter, 2000).

Predictive Considerations

In addition to meeting psychometric criteria, tests designed for use with persons with aphasia should allow for measurement of recovery or progress in treatment. Several researchers have noted that standardized tests are clearly unsuitable measures of language change or recovery (David, 1990; Kay et al., 1990). For example, the subtests of most aphasia batteries include too few items to provide a sensitive and reliable measure of a particular language modality or dimension. Likewise, real change made by a patient in a specific area of language functioning may not be represented in the overall test score. It is possible that a treatment protocol for a patient might result in real and meaningful change in the patient's language performance in daily communication activities; however, the potential lack of corresponding change in test scores would obscure a determination of treatment effectiveness. During the course of treatment an individual is expected to relearn language behavior or develop compensatory behaviors to replace the deficit. Traditional language tests measure current levels of functioning but do not reflect learning that occurred over time (Spreen & Risser, 2003). Furthermore, standardized language tests typically do not allow cueing or probing to "test the limits" of performance or examine learning styles.

Ethnocultural Considerations

It is well regarded that society is becoming increasingly diverse. As such there is an increasing number of patients on speech-language pathologists' caseloads for whom English is not the first or primary language, and Eurocentric culture is not the primary culture. Evaluating these individuals for the presence of a neurogenic communication disorder presents a challenge to clinicians who are not bilingual or multilingual (Baker, 2000). Speen and Risser (2003) suggest that evaluation should include testing in all premorbidly spoken languages of a patient and ideally be conducted by a clinician who is fluent in those languages. Evaluation of ability in one language only may lead to errors in diagnosis, such as failing to detect symptoms that appear in one language but not the other, or assessment bias introduced by using a translator to administer a test. Clearly it may not always be possible for a clinician to evaluate a patient in all languages in which that patient may be fluent; however, it is incumbent upon the clinician to be at least aware of the multilingual nature of a client and to plan as sensitive and thorough an assessment session as possible. Additionally, attitudes on the part of the patient toward the testing process, the clinical setting, or a question-and-answer format may be threats to successful assessment (Baker, 2000).

Culture is "a system of shared beliefs, values, customs, behaviors, and artifacts that members of a group use to cope with their world and one another, and that are transmitted from one generation to another through learning" (Bates & Plog, 1990). Appreciating cultural differences and using culturally competent assessment practices is important to a successful assessment interaction (Mahendra et al., 2005). They describe one framework for achieving cultural competence used by the National Faculty Center at the University of Arizona (National Faculty Center, 2006) that incorporates three stages: awareness, application, and advocacy. As one moves through these stages in one's professional development, one becomes better able to plan and implement an assessment session that is appropriate to the disorder as well as being sensitive to the cultural and linguistic traits of a client.

Ethnocultural considerations have a distinctive role in test selection for a client whose culture or language differs from that of the clinician. Spreen and Risser (2003) suggest that geographic, cultural, and regional considerations should guide test selection for individuals whose first language is not English. Although adaptations of a test may be available (i.e., a Spanish version of the WAB), it is preferable to use tests developed in the country consistent with the premorbid language of the patient (Paradis, 2004). For example, the Aachen Aphasia Test (Huber et al., 1983) would likely be more appropriate for individuals whose native language is German than a German translation of a test written in English (Baker, 2000). However, a client may be from a different geographic region than that in which the test was developed, and thus produce errors that are related to a cultural or linguistic difference rather than a communication disorder. Regional differences, particularly in vocabulary, may induce artificial errors (Barker-Collo, 2001). For example, the Psycholinguistic Assessments of Language Processing in Aphasia (Kay, Lesser, & Coltheart, 1992) contains several items (such as pram) that while recognized in the English language per se, may be unfamiliar to English-speaking individuals living in the United States. Kennedy & Chiou (2005) described 33 assessment tools in languages other than English that are available for use with individuals with communication disorders. They reported that their enthusiasm for the number of available assessment tools was tempered by the lack of adherence to psychometric test-construction principles in many of these tools.

Recently, investigators have begun to examine more closely relationships among test procedures in African-American individuals with aphasia. Ulatowsa et al. (2001) examined performance by African-Americans who were neurologically unimpaired and who had aphasia. They found that using fable and proverb interpretation tasks improved the quality of assessment because those communication items fostered greater communication interaction than standardized tests or functional communication measures. Ulatowska et al. (2001) suggested that the stimuli supported familiar text and discourse styles in the participants' cultures and thus encouraged a quick yet sensitive assessment of natural language. Results from Molrine and Pierce (2002) provided support for this conclusion. Molrine and Pierce administered the Minnesota Test for the Differential Diagnosis of Aphasia (Schuell, 1965), the Western Aphasia Battery (Kertesz, 1982), and the Boston Diagnostic Aphasia Examination (Goodglass & Kaplan, 1983) to 48 individuals who were black or Caucasian and compared group scores. Across all the subtests of the three batteries, only three subtests showed a significant difference between the two groups. Those three subtests required less structured responses and emphasized variety, quantity, and relevance of information. Molrine and Pierce reported that the three test batteries (MTDDA, WAB, and BDAE) are unlikely to yield performance that is influenced by group membership, while the less structured discourse tasks may show performance differences.

Studies of demographic, cultural, and linguistic influences on test performance in individuals without neurologic impairment and with aphasia have also appeared for persons living outside the United States. For example, Kohnert, Hernandez, and Bates (1998) and Pineda et al., (2000) examined cultural and linguistic influences in Spanish versions of the Boston Naming Test and the BDAE. Mansur and colleagues (2005) and Radanovic and Mansur (2002) studied similar influences in Portuguese. While the studies report individual differences according to the dependent variables examined, lessons to clinicians are similar about the importance of considering ethnocutural influences on the assessment process and diagnostic product.

Ethnocultural considerations apply not only to aphasia and language tests administered by clinicians but also to those tests regularly administered by other team members (Garcia & Desrochers, 1997; Tower, 2004). Chapey and Lu (1998) suggested that such important differences in language and the value that a given culture places upon different tasks and priorities are critical considerations for both assessment and intervention. In addition, values such as the duration of residency in the United States, English proficiency, and the value that a given culture places upon different language and cognitive abilities, test stimuli, and tasks all influence an individual's performance (Ardilla, 1995; Jacobs et al., 1997; Kempler et al., 1998; Payne-Johnson, 1992). Consequently, clinicians must be aware of how salient and suitable stimuli and procedures are to individuals from particular cultural groups. Likewise, assessment findings will be more accurate and valid if the normative group for a given aphasia test is representative of the ethnocultural or linguistic group to which a person with aphasia belongs (Spreen & Risser, 2003).

Body Functions and Structure, Activity, and Participation Considerations

The World Health Organization's framework for health and disability (Towards a Common Language for Functioning, Disability and Health, 2002) influences how aphasia is conceptualized and consequently assessed and treated (Simmons-Mackie, 2004; Threats, 2004; Threats & Worrall, 2004). In the ICF, functioning and disability are associated with an individual's health condition (disease or disorder); however, health condition is not the only consideration in assessment. In aphasia or other neurogenic communication disorders, an individual's performance in his or her usual environment will be influenced not only by the degree and nature of impairment in body structure or function and in language, but also by limitations in personal activities and restrictions to participation in society. Therefore, the ICF involves consideration of contextual factors that influence performance, such as social and physical-environmental factors (e.g., social attitudes of individuals in the patient's community, or architectural design of the patient's home) and personal factors (e.g., age, education, or co-existing physical or mental health conditions) that may interact with impairment, activity, and participation. Within ICF, clinicians appraise each of the factors that influence performance since there is not a one-to-one correspondence among these factors and levels of the ICF (Frattali, 1992, 1998a; Ross & Wertz, 1999; 2005; Threats & Worrall, 2004). Estimating the nature and extent of activity and participation assets and limitations, or predicting functional outcome and social reintegration solely on the basis of body functioning and structure is difficult at best (Towards a Common Language for Functioning, Disability and Health, 2002).

Body Functions and Structure

Impairment in body functions and/or structure refers to a loss or anomaly in anatomical, physiologic, or psychological structure or function. Examples of conditions at the impairment level of the ICF include aphasia, hemiparesis, hemianopsia, and dysphagia.

Activity

Within the activity level of ICF, aphasia may impose limitations on the four language modalities of speaking, listening, reading, and writing, as well as tasks necessary for daily living. Such limitations in language-related activities of daily living refer to any communication difficulties that arise in everyday contexts (e.g., using the telephone, writing checks, or reading the newspaper). Therefore, assessment at the activity level can involve the use of comprehensive aphasia tests and tests of specific language functions (e.g., naming or productive syntax ability) as well as functional status measures to assess the extent and type of language with which a person with aphasia may present (Baines, Heeringa, & Martin, 1999; Frattali, 1998b). Additionally, analysis of spontaneous language and communication within the context of activities of daily living (ADLs) and personally meaningful activities is an essential component of assessment (Armstrong, 2000).

The emphasis on functional communication requires clinicians to summarize patient data, often on scales such as the Functional Independence Measure (The FIM System,, 2006; Granger et al., 1993). The Functional Independence Measure (FIM) is a tool for measuring an individual's functional ability across motor, cognitive, and self-care domains and is part of The FIM System®. FIM uses a seven-point rating scale (1, which equals "Total Assist," to 7, which equals "Complete Independence (Timely, Safely.)" The FIM was originally designed to assist in setting reimbursement rates in response to medical cost-containment efforts and to document a patient's performance on a minimum set of skills at intake and discharge (Ottenbacher et al., 1996) and continues to be frequently used, although it is now part of a subscription system (The FIM System, 2006).

A serious drawback to the FIM is the limited number of items used to summarize language abilities. Consequently the brevity of description of communication skills on this rudimentary scale makes it an instrument of questionable reliability, validity, and sensitivity for assessment of persons with aphasia (Bunch & Dvonch, 1994; Gallagher, 1998; Murray & Chapey, 2001; Ravaud, Delcey, & Yelnik, 1999). In fact, Ottenbacher et al., (1996) found the poorest rating reliability for the comprehension item. Although other scales such as the Functional Assessment Measure (Hall, 1997; Wright, 2000), Frenchay Activities Index (Holbrook & Skilbeck, 1983) and the Functional Communication Measure (Functional Communication Measure, 1995) contain more communication-related information, they also are limited in terms of content, sensitivity and/or validity (Golper, 1996; Odell et al., 1997).

Rather than rely on these scales to summarize communication-related activity limitations, clinicians may adopt other longer but more precise functional language inventories. Several commonly used inventories are the Communicative Effectiveness Index (Lomas et al., 1989), the Functional Assessment of Communication Skills for Adults (Ferketic et al., 1995), the Communicative Activities of Daily Living-2 (Holland, Frattali, & Fromm, 1999), the

Amsterdam-Nijmegan Everyday Language Test (Blomert et al., 1994), or the Assessment of Language-Related Functional Activities (Baines et al., 1999).

Participation in Society

Sustained life participation in personally, culturally, and intrinsically valued tasks and goals enhances individual well-being for all human beings (Cantor & Sanderson, 1999). Such participation and concomitant well-being depend in part upon social, personal, and tangible resources that increase or decrease an individual's likelihood of participating in various tasks. These resources should be assessed and when necessary, supported or augmented to facilitate and motivate "continued participation (even) in the face of threat or frustration" (Cantor & Sanderson, 1999) in order to keep individuals "vigilant as they find new ways to participate in life" (p. 230) and thereby gain renewed health and well-being.

Activity and participation often appear together in assessment tasks and cover a full range of life areas (ICF, 2001). They can be examined in terms of performance (a person's activities in his or her current environment) and capacity (a person's ability to act in a uniform environment). Participation restrictions refer to obstacles that limit an individual from fulfilling his or her social, occupational, or personal role or goals. They reflect the difference between an individual's observed and expected performance. For example, persons with aphasia may be unable to return to work, may become socially isolated, and may undergo role changes (i.e., from provider to dependent). These changes may be the result of aphasia or functional communication problems, or because of transportation and access barriers in the community.

To assess participation and any restrictions to participation, clinicians may use measures of psychosocial status or wellness measures. Two psychosocial scales with a linguistic basis are the Stroke Aphasia Depression Questionnaire (SADQ; Sutcliffe & Lincoln, 1998) and the Geriatric Depression Scale (GDS; Yesavage et al., 1983). Visual-analogue mood scales were created to circumvent linguistic requirements in evaluating psychosocial status and detecting depression symptoms. These scales are 100-mm lines anchored by faces representing mood states; clients mark on the lines to indicate their current mood states. Two scales often used with persons with aphasia are the Visual Analogue Dysphoric Scale (VADS; Stern & Bachman, 1991) and the Visual Analogue Mood Scale (VAMS; Stern et al., 1997). Another measure, the Visual Analogue Self-Esteem Scale (VASES; Brumfitt & Sheeran, 1999), assesses psychosocial status from the perspective of self-esteem.

Another approach to assessing activity and participation levels and/or restrictions is through the use of wellness measures. Two examples of such scales are the Sickness Impact

Profile (Bergner et al., 1981) and the Duke-UNC Health Profile (Parkerson, Gehlbach, & Wagner, 1981). Doyle and colleagues (2003) developed the Burden of Stroke Scale (BOSS) to measure communication difficulty and psychological distress in persons following a stroke. The BOSS is a health-status assessment instrument and measures patient-reported functioning and well-being.

Hypothesis Formation

The information obtained during data collection must be organized, systematized, and condensed in a meaningful way (Murray & Chapey, 2001; Nickels, 2005). In this decision-making component of assessment, the clinician sifts through all the information obtained, delicately balancing and blending the data to arrive at a penetrating understanding of a patient's total behavior. Hypothesis formation is a sophisticated clinical judgment applied to the information collected (Lahey, 1988). It is an evaluation of the type, frequency, and pattern of behaviors produced by the patient as well as an exploration of the interrelatedness of various behaviors observed throughout the assessment period. A synthesis of diagnostic findings will aid not only in determining the suitability of the patient for treatment but also in indicating priorities and specific plans for a program of intervention.

Hypothesis formation is also part of the process of evidence-based practice (EBP). One of the steps in EBP is creation of a clinical question to be answered with evidence. A good clinical question should be patient-oriented and practical, and guide an evidence search (Shlonsky & Gibbs, 2004). The question should lead to constructive action that will benefit the patient and his or her family. Three forms of evidence are important to gather to formulate an hypothesis, gather information, and answer the clinical question: published data that represent the best evidence gathered from research; information about assessment values and expectations gleaned from the patent and his or her family; and a clinician's individual experience (Evidence-based practice in communication disorders [Position Statement], 2005; Shlonsky & Gibbs, 2004). Among the hypotheses that may be formed during the assessment process are those about aphasia classification, aphasia severity, and the locus of deficit derived from a model of language processing.

Aphasia Classification

Many classification systems have been developed to characterize adults with aphasia (Basso, 2003; Kertesz, 1979). Some clinicians use one of the dichotomous classifications systems (e.g., fluent vs. nonfluent aphasia, or receptive vs. expressive aphasia), while others use one of the anatomically based classification systems (e.g., Broca's, Wernicke's, or conduction aphasia). Still others use the classification system developed by Schuell and colleagues (Schuell, Jenkins, & Jimenez-Pabon, 1964) to organize and label the results of their assessment. However, there is still no universally acceptable classification system (Holland, Fromm, & Swindell, 1986).

The validity of aphasia classification systems has been called into question for several reasons (Byng et al., 1990; Caplan, 1993; Crary, Wertz, & Deal, 1992; Gordon, 1998; McNeil & Kimelman, 2001; Schwartz, 1984; Varney, 1998; Wertz, Deal, & Robinson, 1984): (1) the language profile of many patients cannot be fit into one of the categories (estimates range from 25% to as many as 70% of patients with aphasia who cannot be successfully classified); (2) patients in these categories cannot be said to be homogeneously impaired; (3) certain aphasia classifications such as receptive/expressive or sensory/motor are misleading since most if not all patients with aphasia display some degree of impairment in both language comprehension and production abilities; (4) a patient can evolve from one classification to another during the course of recovery; (5) the inclusionary criteria for the different aphasia types frequently overlap (e.g., all aphasia types include anomia as a symptom); (6) classification of aphasia type may vary as a function of the aphasia battery used (e.g., BDAE vs. WAB results); (7) discrepancies in interjudge reliability can possibly stem from a lack of agreement about how to assign and weight specific responses; (8) categories convey little information concerning the nature of the underlying language impairment (e.g., which particular level [semantic vs. phonologic] of language processing is impaired); and (9) syndrome classification in itself does not provide the basis for any comprehensive treatment program. Despite these concerns, the use of aphasia classifications remains a common and often useful means of describing language deficits in both clinical and research settings. For example, for some patients, a particular aphasia type may succinctly describe their language profile, and consequently the label may, at times, be useful to include in a medical chart note, clinical report, or research paper. Aphasia types are a clinical "shorthand" system of identifying patient characteristics among clinicians (Bartlett & Pashek, 1994), for scientific inquiry and organizing thinking about aphasia; however, their limitations must be kept in mind.

Severity Classification

Determining the severity of the language impairment in a person with aphasia may guide the clinician in selecting appropriate testing materials. For example, for patients with severe language impairments, clinicians may wish to avoid a frustrating assessment experience for themselves and their patients by selecting shorter tests for the initial assessment or only one test or procedure. Ross and Wertz (1999) reported that severity ratings on two standardized impairment measures, the WAB and PICA, and a standard measure of disability, the CADL, were strongly correlated. Scores on these measures were also strongly correlated to measures of connected speech. The measures are not replacements for one another in terms of content; however, Ross and Wertz (1999) suggested that perhaps administering more than one measure to determine severity of aphasia may be redundant.

In addition to standardized tests other instruments that may be useful in determining aphasia severity are clinical judgment supported by observation, severity rating scales, or a severity score, such as that included on the BDAE. Regardless of the measure used to determine or index overall aphasia severity, clinicians will want to be certain that the measure has been examined with respect to validity and reliability. For example, Lezak et al., (2004) noted that the severity estimate derived from a standardized battery, even the CADL, may underestimate a patient's ability to communicate in everyday situations. Several personal and environmental factors (ICF, 2001) such as contextual cues, routines, familiarity with vocabulary, and well-known communication partner styles, may contribute to underestimation. These factors are unique qualities to everyday interaction and are difficult to replicate in a standardized examination. Aphasia severity rating may also provide a useful guide for assigning patients to language treatment groups (Beeson & Holland, 1994) or selecting treatment goals.

Models of Language Processing: Cognitive Neuropsychological, and Psycholinguistic Information Processing

Rather than summarizing assessment results with two or three test or procedure scores clinicians may use cognitive neuropsychological, psycholinguistic or information processing models to guide assessment and describe clinical findings (Byng et al., 1990; Caplan, 1993; Hillis, 1993, 2002a, 2005; Kay, Lesser, & Coltheart, 1996). Davis (2000) differentiated core aspects of these models in terms of their origin, domain, and principal method of evaluation (p. 70). For example, the origin of cognitive neuropsychological models is the field of cognitive psychology; the domain is mental representation and processes in cognition; and the principle method of assessment is case studies of brain-damaged persons. In these models a particular language behavior (e.g., picture naming or sentence production) is conceptualized as a sequence of operations (e.g., for picture naming: analyze visuoperceptual or auditory input, access semantic stores, access phonologic output lexicon). Figure 4–4 is a cognitive neuropsychological model of the language processing system proposed by Kay, Lesser, and Coltheart (1996). The clinician's task in employing models is to determine the integrity of each of the language operations or components within each language modality in order to localize the level or levels at which the language behavior breaks down. In addition, a model-based approach allows clinicians to assess the types of errors made and the manner in

which a patient completes each language task. For example, according to information-processing approaches, clinicians analyze the underlying processing mechanisms that may be impaired and thus causing surface-level symptoms, in order to understand the nature of the language deficit. Examples of these processes are memory, attention, and executive functions. Using a model of language approach acknowledges that similar behaviors shown by a person with aphasia (i.e., anomia) may result from different underlying processing problems. For example, one patient may have difficulty with written naming because of a breakdown at the semantic level whereas another patient may also be unable to write the name of a target item, but due to a different cause—an inability to access information from the orthographic output lexicon.

Summary

The assessment process supports the need for clinicians to go beyond administering aphasia batteries and labeling aphasia type and severity to describe and summarize the actual cognitive, linguistic (content and form), and pragmatic strengths and weaknesses of each person with aphasia and to hypothesize about contributing factors (Murray & Chapey, 2001; Murray & Clark, 2006). These types of information are essential in clarifying the language and communication breakdown and in guiding the determination of treatment goals and activities. The information can also yield descriptive summaries that indicate the level at which language performance (a) is completely accurate, (b) begins to break down, and (c) breaks down completely. Additionally, such summaries can identify factors that facilitate or impede the patient's language use, help clinicians determine initial goals of therapy, and guide reassessment to monitor progress. The assessment process that results in descriptive language summaries that are accurately written, well-organized, easy to understand, and free of professional jargon, slang, and vague terminology are an asset to hypothesis formation and patient management.

Hypothesis Testing and Reporting

The results of hypothesis formation, and, specifically, the treatment goals that are established, should be considered tentative and flexible enough to change as new evidence emerges (Lahey, 1988; Murray & Chapey, 2001; Whitworth et al., 2005). Hypothesis testing continues throughout a patient's treatment program and enables the clinician to continue to secure additional data about language abilities and impairments in order to determine the validity, accuracy, and appropriateness of the hypotheses that were formulated. Separation of assessment and intervention activities allows for the initial presentation of information in an organized manner in order to begin treatment. However, assessment should be an ongoing part of treatment and occur at every phase of rehabilitation (Murray & Chapey, 2001).

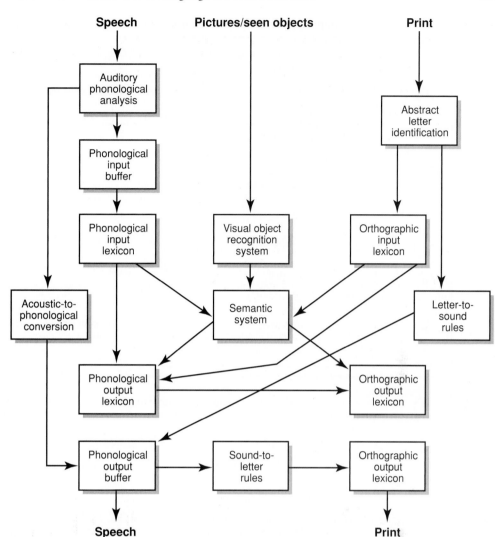

Figure 4–4. A Cognitive Neuropsychological Model of Assessment of Naming[a]

[a]Kay, J., Lesser, R., & Coltheart, M. (1996). Psycholinguistic Assessments of Language Processing in Aphasia (PALPA): An introduction. *Aphasiology, 10, 159–215. Reprinted with Permission.*

At various points during the assessment process—the initial assessment session and other evaluation and/or treatment sessions—a clinician must report the results of the hypothesis testing to other individuals on the assessment team, as well as the patient, family, and significant others. Assessment findings are usually presented when all of the data have been assembled (e.g., unstructured and structured observations, case history, and reports from other team members). The findings may be conveyed verbally at family and/or staff conferences, as well as in the form of a short, concise written report. Frequently, visual illustrations (e.g., a diagram of the brain to assist in describing anatomic areas that have been affected by the patient's stroke or brain injury) help patients, caregivers, and other professionals comprehend the information provided (Shipley & McAfee, 2004). When presenting information it is important to avoid overloading the patient and family with too much informa-

tion at one time. Clinicians should be prepared to repeat and/or paraphrase information across several sessions to assure that the patient and family understand the assessment results (Avent et al., 2005; Luterman, 1996).

A widely used written format for reporting information in a patient's file is the **SOAP note**. SOAP notes are part of the Problem Oriented Medical Records system of reporting and orienting information in a client's file according to specific problems or deficits a patient demonstrates. In this type of reporting format the "S" stands for *subjective*. Comments in this section are the clinician's subjective comments, nonmeasureable observations about the patient or the session, historical information, any other information that is pertinent to the session, or an aspect of the assessment session. "O" stands for *objective* and this section contains data from the assessment activities. This section presents the findings from the assessment session, without interpretation. The

Reporting Assessment results: two examples of a SOAP note

(S) Mr. S was attentive to all tasks and cooperative throughout the session. He demonstrated and commented about frustration with word-finding difficulties.

(O) The test of adolescent/adult word finding was administered. Mr. S achieved the following scores:

Subtest	% correct
Picture naming: nouns	28%
Sentence-completion naming	19%
Description naming	8%
Picture naming: verbs	5%
Category naming	19%
Total naming	17%
Comprehension	90%
Average item response time	12 secs

(A) Mr. S presented with severe (below the first percentile rank) word-finding difficulty across a variety of word types (i.e., nouns and verbs) and word-finding tasks. Additionally, Mr. S. required substantial time to produce the names of the test items.

(P) Bi-weekly, 1-hour therapy sessions to be scheduled. The focus of therapy should be to increase the accuracy and speech of Mr. S's word-finding abilities at the isolated word level and using a cueing hierarchy approach.

(S) 72 yr female sustained LCVA 15 days ago. ST at hosp; referred for Tx upon dc. Pt's daughter reported good progress c̄ word retrieval. Pt. coop during eval and reported frustration with word retrieval difficulties.

(O) 50% accuracy for confrontation naming. BNT 30/60. Y/N response 100% in questions with concrete and familiar elements. Cognition, reading and writing WFL.

(A) Dx: mod-sev anomic aphasia.

(P) Speech therapy 3x/week x 5 weeks to address following goals: 1: ↑ word-retrieval success in structured tasks and conf naming to 80%. 2: ↑ word-retrieval success in conv speech to 50%. Excellent prognosis considering the patient's cognitive status, motivation and stimulability.

Figure 4–5. Two examples of SOAP notes

"A" section of a SOAP note stands for *assessment* and contains the clinician's interpretation of the assessment data and findings, as well as the session performance. The fourth section is "P", which stands for *plan*. In this section the clinician writes the direction—or plan—for future assessment or treatment. A sample of a SOAP note appears in Figure 4-5. SOAP notes, or other clinical or chart notes, are usually written in as succinct a manner as possible. As Golper (1996) noted, "brief notes get read and long narratives do not" (p. 69).

It is important that data are included in a report of assessment sessions as they lay the foundation for the diagnosis. Equally as important is a statement of functional communication, which is derived from the data as well as the patient's overall performance during the session. The WHO ICF provides a useful tool for framing this statement, as does the Life Participation Approach to Aphasia (Chapey et al., 2001; Elman, 2005). A statement of functional communication skills, particularly including interaction with family members and significant others, is particularly useful in setting and prioritizing treatment goals.

GOALS OF ASSESSMENT

Goal 1: Determination of the Presence of Aphasia

One goal of the assessment process is to determine whether a patient presents with aphasia, or a related neurogenic language disorder (e.g.,. right hemisphere disorder or dementia), or whether his or her language and communication skills are within normal limits when compared to peers. Frequently the presence or absence of aphasia can be determined relatively quickly during the initial observation or interaction with the patient. For example, when the language impairment is severe or moderate the presence of aphasia is obvious and a diagnosis can be made quickly. In this case the remainder of the session can be devoted to specifying the nature and extent of the disorder. In contrast, when aphasia symptoms are mild, it may be more difficult to confirm the presence of language or communication impairment. That is, language problems may not be immediately apparent when conversational time is limited and when the responses during conversation are conventional, expected, or routine. In such cases, despite the presence of aphasia as identified by the patient, family, or physician, a person with aphasia may be so mildly impaired that he or she achieves perfect or near-perfect scores on traditional test batteries. In this case, assessment must continue on many levels (e.g., ICF) and include information about cognitive, linguistic, and communicative skills to provide a comprehensive and detailed description of language and communication strengths and weaknesses.

Determining the presence of aphasia may be challenging for many reasons. For example, test norms may not accurately reflect a patient's peer group in terms of age, language, cultural background, linguistic preference, or educational background (Garcia & Desrochers, 1997; Neils-Strunjas, 1998; Spreen & Risser, 2003). The limited range of tasks on some aphasia test batteries may not detect subtle differences in language abilities. For example, Wertz and colleagues (1984) found that using the Western Aphasia Battery, five out of 45 patients were diagnosed with normal language skills; however, using the Boston Diagnostic Aphasia Examination, all 45 patients were diagnosed with aphasia. Language disorders may only appear at complex levels (e.g., employment-related discourse) and/or be a result of impairment in executive functioning skills, such as immediate memory (Davis, 2000). Therefore, at times, the final decision regarding the presence of aphasia in individuals who are mildly impaired may be tentative and must be based on carefully documented observation and clinical judgment (Chapey, 1986).

In addition to determining the presence of aphasia it is often the clinician's responsibility to differentiate between language impairment in aphasia and language impairment that results from a different etiology. Careful analysis of the case history will aid in confirming whether the language symptoms reflect the presence of aphasia or related neurogenic communication disorders of right hemisphere syndrome, dementia, primary progressive aphasia, traumatic brain injury, a neurologic deficit (e.g., schizophrenia), a pharmacologic disorder, a metabolic disorder, or an emo-

tional disorder (e.g., depression). The language impairments associated with these disorders have different underlying sources of disturbance and follow different clinical courses. Consequently they demand different treatment approaches. However, it is important to note that having aphasia does not exempt an individual from also presenting with one or more of the above conditions. Careful observation and differential diagnosis will aid in determining the contribution of any disorders to current language functioning within the communication environment and personal environment of the individual (ICF, 2001; LaPointe, 2005).

Right Hemisphere Syndrome

The communication problems that appear in individuals with right hemisphere syndrome (RHD) are not exclusively language-based. Blake (2005) divided deficits associated with RHD into three general categories: communication, attention/perception, and cognition. Although diagnosis of RHD from the perspective of etiology may be easily evident, diagnosis of the behavior deficit is not often easy for several reasons: there may be overlap among deficits in an individual patient; cognitive deficits may interfere with language performance; no clear definition of RHD exists (Blake, 2005; Blake et al., 2003; Myers, 2001); no clear boundaries separate normal and abnormal behavior for the pragmatic and cognitive deficits often observed in persons with RHD (Blake, 2005); and patients with RHD represent a heterogeneous population in terms of extent and type of deficits (Murray & Chapey, 2001; Myers, 2005). Several test batteries that are appropriate for use with persons with RHD are listed in Table 4–6.

Communication Disorders

The communicative deficits that are common among patients with RHD do not resemble those of patients with aphasia, and become most apparent in prolonged conversation and other open-ended or sophisticated communication tasks (Bartels-Tobin & Hinckley, 2005; Brookshire, 2003;

TABLE 4–6	
Tests for Right Hemisphere Syndrome	
Right Hemisphere Language Battery -2	Bryan (1994)
The Mini Inventory of Right Brain Injury -2	Pimentel & Knight (2000)
Rehabilitation Institute of Chicago Clinical Management of Right Hemisphere Dysfunction, 2nd ed.	Halper et al. (1996)

Brownell et al., 1995; Marini et al., 2005; Myers, 1999; Tompkins, 1995). As communicative tasks or contexts become increasingly abstract or complex patients with RHD are likely to manifest some or all of the following comprehension and production deficits: (a) difficulty organizing and summarizing information in an efficient, meaningful way; (b) a tendency to produce impulsive answers that are tangential and/or provide unnecessary detail; (c) difficulty distinguishing between information that is relevant and irrelevant; (d) an inability to generate and interpret inference; (e) problems in assimilating and using contextual cues; (f) difficulty conveying information in a cohesive and coherent manner; (g) a tendency to overpersonalize external events; (h) a tendency to lend a literal or superficial interpretation to figurative language (e.g., idioms, metaphors, indirect requests); (i) a reduced sensitivity to communicative context and partners, and to the pragmatic or extralinguistic aspects of communication (e.g., turn-taking, topic maintenance, topic shifting); (j) difficulty organizing and maintaining discourse structure (e.g., macrostructure such as main ideas or themes); (k) an inability to comprehend successfully or to produce cohesive ties in discourse; (l) difficulty comprehending or producing prosody in conversational context; and (m) reduced appreciation or altered expression of emotion. Many researchers hypothesize that the variety of perceptual, affective, and/or cognitive deficits that patients with RHD may experience underlie or at least contribute to their higher level of communication disorders (Blake, 2005; Blonder et al., 2005; Myers, 1999; Tompkins et al., 1994).

Attention/Perception Disorders

A number of deficits in attention and/or perception can appear in a person with RHD. These deficits may manifest themselves in several ways, including contributing to a communication deficit. Among the symptoms a person with RHD may experience are (a) anosognosia (denial of illness); (b) inability to focus on internal or external stimuli due to reduced attentional capacity or inability to effectively allocate attentional resources; (c) visuospatial neglect (left hemispatial neglect); (d) visuoperception deficits; (e) prosopagnosia (inability to recognize familiar faces); (f) topographic orientation deficit (inability to relate to the surrounding space); (g) visuoconstruction deficits; (h) verbal or nonverbal memory deficit; (i) executive functioning deficits; and (j) similar auditory perceptual problems (e.g., auditory agnosia, amusia, sound-localization deficits, impaired discrimination of prosody, and music perception difficulty). These perceptual problems are associated with difficulties in appreciating the external context in which the stimulus is embedded and with problems integrating the stimulus with the internal associations. Recent research suggests that the deficits underlying these symptoms may not be straightforward. For example, persons with RHD may not have access to certain types of contextual information, even under reduced processing conditions, and therefore may not be able to use that information sucessfully to comprehend complex linguistic content (Cherney, 2002; Leonard & Baum, 2005). Although many of the problems and agnosias observed in persons with RHD are primarily associated with bilateral lesions, some of them may occur following unilateral right hemisphere brain damage.

Cognitive Deficit

Approximately half of the patients with RHD admitted to rehabilitation centers have cognitive deficits (Blake et al., 2002); however, the pattern of deficits observed is not well-explained, for several reasons. Cognitive abilities are interrelated and cannot often be tested independently (McDonald, 2000a; Monetta & Joanette, 2003). In the general population as well as in the population of persons with RHD there is a range of cognitive abilities, and the manner in which cognitive deficits manifest themselves to interfere with communication varies with the type and severity of RHD. Potentially all cognitive domains (e.g., memory and attention) may be disrupted in RHD; however, it is unlikely that all persons with RHD will display deficits in all areas (Murdoch, 2006). In conducting a thorough evaluation of the cognitive deficits in patients with RHD, as well as the deficits' contribution to communication difficulties, clinicians should use assessment procedures (e.g., RHD battery or memory testing), close observation of behavior, and consultation with family members and significant others to compare current and premorbid levels of functioning.

Dementia

Course of the Disease

Dementia is a condition of acquired, progressive degeneration of intellectual abilities affecting several cognitive domains such as language, memory, visuospatial skills, emotion or personality, and executive functions such as reasoning or abstraction (Disease Definition, Natural History, and Epidemiology, 2006). The diagnosis requires impairment in short- and long-term memory, abstract thinking, judgment, and higher cortical function and intellect, which cause significant social and occupational impairment, and which are not related to delirium. Symptomatology varies from subtle changes during the early stages of the dementing illness that may not be noticeable during daily activities, to profound changes during the later stages that may render the patient unable to function socially or occupationally. Dementia may result from a variety of reversible and irreversible disorders (Kaufer & Cummings, 1997). Table 4–7 lists examples of etiologies of reversible and irreversible dementias. Cognitive symptoms associated with reversible dementias can be remediated by treating the underlying medical condition. The

TABLE 4–7

Examples of Reversible and Irreversible Causes of Dementia

Reversible Causes that Can Resemble Dementia

Depression (pseudodementia)
Drug use (e.g., anticholinergic side effects)
Infection (e.g., meningitis, encephalitis)
Hearing loss
Neoplasm
Normal pressure hydrocephalus
Mental and/or sensory deprivation
Renal failure (dialysis dementia)
Thyroid disease
Toxin exposure (e.g., lead poisoning)
Vitamin deficiency (e.g., pellagra, Wernicke-Korsakoff syndrome)

Irreversible Causes

Alzheimer's disease
Creutzfeld-Jakob disease
Human immunodeficiency virus encephalopathy
Huntington's disease
Multi-infarct dementia
Multiple sclerosis
Parkinson's disease
Pick's disease
Progressive supranuclear palsy
Traumatic brain injury (e.g., dementia pugilistica)
Vascular dementia

prevalence of reversible dementias is much lower than previously thought (Clarfield, 2003). A meta-analysis by Clarfield (2003) showed that potentially reversible dementias comprised only 9% of all dementias, and less than 1% of dementia cases were actually reversed. Nonetheless, it is very important that reversible causes of dementia be ruled out prior to diagnosing a patient with irreversible dementia. In contrast, researchers have yet to identify treatments that will reduce or eliminate the cognitive symptoms associated with irreversible dementing diseases. The most commonly occurring dementias are irreversible: Alzheimer's disease (56% of all dementias) and vascular dementia (20%).

Site of Lesion

Dementia may also be categorized on the basis of neuroanatomic location of the causative lesion (Bourgeois, 2005; Brookshire, 2003; Lezak et al., 2004; Ripich, 1995). In the cortical dementias the pathophysiology affects primarily the cortical brain tissue; examples are Alzheimer's disease, Pick's disease, and frontotemporal dementia. Subcortical dementias are those in which the pathology primarily affects subcortical structures such as the thalamus and basal ganglia; examples are Parkinson's disease, Huntington's disease, and progressive supranuclear palsy. When both cortical and subcortical brain tissue is affected by the disease process, the result is a mixed dementia. An example of a mixed dementia is dementia with Lewy bodies. Vascular dementias arise as a result of thrombotic or embolic occlusions that cause focal neurologic symptoms. Three subgroups are multi-infarct dementia, lacunar state (multiple small infarcts in the subcortex, midbrain, or brain stem), and Binswanger's disease. Some differences exist among the symptom profiles associated with each of these dementia classifications. For example, in terms of communication profiles, patients with cortical dementia may demonstrate logorrhea, empty speech, verbal paraphasias, impaired comprehension, relatively preserved repetition, and topic digression; in contrast, patients with subcortical dementia tend to have decreased output on verbal fluency tests (divergent thinking), agraphia, and motor-speech disturbances such as slow rate, hypophonia, and articulation and intonation difficulties.

Stage of Dementia

Yet another way of understanding dementia and its accompanying behavioral symptoms is in terms of staging over time. Dementia progresses through three stages: early, middle, and late. Despite some differences in symptomatology among patients with varying dementia etiologies (Snowden, 1999), there are similarities in behavior as the dementing disease progresses over time (Bayles & Kaszniak, 1987; Cohan, 1997; Hart & Semple, 1990). Typically, in the early stages of dementia, patients are forgetful and disoriented for time but generally not for place or person. Both their short- and long-term memory abilities are typically already affected. In terms of language abilities, patients may still appear to be successful communicators, especially during casual conversations; however, they may sometimes digress from the topic and ramble at length during conversation. During these stages, patients with dementia may also display periodic word-finding problems and difficulty interpreting higher-level language forms such as humor or sarcasm.

During the middle stages of dementia, patients become further disoriented and have difficulty with both time and place information. Memory abilities become further impaired and patients can no longer manage personal finances, employment, or medication. Conversational problems are now prominent, with patients having difficulty adhering to conversational rules such as turn-taking, topic maintenance, and topic shifting. Language output becomes vague, empty, perseverative, and often irrelevant. Patients will frequently produce semantic paraphasias and may misuse syntactic forms that affect the meaning of an utterance. Problems with auditory and reading comprehension also become prominent during this stage of dementia.

In the later stages of dementia, the patient becomes disoriented for time, place, and person, and is now dependent for most activities of daily living. Language output may be completely void of meaning, and many patients eventually become mute; language comprehension abilities are similarly devastated (Bayles et al., 2000).

Recent research is exploring the notion that there are subtypes of dementia (e.g., Kertesz, 2005) and continuing the process of differential diagnosis among dementia, aphasia, and other progressive disorders. While these disorders are different, a review of the linguistic and cognitive changes that occur in dementia indicates that there are some similarities between patients with aphasia and those with dementia, particularly patients with anomic aphasia and patients in early stages of dementia (Nicholas et al., 1985). However, several linguistic and cognitive features may help distinguish individuals with aphasia from individuals with dementia. For example, errors in language form (i.e., morphology and syntax) are less common in the language output of patients with dementia, whereas perseveration of ideas is less common in the language output of patients with aphasia (Bayles & Kaszniak, 1987). In terms of cognitive symptoms, Bayles and colleagues (1989) reported that patients with mild and moderate dementia performed significantly more poorly on delayed recall compared with their immediate recall performance; in contrast, no such disparity was seen between the delayed and immediate recall performances of patients with aphasia. Patients with dementia also displayed much greater difficulty on memory tests of delayed spatial and verbal recognition than did patients with aphasia. Three assessment measures designed for patients with dementia are the Arizona Battery for Communication Disorders in Dementia (Bayles & Tomoeda, 1993), the Alzheimer's Quick Test (Wiig et al., 2004), and the Functional Linguistic Communication Inventory (Bayles & Tomoeda, 1994).

Traumatic Brain Injury

Traumatic brain injury (TBI) is the result of an external force applied to the head. Brain-tissue damage in a TBI may be discrete and focal; typically, however, injury is diffuse and includes cortical and subcortical structures in multiple lobes of the brain. Patients who sustain discrete lesions may display language impairments that are similar to those that appear in individuals with aphasia following a stroke. Patients with diffuse damage may display cognitive-communicative deficits, perceptual deficits, and disorders of executive functioning. Traumatic brain injury can range from mild to severe, as determined by neurologic findings (e.g., length of loss of consciousness) and by behavioral deficits in one or more of the following areas: attention, perception and recognition, short- or long-term memory, working memory, problem-solving, conceptual organization, abstract reasoning, self-monitoring, and learning as well as comprehension and production of speech and language (Adamovich, 2005; Brookshire, 2003; Davis, 2000; McCullagh & Feinstein, 2005; Murdoch & Theodoros, 2001; Stierwalt, 2002).

Generally, patients who survive their TBI are less likely to present with frank aphasia; instead, they show cognitive-communicative problems that affect multiple aspects of functioning. However, clinicians should plan assessments that examine behavior resulting from both focal and diffuse brain lesions. Few specific assessment tools exist exclusively for patients with TBI (e.g., the Brief Test of Head Injury (Helm-Estabrooks & Hotz, 1991); the Scales of Cognitive Ability for Traumatic Brain Injury (Adamovich & Henderson, 1992)); however, many tests designed to assess language or cognitive function are well suited for use with individuals who sustain a TBI. Sohlberg & Mateer (2001) identified several tests that may be useful in assessing cognitive-communicative behavior in four performance categories: attention; memory/new learning; executive functions; and behavior, adjustment, and outcome measures. Hartley (1995) identified tests in ten categories: attention; memory; visuospatial perception and construction; motor functioning; intelligence; executive functioning; auditory comprehension; verbal learning; oral expression; and verbal integration and reasoning with language (Hartley, 1995, pp. 82–85). Murray and Clark (2006) listed tests in six categories: (1) attention; (2) neglect; (3) nonverbal memory; (4) verbal memory; (5) verbal and nonverbal memory; and (6) executive function (Murray & Clark, 2006, pp. 194–195). Recent evidence reviews have discussed procedures and tools for standardized and nonstandardized assessment of persons with TBI (Coelho et al., 2005; Turkstra, Coelho, & Ylvisaker, 2005; Turkstra et al., 2005). Practice guidelines for standardized assessment as well as tables listing commonly used tests, including detailed reviews, psychometric properties, and expert opinion, can be found in Turkstra, Coelho and Ylvisaker (2005); Turkstra et al., (2005) and Turkstra et al. (2003).

In contrast to the difficulties with content and form frequently observed in patients with aphasia, individuals with cognitive-communicative impairments as a result of TBI display difficulties in pragmatic aspects of language. Examples of these deficits include difficulty organizing verbal and written output so that it is coherent, cohesive, and concise; problems selecting and maintaining appropriate conversational topics; and the frequent production of irrelevant, tangential, or confabulatory verbal and written output (Coelho, 2002; Coelho et al., 2005; Davis, 2000; Hartley, 1995; McDonald, 2000b; Sohlberg & Mateer, 2001). Other higher-level language difficulties seen in patients with TBI, such as problems attending to, comprehending, and/or retaining complex or abstract information (e.g., commands, stories, or other linguistic material) are usually secondary to cognitive impairments of attention, memory, or executive functions (Whyte et al., 2000; Youse & Coelho, 2005). Although both patients with aphasia and patients with TBI may have word-retrieval problems, there are often some qualitative differences between the types of errors produced by these two patient populations (Boles, 1997; Holland, 1982; Holland et al., 1986). Specifically, in addition to the circumlocutions, semantic paraphasias, and reduced word fluency that are typical of both groups, patients with TBI may make naming errors that are related to their personal situation or to the nature of the stimulus, that are errors of confabulation, or that are a product of visual misperception.

Individuals with cognitive-communicative disorders following TBI vary considerably in behavior, and this must be taken into consideration when planning assessment. Sohlberg and Mateer (2001) suggest that eight variables contribute to variability in behavior: (1) nature of brain injury; (2) patient's preinjury history; (3) current demands on the patient's life; (4) environmental supports; (5) premorbid personality; (6) emotional response to injury; (7) coping skills; and (8) patient and family expectations (Sohlberg & Mateer, 2001, p. 89). Paterson and Scott-Findlay (2002) suggest that interviewing individuals with cognitive-communicative disorders following TBI may be difficult if language and cognitive impairments interfere with effective recall and reflection. Given the complex nature of communicative and cognitive deficits in a person following a TBI, clinicians are challenged to create assessment protocols that will reflect typical and traditional assessment practices as well as the individual variability of patients and their families (Hanks, Ricker, & Millis, 2004; Larkins, Worrall, & Hickson, 2000).

Primary Progressive Aphasia

Primary progressive aphasia (PPA) is a clinical syndrome in which patients suffer progressive language deterioration despite unidentifiable stroke, tumor, infection, or metabolic disease, and by the presence of relative preservation of cognition and independence in activities of daily living, at least in the early years of the disease process (Mesulam et al., 2003; Mesulam & Weintraub, 1992; Weintraub, Rubin, & Mesulam, 1990). In addition, Weintraub and colleagues (1990) suggest that patients should present with at least a 2-year history of isolated and progressive language impairment before being diagnosed with PPA. Currently, there is some debate about whether PPA is a separate clinical entity, or a precursor or variant of more generalized dementias such as Alzheimer's or Pick's disease (Clark et al., 2005; Kertesz et al., 2003; Kertesz et al., 1994; Knibb & Hodges, 2005). Subgroups of PPA have been identified on the basis of clinical features such as phonologic disorders and language deficits (Grossman & Ash, 2004; LeRhun, Richard, &

Pasquier, 2005). Grossman and colleagues (2004) suggested that converging evidence supports distinct subgroups of nonfluent PPA and semantic dementia, but not other subgroups.

Although distinguishing PPA from the language impairments caused by progressive dementing diseases remains controversial, differentiating PPA from traditional aphasia can be made on the bases of etiology (i.e., unknown or diffuse versus focal brain damage) and course of the disorder (i.e., progressive versus relatively static presentation of symptoms). The language symptoms of patients with PPA may be quite variable. Aphasia types such as anomic aphasia, Broca's aphasia, conduction aphasia, pure word deafness, nonfluent aphasia, mixed transcortical aphasia, and global aphasia have been reported in persons with PPA (Duffy & Petersen, 1992; Grossman & Ash, 2004; Rogers & Alarcon, 1998; Westbury & Bub, 1997). Despite this variability, the incidence of nonfluent PPA is reported more frequently in the literature than fluent PPA. For patients with nonfluent PPA, specific language symptoms appear to be similar to those associated with traditional aphasia and most frequently include word- finding deficits (the most common initial symptom as well), a semantic interference effect (Vandenberghe et al., 2005), repetition difficulties, and auditory comprehension problems (Westbury & Bub, 1997). Interestingly, in their review of 112 published cases of PPA, Westbury and Bub noted that both reading and writing modalities tended to remain relatively strong for years after the onset of the disorder. Hillis, Oh, and Ken (2004) and Hillis, Tuffiash, and Caramazza (2002) also reported relatively preserved writing abilities and a double differentiating pattern in naming deterioration in patients with PPA. Patients with nonfluent PPA showed greater deterioration on production of verbs than nouns, while patients with fluent PPA showed greater deterioration on nouns.

Psychiatric Disorders

Several psychiatric disorders can negatively affect an individual's communication abilities (Frank, 1998). Of these, schizophrenia generally receives the most attention in the speech and language pathology literature. Schizophrenia is a relatively common, chronic psychotic disorder that most frequently manifests in late adolescence or early adulthood. However, a form of schizophrenia with onset of symptoms in the second half of life has also been reported (Keefe & Harvey, 1994). This disorder is associated with both positive (i.e., the presence of abnormal behavior) and negative (i.e., the absence of normal behavior) symptoms. Positive symptoms include thought disorder, delusions, and hallucinations; negative symptoms include flat affect, apathy, and social withdrawal. Individuals with schizophrenia also present with a variety of neuropsychological problems including memory and attention deficits, and executive function impairments such as anosognosia (i.e., lack of awareness of deficits), perseveration, and difficulties with planning and problem solving (Elliott et al., 1998).

Communication impairment in individuals with schizophrenia may include word-finding difficulties, language output characterized by reduced content, disturbed affective prosody, perseveration, irrelevance, divergent thinking skills, cohesion, and organizational problems (DiSimoni, Darley, & Aronson, 1977; Goren, Tucker, & Ginsberg, 1996; Murdoch, 2006; Nemoto, Mizuno, & Kashima, 2005). Productive morphosyntactic abilities and basic auditory and reading comprehension abilities are typically spared. Although the communication problems of patients with aphasia are generally sufficiently different from those of patients with schizophrenia, difficulty distinguishing between the two may arise in some cases, such as patients with aphasia who presented with premorbid psychotic disorders.

Goal 2: Identification of Complicating Conditions

Many individuals with aphasia and related neurogenic communication disorders also manifest other physiologic or psychosocial deficits that may contribute to, precipitate, or maintain a language problem, or interfere with treatment planning. The diagnosis of a language and communication disorder must be viewed within the context of these complicating conditions. An efficient method of identifying these conditions is through a comprehensive case history and thorough interview of the patient, his or her caregivers, and other individuals who are important in the patient's life (i.e., co-workers and friends).

Case History and Interviews

To identify the precipitating and maintaining factors that affect language and communication deficits, the clinician should complete a thorough and systematic review of a patient's demographic, medical, and behavioral information including a detailed history in several areas: educational, medical, family, mental health, and occupation, as well as past, present, and future communication environments and goals. This information can be gathered by reviewing the patient's medical chart and by asking the patient, family, and significant others to complete pre-interviews or referral forms. It is preferable, but not always possible, for a clinician to obtain a significant amount of information regarding the patient's history before the initial patient contact. Prior knowledge will enable the clinician to formulate an opinion concerning the possible areas that need greater specificity during testing and plan accordingly.

One method for gathering information prior to the initial assessment session is through the use of a patient-history questionnaire. Most textbooks on diagnosis in speech-language pathology or neurogenic communication disorders contain examples of case-history forms or pre-interview questionnaires (Shipley & McAfee, 2004). Individual work settings often develop a form that reflects the needs of the institution (e.g., acute-care facility or rehabilitation hospital). Using the patient history, clinicians can often save time, provide a systematic method for obtaining additional information, and provide a focus and direction for subsequent interviews. An example of a case history appears in Appendix 4-1.

During subsequent interviews and treatment sessions, specific areas that seem unclear from the case history or initial interview, or that need greater specificity, can be explored. Interviews provide an opportunity to verify and clarify information obtained on the referral forms, and to pursue data that may be pertinent to the nature of the patient's communication problem but that were not included on the form. For example, the clinician may attempt to determine the degree to which the verbal and nonverbal behaviors of individuals in the patient's environment facilitate or impede language recovery. Other areas that may be described are the relationships between and among persons in the environment, the social role change of the client and family subsequent to aphasia, patient and family understanding of and attitudes toward aphasia, needs and expectations concerning treatment and treatment outcome, and the realistic or unrealistic nature of these expectations. Families can quickly experience information overload during interview sessions so it is better to uncover information at a pace to match families' needs rather than to "over-help" by presenting an abundance of information at one time (Avent, 2005).

In addition, information can be gained by interviewing or reviewing the reports of other assessment and/or intervention team members who have evaluated some aspect of the patient's physical, psychological, emotional, social, or occupational functioning. Such a team may be composed of the attending physician and nursing staff, a neurologist, a physiatrist, a geriatrician, an occupational therapist, a physical therapist, a neuropsychologist, a social worker, a therapeutic recreational specialist, a dietitian, a rehabilitation counselor, and family members. It is crucial to have good communication among team members, particularly in those clinical settings in which others such as the neuropsychologist or occupational therapist may share the responsibility of determining the cognitive and linguistic abilities of patients with aphasia.

Complicating Conditions

During testing of the patient with aphasia, the clinician should be alert for signs of dysfunction in areas that do not appear to be generally equivalent in severity with overall language or cognitive performance. This is done to determine whether any complicating conditions may interfere with treatment and recovery. Detailed assessment of these areas should be completed prior to the in-depth evaluation of language abilities, as soon as the clinician becomes aware of their presence. Testing included in this category would be procedures designed to discern auditory and visual sensitivity, auditory and visual agnosia, behaviors frequently associated with right hemisphere functions, motoric impairments, medical conditions, and post-stroke psychobehavioral disorders such as clinical depression.

Auditory and Visual Sensitivity

Assessment of auditory sensitivity should include hearing screening at WHO ICF (ICF, 2001) levels of impairment and activity/participation (Guidelines for audiologic screening, 1997). Screening procedures include a case history regarding hearing difficulties or pain in the ear, visual inspection of the outer ear, otoscopic inspection as appropriate, pure-tone hearing screening, and screening tympanometry. While not all these procedures may be available or appropriate in specific circumstances, at the least the clinician should have access to information concerning a patient's threshold for the awareness of sound (impairment level) and reported difficulties in hearing. If an audiologist is part of the assessment team the data that should minimally be available to the clinician are (a) threshold for awareness of sound, (b) pure tone air and bone thresholds, and (c) speech discrimination scores.

Although aphasia is not a problem of auditory sensitivity, hearing loss can negatively affect a patient's auditory comprehension abilities. The necessity of testing hearing sensitivity is made even more obvious by the fact that many patients with aphasia are older and therefore at high risk for hearing disorders (Gates et al., 1990; Yueh et al., 2003). However, testing the hearing acuity of some patients may be difficult if they are severely language-impaired and therefore unable to understand test instructions or to grasp the nature of the response requirements (Wilson, Fowler, & Shanks, 1981; Kelly, 2006). Accordingly, collaboration between the clinician and the audiologist is necessary to assure a valid assessment of hearing abilities. Additionally, for those patients with aphasia who wear hearing aids or rely upon other assistive listening devices, it is important for the clinician to check whether these devices are in working order (e.g., no buildup of cerumen, functional batteries) prior to the language evaluation.

It is equally important to determine that the patient's visual acuity and visual fields are functionally intact so as not to significantly impede assessment and treatment procedures. Examples of disorders that might impede visual acuity are cataracts and myopia, and an example of a visual-field dysfunction is right homonymous hemianopia. Assuring adequate vision is particularly important for clinicians working with older patients with aphasia since at least one-third of the elderly have some degree of vision loss (Quillen, 1999). When a visual defect is suspected, the patient should be referred to an ophthalmologist for testing. For patients with aphasia who have been identified as having visual acuity problems, clinicians should ensure that any assistive devices (e.g., glasses, contact lenses, magnifying glass) are available and in appropriate condition (e.g., clean, most recent prescription) when completing the language assessment. For patients with aphasia who have identified visual-field cuts, the clinician can arrange visual stimuli in a vertical presentation to avoid eliciting visual-based versus language-based errors.

Auditory and Visual Agnosia

Occasionally, patients with aphasia, particularly those who have suffered bilateral brain damage, may present with auditory or visual agnosia (Bauer & Demery, 2003; Burns, 2004; Cummings & Trimble, 2002; Stringer, 1996). Patients with auditory agnosia have difficulties recognizing auditory stimuli even though they may recognize the same stimuli in other modalities and even though they have adequate hearing sensitivity (Bauer & Demery, 2003; Bauer & Zawacki, 1997). Patients with aphasia may demonstrate one or more of the following types of auditory agnosia (Bauer & Demery, 2003; Burns, 2004; Vignolo, 2005): (a) amusia, or the inability to recognize music rhythms, or forms; (b) auditory sound agnosia, or the inability to recognize nonverbal sounds; and (c) pure word deafness, or the inability to recognize and repeat spoken language with a relatively preserved ability to recognize nonverbal sounds.

Visual agnosia refers to impairment in the recognition of visual stimuli despite adequate visual sensitivity (Farah, 2004). Several types of visual agnosia can occur with aphasia (Burns, 2004; DeRenzi, 1997; Farah, 2004; Stringer, 1996): (a) prosopagnosia, or a difficulty in recognizing familiar faces; (b) autopagnosia, or difficulty in recognizing body parts; or (c) visual object agnosia, or a difficulty in recognizing actual or pictured objects. In diagnosing auditory or visual agnosia, it is important to exclude sensory deficits in the affected modality, comprehension deficits, expressive disturbances, and unfamiliarity with the test stimuli (Stringer, 1996).

Right Hemisphere Function

Patients with aphasia may demonstrate nonverbal impairments that are more frequently associated with right hemisphere brain damage and that may directly or indirectly interfere with the therapeutic process. For example, some patients with aphasia present with an apraxia, such as constructional apraxia or difficulties copying or composing drawings of two- or three-dimensional figures (Georgopoulos, 2004; Rothi & Heilman, 1997). Such patients might construct drawings that are oversimplified and reduced in size but that improve with repetition. Therefore, several aphasia batteries (e.g., WAB, PICA) include subtests that examine for the presence of constructional impairments and other apraxias.

Patients with aphasia may also display inattention or neglect to the right side of space. Although neglect is more frequently associated with right hemisphere brain damage, recent research indicates that it is also quite common following left hemisphere brain damage, with incidence rates of between 15% to 65% (Karnath, Milner, & Vallar, 2002; Pedersen et al., 1997). Therefore, during assessment, clinicians may use published tests such as the Behavioral Inattention Test (Wilson, Cockburn & Halligan, 1987), or may develop cancellation, line bisection, copying, and other pencil-and-paper tasks to identify neglect in their aphasic patients. In addition, since neglect may affect any modality, testing should be in other modalities as well.

Motoric Impairments

It is not uncommon for patients with aphasia to present with a variety of motoric impairments that may directly or indirectly affect their functional communicative abilities. Specifically, motoric deficits may impair the speed and accuracy of a patient's motor speech, gestural, and graphomotor abilities. Three frequently co-occurring motoric impairments are apraxia, dysarthria, and hemiparesis.

Apraxia. Apraxia generally refers to impairment in the capacity to position muscles and to plan and sequence muscle movements for volitional purposes (Darley et al., 1975; Duffy, 2005). This motoric performance problem cannot be attributed to muscular weakness, slowness, or incoordination as these same muscles may be used without difficulty in reflexive or automatic motor acts. Likewise, patients who have difficulties performing skilled and purposeful motor acts because of cognitive or motivational problems would not be considered apraxic. Two common forms of apraxia that may co-occur with aphasia and that may negatively impact a patient's communication abilities are apraxia of speech and limb apraxia.

In patients with apraxia of speech, the apraxia involves the speech musculature, resulting in difficulty with the volitional production of phonemes and phoneme sequences (Ballard, Granier, & Robin, 2000; McNeil, Doyle, & Wambaugh, 2000; Ogar et al., 2005; Ogar et al., 2006; Peach, 2004). Consequently, these patients demonstrate articulatory breakdown in the form of variable and inconsistent articulatory substitutions, distortions, omissions, repetitions, or additions. These patients also present with prosodic alterations including abnormal stress patterns, slow speech rate, and pauses that are inappropriate or of increased duration. Some of the speech symptom variability

in apraxia of speech is related to the context in which the utterance is produced, such as word or utterance length, word frequency, the phonetic complexity of the word or utterance, and the nature of the task being performed (e.g., repetition vs. spontaneous production). Since this disorder is frequently associated with damage to premotor cortex or insular regions of the left hemisphere (Dronkers, 1996; Duffy, 2005; Ogar et al., 2006), it is commonly associated with aphasia.

Considering the potential interference of apraxia of speech and its frequent coexistence with aphasia, many aphasia batteries (e.g., BDAE) include subtests to examine for the presence of apraxia of speech. In addition, clinicians may also choose to further examine the motor speech abilities of their patients with aphasia using standardized tests such as the Apraxia Battery for Adults- 2 (Dabul, 2000) or the Comprehensive Apraxia Test (DiSimoni, 1989), or a procedure such as Tasks for Assessing Motor Speech Planning or Programming Capacity (Duffy, 2005).

Limb Apraxia. Limb apraxia refers to an inability to execute acquired and volitional movements of the fingers, wrist, elbow, or shoulder that is unrelated to motoric, sensory, or cognitive deficits (Heilman, Watson, & Rothi, 2006; Maher & Rothi, 2001; Neiman et al., 2000; Ochipa, Rothi, & Leslie, 2000; Rose & Douglas, 2003). Limb apraxia is another frequent correlate of aphasia but may often remain undiagnosed, particularly in patients with hemiparesis who must attempt to perform skilled movements with their non-dominant arm (i.e., their difficulty is attributed to using their nonpreferred arm versus an apraxic disorder). Generally, patients with limb apraxia have more difficulty performing distal versus proximal movements, and transitive (i.e., involving a tool or instrument) versus intransitive movements. Patients with this disorder may make the following types of errors (Rothi et al., 1988): (a) content errors, in which they perform the wrong movement or action (e.g., when asked to show how they brush their teeth, they show how to comb their hair); and (b) production errors, in which the spatial or temporal organization of the movement or action is incorrect (e.g., pantomiming brushing one's teeth by holding the toothbrush vertically versus horizontally).

The assessment of ideomotor praxis should occur prior to administering any language or cognitive tests (Helm-Estabrooks & Albert, 1991). Failure to do so may result in patients with limb apraxia being mistakenly diagnosed with comprehension or other neuropsychological deficits (e.g., memory, attention) because they have difficulty completing commands that require purposeful movements, and also possibly because of problems providing a reliable pointing or yes/no head movement response. Clinicians may assess the presence or absence of limb apraxia by developing a battery of tasks that represent a range of difficulty and complexity (Belanger, Duffy, & Coelho, 1996; Rothi, Raymer, &

TABLE 4–8

Items of Paired-Word Intelligibility Test Listed by Phonetic Contrast

Category of Feature	Pair 1	Pair 2	Pair 3
Initial voicing	bee-pea	do-two	goo-coo
Final voicing	add-at	buzz-bus	need-neat
Vowel duration	eat-it	gas-guess	pop-pup
Stop vs. fricative	see-tea	sew-toe	do-zoo
Glottal vs. null	high-eye	hit-it	has-as
Fricative vs. affricate	shoe-chew	shop-chop	ship-chip
Stop vs. nasal	dough-no	bee-me	buy-my
Alveolar vs. palatal	see-she	sew-show	sip-ship
Tongue height	eat-at	soup-soap	eat-eight
Tongue advancement	hat-hot	tea-two	day-dough
Stop place	pan-can	dough-go	bow-go
Diphthong	buy-boy	high-how	aisle-oil
r/l	ray-lay	rip-lip	raw-law
w/r	way-ray	row-woe	won-run
Liquid vs. vowel	string-stirring	spring-spurring	bring-burring
Cluster with one intrusive vowel	blow-below	plight-polite	claps-collapse

(From Kent, R. D., Weismer, J. F., Kent, J. C., & Rosenbek, J. (1989). Toward phonetic intelligibility testing in dysarthria. *Journal of Speech and Hearing Disorders, 54* (4), 493.)

Heilman, 1997) or by using one of the commercially available apraxia tests such as the Test of Oral and Limb Apraxia (Helm-Estabrooks, 1991) or the Apraxia Battery for Adults- 2 (Dabul, 2000).

Dysarthria. Dysarthria refers to a group of neurologic motor speech disorders that result from impaired control or changes in the tone (i.e., weakness, slowness, imprecision, and/or incoordination) of the speech musculature (Darley et al., 1975; Duffy, 2005; Freed, 2000). Patients with dysarthria have difficulty with one or more of the basic subsystems of motor speech production, including respiration, phonation, resonance, articulation, and prosody. Motor speech symptoms of individual patients tend to be relatively consistent across speaking contexts. However, motor speech symptoms may vary considerably among patients with this disorder due to different etiologies and different muscular involvement. Persistent dysarthria is most likely to be present in patients with aphasia who have suffered bilateral brain damage, since the speech musculature is innervated bilaterally (Duffy, 2005).

Clinicians may use a variety of published tools to quantify and qualify dysarthric speech disturbances, including the Assessment of Intelligibility of Dysarthric Speech (Yorkston, Beukelman, & Traynor, 1984), the Frenchay Dysarthria Assessment (Enderby, 1983), and the Dysarthria Examination Battery (Drummond, 1993). Another assessment option is the word-intelligibility test developed by Kent et al. (1989).

This test is "designed to examine 19 acoustic-phonetic contrasts that are likely to (a) be sensitive to dysarthric impairment, and (b) contribute significantly to speech intelligibility" (p. 482). Table 4–8 lists items of paired-word intelligibility from Kent et al. (1989). Importantly, Kent and colleagues provide a discussion of the therapeutic implications of their test.

Hemiparesis. Many patients with aphasia may present with hemiparesis or muscular weakness of the right side of their body. If the motoric impairment is so severe that the entire side of the body is paralyzed, the term hemiplegia may be used. Weakness of the right hand or a reliance on their non-dominant, left hand may compromise the speed and precision of many patients' writing, typing, drawing, and/or gesturing.

Medical Conditions

Individuals with aphasia may also have a variety of medical conditions that may interfere with assessment and treatment of aphasia. These conditions are not the etiology of aphasia but may contribute to an individual's ability to respond to assessment activities. Examples of such conditions are a vitamin or mineral deficiency, learning disability, high or low blood pressure leading to additional strokes or to loss of consciousness, high cholesterol level, and diabetes. Information about the presence of these disorders should be discussed as part of the history and interview with the patient and family member. Clinicians should be aware of treatment for these disorders and be mindful of any symptoms that may appear as assessment and treatment sessions continue.

Post-Stroke Psychobehavioral Disorders

Many patients suffer from post-stroke psychobehavioral disorders including depression, anxiety, catastrophic reactions, mania, psychosis, adjustment disorder, and behavioral problems such as aggressiveness and sexual inappropriateness (Bishop & Pet, 1995; Craig & Cummings, 1995; Frank, 1998). These psychobehavioral disorders may be the result of one or more of the following (Gupta, Pansari, & Shetty, 2002; Koenig, 1997; Whyte, 2002): a premorbid mood disorder, medications (e.g., depression is a common side effect of certain antihypertensives), brain damage, or a psychological reaction to the stress associated with acquiring communication, as well as other possible cognitive and physical impairments. Such psychobehavioral disorders are viewed as serious medical problems that can compromise the overall assessment and rehabilitative process, including speech and language evaluation and treatment (Patterson, 2002; Swindell & Hammons, 1991).

Because it is the most commonly observed mood disorder subsequent to brain damage, research has focused primarily on issues relating to depression in aphasia. Post-stroke depression (PSD) is a broadly descriptive term (Spencer, Tompkins, & Schultz, 1997) applied to persons who experience depression following left or right hemisphere stroke. PSD occurring in persons with aphasia following left hemisphere stroke has been described as situational depression (Lyon, 1998), mood disorder (Code, Hemsley, & Herrmann, 1999; Craig & Cummings, 1995), part of the grief response (Tanner, Gerstenberger, & Keller, 1989), and reactive (Goldstein, 1948; Währborg, 1991). Hermann and Wallesch (1993) identified three stages of PSD that occur as the rehabilitation process unfolds: primary depression resulting from structural neural change; secondary depression from neuropsychological sequelae of stroke; and tertiary depression arising from maladaptive coping strategies for long-term social change. The variation in these descriptions alludes to the importance of careful assessment and description of depression in persons with aphasia, and appropriate referral to a mental-health professional.

Client self-report, clinical observation, and report by a caregiver are three methods of noting the presence of depression symptoms in patients with aphasia (Swindell & Hammons, 1991; Währborg, 1991). Self-report using a behavior rating scale or through interview is appropriate for clients with mild aphasia who have language and cognitive abilities sufficient to complete the tasks. As aphasia severity increases self-report becomes unreliable and depression symptoms must be identified through clinical observation or report by a caregiver.

Rating Scales. Rating scales are used to judge a client's mood state. Some scales have a heavy linguistic basis, while others present information in pictorial format to avoid the diagnostic dilemma created by using a linguistically based diagnostic task with a person who has moderate to severe aphasia.

Two scales with a linguistic basis are the Stroke Aphasia Depression Questionnaire (Sutcliffe & Lincoln, 1998) and the Geriatric Depression Scale (Yesavage & Brink, 2006; Yesavage et al., 1983). The Stroke Aphasia Depression Questionnaire (SADQ) uses predominantly caregiver-report and, if needed, client report, and was validated with persons with mild and severe aphasia. An advantage of the SADQ is that it was designed for use with persons with aphasia and can be completed by a caregiver; however, it has a heavy linguistic bias. The Geriatric Depression Scale (GDS) uses client self-report. Both the long and short forms of the GDS are internally consistent, sensitive, and predictive instruments, and are used to detect depression (Agrell & Dehlin, 1989). The major disadvantage to the GDS is also its heavy reliance on the linguistic abilities of the client.

Visual-analogue mood scales were created to circumvent linguistic requirements in detecting depression symptoms. These scales are 100-mm lines anchored by faces representing mood states, and clients mark on the lines to indicate their current mood states. Two scales used with persons with aphasia are the Visual Analogue Dysphoric Scale (Stern & Bachman, 1991) and the Visual Analogue Mood Scale (Stern et al., 1997). The Visual Analogue Dysphoric Scale (VADS) is anchored by two poles, happy and sad, and is a valid indicator of mood state in clients with aphasia, even those with severe auditory comprehension deficits (Stern & Bachman, 1991). The Visual Analogue Mood Scale (VAMS) has eight scales, each anchored with a neutral face and a mood face (sad, happy, tense, afraid, confused, tired, energetic, and angry). The VAMS has normative data and cutoff scores to indicate pathologic mood state, and studies have validated the VAMS for use with many types of clients, including persons with aphasia. The Aphasic Depression Rating Scale (Benaim et al., 2004) was created in part from items on the Visual Analogue Mood Scale to examine depression in persons with severe aphasia or those in a hospital setting.

In contrast, the Visual Analogue Self-Esteem Scale (Brumfitt & Sheeran, 1999) assesses mood state from the perspective of self-esteem. Self-esteem is a global characteristic rather than a specific attribute (e.g., sadness) that is related to but not synonymous with depression, and is thought to be consistent over time in contrast to specific attributes that may easily change. The Visual Analogue Self-Esteem Scale has 10 items, each of which contains two pictures and a corresponding descriptor (e.g., pessimistic and optimistic). Clients use a five-point scale to represent their views of themselves.

The Challenge of Identifying Depression Symptoms. Several challenges present themselves when describing depression symptoms in persons with aphasia. The most notable, described by Starkstein and Robinson (1988, p.1) is the "... fundamental paradox of studying a problem (i.e. emotional disorder) when the basic method for assessing the problem (i.e. language) is disturbed." Depression in persons with aphasia may be underestimated in the literature on post-stroke depression because most studies exclude participants with severely impaired linguistic skills.

Client-related factors also pose challenges to identifying depression symptoms. Clients who have compromised cognitive abilities may be unable to reflect on their current mood states, or judge their levels of functioning or outlooks on life, as required by some assessment methods. The presence of neurobehavioral sequelae of stroke such as anosognosia, dysprosodia, apathy, or amnesia can confound, mask, or lead to misdiagnosis of depression (Stern, 1999). Age-related factors, such as sensory changes that may limit the ability to read or hear questions, dementia, memory loss, pseudodementia, and increased use of medication may alter responsivity. Changes in body image or presence of physical disability may also confound the diagnosis of depression after stroke (Dunkle, 1984). Changes in the family or environmental support structure may induce social isolation, functional dependence, or fatigue, further complicating the identification of depression symptoms, particularly in elderly clients with aphasia (King, 1996).

The presence and course of depression symptoms is difficult to predict. No consistent relationship has been observed between PSD and lesion site or size, or type of aphasia. PSD is likely to be both a psychological reaction to life-changing events and a neurochemical result of cortical or subcortical lesion.

Goal 3. Analysis of Cognitive Ability

Cognition is a generic term for any process whereby an organism becomes aware of or obtains knowledge of an object (English & English, 1958). It "refers to all the processes by which sensory input is transformed, reduced, elaborated, stored, recovered, and used" (Neisser, 1967, p. 4). It is a group of processes that we use in a coordinated and integrated manner in order to achieve knowledge and command of our world. That is, cognition is our means of processing and handling information.

Mental Operations

A multitude of specific processes contribute to our overall cognitive proficiency. According to Chapey (1994) these processes of cognition can be operationally defined as the five mental operations of the Guilford Structure of Intellect model (Guilford, 1967, 1988) — namely, recognition/understanding/comprehension (including perception and attention), memory, and thinking (convergent, divergent, and evaluative).

Recognition/Understanding

Recognition/understanding/comprehension involves knowing, awareness, immediate discovery or rediscovery, recognition of information in various forms, perception, attention, and comprehension or understanding. Recognition involves acknowledgment that something has been seen or perceived previously (Guilford, 1967). Several attentional behaviors have been identified and can be assessed, including (a) sustained attention, or the ability to maintain attention and therefore produce consistent performance over a long period; (b) focused or selective attention, or the ability to focus on and prioritize part of our external or internal environment in the presence of competing stimuli; and (c) divided attention, or the ability to attend to and complete more than one task, or to attend and process multiple stimuli simultaneously (Lezak et al., 2004; Murray, 2002; Spreen & Strauss, 1998). Several neuropsychological tests serve to assess perception (Lezak et al., 2004). The area of comprehension has been well researched in terms of assessment procedures and tools (see Goals 4 and 5).

Memory

Memory is the power, act, or process of fixing newly gained information in storage as well as retaining and retrieving this new information at a later time (Guilford, 1967; Klatzky, 1980; Squire, 1987). Memory is both short-term or working memory and long-term. Short-term memory is a capacity-limited arena, and is usually thought to hold seven items plus or minus two (Clark et al., 2005; Miller, 1956). Information is processed in short-term memory and temporarily stored (Baddeley, 1986). This memory structure is hypothesized to contain buffers (e.g., phonologic loop, visuospatial sketchpad) that briefly hold incoming information, as well as an executive component that controls what information is processed and stored. Memory is also long-term, and the repository of factual and relational information stored over one's lifetime.

Impairments of both working memory and long-term memory have been observed in patients with aphasia (Murray, Ramage, & Hopper, 2001). In fact, Allport (1986) proposed that "the dysphasias...are a class of memory disorder" (p. 32). Patients with aphasia demonstrate working memory deficits when completing verbal as well as visuospatial and other nonverbal memory tasks (Tompkins et al., 1994). Additionally, some evidence suggests that there is a relation between patients' working memory and language abilities (Caspar et al., 1998; Tompkins et al., 1994). Wright and Shisler (2005) reviewed several theories of working memory and described how elements of those theories may pertain to aphasia. They concluded that assessing and treating working memory in persons with aphasia is an important area of future research, as current results relating aphasia and working memory, while promising, are inconclusive.

Long-term memory contains Guilford's entire Structure of Intellect (SOI) cube: operations, contents, and products (Chapey, 2001). Information is hypothesized to be stored in different sites or in a different manner depending on the type of memory, rather than in a unitary storage system. Research has identified long-term memory deficits among patients with both verbal and nonverbal information (Beeson et al., 1993; Burgio & Basso, 1997; Ween, Verfaellie, & Alexander, 1996). Although minimal research has been completed to examine the relation between long-term memory deficits and language abilities in aphasia, there is some evidence from other patient populations (e.g., patients having undergone temporal lobectomy) that impairments to certain long-term memory stores may negatively affect vocabulary acquisition skills as well as pragmatic language abilities (Gabrieli, Cohen, & Corkin, 1988; Wilson & Wearing, 1995).

Thinking

There are three types of thinking: convergent thinking, divergent thinking, and evaluative thinking. **Convergent thinking** is the generation of logical conclusions from given information, in which emphasis is on achieving the conventionally best outcomes. Usually, the information given fully determines the outcome (Guilford & Hoepfner, 1971). Convergent production leads to logical deductions or compelling inferences and requires the generation of logical necessities.

Divergent thinking involves the generation of logical alternatives from a set of given information, in which emphasis is on variety, quantity, and relevance of output from one source. Divergent thinking fosters generation of logical possibilities, with the ready flow of ideas, the flexibility to change the direction of one's responses (Guilford, 1967), and suggestion of ideas in situations where a proliferation of ideas on a specific topic is required. Such behavior necessitates the use of a broad search of memory storage, and the production of multiple possible solutions to a problem. It is the ability to extend previous experience and knowledge or to widen existing concepts (Cropley, 1967). Divergent behavior is directed toward new responses — new in the sense that the thinker was not aware of the response before beginning the particular line of thought (Gowan, Demos, & Torrence, 1967). Divergent questions are open-ended and do not have a single correct answer. Responses are scored according to the number of ideas produced (flu-ency), and the variety of ideas suggested (flexibility). They can also be scored according to the originality, frequency, or unusualness of the response, and/or the elaboration or the ability to specify numerous details in planning an event or making a decision (Guilford, 1967). Purdy (2006) examined cognitive flexibility in persons with aphasia and showed that individuals with greater cognitive flexibility are more likely to be successful using compensatory strategies during functional communication tasks than individuals with less flexibility.

According to Guilford (1967), **evaluative thinking** or judgment involves the ability of the individual to use knowledge to make appraisals or comparisons or to formulate evaluations in terms of known specifications or criteria, such as correctness, completeness, identity, relevance, adequacy, utility, safety, consistency, logical feasibility, practical feasibility, or social custom.

Executive-Function Abilities

Various researchers use the term "executive functions" to refer to a collection of cognitive abilities (or composite abilities) that enable us to successfully complete independent, deliberate, and novel behaviors (Dugbartey et al., 1999; Murray, 2002; Purdy, 2002; Ylvisaker & Feeney, 1998). These behaviors allow us to generate, choose, plan, and monitor responses that are goal-directed and adaptive (Borkowski & Burke, 1996; Denckla, 1996; Ylvisaker & Feeney, 1998). Such functions include (a) self-awareness of one's strengths and weaknesses and level of task difficulty (which involves recognition/understanding); (b) inhibition of incompatible responses; and (c) reasoning, problem-solving, strategic thinking, and decision-making. Within the Guilford model, problem-solving, decision-making, and learning are composite abilities that involve many or all of these executive functions. The specific aspects of functioning that are used depend on the problem presented, the decision to be made, the reasoning required, and/or the information to be learned.

Individuals with aphasia may have executive-function difficulties such as problem-solving and decision-making deficits (Chapey, 2001; Purdy, 2002; Ramsberger, 2005; Tatemichi et al., 1994) and preservation or failure to inhibit or shift a response (Albert & Sandson, 1986; Glosser & Goodglass, 1990; Purdy, 2006). Some individuals with aphasia also present with executive-function difficulties thought to be characteristic of sequelae of right hemisphere brain damage, such as lack of awareness or anosognosia (Marshall et al., 1998; Paquier, 2005; Stone, Halligan, & Greenwood, 1993).

Contents of the Guilford SOI Model

According to Guilford (1967, 1988), in the Structure of Intellect model there are five broad, substantive, basic types of information or content that the organism discriminates: visual, auditory, symbolic, semantic, and behavioral (in the original model visual and auditory contents were subsumed under the term "figural"). The two that are most relevant to language are semantic content and behavioral content. Semantic content pertains to "information in the form of conceptions or mental constructs to which words are often applied." Therefore, it involves thinking and verbal communication; however, it need not necessarily be dependent on words (Guilford & Hoepfner, 1971). Behavioral content pertains to the psychological aspects of human interactions or to information that is essentially nonfigural and nonverbal: the attitudes, needs, desires, moods, intentions, perceptions, and thoughts of others and of ourselves. This content pertains to the cues that the human organism obtains about the attention, perception, thinking, feeling, emotions, and intentions of others that come indirectly through nonverbal means.

Products of the Guilford SOI Model

There are six products in the Guilford model. According to Guilford and Hoepfner (1971), products are the manner in which things are associated in the mind and the depth to which they are related. Products are considered on a continuum from simple to complex, or concrete to abstract (Chapey, 2001). The continuum of products begins with units, which combine to enter into *classes*. *Classes* then enter into *relations*, which enter into *systems*, which enter into *transformations*, which ultimately enter into *implications*, the most complex product in the model.

Guilford and Hoepfner (1971) describe the products in the following manner. *Units* are relatively "segregated or circumscribed items" or "chunks" of information having "thing" character. They are items to which nouns are often applied. *Classes* are "conceptions underlying sets of items of information grouped by virtue of their common properties" and involve common properties within sets. *Relations* are meaningful connections "between items of information based upon variables or points of contact that apply to them." *Systems* are organized patterns of information or "complexes of interrelated or interacting parts." *Transformations* are changes of various kinds (such as redefinitions, shifts, transitions, or modifications) in existing information. *Implications* are "circumstantial connections between items of information, as by virtue of contiguity, or any condition that promotes "belongingness." Implications involve information expected, anticipated, suggested, or predicted by other information.

Assessment of Cognition

Since cognition is the process by which language is learned and used, each of the cognitive processes identified in the SOI model should assessed (Wade, 2005). Specifically, the ability to produce semantic and behavioral units, classes (concepts), systems, relations, transformations, and implications under all mental operations (recognition/understanding, memory, thinking, and executive functions) are explored. Tests developed by Guilford and colleagues can be used for this purpose (Chapey, 2001). Many other published tests also tap these abilities (Lezak et al., 2004; Spreen & Strauss, 1998). In addition, recognition/understanding and convergent thinking are assessed on many standard tests of aphasia.

Assessing Attention

The status of the attention abilities in a person with aphasia is evaluated in both unstructured and structured contexts in an attempt to provide information about if and how such problems interfere with activities of daily living (Coslett, 2000). In unstructured observations, the clinician can determine whether the individual appears alert and able to maintain attention over a specific length of time. Patient ability to resist distraction by either external or internal stimuli is also noted. These and other aspects of attention may also be assessed using published tests such as those listed in Table 4–9 and in Lezak et al. (2004), Murray and Clark (2006), and van Zomeren and Spikman (2005). For example, the Test of Everyday Attention (Robertson et al., 1994) contains real-life materials and tasks that target a variety of attentional processes: sustained attention, focused attention, divided attention, and attentional switching skills. The Wisconsin Card Sorting Test (Grant & Berg, 1993) tests abstract behavior and the ability to "shift set." Clinicians may also use rating scales such as the one developed by Ponsford and Kinsella (1991), which are completed by both the clinician and the patient (Fig. 4–6).

Assessing Memory

Unstructured observations may provide some information about patient memory abilities such as whether or not the individual is oriented to place, time, and person. For structured assessment, many commercially available tests of memory are accessible. However, relatively few tests are appropriate for persons with aphasia, since most of the tests rely heavily upon processing of linguistic stimuli, verbal responses, or both (Table 4–9). The Rivermead Behavioral Memory Test (RBMT; Wilson, Cockburn, & Baddeley, 2003) represents an exception and includes subtests such as remembering an appointment or a short route. Cockburn and colleagues (1990) demonstrated that most RBMT subtests can be validly administered to patients with aphasia, since performance of only a few subtests are significantly affected by language impairment. Other appropriate structured evaluations include the Visual Memory Span subtest of the Wechsler Memory Scale-3 (Wechsler, 1997b) to assess working memory abilities (particularly the Backward

TABLE 4–9

Tests to Assess Cognitive Processes and Mental Operations in Persons with Aphasia

Cognitive Function	Instrument	Source
Comprehensive	Burns Brief Inventory of Communication and Cognition	Burns (1997)
	Cognitive Linguistic Quick Test	Helm-Estabrooks (2003)
	Cognistat	Kiernan et al. (1995)
	Mini-Mental Status Examination	Folstein et al. (1975)
	Ross Information Processing Assessment-2	Ross-Swain (1996)
Attention	Behavioral Inattention Test	Wilson et al. (1987)
	Color Trails Test	D'Elia et al. (1996)
	Connors Continuous Performance Test	Connors (2000)
	Criterion-Oriented Test of Attention	Williams (1994)
	d2 Test of Attention	Brickencamp & Zillmer (1998)
	Paced Auditory Serial Addition Test	Gronwall & Sampson (1974)
	SCAN-A: A Test for Auditory Processing Disorders in Adolescents and Adults	Keith (1993)
	Symbol Search subtest of the WAIS-3	Wechsler (1997a)
	Test of Everyday Attention	Robertson et al. (1994)
Memory	Benton Visual Retention Test	Sivan (1992)
	Continuous Visual Memory Test	Trahan & Larrabee (1988)
	Figural Memory subtest of the WMS-3	Wechsler (1997b)
	Rey Complex Figure Test and Recognition Trial	Meyers & Meyers (1995)
	Rivermead Behavioral Memory Test (RBMT-II)	Wilson et al. (2003)
	Spatial Span subtest of the WMS-3	Wechsler (1997b)
	Visual Memory Span subtest of the WMS-3	Wechsler (1997b)
	Visual Reproduction subtests of the WMS-3	Wechsler (1997b)
Executive functions	Behavioral Assessment of the Dysexecutive Syndrome	Wilson et al. (1996)
	Behavior Rating Inventory of Executive Function	Gioia et al. (2000)
	BNVR: The Butt Non-Verbal Reasoning Test	Butt & Bucks (2004)
	Comprehensive Test of Nonverbal Intelligence	Hammill et al. (1996)
	Delis-Kaplan Executive Function System	Delis et al. (2001)
	Executive Control Battery	Goldberg et al. (2002)
	Functional Assessment of Verbal Reasoning and Executive Strategies	MacDonald (1998)
	Matrix Reasoning subtest of the WAIS-3	Wechsler (1997a)
	Picture Arrangement subtest of the WAIS-3	Wechsler (1997a)
	Porteus Maze Test	Porteus (1959)
	Rapid Assessment of Problem Solving (RAPS)	Marshall et al. (2003)
	Raven's Coloured Progressive Matrices	Raven et al. (1995)
	Test of Nonverbal Intelligence-3	Brown et al. (1997)
	Williams Inhibition Test	Williams (2006)
	Wisconsin Card Sorting Test	Grant & Berg (1993)

Tapping portion), and the Rey Complex Figure Test (Meyers & Meyers, 1995) to examine long-term visuospatial recall. Although performance is usually quantified in terms of the number and length of items remembered or the length of time items can be retained, responses may also be analyzed to identify patterns of impairment (such as remembering only the beginning or end of the material or the production of random errors).

Assessing Thinking

Common methods of assessing convergent thinking skills are confrontation naming tasks, matching tasks, sentence-completion tasks, and question-and-answer tasks that obligate a specific response. These tasks appear in comprehensive aphasia test batteries (e.g., WAB), tests of specific function (e.g., TAWF), and in tasks created by clinicians. Several measures also exist to assess divergent thinking skills. These

Questionnaire

Therapist: _____

Discipline: _____   Date: _____

Could you please answer the following questions about _____ by checking the box which most nearly applies to their behavior now:

Has he/she recently?	Not at all (0)	Occasionally (1)	Sometimes (2)	Almost always (3)	Always (4)
1- Seemed lethargic (i.e., lacking energy)	☐	☐	☐	☐	☐
2- Tired easily	☐	☐	☐	☐	☐
3- Been slow in movement	☐	☐	☐	☐	☐
4- Been slow to respond verbally	☐	☐	☐	☐	☐
5- Performed slowly on mental tasks	☐	☐	☐	☐	☐
6- Needed prompting to get on with things	☐	☐	☐	☐	☐
7- Stared into space for long periods	☐	☐	☐	☐	☐
8- Had difficulty concentrating	☐	☐	☐	☐	☐
9- Been easily distracted	☐	☐	☐	☐	☐
10- Been unable to pay attention to more than one thing at a time	☐	☐	☐	☐	☐
11- Made mistakes because he/she wasn't paying attention properly	☐	☐	☐	☐	☐
12- Missed important details in what he/she is doing	☐	☐	☐	☐	☐
13- Been restless	☐	☐	☐	☐	☐
14- Been unable to stick at an activity for very long	☐	☐	☐	☐	☐

Total: _____

Score: _____

Figure 4–6. Rating Scale of Attentional Behaviour[a]

[a]Ponsford, J., & Kinsella, G. (1991). The use of a rating scale of attentional behaviour. *Neuropsychological Rehabilitation, 1(4), 241–257. Reprinted with Permission.*

measures have in common the lack of a predetermined response. Examples of tests that assess divergent thinking skills are word-fluency tasks (e.g., FAS test), creativity tests (Torrance, 1966), tasks requiring a patient to suggest creative uses for common objects (e.g., how many uses can be created for a hammer), or narrative storytelling tasks (e.g., spontaneous speech elicited from the "Cookie Theft" picture in the BDAE). Evaluative thinking can be assessed by asking a patient to predict the outcome of an event (e.g., a television situation comedy or a story), judge the appropriateness of a correct and an incorrect response to a situation (e.g., what to do if one finds a wallet), or self-reflect on previous behavior.

Assessing Executive Functions

The assessment of executive functions also includes observations as well as the administration of psychometrically rigorous tests (see Table 4–9). For example, the Test of Problem Solving (TOPS; Bowers et al., 1991) may be used to explore processes such as explaining inferences, determining causes, answering negative questions, determining solutions, and avoiding problems (note that norms for TOPS are only provided for children). Sohlberg and colleagues' (Braswell et al., 1993) Profile of Executive Control System involves both observation of the individual performing daily tasks as well as a patient interview. Other examples are the Test of Nonverbal Intelligence-3 (Brown, Sherbenou, & Johnson, 1997) and the Williams Inhibition Test (Williams, 2006).

Goal 4: Analysis of Ability to Comprehend Language Content

Language content is the meaning, topic, or subject matter of individual words, individual utterances, and/or conversation (Lahey, 1988; McCauley, 2001). Content also refers to the characterization or conceptualization of topics according to how they relate or are similar to one another in different messages. A topic is the particular idea expressed in a message, such as comments about a specific object (e.g., a pipe); a particular action (e.g., eating lunch); or a specific relation (e.g., the relation between Harry and his wand, or a patient and his shoes) (Lahey, 1988). It is important to note that the meaning of words and concepts may change over time and across cultures, and may depend on the social and experiential context in which they are used.

The ability to comprehend the content of language is always impaired in aphasia (e.g., Webb & Love, 1983) but may not always be evident in connected-speech tasks because of the influence of context (Whitworth et al., 2005). Patients with mild aphasia may successfully use contextual cues and predictable communicative sequences (e.g., greeting) and produce responses that appear to demonstrate comprehension, yet are not derived from full comprehension of

language content. A deficit in content comprehension involves assigning meaning to incoming auditory or written messages and/or to understanding words as they relate to objects, persons, actions, ideas, and experiences. For many patients with aphasia, this impairment is confounded by deficiencies in cognitive abilities such as perception (e.g., visual or auditory discrimination), memory, and thinking. Assessment, therefore, centers on analyzing not only the patient's comprehension of language content but also on perceptual and cognitive abilities that may interfere with comprehension. Comprehension of content should be assessed in both the auditory and reading modalities, and at multiple levels of performance: single words, connected speech (short and long utterances), and gestural communication. These assessments are necessary since in many patients auditory comprehension is better than reading comprehension, some patients display better reading skills than auditory comprehension skills, and for others comprehension at one performance level is better than at other levels (see Appendix 4-2).

Comprehension of Content in Isolated Words

Receptive vocabulary is assessed by asking patients with aphasia to point to real or pictured objects, actions, attributes, and relationships, and categories of objects, actions, numbers, and letters (e.g., "Point to car," "Point to drinking," "Show me yellow"). Knowledge of language categories is assessed by requiring the patient to point to objects, pictures, or words that belong to a specific class or group of words (e.g., "Show me the words that are the names of fruit"), and to identify rhyme words, synonyms, and antonyms. Most aphasia batteries include subtests to examine word-level comprehension of objects, actions, and so forth. However, few of them include subtests to examine understanding of word relationships and categories. Therefore, clinicians must rely upon probe tasks to assess this aspect of word comprehension (see Appendix 4-2). Another option is to use tests such as the Pyramids and Palm Trees test (Howard & Patterson, 1992). During administration of this instrument, patients are asked to match pictures on the basis of a semantic association (e.g., for the target "pyramid," the response choices are "palm tree" and "pine tree"). The six versions of this test allow the clinician to determine whether the patient has a general semantic deficit or a modality-specific problem.

Assessment of content may be difficult to ascertain as the patient may rely on strategies other than meaning comprehension to respond (Raymer & Rothi, 2000). For example, a patient may attend to a superficial feature and use a sophisticated guessing strategy to produce the correct response. Generally, pointing tasks to assess comprehension can be made more difficult by increasing the number of items or words from which the patient must select the target (e.g., increase from two to six distractor items), by increasing the similarity of the target and distractor items (e.g., for the target word "car," printed distractors could be changed from "lemon," "glass," and "toe," to "cab," "bus," and "bar"), or both. The influence of other variables such as word frequency or familiarity, length, and imageability on a patient's understanding can also be examined.

Comprehension of Content in Connected Language

Comprehension of labels for objects, actions, attributes, and relationships and categories of objects, actions, and relationships should be assessed in connected language at both the sentence and discourse levels. At the sentence level, the clinician evaluates the patient's ability to point to common objects by description (e.g., "Read this sentence and point to the object that it describes") or by function (e.g., "Point to something that cuts"), and/or the patient's ability to follow directions or commands (e.g., "Write your address and then underline the name of your street"). Testing also includes assessment of the patient's ability to understand concrete and abstract sentences. For example, in evaluating concrete sentences, the clinician might ask, "Is this a cup?" Items that evaluate more abstract comprehension abilities typically assess the patient's understanding of complex relationships, such as comparative (e.g., "Are grapefruits larger than lemons?"), spatial (e.g., "Is California west of Arizona?"), temporal (e.g., "Does November come before October?"), inferential (e.g., "The man cut the steak. Did the man use a knife?"), cause-and-effect ("Can smoke cause a fire?"), or synonymy (e.g., "Does sob mean the same as cry?") (Wiig & Semel, 1984). Additional examples appear in Appendix 4-2. In addition to manipulating vocabulary characteristics (e.g., word frequency or imageability), clinicians alter variables such as sentence length and/or relational complexity to increase or decrease the difficulty of sentence-level comprehension tasks.

During highly structured assessment of both language content and form, response requirements are carefully controlled to be sure that success or failure is dependent on the stimulus characteristics and not on an inability to respond. For example, requiring a patient to gesture a response (e.g., "Pretend to use a hammer") may be complicated by a co-existing limb apraxia. Therefore, this patient may be required to respond by pointing to a word or picture, or by saying or pointing to a one-word answer such as yes/no, true/false, or right/wrong. Abilities and impairments can then be confidently ascribed to the specific input parameter that is being systematically controlled.

Comprehension of discourse-length spoken or written material is also to be assessed since there may be a difference between sentence-level and discourse-level comprehension abilities (Armstrong, 2000; Brownell & Friedman, 2000; Larfeuil & LeDorze, 1997; Nicholas, MacLennan, &

Brookshire, 1986). Most aphasia batteries include subtests designed to assess auditory and reading comprehension abilities at the discourse level. However, research has revealed that patients with aphasia were able to answer more than half of the reading items from several popular aphasia batteries correctly (e.g., BDAE, WAB) at a significantly greater rate than by chance. This suggests that their responses show relatively low passage dependency and instead are based on some other comprehension strategy. Consequently, when clinicians use these materials they may be assessing reading comprehension levels of information other than those which were planned. In comparison to the reading subtests of aphasia batteries, the Nelson Reading Skills Test (Hanna, Schell, & Schreiner, 1977) was found to have more acceptable passage dependency. That is, patients with aphasia and adults with no brain damage had to read the paragraphs to answer the test questions correctly (Nicholas & Brookshire, 1987) rather than rely on other, unknown strategies to respond. Another assessment option, the Discourse Comprehension Test (Brookshire & Nicholas, 1997), is designed to examine understanding of information that varies in terms of salience (main ideas vs. detailed information), as well as directness (explicitly stated information vs. implied information). Therefore, it can be administered as either a test of listening or reading comprehension.

Lastly, the aphasic patient's ability to understand meaning in unstructured, spontaneous language is determined. This is done by noting the type and amount of content that appears to be understood, as demonstrated by appropriate responses to conversation. For example, if a patient hears the statements "No, this belongs to the nurse. Is this hers?" and "This is mine. Please give it to me" and responds appropriately, the clinician may begin to hypothesize that the patient comprehends the relationship of possession. However, it is important to be cautious when basing judgments about discourse-level abilities on the basis of general conversational speech since patients with aphasia frequently nod or gesture appropriately as a response to social or prosodic cues and may not be comprehending the language content.

Gesture

Clinicians also assess the ability to comprehend gestures or pantomime since, for some patients with severe aphasia, gestures may represent a patent modality for comprehension (Daniloff et al., 1986; Daniloff et al., 1982; Marshall, 2006; Power & Code, 2006; Rose, 2006; Varney, 1982). In particular, patients with severe auditory comprehension impairments but relatively minimal or mild reading impairments have been found to display better gestural recognition abilities than those patients with severe auditory and reading comprehension impairments (Goodwin, 2002). This finding has led some researchers to suggest that reading-comprehension abilities may be a better indicator of the ability to communicate effectively via gestures than of overall aphasia severity (Daniloff et al., 1982; Rose & Douglas, 2003). In contrast, other studies have found a relationship between praxis and pantomime-recognition impairments (Bell, 1994; Wang & Goodglass, 1992). With respect to gestural codes, iconic gestures (e.g., pantomiming the function of objects), and AmerInd signs (i.e., a modification of American Indian hand talk) are easier for naive viewers to discern than American Sign Language (ASL) and consequently may be more suitable for use in assessing and treating aphasia (Campbell & Jackson, 1995; Daniloff et al., 1986; Power & Code, 2006).

Gestural recognition abilities are not typically tested as part of most aphasia batteries. Therefore, clinicians may use a subtest of an aphasia battery, one of the nonstandardized tasks described in the literature (Bell, 1994; Daniloff et al., 1982; Rothi et al., 1997), or a probe task developed by themselves. Generally, gestural comprehension is assessed with videotaped or live presentation of gestures, and the patient points to the correct picture in a multiple-choice format. In addition to assessing gesture comprehension abilities in isolation, clinicians may also examine the effect of providing gestural information in concert with auditory information (Marshall, 2005; Records, 1994; Rose, 2006). That is, clinicians can determine whether gestural information aids auditory comprehension.

Influential Variables

A variety of variables may positively or negatively influence aphasic patients' abilities to comprehend language content as well as language form (see Goal 5 for further information about assessing comprehension of language form). Research indicates that comprehension of both content and form are inversely proportional to the level of intellectual complexity (Shewan & Canter, 1971; Siegel, 1959), length (Shewan & Canter, 1971; Weidner & Lasky, 1976), and degree of semantic similarity among response choices (Baker, Blumstein, & Goodglass, 1981; Duffy & Watkins, 1984; Howland & Pierce, 2004). In contrast, there is believed to be a positive relationship between comprehension abilities and other stimulus variables, such as:

- word frequency (Gerratt & Jones, 1987; Marshall et al., 2001; Nickels & Howard, 1995; Pashek & Tompkins, 2002; Schuell, Jenkins, & Landis, 1961),
- age of acquisition (Hirsch & Ellis, 1994),
- imageability (Cole-Virtue & Nickels, 2004; Kay et al., 1990; Luzzatti et al., 2001),
- emotional content (Boller et al., 1979),
- salience (i.e., main ideas vs. details),
- directness (i.e., stated vs. implied) (Cole-Virtue & Nickels, 2004; Ernest-Baron, Brookshire, & Nicholas,

1987; Laiacona et al., 2000; Nicholas & Brookshire, 1986, 1995a; Nickels & Howard, 1995),
- sentence constraint (Faust & Kravetz, 1998; Puskaric & Pierce, 1997),
- redundancy (Gardner, Albert, & Weintraub, 1975; Huntley, Pindzola, & Weidner, 1986; Stachowiak et al., 1977),
- context (Cannito, Vogel, & Pierce, 1989; Hough et al., 1997; Howland & Pierce, 2004; Nickels & Howard, 1995), and
- personal significance of the material.

Additionally, for some patients with aphasia, the grammatical class or part of speech (e.g., verbs vs. nouns) can influence their comprehension abilities (Berndt, Handiges et al., 2002; Carramazza & Hillis, 1991; Daniloff et al., 1982). However, the effect of these variables is neither consistent nor predictable. Recent research is attempting to tease apart the individual effects of variables (e.g., Berndt, Haendiges et al., 2002), and beginning to suggest that other factors (e.g., age of acquisition) are of greater importance (Hirsch & Ellis, 1994).

Several factors (listed below) related to the presentation of the verbal stimuli also contribute to a patient's success or failure in comprehension (Blumstein et al., 1985; Gardner et al., 1975; Hough et al., 1997; Kimelman & McNeil, 1989; Lasky, Weidner, & Johnson, 1976; Murray, Holland, & Beeson, 1997; Records, 1994; Toppin & Brookshire, 1978). Consequently, the degree to which a patient's comprehension is facilitated or impeded by tone of voice, intensity, stress, attentional demands (e.g., focused vs. divided attention tasks), concomitant gestures or pictorial cues, presentation rate, pauses at intervals, prolongation of words, and imposed response delays can be determined.

Goal 5: Analysis of the Ability to Comprehend Language Form

Language form includes syntax, a system of rules used to order words and relate them to one another in order to express ideas, and morphology, a system of rules used to construct words (Nelson, 1998). In aphasia, impairments in the ability to understand syntax or grammatical morphology are common. Consequently, assessment involves an analysis of the patient's ability to understand language form at both the word and sentence levels (see Appendix 4-3).

Comprehension of Form Words and Morphology

Form words can be of two types: substantive or open-class words (e.g., verbs, nouns, adjectives, adverbs) and relational or closed-class words (e.g., prepositions, conjunctions, and articles) (Allen & Badecker, 2001; Saffran, Berndt, & Schwartz, 1989). Because most aphasia batteries focus primarily on examining comprehension of nouns, clinicians may devise tests of their own or borrow from nonstandardized measures to conduct a broad-based assessment of comprehension of form words. The ability to comprehend the meaning of both substantive and relational words can be assessed through the use of picture-verification tasks in which the patient with aphasia sees a picture, hears or reads a word or phrase, and points to the best picture for that word or phrase. For example, a picture-verification task to evaluate comprehension of prepositions might include stimuli such as "Point to (a) The cup is on the table; (b) The cup is under the table; or (c) The cup is near the table." Because of interest in the patient's ability to comprehend prepositions, the clinician may first ensure that the patient can accurately recognize the substantive words within the test stimuli (e.g., "cup," "table") (see Appendix 4-3). In each instance, responses are analyzed to determine the type and frequency of words the patient is able to understand, the length of the stimulus that can be understood, and the latency or length of time needed to comprehend the material and respond.

In attempts to understand further the nature of form words, researchers are examining aspects of them and how they are compromised in persons with aphasia. For example, some studies have examined the relationship between the phonologic and morphologic forms (Braber et al., 2005; Miceli, Capasso, & Caramazza, 2004) and found inconsistent results regarding the influence of phonologic form on morphologic form. Saffran et al. (1989) developed a procedure for quantitative analysis of narrative speech to examine morphologic and syntactic structure, and reported that aspects of grammatical morphology may dissociate in agrammatism. Kim and Thompson (2000) and Shapiro, Shelton, and Caramazza (2000) suggested that one dimension of lexical organization is by word-form class (nouns or verbs, and verb-argument structure).

Morphology involves the rules used to form words into other words (Caplan, 1993). More specifically, in English, word formation is accomplished via affixing derivational or inflectional morphemes. Addition of a derivational morpheme changes a word into a different form word (e.g., "pain" into "painful"), whereas addition of an inflectional morpheme signifies a certain syntactic relationship (e.g., subject-verb agreement of "read" for "She reads."). Deficits comprehending both types of morphology are observed in patients with aphasia (Badecker & Caramazza, 1987; Braber et al., 2005). However, few assessment tools have been developed to examine such abilities. Two exceptions are the commercially available Psycholinguistic Assessments of Language Processing in Aphasia (Kay et al., 1992), and, in the research literature, a test developed by Caplan and Bub (1990). Caplan and Bub's test includes subtests to assess recognition and comprehension of morphologically complex words. The recognition subtest contains real, affixed words (e.g., "runs") and nonwords (e.g., "runned"), and patients with aphasia make a lexical decision regarding

whether the item heard or read was a real or made-up word. In the comprehension subtest, patients complete a word-picture matching task and a similarity judgment task.

Comprehension of Syntactic Constructions

Processing syntactic structures involves the knowledge of how one orders words within an utterance and how to construct various sentence types, such as active, passive, negative, and negative–passive. To comprehend syntactic information, patients with aphasia need adequate knowledge of syntactic rules (i.e., the ability to parse the structures that organize phrase elements into hierarchically translatable constituents such as subject NP, or object NP). They also need to be able to process quickly a transient auditory signal (if it is a listening situation) and to retain a memory representation of the signal to assure that sentential elements are not missed or misinterpreted (Berndt, 1998; Caplan, 1993; Schwartz, Fink, & Saffran, 1995). Disruption to this temporal aspect of syntactic processing will likely result in slow, labored reading abilities, although in reading there may be multiple opportunities to extract syntactic information from the written material.

Patients with aphasia may have difficulty comprehending the syntactic structure of spoken or written language that range from minimal difficulty, to very selective deficits (i.e., problems interpreting only certain sentence types such as cleft-object sentences), to profound impairments (i.e., patients must rely on semantic and pragmatic knowledge to comprehend sentences) (Chatterjee & Maher, 2000; Dick et al., 2001; Grodzinsky, 2000). Research in recent years has examined syntactic deficits in persons with aphasia from several perspectives: syntactic structure (Friedmann, 2005), availability of word class during syntactic comprehension (Park, McNeil, & Doyle, 2002; ter Keurs, Brown, & Hagoort, 2002), and differences in time post-onset of aphasia (Springer et al., 2000).

In assessing syntactic comprehension abilities and deficits, patients are often asked to respond to basic sentence types. However, aphasia batteries rarely include items that assess a range of syntactic comprehension abilities. Further, other tests have been criticized because they do not allow differentiation between disorders of syntactic comprehension or short-term or working memory limitations (Caplan, 1993; Martin & Miller, 2002). Lacking this distinction, clinicians may make an incorrect diagnosis and potentially plan inappropriate treatment. Three tests assess syntactic deficits in detail: the PALPA (Kay et al., 1992), the Verb and Sentence Test (Bastiaanse et al., 2003), and the Sentence Processing Resource Pack (Marshall et al., 1998). Clinicians may also probe the syntactic processing abilities of their patients with aphasia using commercially available tests such as the Revised Token Test (McNeil & Prescott, 1978), tests from the research literature (Caplan & Bub, 1990; Caplan, Waters, & Hildebrandt, 1997), or probes developed based on these test procedures.

Assessment often takes the form of a picture-sentence verification task in which the patient decides whether a spoken or written phrase or sentence is true or false or if it answers the question "yes" or "no". For example, the patient might be presented with a picture of a boy pushing a girl. Subsequently, he would point to the printed word "true" or "false" after each of the following sentences: "The boy is pushing the girl"; "The girl is pushing the boy"; "The boy is being pushed by the girl," and so forth. Caplan and colleagues (1997) also have patients demonstrate or act out sentence stimuli using the objects provided. The stimuli are constructed so that sentences cannot be interpreted solely on the basis of semantic processing or word knowledge, and so that distractor items represent plausible sentence inter-

pretations (Beretta et al., 1999; Berndt, 1998). During analysis of responses, clinicians attend to accuracy of response as well as to error types.

In determining the complexity of structures that the patient can comprehend, clinicians attend to the following syntactic features of a sentence: (a) **canonicity of thematic role order** (canonical order refers to sentences with the structure of subject-verb-object), (b) the **number of verbs** in a sentence, (c) the **verb argument** structure, and (d) the **number of propositions or thematic roles** played by nouns around a given verb. Table 4–10 contains a list of the sentence types (as well as possible foils) in an order of increasing complexity. Patients with aphasia and comprehension deficits (Caplan et al., 1993; 1997) should respond more

TABLE 4–10

Sentence Types that May Be Used to Probe Syntactic Comprehension

Sentence Structure	Number of			Canonicity of Thematic Roles
	Words	Propositions	Thematic Roles	
Active				
The lion kicked the elephant	5	1	2	Canonical
(Foil: The elephant kicked the lion)				
Active Conjoined Theme				
The pig chased the lion and the cow	8	1	2	Canonical
(Foil: The lion chased the pig and the cow)				
Active with Adjunct				
The elephant pulled the dog to the horse	8	1	3	Canonical
(Foil: The dog pulled the elephant to the horse)				
Passive with Adjunct				
The dog was pulled to the horse by the elephant	9	1	3	Noncanonical
(Foil: The horse pulled the dog to the elephant)				
Truncated Passive (TP)				
The pig was touched	4	1	2	Noncanonical
(Foil: The animal that was depicted as touching the pig was touched)				
Passive (P)				
The elephant was pushed by the cow	7	1	2	Noncanonical
(Foil: The cow pushed the elephant)				
Cleft Object (CO)				
It was the dog that the horse passed	8	1	2	Noncanonical
(Foil: The dog passed the horse)				
Conjoined (C)				
The elephant followed the lion and pulled the dog	9	2	4	Canonical
(Foil: The elephant followed the lion that pulled the dog)				
Object-Subject (OS)				
The horse kicked the elephant that touched the dog	9	2	4	Canonical
(Foil: The horse kicked the elephant and touched the dog)				
Subject-Object (SO)				
The dog that the pig followed touched the horse	9	2	4	Noncanonical
(Foil: The pig that followed the dog touched the horse)				

(From Caplan, D., Waters, G. S., & Hildebrandt, N. (1997). Determinants of sentence comprehension in aphasic patients in sentence-picture matching tasks. *Journal of Speech, Language, and Hearing Research, 40,* 542–555.)

accurately and more quickly to sentence types at the top versus the bottom of the list of items in this table. A clinician can compare his or her patient's understanding of sentence types of active versus truncated passive, active conjoined versus cleft object, active with adjunct versus passive with adjunct, object-subject versus subject-object, and conjoined versus subject-object. This hierarchy of sentence types serves as a possible framework to identify the approximate level at which a patient is functioning and to describe the syntactic features that the patient with aphasia can comprehend.

Goal 6: Analysis of the Ability to Produce Language Content

Impairments in the ability to produce language content are always part of aphasia (Benson, 1979; Goodglass, 1993). Deficiencies are observed in the appropriate selection or use of vocabulary words relating to objects, events, relationships, and content. The person with aphasia may have difficulty in word finding, labeling, and categorizing, and/or in the spontaneous selection or substitution of one appropriate word for another. Therefore, assessment involves an analysis of the ability to provide the spoken and written label or name of objects, actions, events, attributes, and relationships in response to highly structured tasks as well as during connected and spontaneous language. Importantly, clinicians should not assume that a patient's writing deficits will parallel his or her spoken language deficits. Indeed, writing disturbances may differ both quantitatively and qualitatively from disturbances in spoken language (Varney, 1998).

Production of Content in Highly Structured Tasks

An important component of content assessment involves determining the patient's ability to provide the verbal and written label of objects, actions, events, attributes, and relationships at various levels of task and stimulus difficulty. Clinicians routinely use several common, structured word-finding tasks that vary in terms of difficulty to assess production of content: (a) defining referents, (b) superordinate or category naming, (c) verbal fluency, (d) confrontation naming, (e) automatic closure naming, (f) automatic serial naming, (g) recognition naming, and (h) repetition naming (Murray & Chapey, 2001). For each task, a variety of psycholinguistic variables such as word frequency, picturability, length, imageability, age of acquisition, and concreteness can be varied to enable the clinician to specify the nature and extent of the word-finding impairment (Deloche et al., 1997; Nickels, 1995; Nickels & Howard, 1995; Snodgrass & Vanderwoort, 1980; Wilshire & Coslett, 2000). Most aphasia batteries and tests of spoken or written naming, such as the Test of Adolescent and Adult Word Finding (German, 1990), include subtests that examine several if not all of these types of word-finding abilities (see Table 4–5).

Defining Referents

A patient's ability to define words is assessed by asking the patient questions such as "What does anchor mean?" or "What does robin mean?" Responses are analyzed to determine the type of explanation produced, such as definition by usage, by location, or by classification. The ability to name words that are defined can also be explored further with follow-up questions that solicit either more detailed information, or a response that is in a different category (e.g., "A kind of plant that grows in a garden is _____." as a follow up to "What does garden mean?).

Category Naming

The ability to classify semantically related words and concepts is assessed through tasks that require responses at various levels and types of categories. The patient's ability to categorize in his or her own language can be scored according to (a) **perceptual categories**: classifying on the basis of a relevant sensory quality of a stimulus such as shape, size, or color (e.g., banana, lemon, grapefruit are all yellow); (b) **conceptual or semantic categories**: classifying on the basis of a generalized idea of a class of objects (e.g., banana, lemon, grapefruit are all fruit); and (c) **functional categories**: classifying on the basis of an action or function associated with a class of objects (e.g., banana, lemon, grapefruit are all for eating) (Goldstein, 1948). The clinician may also examine the degree of concreteness or abstractness of a patient's category responses. For example, grouping items on the basis of perceptual categories would be considered a more concrete response than grouping on the basis of semantic or functional category. Further, category naming may be examined according to the semantic level of words (Baker & Goodglass, 1976). Objects can be categorized at the superordinate level (e.g., animal), the basic object level (e.g., dog), or the exemplar level (e.g., Labrador Retriever).

To explore the ability to decipher categories, patients may be asked to (a) provide the verbal or written name of an object category (e.g., "Rose, tulip, and carnation are all a type of _____."), (b) name as many words as possible that belong to a certain category (e.g., "Write down the names of as many animals as you can.") (a divergent semantic task), (c) produce word associations (e.g., "What is the first word that you think of when I say school?"), and (d) sort objects into categories and explain the rationale for their sort (e.g., Goldstein's [1948] sort task).

Verbal Fluency

Verbal fluency tasks are category-naming tasks that obligate divergent thinking within one's semantic space. These tasks require patients to name as many words as they can think of within a certain category (as described above) or starting with a particular letter such as P, R, F, or C (Benton et al., 1994). For the letter task, patients are instructed not to use proper nouns. A time limit of at least 60 seconds is typically imposed, and the patient is given more than one test trial. Normative data for these types of naming tasks are available in the research literature (Heaton et al., 1992; Spreen & Strauss, 1998).

Confrontation Naming

Verbal and written naming in response to visual presentation is assessed by presenting objects, actions, events, and relationships, or pictures of these items, that vary in frequency, imageability, degree of abstractness, and type of category. For example, in an assessment of content-production ability, oral and written naming of objects, geometric forms, letters, animals, colors, body parts, and actions is almost always evaluated. For patients with right hemiparesis or other motoric impairments that may affect legibility of a written response, it may also be beneficial to assess writing skills with block letters that can be ordered to spell words (e.g., for a picture of a circle, the clinician gives the patient blocks with the letters "I," "R," "C," "E," "C," and "L" and asks him or her to spell the name of this picture); to make this task more difficult, distractor letter blocks could be added.

Confrontation naming has been criticized for its potential lack of relationship to daily communication activities (Mayer & Murray, 2003). Although confrontation naming is not always a part of conversational exchange, it is a communicative response that is a frequent and regular part of successful communication between individuals. For example, many communication exchanges contain short questions that further the intent of the exchange (e.g., Q: "Where do you want to go for dinner?" R: "Spinnaker"). To address this reasonable criticism, a clinician might carefully select the target items to include some that are familiar to the patient and frequently used by his or her family. Confrontation naming can also be assessed during connected speech tasks (Allchin & Patterson, 2000; Mayer & Murray, 2003; Patterson & Hinnach, 2005).

Automatic-Closure Naming

The capacity to complete an open-ended sentence or phrase stem such as "The sky is _____" is often a component of assessment. These sentence or phrase stems can be varied in terms of constraint or the degree to which a stem generates a particular response (Fischler & Bloom, 1979; Schwanenflugel & Shoben, 1985). For example, the stimulus "It's raining cats and _____" would be considered highly constrained because only one response, "dogs," is appropriate, given the nonliteral interpretation of the sentence. In contrast, the stimulus "He ate the _____" would be minimally constrained because there are numerous plausible responses. For both adults with aphasia and non-brain-damaged adults, automatic-closure naming is facilitated when the sentence or phrase stem is highly constrained or conver-

gent, and there is a limited number, or closed set, of response choices (Breen & Warrington, 1994; McCall et al., 1997; Treisman, 1965).

Automatic Serial Naming

The ability to produce rote or over-learned material may also be appraised. For example, the patient may be asked to count to 20, name the days of the week, write out the letters of the alphabet, and/or recite well-known prayers, nursery rhymes, or poems. It has often been assumed that this ability is intact when other naming abilities are not; however, this is not always the case.

Recognition Naming

When patients are unable to name an item, the correct word can be offered to them to determine whether they are capable of recognizing words they cannot name. For example, for the target stimulus "elephant," a patient may be required to indicate which of three verbal or written choices is the appropriate label (e.g., "giraffe," "elephant," or "telephone"). To increase the difficulty of this task, distractor items can be manipulated to be semantically (e.g., "giraffe") and/or phonologically or orthographically (e.g., "telephone") similar to the target. The most recent version of the Boston Naming Test includes this testing component.

Repetition Naming

Repetition or copying of words is assessed to determine whether the patient can repeat or copy words that he or she cannot verbally name or write, respectively (e.g., the clinician says "Now repeat: elephant.").

Production of Content in Connected Language

The ability to retrieve precise words for objects, events, relationships, and ideas during unstructured, spontaneous language production is important to the communication of meaning. In addition, the ability of a person with aphasia to produce content during highly structured tasks may differ from his or her abilities during less structured communication activities that require greater amounts of verbal or written output and more thinking to prepare the response. Therefore, clinicians analyze samples of their patients' spoken or written connected language to determine the accuracy, responsiveness, completeness, promptness, and efficiency of the content.

Picture description tasks are often used to elicit spoken and written discourse. The data generated can provide a controlled source for analyzing parameters of language content, form, and use (Armstrong, 2000; Shadden, 1998b). Although several aphasia test batteries include spoken and written picture-description tasks, eliciting larger samples using other connected language tasks should improve the

TABLE 4–11

Concepts Elicited from Normal Speakers Describing the "Cookie Theft" Picture

two	little	mother	in the kitchen (indoors)
children	girl	woman (lady)	general statement about disaster
little	sister	children behind her	
boy	standing	standing by sink	
brother	by boy	washing (doing)	lawn
standing	reaching up	dishes	sidewalk
on stool	asking for	drying	house next door
wobbling (off balance)	cookie	faucet on	open windows
3-legged	has finger to mouth	full blast	curtains
falling over	saying "shhh"	ignoring (daydreaming)	
on the floor	(keeping him quiet)	water	
hurt himself	trying to help (not trying to	overflowing	
reaching up	help)	onto floor	
taking (stealing)	laughing	feet getting wet	
cookies		dirty dishes left	
for himself		puddle	
for his sister			
from the jar			
on the high shelf			
in the cupboard			
with the open door			
handing to sister			

(From Yorkston, K. & Beukelman, D. (1980). An analysis of connected speech samples of aphasic and normal speakers. *Journal of Speech and Hearing Disorders, 45,* 27–36.)

reliability and validity of assessment results. In addition, to assure adequate test-retest stability for measures of connected language, clinicians may wish to use at least four or five stimuli to collect language samples that are at least 300 to 400 words in length (Armstrong, 2000; Brookshire & Nicholas, 1994). The stimuli should include more than picture-description tasks since these tend to elicit labeling behavior and potentially limit the number and variety of lexical and pragmatic behaviors produced as well as the complexity of morphosyntactic structures generated by patients (Armstrong, 2000; Armstrong, 2002; Davis, 2000; Li et al., 1996; Olness et al., 2002; Shadden, 1998b; Shadden et al., 1991). Other language tasks that may be used to elicit spoken or written language samples include conversational discourse, sequential events illustrated through multiple pictures, story-retelling, video-narration, providing interpretation of fables or stories, or procedural description tasks (e.g., "How do you change a tire?") (Cherney et al., 1998; Shadden et al., 1991; Ulatowska, Doyel, Freedman-Stern et al., 1983; Ulatowska, Freedman-Stern, Doyel et al., 1983). However, the usefulness of data from these tasks may be moderated by the presence of interfering variables such as motor-speech disorders.

Numerous methods are available to analyze content in connected-language samples (Armstrong, 2000; Shadden, 1998a). For example, one popular scoring system, developed

by Yorkston and Beukelman (1980), requires the clinician to determine the number of content units or "grouping of information that was always expressed as a unit" (p. 30), per unit of time. These researchers provided a list of content units for the "cookie theft" picture-description task of the BDAE (Table 4–11). One limitation of this system, however, is that it only provides responses to this picture. Consequently, Nicholas and Brookshire (1993) expanded on this idea and created a scoring system to analyze content in language samples derived from a variety of stimuli. In their system, rules are provided to help the clinician determine the number of words and "correct information units" (CIUs), or words that are "accurate, relevant and informative relative to the eliciting stimulus" (p. 340). Nicholas and Brookshire recommend that clinicians calculate both words per minute and the percentage of CIUs (i.e., number of CIUs/number of words) to obtain the most information about both the content and efficiency of their patients' connected language. Nicholas and Brookshire (1995b) also described a rule-based system for scoring the presence, completeness, and accuracy of content pertaining to the main concepts or gist in the connected language of patients with aphasia. In addition, they listed the main concepts consistently identified by non-brain-damaged adults in response to the "cookie theft" picture from the BDAE (Nicholas & Brookshire, 1995b) and to their stimulus "the birthday party picture" (Nicholas & Brookshire, 1992). These content measures are excellent predictors of how informative patients with aphasia are as perceived by unfamiliar listeners (Doyle et al., 1996). In addition, changes on these measures over time correlate positively with unfamiliar listeners' perceptions of socially relevant changes in the communicative ability of patients with aphasia (Ross & Wertz, 1999). Doyle, Goda, and Spencer (1995) compared the performance of persons with aphasia on structured-discourse tasks and conversation and noted significant differences in contexts. They reported that despite differences, performance on the structured tasks predicted performance in conversation. This observation is helpful in planning an assessment session in that the time-consuming task of conversational analysis may not be required during an early session in order to determine a diagnosis. Instead, structured-discourse tasks can be included in the initial assessment and conversational analysis (Boles & Bombard, 1998) completed at a later date.

Other measures available to analyze production of content in connected language are described as structural or functional in nature. Examples of structural-content analysis measures are word class, grammatical complexity, semantic diversity, and error pattern. Examples of functional-content analysis measures are speech acts (Searle, 1969), transitional elements, cohesion, and coherence.

Production of Content in Gesture

Although gestural abilities are often impaired in aphasia due to linguistic, cognitive, and/or apraxic deficits, many patients, even those with severe and global aphasia, have been able to acquire simple forms of gestural communication (Helm-Estabrooks, Fitzpatrick, & Barresi, 1982; Lott, 1999; Skelly, 1979). With respect to gestural codes, iconic (e.g., demonstrating how to use a toothbrush), symbolic (e.g., showing how to salute), and AmerInd gestures are often more suitable than American Sign Language (ASL) signs as assessment and treatment stimuli because they can be discerned more easily by unfamiliar viewers, and because they have been created or adapted for one-handed gesturing (Campbell & Jackson, 1995; Daniloff et al., 1982; Skelly, 1979).

Most aphasia batteries (e.g., ADP, PICA) include a subtest that examines ability to produce a limited number of iconic gestures, common symbolic gestures, or both. Another option is to assess the gestural-production skills using one of the several nonstandardized procedures described in the research literature (Alexander & Loverso, 1993; Conlon & McNeil, 1989; Rothi, Raymer et al., 1997; Rose, 2006).

Drawing

For some severely impaired patients with aphasia, it may be useful to examine their ability to reproduce or spontaneously produce drawings in order to communicate content

(Lyon & Helm-Estabrooks, 1987; Ward-Lonergan & Nicholas, 1995). However, before communicative drawing is adapted as a viable option, Lyon and Helm-Estabrooks (1987) suggest that the following abilities be considered as prerequisites: (a) an intact visuosemantic system for the concepts to be drawn, (b) adequate access to the symbols within this visuosemantic system, (c) adequate motoric and praxic abilities to draw these symbols, and (d) the ability to manipulate or augment drawn output "in a communicatively interactive and problem-solving manner" (p. 62). Therefore, assessment may involve determining the integrity of the patient's abilities in each of these areas via probes such as copying and drawing from memory, and via an evaluation of hand and limb motoric and praxic skills. The Daily Mishaps Test, which requires the patient to draw enacted scenarios that contain one- to three-part scenes, may also be used to evaluate patients' drawing abilities (Helm-Estabrooks & Albert, 1991). Although no formal scoring procedures are provided, clinicians can develop their own or borrow from scoring criteria described in the research literature (Murray, 1998). Sacchett (2002) reviewed approaches to the use of drawing in aphasia, and suggested three principles to include in evaluation and treatment: draw economically rather than perfectly; allow the communication partner to contribute to the drawing; and use interactive drawing within natural contexts.

Cognitive Neuropsychological and Neurolinguistic Approaches to Assessment of Content Production

Clinicians who adhere to a neuropsychological or a neurolinguistic approach to assessment attempt to determine the nature of their aphasic patients' language impairment with respect to models of language (Caplan, 1993; Hillis, 2002a, 2005; Kay et al., 1996; Nadeau, Rothi, & Crosson, 2000). That is, the clinician attempts to localize which particular component(s) of the model are impaired (see Fig. 4–4). In terms of word-finding abilities, for example, patients with aphasia have been found to have breakdowns in the word-retrieval process at the semantic and/or phonologic or graphemic output lexicon levels. These symptoms are most frequently characterized as impairments of access to or egress from memory, rather than loss of these respective linguistic representations (Raymer, 2005; Raymer & Rothi, 2002; Wilshire & Coslett, 2000). Patients with aphasia may also display difficulties at the articulatory/graphic planning stage or with the motor realization of that plan, but these difficulties are often viewed as a motoric (e.g., apraxia of speech, apractic agraphia), rather than a linguistic problem.

The research literature contains many articles that provide guidance for performing a neuropsychological or neurolinguistic assessment of disorders of content production (Rothi et al., 1991; Hillis, 1998). Rothi et al. (1991) and Hillis (1998) described how cognitive neuropsychological models guided their assessments of word-retrieval deficits across modalities, tasks, and sessions in order to distinguish impaired access/egress from degradation of linguistic knowledge. Rothi et al. (1991), suggested that access/egress word-retrieval deficits are associated with inconsistent errors, and knowledge impairments are associated with consistent errors. Hillis demonstrated how the pattern of performance in a series of word-retrieval tasks can be used to identify the loci of damaged cognitive mechanisms that underlie the deficit. Raymer (2005), Raymer and Rothi (2002), and Murray and Clark (2006) described several tasks that would be helpful in this type of assessment. For example, an evaluation might vary the stimuli according to psycholinguistic factors (e.g., age of acquisition or imageability), explore error analysis (e.g., paraphasias or neologisms), rate the informativeness of responses, or compare oral and written responses.

Three test batteries also are available that adopt a neuropsychological or neurolinguistic approach to the assessment of aphasia: the Psycholinguistic Assessments of Language Processing in Aphasia (PALPA; Kay et al., 1996), the Psycholinguistic Assessment of Aphasia (PAL; Caplan & Bub, 1990), and LeMo (DeBleser et al., 1997). LeMo is a computer-assisted, expert system for assessment of word-processing impairments; however, it is currently only available in a German version. These batteries include a variety of tasks to help the clinician identify the locus or loci of impairments in producing spoken or written language content and form at the word level. However, only the PAL includes subtests to determine language-production skills at the sentence level; none of these batteries examines language skills at the discourse level. In addition, the batteries are not standardized and do not provide comprehensive normative data.

Error Analysis in Production of Language Content

In addition to observing the accuracy and quantity of content in aphasic patients' verbal and written output, clinicians can analyze the nature and pattern of errors made (Goodglass et al., 1997; Kulke & Blanken, 2001; Schwartz & Brecher, 2000; Wilshire, 2002). In terms of types of paraphasias or naming errors, patients with aphasia frequently produce one or more of the following: (a) **phonemic** or literal paraphasia: the response contains substitution, addition, omission, and/or rearrangement of the target word's phonemes (e.g., "skoon" for the target "spoon"); (b) **semantic** paraphasia: the substituted word is semantically related to the target word (e.g., "fork" for the target "spoon"); (c) **random** paraphasia: the substituted word has no apparent semantic relation to the target word (e.g., "tractor" for the target "spoon"); (d) **circumlocution:** the response is a description or definition of the target word (e.g., "it's metallic and is used to eat soup" for the target "spoon"); (e) **neologism:** the response is a nonsense word (e.g., "clumpter" for the target "spoon"); (f) **indefinite substitution:** the response is a nonspecific word or description (e.g., "a thing for doing stuff" for the target "spoon"); and (g) **no response**.

Several researchers have developed detailed coding systems to describe the word-finding errors of patients with aphasia (Brookshire & Nicholas, 1993; Cuetos, Aguado, & Caramazza, 2000; Kemmerer & Tranel, 2000; Mitchum et al., 1990; Zingeser & Berndt, 1988). For example, Kemmerer and Tranel coded verbs in five categories: verb errors, phrasal errors, nominal errors, adpositional errors, and other errors. Cuetos et al. (2000) coded nouns in six categories: semantic, formal, mixed, unrelated, nonword, and other. Brookshire and Nicholas (1995) described a set of categories to quantify and qualify performance deviations in language output that could not be scored as real words or correct information units (Table 4–12) (see also Nicholas & Brookshire, 1993). These authors used this system to analyze the language of their patients with aphasia and found that they produced a significantly greater proportion of inaccurate words, false starts, and part-words or unintelligible words in comparison to their non-brain-damaged peers. Error analysis may also be a prognostic factor in recovery from stroke-induced aphasia (Davis & Majesky, 2005).

Cohesion Analysis

Cohesion is defined as the relations of meaning that "tie" or "glue" linguistic items together (such as one main clause and all subordinate clausal and nonclausal elements attached or embedded in it), thereby creating meaningful interdependencies among the words in a text or within a discourse sample. Cohesion is achieved linguistically through a variety of cohesive devices that contribute to the overall coherence of the verbal or written output. Various researchers recommend exploring semantic cohesion in the spontaneous connected speech of patients with aphasia (Glosser & Deser, 1990; Glosser, Wiener, & Kaplan, 1988; Liles, 1985; Liles & Coelho, 1998; Lock & Armstrong, 1997). In contrast, Bloom et al., (1996) reported that while coherence was disrupted in their patients with left hemisphere damage, cohesion was not.

Of the numerous types of cohesive devices (Halliday & Hasan, 1976), the following types are most frequently examined in the language of patients with aphasia (Glosser & Deser, 1990; Lemme, Hedberg, & Bottenberg, 1984): (a) **reference:** terms such as personal pronouns (e.g., "he," "us") and demonstrative pronouns (e.g., "these," "here") are used to refer to a previously stated or written, unambiguous antecedent (Armstrong, 2000); (b) **lexical ties:** vocabulary is selected to exemplify previously stated or written information (e.g., repetition of nouns, provision of a synonym or superordinate); (c) **conjunction:** conjunctive devices such as "and" and "then" are included; and (d) **ellipsis:** certain items

TABLE 4–12

Categories of Performance Deviations That May Be Examined in Samples of Connected Language*

Category	Definition	Examples
Nonword		
Part-word or unintelligible production	Word fragments or productions that are intelligible in context	. . . on a *st . . sk . . .* stool . . . on a *frampi*
Nonword filler	Utterances such as "uh" or "um"	. . . on a . . *um* . . stool . . *uh.* . . .
Non-CIU		
Inaccurate	Not accurate with regard to the stimulus, and no attempt to correct	. . . on a *chair* (for stool)
False start	False start or abandoned utterance	. . . on a *chair* . . no, a stool
Unnecessary exact	Exact repetition of words, unless used purposefully for emphasis or cohesion	. . . on a . . *on a* stool
Nonspecific or vague	Nonspecific or vague words lacking an unambiguous referent	. . . on a *thing*
Filler	Empty words that do not communicate information about the stimulus	. . . on a . . *you know* . . stool
And	All occurrences of the word *and*	. . . a boy *and* a stool
Off-task or irrelevant	Commentary on the task or the speaker's performance	*I've seen this one before.* *I can't say it.*

*In the examples, only nonwords and words printed in italics were scored as performance deviations.

(From Brookshire, R.H. & Nicholas, L.E. (1995). Performance deviations in the connected speech of adults with no brain damage and adults with aphasia. *American Journal of Speech-Language Pathology, 4,* 118–123.)

are omitted because they can be presupposed from the previous stated or written text.

During assessment, clinicians may explore the relationship between the clarity of a message and the amount of cohesion it contains (Armstrong, 1987). This is accomplished by identifying the occurrence of these cohesive devices in connected language and determining the degree and accuracy of their use, which may be either appropriate (Coelho et al., 1994), inappropriate (Glosser & Deser, 1990; Liles & Coelho, 1998), complete (the antecedent is easily identified), incomplete (the antecedent was not provided), or inaccurate (an ambiguous antecedent) (Liles, 1985).

Influential Variables

Many variables may facilitate or impede production of language content. Assessment should include analysis of these variables in order to specify the nature and extent of the word-finding impairment. Such analyses yield valuable information not only about patient functioning but also about potential treatment activities and stimuli. Three categories of influential variables are item-related, task-related, and patient-related. Examples of item-related variables that may influence content production are the target words' frequency (Deloche et al., 1996), age of acquisition (Bird, Franklin, & Howard, 2001; Deloche et al., 1997; Hirsch & Ellis, 1994), length (Nickels & Howard, 2004), concreteness (Nickels, 1995), semantic category (Goodglass et al., 1966), grammatical class (Berndt, Haendiges et al., 2002), degree of

certainty (Mills et al., 1979), and operativity (Nickels & Howard, 1995). Examples of task-related influential variables are type of sensory input (Benton, Smith, & Lang, 1972), stimulus novelty (Faber & Aten, 1979), length of trial and intertrial time (Brookshire, 1971; Fridriksson et al., 2005), type of naming task (Berndt et al., 2002), concomitant gesturing (Cunningham & Ward, 2003; Hanlon, Brown, & Gerstman, 1990; Rose & Douglas, 2001), verbal reinforcement (Stoicheff, 1960), attention condition (Murray, 1996), and word-retrieval success rate (Brookshire, 1972; Nickels & Best, 1996). It is important to note that these variables may not only influence the content produced by patients with aphasia during word-level or structured language, but also during connected language. Therefore, during assessment clinicians should introduce conversational topics that vary in terms of abstraction, intellectual complexity, length, and familiarity in order to examine which topics facilitate and which impede the amount of meaningful content, jargon, and/or word-finding errors in their patients' spoken or written language.

Evaluation also includes an analysis of patient-related variables. Examples of these are skills of the communication partner (Hickey & Rondeau, 2005; Linebaugh et al., 2006), and the ability of a patient to use clinician-produced and/or self-generated cues (Freed, Marshall, & Nippold, 1995; Marshall et al., 2002; Pease & Goodglass, 1978). Pease and Goodglass (1978) described a differential effect of cues on production of language content. They demonstrated that cues have potency as aids to word retrieval, but that the

TABLE 4–13

An Example of a Cueing Hierarchy

1. The clinician imposes a delay or the patient requests additional time to produce the word
2. The clinician provides a semantically related word or the patient generates one or more words that are semantically related to the target (e.g., "sugar" or "tea" for the target "coffee")
3. The clinician provides a phonemic cue (e.g., "/k/ for the target "coffee") or the patient produces one or more words that are phonetically similar to the target (e.g., "cost," or "caddy")
4. The clinician or the patient provides a description of the target word (e.g., "I drink this every morning." For the target "coffee").
5. The clinician provides a carrier phrase for the target word (e.g., "A cup of _____.").

potency varies for individuals with aphasia. Cueing hierarchies, such as that displayed in Table 4–13, can be explored to examine word-finding stimulability and to determine what type of self-correction strategies a patient uses (Linebaugh & Lehner, 1977; Linebaugh, Shisler, & Lehner, 2005; Patterson, 2001).

Goal 7: Analysis of Ability to Produce Language Form

Linguistic form includes morphology, syntax, and phonology. Morphology refers to the set of rules that govern the structure of words and the construction of word forms from the basic elements of meaning (i.e., morphemes). Syntax refers to the rule system for ordering words into sentences. Phonology refers to the sound system as well as the rules used to combine those sounds (Nelson, 1998). Aphasia may result in difficulties producing one or more aspects of form; consequently, each should be assessed during an in-depth language evaluation.

Production of Form Words and Morphology

Morphologic and syntactic impairments in verbal production are common in patients with aphasia. Such deficits are observed in the use of relational words such as articles, prepositions, conjunctions, and personal pronouns (Goodglass, Christiansen, & Gallagher, 1993; Kohn & Melvold, 2000). In addition, morphologic inflections such as the plural /-s/, possessive /-s/, or present progressive /-ing/ are frequently omitted or inappropriately used. In aphasia, the occurrence of morphologic and phonological errors is not necessarily correlated (Miceli et al., 2004). Persons with aphasia who make morphologic errors are likely to produce

phonologic errors, but the reverse is not the case. A hierarchy of difficulty for producing these various morphemes has been found to be a function of grammatical rather than phonologic complexity (Goodglass & Berko, 1960; Haarmann & Kolk, 1992; Miceli et al., 2004). Specifically, patients with aphasia tend to display relatively greater difficulty as they shift from producing determiners to prepositions to pronouns to auxiliary verbs for form words, and as they shift from producing plural to adjective to verb inflections for grammatical morphemes.

Most traditional aphasia batteries do not assess this aspect of language. However, both the PALPA (Kay et al., 1997) and the PAL (Caplan & Bub, 1990) include subtests to assess production of morphology. For example, on the PAL, patients are given a word that they insert into a given sentence (e.g., "courage" must be affixed to fit into the sentence "If a man is brave, we say he is _____."). Goodglass and Berko's (1960) sentence-completion test examines a patient's ability to affix several types of grammatical morphemes. For example, to examine the regular past tense /-ed/ morpheme, the clinician reads the stimuli aloud and the patient then supplies the final word with the target morphologic inflection: "He is using the fly swatter to swat flies. Yesterday, several flies were _____."

The above tests elicit form words and morphology via relatively structured or constrained, highly structured tasks. In addition, a number of scoring systems described in the aphasia literature may be used to examine these syntactic features in connected-language samples (Menn, Ramsberger, & Helm-Estabrooks, 1994; Saffran et al., 1989; Thompson et al., 1995). For example, Menn and colleagues developed an Index of Grammatical Support to examine the average number of form words and grammatical morphemes that are correctly used in the spoken output of patients with aphasia.

Production of Syntactic Constructions

Persons with aphasia may experience difficulty in combining words into both simple and complex constructions in order to express relationships (Chatterjee & Maher, 2000). More specifically, patients demonstrate restricted use of syntactic forms and therefore produce incomplete syntactic structures, simple syntactic structures, or both (Bird & Franklin, 1996; Cappa et al., 2000; Edwards, 1998). They may also produce few complex syntactic structures or sentence forms and commit more errors when attempting them.

The goal of assessment of production of syntactic construction is to determine the specific syntactic structures that are available to each patient with aphasia. To examine the production of spoken and written sentences in highly structured contexts, clinicians may choose from one of the few structured tests (see Table 4–5) or subtests that are designed to elicit a variety of syntactic forms (e.g., passives,

TABLE 4–14

Examples of Syntactic Constructions

Construction	Examples
Noun phrase	cookies; the boss
Verb	stealing; hurry up
Adjective	big; warm
Prepositional phrase	in the basket
Expanded noun phrase	cookies in the jar
Expanded verb	get up in the morning
Expanded adjective	sick of the office
Expanded prepositional phrase	in bed in the morning
Subject + auxiliary	so is the woman; aren't they? (tag question)
Subject-verb	the man's running
Subject + predicate	he's the president
Verb-object	dry the dishes
Subject-object	the dog . . . chicken
Topic-comment	boy . . . off stool; burglar . . . policeman
Expanded subject-verb	the guy's running to work
Expanded subject + predicate	the woman's angry with her husband
Expanded verb-object	grab the chicken quickly/from the basket
Expanded subject-object	dog . . . chicken in basket
Expanded topic-comment	burglar policeman outside
Subject-verb-object	the dog stole the chicken
Expanded subject-verb-object	the mother's washing dishes in the kitchen
Complex	I hope he gets to work on time
Multicomplex	he picks the corn to see if it's ripe
Aborted utterance	this boy has . . .
Abandoned utterance	the sink is overflowing on to the . . .

datives, relative clauses). For example, on the PAL (Caplan & Bub, 1990), patients are asked to describe a picture with the constraint that they must begin their description with a certain word such as "bicycle" (e.g., the intent is to elicit the passive sentence, "The bicycle is being pushed by the man.").

Another assessment option is to examine connected, spoken, or written language samples using one of the several syntactic scoring systems described in the aphasia literature (Curtiss et al., 2004; Edwards, 1995; Goodglass, Christiansen, & Gallagher, 1994; Rochon et al., 1998; Saffran et al., 1989; Thompson et al., 1995) (Table 4–14). Although some of these analysis systems were developed to characterize agrammatic language output (e.g., Saffran et al., 1989), other systems were aimed at characterizing structural aspects of fluent or paragrammatic language output (e.g., Edwards, 1995). Most of these scoring systems provide detailed procedures for collecting language samples (typically using picture-description or story retelling tasks), separating samples into utterances or T-units (i.e., an independent main clause and any dependent clauses modifying it), and identifying a variety of syntactic forms and relationships

(e.g., proportion of grammatical sentences, proportion of simple vs. complex grammatical sentences, number and type of sentential constituents). Because the procedures are so explicit, researchers report good inter-rater reliability.

Analysis of Production of Word Forms, Morphology, and Syntactic Construction

Analysis of production responses is typically completed in two broad categories: error analysis, and analysis of frequency and consistency of production. Error analysis typically takes the form of whether the morphologic or syntactic errors are a substitution or omission of target structures. Substitution errors might involve the interchangeability of constituents. For example, the patient might confuse nouns with verbs, or affix the inappropriate morphologic inflection. Substitutions may be further examined to determine whether errors are within-category (e.g., "in" for "with") or across-category (e.g., "her" for "with") substitutions (Haarman & Kolk, 1992). Omission errors might, for example, involve production of verbs in their infinitive form (e.g., without person or number agreement or tense endings), or the omission of a whole group of words such as relational words or auxiliary verbs. Intelligibility analysis is a part of error analysis as it involves determining whether sentences are understandable in spite of omissions and substitutions. Interestingly, in English, word-order violations are relatively uncommon among patients with aphasia (Bates et al., 1988; Menn & Obler, 1990); therefore, identifying word-order violations is not typically a major focus of error analysis.

The frequency and consistency of production of various syntactic structures is evaluated to determine which structures are frequently, infrequently, or never used and which are consistently or inconsistently used correctly. For example, some patients with fluent types of aphasia may produce a variety of syntactic forms but produce complex syntactic forms at a reduced frequency compared with their non-brain-damaged peers (Edwards, 1995; 1998). When patients with aphasia inconsistently use form words, morphologic inflections, or syntactic forms, the clinician tries to identify whether or not there are any influential linguistic or task variables. For example, for some patients with aphasia, a relationship exists between the degree of structure or task constraint (e.g., sentence-completion vs. conversational activities) and the number and type of grammatical errors produced (Hofstede & Kolk, 1994).

Production of Phonology

Phonology refers to the set of sounds in a language as well as the rules used to distribute and sequence those sounds into words (Owens, 2004). Speech and language pathologists typically assess two components of phonology: a segmental component that consists of phonemes and syllables, and a suprasegmental component that includes intonation, stress, and pauses.

Segmental Phonology

Aphasia is frequently accompanied by a segmental phonologic disorder or an impairment in the ability to produce the distinctive sound elements of a word or syllable in the standard manner. In fact, Blumstein (1998) concluded that "nearly all aphasic patients produce phonological errors in their speech output" (p. 162). Often, segmental phonologic disorders are associated with dysarthria or apraxia of speech (Dogil & Mayer, 1998) and consequently with breakdown in terms of phonetic implementation (Aichert & Ziegler, 2004). Both of these disorders are frequent accompaniments of aphasia and have been described above under Goal 2. When either or both of them are present, phonology should be assessed in detail. The data collected should include (a) phonemic errors produced during unstructured spontaneous language and the phonologic context of those errors, (b) errors produced on a standard articulation test, (c) results of stimulability testing or the patient's ability to modify his or her production of error phonemes following auditory and

visual stimulation, (d) a phonetic inventory, and (e) results of an evaluation of the patient's peripheral speech mechanism.

Suprasegmental Phonology

The production of suprasegmental components of phonology may also be problematic for some patients with aphasia (den Ouden & Bastiaanse, 2003; Seddoh, 2000). There are many suprasegmental components, but two that are commonly affected in aphasia are intonation and stress

Intonation refers to modulations of the pitch or musical flow of an utterance and is primarily dependent upon laryngeal control (Blumstein, 1998). Ability to produce typical melodic intonation or prosodic quality is assessed to determine whether the patient has problems using pitch variations to indicate grammatical segmentation or complexity (Goodglass, 1968), such as at the end of a phrase or sentence. Difficulties in the production of intonation have been reported, particularly in patients with Broca's aphasia or anterior left hemisphere lesions (Seddoh, 2004) and may contribute to difficultly in word comprehension.

Stress refers to the force or accentuation of a particular sound or syllable (Blumstein, 1998). In evaluating a patient's ability to produce appropriate stress patterns a clinician determines whether the patient with aphasia uses stress patterns that are typical of his or her linguistic peer group and predictable within linguistic context, or if he or she manifests incorrect stress placement that results in subsequent reduction or omission of vowels or morphemes that would normally have been stressed. Stress is assessed at both the phrase and sentence level (Goodglass, 1968).

A goal of assessment is to determine the specific suprasegmental phonologic variables that the patient with aphasia can produce, or that he or she can be stimulated to produce. This can be accomplished during moderately structured observations or by administering aphasia batteries (e.g., WAB, BDAE) that contain tasks in which suprasegmental features of spoken output are examined, such as tasks that require the clinician to rate the fluency of connected speech. Additionally, those suprasegmental features that can be used to improve the intelligibility of spontaneous speech or the communication of meaning should be identified and incorporated into therapeutic goals.

Goal 8: Analysis of the Ability to Comprehend and Produce Pragmatic Aspects of Communication Interaction

Communication is the reciprocal act of sending and receiving information, and is profoundly influenced by the context in which it is used and the partners who are involved. That is, both the communication environment and the partners are dynamic components of the communication itself. Therefore, language (including content and form) varies with each context and partner (Joanette, Ansaldo, & Stemmer, 1999). Indeed, the language produced or comprehended by an individual at any point in time will be an interactive product of contextual variables and the individual's structural linguistic knowledge (Gallagher, 1983). Communicative competence is the successful interaction of comprehension of language content, language form, and pragmatics (Lahey, 1988).

Pragmatics refers to the system of rules that regulate the use of language in context (Bates, 1976). It involves the interactional aspects of communication and the use of language for communication (Prutting & Kirchner, 1983). The emphasis is not on sentence structure but rather on how meaning is communicated—how units of language function in discourse and as authentic communication within social contexts (Holland & Hinckley, 2002). Pragmatics is a knowledge of who can say what to whom, in what way, where, when, why, and by what means (Prutting, 1979). It is the knowledge of how to converse with different partners and in different contexts, as well as the knowledge of the rights, obligations, and expectations underlying the initiation, maintenance, and termination of discourse.

Pragmatic abilities include a communicator's proficiency in constantly adjusting the content, form, and acceptability of his or her message, in switching or shifting sets of reference as in topic changes, and in being sensitive to the influence of the communication partner's social status and communicative abilities and to the physical context in which communication occurs (Penn, 1999). It also refers to the ability to use language for a variety of functions or intents such as requesting, greeting, warning, and protesting (Lucas, 1980). Penn (1999) identified three knowledge areas that comprise pragmatic competence: (1) knowledge—of language and its structure, of the world and its contents, and social knowledge; (2) adaptation—the speed and ease with which reaction to environment occurs; and (3) processing variables—the "real-time" behaviors required to engage in successful interaction, such as attention and memory.

Pragmatic aspects of language often remain an area of relative strength for many patients with aphasia (Wulfeck et al., 1989). Indeed, most patients with aphasia can communicate better than they can speak. However, "pragmatic skills certainly can be affected by focal brain damage" (Holland, 1996). Consequently, clinicians assess pragmatic skills to determine whether these abilities are an area of strength that may be capitalized upon during treatment, or whether they are problematic and need to be remediated during treatment. Specifically, it is important to examine the comprehension and production of several sources of knowledge about pragmatics and patterns of use, such as speech acts and intents, and discourse rules that govern conversational skills such as turn-taking and topic selection, maintenance, and code switching. It is also important to determine how these factors are influenced by various contexts and partners (Murray & Chapey 2001).

The WHO ICF (ICF, 2001) provides a useful framework for assessing pragmatic comprehension and production. In particular, the activity and participation levels of the ICF guide clinicians to look beyond a patient's abilities and deficits in language content and form, and assess the patient's ability to convey meaning and to communicate in a manner that is functional for that individual (Elman & Bernstein-Ellis, 1999; Holland & Thompson, 1998). "Functional" has a different meaning for each individual with aphasia, and can best be assessed using multiple measures such as direct observation, conversational analysis, and discourse analysis, as well as published tools (Holland & Hinckley, 2002).

Communication Environment

Various communication settings and activities may affect the length, morphosyntactic complexity (e.g., anaphoric pronouns), redundancy, fluency, responsiveness (e.g., elaborations of comments), semantic relatedness, and lexical selections (e.g., technical jargon) of the language that is produced or that is understood (Labov, 1970; Lyon, 1992). For example, clinicians frequently observe variations in production and comprehension of spoken and written language when comparing communicative performance in the therapy room to that observed in more natural environments (Egolf & Chester, 1977). Also, Glosser et al. (1988) found that verbal complexity and language errors vary significantly with different contents and contexts of communication. For example, in conditions that restrict visual contact between the speaker and listener (e.g., communicating over the telephone or through an opaque barrier), patients with aphasia, like non-brain-damaged adults, produce fewer communicative gestures and more complex verbalizations. Hofstede and Kolk (1994) also observed changes in the morphosyntactic output of patients with aphasia across different speaking conditions (e.g., conversation, formal interview, picture description). Further, "aphasic patients show appropriate and predictable linguistic changes in response to nonlinguistic social contextual variables" (Glosser et al., 1988, p. 115). Therefore, assessment involves an analysis of whether or not the patient's linguistic behavior changes with various contexts, and if so, how specific contexts facilitate or hinder the number and variety of his or her communicative behaviors.

Communication Partners

Specific communication partners may also affect the form, content, and intent of language that is produced (Gallagher, 1983). Partner characteristics such as age, sex, familiarity, and authoritative status, as well as internal variables such as world knowledge, values, previous experiences, and emotional status, affect communication (Davis, 2000). Frequently the burden of communication between a person with aphasia and his or her communication partners will shift following aphasia (Linebaugh et al., 2006). Clinicians must analyze such partner variability and note patterns of performance.

Part of successful communication involves having the opportunity to communicate highly personal thoughts and emotions to those who are judged to be important partners, as well as feeling the fulfillment associated with sending and receiving messages (Armstrong, 2005; Denman, 1998; Lubinski, 1995). That is, successful communication gives the individual the feeling of social connectedness to others, the ability to influence other's thoughts and actions, and a means of establishing shared reference (Hengst, 2003). Unfortunately, some patients with aphasia may have few opportunities for successful, meaningful communication due to a lack of sensitivity to the value of interpersonal communication, few reasons to talk, lack of privacy, excessive background noise, no viable communication partner, negative perceptions of their communicative competence, and/or lack of stimulation in general (Kagan, 1995; Lubinski, 1995; McCooey, Toffolo, & Code, 2000; Parr & Byng, 2000; Parr, Byng, & Gilpin, 1997). Therefore, the aphasia assessment should include an evaluation of the communication opportunities afforded the patient and the barriers to such communication using tools such as the Profile of the Communication Environment of the Adult Aphasic (Lubinski, 2001), or Pragmatic Protocol (Prutting & Kirchner, 1987). Part of the assessment is the determination of whether a patient has anyone with whom to talk, the names and relationship to the patient of the frequent and infrequent communicative partners, and how their presence and communication style affect the patient's communicative behavior and the communicative interaction.

Other nonstandardized tools such as the Family Interaction Analysis (Florance, 1981) (Table 4–15) or observational measures of a conversational partner's support and level of participants (Kagan et al., 2004) may also help the clinician identify the psychosocial factors that promote successful communication interaction and those that contribute to a communication-impaired environment. The information gained from these types of analyses may help provide information about the caregivers' and significant others' sensitivity to the patient's communication difficulties, as well as about their successful and unsuccessful strategies for communicating with the patient (Simmons-Mackie & Kagan, 1999). Subsequently, the clinician can help the patient, and significant communication partners, create a positive and rewarding communication environment that contains stimulating activities and a variety of interesting communication partners (Elman, 2005).

Speech Acts and Communicative Intent

Pragmatics is the rule-governed, social use of language and represents the speaker's method of conveying intended meaning. Speech acts are the instantiations of pragmatics. Austin (1962) and Searle (1969) described speech acts as theoretic units of communication between a speaker and listener that are performed in the course of verbal and written interaction, and carry with them an intention on the part of the speaker. According to Searle (1969), the speech act includes what the message-sender means, what the message means, what the message-sender intends, what the message-receiver intends, what the message-receiver understands, and what the rules are governing the linguistic utterance. In Searle's theory, the proposition is the words or sentences produced, and the illocutionary force of this proposition is the message-sender's intent in producing the utterance.

A number of taxonomies have been developed to describe the variety of intentions that can be used in communicating (Austin, 1962; Dore, 1974; Searle, 1969). Frequently identified intents include (a) **response:** the intention to attend to and respond to another's utterance or question; (b) **request:** the intention to address another for help, whether it be to solicit information, action, or perhaps acknowledgment; (c) **greeting:** the intention to convey a conventional greeting; (d) **protesting:** the intention to object to another person's behavior, or to reject or resist the action, statement, or command of another; (e) **description/comment:** the intention to give a mental image of something seen or heard; (f) **assertion:** the intention to point out to another that some statement or proposition is true; this intent includes a subset called affirmation, which includes instances in which the speaker is agreeing with or confirming a proposition; and (g) **informing:** the intention to report on present and past experiences.

Many of these intents are used in one or more of the following four communication categories proposed by Lomas et al. (1989) (see Table 4–2): (a) basic need: communication skills that are needed to accomplish basic needs such as eating and daily hygiene; (b) health threat: communication skills that are needed to maintain physical well-being or health (e.g., calling for assistance after falling, telephoning 911 for emergency help); (c) life skill: communication skills that support the ability to provide or understand information needed to complete daily activities such as shopping, home maintenance, and driving; and (d) social need: communication skills that are needed to participate in social activities such as playing cards, going to church, or writing a letter to a friend.

Intents may be communicated and comprehended through semantic-syntactic utterances and/or by previous or subsequent utterances. In addition, they may be expressed (and comprehended) through facial expression or accompanying actions, gestures, or tone of voice. What is not said may also communicate intent. Further, one can say one thing and mean another. That is, individuals frequently use their knowledge of the communication environment and their partners to help them decipher between what is said and what is meant.

TABLE 4–15

Family Interaction Analysis: Scoring Form

Significant-Other Behaviors	S	U	R
Nonfacilitative			
1. Inattentive posture			
2. Incongruent affect			
3. Lengthy response			
4. Self-focus			
5. Inappropriate topic change			
6. Advice-giving			
7. Judgmental response			
8. Premature confrontation			
9. Interrupting			
10. Guessing			
11. Repeating			
12. Simple language			
13. Loud voice			
14. Abrupt topic change			
15. Speaking for patient			
Facilitative			
16. Closed question			
17. Verbal following			
18. Minimal encouragers			
19. Open question			
20. Paraphrasing content			
21. Reflecting feeling			
22. Summarizing content			
23. Summarizing feeling			
24. Sharing			
25. Confrontation			
26. Interpretation			
27. Verbal cueing			
28. Gesturing			
29. Instruction			
30. Labeling			
31. Modeling			
32. Physical cue			
33. Request for attention			

Key: S = successful; U = unsuccessful; R = rejection.

(From Florance, C. (1981). Methods of communication analysis used in family interaction therapy. *Clinical Aphasiology, 11,* 204–211.)

Patients with aphasia often have a relatively preserved ability to interpret a variety of speech acts and intents, including the ability to respond correctly to indirect requests (Foldi, 1987; Wilcox, Davis, & Leonard, 1978). In terms of production, some patients maintain the ability to produce a variety of speech acts or intents, including requests for clarification, responses to requests for clarification, and greetings (Newhoff et al., 1985; Prinz, 1980; Ulatowska et al., 1992). Despite these preserved pragmatic abilities, however, impairments in other aspects of pragmat-

ics are reported. First, patients with aphasia use a restricted range of speech acts and intents (Armstrong, 2001; Prutting, 1979; Wilcox et al., 1978). For example, Doyle and colleagues (1994) found that patients with aphasia primarily produced responses to direct requests. In contrast, assertions predominated the verbal output of non-brain-damaged adults. Second, different pragmatic impairments are observed among patients with different types of aphasia and different sites of brain damage (Murray & Holland, 1995; Prutting & Kirchner, 1987). Because of these possible pragmatic limitations, examining patients' abilities to communicate and comprehend various speech acts or intents is an important part of a comprehensive aphasia assessment.

Discourse Skills

The pragmatic nature of communicative interaction appears in discourse in the form of verbal and nonverbal speech acts that initiate or maintain a topic, shift topic, repair or revise a previous speech act, or terminate a topic. These speech acts are intended to establish cooperative discourse participation to achieve a mutual communication goal. Grice (1975) proposed that successful discourse is achieved when (a) the message-sender provides a sufficient amount of information (i.e., not too much and not too little); (b) the messages being shared are truthful; (c) the vocabulary used is relevant to the topic and is cohesively related; and (d) the manner in which messages are shared is concise and avoids ambivalence and obscurity.

Initiation of the speech act (as the message-sender) includes topic selection, introduction, and/or change of topic. This communicative act should contain new, relevant, and what is judged to be sincerely wanted information. The message-sender therefore needs to determine what, if any, information is shared by the various message-receivers. Thus, topical or referential identification involves searching one's long-term memory for information that is judged to be relevant, interesting, and wanted or already known by the partner. For some patients with aphasia, inappropriate initiation has been observed (Avent, Wertz, & Auther, 1998; Patterson & Fahey, 1994). Despite this, persons with aphasia have been reported to be relatively good at being sensitive to their partners' interests and previous knowledge (Penn, 1988).

Maintenance of communication involves turn-taking or the variation of roles as message-sender and message-receiver in order to serve the pragmatic function of sustaining the communicative exchange. The role of the message-receiver is to comprehend the message that is communicated. Comprehension can be indicated by one or a combination of the following: nonverbal responses (e.g., nodding the head, leaning forward), a short and usually affirmative verbal response such as "yes," and visual orientation rather than gaze avoidance (Davis, 1981). To assist the message-sender, the message-receiver must also monitor and evaluate the message and provide feedback concerning the effectiveness and acceptability of the communication exchange.

The message-sender may use gaze and hand posture to signal control of the interaction. To retain his or her role, the message-sender may use gaze-avoidance and a hand gesture that is not maintained or not returned to a resting state through a phonetic clause juncture (Rosenfeld, 1978). When a message-sender wants a reaction or response, he or she signals "with a pause between clauses" or "with a rising or falling pitch at the end of a phonemic clause" (Davis, 1981, p. 171). The message-receiver also uses gaze to signal control in an interaction. The message-receiver maintains his or her role by visually orienting toward the message-sender.

Nonverbal cues are usually used by partners to signal a wish to maintain or change roles (Rosenfeld, 1978). Because role-switching typically occurs as a result of the message-sender's desire to relinquish the role, the message-receiver needs to formulate a judgment concerning the message-sender's willingness to switch roles. When role-switching occurs in the absence of the speaker's readiness to switch, it may be accompanied by overloudness and a shift of the head away from the speaker.

Successful maintenance of turn and turn-taking behavior results in a mutually satisfying interaction. When one of the communication partners has aphasia the nature of the turn may change, with the partner who does not have aphasia assuming more of the conversational burden than the partner with aphasia. Maintenance and turn-taking must be appropriate for the communication partners and not attempt to adhere to standards appropriate for conversations when neither partner has aphasia.

As the person with aphasia takes turns in a conversation, the turn may be successful; however, the overall communicative event may be altered. For example, although the pause time in turn-taking may be lengthened for a person with aphasia participating in conversation (Lesser & Milroy, 1993; Prutting & Kirchner, 1987), most patients with aphasia continue to display appropriate turn-taking skills, often relying primarily upon the use of nonverbal behaviors such as nodding or eye gaze (Penn, 1988; Schienberg & Holland, 1980).

Repair and revision are an integral part of discourse maintenance and regulation, and reflect a message-sender's sensitivity to a message-receiver's state of comprehension. Moves by both communication partners identify communication sequences that were unsuccessful and apply repair strategies to assure comprehension of the communicative message. Discourse regulatory devices such as requests for clarification are essential to the maintenance of communication (Fey & Leonard, 1983; Schegloff, Jefferson, & Sacks, 1977). The most common form of repair in normal interactions is the self-initiated self-repair, and it typically occurs within the turn in which the communication breakdown has transpired.

Because of the well-documented difficulties persons with aphasia have in conveying accurate and nonambiguous information (a product of their language-content and form deficits), repair and revision strategies are important and frequently used when communicating with patients with aphasia (Ferguson, 1994; Milroy & Perkins, 1992). Furthermore, the linguistic impairments of patients with aphasia may limit their ability to identify communication breakdowns, to repair them, or both. Although some patients with aphasia retain the ability to initiate and make repairs (Klippi, 1996) this process typically takes longer to resolve than during interactions among non-brain-damaged individuals, and may be accomplished collaboratively rather than solely by one partner (Laasko, 2003). The type of repair used varies in interactions between the person with aphasia and his or her family, and between the person with aphasia and the clinician (Lindsay & Wilkinson, 1999), and among types of discourse activity (Heeschen & Schegloff, 1999). However, some types of repair can be detrimental to communication interactions. For example, the partner may, in a good faith attempt to help the patient with aphasia, use repairs excessively to correct conversational errors, even if these errors have not obscured the meaning of the patient's message (Booth & Perkins, 1999; Murray, 1998). This strategy can foster the perception that the patient with aphasia is not a competent partner as well as change the interactional roles from that of partners to that of a student-teacher or patient-clinician.

Maintenance of communication interaction may also involve a response that sustains a topic. For example, a contingent utterance shares the same topic as the preceding utterance and adds information to the prior communication act. Thus, sequential organization of topics is also a component of communication maintenance (Beeke, Wilkinson, & Maxim, 2001). For example, in procedural and narrative discourse, a sufficient number of steps and episodes, respectively, must be elaborated on or communicated in a logical order (Ulatowska, Doyel et al., 1983) in order to ensure satisfactory exchange of information.

Individuals with aphasia have been shown to demonstrate a variety of difficulties in maintaining communication interactions. Although patients with mild aphasia frequently demonstrate appropriate discourse maintenance skills, patients with more severe language impairments use fewer contingent utterances than do non-brain-damaged adults (Ulatowska et al., 1992). They have also been found to produce somewhat lengthy and digressive or tangential responses (Penn, 1988). In terms of sequential organization, fewer complete episodes and more missing episodes are observed in story retellings by patients with aphasia compared to responses of non-brain-damaged adults (Uryase, Duffy, & Liles, 1991). Although Ulatowska et al. (1983a, 1983b) found that patients with aphasia omitted story episodes and procedural steps, and included some inaccurate information, they also noted that those episodes and steps that were conveyed were those considered essential to the story or procedure. Furthermore, most of these episodes and events were presented in the correct sequence.

In summary, although patients with aphasia show many pragmatic strengths in terms of their ability to communicate successfully in discourse activities, they may also display a variety of impairments that may negatively affect the efficiency and success of their discourse interactions.

Consequently, assessment in adult aphasia involves an analysis of the patient's ability to initiate and maintain discourse in various contexts and with various partners. This is particularly important given the highly individualized role of context in many communicative exchanges.

Assessing Pragmatic Skills and Functional Communication

Although assessing pragmatic abilities and assessing functional communication skills are often viewed as one and the same, there are some notable distinctions between the two assessment approaches (Elman & Bernstein-Ellis, 1999; Lyon, 2000; Manochiopinig, Sheard, & Reed, 1992; Worral, 1995). Pragmatic skills encompass the use of the rules that govern social interaction in a language and culture, while functional communication refers to the ability to operate and interact in real-life situations in response to specific communicative demands. Both reflect the summation of an individual's linguistic, pragmatic, and cognitive skills. Table 4–16 lists a variety of tests and observational profiles that can be used to examine pragmatic abilities, functional communication skills, or both.

Pragmatics

Pragmatic abilities are primarily assessed using observational profiles or checklists in which the clinician identifies the presence and appropriateness of various pragmatic behaviors. Typically these observations are based upon discourse samples, since this level of communication interaction illuminates "the complex associations across linguistic, pragmatic, and cognitive processes as well as the potential dissociations (of) either across or within clinical populations" (Chapman, Highley, & Thompson, 1998, p. 56). Although some clinicians and payors view such analysis as time-consuming, Boles and Bombard (1998) found that such behaviors could be reliably analyzed with 5- to 10-minute discourse samples of patients when these behaviors occurred at a rate of approximately three times per minute. Tools for pragmatic analysis, such as direct observation, discourse analysis, and conversational analysis, offer important information in the assessment process and should be included (Armstrong, 2000; Boles & Bombard, 1998; Holland & Hinckley, 2002).

Tools such as the Pragmatic Protocol (Prutting & Kirchner, 1987), the Communication Profile (Gurland & Gerber, 1982), the Revised Edinburgh Functional Communication Profile (Wirz et al., 1990), and the Profile of Communicative Appropriateness (Penn, 1988) can be used to rate a patient's use of specific pragmatic skills. For example, the clinician can use approximately 15 minutes of conversation between the patient with aphasia and a familiar partner to complete the Pragmatic Protocol and to rate the appropriateness of 30 pragmatic parameters covering a

TABLE 4–16

Tests of Pragmatic and Functional Language Abilities

Instruments	Source
Structured Tests	
Assessment of Language-Related Functional Abilities	Baines et al. (1999)
Communication Activities of Daily Living-2	Holland et al. (1999)
Functional Communication Therapy Planner	Worral (1999)
The Amsterdam-Nijmegan Everyday Language Test	Blomert et al. (1994)
The 'dice' game	McDonald & Pearce (1995)
Rating Scales and Inventories	
A Questionnaire for Surveying Personal and Communicative Style	Swindell et al. (1982)
ASHA Functional Assessment of Communication Skills For Adults (ASHA FACS)	Frattali et al. (1995)
Assessment Protocol of Pragmatic-Linguistic Skills	Gerber & Gurland (1989)
Communication Profile	Gurland et al. (1982)
Communicative Competence Evaluation Instrument	Houghton et al. (1982)
Communicative Effectiveness Index	Lomas et al. (1989)
Communicative Profiling System	Simmons-Mackie & Damico (1996)
Everyday Communicative Needs Assessment	Worrall (1992)
Functional Communication Profile	Klein (1994)
Functional Communication Profile	Sarno (1969)
Functional Outcome Questionnaire for Aphasia	Glueckauf et al. (2003)
Inpatient Functional Communication Interview	O'Halloran et al. (2004)
LaTrobe Communication Questionnaire	Douglas et al. (2000)
Pragmatic Protocol	Prutting & Kirchner (1987)
Profile of Communicative Appropriateness	Penn (1988)
Revised Edinburgh Functional Communication Profile	Wirz et al. (1990)
Social Networks: A Communication Inventory For Individuals With Complex Communication Needs And Their Communication Partners	Blackstone & Berg (2003)
The Communication Profile: A Functional Skills Survey	Payne (1994)
The Speech Questionnaire	Lincoln (1982)

range of speech acts (e.g., requests, comments) and discourse abilities (e.g., topic maintenance, repair/revision skills) across verbal, nonverbal, and paralinguistic domains. When the clinician summarizes Pragmatic Protocol results, he or she compares the overall number of appropriate and inappropriate pragmatic behaviors (i.e., calculates a percentage of appropriate behaviors). These results are interpreted with respect to the number of pragmatic behaviors for which there was no opportunity to observe in the language sample. Such assessment tools clearly provide information that is not obtained from more traditional standardized tests. However, some of the pragmatic tools may have specific psychometric limitations and should be used with caution (Armstrong, 2000; Ball et al., 1991; Hux et al., 1997; Manochiopinig et al., 1992; Penn, 1999; Perkins, Crisp, & Walshaw, 1999).

Functional Communication

Generally two methodologic approaches are used to examine functional communication skills: structured tests, in which performance of test items is evaluated, and observational profiles, based on unstructured or moderately structured communication interactions. Of the structured tests available (see Table 4–16), the Communication Activities of Daily Living-2 (CADL-2; Holland et al., 1999) is probably the best known. The CADL-2 examines a patient's ability to recognize and produce a variety of speech acts and interactions across both spoken and written language modalities. Evaluation of communicative success is based on both verbal and nonverbal responses. The CADL-2 differs from the earlier version of the CADL in that it is slightly shorter (i.e., 50 items that take about 25 minutes to complete versus 68 items that take about 35 minutes to complete), and does not include role-playing items.

Strengths of standardized tests of functional communication include their documented reliability and their use in noting change over time. However, this approach and these tests have been criticized because of the restricted view of the manner in which patients with aphasia spontaneously interact in real-life functional communication situations (Lomas et al., 1989; Manochiopinig et al., 1992) and because administering one of these tests is more time-consuming than completing a rating protocol (Crockford & Lesser, 1994).

A number of observational profiles and rating protocols are available to examine the functional communication abilities of patients with aphasia (see Table 4–16). This group of measures includes the Functional Communication Profile (Sarno, 1969), Communicative Effectiveness Index (Lomas et al., 1989), ASHA Functional Assessment of Communication Skills for Adults (ASHA FACS; Frattali et al., 1995), the Communication Profile: A Functional Skills Survey (Payne, 1994), and the Inpatient Functional Communication Interview (O'Halloran et al., 2004). The ASHA FACS has both qualitative and quantitative scales for scoring a patient's ability to complete a variety of everyday communication activities across four domains: social communication (e.g., "exchanges information on the telephone"), communication of basic needs (e.g., "responds in an emergency"), reading, writing, and number concepts (e.g., "understands simple signs"), and daily planning (e.g., "follows a map"). Unlike several of the other observational profiles, this test has undergone extensive standardization and has good reliability and validity.

Another notable rating scale is Payne's (1994) Communication Profile: A Functional Skills Survey. This protocol uses an interview approach in which the patient rates the relative importance of 26 communication behaviors in his or her daily life related to his or her basic, present health-care and social needs. The normative sample for this instrument includes patients of varying ethnicity, living accommodations, employment history, and income levels, and is therefore culturally sensitive. Several other ratings scales have been created, some of which are widely available and frequently used and others that are available only in research papers. Also, many methods of conversational analysis have been published (Armstrong, 2000; Penn, 1999). Some follow previously published methods of analysis (e.g., Nicholas & Brookshire, 1995a) and others were created anew with respect to a theoretic model (O'Halloran et al., 2004).

Several researchers propose that clinicians should not rely on the results of a single test or observational profile for the assessment of functional communication abilities (Worrall et al., 2002). Within the context of the WHO ICF (ICF, 2001), Worrall et al. (2002) reviewed several measures of functional communication and observed patients with aphasia in functional communication situations. They suggested that the ICF is a valuable model to guide assessment but may oversimplify the real-life communication needs of individuals with aphasia. They proposed that three types of functional communication should be considered in assessment of persons with aphasia: (a) generic (e.g., speech acts for social greeting), (b) population-specific (e.g., for individuals with a specific impairment or communicating within a specific setting), and (c) individualized (particular needs of an individual). Worrall (1995, p. 53) suggested that "the concept of functional communication is too complex for a single test administration" and developed the Everyday Communicative Needs Assessment (Worrall, 1992). This contains a series of tasks, including an interview, to evaluate a patient's communicative needs (Table 4–17); a questionnaire to assess the individual's social-support system; and observations and ratings of the patient's interactions in his or her natural environment and with his or her daily communicative partners. The Communicative Profiling System, developed by Simmons-Mackie and Damico (1996), is similar and also represents a multi-method approach to examining the conversational abilities of patients with aphasia, and the way these skills are influenced by daily communication partners and environments. Social Network Theory (Blackstone & Berg, 2003) examines functional communication within the structure of an individual's communication needs and abilities, and within an expanding circle of family, acquaintances, and unfamiliar partners; it is built upon the model of communication as joint interaction.

Irwin, Wertz, and Avent (2002) compared results of measures of language impairment (PICA; Porch, 1981), functional communication (Rating of Functional Performance; Wertz et al., 1981), and a measure of pragmatic abilities (Pragmatic Protocol; Prutting & Kirchner, 1987) over the course of a year. They reported that severity of language impairment was related to severity of functional communication and pragmatic performance, but the latter two measures were only related in patients in the acute stage of aphasia, not the chronic stage. This work highlights the utility of using multiple tools on multiple assessment dates to assess different aspects of aphasia to obtain a well-rounded assessment.

It is likely that the number of tools for assessing functional communication will increase and become ever more sophisticated (Hartley, 1995). It is unlikely, however, that any one tool will adequately measure the functional communication skills for all patients with aphasia and other neurogenic communication disorders. For many of the tools developed recently, and those that will be created in the future, research is needed to determine whether they possess the following attributes: "sensitivity to change over time; reliability within and across raters, and over time; sufficient range of performance measured to prevent threshold effects; usefulness across different methods of administration;

TABLE 4–17

Example of an Interview Guide, One Aspect of Worrall's (1992) Everyday Communicative Needs Assessment

1. **Finances**
   — checking and paying bills
   — writing checks
   — reading bank statements
   — balancing accounts/budgeting
   — organizing payment of rent/mortgage
   — reading literature (e.g., Social Security/Veterans Affairs)
   — filling in forms (e.g., Social Security, Veterans Affairs, Medicare)
   — using an automatic teller machine

2. **Using the Phone**
   — looking up numbers in phone book
   — using Yellow Pages
   — dialing emergency numbers
   — writing down phone messages
   — making appointments/business calls
   — making social calls

3. **Preparing Food**
   — reading labels on food packets
   — measuring ingredients
   — reading sell by/use by dates and calculating food freshness
   — following recipes
   — making choices at mealtimes
   — using the microwave and oven

4. **General Household Activities**
   — following washing and ironing instructions on clothes
   — following instruction leaflets for household appliances
   — setting washing machine
   — directing workmen (e.g., plumber)
   — dealing with people who come to door (e.g., meter-reader)
   — following written instruction re DIY jobs (e.g., shelves)
   — writing note for milkman, home help, etc.
   — caring for pets
   — following instructions for use of gardening products
   — gardening

Coding for reasons:
1. immobility
2. aphasia
3. other stroke-related problems
4. other

(From Worrall, L. (1995). The functional communication perspective. In C. Code & D. J. Muller (Eds.), *The treatment of aphasia: From theory to practice* (pp. 47–69). San Diego, CA: Singular Publishing. *Reprinted with permission.*)

usefulness during different phases of rehabilitation and relevance to function outside the clinical setting" (Frattali, 1992). Considering the trend for health care to focus on functional outcomes and measures, this task should be one of our highest priorities.

Goal 9: Analysis of Quality of Life in Persons with Aphasia

Quality of life, (QOL) is related to an individual's activity and participation in society, and his or her satisfaction with their physical, emotional and social environment. QOL is defined as "an individual's perception of their position in life in the context of the culture and value systems in which they live and in relation to their goals, expectations, standards and concerns. It is a broad ranging concept affected in a complex way by the person's physical health, psychological state, personal beliefs, social relationships and their relationship to salient features of their environment."(WHOQOL: Measuring Quality of Life, 1997.) QOL has several dimensions, including physical problems, body image, communication, and interpersonal issues (Code, 2003; LaPointe, 1996; Madden, Oelshlaeger, & Damico, 2002; Rolnick & Hoops, 1969) and is typically measured with a self-report.

Threats (2005) described the complex interrelationship between QOL and ICF. Both instruments were developed by the World Health Organization and show overlap in their perspectives yet serve different purposes. The ICF is intended to be used to report observations of an individual's behavior, including the perspective of the person being evaluated. ICF measures list behaviors in categories, and as the assessment progresses the behaviors should be prioritized as to importance in an individual's life. QOL is a perceptual rating that presents an individual's subjective opinions about his or her status or position in life. Several researchers and clinicians support the use of the WHO ICF in assessment of QOL (e.g., Ross & Wertz, 2005), yet there are points of disagreement (Worral & Cruice, 2005).

Cruice and colleagues (2003), using the ICF as a framework, sought to determine which aspects of communication predicted participants' QOL. They reported that in addition to emotional and psychosocial well-being, functional communication was a contributor to positive QOL. They proposed the communication-related QOL (CRQOL) model as an enhanced version of QOL that incorporated functional communication. The CRQOL (Cruice et al., 2003) describes the language and communication behaviors that may be associated with the ICF levels as well as personal and environmental factors that may influence communication, and can be used as a guide when assessing QOL in persons with aphasia.

Another QOL assessment measure designed for use with persons with aphasia is the Stroke and Aphasia Quality of Life Scale (SAQOL and SAQOL-39) (Hilari & Byng, 2001; Hilari et al., 2003). The authors adapted this scale from the Stroke-Specific Quality of Life Scale (SS-QOL) (Williams et al., 1999) in part because they believed the SS-QOL and other QOL scales were difficult for some persons with aphasia to use given the linguistic requirements of the scales. The SAQOL measures QOL in four subdomains: physical, psychosocial, communication, and energy. It was reported to be reliable and valid, but requires additional investigation for successful use in assessment. Finally, the Communication Quality of Life Scale (ASHA CQL) (Paul et al., 1997) provides information about the psychosocial, vocational, and educational effects of a having a communication impairment.

Ross & Wertz (2003) compared responses on three QOL measures: WHOQOL Instrument (WHOQOL, 1997), WHOQOL-BREF (World Health Organization Quality of Life – BREF, 2004), and the Psychosocial Well-Being Index (Lyon et al., 1997). These measures were selected to be consistent with the WHO recommendation of assesing QOL with both general and disease-specific instruments. Ross and Wertz found that three domains—level of independence, social relationships, and environment—were best at distinguishing QOL in persons with and without aphasia. They emphazied two considerations that should guide measurement of QOL in persons with aphasia in the future. First, there is no current single meausre that will best capture QOL for all patients with aphasia, and, given the individual variation in patients, finding one best instrument for all patients may be an unrealistic goal. Second, the importance of measuring QOL does not diminish the importance of assessing impairment-based functions, such as comprehension and producion of language form and content.

One difficulty associated with QOL measures is that they frequently have heavy reliance on linguistic skills in order for an individual to complete the measure (Cruice et al., 2003). Cruice et al. devised an iconic tool to assess QOL in individuals with aphasia to avoid this problem.

QOL can also be examined in terms of burden on a patient and his or her family. Doyle and colleagues (Doyle et al., 2003; Doyle et al., 2004) developed the Burden of Stroke Scale to quantify physical, cognitive, and psychological aspects of the burden of stroke, as reported by the patient. Reponses to a series of questions in several domains provide a clinician with an expansive picture of the effect of stroke on a patient, with or without a communication disorder. Linebaugh et al. (2006) examined burden from the point of view of communication between a person with aphasia and his or her communication partner. They reported that communication burden was indeed reapportioned between a person with aphasia and his or her communication partner, and that factors such as amount of functional communication evinced by the patient influenced the degree of shift.

QOL Reported by Family Members

Cruice and colleagues (2005) examined the relationship between responses about patients' QOL from the patients themselves and proxy respondents. They discovered biases in responding across aspects of the survey tools they used, and called for the development of measures that are accessible to all patients with aphasia. Another example of a QOL

measure developed for completion by a family member as well as the person with a communication disorder is the LaTrobe Communication Questionnaire (Douglas, O'Flaherty, & Snow, 2000). This tool examines communicative behaviors in several conversational domains from the perspectives of the patient and his or her family members. Similar to Cruice et al. (2003), Douglas et al. (2000) found disagreement between rating of patients and of family members. Glueckauf et al. (2003) developed a questionnaire designed to assess functional outcome of treatment in persons with aphasia, as reported by caregivers. Of note with this instrument is that it does not appear to be heavily biased by caregiver strain, which is caused by the daily responsibilities of caring for a person with aphasia and by the compromise to communicative interactions.

Engell and colleagues (2003) examined responses from persons with aphasia and their family members using a pictorial and a written version of the Aachen Life Quality Inventory. The tool examined responses in the physical and psychosocial domains, and the pictorial version used icons (e.g., person on a bench to indicate loneliness, and thumb up or down to indicate opinion) for both the stimulus items and responses. Engell et al. (2003) reported success with this instrument in measuring QOL. Similar to other studies, they found differences between the ratings of patients and family members for many of the items. These results highlight the importance of creatively measuring QOL in individuals with aphasia, particularly those with severe aphasia who likely may be unable to comprehend complex written material or verbally respond in connected speech. In addition, it supports the need to examine psychosocial factors as well as physical factors that influence QOL.

The literature is inconsistent in reporting the reliability and accuracy of informants' rating of communication abilities of their significant other with aphasia. This inconsistency is related both to conditions surrounding the assessment process (e.g., length of questionnaire or method of analysis in the study) as well as observer characteristics (e.g., emotional influence or clarity of observation). The effort to refine instruments and procedures for assessment of QOL by proxy report continues to be of importance, although a single instrument is unlikely to be effective for all patients with aphasia and their families.

Relationship among QOL and ICF Impairment and Activity-Based Measures

A question of interest to clinicians is the degree of relationship of communication disorder among measures of language impairment (such as word-retrieval assessments), measure of activity (such as the CADL-2; Holland et al., 1999), and measures of QOL (such as the CRQOL; Cruice et al., 2003). Ross and Wertz (2002) administered six assessment tools to individuals with chronic aphasia. Two were measures of impairment (WAB; Kertesz, 1982, and PICA; Porch, 1967), two were measures of communication-activity limitation (CADL-2; Holland et al., 1999, and ASHA FACS; Ferketic et al., 1995), and two were measures of QOL (WHOQOL-BREF, 2004, and Personal Wellness Inventory; Lyon et al., 1997). In contrast to the notion that individuals with aphasia might show different results on the three types of measures, Ross and Wertz found no systematic significant relationships. One interpretation of these results is at face value, and suggests no relationship; however, Ross and Wertz chose to look more closely at several factors that might have influenced results, such as experimental method (e.g., sample size) and nature of the instruments (e.g., range of test items). They concluded that at best, the relationship among these levels of measurement is unclear but the importance of QOL and the contribution of communication skills to QOL deserves continued study.

Sarno (1997) examined the performance changes on three measures in two groups of persons with aphasia. The measures were a language-based tool, Neurosensory Center Comprehensive Examination for Aphasia (Spreen & Benton, 1977; Spreen & Strauss, 1998); an activity-based tool, the Functional Communication Profile (Sarno, 1969); and a quality-of-life measure, The Functional Life Scale (Sarno, Sarno, & Levita, 1973). Participants in this study were divided into younger and older age groups; however, age was not a factor in the results. Sarno et al. (1997) reported that improved QOL in persons with aphasia in the first year poststroke was related to aphasia rehabilitation services that included language, communication, and psychosocial goals.

In their editorial on QOL, Worrall and Holland (2003) laid out the importance of measuring QOL in persons who live with aphasia, and also suggested that the challenge in the future would be to refine QOL measurements to capture those elements of an individual's life that reflect quality. Worrall and Holland identified areas of consensus in considering QOL in persons with aphasia and areas about which more information is required to creatively assess and ultimately treat QOL in individuals with aphasia. Assessing QOL and participation in society is of ever-increasing importance as individuals adjust and accommodate to life with aphasia (LaPointe, 1996; Ross & Wertz, 2005).

Goal 10: Determination of Candidacy for Prognosis in Therapy

Formulating prognoses for recovery from aphasia is one of the primary tasks of the speech-language pathologist (Tompkins, Jackson, & Shulz, 1990) and is one of the first questions usually asked by patients with aphasia, their caregivers, and family. Although relevant and reliable predictors and optimal methods of measuring prognoses are still limited, some of the prognostic indicators commonly suggested in the literature include **biographical variables** such as age, gender, education, premorbid intelligence, support systems, usual/necessary activities, and level and type of life participation; **medical variables** such as etiology and duration of aphasia, site and extent of brain lesion, and concomitant physical and mental-health problems; and **language and cognitive variables** such as type and severity of aphasia and language stimulability.

Biographical Variables

Age

Many authors note that age and outcome correlate significantly (Holland & Bartlett, 1985; Marshall, Tompkins, & Phillips, 1982; Sands, Sarno, & Shankwilder, 1969); that is, younger patients with aphasia typically demonstrate greater language recovery than older patients. Ogrezeanu and colleagues (1994) showed such a correlation for patients younger than 71 years of age. However, several researchers have failed to identify a meaningful relationship between age and aphasia recovery (Basso, 1992; de Riesthal & Wertz, 2004; Wertz et al., 1981). Basso (1992) suggested that demographic variables such as age and education play a minor role in prognosis, whereas neurologic factors, such as severity of aphasia, play a major role. Consequently, there are most likely many variables such as personal attitude, available support systems, level and type of life participation, learning style, pharmacologic treatment, and general medical health that confound the influence of age on recovery (Berthier, 2005; Crosson et al., 2005; Darley, 1977; Johnson, George, & Hinckley, 1998; Laganaro, DiPietro, & Schnider, 2006). Indeed, Tompkins et al. (1990) note that physiologic characteristics such as activity level or general health indicators and "psychosocial factors like personality, social involvement, or life satisfaction . . . are more predictive of cognitive ability, life adaptation, and morale than is chronological age" (p. 399).

Gender

Some studies show that gender and outcome correlate significantly, favoring males (Holland et al., 1989). Other studies report mixed findings with respect to the influence of gender on prognosis (Sarno, Buonaguro, & Levita, 1985). Basso (1992) found better recovery of spoken language in female as opposed to male patients with aphasia but did not observe this differential recovery in auditory comprehension skills. However, other researchers have failed to observe any significant differences in the recovery of female and male patients (Ogrezeanu et al., 1994). Consequently, future research is necessary to shed light on the exact nature of gender as a prognostic indicator in language recovery.

Education and Premorbid Intelligence

Although many clinicians use education level as a prognostic factor in aphasia, Tompkins et al. (1990) point out that years of formal education do not necessarily correspond to pre-morbid intellectual ability. Instead, these authors recommend the use of estimates of premorbid intelligence that weigh and enter standard demographic data including age, education, gender, occupational category, and race into specifically developed equations (Barona, Reynolds, & Chastain, 1984; Griffin et al., 2002; Lynch & McCaffrey, 1997; Spreen & Strauss, 1998). These estimates of premorbid functioning may have more predictive power than educational level alone, except in cases in which the patient had been illiterate (Lecours et al., 1988).

Medical Variables

Etiology/Type of Stroke

Prognosis in aphasia is more positive in cases resulting from traumatic as opposed to vascular etiology (Basso, 1992; Kertesz & McCabe, 1977). In terms of the type of stroke, if the patient survives a hemorrhagic stroke, he or she is likely to experience more recovery than the patient who had an ischemic (i.e., thrombotic or embolic) stroke (Holland et al., 1989; Laasko, 2003), and the recovery pattern is often different (Brookshire, 2003).

Time Since Onset

The fastest rate of recovery is typically observed during the first few months post-onset when spontaneous physiologic recovery processes are taking place. However, research and clinical experiences indicate that patients with aphasia can, and do, continue to make measurable progress for many, many years following the onset of aphasia (Davis, 2000). Although Sands et al. (1969) found that the longer the time between the onset of aphasia and the beginning of intervention the poorer the prognosis, more recent research suggests that deferred treatment is not necessarily detrimental to language recovery (Wertz et al., 1987). Indeed, clinical research studies frequently include participants who are many months, even years, post-onset, and many of these participants show change as a result of treatment.

Site and Extent of Lesion

In general, patients with larger dominant-hemisphere lesions or multiple lesions have a poor prognosis (Kertesz, 1979). Relations between site of lesion and aphasia outcome have also been identified. For example, lesions of the central core of the dominant-hemisphere language area, served by the middle cerebral artery, even when they are small, frequently result in severe aphasias (Hillis et al., 2000). Lesions to left temporobasal areas are also associated with less recovery compared to lesions outside of this region (Goldenberg & Spatt, 1994; Naeser & Palumbo, 1994; Thompson, 2000). Darley (1982) noted that some patients with poor prognosis because of the site and extent of lesion have nevertheless

recovered well. As technology to support neural imaging increases in accuracy and efficiency, increasingly finer-grained relationships may be made between site and extent of lesion and prediction for recovery, such as the studies reviewed by Cappa (2005) and by Hillis (2002b).

Physical and Mental Health Problems

The presence of other physical and mental-health problems in addition to aphasia often results in a poor prognosis (Jorgensen et al., 1995). For example, concomitant motor-speech disorders (e.g., apraxia of speech) have been shown to have a negative influence on aphasia recovery (Keenan & Brassell, 1974; Ogrezeanu et al., 1994). In terms of mental health, depression, anxiety, and other psychological problems may negatively affect outcome (Code et al., 1999; Code & Hermann, 2005). In addition, patients with aphasia who have few medical problems tend to have a shorter length of hospital stay, which has also been associated with better recovery (Holland et al., 1989).

Medications

Certain drugs can adversely affect the ability of a person with aphasia to respond to tasks. For example, dysarthria and stuttering are common adverse reactions to certain anti-depressants and anticonvulsant medications (Murray & Clark, 2006; O'Sullivan & Fagan, 1998). Likewise, many anticonvulsant medications may produce undesirable side effects such as confusion, fatigue, and decreased arousal levels, which can affect patient ability to complete language activities (Vogel, Carter, & Carter, 1999). Therefore, the clinician needs to know what medication a patient takes and the impact of each, separately and in combination.

Neuropsychological and Language Variables

Neuropsychological Variables

Although in recent years many studies have described the relationship between cognitive functioning and language deficit in aphasia, most have been with respect to a particular skill or treatment program (Purdy, 2002). Currently, only minimal research has examined the relation between neurocognitive status and language recovery. Results of this research are mixed. That is, some studies, such as that by Goldenberg and Spatt (1994), show a positive relationship between initial neurocognitive test scores and language recovery (Bailey, Powell, & Clark, 1981; Messerli, Tissot, & Rodriguez, 1976). These researchers found that temporobasal lesions are associated with poor aphasia recovery because such lesions cause a disconnection between deep temporal lobe structures associated with memory abilities and cortical areas associated with language abilities. That is, these lesions result in problems in learning language as well as in acquiring compensatory strategies. In contrast, other studies fail to observe a significant correlation between initial cognitive status and subsequent recovery (Basso, 1987; David & Skilbeck, 1984). Despite some null findings, many clinicians believe that the presence of concomitant attention, memory, and/or executive-function deficits negatively affect patients' ability to attend to and remember language, to problem solve, to learn to develop compensatory strategies, and to generalize learned behavior to new communicative situations (de Riesthal & Wertz, 2004; Helm-Estabrooks, 2002). More importantly, clinical research is attempting to identify those neuropsychological factors that may facilitate (or impede) progress in treatment (Purdy, 2006; Ramsberger, 2005; Shuster, 2004).

Aphasia Characteristics

Severity. The initial severity of aphasia is one of the strongest predictors of outcome (Kertesz & McCabe, 1977; Ogrezeanu et al., 1994; Pedersen, Vinter, & Olsen, 2004); that is, patients with severe language impairments tend to show poorer recovery than those with milder language deficits. More specifically, initial ability to speak has been found to share a relationship to the eventual speech performance of the individual with aphasia (Keenan & Brassell, 1974). Similarly, patients who are severely impaired in auditory recognition and comprehension have an unfavorable prognosis compared with those who are less affected in these language areas (Davis, 2000; Robey, 1998).

Language Profile. Type of aphasia may be predictive of the amount of recovery and the residual pattern of language impairment. For example, patients with global aphasia are expected to have the poorest outcome, particularly those who continue to present with global aphasia beyond 3 months post-onset (Laska et al., 2001; Ogrezeanu et al., 1994; Paolucci et al., 1998). In contrast, patients with anomic aphasia are expected to have the best outcome such that approximately half of these patients experience complete recovery by 1 year post-onset (Kertesz, 1979).

The language improvement that most patients experience often results in a change of aphasia type over time. For example, many patients with global aphasia eventually present with Broca's aphasia as their auditory comprehension and language-production abilities recover (Holland, Swindell, & Forbes, 1985). In contrast, Broca's, Wernicke's, conduction, and transcortical (sensory, motor, or mixed) aphasias frequently resolve toward anomic aphasia over time (Goodglass, 1992; Ogrezeanu et al., 1994; Rapcsak & Rubens, 1994).

Stimulability

Self-correction. A patient's awareness of his or her speech difficulty as well as his or her ability to self-correct relate positively to improvements in speaking abilities (Keenan & Brassell, 1974; Oomen, Postma, & Kolk, 2001; Wepman,

1958). That is, patients who have insight into their language disorder as well as an awareness of situations that either enhance or degrade their communication ability have a better prognosis (Marshall & Tompkins, 1982; van Harskamp & Visch-Brink, 1991).

Cuing. Insight into the prognosis for a patient with aphasia may also be gained from examining the degree to which his or her language behaviors can be easily modified. For example, Keenan and Brassell (1974) observe that aphasic patients whose spoken language is initially stimulable to prompts and cues display better recovery of spoken language than do those patients for whom prompting is ineffective. Clinicians might expect that those patients with aphasia who can learn to produce their own cues would have better language outcomes or demonstrate better generalization of target language behaviors than patients who are dependent upon others to provide cues (Freed et al., 1995; Marshall & Freed, 2006; Marshall et al., 2002).

Personality/Social Variables

Personal Attitude

The desire of a patient with aphasia to improve his or her level of motivation, self-efficacy, and determination may influence the course and outcome of aphasia therapy (Darley, 1977; Murray & Chapey, 2001; Rosenbek, LaPointe, & Wertz, 1989; Shill, 1979). As van Harskamp and Visch-Brink (1991) proposed, the "kernal" of therapy is the stimulation of the patient's willingness to participate actively in the learning process and to practice learned skills at every opportunity. These researchers further stated that "the patient's motivation is of utmost importance: patients need to exert themselves to make progress" (p. 533). In addition, the level and type of participation in everyday activities and in life may well have a profound effect on prognosis since patients need something to talk about and since such participation can have a positive effect on motivation (Chapey et al., 2000). Indeed, research indicates that personality variables and social support are linked to health generally, to morbidity and mortality, as well as to prognosis in treatment in a variety of health conditions such as stroke (Tompkins et al., 1990). An excellent example of the supportive effects of personal variables is humor in treatment (Simmons-Mackie & Schultz, 2003). Tompkins and colleagues (1990) suggested that using valid and reliable psychosocial scales to measure a patient's personality variables has the potential for enriching our understanding of patients' responses to treatment and for facilitating prognoses.

Family Attitude

Family interest in the patient with aphasia and their desire to see improvement in language and communication abilities will also contribute to a determination of candidacy for treatment and influence the progress made during intervention. For example, a committed support network is needed to help the patient's treatment attendance as well as to encourage the patient's use of treated language behaviors in his or her daily environment (Blackstone & Berg, 2003; Patterson & Wells, 1995; Payne, 1997; Wells, 1999). Indeed, in an article assessing factors that predict optimal post-stroke progress, Evans et al. (1991) found that a patient does significantly better when the primary support person is not depressed, is married, is knowledgeable about stroke care, and is from a functional rather than dysfunctional family. These authors suggest that caregiver-related problems can have a collective effect on rehabilitation outcome and that treatment should therefore reduce caregiver depression, perhaps through participation in activities and in life (Chapey et al., 2000), minimize family dysfunction, and increase the family's knowledge about stroke care. These goals are often difficult to achieve in modern times with family structures that vary and in the presence of multifaceted, busy lives. Tompkins and colleagues (Tompkins et al., 1990; 1987) also stress the importance of developing more reliable and valid measures of social networks and support resources to facilitate statements concerning prognosis.

Paramount in helping families support their significant others with aphasia is education. Families need differing amounts and types of information at different stages in the course of aphasia (Avent, 2005; Avent et al., 2005; Purdy & Hindenlang, 2005). Families with an adequate amount and type of information will be better able to support assessment and treatment activities, and to learn to live with aphasia within a productive family network.

In summary, it should be noted that no one factor discussed above consistently determines a patient's progress and success in therapy, and despite the best intentions, the optimal recovery environment may not be easily created. Clinicians and families should work cooperatively to construct a positive support network for treatment. If a patient seems to have reached a performance plateau, perhaps changing an element of treatment for a trial period would be appropriate before a final decision is reached about termination or postponement of intervention.

Goal 11: Specification and Prioritization of Intervention Goals

In an excellent chapter entitled "From Assessment to Intervention: Problems and Solutions," Snyder (1983) proposes that making the transition from assessment to intervention is like trying to solve a puzzle. Specifically, she stated that "success in solving puzzles seems to require that we have . . . only the correct pieces" (p. 160). Snyder also noted that the assessment process may be lengthy as ". . . it takes time and effort to identify and discard the wrong pieces.

Further we need to be able to conceptualize how the pieces fit together and operate as a whole. The puzzle is not really solved unless it fits together and works" (p. 160). There is no one solution to the assessment-intervention puzzle, particularly when working with patients with aphasia for whom variability is the norm.

The transition from assessment to treatment must be viewed from several perspectives, one of which is the theoretic model that underlies the communication deficit or the approach to treatment. Four recently published books guide clinicians through the process of assessment and treatment from theoretic bases: Hillis (2002a), Murray & Clark (2006), Nadeau et al. (2000), and Whitworth et al. (2005). Each of these books is written from a different theoretic perspective; however, each considers the transition from assessment to treatment as a dynamic process that is driven by a theoretic model and by data.

During the data-collection phase of assessment, the puzzle pieces are gathered and subsequently assembled into the puzzle frame during attempts to organize, systematize, and condense the data in a meaningful way. The "assembly" phase of assessment involves a sophisticated clinical judgment that is applied to the information collected. It is an evaluation of the type, frequency, and pattern of behaviors produced by the patient, an identification of influential biographic, medical, and social variables, and an exploration of the interrelatedness of these various behaviors and variables to specify and prioritize intervention goals.

Within the context of the WHO ICF (ICF, 2001), both the data-collection and hypothesis-formation phases of assessment target the three components of body structure and function, activities, and participation. Indeed, all three areas are the focus of both assessment and intervention from the onset of a clinician's acquaintance with a patient and should not be viewed merely as carryover goals (Chapey et al., 2000). Treatment goals should be created to address any language deficit, but in addition must assist a person with aphasia in progressing toward his or her life goals (Duchan & Black, 2001). Byng and Duchan (2005) discussed the social model of disability and how it might apply to aphasia therapy. The social model of therapy can be used in conjunction with other treatment models as it is intended to relate to the beliefs and attitudes of the clinician and foster a positive rehabilitation environment between the clinician and the patient. Siegert and Taylor (2004) suggested that recognition of theories of goals and motivation should be part of the rehabilitation planning process in an effort to maximize any treatment gains.

For all three WHO ICF levels, aphasia treatment is a multidimensional process that often requires a succession of treatment techniques and methods (Duchan & Black, 2001; Murray & Chapey, 2001; van Harskamp & Visch-Brink, 1991). However, the usual focus of treatment is on auditory comprehension and spoken-language production since these are the most essential components of daily communication for most people. Reading and writing may be used to facilitate or to cue listening and speaking skills but may not typically be the central focus of therapy. Regardless of the language modality to be targeted in treatment, emphasis is primarily focused on improving comprehension and production of meaning and informational content by the patient with aphasia, and on improving functional use of language in everyday communication activities and environments. Language forms become the focus of therapy only when they are needed to increase the meaning of language and the functions for which language can be used. Indeed, too much attention to the formal linguistic aspects of language may impede the communicative act (van Harskamp & Visch-Brink, 1991). Although a typical session may integrate cognitive, linguistic, and pragmatic goals, the facilitation of meaning, of functional language, of activities, and of life participation should be viewed as the core of language treatment (Murray & Chapey 2001).

Specific treatment goals are formulated by analyzing descriptions of the patient's language and life and determining the area that is most in need of intervention (Chapey et al., 2000). Patterns of strengths and weaknesses are identified to determine behaviors that might be used as a base on which to build more functional and more complex responses (Chapey, 1994). For example, in the activities area, treatment may be initiated at the level at which the patient just begins to experience difficulty in one or more of the following: accuracy, responsiveness, completeness, promptness, and efficiency of behavior (Brookshire, 1972; 1976; Murray & Chapey, 2001). An alternate approach to treatment has been suggested by Kiran and Thompson (2003), who showed that training complex items in treatment facilitated generalization to untrained items that were less complex. Additional research is expanding the goals to which this technique may be applied.

In addition to setting target responses, the stimulus variables and response conditions that facilitate increasingly accurate responses should be defined so that they may be used during therapy (Murray & Chapey, 2001). For example, during assessment, the clinician may note that the patient responds more accurately to visual rather than auditory stimuli, or responds more quickly and accurately when using gestures rather than speech; consequently, the clinician can capitalize upon this information when developing treatment goals and activities. In treatment, the clinician may begin with and build on the patient's strengths to optimize initial success (Chapey, 1986; 1994). As Rosenbek and colleagues (1989) note, once the persons with aphasia's "strengths have been enhanced, they can be used in combination with weaknesses" (p. 138).

Goals and strategies, then, are selected on the basis of assessment results that show communicative behaviors that the patient with aphasia can already produce either consistently or inconsistently, behaviors that he or she can be stimulated to produce, behaviors at the point where he or she begins to have difficulty, or communicative behaviors and activities that he or she values and will need on a daily basis to participate in activities and in life. A task hierarchy is then developed (e.g., recognition of familiar one-word utterances, recognition of less familiar one-word utterances, recognition of two- to three-word familiar phrases and commands, etc.), and specific tasks and stimuli are chosen so that they are simple enough to ensure success and yet complex enough to stimulate learning, and so that they pertain to the patient's daily needs and activities (Chapey, 1986; 1994; Murray & Chapey, 2001).

The actual type of treatment that is selected will depend on what is most appropriate for a specific patient's language and communication deficits, and what is compatible with a clinician's definition of aphasia (Chapey, 1994; Nadeau et al., 2000). By far, the largest number of approaches and the most widely accepted approaches to aphasia therapy can be described as stimulation approaches (Duffy & Coelho, 2001). This concept, first suggested by Schuell et al. (1955), emphasizes that the recovery process is a reorganization and retrieval of disrupted language processes rather than the relearning of highly specific language responses. Specific examples of various approaches to aphasia treatment are presented in subsequent chapters of this text. In many instances, an eclectic, multidimensional approach involving two or perhaps three of these approaches may be used (Byng et al., 1990; Chapey, 1994; Holland & Thompson, 1998; Murray & Chapey, 2001). This viewpoint recognizes the importance of the expertise, the competence, and the judgment of the clinician in using existing knowledge and appropriate tools, and in establishing an individualized regimen for each of his or her patients with aphasia. This viewpoint also acknowledges that patients with aphasia and their caregivers and families may present with a variety of difficulties, and that treatment must not only address language impairments, but also the social, emotional, and vocational activity limitations and participation restrictions that may accompany these language impairments (ICF, 2001; Simmons-Mackie, 2001).

Regardless of approach, the main objective of treatment is to increase a patient's success in using language and related behaviors (e.g., drawing, gestures) to exchange information and ultimately to improve communication and participation in real life (Chapey et al., 2000; van Harskamp & Visch-Brink, 1991). That is, the objective is to enable patients with aphasia to regain as much language and communication as possible, and to accommodate or compensate for their language and communication impairments as best they can, so that they can participate in their daily personal, social, and vocational activities to the fullest extent to which they are capable. The objective of the rehabilitative process, then, is to increase the productive use of cognitive, linguistic, and pragmatic skills in spontaneous communication, activities, and life participation to the optimum level possible.

Future Trends

Development of Assessment Tools

We still have a great deal to learn about assessment. We can begin this journey by developing more assessment tools (tests, protocols, and coding systems for evaluating behavior) that are psychometrically rigorous, accurate, in-depth, efficient, and clinically relevant. These tools should be standardized and nonstandardized; unstructured, moderately structured, and highly structured; and reliable and modifiable. With respect to the WHO framework (ICF, 2001), the majority of existing assessment tools focus on examining the four language modalities of aphasia at the impairment level; new tests and protocols should include assessment of the activity and participation levels as well. Over the past decade several new aphasia measures have been developed that have the aim of identifying personal activity abilities and limitations, and quantifying and qualifying the consequences of aphasia at the society participation level (Chapey et al., 2001; Holland & Thompson, 1998; Simmons-Mackie, 2001; Simmons-Mackie & Damico, 1996; Worrall et al., 2002). Many of these instruments, although theoretically well-founded, lack demonstrated psychometric rigor, such as that obtained from validity and reliability studies. Consequently, there is a need for further development of tools to assess activity and participation-level abilities and restrictions among patients with aphasia. In addition, refinement and continued development of tools to evaluate the adjustment to aphasia by family members and caregivers is important. Development and use of these tools should take into account the psychosocial status and communication patterns and needs of these individuals as well as their perceptions of their quality of life, and the degree of their role limitations while living with an individual with aphasia (Warren, 1999; Zemva, 1999).

Developing and field-testing an assessment measure is a resource-intensive task (Chapey, 1992; Murray & Chapey, 2001). Several factors present obstacles to test development, such as lack of time within a full-time professional position, funding for development, and pressure for accountability brought about by public and insurance funding of habilitation and rehabilitation (Chapey, 1994). The term "accountability" comes from the words "to account" and means "to furnish a justifying analysis or explanation" (Webster's New Collegiate Dictionary, 1977). Being accountable for one's work is laudable. However, the system of accountability that appears to have emerged is "cost accounting," which does not foster meaningful, functional communication, or reflect current definitions of language, communication, learning, and activities and life participation.

Emphasis on economy rather than therapy effectiveness affects current clinical practice. Specifically, government and private health-care agencies designate that the behaviors that will be produced by the patient in treatment must be specified in writing in advance (Murray & Chapey, 2001). That is, goals are usually operationally written, such as "By the end of this session, John will name three kinds of fruit." This leads to what Frattali (1992) called a deficit-oriented approach to intervention. Current accountability, then, often involves assessing whether the patient reached criterion, or the expected level of performance. Within this framework of accountability, assessment and intervention target specific language modalities that are discrete, highly measurable, surface-structure behaviors that can be predicted in advance and that primarily reflect short-term outcomes (Chapey, 1994). Consequently, this practice encourages a "skills approach" (Chapey, 1992; 1994; Frattali, 1992) to treatment rather than targeting functional communication within a meaningful context and/or activity, or rather than addressing changes in patients' and caregivers' life participation, or perceptions and expectations of themselves and their communicative interactions. All of the latter may be more difficult to measure via long-term outcomes but are far more important to the patient and family.

Tools to Reflect Different Perspectives
of Communication Needs

It is clear that future development of assessment instruments must include several perspectives of an individual's communication needs: ICF levels of impairment and activity/participation; functional communication in multiple communication situations; quality-of-life measurements for an individual with aphasia and for his or her family members and /or caregivers; and cognitive deficits underlying communication deficits. There will likely be many assessment tools developed in the coming years (Worrall et al., 2002). Two challenges to the field of speech-language pathology, and to related fields of study such as cognitive neuropsychology, present themselves to persons who accept the challenges of creating new assessment tools. The first challenge is to create a tool that is psychometrically rigorous yet can be easily used in a clinical environment. As discussed previously, many tools are well-constructed yet do not lend themselves to efficient use in a clinical setting. Examples of efforts in this direction are studies that correlate behavior from different tools in an attempt to find the best predictor of behavior that is also most efficient (e.g., Doyle, Goda, & Spencer, 1995).

The second challenge is for clinicians to apply rigorous criteria when evaluating and selecting tools for use in assessment. Clinicians should consider the needs of the patient, constraints of the practice setting (e.g., acute-care facility or home care) and consequences to the patient and to the diagnostic outcome of using the tool (Messick, 1980). Many sources describe psychometric properties and how to use them to evaluate a test (Shipley & McAfee, 2004), and it will be important for clinicians to use these sources.

Tools to Differentiate Disorders and Levels of Performance

Several current tools differentiate types of aphasia (e.g., BDAE); however, disagreement exists among them. Tools to better differentially diagnose aphasia as well as to describe observed behavior in more depth than is often currently possible will be important contributions to clinical practice. Studies that investigate the use of current assessment tools in creative ways will further assist clinicians in conducting appropriate and meaningful assessments. In addition, improved tools to assess cognitive deficits that underlie communication deficits will aid clinicians in understanding and relating the linguistic and nonlinguistic aspects of performance. These activities will lead to increased sensitivity and specificity during assessment, and ultimately assist in treatment planning.

Evidence-Based Practice

Evidence-based practice (EBP) is a method of clinical decision-making that incorporates information from three sources: current, high-quality research literature; clinical experience; and patient values and preferences (Evidence-based practice, 2005; Sackett et al., 1996). It is important to acknowledge that any one of these three areas independently cannot provide sufficient evidence for clinical decisions. The combination of information from three areas viewed as a unit will support clinical decision-making.

Two primary activities contribute to efforts in the first piece of EBP: reading systematic reviews in topic areas and reading individual research articles. Several groups and individuals have published systematic reviews or meta-analyses of topics in neurogenic communication disorders. Four examples of efforts in this direction are the published guidelines from the National Center for Evidence-Based Practice in Communication Disorders, which is part of the American Speech-Language-Hearing Association (The N-CEP Registry of Clinical Practice Guidelines and Systematic Reviews, 2005), practice guidelines from the Academy of Neurologic Communication Disorders and Sciences (Frattali et al., 2003), the Royal College of Speech Language Therapists (Royal College of Speech and Language Therapists: Clinical Guidelines, 2005), and Robey (1998). Using these resources as a starting point allows the clinician to be efficient in finding evidence to support clinical decisions. Currently most of the systematic reviews relate to treatment of communication disorders rather than assessment. Systematic reviews of the various assessment tools used with different populations and in various clinical set-

tings will be important to develop in the future. A cautionary note is appropriate as there is often more evidence available than is published (Elman, 2006; Robey, 1998).

The second piece of EBP is observation from clinical practice. Clinicians recognize the importance to accurate diagnosis of observing and documenting a patient's performance across several activities. Systematically documenting specific aspects of patients' behavior during assessment activities across multiple patients, clinicians, and clinical settings, and collectively sharing this information, will result in a database of clinical opinion that complements published research studies.

Finally, the third piece of EBP is opinions and perspectives from patients and their families. While the manner in which a clinician conducts assessments may remain relatively consistent across patients, data from an individual assessment will be patient-specific. These data will be valuable in further assessment activities for a patient and in treatment planning. Further, any anecdotal information exchanged between clinicians will contribute to the shared knowledge base.

Taken together, the three pieces of evidence-based practice are critical to guide future practices in assessment of persons with aphasia and other neurogenic communication disorders. However, clinicians have reported that obstacles, such as lack of time, may prevent the use of EBP principles (Dollaghan, 2004; Zipolo & Kennedy, 2005).

Functional Communication, Quality of Life, and Living with Aphasia

Future efforts in assessment must continue to refine methods of examining functional communication skills in persons with aphasia as they communicate with family members and others in their environment. While assessment activities at the ICF level of impairment are important to the assessment process, defining language and communication only in terms of measurable and specific surface structures seems to miss the very core of what constitutes language and communication. Meaning is the essence of language, and language and communication are like an iceberg—much of what is meant and communicated is below the surface; only a small portion of the communication is spoken or written or heard or read (Chapey, 1992; 1994). Likewise, this approach to aphasia assessment and treatment minimizes or ignores the many societal factors (e.g., perceptions and actions of family, friends, or co-workers) that may interact with the patient's language and communication abilities, and, consequently, the degree of participation restriction they experience (Simmons-Mackie, 2001; Simmons-Mackie & Damico, 1996).

A positive QOL is an important factor in a person's life. Perceptions of the patients and their caregivers are legitimate outcome measures, and future efforts aimed at refining the measures currently used to quantify and qualify the effects of aphasia on the societal participation of our patients and their families, as well as developing new measures, are important clinical research activities. As a field, we must continue to search for a consensus of which core elements constitute functional communication and contribute to QOL, and create assessment tools that have relevance to communicative functioning in a variety of clinical settings as well as outside clinical settings in daily communicative environments (Frattali, 1998b). Of particular value in achieving this goal is the development of multi-dimensional assessment protocols that are thorough (and therefore measure a range of performance and outcomes), reliable, and sensitive to changes over time.

When a person is diagnosed with aphasia, he or she and his or her family members will live with aphasia. An important direction in developing assessment tools is to advance the notion that it is critical to determine the effects of aphasia and, subsequently, treatments for aphasia, on the communicative abilities of patients with aphasia and their families, as well as on the social well-being of patients and their caregivers. Clinicians must be committed to conveying this message to political and fiscal policy-makers so that we can deliver the first-rate care that our patients with aphasia deserve.

KEY POINTS

1. A thorough assessment of language and communication should include evaluation of an individual's cognitive, linguistic, and pragmatic abilities, and quality of life for the patient and his or her family or caregivers.

2. The goal of assessment is typically multifold in that etiologic (e.g., the determination of the presence of aphasia and concomitant problems), cognitive/linguistic/pragmatic (e.g., the identification of specific language strengths and weaknesses), communicative facilitators and obstacles (e.g., events and persons who support or inhibit communication), social aspects of living with aphasia (e.g., activity and participation limitations or restrictions), quality of life (e.g., life satisfaction for a patient and family), and treatment goals (e.g., the provision of insight into possible treatment candidacy and treatment procedures) should be specified and accomplished.

3. During assessment data should be obtained through reported observations and direct observations, which may be unstructured (e.g., conversation), moderately structured (e.g., procedural discourse task), highly structured (e.g., a traditional aphasia battery) and nonstandardized (e.g., experimental protocols).

4. Prior to administering any test or procedure clinicians should examine its psychometric adequacy in terms of reliability and validity.

5. The integrity of cognitive and executive-function abilities should be determined because deficits in these areas may negatively affect production of language and communication skills as well as acquisition of new knowledge.

6. Comprehension and production of language content (i.e., meaning) and language form (i.e., phonology, morphology, and syntax) must be assessed using stimuli that vary in length, complexity, and familiarity. Listening, speaking, reading, writing, and use of alternative or augmentative communication systems (e.g., drawing, gesturing, or using an electronic device) must be assessed.

7. Pragmatic abilities across a variety of communication contexts and partners and with differing amounts of support must be assessed. Functional communication skills should be assessed to determine the interaction of a patient's cognitive, linguistic, and pragmatic abilities during communication in daily life activities.

8. Factors that contribute to successful or unsuccessful communication activities should be identified in assessment (e.g., medical, neuropsychological, or social supports or hindrances). This evaluation should include quality of life-assessment for both patients and their family members and caregivers.

9. Following data collection, clinicians must synthesize the assessment data to form hypotheses concerning the nature and extent of the patient's language and communication deficits. In particular, clinicians should be able to summarize the nature and extent of a patient's language impairment, personal-activity limitations, and societal-participation restrictions within the context of the WHO model of functioning and disability.

10. Future trends in assessment should focus on developing tools that are psychometrically rigorous and clinically relevant, that reflect different perspectives of communication needs, and that differentiate neurogenic communication disorders and levels of performance. Clinicians should also engage in the principles of evidence-based practice. Finally, as assessment activities become increasingly refined, they should encompass all levels of the WHO ICF to assess the nature and extent of the language impairment as well as the effect on activities and life participation for a patient and his or her family.

1. Pretend that you have been hired to develop a speech-language pathology department in a rehabilitation hospital. In particular, your department will specialize in serving adults with acquired language disorders. Keeping in mind that you have a limited budget to purchase assessment tools and materials, list which unstructured, moderately-structured, highly-structured, and nonstandard observational tools you will purchase. Justify your selection. How and why might this list differ if your department was located in an acute-care hospital or a skilled-nursing facility, or if you were working in home health care?

2. Describe and justify what the assessment battery might be for assessing the cognitive, linguistic, and pragmatic abilities, and quality of life for a patient who was described as "mildly aphasic with reading and writing difficulties" as a result of a bedside evaluation.

3. Imagine you have been given a referral to assess the language and communication abilities of an individual who is 79 years old, who was previously diagnosed with aphasia, and who has a history of bilateral strokes. What complicating conditions might be expected, and how will the assessment process take into consideration their possible effects?

4. Using the WHO ICF model as a guide, design and justify an assessment battery to evaluate the nature and extent of language and communication abilities and quality of life for a person with global aphasia and who is a resident in a skilled-nursing facility. How might this battery differ if the patient lived at home with a spouse who was able to provide appropriate care and companionship?

5. Describe how you would measure outcome of treatment and justify treatment recommendations using data from unstructured, moderately-structured, highly-structured, and nonstandardized observational tools.

6. Review the research literature, consult with colleagues, and review anecdotal information from your clinical practice or experience to determine the presence (or absence) of evidence supporting the use of an assessment tool in the following areas:
   (a) oral naming
   (b) written word finding
   (c) production of spoken morphosyntax
   (d) oral discourse production (conversational and procedural)
   (e) written narrative production
   (f) reading comprehension
   (g) production of speech acts
   (h) depression
   (i) visual neglect
   (j) executive functioning
   (k) quality of life

References

Adamovich, B. L. B. (2005). Traumatic brain injury. In L. L. LaPointe (Ed.), *Aphasia and related neurogenic language disorders* (pp. 225–236). New York: Thieme.

Adamovich, B. L. B., & Henderson, J. (1992). *Scales for Cognitive Ability for Traumatic Brain Injury*. Chicago: Riverside.

Agrell, B., & Dehlin, O. (1989). Comparison of six depression rating scales in geriatric stroke patients. *Stroke, 20*, 1190–1194.

Aichert, I., & Ziegler, W. (2004). Segmental and metrical encoding in aphasia: Two case reports. *Aphasiology, 18*(12), 1201–1211.

Albert, M. L., & Sandson, J. (1986). Perseveration in aphasia. *Cortex, 22*, 103–115.

Alexander, M. P., & Loverso, F. (1993). A specific treatment for global aphasia. *Clinical Aphasiology, 21*, 277–289.

Al-Khawaja, I., Wade, D. T., & Collin, C. F. (1996). Bedside screening for aphasia: A comparison of two methods. *Journal of Neurology, 243*(2), 201–204.

Allchin, J., & Patterson, J. P. (2000). *Effects of a semantic based treatment strategy on naming and discourse skills*. Paper presented at the American Speech-Language-Hearing Association, Washington, D.C.

Allen, M., & Badecker, W. (2001). Morphology: The internal structure of words. In B. Rapp (Ed.), *The handbook of cognitive neuropsychology: What deficits reveal about the human mind* (pp. 211–232). New York: Psychological Press.

Allport, D. A. (1986). Distributed memory, modular subsystems and dysphasia. In S. Newman & R. Epstein (Eds.), *Current perspectives in dysphasia* (pp. 32–60). New York: Churchill Livingstone.

Anastasi, A., & Urbani, F. (1996). *Psychological testing* (7th ed.). New York: Prentice-Hall.

Ardila, A. (1995). Directions of research in cross-cultural neuropsychology. *Journal of Clinical and Experimental Neuropsychology, 17*, 143–150.

Armstrong, E. (1987). Cohesive harmony in aphasic discourse and its significance to listener perception of coherence. *Clinical Aphasiology, 17*, 210–215.

Armstrong, E. (2000). Aphasia discourse analysis: The story so far. *Aphasiology, 14*(9), 875–892.

Armstrong, E. (2001). Connecting lexical patterns of verb usage with discourse meanings in aphasia. *Aphasiology, 15*(10–11), 1029–1045.

Armstrong, E. (2002). Variation in the discourse of non-brain-damaged speakers on a clinical task. *Aphasiology, 16*(4–6), 647–658.

Armstrong, E. (2005). Expressing opinions and feelings in aphasia: Linguistic options. *Aphasiology, 19*(3–5), 285–295.

Austin, J. (1962). *How to do things with words*. Oxford: Oxford University Press.

Avent, J. (2005). *Validation of the importance of information about aphasia*. Paper presented at the Clinical Aphasiology Conference, Sanibel, FL.

Avent, J., Glista, S., Wallace, S., Jackson, J., Nishioka, J., & Yip, W. (2005). Family information needs about aphasia. *Aphasiology, 19*(3–5), 365–375.

Avent, J., Wertz, R. T., & Auther, L. L. (1998). Relationship between language impairment and pragmatic behavior in aphasic adults. *Journal of Neurolinguistics, 11,* 207–221.

Baddeley, A. D. (1986). *Working memory.* New York: Oxford University Press.

Badecker, W., & Caramazza, A. (1987). The analysis of morphological errors in a case of acquired dyslexia. *Brain and Language, 32,* 278–305.

Bailey, S., Powell, G., & Clark, E. (1981). A note on intelligence and recovery from aphasia: The relationship between Raven's Matrices scores and change on the Schuell aphasia test. *British Journal of Disorders of Communication, 16,* 193–203.

Baines, K. A., Heeringa, H. M., & Martin, A. W. (1999). *Assessment of Language-related Functional Activities.* Austin, TX: Pro-Ed.

Baker, E., Blumstein, S. E., & Goodglass, H. (1981). Interaction between phonological and semantic factors in auditory comprehension. *Neuropsychologia, 19,* 1–15.

Baker, E., & Goodglass, H. (1976). Semantic field, naming, and auditory comprehension in aphasia. *Brain and Language, 3*(3), 359–374.

Baker, R. (2000). The assessment of functional communication in culturally and linguistically diverse populations. In L. E. Worrall & C. M. Frattali (Eds.), *Neurogenic communication disorders: A functional approach* (pp. 81–100). New York: Thieme.

Ball, M., Davies, E., Duckworth, M., & Middlehurst, R. (1991). Assessing the assessments: A comparison of two clinical pragmatic profiles. *Journal of Communication Disorders, 24,* 367–379.

Ballard, K. J., Granier, J. P., & Robin, D. A. (2000). Understanding the nature of apraxia of speech: Theory, analysis and treatment. *Aphasiology, 14*(10), 969–995.

Barker-Collo, S. L. (2001). The 60-item Boston Naming Test: Cultural bias and possible adaptations for New Zealand. *Aphasiology, 15,* 85–92.

Barona, A., Reynolds, C., & Chastain, R. (1984). A demographically based index of premorbid intelligence for the WAIS-R. *Journal of Clinical and Consulting Psychology, 52,* 885–887.

Bartels-Tobin, L. R., & Hinckley, J. J. (2005). Cognition and discourse production in right hemisphere disorder. *Journal of Neurolinguistics, 18*(6), 461–477.

Bartlett, C. L., & Pashek, G. V. (1994). Taxonomic theory and practical implications in aphasia classification. *Aphasiology, 8*(2), 103–126.

Basso, A. (1987). Approaches to neuropsychological rehabilitation: Language disorders. In M. Meier, A. L. Benton, & L. Diller (Eds.), *Neuropsychological rehabilitation* (pp. 294–314). London: Churchill Livingstone.

Basso, A. (1992). Prognostic factors in aphasia. *Aphasiology, 6*(4), 337–348.

Basso, A. (2003). *Aphasia and its therapy.* Oxford: Oxford University Press.

Bastiaanse, R., Edwards, S., Mas, E., & Rispens, J. (2003). Assessing comprehension and production of verbs and sentences: The Verb and Sentence Test (VAST). *Aphasiology, 17*(1), 49–73.

Bates, D. G., & Plog, F. (1990). *Cultural anthropology* (3rd ed.). New York: Macgraw Hill.

Bates, E. (1976). *Language in context.* New York: Academic Press.

Bates, E., Friederici, A., Wulfeck, B., & Juarez, L. (1988). On the preservation of syntax in aphasia: Cross-linguistic evidence. *Brain and Language, 33,* 323–364.

Bauer, R. M. (2006). The agnosias. In P. Snyder, P. Nussbaum, & D. Robins (Eds.), *Clinical neuropsychology: A pocket handbook for assessment* (2nd ed.). Washington, DC: American Psychological Association.

Bauer, R. M., & Demery, J. A. (2003). Agnosia. In K. M. Heilman & E. Valenstein (Eds.), *Clinical neuropsychology* (pp. 236–295). New York: Oxford University Press.

Bauer, R. M., & Zawacki, T. (1997). Auditory agnosia and amusia. In T. E. Feinberg & M. J. Farah (Eds.), *Behavioral neurology and neuropsychology* (pp. 267–276). New York: McGraw-Hill.

Bayles, K. A., Boone, D. R., Tomoeda, C. K., Slauson, T. J., & Kaszniak, A. W. (1989). Differentiating Alzheimer's patients from the normal elderly and stroke patients with aphasia. *Journal of Speech and Hearing Disorders, 54,* 74–87.

Bayles, K. A., & Kaszniak, A. W. (1987). *Communication and cognition in normal aging and dementia.* San Diego: College-Hill Press.

Bayles, K. A., Kim, E., Mahendra, N., McKnight, P., Rackley, A., Tomoeda, C. K., et al. (2005). *Summary technical report number 1 - Systematic review and practice recommendations for use of spaced retrieval training with individuals with dementia.* Retrieved July 11, 2006, from http://www.ancds.org/practice.html

Bayles, K. A., & Tomoeda, C. K. (1993). *Arizona Battery for Communication Disorders of Dementia (ABCD).* Austin, TX: Pro-Ed.

Bayles, K. A., & Tomoeda, C. K. (1994). *Functional Linguistic Communication Inventory.* Tucson, AZ: Canyonlands.

Bayles, K. A., Tomoeda, C. K., Cruz, R. F., & Mahendra, N. (2000). Communication abilities of individuals with late-stage Alzheimer disease. *Alzheimer Disease and Associated Disorders, 14*(3), 176–181.

Beeke, S., Wilkinson, R., & Maxim, J. (2001). Context as a resource for the construction of turns at talk in aphasia. *Clinical Linguistics and Phonetics, 15*(1–2), 79–83.

Beeson, P., Bayles, K. A., Rubens, A. B., & Kaszniak, A. W. (1993). Memory impairment and executive control in individuals with stroke-induced aphasia. *Brain and Language, 45,* 253–275.

Beeson, P., & Holland, A. L. (1994). *Aphasia groups: An approach to long-term rehabilitation. Telerounds 19.* Tucson, AZ: National Center for Neurogenic Communication Disorders.

Belanger, S. A., Duffy, R. J., & Coelho, C. A. (1996). The assessment of limb apraxia: An investigation of task effects and their cause. *Brain and Cognition, 32,* 384–404.

Bell, B. D. (1994). Pantomime recognition impairment in aphasia: An analysis of error types. *Brain and Language, 47,* 269–278.

Benaim, C., Bruno, C., Perennou, D., & Pelissier, J. (2004). Validation of the Aphasic Depression Rating Scale. *Stroke, 35,* 1692–1696.

Benson, F. (1979). Neurologic correlates of anomia. In H. Whitaker & H. A. Whitaker (Eds.), *Studies in neurolinguistics* (Vol. 4, pp. 292–328). New York: Academic Press.

Benton, A. L., Hamsher, K., Rey, G. J., & Sivan, A. B. (1994). *Multilingual Aphasia Examination* (3rd ed.). San Antonio, TX: The Psychological Corporation.

Benton, A. L., Hamsher, K., Varney, N. R., & Spreen, O. (1993). *Contributions to neuropsychological assessment.* New York: Oxford University Press.

Benton, A. L., Smith, K., & Lang, M. (1972). Stimulus characteristics and object naming in aphasic patients. *Journal of Communication Disorders, 5,* 19–24.

Beretta, A., Pinango, M., Patterson, J. P., & Harford, C. (1999). Recruiting comparative cross-linguistic evidence to address competing accounts of agrammatic aphasia. *Brain and Language, 67*(3), 149–168.

Bergner, M., Bobbitt, R., Carter, W., & Gilson, B. (1981). The sickness impact profile: Development and final revision of a health status measure. *Medical Care, 19,* 787–805.

Berndt, R. S. (1998). Sentence processing in aphasia. In M. T. Sarno (Ed.), *Acquired aphasia* (3rd ed., pp. 229–268). New York: Academic Press.

Berndt, R. S., Burton, M. W., Haendiges, A. N., & Mitchum, C. C. (2002). Production of nouns and verbs in aphasia: Effects of elicitation context. *Aphasiology, 16*(1–2), 83–106.

Berndt, R. S., Haendiges, A. N., Burton, M. W., & Mitchum, C. C. (2002). Grammatical class and imageability in aphasia word production: Their effects are independent. *Journal of Neurolinguistics, 15*(3–5), 353–371.

Berthier, M. (2005). Post-stroke aphasia: Epidemiology, pathophysiology and treatment. *Drugs & Aging, 22*(2), 163–182.

Bird, H., & Franklin, S. (1996). Cinderella revisited: A comparison of fluent and non-fluent aphasic speech. *Journal of Neurolingustics, 9,* 187–206.

Bird, H., Franklin, S., & Howard, D. (2001). Age of acquisition and imageability ratings for a large set of words, including verbs and function words. *Behavior Research Methods, Instruments and Computers, 33*(1), 73–79.

Bishop, D. S., & Pet, R. (1995). Psychobehavioral problems other than depression in stroke. *Topics in Stroke Rehabilitation, 2,* 56–58.

Bishop, D. V. M. (2003). *Test for Reception of Grammar (TROG-2)* (2nd ed.). San Antonio, TX: Harcourt Assessment.

Bishop, D. V. M. (2005). *Test for Reception of Grammar-Electronic (TROG-E).* San Antonio, TX: Harcourt Assessment.

Blackstone, S., & Berg, M. (2003). *Social networks: A communication inventory for individuals with complex communication needs and their communication partners.* Monterey CA: Augmentative Communication.

Blair, J. R., & Spreen, O. (1989). Predicting premorbid IQ: A revision of the National Adult Reading Test. *The Clinical Neuropsychologist, 3,* 129–136.

Blake, M. L. (2005). Right hemisphere syndrome. In L. L. LaPointe (Ed.), *Aphasia and related neurogenic language disorders* (3rd ed., pp. 213–224). New York: Thieme.

Blake, M. L., Duffy, J. R., Myers, P. S., & Tompkins, C. A. (2002). Prevalence and patterns of right hemisphere cognitive/communicative deficits: Retrospective data from an inpatient rehabilitation unit. *Aphasiology, 16,* 537–548.

Blake, M. L., Duffy, J. R., Tompkins, C. A., & Myers, P. S. (2003). Right hemisphere syndrome is in the eye of the beholder. *Aphasiology, 17*(5), 423–432.

Blomert, L., Kean, M. L., Koster, C., & Schokker, J. (1994). Amsterdam-Nijmegen Everyday Language Test: Construction, reliability, and validity. *Aphasiology, 8,* 381–407.

Blonder, L. X., Heilman, K. M., Ketterson, T., Rosenbek, J., Raymer, A. M., Crosson, B., et al. (2005). Affective facial expression and lexical expression in aprosodic versus aphasic stroke patients. *Journal of the International Neuropsychological Society, 11*(6), 677–685.

Bloom, R. L., Borod, J. C., Santschi-Haywood, C., Pick, L. H., & Obler, L. K. (1996). Left and right hemisphere contributions to discourse coherence and cohesion. *International Journal of Neuroscience, 88*(1–2), 125–140.

Blumstein, S. E. (1998). Phonological aspects of aphasia. In M. T. Sarno (Ed.), *Acquired Aphasia* (3rd ed., pp. 129–151). New York: Academic Press.

Blumstein, S. E., Katz, B., Goodglass, H., Shrier, R., & Dworetsky, B. (1985). The effects of slowed speech on auditory comprehension in aphasia. *Brain and Language, 24,* 246–265.

Boles, L. (1997). A comparison of naming errors in individuals with mild naming impairment following post-stroke aphasia, Alzheimer disease, and traumatic brain injury. *Aphasiology, 11,* 1043–1056.

Boles, L., & Bombard, T. (1998). Conversational discourse analysis: Appropriate and useful sample sizes. *Aphasiology, 12,* 547–560.

Boller, F., Cole, M., Virtunski, P. B., Patterson, M., & Kim, Y. (1979). Paralinguistic aspects of auditory comprehension in aphasia. *Brain and Language, 7,* 164–174.

Booth, S., & Perkins, L. (1999). The use of conversation analysis to guide individualized advice to carers and evaluate change in aphasia: A case study. *Aphasiology, 13,* 283–304.

Borkowski, J. G., & Burke, J. E. (1996). Theories, models, and measurements of executive functioning. In G. R. Lyon & N. A. Krasnegor (Eds.), *Attention, memory, and executive function* (pp. 235–261). Baltimore, MD: Paul H. Brookes.

Bourgeois, M. S. (2005). Dementia. In L. L. LaPointe (Ed.), *Aphasia and related neurogenic language disorders* (3rd ed., pp. 199–212). New York: Thieme.

Bowers, L., Barrett, M., Huisingh, R., Orman, J., & LoGuidice, C. (1991). *TOPS-Adolescent: Test of Problem Solving.* East Moline, IL: LinguiSystems.

Bowers, L., Huisingh, R., LoGiudice, C., & Orman, J. (2005). *The Word Test-2: Adolescent.* Austin, TX: Pro-Ed.

Boyle, M., Coelho, C. A., & Kimbarow, M. L. (1991). Word fluency tasks: A preliminary analysis of variability. *Aphasiology, 5,* 171–182.

Braber, N., Patterson, K., Ellis, K., & Ralph, M. A. L. (2005). The relationship between phonological and morphological deficits in Broca's aphasia: Further evidence from errors on verb inflection. *Brain and Language, 92*(3), 278–287.

Braswell, D., Hartry, A., Noornbeek, S., Johansen, A., Johnson, L., Schultz, J., et al. (1993). *Profile of executive control system.* Puyallup, WA: Association for Neuropsychological Research and Development.

Breen, K., & Warrington, E. K. (1994). A study of anomia: Evidence for a distinction between nominal and propositional language. *Cortex, 30,* 231–245.

Brickencamp, R., & Zillmer, E. (1998). *d2 Test of attention.* Lutz, FL: Psychological Assessment Resources.

Brookshire, R. H. (1971). Effects of trial time and inter-trial interval on naming by aphasic subjects. *Journal of Communication Disorders, 3,* 289–301.

Brookshire, R. H. (1972). Effects of task difficulty on naming performance of aphasic subjects. *Journal of Speech and Hearing Research, 15,* 551–558.

Brookshire, R. H. (1976). Effects of task difficulty on sentence comprehension performance of aphasic subjects. *Journal of Communication Disorders, 9,* 167–173.

Brookshire, R. H. (2003). *Introduction to neurogenic communication disorders* (6th ed.). St. Louis: Mosby.

Brookshire, R. H., & Nicholas, L. E. (1993). A system for quantifying the informativeness and efficiency of the connected speech of adults with aphasia. *Journal of Speech and Hearing Research, 28*(4), 405–410.

Brookshire, R. H., & Nicholas, L. E. (1994). Speech sample size and test-retest stability of connected speech measures for adults with aphasia. *Journal of Speech and Hearing Research, 37,* 399–407.

Brookshire, R. H., & Nicholas, L. E. (1995). Performance deviations in the connected speech of adults with no brain damage and adults with aphasia. *American Journal of Speech-Language Pathology, 4,* 118–123.

Brookshire, R. H., & Nicholas, L. E. (1997). *The Discourse Comprehension Test.* Minneapolis, MN: BRK.

Brown, L., Sherbenou, R. J., & Johnsen, S. K. (1997). *Test of Nonverbal Intelligence* (3rd ed.). Austin, TX: Pro-Ed.

Brown, V. L., Hammill, D. D., & Wiederholt, J. L. (1995). *Test of Reading Comprehension* (3rd ed.). Austin, TX: Pro-Ed.

Brownell, H. H., & Friedman, O. (2000). Discourse ability in patients with unilateral left and right hemisphere brain damage. In R. S. Berndt (Ed.), *Language and aphasia* (2nd ed., Vol. 3, pp. 157–172). Amsterdam: Elsevier.

Brownell, H. H., Gardner, H., Prather, P., & Martino, G. (1995). Language, communication, and the right hemisphere. In H. S. Kirshner (Ed.), *Handbook of neurological speech and language disorders* (pp. 325–349). New York: Marcel Dekker.

Brumfitt, S. M., & Sheeran, P. (1999). The development and validation of the Visual Analogue Self-Esteem Scale (VASES). *British Journal of Clinical Psychology, 38,* 387–400.

Bryan, K. L. (1994). *The Right Hemisphere Language Battery* (2nd ed.). Chichester: Wiley.

Bunch, W. H., & Dvonch, V. M. (1994). The "value" of functional independence measure scores. *American Journal of Medical Rehabilitation, 73*(1), 40–43.

Burgio, F., & Basso, A. (1997). Memory and aphasia. *Neuropsychologia, 35,* 759–766.

Burns, M. (1997). *Burns Brief Inventory of Communication and Cognition.* San Antonio, TX: The Psychological Corporation.

Burns, M. (2004). Clinical management of agnosia. *Topics in Stroke Rehabilitation, 11*(1), 1–9.

Butt, P., & Bucks, R. (2004). *BNVR: The Butt Non-Verbal Reasoning Test.* Bicester, UK: Speechmark.

Buzolich, M. (1995). Empowering system users in peer training. *Augmentative and Alternative Communication, 11*(1), 37–48.

Byng, S., & Duchan, J. (2005). Social model philosophies and principles: Their applications to therapies for aphasia. *Aphasiology, 19*(10–11), 906–922.

Byng, S., Kay, J., Edmundson, A., & Scott, C. (1990). Aphasia tests reconsidered. *Aphasiology, 4,* 67–91.

Campbell, C. R., & Jackson, S. T. (1995). Transparency of one-handed AmerInd hand signals to nonfamiliar viewers. *Journal of Speech and Hearing Research, 38,* 1284–1289.

Cannito, M. P., Vogel, D., & Pierce, R. S. (1989). Sentence comprehension in context: Influence of prior visual stimulation. *Clinical Aphasiology, 18,* 432–443.

Cantor, N., & Sanderson, C. (1999). Life task participation and well-being: The importance of taking part in daily life. In D. Kahneman, E. Diener & N. Schwarz (Eds.), *Well-being* (pp. 230–243). New York: Russell Sage Foundation.

Caplan, D. (1993). Toward a psycholinguistic approach to acquired neurogenic language disorders. *American Journal of Speech-Language Pathology, 2,* 59–83.

Caplan, D., & Bub, D. (1990). *Psycholinguistic assessment of aphasia.* Paper presented at the American Speech-Language-Hearing Association, Seattle, WA.

Caplan, D., Waters, G. S., & Hildebrandt, N. (1997). Determinants of sentence comprehension in aphasic patients in sentence-picture matching tasks. *Journal of Speech, Language and Hearing Research, 40,* 542–555.

Cappa, S. F. (2005). Neuroimaging recovery from aphasia. *Neuropsychological Rehabilitation, 10*(3), 365–376.

Cappa, S. F., Moro, A., Perani, D., & Piatelli-Palmarini, M. (2000). Broca's aphasia, Broca's area, and syntax: A complex relationship. *Behavioral and Brain Sciences, 23,* 27–28.

Carmines, E. G., & Zeller, R. A. (1979). *Reliability and validity assessment.* Newbury Park, CA: Sage.

Carramazza, A., & Hillis, A. (1991). Lexical organization of nouns and verbs in the brain. *Nature (London), 349,* 788–790.

Caspari, I., Parkinson, S. R., LaPointe, L. L., & Katz, R. C. (1998). Working memory and aphasia. *Brain and Cognition, 37,* 205–223.

Chapey, R. (1983). Language-based cognitive abilities in adult aphasia: Rationale for intervention. *Journal of Communication Disorders, 16,* 405–424.

Chapey, R. (1986). Assessment of language disorders in adults. In R. Chapey (Ed.), *Language intervention strategies in adult aphasia* (2nd ed., pp. 81–140). Baltimore: Williams & Wilkins.

Chapey, R. (1992). Functional communication assessment and intervention: Some thoughts on state of the art. *Aphasiology, 6*(1), 85–93.

Chapey, R. (1994). Assessment of language disorders in adults. In R. Chapey (Ed.), *Language intervention strategies in aphasia* (3 ed., pp. 80–120). Baltimore: Williams & Wilkins.

Chapey, R. (2001). Cognitive stimulation: Stimulation of recognition/comprehension, memory, and convergent, divergent and evaluative thinking. In R. Chapey (Ed.), *Language intervention strategies in aphasia and related neurogenic communication disorders* (pp. 397–434). Philadelphia: Lippincott Williams & Wilkins.

Chapey, R., Duchan, J., Elman, R., Garcia, J., Kagan, A., Lyon, L., et al. (2001). Life participation approaches to adult aphasia: A statement of values for the future. In R. Chapey (Ed.), *Language intervention strategies in aphasia and related neurogenic communication disorders* (4th ed., pp. 235–245). Philadelphia: Lippincott Williams & Wilkins.

Chapey, R., Elman, R., Duchan, J., Garcia, J., Kagan, A., Lyon, L., et al. (2000). Life participation approaches to adult aphasia: A statement of values for the future. *ASHA Leader, 5,* 3.

Chapey, R., & Lu, S. (1998). Intercultural variations of specific pragmatic aspects of language: Implications for the assessment and treatment of aphasia: Unpublished document.

Chapman, S., Highley, A. P., & Thompson, J. L. (1998). Discourse in fluent aphasia and Alzheimer's disease: Linguistic and pragmatic considerations. *Journal of Neurolinguistics, 11,* 55–78.

Chatterjee, A., & Maher, L. M. (2000). Grammar and agrammatism. In S. E. Nadeau, L. J. Rothi, & B. Crosson (Eds.), *Aphasia and language: Theory to practice* (pp. 133–156). New York: Guilford Press.

Cherney, L. R. (2002). Unilateral neglect: A disorder of attention. *Seminars in Speech and Language, 23*(2), 117–128.

Cherney, L. R., Shadden, B. B., & Coelho, C. A. (1998). *Analyzing discourse in communicatively impaired adults.* Gaithersburg, MD: Aspen.

Christensen, A. L. (1975). *Luria's neuropsychological investigation.* New York: Spectrum.

Clarfield, A. M. (2003). The decreasing prevalence of reversible dementias: An updated meta-analysis. *Archives of Internal Medicine, 163*(18), 2219–2229.

Clark, D. G., Charuvastra, A., Miller, B., Shapira, J. S., & Mendex, M. F. (2005). Fluent versus nonfluent primary progressive aphasia: A comparison of clinical and functional neuroimaging features. *Brain and Language, 94*(1), 54–60.

Cockburn, J., Wilson, B., Baddeley, A., & Hieorns, R. (1990). Assessing everyday memory in patients with dysphasia. *British Journal of Clinical Psychology, 29*, 353–360.

Code, C. (2003). The quantity of life for people with chronic aphasia. *Neuropsychological Rehabilitation, 13*(3), 379–390.

Code, C., Hemsley, G., & Herrmann, M. (1999). The emotional impact of aphasia. *Seminars in Speech and Language, 20*, 19–31.

Code, C., & Hermann, M. (2005). The relevance of emotional and psychosocial factors in aphasia to rehabilitation. *Neuropsychological Rehabilitation, 13*(1/2), 109–132.

Coelho, C. (2002). Story narratives of adults with closed head injury and non-brain-injured adults. *Journal of Speech, Language and Hearing Research, 45*, 1232–1248.

Coelho, C., Grela, B., Corso, M., Gamble, A., & Feinn, R. (2005). Microlinguistic deficits in the narrative discourse of adults with traumatic brain injury. *Brain Injury, 19*(13), 1139–1145.

Coelho, C., Liles, B. Z., Duffy, R. J., Clarkson, J. V., & Elia, D. (1994). Longitudinal assessment of narrative discourse in a mildly aphasic adult. *Clinical Aphasiology, 22*, 145–155.

Coelho, C., Ylvisaker, M., & Turkstra, L. (2005). Nonstandardized assessment approaches for individuals with traumatic brain injuries. *Seminars in Speech and Language, 26*(4), 223–241.

Cohan, M. (1997). Stages of dementia: An overview. In C. R. Kovach (Ed.), *Late-stage dementia care: A basic guide* (pp. 3–11). Philadelphia: Taylor & Francis.

Cole-Virtue, J., & Nickels, L. (2004). Why cabbage and not carrot?: An investigation of factors affecting performance on spoken word to picture matching. *Aphasiology, 18*(2), 153–179.

Conlon, C. P., & McNeil, M. R. (1989). The efficacy of treatment for two globally aphasic adults using visual action therapy. *Clinical Aphasiology, 19*, 185–195.

Connors, C. K. (2000). *Connor's Continuous Performance Test-II.* Toronto, Canada: Multi-Health Systems.

Cordes, A. K. (1994). The reliability of observational data: I. Theories and methods for speech-language pathology. *Journal of Speech and Hearing Research, 37*, 264–278.

Coslett, H. B. (2000). Language and attention. In R. S. Berndt (Ed.), *Language and aphasia* (2nd ed., Vol. 3, pp. 257–268). Amsterdam: Elsevier.

Craig, A. H., & Cummings, J. L. (1995). Neuropsychiatric aspects of aphasia. In H. S. Kirshner (Ed.), *Handbook of neurological speech and language disorders* (pp. 483–498). New York: Marcel Dekker.

Craig, H. (1983). Applications of pragmatic language models for intervention. In T. Gallagher & C. Prutting (Eds.), *Pragmatic assessment and intervention issues in language* (pp. 101–129). San Diego, CA: College Hill Press.

Crary, M. A., Haak, N. J., & Malinsky, A. E. (1989). Preliminary psychometric evaluation of an acute aphasia screening protocol. *Aphasiology, 3*, 611–618.

Crary, M. A., Wertz, R. T., & Deal, J. L. (1992). Classifying aphasias: Cluster analysis of Western Aphasia Battery and Boston Diagnostic Aphasia Examination. *Aphasiology, 6*(1), 29–36.

Crockford, C., & Lesser, R. (1994). Assessing functional communication in aphasia: Clinical utility and time demands of three methods. *European Journal of Disorders of Communication, 29*(2), 165–182.

Cronbach, L. J. (1990). *Essentials of psychological testing* (4th ed.). New York: Harper and Row.

Cropley, A. (1967). *Creativity.* London: Longman.

Crosson, B., Moore, A., Gopinath, K., White, K., Wierenga, C., Gaiefsky, M., et al. (2005). Role of right and left hemispheres in recovery of function during treatment of intention in aphasia. *Journal of Cognitive Neuroscience, 17*, 392–406.

Croteau, C., Vychytil, A. M., Larfeuil, C., & LeDorze, G. (2004). "Speaking for" behaviors in spouses of people with aphasia: A descriptive study of six couples in an interview situation. *Aphasiology, 18*(4), 291–312.

Cruice, M., Worrall, L., Hickson, L., & Murison, R. (2003). Finding a focus for quality of life with aphasia: Social and emotional health, and psychological well-being. *Aphasiology, 17*(4), 333–353.

Cruice, M., Worral, L., Hickson, L., & Murison, R. (2005). Measuring quality of life: Comparing family members' and friends' ratings with those of their aphasic partners. *Aphasiology, 19*(2), 111–129.

Cuetos, F., Aguado, G., & Caramazza, A. (2000). Dissociation of semantic and phonological errors in naming. *Brain and Language, 75*, 451–460.

Cummings, J. L., & Trimble, M. R. (2002). *Concise guide to neuropsychiatry and behavioral neurology.* Arlington, VA: American Psychiatric Association.

Cunningham, R., Farrow, V., Davies, C., & Lincoln, N. (1995). Reliability of the assessment of communicative effectiveness in severe aphasia. *European Journal of Disorders of Communication, 30*, 1–16.

Cunningham, R., & Ward, C. D. (2003). Evaluation of a training programme to facilitate conversation between people with aphasia and their partners. *Aphasiology, 17*(8), 687–707.

Curtiss, S., MacSwan, J., Schaeffer, J., Kural, M., & Sano, T. (2004). GCS: A grammatical coding system for natural language data. *Behavior Research Methods, Instruments and Computers, 36*(3), 459–480.

Dabul, B. (2000). *Apraxia Battery for Adults (ABA-2)* (2nd ed.). Austin, TX: Pro-Ed.

Damico, J. S., Simmons-Mackie, N., Oelshlaeger, M., Elman, R., & Armstrong, E. (1999). Qualitative methods in aphasia research: Basic issues. *Aphasiology, 13*, 651–666.

Daniloff, J. K., Fritelli, G., Buckingham, H. W., Hoffman, P. R., & Daniloff, R. G. (1986). AmerInd versus ASL: Recognition and imitation in aphasic subjects. *Brain and Language, 28*, 95–1131.

Daniloff, J. K., Noll, J. D., Fristoe, M., & Lloyd, L. L. (1982). Gesture recognition in patients with aphasia. *Journal of Speech and Hearing Disorders, 47*, 43–49.

Darley, F. (1977). A retrospective view: Aphasia. *Journal of Speech and Hearing Disorders, 42*, 161–169.

Darley, F. (1982). *Aphasia*. Philadelphia: W.B. Saunders.

Darley, F., Aronson, A. E., & Brown, J. R. (1975). *Motor speech disorders*. Philadelphia: Saunders.

David, R. M. (1990). Aphasia assessment: The acid test. *Aphasiology, 4*, 103–107.

David, R. M., & Skilbeck, C. E. (1984). Raven IQ and language recovery following stroke. *Journal of Clinical Neuropsychology, 6*, 302–308.

Davidson, B., Worrall, L. E., & Hickson, L. (2003). Identifying the communication activities of older people with aphasia: Evidence from naturalistic observation. *Aphasiology, 17*(3), 243–264.

Davis, C., & Majesky, S. (2005). *Are speech errors produced initially prognostically significant at 8 months post stroke?* Paper presented at the Clinical Aphasiology Conference, Sanibel, FL.

Davis, G. A. (1981). Incorporating parameters of natural conversation in aphasia treatment. In R. Chapey (Ed.), *Language intervention strategies in adult aphasia*. Baltimore, MD: Williams & Wilkins.

Davis, G. A. (2000). *Aphasiology: Disorders and clinical practice*. Needham Heights, MA: Allyn & Bacon.

DeBleser, R., Cholewa, N., Stadie, N., & Tabatabaie, S. (1997). LeMo, an expert system for single case assessment of word processing impairments in aphasic patients. *Neuropsychological Rehabilitation, 7*(4), 339–365.

D'Elia, L. F., Satz, P., Uchiyama, C. L., & White, T. (1996). *Color Trails Test*. Lutz, FL: Psychological Assessment Resources.

Delis, D. C., Kaplan, E., & Kramer, J. H. (2001). *Delis-Kaplan Executive Function System*. San Antonio, TX: Harcourt Assessment.

Deloche, G., Hannequin, D., Dordain, M., Perrier, D., Cardebat, D., Metz-Lutz, M. N., et al. (1997). Picture written naming: Performance parallels and divergencies between aphasic patients and normal subjects. *Aphasiology, 11*, 219–234.

Deloche, G., Hannequin, D., Dordain, M., Perrier, D., Pichard, B., Quint, S., et al. (1996). Picture confrontation oral naming: Performance differences between aphasics and normals. *Brain and Language, 53*, 105–120.

Denckla, M. B. (1996). A theory and model of executive function: A neuropsychological perspective. In G. R. Lyon & N. A. Krasnegor (Eds.), *Attention, memory, and executive function* (pp. 263–278). Baltimore, MD: Paul H. Brookes.

Denman, A. (1998). Determining the needs of spouses caring for aphasic partners. *Disability and Rehabilitation, 20*(11), 411–423.

den Ouden, D. B., & Bastiaanse, R. (2003). Syllable structure at different levels in the speech production process: Evidence from aphasia. In J. van deWeijer, V. J. van Hueven, & H. van derr Hulst (Eds.), *The phonological spectrum* (Vol. II: Suprasegmental Structure, pp. 81–109). Amsterdam: John Benjamins.

DeRenzi, E. (1997). Visuospatial and constructional disorders. In T. E. Feinberg & M. J. Farah (Eds.), *Behavioral neurology and neuropsychology* (pp. 297–307). New York: McGraw-Hill.

DeRenzi, E., & Ferrari, C. (1978). The Reporter's Test: A sensitive test to detect expressive disturbances in aphasics. *Cortex, 14*, 279–293.

de Riesthal, M., & Wertz, R. T. (2004). Prognosis for aphasia: Relationship between selected biographical and behavioural variables and outcome and improvement. *Aphasiology, 18*(10), 899–915.

Development of the World Health Organization WHOQOL-BREF Quality of life assessment. (1998). *Psychological Medicine* (Vol. 28): The WHOQOL Group.

Dick, F., Bates, E., Wulfeck, B., Utman, J., Dronkers, N. F., & Gernsbacher, M. A. (2001). Language deficits, localization, and grammar: Evidence for a distributive model of language breakdown in aphasic patients and neurologically intact individuals. *Psychological Review, 108*(4), 759–788.

Directory of speech-language pathology assessment instruments. (2006). Retrieved May 1, 2006, from http://www.asha.org/members/slp/assessment-directory.htm

Disease definition, natural history, and epidemiology. (2006). Retrieved January 7, 2006, from http://www.psych.org/psych_pract/treatg/pg/pg_dementia_2.cfm

DiSimoni, F. (1989). *Comprehensive Apraxia Test*. Dalton, PA: Praxis House.

DiSimoni, F., Darley, F. L., & Aronson, A. E. (1977). Patterns of dysfunction in schizophrenic patients on an aphasia test battery. *Journal of Speech and Hearing Disorders, 42*, 498–513.

DiSimoni, F., Keith, R., & Darley, F. (1980). Prediction of PICA overall score by short versions of the test. *Journal of Speech and Hearing Research, 23*, 511–516.

Doesborgh, S. J. C., van de Koenderman, W. M. E., Dippel, D. W. J., van Harskamp, F., Koudstaal, P. J., & Visch-Brink, E. G. (2003). Linguistic deficits in the acute phase of stroke. *Journal of Neurology, 250*(8), 977–982.

Dogil, G., & Mayer, J. (1998). Selective phonological impairment: A case of apraxia of speech. *Phonology, 15*, 143–188.

Dollaghan, C. (2004). Evidence-based practice in communication disorders: What do we know, and when do we know it? *Journal of Communication Disorders, 37*(5), 391–400.

Dollaghan, C. A., & Campbell, T. F. (1992). A procedure for classifying disruptions in spontaneous language samples. *Topics in Language Disorders, 12*(2), 56–68.

Dore, J. (1974). A pragmatic description of early language development. *Journal of Psycholinguistic Research, 3*, 343–350.

Douglas, J. M., O'Flaherty, C. A., & Snow, P. A. (2000). Measuring perception of communicative ability: The development and evaluation of the La Trobe communication questionnaire. *Aphasiology, 14*(3), 251–268.

Doyle, P. J., Goda, A. J., & Spencer, K. A. (1995). The communication informativeness and efficiency of connected discourse by adults with aphasia under structured and conversational sampling conditions. *American Journal of Speech-Language Pathology, 4*, 130–134.

Doyle, P. J., McNeil, M. R., Hula, W. D., & Mikolic, J. M. (2003). The Burden of Stroke Scale (BOSS): Validating patient-reported communication difficulty and associated psychological distress in stroke survivors. *Aphasiology, 17*(3), 291–304.

Doyle, P. J., McNeil, M. R., Mikolic, J. M., Prieto, L., Hula, W. D., Lustig, A., et al. (2004). The Burden of Stroke Scale (BOSS) provides valid and reliable score estimates of functioning and well-being in stroke survivors with and without communication disorders. *Journal of Clinical Epidemiology, 57*(10), 997–1997.

Doyle, P. J., Thompson, C. K., Oleyar, K., Wambaugh, J., & Jackson, A. (1994). The effects of setting variables on conversational discourse in normal and aphasic adults. *Clinical Aphasiology, 22*, 135–144.

Doyle, P. J., Tsironas, D., Goda, A. J., & Kalinyak, M. (1996). The relationship between objective measures and listeners' judgments of the communicative informativeness of the connected discourse of adults with aphasia. *American Journal of Speech-Language Pathology, 5*, 53–60.

Dronkers, N. F. (1996). A new brain region for coordinating speech articulation. *Nature, 384*, 159–161.

Druks, J., & Masterson, J. (2000). *An object and action naming battery.* New York: Psychology Press.

Drummond, S. (1993). *Dysarthria Examination Battery.* San Antonio, TX: Harcourt Assessment.

Duchan, J., & Black, M. (2001). Progressing toward life goals: A person-centered approach to evaluating therapy. *Topics in Language Disorders, 22*(1), 37–49.

Duffy, J. R. (2005). *Motor speech disorders: Substrates, differential diagnosis, and management* (2nd ed.). Philadelphia: Elsevier.

Duffy, J. R., & Coelho, C. (2001). Schuell's stimulation approach to rehabilitation. In R. Chapey (Ed.), *Language intervention strategies in aphasia and related neurogenic communication disorders* (4th ed., pp. 341–382). Philadelphia: Lippincott, Williams & Wilkins.

Duffy, J. R., & Petersen, R. C. (1992). Primary progressive aphasia. *Aphasiology, 6*, 1–15.

Duffy, J. R., & Watkins, L. B. (1984). The effect of response choice relatedness on pantomime and verbal recognition ability in aphasic patients. *Brain and Language, 21*, 291–306.

Dugbartey, A. T., Rosenbaum, J. G., Sanchez, P. N., & Townes, B. D. (1999). Neuropsychological assessment of executive functions. *Seminars in Clinical Neuropsychiatry, 4*, 5–12.

Dunkle, R. E. (1984). Differential diagnosis: The key to appropriate treatment. In C. R. Hooper & R. E. Dunkle (Eds.), *The older aphasic person* (pp. 69–127). Rockville, MD: Aspen.

Dunn, L. M., & Dunn, E. S. (1997). *Peabody Picture Vocabulary Test III.* Circle Pines, MN: American Guidance Service.

Edwards, S. (1995). Profiling fluent aphasic spontaneous speech: A comparison of two methodologies. *European Journal of Disorders of Communication, 30*(3), 333–345.

Edwards, S. (1998). Diversity in the lexical and syntactic abilities of fluent aphasic speakers. *Aphasiology, 12*, 99–117.

Egolf, D. B., & Chester, S. L. (1977). A comparison of aphasics' verbal performance in the language clinic with their verbal performance in other program areas of a comprehensive rehabilitation center. *Rehabilitation Literature, 38*(1), 9–11.

Eisenson, J. (1994). *Examining for aphasia* (3rd ed.). Austin, TX: Pro-Ed.

Elliott, R., McKenna, P. J., Robbins, T. W., & Sahakian, B. I. (1998). Specific neuropsychological deficits in schizophrenic patients with preserved intellectual function. *Cognitive Neuropsychiatry, 3*, 45–70.

Ellis, A., & Young, A. (1988). *Human cognitive neuropsychology.* Hillsdale, NJ: Erlbaum.

Elman, R. (2005). Social and life participation approaches to aphasia intervention. In L. L. LaPointe (Ed.), *Aphasia and related neurogenic language disorders* (3rd ed., pp. 39–50). New York: Thieme.

Elman, R. (2006). Evidence-based practice: What evidence is missing? *Aphasiology, 20*(2/3/4), 103–109.

Elman, R., & Bernstein-Ellis, E. (1999). What is functional? *American Journal of Speech-Language Pathology, 4*, 115–117.

Enderby, P. (1983). *Frenchay Dysarthria Assessment.* San Diego: College Hill Press.

Enderby, P., & Crow, E. (1996). Frenchay Aphasia Screening Test: Validity and comparability. *Disability and Rehabilitation, 18*, 238–240.

Enderby, P., Wood, V., & Wade, D. (2006). *Frenchay Aphasia Screening Test* (2nd ed.). Hoboken, NJ: John Wiley & Sons.

Enderby, P., Wood, V., Wade, D., & Langton Hewer, R. (1987). The Frenchay Aphasia Screening Test: A short simple test appropriate for non-specialists. *International Journal of Rehabilitation Medicine, 8*, 166–170.

Engell, B., Hutter, B. O., Willmes, K., & Huber, W. (2003). Quality of life in aphasia: Validation of a pictorial self-rating procedure. *Aphasiology, 17*(4), 383–396.

English, H. B., & English, A. C. (1958). *Comprehensive dictionary of psychological and psychoanalytic terms.* New York: McKay.

Ernest-Baron, C., Brookshire, R. H., & Nicholas, L. E. (1987). Story structure and retelling of narrative by aphasic and non-brain-damaged adults. *Journal of Speech and Hearing Research, 30*, 44–49.

Evans, R., Bishop, D., & Haselkorn, J. (1991). Factors predicting satisfactory home care after stroke. *Archives of Physical Medicine and Rehabilitation, 10*, 144–147.

Evidence-based practice in communication disorders [Position Statement]. (2005). Retrieved March 1, 2006, from http://www.asha.org/members/deskref-journals/deskref/default

Faber, M., & Aten, J. L. (1979). Verbal performance in aphasic patients in response to intact and altered pictorial stimuli. *Clinical Aphasiology, 10*, 177–186.

Farah, M. J. (2004). *Visual agnosia* (2nd ed.). Cambridge, MA: The MIT Press.

Fastenau, P. S., Denburg, N. L., & Mauer, B. A. (1998). Parallel short forms for the Boston Naming Test: Psychometric properties and norms for older adults. *Journal of Clinical and Experimental Neuropsychology, 20*(6), 828–834.

Faust, M., & Kravetz, S. (1998). Levels of sentence constraint and lexical decision in the two hemispheres. *Brain and Language, 2*, 149–162.

Ferguson, A. (1994). The influence of aphasia, familiarity and activity on conversational repair. *Aphasiology, 8*, 143–157.

Ferketic, M., Frattali, C. M., Holland, A. L., Thompson, C. K., & Wohl, C. (1995). *Functional assessment of communication skills for adults.* Rockville, MD: American Speech-Language-Hearing Association.

Fey, M., & Leonard, L. (1983). Pragmatic skills of children with specific language impairment. In T. Gallagher & C. Prutting (Eds.), *Pragmatic assessment and intervention issues in language* (pp. 65–83). San Diego: College Hill Press.

The FIM System. (2006). Retrieved January 10, 2006, from http://www.udsmr.org/fim2_subinfo.php

Fischler, I., & Bloom, P. (1979). Automatic and attentional processes in the effect of sentence contexts on word recognition. *Journal of Verbal Learning and Verbal Behavior, 18*, 1–20.

Fitch-West, J., & Sands, E. S. (1998). *Bedside Evaluation Screening Test (BEST-2)* (2nd ed.). Austin, TX: Pro-Ed.

Florance, C. (1981). Methods of communication analysis used in family interaction therapy. *Clinical Aphasiology, 11,* 204–211.

Foldi, N. S. (1987). Appreciation of pragmatic interpretations of indirect commands: Comparison of right and left hemisphere brain-damaged patients. *Brain and Language, 31,* 88–108.

Folstein, M. F., Folstein, S. E., & McHugh, P. B. (1975). *Mini-Mental Status Examination.* Lutz, Fl: Psychological Assessment Resources.

Fougeyrollas, P., Cloutier, R., Bergeron, H., Cote, J., Cote, M., & St. Michel, G. (1997). *Revision of the Quebec Classification: Handicap creation process.* Quebec: International Network on the Handicap Creation Process.

Frank, C. (1998). Overview of psychiatric disease for the speech-language pathologist. In A. F. Johnson & B. H. Jacobson (Eds.), *Medical speech-language pathology: A practitioner's guide* (pp. 637–654). New York: Thieme.

Frattali, C. (1992). Functional assessment of communication: Merging public policy with clinical views. *Aphasiology, 6,* 63–83.

Frattali, C. (1998a). Measuring modality-specific behaviors, functional abilities, and quality of life. In C. M. Frattali (Ed.), *Measuring outcomes in speech-language pathology* (pp. 55–88). New York: Thieme.

Frattali, C. (1998b). Outcomes assessment in speech-language pathology. In A. F. Johnson & B. H. Jacobson (Eds.), *Medical speech-language pathology: A practitioner's guide* (pp. 685–709). New York: Thieme.

Frattali, C., Bayles, K. A., Beeson, P. M., Kennedy, M. R. T., Wambaugh, J., & Yorkston, K. M. (2003). Development of evidence-based practice guidelines: Committee update. *Journal of Medical Speech Language Pathology, 11*(3), ix–xvii.

Frattali, C., Thompson, C. K., Holland, A. L., Wohl, C. B., & Ferketic, M. M. (1995). *American Speech-Language-Hearing Association Functional Assessment of Communication Skills for Adults.* Rockville, MD: American Speech-Language-Hearing Association.

Freed, D. B. (2000). *Motor speech disorders: Diagnosis and treatment.* San Diego: Singular.

Freed, D. B., Marshall, R. C., & Nippold, M. (1995). Comparison of personalized cueing and provided cueing on the facilitation of verbal labeling by aphasic subjects. *Journal of Speech, Language, and Hearing Research, 38,* 1081–1090.

Fridriksson, J., Holland, A. L., Beeson, P. M., & Morrow, L. (2005). Spaced retrieval treatment of anomia. *Aphasiology, 19*(2), 99–109.

Friedmann, N. (2005). Degrees of severity and recovery in agrammatism: Climbing up the syntactic tree. *Aphasiology, 19*(10/11), 1037–1051.

Functional Communication Measure. (1995). Rockville, MD: American Speech-Language-Hearing Association.

Gabrieli, J. D., Cohen, N. J., & Corkin, S. (1988). The impaired learning of semantic knowledge following bilateral medial temporal lobe resection. *Brain and Cognition, 7,* 157–177.

Gallagher, T. (1983). Pre-assessment: A procedure for accommodating language variability. In T. Gallagher, M., & C. Prutting (Eds.), *Pragmatic assessment and intervention issues in language* (pp. 1–29). San Diego, CA: College-Hill Press.

Gallagher, T. (1998). National initiatives in outcome measurement. In C. M. Frattali (Ed.), *Measuring outcomes in speech-language pathology* (pp. 527–545). New York: Thieme.

Garcia, L. J., & Desrochers, A. (1997). Assessment of language and speech disorders in Francophone adults. *Journal of Speech-Language Pathology and Audiology, 21,* 217–293.

Gardner, H., Albert, M. L., & Weintraub, S. (1975). Comprehending a word: The influence of speed and redundancy on auditory comprehension in aphasia. *Cortex, 11,* 155–162.

Garrett, K., & Lasker, J. (2005). *Multimodal communication screening task for persons with aphasia.* Lincoln, NE: AAC Lab.

Gates, G. A., Cooper, J. C., Kannel, W. B., & Miller, N. J. (1990). Hearing in the elderly: The Framingham cohort. *Ear and Hearing, 11,* 247–256.

Georgopoulos, A. P. (2004). Brain mechanisms of praxis. In M. S. Gazzaniga (Ed.), *The cognitive neurosciences* (3rd ed., pp. 475–484). Cambridge, MA: The MIT Press.

Gerber, S., & Gurland, G. B. (1989). Applied pragmatics in the assessment of aphasia. *Seminars in Speech and Language, 10,* 270–281.

German, D. J. (1990). *Test of Adolescent and Adult Word-Finding.* Austin, TX: Pro-Ed.

Gerratt, B. R., & Jones, D. (1987). Aphasic performance on a lexical decision task: Multiple meanings and word frequency. *Brain and Language, 30*(1), 106–115.

Gioia, G., Isquith, P., Guy, S., & Kenworthy, L. (2000). *Behavior Rating Inventory of Executive Function (BRIEF).* Lutz, FL: Harcourt Assessment.

Glosser, G., & Deser, T. (1991). Patterns of discourse production among neurological patients with fluent language disorders. *Brain and Language, 40,* 67–88.

Glosser, G., & Goodglass, H. (1990). Disorders in executive control functions among aphasic and other brain-damaged patients. *Neuropsychology, 12,* 485–501.

Glosser, G., Wiener, M., & Kaplan, E. (1988). Variations in aphasic language behaviors. *Journal of Speech and Hearing Disorders, 53,* 115–124.

Glueckauf, R., Blonder, L., Ecklund-Johnson, E., Maher, L., Crosson, B., & Rothi, L. (2003). Functional outcome questionnaire for aphasia: Overview and preliminary psychometric evaluation. *NeuroRehabilitation, 18*(4), 281–290.

Goldberg, E., Podell, K., Bilder, R., & Jaeger, J. (2002). *Executive Control Battery.* Melbourne, AU: Psych Press.

Goldenberg, G., & Spatt, J. (1994). Influence of size and site of cerebral lesions on spontaneous recovery of aphasia and on success of language therapy. *Brain and Language, 47*(4), 684–698.

Goldstein, K. (1948). *Language and language disturbance.* New York: Grune and Stratton.

Golper, L. C. (1996). Language assessment. In G. L. Wallace (Ed.), *Adult aphasia rehabilitation* (pp. 57–86). Boston: Butterworth-Heinemann.

Goodglass, H. (1968). Studies on the grammar of aphasics. In S. Rosenberg & J. Koplin (Eds.), *Developments in applied psycholinguistic research* (pp. 177–208). New York: MacMillan.

Goodglass, H. (1992). Diagnosis of conduction aphasia. In S. Kohn (Ed.), *Conduction aphasia* (pp. 39–50). Hillsdale, NJ: Lawrence Erlbaum.

Goodglass, H. (1993). *Understanding aphasia.* San Diego: Academic Press.

Goodglass, H., & Berko, J. (1960). Agrammatism and inflectional morphology in English. *Journal of Speech and Hearing Research, 3,* 257–267.

Goodglass, H., Christiansen, J. A., & Gallagher, R. (1993). Comparison of morphology and syntax in free narrative and structured tests: Fluent vs. nonfluent aphasics. *Cortex, 29,* 377–407.

Goodglass, H., Christiansen, J. A., & Gallagher, R. (1994). Syntactic constructions used by agrammatic speakers: Comparison with conduction aphasics and normals. *Neuropsychology, 8*(4), 598–613.

Goodglass, H., & Kaplan, E. (1983). *Boston Diagnostic Aphasia Examination* (2nd ed.). Philadelphia: Lea Febiger.

Goodglass, H., Kaplan, E., & Baressi, B. (2001). *Boston Diagnostic Aphasia Examination* (3rd ed.). Baltimore: Lippincott, Williams & Wilkins.

Goodglass, H., Klein, B., Carey, P., & Jones, K. J. (1966). Specific semantic word categories in aphasia. *Cortex, 2,* 74–89.

Goodglass, H., Wingfield, A., Hyde, M., Berko Gleason, J., Bowles, N. L., & Gallagher, R. (1997). The importance of word-initial phonology: Error patterns in prolonged naming efforts by aphasic patients. *Journal of the International Neuropsychological Society, 3,* 128–138.

Goodman, P. (1971). *Speaking and language: Defense of poetry.* New York: Random House.

Goodman, R. A., & Caramazza, A. (1986a). *The Johns Hopkins University Dysgraphia Battery.* Baltimore, MD: The Johns Hopkins University.

Goodman, R. A., & Caramazza, A. (1986b). *The Johns Hopkins University Dyslexia Battery.* Baltimore, MD: The Johns Hopkins University.

Goodwin, C. (2002). Conversational frameworks for the accomplishment of meaning in aphasia. In C. Goodwin (Ed.), *Conversation and brain damage* (pp. 90–116). Oxford: Oxford University Press.

Gordon, J. K. (1998). The fluency dimension in aphasia. *Aphasiology, 12,* 673–688.

Goren, A. R., Tucker, G., & Ginsberg, G. M. (1996). Language dysfunction in schizophrenia. *European Journal of Disorders of Communication, 31,* 153–170.

Gorno-Tempini, M. L., Dronkers, N., Rankin, K. P., Ogar, J., Phengrasamy, L., Rosen, H., et al. (2004). Cognition and anatomy in three variants of primary progressive aphasia. *Annals of Neurology, 55*(3), 335–346.

Gowan, J., Demos, G., & Torrence, E. (1967). *Creativity: Its educational implications.* New York: John Wiley and Sons.

Granger, C. V., Hamilton, B. B., Linacre, J. M., Heinemann, A. W., & Wright, B. D. (1993). Performance profiles of the functional independence measure. *American Journal of Medical Rehabilitation, 72*(2), 84–89.

Grant, D. A., & Berg, E. A. (1993). *Wisconsin Card Sorting Test.* Lutz, FL: Psychological Assessment Resources.

Grice, H. P. (1975). Logic and conversation. In P. Cole & J. Morgan (Eds.), *Studies in syntax and semantics* (Vol. 3: Speech Acts, pp. 41–58). New York: Academic Press.

Griffin, S., Rivera Mindt, M., Rankin, E., Ritchie, A., & Scott, J. (2002). Estimating premorbid intelligence: Comparison of traditional and contemporary methods across the intelligence continuum. *Archives of Clinical Neuropsychology, 17*(5), 497–507.

Grill, J. J., & Kirwin, M. M. (1989). *Written language assessment.* Novato, CA: Academic Therapy.

Grober, E., & Sliwinski, M. (1991). Development and validation of a model for estimating premorbid verbal intelligence in the elderly. *Journal of Clinical and Experimental Neuropsychology, 13,* 933–949.

Grodzinsky, Y. (2000). The neurology of syntax: Language use without Broca's area. *Behavioral and Brain Sciences, 23,* 1–21.

Gronwall, D. M. A., & Sampson, H. (1974). *Paced Auditory Serial Additions Test.* Victoria, BC: Neuropsychology Laboratory, University of Victoria.

Grossman, M., & Ash, S. (2004). Primary progressive aphasia: A review. *Neurocase, 10*(1), 3–18.

Guidelines for audiologic screening. (1997). Retrieved November 2, 2005, from http://www.asha.org/NR/rdonlyres/A13D0ECC-684B-4E33-BA0E-CAF6681CEDEB/0/v4GLAudScreening.pdf

Guilford, J. P. (1967). *The nature of human intelligence.* New York: McGraw-Hill.

Guilford, J. P. (1988). Some changes in the structure-of-intellect model. *Educational and Psychological Measurement, 48*(1), 1–4.

Guilford, J. P., & Hoepfner, R. (1971). *The analysis of intelligence.* New York: McGraw-Hill.

Gupta, A., Pansari, K., & Shetty, H. (2002). Post-stroke depression. *International Journal of Clinical Practice, 56*(7), 532–537.

Gurland, G., Chwat, S. E., & Wollner, S. G. (1982). Establishing a communication profile in adult aphasia: Analysis of communicative acts and conversation sequences. *Clinical Aphasiology, 12,* 18–27.

Haaland, K. Y., & Flaherty, D. (1984). The different types of limb apraxia error made by patients with left vs. right hemisphere damage. *Brain and Cognition, 3,* 370–384.

Haarmann, H. J., & Kolk, H. H. J. (1992). The production of grammatical morphology in Broca's and Wernicke's aphasias: Speed and accuracy factors. *Cortex, 28,* 97–112.

Hall, K. M. (1997). The Functional Assessment Measure. *Journal of Rehabilitation Outcomes Measurement, 1*(3), 63–65.

Halliday, M., & Hasan, R. (1976). *Cohesion in English.* London: Longman.

Halper, A. S., Cherney, L. R., & Burns, M. S. (1996). *Rehabilitation Institute of Chicago Clinical Management of Right Hemisphere Dysfunction* (2nd ed.). Gaithersburg, MD: Aspen.

Hammill, D. D., Brown, V. L., Larsen, S., & Wiederholt, J. L. (1994). *Test of Adolescent and Adult Language* (3rd ed.). Circle Pines, MN: AGS.

Hammill, D. D., & Larson, S. C. (1996). *Test of Written Language* (3rd ed.). Austin, TX: Pro-Ed.

Hammill, D. D., Pearson, N. A., & Widerholt, J. L. (1996). *Comprehensive Test of Nonverbal Intelligence.* Lutz, FL: Psychological Assessment Resources.

Hanks, R. A., Ricker, J. H., & Millis, S. R. (2004). Empirical evidence regarding the neuropsychological assessment of moderate and severe traumatic brain injury. In J. H. Ricker (Ed.), *Differential diagnosis in adult neuropsychological assessment* (pp. 218–242). New York: Springer.

Hanlon, R. E., Brown, J. W., & Gerstman, L. J. (1990). Enhancement of naming in nonfluent aphasia through gesture. *Brain and Language, 38,* 298–314.

Hanna, G., Schell, L. M., & Schreiner, R. (1977). *The Nelson Reading Skills Test.* Chicago, IL: Riverside.

Hart, S., & Semple, J. M. (1990). *Neuropsychology and the dementias.* New York: Taylor & Francis.

Hartley, L. L. (1995). *Cognitive-communicative abilities following brain injury.* San Diego, CA: Singular.

Head, H. (1920). Aphasia and kindred disorders of speech. *Brain*, *43*, 87–165.

Heaton, R. K., Grant, I., & Matthews, C. G. (1992). *Comprehensive norms for an expanded Halstead-Reitan Battery: Demographic corrections, research findings and clinical applications with a supplement for the Wechsler Adult Intelligence Scale–Revised*. Lutz, FL: Psychological Assessment Resources.

Heeschen, C., & Schegloff, E. A. (1999). Agrammatism, adaptation theory, conversation analysis: On the role of so-called telegraphic style in talk-in-interaction. *Aphasiology*, *13*, 365–406.

Heilman, K. M., & Rothi, L. J. G. (2003). Apraxia. In K. M. Heilman & E. Valenstein (Eds.), *Clinical neuropsychology* (4th ed., pp. 215–235). New York: Oxford University Press.

Heilman, K. M., Watson, R. T., & Rothi, L. J. G. (2006). Limb apraxias. In P. Snyder, P. D. Nussaum & D. L. Robins (Eds.), *Clinical neuropsychology: A pocket handbook for assessment* (2nd ed., pp. 534–546). Washington, DC: American Psychological Association.

Helm-Estabrooks, N. (1991). *Test of Oral and Limb Apraxia*. Austin, TX: Pro-Ed.

Helm-Estabrooks, N. (1992). *Aphasia Diagnostic Profiles*. Austin, TX: Pro-Ed.

Helm-Estabrooks, N. (2002). Cognition and aphasia: A discussion and a study. *Journal of Communication Disorders*, *35*(2), 171–186.

Helm-Estabrooks, N. (2003). *Cognitive Linguisic Quick Test*. San Antonio: PsychCorp.

Helm-Estabrooks, N., & Albert, M. L. (1991). *Manual of aphasia therapy*. Austin, TX: Pro-Ed.

Helm-Estabrooks, N., Fitzpatrick, P. M., & Barresi, B. (1982). Visual action therapy for global aphasia. *Journal of Speech and Hearing Disorders*, *47*, 385–389.

Helm-Estabrooks, N., & Hotz, G. (1991). *Brief Test of Head Injury*. Chicago: Riverside.

Helm-Estabrooks, N., Ramsberger, G., Morgan, A. R., & Nicholas, M. (1989). *Boston Assessment of Severe Aphasia*. Chicago: Riverside.

Henderson, L. W., Frank, E. M., Pigatt, T., Abramson, R. K., & Houston, M. (1998). Race, gender, and educational level effects on Boston Naming Test scores. *Aphasiology*, *12*, 901–911.

Hengst, J. A. (2003). Collaborative referencing between individuals with aphasia and routine communication partners. *Journal of Speech, Language and Hearing Research*, *46*, 831–848.

Herrmann, M., & Wallesch, C. W. (1993). Depressive changes in stroke patients. *Disability and Rehabilitation*, *150*, 55–66.

Hickey, E. M., & Rondeau, G. (2005). Social validation in aphasiology: Does judges' knowledge of aphasiology matter? *Aphasiology*, *19*(3–5), 389–398.

Hilari, K., & Byng, S. (2001). Measuring quality of life in people with aphasia: The Stroke Specific Quality of Life Scale. *International Journal of Language and Communication Disorders*, *36 Supplement*, 86–91.

Hilari, K., Byng, S., Lamping, D., & Smith, S. (2003). Stroke and Aphasia Quality of Life Scale-39 (SAQOL-39): Evaluation of acceptability, reliability, and validity. *Stroke*, *34*, 1944–1950.

Hillis, A. E. (1993). The role of models of language processing in rehabilitation of language impairment. *Aphasiology*, *7*(1), 5–26.

Hillis, A. E. (1998). Treatment of naming disorders: New issues regarding old therapies. *Journal of the International Neuropsychological Society*, *4*(6), 648–660.

Hillis, A. E. (2002a). *The handbook of adult language disorders: Integrating cognitive neuropsychology, neurology and rehabilitation*. New York: Psychology Press.

Hillis, A. E. (2002b). Mechanisms of early aphasia recovery. *Aphasiology*, *16*(9), 885–895.

Hillis, A. E. (2005). For a theory of cognitive rehabilitation: Progress in the decade of the brain. In P. W. Halligan & D. T. Wade (Eds.), *Effectiveness of rehabilitation for cognitive deficits* (pp. 271–279). New York: Oxford University Press.

Hillis, A. E., Barker, P., Beauchamp, N., Gordon, B., & Wityk, R. (2000). MR perfusion imaging reveals regions of hypoperfusion associated with aphasia and neglect. *American Academy of Neurology*, *55*, 782–788.

Hillis, A. E., Oh, S., & Ken, L. (2004). Deterioration of naming nouns versus verbs in primary progressive aphasia. *Annals of Neurology*, *55*(2), 268–275.

Hillis, A. E., Tuffiash, E., & Caramazza, A. (2002). Modality-specific deterioration in naming verbs in nonfluent primary progressive aphasia. *Journal of Cognitive Neuroscience*, *14*, 1099.

Hirsch, K. W., & Ellis, A. (1994). Age of acquisition and lexical processing in aphasia: A case study. *Cognitive Neuropsychiatry*, *11*(4), 435–358.

Hofstede, B. T. M., & Kolk, H. H. J. (1994). The effects of task variation on the production of grammatical morphology in Broca's aphasia: A multiple case study. *Brain and Language*, *46*, 278–328.

Holbrook, M., & Skilbeck, C. E. (1983). An activities index for use with stroke patients. *Age and Aging*, *12*, 166–170.

Holland, A. L. (1982). When is aphasia aphasia? The problem of closed head injury. *Clinical Aphasiology*, *11*, 345–349.

Holland, A. L. (1996). Pragmatic assessment and treatment for aphasia. In G. L. Wallace (Ed.), *Adult aphasia rehabilitation* (pp. 161–174). Boston: Butterworth-Heinemann.

Holland, A. L., & Bartlett, C. L. (1985). Some differential effects of age on stroke-produced aphasia. In H. K. Ulatowska (Ed.), *The aging brain: Communication in the elderly* (pp.141–155). San Diego, CA: College-Hill Press.

Holland, A. L., Frattali, C. M., & Fromm, D. (1999). *Communication Activities of Daily Living-2* (2nd ed.). Austin, TX: Pro-Ed.

Holland, A. L., Fromm, D., & Swindell, C. (1986). The labeling problem in aphasia: An illustrative case. *Journal of Speech and Hearing Disorders*, *51*, 176–180.

Holland, A. L., Greenhouse, J., Fromm, D., & Swindell, C. S. (1989). Predictors of language restitution following stroke: A multivariate analysis. *Journal of Speech and Hearing Research*, *32*, 232–238.

Holland, A. L., & Hinckley, J. J. (2002). Assessment and treatment of pragmatic aspects of communication in aphasia. In A. Hillis (Ed.), *The handbook of adult language disorders: Integrating cognitive neuropsychology, neurology and rehabilitation* (pp. 413–427). New York: Psychology Press.

Holland, A. L., Swindell, S., & Forbes, M. (1985). The evolution of initial global aphasia: Implications for prognosis. *Clinical Aphasiology*, *15*, 169–175.

Holland, A. L., & Thompson, C. K. (1998). Outcomes measurement in aphasia. In C. M. Frattali (Ed.), *Measuring outcomes in speech-language pathology* (pp. 245–266). New York: Thieme.

Holtzapple, P., Pohlman, K., LaPointe, L. L., & Graham, L. F. (1989). Does SPICA mean PICA? *Clinical Aphasiology*, *18*, 131–144.

Hough, M. S., Vogel, D., Cannito, M. P., & Pierce, R. S. (1997). Influence of prior pictorial context on sentence comprehension in older versus younger aphasic subjects. *Aphasiology, 11,* 235–247.

Houghton, P., Pettit, J. M., & Towey, M. P. (1982). Measuring communication competence in global aphasia. *Clinical Aphasiology, 12,* 28–39.

Howard, D., & Patterson, K. E. (1992). *Pyramids and Palm Trees.* Bury St. Edmunds: Thames Valley Test Company.

Howland, J., & Pierce, R. S. (2004). Influence of semantic relatedness and array size on single-word reading comprehension in aphasia. *Aphasiology, 18*(11), 1005–1013.

Huber, W., Poeck, K., Weniger, D., & Willmes, K. (1983). *Der Aachener Aphasie Test.* Gottingen: Hogrefe.

Huber, W., Poeck, K., & Willmes, K. (1984). The Aachen Aphasia Test. In F. C. Rose (Ed.), *Progress in aphasiology* (pp. 291–303). New York: Raven Press.

Huntley, R. A., Pindzola, R. H., & Weidner, W. E. (1986). The effectiveness of simultaneous cues on naming disturbance in aphasia. *Journal of Communication Disorders, 19*(4), 261–270.

Hux, K., Sanger, D., Reid, R., & Maschka, A. (1997). Discourse analysis procedures: Reliability issues. *Journal of Communication Disorders, 30,* 133–150.

International Classification of Functioning, Disability and Health: ICF. (2001). Geneva: World Health Organization.

Irwin, W., Wertz, R., & Avent, J. (2002). Relationships among language impairment, functional communication, and pragmatic performance in aphasia. *Aphasiology, 16*(8), 823–835.

Ivnik, R. J., Malec, J. F., Smith, G. E., Tangalos, E. G., & Petersen, R. C. (1996). Neuropsychological test norms above age 55: COWAT, BNT, MAE Token, WRAT-R Reading, AMNART, STROOP, TMT, and JLO. *The Clinical Neuropsychologist, 10,* 262–278.

Jackson, S. T., & Tompkins, C. A. (1991). Supplemental aphasia tests: Frequency of use and psychometric properties. *Clinical Aphasiology, 20,* 91–99.

Jacobs, D. M., Sano, M., Albert, S., Schofield, P., Dooneief, G., & Stern, Y. (1997). Cross cultural neuropsychological assessment: A comparison of randomly selected, demographically matched cohorts of English and Spanish-speaking older adults. *Journal of Clinical and Experimental Neuropsychology, 19,* 331–339.

Joanette, Y., Ansaldo, A., & Stemmer, B. (1999). Acquired pragmatic impairments and aphasia. *Brain and Language, 68*(3), 529–534.

Johnson, A. F., George, K. P., & Hinckley, J. (1998). Assessment and diagnosis in neurogenic communication disorders. In A. F. Johnson & B. H. Jacobson (Eds.), *Medical speech-language pathology: A practitioner's guide* (pp. 337–353). New York: Thieme.

Jorgensen, H. S., Nakayama, H., Raaschou, H. O., Vive-Larsen, J., Stoier, M., & Olsen, T. S. (1995). Outcome and time course of recovery in stroke. Part 1: Outcome: The Copenhagen stroke study. *Archives of Physical Medicine and Rehabilitation, 76,* 399–405.

Kagan, A., Winckel, J., Black, S., Duchan, J. F., Simmons-Mackie, N., Square, P., et al. (2004). A set of observational measures for rating support and participation in conversation between adults with aphasia and their conversation partners. *Topics in Stroke Rehabilitation, 11*(1), 67–83.

Kahneman, D., Diner, E., & Schwartz, N. (1999). *Well-being.* New York: Russell Sage Foundation.

Karnath, H. O., Milner, A. D., & Vallar, G. (2002). *The cognitive and neural bases of spatial neglect.* Oxford, UK: Oxford University Press.

Kaufer, D. I., & Cummings, J. L. (1997). Dementia and delirium: An overview. In T. E. Feinberg & M. J. Farah (Eds.), *Behavioral neurology and neuropsychology* (pp. 499–520). New York: McGraw-Hill.

Kaufman, A. S., & Kaufman, N. L. (1994). *Kaufman Functional Academic Skills Test.* Circle Pines, MN: American Guidance Service.

Kay, J., Byng, S., Edmundson, A., & Scott, C. (1990). Missing the wood and the trees: A reply to David, Kertesz, Goodglass and Weniger. *Aphasiology, 4,* 115–122.

Kay, J., Lesser, R., & Coltheart, M. (1996). Psycholinguistic Assessments of Language Processing in Aphasia (PALPA): An introduction. *Aphasiology, 10,* 159–215.

Kay, J., Lesser, R., & Coltheart, R. M. (1992). *Psycholinguistic Assessments of Language Processing in Aphasia.* Hove, East Sussex, UK: Lawrence Erlbaum.

Keefe, R. S. E., & Harvey, P. D. (1994). *Understanding schizophrenia: A guide to the new research on causes and treatment.* New York: Free Press.

Keenan, J. S., & Brassell, E. G. (1974). A study of factors related to prognosis for individual aphasic patients. *Journal of Speech and Hearing Disorders, 39,* 257–269.

Keenan, J. S., & Brassell, E. G. (1975). *Aphasia Language Performance Scales.* Murfreesboro, TN: Pinnacle Press.

Keith, R. W. (1993). *SCANA: A test for auditory processing disorders in adolescents and adults.* San Antonio, TX: The Psychological Corporation.

Kelly, R. J. (2006). A model for assessing hearing loss in older adults with neurogenic communication disorders. *Perspectives on Neurophysiology and Neurogenic Speech and Language Disorders, 16*(3), 22–25.

Kemmerer, D., & Tranel, D. (2000). Verb retrieval in brain-damaged subjects: 2. Analysis of errors. *Brain and Language, 73,* 393–420.

Kempler, D., Teng, E. L., Dick, M., Taussig, I. M., & Davis, D. S. (1998). The effects of age, education, and ethnicity on verbal fluency. *Journal of the International Neuropsychological Society, 4,* 531–538.

Kennedy, M. R. T., & Chiou, H. H. (2005). Assessment tools for adolescents and adults in languages other than English. *Perspectives on Neurophysiology and Neurogenic Speech and Language Disorders, 15*(2), 20–23.

Kent, R. D., Weismer, J. F., Kent, J. C., & Rosenbek, J. (1989). Toward phonetic intelligibility testing in dysarthria. *Journal of Speech and Hearing Disorders, 54*(4), 482–499.

Kertesz, A. (1979). *Aphasia and associated disorders: Taxonomy, localization, and recovery.* New York: Grune and Stratton.

Kertesz, A. (1982). *Western Aphasia Battery.* New York: Grune and Stratton.

Kertesz, A. (2005). Frontotemporal dementia: One disease, or many? Probably one, possibly two. *Alzheimer Disease and Associated Disorders, 19*(Supplement 1), S19–24.

Kertesz, A. (2006). *Western Aphasia Battery–Enhanced.* San Antonio, TX: Psychological Corporation.

Kertesz, A., Davidson, W., McCabe, P., Takagi, K., & Munoz, D. (2003). Primary progressive aphasia: Diagnosis, varieties, evolution. *Journal of the International Neuropsychological Society, 9,* 710–719.

Kertesz, A., Hudson, L., Mackenzie, I. R. A., & Munoz, D. G. (1994). The pathology and nosology of primary progressive aphasia. *Neurology, 44,* 2065–2072.

Kertesz, A., & McCabe, P. (1977). Recovery patterns and prognosis in aphasia. *Brain, 100,* 1–18.

Kiernan, R. J., Mueller, J., & Langston, J. W. (2006). *Cognistat.* Fairfax, CA: NCNG.

Kim, M., & Thompson, C. K. (2000). Patterns of comprehension and production of nouns and verbs in agrammatism: Implications for lexical organization. *Brain and Language, 74,* 1–25.

Kimelman, M. D. Z., & McNeil, M. R. (1989). Contextual influences on the auditory comprehension of normally stressed targets by aphasic listeners. *Clinical Aphasiology, 18,* 407–419.

King, R. B. (1996). Quality of life after stroke. *Stroke, 27,* 467–1472.

Kiran, S., & Thompson, C. K. (2003). The role of semantic complexity in treatment of naming deficits: Training semantic categories in fluent aphasia by controlling exemplar typicality. *Journal of Speech, Language and Hearing Research, 46* (5), 773–787.

Klatzky, R. L. (1980). *Human memory: Structures and Processes* (2nd ed.). San Francisco: W.H. Freeman & Co.

Klein, L. (1994). *Functional Communication Profile.* East Moline, IL: LinguiSystems.

Klippi, A. (1996). *Conversation as an achievement in aphasia.* Helsinki: Finnish Literature Society.

Knibb, J. A., & Hodges, J. R. (2005). Semantic dementia and primary progressive aphasia: A problem of categorization? *Alzheimer Disease and Associated Disorders, 19* (Supplement 1), S7–S14.

Koenig, H. G. (1997). Mood disorders. In P. D. Nussbaum (Ed.), *Handbook of neuropsychology and aging* (pp. 63–79). New York: Plenum Press.

Kohn, S., & Melvold, J. (2000). Effects of morphological complexity on phonological output deficits in fluent and nonfluent aphasia. *Brain and Language, 73*(3), 323–346.

Kohnert, K. J., Hernandez, A. E., & Bates, E. (1998). Bilingual performance on the Boston Naming Test: Preliminary norms in Spanish and English. *Brain and Language, 65*(3), 422–440.

Kulke, F., & Blanken, G. (2001). Phonological and syntactic influences on semantic misnamings in aphasia. *Aphasiology, 15*(1), 3–15.

Kusunoki, T. (1985). A study on scaling of Standard Language Test of Aphasia (SLTA): A practical scale based on a three-factor structure. *Japanese Journal of Behaviormetrics, 12*(23), 8–12.

Laasko, M. (2003). Collaborative construction of repair in aphasic conversation: An interactive view on the extended speaking turns of persons with Wernicke's aphasia. In C. Goodwin (Ed.), *Conversation and brain damage* (pp. 163–188). Oxford: Oxford University Press.

Labov, W. (1970). The study of language in its social context. *Studium Generale, 23,* 30–87.

Laganaro, M., DiPietro, M., & Schnider, A. (2006). What does recovery from anomia tell us about the underlying impairment: The case of similar anomic patterns and different recovery. *Neuropsychologia, 44*(4), 534–545.

Lahey, M. (1988). *Language disorders and language development.* New York: MacMillan.

Laiacona, M., Luzzatti, C., Zonca, G., Guarnaschelli, A., & Capitani, E. (2000). Lexical and semantic factors influencing picture naming in aphasia. *Brain and Cognition, 46*(1–2), 184–187.

Laine, M., Koivuselka-Sallinen, P., Hanninen, R., & Neimi, J. (1993). *Bostonian nimentatestin suomenkielinen versio.* Helsinki: Psykologien Kustannus.

LaPointe, L. L. (1996). Quality of life with aphasia. *Seminars in Speech and Language, 20*(1), 5–16.

LaPointe, L. L. (2005). Foundations: Adaptation, accommodation, aristos. In L. L. LaPointe (Ed.), *Aphasia and related neurogenic language disorders* (3rd ed., pp. 1–18). New York: Thieme.

LaPointe, L. L., & Horner, J. (1978). The Functional Auditory Comprehension Test (FACT): Protocol and test format. *FLASHA Journal, Spring,* 27–33.

LaPointe, L. L., & Horner, J. (1998). *Reading Comprehension Battery for Aphasia* (2nd ed.). Austin, TX: Pro-Ed.

Larfeuil, C., & LeDorze, G. (1997). An analysis of the word-finding difficulties and of the content of the discourse of recent and chronic aphasia speakers. *Aphasiology, 11*(8), 783–811.

Larkins, B. M., Worrall, L., & Hickson, L. (2000). Functional communication in cognitive communication disorders following traumatic brain injury. In L. Worrall & C. Frattali (Eds.), *Neurogenic communication disorders: A functional approach* (pp. 206–219). New York: Thieme.

Laska, A., Hellblom, A., Murray, V., Kahan, T., & Von Arbin, M. (2001). Aphasia in acute stroke and relation to outcome. *Journal of Internal Medicine, 249,* 413–422.

Lasky, E. Z., Weidner, W. E., & Johnson, J. P. (1976). Influence of linguistic complexity, rate of presentation, and interphrase pause time on auditory-verbal comprehension of adult aphasic patients. *Brain and Language, 3,* 386–395.

Lecours, A. R., Mehler, J., Parente, M. A., & Beltrami, M. C. (1988). Illiteracy and brain damage: III. A contribution to the study of speech and language disorders in illiterates with unilateral brain damage. *Neuropsychologia, 26,* 575–589.

LeDorze, G., & Brassard, C. (1995). A description of the consequences of aphasia on aphasic persons and their relatives and friends, based on the WHO model of chronic diseases. *Aphasiology, 9*(3), 239–256.

Lee, L. (1971). *Northwestern Syntax Screening Test.* Evanston, IL: Northwestern University Press.

Lemme, M., Hedberg, N., & Bottenberg, D. (1984). Cohesion in narratives of aphasic adults. *Clinical Aphasiology, 14,* 215–222.

Leonard, C. L., & Baum, S. R. (2005). Research note: The ability of individuals with right-hemisphere damage to use context under conditions of focused and divided attention. *Journal of Neurolinguistics, 18*(6), 427–441.

LeRhun, E., Richard, F., & Pasquier, F. (2005). Natural history of primary progressive aphasia. *Neurology, 65*(6), 887–891.

Lesser, R., & Milroy, L. (1993). *Linguistics and aphasia: Psycholinguistic and pragmatic aspects of intervention.* London: Longman.

Lezak, M. D., Howieson, D. B., & Loring, D. W. (2004). *Neuropsychological assessment* (4th ed.). Oxford: Oxford University Press.

Li, E. C., Ritterman, S., Delta Volpe, A., & Williams, S. E. (1996). Variation in grammatic complexity across three types of discourse. *Journal of Speech-Language Pathology and Audiology, 20,* 180–186.

Liles, B. Z. (1985). Narrative ability in normal and language disordered children. *Journal of Speech and Hearing Research, 28,* 123–133.

Liles, B. Z., & Coelho, C. A. (1998). Cohesion analysis. In L. R. Cherney, B. Shadden, & C. Coelho (Eds.), *Analyzing discourse in communicatively impaired adults* (pp. 65–84). Gaithersburg, MD: Aspen.

Lincoln, N. (1982). The speech questionnaire: An assessment of functional language ability. *International Rehabilitation Medicine, 4,* 114–117.

Lindsay, J., & Wilkinson, R. (1999). Repair sequences in aphasic talk: A comparison of aphasic-speech language therapist and aphasic-spouse conversations. *Aphasiology, 13*(4–5), 305–325.

Linebaugh, C., Kryzer, K. M., Oden, S., & Myers, P. S. (2006). Reapportionment of communicative burden in aphasia: A study of narrative interaction. *Aphasiology, 20*(1), 84–96.

Linebaugh, C., & Lehner, L. (1977). Cueing hierarchies and word retrieval: A therapy program. *Clinical Aphasiology, 7,* 19–31.

Linebaugh, C., Shisler, R. J., & Lehner, L. (2005). CAC Classics: Cueing hierarchies and word retrieval: A therapy program. *Aphasiology, 19*(1), 77–92.

Linscott, R. J. (1996). The Profile of Functional Impairment in Communication (PFIC): A measure of communication impairment for clinical use. *Aphasiology, 10*(6), 397–412.

Lock, S., & Armstrong, E. (1997). Cohesion analysis of the expository discourse of normal, fluent aphasic and demented adults: A role in differential diagnosis? *Clinical Linguistics and Phonetics, 11,* 299–317.

Lomas, J., Pickard, L., Bester, S., Elbard, H., Finlayson, A., & Zoghaib, C. (1989). The communicative effectiveness index: Development and psychometric evaluation of functional communication. *Journal of Speech and Hearing Disorders, 54,* 113–124.

Lott, P. (1999). *Gesture and aphasia.* New York: Peter Lang.

Love, T., & Oster, E. (2003). On the categorization of aphasic typologlies: The SOAP (A test of syntactic complexity). *Journal of Psycholinguistic Research, 31*(5), 503–529.

Lubinski, R. (1995). Environmental considerations for elderly patients. In R. Lubinski (Ed.), *Dementia and communication* (pp. 257–278). San Diego: Singular.

Lubinski, R. (2001). Environmental systems approach to adult aphasia. In R. Chapey (Ed.), *Language intervention strategies in adult aphasia* (3rd ed., pp. 269–296). Philadelphia: Williams & Wilkins.

Lucas, E. (1980). *Semantic and pragmatic language disorders: Assessment and remediation.* Rockville, MD: Aspen.

Luterman, D. M. (1996). *Counseling persons with communication disorders and their families.* Austin, TX: Pro-Ed.

Luzzatti, C., Raggi, R., Zonca, G., Pistarini, A., Contardi, A., & Pinna, G. D. (2001). On the nature of the selective impairment of verb and noun retrieval. *Cortex, 37*(5), 724–726.

Lynch, J., & McCaffrey, R. (1997). Premorbid intellectual functioning and the determination of cognitive loss. In R. McCaffrey, A. Williams, J. Fisher & L. Laing (Eds.), *The practice of forensic neuropsychology: Meeting challenges in the courtroom* (pp. 91–116). New York: Plenum Press.

Lyon, J. (1992). Communication use and participation in life for adults with aphasia in natural settings. *American Journal of Speech-Language Pathology, 1,* 7–14.

Lyon, J. (1998). *Coping with aphasia.* San Diego: Singular Press.

Lyon, J. (2000). Finding, defining, and refining functionality in real life for people confronting aphasia. In L. Worral & C. Frattali (Eds.), *Neurogenic communication disorders: A functional approach* (pp. 137–161). New York: Thieme.

Lyon, J., Cariski, D., Keisler, L., Rosenbek, J., Levine, R., Kumpala, J., et al. (1997). Communication partners: Enhancing participation in life and communication for adults with aphasia in natural settings. *Aphasiology, 11,* 693–708.

Lyon, J., & Helm-Estabrooks, N. (1987). Drawing: Its communicative significance for expressively restricted aphasic adults. *Topics in Language Disorders, 8,* 61–71.

MacDonald, S. (1998). *Functional assessment of verbal reasoning and executive strategies.* Guleph, Canada: Clinical Publishing.

MacGinitie, W. H., MacGinitie, R. K., Maria, K., & Dreyer, L. G. (2000). *Gates-MacGinitie Reading Tests* (4th ed.). Itasca, IL: Riverside.

Madden, M., Oelshlaeger, M., & Damico, J. (2002). The conversational value of laughter for a person with aphasia. *Aphasiology, 16*(12), 119–121.

Mahendra, N., Ribera, J., Sevcik, R., Adler, R., Cheng, L. R. L., Davis-McFarland, E., et al. (2005). Why is yogurt good for you? Because it has live cultures. *Perspectives on Neurophysiology and Neurogenic Speech and Language Disorders, 15*(1), 3–7.

Maher, L. M., & Rothi, L. J. G., (2001). Disorders of skilled movement. In R. S. Berndt (Ed.), *Handbook of neuropsychology* (2nd ed., Vol. 3 Language and aphasia, pp. 269–283). Amsterdam, Netherlands: Elsevier Science.

Manochiopinig, S., Sheard, C., & Reed, V. A. (1992). Pragmatic assessment in adult aphasia: A clinical review. *Aphasiology, 6,* 519–533.

Mansur, L. L., Radanovic, M., Taquemori, L., Greco, L., & Araujo, G. C. (2005). A study of the abilities in oral language comprehension of the Boston Diagnostic Aphasia Examination–Portuguese version: A reference guide for the Brazilian population. *Brazilian Journal of Medical and Biological Research, 38*(2), 277–292.

Marini, A., Carlomagno, S., Caltagirone, C., & Nocentini, U. (2005). The role played by the right hemisphere in the organization of complex textual structures. *Brain and Language, 93*(1), 46–54.

Markwardt, F. C. (1998). *Peabody Individual Achievement Test–Revised.* Circle Pines, MN: American Guidance Service.

Marshall, J. (2005). Aphasia in a bilingual user of British sign language and English: Effects of cross-linguistic cues. *Cognitive Neuropsychology, 22*(6), 719–736.

Marshall, J. (2006). The role of gesture in aphasia therapy. *Advances in Speech-Language Pathology, 8*(2), 110–114.

Marshall, J., Black, M., Byng, S., Chiat, S., & Pring, T. (1998). *The sentence processing resource pack.* Bicester, UK: Speechmark.

Marshall, J., Pring, T., Chiat, S., & Robson, J. (2001). When ottoman is easier than chair: An inverse frequency effect in jargon aphasia. *Cortex, 37*(1), 33–53.

Marshall, J., Robson, J., Pring, T., & Chiat, S. (1998). Why does monitoring fail in jargon aphasia?: Comprehension, judgment, and therapy evidence. *Brain and Language, 63,* 79–107.

Marshall, R. C., & Freed, D. B. (2006). The personalized cueing method: From the laboratory to the clinic. *American Journal of Speech-Language Pathology, 15*, 103–111.

Marshall, R. C., Karow, C. M., Freed, D. B., & Babcock, P. (2002). Effects of personalized cue form on the learning of subordinate category names by aphasic and non-brain-damaged subjects. *Aphasiology, 16*, 763–771.

Marshall, R. C., Karow, C. M., Morelli, C. A., Iden, K. K., & Dixon, J. (2003). A clinical measure for the assessment of problem solving in brain injured adults. *American Journal of Speech-Language Pathology, 12*(3), 333–348.

Marshall, R. C., & Tompkins, C. (1982). Verbal self-correction behaviors of fluent and nonfluent aphasic subjects. *Brain and Language, 15*, 292–306.

Marshall, R. C., Tompkins, C., & Phillips, D. (1982). Improvement in treated aphasia: Examination of selected prognostic factors. *Folia Phoniatrica, 34*(6), 305–315.

Martin, A. D. (1977). Aphasia testing: A second look at the Porch Index of Communicative Ability. *Journal of Speech and Hearing Disorders, 42*, 547–561.

Martin, R. C., & Miller, M. (2002). Sentence comprehension deficits: Independence and interaction of syntax, semantics and working memory. In A. Hillis (Ed.), *The handbook of adult language disorders: Integrating cognitive neuropsychology, neurology, and rehabilitation* (pp. 295–310). New York: Psychology Press.

Mayer, J. F., & Murray, L. L. (2003). Functional measures of naming in aphasia: Word retrieval in confrontation naming versus connected speech. *Aphasiology, 17*(5), 481–497.

Mazaux, J. M., & Orgogozo, J. M. (1981). *Boston Diagnostic Aphasia Examination: Échelle Française*. Paris: Éditions Scientifiques et Psychologiques.

McCall, D., Cox, D. M., Shelton, J. R., & Weinrich, M. (1997). The influence of syntactic and semantic information on picture-naming performance in aphasic patients. *Aphasiology, 11*, 581–600.

McCauley, R. J. (2001). *Assessment of language disorders in children*. Mahwah, NJ: Lawrence Erlbaum.

McCauley, R. J., & Swisher, L. (1984). Use and misuse of norm-referenced tests in clinical assessment: A hypothetical case. *Journal of Speech and Hearing Disorders, 49*, 338–348.

McCooey, R., Toffolo, D., & Code, C. (2000). A socioenvironmental approach to functional communication in hospital in-patients. In L. Worrall & C. Frattali (Eds.), *Neurogenic communication disorders: A functional approach* (pp. 295–311). New York: Thieme.

McCullagh, S., & Feinstein, A. (2005). Cognitive changes. In J. Silver & T. Y. McAllister, S.C. (Eds.), *Textbook of traumatic brain injury* (pp. 321–335). Washington, DC: American Psychiatric.

McDonald, S. (2000a). Exploring the cognitive basis of right-hemisphere pragmatic language disorders. *Brain and Language, 75*(1), 82–107.

McDonald, S. (2000b). Putting communication disorders in context after traumatic brain injury. *Aphasiology, 14*(4), 339–347.

McDonald, S., & Pearce, S. (1995). The 'dice' game: A new test of pragmatic language skills after closed-head injury. *Brain Injury, 9*(3), 255–271.

McNeil, M. R., Doyle, P. J., & Wambaugh, J. L. (2000). Apraxia of speech: A treatable disorder of motor planning and programming. In S. E. Nadeau, L. J. G. Rothi, & B. Crosson (Eds.), *Aphasia and language: Theory to practice* (pp. 221–266). New York: Guilford Press.

McNeil, M. R., & Kimelman, M. D. Z. (2001). Darley and the nature of aphasia: The defining and classifying controversies. *Aphasiology, 15*(3), 221–229.

McNeil, M. R., & Prescott, T. E. (1978). *Revised Token Test*. Austin, TX: Pro-Ed.

McNeil, M. R., Prescott, T. E., & Chang, E. C. (1975). A measure of PICA ordinality. *Clinical Aphasiology, 4*, 113–124.

Meline, T. (2005). *Research in communication sciences and disorders: Methods, applications, evaluation*. Upper Saddle Rive NJ: Pearson Education.

Menn, L., & Obler, L. K. (1990). *Agrammatic aphasia*. Amsterdam: Benjamins.

Menn, L., Ramsberger, G., & Helm-Estabrooks, N. (1994). A linguistic communication measure for aphasic narratives. *Aphasiology, 8*, 343–359.

Messerli, P., Tissot, A., & Rodriguez, R. (1976). Recovery from aphasia: Some factors for prognosis. In Y. Lebrun & R. Hoops (Eds.), *Recovery in aphasics* (pp. 124–135). Amsterdam: Swets and Zeitlinger.

Messick, S. (1980). Test validity and the ethics of assessment. *American Psychologist, 35*(11), 1012–1027.

Mesulam, M. M., Grossman, M., Hillis, A. E., Kertesz, A., & Weintraub, S. (2003). The core and halo of primary progressive aphasia and semantic dementia. *Annals of Neurology, 54*(S5), S11–S14.

Mesulam, M. M., & Weintraub, S. (1992). Primary progressive aphasia. In F. Boller (Ed.), *Heterogeneity of Alzheimer's disease* (pp. 43–66). Berlin: Springer-Verlag.

Meyers, J., & Meyers, K. (1995). *Rey Complex Figure Test and Recognition Trial*. Lutz, FL: Par Resources.

Miami Emergency Neurologic Deficit (MEND) prehospital checklist. (2001). Retrieved April 22, 2006, from http://www.strokeassociation.org/downloadable/stroke/5166_ prehospital_chklist.pdf

Miceli, G., Capasso, R., & Caramazza, A. (2004). The relationship between morphological and phonological errors in aphasic speech: Data from a word repetition task. *Neuropsychologia, 42*(3), 273–287.

Miller, G. (1956). The magical number seven, plus or minus two: Some limits on our capacity for processing information. *Psychological Review, 63*, 81–97.

Miller, N., Willmes, K., & DeBleser, R. (2000). The psychometric properties of the English language version of the Aachen Aphasia Test (EAAT). *Aphasiology, 14*(7), 683–722.

Mills, R., Knox, A., Juola, J., & McFarland, W. (1979). Cognitive loci of impairments of picture naming by aphasic subjects. *Journal of Speech and Hearing Research, 22*, 73–87.

Milroy, L., & Perkins, L. (1992). Repair strategies in aphasic discourse: Towards a collaborative model. *Clinical Linguistics and Phonetics, 6*, 27–40.

Mitchum, C. C., Ritgert, B. A., Sandson, J., & Berndt, R. S. (1990). The use of response analysis in confrontation naming. *Aphasiology, 4*, 261–280.

Molrine, C. J., & Pierce, R. S. (2002). Black and White adults' expressive language performance on three tests of aphasia. *American Journal of Speech-Language Pathology, 11*(2), 139–150.

Monetta, L., & Joanette, Y. (2003). Specificity of the right hemisphere's contributions to verbal communication: The cognitive resources hypothesis. *Journal of Medical Speech-Language Pathology, 11*(4), 203–211.

Muma, J. (1978). *Language handbook: Concepts, assessment, intervention.* Englewood Cliffs, NJ: Prentice-Hall.

Murdoch, B. (2006). *Neurogenic disorders of language: Theory driven clinical practice.* Clifton Park, NY: Thompson Delmar Learning.

Murdoch, B., & Theodoros, D. G. (2001). *Traumatic brain injury: Associated speech, language, and swallowing disorders.* San Diego, CA: Singular Thomson Learning.

Murray, L. (1996). *Relation between resource allocation and word-finding in aphasia.* Paper presented at the American Speech-Language-Hearing Association, Seattle, WA.

Murray, L. (1998). Longitudinal treatment of primary progressive aphasia: A case study. *Aphasiology, 12,* 651–672.

Murray, L. (2002). Attention deficits in aphasia: Presence, nature, assessment and treatment. *Seminars in Speech and Language, 23*(2), 107–116.

Murray, L., & Chapey, R. (2001). Assessment of language disorders in adults. In R. Chapey (Ed.), *Language intervention strategies in aphasia and related neurogenic communication disorders* (pp. 55–126). Philadelphia: Williams & Wilkins.

Murray, L., & Clark, H. (2006). *Neurogenic disorders of language.* Clifton Park, NJ: Thompson Delmar Learning.

Murray, L., & Holland, A. L. (1995). The language recovery of acutely aphasic patients receiving different therapy regimens. *Aphasiology, 9,* 397–405.

Murray, L., Holland, A. L., & Beeson, P. M. (1997). Auditory processing in individuals with mild aphasia: A study of resource allocation. *Journal of Speech, Language, and Hearing Research, 40,* 792–809.

Murray, L., Ramage, A. E., & Hopper, T. (2001). Memory impairments in adults with neurogenic communication disorders. *Seminars in Speech and Language, 22,* 129–138.

Myers, P. (1999). *Right hemisphere damage: Disorders of communication and cognition.* San Diego, CA: Singular.

Myers, P. (2001). Toward a definition of RHD syndrome. *Aphasiology, 15*(10/11), 913–918.

Myers, P. (2005). CAC Classics: Profiles of communication deficits in patients with right cerebral hemisphere damage: Implications for diagnosis and treatment. *Aphasiology, 19*(12), 1147–1460.

Nadeau, S. E., Rothi, L. J. G., & Crosson, B. (Eds.). (2000). *Aphasia and language: Theory to practice.* New York: Guilford Press.

Naeser, M. A., & Palumbo, C. L. (1994). Neuroimaging and language recovery in stroke. *Journal of Clinical Neurophysiology, 11,* 150–174.

National Faculty Center. (2006). Retrieved February 20, 2006, from http://nfc.arizona.edu/

The N-CEP registry of clinical practice guidelines and systematic reviews. (2005). Retrieved April 27, 2006, from http://www.asha.org/members/ebp/registry/N-CEP-Registry.htm

Neils, J., Baris, J. M., Carter, C., Dellaira, A. L., Nordloh, S., Weiler, E., et al. (1995). Effects of age, education, and living environment on Boston Naming Test performance. *Journal of Speech and Hearing Research, 38,* 1143–1149.

Neils-Strunjas, J. (1998). Clinical assessment strategies: Evaluation of language comprehension and production by formal test batteries. In B. Stemmer & H. Whitaker (Eds.), *Handbook of neurolinguistics* (pp. 71–82). New York: Academic Press.

Neiman, M. R., Duffy, R. J., Belanger, S. A., & Coelho, C. (2000). The assessment of limb apraxia: Relationship between performances on single- and multiple- object tasks by left hemisphere damaged patients. *Neuropsychological Rehabilitation, 10*(4), 429–448.

Neisser, U. (1967). *Cognitive psychology.* New York: Appleton-Century-Crofts.

Nelson, H., & Willison, J. (1991). *National Adult Reading Test* (2nd ed.). London: NFER Nelson.

Nelson, N. W. (1998). *Childhood language disorders in context: Infancy through adolescence* (2nd ed.). Needham Heights., MA: Allyn & Bacon.

Nemoto, T., Mizuno, M., & Kashima, H. (2005). Qualitative evaluation of divergent thinking in patiens with schizophrenia. *Behavioral Neurology, 16*(4), 217–224.

Newcombe, F., Oldfield, R. C., Ratcliff, G. G., & Wingfield, A. (1971). Recognition and naming of object-drawing by men with focal brain wounds. *Journal of Neurosurgery and Psychiatry, 34,* 329–340.

Newhoff, M., Tonkovich, J. D., Schwartz, S. L., & Burgess, E. K. (1985). Revision strategies in aphasia. *Clinical Aphasiology, 12,* 83–84.

Nicholas, L. E., & Brookshire, R. H. (1986). Consistency of the effects of rate of speech on brain-damaged adult's comprehension of narrative discourse. *Journal of Speech and Hearing Research, 29,* 462–470.

Nicholas, L. E., & Brookshire, R. H. (1987). Error analysis and passage dependency of test items from a standardized test of multiple-sentence reading comprehension for aphasic and non-brain-damaged adults. *Journal of Speech and Hearing Disorders, 52,* 358–366.

Nicholas, L. E., & Brookshire, R. H. (1992). A system for scoring main concepts in the discourse of non-brain-damaged and aphasic speakers. *Clinical Aphasiology, 21,* 87–99.

Nicholas, L. E., & Brookshire, R. H. (1993). A system for quantifying the informativeness and efficiency of the connected speech of adults with aphasia. *Journal of Speech and Hearing Research, 36,* 338–350.

Nicholas, L. E., & Brookshire, R. H. (1995a). Comprehension of spoken narrative discourse by adults with aphasia, right-hemisphere brain damage, or traumatic brain injury. *American Journal of Speech-Language Pathology, 4,* 69–81.

Nicholas, L. E., & Brookshire, R. H. (1995b). Presence, completeness, and accuracy of main concepts in the connected speech of non-brain-damaged adults and adults with aphasia. *Journal of Speech and Hearing Research, 38,* 145–156.

Nicholas, L. E., MacLennan, D. L., & Brookshire, R. H. (1986). Validity of multiple-sentence reading comprehension tests for aphasic adults. *Journal of Speech and Hearing Disorders, 51,* 82–87.

Nicholas, M., Obler, L. K., Albert, M. L., & Helm-Estabrooks, N. (1985). Empty speech in Alzheimer's disease and fluent aphasia. *Journal of Speech and Hearing Research, 28,* 405–410.

Nickels, L. A. (1995). Getting it right? Using aphasic naming errors to evaluate theoretical models of spoken word production. *Language and Cognitive Processes, 10,* 13–45.

Nickels, L. A. (2005). Tried, tested and trusted?: Language assessment for rehabilitation. In P. Halligan & D. Wade (Eds.), *Effectiveness of rehabilitation for cognitive deficits* (chap. 16). New York: Oxford University Press.

Nickels, L. A., & Best, W. (1996). Therapy for naming deficits (part I): Principles, puzzles and practices. *Aphasiology, 10*(1), 21–47.

Nickels, L. A., & Howard, D. (1995). Aphasia naming: What matters? *Neuropsychologia, 33*(10), 1281–1303.

Nickels, L. A., & Howard, D. (2004). Dissociating effects of number of phonemes, number of syllables, and syllabic complexity on word production in aphasia: It's the number of phonemes that counts. *Cognitive Neuropsychology, 21*(1), 57–78.

NIH Stroke Scale. (2003). Retrieved April 22, 2006, from http://ninds.nih.gov/doctors/NIHStrokeScale.pdf

Nkase-Thompson, R., Manning, E., Sherer, M., Yablon, S. A., Gontkovsky, S. L., & Vickery, C. (2005). Brief assessment of severe language impairments: Initial validation of the Mississippi Aphasia Screening Test. *Brain Injury, 19*(9), 685–691.

Obler, L. K., & Albert, M. L. (1979). *The Action Naming Test.* Boston: VA Medical Center.

Ochipa, C., Rothi, L. J. G., & Leslie, J. (2000). Limb apraxia. In S. E. Nadeau, L. J. G. Rothi, & B. Crosson (Eds.), *Aphasia and language: Theory to practice* (pp. 267–283). New York: Guilford Press.

Odell, K. H., Bair, S., Flynn, M., Workinger, M., Osborne, D., & Chial, M. (1997). Retrospective study of treatment outcome for individuals with aphasia. *Aphasiology, 45*, 415–432.

Ogar, J., Slama, H., Dronkers, N. F., Amici, S., & Gorno-Tempini, M. L. (2005). Apraxia of speech: An overview. *Neurocase, 11*(6), 427–432.

Ogar, J., Willock, S., Baldo, J., Wilkins, D., Ludy, C., & Dronkers, N. F. (2006). Clinical and anatomical correlates of apraxia of speech. *Brain and Language, 97*(3), 343–350.

Ogrezeanu, V., Voinescu, I., Mihailescu, L., & Jipescu, I. (1994). "Spontaneous" recovery in aphasics after single ischaemic stroke. *Romanian Journal of Neurology and Psychiatry, 32*, 77–90.

O'Halloran, R., Worrall, L., Toffolo, D., Code, C., & Hickson, L. (2004). *IFCI: Inpatient Functional Communication Interview.* Bicester, UK: Speechmark.

Olness, G. S., Ulatowska, H. K., Wertz, R. T., Thompson, J. L., & Auther, L. L. (2002). Discourse elicitation with pictorial stimuli in African Americans and Caucasians with and without aphasia. *Aphasiology, 16*(4–6), 623–633.

Oomen, C., Postma, A., & Kolk, H. (2001). Prearticulatory and postarticulatory self-monitoring in Broca's aphasia. *Cortex, 37*(5), 627–641.

O'Sullivan, T., & Fagan, S. C. (1998). Drug-induced communication and swallowing disorders. In A. F. Johnson & B. H. Jacobson (Eds.), *Medical speech-language pathology: A practitioner's guide* (pp. 176–191). New York: Thieme.

Ottenbacher, K. J., Hsu, Y., Granger, C. V., & Fiedler, R. C. (1996). The reliability of the Functional Independence Measure: A quantitative review. *Archives of Physical Medicine and Rehabilitation, 77*, 1226–1232.

Owens, R. (2004). *Language development* (6th ed.). Boston: Allyn & Bacon.

Paolucci, S., Antonucci, G., Pratesi, L., Traballesi, M., Lubich, S., & Grasso, M. G. (1998). Functional outcome in stroke inpatient rehabilitation: Predicting no, low, and high response patients. *Cerebrovascular Diseases, 8*, 228–234.

Paquier, P. F. (2005). A synthesis of the role of the cerebellum in cognition. *Aphasiology, 19*(1), 3–19.

Paradis, M. (2004). *A neurolinguistic theory of bilingualism.* Philadelphia: John Benjamins.

Paradis, M., & Libben, G. (1987). *The assessment of bilingual aphasia.* Hillsdale, NJ: Erlbaum.

Paradis, M., & Libben, G. (1993). *Evaluacion de la afasia en los bilingues.* Barcelona, Spain: Masson.

Park, G. H., McNeil, M. R., & Doyle, P. J. (2002). Lexical access rate of closed-class elements during auditory sentence comprehension in adults with aphasia. *Aphasiology, 16*(8), 801–814.

Parkerson, G. R., Gehlbach, S. H., & Wagner, E. H. (1981). The Duke-UNC Health Profile: An adult health status measure. *Medical Care, 19*, 787–805.

Parr, S., & Byng, S. (2000). Perspectives and priorities: Accessing user views in functional communication assessment. In L. Worrall & C. Frattali (Eds.), *Neurogenic communication disorders: A functional approach* (pp. 55–66). New York: Thieme.

Parr, S., Byng, S., & Gilpin, S. (1997). *Talking about aphasia.* Buckingham: Open University Press.

Pashek, G. V., & Tompkins, C. A. (2002). Context and word class influences on lexical retrieval in aphasia. *Aphasiology, 16*(3), 261–286.

Paterson, B., & Scott-Findlay, S. (2002). Critical issues in interviewing people with traumatic brain injury. *Qualitative Health Research, 12*(3), 399–409.

Patterson, J. (2001). The effectiveness of cueing hierarchies as a treatment for word retrieval impairment. *Perspectives on Neurophysiology and Neurogenic Speech and Language Disorders, 11*(2), 11–18.

Patterson, J. (2002). Post stroke depression in persons with chronic aphasia. *Perspectives on Gerontology, 15*(3), 7–10.

Patterson, J., Delton, C., McIntire, C., Lloyd, C., & Craney, J. (2003). *Semantic therapy: Treatment effeciveness and generalization to connected speech.* Paper presented at the California Speech-Language-Hearing Association, Long Beach, CA.

Patterson, J., & Fahey, K. B. (1994). Design, implementation, and evaluation of a treatment program to improve initiating skills in persons with language impairment. *Rocky Mountain Journal of Communication Disorders, 10*, 19–26.

Patterson, J., & Hinnach, S. E. (2005). *Word familiarity effects during naming and discourse production in aphasia.* Paper presented at the American Speech-Language-Hearing Association, San Diego.

Patterson, K., Coltheart, M., & Marshall, J. C. (1985). *Surface dyslexia.* London, England: Erlbaum.

Patterson, R., & Wells, A. (1995). Involving the family in planning for life with aphasia. *Topics in Stroke Rehabilitation, 2*, 39–46.

Paul, D. R., Frattali, C., Holland, A. L., Thompson, C. K., Caperton, C. J., & Slater, S. *Quality of Communication Life Scale (ASHA-QCL).* Rockville, MD: American Speech-Language-Hearing Association.

Payne, J. C. (1994). *Communication profile: A functional skills survey.* San Antonio, TX: Communication Skill Builders.

Payne, J. C. (1997). *Adult neurogenic language disorders: Assessment and treatment: A comprehensive ethnobiological approach.* San Diego: Singular.

Payne-Johnson, J. C. (1992). An ethnocentric perspective on African American elderly persons and functional communication assessment. *The Howard Journal of Communication, 3*, 194–203.

Peach, R. K. (2004). Acquired apraxia of speech: Features, accounts, and treatment. *Topics in Stroke Rehabilitation, 11*(1), 49–58.

Pease, D. M., & Goodglass, H. (1978). Effects of cueing on picture naming in aphasia. *Cortex, 14,* 178–189.

Pedersen, P., Jorgensen, H. S., Nakayama, H., Raaschou, H. O., & Olsen, T. S. (1997). Hemineglect in acute stroke: Incidence and prognostic implications. *American Journal of Physical Medicine and Rehabilitation, 76,* 122–127.

Pedersen, P., Vinter, K., & Olsen, T. (2004). Aphasia after stroke: Type, severity and prognosis. *Cerebrovascular Diseases, 17,* 35–43.

Penn, C. (1988). The profiling of syntax and pragmatics in aphasia. *Clinical Linguistics and Phonetics, 2,* 179–207.

Penn, C. (1999). Pragmatic assessment and therapy for persons with brain damage: What have clinicians gleaned in two decades? *Brain and Language, 68*(3), 535–522.

Perkins, L., Crisp, J., & Walshaw, D. (1999). Exploring conversation analysis as an assessment tool for aphasia: The issue of reliability. *Aphasiology, 13*(4–5), 259–281.

Pimentel, P. A., & Knight, J. A. (2000). *The Mini Inventory of Right Brain Injury* (2nd ed.). Austin, TX: Pro-Ed.

Pineda, D. A., Roselli, M., Ardila, A., Meija, S. E., Romero, M., & Perez, C. (2000). The Boston Diagnostic Aphasia Examination –Spanish version: The influence of demographic variables. *Journal of the International Neuropsychological Society, 6,* 802–814.

Plante, E., & Beeson, P. (2004). *Communication and communication disorders: A clinical introduction* (2nd ed.). Boston: Allyn and Bacon.

Ponsford, J., & Kinsella, G. (1991). The use of a rating scale of attentional behaviour. *Neuropsychological Rehabilitation, 1*(4), 241–257.

Porch, B. E. (1967). *Porch Index of Communicative Ability. (Vol. 1) Theory and development.* Palo Alto, CA: Consulting Psychologists Press.

Porch, B. E. (1971). Multidimensional scoring in aphasia testing. *Journal of Speech and Hearing Research, 14*(4), 776–792.

Porch, B. E. (1981). *Porch Index of Communicative Ability. (Vol. 2) Administration, scoring, and interpretation* (3rd ed.). Palo Alto, CA: Consulting Psychologists Press.

Porteus, S. D. (1959). *The Maze Test and clinical psychology.* Palo Alto, CA: Pacific Books.

Powell, G. E., Bailey, S., & Clark, E. (1980). A very short form of the Minnesota Aphasia Test. *British Journal of Social and Clinical Psychology, 19,* 189–194.

Power, E., & Code, C. (2006). Waving not drowning: Utilizing gesture in the treatment of aphasia. *Advances in Speech-Language Pathology, 8*(2), 115–119.

Prinz, P. (1980). A note on requesting strategies in adult aphasics. *Journal of Communication Disorders, 13,* 65–73.

Prutting, C. (1979). Process/pra/ses/n: The action of moving forward progressively from one point to another on the way to completion. *Journal of Speech and Hearing Research, 14,* 776–792.

Prutting, C., & Kirchner, D. (1983). Applied pragmatics. In T. Gallagher & C. Prutting (Eds.), *Pragmatic assessment and intervention issues in language* (pp. 29–64). San Diego, CA: College-Hill Press.

Prutting, C., & Kirchner, D. (1987). A clinical appraisal of the pragmatic aspects of language. *Journal of Speech and Hearing Disorders, 52,* 105–119.

Purdy, M. (2002). Executive function ability in persons with aphasia. *Aphasiology, 16*(4–6), 549–557.

Purdy, M. (2006). Prediction of strategy use by adults with aphasia. *Aphasiology, 20*(2–4), 337–348.

Purdy, M., & Hindenlang, J. (2005). Educating and training caregivers of persons with aphasia. *Aphasiology, 19*(3–5), 377–388.

Puskaric, N. J., & Pierce, R. S. (1997). Effects of constraint and expectation on reading comprehension in aphasia. *Aphasiology, 11,* 249–261.

Quillen, D. A. (1999). Common causes of vision loss in elderly patients. *American Family Physician, 60*(1), 99–108.

Radanovic, M., & Mansur, L. L. (2002). Performance of a Brazilian population sample in the Boston Diagnostic Aphasia Examination: A pilot study. *Brazilian Journal of Medical and Biological Research, 35*(3), 305–317.

Ramsberger, G. (2005). Achieving conversational success in aphasia by focusing on non-linguistic cognitive skills: A potential promising new approach. *Aphasiology, 19*(1011), 1066–1073.

Rapcsak, S. Z., & Rubens, A. B. (1994). Localization of lesions in transcortical aphasia. In A. Kertesz (Ed.), *Localization and neuroimaging in neuropsychology* (pp. 297–329). San Diego: Academic Press.

Ravaud, J. F., Delcey, M., & Yelnik, A. (1999). Construct validity of the Functional Independence Measure (FIM): Questioning the unidimensionality of the scale and the "value" of FIM scores. *Scandinavian Journal of Rehabilitation Medicine, 31*(1), 31–41.

Raven, J., Raven, J. C., & Court, J. H. (1995). *Raven's Colored Progressive Matrices.* San Antonio, TX: Harcourt Assessment.

Raymer, A. M. (2005). Naming and word-retrieval problems. In L. L. LaPointe (Ed.), *Aphasia and related neurogenic language Disorders* (pp. 68–82). New York: Thieme.

Raymer, A. M., Maher, L. M., Greenwald, M. L., Morris, M., Rothi, L. J. G., & Heilman, K. M. (1990). *The Florida Semantics Battery: Experimental edition.* Gainesville, FL: University of Florida Department of Neurology.

Raymer, A. M., & Rothi, L. J. G. (2000). The semantic system. In S. E. Nadeau, L. J. G. Rothi, & B. Crosson (Eds.), *Aphasia and language: Theory to practice* (pp. 108–132). New York: The Guilford Press.

Raymer, A. M., & Rothi, L. J. G. (2002). Clinical diagnosis and treatment of naming disorders. In A. E. Hillis (Ed.), *The handbook of adult language disorders: Integrating cognitive neuropsychology, neurology and rehabilitation* (pp. 163–182). New York: Psychology Press.

Records, N. L. (1994). A measure of the contribution of a gesture to the perception of speech in listeners with aphasia. *Journal of Speech and Hearing Research, 37,* 1086–1099.

Reitan, R. M. (1991). *Reitan-Indiana Aphasia Screening Test.* Tucson, AZ: Reitan Neuropsychology Laboratory.

Rey, G. J., & Benton, A. L. (1991). *Examen de Afasia Multilingue: Manual de instrucciones.* Iowa City, IA: AJA Associates.

Ripich, D. N. (1995). Differential diagnosis and assessment. In R. Lubinski (Ed.), *Dementia and communication* (pp. 188–222). San Diego: Singular.

Robertson, I. H., Ward, T., Ridgeway, V., & Nimmo-Smith, I. (1994). *The Test of Everyday Attention.* San Antonio, TX: Harcourt.

Robey, R. (1998). A meta-analysis of clinical outcomes in the treatment of aphasia. *Journal of Speech, Language and Hearing Research, 41,* 172–187.

Rochon, E., Saffran, E., Berndt, R., & Schwartz, M. (1998). Quantitative production analysis: Norming and reliability data. *Brain and Language, 65*, 10–13.

Rogers, M. A., & Alarcon, N. B. (1998). Dissolution of spoken language in primary progressive aphasia. *Aphasiology, 12*(7/8), 635–650.

Rolnick, M., & Hoops, H. (1969). Aphasia as seen by the aphasic. *Journal of Speech and Hearing Research, 34*, 48–53.

Rose, M. (2006). The utility of arm and hand gestures in the treatment of aphasia. *Advances in Speech-Language Pathology, 8*(2), 92–109.

Rose, M., & Douglas, J. M. (2001). The differential facilitatory effects of gesture and visualization processes on object naming in aphasia. *Aphasiology, 15*(10–11), 977–990.

Rose, M., & Douglas, J. M. (2003). Limb apraxia, pantomime, and lexical gesture in aphasic speakers: Preliminary findings. *Aphasiology, 17*(5), 453–464.

Rosenbek, J., LaPointe, L., & Wertz, R. (1989). *Aphasia: A clinical approach*. Austin, TX: Pro-Ed.

Rosenfeld, N. (1978). Conversational control function of nonverbal behavior. In A. Siegman & S. Feldstein (Eds.), *Nonverbal behavior and communication*. Hillsdale, NJ: Lawrence Erlbaum.

Ross, K. B., & Wertz, R. T. (1999). Comparison of impairment and disability measures for assessing severity of, and improvement in, aphasia. *Aphasiology, 13*, 113–124.

Ross, K. B., & Wertz, R. T. (2002). Relationships between language-based disability and quality of life in chronically aphasic adults. *Aphasiology, 16*(8), 791–800.

Ross, K. B., & Wertz, R. T. (2003). Quality of life with and without aphasia. *Aphasiology, 17*(4), 355–364.

Ross, K. B., & Wertz, R. T. (2005). Advancing appraisal: Aphasia and the WHO. *Aphasiology, 19*(9), 860–900.

Ross-Swain, D. (1996). *Ross Information Processing Assessment* (2nd ed.). Austin, TX: Pro-Ed.

Rothi, L. J. G., & Heilman, K. M. (1997). *Apraxia: The neuropsychology of action* (pp. 61–73). Hove, UK: Psychology Press/Erlbaum.

Rothi, L. J. G., Mack, L., Verfaellie, M., Brown, P., & Heilman, K. M. (1988). Ideomotor apraxia: Error pattern analysis. *Aphasiology, 2*, 381–387.

Rothi, L. J. G., Raymer, A. M., & Heilman, K. M. (1997). Limb praxis assessment. In L. J. G. Rothi & K. M. Heilman (Eds.), *Apraxia: The neuropsychology of action*. Hove, UK: Psychology Press/Erlbaum.

Rothi, L. J.G, Raymer, A. M., Maher, L., Greenwald, M., & Morris, M. (1991). Assessment of naming failures in neurological communication disorders. *Clinics in Communication Disorders, 1*, 7–20.

Royal College of Speech and Language Therapists: Clinical Guidelines. (2005). Retrieved April 20, 2006, from http://www.rcslt.org/resources/clinicalguidelines

Ruff, R. M., Light, R. H., Parker, S. B., & Levin, H. S. (1996). Benton Controlled Oral Word Association Test: Reliability and updated norms. *Archives of Neuropsychology, 11*(4), 329–338.

Ryff, C., & Singer, B. (1998). The contours of positive human health. *Psychological Inquiry, 9*(1), 1–29.

Sacchett, C. (2002). Drawing in aphasia: Moving towards the interactive. *International Journal of Human-Computer Studies, 57*(4), 263–277.

Sackett, D. L., Rosenberg, W. M., Gray, J. A. M., Haynes, R. B., & Richardson, W. S. (1996). Evidence-based medicine: What it is and what it isn't. *British Medical Journal, 312*, 71–72.

Saffran, E. M., Berndt, R. S., & Schwartz, M. F. (1989). The quantitative analysis of agrammatic production: Procedure and data. *Brain and Language, 37*, 440–479.

Salter, K., Jutai, J., Foley, N., Hellings, C., & Teasel, R. (2006). Identification of aphasia post stroke: A review of screening assessment tools. *Brain Injury, 2*(6), 559–568.

Sands, E., Sarno, M., & Shankwilder, D. (1969). Long term assessment of language function in aphasia due to stroke. *Archives of Physical Medicine and Rehabilitation, 50*, 202–207.

Sarno, J., Sarno, M., & Levita, E. (1973). The functional life scale. *Archives of Physical Medicine and Rehabilitation, 54*(5), 214–220.

Sarno, M. (1969). *The Functional Communication Profile: Manual of directions*. New York: Institute of Rehabilitation Medicine.

Sarno, M. (1997). Quality of life in aphasia in the first post-stroke year. *Aphasiology, 11*(7), 665–679.

Sarno, M., Buonaguro, A., & Levita, E. (1985). Gender and recovery from aphasia after stroke. *Journal of Nervous and Mental Disorders, 173*(10), 605–609.

Schegloff, E., Jefferson, G., & Sacks, H. (1977). The preference for self-correction in the organization of repair in conversation. *Language and Cognitive Processes, 53*, 361–382.

Schienberg, S., & Holland, A. L. (1980). Conversational turn-taking in Wernicke's aphasia. *Clinical Aphasiology, 10*, 106–110.

Schuell, H. (1965). *The Minnesota Test for Differential Diagnosis of Aphasia*. Minneapolis, MN: University of Minnesota Press.

Schuell, H., Carroll, V., & Street, B. (1955). Clinical treatment of aphasia. *Journal of Speech and Hearing Disorders, 20*, 43–53.

Schuell, H., Jenkins, J., & Jimenez-Pabon, E. (1964). *Aphasia in adults*. New York: Harper and Row.

Schuell, H., Jenkins, J., & Landis, L. (1961). Relationship between auditory comprehension and word frequency in aphasia. *Journal of Speech and Hearing Research, 4*, 30–36.

Schwanenflugel, P., & Shoben, E. (1985). The influence of sentence constraint on the scope of facilitation for upcoming words. *Journal of Memory and Language, 24*, 232–252.

Schwartz, M. F. (1984). What the classical aphasia categories can't do for us, and why. *Brain and Language, 21*(1), 3–8.

Schwartz, M. F., & Brecher, A. (2000). A model-driven analysis of severity, response characteristics, and partial recovery in aphasics' picture naming. *Brain and Language, 73*(1), 62–91.

Schwartz, M. F., Fink, R. B., & Saffran, E. M. (1995). The modular treatment of agrammatism. *Neuropsychological Rehabilitation, 5*(97), 127.

Schwartz, R. L., Adair, J. C., & Raymer, A. M. (2000). Conceptual apraxia in probable Alzheimer's disease as demonstrated on the Florida Action Recall Test. *Journal of the International Neuropsychological Society, 6*, 265–270.

Searle, J. (1969). *Speech acts: An essay in the philosophy of language*. London: Cambridge University Press.

Seddoh, S. (2000). Basis of intonation disturbance in aphasia: Production. *Aphasiology, 14*(11), 1105–1126.

Seddoh, S. (2004). Prosodic disturbance in aphasia: Speech timing versus intonation production. *Clinical Linguistics and Phonetics, 18*(1), 17–38.

Shadden, B. (1998a). Information analysis. In L. R. Cherney, B. B. Shadden, & C. Coelho (Eds.), *Analyzing discourse in communicatively impaired adults* (pp. 85–114). Gaithersburg, MD: Aspen.

Shadden, B. (1998b). Obtaining the discourse sample. In L. R. Cherney, B. B. Shadden, & C. Coelho (Eds.), *Analyzing discourse in communicatively impaired adults* (pp. 9–34). Gaithersburg, MD: Aspen.

Shadden, B., Burnette, R., B., Eikenberry, B. R., & DiBrezzo, R. (1991). All discourse tasks are not created equal. In T. Prescott (Ed.), *Clinical Aphasiology* (Vol. 20, pp. 327–241). Austin, TX: Pro-Ed.

Shapiro, K., Shelton, J., & Caramazza, A. (2000). Grammatical class in lexical production and morphological processing: Evidence from a case of fluent aphasia. *Cognitive Neuropsychology, 17*(8), 665–682.

Shewan, C. M. (1979). *Auditory Comprehension Test for Sentences.* Chicago: Biolinguistics Clinical Institutes.

Shewan, C. M. (1988a). Expressive language recovery in aphasia using the Shewan Spontaneous Language Analysis (SSLA) system. *Journal of Communication Disorders, 21,* 155–169.

Shewan, C. M. (1988b). The Shewan Spontaneous Language Analysis (SSLA) system for aphasic adults: Description, reliability, and validity. *Journal of Communication Disorders, 21,* 103–138.

Shewan, C. M., & Canter, G. (1971). Effects of vocabulary, syntax and sentence length on auditory comprehension in aphasic patients. *Cortex, 7,* 209–226.

Shewan, C. M., & Kertesz, A. (1984). Effects of speech and language treatment on recovery from aphasia. *Brain and Language, 23,* 272–299.

Shill, M. (1979). Motivational factors in aphasia therapy: Research suggestions. *Journal of Communication Disorders, 12*(6), 503–517.

Shipley, J. G., & McAfee, J. G. (2004). *Assessment in speech-language pathology* (3rd ed.). Clifton Park, NY: Thompson Delmar Learning.

Shlonsky, A., & Gibbs, L. (2004). Will the real evidence-based practice please stand up? Teaching the process of evidence-based practice to the helping professions. *Brief Treatment and Crisis Intervention, 4,* 137–153.

Shuster, L. (2004). Resource theory and aphasia reconsidered: Why alternative theories can better guide our research. *Aphasiology, 18*(9), 811–830.

Siegel, G. (1959). Dysphasic speech responses to visual word stimuli. *Journal of Speech and Hearing Research, 2,* 152–160.

Siegert, R., & Taylor, W. (2004). Theoretical aspects of goal-setting and motivation in rehabilitation. *Disability and Rehabilitation, 26*(1), 1–8.

Simmons-Mackie, N. (2001). Social approaches to intervention. In R. Chapey (Ed.), *Language intervention strategies in aphasia and related neurogenic communication disorders* (4th ed., pp. 246–268). Philadelphia: Lippincott Williams & Wilkins.

Simmons-Mackie, N. (2004). Using the ICF framework to define outcomes. *Perspectives on Neurophysiology and Neurogenic Speech and Language Disorders, 14,* 9–11.

Simmons-Mackie, N., & Damico, J. S. (1996). Accounting for handicaps in aphasia: Communicative assessment from an authentic social perspective. *Disability and Rehabilitation, 18,* 540–549.

Simmons-Mackie, N., & Kagan, A. (1999). Communication strategies used by 'good' versus 'poor' speaking partners of individuals with aphasia. *Aphasiology, 13*(9–11), 807–820.

Simmons-Mackie, N., & Schultz, M. (2003). The role of humor in therapy for aphasia. *Aphasiology, 17*(8), 751–766.

Sivan, A. B. (1992). *Benton Visual Retention Test* (5th ed.). Lutz, FL: Psychological Assessment Resources.

Skelly, M. (1979). *AmerInd gestural code based on universal American Indian hand talk.* New York: Elsevier.

Skenes, L., & McCauley, R. (1985). Psychometric review of nine aphasia tests. *Journal of Communication Disorders, 18*(6), 461–474.

Sklar, M. (1983). *Sklar Aphasia Scale.* Los Angeles, CA: Western Psychological Services.

Snodgrass, J., & Vanderwoort, M. (1980). A standardized set of 260 pictures: Norms for name agreement, image agreement, familiarity, and visual complexity. *Journal of Experimental Psychology: Human Learning and Memory, 6,* 174–215.

Snowden, J. S. (1999). Neuropsychological evaluation and the diagnosis and differential diagnosis of dementia. *Reviews in Clinical Gerontology, 9,* 65–72.

Snyder, L. S. (1983). From assessment to intervention: Problems and solutions. In J. Miller, D. Yoder, & R. Schiefelbush (Eds.), *Contemporary issues in language intervention* (pp.147–164). Rockville, MD: American Speech-Language-Hearing Association.

Sohlberg, M. M., & Mateer, C. A. (2001). *Cognitive rehabilitation: An integrative neuropsychological approach.* New York: The Guilford Press.

Spellacy, F. J., & Spreen, O. (1969). A short form of the Token Test. *Cortex, 5*(4), 391–397.

Spencer, K. A., Tompkins, C. A., & Schultz, R. (1997). Assessment of depression in patients with brain pathology: The case of stroke. *Psychological Bulletin, 122,* 132–152.

Spreen, O., & Benton, A. L. (1977). *Neurosensory center comprehensive examination for aphasia.* Victoria, BC: University of Victoria, Neuropsychology Laboratory.

Spreen, O., & Risser, A. H. (2003). *Assessment of aphasia.* Oxford: Oxford University Press.

Spreen, O., & Strauss, E. (1998). *A compendium of neuropsychological tests* (2nd ed.). New York: Oxford University Press.

Springer, L., Huber, W., Schlenck, K. J., & Schlenk, C. (2000). Agrammatism: Deficit or compensation? Consequences for therapy. *Neuropsychological Rehabilitation, 10*(3), 279–309.

Squire, L. R. (1987). *Memory and brain.* New York: Oxford University Press.

Stachowiak, F. J., Huber, W., Poeck, K., & Kerschensteiner, M. (1977). Text comprehension in aphasia. *Brain and Language, 4,* 177–195.

Starkstein, S. E., & Robinson, R. G. (1988). Aphasia and depression. *Aphasiology, 2,* 1–20.

Stern, R. (1999). Assessment of mood states in aphasia. *Seminars in Speech and Language, 20,* 33–49.

Stern, R., Arruda, J. E., Hooper, C. R., Wolfner, G. D., & Morey, C. E. (1997). Visual analogue mood scales to measure internal mood state in neurologically impaired patients: Description and initial validity studies. *Aphasiology, 11*(1), 40–59.

Stern, R., & Bachman, D. L. (1991). Depressive symptoms following stroke. *American Journal of Psychiatry, 148,* 351–356.

Stierwalt, J. A. G. (2002). Attention impairment following traumatic brain injury. *Seminars in Speech and Language, 23*(2), 129–138.

Stoicheff, M. L. (1960). Motivating instructions and language performance of dysphasic subjects. *Journal of Speech and Hearing Research, 3,* 75–85.

Stone, S. P., Halligan, P. W., & Greenwood, R. J. (1993). The incidence of neglect phenomena and related disorders in patients with an acute right or left hemisphere stroke. *Age and Ageing, 22,* 46–52.

Strauss, E., Sherman, E. M. S., & Spreen, O. (2006). *A compendium of neuropsychological tests* (3rd ed.). Oxford: Oxford University Press.

Strauss, E., Spreen, O., & Hunter, M. (2000). Implications of test revisions for research. *Psychological Assessment, 12,* 237–244.

Stringer, A. Y. (1996). *A guide to adult neuropsychological diagnosis.* Philadelphia, PA: F.A. Davis.

Stroke scales. (2006). Retrieved April 22, 2006, from http://www.stroke-site.org/stroke_scale/stroke_scales.html

Sugishita, M. (1988). *WAB Aphasia Test in Japanese.* Tokyo: Igaku Shoin.

Sutcliffe, L. M., & Lincoln, N. B. (1998). The assessment of depression in aphasic stroke patients: The development of the Stroke Aphasic Depression Questionnaire. *Clinical Rehabilitation, 12,* 506–513.

Swinburn, K., Porter, G., & Howard, D. (2004). *Comprehensive Aphasia Test.* Hove, East Sussex, UK: Psychology Press.

Swindell, C. S., & Hammons, J. (1991). Post-stroke depression: Neurologic, physiologic, diagnostic, and treatment implications. *Journal of Speech and Hearing Research, 34,* 325–333.

Swindell, C. S., Pashek, G. V., & Holland, A. L. (1982). A questionnaire for surveying personal and communicative style. *Clinical Aphasiology, 12,* 50–63.

Syder, D., Body, R., Parker, M., & Boddy, M. (1993). *Sheffield Screening Test for Acquired Language Disorders.* Windsor: NFER-NELSON.

Tanner, D., & Culbertson, W. (1999). *Quick Assessment for Aphasia.* Oceanside, CA: Academic Communication Associates.

Tanner, D., Gerstenberger, D. L., & Keller, C. S. (1989). Guidelines for treatment of chronic depression in the aphasic patient. *Rehabilitation Nursing, 14,* 77–80.

Tatemichi, T. K., Desmond, D. W., Stern, Y., Paik, M., Sano, M., & Bagiella, E. (1994). Cognitive impairment after stroke: Frequency, patterns, and relationship to functional abilities. *Journal of Neurology, Neurosurgery, and Psychiatry, 57,* 202–207.

ter Keurs, M., Brown, C. M., & Hagoort, P. (2002). Lexical processing of vocabulary class in patients with Broca's aphasia: An event-related brain potential study on agrammatic comprehension. *Neuropsychologia, 40*(9), 1547–1561.

Tetnowski, J. A., & Franklin, T. C. (2003). Qualitative research: Implications for description and assessment. *American Journal of Speech-Language Pathology, 12,* 155–164.

Thompson, C. (2000). The neurobiology of language recovery in aphasia. *Brain and Language, 71,* 245–248.

Thompson, C., Shapiro, L. P., Tait, M. E., Jacobs, B. J., Schneider, S. L., & Ballard, K. J. (1995). A system for the linguistic analysis of agrammatic language production. *Brain and Language, 51,* 124–129.

Threats, T. (2004). The use of the ICF in intervention for persons with neurogenic communication disorders. *Perspectives on Neurophysiology and Neurogenic Speech and Language Disorders, 14,* 1–8.

Threats, T. (2005). ICF and QOL: A partnership. *Perspectives on Neurophysiology and Neurogenic Speech and Language Disorders, 15* (4), 4–6.

Threats, T., & Worrall, L. (2004). Classifying communication disability using the ICF. *Advances in Speech-Language Pathology, 6*(1), 53–62.

Thurstone, L. L., & Thurstone, T. G. (1962). *Primary mental abilities–Revised.* Chicago: Science Research Associates.

Tombaugh, T. N., & Hubley, A. M. (1997). The 60-item Boston Naming Test: Norms for cognitively intact adults aged 25 to 88 years. *Journal of Clinical and Experimental Neuropsychology, 19,* 922–932.

Tompkins, C. A. (1995). *Right hemisphere communication disorders: Theory and management.* San Diego: Singular.

Tompkins, C. A., Bloise, C. G. R., Timko, M. L., & Baumgaertner, A. (1994). Working memory and inference revision in brain-damaged and normally aging adults. *Journal of Speech and Hearing Research, 37,* 896–912.

Tompkins, C. A., Jackson, S., & Shulz, R. (1990). On prognostic research in adult neurologic disorders. *Journal of Speech and Hearing Research, 33,* 398–401.

Tompkins, C. A., Rau, M., Schulz, R., & Rhyne, C. (1987). Post-stroke depression in primary support persons: Predicting those at risk. *ASHA, 29,* 79.

Toppin, C. J., & Brookshire, R. H. (1978). Effects of response delay and token relocation on Token Test performance of aphasic subjects. *Journal of Communication Disorders, 2,* 57–68.

Torrance, E. P. (1966). *Torrance Test of Creative Thinking.* Princeton, NJ: Personnel Press.

Towards a common language for functioning, disability and health. (2002). Retrieved February 2, 2006, from http://www.designfor21st.org/documents/who_icf_2002.pdf

Tower, C. D. (2004). Disability through the lens of culture. *Journal of Social Work in Disability and Rehabilitation, 2*(2/3), 5–22.

Trahan, D. E., & Larrabee, G. J. (1988). *Continuous Visual Memory Test.* Lutz, FL: Psychological Assessment Resources.

Treisman, A. (1965). Effect of verbal context on latency of word selection. *Nature, 206,* 218–219.

Turkstra, L., Coelho, C., & Ylvisaker, M. (2005). The use of standardized tests for individuals with cognitive-communication disorders. *Seminars in Speech and Language, 26*(4), 215–222.

Turkstra, L., Coelho, C., Ylvisaker, M., Kennedy, M., Sohlberg, M. M., Avery, J., et al. (2005). Practice guidelines for standardized assessment for persons with traumatic brain injury. *Journal of Medical Speech Language Pathology, 13*(2), ix–xxviii.

Turkstra, L., Ylvisaker, M., Coelho, C., Kennedy, M., Sohlberg, M. M., Avery, J., et al. (2003). *Standardized assessment for persons with traumatic brain injury.* Retrieved February 12, 2006, from http://www.ancds.org/pdf/CogComStandardized_Tech_report.pdf

Ulatowska, H. K., Allard, L., Reyes, B. A., Ford, J., & Chapman, S. (1992). Conversational discourse in aphasia. *Aphasiology, 6,* 325–331.

Ulatowska, H. K., Doyel, A. W., Freedman-Stern, R. F., Macaluso-Haynes, S., & North, A. J. (1983). Production of procedural discourse in aphasia. *Brain and Language, 18,* 315–341.

Ulatowska, H. K., Freedman-Stern, R. F., Doyel, A. W., Macaluso-Haynes, S., & North, A. J. (1983). Production of narrative discourse in aphasia. *Brain and Language, 19,* 317–334.

Ulatowska, H. K., Wertz, R. T., Chapman, S. B., Hill, C. L., Thompson, J., L., Keebler, M. W., et al. (2001). Interpretation of fables and proverbs by African Americans with and without aphasia. *American Journal of Speech-Language Pathology, 10,* 40–50.

Uryase, D., Duffy, R. J., & Liles, B. Z. (1991). Analysis and description of narrative discourse in right-hemisphere-damaged adults: A comparison with neurologically normal and left-hemisphere-damaged aphasic adults. *Clinical Aphasiology, 19,* 125–137.

Vandenberghe, R. R., Vandenbulcke, M., Weintraub, S., Johnson, N., Porke, K., Thompson, C. K., et al. (2005). Paradoxical features of word finding difficulty in primary progressive aphasia. *Annals of Neurology, 57*(2), 204–209.

van Harskamp, F., & Visch-Brink, E. (1991). Goal recognition in aphasia therapy. *Aphasiology, 5,* 529–539.

van Heutgen, C. M., Dekker, J., & Deelman, B. G. (1999). A diagnostic test for apraxia with stroke patients: Internal consistency and diagnostic value. *The Clinical Neuropsychologist, 13,* 182–192.

van Zomeren, A. H., & Spikman, J. M. (2005). Testing speech and control: The assessment of attentional impairments. In P. Halligan & D. Wade (Eds.), *Effectiveness of rehabilitation for cognitive deficits* (chap. 8). New York: Oxford University Press.

Varney, N. R. (1982). Pantomime recognition defect in aphasia: Implications for the concept of asymbolia. *Brain and Language, 15,* 32–39.

Varney, N. R. (1998). Neuropsychological assessment of aphasia. In G. Goldstein, P. D. Nussbaum & S. R. Beers (Eds.), *Neuropsychology* (pp. 357–378). New York: Plenum Press.

Vignolo, L. A. (2005). Music agnosia and auditory agnosia: Dissociations in stroke patients. In A. Guiliano, C. Faienza, D. Minciacchi, L. Lopez & M. Manjo (Eds.), *The neurosciences and music* (pp. 50–57). New York: New York Academy of Sciences.

Vogel, D., Carter, P., & Carter, J. (1999). *Effects of drugs on communication disorders* (2nd ed.). Clifton Park, NJ: Thomson Delmar Learning.

Wade, D. T. (2005). Applying the WHO ICF framework to the rehabilitation of patients with cognitive deficits. In P. W. Halligan & D. T. Wade (Eds.), *Effectiveness of rehabilitation for cognitive deficits* (chap. 5). New York: Oxford University Press.

Währborg, P. (1991). *Assessment and management of emotional and psychosocial reactions to brain damage and aphasia.* San Diego: Singular.

Wallace, G., & Hammill, D. D. (2002). *Comprehensive Receptive and Expressive Vocabulary Test-Adult* (2nd ed.). Austin, TX: Pro-Ed.

Wang, L., & Goodglass, H. (1992). Pantomime, praxis, and aphasia. *Brain and Language, 42,* 402–418.

Warden, M. R., & Hutchinson, T. J. (1993). *The Writing Process Test.* Austin, TX: Pro-Ed.

Ward-Lonergan, J., & Nicholas, M. (1995). Drawing to communicate: A case report of an adult with global aphasia. *European Journal of Disorders of Communication, 30,* 475–491.

Warren, R. G. (1999). Creating value with measurement: Moving toward the patient. *Topics in Stroke Rehabilitation, 5,* 17–37.

Webb, W. G., & Love, R. J. (1983). Reading problems in chronic aphasia. *Journal of Speech and Hearing Disorders, 48,* 164–171.

Webster's New Collegiate Dictionary. (1977). Springfield: Merriam-Webster.

Wechsler, D. (1997a). *Wechsler Adult Intelligence Scale* (3rd ed.). San Antonio, TX: The Psychological Corporation.

Wechsler, D. (1997b). *Wechsler Memory Scale* (3rd ed.). San Antonio, TX: The Psychological Corporation.

Wechsler, D. (2001). *Wechsler Test of Adult Reading.* San Antonio TX: Harcourt Assessment.

Ween, J. E., Verfaellie, M., & Alexander, M. P. (1996). Verbal memory function in mild aphasia. *Neurology, 47,* 795–801.

Weidner, W. E., & Lasky, E. Z. (1976). The interaction of rate and complexity of stimulus on the performance of adult aphasic subjects. *Brain and Language, 3,* 34–40.

Weintraub, S., Rubin, N. P., & Mesulam, M. M. (1990). Primary progressive aphasia: Longitudinal course, neuropsychological profile, and language features. *Archives of Neurology, 47,* 1329–1335.

Welch, L. W., Doineau, D., Johnson, S., & King, D. (1996). Educational and gender normative data for the Boston Naming Test in a group of older adults. *Brain and Language, 53,* 260–266.

Wells, A. (1999). Family support systems: Their role in aphasia. *Aphasiology, 13*(12), 911–914.

Weniger, D. (1990). Diagnostic tests as tools of assessment and models of information processing: A gap to bridge. *Aphasiology, 4,* 109–113.

Wepman, J. (1958). The relationship between self-correction and recovery from aphasia. *Journal of Speech and Hearing Disorders, 23,* 302–305.

Wertz, R. T., Collins, M., Weiss, D., Kurtzke, J., Friden, T., Brookshire, R., et al. (1981). Veterans Administration cooperative study on aphasia: A comparison of individual and group treatment. *Journal of Speech and Hearing Research, 2,* 580–594.

Wertz, R. T., Deal, J. L., & Robinson, A. J. (1984). Classifying the aphasias: A comparison of the Boston Diagnostic Aphasia Examination and the Western Aphasia Battery. *Clinical Aphasiology, 14,* 40–47.

Wertz, R. T., Weiss, D., Aten, J., Brookshire, R. H., Garcia-Bunuel, L., Holland, A. L., et al. (1987). A comparison of clinic, home and deferred language treatment for aphasia: A VA cooperative study. *Archives of Neurology, 43,* 653–658.

Westbury, C., & Bub, D. (1997). Primary progressive aphasia: A review of 112 cases. *Brain and Language, 60,* 381–406.

Whitworth, A., Webster, J., & Howard, D. (2005). *Assessment and intervention in aphasia.* Hove and New York: Psychology Press.

WHOQOL: Measuring quality of life. (1997). Retrieved January 29, 2006, from http://www.who.int/mental/media/68.pdf

Whurr, R. (1996). *The Aphasia Screening Test (2nd ed.).* San Diego: Singular.

Whyte, E. M. (2002). Post stroke depression: Epidemiology, pathophysiology, and biological treatment. *Biological Psychiatry, 52*(3), 253–264.

Whyte, J., Schuster, K., Polansky, M., Adams, J., & Coslett, H. B. (2000). Frequency and duration of inattentive behavior after traumatic brain injury: Effects of distraction, task and practice. *Journal of the International Neuropsychological Society, 6,* 1–11.

Wiederholt, J. L., & Bryant, B. R. (2002). *Gray Oral Reading Tests* (4th ed.). Austin, TX: Pro-Ed.

Wiig, E., Neilsen, N. P., Minthorn, L., & Warkentin, S. (2004). *Alzheimer's Quick Test.* San Antonio, TX: PsychCorp.

Wiig, E., & Semel, E. (1984). *Language assessment and intervention for the learning disabled* (2nd ed.). Columbus, OH: Charles E. Merrill.

Wilcox, M. J., Davis, G. A., & Leonard, L. L. (1978). Aphasic's comprehension of contextually conveyed meaning. *Brain and Language, 6*, 362–377.

Wilkinson, G. S. (1993). *Wide Range Achievement Test* (3rd ed.). Wilmington, DE: Wide Range.

Williams, J. M., & Shane, B. (1986). The Reitan-Indiana Aphasia Screening Test: Scoring and factor analysis. *Journal of Clinical Psychology, 42*(1), 156–160.

Williams, L. S., Weinberger, M., Harris, L., Clark, D., & Biller, J. (1999). Development of a stroke-specific quality of life scale. *Stroke, 30*, 1362–1369.

Williams, M. (1994). *Criterion-Oriented Test of Attention.* Woodsboro, MD: Cool Spring Software.

Williams, M. (2000). *The Naming Test.* Drexel Hill, PA: BrainMetric.

Williams, M. (2006). *Williams Inhibition Test.* Retrieved April 10, 2006, from http://digibuy.com/cgi-bin/product.html?97736441415

Wilshire, C. E. (2002). Where do aphasic phonological errors come from? Evidence from phoneme movement errors in picture naming. *Aphasiology, 16*(1–2), 169–197.

Wilshire, C. E., & Coslett, H. B. (2000). Disorders of word retrieval in aphasia: Theories and potential applications. In S. E. Nadeau, L. J. G. Rothi, & B. Crosson (Eds.), *Aphasia and language: Theory to practice* (pp. 82–107). New York: The Guilford Press.

Wilson, B. A., Alderman, N., Burgess, P., Emslie, H., & Evans, J. J. (1996). *Behavioral Assessment of the Dysexecutive Syndrome.* Gaylord, MI: Northern Rehabilitation Services.

Wilson, B. A., Cockburn, J., & Baddeley, A. D. (2003). *Rivermead Behavioral Memory Test (RBMT-II).* San Antonio, TX: Harcourt Assessment.

Wilson, B. A., Cockburn, J., & Halligan, P. (1987). *The Behavioral Inattention Test.* Gaylord, MI: Northern Rehabilitation Services.

Wilson, B. A., & Wearing, D. (1995). Prisoner of consciousness: A state of just awakening following herpes simplex encephalitis. In R. Campbell & M. A. Conway (Eds.), *Broken memories: Case studies of memory impairment* (pp. 14–30). Cambridge, MA: Blackwell.

Wilson, R. H., Fowler, C. G., & Shanks, J. E. (1981). Audiological assessment of the aphasic patients. *Seminars in Speech, Language, and Hearing, 2*, 299–300.

Wirz, S., Skinner, C., & Dean, E. (1990). *Revised Edinburgh Functional Communication Profile.* Tucson, AZ: Communication Skill Builders.

Woolfolk, E. (1999). *Comprehensive Assessment of Spoken Language.* Austin, TX: Pro-Ed.

World Health Organization Quality of Life (WHOQOL-BREF). (2004). Retrieved March 17, 2006, from http://www.who.int/mental_health/evidence/who_gol_user_manual_98.pdf.

Worrall, L. (1992). Functional communication assessment: An Australian perspective. *Aphasiology, 6*, 105–110.

Worrall, L. (1995). The functional communication perspective. In C. Code & Muller, D (Eds.), *The treatment of aphasia: From theory to practice* (pp. 47–69). San Diego: Singular.

Worrall, L. (1999). *Functional communication therapy planner.* Bicester, England: Speechmark.

Worrall, L., & Cruice, M. (2005). Why the WHO ICF and QOL constructs do not lend themselves to programmatic appraisal for planning therapy for aphasia: A commentary on Ross and Wertz, "Advancing appraisal: Aphasia and the WHO". *Aphasiology, 19*(9), 885–893.

Worrall, L., & Holland, A. L. (2003). Editorial: Quality of life in aphasia. *Aphasiology, 17*(4), 329–332.

Worrall, L., McCooey, R., Davidson, B., Larkins, B., & Hickson, L. (2002). The validity of functional assessment of communication and the activity/participation components of the ICIDH-2: Do they reflect what really happens in real life? *Journal of Communication Disorders, 35*(2), 107–137.

Wright, H. H., & Shisler, R. J. (2005). Working memory and aphasia: Theory, measures, and clinical implications. *American Journal of Speech-Language Pathology, 14*, 107–118.

Wright, J. (2000). *The Functional Assessment Measure.* Retrieved January 10, 2006, from http://www.tbims.org/combi/FAM

Wulfeck, B., Bates, E., Juaraez, L., Opie, M., Friederici, A., MacWhinney, B., et al. (1989). Pragmatics in aphasia: Cross-linguistic evidence. *Language and Speech, 32*, 315–336.

Yesavage, J. A., & Brink, T. L. (2006). *Geriatric Depression Scale.* Retrieved March 31, 2006, from http://www.stanford.edu/~yesavage/GDS.html

Yesavage, J. A., Brink, T. L., Rose, T. L., Lunn, O., Huang, V., Adey, M., et al. (1983). Development and validation of a geriatric depression screening scale: A preliminary report. *Journal of Psychiatric Research, 17*, 37–49.

Ylvisaker, M., & Feeney, T. J. (1998). *Collaborative brain injury intervention: Positive everyday routines.* San Diego: Singular.

Yorkston, K. M., & Beukelman, D. (1980). An analysis of connected speech samples of aphasic and normal speakers. *Journal of Speech and Hearing Disorders, 45*, 27–36.

Yorkston, K. M., Beukelman, D. R., & Traynor, C. (1984). *Assessment of Intelligibility of Dysarthric Speech.* Austin, TX: Pro-Ed.

Youse, K., & Coelho, C. (2005). Working memory and discourse production abilities following closed-head injury. *Brain Injury, 19*(12), 1001–1009.

Yueh, B., Shapiro, N., MacLean, C. H., & Shekelle, P. G. (2003). Screening and management of adult hearing loss in primary care: Scientific review. *Journal of the American Medical Association, 289*(15), 1976–1985.

Zemva, N. (1999). Aphasic patients and their families: Wishes and limits. *Aphasiology, 13*, 219–224.

Zingeser, L. B., & Berndt, R. S. (1988). Grammatical class and context effects in a case of pure anomia: Implications for models of language production. *Cognitive Neuropsychology, 5*, 473–516.

Zipoli, R. P., & Kennedy, M. (2005). Evidence-based practice among speech-language pathologists: Attitudes, utilization, and barriers. *American Journal of Speech-Language Pathology, 14*, 208–220.

APPENDIX 4.1
Pre-interview or Referral Form for Collecting Family and Medical History and Status Information

Information About the Respondent

Name _____ Date of Report _____

Phone number_____ e-mail _____

Relationship to patient _____

Information About the Patient

Name _____ Birth place _____

Address _____ Birth date _____

Phone Number _____ e-mail _____

Dear Respondent:

We are asking you the following questions to help us understand the above person, and to plan assessment and treatment activities. Please answer them as fully as possible. If you need more space, use the back of the sheet. Thank you in advance for your time and assistance.

1. What do you feel is the patient's problem? _____

   _____

2. What caused the aphasia (head injury, stroke, illness)? _____

   _____

3. What was the date of injury or of the onset of the illness (head injury, stroke, illness)? _____

   _____

4. Who is the patient's physician? _____

   What is the physician's address? _____

   What is the physician's phone number ? (_____) _____

5. What was the patient's handedness (before stroke or disease onset)? Right _____

   Left _____ Ambidextrous _____

6. Does the patient wear glasses? _____

   Can the patient see well enough to read?

   with glasses _____ without glasses _____

   Does the patient have any other visual problems, such as right or left visual-field cut or

   cataracts? _____

7. Does the patient have a hearing loss? _____

   Does the patient wear a hearing aid? _____.

   If yes, in the right ear _____, left ear _____, or both _____?

8. How would you describe the patient's general health? _____

_____

_____

9. Please list the patient's current medications and dosages (if known):

_____

_____

_____

_____

10. Does the patient have a history of any of the following?

Onset Date and Current Status

Stroke	Yes	No	_____
Aphasia	Yes	No	_____
Other communication disorder	Yes	No	_____
Right- or left-sided weakness	Yes	No	_____
Dementia (e.g., Alzheimer's disease)	Yes	No	_____
Memory impairment	Yes	No	_____
Other neurologic disease	Yes	No	_____
Head injury	Yes	No	_____
Seizure disorder	Yes	No	_____
Clinical depression	Yes	No	_____
Psychiatric problems	Yes	No	_____
Alcohol abuse/problems	Yes	No	_____
Other substance abuse	Yes	No	_____
Other major illness	Yes	No	_____

11. List members of the immediate family:

Name	Age	Relationship	Phone number	Check if living in same environment as patient
_____	___	_____	_____	_____
_____	___	_____	_____	_____
_____	___	_____	_____	_____
_____	___	_____	_____	_____

12. If the patient is living at home, are there others living in the home besides the immediate family?

_____

_____

If the patient is not living at home, where does he or she live?

_____

_____

_____

13. Are there relatives on the patient's side of the family who have had a similar problem with speech and language? If so, who? _____

14. What is the patient's native language? _____

 If not English, at what age did the patient learn English? _____

 What other languages does the patient speak? _____

 What is the preferred language in the home? _____

15. What is the patient's highest level of education? _____

16. What (is/was) the patient's primary occupation? _____

 Who (is/was) the patient's employer? _____

 Is the patient presently working? _____

 Describe the patient's work history (for example, kind of employment and approximate dates).

 _____

 _____

17. Patient's mother's name _____ Living _____ Deceased _____

 Patient's father's name _____ Living _____ Deceased _____

18. Marital status: single _____ widowed _____ separated _____

 married _____ divorced _____ remarried _____

19. Does the patient have children _____ or grandchildren _____?

Children	Name	City of residence	Age
	_____	_____	_____
	_____	_____	_____
	_____	_____	_____
	_____	_____	_____

Grandchildren			
	_____	_____	_____
	_____	_____	_____
	_____	_____	_____
	_____	_____	_____
	_____	_____	_____

20. (Answer Question 20 if appropriate.) What is the spouse's name? _____

 What (is/was) the spouse's occupation? _____

 Who (is/was) the spouse's employer? _____

 Is the spouse presently working? _____

 What is the spouse's native language? _____

 If not English, when did the spouse learn English? _____

 What other languages does the spouse speak? _____

 What is the preferred language to communicate with the spouse? _____

21. Does the patient need to be taken care of at all times? _____

 If so, who performs this function? _____

22. To what extent can the patient care for himself (dress, feed, and wash himself)? _____

23. Has the patient's speech and language problem affected the family in any way? If so, how? _____

 _____

24. Describe the patient's ability to communicate in general and with family members.

_____

_____

25. When did you first notice that the patient had difficulty talking or understanding? _____

_____

26. How much does he or she talk or write now? _____

_____

27. How much of this speech or writing does the family understand? _____

_____

28. To what degree do other adults understand the patient's communication? _____

_____

29. How do you think he or she feels about his or her communication abilities? _____

_____

30. What strategies have you found useful to help with the patient's communication? _____

_____

31. Is he or she attempting to communicate verbally?   Yes   No
    Is he or she attempting to communicate in writing?   Yes   No
    Is he or she attempting to communicate using gestures?   Yes   No
    Can he or she tell you his or her name and address?   Yes   No
    Can he or she write his or her name and address?   Yes   No
    Is his or her speech intelligible?   Yes   No
    Is his or her writing intelligible?   Yes   No
    Can he or she say short sentences?   Yes   No
    Can he or she write short sentences?   Yes   No
    Can he or she repeat or copy words?   Yes   No
    Is there automatic speech (e.g., "Hello," "Thank you," "I'm fine.")?   Yes   No
    Can he or she understand conversational speech?   Yes   No
    Can he or she read and understand the newspaper?   Yes   No

32. Below are words that describe a person's personality and behavior. Circle those words that you feel apply to the patient's present status.

happy	fights often	sad	enthusiastic	patient
very friendly	warm	independent	energetic	intense
moody	critical	dependent	prefers to be alone	jealous
authoritarian	supportive	impatient	shy	receptive
bossy	at ease	responsive	cooperative	relaxed
active	indifferent	distractible	outgoing	directive
tense	listless	cold	can't sleep	affectionate
even-tempered	quarrelsome	vigorous	easily fatigued	curious
has temper tantrums		exhibits control of emotions		
follows the lead of others		exhibits self-help		
waits for recognition		has many fears		
has few fears		initiates activities		
walks in sleep		seeks social relationships		
demands attention		willing to try unknown		
stays with an activity				

33. In general, the (spouse-patient) or (family-patient) relationship is (circle one):

   comfortable   strained   hostile   indifferent

34. Have you read or heard anything about aphasia/head injury/illness? _____ If yes, what did you hear and where did you hear it?

_____

_____

What has your doctor talked to you about aphasia/head injury/illness? _____

What kind of information do you think you need about aphasia/head injury/illness?

_____

35. What are the patient's interests or favorite activities? _____

_____

_____

Can the patient engage in these activities as he or she did before aphasia/head injury/illness? _____

Does the patient show the same interest level in these activities? _____

Are the patient's favorite activities the same now or different than before the aphasia/head injury/illness?

_____

36. Does the patient watch TV? _____ If so, what are his or her favorite programs?

_____

_____

37. Does the patient read much? _____ If so, what type of reading material does he or she enjoy? _____

_____

Did the patient like to read before the aphasia/head injury/illness? _____

Is his or her level of reading the same now or different than it was before the aphasia/head injury/illness?

_____

38. Does the patient write notes or letters? _____ If so, how much writing does he or she do?

_____

_____

Did the patient like to write before the aphasia/head injury/illness? _____

Is his or her level of writing the same now or different than it was before the aphasia/head injury/illness?

_____

39. Has the patient been seen for:

	Dates	Agency	Address
a. Speech therapy	_____	_____	_____
b. Audiology	_____	_____	_____
c. Physical therapy	_____	_____	_____
d. Occupational therapy	_____	_____	_____
e. Psychological counseling	_____	_____	_____
f. Other rehabilitation	_____	_____	_____

APPENDIX 4.2
Examples of Auditory Retention and Comprehension Tasks

Task	Example	Input[a]	Output
Auditory Retention Tasks			
Recognition or repetition of digits	Point to: 8, 4, 2	A	G
	Say after me: 9, 3, 7	A	V
Recognition or repetition of words	Touch the red square and blue circle	A	G
	Say after me: man, cup, hat, dog	A	V
Recognition or repetition of noun phrases	Point to: The man	A	G
	Say after me: The man	A	V
Recognition or repetition of verb phrases	Point to: Ate the lunch	A	G
	Say after me: Ate the lunch	A	V
Recognition or repetition of sentences	Point to: The man ate the sandwich.	A	G
	Say after me: The man ate the sandwich.	A	V
Auditory Comprehension Tasks			
Recognition of objects named	Point to the hat	A	G
Recognition of events named	Point to running	A	G
Recognition of relationships named	Point to family	A	G
Recognition of two or more objects, two or more events, or two or more relationships named	Point to the quarter and the comb	A	G
	Point to washing and to eating		
	Point to family and to in front of		
Recognition of categories named	Point to fruit	A	G
Recognition of two or more categories named	Point to clothing and to food	A	G
Recognition of objects when given the function of the object	Point to the one that is used for writing	A	G
Recognition of two objects when given the function of the objects	Point to the one that is used to buy things and the one that is used to comb hair	A	G
Recognition of an event described	Point to the one that shows what we do every night (sleep)	A	G
Recognition of two events described	Point to the one that shows food being prepared and the one that shows going to work	A	G
Recognition of semantically similar objects, events, relationships (2, 3, 4)	Point to the ones that go together: shopping, walking, cooking	A	G
Recognition of rhyme words	Point to a picture that rhymes with the word peas	A	G
Recognition of antonyms	Point to the opposite of up	A	G
Recognition of synonyms	Point to a word that means the same as sob	A	G
Following directions	Ring the bell	A	G
Understanding concrete sentences	Is this a cup?	A	G
Understanding abstract sentences	Will a stone sink in water?	A	G
Understanding complex or abstract relationships in sentences (adapted from Wiig and Semel [1976])			
a. Comparative relationship	Are towns larger than cities?	A	G/V
b. Possessive relationship	Does the hat belong to the girl?	A	G/V
c. Spatial relationship	Is the man walking in front of the cat?	A	G/V
d. Temporal relationship	Does lunch come before breakfast?	A	G/V
e. Inferential relationship	The man cut the steak. Did the man use a knife?	A	G/V
f. Familial relationship	Is your mother's brother your aunt?	A	G/V
g. Part-whole relationship	Does milk come from cows?	A	G/V

Task	Example	Input[a]	Output
h. Object-to-action relationship	Can a car be driven?	A	G/V
i. Cause-effect relationship	Can smoke cause fire?	A	G/V
j. Sequential relationship	Were the Indians in this country before the white men came?	A	G/V
k. Degree relationship	Are inches larger than feet?	A	G/V
l. Antonym relationship	Is day the opposite of night?	A	G/V
m. Synonym relationship	Does sob mean the same as cry?	A	G/V
Comprehension of Content Categories			
a. Existence	Point to the hat	A	G/V
b. Nonexistence	Point to: "The pie is all gone"	A	G/V
c. Recurrence	Point to: "The man returns"	A	G/V
d. Rejection	Point to: "He doesn't want a bath"	A	G/V
e. Denial	Point to: "The cup is not yellow"	A	G/V
f. Possession	Point to the woman's coat	A	G/V
g. Attribution	Point to the large red circle	A	G/V
Understanding paragraphs	(Read paragraph) Questions: In this story, did Lucky find a bird?	A	G/V

Key: A = auditory; G = gestural; V = verbal.
(From Chapey, 1994; Murray & Chapey, 2001)

APPENDIX 4.3
Various Tasks Used to Assess Auditory Comprehension of Syntax

Task	Example	Input	Output
Understanding Substantive Words			
Pronouns			
a. Personal	Point to: "She ate the cake."	A	G
b. Reflexive personal	Point to: "She kept it to herself."	A	G
c. Indefinite	Point to: "Is there any left?"	A	G
d. Demonstrative	Point to: "This is the cake."	A	G
e. Interrogative	Point to: "Which one won the race?"	A	G
f. Negative	Point to: "Nobody is interested."	A	G
Adjectives (attribution)			
a. Color	Point to the blue one	A	G
b. Size	Point to the large one	A	G
c. Shape	Point to the square one	A	G
d. Length	Point to the short one	A	G
e. Height	Point to the tall one	A	G
f. Width	Point to the narrow one	A	G
g. Age	Point to the new one	A	G
h. Taste	Point to the sour one	A	G
i. Speed	Point to the slow one	A	G
j. Temperature	Point to the cold one	A	G
k. Distance	Point to the one that is near	A	G
l. Comparatives	Point to the larger one	A	G
m. Superlatives	Point to the largest one	A	G
Adverbs			
a. 'ly' adverbs	Point to the friendly one	A	G
Understanding Relational Words			
Prepositions			
a. Locative	Put the hat in the box	A	G
b. Directional	Push the book under the table	A	G
c. Temporal	Do you go to church on Sunday?	A	G
Conjunctions	Point to ice cream and cake	A	G
Articles	Point to a cake	A	G
(Picture of a boy hitting a girl)			
a. Active declarative	The boy has hit the girl.	A	G/V
b. Yes/no question	Did the boy hit the girl?	A	G/V
c. Who question	Whom has the boy hit?	A	G/V
d. Negative	The boy has not hit the girl.	A	G/V
e. Negative question	Has the boy not hit the girl?	A	G/V
f. Passive	The girl has been hit by the boy.	A	G/V
g. Passive question	Has the girl been hit by the boy?	A	G/V
h. Negative passive	The girl has not been hit by the boy.	A	G/V
i. Negative passive question	Has the girl not been hit by the boy?	A	G/V
j. Complex sentences	Is this sentence complete or incomplete: "The nurse who comes in the morning"	A	G/V

Key: A = auditory; G = gestural; V = verbal.
(From Chapey, R., (1994). Assessment of language disorders in adults. In R. Chapey (Ed.),
Language intervention strategies in aphasia (3rd ed., pp. 80-120). Baltimore: Williams & Wilkins.)

Section II

Principles of Language Intervention

Chapter 5

Research Principles for the Clinician

Connie A. Tompkins, April Gibbs Scott, and Victoria L. Scharp

OBJECTIVES

Most clinicians value the intuitive, artistic nature of their endeavors. Most also recognize that effective clinical management cannot proceed by intuition alone. As Kearns (1993) suggests, "failure to apply scientific thinking and measurement during the clinical process is surely as misguided as leaving our empathy, clinical intuition, and caring attitudes behind as we enter the clinical arena" (p.71). This chapter advocates a scientific approach to clinical decision-making, emphasizing primarily the clinician's role as a consumer of research information. Other sections recount the advantages of a systematic approach to treatment planning and implementation, and suggest ways in which clinicians can contribute to the professional evidence base. Finally, some future trends are considered in the application of research principles to clinical intervention.

PERSPECTIVES AND DEFINITIONS

Setting the Stage: Some Key Concepts and Terms

The Research Process

For the purposes of this chapter, **research** can be viewed as a process of asking and answering questions, which is structured by a set of criteria and procedures for maximizing the probability of attaining **reliability**, **validity**, and **generality** of results (Silverman, 1985). Each of these factors affects the confidence one can have in the findings and conclusions of a research effort.

Reliability refers to the stability, consistency, or repeatability of results. Among the most well-known types are inter- and intra-observer reliability, and test-retest reliability. When standardized instruments or nonstandard probes are used to document performance, these or related indicators (e.g., parallel/alternate-forms reliability) should be reported and evaluated. Standard error has an important role in the measurement of reliability. Standard error reflects the precision of any particular statistic (mean, median, correlation, proportion, difference between means, etc.) by estimating the random fluctuations that would be obtained if that same index were derived on repeated occasions. A statistic called the "standard error of measurement" estimates the consistency with which a particular test would measure performance on repeated administrations. The larger the standard error relative to the magnitude of obtained scores, the more difficult it is to tell whether any single score is truly different from some other score (e.g., whether there is a change after treatment). It is beyond the scope of this chapter to elaborate on the calculation and interpretation of standard error statistics, but Kerlinger (1973) is a good source for those who want more information.

Two less familiar forms of reliability also require brief mention. The first, **internal consistency reliability**, reflects the homogeneity of test items, and by inference, the extent to which those items measure the same construct. Items that are summed to generate a "total score" index of a single construct, such as "word-finding ability" or "communicative adequacy," should have acceptable levels of internal consistency. If the items that are added together do not measure the same thing, combining them into a single score is like comparing the proverbial apples and oranges. Second, **procedural reliability** data reflect the consistency of implementation of the experimental conditions or treatment procedures in a research study. Also known as "reliability of the independent variable," procedural reliability is often neglected in the language intervention literature. We will return to this concept in another section of the chapter.

Validity refers to "truth" of measurement. The definition of validity is illustrated by the following question: Are we measuring what we think we are measuring? Although many assume that validity is a fixed property of tests and measures, inferences about a measure's validity will vary with its application. That is, claims of validity for any particular measure will be influenced by factors such as the conclusions one wishes to draw, the individuals who are tested, and the procedures that are employed.

For tests and other measurement instruments, the familiar types of validity are content, criterion (predictive and concurrent), and construct validity. Two other validity concepts are important for designing and evaluating research. **Internal validity** reflects how confidently one can attribute observed changes to the experimental treatments or conditions themselves, rather than to artifacts or confounding variables (Campbell & Stanley, 1966). **External validity** involves the generality or representativeness of results and conclusions (Campbell & Stanley, 1966), and concerns the extent to which findings can be expected to apply to particular populations, settings, or measurement and treatment variables.[1] It is important to remember that reliability is necessary for, but does not guarantee, validity. Ventry and Schiavetti (1980) give an example of a scale that is consistently off by 1/2 pound: it is a reliable (consistent) instrument, but not a valid one.

Treatment Outcomes and Their Measurement

In recent years, outcomes measurement has seen increasing emphasis on the multi-dimensional consequences of health problems and health-care provision. The idea is that a positive *outcome* (which can be defined simply as the result of any intervention) encompasses social, psychological, and attitudinal changes in addition to the traditional concerns with physical and physiologic improvements (Donabedian, 1980). Probably the best-known working framework for outcomes measurement is the World Health Organization's (WHO) International Classification of Functioning, Disability and Health (WHO, 2001). This framework distinguishes among three levels of functioning: body structure and function (formerly, "impairment"), activity (formerly, "disability"); and participation (formerly, "handicap"). Measurement at the level of body structure and function addresses specific anatomical, physiologic, or psychological impairments, such as agrammatic output in aphasia. The activity level is concerned with the influence of an impairment on an individual's activities and daily-life skills (e.g., agrammatism, apraxia of speech, and dysarthria may affect the ability to talk on the phone, to order a meal in a restaurant, or to read aloud to grandchildren). And assessment of participation reflects the effects of a health condition on social roles and life situations—for example, severely dysarthric speech restricts a teacher's ability to perform his or her job or diminishes a grandmother's ability to bond with her grandchildren.

According to Frattali (1998a), both efficacy research and outcomes research contribute to outcomes measurement. **Efficacy research** uses rigorously specified, well-controlled protocols to evaluate a treatment under optimal conditions, whereas **outcomes research** is conducted in typical or routine circumstances. Because well-designed efficacy research minimizes potential confounds, its internal validity can be strong, rendering a high degree of confidence in its results. Outcomes research yields a lesser degree of confidence but may provide insights into processes and phenomena that cannot easily or validly be isolated and controlled.

Finishing this terminological survey, outcomes measurement can be aimed at documenting the efficacy, efficiency, effectiveness, and/or effects of treatment (see Frattali, 1998a, for a full discussion). There is little consensus about the meanings of these terms. Some link the terms "treatment effectiveness" and "treatment efficacy" with the conditions under which the data are gathered, suggesting that outcomes research yields evidence on the effectiveness of treatment, and only efficacy research can meet the standard for treatment efficacy data (see Frattali, 1998a). Robey and Schultz (1998) fold in another distinction, using the term "efficacy" to refer to the benefits derived from treating an individual patient (under ideal conditions), and "effectiveness" to indicate the benefits for a broader population (under typical conditions). So, for Robey and Schultz, demonstrating treatment efficacy is a prerequisite for establishing treatment effectiveness. However, in this chapter we follow Frattali and others in using the term **treatment effectiveness** as a higher-order concept concerning whether a treatment works (Kendall & Norton-Ford, 1982), regardless of the research method used to generate the evidence. From this perspective, both efficacy and outcomes research can be used to investigate treatment effectiveness, but with different degrees of control and consequent confidence in results (Frattali, 1998a).

Science as a State of Mind

Knowledge of methods used to maximize reliability and validity is essential for conducting and evaluating research, and a later section of this chapter examines some reliability and validity concerns related to language intervention studies. But as Chial (1985) reminds us, a commitment to science is also a state of mind. Some principles at the heart of a scientific orientation are summarized in Table 5–1.

An additional principle, central to a discipline such as clinical aphasiology, is a concern for **practical** or **clinical significance**, which calls for evaluating the relevance or meaningfulness of changes that are reported for research and treatment efforts. Is a statistically significant pre-post treatment change of 5% a clinically important difference? What about a two-fold increase in the number of times a client initiates a conversation with an unfamiliar person? There is no easy answer, as the importance of a change depends on factors such as the specific processes or behaviors

---

[1] The factors that compromise internal and external validity in research also affect the validation of a test instrument; for examples, consult Franzen (1989).

TABLE 5–1

Some Key Principles and Values of Science

Testability: Propositions and questions are specific enough to be evaluated

Replicability: Procedural specificity and detail are sufficient to allow findings to be reproduced

Objectivity: Dogmatism and bias are rejected; counterevidence and alternative interpretations are sought

Systematicity: Theories and experiments are evaluated and developed in a logical, orderly way

Tentativeness: The possibility and sources of error are recognized; the elusiveness of answers is understood

Concern for protection of human subjects: The welfare of those participating in research projects is paramount

being targeted, the client's needs and level of functioning, and the nature of the treatment goals.

The question of clinical significance can be formalized to some extent with reference to the WHO model (WHO, 2001). Improvements at the level of activity or participation are more relevant, meaningful, and important than changes that are limited to the level of body structure and function. We return to these issues later in the chapter.

Science and Clinical Decision-Making

While some clinicians may shudder at the thought of "doing research," effective diagnosis and treatment are modeled on the principles that guide scientific inquiry. Silverman (1985) emphasizes four principles in a scientific approach to clinical management: specifying clear objectives; posing answerable hypotheses and questions; observing systematically; and remaining aware of the tentative nature of the findings. We add a fifth: justifying the choice of measures and treatments as appropriate to clients' needs and clinical goals.

Parallels often have been drawn between research and clinical processes (e.g., Kent, 1985b; Silverman, 1985; Warren, 1986). For example, Nation and Aram (1984) suggest that careful diagnosis is like conducting a "mini research project" (p. 54). Table 5–2 illustrates the scientific nature of the diagnostic process (after Nation & Aram) by

TABLE 5–2

Some Useful Descriptive Information About Neurologically Impaired Persons

Brookshire (1983):	Age	Etiology
	Education	Time post-onset
	Gender	Severity of aphasia
	Premorbid handedness	Type of aphasia
	Source of subjects	Lesion location
Rosenbek (1987):	*Risk factors*	*Other medical factors*
	Smoking	Medications
	Drinking	Seizures
	Obesity	
	Diabetes	
	Hypertension	
Rosenbek et al. (1989):	Willingness to practice	
	Ability to learn	
	Ability to generalize	
	Ability to retain	
Tompkins et al. (1990):	Physiologic indices of aging	Personality/attitudinal
	Estimated premorbid intelligence	variables
	Auditory processing abilities	Social integration/social support

setting out the chain of diagnostic steps that correlate with scientific problem-solving. The diagnostic literature has underscored this theme for decades. Johnson, Darley, and Spriestersbach (1963), for instance, emphasized diagnosis as a hypothesis-testing process, guided by principles of critical thinking, special observation skills, and impartial, precise, and reliable observation.

Clinically accountable treatment, which can be documented as efficacious and/or effective, is guided by these same procedures and principles. Using a hypothesis-testing model we would postulate what can be done to ameliorate a client's weaknesses and/or to compensate, modify, or accommodate other communicative obstacles the client may face. Then we would test and refine these clinical hypotheses as we evaluate our client's progress. Evidence-based practice (EBP), a recent emphasis in clinical practice, provides one framework and a set of procedures to help us make the best possible clinical decisions. EBP has been defined as "the conscientious, explicit, and judicious use of current best evidence in making decisions about the care of individual patients . . . [by] integrating individual clinical expertise with the best available external clinical evidence from systematic research" (Sackett, Rosenberg, Muir Gray, Haynes, & Richardson, 1996). Individual client characteristics, preferences, and values are part of the EBP framework as well (Sackett, Straus, Richardson, Rosenberg, & Haynes, 2000). As the definition implies, clinicians need to learn how to locate, evaluate, and apply the available research in order to engage in EBP. This further underscores the value of science to clinicians, a topic we elaborate next.

The Value of Science to Clinicians

So why should clinicians care about research and science? At least five reasons are immediately evident. First, as discussed just above, the principles and skills of science are essential to accountable clinical practice, including EBP. Second, all of us must think critically to be wise consumers in life. For the purposes of this chapter, the need for critical thinking applies to the published data and continuing-education information that we consume professionally, and to the information we find on the Internet. Without critical evaluation, it is too easy to accept at face value anything that is published or presented at a professional conference, or located in an Internet search, especially when the author or presenter is known as an authority. Third, clinicians always have had an ethical responsibility to evaluate the impact of their services. In this vein, Rosenbek, LaPointe, and Wertz (1989) assert that "untested treatments are immoral, therefore clinical practice must include clinical experimentation" (p. 12). Fourth, and relatedly, clinicians can make important contributions to the evidence base that should form the foundation of diagnostic and treatment activities. Research is sorely needed to evaluate the effects, effectiveness, and efficiency of various assessment and treatment approaches, with results documented at multiple outcome levels. Drastic reductions in reimbursement for services and increasing requirements to collect and report outcomes data (e.g., HCFA Outcomes and Assessment Information Set [OASIS] for home-care patients; JCAHO ORYX initiative for the accreditation of hospitals and long-term-care facilities, and for collecting core performance data and hospital quality measures) only underscore the urgency of generating a solid evidence base to justify clinical interventions. Finally, a scientific approach kindles informed curiosity, and keeps us thinking and growing professionally. A scientific attitude may help to stave off "burnout"; searching for another question or pursuing a different hypothesis definitely help to keep life interesting. The next sections of this chapter will highlight clinicians as both consumers and potential producers of research.

THE CLINICIAN AS RESEARCH CONSUMER

As clinicians, the research-consumer role is one of the most important that we can adopt. Participating in continuing-education efforts or scouring the Internet for the latest developments, while laudable, are worth little if we simply soak up or disseminate the information without critical evaluation.

Some Questions to Ask in Evaluating Research

The literature is replete with contributions that describe general principles for evaluating published material and presentations. Some of the most important considerations are recapitulated here, in the form of 12 questions for the consumer, with examples and elaboration specific to neurologic or aging populations. Most of these questions can be asked of both "basic" and "treatment efficacy" research. They are culled primarily from Kent (1985a), Silverman (1985), and Ventry and Schiavetti (1980),[2] but are represented in similar form in contemporary writings on the subject of research evaluation (e.g., Schiavetti & Metz, 2005). The order of the questions reflects the order in which a research consumer could answer them, when reading a research article. The American Speech-Language-Hearing Association (ASHA) Web site also provides excellent information about how to assess both the level and quality of evidence provided by any single study (www.asha.org/members/ebp/assessing.htm).

1. Are rationales and hypotheses provided, and are they convincing? The weight one gives to rationales and hypotheses will vary depending on their sources, which can include critical examination of literature,

---

[2] Some of these issues have been elaborated further by Tompkins (1992).

knowledge of normal and disordered processes, and clinical observation and intuition. Sound rationales and hypotheses most often originate from more than one of these roots. A rationale such as "I wonder what would happen if..." is, on its own, far from substantial and needs support and development from other sources. In most other instances, though, the value of a rationale will not be so clear-cut. Each of us must decide whether a convincing case is made for the study questions or hypotheses, whether they are explicitly posed or implied.

2. Are the research questions answerable? From the perspective of research evaluation, an answerable question is one that is explicitly specified. A well-specified question is like an appropriately written behavioral objective. There is an obvious difference between clinical goals such as "improving auditory comprehension" and "achieving 85% comprehension of Yes/No questions about implied main ideas in spoken eighth-grade level paragraphs." The latter is measurable. To take another example, the generic efficacy question, "Does aphasia treatment work?" lacks operational specificity, and is impossible to answer in any one or even several studies. A more answerable question would indicate the nature of the treatment, the characteristics of patients to whom it is to be applied, and the criteria for determining if it has "worked."

3. Do the participants represent the group(s) they are meant to represent? Using an example from aphasia, Darley (1972) emphasized long ago that researchers must define and operationalize what they mean by "aphasia." The occurrence of one or more dominant hemisphere "strokes" certainly is not sufficient evidence to render the diagnosis of aphasia. Neither, alone or in combination with etiologic information, is poor performance on an aphasia test; low scores could reflect a number of other pre- or post-morbid conditions. Damage to the central nervous system also causes several varieties of non-aphasic language disturbance (e.g., language of confusion; language of generalized intellectual impairment in dementia; Wertz, 1985). This diagnostic distinction is more than a simple semantic one. We would not expect traditional aphasia treatments to benefit someone with an isolated dysarthria, or someone whose language impairments are embedded in an assortment of other cognitive problems such as confusion and severe memory disorder. To address this question, a research report should describe the criteria, rationales, and reliability for judgments about the essential communicative diagnoses and client characteristics. For qualitative or subjective judgments in particular, it is desirable to have independent verification by someone who is unaware of, or "blind" to, each participant's specific status, and who does not have a stake in the outcome of the study.

4. Are the participants sufficiently described for the reader to assess the believability, replicability, and generalizability of results? Again drawing on aphasia to illustrate, a number of variables may influence results in treatment studies, such as duration of aphasia, severity of deficits, aphasia type, etiology, prior neurologic and psychiatric history, sensory and motor status, and literacy (Rosenbek et al., 1989; Shewan, 1986). Similar sets of factors affect research with other neurologically impaired populations, and some of the same variables are relevant for characterizing communication behaviors of normally aging adults. Of course, it is also important that component skills or prerequisites for processing and responding to treatment or probe stimuli (e.g., visual and auditory perceptual abilities) are specified and measured.

Brookshire (1983) suggests a minimum list of descriptors for clients with aphasia in his treatise on the subject of subjects. Others (e.g., Rosenbek, 1987; Rosenbek et al., 1989; Tompkins, Jackson, & Schulz, 1990) have offered additional possibilities and discussed novel ways to operationalize some of the tried-and-true descriptors (see Table 5–3). It is not practical, or even necessary, to expect all of these variables to be described in every study. However, having a greater number of well-operationalized descriptors such as these may make it easier for consumers to determine how to apply results, and for investigators to attempt replication and extension of reported findings. As Brookshire (1983) notes, including characteristics such as those discussed here also is important for the internal validity of a study. If such factors are not reported, readers cannot rule out the possibility that the results have been influenced in unintended ways. Detailed subject information is critical as well to begin formulating hypotheses about why certain participants do not respond as expected, or about which individuals might benefit most from particular interventions.

TABLE 5–3

Scientific Steps in the Diagnostic Process

1. Define and delimit the problem
2. Develop hypotheses to be tested; know what evidence is needed to evaluate them
3. Develop procedures to test hypotheses systematically
4. Collect the data: minimize bias and maximize validity
5. Analyze the data: score and organize objectively
6. Interpret the data: evaluate meaningfulness and support or reject hypotheses
7. Generalize from data: reason from the evidence to draw tentative conclusions

5. Are the procedures, conditions, and variables adequately specified? This question most obviously refers to the issue of replicability, but inadequate specification also may raise internal-validity concerns that diminish confidence in the results. Research reports should clearly present the essential aspects of procedures and conditions, and the operational definitions of the dependent (outcome) and independent (predictor) variables. For aphasia treatment trials, some important characteristics of the independent variable (the treatment) include the type and training of the clinician, amount and frequency of treatment, type of treatment, intensity of treatment, and nature of the no-treatment comparison condition (Rosenbek et al., 1989; Shewan, 1986). Treatment procedures, criteria or decision rules, and responses also should be described as precisely as possible. In addition, if several conditions are contrasted, clear operational distinctions should be provided and validated.

6. Are the procedures, conditions, and variables reliable and valid? Let us focus first on *reliability* issues. As noted earlier, the reliability (and validity) question can be asked of standardized measures. But often, psychometrically sound measures are not appropriate or available, and investigators develop or modify dependent measures of their own. When these specialized measures are used, researchers should provide the best data they can to address reliability concerns. Test-retest and standard-error information are crucial. Without them, it is impossible to determine whether changes on an outcome measure might be due to unstable (unreliable) measurements rather than an intervention. An estimate of test-retest characteristics can be made from multiple assessments taken in a baseline (pre-intervention) phase of single-subject experiments, and repeated measures can be taken for a similar purpose prior to implementing experimental procedures or treatments in a group study. The appropriate standard-error statistic can be calculated and evaluated as well.

Just as crucial are inter-observer and intra-observer reliability for dependent and independent variables, to be assessed in each phase of a study. Dependent-variable reliability data are needed to ensure that the scoring of outcome measures is objective and repeatable. Without evidence of acceptable agreement between independent judges, and of consistent scoring by the same judge, the research consumer has to question whether idiosyncratic decisions or unintentional bias could have affected the results. Independent-variable reliability data also are essential, to demonstrate that all aspects of the independent variable (in this case, the treatment) have been delivered consistently and as intended. Thus, research reports should document evidence of procedural reliability for various aspects of an intervention, such as the timing and selection of cues or prompts, and

the accuracy and delivery of feedback (see examples in Bourgeois, 1992; Massaro & Tompkins, 1993).

A variety of issues and procedures in observer reliability assessment have been discussed by Kearns and his colleagues (Kearns, 1990, 1992; Kearns & Simmons, 1988; McReynolds & Kearns, 1983). One caveat is that certain well-known correlation coefficients that often are reported to document reliability (e.g., Pearson r, Spearman ρ) are not the best choices for this purpose. These statistics only index the degree of association between two sets of scores, without taking into account exact score agreement. But two sets of scores can be highly associated (i.e., people who score high one time also score high the second time) and still be significantly different (see, e.g., Wertz, Shubitowski, Dronkers, Lemme, & Deal, 1985). If exact score agreement is of concern, as would be the case for reliability assessment, several other correlations are appropriate, including variants of the intraclass correlation coefficient (Shrout & Fleiss, 1979). Some other points to keep in mind are that levels of chance agreement should be considered when evaluating the acceptability of reliability indices (see Kearns, 1990, 1992), and that ceiling effects can skew reliability results.

We turn now to *validity* issues to continue illustrating Question 6. One specific concern relates again to the abundance of specially designed, nonstandardized measures in aphasiology research and treatment. It is unreasonable to expect such measures to have known validity, but readers should expect at minimum some evidence and logical arguments about the choice of items included, and about their internal-consistency reliability. From a broader perspective, a validity assessment should ask whether the reported observations were appropriate for answering the questions asked, and whether the investigator observed and described what he or she wished to[3] (Silverman, 1985). Along these lines, readers should scrutinize the choice of outcome measures in light of the stated research goals. For example, if the goal of a study is to assess knowledge of particular syntactic constructions in aphasia, how appropriate would it be to rely on a test that requires spoken production of those constructions? The answer depends on a lot of factors, but one might question the validity of this plan because problems of response formulation and execution could mask intact syntactic knowledge. The validity of the connection between treatment and outcome measures also is paramount. As a hypothetical example, one might question whether reading comprehension, as an

---

[3] Under these guidelines, it should be clear that Question 3 above bears on the validity of subject selection.

outcome goal, would be expected to improve after a treatment that focused on oral reading of single words. Readers should look for investigators to justify the link between their independent and dependent variables.

Let us return for a moment to an earlier maxim: reliability is necessary (though not sufficient) to ensure validity. The validity of a treatment also depends in part on demonstrating procedural reliability, or compliance with the experimental protocol.[4] Wertz (1992) raises the issue of compliance in treatment studies, but his point applies to other kinds of research as well. Deviations from a protocol part way through a study, such as modifying selection criteria to include more participants, relaxing the amount of treatment or practice provided, or changing the clinician, can vitiate the validity of a research effort.[5]

A special validity problem in studies of people with aphasia and related impairments is how to account for "spontaneous recovery" in evaluating treatment outcome. This is discussed in Question 9 below.

7. Is the behavior sample adequate? Four senses of "adequacy" are considered here. The first concerns repeated measurement with the same instrument or task, which was emphasized above. Typically, one-shot measurement is not sufficient. Repeated measurements may be needed to assess the stability of the participants' pre-treatment baseline performance, to gather data to approximate test-retest reliability before initiating a treatment or experimental manipulation, and/or to observe the timing or pattern of changes over the course of a study. The second sense of adequacy refers to the number of observations in each task. Generally, the more observations or items included in a measure, the more reliable that measurement will be. Brookshire and Nicholas (1994) demonstrate this point, showing that discourse measures based on single (short) speech samples are less stable than those based on a combination of samples. The third sense of adequacy refers to collecting multiple indicators at each measurement occasion, including measures that index treated behaviors and conditions as well as untreated behaviors and conditions. For example, multiple measurements are needed in treatment studies to assess whether an effect has generalized beyond that which is specifically trained (and perhaps as a control for "spontaneous recovery"; see Question 9). Finally, comprehensive assessments in multiple environments or contexts will enhance the generalizability of results.

8. Are precautions taken to reduce potential, even unknowing, bias? It is well-documented that both examiners' and participants' expectations can introduce critical biases in a research investigation. Hence the emphasis in medical research on "double-blind" studies, which keep both investigators and participants unaware of whether any individual participant is assigned to a treatment or control group. In language intervention studies, beyond keeping investigators blind to each participant's group (and even diagnosis) whenever possible, another control for experimenter bias is to have different examiners provide treatment and evaluate treatment data. An additional check on examiner bias is achieved when independent inter-observer reliability is demonstrated to be high for selecting participants, adhering to procedures, scoring outcomes, and judging the existence and magnitude of treatment effects. The influence of participant expectations ("placebo effects") can be evaluated through simultaneous measurement of treated and untreated "control" behaviors. If all behaviors respond similarly over the course of treatment, it is possible that something other than the treatment was responsible for the changes. Question 9 elaborates on this approach as a check on the influence of spontaneous recovery.

9. Are the data interpreted appropriately? Two facets of this question are considered. One element concerns whether the results could be due to something other than the factors that interest the investigator. This is an issue of internal validity. Threats to internal validity probably can never be ruled out entirely, but an investigator should acknowledge and discuss their possible influence, and be appropriately cautious in providing interpretations and conclusions.

It is beyond the scope of this chapter to review all threats to internal validity (see discussions in Campbell & Stanley, 1966; Ventry & Schiavetti, 1980; and Schiavetti & Metz, 2005; and for a more general reference on alternative interpretations, see Huck & Sandler, 1979). However, several major internal-validity threats are discussed here from the perspective of language-intervention research. One that is important in group-treatment trials is the composition of no-treatment control groups. A randomly assigned control group is essential for demonstrating efficacy in group studies (Wertz, 1992). But since it has generally been believed that it is unethical to deny treatment, this crucial condition is rarely met.[6] Rather, control

---

[4] Assessing procedural reliability also would be important for studies comparing treatments; treatment delivery would need to be monitored to ensure that the treatments retained their intended distinctions.

[5] But a later section of this chapter will point out the flexibility of single-subject experimental designs, as long as modifications are analytically motivated and systematically applied.

---

[6] Wertz et al. (1986) solved this dilemma by including a deferred treatment group, whose progress during the no-treatment phase could be analyzed as control data. Elman and Bernstein-Ellis (1999) used a similar approach in a study of the efficacy of group treatment for aphasia.

groups typically are self-selected, consisting of patients who, for example, live in remote areas without access to treatment, elect not to participate, or cannot pay for treatment. A self-selected control group may differ from the treatment group in critical ways that are relevant to the response to treatment. The consequence is that differences in outcome between treatment and control groups may be attributable to these pre-treatment inequalities and not to the treatment per se. A related difficulty centers around differential dropout from a study. There are a variety of reasons that clients drop out of treatment studies: they may be too ill or too severely impaired to participate; they may have improved enough that they no longer want treatment; they may not be aware of a continued need for treatment; they may not like the treatment they are receiving. Any of these sorts of factors may make the groups unequal, biasing the results of the study.

Another difficult problem for the internal validity of language intervention research is a possibility of concurrent other treatments and/or prior treatments interacting with the treatment of interest. Perhaps the other treatments paved the way, bringing the client to the point at which he or she was ready to profit from the intervention under study. This is one example of an order effect. More generally, the order and sequence with which conditions are applied in a study may influence the reported results. Sequence and order effects may even affect results on a day-to-day basis. For example, if conditions are arranged in a fixed order or sequence, fatigue or warm-up effects may adversely affect some performances and not others. Conditions should be randomized or counterbalanced in group studies, and in across-subject replications of single-subject experimental designs.

The influence of spontaneous or physiologic recovery is nature's version of an "interacting treatments" problem. Physiologic improvement brings about behavior changes that can be extremely difficult to separate from changes we would like to attribute to our treatments. Some researchers have tried to skirt the issue by conducting their treatment investigations in neurologically stable patients, years beyond the presumed effects of spontaneous recovery. One limitation of this approach is that no one knows the duration and timeline of spontaneous recovery (particularly for those with traumatic brain injuries). Another concern is that most language and communication treatment is delivered in the period shortly after onset of the disabling condition, so it is imperative to evaluate interventions for those who may still be undergoing neurologic restitution.

For a large group-treatment trial, random assignment to treatment and control groups is one solution.

Then the effects of spontaneous recovery are assumed not to differ between groups (Wertz, 1992). However, random assignment does not ensure group equality, particularly for the small sample studies that tend to populate the literature on aphasia and related disorders. Another approach is to measure several "control behaviors" that are approximately equal in difficulty to the target behaviors, but that the treatment is not expected to influence. If the recovery curve is steeper for treated than for untreated functions, treatment may be responsible for the changes.[7] Multiple baseline designs (McReynolds & Kearns, 1983), which track untreated behaviors while others are treated, can provide evidence of this sort for individual participants. Each time treatment is applied to a previously untreated behavior, the slope of change for that behavior should accelerate if treatment is exceeding the influence of spontaneous recovery. Single-subject experimental designs that allow reversal and reinstitution of treatment effects for the same behavior in the same individuals (McReynolds & Kearns, 1983) also can provide convincing evidence of the influence of treatment over spontaneous recovery.

A related issue in interpreting the results of intervention studies is that apparent treatment effects might have resulted from the time and attention given to the client, rather than from the content and/or process of treatment. Again, the simultaneous measurement of treated and untreated behaviors can help to address this issue. This problem also can be diluted by taking repeated measurements in a pre-treatment baseline phase, where participants are being given time and attention.

Another set of potential problems in attributing results to the experimental conditions involves the influence of factors that have demonstrated relationships to language and cognitive performance in non-neurologically-impaired individuals. Some of these include age, hearing ability, medical risk factors, education/premorbid intelligence, and literacy (see Tompkins, 1992, for elaboration). It is important to remember that not all "errors" are due to a patient's neurologic condition. A good example of this point comes from Yorkston and her colleagues (Yorkston, Farrier, Zeches, & Uomoto, 1990; Yorkston, Zeches, Farrier, & Uomoto, 1993), who demonstrated that certain measures of word usage and grammatical complexity differed according to socioeconomic status in

---

[7]However, another dilemma is that it is not known whether the rate, timing, or extent of spontaneous recovery is comparable for different behaviors or functions. Lesser change in an untreated function may simply represent a difference in the "recovery schedule," or in the complexity of the treated and untreated behaviors.

non-brain-damaged adults. Similarly, Tompkins et al. (1993) reported that several connected speech attributes thought to characterize adults with right hemisphere brain damage did not distinguish their speech samples from those of normally aging adults. And, in a study of 180 normal native Spanish speakers, Ardila and Rosseli (1996) found significant relationships between performance on a picture-description task and the variables of age, gender, and education. The lesson is that findings for people with neurologic impairments must be evaluated against the appropriate control data and expectations.

The last statement exemplifies the second facet of Question 9: given what we already know, does the interpretation ring true? Evaluating interpretations at this level requires knowledge of or access to current theory and data, and a sense of their validity and replicability.

10. Are maintenance and generalization programmed and probed in treatment studies? This question is related to issues of adequate behavior samples and multi-dimensional outcomes. It is important to plan treatments to maximize the likelihood of their generalizing (see Kearns, 1989; Thompson, 1989), and to assess whether treatment effects in fact do generalize to untrained exemplars and to other ecologically valid measures, situations, and conversational partners. Kearns (1993) indicates that generalization planning involves "comprehensive, multifaceted evaluation; the establishment of generalization criteria; incorporation of treatment strategies that might facilitate generalization; continuous measurement and probing for functional, generalized improvements; and, when necessary, extending treatments to additional settings, people and conditions until targeted levels of generalization occur" (p.71). If generalization beyond the treated tasks is not apparent, the practical significance of treatment effects is in doubt. Similarly, maintenance of treatment gains should be assessed. It is rare for long-term maintenance data, much more than a few weeks after the end of treatment, to be provided in language-intervention studies. One exception is found in Freed, Marshall, & Frazier (1997), who monitored maintenance of intervention gains for 13 weeks after the end of treatment (see also Marshall & Freed, 2006). Evaluating maintenance of gains over extended time intervals should become a priority.

11. Are individual participant characteristics related to the reported outcomes? Individual performance can be analyzed in group data, and factors that appear to contribute to success or failure can be evaluated. Most clinical manipulations, such as inserting pauses to improve a client's auditory language comprehension, affect some individuals and not others (e.g., Nicholas & Brookshire, 1986). In order to apply findings to other individuals, it is important to try to identify what characterizes those with good and poor response.

12. Is there some attempt to evaluate the meaningfulness or importance of changes attributed to the experimental manipulations? We return to the issue of practical significance here, and raise the related concept of "effect size." Metter (1985) suggested that some neurologists' skepticism about aphasia treatment stems from concerns about the relevance of specific improvements in treated deficits to real-life, functional goals. Goldstein (1990) reviews several approaches for examining clinical significance, including normative comparisons of target performance, and subjective evaluations of changes effected. Results of these types of assessments currently appear in some language intervention research. For example, normative comparison data in the aphasia literature have been gathered by assessing the frequency of requests for information by neurologically intact adults in conversations with unfamiliar partners (Doyle, Goldstein, Bourgeois, & Nakles, 1989), and by examining non-brain-damaged adults' usage of social conventions (Thompson & Byrne, 1984). Studies by Doyle, Goldstein, and Bourgeois (1987) and Massaro and Tompkins (1993) exemplify two varieties of subjective evaluation, assessing listeners' ratings of the adequacy of selected communication parameters following language intervention. Whitney and Goldstein (1989) used a hybrid approach, in which subjective evaluations were made of aphasic adults' speech samples intermixed with samples from non-brain-damaged control speakers.

When a research procedure or clinical intervention is not expected to lead directly to a functional outcome, several other measures of "importance" can be reported. Analysis of effect size has a precise statistical meaning (e.g., Cohen, 1977), but the idea is to determine how "large" or meaningful some statistically significant difference really is. Wertz (1991) suggests evaluating the size of a difference between groups of scores by examining their distributions for overlap or separation. This could be done by calculating the 95% confidence intervals for each set of scores, using standard-error estimates. Another way to assess the importance or strength of an experimental effect is to set a predetermined difference criterion; for example, designating a change of at least one standard-deviation unit, or a doubling or tripling of baseline performance, as clinically meaningful. To convey some indication of the strength of an observed group effect, researchers can report the number or percentage of participants in a group study whose performance conforms to the overall, average pattern, and/or who achieve the designated criterion for meaningful change.

THE CLINICIAN AS INVESTIGATOR

As a prelude to this section, it is important to acknowledge that recent changes in the service-delivery climate have made it virtually impossible for most clinicians to participate in research efforts. But despite some very real practical limitations, we think there is value in the perspective and information that follows. We are convinced that the most important thing we can do as a discipline to garner both credibility and reimbursement for our services is to appeal to the soundest evidence base possible to justify their efficacy and effectiveness. While it is clearly necessary to collect outcomes data for treatments as they are typically delivered, it also is critical to conduct treatment research that goes beyond what is dictated by the current clinical climate, as a means to determine what would be possible under less constrained circumstances (e.g., with more intense treatment, or more sessions to establish overlearning). The small number of researchers in our discipline simply cannot tackle these problems alone. Thus we hope that clinicians who read this will be inspired to take part, at some level, in these crucial evidence-gathering efforts.

Contributing to the Scientific Data base

Clinicians can contribute meaningfully to their professional literature, although there will almost certainly be obstacles along the way (see, e.g., Schumacher & Nicholas, 1991; Warren, Gabriel, Johnston, & Gaddie, 1987). A collaborative relationship with established investigators will be a crucial source of guidance and support. One goal of ASHA's focused initiative on evidence-based practice (EBP) is to provide a Web-based environment to link clinicians and researchers for collaborative investigations (www.asha.org/members/ebp/fi-06-ebp.htm). Exploring such connections, clinicians might, for example, find an opportunity to become an important part of a data-gathering team for a relatively large investigation initiated by someone other than themselves. Interested clinicians also may be able to initiate collaborative investigations on topics of their own choosing. For example, with the support of established researchers, clinicians may be able to evaluate the outcomes of their own interventions—in some cases through efficacy research but more likely by collecting outcomes data. Alternatively, clinicians may be able to contribute more generally to information in the field, helping to provide much-needed data through original studies or replications and extensions of existing work. The next sections of this chapter focus on clinician-initiated research, but the information is also relevant for interested clinicians who would rather assume a more peripheral research role.

Clinicians Evaluating Their Own Interventions

Treatment-Efficacy Investigations

Single-subject or within-subject experimental designs (e.g., McReynolds & Kearns, 1983) are probably the most appropriate designs for clinicians who wish to become involved in evaluating the efficacy of their own treatments. While the EBP movement emphasizes evidence from systematic research and large randomized controlled trials, single-subject experimental designs will remain important whenever sufficient evidence is lacking (e.g., for atypical or rare client profiles, for understudied populations such as individuals with bilingual/multilingual aphasia, for newer service-delivery models such as telerehabilitation, or for relatively new additions to the scope of practice such as right hemisphere language disorders).

Derived from behavioral psychology, single-subject experimental designs are not glorified case studies. Well-conceived single-subject experimental designs are built around important components of scientific inquiry, such as operational definitions, attention to reliability and validity, and control of extraneous variables. The designs incorporate repeated measurements of observable, operationally-defined target behaviors, with independent scoring of a portion of those behaviors by more than one examiner, to demonstrate objectivity and consistency. Stable pre-intervention baseline data, collected on the clearly specified dependent variables, are used as reference points for evaluating the efficacy of replicable interventions conducted with well-defined participants. The effects of these interventions are evaluated continuously within and across design phases (e.g., baseline, treatment, return to baseline or maintenance); across behaviors; and/or across patients. Although tightly controlled and well suited to maximize internal validity, the designs allow flexibility in treatment when a need for modification becomes apparent (Connell & Thompson, 1986; Kearns, 1986a; McReynolds & Thompson, 1986).

Those unfamiliar with single-subject experimental designs may equate them with pretest-posttest studies, but the two are quite dissimilar. In a pretest-posttest design, a target behavior (e.g., some aspect of reading comprehension) is assessed once prior to treatment, an intervention is applied, and then the target behavior is measured again. While this design often is used to gather "outcomes data," it generates only a weak form of evidence about a treatment's effects because of inherent threats to internal validity; any number of factors other than the treatment of interest could have caused a change from the first measurement to the second. In fact, some would not grant the status of "evidence" to the results of pretest-posttest studies (for further discussion, see Campbell & Stanley, 1966; Ventry & Schiavetti, 1980).

Single-subject experimental designs are discussed in detail in a number of sources (e.g., Connell & Thompson,

1986; Kearns, 1986a; McReynolds & Kearns, 1983; McReynolds & Thompson, 1986). Kent (1985a) provides a useful table illustrating a variety of research questions, along with some of the single-subject designs that are appropriate for addressing those questions. Examples of studies using these designs with neurologically-impaired adults also are available in the aphasiology literature (e.g., Ballard & Thompson, 1999; Doyle, Oleyar, & Goldstein, 1991; Edmonds & Kiran, 2006; Feeney & Ylvisaker, 2003; Freed et al., 1997; Garrett & Huth, 2002; Kearns & Potechin Scher, 1989; Kiran & Thompson, 2003; Massaro & Tompkins, 1993; McNeil et al., 1998; Moss & Nicholas, 2006; Thompson & Shapiro, 1995; Whitney & Goldstein, 1989; Yoshihata, Toshiko, Chujo, & Kaori, 1998).

Despite the strengths of these designs, there remain relatively few published examples. The difficulty of implementing controlled research in a clinical environment is no doubt largely responsible for this situation. In describing their efforts to evaluate a treatment approach for a patient with fluent aphasia, clinicians Schumacher and Nicholas (1991) recount a variety of problems that they faced when conducting research in their clinical setting. They question the feasibility of single-subject research in the clinical arena, unless a clinician is provided with release time for research, or with assistance for collecting and analyzing data. Warren et al. (1987) suggest that the major difference between typical clinical procedure and rigorous study is the time required to conduct behavior probes for no-treatment tasks and phases. In addition, designing and implementing generalization probes outside the treatment setting takes time and planning. Beyond feasibility problems, the often highly-specific treatments used in single-subject research do not necessarily generalize to the needs of other clients (e.g., Franklin, 1997).

These barriers notwithstanding, we agree with Schumacher and Nicholas (1991) and Warren et al. (1987), who clearly believe that clinicians can generate worthwhile research in certain conditions. Those who have the drive to tackle a research problem, and who consult with knowledgeable researchers before starting, could probably evaluate a number of questions in their clinical settings, particularly if they enlist assistance in scoring, checking scoring reliability, and the like. If several clinicians in one location are interested, they can share these tasks, or graduate students from local university programs can be recruited and trained to assist. Some of the kinds of studies that clinicians can probably implement most readily are described below.

Treatment-Outcomes Research

In an ideal world, ethical considerations would motivate and support the collection of credible evidence about treatment effectiveness. In the real world, emerging regulations and accreditation requirements will ensure the accumulation of at least some level of treatment-outcomes data. ASHA's National Outcomes Measurement System (NOMS) has provided one vehicle for collecting and analyzing outcomes data. With a goal of developing a national database for speech-language pathologists and audiologists, the NOMS project advocated the use of 11 pre- and post-treatment functional measures, scored on 7-point scales, to provide some estimate of treatment effectiveness. Demographic and consumer satisfaction data also have been collected. The NOMS database was intended to serve as a resource for selecting interventions and advocating for or justifying reimbursement for clinical services. ASHA's recent EBP initiative (www.asha.org/members/ebp/default) has in large part subsumed these goals, bringing ASHA practices in line with those in the broader community of clinical service providers around the world.

As indicated above, treatment outcome studies are conducted in the typical setting without stringent controls, yielding less confidence in results than would rigorously-designed studies. However, clinicians can enhance the rigor of their treatments, their data-gathering efforts, and the resultant outcomes data by attending to the scientific principles discussed thus far.[8] To recapitulate, these include operationally specifying the nature of the client's abilities and the treatment plans; maximizing reliability and validity of measurement and treatment implementation; collecting an adequate behavior sample, including repeated measurements; attempting to control or account for extraneous factors such as spontaneous recovery; programming for and measuring generalization to untreated behaviors and settings; assessing the maintenance of behavior change after treatment ends; examining potential factors related to success or failure; and assessing social validity to determine whether any changes effected have "made a difference."

Clinicians Contributing More Generally to the Professional Literature

Several avenues are probably most feasible for clinicians who wish to contribute to our clinical evidence base: evaluating outcomes (or efficacy) related to established treatment programs; replicating or extending existing studies; analyzing factors that may be important in interpreting assessment data or in implementing treatments; and gathering comparative performance data from persons without neurologic impairments. Each of these is considered briefly below.

Evaluating Outcomes of Established Programs

Numerous treatment programs exist, and are recommended to clinicians, with only a cursory evidence base, if any.

---

[8] Of course, as Kent and Fair (1985) warn, equating science with effective clinical problem-solving may dilute or trivialize the meaning of the former, and misrepresent or overlook some of what occurs in the latter.

Clinicians are well-situated to evaluate these sorts of programs. One model of this kind of work is provided by Conlon and McNeil (1991), who examined the efficacy of Visual Action Therapy (Helm-Estabrooks, Fitzpatrick, & Barresi, 1982) for adults with global phasia. Another example comes from Freed and colleagues (1997), who assessed the long-term effectiveness of PROMPT treatment (Chumpelik, 1984) for a client with apraxia of speech and aphasia. When attempting to evaluate these kinds of programs, clinicians may note that the specification of treatment procedures is inadequate to allow consistent treatment delivery. In this case, a good deal of planning and work must go into the project up front to specify stimulus choices, cueing/prompting criteria and hierarchies, scoring procedures, and the like. However, after that it becomes a much simpler matter to carry out the treatment program and to use it with other potential candidates. An example of this approach can be found in Massaro and Tompkins (1993), who operationalized a Feature Analysis treatment program (Szekeres, Ylvisaker, & Cohen, 1987) that has been recommended for traumatically brain-injured patients, and gathered some data about the program's efficacy with two patients.

Conducting Replication and Extension Studies

Replication and extension studies are particularly lacking in the speech-language pathology research base. But they are important in part because so much of our research has been done on small samples of participants, who exhibit a limited range of characteristics. Attempting to replicate the findings from an already published project with another sample of participants, or to extend the study using different participants, stimuli, or settings, is an excellent way for a clinical researcher to begin. Some examples of replication and extension studies can be found in Beard and Prescott (1991); Bloise and Tompkins (1993); and Kimelman and McNeil (1987). Bastiaanse, Bosje, & Franssen (1996) also reported a study replicating a treatment approach used in two previous investigations for word-finding problems. The work of Kearns and Potechin Scher (1989) and Byng, Nickels, and Black (1994) presents an even less-frequent phenomenon: replication and extension by the original investigators. Typically, page limits on publications preclude researchers from providing complete methodological detail, so anyone who wishes to replicate a study would need to contact the original authors for specific materials and procedures.

Analyzing Factors that Influence Delivery and Interpretation of Assessments of Treatments

Questions about the content, procedures, or interpretation of assessment tools have motivated a variety of clinical research. These kinds of questions typically stem from clinical observation; as such, they are good candidates for the interested clinical investigator. In one example, Nicholas,

MacLennan, and Brookshire (1986) evaluated a number of reading-comprehension batteries, and documented the extent to which the comprehension questions could be answered without reading the associated passages. In other work, Nicholas, Brookshire, MacLennan, Schumacher, & Porazzo (1989) revised and standardized the administration and scoring procedures for the Boston Naming Test, to improve their specification. The authors reported extended normative data for their revision as well. Investigations also have focused on determining the psychometric properties of abbreviated versions of standardized assessment instruments, such as DiSimoni, Keith, & Darley's (1980) evaluation of a shortened form of the Porch Index of Communicative Ability (Porch, 1981). Another set of inquiries has focused on whether hypothetically important elements of treatment programs have an effect in practice. For example, several studies have examined whether the "new information" principle of PACE therapy (Promoting Aphasics' Communicative Effectiveness; Davis & Wilcox, 1985) has observable effects on narratives elicited from adults with aphasia (Bottenberg & Lemme, 1991; Brenneise-Sarshad, Nicholas, & Brookshire, 1991).

Gathering Normal Comparison Data

Judgments of our clients' abilities and performance should be made against a backdrop of knowledge about the non-neurologic factors that may influence performance on language and cognitive tasks. Among the possible influences, noted earlier, are factors such as age, education, literacy, socioeconomic status, physical health, or hearing impairment; however, few relevant data are available. Clinicians can design protocols to gather group data as a partial response to this need. Some examples are provided by Parr (1992), who examined everyday reading and writing practices of normal adults; Hansen and McNeil (1986), who studied writing with the nondominant hand; Elman, Roberts, & Wertz (1991), who documented the influence of education on judgments of non-neurologically-impaired adults' writing and drawing samples; Tompkins et al. (1993), who assessed some characteristics of performance in normally aging adults' picture descriptions; and Yorkston et al. (1990; 1993) who reported on the discourse performance of non-brain-damaged participants who were similar in terms of socioeconomic status to the "typical" traumatically brain-injured patient.

In any context, practical concerns affect the kinds of questions or problem areas that one can study. Time-demands and the need for consultation and support personnel have already been emphasized; having equipment and facilities on hand also is important. For group data-collection, the availability of appropriate participants is a major issue. Funding also is a likely concern, but it may be possible to run some studies, particularly those evaluating established treatments, as part of routine clinical practice (see, e.g., Kearns, 1986b; and Massaro & Tompkins, 1993)—particularly if the clinician is willing and able to spend some extra time in the workplace. In the end, personal interests and the perceived value of the research may be the most important motivators for clinicians deciding to embark on the research enterprise.

Some Competencies for Researching Clinicians

With assistance from expert collaborators as needed, a clinician-investigator should be able to formulate answerable questions that have practical significance, and to make the necessary observations — with acceptable levels of validity and reliability — to offer tentative answers. These skills presume current knowledge in the content area (e.g., the nature of neurologic disorders and their treatment; the nature of normal language and cognition) as well as familiarity with guidelines for evaluating research. Persistence and tolerance for imperfection are important personality characteristics, because, as Warren (1986) reminds us, there is no perfect design for any study. Compromises are always necessary, in research as well as in clinical endeavors.

Initiating a Research Project

When clinicians decide that they have the appropriate interests, competencies, and supports, they can begin developing a research project. The first step is to hone the idea that sparked interest in the investigation. This can be accomplished by consulting with experts and by reviewing the available literature, to see what aspects of the research problem have not been addressed adequately, or at all. Computerized databases such as PsycLIT, PsychINFO, and Medline, and abstract journals such as *Psychological Abstracts* and *Index Medicus* will help interested readers locate the relevant literature. Google Scholar (http://scholar.google.com) is also a good source for a discerning eye; the National Institutes of Health's CRISP database (http://crisp.cit.nih.gov) provides abstracts of funded research projects; and the ASHA Web site (www.asha.org/default.htm) allows ASHA members to search the main speech-language pathology and audiology journals. For those who wish to study neurologic disorders of language and communication, particularly in adults, publications from the Clinical Aphasiology Conference (e.g., Lemme, 1993; Prescott, 1989, 1991a, 1991b; and more recently in dedicated issues of the journal *Aphasiology*) are all available at http://aphasiology.pitt.edu, and are particularly valuable references. *Aphasiology* (www.ingentaconnect.com/content/02687038/) also periodically dedicates an entire issue to a feature called a "Forum", which presents a lead article on a topic, and subsequent commentary by other investigators. This format alerts readers to subject matter and questions of

current interest. Gaps in the evidence-base can also be identified by searching current compendia of treatment evidence and/or treatment guidelines. For aphasiology and related disorders, some such information resides at the ANCDS Web site (www.ancds.org/practice.html). ASHA's National Center for Evidence-Based Practice also provides a searchable registry of systematic evidence reviews (www.asha.org/members/ebp/compendium) and links to other relevant sites (e.g., the Royal College of Speech-Language Therapists site, www.rcslt.org). It is worth noting that some relevant evidence will be overlooked in such compendia, due to various potential biases in the EBP review process (e.g., publication bias, funding bias; Elman, 2006).

While reviewing the relevant literature, the reader should try to determine what factors point to the need for further investigation in an area of interest. For example, the quality of the study may be at issue: control for spontaneous recovery or examiner bias may be in doubt; the operationalization of the dependent measures may be debatable; the findings may have limited generalizability given the size and characteristics of the participant sample; or the durability and meaningfulness of results may not be addressed. A project can be developed to rectify particular issues of concern, or to replicate and extend findings in research that is essentially sound.

Planning can proceed by focusing on the questions that have been outlined above, for research consumers. Brainstorming with others about the best ways to operationalize and measure variables, or about how to minimize factors that might confound the results, is a valuable activity. And again, it is probably wise to check preliminary ideas and plans with someone who has research expertise. Doing so before a study is initiated can help avoid later problems of interpretation. It is also recommended that the methods be pilot-tested on at least a few people before the actual data collection begins. Even experienced investigators generally identify wrinkles that remain to be ironed out during initial feasibility testing.

Finally, in the planning phase, clinician-investigators should ascertain the requirements and procedures of their institution's Research and Human Rights Committee, Institutional Review Board, or similar committee. These committees are responsible for reviewing all planned research protocols in order to protect the rights of research participants and to minimize research risk in relation to projected benefits. Typically, these committees ask for a description of the aims, procedures, and risks and benefits of the proposed research, along with specific precautions taken to protect participants' research rights and the privacy of their personal information and research data. A detailed consent form, spelling out these elements for the participants, also is essential.

Often an investigator has to make modifications to a research protocol after the research committee's initial review, and in general, it can take quite a while for such committees to grant final approval. As a result, an investigator's goals may have to be modified to some extent unless and until there is an already-approved research protocol. For example, it may not be possible to investigate changes for an individual client during the typical period of spontaneous recovery from stroke. With help from a research collaborator, the clinician-investigator may be able to frame a research question and appropriate methods prospectively, in a way that can be applied to the next patient(s) who fit the study criteria.

Opportunities for Funding and Consultation Assistance

Funding may be an important consideration, either for partial salary coverage in order to obtain release time to plan and conduct a project, or for paying research assistants or participants. A variety of funding opportunities may be available for clinician-investigators, depending on their level of expertise. Several are outlined below.

1. The American Speech-Language-Hearing Foundation (ASHF) has for a number of years sponsored New Investigator research grants for those who have recently completed their latest degree program. ASHF also awards New Century Scholars grants, which have two funding elements: one for doctoral students who plan to work in an academic setting in the United States after graduation, and one for teacher-investigators. Information about each of these opportunities is available at http://www.asha.org/foundation/grants/.

2. ASHA provides a range of information, and even some funding. For example, (a) the ASHA Research Listserv (www.asha.org/members/research/reports/research_list .htm) gives a weekly update on opportunities for funding, fellowships, conferences, and workshops. Requests to subscribe to this on-line mailing list can be sent to asha-research-digest-request@lists.asha.org. (b) A section of the ASHA Web site called "Grants and Funding for Researchers" (www.asha.org/members/research/ grants/) includes topics such as "Grants and Grantsmanship," which primarily gives information about grants available from the National Institutes of Health (NIH), including those for new investigators; and "Resources for Grantwriting and Funding," which provides a directory of grants, foundations, and agencies that have funded clinical-research efforts in communication disorders, as well as a list of relevant publications and Web sites. (c) ASHA's Special Interest Division 2 (Neurophysiology and Neurogenic Disorders) offers a small grant to supplement ASHF New Investigator awards. (d) For students of all levels, ASHA publishes a manual called "Funding Sources: A Guide for Future

Audiologists, Speech-Language Pathologists, and Speech, Language, and Hearing Scientists." This manual provides information on funding assistance and is sold in ASHA's on-line store (www.asha.org/shop).

3. Governmental funding may be available, as well, through highly competitive grants. For example, the NIH offers a variety of opportunities. The NIH Small Grants Program (R03; www.nidcd.nih.gov/funding/ types/researchgrants.asp) provides 2 years of funding to support pilot projects and feasibility research for investigators with limited research experience. NIH Career Development Awards, or K-awards, are intended for people who hold a doctoral degree, but who have primarily clinical training (http://grants1.nih.gov training/careerdevelopmentawards.htm). For predoctoral or postdoctoral student-investigators, the NIH also funds individual fellowship grants (F31, F32 awards, http://grants1.nih.gov/grants/funding/funding_program. htm). Language researchers would most likely apply for NIH funding from the National Institute on Deafness and Other Communication Disorders (NIDCD, www.nidcd.nih.gov/index.asp), but some projects might be fundable by the National Institute on Aging (NIA, www.nia.nih.gov) or the National Institute of Mental Health (NIMH, www.nimh.nih.gov). For those who wish to have more information about the grants process, the NIH offers regional seminars on program funding and grants (see http://grants1.nih.gov/grants seminars.htm). Other governmental sources of funding include (a) the U.S. Department of Veteran's Affairs Merit Review program (www1.va.gov/resdev/funding/ professional_ dev.cfm), which provides funds for initiating research efforts to new investigators both inside and outside that system; and (b) the Canadian Institutes of Health Research (http://www. cihr-irsc.gc.ca/e/780.html, formerly Medical Research Council of Canada), which lists opportunities for research in Canada and supports training awards for clinician-scientists and new-investigator salary awards, among others.

4. Internal institutional funding may be available in some cases. Some hospitals and rehabilitation centers sponsor competitions for funding, or release time, to encourage staff research efforts. Many universities grant seed monies for pilot projects that are expected to lead to larger efforts; a clinician-investigator's project, sponsored by a faculty member, might be partially fundable in this way. Universities also may have funds to help support dissertation research. Universities also offer courses on grantsmanship.

5. Individual grant support may be available from private foundations associations and foundations, such as the Alzheimer's Disease and Related Disorders Association (www.alz.org/professionals_and_researchers_research ers.asp), the American Association of University

Women (www.aauw.org/education/fgaindex.cfm), and the Sigma Xi Research Society (www.sigmaxi.org/programs/giar/index.shtml).

The value of consulting assistance has been emphasized repeatedly in this chapter. The way to get the most out of a consultative relationship is to consult before beginning a project, rather than trying to salvage mistakes later. But best-laid plans being what they are, a good consultant also may be able to help rescue some elements of an errant project after the fact. A clinician-investigator should not be afraid to seek help with a project by contacting people with the appropriate expertise.

There are a variety of avenues for identifying potential consultants. As noted previously, ASHA is creating an Internet resource to link clinicians and researchers for collaborative research (www.asha.org/members/ebp/fi-06-ebp.htm). Conferences and workshops provide another venue. The AHSF has put on several workshops on treatment-efficacy research, and in recent years, ASHA has sponsored travel fellowships that give new and minority investigators the opportunity to present research, completed or in progress, at the Science and Research Career Forum and the Research Symposium that coincide with ASHA's annual convention. The Academy of Neurologic Communication Disorders and Sciences (ANCDS, www.ancds.org) provides its members with opportunities to exchange information and ideas, and with an annual education and scientific meeting the day before the ASHA convention. A clinician-investigator who is the first author on a research effort can secure an invitation to the Clinical Aphasiology Conference (www.clinicalaphasiology.org) by submitting a research abstract for evaluation by the program committee, whether or not the paper is accepted for presentation; two authors can attend if the paper is accepted. Student investigators also have an opportunity to compete for funding to attend the Clinical Aphasiology conference, thanks to a conference grant from the NIDCD. Attending such conferences is valuable for both continuing education and networking purposes, but simply reading published conference proceedings or consensus reports can also point clinicians towards experts who might be willing to serve as research consultants.

University faculty members or master clinicians who publish their work would be good contacts as well. Other sources of possible expert consultants are professional journals, which list their authors and reviewers, and Web sites associated with specific disorders (e.g., www.aphasia.org; www.strokeassociation.org; www.parkinson.org) that provide information and links about relevant research. Information and consultants for interdisciplinary investigations also can be culled from the national and international governing bodies for related disciplines (e.g., occupational therapy: http://www.aota.org/; physical therapy: http://www.apta.org/; neurology: http://www.aan.com/). The ASHA Web site provides its members with helpful information for establishing interdisciplinary collaborations (www.asha.org), which applies to initiating and sustaining any types of collaborative relationships.

Selling the Administration on Your Research Plans

Investigators in most clinical settings would need administrative approval and support for their research efforts. Silverman (1985) provides arguments related to increasing the institution's accountability to various consumers, such as clients, payers, and the community; maximizing the effectiveness of service delivery; and garnering recognition and grant support. Warren (Warren et al., 1987), a clinician and an administrator, also points out the value of efficacy data for demonstrating accountability to quality-assurance evaluators and third-party payers. The costs involved are justifiable with relation to the enhanced confidence with which outcomes can be linked to treatments provided.

FUTURE TRENDS IN THE CLINICAL APPLICATION OF RESEARCH PRINCIPLES
Level of Outcome and Clinical Significance

Clinical significance and meaningfulness of outcomes have been recurrent themes in this chapter. Third-party payers' requirements for functional treatment goals indicate that these concerns are paramount from a reimbursement perspective as well. It is anticipated that the future will see much more attention to documenting the clinical importance of changes effected by interventions.

To date, research and clinical intervention in aphasia and related disorders has focused most often at the level of body structure and function (impairment) rather than on social communicative functioning (but see, e.g., Brown et al., 2006). As suggested earlier, this may have contributed to the poor opinion of our profession held by some neurologists and other medical personnel. It is certainly critical to implement and evaluate interventions that target more ecologically valid outcomes, such as conversational proficiency, whenever possible. But one obvious dilemma in doing so is that there are almost assuredly intermediate or prerequisite steps to clinically-relevant outcomes. As such, it is probably legitimate to focus for some period of time on the impairment level, especially in the initial stages of treatment. When treatments are not intended or expected to result immediately in clinically significant gains, it will be incumbent upon investigators to specify the eventual pathway from their treatment focus to the desired end result, indicating why or how their treatment goal should be an important step along the way to some meaningful outcome.

Another problem in targeting ecologically valid outcomes is that they can be difficult to operationalize, and consequently to measure. A variety of generic rating scales have been used to quantify "functional outcome" (see Frattali, 1998b), but in many cases, their reliability, validity, and sensitivity to change have been questioned. The ASHA-FACS (Functional Assessment of Communication Skills; Frattali, Thompson, Holland, Wohl, & Ferketic, 1995), which provides a more extensive and specific evaluation of communicative disability for adults with aphasia and traumatic brain injury, is a good supplement to these general assessments. Recent research has expanded the value of the ASHA-FACS Social Communication Scale (Donovan, Rosenbek, Ketterson, & Velozo, 2006). Donovan and colleagues found that a 4-point rating could be substituted for the original 7-point rating; that caregivers could rate items reliably on this subscale; and that the Key form can be used to demonstrate treatment progress. These investigators also cautioned that the Social Communication subscale measures two constructs (understanding and conversing) instead of just one. The Communicative Activities in Daily Living (CADL-2; Holland, Frattali, & Fromm, 1999) is another option for assessing functional communication. More recently, the Burden of Stroke Scale (BOSS; Doyle, 2002; Doyle, McNeil, Hula, & Mikolic, 2003) was established as a valid and reliable patient self-report measure of function and well-being (Doyle et al., 2004). The BOSS allows assessment of communication difficulty and distress, among other measures.

Two additional means for demonstrating the functionality of treatment outcomes are to achieve generalization to everyday settings and tasks and to document the social validity of treatment outcomes. And if effects that are generalized and meaningful can be shown to have staying power, so much the better. To examine the durability of clinically important changes, investigators should begin to assess clinical significance or social validity using data from several phases of treatment studies, including that collected during maintenance probes.

Social-validity assessments are relatively new and infrequently used, so standards and criteria for conducting them are still evolving. The future should see more attempts to develop a rigorous technology for determining social validity. The concerns of reliability, validity, and generalizability are paramount here as they are in any measurement effort. Questionnaires and rating scales should be constructed so that the resulting data are sound.

Silverman (1985) discusses several other critical factors such as the design of the social validity tasks; numbers and characteristics of raters, including their knowledge of subject group or time of sample; and selection of the scaling method. One of the salient questions (Campbell & Dollaghan, 1992; Goldstein, 1990; Tompkins, 1992) has to do with the choice of the "gold standard" for a normative comparison approach to determining clinical significance. When patients are severely impaired, an appropriate standard might be one that approximates the communicative performance of a milder, but functional, aphasic communi-

cator. For mildly involved patients, a normal criterion may be appropriate. Whatever the comparison group, though, we foresee more care in specifying individual participant variables that should be relevant, including some of those identified above. The common practice of matching comparison and treatment subjects only for chronologic age and gender will be recognized as insufficient.

As procedural issues are being sorted out, much more work also will be needed to assess the correspondence between these sorts of social-validity data and other measures of communication performance in natural environments. The assessment of real-life behaviors, experiences, and phenomena is at the core of a nontraditional research approach that complements the scientific orientation described earlier in this chapter. This "qualitative research" approach (see, e.g., Denzin & Lincoln, 1998; Strauss & Corbin, 1998) involves detailed data-gathering through extensive interviewing and observation of communicative behaviors and social interactions in a variety of authentic contexts. The investigator relies on "disciplined subjectivity" (Heron, 1996, p. 143) to interpret the accumulated information and generate hypotheses about processes that are at work. Simmons-Mackie & Damico (1996) emphasize the goodness-of-fit between the qualitative research perspective and the assessment of "participation" (WHO, 2001) in aphasia. They describe a Communicative Profiling System that uses qualitative methods to evaluate communication behaviors and strategies, contextual influences on communication, and the available network of communication partners. Conversation Analysis (Goodwin & Heritage, 1990; Shiffrin, 1994), a qualitative research method derived from discourse studies, provides another frame of reference for evaluating communicative success in aphasia. This approach has been used in several investigations (e.g., Ferguson, 1993; Milroy & Perkins, 1992) to explore dynamic aspects of conversational collaboration, and has been adapted for clinical use in such programs as SPPARC: Supporting Partners of People with Aphasia in Relationships and Conversation (Lock, Wilkinson, Bryan, Maxim, Edmundson, Bruce, et al., 2001). Some treatment studies (e.g., Perkins, 1995; Perkins, Crisp, & Walshaw, 1999) have combined quantitative and qualitative methods in an effort to establish a more complete clinical picture than would be obtained by either approach alone. While lacking elements of rigor identified earlier in this chapter and particularly susceptible to (unintended) examiner bias, qualitative approaches can provide a rich source of ideas for those who are interested in documenting, describing, and characterizing meaningful outcomes.

Developing the Evidence Base in Bilingual/Multilingual Aphasia

Growing numbers of people across the United States have diverse language backgrounds, and more than half of the world's population is at least bilingual. Yet there are very few systematic, theoretically, and methodologically sound studies that examine within- and across-language treatment for bilingual/multilingual aphasia. Edmonds and Kiran (2006) recently published an admirable investigation with a single-subject experimental design that provides a useful model for future work. The difficulties in this area of study are many: e.g., a lack of conceptual models of bilingual/multilingual language processing, of assessment tools with adequate psychometric properties, of clinicians with diverse language backgrounds, and of access to interpreters. Nonetheless, this area of clinical investigation is vital, and is fully expected to receive increasing attention in the future.

Evaluating Effectiveness of Nontraditional Treatment Approaches

Even before funding pressures prompted increasing exploration of alternatives to direct individual language treatment, some interest in nontraditional options was evident. We expect to see heightened attention to establishing the effectiveness of nontraditional intervention approaches, including those that involve communication partners, provide therapy in a group context, rely on computerized treatment delivery, involve telerehabilitation, or incorporate pharmacotherapy.

Targeting communication-partner behaviors, instead of or in addition to those of the individuals with communication disorders, remains a relatively untapped but potentially important direction in treatment research (see Turner & Whitworth, 2006, for a recent review). After all, communication is an interactive process, and its success hinges on the interplay between participants. Turning some attention to the neurologically intact member of a communicative dyad would have considerable ecological validity. And with clients receiving less direct treatment, it will become more imperative to rely on communication partners as intervention agents.

Some research has already explored interventions that focus on the communication partner rather than the person with aphasia (e.g., Kagan, Black, Duchan, Simmons-Mackie, & Square, 2001; Purdy & Hindenlang, 2005; Simmons-Mackie, Kearns, & Potechin, 2005). For example, Simmons, Kearns, and Potechin (1987; see also Simmons-Mackie et al., 2005) evaluated an intervention to diminish inappropriate partner behaviors, such as interrupting before the participant with aphasia has time to respond. Additionally, Flowers and Peizer (1984), and Simmons-Mackie & Kagan (1999) reported systems designed to quantify partner strategies and to identify those that were more or less successful in communicative exchanges, so that they could be addressed in treatment. Measures of conversational burden (e.g., Marshall, Freed, & Phillips, 1997; Packard & Hinckley, 1999) also have been used to describe dynamic partner interactions, and to isolate variables such as topic initiation

that can be manipulated in therapy. In their recent review, Turner and Whitworth (2006) underscore in particular the limited available information about the influence of a conversation partner on the outcomes of a person with aphasia. And in a twist on this theme that emphasizes the level of participation, Cruice, Worrall, and Hickson (2006) recommend training the friends of people with aphasia on how to maintain social relationships with their aphasic friends. In short, the area of conversation-partner training remains ripe for further investigation and evaluation.

Relatedly, the future also may see more efforts to train communication partners as intervention agents (e.g., Bourgeois, 1991; Burgio et al., 2001; Kagan et al., 2001). This approach may accomplish several goals simultaneously: it can bring the intervention to the natural environment, free some of the clinician's time, and allow more treatment to be delivered than would otherwise be feasible or affordable. It also may empower communication partners by giving them some specific things to do in the event of communication breakdown. One such model, Supported Conversation for Adults with Aphasia (SCA), has been developed by Kagan (1995, 1998). SCA offers individuals, including those with severe aphasia, the opportunity to interact with volunteer partners who are trained to support conversational-level communication using a range of methods and expressive modalities. In a randomized, single-blind, controlled study, Kagan et al. (2001) demonstrated the effectiveness of SCA in improving the conversational skills of trained communication partners. After training, the adults with aphasia who conversed with these trained partners were also improved, on both information transfer and interactional variables.

Obviously, either of these approaches can have a number of pitfalls. A clinician would have to invest time to train the communication partners, and to monitor delivery of treatment and/or evaluation of responses. Personalities and prior patterns of interaction between communication partners also may mitigate against these methods, or diminish their effectiveness. In addition, it may be difficult to get reimbursement for services that target communication partners, unless creative outcome measures are employed or until sufficient high-quality evidence is available. And of course, rigorous evaluation of effectiveness will be necessary, as it is for any language-intervention approach. Despite these possible drawbacks, the potential benefits of interventions that involve the neurologically-intact communication partner are likely to spur further exploration in the future.

Another nontraditional intervention approach, group treatment, has the potential to enhance generalization of treatment gains because the group context provides a relatively natural setting within which to target both linguistic and communicative goals. Group therapy for aphasia is increasingly being considered a viable adjunct to individual treatment, and in many cases may serve as the primary therapeutic milieu. This undoubtedly is due in part to reimbursement constraints, but evidence is emerging that group aphasia therapy can effect positive outcomes. The seminal Veteran's Administration cooperative study comparing the effects of individual and group aphasia treatment (Wertz et al., 1981) as well as other more recent studies (e.g., Avent, 1997; Bollinger, Musson, & Holland, 1993; Elman & Bernstein-Ellis, 1999; Marshall, 1993) have demonstrated improvements on both standardized and referential language measures, as well as in functional communication abilities, for individuals at all severity levels in various group-treatment approaches. Kearns (1994) reviews factors to be considered in providing and evaluating group therapy for individuals with aphasia, and a number of other current references discuss methods for delivering and assessing group treatment of patients with aphasia (e.g., Elman, 1999; Marshall, 1999). Group-treatment approaches have also been used with the relatives of people with aphasia, with or without the aphasic partners in attendance. A few recent examples are provided by Hinckley and Packard (2001) and van der Gaag et al., (2005). These studies have demonstrated improvements for the person with aphasia at the levels of impairment (communication skills), (van der Gaag et al., 2005), functional activities (Hinckley & Packard, 2001), and family relationships/quality of life (Hinckley & Packard, 2001; van der Gaag et al., 2005). Group treatment also has been evaluated in other populations, such as traumatic brain injury (Rath, Simon, Langenbahn, Sherr, & Diller, 2003). One obstacle to analyzing the effectiveness of group treatment specifically is the complexity of implementing rigorous data-collection for multiple participants, who may have multiple goals.

Computer-aided approaches to language treatment are also burgeoning, and the future promises to see expansion of efforts in this area as well. The accumulating evidence in aphasia (e.g., Fink, Brecher, Schwartz, & Robey, 2002; Katz & Wertz, 1997; Laganaro, Di Pietro, & Schnider, 2003; Raymer, Kohen, & Saffell, 2006; Wallesch & Johannsen-Horbach, 2004) shows some promise of improvements in language performance with computer-delivered therapy, as well as generalization of learned skills to noncomputer language contexts, mostly when a clinician is also involved. The potential advantages of group treatment, such as cost-effectiveness and the opportunity to tailor tasks for individual patients, must be weighed against possible disadvantages such as a lack of procedural flexibility and limited opportunities for communicative interaction and exchange for the person with aphasia. A more complete discussion of the merits and drawbacks of computer-aided aphasia rehabilitation was published by Roth and Katz (1998). As with the other nontraditional treatment approaches that are discussed here, computer-delivered aphasia therapy must be subjected to rigorous evaluation over time to establish its effectiveness and efficacy. Wertz & Katz (2004) recently provided an evaluation of selected studies in the area, along with their thoughts about improving the evidence base.

Telerehabilitation is another clinical service model that is on the rise (see, e.g., www.atmeda.org, the Web site of the American Telemedicine Association). ASHA recently held a grant competition for model telepractice programs as part of its initiative to increase Web-based service delivery (www.asha.org/about/publications/leader-online/archives/2003/q2/030415d.htm). This initiative was designed to facilitate the delivery of quality health-related information and clinical services to those who face access barriers, such as lack of availability of clinicians with appropriate and specialized expertise. The aphasiology literature is beginning to include some examples of studies that use telepractice methods to measure performance in aphasia and related disorders (e.g., Brennan, Georgeadis, Baron, & Barker, 2004), but there is a long way to go to document the effectiveness and efficacy of treatment thus delivered. To the extent that specific telepractice models and methods can be conceptualized as subsets of the area of computer-assisted intervention, recommendations for improving the evidence base on computer-aided treatment (e.g., Wertz & Katz, 2004) will be highly relevant to telerehabilitation as well.

Lastly, two forms of biologic intervention may have promise as nontraditional approaches to treating aphasia. One, still in its infancy, involves artificially implanting tissue into the brain to increase the number of synaptic connections among or between residual intact regions. Research that uses tissue or cell transplantation aims to reorganize neural circuitry to help the recipient regain function (Small, 2004). Pharmacotherapy is another biologic approach for which definitive benefits remain unknown. Some critical reviews of pharmacotherapy in aphasia (e.g., Small, 1994; Small, 2004) document the spectrum of its use and reported effectiveness, which ranges from no benefit to some positive results when administered as an adjunct to traditional language therapy. Pharmacologic intervention has been investigated for several decades now, but further research is necessary to determine its value for aphasia and related language disorders.

KEY POINTS

1. Research and clinical decision-making processes have a number of parallels.
2. A scientific orientation to clinical management has value for a variety of reasons; among these are that clinical accountability is enhanced by following the hypothesis-testing approach that guides scientific inquiry, and that reimbursement decisions for treatment will rest increasingly on a clinician's knowledge and application of high-quality evidence.
3. Clinicians should become critical consumers of the relevant evidence base, regardless of the format in which it is provided (e.g., EBP reviews, individual studies, conference presentations, continuing-education coursework).

4. Reliability, validity, and generalizability of results are important concepts in the evaluation of research. Clinical significance should be addressed as well in evaluating research and treatment efforts.

5. Outcomes measurement comprises both "efficacy research," which involves rigorous, controlled experimental documentation of the effects of treatment, and "outcomes research," which documents the results of treatment in typical circumstances. Outcomes research yields less confidence in results but is important for evaluating phenomena that cannot easily be isolated or controlled.

6. As used in this chapter, the term "treatment efficacy" refers to evidence that is generated from efficacy research, while "treatment effectiveness" refers more broadly to evidence about how well a treatment works, regardless of the rigor of the research method.

7. Outcomes assessment also can be characterized with reference to a multi-dimensional model of the consequences of health conditions, such as the World Health Organization classification scheme of body structure and function, activity limitation, and participation restriction.

8. A set of principles, reviewed and illustrated in the chapter, can be used to evaluate both basic and applied research. These focus on issues germane to study rationale, design, and interpretation.

9. Clinicians can satisfy empirical, ethical, and practical concerns by becoming involved in clinical research, and their participation in this process is crucial to the development of a sufficient evidentiary basis for treatment. Clinicians may best be able to contribute by collecting treatment-outcomes data, participating in treatment-efficacy studies, replicating and extending existing studies, evaluating published assessment tools and treatment approaches, and/or gathering normative comparison data.

10. Several public and private funding resources are available to both new and experienced clinician-investigators.

11. Established researchers can offer valuable consultation and collaboration to support clinician-investigators in their research endeavors.

12. The future is expected to see increasing emphasis on evaluating the functional and social consequences of treatment, increasing the evidence base in bilingual/multilingual aphasia, and documenting the effectiveness of nontraditional treatment approaches involving communication/conversation partners, group treatment, computer-based interventions, telerehabilitation, and pharmacotherapy.

ACTIVITIES FOR REFLECTION AND DISCUSSION

1. Discuss the benefits of a scientific approach to clinical decision-making. Are there any drawbacks?
2. Debate Rosenbek, LaPointe, & Wertz's (1989) opinion that "untested treatments are immoral. . ." (p. 12).
3. Which of the threats to internal validity of a treatment study would be the easiest to solve or avoid? Why? Which would be the most difficult, and why?
4. (a) Evaluate a published treatment study, using the 12 criteria in this chapter. (b) Keeping in mind that no research effort can be, or is, perfect, and using your treatment-study evaluation as a guide, discuss how your confidence in the outcome has been affected.
5. Discuss how the concepts related to internal validity could be applied to improve your clinical work.
6. Can you see yourself contributing to the scientific data base in some way? Why or why not? And if "Yes," how?

References

Ardila, A., & Rosselli, M. (1996). Spontaneous language production and aging: Sex and educational effects. *International Journal of Neuroscience, 87*(1–2), 71–78.

Avent, J. (1997). Group treatment in aphasia using cooperative learning methods. *Journal of Medical Speech-Language Pathology, 5,* 9–26.

Ballard, K. J., & Thompson, C. K. (1999). Treatment and generalization of complex sentence production in agrammatism. *Journal of Speech, Language, and Hearing Research, 42,* 690–707.

Bastiaanse, R., Bosje, M., & Franssen, M. (1996). Deficit-oriented treatment of word-finding problems: Another replication. *Aphasiology, 10,* 363–383.

Beard, L. C., & Prescott, T. E. (1991). Replication of a treatment protocol for repetition deficit in conduction aphasia. *Clinical Aphasiology, 19,* 197–208.

Bloise, C. G. R., & Tompkins, C. A. (1993). Right brain damage and inference revision, revisited. *Clinical Aphasiology, 21,* 145–155.

Bollinger, R. L., Musson, N. D., & Holland, A. L. (1993). A study of group communication intervention with chronically aphasic persons. *Aphasiology, 7,* 301–313.

Bottenberg, D., & Lemme, M. L. (1991). Effect of shared and unshared listener knowledge on narratives of normal and aphasic adults. *Clinical Aphasiology, 19,* 109–116.

Bourgeois, M. S. (1991). Communication treatment for adults with dementia. *Journal of Speech and Hearing Research, 34,* 831–844.

Bourgeois, M. S. (1992). Evaluating memory wallets in conversations with patients with dementia. *Journal of Speech and Hearing Research, 35,* 1344–1357.

Brennan, D. M., Georgeadis, A. C., Baron, C. R., Barker, L. M. (2004). The effect of videoconference-based telerehabilitation on story retelling performance by brain-injured subjects and its implications for remote speech-language therapy. *Telemedicine and E-Health Journal, 10*(2), 147–154.

Brenneise-Sarshad, R., Nicholas, L. E., & Brookshire, R. H. (1991). Effects of apparent listener knowledge and picture stimuli on aphasic and non-brain-damaged speakers' narrative discourse. *Journal of Speech and Hearing Research, 34,* 168–176.

Brookshire, R. H. (1983). Subject description and generality of results in experiments with aphasic adults. *Journal of Speech and Hearing Disorders, 48,* 342–346.

Brookshire, R. H., & Nicholas, L. E. (1994). Test-retest stability of measures of connected speech in aphasia. *Clinical Aphasiology, 22,* 119–134.

Brown, K., McGahan, L., Alkhaledi, M., Seah, D., Howe, T., & Worrall, L. (2006). Environmental factors that influence the community participation of adults with aphasia: The perspective of service industry workers. *Aphasiology, 20*(7), 595–615.

Burgio, L. D., Allen-Burge, R., Roth, D. L., Bourgeois, M. S., Dijkstra, K., Gerstle, J., et al. (2001). Come talk with me: Improving communication between nursing assistants and nursing home residents during care routines. *Gerontologist, 41*(4), 449–460.

Byng, S., Nickels, L., & Black, M. (1994). Replicating therapy for mapping deficits in agrammatism: Remapping the deficit? *Aphasiology, 8,* 315–341.

Campbell, D. T., & Stanley, J. C. (1966). *Experimental and quasi-experimental designs for research*. Chicago: Rand McNally.

Campbell, T. F., & Dollaghan, C. (1992). A method for obtaining listener judgments of spontaneously produced language: Social validation through direct magnitude estimation. *Topics in Language Disorders, 12,* 42–55.

Chial, M. R. (1985). Scholarship as process: A task analysis of thesis and dissertation research. *Seminars in Speech and Language, 6,* 35–54.

Chumpelik, D. (1984). The PROMPT system of therapy: Theoretical framework and applications for developmental apraxia of speech. *Seminars in Speech and Language, 5,* 139–156.

Cohen, J. (1977). *Statistical power analysis for the behavioral sciences*. New York: Academic Press.

Conlon, C. P., & McNeil, M. R. (1991). The efficacy of treatment for two globally aphasic adults using visual action therapy. *Clinical Aphasiology, 19,* 185–195.

Connell, P. J., & Thompson, C. K. (1986). Flexibility of single-subject experimental designs. Part III: Using flexibility to design or modify experiments. *Journal of Speech and Hearing Disorders, 51,* 214–225.

Cruice, M., Worrall, L., & Hickson, L. (2006). Perspectives of quality of life by people with aphasia and their family: Suggestions for successful living. *Topics in Stroke Rehabilitation, 13*(1), 14–21.

Darley, F. L. (1972). The efficacy of language rehabilitation in aphasia. *Journal of Speech and Hearing Disorders, 37,* 3–21.

Davis, G. A., & Wilcox, M. J. (1985). *Adult aphasia rehabilitation: Applied pragmatics*. San Diego: College-Hill.

Denzin, N. K., & Lincoln, Y. S. (Eds.) (1998). *The landscape of qualitative research: Theories and issues*. Thousand Oaks: Sage.

DiSimoni, F. G., Keith, R. L., & Darley, F. L. (1980). Prediction of PICA overall score by short versions of the test. *Journal of Speech and Hearing Research, 23,* 511–516.

Donabedian, A. (1980). *Explorations in quality assessment and monitoring. Volume 1: The definition of quality and approaches to its assessment*. Ann Arbor, MI: Health Administration Press.

Donovan, N. J., Rosenbek, J. C., Ketterson, T. U., & Velozo, C. A. (2006). Adding meaning to measurement: Initial Rasch analysis of the ASHA FACS Social Communication subtest. *Aphasiology, 20*(2–4), 362–373.

Doyle, P. J. (2002). Measuring health outcomes in stroke survivors. *Archives of Physical Medicine and Rehabilitation, 83*(12 Suppl 2), 39–43.

Doyle, P. J., Goldstein, H., & Bourgeois, M. S. (1987). Experimental analysis of syntax training in Broca's aphasia: A generalization and social validation study. *Journal of Speech and Hearing Disorders, 52,* 143–155.

Doyle, P. J., Goldstein, H., Bourgeois, M. S., & Nakles, K. (1989). Facilitating generalized requesting behavior in Broca's aphasia: An experimental analysis of a generalization training procedure. *Journal of Applied Behavior Analysis, 22,* 157–170.

Doyle, P. J., McNeil, M. R., Hula, W. D., & Mikolic, J. M. (2003). The Burden of Stroke Scale (BOSS): Validating patient-reported communication difficulty and associated psychological distress in stroke survivors. *Aphasiology, 17*(3), 291–304.

Doyle, P. J., McNeil, M. R., Mikolic, J. M., Prieto, L., Hula, W., Lustig, A., et al. (2004). The Burden of Stroke Scale (BOSS) provides valid and reliable score estimates of functioning and well-being in stroke survivors with and without communication disorders. *Journal of Clinical Epidemiology, 57*(10), 997–1007.

Doyle, P. J., Oleyar, K. S., & Goldstein, H. (1991). Facilitating functional conversational skills in aphasia: An experimental analysis of a generalization training procedure. *Clinical Aphasiology, 19,* 229–241.

Edmonds, L., & Kiran, S. (2006). Effect of semantic naming treatment on cross-linguistic generalization in bilingual aphasia. *Journal of Speech, Language, and Hearing Research, 49,* 729–748.

Elman, R. (1999). *Group treatment of neurogenic communication disorders: The expert clinician's approach*. Boston: Butterworth-Heinemann.

Elman, R. (2006). Evidence-based practice: What evidence is missing? *Aphasiology, 20*(2–4), 103–109.

Elman, R. J., & Bernstein-Ellis, E. (1999). The efficacy of group treatment in adults with chronic aphasia. *Journal of Speech, Language, and Hearing Research, 42,* 411–419.

Elman, R. J., Roberts, J. A., & Wertz, R. T. (1991). The effect of education on diagnosis of aphasia from writing and drawing performance by mildly aphasic and non-brain-damaged adults. *Clinical Aphasiology, 20,* 101–110.

Feeney, T., & Ylvisaker, M. (2003). Context-sensitive behavioral supports for young children with TBI: Short-term effects and long-term outcome. *The Journal of Head Trauma Rehabilitation, 18*(1), 33–51.

Ferguson, A. (1993). Conversational repair of word-finding difficulty. *Clinical Aphasiology, 21,* 299–310.

Fink, R. B., Brecher, A., Schwartz, M. F., & Robey, R. R. (2002). A computer-implemented protocol for treatment of naming disorders: Evaluation of clinician-guided and partially self-guided instruction. *Aphasiology, 16*(10–11), 1061–1086.

Flowers, C. R., & Peizer, E. R. (1984). Strategies for obtaining information from aphasic persons. In R. H. Brookshire (Ed.), *Clinical aphasiology: Conference proceedings 1984*. Minneapolis: BRK.

Franklin, S. (1997). Designing single case treatment studies for aphasic patients. *Neuropsychological Rehabilitation, 7,* 401–418.

Franzen, M. D. (1989). *Reliability and validity in neuropsychological assessment.* New York: Plenum.

Frattali, C. M. (1998a). Outcomes measurement: Definitions, dimensions, and perspectives. In C. M. Frattali (Ed.), *Measuring outcomes in speech-language pathology* (pp. 1–27). New York: Thieme.

Frattali, C. M. (1998b). Measuring modality-specific behaviors, functional abilities, and quality of life. In C. M. Frattali (Ed.), *Measuring outcomes in speech-language pathology* (pp. 55–88). New York: Thieme.

Frattali, C. M., Thompson, C. K., Holland, A. L., Wohl, C. B., & Ferketic, M. M. (1995). *Functional assessment of communication skills for adults.* Rockville, MD: American Speech-Language Hearing Association.

Freed, D. B., Marshall, R. C., & Frazier, K. E. (1997). Long-term effectiveness of PROMPT treatment in a severely apractic-aphasia speaker. *Aphasiology, 11,* 365–372.

Garrett, K. L., & Huth, C. (2002). The impact of graphic contextual information and instruction on the conversational behaviours of a person with severe aphasia. *Aphasiology, 6*(4–6), 523–536.

Goldstein, H. (1990). Assessing clinical significance. In L. B. Olswang, C. K. Thompson, S. F. Warren, & N. J. Minghetti (Eds.), *Treatment efficacy research in communication disorders* (pp. 91–98). Rockville, MD: American Speech-Language-Hearing Foundation.

Goodwin, C., & Heritage, J. (1990). Conversation analysis. *Annual Review of Anthropology, 19,* 283–307.

Hansen, A. M., & McNeil, M. R. (1986). Differences between writing with the dominant and nondominant hand by normal geriatric subjects on a spontaneous writing task: Twenty perceptual and computerized measures. *Clinical Aphasiology, 16,* 116–122.

Helm-Estabrooks, N., Fitzpatrick, P. M., & Barresi, B. (1982). Visual action therapy for global aphasia. *Journal of Speech and Hearing Disorders, 47,* 385–389.

Heron, J. (1996). *Cooperative inquiry: Research into the human condition.* London: Sage.

Hinckley, J. J., & Packard, M. E. (2001). Family education seminars and social functioning of adults with chronic aphasia. *Journal of Communication Disorders, 34*(3), 241–254.

Holland, A., Frattali, C., & Fromm, D. (1999). *Communication activities of daily living* (2nd ed.). Austin, TX: Pro-Ed.

Huck, S. W., & Sandler, H. M. (1979). *Rival hypotheses: Alternative interpretations of data based conclusions.* New York: Harper & Row.

Johnson, W., Darley, F. L., & Spriestersbach, D. C. (1963). *Diagnostic methods in speech pathology.* New York: Harper & Row.

Kagan, A. (1995). Revealing the competence of aphasic adults through conversation: A challenge to health professionals. *Topics in Stroke Rehabilitation, 2,* 15–28.

Kagan, A. (1998). Supported conversation for adults with aphasia: Methods and resources for training conversational partners. *Aphasiology, 12,* 816–830.

Kagan, A., Black, S. E., Duchan, F. J., Simmons-Mackie, N., & Square, P. (2001). Training volunteers as conversation partners using "Supported Conversation for Adults with Aphasia" (SCA): A controlled trial. *Journal of Speech Language & Hearing Research, 44*(3), 624–638.

Katz, R. C., & Wertz, R. T. (1997). The efficacy of computer-provided reading treatment for chronic aphasic adults. *Journal of Speech & Hearing Research, 40,* 493–507.

Kearns, K. P. (1986a). Flexibility of single-subject experimental designs. Part II: Design selection and arrangements of experimental phases. *Journal of Speech and Hearing Disorders, 51,* 204–214.

Kearns, K. P. (1986b). Systematic programming of verbal elaboration skills in chronic Broca's aphasia. In R. C. Marshall (Ed.), *Case studies in aphasia rehabilitation* (pp. 225–244). Austin, TX: Pro-Ed.

Kearns, K. P. (1989). Methodologies for studying generalization. In McReynolds, L. V. & Spradlin, J. (Eds.), *Generalization strategies in the treatment of communication disorders.* Toronto: B. C. Decker.

Kearns, K. P. (1990). Reliability of procedures and measures. In L. Olswang, C. Thompson & S. Warren (Eds.), *Treatment efficacy research in communication disorders* (pp. 71–90). Rockville, MD: American Speech-Language-Hearing Foundation.

Kearns, K. P. (1992). Methodological issues in treatment research: A single-subject perspective. *Aphasia treatment: Current approaches and research opportunities* (pp. 7–16). Washington, D.C.: National Institute on Deafness and Other Communication Disorders.

Kearns, K. P. (1993). Functional outcome: Methodological considerations. *Clinical Aphasiology, 21,* 67–72.

Kearns, K. P. (1994). Group therapy for aphasia: Theoretical and practical considerations. In R. Chapey (Ed.), *Language intervention strategies in adult aphasia* (3rd ed., pp. 304–321). Baltimore: Williams & Wilkins.

Kearns, K. P., & Potechin Scher, G. (1989). The generalization of response elaboration training effects. *Clinical Aphasiology, 18,* 223–245.

Kearns, K. P., & Simmons, N. N. (1988). Interobserver reliability and perceptual ratings: More than meets the ear. *Journal of Speech and Hearing Research, 31,* 131–136.

Kendall, P., & Norton-Ford, J. (1982). Therapy outcome research methods. In P. Kendall & J. Butcher (Eds.), *Handbook of research methods in clinical psychology* (pp. 429–460). New York: John Wiley and Sons.

Kent, R. D. (1985a). Science and the clinician: The practice of science and the science of practice. In R. D. Kent (Ed.), *Seminars in speech and language: Vol. 6. Application of research to assessment and therapy* (pp. 1–12). New York: Thieme-Stratton.

Kent, R. D. (Ed.). (1985b). *Seminars in speech and language: Vol. 6. Application of research to assessment and therapy.* New York: Thieme-Stratton.

Kent, R. D., & Fair, J. (1985). Clinical research: Who, where, and how? In R. D. Kent (Ed.), *Seminars in speech and language: Vol. 6. Application of research to assessment and therapy* (pp. 23–34). New York: Thieme-Stratton.

Kerlinger, F. N. (1973). *Foundations of behavioral research* (2nd ed.). New York: Holt, Rinehart & Winston.

Kimelman, M. D. Z., & McNeil, M. R. (1987). An investigation of emphatic stress comprehension in adult aphasia: A replication. *Journal of Speech and Hearing Research, 30,* 295–300.

Kiran, S., & Thompson, C. K. (2003). The role of semantic complexity in treatment of naming deficits: Training semantic categories in fluent aphasia by controlling exemplar typicality, *Journal of Speech Language and Hearing Research, 46,* 773–787.

Laganaro, M., Di Pietro, M., & Schnider, A. (2003). Effects of phonological neighbourhood in recovery from word-finding impairment: A case study. *Brain and Language, 87*(1), 169–170.

Lemme, M. L. (Ed.). (1993). *Clinical aphasiology* (pp. 21). Austin, TX: Pro-Ed.

Lock, S., Wilkinson, R., Bryan, K., Maxim, J., Edmundson, A., Bruce, C., et al. (2001). Supporting partners of people with Aphasia in relationships and conversation (SPPARC). *International Journal of Language and Communication Disorders, 36*, 24–30.

Marshall, R. C. (1993). Problem-focused group treatment for clients with mild aphasia. *American Journal of Speech-Language Pathology, 3*, 31–37.

Marshall, R. C. (1999). *Introduction to group treatment for aphasia: Design and management.* Boston: Butterworth-Heinemann.

Marshall, R. C., & Freed, D. B. (2006). The personalized cueing method: From the laboratory to the clinic. *American Journal of Speech-Language Pathology, 15*, 103–111.

Marshall, R. C, Freed, D. B, & Phillips, D. S. (1997). Communicative efficiency in severe aphasia. *Aphasiology, 11*, 373–384.

Massaro, M., & Tompkins, C. A. (1993). Feature analysis for treatment of communication disorders in traumatically brain-injured patients: An efficacy study. *Clinical Aphasiology, 22*, 245–256.

McNeil, M. R., Doyle, P. J., Spencer, K. A., Goda, A. J., Flores, D., & Small, S. L. (1998). Effects of training multiple form classes on acquisition, generalization and maintenance of word retrieval in a single subject. *Aphasiology, 12*, 561–574.

McReynolds, L., & Kearns, K. P. (1983). *Single-subject experimental design in communicative disorders.* Baltimore: University Park Press.

McReynolds, L. V., & Thompson, C. K. (1986). Flexibility of single-subject experimental designs. Part I: Review of the basics of single-subject designs. *Journal of Speech and Hearing Disorders, 51*, 194–203.

Metter, E. J. (1985). Issues and directions for the future: Speech pathology: A physician's perspective. *Clinical Aphasiology, 15*, 22–28.

Milroy, L., & Perkins, L. (1992). Repair strategies in aphasic discourse: Towards a collaborative model. *Clinical Linguistics & Phonetics, 6*, 27–40.

Moss, A., & Nicholas, M. (2006). Language rehabilitation in chronic aphasia and time postonset: A review of single-subject data. *Stroke, 37*(12), 3043–3051.

Nation, J. E., & Aram, D. M. (1984). *Diagnosis of speech and language disorders* (2nd ed.). Boston: College-Hill.

Nicholas, L. E., & Brookshire, R. H. (1986). Consistency of the effects of rate of speech on brain-damaged adults' comprehension of narrative discourse. *Journal of Speech and Hearing Research, 29*, 462–470.

Nicholas, L. E., Brookshire, R. H., MacLennan, D. L., Schumacher, J. G., & Porazzo, S. A. (1989). Revised administration and scoring procedures for the Boston Naming Test and norms for non-brain-damaged adults. *Aphasiology, 3*, 569–580.

Nicholas, L. E., MacLennan, D. L., & Brookshire, R. H. (1986). Validity of multiple-sentence reading comprehension tests for aphasic adults. *Journal of Speech and Hearing Disorders, 51*, 82–87.

Packard, M., & Hinckley, J. J. (1999). *Measuring conversational burden in adults with moderate and severe aphasia.* Poster presentation, Clinical Aphasiology Conference, Key West, FL.

Parr, S. (1992). Everyday reading and writing practices of normal adults: Implications for aphasia assessment. *Aphasiology, 3*, 273–284.

Perkins, L. (1995). Applying conversation analysis to aphasia: Clinical implications and analytic issues. *European Journal of Disorders of Communication, 30*, 372–383.

Perkins, L., Crisp, J., & Walshaw, D. (1999). Exploring conversation analysis as an assessment tool for aphasia: The issue of reliability. *Aphasiology, 13*, 259–281.

Porch, B. (1981). *The Porch index of communicative ability.* Palo Alto: Consulting Psychological Press.

Prescott, T. E. (Ed.). (1989). *Clinical aphasiology, 18.* Boston: College-Hill.

Prescott, T. E. (Ed.). (1991a). *Clinical aphasiology, 19.* Austin, TX: Pro-Ed.

Prescott, T. E. (Ed.). (1991b). *Clinical aphasiology, 20.* Austin, TX: Pro-Ed.

Purdy, M., & Hindenlang, J. (2005). Educating and training caregivers of persons with aphasia. *Aphasiology, 19*(3–5), 377–388.

Rath, J. F., Simon, D., Langenbahn, D. M., Sherr, R. L., & Diller, L. (2003). Group treatment of problem-solving deficits in outpatients with traumatic brain injury: A randomised outcome study. *Neuropsychological Rehabilitation 13*(4), 461–488.

Raymer, A. M., Kohen, F. P., & Saffell, D. (2006). Computerised training for impairments of word comprehension and retrieval in aphasia. *Aphasiology, 20* (02–04), 257–268.

Robey, R. R., & Schultz, M. C. (1998). A model for conducting clinical-outcome research: An adaptation of the standard protocol for use in aphasiology. *Aphasiology, 12*, 787–810.

Rosenbek, J. C. (1987). Unusual aphasias: Some criteria for evaluating case studies in aphasiology. *Clinical Aphasiology, 17*, 357–361.

Rosenbek, J. C., LaPointe, L. L., & Wertz, R. T. (1989). *Aphasia: A clinical approach.* Austin, TX: Pro-Ed.

Roth, V. M., & Katz, R. C. (1998). The role of computers in aphasia rehabilitation. In B. Stemmer & H.A. Whitaker (Eds.), *Handbook of neurolinguistics* (pp.585–596). San Diego: Academic Press.

Sackett, D. L., Rosenberg, W., Muir Gray, J. A., Haynes, R. B., & Richardson, W. S. (1996). Evidence based medicine: What it is and what it isn't. *British Medical Journal, 312*, 71–72.

Sackett. D. L., Straus, S., Richardson, W. L., Rosenberg, W., & Haynes, R. B. (2000). *Evidence-based medicine: How to practice and teach EBM* (2nd ed.). New York: Churchill Livingstone.

Schiavetti, N., & Metz, D. E. (2005). *Evaluating research in communicative disorders* (5th Ed.). Boston: Allyn and Bacon.

Schumacher, J. G., & Nicholas, L. E. (1991). Conducting research in a clinical setting against all odds: Unusual treatment of fluent aphasia. *Clinical Aphasiology, 19*, 267–277.

Shewan, C. M. (1986). The history and efficacy of aphasia treatment. In R. Chapey (Ed.), *Language intervention strategies in adult aphasia* (2nd ed.), (pp. 28–43). Baltimore: Williams & Wilkins.

Shiffrin, D. (1994). *Approaches to discourse.* Oxford: Blackwell.

Shrout, P. E., & Fleiss, J. L. (1979). Intraclass correlations: Uses in assessing rater reliability. *Psychological Bulletin, 86*, 420–428.

Silverman, F. H. (1985). *Research design and evaluation in speech-language pathology and audiology* (2nd ed.). Englewood Cliffs, NJ: Prentice-Hall.

Simmons, N. N., Kearns, K. P., & Potechin, G. (1987). Treatment of aphasia through family member training. *Clinical Aphasiology, 17*, 106–116.

Simmons-Mackie, N., & Damico, J. S. (1996). Accounting for handicaps in aphasia: Communicative assessment from an authentic social perspective. *Disability & Rehabilitation, 18*, 540–549.

Simmons-Mackie, N., & Kagan, A. (1999). Communication strategies used by 'good' versus 'poor' speaking partners of individuals with aphasia. *Aphasiology, 9–11*, 807–820.

Simmons-Mackie, N. N., Kearns, K. P., & Potechin, G. (2005). Treatment of aphasia through family member training, *Aphasiology, 19*(6), 583–593.

Small, S. L. (1994). Pharmacotherapy of aphasia. A critical review. *Stroke, 25*(6), 1282–1289.

Small, S. L. (2004). A biological model of aphasia rehabilitation: Pharmacological perspectives. *Aphasiology, 18*(5/6/7), 473–492.

Strauss, A., & Corbin, J. (1998). *Basics of qualitative research: Techniques and procedures for developing grounded theory.* Thousand Oaks: Sage.

Szekeres, S. F., Ylvisaker, M., & Cohen, S. B. (1987). A framework for cognitive rehabilitation therapy. In M. Ylvisaker & E. R. Gobble (Eds.), *Community re-entry for head injured adults* (pp. 87–136). Boston: College Hill Press.

Thompson, C. K. (1989). Generalization research in aphasia: A review of the literature. *Clinical Aphasiology, Vol. 18*, 195–222.

Thompson, C. K., & Byrne, M. E. (1984). Across setting generalization of social conventions in aphasia: An experimental analysis of "loose training." In R. H. Brookshire (Ed.), *Clinical aphasiology: Conference proceedings 1984* (pp. 132–144). Minneapolis: BRK.

Thompson, C. K., & Shapiro, L. P. (1995). Training sentence production in agrammatism: Implications for normal and disordered language. *Brain & Language, 50*, 201–224.

Tompkins, C. A. (1992). Improving aphasia treatment research: Some methodological considerations. In *Aphasia treatment: Current approaches and research opportunities* (pp. 37–46). Washington, D.C.: National Institute on Deafness and Other Communication Disorders.

Tompkins, C. A., Boada, R., McGarry, K., Jones, J., Rahn, A. E., & Ranier, S. (1993). Connected speech characteristics of right hemisphere damaged adults: A re-examination. *Clinical Aphasiology, 21*, 113–122.

Tompkins, C. A., Jackson, S. T., & Schulz, R. (1990). On prognostic research in adult neurogenic disorders. *Journal of Speech and Hearing Research, 33*, 398–401.

Turner, S., & Whitworth, A. (2006). Conversational partner training programmes in aphasia: A review of key themes and participants' roles. *Aphasiology, 20*(6), 483–510.

van der Gaag, A., Smith, L., Davis, S., Moss, B., Cornelius, V., Laing, S., et al. (2005). Therapy and support services for people with long-term stroke and aphasia and their relatives: A six-month follow-up study. *Clinical Rehabilitation. 19*(4), 372–80.

Ventry, I. M., & Schiavetti, N. (1980). *Evaluating research in speech pathology and audiology: A guide for clinicians and students.* Reading, MA: Addison-Wesley.

Wallesch, C. W., & Johannsen-Horbach, H. (2004). Computers in aphasia therapy: Effects and side-effects. *Aphasiology, 18*(3), 223–228.

Warren, R. L. (1986). Research design: Considerations for the clinician. In R. Chapey (Ed.), *Language intervention strategies in adult aphasia* (2nd ed., pp. 66–80). Baltimore: Williams & Wilkins.

Warren, R. L., Gabriel, C., Johnston, A., & Gaddie, A. (1987). Efficacy during acute rehabilitation. *Clinical Aphasiology, 17*, 1–11.

Wertz, R. T. (1985). Neuropathologies of speech and language: An introduction to patient management. In D. F. Johns (Ed.), *Clinical Management of Neurogenic Communication Disorders* (2nd ed., pp. 1–96). Boston: Little-Brown.

Wertz, R. T. (1991). Predictability: Greater than p < .05. *Clinical Aphasiology, 19*, 21–30.

Wertz, R. T. (1992). A single case for group treatment studies in aphasia. *Aphasia treatment: Current approaches and research opportunities* (pp. 25–36). Washington, D.C.: National Institute on Deafness and Other Communication Disorders.

Wertz, R. T., Collins, M. J., Weiss, D., Kurtzke, J. F., Friden, T., Brookshire, R.H., et al. (1981). Veterans Administration cooperative study on Aphasia: A comparison of individual and group treatment. *Journal of Speech and Hearing Research, 24*, 580–594.

Wertz, R. T., & Katz, R. C. (2004). Outcomes of computer-provided treatment for aphasia. *Aphasiology, 18*(4), 229–244.

Wertz, R. T., Shubitowski, Y., Dronkers, N. F., Lemme, M. L., & Deal, J. L. (1985). *Word fluency measure reliability in normal and brain damaged adults.* Paper presented at the American Speech-Language-Hearing Association convention, Washington, DC.

Wertz, R. T., Weiss, D. G., Aten, J. L., Brookshire, R. H., Garcia-Bunuel, L., Holland, A., et al. (1986). Comparison of clinic, home, and deferred language treatment for aphasia: A Veterans Administration cooperative study. *Archives of Neurology, 43*, 653–658.

Whitney, J. L., & Goldstein, H. (1989). Using self-monitoring to reduce disfluencies in speakers with mild aphasia. *Journal of Speech and Hearing Disorders, 54*, 576–586.

World Health Organization (2001). *International Classification of Functioning, Disability and Health*: ICF. Geneva.

Yorkston, K. M., Farrier, L., Zeches, J., & Uomoto, J. M. (1990). *Discourse patterns in traumatically brain injured and control subjects.* Paper presented at the American Speech-Language-Hearing Association convention, Washington, DC.

Yorkston, K. M., Zeches, J., Farrier, L., & Uomoto, J. M. (1993). Lexical pitch as a measure of word choice in narratives of traumatically brain injured and control subjects. *Clinical Aphasiology, 21*, 165–172.

Yoshihata, H., Toshiko, W., Chujo, T., & Kaori, M. (1998). Acquisition and generalization of mode interchange skills in people with severe aphasia. *Aphasiology, 12*, 1035–1045.

Chapter 6

Aphasia Treatment: Recovery, Prognosis, and Clinical Effectiveness

Leora R. Cherney and
Randall R. Robey

OBJECTIVES

The objectives of this chapter are to (1) describe the typical time course and pattern of recovery in individuals with aphasia; (2) review current information regarding the neuroanatomical and neurophysiologic mechanisms underlying recovery and rehabilitation; (3) identify neurologic and personal factors affecting prognosis; and (4) review scientific evidence regarding clinical outcomes of treatments provided by speech-language pathologists.

Clinicians who treat individuals with aphasia have frequently sought to uncover indicators of recovery. Reliable information regarding factors associated with positive recovery as well as factors associated with negative recovery impact several clinical decisions and actions, including determining prognosis, counseling significant others, and identifying candidates for treatment. Basso (1992) has differentiated between neurologic factors and anagraphic factors. Neurologic factors are related to etiology, size and site of lesion, and severity and type of aphasia. In addition, through modern neuroimaging technologies, there has been an increased focus on pathophysiologic indicators of recovery, the long-term cerebral changes related to resolving aphasia, and the neurophysiologic consequences of therapeutic interventions. Anagraphic factors include personal characteristics such as age, sex, handedness, and health status. One of the difficulties encountered in research on recovery from aphasia and prognosis is that many of these factors are interrelated. For example, site of lesion determines to some extent the type of aphasia; size of lesion and type of aphasia have some implications for severity; and type of aphasia may not be independent of age. Nonetheless, clinicians have relied on the extensive literature examining the effects of these factors on recovery to guide their clinical decision-making.

The range of clinical decisions extends beyond prognosis and candidate identification. Once the decision to treat is warranted, clinicians must settle on justifiable treatment(s), a weekly schedule of treatment, and the duration of treatment. The purpose of this chapter is to review the information base underpinning the broad range of clinical decisions, from prognosis to treatment schedules. The chapter proceeds in two major sections. First, studies related to recovery are summarized, with particular emphasis on the factors that may be considered when determining prognosis. Second, the scientific base underlying treatment-related decisions is reviewed. However, the sectioning has been imposed merely for organization purposes and it will be readily apparent that these topics are not mutually exclusive, and, in fact, interact with one another.

RECOVERY

Time Course of Recovery

Two stages in the recovery of function have been differentiated, an early stage and a late stage (Kertesz, 1988). The early stage, when maximum language recovery takes place, coincides with the period of spontaneous recovery, and is considered by investigators to occur within 1 to 3 months post-onset of aphasia (Kertesz & McCabe, 1977; Vignolo, 1964). Spontaneous recovery drops precipitously by 6 to 7 months post-onset (Vignolo, 1964), with little or no spontaneous recovery occurring after 1 year (Kertesz, Harlock, & Coates, 1979; Kertesz & McCabe, 1977). Therefore, spontaneous recovery has a decelerating curve, steepest in the first month post-onset, subsequently flattening out, and finally reaching a plateau between 6 and 12 months post-onset (Basso, 1992; Benson & Ardila, 1996).

A prospective study of 330 patients with aphasia supports a pattern of recovery from aphasia consistent with that of spontaneous recovery (Pederson, Jorgensen, Nakayama, Raaschou, & Olsen, 1995). Patients with aphasia were evaluated on admission to the hospital, weekly during their hospital stay, and then at 6 months post-discharge. The investigators found that stationary language function was reached in 84% of the patients within 2 weeks, and in 95% of the patients within 6 weeks from onset of stroke. Similarly, Pashek and Holland (1988), in their longitudinal study of 43 individuals with aphasia, noted that improvement most frequently began at about 1 to 2 weeks post-onset; furthermore, by 3 months, the clinical status of most of the patients approximated the clinical status that was measured at 12 months.

Late or long-term recovery may take place months or even years after onset of stroke. However, the degree of recovery can vary greatly from patient to patient. For example, Hanson, Metter, and Riege (1989) conducted a retrospective study that followed 35 males with aphasia from 3 to 55 months post-onset. Patients were evaluated with the Porch Index of Communicative Abilities (PICA) on five factors—speaking, writing, comprehension, gesturing, and copying. Language performance continued to evolve over years, with some patients improving significantly, others stabilizing, and others (10 of 35) regressing. No medical factor could be found to account for the regression, but it was noted that language decline occurred in those patients with relatively milder aphasia.

Pattern of Recovery

Despite individual variation in rate and extent of recovery, there seem to be some general patterns of recovery that have been identified for each type of aphasia. Kertesz and McCabe (1977) studied the evolution of aphasia using the Western Aphasia Battery aphasia quotients obtained serially at 45 days, and at 3, 6, and 12 months. They found that 39 of 93 patients (41.9%) changed aphasia type as they recovered. Similarly, Pashek and Holland (1988) followed 43 subjects from the acute stage (within 5 days post-onset) and subsequently at 3, 6, and 12 months post-onset. Using descriptive criteria to define aphasia type, they found that approximately 60% of the sample evolved and were reclassified, with each type of aphasia showing a pattern of evolution. They noted that change most frequently began at about 2 weeks post-onset, with most types of aphasia evolving within the first month (except conduction aphasia, which typically showed a change at about 6 months post-onset) to that of anomic aphasia. Patients who presented initially with a fluent aphasia continued to demonstrate a fluent type of aphasia. Anomic aphasia was often the end-point attained by patients regardless of whether they initially presented with fluent or nonfluent aphasia (Kertesz & McCabe, 1977; Pashek & Holland, 1988).

McDermott, Horner, and DeLong (1996) have provided further information about the evolution of the different aphasia types. They followed 39 patients and evaluated them regularly with the Western Aphasia Battery. They confirmed

that the direction of evolution appears to operate under some constraints, and that aphasia subtypes differ in their evolution. Like Pashek and Holland (1988), they found that patients who presented initially with a fluent aphasia continued to demonstrate a fluent type of aphasia.

The investigators also noted that aphasia severity may interact with the evolution of aphasia (McDermott et al., 1996). Patients with nonfluent or fluent aphasia who evolved from one aphasia type to another were less severely affected than those who did not evolve. However, magnitude of change, and not initial severity, was the critical variable underlying aphasia evolution. Those patients who evolved from one aphasia type to another had greater aphasia quotient changes from the first test session to the second than those who did not, suggesting that improvement in language performance is a necessary condition for evolution of aphasia type. Specifically, it was found that an aphasia quotient change of 20 points or more predicated aphasia type evolution in about two-thirds of the patients with both fluent and nonfluent aphasia.

Several studies have investigated the evolution of typology in patients with severe or global aphasia. Pashek and Holland (1988) found that age was a factor in the evolution from global aphasia. There was a trend for younger patients to evolve to a Broca's aphasia, while older patients remained global or evolved to a Wernicke's aphasia.

Nicholas, Helm-Estabrooks, Ward-Lonergan, and Morgan (1993) followed 24 subjects with severe aphasia, of which 17 were global. Patients were evaluated with the Boston Assessment of Severe Aphasia (BASA) at 1 to 2 months, 6, 12, 18, and 24 months post-onset. The greatest amount of improvement occurred in the first 6 months. While most of the patients with global aphasia showed improvements on the BASA, they did not change classification and remained global.

From a study of 54 patients with global aphasia, Ferro (1992) concluded that there are five different types of global aphasia, depending on the site of lesion, and that each type has a different outcome. Patients with global aphasia resulting from large fronto-temporoparietal lesions with or without subcortical damage had the poorest prognosis and remained global at follow-up. In contrast, the best prognosis was found for those patients with large subcortical infarcts. None of these patients remained global; one patient was not aphasic at follow-up, while the others evolved to transcortical motor aphasia or anomic aphasia. The other three possible localizations for the infarcts that cause acute global aphasia are (a) frontal lesions with or without subcortical involvement; (b) posterior parietal infarct, with or without subcortical involvement; and (c) a double lesion composed of a frontal and temporal cortical infarct. These patients showed a variable degree of recovery, improving to Broca's or transcortical aphasia. Ferro (1992) also found that the first 3 months was the crucial period for improvement, in contrast to the findings of Sarno and Levita (1971), who suggested that the greatest changes for global aphasia were evident in the 6- to 12-month period post-stroke.

Several longitudinal studies have considered the pattern of recovery as it relates to the individual language modalities, and a consistent trend has emerged. Typically, a higher percentage of patients improve in comprehension as opposed to production, and a higher percentage improve in oral as opposed to written language (Hanson & Cicciarelli, 1978; Kenin & Swisher, 1972; Lomas & Kertesz, 1978; Prins, Snow, & Wagenaar, 1978). Basso, Capitani, and Moraschini (1982) found that improvements of oral and written comprehension and production were usually associated. However, in some patients who do not receive rehabilitation, comprehension may be the only modality to improve.

These results are supported by Mazzoni et al. (1992), who assessed a selected sample of 45 patients, none of whom received language therapy, over a 7-month period. The investigators found that comprehension had the best recovery, independent of type and severity of aphasia. In addition, differences in language recovery were evident in relation to type of aphasia. For patients with fluent aphasia, oral expression and written expression improved steadily throughout the 7 months. Auditory comprehension improved for 4 months, while reading comprehension improved over the first month. For patients with nonfluent aphasia, significant improvement was evident in auditory comprehension over a 4-month period. Expression showed less recovery, often because it was negatively influenced by the presence of oral apraxia, while no significant changes were evident in written language. Similarly, Hanson et al. (1989) contend that recovery of language modalities may be dependent on the category of the aphasia. However, they caution that differences in recovery between aphasia categories may become apparent only after 2 years post-onset.

Severity of Aphasia

The initial severity of the aphasia is an important factor to consider in the recovery from aphasia, not only because of its direct impact on outcome (Basso, 1992; Marshall & Phillips, 1983; Marshall, Tompkins, & Phillips, 1982, Paolucci et al., 1996), but also because of its interaction with other factors affecting recovery. Indeed, Pederson et al. (1995) have stated that initial aphasia severity is the single most important factor for ultimate language function. In their investigation of the time course of recovery, they found that patients with more severe aphasia demonstrated a longer period of language recovery than patients with less severe aphasia. More specifically, 95% of patients with severe aphasia reached maximum function within 10 weeks; 95% of patients with moderate aphasia reached maximum function within 6 weeks; while only 2 weeks was required for 95% of those with a mild aphasia to achieve maximum function.

Mazzoni et al. (1992) also found that initial severity was related to outcome of each language modality. For a moderately severe group of 21 patients, both oral expression and written expression improved uniformly over 7 months; auditory and reading comprehension showed no significant improvement, because performance on these modalities was initially at a near normal level. For a severely impaired group of 24 patients, auditory comprehension and, to a lesser extent, reading comprehension improved significantly, while no significant improvement was observed for oral or written expression. Similarly, Mark, Thomas, and Berndt (1992) found that initial severity as measured by performance on language tests, rather than neuroradiologic characteristics, correlated strongly with outcome for a group of patients with global aphasia.

Neural Mechanisms of Recovery

The preceding discussion has focused primarily on descriptive accounts of the behavioral changes that occur during recovery from aphasia. However, it is important to consider, also, the neuroanatomical and neurophysiologic mechanisms contributing to recovery. While these are not completely understood, technologic advances in the area of brain imaging have allowed researchers to address those factors that play a role in early and long-term recovery.

Spontaneous recovery, which occurs naturally without special treatment, may be due, in part, to the resolution of local factors such as the reduction of cerebral edema, the absorption of damaged tissue, and improvement of local circulation. However, these factors probably do not play a role in long-term recovery of function (Bach-Y-Rita, 1990).

Rather, of greater interest to the rehabilitation professional, are those factors associated with brain plasticity. Brain plasticity, which permits enduring functional changes to occur, refers to the capacity to modify structural organization and functioning. According to Bach-Y-Rita (1990), several mechanisms may contribute to brain plasticity: (1) Diaschisis refers to depressed function or hypometabolism of structurally normal cortical regions remote from the lesion, due to the sudden interruption of synaptic connections with the region. Diaschisis may occur within the damaged left hemisphere as well as in the contralateral right hemisphere (Andrews, 1991; Feeney & Baron, 1986). Some long-term recovery may occur with the dissipation of diaschisis, although its mechanisms are not well understood. (2) Regenerative and collateral sprouting refers to changes in connections between neurons from intact cells to denervated regions. Collateral sprouting has been demonstrated in some neural structures, including the thalamus and the cerebellum. While collateral sprouting may be a mechanism of functional recovery, it also may be a maladaptive response, leading to abnormal function. Further studies are needed to clarify its importance to recovery from central-nervous-system lesions.

(3) Unmasking of preexisting but functionally depressed pathways or substitution may be the most important mechanism for recovery. This cortical reorganization occurs when axons and synapses that are present but not used for the particular function under study can be called on when the usually dominant system fails.

Hillis and Heidler (2002) also hypothesize that functional recovery from aphasia involves at least three overlapping stages. The acute stage, occurring in the first few days after stroke, involves the recovery of transiently impaired neural tissue in the ischemic penumbra, the area of the brain surrounding the core infarct. Although this area receives sufficient blood to survive, it is not enough to function. Restoration of function occurs only following increased blood flow to this area. The second stage of recovery begins within days of the stroke, continues for weeks, months, or possibly years after onset, and involves reorganization of structure and function relationships. When the reorganization is complete, further recovery (the third stage) depends on establishing new pathways for processing components that were "cut off" by the brain damage as well as learning compensatory strategies to facilitate more effective communication.

Neuroanatomical Factors: Lesion Size and Site

A basic assumption about recovery from aphasia has been that lesion size exerts a negative influence on recovery (Demeurisse & Capon, 1987; Ferro, 1992; Goldenberg & Spatt, 1994; Kertesz et al., 1979; Kertesz, Lau, & Polk, 1993; Ludlow et al., 1986; Mazzoni et al., 1992; Selnes et al., 1983). Furthermore, lesion size may affect each modality differentially. For example, Selnes, Knopman, Niccum, Rubens, & Larson (1983) found that there was a significant negative correlation between lesion volume and recovery of comprehension for large but not smaller lesions. According to Mazzoni et al. (1992), patients with small lesions demonstrated significant recovery in oral and written expression; comprehension changes were not significant because comprehension was relatively unimpaired initially. Patients with medium-sized lesions improved significantly in all modalities except written expression, while those with large lesions demonstrated improvement in auditory comprehension only. However, Basso (1992) asserts that while the negative effect of extent of lesion on initial severity of aphasia is unquestionable, once initial severity has been taken into account, the effect of lesion size on recovery is not clearcut.

In a series of studies that looked at location and extent of lesion on CT scans and the severity of impairment in different groups of individuals with aphasia, Naeser and colleagues (1987, 1989, 1990) indicated that rather than total lesion size, it is the size of the lesion within specific areas that may affect recovery from aphasia. In their study of 10 patients with Wernicke's aphasia (Naeser et al., 1987), there

was no correlation between total temporoparietal lesion size and severity of auditory comprehension. However, a correlation was found between the amount of temporal-lobe damage within Wernicke's area and severity of auditory comprehension. If the damage was in half or less of Wernicke's area, patients exhibited good comprehension at 6 months post-onset. If the lesion involved more than half of Wernicke's area, patients exhibited poor comprehension, even at 1 year post-onset. Furthermore, anterior-inferior temporal-lobe extension into the middle temporal gyrus area was associated with particularly poor recovery.

Similarly, Kertesz et al. (1993) correlated outcome measures of aphasia severity and comprehension with lesion extent in 22 patients with Wernicke's aphasia. Like Naeser et al. (1987), they found that the extent of involvement within specific structures, rather than overall lesion size, contributed to the prediction of language recovery. The angular gyrus and the anterior mid-temporal area were important for overall language recovery, while the extent of involvement of the angular gyrus contributed most significantly to recovery of auditory comprehension at 1 year. With regard to rate of recovery, involvement of the supramarginal gyrus was associated with poor recovery rates of both overall language and auditory comprehension. Partial sparing of the posterior superior temporal gyrus was associated significantly with the highest recovery rates for comprehension.

The importance of lesion extent within specific structures has also been demonstrated with regard to spontaneous language output (Naeser et al., 1989). Twenty-seven patients with aphasia were divided into two groups based on the severity of their spontaneous speech. The more severe group presented with no speech or only stereotypes in which no meaningful verbal information was conveyed; the less severe group presented with Broca's aphasia characterized by reduced, hesitant, poorly articulated, agrammatic speech. CT scan analysis revealed no single neuroanatomical area that contained an extensive lesion that could be used to distinguish the more-severe from the less-severe group. However, the two groups were separable on the basis of the CT scan when extent of lesions in two subcortical whitematter areas were combined. The two subcortical whitematter pathway areas which, when damaged, severely limited spontaneous speech were the most medial and rostral portion of the subcallosal fasciculus, and the periventricular white matter near the body of the lateral ventricle, deep to the lower motor/sensory cortex area for the mouth.

The involvement of Wernicke's area is also an important factor to consider in recovery from global aphasia. Naeser et al. (1990) examined CT scans of 14 patients with global aphasia. Based on the CT scan information, patients were divided into two groups. One group had large cortical/subcortical frontal, parietal, and temporal lobe lesions that included more than half of Wernicke's area. The other group had large cortical/subcortical frontal and parietal lesions; Wernicke's area was spared, although the lesion extended to the subcortical temporal lobe including the temporal isthmus. Language assessment was conducted initially at 1 to 4 months post-onset and then again 1 year post-onset. Significantly more recovery in auditory comprehension had taken place at 1 to 2 years post-onset for the group that did not have lesions involving Wernicke's area. There was no significant difference between the two groups in recovery of spontaneous speech, word repetition, and naming, where severe deficits continued.

None of the studies discussed above have examined the effects of lesion size in patients who are more than 3 years post-onset. However, two studies have shown that in some patients with aphasia, a visible expansion in lesion size can be observed on CT scans after at least 3 years (Naeser et al., 1998; Van Zagten, Boiten, Kessels, & Lodder, 1996). The increase in lesion size in the left hemisphere had no adverse effect on language, as long as the expansion was unilateral and gradual (Naeser et al., 1998). While the physiologic mechanisms underlying the lesion expansion are not understood, these results provide further support for the contention that lesion size alone is not necessarily an important factor to consider for recovery (Heiss, Kessler, Karbe, Fink, & Pawlik, 1993; Heiss, Kessler, Thiel, Ghaemi, & Karbe, 1999).

Most studies on the effects of lesion size and location have not considered how these factors impact language therapy outcome. However, Goldenberg & Spatt (1994) investigated whether size and site of lesion had differential effects during spontaneous recovery as compared to a period of intensive treatment (since language therapy may employ mechanisms that are different from those at work during spontaneous recovery). They followed 18 patients with aphasia across a period of 8 weeks of spontaneous recovery, 8 weeks of intensive language therapy, and a follow-up period of 8 weeks without treatment. Consistent with previous findings, they found that lesion size negatively influenced recovery in all phases, but lesion location was more important to consider. Patients with lesions to the temporobasal regions showed a similar amount of spontaneous recovery than patients without such lesions, but less improvement during therapy and less total recovery.

Neurophysiologic Studies of Recovery

The neuroimaging CT and MRI studies discussed previously have allowed quantification of site and size of lesions, focusing primarily on the structural damage related to the aphasia. More recently, technologic advances such as PET, SPECT, and functional MRI (fMRI) have permitted investigators to focus on the functional consequences of the lesion.

Results of these neurophysiologic studies are not always comparable because of differences in the imaging techniques and the task paradigms that are used. For example,

task paradigms have included reading sentences (Thulborn, Carpenter, & Just, 1999), verb retrieval (Warburton, Price, Swinburn, & Wise, 1999), and word repetition (Ohyama et al., 1996). Furthermore, patient differences in the size and location of the lesion, and variability in time post-onset and type and severity of aphasia also prevent direct comparison of study results (Cherney & Small, 2006). Despite the rapidly accumulating body of literature, understanding of the complex process of cortical reorganization of language-related brain regions during recovery from aphasia remains limited. More poorly understood is the way in which therapeutic interventions change brain systems responsible for language.

A critical issue relates to whether language improvement during recovery and rehabilitation is supported by left hemisphere zones spared by the lesion, by recruitment of homologous right hemisphere regions, or both. Several studies in patients recovering from aphasia have reported shifts in activation to the contralateral undamaged right hemisphere and have interpreted these as a compensatory function (Buckner, Corbetta, Schatz, Raichle, & Petersen., 1996; Cardebat et al., 1994; Ohyama et al., 1996; Thulborn et al., 1999; Weiller et al., 1995). However, more recently, it has been suggested that right hemisphere homologous activation is a maladaptive response reflecting loss of active transcallosal inhibition (Belin et al., 1996; Blank, Bird, Turkheimer, & Wise, 2003; Rosen et al., 2000) and that it stands in the way of more complete recovery.

Evidence supporting an anomalous role for the right hemisphere during recovery comes from several sources. Naeser and colleagues (2005) demonstrated improved naming in four subjects with chronic nonfluent aphasia when slow rTMS was used to inhibit activation in the anterior portion of right Broca's homologue. They postulated that suppression of this maladaptive right-hemisphere response with subsequent reduction of hyperactivity had a beneficial effect on the more widespread bi-hemispheric neural network for naming, promoting better modulation in both the right hemisphere and the remaining left hemisphere temporoparietal language structures important for picture naming. Other studies have demonstrated that the levels of activation in the right homologous regions do not correlate with measures of verbal production (Fernandez et al., 2004; Naeser et al., 2004; Perani et al., 2003; Rosen et al., 2000) or comprehension (Breier et al., 2004; Fernandez et al., 2004). Rather, better recovery has been associated with greater left-hemisphere activation (Karbe et al., 1998a, 1998b; Miura et al., 1999; Warburton et al., 1999).

The relative contribution of right and left hemisphere activity to language recovery may depend on the length of time following stroke onset. Several imaging studies support the notion that right-hemisphere activation occurs early during recovery (Fernandez et al 2004; Xu et al., 2004). However, Heiss et al. (1999) showed that activation in the right inferior frontal gyrus was temporary and decreased within 8 weeks after stroke onset. In contrast, perilesional left-hemisphere activation may represent sparing or restoration of normal function in tissue around the infarction that was inactive early on after injury (Heiss et al., 1999; Heiss, Thiel, Kessler, & Herholz, 2003; Rosen et al., 2000).

Further support for a pattern of increased right-hemisphere activation followed by reshifting of activation to the left hemisphere is provided by Saur and colleagues (2006). Fourteen patients with aphasia were studied using fMRI and an auditory comprehension task at three time points after left-hemisphere stroke: in the acute phase (mean 1.8 days after stroke onset); in the subacute phase (mean 12.1 days post stroke onset; and in the chronic phase (mean 321 days post stroke). Distinct patterns of activation were apparent at each time point, with strongly reduced activation of remaining left language areas in the acute phase, followed by an up-regulation with recruitment of homologous right-hemisphere language zones. Thereafter, when language comprehension had mostly recovered, there was a return to the normal pattern of activation, with greatest activation in the left hemisphere, particularly Wernicke's area.

The extent to which right-hemisphere activation occurs during early recovery may depend on the site and size of the left-hemisphere lesion. Abo et al. (2004) observed right frontal activation during repetition in a patient with a left frontal lesion; right inferior parietal activation occurred in a patient with left temporoparietal damage. Similarly Xu et al. (2004) observed right inferior frontal activation during a covert word-generation task in a patient with left frontal damage, but not in two patients with left temporoparietal damage. These observations suggest that the site of the right-hemisphere activation depends on the site of the lesion, at least for the types of tasks used in these functional imaging studies. Other investigations have suggested that right-hemisphere participation is present when there is greater damage to the left-hemisphere language areas (Cao, Vikingstad, George, Johnson, & Welch, 1999; Heiss et al., 1999; Karbe et al., 1998a, 1998b).

Neurophysiologic Studies Following Rehabilitation

Studies that directly assess the functional anatomical changes that occur as a consequence of language therapy are beginning to emerge; however, results differ across studies and there is no consensus about our understanding of the way in which therapeutic interventions may change brain systems responsible for language. Even the simpler question regarding the relative contributions of the intact portions of the damaged left hemisphere versus homologous and other regions of the right hemisphere remains unanswered. New left-hemisphere activation may be particularly important when a positive response to the intervention has been observed. Left-sided activations have been reported following

treatment with Melodic Intonation Therapy (MIT) (Belin et al., 1996), phonologic training via reading aloud (Small, Flores, & Noll, 1998), repetitive naming of semantically related pictures (Cornelissen et al., 2003), and memorization of articulatory gestures followed by repetition, reading aloud, and picture naming of a core of words (Leger et al., 2002).

The MIT study was particularly notable since one of the original rationales of this therapy was that it would help the "transfer" of language functions from the dominant but injured left hemisphere to the musically adept right hemisphere (Sparks, Helm, & Albert, 1974). Yet it seemed to do the exact opposite, increasing activation in the damaged left hemisphere. In the study by Leger et al. (2002), not only did left-hemisphere activation increase, but the pattern of activation following treatment was more similar to the pattern seen in normal controls, with activations noted in Broca's area (left inferior frontal gyrus) and the superior part of the left supramarginal gyrus. Interestingly, Cornelissen et al. (2003) found that all three of their subjects behaved in a similar way, with a single perilesional area in the left inferior parietal area displaying statistically significant training-induced changes.

In contrast, Musso et al. (1999) demonstrated a correlation between increased activity in the right temporal cortex and comprehension scores in four subjects with Wernicke's aphasia following brief intensive training of comprehension between scanning sessions. In addition, Thompson (2000) described changes in the right hemisphere homologues of both Wernicke's and Broca's area during a sentence-picture matching task following a sentence-processing therapy.

It should be noted that most of these studies report on just one or two patients. Thus the caveat that must accompany interpretations of all case studies in aphasia recovery is that there is significant individual variability in anatomy and functionality, and the patterns observed in one patient may not be relevant to those observed in another. For example, Cherney and Small (2006) studied two patients with chronic aphasia and compared their functional neuroanatomical responses to a younger control group on two tasks, an oral-reading task involving overt speech and a "passive" audiovisual story-comprehension task. Following identical therapy, behavioral (language) and functional neuroanatomical changes were reexamined using the same fMRI tasks. For the participant with a frontal lesion who was most responsive to therapy, brain activation increased in the right hemisphere during oral reading, but decreased bilaterally in most regions on story comprehension. The other participant with a temporoparietal lesion showed decreased activation, particularly in the right hemisphere, during oral reading but increased activation bilaterally on story comprehension. Results highlight individual variability following language therapy, with brain-activation changes depending on lesion site and size, language skill, type of intervention, and the nature of the fMRI task. Combining individual differences with task differences leads to a wide variety of possible outcomes. Therefore, it may not be sufficient to characterize observed changes in language-related activity patterns after stroke as "left" or "right," when in fact they are highly task-dependent and individually different (Cherney & Small, 2006).

Clearly, many questions remain regarding the effect of rehabilitation on patterns of language organization. In particular, research is needed to address the various factors that potentially influence recovery patterns, such as the type of aphasia, the site and size of the lesion, and the focus of the intervention; further, investigation is also needed in interpreting the relationship between observed changes and the nature of the language task. In particular, the behavioral outcomes associated with different types of treatment may be reflected in differential reorganization of the language network.

As further studies yield new information or confirm previous information, we will move closer to understanding the neural mechanisms that mediate recovery and rehabilitation. This is an important issue because better knowledge of these mechanisms may lead to better management of the patient with aphasia and better prediction of outcome.

Personal Factors Affecting Prognosis

Although personal and biographic factors appear to play only a minor role in recovery from aphasia as compared to neurological factors (Benson & Ardila, 1996), these factors should not be ignored. Indeed, factors of age, handedness, and gender have been studied experimentally, with some conflicting evidence regarding their effects.

Age

Some studies that have addressed the effects of age on recovery suggest that younger patients have a more favorable outcome than older ones (Gloning, Trappl, Heiss, & Quatember, 1976; Holland, Greenhouse, Fromm, & Swindell, 1989; Marshall et al., 1982; Sands, Sarno, & Shankweiler, 1969; Vignolo, 1964). Other studies have not found age to have a significant effect on recovery (Basso, Capitani, & Vignolo, 1979; de Riesthal & Wertz, 2004; Heiss et al., 1993; Keenan & Brassell, 1974; Kertesz & McCabe, 1977; Messerli, Tissot, & Rodriguez, 1976; Pederson et al., 1995; Sarno, 1992; Sarno & Levita, 1971; Wertz & Dronkers, 1990).

In a review of prognostic factors in aphasia, Basso (1992) cautions that the interaction of age with type of aphasia must be considered because patients with fluent aphasia may be older than patients with nonfluent aphasia (Basso, Capitani, Laiacona, & Luzzatti, 1980; Code & Rowley, 1987; de Renzi, Faglioni, & Ferrari, 1980; Ferro & Madureira, 1997;

Miceli et al., 1981; Obler, Albert, Goodglass, & Benson, 1978). Since type of aphasia may be the prognostic factor rather than age, any studies of the effects of age on recovery must control for type of aphasia.

Similarly, the effects of age on recovery must be considered in relation to etiology. Advanced age may be associated with etiologic factors predicting poor outcome (Henley, Pettit, Todd-Pokropek, & Tupper, 1985). For example, patients with aphasia resulting from open or closed head injury appear to recover better than patients with aphasia resulting from stroke (Kertesz & McCabe, 1977; Basso et al., 1982; Benson & Ardila, 1996). This may be explained in part by age differences, since trauma usually affects younger individuals. Individuals with hemorrhagic strokes, who usually are somewhat younger than patients with occlusive strokes, typically have a good prognosis for language recovery after the mass effect is eliminated; in contrast, the prognosis for occlusive strokes is more limited depending on the site of the infarction (Basso, 1992; Benson & Ardilla, 1996; Rubens, 1977).

The effects of age on recovery should also be considered in relation to general health status. For example, in a prospective study of outcome following ischemic stroke, older individuals with a more severe initial stroke demonstrated poorer general outcome at 3 months post-onset (Macciocchi, Diamond, Alves, & Mertz, 1998). The study also indicated that there was a correlation of age with co-morbidities such as medical, psychosocial, and psychiatric disorders, which may not emerge as independent predictors of outcome. Such factors as history of prior stroke, as well as history of hypertension, diabetes, or cardiac disease, have been associated with poorer outcome after stroke, and the impact of these co-morbid disorders may be greater in older persons. These findings are consistent with those of Marshall et al. (1982) and Marshall and Phillips (1983) who found that general health was a predictive variable of speech and language performance, and with Hilari, Wiggins, Roy, Byng, and Smith (2003) who identified number of co-morbid conditions rather than age as a significant predictor of health-related quality of life in a large group of individuals with chronic aphasia. Similarly, duration of hospitalization may be related to age and general health status, and therefore indirectly related to language outcome (Holland et al., 1989).

Gender

It has been proposed that gender differences may influence the pattern of recovery in patients with aphasia (McGlone, 1977, 1980). In two studies investigating the effects of sex on recovery from aphasia, females had a better prognosis than males for oral expression (Basso et al., 1982) and for auditory comprehension (Pizzamiglio, Mammucari, & Razzano, 1985). However, other studies have found no significant difference in recovery for males and females (Kertesz & McCabe, 1977; Pederson et al., 1995; Pickersgill & Lincoln, 1983; Sarno, Buonaguro, & Levita, 1985). Therefore, at this time, there appears to be no converging evidence favoring either gender (Basso, 1992).

Handedness

Some authors have proposed that left-handers and ambidextrous and mixed-handers have a more bilateral representation for language processing, and therefore recover more rapidly from aphasia, than right-handers (Gloning, 1977; Luria, 1970; Subirana, 1958). Furthermore, it has been suggested that recovery from aphasia is more frequent among patients with familial sinistrality (Luria, 1970). However, better prognosis for non-right-handers is not supported by the data from later studies (Basso, Farabola, Grassi, Laiacona, & Zanobia, 1990; Borod, Carper, & Naesser, 1990; Pickersgill & Lincoln, 1983). An issue affecting the interpretation of these studies is that handedness may be evaluated by different methods, and that different criteria may be adopted for considering a hand as dominant. Therefore, like gender, the findings about the effect of handedness on recovery are inconclusive.

Psychosocial Factors

Emotional and psychosocial changes accompany aphasia (Hemsley & Code, 1996; Hermann & Wallesch, 1993; Starkstein & Robinson, 1988). For example, post-stroke depression was found in 25% of patients with stroke during the acute stages; this incidence rose to 31% at 3 months post-onset, decreased to 16% by 12 months post-onset, and then rose again over the next 2 years to 29%, a proportion higher than that at the acute stage (Astrom, Adolfsson, & Asplund, 1993). However, little is known of the interactions between these changes and recovery from aphasia. Many factors, such as motivation, are not easily amenable to experimental study. Nonetheless, emotional and psychosocial well-being may play a significant role in recovery from aphasia, and preliminary evidence suggests a relationship between mood state, progress in rehabilitation, and functional communication (Code & Muller, 1992; Fucetola et al., 2006; Hermann & Wallesch, 1993; Starkstein & Robinson, 1988). However, Hemsley and Code (1996) found unique patterns of individual emotional and psychosocial adjustment over time in patients with aphasia and their significant others, even in patients where aphasia type and severity were similar. Therefore, they caution that psychosocial and emotional adjustment and its prognostic impact on communication and rehabilitation progress cannot be anticipated.

In summary, many studies have focused on the prognostic indicators that may help predict outcome in patients with aphasia. Several of these studies and their key findings have been discussed. Since it appears that no single factor alone can predict outcome, clinicians must assess the information about each variable and make inferences about how they, in combination, affect the extent to which language recovery will occur. Additionally, clinicians must be cognizant of the various ways that outcomes can be measured and, in determining prognosis, consider not only language-impairment and functional-communication measures, but also consider quality-of-life-measures. Clinicians also must decide if the expectation that treatment will effect positive change is justified. The next section reviews the information base for warranting these treatment decisions.

OUTCOMES OF TREATMENTS FOR APHASIA
The Current Context for a Review of Scientific Evidence

Three important factors influence any assay of scientific evidence on clinical outcomes of treatment protocols. The first influential factor is a logical and broadly recognized system for assessing clinical treatments. That system begins in Phase I, with discovery-oriented research for the purpose of uncovering new treatment protocols. The system progresses through Phase II research in which new protocols are developed and tested for their basic properties. A successful outcome in Phase II may warrant a Phase III clinical trial for testing the *efficacy* of a treatment. That is, Phase III research puts to test the general expectation of benefit among persons in a specific clinical population. A successful clinical trial justifies Phase IV research for assessing specific outcomes in day-to-day clinical practice, which is also known as the *effectiveness* of a treatment (Robey, 2004a; Robey & Schultz, 1998). In the last phase of clinical research, Phase V, the focus of research moves from clinical outcomes and the decisions of speech-language pathologists to public-health issues and the decisions of public-health analysts, economists, and policy makers.

The five phases of treatment research represent a normal progression of development and knowledge building. For a developing treatment protocol, one would expect to find some Phase I and Phase II studies. Only for a mature treatment protocol is a record of Phase III, IV, and V studies a reasonable expectation. Therefore, in the normal course of events, a broadly recognized treatment protocol with a substantial record of development and widespread application in general practice is associated with a literature base that includes several studies in each of the phases of clinical research.

In clinical aphasiology, the majority of treatment research findings come from Phase I and Phase II studies. A large proportion of the scientific evidence on treatment outcomes for aphasia has been obtained through studies having the characteristics of Phase IV treatment-effectiveness research. A relatively small fraction of the scientific evidence on treatments for aphasia has been obtained through Phase III clinical trials. That is, the distribution of the scientific-evidence base in clinical aphasiology doesn't completely conform to the expected distribution when clinical research unfolds in a structured developmental sequence of clinical research.

Why the discrepancy? Although the five-phase system for the sequential development of clinical research is recognized in the broader clinical-outcome research community, only within the past few years have aphasiologists been thinking about the system for (a) conducting evidence-based reviews (EBRs) of past research, and (b) designing and implementing new research studies. It is not surprising, then, that the historical record of research findings doesn't conform completely with a system, that for all intents and purposes, didn't exist for the researchers who were making large and important contributions.

Should the body of clinical research completed prior to the application of a certain set of ground rules be held strictly accountable to those ground rules? Should findings coming from studies that do not uniformly conform to the new structure be dismissed? For both questions, the answer is straightforward: of course not. The fact is that many high-quality studies inform researchers and practitioners about the best clinical practices. Prudence and good sense move scientists and practitioners to extract the value contained in the existing body of valid scientific evidence and then build on that record within the broadly recognized system.

The second influential factor in reviewing clinical scientific evidence is the recent advent of evidence-based practice in speech and language pathology. EBP embraces many research designs for investigating the effects of treatment protocols: case studies, case series, case-control studies, cohort studies, cross-sectional studies, parallel-groups studies, and single-subject studies, among others. These are the research designs of Phases I and II clinical research. In a developmental sense, they establish the basic research underpinning the ultimate EBP research design: a clinical trial. Sometimes, however, the scientific evidence produced through Phase I and Phase II research designs are discounted as being less scientifically valid than the evidence produced through clinical trials that must preserve internal validity (Cook & Campbell, 1979) through rigorous experimental controls such as random assignment.

The notion that inherent properties endow certain research designs with greater or lesser degrees of scientific validity, or value, misdirects attention from the essential questions: (a) What form of research is most appropriate for testing the salient hypothesis at a particular point in the developing line of clinical research, and (b) How validly was it carried out? Unfortunately, the practice of appraising the value of scientific evidence based solely on the name of the research design producing it is a natural consequence of appraising literature only through levels-of-evidence tables

commonly found in EBP (Dollaghan, 2006).[1] However, no research design possesses inherent properties conferring (or not) scientific validity to the observed result. The quality of evidence produced through any research design is directly linked to the quality of operational definitions (purposefully determined and otherwise) for implementing that design. Within a structured system of clinical research, certain research designs are appropriate and essential within each phase of experimentation and the quality of any result derives from the experimental rigor that went into producing it.

Taken in isolation, a tabulated hierarchy of research designs does not establish *more or less scientific validity* for the findings arising out of each level in the hierarchy. Rather, presuming scientific validity at all levels in the hierarchy, evidence produced through a certain level may be *more or less influential* for informing clinical practice (e.g., When may a practitioner ethically provide a treatment protocol in general practice based on best-quality evidence?). The notion advanced here is not that experimental rigor doesn't matter; indeed, it is the crux of the matter. Scientific rigor is assessed through the usual means at all levels (e.g., statistical power, effect size, the bandwidth of confidence intervals, a lack of bias, treatment fidelity and compliance, construct validity, and so forth in the long and familiar listing of validity issues). Neither is any of this to say that clinical trials are irrelevant. Indeed, they are absolutely essential for their purpose and render highly valued results when great care is evident in all aspects of experimental rigor and scientific validity.

The third factor influencing a review of scientific evidence on clinical outcomes of treatment protocols is directly related to EBP: the randomized controlled clinical trial (RCT). Because RCTs nominally embody experimental controls exceeding other research designs, they are often thought to produce experimental results constituting the gold standard for influencing clinical practice. Presuming scientific validity and all other things held constant, a successful RCT does establish the assertion of treatment efficacy. However, a RCT is not always possible or desirable in clinical research on behavioral treatments. At one time, many clinical aphasiologists objected to randomized assignment of individuals with aphasia to no-treatment control groups on ethical grounds. As will become evident in the following sections, the question for researchers has moved beyond "Is treatment better than doing nothing at all?" to "Does protocol X bring out greater change than protocol Y?"

---

[1]The fundamental ideas underpinning this and the next paragraphs are attributed to the scholarship of Dr. Christine A. Dollaghan in her roles as Chair of the Advisory Committee on Evidence-Based Practice (American Speech, Language, Hearing Association), and author of a forthcoming text on evidence-based practice.

Basing random allocation to one of two (or more) competing treatments eliminates the original concern.

Systematic Reviews and Meta-Analyses

A review of scientific clinical evidence begins with existing systematic reviews and meta-analyses. In the aphasia-treatment literature, a small corpus of these reviews is available for inspection.

In a Cochrane systematic review, Greener, Enderby, and Whurr (2006a) examined pharmacologic treatments for aphasia. Ten clinical trials met their inclusion and exclusion criteria. The pharmacologic agents in these trials included Piracetam, Bifemelane, Pribedil, Bromocriptine, Idebenone, and Dextran. Greener et al. (2006a) concluded that design constraints combined with absent or unclear information in the manuscripts made thorough assessments of scientific quality unattainable. That complication in a relatively small set of studies rendered the interpretations, conclusions, and generalizations coming out of the review equivocal on many important points. Nonetheless, for one agent, Piracetam, a small treatment effect was detected for improved language performance.

In a different Cochrane systematic review, Greener, Enderby, and Whurr (2006b) examined randomized controlled trials of behavioral treatments for aphasia by speech-language pathologists. Notably, only twelve studies met the entrance criteria for review. Of those, several were relatively dated, and all were characterized by limitations in either (a) research methodology (e.g., design characteristics, sample characteristics), or (b) the incompleteness with which important operational definitions and outcomes were communicated. Greener et al. (2006b) concluded that randomized controlled trials have demonstrated neither the efficacy of treatments for aphasia nor the lack of efficacy.

The highlights of another systematic review of treatments for aphasia (among other communication disorders) was reported in Enderby (1996). Enderby found that treatments were generally effective when treatment protocols were (a) matched carefully with the characteristics of a certain clinical presentation, and (b) provided intensively.

A handful of meta-analyses have been conducted on aphasia-treatment research findings. In a meta-analysis, estimates of effect size are calculated for each study assessing a common research hypothesis; those estimates are then averaged, or synthesized, to achieve a single result that incorporates all tests of that research hypothesis. An estimate of effect size is a quantity for measuring the degree of departure from the null state (e.g., no change from pre-treatment to post-treatment). When an effect size equals zero, no change is evident. As the degree of change brought about by a treatment protocol increases, the value of the corresponding effect size increases.

It is important to note that these meta-analyses have not been restricted to clinical trials. Rather, they have included a variety of aphasia-treatment studies. Greenhouse and colleagues (1990) reported the first meta-analysis of aphasia-treatment literature. They analyzed 13 pre-post tests of aphasia treatment and found an average weighted effect size of 0.80, corresponding to a medium-to-large effect.

Whurr, Lorch, and Nye (1992) conducted a meta-analysis of 45 aphasia-treatment studies and obtained an average effect size of 0.59 separating treated and untreated populations. Although many studies were characterized by methodologic limitations, they concluded that treatments were generally effective.

Robey (1994) conducted a meta-analysis of between-subject effects (i.e., treatment versus control) and within-subjects effects (i.e., pre-test versus post-test) with time-post-onset controlled for each set of effects. The results indicated that the recovery of treated individuals was, on average, nearly twice as extensive as the recovery of untreated individuals when treatment was begun before 3 months post-onset (MPO). Furthermore, treatment brought about an appreciable improvement in performance when begun after the third MPO. Robey (1994) also found that the effect sizes for treated-versus-untreated comparisons exceeded Cohen's (1988) criterion for a medium-sized effect when treatment was initiated before the third MPO and exceeded the criterion for a small-sized effect in the chronic stage when treatment was initiated after 12 MPO.

In a meta-analysis of 55 studies, Robey (1998) obtained results confirming the 1994 findings. Furthermore, Robey found that, in general, (a) greater amounts of treatment brought about larger treatment effects, (b) the average effect size for Schuell-Wepman-Darley Multimodal-stimulation (SWDM) was larger than the overall average, and (c) large gains were achieved by persons with severe aphasia.

Robey, McCallum, and Francois (1999) and Robey, Schultz, Crawford, and Sinner (1999) reported analyses of effect sizes obtained through 12 single-subject research studies. The estimates of effect size indicated generally large and robust treatment effects.

The convergence of this combined evidence leads to the conclusion that treatments for aphasia are generally effective (Albert, 1998). In the past, efficacy per se has not always been demonstrated through valid clinical trials in the modern sense. Nevertheless, the weight of scientific evidence warrants the conclusion that treatments (generally considered) are effective in bringing about desired outcomes.

As Enderby (1996) points out, historically, most dependent variables in aphasia treatment research have been improvements in impairments (WHO, 1980). More recently, treatment studies have begun reporting essential outcomes expressed in terms of activity limitation, social validity, and quality of life.

TABLE 6–1

Number of Aphasia-Treatment Studies at Each Phase of Clinical Research

Clinical Outcome Domain	Phase of Clinical Research				
	I	II	III	IV	V
Overall language performance	12	8	12	—	—
Lexical retrieval	83	37	1	—	—
Syntax	35	26	—	—	—
Speech production/fluency	44	11	1	—	—
Language comprehension	14	—	—	—	—
Reading	39	7	1	—	—
Writing	30	8	2	—	—

Primary Studies

In the past several decades, hundreds of research reports have been published regarding treatments for aphasia. Many of these papers have been considered by the Aphasia Treatment Writing Committee of the Academy of Neurologic Communication Disorders and Sciences (ANCDS), which is conducting meta-analyses for each of several treatment-outcome domains. Building upon the work of the Veterans Affairs Field Advisory Council (Daniels, Stach, & Maher, 2001) and Robey (1998), the committee organized studies for which estimates of effect size were available by six clinical-outcome domains: overall language performance, lexical retrieval, syntax, speech production/fluency, language comprehension and reading and writing (Robey & Beeson, 2005). Table 6–1, a cross-tabulation of those clinical-outcome domains with the number of treatment studies at each phase of clinical research, illustrates the maturity of lines of inquiry in aphasia-rehabilitation research.

Clearly, the line of scientific inquiry on treatment protocols in which the outcome domain is overall language performance (i.e., a test battery for compiling a broad spectrum of language impairments) has advanced to clinical trials more frequently than any of the other domains. This likely reflects a long history of research in this outcome domain. Just as clearly, researchers (a) have established a relatively extensive base of pre-trial research in the remaining domains, and (b) are beginning to take some of their treatment protocols to trial. Indeed, clinical trials seem a next logical step, particularly for treatment protocols to improve lexical retrieval and syntax.

Specific Treatments

The next sections review a few examples of studies in each clinical-outcome domain. These examples are certainly not intended as exhaustive. Examples were selected for their capacity for efficiently illustrating as much information as possible. Indeed, with each category, some studies are associated with greater magnitudes of effect size than those selected for presentation, and other studies are associated with lesser magnitudes. A full treatment of these data will appear in the report of the ANCDS Writing Committee.

Overall Language Performance

Many studies assessing overall language performance as a dependent variable report a general index of aphasia severity taken from a comprehensive test of aphasia such as the Boston Diagnostic Aphasia Examination (BDAE; Goodglass, Kaplan, & Barresi, 2001), the Porch Index of Communicative Abilities (PICA; Porch, 1981), or the Western Aphasia Battery (WAB; Kertesz, 1982). The treatment protocol is often some variation of the Schuell-Wepman-Darley Multimodality (SWDM) treatment (see Duffy, 1994). An innovative exception is a clinical trial testing Computer Reading Treatment provided over a 26-week period (Katz & Wertz, 1997). Using Cohen's (1988) estimator of effect size for within-subject effects ($d_{pre,post}$; see Robey, 2004b, p. 315), the magnitude of change from pre-treatment to post-treatment was $d_{pre,post} = .51$ for the PICA Overall results and $d_{pre,post} = .21$ for the WAB AQ results. Estimates of effect size for the two corresponding control conditions, computer stimulation and no treatment, were $d_{pre,post} = .14$ and $d_{pre,post} = .06$ respectively. For context, these estimates of effect size may be compared to the average effect sizes reported by Robey (1998) for individuals with aphasia in the chronic stage of recovery who were treated (i.e., $\bar{d}_{pre,post} = .66$) and untreated (i.e., $\bar{d}_{pre,post} = .05$). In each case, the Katz and Wertz (1997) estimates are within the confidence intervals for the averaged values.

Syntax

Treatment protocols for improving syntactic production are many and varied. Frequently encountered examples include linguistic-specific treatment (Thompson, 2001) and syntactic stimulation (Davis & Tan, 1987). Jacobs and Thompson (2000) tested a protocol for increasing the accuracy of object-cleft and passive sentences with four persons with Broca's aphasia. Using Busk and Serlin's (1992) first estimator of effect size for single-subject data,[2] d_{BS-1}, the magnitude of change brought about in each participant can be quantified. Combining the estimates of effect size for each of the direct treatment effects (i.e., response to trained tokens) yields an average effect size of $d_{BS-1} = 27.73$. A similar averaging of effect sizes for untrained tokens across the

---

[2]Note that values of Cohen's $d_{pre,post}$ for group data and values of d_{BS-1} for single-subject data are not directly comparable. The equations differ importantly.

four participants provides a means for quantifying the magnitude of change in terms of generalization. In this case, d_{BS-1} for generalization equaled 1.41. For context, in a small meta-analysis of single-subject studies, Robey et al. (1999) found a median effect size for direct treatments of $d_{BS-1} = 3.98$. An average effect size for generalization effects has not yet been established.

The grouped data for four aphasic individuals studied by Thompson, Shapiro, Kiran, & Sobecks (2003) provides insight to another dimension of generalization. Combining the estimates of effect size for three standardized tests resulted in a value of $d_{pre,post}$ equaling 1.02. The comparison value from extant literature is again $\bar{d}_{pre,post} = .66$ from Robey (1998).

Word Retrieval

Treatment protocols for phonologic cueing, semantic cueing, or combined phonologic and semantic cueing are found throughout the research literature on improving word retrieval. Wambaugh, Doyle, Martinez, and Kalinyak-Fliszar (2002) studied both forms of treatment using cueing hierarchies with each of three participants in a single-subject research design. The magnitude of change for both treatment protocols combined over all three participants was $d_{BS-1} = 4.53$. The corresponding magnitude of change for generalization was $d_{BS-1} = 3.27$. Each of these direct treatment effects is referenced to the median value of $d_{BS-1} = 3.98$ reported by Robey et al. (1999). Using a group research design, Hickin, Best, Herbert, Howard, & Osborne (2002) studied the response of eight individuals with aphasia to a treatment protocol combining phonologic and orthographic cues. The direct treatment effect was $d_{pre,post} = .86$; the generalization effect for untreated tokens was $d_{pre,post} = .18$. Once again, the comparison value is $\bar{d}_{pre,post} = .66$ from Robey (1998).

Language Comprehension

Treatment protocols for improving language comprehension take many and varied forms. A particularly well-developed protocol by Crerar, Ellis, and Dean (1996), termed the "Computer Based Microword" has individuals with aphasia make decisions about a closed set of tokens and their relationships with one another. Crerar et al. measured improvements in accuracy rates for prepositions and verbs among 14 participants. The resulting estimates of effect size were $\bar{d}_{pre,post} = .81$ for prepositions and $\bar{d}_{pre,post} = 2.41$ for verbs. Both values exceed the corresponding reference value from Robey (1998) of $\bar{d}_{pre,post} = .66$.

Speech Production or Fluency

Treatment protocols in this category comprise Response Elaboration Training (Kearns, 1985, 1997), Constraint-Induced Therapy (Pulvermüller et al., 2001), Voluntary Control of Involuntary Utterances (Helm-Estabrooks & Albert, 2004), and Melodic Intonation Therapy (Helm-Estabrooks & Albert, 2004), among others.

Wambaugh and Martinez (2000) conducted a single-subject study of three individuals using a variation of Response Elaboration Training. The averaged estimate of effect size was $d_{BS-1} = 5.95$ for a direct treatment effect using correct information units as the dependent variable (reference value from Robey et al., 1999: $d_{BS-1} = 3.98$).

Pulvermüller et al. (2001) reported a group study comparing the effects of Constraint-Induced Therapy (CIT) with those of conventional treatment. The estimate of effect size for the 10 individuals receiving CIT was $d_{pre,post} = .62$ using a value derived from a battery of standardized tests as the dependent variable (reference value in Robey et al., 1999: $\bar{d}_{pre,post} = .66$). Furthermore, the comparison of the two forms of treatment resulted in a between-subjects effect size of $d_{CIT\ vs\ Conventional} = .513$. The closest value in Robey (1998) for serving as a corresponding reference value is $d_{Tx\ vs\ No-Tx} = .31$ for studies comparing treatment to no-treatment in post-acute aphasic individuals.

Reading and Writing

The literature contains relatively few reports of treatment protocols having a primary outcome of improved writing or improved reading. An example of a treatment protocol for improving reading comprehension is found in Cherney, Merbitz, and Grip (1986). These authors administered Oral Reading for Language in Aphasia (ORLA) to a heterogeneous group of persons with aphasia 3 to 5 times per week for 20 to 80 sessions. The estimate of effect size for reading comprehension was $d_{pre,post} = .525$ (reference value is $\bar{d}_{pre,post} = .66$).

An example of a treatment protocol for improving writing is provided by Beeson, Hirsch, & Rewega (2002), who studied four individuals with aphasia and severe agraphia. Two participants received Anagram and Copy Treatment (ACT) and Copy and Recall Treatment (CART), which were completed as a home assignment. Two participants received the CART home-assignment only. Multiple-baseline single-subject data with the number of correctly written words was the dependent measure. The average effect size for the two participants receiving both forms of treatment was $\bar{d}_{BS-1} = 24.03$ (reference value: $\bar{d}_{BS-1} = 3.98$).

Conclusion

Although a great portion of the external evidence for informing clinical practice was published before the conventions of evidence-based practice were broadly recognized, the available scientific evidence supports the conclusion that treatments for aphasia, generally considered, bring about large and beneficial changes. In fact, the evidence on the general question of efficacy/effectiveness of treatments by speech-language pathologists is compelling: treatments by speech-language pathologists bring about desired outcomes (Albert, 2003; Basso, 2005). Furthermore, researchers are producing evidence that opens insight into differential forms of treatment effects: multiple dimensions of outcome obtained through a certain treatment protocol associated with a certain clinical population.

Two large and important challenges confront clinical aphasiologists. The first challenge is describing scientific evidence more fully than has largely occurred in the past. High-quality scientific evidence produced through high-quality clinical research can only be recognized as such if the manuscript contains the quality indicators required by readers for rendering those assessments. Fortunately, guidance in this regard is readily available. For instance, quality indicators for manuscripts reporting randomized controlled trials is the substance of the Consolidated Standards of Reporting Trials Statement (CONSORT; http://www.consort-statement.org/statement/revisedstatement.htm). Similarly, for manuscripts describing non-randomized controlled trials, quality indicators are listed and described in the Transparent Reporting of Evaluations with Nonrandomized Designs Statement (TREND; http://www.trend-statement.org/asp/trend.asp). Meeting this first challenge is certainly not beyond the means of researchers.

The second challenge is testing focused clinical-research questions through precise experimental designs. Presently, we are experiencing a period of transition in which increasingly more focused hypotheses (e.g., a certain treatment protocol is tested in a certain clinical population using clinically relevant measures of outcome) are tested in progressively more precise experiments (e.g., narrow confidence intervals). As Greener, Enderby, and Whurr (2006a) point out, much needs to be done in this regard, but the work is underway.

FUTURE TRENDS

1. Progressive refinements and advancements in imaging technology make possible ever more detailed assessments of pathology, surviving anatomy, and neurophysiology. In large samples, those forms of information, combined with salient history and thorough assessments of communication behavior at certain points in recovery, will undoubtedly clarify indicators and moderators of recovery and rehabilitation.
2. That concert of information will enhance the clinical decisions of aphasiologists regarding prognosis and treatment scheduling.
3. Demonstrated efficacy and effectiveness is an imperative of funding for clinical services and clinical research. From that perspective, aphasiologists must test the efficacy and effectiveness of well-defined treatment protocols through well-controlled experiments that are appropriate for the particular point in the developing line of clinical research. Documentation of quality indicators in the resulting manuscripts will facilitate recognition of the research as high quality.
4. The test of a certain protocol must focus not only on changes in impairment from pre-test to post-test, but also on the effects of certain treatment schedules, certain models of service delivery, direct comparisons of specific treatment protocols, indications and contraindications of candidacy for a protocol, and the permanence of change brought about by a protocol.
5. The scope of clinical experiments must continue to broaden through assessments of treatment effects expressed in terms of direct treatment effects, generalization effects, and maintenance effects, and the social validity of change expressed in terms of activity limitation, participation limitation, quality of life, consumer satisfaction, and costs versus benefits.
6. As in all forms of scientific inquiry, initial findings will be strengthened through independent replications of critical tests.

KEY POINTS

1. Despite individual variation in rate and extent of recovery, there seem to be some general patterns of recovery that have been identified for each type of aphasia. Furthermore, there is a consistent trend in the pattern of recovery as it relates to the individual language modalities.
2. The neural mechanisms contributing to recovery from aphasia are not completely understood. Technologic advances in the area of brain imaging (e.g., PET, SPECT, fMRI) have moved researchers closer to understanding the neural mechanisms that mediate early and late recovery.
3. It is not clear whether language improvements during recovery and rehabilitation are supported by left-hemisphere regions spared by the lesion, by recruitment of homologous right-hemisphere regions, or both. Brain-activation changes during recovery and rehabilitation show individual variability and may be affected by several factors, including lesion size and site, time post-onset, type of language intervention, and fMRI task.
4. There appears to be no single factor alone that can predict outcome in patients with aphasia. Personal and biographical factors such as age, handedness, and gender have been studied experimentally, with some conflicting evidence regarding their effects.

5. The body of scientific evidence supports the conclusion that treatments for aphasia, generally considered, are effective.

6. For many treatment protocols, pre-trial research has established a firm basis for moving on toward conducting clinical trials. That is, in many areas, aphasia-treatment research is poised to advance within the five-phase model of clinical research.

7. Future research, and particularly manuscripts describing clinical research, should conform to the broadly recognized conventions regarding the quality of research findings for informing evidence-based practice.

References

Abo, M., Senoo, A., Watanabe, S., Miyano, S., Doseli, K., Sasaki, N., et al. (2004). Language-related brain function during word repetition in post-stroke aphasics. *Neuroreport, 15*, 1891–1894.

Albert, M. L. (1998). Treatment of aphasia. *Archives of Neurology, 55*, 1417–1419.

Albert, M. L. (2003). Aphasia therapy works! *Stroke, 34*, 992–993.

Andrews, R. J. (1991). Transhemispheric diaschisis: A review and comment. *Stroke, 22*, 943–949.

Astrom, M., Adolfsson, R., & Asplund, K. (1993). Major depression in stroke patients: A three year longitudinal study. *Stroke, 24*, 976–982.

Bach-Y-Rita, P. (1990). Brain plasticity as a basis for recovery of function in humans. *Neuropsychologia, 28*(6), 547–554.

Basso, A. (1992). Prognostic factors in aphasia. *Aphasiology, 6*, 337–348.

Basso, A. (2005). How intensive/prolonged should an intensive/prolonged treatment be? *Aphasiology, 19*, 975–984.

Basso, A., Capitani, E., Laiacona, M., & Luzzatti, C. (1980). Factors influencing type and severity of aphasia. *Cortex, 16*, 631–636.

Basso, A., Capitani, E., & Moraschini, S. (1982). Sex differences in recovery from aphasia. *Cortex, 18*, 469–475.

Basso, A., Capitani, E., & Vignolo, L. A. (1979). Influence of rehabilitation language skills in aphasia. *Archives of Neurology, 36*, 190–196.

Basso, A., Farabola, M., Grassi, M. P., Laiacona, M., & Zanobia, M. E. (1990). Aphasia in left-handers: Comparison of aphasia profiles and language recovery in non-right-handed and matched right-handed patients. *Brain and Language, 38*, 233–252.

Beeson, P. M., Hirsch, F. M., & Rewega, M. A. (2002). Successful single-word writing treatment: Experimental analyses of four cases. *Aphasiology, 16*, 473–491.

Belin, P., Van Eeckhout, P., Zilbovicious, M., Remy, P., Francois, C., Guillaume, S., et al. (1996). Recovery from nonfluent aphasia after melodic intonation therapy: A PET study. *Neurology, 47*, 1504–1511.

Benson, D. F., & Ardila, A. (1996). *Aphasia: A clinical perspective.* New York: Oxford University Press.

Blank, S. C., Bird, H., Turkheimer, F., & Wise, R. J. (2003). Speech production after stroke: The role of the right pars opercularis. *Annals of Neurology, 54*, 310–320.

Borod, J. C., Carper, J. M., & Naesser, M. (1990). Long-term language recovery in left-handed aphasic patients. *Aphasiology, 4*, 561–572.

Breier, J. I., Castillo, E. M., Boake, C., Billingsley, R., Naher, L., Francisco, G., et al. (2004). Spatiotemporal patterns of language-specific brain activity in patients with chronic aphasia after stroke using magnetoencephalography. *NeuroImage, 23*, 1308–1316.

Buckner, R. L., Corbetta, M., Schatz, J., Raichle, M. E., Petersen, S. E. (1996). Preserved speech abilities and compensation following prefrontal damage. *Proceedings of the National Academy of Science USA, 93*, 1249–1253.

Busk, P. L., & Serlin, R. (1992). Meta-analysis for single case research. In T. R. Kratochwill & J. R. Levin (Eds.), *Single-case research design and analysis: New directions for psychology and education.* Hillsdale, NJ: Lawrence Erlbaum.

Cao, Y., Vikingstad, E. M., George, K. P., Johnson, A, F., & Welch, K. M. (1999). Cortical language activation in stroke patients recovering from aphasia with functional MRI. *Stroke, 30*, 2331–2340.

Cardebat, D., Demonet, J. F., Celsis, P., Puel, M., Viallard, G., & Narc-Vergnes, J. P. (1994). Right temporal compensatory mechanisms in a deep dysphasic patient: A case report with activation study by SPECT. *Neuropsychologia, 32*, 97–103.

Cherney, L. R., Merbitz, C. T., & Grip, J. C. (1986). Efficacy of oral reading in aphasia treatment outcome. *Rehabilitation Literature, 47*, 112–118.

Cherney, L. R., & Small, S. L. (2006). Task-dependent changes in brain activation following therapy for nonfluent aphasia: Discussion of two individual cases. *Journal of the International Neuropsychological Society, 12*, 1–15.

Code, C., & Muller, D. J. (1992). *The Code-Muller Protocols: Assessing perceptions of psychosocial adjustment to aphasia and related disorders.* London: Whurr.

Code, C., & Rowley, D. (1987). Age and aphasia type: The interaction of sex, time since onset and handedness. *Aphasiology, 1*(4), 339–345.

Cohen, J. (1988). *Statistical power analysis for the behavioral sciences* (2nd ed.). Hillsdale, NJ: Lawrence Erlbaum.

Cook, T. D., & Campbell, D. T. (1979). *Quasi-experimentation: Design and analysis issues for field settings.* Boston: Houghton Mifflin.

Cornelissen, K., Laine, M., Tarkianen, A., Jarvensivu, T., Martin, N., & Salmelin, R. (2003). Adult brain plasticity elicited by anomia treatment. *Journal of Cognitive Neuroscience, 15*, 444–461.

Crerar, M. A., Ellis, A. W., & Dean, E. C. (1996). Remediation of sentence processing deficits in aphasia using a computer-based microworld. *Brain and Language, 52*, 229–275.

Daniels, S., Stach, C., & Maher, L. (2001). *Treatment of aphasia: An annotated review of the research literature, 1946–2001.* Internal Veterans Affairs Report.

Davis, G. A., & Tan, L. L. (1987). Stimulation of sentence production in a case with agrammatism. *Journal of Communication Disorders, 20*, 447–457.

Demeurisse, G., & Capon, A. (1987). Language recovery in aphasic stroke patients: Clinical, CT, and CBF studies. *Aphasiology, 1*, 301–315.

De Renzi, E., Faglioni, P., & Ferrari, P. (1980). The influence of sex and age on the incidence and type of aphasia. *Cortex, 16,* 627–630.

De Riesthal, M., & Wertz, R. T. (2004). Prognosis for aphasia: Relationship between selected biographical and behavioral variables and outcome and improvement. *Aphasiology, 18,* 899–915.

Dollaghan, C. (2006). Personal communication.

Duffy, J. R., & Coelho, C. A. (2001). Schuell's stimulation approach to rehabilitation. In R. Chapey (Ed.), *Language intervention strategies in adult aphasia* (4th ed.). Baltimore: Williams and Wilkins.

Enderby, P. (1996). Speech and language therapy–does it work? *British Medical Journal, 321*(7047), 1655–1658.

Feeney, D. M., & Baron, J. C. (1986). Diaschisis. *Stroke, 17,* 817–830.

Fernandez, B., Cardebat, D., Demonet, J. F., Joseph, P. A., Mazaux, J-M, Barat, M., et al. (2004). Functional MRI follow-up study of language processes in healthy subjects and during recovery in a case of aphasia. *Stroke, 35,* 2171–2176.

Ferro, J. M. (1992). The influence of infarct location on recovery from global aphasia. *Aphasiology, 6*(4), 415–430.

Ferro, J. M., & Madureira, S. (1997). Aphasia type, age and cerebral infarct localisation. *Journal of Neurology, 244*(8), 505–509.

Fucetola, R., Connor, L. T., Perry, J., Leo, P., Tucker, F. M., & Corbetta, M. (2006). Aphasia severity, semantics, and depression predict functional communication in acquired aphasia.

Gloning, K. (1977). Handedness and aphasia. *Neuropsychologia, 15,* 355–358.

Gloning, K., Trappl, R., Heiss, W. D., & Quatember, R. (1976). Prognosis and speech therapy in aphasia. In Y. LeBrun & R. Hoops (eds.), *Recovery in aphasia* (pp. 57–64). Amsterdam: Swets & Zeitlinger.

Goldenberg, G., & Spatt, J. (1994). Influence of size and site of cerebral lesions on spontaneous recovery of aphasia and on success of language therapy. *Brain and Language, 47,* 684–698.

Goodglass, H., Kaplan, E., & Barresi, B. (2001). *The assessment of aphasia and related disorders* (3rd ed). Philadelphia: Lippincott, Williams, and Wilkins.

Greener, J., Enderby, P., & Whurr, R. (2006a). Pharmacological treatment for aphasia following stroke. *Cochrane Stroke Group Cochrane Database of Systematic Reviews, 3.*

Greener, J., Enderby, P., &Whurr, R. (2006b). Speech and language therapy for aphasia following stroke. *Cochrane Stroke Group Cochrane Database of Systematic Reviews, 3.*

Greenhouse, J. B., Fromm, D., Iyengar, S., Dew, M. A., Holland, A. L., & Kass, R. E. (1990). The making of a meta-analysis: A quantitative review of the aphasia treatment literature. In K. W. Wachter & M. L. Straf (Eds.), *The future of meta-analysis.* New York: Russell Sage Foundation.

Hanson, W. R., & Cicciarelli, A. W. (1978). The time, amount, and pattern of language improvement in adult aphasics. *British Journal of Disorders of Communication, 13,* 59–63.

Hanson, W. R., Metter, E. J., & Riege, W. H. (1989). The course of chronic aphasia. *Aphasiology, 3*(1), 19–29.

Heiss, W-D, Kessler, J., Karbe, H., Fink, G. R., & Pawlik, G. (1993). Cerebral glucose metabolism as a predictor of recovery from aphasia ischemic stroke. *Archives of Neurology, 50,* 958–964.

Heiss, W-D, Kessler, J., Thiel, A., Ghaemi, M., & Karbe, H. (1999). Differential capacity of left and right hemispheric areas for compensation of poststroke aphasia. *Annals of Neurology, 45,* 430–438.

Heiss, W-D, Thiel, A., Kessler, J., & Herholz, K. (2003). Disturbance and recovery of language function: Correlates in PET activation studies. *NeuroImage, 20*(Suppl. 1), S42–S49.

Helm-Estabrooks, N., & Albert, M. L. (2004). *Manual of aphasia and aphasia therapy* (2nd ed.). Austin, TX: Pro-Ed.

Hemsley, G., & Code, C. (1996). Interactions between recovery in aphasia, emotional and psychosocial factors in subjects with aphasia, and their significant others and speech pathologists. *Disability and Rehabilitation, 18*(11), 567–584.

Henley, S., Pettit, S., Todd-Pokropek, A., & Tupper, A. (1985). Who goes home? Predictive factors in stroke recovery. *Journal of Neurology, Neurosurgery, and Psychiatry, 48*(1), 1–6.

Herrmann, M., & Wallesch, C. W. (1993). Depressive changes in stroke patients. *Disability and Rehabilitation, 15,* 55–66.

Hickin, J., Best, W., Herbert, R., Howard, D., & Osborne, F. (2002). Phonological therapy for word-finding difficulties: A re-evaluation. *Aphasiology, 16,* 981–999.

Hilari, K., Wiggins, R. D., Roy, P., Byng, S., & Smith, S. C. (2003). Predictors of Health-related Quality of Life (HRQL) in people with chronic aphasia. *Aphasiology, 17* (4), 365–381.

Hillis, A, E., & Heidler, J. (2002). Mechanisms of early aphasia recovery. *Aphasiology, 16,* 885–895.

Holland, A. L., Greenhouse, J. B., Fromm, D., & Swindell, C. S. (1989). Predictors of language restitution following stroke: A multivariate analysis. *Journal of Speech and Hearing Research, 32,* 232–238.

Jacobs, B. J., & Thompson, C. K. (2000). Cross-modal generalization effects of training noncanonical sentence comprehension and production in agrammatic aphasia. *Journal of Speech, Language, and Hearing Research, 43,* 5–20.

Karbe, H., Thiel, A., Luxenburger, G. W., Herholz, K., Kessler, J., & Heiss, W-D. (1998a). Brain plasticity in post-stroke aphasia: What is the contribution of the right hemisphere? *Brain and Language, 64,* 215–230.

Karbe, H., Thiel, A., Weber-Luxenburger, G., Kessler, J., Herholz, K., & Heiss, W. D. (1998b). Reorganization of the cerebral cortex in post-stroke aphasia studied with positron emission tomography. *Neurology, 50,* A321.

Katz, R. C., & Wertz, R. T. (1997). The efficacy of computer-provided reading treatment for chronic aphasic adults. *Journal of Speech, Language, and Hearing Research, 40,* 493–507.

Kearns, K. P. (1985). Response elaboration training for patient initiated utterances. In R. H. Brookshire (Ed.), *Clinical aphasiology*: Vol. 15 (pp. 196–204). Minneapolis, MN: BRK.

Kearns, K. P. (1997). Broca's aphasia. In L.L. LaPointe (Ed.) *Aphasia and related neurogenic language disorders* (2nd ed). New York: Thieme, pp. 1–41.

Keenan, J., & Brassell, E. (1974). A study of factors related to prognosis for individual aphasic patients. *Journal of Speech and Hearing Disorders, 39,* 257–269.

Kenin, M., & Swisher, L. (1972). A study of pattern of recovery in aphasia. *Cortex, 8,* 56–68.

Kertesz, A. (1982). *Western Aphasia Battery.* New York: Grune and Stratton.

Kertesz, A. (1988). Recovery of language disorders: Homologous contralateral or connected ipsilateral compensation? In S. Finger,

T.E. LeVere, C.R. Almli, & D.G. Stein (eds.), *Brain recovery: Theoretical and controversial issues* (pp. 307–321). New York: Plenum.

Kertesz, A., Harlock, W., & Coates, R. (1979). Computer tomographic localization, lesion size and prognosis in aphasia and nonverbal impairment. *Brain and Language, 8,* 34–50.

Kertesz, A., Lau, W. K., & Polk, M. (1993). The structural determinants of recovery in Wernicke's aphasia. *Brain and Language, 44,* 153–164.

Kertesz, A., & McCabe, P. (1977). Recovery patterns and prognosis in aphasia. *Brain, 100,* 1–18.

Leger, A., Demonet, J-F., Ruff, S., Aithamon, B., Touyeras, B., Puel, M., et al. (2002). Neural substrates of spoken language rehabilitation in an aphasic patient: An fMRI study. *NeuroImage, 17,* 174–183.

Lomas, J., & Kertesz, A. (1978). Patterns of spontaneous recovery in aphasic groups: A study of adult stroke patients. *Brain and Language, 5,* 388–401.

Ludlow, C. L., Rosenberg, J., Fair, C., Buck, D., Schesselman, S., & Salazar, A. (1986). Brain lesions associated with nonfluent aphasia fifteen years following penetrating head injury. *Brain, 109*(Pt 1), 55–80.

Luria, A. R. (1970). *Traumatic aphasia.* The Hague: Mouton.

Macciocchi, S. N., Diamond, P. T., Alves, W. M., & Mertz, T. (1998). Ischemic stroke: Relation of age, lesion location, and initial neurologic deficit to functional outcome. *Archives of Physical Medicine and Rehabilitation, 79*(10), 1255–1257.

Mark, V. W., Thomas, B. E., & Berndt, R. S. (1992). Factors associated with improvement in global aphasia. *Aphasiology, 6*(2), 121–134.

Marshall, R. C., & Phillips, D. S. (1983). Prognosis for improved verbal communication in aphasic stroke patients. *Archives of Physical Medicine and Rehabilitation, 64*(12), 597–600.

Marshall, R. C., Tompkins, C. A., & Phillips, D. S. (1982). Improvement in treated aphasia: Examination of selected prognostic factors. *Folia Phoniatrica, 34,* 305–315.

Mazzoni, M., Vista, M., Pardossi, L., Avila, L., Bianchi, F., & Moretti, P. (1992). Spontaneous evolution of aphasia after ischaemic stroke. *Aphasiology, 6,* 387–396.

McDermott, F. B., Horner, J., & DeLong, E. R. (1996). Evolution of acute aphasia as measured by the Western Aphasia Battery. *Clinical Aphasiology, 24,* 159–172.

McGlone, J. (1977). Sex differences in the cerebral organization of verbal function and cognitive impairment in stroke: Age, sex, aphasia type and laterality differences. *Brain, 100,* 775–793.

McGlone, J. (1980). Sex differences in human brain asymmetry: A critical survey. *Behavioral Brain Sciences, 3,* 215–263.

Messerli, P., Tissot, A., & Rodriguez, J. (1976). Recovery from aphasia: Some factors of prognosis. In Y. LeBrun & R. Hoops (eds.), *Recovery in aphasia* (pp. 124–135). Amsterdam: Swets & Zeitlinger.

Miceli, G., Caltagirone, C., Gainotti, G., Masullo, C., Silveri, C., & Villa, G. (1981). Influence of age, sex, literacy and pathologic lesion on incidence, severity and type of aphasia. *Acta Neurologica Scandinavica, 64,* 370–382.

Miura, K., Nakamura, Y., Miura, F., Yamada, I., Takahashi, M., Yoshikawa, A., et al. (1999). Functional magnetic resonance imaging to word generation task in a patient with Broca's aphasia. *Journal of Neurology, 246,* 939–942.

Moher, D., Schulz, K. F., & Altman, D. G. (2001). The CONSORT Statement: Revised recommendations for improving the quality of reports of parallel-group randomized trials. *Annals of Internal Medicine, 134,* 657–662.

Musso, M., Weiller, C., Kiebel, S., Muller, S. P., Bulau, P., & Rijntjes, M. (1999). Training-induced brain plasticity in aphasia. *Brain, 122,* 1781–1790.

Naeser, M., Martin, P. I., Baker, E. H., Hodge, S. M., Sczerzenie, S. E., Nicholas, M., et al. (2004). Overt propositional speech in chronic nonfluent aphasia studied with the dynamic susceptibility contrast fMRI method. *NeuroImage, 22,* 29–41.

Naeser, M., Martin, P. I., Nicholas, M., Baker, E. H., Seekins, H., Kobayashi, M., et al. (2005). Improved picture naming in chronic aphasia after TMS to part of right Broca's area: An open protocol study. *Brain and Language, 93,* 95–105.

Naeser, M. A., Gaddie, A., Palumbo, C. L., & Stiassny-Eder, D. (1990). Late recovery of auditory comprehension in global aphasia. *Archives of Neurology, 47,* 425–432.

Naeser, M. A., Helm-Estabrooks, N., Haas, G., Auerbach, S., & Srinivasan, M. (1987). Relationship between lesion extent in 'Wernicke's area' on computed tomographic scan and predicting recovery of comprehension in Wernicke's aphasia. *Archives of Neurology, 44,* 73–82.

Naeser, M. A., Palumbo, C. L., Helm-Estabrooks, N., Stiassny-Eder, D., & Albert, M. L. (1989). Severe nonfluency in aphasia. *Brain, 112,* 1–38.

Naeser, M. A., Palumbo, C. L., Prete, M. N., Fitzpatrick, P. M., Mimura, M., Samaraweera, R., et al. (1998). Visible changes in lesion borders on CT scan after five years poststroke, and long-term recovery in aphasia. *Brain and Language, 62,* 1–28.

Nicholas, M. L., Helm-Estabrooks, N., Ward-Lonergan, J., & Morgan, A.R. (1993). Evolution of severe aphasia in the first two years post onset. *Archives of Physical Medicine and Rehabilitation, 74,* 830–836.

Obler, L. K., Albert, M., Goodglass, H., & Benson, D. F. (1978). Aphasia type and aging. *Brain and Language, 6,* 318–322.

Ohyama, M., Senda, M., Kitamura, S., Ishii, K., Mishina, M., & Terashi, A. (1996). Role of the nondominant hemisphere and undamaged area during word repetition in post-stroke aphasia. A PET activation study. *Stroke, 27,* 897–903.

Paolucci, S., Antonucci, G., Gialloreti, L. E., Traballesi, M., Lubich, S., Pratesi, L., et al. (1996). Predicting stroke inpatient rehabilitation outcome: The prominent role of neuropsychological disorders. *European Neurology, 36*(6), 385–390.

Pashek G. V., & Holland, A. L. (1988). Evolution of aphasia in the first year post-onset. *Cortex, 24*(3), 411–423.

Pederson, P. M., Jorgensen, H. S., Nakayama, H., Raaschou, H. O., & Olsen, T. S. (1995). Aphasia in acute stroke: Incidence, determinants, and recovery. *Annals of Neurology, 38,* 659–666.

Perani, D., Cappa, S. F., Tettamanti, M., Rosa, M., Scifo, P., Miozzo, A., et al. (2003). A fMRI study of word retrieval in aphasia. *Brain and Language, 85,* 357–368.

Pickersgill, M. J., & Lincoln, N. B. (1983). Prognostic indicators and the pattern of recovery of communication in aphasic stroke patients. *Journal of Neurology, Neurosurgery and Psychiatry, 46*(2), 130–139.

Pizzamiglio, L., Mammucari, A., & Razzano, C. (1985). Evidence for sex differences in brain organization in recovery in aphasia. *Brain and Language, 25,* 213–223.

Porch, B. E. (1981). *Porch index of communicative abilities, Vol. II: Administration, scoring, and interpretation* (3rd ed.). Palo Alto, CA: Consulting Psychologists Press.

Prins, R. S., Snow, C. E., & Wagenaar, E. (1978). Recovery from aphasia: Spontaneous language versus language comprehension. *Brain and Language, 6*, 192–211.

Pulvermüller, F., Neininger, B., Elbert, T., Mohr, B., Rockstroh, B., Koebbel, P., et al. (2001). Constraint-induced therapy of chronic aphasia after stroke. *Stroke*, 1621–1621.

Robey, R. R. (1994). The efficacy of treatment for aphasic persons: A meta-analysis. *Brain and Language, 47*, 585–608.

Robey, R. R. (1998). A meta-analysis of clinical outcomes in the treatment of aphasia. *Journal of Speech, Language, and Hearing Research, 41*, 172–187.

Robey, R. R. (2004a). A five-phase model for clinical-outcome research. *Journal of Communication Disorders, 37*, 401–411.

Robey, R. R. (2004b). Reporting point and interval estimates of effect-size for planned contrasts: fixed within effect analyses of variance. *Journal of Fluency Disorders, 29*, 307–341.

Robey, R. R., & Beeson, P. (2005). *Aphasia treatment: Examining the evidence*. A paper presented before the annual meeting of the American Speech-Language-Hearing Association, San Diego.

Robey, R. R., McCallum, A. F., & Francois, L. K. (1999). *A meta-analysis of single-subject research on treatments for aphasia*. A paper presented before the 1999 Clinical Aphasiology Conference, Key West, FL.

Robey, R. R., & Schultz, M. C. (1998). A model for conducting clinical outcome research: An adaptation of the standard protocol for use in aphasiology. *Aphasiology, 12*, 787–810.

Robey, R. R., Schultz, M. C., Crawford, A. B., & Sinner, C. A. (1999). Single-subject clinical-outcome research: Designs, data, effect sizes, and analyses. *Aphasiology, 13*, 445–473.

Rosen, H. J., Petersen, S. E., Linenweber, M. R., Snyder, A. Z., White, D. A., Chapman, L., et al. (2000). Neural correlates of recovery from aphasia after damage to left inferior frontal cortex. *Neurology, 55*, 1883–1894.

Rubens, A. B. (1977). The role of changes within the central nervous system during recovery from aphasia. In M. A. Sullivan & M. S. Kommers (Eds.), *Rationale for adult aphasia therapy* (pp. 28–43). University of Nebraska Medical Center.

Sands, E., Sarno, M. T., & Shankweiler, D. (1969). Long-term assessment of language function in aphasia due to stroke. *Archives of Physical Medicine and Rehabilitation, 50*, 202–206.

Sarno, M. T. (1992). Preliminary findings in a study of age, linguistic evolution and quality of life in recovery from aphasia. *Scandinavian Journal of Rehabilitation Medicine Supplement, 26*, 43–59.

Sarno, M. T., Buonaguro, A., & Levita, E. (1985). Gender and recovery from aphasia after stroke. *Journal of Nervous and Mental Disease, 173*, 605–609.

Sarno, M. T., & Levita, E. (1971). Natural course of recovery in severe aphasia. *Archives of Physical Medicine and Rehabilitation, 52*, 175–178.

Saur, D., Lange, R., Baumgaertner, A., Schraknepper, V., Willmes, K., Rijntjes, M., et al. (2006). Dynamics of language reorganization after stroke. *Brain, 129*, 1371–1384.

Selnes, O. A., Knopman, D. S., Niccum, N., Rubens, A. B., & Larson, D. (1983). Computed tomographic scan correlates of auditory comprehension deficits in aphasia: A prospective recovery study. *Annals of Neurology, 5*, 558–566.

Small, S. L., Flores, D. K., & Noll, D. C. (1998). Different neural circuits subserve reading before and after therapy for acquired dyslexia. *Brain and Language, 62*, 298–308.

Sparks, R., Helm, N., & Albert, M. (1974). Aphasia rehabilitation resulting from melodic intonation therapy. *Cortex, 10*, 303–316.

Starkstein, S. E., & Robinson, R. G. (1988). Aphasia and depression. *Aphasiology, 2*, 1–20.

Subirana, A. (1958). The prognosis of aphasia in relation to the factor of cerebral dominance and handedness. *Brain, 81*, 415–425.

Thompson, C. K. (2000). Neuroplasticity: Evidence from aphasia. *Journal of Communication Disorders, 33*, 357–366.

Thompson, C. K. (2001). Treatments of underlying forms: A linguistic specific approach to sentence production deficits in agrammatic aphasia. In R. Chapey (Ed.), *Language intervention strategies in adult aphasia* (4th ed.). Baltimore: Williams and Wilkins.

Thompson, C. K., Shapiro, L. P., Kiran, S., & Sobecks, J. (2003). The role of syntactic complexity in treatment of sentence deficits in agrammatic aphasia: The complexity account of treatment (CATE). *Journal of Speech, Language, Hearing Research, 46*, 591–607.

Thulborn, K. R., Carpenter, P. A., & Just, M. A. (1999). Plasticity of language-related brain function during recovery from stroke. *Stroke, 30*(4), 749–754.

Van Zagten, M., Boiten, J., Kessels, F., & Lodder, J. (1996). Significant progression of white matter lesions and small deep (lacunar) infarcts in patients with stroke. *Archives of Neurology, 53*, 650–655.

Vignolo, L. A. (1964). Evolution of aphasia and language rehabilitation: A retrospective exploratory study. *Cortex, 1*, 344–367.

Wambaugh, J. L., Doyle, P. J., Martinez, A. L., & Kalinyak-Fliszar, M. (2002). Effects of two lexical retrieval cueing treatments on action naming in aphasia. *Journal of Rehabilitation Research and Development, 39*, 455–466.

Wambaugh, J. L., & Martinez, A. L. (2000). Effects of modified response elaboration training with apraxic and aphasic speakers. *Aphasiology, 14*, 603–617.

Warburton, E., Price, C. J., Swinburn, K., & Wise, R. J. (1999). Mechanisms of recovery from aphasia: Evidence from positron emission tomography studies. *Journal of Neurology, Neurosurgery, and Psychiatry, 66*(2), 155–161.

Weiller, C., Isensee, C., Rijntjes, M., Huber, W., Muller, S., Bier, D., et al. (1995). Recovery from Wernicke's aphasia: A positron emission tomographic study. *Annals of Neurology, 37*, 723–732.

Wertz, R. T., & Dronkers, N. F. (1990). Effects of age on aphasia. In E. Cherow (Ed.), *Proceedings of the research symposium on communication sciences and disorders and aging. ASHA reports* (pp. 88–98). Rockville, MD: American Speech-Language-Hearing Association.

Whurr R., Lorch M. P., & Nye, C. (1992) A meta-analysis of studies carried out between 1946 and 1988 concerned with the efficacy of speech and language therapy treatment for aphasic patients. *European Journal of Disorders of Communication, 27*, 1–17.

World Health Organization. (1980). *International classification of impairments, disabilities, and handicaps*. Geneva: Author.

Xu, X. J., Zhang, M. M., Shang, D. S., Wang, Q. D., Luo, B. Y., & Weng, X. C. (2004). Cortical language activation in aphasia: A functional MRI study. *Chinese Medical Journal (English), 117*, 1011–1016.

Chapter 7

Delivering Language Intervention Services to Adults with Neurogenic Communication Disorders

Brooke Hallowell and
Roberta Chapey

OBJECTIVES

The objectives of this chapter are to (1) describe the contexts in which clinicians serve adults with neurogenic communication disorders; (2) explore the gerontologic context of aphasia intervention; (3) describe the many professional roles of the aphasiologist; (4) discuss key legislative issues that affect service delivery; (5) present an overview of the means by which clinicians and service-providing agencies are reimbursed for services; (6) stimulate discussion of the active ways in which clinicians may serve as advocates for patients in the current service-delivery climate; and (7) discuss future trends in service delivery.

At no other time in the history of aphasiology has the context in which clinicians work so influenced the delivery of intervention-services to persons with neurogenic communication disorders. Throughout the world, changes in healthcare policy, reimbursement schemes, national health plans, political climates, insurance mechanisms, clinical licensure, and professional training are having dramatic impacts on our access to patients, as well as on the services we may deliver to them. In the United States, particularly, recent impacts of managed-care in the private sector and evolving federal health policies are significantly impacting the practice of aphasiology.

In this chapter we discuss the contexts in which aphasiologists work and the multiple roles they play. Legislative issues and other factors affecting reimbursement for clinical services are then presented in terms of their implications for the delivery of services to persons with aphasia. Strategic actions in which aphasiologists may engage to further the effectiveness of services, patients' access to care, and the financial stability

of service-providing agencies are highlighted. The nature of the "ultimate excellent clinical aphasiologist" is explored in light of the demands of the current health care climate.

SERVICE DELIVERY CONTEXTS FOR LANGUAGE INTERVENTION

Speech-language pathologists rehabilitate adult patients with aphasia in a variety of settings, such as hospitals, rehabilitation centers, skilled-nursing facilities, nursing homes, clinics, private offices, and the patient's own home.

Hospitals

Most major community hospitals have a comprehensive program for stroke rehabilitation, including a basic rehabilitation team comprised of a physician, a rehabilitation nurse, a social worker, a physical therapist, an occupational therapist, and a speech-language pathologist. Optimally, a physiatrist, a psychologist, and a rehabilitation counselor are also members of this team. The immediately post-stroke or post-trauma patient is frequently placed in an acute medical area and may receive speech-language evaluation, intervention, and counseling at the bedside. Recent trends in reducing the length of time patients are allowed to remain in acute-care contexts, however, have limited acute-care clinicians to a primary focus on screening and diagnostic services rather than on concerted intervention (Katz et al., 2000). Acute-care clinicians are also involved in educating patients' significant others about the nature of aphasia.

In most instances, convalescent stroke and trauma patients are placed near rehabilitation services, in a specific area that is properly equipped for rehabilitation and staffed by personnel with special training in rehabilitation. Adequate space and equipment are usually provided to ensure high-quality evaluation, treatment, and counseling services, which are rendered for both inpatients and outpatients. The advantage of providing speech-language services in this setting is that a hospital may provide integrated, coordinated, comprehensive team management for patients with stroke and aphasia. The same may be said for rehabilitation centers.

Rehabilitation Centers

A rehabilitation center may be a component of a hospital or may exist as a separate, independent facility that has a close working relationship with one or more hospitals. In either case, there are usually both inpatient and outpatient services that provide comprehensive team rehabilitation. For patients who have recovered from the acute stages of stroke or trauma, the decision as to whether they should receive subacute rehabilitation as outpatients or inpatients or be transferred to another facility depends on several variables, such as the extent of disability; overall health status; geographic location of potential placement sites and access to transportation; the degree of need for integrated comprehensive intervention in nursing, speech-language pathology, physical therapy, and occupational therapy; insurance coverage; the patient's financial resources; and the degree of family support and involvement.

Skilled Nursing Facilities

The distinctions among terms such as long-term-care center, nursing home, skilled-nursing facility, and even rehabilitation center have become less and less clear in recent years (Gill, 1995). Since the late 1980s, rehabilitative care has gravitated away from acute-care hospitals, and toward facilities that were once merely considered long-term-care centers or "rest homes" (facilities to which most residents traditionally had been admitted with the anticipation that they would stay there for the rest of their lives). Rather than staying in the hospital until they are rehabilitated to the point of being able to return to their homes, most stroke and trauma patients are now discharged from acute-care centers to subacute care centers, often outside the hospital context. A majority of skilled nursing facilities now offer comprehensive rehabilitative services, both for short-term patients who are expected to return to their homes, as well as for long-term residents. Consequently, over the past 20 years, most United States residents have seen the signs for "nursing homes" in their local neighborhoods change to signs for "skilled nursing and rehabilitation centers" and the like.

Nursing Homes and Long-Term-Care Centers

Even in long-term-care contexts that do not specialize in short-term rehabilitation, speech-language therapy, occupational therapy, and physical therapy services are generally offered. In most instances, these homes also provide ongoing environmental stimulation and attempt to meet the patient's social and emotional needs. Speech-language clinicians in these contexts often work on a contractual basis with the nursing home, either as independent professionals or as employees of a rehabilitation company that contracts with multiple nursing homes in a given area. Thus, nursing-home clinicians frequently work on an itinerant basis, providing speech-language services to two or more facilities.

Many long-term-care centers have varied types of residential facilities that differ according to the levels of care needed by residents. They range from apartments, for adults capable of living independently but wishing to be close to central social and medical facilities, to nursing home rooms, in which residents are provided constant skilled medical and rehabilitative care. In the United States, federal programs do not generally cover the cost of long-term care. Some Medicaid programs cover long-term nursing-home expenses, but only for individuals whose savings are minimal enough to qualify for such programs. Thus, financial concerns are often at the forefront for residents of long-term-care facilities and their adult children. During the past 10 years, many new long-term-care insurance programs have become available. Although potentially costly, they do help individuals plan carefully for long-term-care expenses they may incur as they grow older. Routine help in the home and in adult day care centers can forestall or eliminate institutionalization for many elderly people.

Independent Language, Speech, and Hearing Centers

One type of independent speech and hearing clinic is the freestanding not-for-profit agency. Another is the communication disorders clinic housed within a university training program in communication sciences and disorders, in which student-clinicians are supervised in the provision of services. A third type of speech and hearing center is the office of the independent speech-language pathologist in private practice.

In all of these settings, services are provided for persons of all ages with any of a variety of communication disorders. Typically, all three types of settings have suitable rooms and proper equipment to provide appropriate assessment, intervention, and counseling services to patients. Outpatient services are the primary offering, although many free-standing agencies provide contractual services through hospitals, nursing homes, rehabilitation centers, and home-health agencies as well. Although independent agencies do not generally have formal rehabilitation teams, individual speech-language clinicians often refer patients to other rehabilitation professionals when appropriate and establish close communication with other professionals who are working with a given patient. In addition, many private practices are established in partnership with other rehabilitation personnel, or are located in buildings that house such personnel.

University Clinics

Most clinical academic programs in the field of communication sciences and disorders provide on-campus clinical services that may serve individuals with aphasia. Many programs also provide services through contracts with outside agencies, such as hospitals, nursing homes, and rehabilitation centers. The mission of university-based clinics involves not only the delivery of quality services but also the provision of quality mentored clinical education for student-clinicians. Models for the operation of university-based clinical services vary widely, with some supported through university funds, some depending on self-support through clinical revenues and grant funds, some depending on partnerships with agencies and supervisors who are not employed by the university, and many relying on a combination of such supports. Depending upon the availability of qualified supervision and allowance for free or discounted services, some university-based clinics are able to offer long-term services to people with chronic communication challenges. In such cases this is especially helpful to patients who have exhausted insurance coverage for diagnostic and treatment services but still benefit from continued intervention. Likewise, it is helpful to students, who benefit from the enhanced experience this provides. Special opportunities for expert consultations with faculty members, input from experienced clinical supervisors, and participation in clinical research are additional advantages available to people with aphasia in university contexts.

Home Health

Many patients with stroke and aphasia return to their homes after the acute medical emergency has subsided, or after a period of therapy at a rehabilitation center. When this happens, community-based home health agencies provide a variety of services to the patient through a well-structured, closely coordinated program. Indeed, home-care services to the elderly have grown rapidly because of the pressure on hospitals to reduce costs (Whitten, 2006). Insurers like such services because they are cost-effective and often more efficacious, and many elderly adults prefer to receive services in their own home (Leff et al., 2005; Whitten, 2006). Community-based programs provide reasonable prices and high-quality care and have better long-term results than residential facilities (Kerr, 1992; Whitten, 2006). Skills mastered in treatment programs do not have to be transferred to the home environment because they are taught where they will be used. In addition, independence and self-reliance are fostered.

There is a growing trend in the United States for older people to move in with their children, and to move to homes on properties of their children, especially after the onset of major health concerns. However, as the general population continues to age, the number of adult children available to provide such care will be reduced. Another growing trend is for elderly adults to develop formal or informal co-housing communities. In addition, many belong to naturally occurring retirement communities, which allow individuals to remain at home with the help of programs and resources shared among the residents. This helps the residents to coordinate transportation, health monitoring, and social activities. Aphasiologists are increasingly likely to be engaged in serving individuals living within such communal arrangements.

The range of home health services may include speech-language pathology, physical therapy, occupational therapy, visiting nurse and physician care, and psychiatric, psychological, and social work evaluation and therapy. Additionally, dietary counseling, homemaker or household assistance, and special assistive devices and financial assistance may be available.

Telehealth

Telehealth is the "use of electronic information and communications technologies to provide and support health care services when there is a distance between participants" (Hallowell & Henri, 2007). Telehealth applications hold increasingly greater promise for improving access to care in remote geographic areas where skilled service providers may be scarce or absent. They also are helpful in cases in which transportation to and from service providers is limited or financial resources (including insurance coverage or directly subsidized services) to support one-on-one in-person services are insufficient (Berman & Fenaughty, 2005; Field, 1996; Myers, Luecke, Longan, & Revell, 1998). In addition to expanding access for disadvantaged and rural populations, opportunities are emerging for expansion of home-health services through distance technology (Brown, 2005; Hickman & Dyer, 1998; Martinez, Villarroel, Seoane, & del Pozo, 2004; Ogasawara et al., 2003; Whitten, 2006). An additional advantage of telehealth is that it may expand access to services for people who live in areas that are unsafe, such as in high-crime urban neighborhoods and active international war zones (Doolittle, Otto, & Clemens, 1998; Khazei, Jarvis-Sellinger, Ho, & Lee, 2005).

Much of what is known about the potential for remote service delivery for diagnosis and treatment in communication disorders is derived from research on applications in other disciplines. New developments in technologic access will be shaped by ongoing developments in health policy as it affects telehealth. In the United States, cases in which states have developed regulations for the delivery of services of medical practitioners between states (Scott, 2004) may also be applied to speech-language pathologists.

Few published empirical studies directly address the effectiveness of telehealth delivery specifically related to aphasia. Several studies comparing face-to-face and telehealth assessments support the reliability, feasibility, and acceptability of telehealth evaluations of speech and language disorders (Duffy, Werven, & Aronson, 1997; Glykas & Chytas, 2004; Mashima et al., 2003; Sicotte, Lehoux, Fortier-Blanc, & Leblanc, 2003; Wertz et al., 1992; Wilson & Onslow, 2004).

According to a review by Hallowell and Henri (2007), the factors that will be most influential in continuing efforts to expand service delivery options in speech-language pathology include:

- Licensure issues, especially for services provided between states,
- Training in use of telehealth technology,
- Establishment of standards,
- Reimbursement issues,
- Patient confidentiality issues,
- Attitudes of providers and patients,
- Means of ensuring quality of clinician-patient relationships,
- Potential cost savings,
- Demonstration of clinical outcomes, and
- Telecommunications infrastructure and cost.

GERONTOLOGY AND APHASIA

Life expectancy has increased by more than 20 years since 1901. Life expectancy in the United States is between 74 and 77 years for men and 80 to 82.5 years for women. For those 65 years old, men can expect to live over 17 additional years and women almost another 21 years (Qu & Weston, 2003). The United States will continue to age rapidly as baby boomers (people born between 1946 and 1964) reach age 65 (after 2010). In 2050, over 20% of the population is expected to be age 65 and over (compared with about 13% today) (Kinsella & Velkoff, 2001). Given the rapid growth of the aging population worldwide, the extension of life-expectancy, and the fact that aphasia tends to occur in older adults, understanding the gerontologic context of aphasia intervention is crucial. It is important that clinical aphasiologists understand the process of aging, the multiple dimensions of age-related health concerns and challenges, and the hallmarks of successful aging and wellness. It is also important that they apply this information to their clinical interactions.

Aging is the sum total of all experiences, adaptations, and changes, both physical and emotional, that an individual undergoes during his or her lifetime. Three types of aging are commonly described in the gerontology literature: chronological, biological, and behavioral (Bergeman, 1997; Wei & Levkoff, 2000). Chronologic age is the number of years an individual has lived. Biological age is the relationship between aging and programmed cell death or an individual's susceptibility to disease. Behavioral age relates to how old an individual acts and thinks. It is the ability to function independently and perform activities of daily living (ADLs). A plethora of genetic, social, and cultural factors shape the experience of being old. As clinicians, we assess which specific factors may impact each patient.

Gender and Aging

Given that women live, on average, 7 years longer than men (Cruickshank, 2003), sensitivity to the multiple possible challenges to gender issues in older women is important. Since men tend to become ill and die earlier than women, women often provide for their care. Also, heterosexual women tend to marry a person older than themselves, leaving a large number of women widowed and living alone during their last years. In a study by Wachterman and Sommers (2006), 56.2% of women were widowed at the time they died, compared to 19.5% of men. Also, 23.2% of women compared to 11.5% of men spent the last year of life in nursing homes. The dedication of a couple's financial resources to the first one to be sick leaves many women with fewer financial resources at the end of their lives (AARP Public Policy Institute, 2002). These factors all make aging a critical women's issue.

For elderly individuals who receive care from a family member, approximately half of their assistance is provided by a spouse and half from adult children such as a daughter or daughter-in-law. Although estimates of the proportion of men versus women who serve as caregivers are variable across research studies and across cultures, a large majority of caregivers worldwide are women. Up to about 75% of adult caregivers in the United States are women (Dettinger & Clarkberg, 2002; Family Caregiver Alliance, 2006; Marks, Lambert, & Choi, 2002).

Ageism and Civil Rights

Applicable knowledge about cultural aspects of aging and means of countering ageism in clinical practice is essential. Ageism is a process of systematic stereotyping and discriminating against people because of their age (Butler, Carpenter, Kay, & Simmons, 1969). It is the notion or mindset that people are less human, inferior, less worthy, incompetent, selfish, a threat to the economic security of others, poor, disabled, isolated, decrepit, grumpy, frumpy, sexless, uninteresting, needy, neurotic, comical, powerless, temperamental, mentally unstable, or not the same people they once were— all due to the number of years they have lived (Andrews, 1999; Comfort, 1976; Copper, 1988; Levin & Levin, 1980; Perry, 1999; Quadagno, 1999; Russo, 1999).

Some older people experience prejudice not only from others but from themselves. Many express a sense of shame, failure, and unworthiness related to their age. The message that being old is funny or embarrassing is so ingrained that many take this view of themselves, a phenomenon known as internalized ageism. Primary bases of age discrimination have been said to include:

- irrational fears of an aging population,
- the association of age with sickness and frailty,
- cultural values demanding that one work and have demonstrable productivity in order to prove one's worth,
- common negative portrayals of older people on television and in other media, and
- a Western cultural focus on appearance as a critical human value (Cruickshank, 2003; Schlesinger, 2006).

The harmful impact of such prejudice reinforces discriminatory practices in health care, employment, housing, law, education, and in family interactions. It also sets a fertile stage for elder abuse. Schlesinger (2006) reports the alarming statistic that one to three million Americans over age 65 have been injured, exploited, or otherwise mistreated by someone on whom they depend for care or protection. Health-care professionals are not immune to ageist practices. For example, Williams and Giles (1998) report that the results of a study comparing physician interaction with young versus old patients demonstrate that the old are addressed with less respect and less patience, given less precise information, and asked fewer open-ended questions. They note that patronizing speech to older patients in medical settings occurs in the tone, simplicity, or brevity of the communication. Older patients with aphasia are especially susceptible to these and additional communication problems in medical settings (Murphy, 2006).

Ageism and Women

A good deal of age-related discrimination targets older women (Cruickshank, 2003). The roots of societal prejudice against older women in Western culture have been related to:

- Masculine performance values emphasized at the expense of human, loving, psychosocial, and more feminine values in Western culture;
- The extremely low proportion of visible role models for women over 60 in politics, the media, and business;
- The common preference among older men to be with much younger female companions;
- Portrayal of women as objects and within the context of sex and violence through many media;
- A much stronger contrast of beauty versus the effects of the destructive ravages of time encoded in many daily advertising, news, and entertainment media involving women compared to those involving men (Copper, 1988; Markson & Taylor, 2000; Mellancamp, 1999; Palmore, 1999).

There are two critical reasons for which it is incumbent upon clinical professionals in our field to be proactive in counteracting negative societal values related to gender. First, the fact that the older an individual is, the greater the likelihood that person is a woman, suggests that our older patients are often susceptible to female gender bias. Second, the fact that the number of practicing clinical aphasiologists, in particular, and of practicing speech-language pathologists in general, is comprised of females, makes the body of practicing clinicians a strong force for gender-related advocacy.

Financial Aspects of Aging

Due to increasing longevity and a variety of other social factors, many seniors in the United States live below the poverty line and most others are concerned about money. Many seniors in the country believe that they will be able to live on interest generated from tax-deferred savings but quickly learn that they must begin to withdraw these savings at the age of 70.5 at a substantial yearly rate. Indeed, approximately three-quarters of the principle must be withdrawn by the age of 85, leaving those who live beyond 85 at a significant financial disadvantage (Anderson & Anderson, 2003).

Successful Aging and Wellness

Another factor affecting older adults is wellness. Anderson and Anderson (2003) identify crucial links between six dimensions of health and their impact on how long we live and our vulnerability to chronic illnesses:

- biological well-being,
- psychological and behavioral well-being (thoughts and actions),
- environmental and social well-being (environment and relationships),
- economic well-being (personal achievement and equality),
- existential, religious, and spiritual well-being (faith and meaning), and
- emotional well-being.

Each of these dimensions is linked to the others such that changes in one dimension can precipitate changes in another. Health and longevity may thus depend upon risk and protective factors from across several of the interacting dimensions. Given that aging well involves living well, clinical aphasiologists ideally embrace the characteristics of successful aging and quality of life and appreciate health as more than the absence of disease and disability. A list of recommended readings in this important area is given in Appendix 7-1.

THE MANY ROLES OF THE APHASIOLOGIST

The clinical aphasiologist performs many of the same functions regardless of the professional setting in which he or she is employed. The most common functions of this clinician are identification and selection of clients; assessment; intervention; consultation and collaborative care; counseling; administration; quality assurance; contract negotiation; education; marketing; fundraising; advocacy; ethical decision-making; and research.

Identification and Selection of Clients

The ways in which patients are located or referred vary from setting to setting. In most instances, persons with aphasia are identified when a physician or another member of a rehabilitation team refers them to the aphasiologist. Such referrals are dependent on team members' abilities to recognize the language impairment, and their interest in reporting the problem to the speech-language clinician.

In some residential settings, the clinician screens each individual who enters the facility. The purpose of screening is generally to identify those who have language, speech, and/or swallowing problems. Once persons with aphasia have been identified, a more detailed assessment is performed. Enrollment in a diagnostic and/or treatment program depends on many factors, including the patient's willingness and desire to participate; the attitudes and support of the patient's significant others; authorization from the patient's primary physician; the clinician's existing caseload demands; transportation to and from the clinical setting; and insurance coverage and other economic factors.

Assessment

Assessment and intervention are the most important functions of the aphasiologist. The purpose of assessment is to provide an in-depth description of each client's cognitive, linguistic, and communicative behavior, and to define the factors that should be taken into account in order to stimulate the patient's use of language. The diagnostic process, as well as some of the influences of health-care reform on the way we engage in the diagnostic process, are discussed in detail elsewhere in this text.

Intervention

Rehabilitation, ideally, is a complex, dynamic, comprehensive process of patient care, beginning at the time of onset of the trauma and continuing until the "maximum physical, psychological, social (language), and vocational functions for each individual have been achieved" (Sahs & Hartman, 1976, p. 205). The term "intervention" is frequently used to refer to the process of facilitating rehabilitation through skilled treatment, or therapy.

Through intervention, aphasiologists attempt to heighten each patient's potential to function maximally within his or her environment, to facilitate meaningful relationships, and to restore self-esteem, dignity, and independence. As we will consider in this chapter, many factors in the service-delivery arena may interfere with patients' access to intervention. Thus, the maximum benefits for which patients have potential are not always achieved. Persons with neurogenic communication disorders, like all persons with disabilities, should be treated by highly-qualified clinicians using the best techniques available to meet their holistic needs with quality and dignity.

Language intervention is also a complex, flexible, organized, goal-directed, dynamic process, aimed at restoring the individual's previously learned language through treatment and/or training. Intervention "must be individually patterned, uniquely presented, and continuously tailored to signs of progress and signs of failure" (Darley, 1982, p. 238). It is a process that is designed to change communicative behavior, not just within the domain of the clinical setting, but in all communicative contexts and with all communicative partners.

Intervention is not confined to language and communication alone. The clinician helps patients to maintain and strengthen activities, participation in life, and social contacts; set and achieve life goals; gain a positive attitude; increase morale; gain insight into impairments; and develop feelings of acceptance, optimism, and emotional stability. Intervention is an innovative process that responds to the neurologic, linguistic, and social and life-participation goals and needs of each client, with a focus on the regaining of functional skills for communication in everyday life.

Due to increasing restrictions on frequency and duration of treatment for many patients requiring rehabilitation services, there is a growing need for stimulation and facilitation of communication outside the clinical environment from the earliest stages of treatment. Likewise, it is increasingly important to include caregivers and patients' significant others in direct treatment sessions. Numerous technologic tools are now available to supplement skilled treatment sessions (Katz & Hallowell, 1999) and by Katz (see Chapter 34). While such tools may help to enrich the intervention process, it is essential to recognize that their limitations, when used without a clinician, preclude their use as a solution to problem of reduced frequency and duration of skilled intervention.

Consultation and Collaborative Care

Most clinical aphasiologists function as members of rehabilitative assessment-intervention teams. In this capacity, they share knowledge and information with other professionals, such as occupational therapists, physical therapists, physicians, nurses, social workers, and dietitians, as well as with patients' family members. This necessitates team development and collaborative decision-making (see Chapter 8). Interdisciplinary consultation includes in-service training programs and presentations to professional groups. Team discussions may be related to the coordination or execution of clinical services; the case-management of specific clients; the nature of the patient's aphasia and other co-existing conditions; assessment and intervention related to medical, behavioral, and/or psychological problems; documentation of findings; insurance coverage; personal, occupational, and community activities; life participation; and discharge planning. True collaboration, in which the expertise of all team members is oriented toward holistically rehabilitating individuals to their fullest potential, improves case management through knowledge, understanding, and cooperation.

Referral for Additional Services and Resources

Given the common multiplicity of needs for medical, psychological, financial, legal, and social services among people with aphasia and their significant others, clinical aphasiologists often act as referral sources. It is important to have a deep well of information about specialists, community resources, and support services from which to draw when a patient or family member expresses a particular need. Many organizations worldwide have been designed to help connect people with aphasia to a range of support, networking, and training opportunities. Additionally, there are many centers for clinical treatment and social networking for people with aphasia. Still, access to such resources is limited or nonexistent in many geographic regions of the world. There remains a need not only to create more community resources, but also to assist people with aphasia and their families in identifying additional alternative resources at the local level. Local senior centers, lifelong learning institutes, exercise groups, support groups, respite programs, and elderhostel programs are some examples of resources that may not be designed specifically for people with aphasia, but that may offer wonderful opportunities for those affected by aphasia.

Many persons with aphasia and their significant others have Internet access; informing them of helpful links to sites offering support and information-exchange related to aphasia are often greatly appreciated. There is an ever-growing set of helpful Internet resources to aid clinicians, patients, and significant others make connections related to services, information, and support. The ASHA Web site has a continually updated list of such resources, and a simple Internet search results in numerous resources that may be helpful. Of course, it is important that users scrutinize carefully the validly and quality of Web-based materials.

Counseling

The role of counselor or adviser involves exchanging ideas or opinions and conducting discussions with the patient, members of the family, other professionals, or the community. The specific content of individual or group counseling depends on the individuals involved, but most often involves patients and their significant others. Topics such as the causes of stroke, the life-affecting impacts of stroke and aphasia, types of rehabilitation services available, and death and dying may be discussed.

Administration

Traditionally, administration or management has encompassed record keeping and report writing, scheduling clients, and ordering supplies. In the past, many aphasiologists practiced in clinical capacities with few other management responsibilities. In most of today's service-delivery environments, though, clinicians play greatly expanded administrative roles. Even those without administrative or management titles per se are expected to engage in other activities that are not strictly clinical, such as marketing, advocacy, and quality assurance.

Documentation

Records and reports play a significant role in an aphasiology treatment program. The primary purposes for keeping records are to generate an account of the clinical services provided, to support the planning of future assessment and intervention goals, and to justify reimbursement for services provided. The system of record keeping chosen should be one that can be interpreted easily by other professionals. Some of the specific types of records and reports that may be used are assessment records, session plans (including goals, methods, type of therapy, and an evaluation of the client's responses), conference records, release-of-information forms, referral forms, master schedules, statistical summaries of cases, progress reports, and periodic disposition reports. The primary purpose of preparing reports is to disseminate and maintain information. Accurate, clear, and timely records and reports are essential to (1) providing continuity of service; (2) maintaining a cumulative account of each individual's assets, limitations, and progress in therapy; (3) evaluating the effectiveness, quality, efficiency, and productivity of clinicians and treatment programs; (4) monitoring consumer satisfaction; (5) developing and justifying programs; and (6) ensuring that clinicians and their employers are financially reimbursed for their services.

Thorough documentation is the vehicle that permits authorization (and sometimes pre- and re-authorization) for diagnosis and treatment, and that determines reimbursement by third-party payers (e.g., insurance companies, managed-care organizations, and federal health programs). Thus, clinical aphasiologists should be competent writers and should be well-trained in the fine art of clinical documentation. Speech-language documentation must contain (1) a complete history; (2) a clear statement of the problem; (3) a plan of action to address the problem, including short-term and long-term goals that are describable and quantifiable; (4) descriptions of tasks and modalities to be used in treatment; and (5) a prognostic statement and indication of expected results of intervention—preferably in terms of skills and abilities that facilitate functional behavior, independence, and improved quality of life. No matter how excellent the actual clinical services may be, clinicians and/or their employing agencies are regularly denied reimbursement from insurance companies or other third-party payers when documentation does not address each of these areas.

As treatment continues, progress should be recorded in detail. Changes in an individual's intellectual, emotional, life-participation, and social status as they relate to communicative improvement should be described. Has motivation changed? Have there been changes in pre-existing conditions?

Documentation should be logical and sequential. Each report should be strongly tied to preceding and subsequent reports. Whenever possible, statements from patients and their families or significant others should be a component of progress notes or revisions of goals and procedures. Visual aids such as graphs and charts may add clarity to reports.

In most managed care contexts, and in contexts serving Medicare and Medicaid patients, standardized diagnostic and treatment reporting and billing forms are becoming the norm. Responses to these forms require clinicians to summarize vast amounts of information related to patient care in small designated spaces on pre-printed forms. In some cases clinicians from many disciplines are required to input their data on the same form. Such interdisciplinary coordination requires concerted effort to complete treatment and diagnostic records in a timely manner.

Aphasiologists, like clinicians in most health-care disciplines, may enjoy the advantages of new technologic developments that facilitate report writing and record keeping. For example, report writing templates may be generated through word-processing programs or commercially available programs. Further, in some settings, voice-activation report writing software now allows for hands-free dictation of reports, notes, and letters. Additionally, computerized versions of forms enable efficient form completion, cross-referencing with data base information, and easy transfer of information from one form to another. Some large hospitals and rehabilitation centers use report-writing software that links multiple workstations and integrates input from multiple disciplines. Such software may also be used to coordinate diagnostic, treatment, billing, and patient scheduling functions within and across disciplines (Hallowell & Katz, 1999).

Billing and Coding

Financial reimbursement from third-party payers depends on thoughtful, strategic billing practices. Clinicians are often responsible for the primary billing practices, including the tracking of time spent in treatment and diagnostic services, the coding of services according to coding schemes acceptable to each third-party payer, the completion of billing forms, and the submission of billing forms along with diagnostic and treatment reports to third-party payers. Even in those hospitals, rehabilitation centers, and other agencies that employ clerical professionals who are responsible for billing paperwork, clinicians must provide the factual input that will determine the content of billing records.

In most employment contexts, it is important that clinicians be familiar with numerical coding systems used by third-party payers and with related policies. The two coding systems most commonly used in speech-language pathology are the International Classification of Diseases, 9th rev., Clinical Modification (ICD-9-CM; National Center for Health Statistics, 2006), and the Physicians Current Procedural Terminology, 4th ed. (CPTM; American Medical Association, 1999). Most public and private payers require ICD-9 codes for diagnoses and CPT codes for "procedures," or specific services rendered. These codes serve to standardize billing codes for uniformity among service providers and third-party payers.

ICD-9 diagnostic codes are used to classify medical diagnoses across disciplines and clinical settings. They are required by most insurance companies and by all programs of the U.S. Public Health Service and the Center for Medicare and Medicaid Services (CMS). ICD-9 codes consist of three digits. Sometimes, additional information is conveyed by adding two more digits to the right of a decimal point. A new edition of ICD codes, the ICD-10 codes, are in draft status and are under review by users and CMS at the time of publication of this text. The diagnostic codes currently in use may be obtained through CMS and are also available on the ASHA Web site.

CPT codes are used to standardize the coding of health-care services across disciplines and clinical settings. They consist of five digits. The codes are published annually by the American Medical Association (AMA), and are also available through the ASHA Web site. Numerous software packages and Internet resources are available for help in automation of billing and coding practices.

Appealing Denials for Treatment Authorization or Reimbursement

In many cases, requests for treatment authorization or for reimbursement of services already provided are denied by third-party payers. As managed care practices have expanded dramatically over the past few years, many agencies have seen their denial rates for evaluation and treatment authorizations grow significantly (Henri & Hallowell, 1999b). Typical reasons for which an insurance company may deny authorization or reimbursement include: (1) lack of a physician's order for services; (2) improper documentation or coding of diagnostic and/or treatment information; (3) failure to demonstrate that the patient has adequate rehabilitation potential to justify services; (4) failure to demonstrate the functional impacts that treatment will have on the functional communication, medical management, independence, and quality of life of the individual being served; (5) noncoverage of certain services by the patient's specific health care plan; and (6) exhaustion of services allowed by a given health care plan.

Whenever authorization or reimbursement is denied, clinicians may make an appeal to reverse the denial. In a majority of the cases reported in the United States, appeals for reimbursement are successful (Henri & Hallowell, 1999b). Documentation that supports a letter of appeal may include a copy of written diagnostic or treatment authorization from the primary-care physician, progress notes, and discharge reports. The likelihood of success in the appeals process depends, in large part, on the quality of documentation, as well as in the persistence of the clinician or other professionals pursuing the appeal. Excellent documentation, and ongoing educational and advocacy efforts between clinicians and third-party payers, may help to reduce the likelihood of denials occurring in the first place.

If an appeal to overturn a denial for treatment authorization or reimbursement is unsuccessful, the clinician may be instrumental in having the patient or his or her significant other(s) file a complaint with the insurance company. Likewise, individuals with employer-sponsored insurance may file complaints with the human resources department of their employers. A more confrontational measure is to inform the third-party payer that a complaint will be filed with the state's insurance commissioner. It is important to avoid undermining relationships with insurers, though, and to maintain a cooperative, rather than adversarial, spirit throughout the process of reversing a denial whenever possible (Henri & Hallowell, 1999b).

Scheduling

Scheduling involves preparing a timed plan for the week, month, and/or year. Scheduling for the year involves accounting for legal holidays and professional conventions and conferences, and providing time for in-service training sessions and vacation time for staff members. In planning a weekly schedule, time must be reserved for traveling, holding conferences, writing reports, preparing sessions, coordinating activities, performing in-service education, and reading current professional literature. For most clinicians, the largest amount of time is ideally invested in patient assessment and intervention. Scheduling individual patients depends on such things as the patient's health and prognosis, transportation, clinicians' expertise, current clinical caseloads, insurance coverage, and additional financial considerations.

Ordering Supplies

Relevant equipment, materials, and supplies are often ordered by the clinician, depending on their perceived usefulness and the availability of funds for such purchases. Items that are frequently obtained include standard tests, textbooks, workbooks, prepared treatment materials, tape recorders and audiotapes, videotape recorders and videotapes, computers, software, and paper.

Negotiating Contracts with Third-Party Payers

To be listed on an insurance company's preferred-provider list, or to provide services for members of a preferred-provider plan, clinicians must have a contract with the corresponding insurance company. In many cases, professionals with administrative titles are the designated officials who engage in developing and negotiating the details of such contracts. Sometimes clinicians negotiate contracts, too, especially those who work in private practice, small speech-language hearing centers, community agencies, and university clinics (Henri, Hallowell, & Johnson, 1996).

Currently, many clinicians are keenly interested in joining specialty provider networks. Provider networks enable clinicians to team together, thus expanding patient and referral bases for network members, and decreasing the costs of marketing, billing, and other management functions through shared expenses (Davolt, 1999). Like contracting with HMOs, contracting with networks may be highly beneficial, and even necessary to some clinicians' and agencies' fiscal survival; but it involves complex professional risks, and requires keen business savvy on the part of clinicians. The employment of professional consultants for help in this arena is often well worth its cost.

Education

In the role of educator, the aphasiologist may supervise student-clinicians and paraprofessionals and/or teach in university training programs. The aphasiologist may also present in-service training to administrators, home-health aides, other health-care staff, and family members. Further, continuing self-education is essential to advanced professional competence. Reading professional journals and attending conferences, workshops, and courses helps to enrich professional development. Patient education may involve empowering individuals by informing them about the array of medical, communicative, activity, life-participation, environmental, and social choices available to them. The more individuals are involved in making decisions about their own care, the more positive and participatory they become. In addition, informing patients about their rights and discussing issues such as a positive outlook and its role in recovery, stress management, and self-esteem may be beneficial to treatment.

Ideally, the clinical aphasiologist also educates the public, fostering awareness of means of preventing stroke and traumatic brain injury. "Every year millions of people suffer and die of illnesses that could be cured or eliminated by altering patterns of personal behavior" (Ewart, 1991, p. 931). Clinicians may empower individuals for improvement by stimulating a sense of self-control, mastery, and power to effect change. Through education, they also encourage collective empowerment within the community, and development of strategies to promote better health patterns.

Marketing

Marketing is the process of defining what a potential customer wants or needs, producing that service, and letting others know the service is for sale. It involves (1) detailed analysis of the customers' perceptions, wants, and needs; (2) analysis of the competition and other external factors that will affect service delivery; (3) development of products and services to address customers' wants and needs; (4) fostering an excellent local and regional reputation through assurance of top-quality service and demonstrable outcomes; (5) publicity and advertising (through Web sites, brochures, newsletters, education pamphlets, slide shows, and paid advertising in a variety of media); and (6) networking and successful collaboration with other health professionals.

In this era of health-care reform, few service-providing agencies, be they hospitals, long-term-care facilities, rehabilitation centers, not-for-profit clinics, home-health agencies, university- or college-based clinics, or private practices, have a steady flow of patients who can pay for diagnostic and treatment services. Service providers must now dedicate resources to marketing efforts to ensure that their agencies remain fiscally stable, that patients with communication disorders have access to treatment, and that communication-disorders professionals continue to be employed (ASHA, 1997; Cohn, 1994; Henri & Hallowell, 1997). Clinicians often participate in collaborative marketing efforts, including the development and dissemination of publicity materials, meetings with physicians and other referral sources, conferences with insurance-company representatives, and offering of in-services to the case managers and reviewers who make coverage and reimbursement decisions for managed-care organizations (MCOs).

Quality Assurance

Deep budget cuts and increased competitiveness require health-care professionals to deliver better products and services with greater efficiency. Quality is a competitive advantage. While quality-assurance programs were once considered to be in the domain of management staff, most service-providing agencies now depend on the contributions of all staff members in holistic, strategic quality-assurance efforts (Underhill, 1991). Total quality management (TQM) is a notion that has received a great deal of attention in all types of businesses throughout the world over the past three decades. It involves delivering a service or making a product, engaging employees in every process, assessing customer satisfaction, and modifying operations strategically based on outcomes and consumer feedback. The emphasis is on productivity, flexibility, efficiency, effective communication, and consumer-driven services.

TQM involves building quality into the whole of an organization, not just in specific aspects, components, or departments (Labovitz, 1991). Enterprises with successful TQM programs have well-defined objectives and guidelines for every participant, and are led by informed and active people. Ideally, these institutions invest in the notions that (1) it is

people who are critical to success, thus employees at all levels should be empowered; (2) customers must receive the best possible services; (3) excellence must be pursued in all areas of operation; and (4) strong investments in research and development are essential to quality, as are high readiness and receptiveness to change.

Regulatory agencies, including the Joint Commission on Accreditation of Healthcare Organizations (JCAHO), require accredited clinical facilities to demonstrate continuous quality-improvement programs (Roth, 1999). Regulatory agencies that accredit MCOs (e.g., the National Committee on Quality Assurance (NCQA) also require quality assurance programs on the part of MCOs (Goplerud, 2004). Such programs, generally employing multiple facets of TQM and related quality-management strategies, involve the ongoing and systematic monitoring, analysis, and improvement of services to yield improved patient outcomes. Although ASHA no longer certifies service-delivery programs, the association does offer specific guidelines for quality assurance (ASHA, 2005). Good communication is vital to the success of any total quality process (McLaurin & Bell, 1991; Varian, 1991).

Within health care in general and speech-language pathology in particular, there is a need to define what makes a TQM program. We must define our customers in very specific terms. Who are we serving? Insurance companies, facilities, the state, the patient? What are their specific needs? How can we become more responsive to these needs? What constitutes success in a TQM facility? What is our vision? What are our goals? To be excellent, we must stay close to our customers, learn their preferences, and cater to them (Peters & Waterman, 1982). We must assess consumer satisfaction and ask our patients how we can make their schedules more workable, how we can better use our facilities for their benefit, and how we can improve our human resources in order to be the preferred provider of cognitive, linguistic, and communicative services.

In the field of communication sciences and disorders we must create reliable and valid quality-assurance measures to assess patients' perceptions of the outcomes and efficacy of our treatments. In addition, we need to advocate for our professional integrity by promoting the importance of adequate professional training, certification, and licensure for professionals who work in the area of neurogenic communication disorders. Our clients have complex, multifaceted disabilities and deserve to interact with qualified professionals.

Health care and containment of health-care costs will continue to be a prime political issue in the upcoming decades. The winners in service-delivery competition "will not necessarily be the cheapest health care facilities, but those that meet customer needs by delivering quality care" (Labovitz, 1991, p. 46). It is important that we integrate TQM into our decisions regarding the kind of changes we believe are essential to the highest quality service.

Fundraising

Reduced rates for clinical services under managed care, in combination with reduced frequency and intensity of many covered services, is resulting in generally decreased revenues associated with clinical services. Thus, many service-providing agencies are increasingly reliant on finding additional means of financial support. Not-for-profit agencies, in particular, which are charged with providing services to clients regardless of their ability to pay, are dependent on alternative means of generating income to support clinical revenues. Many for-profit agencies have established their own not-for-profit foundations, or are partnering with existing foundations that help support the provision of services to persons whose access might otherwise be limited. Thus, clinicians are often involved in initiating or supporting fundraising efforts.

Fundraising efforts may include collaboration in developing fundraising materials; establishing and expanding a donor base of individuals, clients, foundations, and corporations that support the concerns of people with communication disorders; participating in annual fundraising campaigns and special events (e.g., benefit concerts, dinners, and sporting events); meeting with donors and potential donors about special clinical programs and needs; collaborating with fundraising professionals on planned-giving programs; and establishing partnerships with corporations and fraternal organizations (Henri & Hallowell, 1999a, 1999b).

Ethical Decision-Making

During the 21st century, health-care workers will increasingly be interacting with patients, family, and other health-care workers, and making decisions about the right to life, euthanasia, do-not-resuscitate (DNR) orders, the quality of life, and the right to health-care access. Agonizing questions we will have to face include: Who has the right to decide how long a patient lives? How much of our limited financial resources should be used to delay death? Should we provide rehabilitative services to people who are near death? How much emphasis should we give a patient's estimated prognosis when we decide whether or not to provide services?

In addition, clinicians face other conflicts of interest related to their own financial gains (Council on Ethical and Judicial Affairs, American Medical Association, 1995). During the past two decades, many rehabilitation companies in the United States have offered financial bonuses to clinicians based upon the amount of time they have engaged in billable service. Henri and Hallowell (1997) enumerate and describe the ways in which incentive systems may affect the quality and ethics of patient care by speech-language pathologists:

- Seeing high-fee patients too long or beyond the point of expecting further reasonable progress;
- Seeing low-fee patients too briefly or at such a frequency and intensity that progress is unlikely;
- Admitting patients to treatment who are unlikely to benefit from skilled therapy (i.e., patients who have limited rehabilitation potential) and overstating the likelihood of improvement to justify admitting persons to treatment;
- When documenting progress for billing, "stretching the truth" (e.g., misrepresenting actual progress or other forms of dishonesty);
- Misrepresenting the actual time spent in treatment; and
- Avoiding or limiting non-billable activities that are important to quality of service (e.g., in-services, informal discussions with team members, staff meetings).

Although an enormous amount of research across disciplines and industries documents the effectiveness of incentive systems, ethical implications of incentive systems are virtually ignored in most of the research literature. One study (Henri & Hallowell, 1997) suggests that students exiting graduate school and entering the clinical workforce are susceptible to such conflicts of interest, which appear to be related to the students' sense of financial need. The study also demonstrates that practicing clinicians across the country confront a multitude of ethical conflicts related not only to financial bonuses, but also to more dire personal needs. For example, an increasing number of clinicians are threatened with the loss of their jobs if they do not achieve a certain minimum level of billable clinical productivity per week. Consequently, many report a sense of ongoing ethical pressure in balancing their needs for job security with the ethical nature of treatment, billing, and caseload-management decisions. As recent worldwide trends in health-care restructuring have reduced financial gains through the provision of rehabilitation services (Katz et al., 2000), clinicians must be well prepared to face with solid moral fortitude personal conflicts of interest related to professional decisions.

Research

Some aphasiologists pursue careers in research at colleges, universities, or at private, state, or federal research agencies. A national shortage of doctoral-level personnel in communication sciences and disorders in the United States is now yielding rich opportunities for careers in higher education (Gallagher, 2006; Geffner, 1997). Furthermore, the need for faculty members who specialize in neurogenic communication disorders is greater than the need for those in other specialties within the profession. According to the results of annual surveys of graduate programs in communication sciences and disorders in the United States (Petrosino, Lieberman, & McNeil, 1997), the anticipated doctoral faculty openings in adult neurogenic disorders outnumbered those in every other specialty within speech-language pathology from 1991 through 1998. Again, in a survey completed in 2002, the number of new doctoral-program graduates in adult neurogenic disorders was far below the number needed to fill the corresponding open positions (Shinn, Goldberg, Kimelman, & Messick, 2001). Adult neurogenic communication disorders continues to be the area of faculty specialty in greatest demand (Shinn et al., 2001).

Many clinicians with interests in scholarly work find personal and professional rewards in continuing their graduate and post-graduate training in research. For some seasoned clinicians, those interests lead to significant career changes as they return to school for doctoral study. Others know from the start of their graduate studies that they want to engage in academic careers, and thus continue their doctoral studies soon after their masters-level training.

Even clinicians who are not invested in research careers should be good consumers of and contributors to research. Minifie (1983) aptly claims that the destiny of our field is imminently tied to practitioners assuming a greater role in developing the clinical science, and that mediocrity comes from a division between clinical and research programs. Research is inseparable from clinical service.

There is a greater need now than in any time in the history of aphasiology to demonstrate the effectiveness of our interventions. It is essential to establish "how much and what kind of treatment is best and what changes constitute important treatment outcomes" (Thompson & Kearns, 1991, p. 52). As third-party payers are demanding published, empirically-based evidence of treatment efficacy and functional treatment outcomes to justify reimbursement for our services, every clinical aphasiologist has a responsibility to document his or her clinical successes and failures. Consequently, clinicians must be familiar with the techniques of scientific research design, measurement, and analysis, and with specific behavioral, cognitive, communicative, and/or linguistic models of intervention (Thompson & Kearns, 1991). Clinicians who are not well-versed in research design, and those whose schedules do not permit time to perform extensive literature reviews, collect data, and write for publication, may establish constructive partnerships with doctoral-level researchers in nearby academic institutions.

While the kind and quality of research that is undertaken depends on the availability of facilities and subjects and on the cooperative atmosphere provided by the administration and staff, it also largely depends on the commitment of the individual clinician to analyze the effectiveness of his or her work. An essential component of quality research is the creation of an environment that is conducive to risk-taking. Thus, the quality, motivation, and personal relationships of the research staff, and the style of management that is either supportive of creativity or critical of new ideas, will influence the quality of research that is conducted (Ringel, 1982).

Advocacy

Increasing competition for limited health-care resources requires that speech-language pathologists be active advo-

cates on behalf of their profession and their patients. Some specific means by which aphasiologists may advocate for their patients were discussed above in terms of appealing denials for authorization and reimbursement, marketing, quality assurance, education, negotiating contracts, and participating in research. Although it may seem obvious to the aphasiologist that speech and language services are essential to the total care of a patient, it is often necessary to demonstrate that fact to consumers and their significant others, colleagues in other disciplines, referral sources, insurance-company representatives, and legislators. Consumer advocacy is usually effective. However, consumers who have communication disorders, especially aphasia, are often unable to advocate independently for the services they need. It is important for the clinician to provide patients and their significant others the information necessary to be effective self-advocates. Aphasiologists may provide guidance concerning how to approach primary-care physicians and insurers, reverse prior authorization or treatment denials, write letters to legislators and insurance commissioners, or even testify before state and regional committees that monitor the performance of MCOs (Hallowell & Henri, in press; 1999b).

In the United States, numerous legislative advocacy campaigns to support the provision of services to persons with communication disorders are supported by ASHA, which provides free advocacy materials on the Internet and through mailings. Numerous state and local professional organizations also provide training and materials to support legislative advocacy. Although it is not often part of clinicians' job descriptions to be engaged in local, regional, and national advocacy, many clinicians feel compelled to do so, recognizing its importance. They may participate in letter-writing campaigns to legislators, election campaigns to support political representatives who support the provision of services to persons with communication disorders, and consumer education projects. Each individual's advocacy efforts contribute to the gains of all patients and professionals in our discipline.

LEGISLATIVE ISSUES AFFECTING SERVICE DELIVERY

Legislation Affecting Access to Care

In the United States, several pieces of federal and state legislation have been passed to ensure that persons of all ages with special conditions have access to adequate and appropriate levels of service. It is important for speech-language clinicians to be familiar with federal and state laws and rules and regulations that support access to special services. The Social Security Act, for example, contains several titles (i.e., chapters or subsections) that ensure reimbursement for speech-language pathology and audiology services (Hallowell & Henri, 2007). Those pertinent to serving adults with aphasia include Title 18 (Medicare), Title 19 (Medicaid),

Title 20 (the Social Services Subsidy, which supports social-work services that, in turn, may help families access speech-language pathology and audiology services). Many of these reimbursement mechanisms have mixed histories serving populations with chronic or degenerative conditions (Smith & Ashbaugh, 1995).

Several other pieces of federal legislation also support services to adults with aphasia. The Americans with Disabilities Act does not ensure funding, but may require employers to make available certain resources in cases where communication disorders have demonstrable impacts on an individual's ability to perform job duties. Other such federal acts include the Individuals with Disabilities Education Act, the primary funding vehicle for states' special-education programs, and the Rehabilitation Act, which funds rehabilitation services, including speech-language pathology and audiology, for persons ranging in age from 16 to 64 (Hallowell & Henri, 2007).

Legislation Affecting Patient Privacy

In the United States, the Health Insurance Portability and Accountability Act (HIPAA) requires that health plans standardize, streamline, and safeguard the transmission of individually identifiable health information among carriers and providers. All health-care professionals, including aphasiologists, and all support staff and student-clinicians in the U.S. are expected to be familiar with HIPAA regulations.

THE ECONOMICS OF LANGUAGE-INTERVENTION SERVICES

The delivery of diagnostic and intervention services is heavily influenced by economics. Professional clinicians are paid for the services they provide. Income generated through clinical services very rarely comes from fees paid by patients directly to providers. Rather, provider agencies are reimbursed by third-party payers. Third-party payers are usually insurance companies, federal health-care plans, or special not-for-profit foundations. Most often, clinicians receive salaries or hourly wages from their employers. Those who are self-employed generally pay themselves a fixed salary or a portion of the profits from their practice's annual revenues.

Third-Party Payers

In most countries, health-care services are covered through nationalized health programs. In the United States, however, individuals are insured primarily through private health-insurance programs, the majority through plans offered by employers as part of a benefits package. In many cases, those who are insured by their employers make some financial contribution to maintain their insurance plans. Often, employees have some choices regarding the type and extent of medical coverage they would like, with less costly plans providing fewer medical benefits.

In addition to private insurance programs, there are two federal health programs that influence service delivery to adults in the United States: Medicare and Medicaid. Medicare provides coverage for speech and language pathologists' services to adults over 65 years of age and for persons under the age of 65 who have long-term disabilities (those lasting more than 2 years). Medicare plans are generally administered through private insurance companies that serve as interfaces between service providers and the Medicare program. Medicaid provides for services to persons who meet definable levels of low-income and specific asset standards. Medicaid programs are administered by individual states. Additionally, individuals who have served in the United States armed forces are eligible for health-care services provided through the Veterans Health Administration in the Department of Veterans Affairs (VA), most often at VA hospitals and clinics.

Reimbursement Schemes

Prior to about 1996, most insurance companies throughout the United States reimbursed service providers for specific services rendered and/or for units of time during which clinicians engaged in billable services with covered individuals. This reimbursement arrangement is known as "fee-for-service." Now, however, far-reaching measures known collectively as "managed care" have modified the traditional modes of reimbursement. Some of these managed-care modes have existed for a long time, especially in certain geographic pockets of the United States. They now characterize the majority of reimbursement arrangements in the United States. Examples of alternative reimbursement modes are discounted fee-for-service, case rate, per diem, and capitation. There are many permutations to each of these modes.

Discounted fee-for-service arrangements involve the establishment of reduced rates for patients who are members of a specific plan. In order to provide services to a plan's members, providers must agree to those rates. Third-party payers are billed for units of billable time or for specific services rendered.

In a *case rate* arrangement, the provider is paid a specific fee for treating a patient with a particular diagnosis, regardless of the duration of care or the number of services rendered. The case rate is based on actuarial analyses of the likely needs of patients according to their diagnoses. The standard Medicare diagnosis-related group (DRG) system and the new Medicare prospective-payment system (PPS) are examples of this type of arrangement.

In a *per diem* arrangement, the third-party payer pays the provider a specific amount of money for each day during which a patient is in the provider's care. The type and number of services does not generally influence the per diem rate.

Capitation involves a fixed amount of money that is paid to a provider, based on the number of people enrolled in a specific plan, not on the actual services rendered. Capitation rates are based on actuarial analyses of the likely needs of individuals who are insured through a specific plan. If those individuals require more services than are covered by the capitation revenue, then providers must absorb the remaining cost of caring for the enrolled individuals. Thus, capitation arrangements can be highly risky for providers. Still, capitation is a fast-growing type of payment system.

Managed Care

The rapid proliferation of managed-care practices in the United States is having a dramatic influence on virtually all aspects of service delivery to persons with aphasia and other communication disorders. Managed care has been defined in myriad ways in the health-care literature. Sometimes it is defined with a focus on managed-care's goals of preventing illness, maximizing health outcomes, coordinating care, and reducing unnecessary care (Henri & Hallowell, 1999b). Other definitions highlight specific cost-control and cost-cutting tactics that are characteristic of managed-care modes of service delivery. Regardless of the specific way one defines managed care, the three main goals most frequently stated are (1) assurance of the quality and coordination of care, (2) access to care for persons who need it, and (3) cost control (Henri & Hallowell, 1999b). Unfortunately, the health-care literature and the popular media are replete with accounts of how the overwhelming focus on cost control in managed care often leads to compromises in quality and access.

Because of great variability in managed-care proliferation according to geographic location within the country, and because of variability in the definition of what constitutes managed care, specific estimates of managed-care market penetration in the United States are variable. A majority of privately insured citizens receive service though a managed-care arrangement. Likewise, a large and growing proportion of Medicare and Medicaid patients receive federally sponsored benefits through managed-care plans. If one considers the cost-control mechanisms that are implemented across virtually all health-care contexts, the actual rate of managed-care penetration across the country is now near 100%. These cost-control mechanisms, enumerated by Henri and Hallowell (1999b), include:

- Increasingly stringent utilization review;
- Preadmission certification for hospital stays;
- Required pre-authorization for services;
- Negotiated reduced reimbursement rates;
- Designation of a restricted list of "preferred providers";
- Designation of physicians as "gatekeepers" of patients' health-care expenditure allotments;
- Salaried employment of physicians by payer organizations;
- Payment of incentives to physicians not to refer patients for specialty (e.g., rehabilitation) services;
- Use of red-flag diagnostic or treatment categories to deny reimbursement; and
- Restrictions on frequency, intensity, and duration of care (p. 4).

During the expansion of managed care in the U.S., there has been a general, parallel trend in health care restructuring all over the globe. Even in those countries that rely extensively on nationalized health-care systems, there have been upheavals in organizational structures and a proliferation of severe cost-cutting tactics in both federal and private programs (Katz et al., 2000).

Managed-Care Organizations

Managed-care organizations (MCOs) are insurance companies or programs that operate in managed-care modes. Given that the definition of managed care varies according to one's professional context and point of view, one might argue that the definition of an MCO does too. Generally, though, MCOs are characterized by (1) use of specific types of cost-saving reimbursement schemes, as described above; (2) promotion of health and wellness through preventive care and patient education; (3) concerted efforts to coordinate the type and number of services received by each enrollee; and (4) reduced enrollment fees for enrollees and/or the employers who pay for enrollees' insurance coverage.

There are many types of MCOs. The two most common examples are preferred-provider organizations and health-maintenance organizations. A preferred provider organization (PPO) is one that contracts with specific providers who agree to offer services to the PPO's enrollees at rates that are significantly below what the same providers would normally charge in a fee-for-service arrangement. Providers generally agree to reduced rates in the form of discounted fees-for-service, capitation schemes, case rates, or per diem allowances. Very low fees, usually in the form of co-payments, serve as an incentive for enrollees to use preferred providers. Members of a plan may use "out-of-network" providers, but at much higher rates and with greater restrictions on the type and extent of services allowable.

A health-maintenance organization (HMO) is a type of MCO in which comprehensive services are provided through one health-care facility or a network of facilities. Many of the clinicians who work for HMOs, including physicians, nurses, rehabilitation therapists, social workers, and others, are salaried by the HMO. They generally do not bill a third-party payer for services. Reimbursement schemes in HMOs are generally based on prospective payment models. The primary-care physician of each enrollee is considered a gatekeeper of all health-care resources, having the authority to determine the frequency, intensity, and duration of any services allowable for each patient. Since the gatekeeper almost always receives financial rewards for spending less of the available financial resources on services to patients, he or she has inherent conflicts of interest related to the determination of services to be provided (Begley, 1987; Grey, 1990a, 1990b; Rodwin, 1995).

Consequences of Managed Care for Intervention in Aphasia

Restructuring of health-care systems to reduce costs has transferred control of the access to, and the duration of, care from clinicians to administrators. Although efforts to control rising health-care costs are laudable, such efforts often threaten patients' access to care and the quality of care they receive (Henri & Hallowell, 1996; Purtillo, 1995; Randall, 1994).

The key challenges to professional practitioners in neurogenic communication disorders are the same as those summarized by Henri and Hallowell (1999b) for the professions of speech-language pathology and audiology in general:

- Consumers' access to our services;
- The quality, intensity, duration, and frequency of care that we can provide;
- The fiscal stability of our service-providing agencies;
- The livelihood of our professionals;
- The maintenance of our professional integrity; and
- Problems of consumers' access to our services (p. 4).

Let us briefly review each of these key areas as they pertain to adults with neurogenic communication disorders.

Consumer Access

Consumers' access to diagnostic and treatment services is threatened by decreased referrals from managed-care's gatekeepers, usually physicians, who often receive financial incentives to decrease the amount of services offered. For persons with neurogenic disorders, managed care's emphasis on acute-care service-delivery models is particularly troublesome. One of the principal ways in which clinicians are held accountable for the outcomes of their services in such models is through the documentation of patients' ongoing improvements throughout treatment, with a logical point of discharge based on maximal progress (Henri & Hallowell, 1999b). Since elderly people and people with chronic health problems, degenerative conditions, and multiple disabilities often do not fit the acute-care patterns of quick and steady gains toward recovery and discharge, such individuals are experiencing more and more difficulty in receiving our services (Clement, Retchin, Brown, & Stegall, 1994; Fox, Wicks, & Newacheck, 1993; Oberlander, 1997; Smith & Ashbaugh, 1995). Furthermore, MCOs are less likely to provide full coverage for such persons (Inglehart, 1995). Restrictions on coverage for conditions diagnosed prior to

enrollment enable MCOs to reduce expenditures associated with the care of costly conditions (Clement, Retchin, Brown, & Stegall, 1994; Fisher, 1994; Hallowell & Henri, 2007; Henri & Hallowell, 1999a; Hiller & Lewis, 1995; Perkins, 1998).

Members of cultural and ethnic minorities and of low-income populations have restricted access to care as well (Daw, 2001; Hallowell & Henri, 2007; Leigh, 1994; Stenger, 1993), perhaps because they are less likely to have health-care coverage through employers, are less likely to be able to afford their own health-insurance coverage, and may be less likely to advocate for their own health-care needs (Henri & Hallowell, 1999b). Ironically, such individuals tend to have disproportionately greater needs for rehabilitation services (Screen & Anderson, 1994).

MCO clauses emphasizing the relatively new concept of "evidence-based medical necessity" further threaten patient access to speech-language services. Under such clauses, if providers cannot present a solid body of well-controlled research to support the effectiveness of any intervention administered, then they will not be reimbursed for providing that intervention. An additional repercussion of medical-necessity clauses is the emphasis on the importance of treatment of medical impairments rather than of disabling conditions that influence quality of life. A disconcerting example of this repercussion is that many clinicians are finding it easier to obtain authorization and reimbursement for dysphagia services than for language intervention. Given that many clinicians who treat aphasia also treat dysphagia, there is an alarming trend to prioritize treatment for swallowing problems over problems of communication (Hallowell & Clark, 2002).

Quality, Intensity, Duration, and Frequency of Care

Despite the supposed focus on "quality" in MCOs, several factors related to managed-care modes of delivery have eroded the quality of care clinicians can deliver. First, a prominent cost-containment feature of managed-care plans is the restriction on duration and frequency of treatments, which limits clinicians' abilities to foster significant functional gains, even in patients with good rehabilitation potential. Second, insurance companies are increasingly intervening in matters that traditionally have been in the hands of clinicians, such as treatment planning and discharge decision-making. This trend has led to decision-making that is more financially driven than clinically sound. Third, interruptions in the continuity of care have increased due to delays in authorization and re-authorization for services. Fourth, although the use of assistants and aides in the treatment of communication and swallowing disorders is relatively new in the United States, concerns about the overuse and misuse of these less expensive (but less qualified) personnel and the potential consequences for further reductions in the quality and outcomes of care are growing (Hallowell & Henri, 2007).

Quality assurance is a stated aim in the literature of virtually every MCO. MCO-accrediting agencies, such as the NCQA, require that MCOs meet high standards of quality-assurance and quality-improvement practices. How can it be, then, that there is such a preponderance of complaints about managed care in the popular media, as well as evidence of decreasing quality in the research literature? One reason is that overall comparative standards among HMOs may be lower than standards under more traditional models. Another is that MCOs tend to minimize their quality under pressure to reduce their own administrative cost-improvement efforts. Recent research on the quality of health care suggests accreditation of HMOs may be misleading because a large proportion of enrollees who are not satisfied with their care withdraw from membership, thus eliminating their participation in consumer satisfaction surveys (Health Advocate, 1998).

Fiscal Stability of Service-Providing Agencies

Many of the features that characterize managed care threaten the fiscal stability of the agencies that support the delivery of care. Reduced reimbursement levels, increased reimbursement processing time, increases in the frequency of reimbursement denials, increased administrative costs, reductions in coverage, and reduced access for some patient populations are all factors that threaten agencies' clinical revenues. A recent surge in staffing reductions, modifications of salaried contracts to hourly contracts based on billable services, implementation of rigorous clinical-productivity standards, and dramatic dissolution of numerous rehabilitation companies and private practices is indicative of the current fiscal pressure on providers.

Because the majority of persons with aphasia are older than the age of 65, two of the most drastic threats to U.S. agencies that support intervention for aphasia have been Medicare's prospective-payment system (PPS), implemented in varied forms since 1983, and Medicare's payment cap for outpatient rehabilitation services, implemented in varied forms since 1999 (Moore, 1999). Both of these measures were implemented by the Center for Medicare and Medicaid Services.

Prospective-payment systems affect inpatient services in inpatient rehabilitation and long-term-care facilities in particular. Rather than being reimbursed for actual costs incurred, or for actual services rendered, facilities are paid a flat daily rate based on the conditions of individual residents. The rates are calculated with complex formulas involving resource-utilization group (RUG) classifications and case-mix data. RUG classifications are based on studies of the actual time clinicians from multiple disciplines spent caring for patients with a variety of conditions as assessed through a standardized assessment scheme, known as the Minimum Data Set (MDS) (regularly updated). Case-mix data are based on RUG classifications of a facility's residents. Applying what is known as the "75% rule," CMS requires that at least 75% of patients admitted to inpatient rehabilitation hospitals have one of 13 qualifying diagnoses (updated from 10 in 2004). While the intent is reasonable to prevent rehabilitation centers from providing services that could be provided through less costly means in less-intensive care environments, the effect on quality of care is compromised. Having government fiscal policy rather than qualified medical providers determine which patients may receive which services is far from an optimal means of clinical decision-making. Worse, even when the latest CMS plan was first being phased in during 2005 (with only 50% compliance expected), patients had dramatically reduced access to rehabilitation hospitals (Moran Company, 2005).

Inpatient rehabilitation hospitals are vital to the restoration of health, independence, and functional abilities of many patients discharged from acute-care hospitals but not ready to return home. Patients who do not have one of the 13 allowable diagnoses now have longer acute-care stays, are transferred to nursing homes, or are discharged to their homes. Many nursing homes and home-health-care agencies do not have the equipment, staff, or expertise to address the medical or rehabilitation needs of patients with complex medical conditions, including cognitive and communicative disorders. Even the financial savings targeted through the CMS policy are not assured. The savings involved in reduced cost-of-care in the short term does not stem the long-term costly needs for care of patients who have not had appropriate care and rehabilitation to begin with (U.S. Government Accountability Office, 2005). Given the frequently complex medical conditions and the common need for intensive rehabilitation of persons with neurogenic communication disorders, the advocacy role of clinical aphasiologist's in light of such managed care trends is vital.

Medicare's payment cap for outpatient rehabilitation services (Medicare Part B) involves a limit ($1,740 at the close of 2006) on payments for both speech-language pathology and physical therapy services, combined. Originally initiated in 1999, the cap dramatically reduces the frequency and duration of treatment that clinicians can provide, and requires clinicians across disciplines to make difficult and often arbitrary decisions about the priority of one treatment over another. Tremendous financial losses have consequently been experienced by long-term-care facilities and rehabilitation providers throughout the United States. The decrease in access to services for persons with neurogenic communication disorders has been equally, if not more, devastating. Following a strong advocacy campaign, this cap was temporarily rescinded in November 1999, but later reinstated. In 2006, an "exceptions" process was implemented, enabling speech-language pathologists to appeal for additional reimbursable treatment based on documentation of a patient's need for additional services. It is incumbent upon clinical aphasiologists to provide sufficient and appropriate documentation to boost patient access to needed rehabilitation services for people with aphasia and related disorders.

Livelihood of Professionals

Given the financial losses to service-providing agencies discussed above, it is not surprising that clinicians, too, are experiencing the effects of managed care in terms of reduced salaries and employment opportunities. Restructuring, re-engineering, consolidation, and down-sizing movements in hospitals, speech and hearing centers, private practices, and rehabilitation companies have had direct and personal impacts on many speech-language clinicians (Henri & Hallowell, 1999b; 2007).

Professional Integrity

Under managed care, many insurance companies, as well as service-providing agencies, are attempting to reduce costs by addressing the expense of employing highly educated and skilled clinicians, such as fully certified and licensed speech-language pathologists. One way they may do this is to employ less costly assistants, technicians, and aides (ASHA, 1996a; Gerard, 1990; Holzemer, 1996). Another is to employ "multiskilled" or "transdisciplinary" professionals who are trained in a variety of medical and rehabilitative diagnostic and treatment methods that were once exclusively in the domain of specific clinical disciplines (ASHA, 1996c). Both of these strategies have resulted in a decrease in the level of skill, education, training, licensure, certification, and overall competence of clinical practitioners, and have yielded tremendous inconsistencies in the quality of care across treatment settings. Although there are merits to some of the arguments for the use of support and/or cross-trained personnel in some environments, it is essential that clinicians advocate for the integrity of their professions (Henri & Hallowell, 1999b), as well as for their specialized expertise in such areas as aphasiology.

Positive Impacts of Managed Care

Not all of managed-care's influences on services available to persons with neurogenic communication disorders are negative. Some of its touted virtues of prevention, cost-saving, accessibility, and accountability have, in fact, impacted our professional practices in positive ways.

Prevention, Access, and Cost

The emphasis of most MCOs on preventive care and health maintenance should ideally reduce the number of people who are affected by stroke, traumatic brain injury, infectious processes, and so on, and thus may help to prevent some communication disorders. Additionally, the reduced cost of insurance coverage for most people who enroll in MCOs enhances the accessibility of coverage. While we lament the decline in revenues for our clinical services, we must also recognize that the continuous escalation of health-care costs from the 1960s through the early 1990s could not continue. Many practitioners and agencies representing the whole array of health-care disciplines are known to have abused the lucrative insurance-billing opportunities within the traditional indemnity fee-for-service modes of operation. Certainly, some reductions in reimbursement and coverage are truly outrageous, having no relevance to patients' actual needs or to actual expenses incurred in offering our services; the Medicare cap shared among speech-language pathologists and physical therapists is a good but unfortunate example. Even in the realm of aphasiology, there have been ongoing abuses of systems that allow for continuous high-cost hourly billing for frequent sessions, and long-lasting treatment programs that are not necessarily optimal in terms of achieving positive functional outcomes.

Accountability and Enhancement of Research

A related and critically important positive impact of health-care restructuring is that it demands increased accountability of clinicians, service-providing agencies, and clinical professions. Scientific evidence of our treatment efficacy and treatment outcomes is being far more carefully scrutinized than ever. This scrutiny has increased awareness of our great need for a richer empirical base of research with which to justify our interventions. Thus, we have been driven to improve the quantity and quality of clinical research in our discipline (Boston, 1994; Sarno, 1998).

Another facet of our heightened accountability is that clinicians are now required to ensure that services provided address important life-affecting changes in clients and patients, and that those services are necessary. Clinicians were once typically trained to think of treatment in terms of clinical performance–based objectives (e.g., those pertaining to grammatical structures, articulator placement, or speech sound discrimination), remote from practical communication in real-world contexts. Now we have been challenged to reformulate our diagnostic and treatment methods to better address "functional outcomes," a concept that is addressed repeatedly in this book.

It is troublesome that the new evidence-based medical-necessity clauses of some MCOs impose unreasonable restrictions on the types of evidence required to justify treatments. It is also troublesome that such clauses often encourage denial of the communicative, cognitive, and psychosocial needs of patients, in favor of the treatment of physical impairments that are not always as life-affecting. Still, clinicians in the past were probably far too liberal in providing services that were not necessarily based in solid scientific research and theory. Further, the resources they had in the treatment-outcomes and efficacy literature to support their treatment approaches were lacking.

The fact that third-party payers and government-sponsored health-care plans now require solid evidence to justify reimbursement has stimulated concerted research and publication efforts on the part of our professional organizations, researchers, and clinicians. Some university research and teaching programs in communication sciences and disorders have reorganized research priorities over the past 10 years, such that clinical research is valued in academic cultures more than it had been previously. Likewise, private, state, and federal funding opportunities for research involving treatment outcomes and treatment efficacy have increased. The continued expansion of controlled research regarding our clinical practices will undoubtedly help us not only justify our services, but also learn better ways to diagnose, treat, and make valid prognostic statements about neurogenic communication disorders.

One additional benefit of managed care, reported by health-care administrators, is that clinical professionals are increasingly aware of the financial impact of their individual and agency-wide services on the financial well-being of their employing agencies. In contexts in which clinicians once performed clinical duties without engaging in the monitoring of clinical revenues, clinicians now frequently play a vital role in business and financial-planning teamwork within their agencies. This change appears to have increased clinicians' sense of ownership for their agencys' operations. Likewise, employers report being impressed with the improved business savvy of their clinical employees (Henri & Hallowell, 1997, 1999b).

Gender Influences on Salary and Status

Wage rates are influenced primarily by the gender composition of specific occupations; low salary and low status are linked to the preponderance of women in a profession (U.S. Government Accountability Office, 2003). Women consistently make less money than men in almost every industry (Bayard, Hellerstein, Newmark, & Troske, 2003; Isaacs, 1995; Schwartz, 1988; Signer, 1988). According to a recent Department of Labor report, women's median weekly full-time wage and salary earnings in 2001 were about 75% of those of men with the same experience (U.S. Government Accountability Office, 2003). Since women make up 75% of the health-care work force, salaries are low throughout the health-care professions.

Not surprisingly, there is also a strong relationship between gender and status. The health-care labor force is notorious for its hierarchical status and power differences between high-ranking and low-ranking workers. For example, despite the long-time predominance of women (over 90%) in the field of communication sciences and disorders (ASHA, 2006), men have continued to represent the majority of directors and heads of programs in the field (c.f., Signer, 1988).

Because women sometimes contribute only secondarily to income, they may not assert their right to a salary commensurate with their training and professional status. The lower salaries in our profession are also tied to inadequate marketing of our scope of practice and the perceived value of our services (Holley, 1988).

THE ULTIMATE EXCELLENT APHASIOLOGIST

What constitutes the ultimate excellent clinical aphasiologist? What factors characterize the very best clinicians? There certainly are not definitive answers to these questions, as the skills and qualities needed for excellence differ according to the contexts in which we work, the patients and colleagues with whom we work, and the nature of our specific professional responsibilities. One must recognize that the degree of excellence perceived is relative to the person who perceives it. A list of prescriptive features indicating what constitutes the "best" aphasiologist may not be appropriate, as diversity in expertise, skills, knowledge, effect, and culture among clinicians is certainly desirable. Still, there are numerous ideal characteristics that we might all aspire to possess.

The excellent aphasiologist is competent. Competent clinicians have a graduate education, national and regional certification in speech-language pathology (in the United States, this means a Certificate of Clinical Competence (CCC) granted by ASHA and, where appropriate, a state license as a speech-language pathologist). They have clinical-practice experience under the supervision and mentorship of seasoned excellent aphasiologists (Kovach & Moore, 1992). They also demonstrate outstanding oral and written communication skills; use only high-caliber assessment and intervention techniques; foster maximum self-determination on the part of patients (Cormier & Cormier, 1991); maintain an effective climate that contributes positively to the therapeutic relationship (Rogers, 1969); provide inspiration, motivation, encouragement, and leadership to patients and their significant others as well as to colleagues; are flexible and adapt well to change; and integrate the personal, scientific, and artistic parts of themselves to achieve a balance of interpersonal, intellectual, and technical competence.

The excellent aphasiologist is knowledgeable. Knowledgeable clinicians are able to reason scientifically, incorporate new findings, and generate new applications. They use knowledge effectively and think and learn independently. They are committed to interdisciplinary study, and have formal and informal training in the arts and sciences, including not only speech-language pathology and audiology, but also cognitive sciences, psychology, linguistics, education, medicine (especially neurology), statistics, computer science, manual communication and other modern languages, business and health administration, economics, gerontology, sociology, anthropology, music, and counseling. They have training and experience in the effective management of communication problems resulting not only from stroke, but also those associated with traumatic brain injury, dementia, movement disorders, infectious processes, neoplasms, and confusional states. Likewise, knowledgeable clinicians are familiar with multiple aspects of aging, and are abreast of the latest research regarding "normal" versus "disordered" aspects of language, conversational discourse, speech, voice, and hearing (Worrall & Hickson, 2003). Their knowledge base is constantly expanding as they read the current professional literature, take advantage of continuing-education opportunities, and learn from their colleagues and patients. They have a profound sense of inquiry, and are open to questioning and exploration (Rogers, 1969). They complement their knowledge with keen insight in managing simple and complex cases.

The excellent aphasiologist is sensitive to issues of gender, age, culture, race, sexual orientation, and socioeconomic status. Sensitive clinicians appreciate multiculturalism and multilingualism, and familiarize themselves with, and celebrate, differences and similarities among their patients and colleagues. Some have been raised in bilingual or multilingual environments. Others strive to learn additional languages in order to expand opportunities for communication and, when possible, to provide services in more than one language. They are aware of the relative lack of persons from culturally diverse populations in the profession of communication sciences and disorders and support strategic efforts to recruit, educate, mentor, support, and retain multicultural clinicians (Wallace & Freeman, 1991). Sensitive clinicians are aware of biases—their own and those of others—and examine the basis for any unreasoned distortion of judgment. They strive to resolve their own prejudices through education, exposure, and sensitivity training.

The excellent aphasiologist is ethical. Ethical clinicians are aware of conflicts of interest and work to resolve personal wants and needs without compromising the appropriateness of their actions (Hirsch, 1994). They are unfailingly honest. They follow their professional codes of ethics, obey all laws, and adhere to their own personal solid moral codes.

The excellent aphasiologist is professional. His or her primary goal is high-quality, first-rate patient care. Effective clinicians have a rationale for everything they do, and communicate that rationale, whenever possible, to patients and the patients' clinicians from other disciplines. They foster responsible participation in the selection of goals, in ways of reaching those goals, and in the development of appropriate attitudes and skills, such as personal responsibility for learning and improvement. They critique, assess, monitor, and

edit their own behavior. They interact effectively with the entire rehabilitation team. They treat colleagues with respect, courtesy, fairness, and good faith (Cormier & Cormier, 1991). They maintain records and reports accurately and completely and keep them up-to-date. They consistently protect clients' privacy and confidentiality, initiate proper referrals and recommendations, and exhibit proper follow-through. They have definite but malleable professional and personal goals and defined ways of reaching those goals.

The excellent aphasiologist is warm, caring, patient, empathetic, and compassionate. The ultimate excellent clinical aphasiologist is sensitive to client-centered and significant-other-centered needs in providing maximally effective services. His or her empathetic and compassionate nature helps to foster feelings of comfort, safety, and confidence among patients, significant others, and collaborating professionals. He or she addresses current events in clients' and families' lives, honors each significant other, listens thoughtfully to their needs, and tailors sessions to meet those needs (Brown, 2005). He or she has effective listening skills (Brownell, 2002). He or she is aware of nonverbal communication messages and is skilled in interpreting them.

The excellent aphasiologist is a thoughtful, motivated, interesting person. Excellent clinicians fit Ringel's definition of "gifted scientists" who are "individualistic, open-minded, freedom-loving, highly motivated, fiercely independent, imaginative, nonconformist and usually critical of the status quo" (Ringel, 1982, p. 401). They are also genuinely motivated to help others (Minifie, 1983), and have a terrific sense of humor, a love of people, a commitment to service, and a passion for patient and professional advocacy. They have weaknesses and failures, and acknowledge and grow through them with grace. Although aware of their assets, they are humble.

The excellent aphasiologist is emotionally healthy. Healthy clinicians serve as role models to clinicians in training, colleagues, consumers, and others in terms of health maintenance, stress management, life-style balance, and self-esteem. They have familiarized themselves with books on healthy interpersonal interaction and intimacy, and understand the fundamentals of interpersonal relationships, which include communication, active listening, previous familial patterning, emotional expression, and the development of compassion and understanding for another. They continue to learn how to cultivate healthy relationships and to love and be loved unconditionally. They avoid professional burnout, actively balancing their psychological resources with the demands of their jobs.

FUTURE TRENDS

Demographic trends will certainly continue to play an important role in aphasia intervention. With post-World War generations growing older and living longer than ever before, and with fewer children being born, attention to issues affecting older adults is steadily growing. Public and private retirement and medical programs will necessarily evolve with increasing focus on the elderly over the next few decades (Mechanic, 1999). The aging of the population brings with it increased risks for catastrophic disease, illness, and disability (Kaplan, Haan, & Wallace, 1999), including adult aphasia. Enhanced consumer education and new methods to prevent stroke and traumatic brain injury will help address these risks.

Other demographic trends, such as the growth of racial, ethnic, and linguistic minority populations in the United States, will continue to stimulate our constructive actions to meet the needs of the members of such populations. Increases in certain patient populations, such as those with HIV/AIDS, in our caseloads (ASHA, 1989; ASHA Committee on Quality Assurance, 1990; Flower & Sooy, 1987; Larsen, 1998) will require that we engage in ongoing research pertaining to relatively new areas of clinical practice.

As new formulae for practice under changing modes of service delivery continue to evolve, we will continue to see further positive effects on our professions, such as more efficient and increasingly outcomes-focused treatments, new types of employment opportunities, and improved interdisciplinary teamwork in the coordination of patient care, co-treatment, and discharge planning. At the same time, we are likely to see more women in leadership roles.

Over the next few decades, we will draw on the evolving empirical research base to enhance our methods for improving our patients' quality of life, independence, and medical management. We will take advantage of technologic advancements that will influence virtually every one of our many professional roles. We will also continue to adapt constructively to reduced patient access, both through advocacy for improved access and through the use of alternative models of intervention and caregiver training.

As the research base on treatment efficacy, cost-effectiveness, and outcomes continues to grow, we will become increasingly sophisticated about the appropriate patterns of practice associated with patients' specific diagnostic characteristics. More and more clinical agencies will implement "clinical pathways," or optimal plans for diagnostic and treatment services that take into account the nature and severity of patients' deficits and time post-onset. Likewise, guidelines concerning the common best practices given a patient's diagnosis, such as ASHA's "Preferred Practice Patterns" (ASHA 1993, 1996b), will undoubtedly continue to be refined.

The specialty of neurogenic communication disorders will benefit from clinicians who are dedicated to fostering all of the characteristics that constitute the "ultimate excellent aphasiologist." The active role that aphasiologists play as advocates for our clients and profession is critical to maximizing our effectiveness.

KEY POINTS

1. Throughout the world, changes in health-care policy, reimbursement schemes, national health plans, political climates, insurance mechanisms, clinical licensure, and professional training are having dramatic impacts on access to patients and the services we deliver to them.

2. Gerontologic issues that affect aphasia intervention include the rapid growth of the aging population worldwide, the extension of life expectancy, and the fact that women live an average of 7 years longer than men. Multiple dimensions of age-related health concerns are discussed, including chronological, biological, and behavioral age and successful ageing and wellness. Ageism is seen as the systematic stereotyping and discriminating against people because of age. The cultural roots and harmful impact of ageism, internalized ageism, and ageism and Civil Rights are explored. Gender and ageism, or the fact that a good deal of age-related discrimination targets older women, and the financial aspects of aging, are explored.

3. Speech-language pathologists rehabilitate patients with aphasia in a variety of contexts such as hospitals, rehabilitation centers, skilled-nursing facilities, nursing homes, clinics, private offices, and the patient's own home. In addition, "telehealth," or the use of electronic communications technologies, may provide and/or support health-care services.

4. The clinical aphasiologist performs many of the same functions regardless of professional setting, such as the identification and selection of clients; assessment; intervention; consultation and collaborative care; counseling; administration; quality assurance; contract negotiation; education; marketing; fundraising; advocacy; ethical decision-making; and research.

5. Legislative issues affecting service delivery in the United States include several pieces of legislation to ensure that persons of all ages with special conditions have access to adequate and appropriate levels of service. In the United States, the Health Insurance Portability and Accountability Act (HIPAA) requires that health plans standardize, streamline, and safeguard the transmission of individually identifiable health information among carriers and providers.

6. The delivery of diagnostic and intervention services is heavily influenced by economics. In the U.S., recent impacts of managed care in the private sector and

evolving federal health policies are significantly impacting the practice of aphasiology. For example, in the U.S., individuals are insured primarily through private health insurance programs, the majority through plans offered by employers as part of a benefits package. In addition to private insurance programs, two federal health programs, Medicare and Medicaid, influence service delivery to adults in the United States. Managed-care practice is having a dramatic influence on service delivery. The three main goals most frequently stated are assurance of the quality and coordination of care, access to care for persons who need it, and cost control. Specific cost-control mechanisms are discussed. Unfortunately, the literature is replete with accounts of how the overwhelming focus on cost control in managed care often leads to compromises in quality and access.

7. Managed care organizations (MCOs) are insurance companies or programs that operate in managed-care modes and are characterized by the use of specific types of cost-saving reimbursement schemes, the promotion of health and wellness through preventive care and education; a concerted effort to coordinate the type and number of services received by each enrollee; and reduced enrollment fees for enrollees and/or the employers who pay for enrollees' insurance coverage. There are many types of MCOs. The two most common examples are preferred-provider organizations (PPOs) and health-maintenance organizations (HMOs).

8. Restructuring of health-care systems to reduce costs has transferred control of the access to, and duration of, care from clinicians to administrators. Although efforts to control rising health-care costs are laudable, such efforts often threaten patients' access to care and the quality of care they receive.

9. Key challenges to professional practice in neurogenic communication disorders are consumers' access to our services; the quality, intensity, duration, and frequency of care that we can provide; the fiscal stability of our service-providing agencies; the livelihood of our professionals; the maintenance of our professional integrity; and problems of consumers' access to our services.

10. The ultimate excellent aphasiologist is seen as one who is competent, knowledgeable, ethical, professional, warm, caring, patient, empathetic, and compassionate, and a thoughtful, motivated, interesting person who is emotionally healthy.

1. Compare and contrast the type of collaborative care and teamwork in which aphasiologists are likely to be engaged within their varied employment contexts.

2. For each of the varied employment contexts, consider which of the many roles of the aphasiologist are most emphasized.

3. Discuss the ways in which employment in each of the different service delivery contexts might affect the quality of life of clinicians.

4. Develop a Web page, flier, or brochure to provide information about community resources available to people with aphasia and their significant others in your local community. Be sure to think broadly about the types of referrals for information, support, and clinical-care options from which your patients might benefit.

5. Imagine that you are team-teaching a graduate course on neurogenic communication disorders and that you have agreed to teach the component addressing the importance and relevance of gerontology to aphasia intervention. Outline the key topics that you would cover in your component on the course. Given time constraints, which topics would you prioritize as most important?

6. Develop a position statement for aphasiologists stating how changing the way that older women are viewed and valued may reduce the prejudice experienced by female patients.

7. In what ways is excellence in documentation critical to the success of the aphasiologist?

8. Describe the ways in which recent service-delivery trends have influenced where (in what type of service-delivery context) persons with neurogenic communication disorders receive treatment.

9. How do reductions in stays in acute-care hospitals impact what the speech-language clinician accomplishes in the acute care context?

10. How do reductions in the frequency and duration of treatment programs for patients with aphasia influence intervention?

11. List specific ways in which aphasiologists may engage actively in quality assurance, marketing, contract negotiation, and fundraising.

12. Describe what you think are the most critical ethical issues for aphasiologists. What might be done to alleviate some of the ethical dilemmas and conflicts of interest that clinicians face in the workplace?

13. In what ways might the full-time clinician without doctoral training participate in research?

14. Make an outline of both positive and negative service-delivery trends that are influencing intervention for adults with aphasia and related disorders. For each of the negative trends, list and discuss specific ways in

which you may act strategically as an advocate to lessen the negative effects for your patients and your profession. List and discuss the specific ways in which you might capitalize on each of the positive trends to improve service for your patients.

15. Consider this hypothetical case: You are an SLP who is treating Mr. Comet, a 48-year-old man who recently suffered a CVA. He is enrolled in an HMO. Mr. Comet's physician, his primary medical provider, has a contract with the patient's HMO. She had authorized one evaluation and six treatment sessions to address speech and language problems secondary to the CVA. You have exhausted those authorized sessions. Now the physician refuses to authorize any further treatment from your discipline. You have ample evidence that Mr. Comet's communication deficits are having a significant impact on his safety, his medical management, his ability to live independently, and his quality of life. You are confident that he is an appropriate candidate for treatment and that you have effective strategies to implement in a treatment program for him. What specific steps will you take to advocate effectively for Mr. Comet's continued access to your services?

16. How would you describe the ultimate excellent clinical aphasiologist? What are your own strengths and weaknesses relative to your view of the ideal clinician?

▶ *Acknowledgment*—This work was supported in part by a grant DC00153-01A1 from the National Institute on Deafness and Other Communication Disorders. Thanks to Meggan Moore and Laurie Turner for editorial assistance.

References

AARP Public Policy Institute. (2002). Women and long-term care (Fact Sheet). Washington, DC: Author.

American Medical Association. (1999). *Coding Current Procedural Terminology, CPT™ 2000*. Chicago, IL: American Medical Association.

American Speech-Language-Hearing Association. (1986). The delivery of speech-language and audiology services in home care. *ASHA, 28*(5), 49–52.

American Speech-Language-Hearing Association. (1989). AIDS/HIV: Implications for speech-language pathologists and audiologists. *ASHA, 31*(6–7), 33–37.

American Speech-Language-Hearing Association. (1993). Preferred practice patterns for the professions of speech-language pathology and audiology. *ASHA, 35*(3), (Suppl. 11).

American Speech-Language-Hearing Association (1996a). Guidelines for the training, credentialing, use, and supervision of speech-language pathology assistants. *ASHA, 38*(Suppl. 16), 21–34.

American Speech-Language-Hearing Association. (1996b). *Preferred practice patterns for the professions of speech-language pathology and audiology*. Rockville, MD: American Speech-Language Hearing Association.

American Speech-Language-Hearing Association. (1996c). Technical report of the Ad Hoc Committee on Multiskilling. *ASHA, 38* (Suppl. 16), 53–61.

American Speech-Language-Hearing Association. (1997). *Marketing manual: A reference guide*. Retrieved October 24, 2006, from http://www.asha.org/NR/rdonlyres/A8E40FD8-F3EE-4207-8D65-D2ABEC15C5C6/0/MarketingManual.pdf

American Speech-Language-Hearing Association. (2005). Quality indicators for professional service programs in audiology and speech-language pathology standards [Quality Indicators]. Retrieved October 1, 2007 from asha.org/policy.

American Speech-Language-Hearing Association. (2006). *Highlights and trends: ASHA member counts*. Retrieved October 20, 2006, from http://asha.org/about/membership-certification/member-counts.htm

American Speech-Language-Hearing Association Committee on Quality Assurance. (1990). AIDS/HIV: Implications for speech-language pathologists and audiologists. *ASHA, 32*, 46–48.

Anderson, N., & Anderson, P. E. (2003). *Emotional longevity: What really determines how long you live*. New York: Viking.

Andrews, M. (1999). The seductiveness of agelessness. *Ageing and Society, 19*, 301–318.

Bayard, K., Hellerstein, J., Newmark, D., & Troske, K. (2003). The new evidence on sex segregation and sex differences in wages from matched employee–employer data. *Journal of Labor Economics, 21*.

Begley, C. E. (1987). Prospective payment and medical ethics. *Journal of Medicine and Philosophy, 12*, 107–122.

Bergeman, C. S. (1997). *Aging: Genetic and environmental influences*. Thousand Oaks, CA: SAGE.

Berman, M., & Fenaughty, A. (2005). Technology and managed care: patient benefits of telemedicine in a rural health care network. *Health Economics, 14*, 559–573.

Boston, B. O. (1994). Destiny is in the data: A wake-up call for outcome measures. *American Speech-Language and Hearing Association, 36*, 35–38.

Brown, N. A. (2005). Information on telemedicine. *Journal of Telemedicine and Telecare, 11*, 117–126.

Brownell, J. (2002). *Listening: Attitudes, principles, and skills*. Boston: Allyn and Bacon.

Butler, I., Carpenter, E., Kay, B., & Simmons, R. (1969). *Sex and status in the workforce*. Washington, DC: American Public Health Association.

Clement, D. G., Retchin, S. M., Brown, R. S., & Stegall, M. H. (1994). Access and outcomes of elderly patients enrolled in managed care. *Journal of the American Medical Association, 271*(19), 1487–1492.

Cohn, R. (1994). Strategies for positioning in the managed health care marketplace. *Journal of Hand Therapy, 7*, 5–9.

Comfort, A. (1976). *A good age*. New York: Crown.

Copper, B. (1988). *Over the hill: Reflections on ageism between women*. Freedom, CA.: Crossing Press.

Cormier, W. H., & Cormier, L. S. (1991). *Interviewing strategies for helpers*. Pacific Grove, CA: Brooks/Cole.

Council on Ethical and Judicial Affairs, American Medical Association. (1995). Ethical issues in managed care. *Journal of the American Medical Association, 273*(4), 330–335.

Cruickshank, M. (2003). *Learning to be old: Gender, culture and aging.* New York: Rowman and Littlefield.

Darley, F. L. (1982). *Aphasia.* Philadelphia: W.B. Saunders.

Davolt, S. (1999). Network providers find strength in numbers. *ASHA Leader, 4*(10), 1, 8.

Daw, J. (2001). Culture Counts in mental health services. *Monitor on Psychology, 32*(11).

Dettinger, E., & Clarkberg, M. (2002). Informal caregiving and retirement timing among men and women: Gender and caregiving relationships in late midlife. *Journal of Family Issues, 23*(7), 857–879.

Doolittle, G. C., Otto, F., & Clemens, C. (1998). Hospice care using homebased telemedicine systems. *Journal of Telemedicine and Telecare, 4*, 58–59.

Duffy, J. R., Werven, G. W., & Aronson, A. E. (1997). Telemedicine and the diagnosis of speech and language disorders. *Mayo Clinic Proceedings, 72*, 1116–1122.

Ewart, C. (1991). Social action theory for a public health psychology. *American Psychologist, 46*(9), 931–942.

Family Caregiver Alliance (2006). *Women and caregiving: Facts and figures.* Retrieved October 16, 2006: http://www.caregiver.org/caregiver/jsp/content_node.jsp?nodeid=892.

Field, M. J. (Ed.). (1996). *Telemedicine: A guide to assessing telecommunications in health care.* Washington, DC: National Academy Press.

Fisher, R. S. (1994). Medicaid managed care: The next generation? *Academic Medicine, 69*(5), 317–322.

Flower, W., & Sooy, D. (1987). AIDS: An introduction for speech-language pathologists and audiologists. *ASHA, 29*, 25–30.

Fox, H. B., Wicks, L. B., & Newacheck, P. W. (1993). State Medicaid health maintenance organization policies and special-needs children. *Health Care Financing Review, 15*, 25–37.

Gallagher, T. (2006). US doctoral education: Critical shortages and plans for reshaping the future. *Folia Phonoiatrica et Logopaedica, 58*(1), 32–35.

Geffner, D. (1997). Growing the field: Who will teach future generations? *ASHA, 39*(37–38), 40–42.

Gerard, R. (1990). Preparing a multiskilled work force for the 21st century hospital. *Journal of Biocommunication, 17*(4), 24–26.

Gill, H. S. (1995). The changing nature of ambulatory rehabilitation programs and services in a managed care environment. *Archives of Physical Medicine and Rehabilitation, 76*, SC10–SC15.

Glykas, M., & Chytas, P. (2004). Technology assisted speech and language therapy. *International Journal of Medical Informatics, 73*, 529–541.

Goplerud, E. (2004). Performance measurement likely to improve quality of care. *Alcoholism and Drug Abuse Weekly, 16*(31), 5–6.

Grey, J. E. (1990a). Conflict of interest (part 1). *Healthcare Forum, 33*, 25–28.

Grey, J. E. (1990b). Conflict of interest (part 2). *Healthcare Forum, 33*, 96–99.

Hallowell, B., & Clark, H. (2002, May). Dysphagia is taking over: Lowered priorities for aphasia services under managed care. Paper presented at the Clinical Aphasiology Conference. Ridgedale, MO.

Hallowell, B., & Henri, B. (2007). Strategically promoting access to speech-language pathology and audiology services. In Lubinski, R., Golper, L. A. C., & Frattali, S. (Eds.), *Professional issues in speech-language pathology and audiology* (2nd Ed). San Diego: Singular, pp. 387–408.

Hallowell, B., & Katz, R. C. (1999). Technological applications in the assessment of acquired neurogenic communication and swallowing disorders in adults. *Seminars in Speech, Language, and Hearing, 20*(2), 149–167.

Health Advocate (1998, Winter). Medicare HMOs with high rates of voluntary disenrollment fully accredited. *Health Advocate, 191*, Los Angeles, CA: National Health Law Program, 8.

Henri, B. P., & Hallowell, B. (1996). Action planning for advocacy: Issues for speech-language pathologists and audiologists in the face of the expansion of managed care. HEARSAY: *Journal of the Ohio Speech and Hearing Association, 11*(1), 61–64.

Henri, B. P., & Hallowell, B. (1997). Ethics and clinical productivity pressures under managed care. *Newsletter of Special Interest Division 11 (Administration and Supervision) of the American Speech-Language-Hearing Association.* Rockville, MD: American Speech-Language-Hearing Association.

Henri, B. P., & Hallowell, B. (1999a). Funding alternatives to offset the consequences of managed care. *Newsletter of Special Interest Division 2 (Neurophysiology and Neurogenic Speech and Language Disorders) of the American Speech-Language-Hearing Association.* Rockville, MD: American Speech-Language-Hearing Association.

Henri, B. P., & Hallowell, B. (1999b). Relating managed care to managing care. In B.S. Cornett (Ed.), *Clinical practice management in speech-language pathology: Principles and practicalities.* Gaithersburg, MD: Aspen, pp. 3–28.

Henri, B. P., Hallowell, B., & Johnson, C. (1996). Advocacy and marketing to support clinical services. In R. Kreb (ed.), *A practical guide to treatment outcomes and cost effectiveness* (pp. 39–48). Rockville, MD: American Speech-Language-Hearing Association Task Force on Treatment Outcomes and Cost Effectiveness.

Hickman, C. S., & Dyer, W. M. (1998). Improving telemedicine consultation with TeleDoc and the emergent technologies. In M. L. Armstrong (Ed.), *Telecommunications for health professionals* (pp. 204–214). New York: Springer.

Hiller, M. D., & Lewis, J. B. (1995). Managed health care benefit plans: What are the ethical issues? *Trends in Health Care, Law & Ethics, 10*(1, 2), 109–112, 118.

Hirsch, B. D. (1994). Risky business: Financial incentives in managed care warrant regulation. *Texas Medicine, 90*(12), 30–33.

Holley, S. (1988). Marketing your services. *ASHA, 30*(9), 37–38.

Holzemer, W. L. (1996). The impact of multiskilling on quality of care. *International Nursing Review, 41*(1), 21–25.

IBM (1999). *About IBM.* [on-line]. Available: http://www.ibm.com/ibm/

Inglehart, J. K. (1995). Health policy report—Medicaid and managed care. *The New England Journal of Medicine, 332*(25), 1727–1731.

Isaacs, E. (1995). Gender discrimination in the workplace: A literature review. *Communications of the ACM, 38*(1), 58–59.

Kaplan, G. A., Haan, M. N., & Wallace, R. B. (1999). Understanding changing risk factor associations with increasing age in adults. *Annual Review of Public Health, 20*, 89–108.

Katz, R. C., & Hallowell, B. (1999). Technological applications in the treatment of acquired neurogenic communication and swallowing disorders in adults. *Seminars in Speech, Language, and Hearing, 20*(3), 251–269.

Katz, R., Hallowell, B., Code, C., Armstrong, E., Roberts, P., Pound, C., & Katz, L. (2000). A multinational comparison of aphasia management practices. *International Journal of Language and Communication Disorders, 35*(2), 303–314.

Kerr, P. (1992, April 3). Cutting costs of brain injuries. *New York Times*, p. D1–D2.

Khazei, A., Jarvis-Selinger, S., Ho, K., & Lee, A. (2005). An assessment of the Telehealth needs and health-care priorities of Tanna Island: A remote, under-served and vulnerable population. *Journal of Telemedicine and Telecare, 11*, 35–40.

Kinsella, K., & Velkoff, V. (2001). *An aging world: 2001.* Washington, D.C.: U.S. Government Printing Office.

Kovach, T., & Moore, S. (1992). Leaders are born through the mentoring process. *ASHA, 34*(1), 33–34.

Labovitz, G. (1991). The total quality health care revolution. *Quality Process, 24*(9), 45–50.

Larsen, C. R. (1998). *HIV-1 and communication disorders: What speech and hearing professionals need to know.* San Diego: Singular.

Leff, B., Burton, L, Mader, S. L. Naughton, B., Burl, J., Inouye, S. K., Greenought, W. B., Guido, S., Langston, C., Frick, K. S., Steinwachs, D., & Burton, J. (2005). Hospital at home: Feasibility and outcomes of a program to provide hospital-level care at home for acutely ill older patients. *Annals of Internal Medicine, 143*(11), 798–808.

Leigh, W. A. (1994). Implications of health-care reform proposals for Black Americans. *Journal of Health Care for the Poor and Underserved, 5*(1), 17–32.

Levin, J., and Levin, W. (1980). *Ageism.* Belmont, CA.: Wadsworth.

Marks, N. Lambert, J. D., & Choi, H. (2002). Transitions to caregiving, gender, and psychological well-being: A prospective U.S. national study. *Journal of Marriage and Family, 64*, 657–667.

Markson, E., & Taylor, C. (2000). The mirror has two faces. *Aging and Society, 20*, 137–160.

Martinez, A., Villarroel, V., Seoane, J., & Del Pozo, F. (2004). A study of a rural telemedicine system in the Amazon region of Peru. *Journal of Telemedicine and Telecare, 10*, 219–225.

Mashima, P. A., Birkmire-Peters, D. P., Syms, M. J., Holtel, M. R., Burgess, L. P. A., & Peters, L. J. (2003). Telehealth: Voice therapy using telecommunications technology. *American Journal of Speech-Language Pathology, 12*, 432–439.

McLaurin, D., & Bell, S. (1991). Open communication lines before attempting total quality. *Quality Process, 24*(6), 25–28.

Mechanic, D. (1999). The changing elderly population and future health care needs. *Journal Of Urban Health, 76*(1), 24–38.

Mellancamp, P. (1999). From anxiety to equanimity: Crisis and generational continuity on TV and the movies, in life and in death. In Woodwood, K. (Ed.), *Figuring Age: Women, Bodies, Generations.* Bloomington, IN: Indiana University Press.

Minifie, F. (1983). ASHA from adolescence onward. *ASHA, 25*, 17–24.

Moore, M. (1999). Nursing homes shaken from effects of Medicare reform. *ASHA Leader, 4*(10), 1–4.

The Moran Company. (2005). *New Estimates of the Impact of Enforcement of the "75% Rule" on Inpatient Rehabilitation Services Volume.* Arlington, VA: Report Commissioned by the Federation of American Hospitals and the American Hospital Association.

Murphy, J. (2006). Perceptions of communication between people with communication disability and general practice staff. *Health Expectations, 9*, 49–59.

Myers, M. K. S., Luecke, J., Longan, D., & Revell, T. (1998). Practical aspects of telemedicine from the user's perspective: Neonatology, general medicine, and inmate health care. In M. L. Armstrong (Ed.), *Telecommunications for Health Professionals* (pp. 215–229). New York: Springer.

National Center for Health Statistics (2006). *International Classification of Diseases, 9th Revision, Clinical Modification (ICD-9-CM).* Retrieved October, 24, 2006, from http://www.cdc.gov/nchs/about/otheract/icd9/abticd9.htm.

Oberlander, J. B. (1997). Managed care and Medicare reform. *Journal of Health Politics, Policy and Law, 32*(2), 595–627.

Ogasawara, K., Ito, K., Jiang, G., Endoh, A., Sakurai, T., Sato, H., Okuhara, Y., Adachi, T., & Hori, K. (2003). Preliminary clinical evaluation of a video transmission system for home visits. *Journal of Telemedicine and Telecare, 9*, 292–295.

Palmore, E. (1999). *Ageism* (2nd Ed). NY: Springer.

Perkins, J. (1998). *Managed Care Update.* Los Angeles, CA: National Health Law Program.

Perry, M. (1999). Animated gerontophobia: Ageism, sexism, and the Disney villainess. In S. Deats & L. Kenker, *Ageing and identity: A humanities perspective.* Westport, CT: Praeger.

Peters, T., & Waterman, R. (1982). *In search of excellence.* New York: Warner Books.

Petrosino, L., Lieberman, R. J., & McNeil, M. R. (1997). *1996-97 National Survey of Undergraduate and Graduate Programs.* Minneapolis, MN: Council of Graduate Programs in Communication Sciences and Disorders.

Purtillo, R. B. (1995). Managed care: Ethical issues for the rehabilitation professions. *Trends In Health Care, Law & Ethics, 10*(1/2), 105–108.

Qu, L., & Weston, R. (2003). Ageing, living arrangements, and subjective well-being. *Family Matters, 66*, 26–33.

Quadagno, J. (1999). *Aging and the life course.* Boston: McGraw Hill.

Randall, V. R. (1994). Impact of managed care organizations on ethnic Americans and underserved populations. *Journal of Health Care for the Poor and Underserved, 5*(3), 224–236.

Ringel, R. (1982). Some issues facing graduate education. *ASHA, 24*, 399–404.

Rodwin, M. A. (1995). Conflicts in managed care. *The New England Journal of Medicine, 332*(9), 604–607.

Rogers, C. (1969). *Freedom to Learn.* Columbus, OH: Charles E. Merrill.

Roth, C. R. (1999). Developing and implementing a quality improvement plan in an acute care hospital setting. *Newsletter of Special Interest Division 2 (Neurophysiology and Neurogenic Speech and Language Disorders) of the American Speech-Language-Hearing Association, 9*(2), 24–28.

Russo, M. (1999). Aging and the scandal of anachronism. In K. Woodward (Ed.), *Figuring Age.* Bloomington, IN: Indiana University Press.

Sahs, A. L., & Hartman, E. C. (1976). *Fundamentals of stroke care.* Washington, DC: U.S. Department of Health, Education and Welfare.

Sarno, M. T. (1998). Recovery and rehabilitation in aphasia. In M. T. Sarno (Ed.), *Acquired Aphasia* (pp. 595–631). San Diego: Academic Press.

Schlesinger, R. (2006, June). An expert's view of ageism: Things aren't any better. *AARP Bulletin, 6*.

Schwartz, J. (1988). Closing the gap. *American Demographics, 10*, 56.

Scott, R. (2004). Investigating e-health policy-tools for the trade. *Journal of Telemedicine and Telecare, 10*, 246–248.

Screen, M. R., & Anderson, N. B. (1994). Legal and ethical issues in communication disorders affecting multicultural populations. In *Multicultural perspectives in communication disorders* (pp. 51–64). San Diego: Singular.

Shinn, R., Goldberg, D., Kimelman, M., & Messick, C. (2001). *2000-01 Demographic Survey of Undergraduate and Graduate Programs in Communication Sciences and Disorders.* Retrieved October, 24, 2006, from http:// www.capcsd.org /survey/2002/2000-01DemographicsSurvey.pdf

Sicotte, C., Lehoux, P., Fortier-Blanc, J., & Leblanc, Y. (2003). Feasibility and outcome evaluation of a telemedicine application in speech-language pathology. *Journal of Telemedicine and Telecare, 9*, 253–258.

Signer, M. (1988). The value of women's work. *ASHA, 30*, 24–25.

Smith, G., & Ashbaugh, J. (1995). *Managed care and people with developmental disabilities: A guidebook.* Alexandria, VA: National Association of State Directors of Developmental Disabilities Services.

Stenger, A. (1993). Who will advocate for patients? *Postgraduate Medicine, 94*(7), 108–110.

Thompson, C., & Kearns, K. (1991). Analytical and technical directions in applied aphasia analysis: The Midas touch. In T. Prescott (ed.), *Clinical Aphasiology* (pp. 41–54). Austin, TX: Pro-Ed.

Underhill, B. (1991). "Total" remains bread and butter of total quality management. Letter to editor. *Quality Process, 24*, 8.

U.S. Government Accountability Office (2003). *Women's Earnings: Work Patterns partially explain differences between men's and women's earnings.* Retrieved October 26, 2006, from http:// clk.about.com/?zi=1/XJ&sdn=usgovinfo&zu=http%3A%2F%2Fwww.gao.gov%2Fnew.items%2Fd0435.pdf

U.S. Government Accountability Office (2005). *Little progress made in targeting outpatient therapy payments to beneficiaries' needs.* Retrieved October 28, 2006, from http://www.gao.gov/new.items/d0659.pdf

Varian, T. (1991). Communicating total quality inside the organization. *Quality Progress, 6*, 30–31.

Wachterman, M., & Sommers, B. (2006). The impact of gender and marital status on end-of-life care: Evidence from the national mortality follow-back. *Journal of Palliative Medicine, 9*(2), 343–352

Wallace, G., & Freeman, S. (1991). Adults with neurological improvement from multicultural populations. *ASHA, 33*(67), 58–60.

Wei, J.Y., & Levkoff, S. (2000). *Aging well: The complete guide to physical and emotional health.* New York: John Wiley and Sons, Inc.

Wertz, R. T., Dronkers, N. F., Bernstein-Ellis, E., Sterling, L. K., Shubitkowski, Y., & Elman, R. (1992). Potential of telephonic and television technology for appraising and diagnosing neurogenic communication disorders in remote settings. *Aphasiology, 6*, 195–202.

Whitten, P. (2006). Telemedicine: Communication technologies that revolutionize healthcare services. *Generations, 30*(2), 20–24.

Williams, A., & Giles, H. (1998). Communication of ageism. In M. Hecht (Ed.), *Communicating prejudice.* Thousand Oaks, CA: Sage.

Wilson, L., & Onslow, M. (2004). Telehealth adaptation of the Lidcombe program of early stuttering intervention: Five case studies. *American Journal of Speech-Language Pathology, 13*, 81–93.

Wolfe, S. M. (1994). Quality assessment of ethics in health care: The accountability revolution. *American Journal of Law and Medicine, 20*(1 & 2), 105–128.

Woodward, K. (Ed.) (1999). *Figuring age.* Bloomington, IN: Indiana University Press.

Worrall, L., & Hickson, L. (2003). *Communication disability in aging: From prevention to intervention.* CA: Thomson-Delmar Learning Systems.

APPENDIX 7.1
Selected Helpful References on Aging ·

Albom, M. (1997). *Tuesdays with Morrie: An old man, a young man, and life's greatest lessons*. New York: Doubleday.

Butler, R. (1969). Ageism: Another form of bigotry. *Gerontologist, 9,* 243-246.

Bytheway, B. (1995). *Agism*. Bristol, PA: Open University Press.

Comfort, A. (1976). *A good age*. New York: Crown.

Copper, B. (1988). *Over the hill: Reflections on ageism between women*. Freedom, CA: Crossing Press.

Cruickshank, M. (2003). *Learning to be old: Gender, culture and aging*. New York: Rowman and Littlefield.

Kubler-Ross, E. (1970). *On death and dying*. New York: MacMillan.

Kushner, H. (2001). *When bad things happen to good people*. New York: Schochen Books.

Levin, J. & Levin, W. (1980). *Ageism*. Belmont, CA.: Wadsworth.

Macdonald, B. with Rich, C. (2001). *Look me in the eye: Old women, aging and ageism*. 3rd ed. Minneapolis, MN.: Spinsters Inc.

Palmore, E. (1999). *Ageism*, 2nd ed. New York: Springer.

Quadagno, J. (1999). *Aging and the life course*. Boston: McGraw Hill.

Sheehy, G. (1976). *Passages: Predictable crises of adult life*. New York: E. P. Dutton.

Sheehy, G. (1982). *Pathfinders: Overcoming the crises of adult life and finding your own well-being*. New York: Bantam Books.

Sheehy, G. (1995). *The silent passage: Menopause*. New York: Pocket Books.

Sheehy, G. (1995). *New passages: Mapping your life across time*. New York: Random House.

Walker, B. (1985). *The crone: Women of age, wisdom, and power*. San Francisco: Harper and Row.

Wei, J. Y., & Levkoff, S. (2000). *Aging well: The complete guide to physical and emotional health*. New York: John Wiley and Sons, Inc.

Woodward, K. (1999). *Figuring age*. Bloomington, IN: Indiana University Press.

Worrall, L. & Hickson, L. (2003). *Communication disability in aging: From prevention to intervention*. CA: Thomson-Delmar Learning Systems.

Chapter 8

Teams and Partnerships in Aphasia Intervention

Lee Ann C. Golper

OBJECTIVES

The objectives of this chapter are (1) to define and examine typical team organization designs found in health care delivery; (2) to review basic elements in group processes that lead to successful teams and some of the potential barriers to developing effective teams; (3) to consider how the team designs may differ depending upon the setting and how priorities and the primary decision-makers change across the continuum of recovery from aphasia; (4) to examine related issues, including collaborative evaluations, documentation, outcomes studies, family and patient education, professional education, and research; and (5) to suggest that the overriding aim of the rehabilitation team throughout the recovery continuum with adult aphasia should be directed at educating and empowering patients and families to become collaborative partners, to make use of community and national resources, and ultimately to lead their own "team aphasia."

IT TAKES A VILLAGE

In almost every service arena throughout the world—from emergency rooms to community mental-health clinics—team intervention with a patient-centered emphasis has long been recognized as the optimal approach to health-services delivery (Billups, 1987; Cifu & Stewart, 1999; Collins, Moore, Mitchell, & Alpress, 1999; Davis, Cornman, Lane, & Patton, 2005; Gibbon, 1999; Heikkila, Korpelainen, Turkka, Lallanranta, & Summala, 1999; Hogh et al., 1999; Lott, Hennes, & Dick, 1999; Rosin et al., 1996). This approach necessitates bringing together the knowledge and skills of individuals from many disciplines in order to ensure that complex problems receive the comprehensive attention they require (Allen, Holm, & Scheifelbusch, 1978). As individuals with aphasia move from their hospital beds to their homes, their concerns often shift from surviving the acute event to issues related to finances or changes in their family dynamics. No one discipline can

encompass the whole life-changing condition known as "aphasia." It takes a village. Developing collaborations with others is particularly important throughout the recovery continuum following the onset of aphasia since many patients with aphasia have medical, physical, psychosocial, emotional, recreational, vocational, and financial concerns that may or may not be directly complicated by their communication impairment. Indeed, such issues can supersede the language deficits. Those of us who work with individuals who have communication disorders have long been proponents of family-centered team intervention (Rosin et al., 1996). We rarely evaluate or treat any type of communication disorder without having some amount of collaboration with the patients' families and with other disciplines. Unfortunately, evidence-based guidelines help us determine how to optimally integrate patients and families into the health-care team are largely lacking (D'Amour, Ferrada-Videla, Rodriguez, & Beaulieu, 2005).

WHAT IS A TEAM?

Teams are groups of people collaborating in some way to reach a common goal. Teams can be made up of two people or fifty people. They can have face-to-face meetings or use more indirect communication methods. They can be a formal, structured hierarchy, or a loosely organized group of peers. Usually, teams have at least one designated leader. Teams may have leaders who are authoritarian, controlling the team's actions, or have leaders who function more as facilitators, advising from the sidelines. They may be made up of people from a single discipline or multiple disciplines and can have professional and nonprofessional members. They can be designed to include the patient and family as active participants or can be restricted to an exclusive panel of specialist-consultants. Teams can have smaller teams within them, such as the nursing care team within the rehabilitation care team. Whatever the composition, structure, or purpose, it is important to remember that teams are human enterprises. Teams are made up of people and personalities and they are often "caldrons of bubbling emotions." (Goleman, 1998, p. 101). No team looks or functions exactly like any other. Appreciating that there is no ideal blueprint for teams and that the team design can vary depending on the setting, let's examine a couple of typical models for team processes in health services delivery.

MODELS

The models of team processes most commonly found in health care delivery are either *multidisciplinary* or *interdisciplinary* teams. In education, particularly early intervention, *transdisciplinary* teams are more common. These team models mainly differ in their role delineations and communication processes. Occasionally, the terms multidisciplinary, interdisciplinary, and transdisciplinary seem to be used interchangeably. Thus, it may be helpful to consider the differences between them. In a multidisciplinary model, specialists with clearly defined roles work side by side, each addressing different problems, or different aspects of a given problem. Multidisciplinary teams are probably a good way to characterize how disciplines typically function in an acute care setting, such as on an inpatient medicine or surgery unit. In that setting, various disciplines have defined roles and work cooperatively together, but for the most part they work in parallel, rather than in partnership, with one another. In multidisciplinary teams, individual members bring discipline-specific skills, and the members' responsibilities are clearly defined and understood (Tuchman, 1996). Opportunities for communication between and among the disciplines may be cursory, and shared goals may be lacking (Allen et al., 1978).

Interdisciplinary teams are, by contrast, intended to be interactive and highly collaborative. There is greater emphasis on communication processes in interdisciplinary teams as compared with multidisciplinary teams (Tuchman, 1996). True interdisciplinary teams allow for at least some amount of blurring between traditional professional boundaries. In interdisciplinary teams, different professional disciplines not only work together in a cooperative manner, they also collaborate in partnerships to implement the treatment procedures. In an interdisciplinary format, goals are discussed as "our goals," rather than "OT goals" or "PT goals."

There is very good evidence to suggest that the most effective model for rehabilitation-services teams is an interdisciplinary design. In their review of 79 studies looking at factors affecting outcomes in stroke, Cifu and Stewart (1999) examined the effects of interdisciplinary versus multidisciplinary teams on patient outcomes. They conducted a meta-analysis of 11 well-defined Level I studies, including eight studies in which patients were randomized to either a multidisciplinary medical stroke unit or an interdisciplinary rehabilitation unit. These analyses demonstrate that interdisciplinary team intervention is associated with decreased mortality, improved functional outcomes, shorter lengths of stays, and decreased costs (Cifu & Stewart, 1999). It may be that a key feature to successful outcomes in stroke rehabilitation is not so much having several different disciplines involved in patient care but, rather, establishing good communication and intervention partnerships.

Teams that are truly transdisciplinary tend to be more common in early childhood intervention settings (Rosin et al., 1996). In these settings team members have had specific transdisciplinary orientation and training and are encouraged to practice *role release*. Role release refers to the elimination of traditional professional boundaries in intervention practices (Tuchman, 1996). A transdisciplinary approach to intervention requires incorporating the knowledge and skills from many discipline areas into one multi-skilled practice (Allen et al., 1978). Transdisciplinary teams are most advantageous when intervention requires interfacing a number of related professional disciplines. Although true transdisciplinary teams are rare in hospitals and other health care settings, the transdisciplinary team model is promoted by the Individuals with Disabilities Education Act (IDEA) of 1990, PL 101-476 (Rosin, 1996).

In health-services settings issues such as clinical privileges and licensure restrictions may interfere with forming transdisciplinary teams. In addition, there may be resistance from staff who are not in favor of "cross-training." There was a movement in health service delivery in the past toward encouraging *cross-training* between disciplines and *multi-skilling* within disciplines. Cross-training refers to situations in which staff members are trained to do all or parts of each other's jobs. Cross-training discourages "that's not my job" thinking and encourages staff to feel a part of a team process. For example, ward clerks may be cross-trained with patient-transport personnel so they can cover for each other when needed. Multi-skilling implies having skills that exceed the boundaries of the traditional scopes of practice within a given discipline (Brown & Handlesman, 2006). An example would be training a speech-language pathologist to draw blood, perform range-of-motion exercises, or take blood pressures. Multi-skilling is sometimes viewed as creating minimally skilled technicians with specific skill sets across several areas but without the depth of knowledge needed to make independent decisions. Cross-training and multi-skilling, unfortunately, are concepts that developed in an attempt to save costs. Thus, the notions of cross-training and multi-skilled staff are sometimes viewed with skepticism among licensed professionals and have fallen out of favor in recent years.

TEAM PROCESSES

Group Communication

Much of what we call "interdisciplinary patient care" is just group problem-solving to develop partnerships in interventions through good communication. The key element is communication. Eliciting group problem-solving and group actions involves more than getting together people who have mutually supportive "roles and goals" in patient care.

How well a group of people work together to help one another help patients and their families depends largely on how well communication is managed within the team. Groups of people work together most effectively when two basic elements are in place: (1) group communication processes that encourage interactions, cooperation, and mutual respect, and (2) focused activities aimed at meeting specific objectives or performance measures (Manion, Lorimer, & Leander, 1996).

Researchers looking at small group communication in health-care settings have found the communication characteristics will vary along a continuum, depending upon the nature and purpose of the group (Northouse & Northouse, 1998). Our behavior and the manner in which we participate in groups shifts when the focus of the group is more toward *content-oriented* activities as opposed to *process-oriented* activities (Loomis, 1979). A content-oriented activity is one that is directed toward some *objective* (e.g., discharge planning) or some *performance measure* (e.g., improved functional rating scores). Team activities that are skewed toward content over process are common in health care settings, where everyone feels pressured to make an economic use of time, or in situations where weekly patient care team conferences are viewed by the participants as merely a mandated necessity. Typically, content-oriented patient care teams spend little time in idle chatting or group process, but move directly to the objectives of the meeting. In these settings, reporting information to the group to ensure everyone has a general notion about what the various disciplines are doing with the patient is essentially the extent of the communication. There is not much attention paid to processes that promote good interactions among team members. At meetings that are highly content-oriented, the team members might make their reports in turn, take their respective notes, and then move on to the next task. When communication is focused more on tasks, without attending to group participation, it is difficult to engender good interactive collaborations within the team.

At the other end of the continuum, process-oriented communication is directed toward developing relationships, cooperation, or mutual goals. Process-oriented communication includes group activities such as sharing feelings, brainstorming solutions, supporting one another, and building alliances. Communication itself may be the main purpose. Therapy groups, such as aphasia group therapy or various support groups, are good examples of groups engaged mostly in process-oriented activities.

Interdisciplinary teams need to strike a balance between content and process. Although interdisciplinary patient-care teams are not "support groups," intervention plans often require negotiations between or among disciplines. Consequently, it is important to incorporate process-oriented communication into the group's activities, even when time is limited and several tasks must be accomplished in a short amount of time. In interdisciplinary management, trust and collaboration are essential. Developing good communication processes at the outset of team development tends to discourage polarities. The team members may refer to these activities, affectionately, as "sharing and caring." Time spent building and maintaining mutual trust and open communication between team members is absolutely essential to a successful interdisciplinary team.

CREATING A COHESIVE TEAM

Developing Cohesion

One of the ways corporations and other groups develop a sense of cohesion within a team is to do things like take periodic retreats or engage in similar activities to promote good interpersonal relationships. Team retreats can be anything from wilderness-survival treks to an afternoon away from the office. Usually, retreats are intended to accomplish both group relationship building and goal setting. Managers and group-process facilitators also use devices like personality inventories, such as the Meyers-Briggs Inventory (Meyers-Briggs & Briggs, 1980) as a way for the group members to identify and inventory their individual work styles and consider how these styles differ from one another. Another method to aid in developing group cooperation and reliance is to involve the members in problem-solving games that require teamwork for solutions. Here is an example: A group of health-care providers is divided into teams of four members and each team is given five sheets of standard, 8½″ × 11″ paper. Each team is then asked to solve this problem, "Imagine that the carpet in this room is a raging river and each of your pieces of paper is a stepping stone. Using only your five 'stepping stone' sheets of paper, how can all the members of your team cross the river?" Since just laying down the five sheets of paper end to end would not allow the group to reach the other side of the room, the solution to the problem requires teamwork. The four-member teams solve the problem and cross the room by laying down the sheets of paper ahead of them in a row; and as each member moves forward one step, the last sheet rotates from the member at the tail of the line to the member at the front to take the next step. Thus, each team member moves forward until everyone has reached the opposite "shore." These activities are intended to convey a simple message about teamwork, which is plan together, work together, look out for one another, and we will get to the goal.

In most health care teams, retreats, personality assessments, and group problem-solving games may not be very practical, but there are less elaborate ways to create a sense of membership and trust within the group. Simply engaging in "ice breakers" during the formative team meetings may be sufficient. For example, have members tell the group something about themselves, like: What is the one junk food they would want to have if stranded on a desert island? What was their greatest achievement in high school? What is one of their most embarrassing moments? Just taking a few minutes to get the group talking to one another and revealing personal information helps to set aside the roles and goals of the team to create a degree of familiarity and comfort among team members and improve interactions in patient care.

Effective Team Leaders

What makes a good leader? There are volumes of answers to that question in management texts and articles, but the general consensus is that effective leaders have an ability (either innate or acquired) to get others to focus their energies on a goal. That ability is not necessarily endowed by status, degrees, or intelligence. Some have suggested the most important characteristic of a good leader is "emotional intelligence" (Goleman, 1998). Goleman lists five components of emotional intelligence that he believed were more important to effective leadership than the individual's intelligence, technical skills, and other cognitive abilities. These traits include *self-awareness* (the ability to recognize your own mood, emotions, and drives); *self-regulation* (the ability to control impulses and moods); *motivation* (having a passion for work beyond money or status); *empathy* (the ability to understand the emotions of others); and *social skill* (a special proficiency in managing interpersonal relationships). Golper and Brown (2004) remind us that leaders have empowerment that can come from a variety of sources. Some leaders draw on the power inherent in their position; that is, empowerment comes from the title of their position (chair, manager, supervisor, director). Some leaders use rewards or coercion (punishment) to exert power. Power can also come from having expertise in a given area. Having knowledge and skills in a particular area of practice can provide an avenue for empowerment in a leadership role. Managers who have experience and expertise in their clinical area lend themselves well to leadership roles in health care. The final source of power is personal power. Personal power in leadership comes from the charisma of the individual and his or her communication skills and general "likeability," which engenders trust in the individual's decision-making and empowers his or her leadership.

BARRIERS TO COMMUNICATION

We have made a case for infusing non-task-directed communication ("sharing and caring") processes into team meetings as helpful when developing a cohesive interdisciplinary team. What are some of the barriers to maintaining good communication? Aside from time—never having enough of it to maintain good group-communication processes—a couple of factors inherent to medical settings specifically can present problems. First is the traditional top-down professional hierarchies that exist in health service delivery, with physicians sitting at the capstone of the pyramid

(Northouse & Northhouse, 1998). The second relates to the ethnocentrisms and fears of encroachment that exist between professions (Ducanis & Golin, 1979).

Decision-Makers Versus Leaders

Physicians

When physicians are a part of the health-service team, they often assume a de facto leadership of the group because they are the primary decision-makers in the health care world. That primacy is appropriate in hospitals during the acute and subacute phase of recovery, where concerns center mainly on the medical status of the patient. But when medical issues are no longer a major concern, the physician's hold on the decision-making processes ought to diminish. Unfortunately, for several reasons related to medical and legal responsibilities and their "gatekeeping" role in health care coverage plans, physicians maintain decision-making power even when they are no longer directly treating the patients.

Throughout the continuum of care, physicians are expected to take the ultimate legal responsibility for patient-care decisions. Additionally, the adult aphasic patient's primary-care physicians are usually the "gatekeepers" for insurance-coverage decisions, or are required to "certify" or "authorize" the need for rehabilitation services on behalf of the payer, such as Medicare. Because these payer groups nearly always require a physician's order for a patient to receive covered therapy services by a non-physician, physicians continue to be the decision-makers long after the medical issues have resolved. Even when the team members consider themselves to work on a par with one another, or when a non-physician heads up the team, typically the only member empowered to authorize the care plan is the physician. And, even though facility policies may say something like "the values, goals, and wishes of the patient and families must be addressed in the care plan," in practice, the values, goals, and wishes of the person writing the orders can intrude. How physicians view their role with relation to the team can help or hinder good group cohesion and communication; any positive or negative attitudes the physician has toward the effectiveness of rehabilitation will also be a factor.

Professional Ethnocentrism

Good interdisciplinary teams are those with members who appreciate and respect the competencies of other disciplines (Sampson & Marthas, 1977). Mutual respect is the cornerstone of successful partnerships with other disciplines. Most of us bring fairly ingrained notions about our professional boundaries, and we often have prejudices about the training and professional standards of others. To work together collaboratively, we may have to reexamine and relinquish some of the notions established during our professional training.

Just like developing good group-communication processes, breaking down professional ethnocentrisms may require specific attention. Ducanis and Golin (1979) discuss the problems with interprofessional ethnocentrisms as a major obstacle to interdisciplinary teams. They suggested teams engage in an explicit examination of attitudes and develop an ongoing dialogue aimed at maintaining good relationships. They designed an instrument referred to as the "Interprofessional Perception Scale," which requires members of different disciplines to examine their interprofessional attitudes. A modification of this scale has been applied in investigation of attitudes within the rehabilitation teams in the Department of Veterans Affairs medical centers (Strasser, Stanley, Falconer, Herrin, & Bowen, 2002). Another modification of Ducanis and Golin's (1979) original instrument is the Revised Interprofessional Attitude Scale (RIPS) described by Skoloda and Angelini (1998). Essentially, this instrument in its various forms allows members of different professional groups (such as physical therapy, speech-language pathology, nursing, respiratory therapy, etc.) to assess their preconceived notions of another professional group by responding to a list of subjective statements and relating them to that group. These include statements such as, for example, "physical therapists are well trained," "physical therapists have good relations with my profession," "physical therapists are very defensive about their professional prerogatives," and so forth (Ducanis & Golin, 1979, p. 34). The members of the various professional groups represented on the team, other than the target group (in this example, physical therapists), indicate whether each statement is "true" or "false." In addition, they indicate how they think members of the target group (physical therapy) would answer about themselves, and then how the members of that profession would say the other professional-group respondents answered. What Ducanis and Golan are suggesting is that it is important to acknowledge our prejudices and appreciate that we all have preconceived attitudes, not necessarily justified by fact or experience, and that these attitudes can hinder the development of open communication, mutual trust, and cooperation in teams. Interdisciplinary teams function best when each member discipline appreciates not only their own strengths and limitations but also appreciates the contributions other disciplines bring (Allen et al., 1978).

Communication Patterns

In their review of group process in the health professions, Sampson and Marthas (1977) found three types of communication channels to be common in health services. The most common type of communication pattern was referred to as the "chain structure," in which communication occurs up and down a line in some established professional hierarchy. In this structure the physician is at the top of the chain and ward clerks, therapy aides, and patient care technicians

are at the bottom. This type of communication structure discourages much direct contact with decision-makers. The second pattern is referred to as the "wheel structure," in which information is fed to a central person, typically the unit's head nurse or the physician. In this structure, the central conduit of information (a nurse, social worker, physician, or ward clerk) is the only person to have the whole picture at any one time. The wheel structure is probably a good way to describe much of the communication that occurs with multidisciplinary teams. Last is the "circle structure," in which messages flow within a connected circle of disciplines. This pattern is most consistent with the type of communication needed to maintain effective interdisciplinary and transdisciplinary teams.

Weak Links and Poor Team Processes

There are several other potential barriers to successful communication and team intervention. Specifically, since teams are made up of human beings, individual members will vary in their ability to be open, receptive, cooperative, and professionally dedicated to the goals of the team. Therefore, there will probably be at least one or two "weak links" in any team. For example, if the speech-language pathologist (SLP) collaborates with the recreational therapist to work on functional-communication abilities during recreation activities, but the recreation therapist is the sort of employee who frequently calls in sick, the SLP will have difficulty implementing his or her goals effectively. Weak links deplete the energies of the group and create resentments. Poor team processes can also present problems. Other examples of poor processes include planning meetings at times when key members cannot be present, or trying to cover too much at one meeting. Not having adequate background information provided to team members before a meeting can lead to inefficiencies. Teams may be too large or too small for the demands placed on them. Teams can have the wrong mix of members or may not have the right combination of expertise and shared responsibilities. Teams also need to be designed to shift activities among members fluidly and to adjust to changes in workload and priorities (Sampson & Marthas, 1977). When process problems are apparent, it may be a good idea to charter a team just to figure out what's wrong with the team. By using tools from a "continuous quality improvement" (CQI) or a "total quality improvement" (TQI) problem-solving approach, the team can identify and correct process problems.

WHO ARE YOUR PARTNERS?

The Patient's Primary Physician

Patients with aphasia may have various physician-specialists involved in their care. Their primary-care physician could be an internist (specialist in internal diseases), neurologist (specialist in diseases of the nervous system), cardiologist (specialist in diseases of the heart and vascular system), physical medicine and rehabilitation physician, also called a physiatrist (specialist in rehabilitation medicine), neurosurgeon (specialist in neurologic surgery), geriatrician (specialist in geriatric medicine), family practice physician, general practitioner, or some other physician coming from a general or specialized area of medicine or surgery. Even though the interests, background, and training of physicians will vary, they bring to the interdisciplinary team a comprehensive knowledge of diseases, disease processes, and disease treatment. They understand how biologic functions and diseases involving one organ system can impair another. They can interpret laboratory data and other findings. They can determine when findings are within normal limits or are abnormal for a given individual. They prescribe drugs and perform invasive procedures for which there may be some risk of injury to the patient. In most situations physicians are given the medical-legal responsibility for care decisions, as well as financial-oversight authority. Physicians may have a good or a not-so-good grasp of the linguistic and other cognitive problems the patient with aphasia has, and they may have a good or a not-so-good sense of the psychosocial issues the adult individual with aphasia and his or her family are likely to face. There is very little in medical training that specifically prepares physicians to characterize the psycholinguistic deficits, quality-of-life changes, or the functional-communication handicap brought on by aphasia. Although the physician may know the patient and family well (which is perhaps not as likely in today's health-care delivery systems as it was previously), he or she may not have spent any time in conversation with the family about what their priorities are, much less in conversation with the patient with aphasia. The physician is the team member best prepared to identify and manage the medically related issues. Physicians will rely on the other specialists, such as speech-language pathologists, to characterize and plan remediation in the arenas in which the patient's physician lacks sufficient familiarity.

Nurses

Nurses come in a lot of varieties. Some may have postgraduate degrees in some specialty area (doctorates, masters degrees, or advanced-practice degrees). They may be Registered Nurses (RNs) with or without bachelors degrees. They may be Licensed Practical Nurses (LPNs), or nurses' aides, personal-care aides, or personal care technicians. Rehabilitation nurses have specific training and expertise in developing and implementing a rehabilitation nursing-care plan. Depending upon where they fit in the hierarchy of skills and training, as well as which state they are licensed in, nursing staff are the professionals who will administer the prescribed medications and perform medical procedures according to the physician's order or oversight. They maintain ongoing monitoring of the patient's vital signs and the patient's general mental and physical status. They also ensure that all of the patient's basic-care needs (nutrition, hydration, elimination, comfort, hygiene, and so forth) are met. In an inpatient facility, nurses have the most ongoing and frequent contact with the patients and families. As a group, nurses are with patients more than any other member of the team, 24 hours a day. Nurses are also trained and skilled in teaching the patient and family to manage their own care, and they are especially good at reinforcing both the team's instructions to the patient and family and the team's goals of functional independence.

Case-Managers and Medical Social Workers

Case-managers are usually nurses and most often are RNs. In general, case-managers are interested in ensuring that the requirements of the patient's health care coverage are met (insurance, managed-care, Medicare, etc.). If coverage requires a certain number of hours or minutes of therapy per week, or that the patient is seen "daily," meaning 7 days a week, the case-manager makes sure the therapy team can provide that level of service. When the speech-language pathologist sees a therapy need that exceeds the patient's insurance coverage, the case manager can be a very helpful advocate for the patient and the team.

Medical social workers sometimes have responsibilities in case management. Usually, however, their primary roles are (1) to provide counseling to patients and families for the psychosocial issues that arise, (2) to provide assistance with practical matters, such as financial concerns, and (3) to arrange for discharges appropriate to the needs of the patient and the family. The medical social worker is often the first person the speech-language pathologist will turn to when family adjustment and coping problems are apparent, or when financial assistance is needed.

Pharmacists

Not all facilities or settings will have pharmacists as participants on their care teams. Hospitals are probably the places where pharmacists are most likely to be involved as formal members of unit teams. In hospitals, pharmacists routinely participate in care-planning meetings and ward rounds. Pharmacists have a key role in determining appropriate therapeutic drug dosages for individual patients based on age, gender, weight, and other medical conditions. They monitor for errors in medication orders, for potential drug complications and side effects, and for polypharmacy effects (taking too many drugs and potentially causing negative interaction effects). They participate in teaching the patient and family self-management of medications, and can work with the speech-language pathologist to address safe self-medication.

Dietitians

Inpatient facilities typically have a dietitian or dietary technician attached to their care team. They follow the patient's nutrition and hydration status, monitoring parameters such as body weight, renal chemistry panels, serum albumin, daily intake of food and water, and general appetite. They also monitor the patient's alertness and well-being. The speech-language pathologist may work with the dietitian, particularly if the patient with aphasia has a concomitant problem managing oral intake, or if there are other issues related more directly to the aphasia, such as difficulties ordering preferred items from the facility menu.

Psychologists

Neuropsychologists, geropsychologists, or general clinical psychologists may be a part of the core care team, or may be consultants to the team. In comprehensive rehabilitation facilities, psychologists are an integral part of the rehabilitation team. In units such as head injury programs, where cognitive and behavioral issues tend to be principal concerns, psychologists may be the team leaders. Psychologists conduct and participate in the team assessments of cognitive, emotional, and behavioral areas. They collaborate with the team to design and implement the cognitive, emotional, and behavioral therapies. They work with families and, when needed, collaborate with medical social workers to link families and patients to community mental health services. Depending upon the individual's training and specialty area, the psychologist can be a very close partner with the speech-language pathologist in developing a profile of the cognitive and other deficits and collaborating on interpretations of test findings.

Recreation Therapy

Rehabilitation units and other facilities, such as skilled-nursing units, are usually required to have someone on staff to conduct a recreation and resident activities program. These individuals may have Bachelor or associate degrees in recreation therapy or may be Certified Activities Directors, who may not have completed professional degrees but have completed a course and passed a state-certifying examination in this area. These individuals are responsible for planning and scheduling the daily-activity calendar of patients. Speech-language pathologists will work closely with the recreation-therapy staff to ensure that the patients can engage as fully as possible in the unit's recreation activities, without experiencing a communication disadvantage. Recreation therapy is more than just keeping patients busy. Recreation-therapy

groups can be the first place where the patient with aphasia and the family resume shared activities; thus, these groups offer excellent opportunities for partnerships with the speech-language pathologist. By engaging patients together with their families in recreation activities that do not require much language facility (such as playing cards or dominoes) the team can demonstrate to the family the patient's residual non-language abilities. By involving patients with aphasia in recreation tasks that have some demand for communication (targeted to be just within the patient's ability range) the speech-language pathologist can demonstrate the value of applying the communication-facilitating strategies they are developing in therapy to everyday social activities.

Occupational Therapists and Physical Therapists

Occupational therapists (OTs) and physical therapists (PTs) have uniquely different professional preparation and perspectives on rehabilitation, but also have some overlapping areas in their scopes of practice. This sometimes leads the general public and health-care personnel to refer to all therapies (including speech-language therapy) as "Physical Therapy." In general, occupational therapists are concerned with the patient's functional daily-living abilities, safety, and independence in self-care and related areas. OTs ensure that patients can take care of their grooming and hygiene, can don and doff clothes, and can functionally transfer in and out of a wheelchair, in and out of bed, in and out of a tub or shower, and so on, for optimal independence and self-care. Most OTs have experience in the assessment and treatment of perceptual-motor abilities and the visuospatial abilities and visuoperceptual abilities associated with brain injuries. Some OTs have had specialized training in "Low Vision Rehab" with patients who have visuosensory losses. They are a valuable partner for the speech-language pathologist in designing a plan for improving a patient's functional impairments involving visual, visuoperceptual, visuomotor, visual recognition, or perceptual-motor deficits, as with conditions such as apraxias and neglect syndromes, or with visual-field cuts. OTs also are very adept at designing or providing assistive devices to improve functional independence. In some settings, OTs may be involved in kitchen and recreation evaluations, or they may be involved in an assessment of the patient's ability to return safely to driving. Many of these areas are going to be crucial for the patient to return to a maximal level of independence. The speech-language pathologist and OT often work in partnership when communication problems interact with other functional losses, or to combine the objectives of both therapies into treatment sessions. For example, the OT might be asked to have the patient point to the items of clothing he or she names before beginning the dressing routine.

Physical therapists (PTs) have a key role with stroke rehabilitation whenever weakness, incoordination, or balance problems are present. For the most part PTs are focused on the patient's mobility, strength, balance, transfers, endurance, range of movement, and exercise or activity tolerance. PTs and OTs may also be involved in other areas of rehabilitation, such as splinting, cardiac rehabilitation, or bladder-continence control. Physical therapists, like all other members of the team, are concerned with maximizing functional independence. Physical therapy addresses not only the neuromuscular weakness, coordination, and balance problems found in patients with neurologic damage, but also the associated functional living problems. For example, the goal of physical therapy may be something like "the patient will walk 50 feet without assistance," but in addition, "the patient will be able to carry a basket of clothes the distance from his bedroom to the laundry room." Speech-language pathologists might partner with the PT to incorporate functional language-facilitating activities into the physical therapist's directions and requests. Similarly, the SLP might incorporate a PT objective into therapy sessions, such as asking the patient to transfer from the bed to a chair before beginning therapy.

Speech-Language Pathologist

The speech-language pathologist (SLP) brings to the team knowledge and skills in the evaluation and remediation of the aphasic person's communication and related cognitive impairments. This text provides a comprehensive review of the breadth of the SLP's expertise in aphasia intervention. The SLP is the member of the team who provides theory-driven and evidence-based language intervention. The SLP evaluation usually includes a psycholinguistic assessment of the patient's language deficits, and an assessment of related cognitive impairments. Test findings, along with all of the evaluations, behavioral data, and observational input provided by other members of the care team—in collaboration with the patient and family in identifying the communication goals—forms the basis of the SLP's intervention program.

Support Personnel

In rehabilitation, it is increasingly common to find support personnel. Certified Occupational Therapy Assistants (COTAs), Physical Therapist Assistants (PTAs), Speech-Language Pathology Assistants (SLP-As), and trained volunteers may be a part of the team, working under the supervision of the licensed/certified professional therapists. In several states these individuals have to have met qualifying examinations to be licensed in their discipline area after completing required education and training (usually either a bachelors degree or an associates degree). The requirements and standards vary by state and by discipline. For example, in Tennessee, the basic requirement for Speech-Language Pathology Assistants is a high-school diploma or equivalent.

Therapy assistants usually are restricted by the State Boards of Examiners to the implementation of treatment procedures only under specific conditions, including under the supervision and direction of professional therapists. Therapy assistants sometimes are viewed as "therapy extenders"—implementing the plans that are established by the physical therapists, occupational therapists, or speech-language pathologists; payers typically do not reimburse services provided by assistants. Evidence supports the role of trained and supervised nonlicensed individuals, such as assistants and volunteers, in aphasia intervention (Kagan, Black, Duchan, Simmons-Mackie, & Square, 2001; Marshall et al., 1989; Paul & Sparks, 2006; Wertz et al., 1986). Assistants and aides do not conduct new patient evaluations, make differential diagnoses, or design the treatment plans. Therapy assistants have to demonstrate specific competencies before they can treat patients independently. In addition to assistants, therapy aides, or "rehab techs," are fairly common in rehabilitation settings. These individuals may be students or others without degrees in rehabilitation therapy specialties but with specific training to lend help to the therapists and assistants in patient care and other clinical duties (e.g., setting up equipment).

Other Allied Professionals

Professionals from a variety of disciplines, such as audiologists, biomedical engineers, assistive technologists, vocational counselors, and chaplains, may be members of the heath-care team with adults with aphasia. If the patient has a hearing impairment, the audiologist can become a central member of the team. If the patient requires special adaptive equipment or augmentative communication systems or equipment for other purposes, the assistive technologist (AT) will help the team select the instruments and design the access switches. If there is potential for the adult with aphasia to return to a previous vocation, similar vocation, or even a new vocation, a rehabilitation vocation counselor is the individual best equipped to direct the patient and family toward potential alternatives. When the patient and family have spiritual needs that require specialized attention, a member of the facility's pastoral care or chaplaincy service will help the team address those concerns.

TEAMS ACROSS THE CONTINUUM
Changing Priorities

As persons with aphasia move from the crisis of the acute event through various care settings, and eventually, hopefully, reentering their home life and community, there will be shifts in primary concerns and priorities for intervention, and correspondingly there will be changes in the major decision-makers.

TABLE 8–1

Shifts in Priorities Across Settings and the Recovery Continuum with Adults with Aphasia

Setting	Typical Priorities
Acute-care	1. Physiologic and medical stability 2. Emotional issues 3. Physical limitations 4. Communicative and other cognitive limitations 5. Discharge plan
Subacute nursing	1. Physiologic and medical status 2. Physical limitations 3. Communicative and other cognitive limitations 4. Functional independence 5. Discharge plan
Inpatient rehabilitation	1. Communication and other cognitive limitations 2. Physical limitations 3. Functional independence 4. Psychosocial and emotional issues 5. Discharge plan
Outpatient rehabilitation	1. Functional independence 2. Communication and other cognitive limitations 3. Physical limitations 4. Psychosocial and emotional issues 5. Financial and vocational issues
Home-health-care	1. Functional independence 2. Communication and other cognitive limitations 3. Physical limitations 4. Financial and vocational issues 5. Psychosocial and emotional issues
Home and community reentry	1. Psychosocial and emotional issues 2. Financial and vocational issues 3. Functional independence 4. Physical limitations 5. Communication and other cognitive limitations

Table 8–1 illustrates how priorities can change across settings and through the continuum of recovery with adult aphasia. Team designs and the primacy of different individuals in the hierarchy of decision-making will also change (Table 8–2). Obviously, these scenarios are intended to illustrate a point. Not every facility, setting, or individual patient will necessarily follow this pattern. Shifts in priorities, team designs, and decision-makers across the recovery continuum are considered here merely to emphasize that intervention extends beyond any one setting or team. Intervention rolls through many settings, from the hospital bed to the nursing home or rehabilitation facility, from outpatient therapy to home-health-care, from the rehabilitation team to independent living. In fairly short order the support systems provided by the multidisciplinary or interdisciplinary teams will end. Patients and families need to be prepared for the time when decision-making responsibilities will fall squarely on their shoulders. As soon as the patient's medical condition has stabilized and the patient enters rehabilitation, the overarching goal of all of the rehabilitation professionals they encounter should be directed toward functional independence and encouraging the patient with aphasia, with his or her family, to take control of their own lives.

Changing Rehabilitation Outcome Goals

As illustrated by a schema described by Sundance and Cope (1995), rehabilitation outcome goals move through a continuum as the patient progresses from a destabilized state during the acute phase up through later phases of community reintegration and productive activity. These authors conceptualized the continuum of treatment to span the following stages.

Level 0 = Physiologic Instability. The acute onset of illness in which medical stabilization is the main concern and diagnostic evaluations are completed.

Level I = Physiologic Stability. Limited attention is given to functional rehabilitation restoration; medical stabilization continues to be addressed.

Level II = Physiologic Maintenance. Rehabilitation primarily is aimed at establishing adequate and safe systems of nutrition and hydration, and prevention of complications, such as aspiration pneumonia, skin breakdown, joint-mobilization problems, and bowel- and bladder-control problems. Secondarily, rehabilitation at this phase will be aimed at communication, self-care, mobilization, and cognitive and behavioral issues, depending on the patient's responsiveness.

Level III = Primary Functional Goals. Functional-deficit-specific goals are established to facilitate discharge to home or to improve residential integration.

Level IV = Advanced Functional Goals. Rehabilitation is directed toward community reintegration.

Level V = Productive Activity. Rehabilitation outcomes are directed at returning the adult with aphasia adult to productive activities within his or her level of ability (Landrum, Schmidt, & McLean, 1995; Paradigm Health Corporation, 1993; Sundance & Cope, 1995).

Changing Settings

Acute Care Setting

Initially, the team's efforts are directed toward moving the patient out of physiologic instability toward a level of

TABLE 8-2

Team Designs and Decision-Makers Across Settings and the Recovery Continuum with Adults with Aphasia

Setting	Team Design	Primary Decision-Makers
Acute-care	Multidisciplinary	1. Physician
Subacute unit	Interdisciplinary	1. Physician
		2. Patient-care team
		3. Patient and family
Inpatient rehabilitation	Interdisciplinary	1. Physician
		2. Rehabilitation team
		3. Patient and family
Outpatient rehabilitation	Multidisciplinary	1. Physician
	Community support networks and partnerships	2. Rehabilitation team
		3. Patient and family
Home-health-care	Multidisciplinary	1. Physician
	Community support networks and partnerships	2. Home-health rehabilitation team
		3. Patient and family
Home and community reentry	Community support networks and partnerships	1. Patient and family

physiologic stability and maintenance (Sundance & Cope, 1995). In the acute setting, the first priorities are (1) ensuring the patient survives the acute event with minimal residual neurologic damage and (2) diminishing the risks for complications. Some patients are ready to participate in rehabilitation services within a few days of the acute event and onset of aphasia. Unfortunately, most acute-stroke clinical care pathways anticipate discharge in 3 to 5 days from admission, making interdisciplinary team rehabilitation virtually impossible. With just a few days' involvement with the patient before discharge, the team's emphasis tends to be on patient and family education and appropriate discharge planning. As is the case with nearly any hospitalization with an acute event, the aphasic person's family is under tremendous emotional stress. They may not be in the best frame of mind to absorb new information or make decisions. The family will, however, be sensitive to the verbal messages, body language, and attitudes of all the team members participating in caring for the patient. It is especially important that family and patients be approached with a professional, supportive, and reassuring attitude (van Vendendaal, Grinspin, & Andriaanse, 1996). Education and verbal messages need to be brief and consistent. Information needs to guide, and not overwhelm. The family should not be expected to fully grasp the consequences of the neurologic damage, so a supercilious lecture on recovery from aphasia full of grim predictions intended to correct the family's "unrealistic expectations" is completely inappropriate and unnecessary at this point. The messages must be accurate but also hopeful.

As we suggested earlier, unless the patient is admitted to an acute "stroke unit," where an interdisciplinary team is in place, the typical model for team care in an acute setting is more likely to look like a multidisciplinary than interdisciplinary model. Consequently, care planning discussions, if they take place at all, focus on sharing assessment findings with other team members, and making discharge recommendations to the physician and medical social worker. Group discussions of observations of the patient are an important part of decision-making during this time. Often, the patient's responsiveness will vary during the day, so team discussions of observations on cognitive and communicative status will help the speech-language pathologist gauge the reliability of communication assessments. Finally, because the patient and family are under stress, it may be better to channel information through as few people as possible, principally through the physician, the primary nurse, or the social worker, and allow them to work with the family. Other professionals should be available to address their particular concerns; however, it is important for the team to keep messages consistent and to not overwhelm the patient or family.

Subacute Nursing Setting

Usually, after the medical and acute physiologic conditions have stabilized, patients are transferred to some kind of subacute setting, where physiologic maintenance may still be the main outcome goal. These settings can be a skilled nursing facility, recuperative care unit, transitional care unit, or the like. Prevention of complications continues to be a concern along with communication, cognitive and emotional issues, mobility, and independence. Emotional issues, such as anxiety and depression on the part of the family, continue to be major concern, and the psychosocial effects of the aphasia and other impairments will begin to be felt by the patient and the family. Psychosocial concerns can include such things as changes in body image and losses in the level of independence; uncertainties about the future and the recovery processes; frustration with communication and impaired movement; emotional lability; changes in family dynamics and a sense of a lack of control over events happening to them; irritability; self-centeredness; unrealistic expectations or denial; and dependency (Churchill, 1993; Flick, 1999). Patients also may display post-stroke depression and anxiety. These emotional problems usually respond to a combination of medication and reassurance. At the subacute phase, the patient's residual physical impairments, if any, often are more of a concern to the family and the patient than communication and other cognitive impairments, possibly because mobility is linked to independence. Integral to improving the patient's psychosocial and emotional status is the implementation of rehabilitation for physical, self-care, and cognitive/communicative problems. If the patient's physical tolerance and cognitive status allow, the earliest possible involvement in rehabilitation should be encouraged (Flick, 1999). Intervention at this phase usually takes place in a residential-program setting where teams tend to be interdisciplinary (Cifu & Stewart, 1999). It is important that everyone working with the patient and family have the same goals in mind and that no one professional group exerts ownership over their goals or procedures. Although different members of the team have a slightly different center of concern, the entire team is responsible for achieving the intervention goals. When possible, intervention procedures are shared and implemented in partnerships between team and family members.

Inpatient Rehabilitation Setting

Some patients transfer directly to a rehabilitation facility from their acute-care ward, and some continue rehabilitation in a skilled nursing facility or following a stay in a subacute nursing unit. Typically, once the patient reaches the rehabilitation setting the major medical issues have resolved and some of the acute emotional reactions and psychosocial issues have become slightly less of a priority than the residual effects of the stroke (such as hemiparesis, aphasia, and other cognitive problems). There may be significant, chronic medical issues to consider, such as pain management, depression, blood pressure management, blood-coagulation management, seizure control, or incontinency, but the patient is typically believed to be generally medically stable. Typically, on an inpatient rehabilitation unit the family sees the patient working for several hours a day with a team of experts attempting to maximize the patient's functional status. Also, most likely, the patient has experienced some amount of recovery at this point. In such settings, the family and the patient are usually highly confident that some improvement will result; consequently, concerns about psychosocial and emotional issues may temporarily be set aside, or at least become less severe. In a rehabilitation setting there is a "full-court press" to address the specific deficit-effects of the stroke. Aggressive speech-language therapy for the aphasia will be implemented, in addition to 3 or 4 hours daily of occupational and physical therapy. The focus on everyone's part is placed on maximizing the patient's abilities to return either to his or her home or to a residential facility, with the overriding goal of maximizing independence. Again, inpatient team intervention tends to be interdisciplinary, and collaborative goals are emphasized. Because all the intensive therapy and team activity leads to an expectation for positive results, one of the problems that arises with the inpatient rehabilitation setting is that patients and families may see the end of rehabilitation as the end of recovery (Flick, 1999). Therefore, psychological stresses may begin to emerge at about the time the inpatient rehabilitation stay is nearing its end. The end of formal treatment can signal a concern for "is this is as good as it gets?," which creates anxiety for both the family and the patient.

Outpatient Rehabilitation Setting

In this setting daily contact with non-therapist, allied disciplines such as pharmacists, social workers, dieticians, nurses, and even physicians is not typical. Therapists from different disciplines may work in the same clinic area, but the team-intervention model is more likely to be closer to the multidisciplinary design. Much like the hierarchy of concerns when patients enter inpatient rehabilitation facilities, the interventions in outpatient rehabilitation settings are impairment-specific, for the most part. However, the overriding goal to improve self-care and independence for home and community integration and toward some resumption of productive activity is still primary. Because the patient is typically coming to therapy from home at this juncture, psychosocial, emotional, financial, and vocational concerns may be uppermost on the minds of the patient and family. In this setting especially, caregivers are likely to express frustration with communicating with the person with aphasia in addition to sadness over the loss of companionship. Issues such as lifestyle changes, social isolation, and financial difficulties may surface after the patient goes home (Flick, 1999); thus, these should be addressed as part of the outpatient rehabilitation program. Since this arena of treatment can tend to be more multidisciplinary than interdisciplinary, due mostly to difficulties with scheduling collaborative therapies and the unavailability of support professionals, a mechanism to address these special issues easily may be lacking. Explicit referrals to a psychologist and other professionals will need to be set up. Similar to a home health based setting, encouraging the patient and family to link with community support networks well ahead of the completion of formal outpatient therapy is essential.

RELATED ISSUES

Team Evaluations and Team Treatments

One of the frequent concerns expressed when team evaluations and treatments are considered is the belief that "only one discipline can bill for this time." That may be the case in any fee-for-service visits, where charges are made per procedure and payers usually will not pay for two procedure charges in the same unit of time. Other types of reimbursement schemes, however, might support collaborative interdisciplinary team evaluations and treatment. For example, when a pre-established payment is made for a certain amount of treatment time (as with Medicare's DRGs or prospective-payment system for Part A coverage, or with inpatient insurance per diem), there are no payer restrictions on having more than one discipline involved in a given evaluation or therapy session. The issue may be provider costs. The facility may resist having more people involved in patient care than are necessary. Increased staff time translates to increased costs to the provider facility; therefore, it may be necessary to justify collaborative evaluations and interventions and nonbillable staff time (such as team meetings) as a facility cost *savings*. Collaborative evaluations may accomplish a more comprehensive assessment in a shorter time frame than evaluations that are done independently. In the earlier discussion of "who are your partners," several examples of collaborative evaluations and interventions were mentioned. It's a bit like the parable of the seven blind men and the elephant, in which a different interpretation emerges depending upon which part of the elephant you are touching. Team evaluations with more than one discipline participating can yield a much better composite picture than independent assessments.

Collaborative interventions can reduce redundancies, reduce the time taken for communications, and more efficiently ease transfers and discharges, which reduce the lengths of stays. Reducing the lengths of stays often saves costs to the facility; it has the added benefit of reducing the risks of nosocomial infections and other hospital stay related complications.

Documentation

Documentation is another important area for collaboration. Some of the current practices in health care in the U.S. today strongly encourage multidisciplinary documentation. For example, Clinical Care Pathways may be used to guide day-to-day care plans, particularly in inpatient facilities. The documentation for these pathways flows across multiple disciplines, and some of the care objectives may be shared between or among disciplines (e.g., patient education) (Ignativicius & Housman, 1995). To be in compliance with the standards of the Joint Commission on Accreditation of Healthcare Organizations (JCAHO) (JCAHO, 2006) or CARF, the Commission on Accreditation of Rehabilitation Facilities (CARF, 2005), it is expected that family and patient education be conducted in a multidisciplinary manner.

Clinical Preparation and Research

Training programs and research are ripe for interdisciplinary collaborations. Emphasis on interdisciplinary education and collaboration in patient care is primarily evident in literature coming out of Canada and the United Kingdom (Cook, 2005; D'Amour et al., 2005; Gibbon, 1999). The time to initiate good interdisciplinary relations to prevent potential problems related to professional ethnocentrisms, discussed earlier, is during the professional clinical preparation. It is important that students have a good exposure to different team interventions as a part of their professional training. Collaborative research also has exciting possibilities. When different disciplines collaborate in research we discover a new way of looking at old notions, and test the extent to which our data apply to other areas.

COMMUNITY AND NATIONAL SUPPORT NETWORKS AND PARTNERSHIPS

Every adult with aphasia who completes formal therapy under the care of either an array of disciplines or just a few eventually reaches an outcome: the rest of life. In outcome-oriented rehabilitation (Landrum et al., 1995; Schmidt, 1999), the intervention services of the health care delivery team are, from the initiation of care, conceptualized, organized, and delivered with an eye on the quality of the rest of life for that person. Landrum et al. (1995) and Schmidt (1999) observe that all too often the team fails to consider until the end of the patient's stay the resources the patient and family have available to them, much less how to incorporate those resources and social support networks into their future.

Schmidt (1999) suggests the following resources should be identified with the patient and family very early in the continuum of rehabilitation therapy services: (1) *Health services funding resources* (what will the insurance coverage provide for this person to support his or her needs now and in the future?); (2) *financial resources* (what are the additional financial resources available to this patient and family?); (3) *family resources* (what are the caregiver and other resources available to this family unit?); and (4) *community resources* (what community and social support services are available to this family?). It is important that every member of the rehabilitation team understand the global impact that aphasia and other problems resulting from brain damage will have on the individual and the family unit. The intervention team should anticipate and incorporate that perspective into each phase of therapy. The team needs to be focused on the future and also keep the patient and family focused on the future. Schmidt (1999) suggests starting with the end-point and aligning expectations throughout the continuum of recovery. The team should be supportive and should encourage and empower aphasic adults and their families to use their available resources to reintegrate into their homes and communities and return to productive activity. One of the projects for the team can be to help the family develop an individualized resource directory for community services. This can include such things as elder care services, day treatment programs, Meals on Wheels, community- or university-based aphasia therapy programs, church activities, support groups, recreation opportunities, and the like. The team can also help the patient and family plan post therapy goals, such as continuing language-reinforcing tasks at home (e.g., word-processor letters, reading selected sections of the newspaper) and family or community activities (e.g., attending a reunion, participating in a church project). These kinds of planned activities may help to carry forward formal treatment into functional living in the future.

The outcome of *survival* following a major neurologic event, such as a stroke, is, literally, life. After formal therapy ends, the patient and the family may need to maintain contact with a support team, and that should not be discouraged. However, one of the overarching goals of rehabilitation should be to identify the potential risks and concerns prior to the end of treatment and help the patient and family establish the community support networks they will need and to then be prepared to lead their own "team aphasia."

National Support Groups

The National Stroke Association (NSA)

The National Stroke Association (NSA) was founded in 1984 as a nonprofit organization dedicated to educating surviors of stroke, their families, health-care professionals, and the general public about stroke. The NSA's focus is on reducing the incidence and impact of stroke through activities related to prevention, medical care, research, resocialization, and rehabilitation. This organization develops and distributes educational materials and publishes a magazine, *Stroke Smart*, and a journal. The NSA provides guidance in developing stroke clubs and stroke support groups; operates a Stroke Center Network program and encourages conducting clinical trials in the prevention and management of stroke and its consequences.

The National Aphasia Association

The National Aphasia Association (NAA) is a nonprofit organization governed by a Board of Directors made up of individuals with professional interests in aphasia (speech-language pathologists, physiatrists, neurologists) and individuals with aphasia and their co-survivors. This organization was charted in nearly two decades ago, and has continued to advocate for and serve the interests of individuals with aphasia and their co-survivors, through its "hot line," Web site, and published materials, including *The Aphasia Handbook* (Sarno & Peters, 2005), and by sponsoring conferences, such as its "Speaking Out" conferences held biennially. The NAA's mission is "to educate the public to know that the word aphasia describes an impairment of the ability to communicate, not an impairment of intellect. The NAA makes people with aphasia, their families, support systems, and health care professionals aware of resources to recover lost skills to the extent possible, to compensate for skills that will not be recovered and to minimize the psychosocial impact of the language impairment" (www.aphasia.org). To that end, the NAA has developed and endorsed the adoption of the Aphasia Bill of Rights (www.aphasia.org), which states: people with aphasia have the right to:

1. Be told, as soon as it is determined, preferably by a qualified speech-language pathologist (SLP), both orally and in writing, that they have "aphasia" and given an explanation of the meaning of aphasia.
2. Be provided, upon release from the hospital, with written documentation that "aphasia" is part of their diagnosis.
3. Be told, both orally and in writing, that there are local resources available to them, including Aphasia Community Groups in their areas, as well as national organizations such as the National Aphasia Association (NAA).
4. Have access to outpatient therapy to the extent deemed appropriate by a qualified speech-language pathologist (SLP).
5. Give their informed consent in any research project in which they are participating.
6. Demand that accrediting health-care agencies and health care facilities establish requirements for and competency in caring for people with aphasia.

SUMMARY

This chapter examined concepts in team collaborations mainly within the context of therapeutic interventions for aphasia in health care facilities and other rehabilitation settings. The notion of team intervention is extended to family-centered partnerships as early as possible and throughout the continuum of care and into community-supported partnerships after formal therapy has ended. In an examination of the differences between *interdisciplinary*, *multidisciplinary*, and *transdisciplinary* teams in health care settings, the importance of good communication is stressed. We have also emphasized how becoming comfortable with a certain amount of blurring of professional scopes of practice may be necessary for the success of interdisciplinary teams. In team dynamics, there needs to be a balance of both content (activities, goals, and products) and process (communication, affiliation, and collaboration). We considered how team processes may be hindered by a number of factors that can be barriers to communication. We looked at how professional hierarchies in health care settings tend to place the physician in the role of primary decision-maker, especially in the more acute phases of care. We considered how the structure of teams tends to vary in different settings, and how the priorities and primary decision-makers might shift over the recovery continuum. The principal goal of this chapter is to emphasize the value of team collaborations and partnerships, both in the formal rehabilitation program itself and in the transition to the home and community. We suggest that one of the overarching goals of therapy should be to empower patients and families to become independent decision-makers. When therapy has ended, the leaders in "team aphasia" are ultimately the patient and the family.

FUTURE TRENDS

Teams and family-centered and community partnerships have an important future in patient care in all arenas, but especially in aphasia intervention. An interdisciplinary team approach is supported by research examining evidence-based treatment (Cifu & Stewart, 1999). Team intervention is also strongly encouraged by legislative and certifying bodies (CARF, 2005; JCAHO, 2006; Rosin et al., 1996), by third-party payers, and as a standard of care preferred by providers (Davis et al., 2005; Gibbon, 1999; Malone & McPherson, 2004; Strasser et al., 2005). All of the current trends and influences in health care delivery today suggest the "lone professional" practice is diminishing and collaborations in patient care are here to stay.

KEY POINTS

1. No team will look or function exactly like any other, but health-care teams in general tend to be organized as multidisciplinary, interdisciplinary, and transdisciplinary models.
2. Multidisciplinary teams are common in inpatient settings. Interdisciplinary teams, common in rehabilitation settings, share common goals. Transdisciplinary

teams, a model applied in early intervention, require "role release," and less distinctive discipline-specific boundaries.
3. Group communication, creating cohesion, and establishing effective leadership are key elements to successful team processes.
4. Professional ethnocentricism can influence how we perceive other professions and diminish the team's ability to work collaboratively and effectively.
5. There are a number of challenges to interdisciplinary team management, including problems with conducting "billable" team evaluations and implementing interdisciplinary team documentation.
6. Presuming our ultimate goal is to bring about the best quality of life after the onset of aphasia, the patient and family are, ultimately, the most important members of the health care team; thus, one objective of management throughout the continuum is to prepare the family to lead "team aphasia" after therapy has ended.

ACTIVITIES FOR REFLECTION AND DISCUSSION

1. What are the advantages and disadvantages of having more than one discipline involved in intervention in patients with aphasia?
2. What are the similarities and differences between multidisciplinary, interdisciplinary, and transdisciplinary teams?
3. Which professional group tends to be the decision-makers in health care in the U.S., and why?
4. What do case-managers and social workers bring to the team?
5. How might teams differ in the acute phase of rehabilitation as compared with the subacute and chronic phases of recovery?
6. During which time frames are patients and families most likely to become more concerned about psychosocial and financial issues than medical issues?
7. List the ways team intervention is encouraged by trends and influences in health service delivery.
8. What is the evidence in support of the benefit of team-based, collaborative services for patients with aphasia?
9. Describe some specific objectives teams might incorporate into the therapy plan to empower patients and families ultimately to take control of "team aphasia" after formal rehabilitation has ended.

References

Allen, K. E., Holm, V. A., & Scheifelbusch, R. L. (1978). *Early intervention—A team approach.* Baltimore, MD: University Park Press.

Billups, J. J. (1987). Interprofessional team process. *Theory Into Practice, 26*(2), 146–152.

Brown, J. E., & Handlesman, J. A. (2006). Professional autonomy and collaboration. In Lubinski, R., Golper, L. A. C., & Frattali, C. M. (Eds.), *Professional issues in speech-language pathology and audiology* (3ʳᵈ Ed.). New York: Thomson-Delmar.

Cifu, D. X., & Stewart, D. G. (1999). Factors affecting functional outcome after stroke: A critical review of rehabilitation interventions. *Archives of Physical Medicine and Rehabilitation, 80*(5 Suppl. 1), S-35–39.

Churchill, C. (1993). Social problems after stroke. *Physical Medicine Rehabilitation: State of the Art Review, 7*(1), 213–223.

Collins, D., Moore, P., Mitchell, D., & Alpress, F. (1999). Role and confidentiality in multidisciplinary athlete support programs. *British Journal of Sports Medicine, 33*(3), 208–211.

Commission on Accreditation of Rehabilitation Facilities (2005). *Medical Rehabilitation Accreditation Manual.* Tucson, AZ: CARF.

Cook, D. A. (2005). Models of interprofessional learning in Canada. *Journal of Interprofessional Care, Supplement 1,* 107–115.

D'Amour, D., Ferrada-Videla, M., Rodriquez, L. S. M., & Beaulieu, M-D. (2005) The conceptual basis for interprofessinal collaboration: Care concepts and theoretical frameworks. *Journal of Interprofessional Care, 19*(1), 116–131.

Davis, C. G., Cornman, C. B., Lane, M. J., & Patton, M. (2005). Person-centered planning training for consumer-directed care for the elderly and disabled. *Care Management Journal, 6*(3), 122–130.

Ducanis, A. J., & Golin, A. K. (1979). *The Interdisciplinary Health Care Team: A Handbook.* Rockville, MD: Aspen.

Flick, C. L. (1999). Stroke rehabilitation: 4. Stroke outcome and psychosocial consequences. *Archives of Physical Medicine and Rehabilitation, 80*(5 Suppl. 1), S-21–26.

Gibbon, B. (1999). An investigation of interprofessinal collaboration in stroke rehabilitation team conferences. *Journal of Clinical Nursing. 8,* 246–252.

Goleman, D. (1998). What makes a leader? *Harvard Business Review, Nov-Dec,* 93–102.

Golper, L. A. C., & Brown, J. (Eds.) (2004). *Business matters.* Rockville, MD: American Speech-Language-Hearing Association.

Heikkila, V. M., Korpelainen, J., Turkka, J., Lallanranta, T., & Summala, H. (1999). Clinical evaluation of driving in stroke patients. *Acta Neurologica Scandinavia, 99*(6), 349–399.

Hogh, P., Waldmar, G., Knudsen, G.M., Bruhn, P., Mortensen, H., Wildschiodtz, G., Bech, R. A., Juhler, M., & Paulson, O. B. (1999). A multidisciplinary memory clinic in a neurologic setting. *European Journal of Neurology, 6*(3), 279–288.

Ignativicius, D. D., & Housman, K. A. (1995). *Clinical pathways for collaborative practice.* Philadelphia: W. B. Saunders.

Joint Commission on Accreditation of Healthcare Organizations. (2006). *JCAHO Standards for Hospitals.* Oakbrook, IL: JCHAO.

Kagan, A., Black, S. E., Duchan, J. F., Simmons-Mackie, N., & Square, P. (2001). Training volunteers as conversational partners using "supported conversation for adults with aphasia" (SCA): A controlled trial. *Journal of Speech, Language, and Hearing Research, 44,* 624–638.

Landrum, P. K., Schmidt, N. D., & McLean, A. Jr. (Eds.) (1995). *Outcome-oriented rehabilitation: Principles, strategies, and tools for effective program management.* Gaithersburg, MD: Aspen.

Loomis, M. E. (1979). *Group processes for nurses.* St. Louis: C. V. Mosby.

Lott, C., Hennes, H. J., & Dick, W. (1999). Stroke—a medical emergency. *Journal of Accident and Emergency Medicine, 16*(1), 2–7.

Malone, D. M., & McPherson, J. R. (2004). Community-and hospital-based early intervention team members' attitudes and perceptions of teamwork. *International Journal of Disability, Development and Education, 51*(1), 99–116.

Manion, J., Lorimer, W., & Leander, W. J. (1996). *Team-based health care organizations: Blueprint for success.* Gaithersburg, MD: Aspen.

Marshall, R. C., Wertz, R. T., Weiss, D. G., Aten, J. L., Brookshire, R. H., Garcia-Bunuel, L. et al. (1989). Home treatment for aphasic patients by trained nonprofessionals. *Journal of Speech and Hearing Disorders, 54,* 462–470.

Meyers-Briggs, I., & Briggs, P. (1980). *Gifts differing: Understanding personality type.* Palo Alto, CA: Consulting Psychologists Press.

National Aphasia Association: www.aphasia.org.

National Stroke Association: www.stroke.org.

Northouse, L. L. & Northouse, P. G. (1998). *Health communication: Strategies for health professionals.* Stamford, CT: Appleton & Lange.

Paradigm Health Corporation Publications (1993). Paradigm Health Corp., 1001 Galaxy Way, Suite Number 400, Concord, CA 94520.

Paul, D. R., & Sparks, S. (2006) Support personnel in communication sciences and disorders. In Lubinski, R., Golper, L. A. C., & Frattali, C. M. (Eds.), *Professional issues in speech-language pathology and audiology* (3ʳᵈ Ed.). New York: Thomson-Delmar.

Rosin, P., Whitehead, A. D, Tuchman, L. I., Gesien, G. S., Begun, A. L., & Irwin, L. (1996). *Partnerships in family-centered care: A guide to collaborative early intervention.* Baltimore: Paul H. Brookes.

Rosin, P. (1996). The diverse American family. In P. Rosin, A. D. Whitehead, L. I. Tuchman, G. S. Gesien, A. L. Begun, & L. Irwin. *Partnerships in family-centered care: A guide to collaborative early intervention.* Baltimore: Paul H. Brookes.

Sampson, E. E., & Marthas, M. S. (1977). *Group process for the health professions.* New York: John Wiley & Sons.

Sarno, M. T., & Peters, J. (2005). *The Aphasia Handbook.* New York: National Aphasia Association.

Schmidt, N. D. (1999). Predicting the future. *Advance for Directors of Rehabilitation, 8*(8), 31–33.

Skoloda, T. E., & Angelini, F. J. (1998). Psychometric properties of the Revised Interprofessional Perception Scale (RIPS). Conference Paper: 20ᵗʰ Annual Interdisciplinary Health Care Teams Conference, International Conference: 1998: Williamsburg, VA.

Strasser, D. C., Stanley, J. M., Falconer, J. A., Herrin, J. S., & Bowen, S. E. (2002). The influence of hospital culture on rehabilitation team functioning in VA hospitals. *Journal of Rehabilitation Research & Development, 39*(1), 115–126.

Sundance, P., & Cope, D. N. (1995). Outcome Level I: Physiologic stability—acute management. In P. K. Landrum, N. D. Schmidt, & A. McLean Jr., (Eds.) *Outcome-oriented rehabilitation: Principles, strategies, and tools for effective program management.* Gaithersburg, MD: Aspen.

Tuchman, L. I. (1996). The team and models of teaming. In P. Rosin, A. D. Whitehead, L. I. Tuchman, G. S. Gesien, A. L. Begun, & L. Irwin (Eds.). *Partnerships in family-centered care: A guide to collaborative early intervention.* Baltimore: Paul H. Brookes.

van Vendendaal, H., Grinspin, D. R., & Andriaanse, H. P. (1996). Educational needs of stroke survivors and their family members as perceived by themselves and by health professionals. *Patient Education Council, 28,* 265–276.

Wertz, R. T., Weiss, D. G., Aten, J. L., Brookshire, R. H., Barcia-Bunuel, L., Holland, A. L. et al. (1986). Comparison of clinic, home, and deferred language treatment for aphasia. A Veterans Administration cooperative study. *Archives of Neurology, 43,* 653–658.

Chapter 9

Issues in Assessment and Treatment for Bilingual and Culturally Diverse Patients

Patricia M. Roberts

OBJECTIVES

The goals of this chapter are as follows:

1. To highlight how culture may influence the clinical process, and to provide references and a framework for detailed study of this area;
2. To provide a brief overview of the key terminology and concepts in bilingualism and bilingual aphasia;
3. To summarize some of the findings from psycholinguistic studies that are most relevant for clinical work with bilingual adults with aphasia;
4. To outline issues in the assessment and treatment of bilingual aphasia. These include test reliability and interpretation; available tests in different languages; patterns of impairment and recovery; setting treatment goals; choice of language(s) for treatment; use of interpreters; and generalization across languages.

In all areas, the goal is to highlight key issues. A single chapter cannot provide a comprehensive literature review on each topic. The focus is on issues most closely linked to clinical work and on issues that have received little attention in the speech pathology literature to date. In some cases, only recent work is cited. In these recent studies and review articles, the reader will find additional references. While language and culture are closely related, the challenges they present to clinicians working with clients with aphasia are quite different. Therefore, in this chapter they will be considered separately.

As awareness of the needs of patients from various cultural and linguistic backgrounds has grown, so has the awareness that clinicians require specific types of knowledge to work with these types of patients. This knowledge draws on at least three fields: (1) bilingualism, (2) culture, and (3) comparative aphasiology. Studies of bilingualism/multilingualism examine how people learn and use two or more languages or dialects, often comparing their performance to that of unilingual speakers. The literature on culture and cultural diversity examines the customs, beliefs, and behaviors of different groups defined by race, national origin, socioeconomic status (SES), or other common factor, and their impact on the clinical process or outcome. Comparative aphasiology refers to the study of aphasia in different languages. All three fields are relevant to the study of culturally and linguistically diverse (CLD) patients. A specialty within the CLD field is CLD neurogenics, or multicultural neurogenics, which focuses on neurogenic communication disorders. This chapter addresses CLD issues in aphasia, those relating to culture and also to bilingualism.

Some authors now use the term "multilingual" to mean speakers of two or more languages. In some studies, the authors fail to provide sufficient information and readers do not know whether the participants were bilingual (two languages) or multilingual (more than two). In the present chapter, we have used one or the other, as seemed appropriate, but the line between the two remains fuzzy. New studies are now probing for potential differences between bilinguals and multilinguals (Dewaele, 2001; Goral, Levy, Obler, & Cohen, 2006; Goral & Obler, in press; Lemhöfer, Dijkstra, & Michel, 2004).

Prior to 1990, bilingual aphasia is rarely mentioned in English textbooks, and cultural issues, if mentioned at all, are given little attention. Yet, "bilingualism, far from being exceptional, is a problem which affects the majority of the world's population" (Mackey, 1967, p. 11).[1] Paradis echoed this view, within a clinical perspective: "Bilingualism is not just a rare, occasional occurrence in the language/speech pathology clinic, but a phenomenon every clinic must be prepared to cope with" (1995c, p. 219).

In recent years, there has been a growing recognition in the English-language aphasiology literature of the importance of addressing the needs of patients from all linguistic and cultural backgrounds. This may reflect both greater

---

[1] In the French version of the same paper, Mackey refers to bilingualism as a "phenomenon." The English wording may or may not express his intended meaning and serves as an example of the potential for distortions of meaning that can occur in translation!

awareness of indigenous minority populations in many countries and the growing numbers of non-native English speakers in countries such as the United States, the United Kingdom, Canada, and Australia. Policy statements by several influential bodies have drawn attention to CLD issues (ASHA, 1985, 1989, 1991; Australian Association of Speech and Hearing, 1994; Australian Institute of Multicultural Affairs, 1985; Cole, 1989; Martin et al., 1998). Professional associations have prepared guidelines or standards for clinicians working with CLD populations (e.g., ASHA, 2004; Crago & Westernoff, 1997). Publications in medicine and (neuro)psychology have also called for more study of CLD groups (e.g., Ardila, 1995; Frayne, Burns, Hardt, Rosen, & Moskowitz, 1996; National Institutes of Health, 1990; NIDCD, 1992).

In the 1980s and 1990s researchers found that language and cultural background have an impact on performance on some neuropsychological tests (Ellis, 1992; Mungas, 1996; Puente & McCaffrey, 1992). In the same period, it became clear that aphasia in languages other than English and aphasia in bilinguals presented features not addressed in the English aphasiology literature.

CULTURE

Avoiding Stereotypes while Recognizing Differences

According to Grosjean (1982): "anthropologists commonly agree that culture consists of a number of components: the human's way of maintaining life, and perpetuating the species, along with habits, customs, ideas, sentiments, social arrangements, and objects. Culture is the way of life of a people or a society, including its rules of behavior; its economic, social and political systems; its language; its religious beliefs; its laws; and so on. Culture is acquired, socially transmitted, and communicated in large part by language." (p. 157).

Cultural background can influence many aspects of communication. Figure 9–1 illustrates how cultural factors, domains/topics, pragmatics, and linguistic knowledge all combine to produce communication. The items within each ring are examples of relevant factors, not a complete list. Depending on the communicative situation, the importance of each ring may grow or shrink. For example, asking someone what time it is has far less cultural content than asking someone out for dinner.

Most discussions of culture focus at a macro level. That is, they look at cultures as a whole. There are many books that describe various cultures, to assist health-care workers and/or teachers in working with people from these cultures (for example: Asante & Gudykunst, 1989; Battle, 1998; Brislin, 1994; Brislin, Cushner, Cherrie, & Yong, 1986; Fawcett & Carino, 1987; Galens, Sheets, & Young, 1995; Goldstein, 2000; Lynch & Hanson, 1992). These books describe various societies or cultural groups in terms of specific characteristics, often prefaced by a historical sketch of how a particular group came to

live in a given country or region. Most sketches include information on (1) health and wellness; (2) disability; (3) family structure and roles within the family; (4) how status is determined; (5) time; (6) religion; (7) food preferences and customs; (8) the language(s) and dialect(s) spoken and some of their key characteristics; and (9) nonverbal aspects of communication.

There are many sources of information on different cultures, and many different cultures that could be relevant for readers in different settings. Therefore, specific cultural profiles will not be presented here. Instead, the following section offers some caveats and comments for clinicians to consider as they read these cultural guidebooks.

The problem with brief cultural sketches is that they tend not to recognize individual variations. Therefore, they can easily create or reinforce ethnic and racial stereotypes. One author, for example, describes the Japanese immigrant family as characterized by interdependency, hierarchical relationships, and empathy, and contrasts this with Anglo-American families which, the author implies, do not share these characteristics (Tempo & Saito, 1996). But not all Anglo-American families are the same. Another cultural guide states that some devout Muslims do not plan more than a few weeks ahead because they believe that only Allah knows the future (Davis, Gentry, & Hubbard-Wiley, 1998). There is no indication of how many Muslims might share this fatalistic approach. Nor does the author remind us that some people of other faiths share a similar fatalistic view of the future. Such inaccurate, sweeping generalizations do little to help us understand each other.

A different approach to culture can help to minimize stereotyping. Gollnick and Chin (1990) suggest viewing individuals as coming from individual (micro) cultures within a broader (macro) culture. This view encourages clinicians to look beyond race or ethnicity to see what factors influence a specific patient's behavior. The microculture variables Gollnick and Chin identify are (1) ethnic or national origin; (2) religion; (3) gender/sex; (4) age; (5) exceptionality; (6) urban-suburban-rural; (7) geographic region; and (8) social class. These eight factors and the individual patient's views and behavior can help us to look beyond ethnic groups and see that, despite their different race and nationality, a 55-year-old Chinese lawyer from Hong Kong may have more in common with a 52-year-old Anglo architect from Chicago than he does with a 22-year-old Hong Kong street vendor. A number of authors have reminded us of the importance of individual differences within cultural groups (e.g., Kayser, 1998; Pontón & Ardila, 1999; Wallace, 1997) but this point is often neglected. We must be particularly careful to guard against cultural stereotypes and generalizations when a patient's appearance (skin color, hair, features) identifies them as having a specific background.

The descriptions in many books stress the differences between CLD groups and the so-called mainstream culture. While these differences can be important, we must not lose sight of the many similarities across cultures, and of individ-

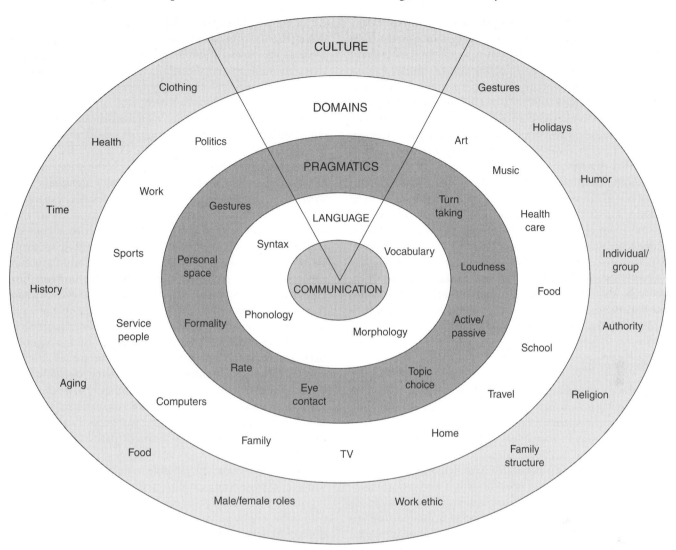

Figure 9–1. Communication within a cultural context.

ual variability within each cultural group. Holland and Penn (1995) describe Native American and African views in which disability is due to evil spirits. These views may lead some patients and families to reject rehabilitation efforts. The cases are used to support Holland and Penn's recommendation that treatment "should [not] be imposed upon patients whose cultural belief systems do not recognize therapy as a need" (p. 154). This is true, not only for CLD patients but for all patients. Some white, middle-class, Anglo-Saxon clients also reject therapy. What are often cited as "cultural variables" apply to all patients. They are factors clinicians can use to assess their possible impact on the clinical process. They allow us to tailor the assessment and treatment to meet the individual needs of each patient, not only those labeled CLD.

Acculturation is another factor in working with CLD patients. Acculturation refers to the process by which people from one cultural background adopt the cultural values and practices of a different culture. Usually, it applies to immigrants adopting the prevailing culture of their new country. Some authors propose seeing people as being on a continuum of acculturation or a series of levels of acculturation (Langdon, 1992b; Marin, 1992; Valle, 1994). Culture is a multilayered, multifaceted thing. A given person may be at a different level of acculturation in different areas of their lives, adopting "mainstream" values and habits around work and retaining more customs and values from their national group around religious or family matters. Within the same family, different members may be at different levels of acculturation. For some adults, proficiency in the mainstream language correlates strongly with their level of acculturation (Burr & Mutchler, 2003; Kang, 2006).

Finally, many immigrants, especially those who have chosen to leave their country of birth, reject aspects of its prevailing culture and embrace the values of their new country. Thus, knowing that someone is a recent immigrant from Haïti, Pakistan, or Russia does not mean that they share the prevailing religious, political, or family values of those countries. This is demonstrated in a study by Erickson, Devlieger, and Sung (1999). Thirty young women, all born in Korea but living in the United States, identified many folk beliefs about illness and disability as being typical of Korean culture. However, their own beliefs closely matched those of the mainstream American culture.

It is important for clinicians working with CLD clients to read about and learn about the cultural backgrounds of their patients. These descriptions provide tools for problem-solving and clues about what to watch for in our interactions. These descriptions suggest questions: Why is this client late? Does the patient want a relative to be in the room during our sessions? Should I shake hands with family members? Can the patient attend an appointment on Friday? However, descriptions about racial, linguistic, or political groups cannot be used to predict what any individual may believe or do.

The Need for Data

Many recommendations in the CLD literature are based on the author's clinical experience, or their opinion. While some provide valuable insights, others are incorrect. For example, one writer stated that the phrase "no if's and's or but's" probably cannot be translated into any other language (Teng, 1996, p. 78). It is possible to translate this into a number of languages (French is one), though it would not necessarily have the status of a fixed expression as it does in English. Many recommendations in the CLD literature are untested. Suggestions such as "Better clinical results may be obtained if music consistent with the African-American culture is played while the client waits" (Terrell, Battle, & Grantham, 1998, p. 37) need to be tested. The clinician should also weigh the possible benefits of suggested changes in the clinical environment or clinical process in relation to their cost, and try to separate politically motivated claims and recommendations from those that have a clinical, patient-focused foundation. Clinicians will find valuable information in journals such as the *Journal of Cross-cultural Psychology* and the *Journal of Cross-cultural Gerontology*, as well as in books written for health-care providers (e.g., Paniagua, 2005). There are also studies and books on areas now called "ethnogerontology" and "gerontolinguistics" (e.g., de Bot & Makoni, 2005). These are relevant to aphasia, given the age of many adults with aphasia.

Clinical Chameleons?

In some cases, a center may serve a single client group, such as Hispanic, African-American, or Chinese. This makes it possible to link the clinical environment to that culture (e.g.,

decor, music, clinical tools). In many cities, however, a clinic serves clients from different cultures. This makes it impossible to tailor the environment to any one group. It also means that the clinician and the client will often not be from the same linguistic or cultural background. Therefore, compromises will have to be made.

To work with CLD clients, clinicians should be as knowledgeable as possible about customs and views that may affect the clinical process. It is possible to change many aspects of our testing and treatment. Possible changes include using appropriate greetings, having other family members attend with the patient, asking the appropriate person in the family group when decisions must be made, asking indirect questions, and allowing more or less time for informal conversation as part of each appointment. It is also possible to learn to interpret signals such as eye contact or punctuality within a range of cultural contexts. It is not possible, however, for a clinician to fully master all the culture-specific behaviors needed in a setting where a wide range of people are seen. Inevitably, when clinical services are offered by a professional who does not share the patient's macro- or microcultural background, some things may seem "foreign." The client, family, and clinician can all work to avoid misunderstandings. The clinician can do this by stating explicitly what the assessment or treatment involves; what role the patient, family, and clinician will each play; asking the patient and family what is important to them (as we do with any patient, but recognizing that for CLD patients the answers may vary more); and giving choices where it is possible to do so. If read with a critical eye, the literature on different cultures provides a starting point for clinical problem-solving. It provides the clinician with tools for his or her work with patients from different backgrounds. It does not and cannot provide step-by-step instructions or rules for any given type of patient.

BILINGUALISM

Debates about Defining Bilingualism

The word "bilingual" has different meanings for different people. In fact, Hakuta has said that the difficulty defining bilingualism makes it "fruitless to estimate the proportion of the world's population that is bilingual" (Hakuta, 1986, p. 4). Other authors have stated that at least half the world's population is bilingual (Grosjean, 1997; Harris & Nelson, 1992). Perhaps surprisingly, in bilingualism research, there is no consensus about the definition of "bilingual." In some studies, the bilingual subjects are in the process of learning a second language, while in others, the subjects have spoken both languages well since early childhood (see Edwards, 2006, for an entertaining discussion of the problem of defining bilingualism).

The lack of consensus about the definition of the word *bilingualism* leads to differences in how the term is used. For some authors, one can speak two languages but not be bilingual if the second language (L2) is a "foreign" language that is not needed for day-to-day life (Baker, 1993; Duncan, 1989; Grosjean, 1992; Paradis, 1997). Thus, Americans who speak French are seen as bilingual by some authors (Frenck-Mestre & Pynte, 1997), but would be called L2 speakers by others. For other authors (see Baetens Beardsmore, 1982), bilingualism is defined in terms of language use, not in terms of knowledge. The problem in basing definitions in bilingualism on patterns of use is that these can change, while the level of knowledge of the language does not. For example, if a bilingual speaker moved from Texas, where she regularly used English and Spanish, to South Dakota, where she only spoke English, would she stop being bilingual a week after she moved? A month after?

This lack of consensus about what *bilingual* means is important to keep in mind when interpreting and comparing studies, and when deciding to whom the results of a particular study apply. If the participants were in the process of learning a second language, the results may nor may not apply to proficient L2 speakers, even though they may all be called bilingual.

Most authors, especially in studies of adult bilinguals, define bilingualism in terms of level of linguistic knowledge. They see bilingualism as a continuum, not a bilingual/unilingual dichotomy (Hakuta, 1986; Paradis, 1998). Many studies refer to more-fluent or less-fluent bilinguals or compare groups with different levels of bilingualism. Furthermore, the bilingualism continuum is multidimensional. A person may have different levels of proficiency in the different language modalities (auditory and written comprehension, verbal expression, and written expression) and in different linguistic components (morphology, syntax, phonology, lexical semantics). Although some authors have viewed "true" bilinguals as those who have equal proficiency in their two languages, such people are the exception, if they exist at all. Even people who appear to have native or near-native proficiency in their second language display subtle differences in their performance on both production and comprehension tasks (Cutler, Mehler, Norris, & Segui, 1992; Hyltenstam, 1992) because each language may influence the other in speech perception (Flege, MacKay, & Meador, 1999; Levey, 2004), vocabulary (Bettoni, 1991; Chitiri & Willows, 1997), and syntax (Dijkstra et al., 2005; Frenck-Mestre & Pynte, 1997; Grosjean & Py, 1991; Hohenstein, Eisenberg, & Naigles, 2006; Kilborn, 1992; MacWhinney, 2002; Oesch-Serra, 1992; Pavlenko, 2000; Pavlenko & Jarvis, 2002; Salamoura & Williams, 2006; Van Hell & Dijkstra, 2002; Van Wijnendaele & Brysbaert, 2002). Bilingualism creates a unique speaker-hearer, unlike a unilingual speaker of either language (Fishman, 1965; Grosjean, 1989, 1998; Hyltenstam, 1992; Selinker, 1992). The most obvious lexical changes occur when words from L2 become accepted as words within L1. In North America, for example, English

terms such as "modem" or "back-up" are often used in Spanish or French conversations about computers. Several models attempt to explain this cross-language interference, including Selinker's interlanguage, the competition model of MacWhinney and Bates (1989), and models derived from Levelt's work. The key point for clinicians to remember about these studies is that, while there is still debate about how and why the interference between languages occurs, it is clear that it does occur for phonology, lexical items, and syntax, and in both comprehension and production. So clinicians should expect to see features of one language in the other, even in neurologically intact adults. For some patients, this makes it difficult to know what is a symptom of the aphasia and what reflects normal language patterns. The processing strategy some patients use for a particular task may not be the one the clinician is targeting.

People rarely experience all activities and all types of interactions in both their languages. Therefore, their vocabulary, use of idioms, and mastery of formal and informal registers is rarely equivalent in the two languages. There are domains of use such as family, religion, and work, each with its own vocabulary and linguistic patterns (Baker, 1995; Fishman, 1965; Miller, 1984; Reyes, 1998). Someone who uses only one language at work may not know work-related vocabulary in his other language. Grosjean (1997, 1998) has termed this the **complementarity principle**—each language is used for certain purposes in specific situations and vocabulary and other types of knowledge only exist in both or all languages if that individual has needed to use both languages in a particular context.

Another feature of bilingualism is its instability over time. A person's level of bilingualism may increase or decrease with use or disuse. Language **attrition**—also called language loss—is a common process (Seliger & Vago, 1991). Attrition may affect different language modalities and linguistic components differently. Expressive use of vocabulary is particularly vulnerable to forgetting (Weltens & Grendel, 1993), while comprehension is less so. The type and degree of attrition vary, in ways not yet well-documented or understood, with the age of acquisition, amount of use, and level of proficiency attained in each language and not simply with years of residency in a particular country (Bahrick, Hall, Goggin, Bahrick, & Berger, 1994; Bettoni, 1991; Goral, 2004; Montrul, 2002). Some aspects of linguistic knowledge that may be particularly vulnerable to attrition are infrequently used words, distinctions that exist in the weakening language but not in the increasingly dominant language, bound items (as opposed to free), and irregularities (Seliger & Vago, 1991; Sharwood Smith, 1989; Weltens & Grendel, 1993). Because of language attrition, a person's first language (L1) or native language is not always their stronger language.

In considering how to define bilingualism, it is important to acknowledge **dialects**. There is no standard for determining at what point a dialect is different enough from its base language to become a language in its own right. Some pairs of languages are more similar and more mutually intelligible than are some language/dialect pairs. In some cases, a speaker of two dialects of the same language may be seen as bilingual, especially when the dialects are not mutually intelligible, as is the case for some dialects of Italian, Arabic, and Chinese, for example. Some authors consider speakers of African-American English and standard English to be bilingual (de Bot & Makoni, 2005), while most do not.

Another factor to keep in mind is that, in regions with a history of extensive interaction between speakers of different languages, the languages themselves change. For example, there are different "world Englishes" learned by native English speakers in Singapore, Hawaii, India, Canada, and Scotland. Within the United States and the United Kingdom, there are also many varieties of English spoken, often linked to regional, racial, or socioeconomic differences. The same is true of Spanish, French, and Arabic, all of which have creole, pidgin, and regional varieties. Clinical assessments must measure language abilities in relation to the patient's dialect.

Code-switching is one feature of how some bilinguals communicate. Code-switching is the use of a word, phrase, or sentence in one language when speaking another. It is sometimes used when the speaker does not know how to say what he wants to in the language being spoken or when one language has a word or phrase which expresses his or her intended meaning better than the other. Code-switching is also triggered by the topic, by shared group membership or experiences, and by other factors. Code-switching occurs more often in some speakers and some groups than in others, and follows different patterns (Jacobson, 1998, 2001; Myers-Scotton, 2005; Myers-Scotton & Jake, 2001). Aphasia may lead to an increase in code-switching (Hyltenstam, 1992). Selinker and Seliger (1972, 1992) coined the term **interlanguage** to refer to the influence of one language on another. Interlanguage refers to errors made by L2 speakers that can be linked to the influence of their L1 (for a review of interlanguage during acquisition, and how interlanguage becomes permanent, see Gass & Selinker, 1994). The most well-known examples of interlanguage are perhaps in pronunciation. For example, some Spanish-speakers roll their R's when speaking English, and some native Chinese speakers substitute /r/ for /l/.

Types of Bilingualism

Many typologies of bilingualism have been proposed. Overly simple models such as the compound/coordinate/subordinate distinction (for overviews see Baetens Beardsmore, 1982, or Hamers & Blanc, 1989) have been discarded by most researchers (Durgunoglu & Roediger, 1987; Grosjean, 1998; Kirsner, Lalor, & Hird, 1993; Paradis, 1995a). Recent studies also suggest that different types of

lexical representations may exist for different types of words, with concrete nouns, for example, sharing more of the elements of their representations than other types of words (Costa, 2005; de Groot, 1993). Most studies group their subjects by age of acquisition of the two languages and by level of proficiency in each language because these two factors influence performance on a wide range of tasks. In clinical work, too, when and how well patients learned their languages are key factors.

Various models of how the two languages are organized and processed have been proposed (Cenoz, Hufeisen, & Jessner, 2003; de Bot, 1992; de Bot & Schreuder, 1993; Dijkstra & Van Heuven, 2002; Green, 1998; Grosjean, 1997; Kroll & de Groot, 1997, 2005; MacWhinney, 2002; Paradis, 1997, 2004). Experimental evidence is still being gathered on these models. It seems clear, however, that the question "do bilinguals store their languages in one system or two?" is overly simple. Research is now focused on the types and strengths of links between languages, the processing strategies used during comprehension and production, and whether these links and strategies vary with level of proficiency in each language, the type of word, the degree of similarity between the two languages, and other factors. Although each model has studies supporting it (and others potentially contradicting it), there is now substantial converging evidence that the two languages are connected. This finding has direct consequences for clinical work, as described below.

Age of Acquisition

Recent work shows sensitive periods of varying length for optimal acquisition of different language components, such as syntax and phonology. During these sensitive periods, children can acquire native-like proficiency in a second language (L2), although not all of them will reach this high level (Pallier, Bosch, & Sebastián-Galles, 1997). Language-learning is still possible later, but more conscious effort is required and the L2 is more likely to show the influence of L1, in at least some linguistic components (Harley & Wang, 1997; Hurford, 1991; Scovel, 1989).

On a clinical level, this means that the later a patient began to learn a given language, the more imperfect their mastery of that language is likely to be. We can expect to see more interlanguage, more influence of L1 on L2, in late learners. However, individual differences in language-learning ability and patterns of use of each language over time will influence the level of proficiency attained.

Localization of Languages in Bilinguals

Localization of language in multilingual speakers has been studied in a series of cases (see Abutalebi, Cappa, & Perani, 2005, for a recent review). It is now clear that functions that are in the left hemisphere of unilinguals are also in the left hemisphere of bilinguals (Paradis, 1990, 1998). This is apparently the case even for tone languages such as Chinese and Thai (Gandour, 1998; Naeser & Chan, 1980). Damage to the left hemisphere affects linguistic tones, which serve a lexical role. Comprehension and production of tones are dissociable (Gandour, 1998; Packard, 1986), just as comprehension and expression for non-tonal elements can be.

Subcortical aphasia similar to that reported in unilinguals has been documented following lesions in the left putamen, left caudate nucleus, internal capsule, and thalamus in several Italian patients (Abutalebi, Miozzo, & Cappa, 2000; Aglioti & Fabbro, 1993; Fabbro & Paradis, 1995; Moretti, Torre, Antonello, Cazzato, & Bava, 2003). There are also cases of subcortical, bilingual aphasia in Mandarin, Cantonese, and Thai (Gandour, 1998). Some authors have linked subcortical lesions, including those in the left caudate nucleus, to control of selecting and switching appropriately between languages (Abutalebi, Miozzo, & Cappa, 2000; Crinion et al., 2006).

Initial PET studies of English/French bilingual adults who learned French at an average age of 7 years found that the two languages activate overlapping regions in the left hemisphere (Klein, Zatorre, Milner, Meyer, & Evans, 1994, 1995). "Within- and across- language searches [synonym generation, translation of single words] involve similar distributed networks even when there are differences in the accuracy and latencies across the tasks, strongly suggesting that word generation in the two languages makes demands on overlapping neural substrates (Klein et al., 1995, p. 31). Hernandez, Dapretto, Mazziotta, and Bookheimer (2001) found no difference in the left-hemisphere areas activated during a naming task in English and Spanish in proficient bilinguals. Translation from L1 (English) to L2 (French) activated the putamen, but backward translation (L2 to L1) did not (Klein et al., 1995).

A similar but not identical result is reported by Kim, Relkin, Lee, and Hirsch (1997) using 12 adults who spoke six different pairs of languages. Using fMRI, they found overlapping areas of activation for L1 and L2 in Wernicke's area for all subjects. For the six early bilinguals, the two languages also activated similar regions in and near Broca's area. Less overlap in Broca's area was observed for the six subjects who began L2 acquisition later (mean age 11). Also using fMRI, Chee, Tan, and Thiel (1999) found that single-word production in Mandarin/English bilingual adults activated the same regions within the left hemisphere in both languages. This was true for early bilinguals (began L2 by age 6) and for late bilinguals (began L2 after age 12).

Somewhat different patterns of results have also been found. Chee, Soon, and Lee (2003) found some overlapping areas of activiation but also differences in activation in the L prefrontal and L temporal regions during a word repetition task (fMRI) by 22 English-Chinese bilinguals. Halsband,

Krause, Sipilae, Teraes, & Laihinen (2002) studied Finnish-English bilingual men with PET scans. During a memory task for pairs of words, the two languages activated some different regions around Broca's area, the left angular and supra-marginal gyri, and the cerebellum. Perani and colleagues (2003) tested two groups of men (all very proficient bilinguals) who spoke either primarily Spanish ($n = 6$) or primarily Catalan ($n = 5$) in their daily lives. There were differences in activation in the left frontal and parietal temporal lobes during a verbal-fluency task for the two groups. Perani and colleagues interpret these differences as being due to a combination of exposure to L2 and to age of acquisition. However, the verbal-fluency task activates a wide range of areas, in both hemispheres; the groups were small, and relatively diverse in their patterns of language use; and no mention is made of knowledge of additional languages. Therefore, other explanations for the results cannot be ruled out.

There are fewer fMRI studies of comprehension tasks. Perani and colleagues used a receptive language task in a series of studies. Using French/English and Italian/English bilingual adults, these studies have shown that the left-hemisphere areas activated when listening to stories in L1 and L2 vary with the age of acquisition and with the level of proficiency in L2 (Dehaene et al., 1997; Perani et al., 1996; Perani et al., 1998).

In at least one study there is evidence that learning a second language can increase gray-matter density in the left hemisphere (left inferior parietal cortex), and that these changes correlate with both age of L2 acquisition and overall proficiency in L2 (Mechelli et al., 2004). Activation of overlapping areas during language tasks does not mean that the same neuronal networks are involved in both languages. Clinically, there is evidence that the vocabulary or the syntax of only one language may be available at certain times, suggesting that different languages draw on different micro-anatomical regions or circuits. This variability is similar to what we see in unilingual patients who can produce some words or sentence types (inconsistently from day to day) but not others.

We are only beginning to map the localization of the bilingual's two languages. The range of tasks used in the brain-mapping studies to date is limited. Few language pairs, and relatively few individuals, have been studied with fMRI and PET. Individual differences in anatomy and localization may be incorrectly interpreted (Dehaene et al., 1997; Steinmetz & Seitz, 1991). Most studies that compare areas activated in two or more languages fail to consider what the difference in activation might have been if participants were retested in the same language. Mahendra, Plante, Magloire, Milman, and Trouard (2003) draw attention to this point in a study that found that the degree of non-overlap for participants' L1 and L2 was no greater than what they call the "run-to-run variability" inherent in fMRI testing. Most studies fail to provide adequate descriptions of the participants' language history and proficiency to allow comparisons across studies. The linguistic demands and neurologic activity associated with the experimental task(s) in unilingual speakers are still being identified and debated (Grosjean, Li, Münte, & Rodriguez-Fornells, 2003; Dijkstra & Van Heuven, 2006). Van Lancker Sidtis goes so far as to say that in fMRI studies "the cognitive meaning of the signal remains uncertain" (2006, p. 285). How neural representation of the two languages relates to symptoms, prognosis, or rehabilitation for aphasia has not yet been addressed.

Functional Links Between Languages

Understanding how languages are stored neuroanatomically is important. Just as important for clinical work is understanding how the two languages are functionally connected. What are the links or relationships between languages that may be exploited in treatment?

In exploring how the two languages are organized, researchers have studied cross-language priming (facilitation) and cross-language interference. These studies use single words, usually nouns. Therefore, the results apply to part of the bilingual lexicon, and not necessarily to other aspects of language. Nonetheless, dozens of studies show that reading or hearing a word in one language can facilitate or interfere with responses in another language. The tasks studied include reading aloud, lexical decision, translating single words, and categorizing words (Altarriba, 1992; Chen, 1992; Costa, Miozzo, & Caramazza, 1999; de Groot, Borgwaldt, Bos, & Van den Eijnden, 2002; Lemhöfer & Dijkstra, 2004; Snodgrass, 1993; Van Hell & de Groot, 1998). In most studies, the priming or interference is stronger in one direction than the other. The strength and the direction of between-language effects are influenced by factors such as the length of time (in milliseconds) between the prime and the target, the level of proficiency of the subjects in each language, age of acquisition, and the stimuli used. All of these factors, except the first, come into play in clinical work.

In addition to the usual factors that make stimuli easier or harder, such as frequency or length of the words, factors specific to bilinguals have been identified. First, the number of "**neighbors**" (words with similar spelling and/or pronunciation) in one language affects lexical decision speed in the other language (Grainger & Dijkstra, 1992). Second, the similarity of the words in each language is a factor. Synonyms with a very similar form in different languages are called "cognates" (e.g. lemon and limòn). Several studies show that priming between languages is greater for cognates than for non-cognates (see above reviews) and processing of cognates is faster and/or more accurate than it is for non-cognates (Lemhöfer & Dijkstra, 2004). Naming of cognates is more accurate than non-cognates for both normal adults and those with aphasia (Ferrand & Humphreys, 1996;

Kohnert, 2004; Roberts & Deslauriers, 1999; Sanchez-Casas & García-Albea, 2005; Stadie, Springer, de Bleser, & Burk, 1995), but individual patients do not necessarily achieve higher scores on cognate words than on non-cognates for all tasks (Goral et al., 2006).

Clinically, these findings suggest that cues in one language may assist word-finding in the other, that interference across languages should be monitored, and that in selecting stimuli, the clinician should be aware of possible cross-language phenomena, including the bilingual neighborhood effect and the influence of cognates.

The literature on culture and on bilingualism has implications for clinical work. The remainder of this chapter will outline these, and examine the challenges facing clinicians who assess and treat bilingual aphasia.

ISSUES IN ASSESSING BILINGUAL APHASIA

To plan appropriate treatment, one must conduct a valid, comprehensive, and reliable assessment. This is difficult to do in bilingual aphasia. There are problems related to culture, level of bilingualism, available tests, interpreters, and test-retest reliability, as outlined below. The assessment of bilingual patients also includes determining the impact of the aphasia on each language.

Culture

Cultural factors can influence the level of cooperation with the assessment. These factors may include the perceived appropriateness of the clinician's age, gender, race, body language, tone of voice, or dress. How the testing tasks are presented (direct versus indirect commands), the patient's understanding of why he or she is being tested, and what is expected of him or her are also important.

Prior to the assessment, the clinician should learn enough about a patient's background to know which aspects of the clinical process might be problematic. For inpatients, it is often helpful to observe the patient and family, and to consult with the social worker and nurses to learn more about the macro- and microcultural history of the patient and about the patient's and family's reaction to the communication disorder. During the assessment and treatment, give the patient and family members choices, when possible, based on cultural factors.

The assessment is a cyclical process of observing, then interpreting, the client's behavior. Before interpreting behaviors, especially apparently negative ones, consider all possible reasons for the behavior, including cultural ones. Being late may indicate a lack of motivation, transportation problems, anxiety about coming to the clinic, executive-function problems, or simply a different view of time. Other behaviors that are easily misunderstood include eye contact, greetings, notifying the clinic to cancel an appointment, asking or not asking questions, indicating yes/no, accepting or refusing food, giving/receiving gifts, gestures, choice of topics for conversation, and being active or passive in the treatment process.

Dealing with CLD patients and families can be a wonderful experience. Flexibility, a nonjudgmental view, and good clinical problem-solving skills are essential qualities. Cheng (1996) emphasizes how difficult intercultural communication is, and how easily misunderstandings can occur. But working with CLD clients can, with a little flexibility on all sides, work well. Published case summaries demonstrate this (Holland & Penn, 1995; Wallace, 1997; Whitworth & Sjardin, 1993). For aphasia assessment and treatment to work, the clinician need not master all aspects of the patient's culture. The clinician and the patient do not have to be from the same culture. Our goals should be to understand the aspects of each patient's beliefs, values, and communication style that will have the most impact on the clinical process. We can then be creative in developing ways of interacting that the patient finds culturally acceptable, while still allowing the clinician to offer assessment and treatment that are clinically appropriate. This goal applies to all patients no matter what their language, cultural background, race, or ethnic origins.

Level of Bilingualism

Decisions about testing and treatment must take into account the patient's premorbid level of bilingualism. The psycholinguistic studies of bilingualism show that the speed and accuracy on many language tasks, the effects of cues, and the amount of interference between languages are all influenced by the level of proficiency in each language. Unfortunately, it is impossible to know precisely what the patient's premorbid abilities were. Using the psycholinguistic literature as a guide, one can use four types of information to arrive at an estimate.

1. Self-ratings: Adults can rate their abilities in each language for various types of tasks (Albert & Obler, 1978; Hamers & Blanc, 1989, 2000) with reasonable levels of accuracy. Some authors use a five-point or seven-point scale, obtaining separate ratings for each language (Langdon, Wiig, & Nielsen, 2005). Others ask subjects to directly compare their abilities in each language (de Groot & Poot, 1997; Roberts & Le Dorze, 1997, 1998). Both types of self-rating correlate with group performance on a number of tasks used in clinical work, including verbal fluency (Lafaury & Roberts, 1998; Langdon et al., 2005; Roberts & Le Dorze, 1997) and picture naming (Kohnert, Hernandez, & Bates, 1998; Roberts & Bois, 1999).

   One group study has used self-rating of premorbid abilities by adults with aphasia (Roberts & Le Dorze, 1998). While this identified groups of balanced bilin-

guals, how well self-ratings correlate with individual performance on a given task or aphasia test has not been adequately examined.

2. Ratings by family members: Information provided by the patient can be supplemented by asking the family to assess the patient's level of bilingualism. Ratings of the patient's abilities may be influenced by the family member's own level of bilingualism. To obtain an accurate view, ask more than one person, and take their own bilingualism into account in interpreting their ratings. A wife who speaks little English may overestimate her husband's abilities. A child who grew up speaking English may be very critical of an immigrant parent's less-than-perfect abilities.

   In trying to establish the patient's premorbid level of bilingualism, it is best to avoid the use of the word "bilingual." For many people, bilingual means perfect and equal proficiency in both languages. When asked if the patient is bilingual, they will say "No," and the patient will be incorrectly identified thereafter as unilingual. It is important to ask sufficiently detailed questions before deciding on a rating, and to ask the questions in terms the patient and family can understand. Instead of "How was his auditory comprehension in ___," ask "Could he understand the news on the radio? people talking at work? people who spoke quickly? people with different accents?..."

3. Patterns of use for each language: Knowing which language was used in which situation helps to determine the importance of each language for the patient, what language(s) will be needed poststroke, and what vocabulary may be used for which types of treatment tasks.

   Baker (1995) has shown the importance of assessing domains of use. In a study of 72 immigrants from six different countries, most of whom had lived in Australia for over 10 years, there was a wide range of patterns of use of L1 and English. Length of residence in Australia and even level of ability in English did not correlate with patterns of use. Subjects identified 10 domains of use: family, friends, shopping, religion, medical, dealing with tradespeople, hobbies, business/work, dealing with the legal/government system, and public transportation. Within these domains, 38 specific tasks were identified. Baker's list of tasks makes a good starting point for a language-use questionnaire.

4. Acquisition history: Knowing how and at what age the patient was exposed to each language may suggest treatment approaches. For example, one might refer to "grammar rules" or the names of verb tenses if English (L2) was learned in a classroom but not if it was acquired informally. The acquisition history and patterns of use both provide indirect evidence about level of proficiency. Early acquisition and extensive use across different domains often suggest a high level of

proficiency. If there are discrepancies between the family's assessment of the patient's abilities, and the patient's use of his languages, these can be explored. For example, if the family or patient claim that the patient "spoke ___ perfectly before his stroke," but this language was rarely used, this discrepancy should be explored, especially given the potential attrition of little-used languages.

Information on language proficiency, use, and acquisition is important in deciding what areas to assess, interpreting the results (separating premorbid characteristics from the effects of the aphasia), and in planning treatment (see Roberts & Shenker (in press) for a language-history questionnaire covering all three of these dimensions). For example, if a patient says "now talk hard - no talk good," this could indicate nonfluent aphasia or could be close to his prestroke level of English. Only by gathering information about the patient's premorbid bilingualism can the clinician estimate their poststroke language impairment and plan appropriate treatment. This information, however, does not allow us to predict patterns of impairment (L1 vs. L2) or recovery, nor to establish a prognosis specifically focused on the bilingualism. "No correlation has been found between pattern of recovery and neurological, etiological, experimental or linguistic parameters: not site, size or origin of lesion, type or severity of aphasia, type of bilingualism, language structure type, or factors related to acquisition or habitual use" (Paradis, 1995b, p. 211).

Using Interpreters

When a patient must be assessed or treated in a language that the clinician does not master (see ASHA 1989 guidelines for the level of proficiency needed for clinical work), an interpreter can be used. Interpreters should be used only if there is no speech-language pathologist (SLP) available who speaks the patient's language(s). This is because of the disadvantages associated with using interpreters. These include difficulties locating an interpreter who is able to spend the time required and who is able to fit into the constraints of the patient's schedule, and the time needed to train interpreters in test administration, interviewing, and therapy techniques. Even with training, interpreters may inadvertently alter the test stimuli or protocol or fail to convey relevant details of the patient's response. Because the SLP does not speak the language being tested, he or she may not always be aware that this has happened. Furthermore, the clinician cannot be certain that the interpreter is reporting all the relevant aspects of the patient's performance, such as the nature of errors. There may be direct costs for the interpreter's time, which are not covered by health insurance.

When demand justifies it, a clinic may hire interpreters for specific languages as full- or part-time staff. Before working with interpreters—either volunteers or paid staff—clinicians should familiarize themselves with the process, its requirements, its pitfalls, its limitations, and any relevant legal restrictions or policies (Gentile, Ozolins, & Vasilakakos, 1996; Kayser, 1995; Langdon, 1992a; Langdon & Cheng, 2002; Martin et al., 1998).

When a professional interpreter or aide trained to fill this role is not available, members of the patient's community or family can be used if they are trained by the SLP for this role. Family members who have close ties to the patient may find it distressing to see the full extent of the deficits exposed. They may also be more inclined to provide cues or assistance to the patient. Friends or members of the patient's religious or community groups can often be more detached. The person chosen as interpreter must also be acceptable to the patient, available for the time needed to complete the assessment, and available for regular treatment sessions.

Given the time and expense required, and given the problems in achieving reliable results in assessment, is it worth using an interpreter? The consensus in the current literature is that patients must be assessed in all languages they use on a regular basis, or for a specific purpose. Without this assessment, the diagnosis, as well as the treatment goals set for the patient, may be inappropriate. The resources and policies of each clinic will determine whether this standard is reached for all patients.

Testing in Various Languages

To adequately assess patients with bilingual aphasia, we need a range of tests that are reliable and valid with demonstrated sensitivity (to detect changes over time and to discriminate between levels of impairment), and with norms for specific groups. Such tests should be as free of cultural bias as possible. Unfortunately, we do not yet have such a range of tests.

It is important to remember that the basic principles of test design (validity, reliability, adequacy of norms, etc.) apply to all aphasia tests, including translations of existing tests that attempt to meet the needs of CLD patients. The (American) Agency for Health Care Research and Quality has identified the need for development of better tests for communication disorders, stating: "With the increasing cultural, linguistic, and racial diversity of the U.S. population, the applicability of assessment instruments to individuals who are members of different subpopulations is of crucial importance to clinical diagnosis and the process of disability determination. Despite the existence of a large number of speech and language assessment instruments, we still lack appropriate instruments for reliably and validly assessing speech and language in many subgroups defined in terms of language, dialect, or cultural differences. Thus, future research funding and priorities should be directed at addressing these serious deficiencies." (2002) (http://www.ahrq.gov/clinic/epcsums/spdissum.htm)

Many clinics and many published studies use in-house translations of published tests (e.g., Radanovic, Mansur, & Scaff, 2004). Thus, studies are published that present data on tests such as the BDAE or the WAB but with no reference for the test in the language of the study. This state of affairs is due partly to the reluctance of publishing houses to accept tests that will have relatively small potential markets. Clinicians and researchers have little choice but to develop their own tests, or their own translations of published tests. However, too often, clinicians and authors then use these tests to compare the severity of the aphasia across languages or to measure improvement over time. Without even basic reliability, validity, and sensitivity data on these instruments, there is no way to interpret the obtained scores, beyond a very general patterns such as "seemed to do well on these tasks" or "low score on this set of items." It is inappropriate to use them to diagnose aphasia or to identify a type of aphasia. On the other hand, faced with the need to assess patients, clinicians may have little choice, particularly in countries where no one has developed aphasia tests in the range of languages needed for patients in that country.

Published Tests in Various Languages

To assess the patient's or family's perception of the impact of the aphasia on the patient's communication, the ASHA Functional Assessment of Communication Skills (FACS; Frattali, Thompson, Holland, Wohl, & Ferketic, 1995) may be used. Its test items are designed to be suitable for use with patients from a wide range of cultural backgrounds. It falls to the individual clinician, however, to translate the questions, with the potential for poor translations and changes in meaning or nuance across the different languages.

To assess the linguistic abilities of bilingual patients, clinicians in North America have limited choices: the Boston Diagnostic Aphasia Examination, the Bilingual Aphasia Test, the Multilingual Aphasia Examination, and the Aachen Aphasia Test all have published versions in various languages. In-house translations of these and other tests are often available in clinics that see patients from different language backgrounds. In all cases (published or unpublished tests), clinicians need to be aware of the widely varying reliability and validity of these tests.

The Boston Diagnostic Aphasia Examanation (BDAE)

The BDAE is widely used in English. Its revised versions have provided additional normative data (Goodglass, Kaplan, & Barresi, 2000). Nonetheless, it is not necessarily an ideal test in its design and performance and was judged unsatisfactory on psychometric grounds in a recent review (http://www.ahrq.gov/clinic/epcsums/spdissum.htm). Spanish versions have been published over the past 15 years by Editorial Medical Panamericana in Argentina and by Masson in

Spain, but its availability has varied. It is currently available from http://www.medicapanamericana.com/.

A French version of the BDAE, published in 2005, is available from ECPA (Editions du Centre de Psychologie Appliquée, a section within Harcourt Assessment/The Psychological Corporation). The manual provides information on a normative sample of 207 adults.

The Bilingual Aphasia Test

The Bilingual Aphasia Test (BAT) developed by Paradis and his colleagues is specifically designed for bilinguals. It exists in over 60 languages, and tests all language modalities. It also has a section that tests translation abilities between more than 100 pairs of languages. Detailed descriptions of the BAT's rationale, development, and administration instructions are available in English (Paradis & Libben, 1987; Paradis, 2004) and in Spanish (Paradis & Libben, 1993). No longer commercially published, it is available directly from its author (see Appendix 9-1).

Each version of the BAT uses vocabulary and pictures that the authors consider culturally appropriate. The content is modified somewhat to assess different features in different languages. Each version has been "normed" on a sample of native speakers of each language; however, published normative data for most languages are not available in English-language journals (or in the other languages included in data bases such as PsychInfo and Medline).

According to Paradis and Libben (1987), normal speakers of each language, or L2 speakers with 400 or more hours of instruction, should score 100% on most subtests. However, two studies of Spanish-English bilingual speakers in Texas and in Florida suggest that this may not be the case. In one study, a group of 14 Spanish-English bilingual adults (mean education 14.5 years, Cuban background) did not score within the expected range for normals on six of 24 subtests in Spanish (L1) and on two subtests in English (L2) (Manuel-Dupont, Ardila, Rosselli, & Puente, 1992). Similar results are reported by Muñoz and Marquardt (in press) with a group of 22 Spanish-English bilingual older adults. The mean group scores were below 70% on 54 items of the short version of the BAT, 22 on the Spanish section of the test. There are no studies documenting the equivalent difficulty of various versions of the test in different languages or its test-retest reliability.

The Multilingual Aphasia Examination

This test, despite its name, is available only in Spanish (MAE-S) (Rey & Benton, 1991) and English (MAE-E) (Benton, Hamsher, & Sivan, 1994; Rey, Feldman, Rivas-Vazquez, Levin, & Benton, 1999). Its manual and a series of publications provide data on its reliability, discrimination, sensitivity, and split-half performance with children (Schum, Sivan, & Benton, 1989) and with English-speaking adults

(Elias, Elias, D'Agostino, Silbershatz, & Wolf, 1997; Ivnik et al., 1996; Schum & Sivan, 1997). The Spanish version was standardized on 234 North American Spanish speakers (Spreen & Strauss, 1998). There are also a number of studies of its psychometric properties in Spanish (e.g., Rey et al., 2001).

The Aachen Aphasia Test

The AAT is not familiar to most clinicians in North America, but it has demonstrated validity and reliability, including test-retest reliability. Published versions exist in German (Huber, Poeck, Weniger, & Willmes, 1983; see www.testzentrale.de), Dutch (Graetz, de Bleser, & Willmes, 1992), and Italian (Luzzatti, Willmes, & de Bleser, 1992, 1996) (see www.osnet.it). An experimental version in English was developed and its properties found to be satisfactory (Miller, Willmes, & de Bleser, 2000), but the English version has not been published. There is also an unpublished Portuguese version of the test. The equivalence of this test across languages and, therefore, its suitability for use with bilingual adults remain untested. However, the results of each patient can be converted to stanine scores, T-scores, and to percentile ranks, allowing comparison of each patient to the (unilingual) normative sample the test was based on, for each language.

Tests in Other Languages and Dialects

Clinicians assessing aphasia in unilingual patients can draw on a wide range of tests, some aimed at detecting mild impairments, others at severe ones. Some tests assess a specific aspect of language, such as reading, in detail. No such range of tests exists for bilingual aphasia. However, there are tests developed in different languages, some of which have versions in more than one language. A list of a number of these tests, and studies reporting results obtained with unpublished, experimental versions, was included in the previous version of the current chapter (Roberts, 2001). However, many of these tests are not available commercially, were never published, and/or go out-of-print rapidly, making it difficult to compile an accurate listing at any point in time.

To use tests designed for one group to assess members of another group (for example, a test from Italy to test Italian-English speaking immigrants in North America or Australia), clinicians need studies of their reliability and validity (Ardila, 1995; Baker, 1993). A number of studies have been done; they illustrate how complex this area is and how much is yet to be done. The following (incomplete) review highlights some of the issues.

Armstrong, Borthwick, Bayles, and Tomoeda (1996) found that the Arizona Battery for Communication Disorders in Dementia (Bayles & Tomoeda, 1991) is suitable for use with speakers of British English. The authors do not recommend changing any stimulus items. They recommend using the American norms.

There are many studies on the Boston Naming Test (BNT) (Kaplan, Goodglass, & Weintraub, 1983) in various languages (see Roberts & Kiran, 2007). In Spanish and French versions of the BNT, the item difficulty is not the same as in the English version (Roberts, Garcia, Desrochers, & Hernandez, 2002).

When the BNT is used in English with different cultural groups, results are mixed. Worrall, Yiu, Hickson, and Barrett (1995) found two of the 60 items are not familiar to Australians, but Tallberg (2005) found no items had to be removed for cultural reasons for Swedish adults. A Greek version of the test has, apparently, retained all 60 items (Tsolaki, Tsantali, Lekka, Kiosseoglu, & Kazis, 2003). The Korean "BNT" has so many changed items that it no longer resembles the original test (Kim & Na, 1999). In each case, authors used different definitions of "culturally appropriate," further complicating comparisons across these and other studies.

The unmodified BNT was sensitive to age and education in English-speaking Australian subjects (Worrall et al., 1995) and in 45 unilingual French Canadian subjects (Doucet & Roberts, 1999). Scores differed significantly with age, education, and gender in elderly Dutch-speaking Belgians (many of whom were likely to be multilingual, although this is not noted) (Mariën, Mampaey, Vervaet, Saerens, & De Deyn (1998). In Swedish-speaking adults, Tallberg (2005) found a significant effect for education. This suggests that despite cultural factors and problems with name-agreement for some stimuli, the test is fairly robust. However, studies of bilingual adults (Kohnert et al., 1998; Roberts et al., 2002) show that the unilingual norms clearly do not apply. Thus, different cut-off scores must be established for different age and education levels within each linguistic group.

Of those studies of African-American performance on the BNT, some have shown no difference in BNT scores across races when age and education are controlled (Henderson, Frank, Pigatt, Abramson, & Houston, 1998). Other studies find that African-Americans score below Caucasians (e.g., Lichtenberg, Ross, & Christensen, 1994). However, small sample size and failure to control for or to report education limit the usefulness of these findings.

There are fewer studies of other tests, but some work has been done. Molrine and Pierce (1998) found that on the Boston Diagnostic Aphasia Examination (BDAE) (Goodglass & Kaplan, 1983) the Western Aphasia Battery (WAB) (Kertesz, 1982), and the Minnesoa Test for Differential Diagnosis of Aphasia (MTDDA) (Schuell, 1965), the scores of African-Americans were below those of Caucasian-Americans (*n* = 24 of each) on only three of 26 subtests of expressive language. For upper-SES subjects, these were Animal Naming (BDAE, WAB), and paragraph retelling (MTDDA), and, for middle-SES, word reading (BDAE). With 12 subjects for each SES level and only a single category used in the verbal-fluency test (Animal Naming), these results are preliminary. Huntress (1979), quoted in Wallace & Tonkovich, 1997, p. 153) found statistically significant but not clinically significant differences in performance on the MTDDA in a group of 15 African-Americans, matched for age, education, and income to a group of white subjects. If credit had been given for responses that were correct, but given in nonstandard English, the scores for the African-American group would have been higher. Thus, this study also suggests that test performance can be very similar across CLD groups.

More studies of CLD test performance are needed, with complete data on the age, education, and language history of participants. This information is essential to allow readers to know to whom the results of a particular study may apply and to permit comparison across studies and appropriate generalization of the findings. The studies done to date illustrate that the answer to the question "can existing tests be used with CLD populations?" is complex. We cannot reject all tests initially normed on white, middle-class, native English speakers as unsuitable for use with other groups. Some tests, and many subtests in existing batteries, are proving to be appropriate. Other tests need specific stimuli, or scoring procedures, changed. Still others may prove entirely inappropriate. Through rigorous validation and normative studies, we will learn which is which.

Informal Assessments and In-House Translations

Until we have more data and more norms for various patient groups, clinicians will continue their current practice of using their own translations of published tests or in-house translations of various tasks on CLD patients, without norms to guide them. The use of nonstandardized evaluation tools is widespread (Katz et al., 2000) and is not limited to CLD patients. Clinical judgment is an important component in interpreting these results. There are, however, pitfalls associated with using ad hoc translations of subtests or tasks.

Tasks can change in nature and in difficulty when they are translated. For example, counting and reciting the months of the year are different tasks in English, but not in Mandarin (Chinese), since the months are called "one-month, two-month, three-month..." (Naeser & Chan, 1980). Spelling is a challenge, and a very familiar task in English, but not in Spanish or Italian because of their highly regular phoneme-grapheme correspondence (Ardila, 1998). Spelling, of course, exists only in languages that use an alphabet-based writing system. In naming, or auditory discrimination tasks, nouns that are high-frequency and short in one language can be low-frequency and multisyllabic in another language, changing several dimensions of the task. For bilinguals, frequency of use may be much more idiosyn-

cratic and less predictable than in unilinguals. At least one study has found that the frequency effects so well documented in unilinguals may be absent for bilingual speakers (Lehtonen & Laine, 2003). Because knowledge is dependent on domains of use, we cannot assume that all bilinguals know "simple" vocabulary in both languages. Name agreement is lower for bilingual speakers than for unilingual speakers (Goggin, Estrada, & Villarreal, 1994; Roberts et al., 2002), which may have implications for how naming and other lexical retrieval tasks are scored. In an innovative study, Croft, Marshall, and Pring (2006) devised a naming test for Bengali-English bilingual aphasic adults by selecting 30 pictures out of a possible of 150 based on naming-latency and name-agreement data obtained from a control group of 20 nonaphasic members of the same community. In a sense, they used the patients' cultural peers as context for assessing and interpreting the naming deficits of their six patients, given the unavailability of a published naming test for Bengali-English speakers in England.

A further challenge in assessing CLD patients is that some symptoms of aphasia vary across languages (Menn, 2001). This has been shown in syntactic deficits (Bates & Wulfeck, 1989; Bates, Wulfeck, & MacWhinney, 1991; Menn, 1989; Menn & Obler, 1990; Menn, O'Connor, Obler, & Holland, 1995; Nilipour & Paradis, 1995; Sasanuma, 1986) and for deep and surface dyslexia (Ardila, 1998; Luzzatti, Laiacona, Allamano, De Tanti, & Inzaghi, 1998; Sasanuma, 1986).

The noun/verb dissociation, commonly seen in aphasia in English and several European languages, is difficult to assess in Chinese, where many words are noun-verb compounds (Bates, Chen, Tzeng, Li, & Opie, 1991; Chen & Bates, 1998; Law & Leung, 2000). There are also studies of reading deficits that suggest that the frequency and/or the types of errors vary across languages, making the deep-dyslexia and surface-dyslexia patterns described for English inapplicable to some other languages (Ardila, 1998; Ferreres & Miravalles, 1995; Sasanuma, 1986). Other studies report patterns similar to those reported in English-speaking patients (Weekes et al., 1998), including acquired dyslexia (Toraldo, Cattani, Zonca, Saletta, & Luzzatti, 2006). These studies demonstrate that one cannot apply all English-based definitions of symptoms or syndromes to other languages. Some apply, some do not. Assessment results must be interpreted with caution, and must take into account the features of the patient's (other) language or dialect. For bilinguals, competition between the processing strategies or the elements of the two languages and interlanguage must both be considered when determining what is a clinical symptom and what is a premorbid feature of bilingualism. There are also error types that are possible in some languages but not in others (correct phonemes, but incorrect tones; wrong gender or case for nouns; creating a false cognate word to cover a word-finding problem). Symptom lists generated to describe one language do not address many possible symptoms in other languages.

Test-Retest Reliability

When a patient is tested twice or more, once in each language, the question of test-retest (TRT) reliability arises. To interpret possible between-language differences, we need to know the normal variability on retesting within a single language. On the BNT, most unilingual English speakers scored within 1 point on retesting, but some changed by 3 or 4 points (Roberts et al., 2002). On the Graded Naming Test, Roberts (2003) found less individual variability and a group mean improvement of 1 point (out of a score of 30). Roberts and Le Dorze (1994) have shown that on semantic verbal fluency, individual scores may increase or decrease by more than 30%. Brookshire and Nicholas (1994) found significant variability on retesting using the picture-description task from the BDAE. More accurate scores and less TRT variability are obtained when results of several connected-speech tasks or several verbal-fluency categories are combined (Brookshire & Nicholas, 1994; Monsch et al., 1992). Until there are more data on the variability of individual scores within a given language, clinicians should be cautious in interpreting different scores between languages (see Roberts (1998) and Roberts and Kiran (2007) for more on this). Interpretation/comparison of scores on different languages is particularly difficult when using tests with unknown test-retest reliability for individual scores, and tests with no published norms, or norms based on samples with different educational, age, and cultural/linguistic backgrounds than the patient being tested.

Clinicians can sample or test some tasks twice in each language for each patient to provide an indication of within-language variability that can guide the interpretation of between-language differences. Using the complete test, not the shortened version, a longer sample, and more exemplars in informal evaluations will often yield more reliable results.

The Test Mess

There is a lack of culturally and psycholinguistically appropriate, rigorous tests of aphasia in the range of languages spoken by people living in many countries, including the U.S., Canada, the U.K., and India. Some have even speculated that it may be impossible to devise any kind of meaningful norms, given the impact of language proficiency and dialect on each individual's (prestroke) performance. The individual variability that is part and parcel of bilingualism combines with the idiosyncrasies of the aphasia each patient experiences. One possible (pessimistic) conclusion is that it will be impossible to develop rigorous tests for bilingual adults with aphasia. The best we can hope for is to develop a range of tasks that allows clinicians to explore various language functions, without seeking to draw strong conclusions

about the severity of the aphasia or to classify it. On the other hand, governments, insurance companies, and employers raise the need to identify, accurately diagnose, and quantify the language impairment in order to support funding for therapy and disability claims. The calls for evidence-based practice (EBP) motivate clinicians to base their therapy on the most valid (accurate) test results possible. Thus, a debate is going on between the optimists, who argue that psychometrically sound tests are possible, at least for large subgroups of bilingual individuals, if we, as a profession, invest the time to develop and assess them adequately, and the pessimists, who argue that the combined complexities of bilingualism and aphasia make it unrealistic to attempt to develop such tests.

Patterns of Impairment and Recovery in Bilingual Aphasia

One purpose of the assessment is to determine the impact of the aphasia on each language. The patterns of impairment and recovery in bilingual aphasia have been described in individual, usually exceptional, patients since the 19th century (Paradis, 1983). Paradis has identified and labeled these patterns (Paradis, 1989, 1993a, 1998; Paradis & Libben, 1987). To facilitate clinical use of these patterns, I have modified Paradis' list somewhat, separating impairment from recovery, and expanding and commenting on the definitions.

Reported Types of Impairment in Bilingual Aphasia

1. Parallel impairment: the two languages are impaired in the same manner and to the same degree. Parallel impairment is determined in relation to premorbid proficiency. If the patient mastered both languages equally premorbidly, the level of ability will be equal post-onset. If one language was stronger than the other, it remains so in cases of parallel impairment. Because aphasia can affect some aspects of language more than others (comprehension vs. expression, or oral vs. written language), the most accurate way to use this label is to rate each modality separately. There may be parallel impairment in auditory comprehension, but differential impairment in reading comprehension, for example.
2. Differential impairment: one language is more severely damaged by the aphasia than the other one. Thus, a difference in proficiency may exist between languages that were approximately equal premorbidly. Or, a premorbid difference may have been erased by the stroke. For example, Spanish may have been stronger than English prestroke, but poststroke, the two are equal. This is not parallel impairment, because the aphasia has had a greater impact on Spanish.
3. Differential aphasia: this refers to the type of aphasia, not to the degree of deficit. Differential aphasia exists

when symptoms differ across languages. In a case reported by Albert and Obler (1978), a multilingual patient appeared to have Broca's aphasia in one language and Wernicke's aphasia in another. Chengappa, Bhat, and Padakannaya (2004), using in-house translations of the WAB, found their 70-year-old patient had global aphasia in Hindi and Kannada, and Wernicke's aphasia in English and Tamil. The validity of published reports of differential aphasia has been questioned (Dronkers, Yamasaki, Webster Ross, & White, 1995; Paradis, 1997, 1998).

4. Blended or mixed pattern: "patients systematically mix or blend features of their languages at any or all levels of linguistic structure (i.e., phonological, morphological, syntactic, lexical and semantic) inappropriately" (Paradis, 1989, p. 117). In these cases, it is as if the patient no longer recognizes what words or features belong in each language, and blends both languages. The patient uses this blended language even when speaking to unilinguals. This is not the same as code-switching or mixing, which is normal behavior in many bilinguals when speaking to another bilingual. Initially called "mixed impairment," Paradis now labels this as blending (1998), to avoid possible confusion with mixed aphasia.

5. Selective aphasia: only one language is affected; the other remains at its premorbid level (Paradis & Goldblum, 1989).

Reported Types of Recovery in Bilingual Aphasia

1. Parallel recovery: both languages improve at the same rate and to the same degree, relative to premorbid levels.

2. Differential recovery: one language recovers better than the other.

3. Successive recovery: "one language does not begin to reappear until another has been maximally recovered" (Paradis, 1989, p. 117). In practice, one cannot determine when maximum recovery has been reached, but the label of successive recovery applies when one language appears to have reached a plateau before any real progress occurs in the other language.

4. Antagonistic recovery: as one language improves, the other regresses. In some cases, the pattern alternates, with first one language improving, then the other (Nilipour & Ashayery, 1989; Paradis, Goldblum, & Abidi, 1982; Paradis & Goldblum, 1989). This variant is also called "alternating antagonism," or see-saw recovery.

5. Selective recovery: only one language shows improvement (Aglioti & Fabbro, 1993).

In theory, these types seem clear. In practice, because of the problems inherent in testing bilingual aphasia and in determining the premorbid mastery of each language, it can be difficult to distinguish among the first three types of impairment. Some authors use the label "differential impairment" when one language is better than the other, even when this reflects premorbid proficiency (Nilipour, 1988). According to Paradis' definition, these should be labeled as parallel. Some published cases of differential aphasia have been reclassified since the authors failed to take into account different symptom presentation in different languages, or did not use appropriate tests and bilingual norms (see Gomez-Tortosa, Martin, Gaviria, Charbel, & Ausman, 1995; Kohnert et al., 1998; Paradis, 1993b, 1997; Silverberg & Gordon, 1979). In at least one published case, impairment that is similar to Paradis' antagonistic pattern was due to the occurrence of additional lesion(s) (Moretti et al., 2003).

Before labeling a recovery or impairment pattern, one must carefully consider the symptom pattern of the specific languages, the patient's dialect, sociocultural factors (what is a normal pattern for the patient's peer group), and the nature of the test used (Paradis, 1995b). Given the complementarity principle, and given that bilinguals usually have different premorbid levels of proficiency in their languages, and different levels in different language modalities, and given that aphasia can differentially affect each language modality, ratings of impairment should be done separately for auditory comprehension, reading, verbal expression, and written expression. The case of an English-Nepalese bilingual illustrates how the "strong" language can vary across tasks (Byng, Coltheart, Masterson, Prior, & Riddoch, 1984).

The few studies done thus far also highlight the need to proceed cautiously in classifying bilingual aphasia by syndrome type. Dronkers and colleagues (1995) have shown that the aphasia classification of a patient can change when credit is given for regional dialect. The issue of classifying aphasia is complex. Non-CLD patients are assigned to different syndromes using the WAB and the BDAE in English (Crary, Wertz, & Deal, 1992). It is not surprising, therefore, that attempts to classify CLD patients by syndrome will often lead to unreliable results. Of course, it is not necessary to label an aphasia syndrome or patterns of bilingual impairment or recovery. Treatment and counseling generally target symptoms and language processing, and/or maximize the use of residual abilities, not labels. Still, to the extent that labels are used, they must be used cautiously, and seen as representing tendencies or general patterns, not absolute truths.

The syndrome types described in English-, Italian-, French- and German-speaking patients appear to exist in a wide range of languages. There is no data about whether the incidence of these syndromes in bilingual patients is similar to that in unilingual patients.

Many authors have attempted to explain nonparallel recovery. The literature contains proposals usually based on speculation, or on observation of a few, nonrandomly selected patients. After reviewing the various theories and their supporting case reports, Paradis (1989) concludes: "no single principle or hierarchy of principles has emerged to explain the whole array of recovery patterns. Neither primacy, nor automaticity, habit strength, stimulation pre- or post-onset, appropriateness, need, affectivity, severity of the aphasia, type of bilingualism or type of aphasia could account for the non-parallel recovery patterns observed" (p. 127).

The literature offers little information on the incidence of each type of impairment. Clinical experience suggests that parallel impairment and parallel recovery are by far the most common patterns, especially after the first few weeks. There is some support for this view in the literature (Chary, 1986 quoting Nair & Virmani; Junqué, Vendrell, & Vendrell, 1995; Lhermitte, Hécaen, Dubois, Culioli, & Tabouret-Kelly, 1966; Paradis, 1977; Vaid & Genesee, 1980). There are also a number of published cases of parallel impairment and recovery (Dronkers et al., 1995; Mimouni, Béland, Danault, & Idrissi, 1995; Nilipour, 1988; Roberts et al., 1997; Sasanuma & Park, 1995). There are more published reports of nonparallel patterns, because of a tendency to write-up the unusual or interesting patterns. We need studies of unselected, consecutive cases with detailed language histories and thorough testing to determine the incidence of parallel and nonparallel recovery.

ISSUES IN INTERVENTION

Treatment for bilingual aphasia has been neglected in the literature. Little published information exists on the effects of treatment and even less on appropriate methods. Two types of studies provide some guidance: studies of the effects of treatment in various languages; and a small number of studies of the symptoms of bilingual aphasia. The principles that guide unilingual treatment are also relevant to bilingual treatment. The following section presents these, along with a liberal dose of suggestions based on clinical experience and a review of published treatment studies (Table 9–1). Most findings and suggestions presented below have not yet been tested formally, though they have proved effective in clinical practice.

Effects of Treatment in Bilinguals

One the one hand, bilingual treatment studies are few in number, and vary widely in the level of detail and hence in their value in supporting clinical practice. On the other hand, the studies that have been done, and the unilingual treatment studies in a range of languages, suggest that treatment principles that work in unilinguals often work in bilinguals as well. A study by Wiener, Obler, and Taylor-Sarno (1995) documented the treatment outcomes, length-of-stay, and reasons for discharge for 54 unilingual and 55 bilingual patients in a New York City rehabilitation center. The

authors expected to find that the bilingual patients were underserved (shorter treatment, fewer types of treatment) and made less improvement than the unilingual patients. Instead they found that "bilingual patients showed recovery that was virtually equivalent to that of unilinguals" (p. 55).

There are reports that when only one language is used in treatment or practice, one or more of the patient's untreated languages improve (Edmonds & Kiran, 2006; Holland & Penn, 1995; Penn & Beecham, 1992). The treated language may improve more than the untreated one (de Luca, Fabbro, Vorano, & Lovati, 1994; Fredman, 1975; Laganaro & Overton Venet, 2001; Wender, 1989), especially for expressive language tasks (Sasanuma & Park, 1995). This finding has been replicated in single case studies (Edmonds & Kiran, 2006; Roberts et al., 1997; Watamori & Sasanuma, 1976, 1978) and in group studies (Junqué, Vendrell, & Vendrell-Brucet, 1989; Junqué et al., 1995).

Other studies, however, have found equal improvement in two or more languages following treatment in one language on expressive tasks (Edmonds & Kiran, 2006; Penn, 2003), or equal improvement in receptive language (Sasanuma & Park, 1995), or greater gains in the untreated language (L2) (Roberts, 1992). The participants in two of these studies (*n* = 2 in Sasanuma and Park, and *n* = 1 in Roberts) were 3 months or less post-CVA when treatment began. Therefore, the effects of spontaneous recovery cannot be separated from treatment effects. There are at least two other reports of greater gains in the untreated language (L1) (Durieu, 1969 and Linke, 1979 cited in Paradis, 2004 p. 91). Hinckley (2003) provided roughly equal amounts of therapy in Spanish and English, but found greater gains in Spanish, the patient's first-learned and stronger language. Kohnert (2004) provided very brief treatment in Spanish, then in English, to a patient and found that while both languages improved, the between-language generalization and the maintenance of gains were both greater for cognate words than for non-cognate words in a patient approximately 15 months post-CVA. Given that only four treatment sessions were given, these results should be interpreted very cautiously.

Some authors have interpreted a lack of generalization from one language to another as support for the view that the two languages are stored in separate systems. However, we know that some unilingual patients do not generalize from treated to untreated stimuli. This does not mean that the two sets of stimuli are stored in "different systems." Nor does it mean that the two languages are processed in different areas of the brain. As we learn more about within-language generalization, we will be better able to interpret between-language generalization, and vice versa.

Roberts and Kiran (2007) point out a recurring flaw in the body of studies of treatment effects. Patients are often identified as having different patterns of bilingualism (e.g., late vs. early acquisition; or fairly equal proficiency vs. one-language dominant). If their response to treatment is different,

TABLE 9–1

Studies of Bilingual Aphasia Treatment
Greater Gains in Treated Language or Gains Associated in Time with Language of Treatment

Authors, Date	n and Age, Education; Time Post-onset	Languages Known and Ages Learned or First Exposure	Information on Language of Birth	Focus/Method of Treatment	Design	Dependent Variable(s)	Length and Frequency of Treatment/ Previous Treatment	Results
Roberts, de la Riva, & Rhéaume, 1997	n = 1, 46 years old; MA linguistics; 4 years post-CVA	French L1, English L2 by age 8; constant use of both from age 5 or 6 onward	Slightly stronger French in all 4 modalities, by self-report	Anomia; Howard 1985 phonol cues	Treatment in French only; multiple baselines	% correct on 3 sets of 10 words; also BAT, BDAE French and English	3 times per week; total of 12 sessions; no treatment for past 2 years	For treatment stimuli: strong gains in TL; equal and limited generalization to UL and to other stimuli in TL; little change in standard tests
Watamori & Sasanuma, 1976	n = 1; 65 years old; 1 university degree, plus additional studies; approx. 3 months post-CVA	Japanese L1, English L2 from early childhood	"used with equal proficiency" but no rating reported	Treatment in English only (after 2-week trial in Japanese); stimulation method	Pretest-posttest	Scores on MTDDA and modified PICA	Approx. 1 year	Approx. equal gains in TL and UL for auditory comp. and reading; greater gains in TL (English) on verbal and written expression
Laganaro & Overton Venet, 2001	n = 1, 50 years old; university, including unspecified post-grad studies; engineer; 8 months post-gunshot wound	Spanish L1, English L2, French L3— not listed but deduced	None	Alexia; computer ex on spelling, lexical decision, categorization, rhymes, word-building	Alternating treatment design; alternating blocks in Spanish and English	% correct and speed on lexical decision and reading tasks devised for this patient. No formal tests.	Once per week with daily home practice of approx. 1 hr; 8 weeks of treatment	Gains in both Ls, with slight advantage for TL in most blocks of 2 weeks

(continued)

TABLE 9–1

Studies of Bilingual Aphasia Treatment
Greater Gains in Treated Language or Gains Associated in Time with Language of Treatment (Continued)

Authors, Date	n and Age, Education; Time Post-onset	Languages Known and Ages Learned or First Exposure	Information on Language of Birth	Focus/Method of Treatment	Design	Dependent Variable(s)	Length and Frequency of Treatment/ Previous Treatment	Results
Galvez & Hinckley, 2003	n = 1; 71 years old; 6 months post-R CVA	Spanish L1, English L2, age at first exposure unknown	Very incomplete LOB info; born in unnamed country outside U.S.; overall self-rating "equally proficient"	Semantic treatment for anomia	Treatment in Spanish only until reached 80% on treatment stimuli; then English treatment	BAT Spanish and English	Unknown frequency and unknown no. of sessions; No info on previous or simultaneous treatment	Spanish naming and English naming improved after Spanish treatment; no other scores reported; at end of study, BAT in both Ls improved scores
Gains Do Not Match Pattern of Treatment								
Hinckley, 2003	n = 1; Age not given; "highly educated"; 4 months post-CVA	Spanish L1, English L2, learned "as a teenager"	none	anomia	Alternating treatment design; L changed every session; equal time on each language	BAT; PALPA	7 weeks; frequency not stated; semantic and phonemic cues and repetition; recent or simultaneous treatment unknown	No scores given for pre/post naming task; gains on BAT and PALPA much greater in Spanish than English
Penn & Beecham, 1992 (same patient)	n = 1; 38 years old; 19 years school; lawyer; 9 months after his 2nd CVA (prior CVA 3 years previously)	Ndebele L1; Pedi L1 or L2; Afrikaans, English, Zulu; and 5 others; age of first exposure not given; Ndebele earliest; English at school	Best Ls Ndebele and Pedi; 3rd best Zulu, most-used Afrikaans; English 6th best; no modality-specific ratings	Discourse structure	Treatment in English only; pretest-posttest	Score on Profile of Communicative Appropriateness; qualitative analysis of discourse; rate of speech	9 sessions in 14 weeks; no info provided on previous treatment	Scores not given; description of improvement in all Ls spoken and better organized and more appropriate discourse

Mixed Results

Galvez & Hinckley, 2003	*n* = 1; 71 yrs old; 6 mo post-onset	Spanish L1; English L2 w/ "little exposure" to Engligh up to age 18	"Equally proficient" by self-report; no breakdown by modality	Anomia skill-based tx, semantic and phonemic cues	"Multiple-baseline across behaviors"; tx in Spanish up to 80% criterion, then in English	Scores on target stimuli not provided; score on short BAT, naming and other modalities	Unknown	Recent or simult. tx: unknown	Unclear; text contradicts figures in Table 1; both languages treated; both improved approx. equally
Edmonds & Kiran, 2006	*n* = 3; 53, 53, and 56 years old; 8 to 9 months post-CVA; 10 or 12 years education	P1: L1 Spanish, L2 English starting at age 21; P2 and P3: both Ls from birth	P1: slightly better in Spanish; P2 and P3: stronger in English	Semantic feature analysis treatment for anomia	Train each list of 10 to criterion level; "multiple baseline across participants and behaviors"	Scores on target stimuli, related and unrelated words; WAB, BNT, PALPA, BAT	13 to +40 sessions; no info provided on previous treatment		Varying levels of progress and generalization within and between languages

Key: TL = treated language; UL = untreated language.

most authors conclude that their different bilingualism levels are the cause of the observed differences. Given the variable (and still unpredictable) patterns of response to treatment, and given that some unilingual patients fail to generalize gains to untreated stimuli and/or modalities, this leap of logic is surprisingly naïve. Roberts and Kiran (2007) identify other methodologic flaws or challenges all authors (and clinicians) face in trying to devise bilingual aphasia treatment and understand its results. They propose a number of concrete solutions to meet these challenges. We need better-designed studies and more complete descriptions of patients (see also Roberts, Code, & McNeil, 2003), especially their language background. Authors and readers need to be much more cautious in how they interpret results. Some unilingual adults with aphasia generalize treatment gains to untreated stimuli and/or modalities, while others do not. So, when a bilingual patient either generalizes or fails to generalize gains, we should not be too quick to assume that the explanation for the results must be the patient's bilingualism.

Treatment

Treatment Methods

The studies just cited show that a general stimulation approach can be used in bilingual patients who speak English and Japanese (Watamori & Sasanuma, 1976, 1978) and Japanese and Korean (Sasanuma & Park, 1995). Howard's phonemic cueing technique was used with a French-English bilingual patient with chronic aphasia (Roberts et al., 1997). Other studies give little information about the treatment method (de Luca et al., 1994; Junqué et al., 1989; Junqué et al., 1995) or describe activities or examples of types of tasks (Fredman, 1975; Wender, 1989).

Other sources, however, show that a number of aphasia treatment methods have been used in a range of different languages. These include PACE therapy (Carlomagno, 1994; Sasanuma, 1993), Melodic Intonation Therapy (Belin, Van Eeckhout, Zilbovicius, & Remy, 1996; Van Eeckhout, Pillon, Signoret, Deloche, & Seron, 1992; Visch-Brink, van Harskamp, Van Amerongen, Wielaert, & van de Sandt-Koenderman, 1993). Examples of cognitive neuropsychological approaches, cueing techniques, and Blissymbols in a range of languages can be found in sources specifically highlighting international work (e.g., Holland & Forbes, 1993), but also scattered throughout the published aphasia-treatment literature.

In adapting a technique developed in one language for use in another, the specific characteristics of each language must be borne in mind. Some cues that have great value in one language, such as word order in English, may have little value in another. Also, cues that are not possible in English may be important to use in other languages. The gender of

nouns in Spanish, for example, to assist word retrieval, or the auxiliary used to conjugate verbs in French or Italian. In some languages, rehabilitation strategies unique to that language must be developed, as for kana/kanji reading and writing in Japanese (see Sasanuma, 1993).

Another possible pitfall in adapting therapy techniques is establishing appropriate hierarchies of difficulty for tasks and stimuli. The syntactic difficulty of different sentence types must be determined in a language-specific context. In choosing stimuli, based on word frequency, cultural variations can be important. Also, controlling for cognate words in a naming or other lexical task is important for some language pairs (see earlier section). A task may be easier if it involves cognate words than if there are no cognates, at least for some patients (Ferrand & Humphreys, 1996; Kohnert, 2004; Roberts & Deslauriers, 1999; Stadie et al., 1995). Word-frequency lists are of unknown validity for bilingual speakers, as are age-of-acquisition norms, for reasons outlined above. This means that the selection of stimuli and assessment of task difficulty for each patient will depend to a great extent on the clinician's ability to observe patterns, and experiment with various dimensions of a task to adjust its difficulty on a patient-by-patient basis.

The fact that a treatment approach has been used with speakers of different languages does not guarantee that it is appropriate for bilingual speakers of two of those languages. Studies are needed. Until these studies are done, unilingual-treatment studies offer some guidelines about changes needed to adapt a method from one language to another. They also demonstrate that the principles the method is based on can apply to both languages. A high level of linguistic competence is needed to adapt most treatment strategies into different languages.

Setting Goals in Treatment

The principles for unilingual treatment apply also to bilinguals: goals should be realistic, meaningful to the patient, and tailored to the individual patient's deficits. The factors relevant in unilingual work apply to bilinguals. Some additional factors must be considered, however.

Realistic goals are based on the patient's pre- and post-morbid proficiency and patterns of use. Improving a patient's L2 or reversing the attrition that has occurred in a little-used L1 are not part of our clinical mandate. Given how little is known about prognosis in bilinguals, our goals must be even more modest, and our comments to the family about prognosis more guarded than for unilinguals. As the recovery progresses, as the treatment brings changes or fails to bring changes in targeted aspects of communication, our goals will change, and our prognosis along with them.

The patient's need for each language in various situations is a key factor in setting goals. Even when therapy is carried out in both languages, this does not mean that all tasks should be. For example, if the patient used only one language for reading, the treatment goals should reflect this.

In tailoring treatment goals to the patient's deficits, processing and self-cueing strategies are important factors. These often reflect the interaction of the two languages. Some bilinguals use processing strategies from one language to interpret the other (Heredia & Altarriba, 2002). An L1 English speaker may rely on word order as a cue for thematic roles when processing sentences in L2, even when L2 does not use word order to mark them (Liu, Bates, & Li, 1992, for example). It is important for the clinician to consider factors from both languages, and the possible interaction of languages, in interpreting error patterns.

In overcoming word-retrieval problems, there are strategies that are unique to bilinguals. First, when unable to say what he wants to in one language, the patient may simply switch to his other language. This is an obvious and appropriate strategy, if the listener is bilingual. Some patients use it spontaneously. For others, explicit teaching may be needed. If the listener has even some grasp of this other language, the message may be understood, or enough of it to move the exchange along. In language pairs with cognates, saying or writing a cognate word in one language will often allow even a unilingual speaker of the other language to understand the word. This switching behavior when talking to a bilingual listener has been documented in patients with aphasia (Marty & Grosjean, 1998; Springer, Miller, & Bürk, 1998), and is seen daily in clinical settings.

A second strategy that bilinguals use spontaneously is producing a word from one language to self-cue its retrieval from another (Roberts & Deslauriers, 1999; Roberts et al., 2002). This can be encouraged or explicitly taught if it is an effective strategy for the patient and not pathological or uncontrolled switching (see Grosjean, 1984).

Choice of Language(s) of Treatment

Regardless of the treatment goals and methods, the languages used in treatment should reflect premorbid use and proficiency. Although anecdotal reports suggest that treatment in more than one language is harmful (e.g., Chlenov, 1948; Wald, 1958, 1961 cited in Paradis, 1993b; Paradis, 2004), there is no recent, controlled study on this issue. Case studies in which treatment has been offered in two or more languages, with positive outcomes (e.g., Edmonds & Kiran, 2006; Hinckley, 2003), provide support for clinical impressions that most patients can keep their languages separate and that, if they regularly use more than one language in their daily lives, they benefit from treatment that targets these languages. The only exceptions to this are the rare cases that display a blended pattern of impairment. For these patients, treatment may need to be restricted to one language. For most patients, in light of the research showing that the two languages interact, and that bilinguals regularly use their languages as a whole system, with both languages always active to some degree, there is little support for limiting treatment to one language. Clinical experience shows that most patients can work in one of three ways:

1. Working on one language with the clinician, and the other language at home or with a volunteer. This may be the only way to work with a language the clinician does not speak.
2. Alternating languages. This involves a block of sessions in one language, followed by a block in the other. Each block can be a certain number of consecutive sessions or can be measured in weeks, with regular probes to see whether treatment gains in one language are generalizing to the other language(s).
3. Separate the languages by modality, reflecting the patient's premorbid patterns of use. For example, work on writing in one language and auditory comprehension in both languages.

In the rare cases where a patient "loses" a language they used extensively, they may want to work on this language but be unable to. Clinical experience suggests that it is pointless to attempt to work in a language until the patient can access it fairly consistently. Work in the other language(s), provide passive exposure to the "lost" language, and probe it regularly to see if it reappears. When and if it does, the balance of languages in treatment can be adjusted to include this language. The case described by Roberts (1998) illustrates this approach.

The questions of what pattern of languages to use in treatment and of generalization between languages are closely linked. Both are complex and both require study. To the extent that treatment generalizes from one language to another, treatment in only one language may be ethically appropriate. However, when generalization does not occur, treatment may be necessary in both languages needed by the patient.

FUTURE TRENDS

It seems safe to predict that interest in bilingual aphasia will continue to grow as more clinicians and researchers recognize its importance. There has been a surge of interest in bilingual/multilingual language processing in nonimpaired speakers. The findings from these studies of language-localization and word and sentence processing are shedding light on the psycholinguistics of bilingualism. Models of bilingual language processing, an arcane and very tiny field 10 years ago, are the focus of considerable interest and are being revised in light of these new experimental results. Logically, studies of speakers with aphasia can contribute to our understanding of multilingual language processing, although this line of research remains relatively undeveloped.

Aphasia-treatment studies will continue to grow in both number and sophistication, using designs that are now common in the unilingual aphasia-treatment literature. For these studies of treatment to coalesce into a body of knowledge that can be interpreted and applied to clinical practice, it is vital that authors and reviewers insist on greater consistency across studies in how patients are described. Authors and readers must also learn to be more cautious in drawing conclusions from studies with small numbers of patients.

The most uncertain area may be assessment. Existing tests need to undergo thoughtful, objective review according to established psychometric standards; their suitability for use with bilingual speakers must be explored. It means very little to say that a patient scored 12 in Spanish and 14 in English if we do not know whether the Spanish and English tests are all of equal difficulty and if we do not know what the normal range of variability might be for retesting a single patient using the same tests or task.

Other future trends will depend, in part, on how we meet the challenges inherent in studying CLD patients. The first challenge is objectivity. We must be open to results that contradict our own, or society's, expectations about a particular group. Test performance and treatment outcomes for some CLD patients may be better than for other patients, or worse, or there may be no difference beyond minor sampling differences. As the calls for more focus on CLD issues are answered by studies with hard data, we must interpret this data objectively. We must give equal weight to the similarities across groups as well as to the differences. We must be very cautious in saying why a result was obtained.

The second challenge is experimental rigor. Factors related to bilingualism and culture are difficult to control in studies already complex because of the many neurologic and linguistic variables related to the aphasia. Given the difficulty in finding patients with similar linguistic, cultural, and neurologic status, collaborative studies (across centers and in different countries) will help ensure adequate sample sizes and representative results. As discussed by Roberts and Kiran (2007), appropriate experimental control and the publication of replications will be essential to allow correct interpretation of the results.

The third challenge is cultural and linguistic competence. With study, and interaction with people of various cultures, clinicians can become culturally aware, and learn to adapt their methods to reduce cultural stumbling blocks on the clinical path. Linguistic competence represents a greater challenge. A significant challenge for the profession is to recruit and train people who meet the required standards.

The final challenge is time. A bilingual patient takes more time than a unilingual one. Finding, adapting, or developing tests and treatment material, finding and training interpreters, and testing in two languages instead of one are among the factors that take more time. Working in two languages in treatment also adds to the time required, especially for cases in which the gains in one language do not generalize to the other and the patient needs to regain use of both languages. Given the increased interest in CLD issues, we may hope to

see experimental support for specific treatment methods, and more tests to support our clinical work. However, without adequate time, these positive developments will not benefit the patients. Clinicians in many settings are subject to limits in the number of sessions they may provide, or the length of stay the patient is allowed. These constraints and pressures to see more patients in shorter times will make it increasingly difficult to give bilingual patients the care they need. Research documenting the best methods and their impact will support our efforts to obtain essential services for CLD patients.

KEY POINTS

Clinicians who work with CLD patients should read as widely as possible in the literature on culture and on bilingualism. Among the points that are clinically important are the following:

1. Language and culture are closely tied.
2. It is important to consider the possible influence of cultural factors on clinical work, using the patient's background to suggest factors that may be relevant, and interpreting behavior within the appropriate cultural context. It is equally important to avoid cultural stereotypes and assumptions. Each client is a unique individual from a specific microculture, within a macroculture.
3. Bilingualism is a continuum, with different levels of ability for different linguistic tasks and different domains of use. Bilingual abilities change over time with patterns of use or disuse.
4. A bilingual person is a unique speaker-hearer, with abilities in each language that often reflect the influence of the other.
5. The languages of a bilingual are (usually) stored in the left hemisphere, as they are for unilinguals, in largely but perhaps not completely overlapping cortical and subcortical regions.
6. Lexical items are connected across languages, with between-language facilitation and interference both occurring in neurologically intact adults. Cognates appear more closely linked than non-cognates. These between-language factors should be considered in interpreting aphasic error patterns and in planning treatment.
7. It can be difficult to assess bilingual patients for many reasons, including availability of tests, local norms, the need for interpreters, and a lack of data on individual test-retest reliability on aphasia tests.
8. Interpretation of test results should be done in light of the patient's premorbid level of bilingualism, dialect(s), patterns of use, and the features and unique symptom hierarchy of each language tested.

9. Five patterns of impairment and five patterns of recovery have been identified, with parallel patterns believed to be the most common.

10. A number of treatment principles and methods have been successfully used with a range of languages. However, we need much more research into treatment methods for bilingual patients with aphasia and into cross-language generalization.

ACTIVITIES FOR REFLECTION AND DISCUSSION

1. Review the definitions for:
   bilingualism; domains of use; microculture; level of bilingualism; parallel recovery; differential recovery; types of impairment vs. types of recovery.

2. Can you think of two domains of use for language that are not listed in this chapter?

3. a) Estimate your own level of bilingualism in each of the four language modalities on a scale of 1 to 7.
   b) Then ask someone else to rate your proficiency in each of the modalities. Are the ratings the same?
   c) Explore the reasons for each rating with the person rating you.

4. Why is bilingualism so difficult to define?

5. Assessment: obtain a copy of the Multilingual Aphasia Examination, the Bilingual Aphasia Test, or the Aachen Aphasia Test.
   a) Compare the sections and number of items per test with the Boston Diagnostic Aphasia Examination or the Western Aphasia Battery. Compare the ease of scoring and the instructions given for administering and scoring the test. How important are the ease of scoring and clarity of the recording forms?
   b) Prepare a short paper or a presentation for your class/rehabilitation team/continuing-education discussion group about what makes a good aphasia test, and how close each test you have examined comes to meeting the standards. It may be helpful to obtain a chapter on how to assess the quality of a test; psychology textbooks and research-methods textbooks (e.g., Kazdin's *Research Design in Clinical Psychology*) often contain succinct overviews of the criteria an ideal test would meet (validity, reliability, sensitivity, etc.)

6. Do you think it will be possible to develop a valid and reliable test for naming abilities in bilingual speakers? Pick a specific type of speaker that you often see or that is common in your country or city to help you imagine the kinds of challenges that might arise. How would you go about developing such a test?

7. Imagine you want to present treatment results for your next bilingual patient at clinical rounds or a small con-ference. What testing or tasks would you need to add to your usual clinical procedures to be able to do this? These might include obtaining a baseline for one of the behaviors you will work on in therapy by testing two or three times instead of just once before starting treatment; recording treatment sessions (video and/or audio) so you can rescore the patient's answers; retesting the patient on the same stimuli used during the pretherapy baseline tasks. How will you measure generalization between languages?

8. What do you think is the biggest challenge in improving service to bilingual adults with aphasia in your city/region/country? Suggest specific strategies to meet this challenge.

9. Identify three small, practical steps that you, your university, or your treatment center could take to improve service for bilingual patients with aphasia. Discuss the feasibility of implementing each of these steps.

References

Abutalebi, J., Cappa, S. F., & Perani, D. (2005). What can functional neuroimaging tell us about the bilingual brain? In J. F. Kroll & A. M. B. De Groot (Eds.), *Handbook of bilingualism: Psycholinguistic approaches* (pp. 497–515). New York: Oxford University Press.

Abutalebi, J., Miozzo, A., & Cappa, S. F. (2000). Do subcortical structures control language selection in bilinguals? Evidence from pathological language mixing. *Neurocase, 6,* 51–56.

Aglioti, S., & Fabbro, F. (1993). Paradoxical selective recovery in a bilingual aphasic following subcortical lesions. *Cognitive Neuroscience and Neuropsychology, 4,* 1359–1362.

Albert, M., & Obler, L. (1978). *The bilingual brain.* New York: Academic Press.

Altarriba, J. (1992). The representation of translation equivalents in bilingual memory. In R. J. Harris (Ed.), *Cognitive processing in bilinguals* (pp. 157–174). New York: Elsevier.

American Speech-Language-Hearing Association. (1985). Clinical management of communicatively handicapped minority language populations. *ASHA, 27,* 29–32.

American Speech-Language-Hearing Association (1991). Multicultural action agenda. *ASHA, 33*(5), 39–41.

American Speech-Language-Hearing Association (2004). Knowledge and skills needed by speech-language pathologists to provide culturally and linguistically appropriate services. *ASHA, Supplement 4.*

American Speech-Language-Hearing Association: Committee on the Status of Racial Minorities. (1989). Bilingual speech-language pathologists and audiologists. *ASHA, 31,* 93.

Ardila, A. (1995). Directions of research in cross-cultural neuropsychology. *Journal of Clinical an Experimental Neuropsychology, 17,* 143–150.

Ardila, A. (1998). Semantic paralexias in the Spanish language. *Aphasiology, 12,* 885–900.

Armstrong, L. Borthwick, S. E., Bayles, K. A., & Tomoeda, C. K. (1996). Use of the Arizona Battery for Communication Disorders of Dementia in the UK. *European Journal of Disorders of Communication, 31,* 171–180.

Asante, M. K., & Gudykunst, W. B. (1989). *Handbook of international and intercultural communication.* Newbury Park: Sage.

Australian Association of Speech and Hearing (1994). *Speech pathology in a multicultural, multilingual society.* Melbourne: AASH.

Australian Institute of Multicultural Affairs. (1985). *Ageing in a multicultural society.* Canberra: AIMA.

Baetens Beardsmore, H. (1982). *Bilingualism: Basic principles.* Clevendon: Multilingual Matters.

Bahrick, H. P., Hall, L. K., Goggin, J. P., Bahrick, L. E., & Berger, S. A. (1994). Fifty years of language maintenance and language dominance in bilingual Hispanic immigrants. *Journal of Experimental Psychology: General, 123,* 264–283.

Baker, R. (1993). The assessment of language impairment in elderly bilinguals and second language speakers in Australia. *Language Testing, 10,* 255–276.

Baker, R. (1995). Communicative needs and bilingualism in elderly Australians of six ethnic backgrounds. *Australian Journal on Ageing, 14*(2), 81–88.

Baker, R. (2007). The assessment of functional communication in culturally and linguistically diverse populations. In L. Worrall & C. Frattali (Eds.), *Neurogenic communication disorders: A functional approach* (pp. 81–100). New York: Thieme Medical.

Bates, E., Chen, S., Tzeng, O., Li, P., & Opie, M. (1991). The noun-verb problem in Chinese aphasia. *Brain and Language, 41,* 203–233.

Bates, E., & Wulfeck, B. (1989). Comparative aphasiology: A cross-linguistic approach to language breakdown. *Aphasiology, 3*(2), 111–142.

Bates, E., Wulfeck, B., & MacWhinney, B. (1991). Cross-linguistic research in aphasia: An overview. *Brain and Language, 41,* 123–148.

Battle, D. E. (Ed.) (1998). *Communication disorders in multicultural populations.* (2nd ed.). Newton, MA: Butterworth-Heinemann.

Bayles, K. A., & Tomoeda, C. K. (1991). *Arizona Battery for Communications Disorders of Dementia.* Tucson, AZ: Canyonlands.

Belin, P., Van Eeckhout, P., Zilbovicius, M., & Remy, P. (1996). Recovery from non-fluent aphasia after melodic intonation therapy: A PET study. *Neurology, 47,* 1504–1511.

Benton, A. L., Hamsher, K., & Sivan, A. B. (1994). *Multilingual Aphasia Examination.* (3rd ed.). Iowa City: AJA.

Bettoni, C. (1991). Language variety among Italians: Anglicisms, attrition, and attitudes. In S. Romaine (Ed.), *Language in Australia.* Cambridge: Cambridge University Press.

Brislin, R. W. (1994). *Intercultural training: An introduction.* Thousand Oaks, CA: Sage.

Brislin, R. W., Cushner, K., Cherrie, C., & Yong, M. (1986). *Intercultural interactions: A practical guide.* Beverly Hills, CA: Sage.

Brookshire, R. H., & Nicholas, L. E. (1994). Test-retest stability of measures of connected speech in aphasia. In M. L. Lemme (Ed.), *Clinical aphasiology* (Vol. 22, pp. 119–134). Austin, TX: Pro-Ed.

Burr, J. A., & Mutchler, J. E. (2003). English language skills, ethnic concentration, and household composition: Older Mexican immigrants. *Journal of Gerontology: Series B: Psychological Sciences and Social Sciences, 58B,* S83–S92.

Byng, S., Coltheart, M., Masterson, J., Prior, M., & Riddoch, J. (1984). Bilingual biscriptal deep dyslexia. *Quarterly Journal of Experimental Psychology, 36A,* 417–433.

Carlomagno, S. (1994). *Pragmatic approaches to aphasia therapy* (Hodgkinson, G., Trans.). London: Whurr.

Cenoz. J., Hufeisen, B., & Jessner, U. (Eds.) (2003). *The multilingual lexicon.* Boston: Kluwer Academic.

Chary, P. (1986). Aphasia in a multi-lingual society. In J. Vaid (Ed.), *Language processing in bilinguals: Psycholinguistic and neurolinguistic perspectives.* (pp. 183–197). Hillsdale, NJ: Lawrence Erlbaum.

Chee, M. W. L., Soon, C. S., & Lee, H. L. (2003). Common and segregated neuronal networks for different languages revealed using functional magnetic resonance adaptation. *Journal of Cognitive Neuroscience, 15,* 85–97.

Chee, M. W. L., Tan, E. W. L., & Thiel, T. (1999). Mandarin and Chinese single word processing studied with functional magnetic resonance imaging. *Journal of Neuroscience, 19,* 3050–3056.

Chen, H. C. (1992). Lexical processing in bilingual or multilingual speakers. In R. J. Harris (Ed.), *Cognitive processing in bilinguals* (pp. 253–264). New York: Elsevier.

Chen, S., & Bates, E. (1998). The dissociation between nouns and verbs in Broca's and Wernicke's aphasia: Findings from Chinese. *Aphasiology, 12,* 5–36.

Cheng, L. L. (1996). Beyond bilingualism: A quest for communicative competence. *Topics in Language Disorders, 16,* 9–21.

Chengappa, S., Bhat, S., & Padakannaya, P. (2004). Reading and writing skills in multilingual/multilingual aphasics: Two case studies. *Reading and Writing, 17,* 121–135.

Chitiri, H.- F., & Willows, D. M. (1997). Bilingual word recognition in English and Greek. *Applied Psycholinguistics, 18,* 138–156.

Cole, L. (1989). E pluribus unum: Multicultural imperatives for the 1990's and beyond. *ASHA, 31*(2), 65–70.

Costa, A. (2005). Lexical access in bilingual production. In J. F. Kroll & A. M. B. De Groot (Eds.), Handbook of bilingualism: Psycholinguistic approaches (pp. 308–325). New York: Oxford University Press.

Costa, A., Miozza, M., & Caramazza, A. (1999). Lexical selection in bilinguals: Do words in the bilingual's two lexicons compete for selection? *Journal of Memory and Language, 41,* 365–397.

Crago, M. B., & Westernoff, F. (1997). *Canadian Association of Speech Language Pathologists and Audiologists.* Position Paper on speech-language pathology and audiology in the multicultural, multilingual context. *Journal of Speech Language Pathology and Audiology, 21*(3), 35–44. Also online at: www.caslpa.ca

Crary, M. A., Wertz, R. T., & Deal, J. L. (1992). Classifying aphasia: Cluster analysis of Western Aphasia Battery and Boston Diagnostic Examination results. *Aphasiology, 6,* 29–36.

Crinion, J., Turner, R., Grogan, A., Hanakawa, T., Noppeney, U., Devlin, J., et al. (2006). Language control in the bilingual brain. *Science, 312*(5779), 1537–1540.

Croft, S., Marshall, J., & Pring, T. (2006). Assessing noun naming impairments in bilingual aphasia. *Brain and Language, 99,* 21–22.

Cutler, A., Mehler, J., Norris, D., & Segui, J. (1992). The monolingual nature of speech segmentation by bilinguals. *Cognitive Psychology, 24,* 381–410.

Davis, P. N., Gentry, B., & Hubbard-Wiley, P. (1998). Clinical practice issues. In D. E. Battle (Ed.), *Communication disorders in multicultural populations* (2nd ed., pp. 427–452). Boston: Butterworth-Heinemann.

de Bot, K. (1992). A bilingual production model: Levelt's "speaking" model adapted. *Applied Linguistics, 13*(1), 1–24.

de Bot, K., & Makoni, S. (2005). *Language and aging in multilingual contexts.* In N. H. Hornberger & C. Baker (Series Eds.), *Bilingual Education and Bilingualism* (Vol 53). Toronto: Multilingual Matters.

de Bot, K., & Schreuder, R. (1993). Word production and the bilingual lexicon. In R. Schreuder & B. Weltens (Eds.), *The bilingual lexicon* (pp. 191–214). Philadelphia: John Benjamins.

de Groot, A. M. B. (1993). Word-type effects in bilingual processing tasks: Support for a mixed-representational system. In R. Schreuder & B. Weltens (Eds.), *The bilingual lexicon* (pp. 27-52). Philadelphia: John Benjamins.

de Groot, A. M. B., & Borgwaldt, S., Bos, M., & Van den Eijnden, E. (2002). Lexical decision and word naming in bilinguals: Language effects and task effects. *Journal of Memory and Language, 47*, 91–124.

de Groot, A. M. B., & Poot, R. (1997). Word translation at three levels of proficiency in a second language: The ubiquitous involvement of conceptual memory. *Language Learning, 47*(2), 215–264.

Dehaene, S., Dupoux, E., Mehler, J., Cohen, L., Paulesu, E., Perani, D., et al. (1997). Anatomical variability in the cortical representation of first and second language. *NeuroReport, 8*, 3809–3815.

de Luca, G., Fabbro, F., Vorano, L., & Lovati, L. (1994). *Valuazione con il Bilingual Aphasia Test (BAT) della rieducazione dell'afasico multilingue.* Paper presented to the 4th meeting on Disturbi cognitivi, comportamentali e della communicazione nelle lesioni cerebrali acquisite. Udine, Italy. July Proceedings. pp. 51–68.

Dewaele, J. M. (2001). Activation or inhibition? The interaction of L1, L2 and L3 on the language mode condinuum. In J. Cenoz, B. Hufeisen, & U. Jessner (Eds.), *Cross-linguistic influence in third language acquisition: Psycholinguistic perspectives* (pp. 69–89). Oxford: Oxford University Press.

Dijkstra, T., del Prado Martin, F. M., Schulpen, B., Schreuder, R., & Baayen, R. H. (2005). A roommate in cream: Morphological family size effects on interlingual homograph recognition. *Language and Cognitive Processes, 20*, 7–41.

Dijkstra, T., & Van Heuven, W. (2002). The architecture of the bilingual word recognition system: From identification to decision. *Bilingualism: Language and Cognition, 5*, 175–197.

Dijkstra, T., & Van Heuven, W. (2006). On Language and the Brain—Or on (Psycho)linguists and Neuroscientists? Commentary on Rodriguez-Fornells et al. *Language Learning, 56*(Suppl 1), 191–198.

Doucet, N., & Roberts, P. M. (1999, May). *Performance des adultes francophones québécois au Boston Naming Test.* Presented to the Association canadienne française pour l'avancement des sciences. Ottawa, Canada.

Dronkers, N., Yamasaki, Y., Webster Ross, G., & White, L. (1995). Assessment of bilinguality in aphasia: issues and examples from multicultural Hawaii. In M. Paradis (Ed.), *Aspects of bilingual aphasia.* (pp. 57–66). Tarrytown, NY: Elsevier.

Duncan, D. M. (1989). Issues in bilingualism research. In D. M. Duncan (Ed.), *Working with bilingual language disability* (pp. 18–35). New York: Chapman and Hall.

Durgunoglu, A. Y., & Roediger, H. L. (1987). Test differences in accessing bilingual memory. *Journal of Memory and Language, 26*, 377–391.

Edmonds, L. A., & Kiran, S. (2006). Effect of semantic based treatment on cross linguistic generalization in bilingual aphasia. *Journal of Speech, Language, and Hearing Research, 49*, 729–748.

Edwards, J. (2006). Foundations of bilingualism. In T.K. Bhatia & W.C. Ritchie (Eds.) *The handbook of bilingualism* (pp. 7–31). Oxford: Blackwell.

Elias, M. F., Elias, P. K, D'Agostino, R. B., Silbershatz, H., & Wolf, P. A. (1997). Role of age, education, and gender on cognitive performance in the Framingham Heart Study: Community-based norms. Experimental Aging Research, 23, 201–235.

Ellis, N. (1992). Linguistic relativity revisited: the bilingual word length effect in working memory during counting, remembering numbers and mental calculation. In R. J. Harris (Ed.), *Cognitive processing in bilinguals* (pp. 137-156). New York: Elsevier.

Erickson, J. G., Devlieger, P. J., & Sung, J. M. (1999). Korean-American female perspectives on disability. *American Journal of Speech-Language Pathology, 8*, 99–108.

Fabbro, F., & Paradis, M. (1995). Differential impairments in four multilingual patients with subcortical lesions. In M. Paradis (Ed.), *Aspects of bilingual aphasia.* (pp. 139–176). Tarrytown, NY: Elsevier.

Fawcett, J. T., & Carino, B. V. (1987). *Pacific bridges: The new immigration from Asia and the Pacific Islands.* New York: Center for Migration Studies.

Ferrand, L., & Humphreys, G. W. (1996). Transfer of refractory states across languages in a global aphasic patient. *Cognitive Neuropsychology, 13*, 1163–1191.

Ferreres, A. R., & Miravalles, G. (1995). The production of semantic paralexias in a Spanish-speaking aphasic. *Brain and Language, 49*, 153–172.

Fishman, J. A. (1965). Who speaks what language to whom and when? *Linguistics, 2*, 67–88.

Flege, J. E., MacKay, I. R. A., & Meador, D. (1999). Native Italian speakers' perception and production of English vowels. *Journal of the Acoustical Society of America, 106*, 2973–2987.

Frattali, C. M., Thompson, C. K., Holland, A. L., Wohl, C. B., & Ferketic, M. M. (1995). *The American Speech-Language-Hearing Association functional assessment of communication skills for adults (ASHA FACS).* Rockville, MD: ASHA.

Frayne, S. M., Burns, R. B., Hardt, E. J., Rosen, A. K., & Moskowitz, M. A. (1996). The exclusion of non-English-speaking persons from research. *Journal of General Internal Medicine, 11*, 39–43.

Fredman, M. (1975). The effect of therapy given in Hebrew on the home language of the bilingual or polyglot adult aphasic in Israel. *British Journal of Disorders of Communication, 10*, 61–69.

Frenck-Mestre, C., & Pynte, J. (1997). Syntactic ambiguity resolution while reading in second and native languages. *Quarterly Journal of Experimental Psychology, 50A*, 119–148.

Galens, J., Sheets, A., & Young, R. V. (1995). *Gale encyclopedia of multicultural America.* New York: Gale Research.

Galvez, A., & Hinckley, J. J. (2003). Transfer patterns of naming treatment in a case of bilingual aphasia. *Brain and Language, 87,* 173–174.

Gandour, J. (1998). Aphasia in tone languages. In P. Coppens, Y. Lebrun, & A. Basso (Eds.), *Aphasia in atypical populations* (pp. 117–142). Mahwah, NJ: Lawrence Erlbaum.

Gass, S. M., & Selinker, L. (1994). *Second language acquisition.* Hillsdale, NJ: Lawrence Erlbaum.

Gentile, A., Ozolins, U., & Vasilakakos, M. (1996). *Liaison interpreting: A handbook .* Melbourne: Melbourne University Press.

Goggin, J. P., Estrada, P., & Villarreal, R. P. (1994). Picture-naming agreement in monolinguals and bilinguals. *Applied Psycholinguistics, 15,* 177–193.

Goldstein, B. (2000). *Cultural and linguistic diversity resource guide for speech-language pathologists.* San Diego: Singular.

Gollnick, D., & Chinn, P. (1990). *Multicultural education in a pluralistic society.* Colombus, OH: Merrill.

Gomez-Tortosa, E., Martin, E. M., Gaviria, M., Charbel, F., & Ausman, J. I. (1995). Selective deficit of one language in a bilingual patient following surgery in the left perisylvian area. *Brain and Language, 48,* 320–325.

Goodglass, H., & Kaplan, E. (1983). *The assessment of aphasia and related disorders.* (2nd ed.). Philadelphia: Lea and Febiger.

Goodglass, H., Kaplan, E., & Barresi, B. (2000). *The Boston Diagnostic Aphasia Examination.* (3rd ed.). Austin, TX: Pro-Ed.

Goral, M. (2004). First-language decline in healthy aging: Implications for attrition in bilingualism. *Journal of Neurolinguistics, 17,* 31–52.

Goral, M., Levy, E. S., Obler, L. K., & Cohen, E. (2006). Cross-language lexical connections in the mental lexicon: Evidence from a case of trilingual aphasia. *Brain and Language, 98,* 235–247.

Goral, M., & Obler, L. K.(in press) Two's company, three's a crowd? Recent advances in psycholinguistic and neurolingustic study of multilingual speakers. In A. Stavans & I. Kupferberg (Eds.), *Studies in language and language education: Essays in honor of Elite Olshtain.* Jerusalem: The Hebrew University Magnes Press.

Graetz, P., de Bleser, R., & Willmes, K. (1992). *Akense afasie test.* Lisse, The Netherlands: Swetz and Zeitlinger.

Grainger, J., & Dijkstra, T. (1992). On the representation and use of language information in bilinguals. In R. J. Harris (Ed.), *Cognitive processing in bilinguals* (pp. 207–220). New York: Elsevier.

Green, D. W. (1998). Motor control of the bilingual lexico-semantic system. *Bilingualism: Language and Cognition, 1,* 67–81.

Grosjean, F. (1982). *Life with two languages: An introduction to bilingualism.* Cambridge: Harvard University Press.

Grosjean, F. (1984). Polyglot aphasics and language mixing: A comment on Perecman. *Brain and Language, 26,* 349–355.

Grosjean, F. (1989). Neurolinguists beware! The bilingual is not two monolinguals in one person. *Brain and Language, 36,* 3–15.

Grosjean, F. (1992). Another view of bilingualism. In R. J. Harris (Ed.), *Cognitive processing in bilinguals* (pp. 51–62). New York: Elsevier.

Grosjean, F. (1997). The bilingual individual. *Interpreting, 2,* 163–187.

Grosjean, F. (1998). Studying bilinguals: Methodological and conceptual issues. *Bilingualism: Language and Cognition, 1,* 131–149.

Grosjean, F., Li, P., Münte, T. F., & Rodriguez-Fornells, A. (2003). Imaging bilinguals: When the neurosciences meet the language sciences. *Bilingualism: Language and Cognition, 6,* 159–165.

Grosjean, F., & Py, B. (1991). La restructuration d'une première langue: l'intégration de variantes de contact dans la compétence des migrants bilingues. *La linguistique, 27*(2), 35–60.

Hakuta, K. (1986). *Mirror of language.* New York: Basic Books.

Halsband, U., Krause, B. J., Sipilae, H., Teraes, M., & Laihinen, A. (2002). PET studies on the memory processing of word pairs in bilingual Finnish-English subjects. *Behavioural Brain Research, 132,* 47–57.

Hamers, J., & Blanc, M. (1989). *Bilinguality and bilingualism.* Cambridge: Cambridge University Press.

Hamers, J., & Blanc, M. (2000). *Bilinguality and bilingualism.* (2nd ed.). Cambridge: Cambridge University Press.

Harley, B., & Wang, W. (1997). The critical period hypothesis: Where are we now? In A. M. B. de Groot & J. F. Kroll (Eds.), *Tutorials in bilingualism.* (pp. 19–52). Mahwah, NJ: Lawrence Erlbaum.

Harris, R. J., & Nelson, E. M. (1992). Bilingualism: Not the exception any more. In R. J. Harris (Ed.), *Cognitive processing in bilinguals* (pp. 3–14). New York: Elsevier.

Henderson, L. W., Frank, E. M., Pigatt, T., Abramson, R. K., & Houston, M. (1998). Race, gender, and educational level effects on Boston Naming Test scores. *Aphasiology, 12,* 901–911.

Heredia, R. R., & Altarriba, J. (Eds.). (2002). *Bilingual sentence processing.* New York: Elsevier.

Hernandez, A. E., Dapretto, M., Mazziotta, J., & Bookheimer, S. (2001). Language switching and language representation in Spanish-English bilinguals: An fMRI study. *Neuroimage, 14,* 510–520.

Hinckley, J. J. (2003). Picture naming treatment in aphasia yields greater improvement in L1. *Brain and Language, 87,* 171–172.

Hohenstein, J., Eisenberg, A., & Naigles, L. (2006). Is he floating across or crossing afloat? Cross-influence of L1 and L2 in Spanish-English bilingual adults. *Bilingualism: Language and Cognition, 9,* 249–261.

Holland, A. L., & Forbes, M. M. (1993). *Aphasia treatment: World perspectives.* San Diego: Singular.

Holland, A. L., & Penn, C. (1995). Inventing therapy for aphasia. In L. Menn, M. O'Connor, L. K. Obler, & A. Holland (Eds.), *Non-fluent aphasia in a multilingual world.* (pp. 144–155). Philadelphia: John Benjamins.

Huber, W., Poeck, K., Weniger, D., & Willmes, K. (1983). *Der Aachener Aphasie Test.* Gottingen: Verlag fur Psychologie Hogrefe.

Hurford, J. R. (1991). The evolution of the critical period for language acquisition. *Cognition, 40,* 159–201.

Hyltenstam, K. (1992). Non-native features of near-native speakers: On the ultimate attainment of childhood L2 learners. In R. J. Harris (Ed.), *Cognitive processing in bilinguals* (pp. 351–368). New York: Elsevier.

Ivnik, R. J., Malec, J. F., Smith, G. E., Tangalos, E.G. et al. (1996). Neuropsychological tests' norms above age 55: COWAT, BNT, MAE Token, WRAT-R Reading, AMNART, STROOP, TMT, and JLO. *Clinical Neuropsychologist, 10,* 262–278.

Jacobson, R. (1998) (Ed.), *Code-switching worldwide.* New York: Mouton de Gruyter.

Jacobson, R. (2001) (Ed.). *Code-switching worldwide II.* New York: Mouton de Gruyter.

Junqué, C., Vendrell, P., & Vendrell, J. (1995). Differential impairments and specific speech phenomena in 50 Catalan-Spanish bilingual aphasic patients. In M. Paradis (Ed.), *Aspects of bilingual aphasia* (pp. 177–210). Tarrytown, NY: Pergamon.

Junqué, C., Vendrell, P., & Vendrell-Brucet, J. (1989). Differential recovery in naming in bilingual aphasics. *Brain and Language, 36*, 16–22.

Kang, S.-M. (2006). Measurement of acculturation, scale formats and language competence: Their implications for adjustment. *Journal of Cross-cultural Psychology, 37*, 669–693.

Kaplan, E., Goodglass, H., Weintraub, S. (1983). *The Boston Naming Test*. Philadelphia: Lea & Febiger.

Katz, R. C., Hallowell, B., Code, C., Armstrong, E., Roberts, P. M., Pound, C., & Katz, L. (2000). A multi-national comparison of aphasia management practices. *International Journal of Language and Communication Disorders. 35*, 303–314.

Kayser, H. (1995). Interpreters. In H. Kayser (Ed.), *Bilingual speech-language pathology: An Hispanic focus* (pp. 207–221). San Diego: Singular.

Kayser, H. (1998). Outcome measurement in culturally and linguistically diverse populations. In C. M. Frattali (Ed.), *Measuring outcomes in speech-language pathology* (pp. 225–244) New York: Thieme.

Kertesz, A. (1982). *The Western Aphasia Battery*. New York: Grune and Stratton.

Kilborn, K. (1992). On-line integration of grammatical information in a second language. In R. J. Harris (Ed.), *Cognitive processiong in bilinguals* (pp. 337–350). New York: Elsevier.

Kim, H., & Na, D. L. (1999). Normative data on the Korean version of the Boston Naming test. *Journal of Clinical and Experimental Neuropsychology, 21*, 127–133.

Kim, K. H. S., Relkin, N. R., Lee, K.-M., & Hirsch. J. (1997). Distinct cortical areas associated with native and second languages. Nature, 388, 171–174.

Kirsner, K., Lalor, E., & Hird, K. (1993). The bilingual lexicon: Exercise, meaning and morphology. In R. Schreuder & B. Weltens (Eds.), The bilingual lexicon (pp. 215–248). Philadelphia: John Benjamins.

Klein, D., Zatorre, R. J., Milner, B., Meyer, E., & Evans, A. C. (1994). Left putaminal activation when speaking a second language: Evidence from PET. *NeuroReport, 5*, 2295–2297.

Klein, D., Zatorre, R. J., Milner, B., Meyer, E., & Evans, A. C. (1995). The neural substrates of bilingual language processing: Evidence from positron emission tomography. In M. Paradis (Ed.), *Aspects of bilingual aphasia* (pp. 23–36). Tarrytown, New York: Pergamon.

Kohnert, K. (2004). Cognitive and cognate-based treatments for bilingual aphasia: A case study. *Brain and Language, 91*, 294–302.

Kohnert, K. J., Hernandez, A. E., & Bates, E. (1998). Bilingual performance on the Boston Naming Test: Preliminary norms in Spanish and English. *Brain and Language, 65*(3), 422–440.

Kroll, J. F., & de Groot, A. M. B. (1997). Lexical and conceptual memory in the bilingual: Mapping form in two languages. In A. M. B. de Groot & J. F. Kroll (Eds.), *Tutorials in bilingualism: Psycholinguistic perspectives* (pp. 169–199). Mahwah, NJ: Lawrence Erlbaum.

Kroll, J. F., & de Groot, A. M. B. (2005). *Handbook of bilingualism: Psycholinguistic approaches*. New York: Oxford University Press.

Lafaury, P. J., & Roberts, P. M. (1998, November). *Cognate words in a verbal fluency task*. Paper presented to the annual conference of the American Speech-Language-Hearing Association. San Antonio, TX.

Laganaro, K. M., & Overton Venet, M. (2001). Acquired alexia in multilingual aphasia and computer-assisted treatment in both languages: Issues of generalization and transfer. *Folia Phoniatrica et Logopaedica, 53*, 135–144.

Langdon, H. W. (1992a). *Interpreter/translator process in the educational setting: A resource manual*. Sacramento, CA: Resources in Special Education.

Langdon, H. W. (1992b). The Hispanic population: Facts and figures. In H.W. Langdon (Ed.), *Hispanic children and adults with communication disorders* (pp. 20–56). Gaithersburg, MD: Aspen.

Langdon, H. W., & Cheng, L. L. (2002). *Collaborating with interpreters and translators: A guide for communication disorders professionals*. Eau Claire, WI: Thinking.

Langdon, H. W., Wiig, E. W., & Nielsen, N. P. (2005). Dual-dimension naming speed and language dominance ratings by bilingual Hispanic adults. *Bilingual Research Journal, 29*, 319–336.

Law, S. P., & Leung, M. T. (2000). Sentence processing deficits in two Cantonese aphasic patients. *Brain and Language, 72*, 310–342.

Lehtonen, M., & Laine, M. (2003). How word frequency affects morphological processing in monolinguals and bilinguals. *Bilingualism: Language and Cognition, 6*, 213–225.

Lemhöfer, K., & Dijkstra, T. (2004). Recognizing cognates and interlingual homographs: Effects of code similarity in language-specific and generalized lexical decision. *Memory and Cognition, 32*, 533–550.

Lemhöfer, K., Dijkstra, T., & Michel, M.-C. (2004). Three languages, one ECHO: Cognate effects in trilingual word recognition. *Language and Cognitive Processes, 19*, 585–611.

Levey, S. (2004). Discrimination and production of English vowels by bilingual speakers of Spanish and English. *Erceptual and Motor Skills, 99*, 445–462.

Lhermitte, R., Hécaen, H., Dubois, J., Culioli, A., & Tabouret-Kelly, A. (1966). Le problème de l'aphasie des polyglottes: Remarques sur quelques observations. *Neuropsychologia, 4*, 315–329.

Lichtenberg, P. A, Ross, T., & Christensen, B. (1994). Preliminary normative data on the Boston Naming Test for an older urban population. *The Clinical Neuropsychologist, 8*, 109–111.

Liu, H., Bates, E., & Li, P. (1992). Sentence interpretation in bilingual speakers of English and Chinese. *Applied Psycholinguistics, 13*, 451–484.

Luzzatti, C., Laiacona, M., Allamano, N., De Tanti, A., & Inzaghi, M. G. (1998). Writing disorders in Italian aphasic patients: A multiple single-case study of dysgraphia in a language with shallow orthography. *Brain, 121*, 1721–1734.

Luzzati, C., Willmes, K., & de Bleser, R. (1992). *Aachener Aphasie Test: Versione italiana*. Firenze: O. S. Organizzazioni Speciali.

Lynch, E. W., & Hanson, J. (1992). *Developing cross-cultural competence: A guide for working with young children and their families*. Baltimore: Brookes.

Mackey, W. F. (1967). *Bilingualism as a world problem/Le bilinguisme: Phénomène mondial*. Montreal: Harvest House.

MacWhinney, B. (2002). Extending the competition model. In R. R. Heredia & J. Altarriba (Eds.), *Bilingual Sentence Processing* (pp. 31–58). Vol. 134 of G. E. Stelmach (Series Ed.) Advances in Psychology. New York: Elsevier.

MacWhinney, B., & Bates, E. (1989). *The cross-linguistic study of sentence processing.* New York: Cambridge University Press.

Mahendra, N., Plante, El., Magloire, J., Milman, L., & Trouard, T. P. (2003). fMRI variability and the localization of languages in the bilingual brain. N*euroReport, 14,* 1225–1228.

Manuel-Dupont, S., Ardila, A., Rosselli, M., & Puente, A. E. (1992). Bilingualism. In A. E. Puente & R. J. McCaffrey (Eds.), *Handbook of neuropsychological assessment* (pp. 193–210). New York: Plenum Press.

Mariën, P. M., Mampaey, E., Vervaet, A., Saerens, J., & De Deyn, P. P. (1998). Normative data for the Boston Naming Test in native Dutch-speaking Belgian elderly. *Brain and Language, 65,* 447–467.

Marin, G. (1992). Issues in the measurement of acculturation among Hispanics. In K. F. Geisinger (Ed.), *Psychological testing of Hispanics, APA Science Volumes* (pp. 235–251). Washington, DC: APA.

Martin, D., Anderson, S., Chaudry, N., Clark, C., Hooke, E., Little, C., et al. (1998). *Good practice for speech and language therapists working with clients from linguistic minority communities: Guidelines of the Royal College of Speech and Language Therapists.* London: RCSLT.

Marty, S., & Grosjean, F. (1998). Aphasie, bilinguisme et modes de communication. *Aphasie und verwandte, 12*(1), 8–28.

Mechelli, A., Crinion, J. T., Noppeney, U., O'Doherty, J., Ashburner, J., Frackowiak, R. S., et al. (2004). Structural plasticity in the bilingual brain: Proficiency in a second language and age at acquisition affect grey-matter density. *Nature, 431*(7010), 757.

Menn, L. (1989). Comparing approaches to comparative aphasiology. *Aphasiology, 3*(2), 143–150.

Menn, L. (2001). Comparative aphasiology: Cross-language studies of aphasia. In R.S. Berndt (Ed.). *Handbook of Neuropsychology* (2nd ed., pp. 51–68). Vol. 3: Language and Aphasia. Amsterdam: Elsevier.

Menn, L., & Obler, L. K. (1990). *Agrammatic aphasia: A cross-language narrative sourcebook.* Philadelphia: John Benjamins.

Menn, L., O'Connor, M., Obler, L. K., & Holland. (1995). *Nonfluent aphasia in a multilingual world.* Philadelphia: John Benjamins.

Miller, N. (1984). Language use in bilingual communities. In N. Miller (Ed.), *Bilingualism and language disability: Assessment and remediation* (pp. 3–25). San Diego, CA: College-Hill Press.

Miller, N., Willmes, K., & de Bleser, R. (2000). The psychometric properties of the English language version of the Aachen Aphasia Test (EAAT). *Aphasiology, 14,* 683–722.

Mimouni, Z., Béland, R., Danault, S., & Idrissi, A. (1995). Similar language disorders in Arabic and French in an early bilingual aphasic patient. *Brain and Language, 51,* 132–134.

Molrine, C. J., & Pierce, R. S. (1998, November). *African American and European American adults' expressive language performance on three aphasia tests.* Paper presented to annual American Speech-Language-Hearing conference. San Antonio, TX.

Monsch, A., Bondi, M., Butters, N., Salmon, D., Katzman, R., & Thal, L. (1992). Comparison of verbal fluency tasks in the detection of dementia of the Alzheimer type. *Archives of Neurology, 49,* 1253–1258.

Montrul, S. (2002). Incomplete acquisition and attrition of Spanish tense/aspect distinctions in adult bilinguals. Bilingualism: Language and Cognition, 39–68.

Moretti, R., Torre, P., Antonello, R. M., Cazzato, G., & Bava, A. (2003). Subcortical-cortical lesions and two-step aphasia in a bilingual patient. In S.P. Shohov (Ed.). *Advances in psychology research.* (Vol 23, pp. 33–44). New York: Nova Science.

Mungas, D. (1996). The process of development of valid and reliable neuropsychological assessment measures for English- and Spanish-speaking elderly persons. In G. Yeo & D. Gallagher-Thompson (Eds.), *Ethnicity and the dementias* (pp. 33–46). Washington, DC: Taylor & Francis.

Muñoz, M. L., & Marquardt, T. P. (in press). The performance of neurologically normal bilingual speakers of Spanish and English on the short version of the Bilingual Aphasia Test. *Aphasiology,* 1–17.

Myers-Scotton, C. (2005). Supporting a differential access hypothesis: Code switching and other contact data. In J.F. Kroll & A.M.B. de Groot (Eds*.) Handbook of bilingualism: Psycholinguistic approaches* (pp. 326–348). New York: Oxford University Press.

Myers-Scotton, C., & Jake, J. (2001). Explaining aspects of codeswitching and their implications. In J. Nicol (Ed.), *One mind, two languages: Bilingual language processing* (pp. 84–116). Oxford: Blackwell.

Naeser, M. A., & Chan, S. W.- C. (1980). Case study of a Chinese aphasic with the Boston Diagnostic Aphasia Exam. *Neuropsychologia, 18,* 389–410.

National Institute of Deafness and other Communication Disorders (1992). *Report from the working group: Research and research training needs of minority persons and minority health issues.* Bethesda, MD: National Institutes of Health.

National Institutes of Health (1990). *National Institutes of Health Guide, 35*(19), 1–2.

Nilipour, R. (1988). Bilingual aphasia in Iran: A preliminary report. *Journal of Neurolinguistics, 3*(2), 185–232.

Nilipour, R., & Ashayery, H. (1989). Alternating antagonism between two languages with successive recovery of a third in a trilingual aphasic patient. *Brain and Language, 36,* 23–48.

Nilipour, R., & Paradis, M. (1995). Breakdown of functional categories in three Farsi-English bilingual aphasic patients. In M. Paradis (Ed.), *Aspects of bilingual aphasia* (pp. 123–138). Tarrytown, NY: Elsevier.

Oesch-Serra, C. (1992). Code-switching et marqueurs discursifs: Entre variation et conversation. *Travaux neuchâtelois de linguistique, 18,* 155–171.

Packard, J. (1986). Tone production deficits in nonfluent aphasic Chinese speech. *Brain and Language, 29,* 212–223.

Pallier, C., Bosch, L., & Sebastián-Galles, N. (1997). A limit on behavioral plasticity in vowel acquisition. *Cognition, 64,* B9–B17.

Paniagua, F. A. (2005). *Assessing and treating culturally diverse clients: a practical guide.* (3rd ed). Thousand Oaks, CA: Sage.

Paradis, M. (1977). The stratification of bilingualism. In M. Paradis (Ed.), *Aspects of bilingualism* (pp. 165–175). Columbia, SC: Hornbeam Press.

Paradis, M. (1983). *Readings on aphasia in bilinguals and polyglots.* Montreal: Didier.

Paradis, M. (1989). Bilingual and polyglot aphasia. In F. Boller & J. Grafman (Eds.), *Handbook of Neuropsychology* (Vol. 2, pp. 117–140). New York: Elsevier.

Paradis, M. (1990). Language lateralization in bilinguals: Enough already! *Brain and Language, 39,* 576–586.

Paradis, M. (1993a). Multilingualism and aphasia. In G. Blanken (Ed.), *Linguistic disorders and pathologies. An international handbook* (pp. 278–288). New York: Waller de Gruyter.

Paradis, M. (1993b). Bilingual aphasia rehabilitation. In M. Paradis (Ed.), *Foundations of aphasia rehabilitation* (pp. 423–419). New York: Pergamon.

Paradis, M. (1995b) The need for distinctions. In M. Paradis (Ed.), *Aspects of bilingual aphasia* (pp. 1–9). Tarrytown, NY: Elsevier.

Paradis, M. (1995c). Bilingual aphasia 100 years later: consensus and controversies. In M. Paradis (Ed.), *Aspects of bilingual aphasia* (pp. 211–223). Tarrytown, NY: Elsevier.

Paradis, M. (1997). The cognitive neuropsychology of bilingualism. In A.M.B. de Groot & J. F. Kroll (Eds.), *Tutorials in bilingualism: Psycholinguistic perspectives* (pp. 331–354). Mahwah, NJ: Lawrence Erlbaum.

Paradis, M. (1998). Acquired aphasia in bilingual speakers. In M. Taylor-Sarno (Ed.), *Acquired aphasia* (3rd ed., pp. 531–549). New York: Academic Press.

Paradis, M. (2004). *A neurolinguistic theory of bilingualism.* Philadelphia: John Benjamins.

Paradis, M., & Goldblum, M. C. (1989). Selective crossed aphasia followed by reciprocal antagonism in a trilingual patient. *Brain and Language, 36,* 62–75.

Paradis, M., Goldblum, M. C., & Abidi, R. (1982). Alternate antagonism with paradoxical translation behaviour in two bilingual aphasic patients. *Brain and Language, 15,* 55–69.

Paradis, M., & Libben, G. (1987). *The assessment of bilingual aphasia.* Hillsdale, NJ: Lawrence Erlbaum.

Paradis, M., & Libben, G. (1993). *La evaluación de la afasie en los bilingues.* Barcelona: Masson.

Pavlenko, A. (2000). L2 influence on L1 in late bilingualism. *Issues in Applied Linguistics, 11,* 175–205.

Pavlenko, A., & Jarvis, S. (2002). Bidirectional transfer. *Applied Linguistics, 23,* 190–214.

Penn, C., & Beecham, R. (1992). Discourse therapy in multilingual aphasia: A case study. *Clinical Linguistics & Phonetics, 6,* 11–25.

Perani, D., Abutalebi, J., Paulesu, E., Brambati, S., Scifo, P., Cappa, S. F., et al. (2003). The role of age of acquisition and language usage in early, high-proficient bilinguals: An fMRI study during verbal fluency. *Human Brain Mapping, 19,* 170–182.

Perani, D., Dehane, S., Grassi, F., Cohen, L., Cappa, S., Paulesu, E., et al. (1996). Brain processing of native and foreign languages. *NeuroReport, 7,* 2439–2444.

Perani, D., Paulesu, E., Galles, N. S., Dupoux, E., Dehaene, S., Bettinardi, V., et al. (1998). The bilingual brain: Proficiency and age of acquisition of the second language. *Brain, 121,* 1841–1852.

Pontón, M. O., & Ardila, A. (1999). The future of neuropsychology with Hispanic populations in the United States. *Archives of Clinical Neuropsychology, 14,* 565–580.

Puente, A. E., & McCaffrey (Eds.) (1992). *Handbook of neuropsychological assessment: A biopsychosocial perspective.* NY: Plenum Press.

Radanovic, M., Mansur, L. L., & Scaff, M. (2004). Normative data for the Brazilian population in the Boston Diagnostic Aphasia Examination: Influence of schooling. *Brazilian Journal of Medical and Biological Research, 37*(11), 1731–1738.

Rapport, R. L., Tan, C. T., & Whitaker, H. A. (1983). Language function and dysfunction among Chinese- and English-speaking polyglots: Cortical stimulation, Wada testing and clinical studies. *Brain and Language, 18,* 342–366.

Rey, G. J., & Benton, A. (1991). *Multilingual Aphasia Examination-Spanish.* Iowa City: AJA.

Rey, G. J., Feldman, E., Hernandez, D., Levin, B. E., Rivas-Vazquez, R., Nedd, K. J., et al. (2001). Application of the Multilingual Aphasia Examination-Spanish in the evaluation of Hispanic patients post closed-head trauma. *The Clinical Neuropsychologist, 15,* 13–18.

Rey, G. J., Feldman, E., Rivas-Vazquez, R., Levin, B. E., & Benton, A. (1999). Neuropsychological test development and normative data on Hispanics. *Archives of Clinical Neuropsychology, 14,* 593–601.

Reyes, B. A. (1998). Bilingual aphasia: A case study. Communication disorders and sciences in culturally and linguistically diverse populations. Rockville, MD: ASHA SID 14, 2–7.

Roberts, P. M. (1992, October). *Therapy and spontaneous recovery in a bilingual aphasic.* Paper presented to the Academy of Aphasia. Toronto, Canada.

Roberts, P. M. (1998). Clinical research needs in bilingual aphasia. *Aphasiology, 12,* 119–130.

Roberts, P. M. (2001). Aphasia assessment and treatment for bilingual and culturally diverse patients. In R. Chapey (Ed.) Language intervention strategies for aphasia and related neurogenic communication disorders (pp. 208–232). Baltimore: Lippincott Williams & Wilkins.

Roberts, P. M. (2003). Performance of Canadian adults on the Graded Naming Test. *Aphasiology, 17,* 933–946.

Roberts, P. M., & Bois, M. (1999). Picture-name agreement for French-English bilingual adults. *Brain and Cognition, 40,* 238–241.

Roberts, P. M., Code, C. F. S., & McNeil, M. R. (2003). Describing participants in aphasia research. Part 1: Audit of current practices. *Aphasiology, 17,* 911–932.

Roberts, P. M., de la Riva, J., & Rhéaume, A. (1997, May). *Effets de l'intervention dans une langue pour l'anomie bilingue.* Paper presented at the annual meeting of the Canadian Association of Speech-Language Pathology and Audiology. Toronto.

Roberts, P. M., & Deslauriers, L. (1999). Picture naming of cognate and non-cognate nouns in bilingual aphasia. *Journal of Communication Disorders, 32,* 1–23.

Roberts, P. M., Garcia, L. J., & Desrochers, A., & Hernandez, D. (2002). English performance of proficient bilingual adults on the Boston Naming Test. *Aphasiology, 16,* 635–645.

Roberts, P. M., & Kiran, S. (2007). Bilingual aphasia and anomia. In A. Ardila & E. Ramos (Eds.), *Speech and language disorders in bilinguals* (pp. 109–130). New York: Nova Science.

Roberts, P. M., & Le Dorze, G. (1994). Semantics verbal fluency in aphasia: a quantitative and qualitative study in test-retest conditions. *Aphasiology, 8,* 569–582.

Roberts, P. M., & Le Dorze, G. (1997). Semantic organization, strategy use and productivity in bilingual semantic verbal fluency. *Brain and Language, 59*, 412–449.

Roberts, P. M., & Le Dorze, G. (1998). Bilingual aphasia: semantic organisation, strategy use, and productivity in semantic verbal fluency. *Brain and Language, 65*, 287–312.

Roberts, P. M., & Shenker, R. C. (in press). Assessment and treatment of stuttering in bilingual speakers. In E. G. Conture & R. F. Curlee (Eds.) *Stuttering and related disorders of fluency.* (3rd ed.). New York: Thieme.

Salamoura, A., & Williams, J. N. (2006). Lexical activation of cross-language syntactic priming. *Bilingualism: Language and Cognition, 9*, 299–307.

Sanchez-Casas, R., & García-Albea, J. E. (2005). The representation of cognate and noncognate words in bilingual memory: Can cognate status be characterized as a special kind of morphological relation? In J. F. Kroll & A. M. B. De Groot (Eds.) *Handbook of bilingualism: Psycholinguistic approaches* (pp. 226–250). New York: Oxford University Press.

Sasanuma, S. (1986). Universal and language specific symptomatology and treatment of aphasia. *Folia Phoniatrica, 38*, 121–175.

Sasanuma, S. (1993). Aphasia treatment in Japan. In A. L. Holland & M. M. Forbes (Eds.), *Aphasia treatment: World perspectives* (pp. 175–198). San Diego: Singular.

Sasanuma, S., & Park, H. S. (1995). Patterns of language deficits in two Korean-Japanese bilingual aphasic patients: A clinical report. In M. Paradis (Ed.), *Aspects of bilingual aphasia.* (pp. 111–123). New York: Elsevier.

Schuell, H. (1965). *The Minnesota Test for Differential Diagnosis of Aphasia.* Minneapolis: University of Minnesota Press.

Schum, R. L., Sivan, A. B. (1997). Verbal abilities in healthy elderly adults. *Applied Neuropsychology, 4*(2), 130–134.

Schum, R. L., Sivan, A. B., & Benton, A. (1989). Multilingual Aphasia Examination: Norms for children. *Clinical Neuropsychologist, 3*, 375–383.

Scovel, T. (1989). *A time to speak: A psycholinguistic inquiry into the critical period for human speech.* Cambridge: Newbury House.

Seliger, H. W., & Vago, R. M. (1991). The study of first language attrition: An overview. In H. W. Seliger & R. M. Vago (Eds.), *First language attrition.* (pp. 1–15). New York: Cambridge University Press.

Selinker, L. (1972). Interlanguage. *International Review of Applied Linguistics, 10*, 209–231.

Selinker, L. (1992). *Rediscovering interlanguage.* New York: Longman.

Sharwood Smith, M. A. (1989). Cross-linguistic influence in language loss. In K. Hyltenstam & L. K. Obler (Eds.), *Bilingualism across the lifespan: Aspects of acquisition, maturity, and loss* (pp. 185–201). New York: Cambridge University Press.

Silverberg, R., & Gordon, H. (1979). Differential aphasia in two bilingual individuals. *Neurology, 29*, 51–55.

Snodgrass, J. G. (1993). Translating versus picture naming: Similarities and differences. In R. Schreuder & B. Weltens (Eds.), *The bilingual lexicon* (pp. 83–114). Philadelphia: John Benjamins.

Spreen, O., & Strauss, E. (1998). *A compendium of neuropsychologicial tests: Administration, norms and commentary.* (2nd ed.). New York: Oxford University Press.

Springer, L., Miller, N., & Bürk, F. (1998). A cross language analysis of conversation in a trilingual speaker with aphasia. *Journal of Neurolinguistics, 11*, 223–241.

Stadie, N., Springer, L., de Bleser, R., & Burk, F. (1995). Oral and written naming in a multilingual patient. In M. Paradis (Ed.), *Aspects of bilingual aphasia* (pp. 85–100). New York: Elsevier Science.

Steinmetz, H., & Seitz, R. J. (1991). Functional anatomy of language processing: Neuroimaging and the problem of individual variability. *Neuropsychologia, 29*, 1149–1161.

Tallberg, I. M. (2005). The Boston Naming Test in Swedish: Normative data. *Brain and Language, 94*, 19–31.

Tempo, P. M., & Saito, A. (1996). Techniques of working with Japanese American families. In G. Yeo & D. Gallagher-Thompson (Eds.), (1996). *Ethnicity and the dementias.* Washington, DC: Taylor and Francis.

Teng, (1996). Cross-cultural testing and the Cognitive Abilities Screening Instrument. In G. Yeo & D. Gallagher-Thompson (Eds.), (pp. 109–122). *Ethnicity and the dementias.* Washington, DC: Taylor and Francis.

Terrell, S. L., Battle, D. E., & Grantham, R. B. (1998). African American cultures. In D. E. Battle (Ed.). *Communication disorders in multicultural populations* (2nd ed., pp. 31–71). Newton, MA: Butterworth-Heinemann.

Toraldo, A., Cattani, B., Zonca, G., Saletta, P., & Luzzatti, C. (2006). Reading disorders in a language with shallow orthography: A multiple single-case study in Italian. *Aphasiology, 20*, 823–850.

Tsolaki, M., Tsantali, S., Lekka, G., Kiosseoglu, G., & Kazis, A. (2003). Can the Boston Naming Test be used as a clinical tool for differential diagnosis in dementia. *Brain and Language, 87*, 185–186.

Vaid, J., & Genesee, F. (1980). Neuropsychological approaches to bilingualism: A critical review. *Canadian Journal of Psychology, 34*(4), 417–445.

Valle, R. (1994). Culture-fair behavioral symptom differential assessment and intervention in dementing illness. *Alzheimer Disease and Associated Disorders, 8*(3), 21–45.

Van Eeckhout, P., Pillon, B., Signoret, J.-L., Deloche, G., & Seron, X. (1992). Rééducation des réductions sévères de l'expression orale: La thérapie mélodique et rythmée. In X. Seron & C. Laterre (Eds.), *Rééduquer le cerveau: Logopédie, psychologie, neurologie.* (pp. 109–121). Brussels: Pierre Mardaga.

Van Hell, J. G., & de Groot, A. M. B. (1998). Conceptual representation in bilingual memory: Effects of concreteness and cognate status in word association. *Bilingualism: Language and Cognition, 1*, 193–212.

Van Hell, J., & Dijkstra, T. (2002). Foreign language knowledge can influence native language performance in exclusively native contexts. *Psycholinguistic Bulletin and Review, 9*, 780–789.

Van Lancker Sidtis, D. (2006). Does functional neuroimaging solve the questions of neurolinguistics? *Brain and Language, 98*, 276–290.

Van Wijnendaele, I., & Brysbaert, M. (2002). Visual word recognition in bilinguals: Phonological priming from the second to the first language. *Journal of Experimental Psychology: Human Perception & Performance, 28*, 616–627.

Visch-Brink, E. G., van Harskamp, F., Van Amerongen, N. M., Wielart, S. M., & van de Sandt-Koenderman, M. E. (1993). A multidisciplinary approach to aphasia therapy. In A. L. Holland & M. M. Forbes (Eds.), *Aphasia treatment: World perspectives* (pp. 227–262). San Diego: Singular.

Wallace, G. L. (1997). *Multicultural neurogenics: A resource for speech-language pathologists providing services to neurologically impaired adults from culturally and linguistically diverse backgrounds.* San Antonio: The Psychological Corporation.

Wallace, G. L., & Tonkovich, J. D. (1997). African Americans: Culture, communication, and clinical management. In G. L. Wallace (Ed.), *Multicultural neurogenics* (pp. 133–164). San Antonio: Communication Skill Builders.

Watamori, T., & Sasanuma, S. (1976). The recovery process of a bilingual aphasic. *Journal of Communication Disorders, 9,* 157–166.

Watamori, T., & Sasanuma, S. (1978). The recovery process of two English-Japanese bilingual aphasics. *Brain and Language, 6,* 127–140.

Weekes, B. S., Chen, M. J., Qun, H. C., Lin, Y. B., Yao, C., & Xiao, X. Y. (1998). Anomia and dyslexia in Chinese: A familiar story? *Aphasiology, 12,* 77–98.

Weltens, B., & Grendel, M. (1993). Attrition of vocabulary knowledge. In R. Schreuder & B. Weltens (Eds.), *The bilingual lexicon* (pp. 135–156). Philadelphia: John Benjamins.

Wender, D. (1989). Aphasic victim as investigator. *Archives of Neurology, 46,* 91–92.

Whitworth, A., & Sjardin, H. (1993). The bilingual person with aphasia. In D. Lafond, Y. Joanette, R. Ponzio, R. Degiovani, & M. T. Sarno (Eds.), *Living with aphasia: Psychosocial issues* (pp. 129–149). San Diego: Singular.

Wiener, D., Obler, L. K., & Taylor-Sarno, M. (1995). Speech/language management of the bilingual aphasic in a U.S. urban rehabilitation hospital. In M. Paradis (Ed.), *Aspects of bilingual aphasia* (pp. 37–56). Tarrytown, NY: Elsevier.

Worrall, L. E., Yiu, E. M.- L., Hickson, L. M. H., & Barrett, H. M. (1995). Normative data for the Boston Naming Test for Australian elderly. *Aphasiology, 9,* 541–551

APPENDIX 9.1
Addresses for Ordering Tests (subject to change)

Spanish version of the BDAE
Editorial Medica Panamericana
Alberto Alcocer, 24-6a
28036 Madrid
Spain
(tel: 011 3491 457 0203)
http://www.medicapanamericana.com/

sgonzalez@medicapanamericana.com

Bilingual Aphasia Test
The administration manual is available in Spanish:
Evaluación de la afasia en los bilingües, Barcelona: Masson (ISBN 84-311-0644-1).
Masson, S.A.
Avda Príncipe de Asturias, 20
08012 Barcelona Spain

and in Italian:
Valutazione dell'afasia bilingue, Bologna: EMS s.r.l.
EMS s.r.l.

Via P. Fabbri, 72
43138 Bologna Italy

The Chinese version: *Shuangyu shiyuzheng de pinggu*. Guangzhou: Jinan daxue chubanshe is available from Jinan University Press, Guangzhou, P.R. China.
Contact person:
Dr. Lin Gu-Hui
R201 Nanhu Yuan #7
Jinan University
Guangdong,
P.R. China 510630

The Aachen Aphasia Test—English
For the English version contact:
Dr. N. Miller
Speech and Language Sciences
George VI Building
University of Newcastle
GB Newcastle NE1 7RU
England

Section III

Psychosocial/Functional Approaches to Intervention: Focus on Improving Ability to Perform Communication Activities of Daily Living

Chapter 10

Life-Participation Approach to Aphasia: A Statement of Values for the Future

LPAA Project Group (in alphabetical order): Roberta Chapey, Judith F. Duchan, Roberta J. Elman, Linda J. Garcia, Aura Kagan, Jon G. Lyon, and Nina Simmons-Mackie

Unprecedented changes are occurring in the way treatment for aphasia is viewed—and reimbursed. These changes, resulting from both internal and external pressures, are influencing how speech-language pathologists carry out their jobs.

Internal influences include a growing interest in treatments that produce meaningful real life outcomes leading to enhanced quality of life. Externally, we are influenced by disability rights activists encouraging adjustments in philosophy and treatment and by consumers frustrated by unmet needs and unfulfilled goals. Most recently, a strong external influence is emanating from the curtailment of funding for our work, which has caused a significant reduction in available services to people affected by aphasia.

To accommodate these varied influences on service delivery, it is important to take a proactive stance. We therefore propose a philosophy of service delivery that meets the needs of people affected by aphasia and confronts the pressures from our profession, providers, and funding sources. Our statement of values has been guided by the ideas and work of speech-language pathologists as well as by individuals in psychology, sociology, and medicine (see the ASHA Web site, www.asha.org/public/speech/disorders/LPAA.htm, for a detailed reference list). We intend neither to prescribe exact methods for achieving specific outcomes, nor to provide a quick fix to the challenges facing our profession. Rather, we offer a statement of values and ideas relevant to assessment, intervention, policy making, advocacy, and research that we hope will stimulate discussion related to restructuring of services and lead to innovative clinical methods for supporting those affected by aphasia.

DEFINING THE APPROACH

The "Life Participation Approach to Aphasia" (LPAA) is a consumer-driven service delivery approach that supports individuals with aphasia and others affected by it in achieving their immediate and long term life goals (note that "approach" refers here to a general philosophy and model of service delivery, rather than to a specific clinical approach). LPAA calls for a broadening and refocusing of clinical practice and research on the consequences of aphasia. It focuses on reengagement in life, beginning with initial assessment and intervention, and continuing, after hospital discharge, until the consumer no longer elects to have communication support.

LPAA places the life concerns of those affected by aphasia at the center of all decision making. It empowers the consumer to select and participate in the recovery process and to collaborate on the design of interventions that aim for a more rapid return to active life. These interventions thus have the potential to reduce the consequences of disease and injury that contribute to long-term health-care costs.

THE ESSENCE OF LPAA

We encourage clinicians and researchers to focus on the real-life goals of people affected by aphasia. For example, in the initial stages following a CVA, a goal may be to establish effective communication with the surrounding nursing staff and physicians. At a later stage, a life goal may be to return to employment or participation in the local community. Regardless of the stage of management, LPAA emphasizes the attainment of reengagement in life by strengthening daily participation in activities of choice.

Residual skill is thus seen as only one of many requisites. For example, full participation depends on motivation and a consistent and dependable support system. A highly supportive environment can lessen the consequences of aphasia on one's life, whatever the language impairment. A nonsupportive environment, on the other hand, can substantially increase the chance of aphasia affecting daily routines. Someone with mild aphasia in a nonsupportive environment

TABLE 10–1

Examples of the Shift in Focus of Life-Participation Approach to Aphasia

LPAA	Examples of Shift in Focus
Assessment includes determining relevant life participation needs and discovering clients' competencies	In addition to assessing language and communication deficits, clinicians are equally interested in assessing how the person with aphasia does *with support*
Treatment includes facilitating the achievement of life goals	In addition to work on improving and/or compensating for the language impairment, clinicians are prepared to work on anything in which aphasia is a barrier to life participation (even if the activity is not directly related to communication)
Intervention routinely targets environmental factors outside of the individual	In addition to working with the individual on language or compensatory functional-communication techniques, clinicians might train communication partners or work on other ways of reducing barriers to make the environment more "aphasia-friendly"
All those affected by aphasia are regarded as legitimate targets for intervention	In addition to working with the individual who has aphasia, clinicians would also work on life-participation goals for family and others who are affected by the aphasia, including friends, service providers, work colleagues, etc.
Clinician roles are expanded beyond those of teacher or therapist	In addition to doing therapy, clinicians might take on the role of: • "communication partner," and give the person with aphasia the opportunity to engage in conversation about life goals, concerns about the future, barriers to life participation, etc. • "coach," "problem solver," or "support person" in relation to overcoming challenges in reengaging in a particular life activity
Outcome evaluation involves routinely documenting quality of life and life participation changes	In addition to documenting changes in language and communication, clinicians would routinely evaluate the following in partnership with clients: • life activities and how satisfying they are • social connections and how satisfying they are • emotional well-being

might experience greater daily encumbrances than another with severe aphasia who is highly supported.

In this broadening and refocusing of services, LPAA recommends that clinicians and researchers consider the dual function of communication: transmitting and receiving messages and establishing and maintaining social links. Furthermore, life activities do not need to be in the realm of communication to deserve or receive intervention. What is important is to judge whether aphasia affects the execution of activities of choice and one's involvement in them (see Table 10–1 (www.asha.org/public/speech/disorders/LPAA.htm) for a few examples of how LPAA may lead to a broadening and refocusing of services).

THE ORIGINS OF LPAA

Functional and Pragmatic Approaches

LPAA draws on ideas underlying functional and pragmatic approaches to aphasia and shares some common values with

those who take a broad approach to functional communication treatment by focusing on life-participation goals and social relationships. In our view, however, the term "functional" does not do justice to the breadth of this work. In addition, the term is often used narrowly to mean "functional independence in getting a message across." Although LPAA recognizes the value of this type of impairment-level work, it should form part of a bigger picture where the ultimate goal for intervention is reengagement into everyday society.

Human Rights Issues and Consumers' Goals

LPAA is a means of addressing the unmet needs and rights of individuals with aphasia and those in their environment. Indeed, the Americans with Disabilities Act (ADA), signed into law on July 26, 1990, requires that physical and communication access be provided for individuals with aphasia and other disabilities and allows them legal recourse if they are blocked from accessing employment, programs, or services in the public and private sectors.

In 1992, ASHA provided guidelines for a "communication bill of rights" (National Joint Committee for the Communicative Needs of Persons with Severe Disabilities). Its preface states that "all persons, regardless of the extent or severity of their disabilities, have a basic right to affect, through communication, the conditions of their own existence." Communication is defined as "a basic need and basic right of all human beings" (p. 2). ASHA thus views communication as an integral part of life participation.

Emphasis on Competence and Inclusion

LPAA philosophy embraces a view of treatment that emphasizes competence and inclusion in daily life, focusing as much on the consequences of chronic disorders as on the language difficulty caused by the aphasia. Along with other movements in education and health care, LPAA shifts from a focus on deficits and remediation to one of inclusion and life participation (see Fougeyrollas et al., 1997; WHO, 1997). Such international changes in focus point to the need to address the personal experience of disability and promote optimal life-inclusion and reintegration into society.

Changes in Reimbursement and Service Delivery

Health care and its reimbursement system have undergone an unprecedented overhaul in America. Financial exigencies have led to an emphasis on medically essential treatments and others seen as likely to save on future health care costs. Many of the incentives in this model result in the provision of efficient short-term minimal care, rather than the longer term, fuller care supported in the past.

LPAA represents a fundamental shift in how we view service delivery for people confronting aphasia. Since LPAA focuses on broader life-related processes and outcomes starting from the onset of treatment, service delivery and its reimbursement will require novel means that stand outside most current practices. We are confident that cost-sensitive and therapeutically effective models are possible. Our purpose in this introductory article is to prompt a discussion with providers and consumers as to whether life participation principles and values should play a more central role in the delivery and reimbursement of future service delivery for all those affected by aphasia.

THE CORE VALUES OF LPAA

LPAA is structured around five core values that serve as guides to assessment, intervention, and research.

The Explicit Goal Is Enhancement of Life Participation

In the LPAA approach, the first focus of the client, clinician, and policy-maker is to assess the extent to which persons affected by aphasia are able to achieve life participation goals, and the extent to which the aphasia hinders the attainment of these desired outcomes. The second focus is to improve short- and long-term participation in life.

All Those Affected by Aphasia Are Entitled to Service

LPAA supports all those affected directly by aphasia, including immediate family and close associates of the adult with aphasia. The LPAA approach holds that it is essential to build protected communities within society where persons with aphasia are able not only to participate but are valued as participants. Therefore, intervention may involve changing broader social systems to make them more accessible to those affected by aphasia.

The Measures of Success Include Documented Life-Enhancement Changes

The LPAA approach calls for the use of outcome measures that assess quality of life and the degree to which those affected by aphasia meet their life participation goals. Without a cause to communicate, we believe, there is no practical need for communication. Therefore, treatment focuses on a reason to communicate as much as on communication repair. In so doing, treatment attends to each consumer's feelings, relationships, and activities in life.

Both Personal and Environmental Factors Are Targets of Intervention

Disruption of daily life for individuals affected by aphasia (including those who do not have aphasia themselves) is evident on two levels: personal (internal) and environmental (external). Intervention consists of constantly assessing, weighing, and prioritizing which personal and environmental factors should be targets of intervention and how best to provide freer, easier, and more autonomous access to activities and social connections of choice. This does not mean that treatment comprises only life resumption processes, but rather that enhanced participation in life "governs" management from its inception. In this fundamental way, the LPAA approach differs from one in which life enhancement is targeted only after language repair has been addressed.

Emphasis Is on the Availability of Services as Needed at All Stages of Aphasia

LPAA begins with the onset of aphasia and continues until consumers and providers agree that targeted life enhancement changes have occurred. However, LPAA acknowledges that life consequences of aphasia change over time and should be addressed regardless of the length of time post-onset.

Consumers are therefore permitted to discontinue intervention, and reenter treatment when they believe they need to continue work on a goal or to attain a new life goal.

CONCLUSIONS

Our health-care systems are undergoing change and, as a result, so are our professions. How we allow this change to affect our clinical practice, our research directions, and our response to consumer advocacy is up to us. We need to educate policy-makers that being fiscally responsible means having a consumer-driven model of intervention focusing on interventions that make real-life differences and minimize the consequences of disease and injury.

While it is clear that the implicit motivation underlying all clinical and research efforts in aphasia is related to increased participation in life, the path to achieving that goal is often indirect. Because LPAA makes life goals primary and explicit, it holds promise as an approach in which such goals are attainable. We invite other speech-language pathologists to join us in discussing and developing life participation approaches to aphasia.

References

Short List of References

Please refer to the ASHA Web site (www.asha.org/publications/ashalinks.htm) for a detailed reference list of the important prior work that has influenced and guided creation of LPAA. The following references are cited in this chapter.

Fougeyrollas, P., Cloutier, R., Bergeron, H., Cote, J., Cote, M., & St. Michel, G. (1997). *Revision of the Quebec Classification: Handicap creation process.* Lac St-Charles, Quebec: International Network on the Handicap Creation Process.

National Joint Committee for the Communicative Needs of Persons with Severe Disabilities. (1992). Guidelines for meeting the communication needs of persons with severe disabilities. *ASHA, 34* (March, Suppl. 7), 1–8.

World Health Organization. (1997). *International classification of impairments, activities and participation: A manual of dimensions of disablement and functions. Beta-1 draft for field trials.* Geneva, Switzerland: WHO.

Detailed List of References

Alexander, M. (1988). Clinical determination of mental competence: A theory and retrospective study. *Archives of Neurology, 45,* 23–26.

Angeleri, F., Angeleri, V., Foschi, N., Giaquinto, S., & Nolfe, G. (1993). The influence of depression, social activity, and family

This chapter was previously published as an article in *The ASHA Leader* (February 15, 2000, pp. 4–6). Reprinted with permission from the American Speech-Language-Hearing Association.

stress on functional outcome after stroke. *Stroke, 24,* 1478–1483.

Armsden, G., & Lewis, F. (1993). The child's adaptation to parental medical illness: Theory and clinical implications. *Patient Education and Counseling, 22,* 153–165.

Amstrong, E. (1993). Aphasia rehabilitation: A sociolinguistic perspective. In A. Holland & M. Forbes (Eds.), *Aphasia treatment: World perspectives* (pp. 263–290). San Diego: Singular.

Astrom, M., Asplund, K., & Astrom, T. (1992). Psychosocial function and life satisfaction after stroke. *Stroke, 23,* 527–531.

Aten, J. (1986). Functional communication treatment. In R. Chapey (Ed.), *Language intervention strategies in adult aphasia* (pp. 292–303). Philadelphia: Williams & Wilkins.

Aten, J., Cagliuri, M., & Holland, A. (1982). The efficacy of functional communication therapy for chronic aphasic patients. *Journal of Speech and Hearing Disorders, 47,* 93–96.

Banigan, R. (1998). *A family-centered approach to developing communication.* Boston: Butterworth-Heinemann.

Bastiaanse R., & Edwards, S. (1998). Diversity in aphasiology: A crisis in practice or a problem of definition? *Aphasiology, 12,* 447–452.

Becker, G. (1997). *Disrupted lives: How people create meaning in a chaotic world.* Los Angeles: University of California Press.

Becker, G. (1980). Continuity after a stroke: Implications for life-course disruption in old age. *The Gerontologist, 33,* 148–158.

Becker, G., & Nachtigall, R. (1995). Managing an uncertain illness trajectory in old age: Patients' and physicians' views of stroke. *Medical Anthropology Quarterly, 9,* 165–187.

Bernstein-Ellis, E., & Elman, R. (1999). Aphasia group communication treatment: The Aphasia Center of California approach. In R. Elman (Ed.), *Group treatment of neurogenic communication disorders* (pp. 47–56). Woburn, MA: Butterworth-Heinemann.

Bethoux, R., Calmels, P., Gautheron, V., & Minaire, P. (1996). Quality of life of the spouses of stroke patients: A preliminary study. *International Journal of Rehabilitation Research, 19,* 291–299.

Beukelman, D., & Mirenda, P. (1992). *Augmentative and alternative communication: Management of severe communication disorders of children and adults.* Baltimore, MD: Paul H. Brookes.

Biegel, D., Sales, E., Schulz, R., & Rau, M. (1991). *Family caregiving in chronic illness* (pp. 129–146). London: Sage.

Bindman, B., Cohen-Schneider, R., Kagan, A., & Podolsky, L. (1995). Bridging the gap for aphasic individuals and their families: Providing access to service. *Topics in Stroke Rehabilitation, 2,* 46–52.

Blackford, K. (1988). The children of chronically ill parents. *Journal of Psychosocial Nursing and Mental Health Services, 26,* 33–36.

Black-Schaffer, R., & Osberg, J. (1990). Return to work after stroke: Development of a predictive model. *Archives of Physical Medicine and Rehabilitation, 71,* 285–290.

Blomert, L. (1990). What functional assessment can contribute to setting goals for aphasia therapy. *Aphasiology, 4,* 307–320.

Bogdan, R., & Biklen, D. (1993). Handicapism. In M. Nagler (Ed.), *Perspectives on disability* (pp. 69–76). Palo Alto, CA: Health Markets Research.

Boland, J., & Follingstad, R. (1987). The relationship between communication and marital satisfaction: A review. *Journal of Sex and Marital Therapy, 13,* 286–313.

Boles L. (1997). Conversation analysis as a dependent measure in communication therapy with four individuals with aphasia. *Asia Pacific Journal of Speech, Language, and Hearing, 2,* 43–61.

Bouchard-Lamothe, D., Bourassa, S., Laflamme, B., Garcia, L., Gailey, G., & Stiell, K. (1999). Perceptions of three groups of interlocutors of the effects of aphasia on communication: An exploratory study. *Aphasiology, 13*, 839–855.

Bourgeois, M. (1997). Families caring for elders at home: Caregiver training. In B. Shadden & M. A. Toner (Eds.), *Aging and communication* (pp. 227–249). Austin, TX: Pro-Ed.

Bradburn, N. M. (1969). *The structure of well-being.* Chicago: Aldine.

Brookshire, R. (1994). Group studies of treatment for adults with aphasia: Efficacy, effectiveness, and believability. *ASHA Special Interest Division 2 Newsletter, 4*, 5–13.

Brumfitt, S. (1993). Losing your sense of self: What aphasia can do. *Aphasiology, 7*(6), 569–591.

Brumfitt, S., & Clark P. (1983). An application of psychotherapeutic techniques to the management of aphasia. In C. Code & D. Müller (Eds.), *Aphasia therapy.* London: Whurr.

Byng, S. (1995). What is aphasia therapy? In C. Code & D. Müller (Eds.), *The treatment of aphasia: From theory to practice* (pp. 3–17). London: Whurr.

Byng, S., & Black, M. (1995). What makes a therapy? Some parameters of therapeutic intervention in aphasia. *European Journal of Disorders of Communication, 30*, 303–316.

Byng, S., Kay, J., Edmundson, A., & Scott, C. (1990). Aphasia tests reconsidered. *Aphasiology, 4*, 67–91.

Byng, S., Pound, C., & Parr, S. (in press). Living with aphasia: A framework for therapy interventions. In I. Papathanasiou (Ed.), *Acquired neurological communication disorders: A clinical perspective.* London: Whurr.

Caplan, D. (1993). Toward a psycholinguistic approach to acquired neurogenic language disorders. *American Journal of Speech-Language Pathology, 2*(1), 59–83.

Carriero, M. R., Faglia, Z., & Vignolo, L. A. (1987). Resumption of gainful employment in aphasics: Preliminary findings. *Cortex, 26*, 667–672.

Chapey, R. (1992). Functional communication assessment and intervention: Some thoughts on the state of the art. *Aphasiology, 6*, 85–93.

Christensen, J. M., & Anderson, J. D. (1989). Spouse adjustment to stroke: Aphasic versus nonaphasic partners. *Journal of Communication Disorders, 22*, 225–231.

Clark, L. (1997). Communication intervention for family caregivers and professional health care providers. In B. Shadden & M. Toner (Eds.), *Aging and communication* (pp. 251–274). Austin, TX: Pro-Ed.

Clinical Forum. (1998). Beyond the "plateau": Discharge dilemmas in chronic aphasia. *Aphasiology, 12*, 207–243.

Cochrane, R., & Milton, S. (1984). Conversational prompting: A sentence building technique for severe aphasia. *The Journal of Neurological Communication Disorders, 1*, 4–23.

Code, C., & Müller, D. (1992). *The Code-Müller protocols: Assessing perceptions of psychosocial adjustment to aphasia and related disorders.* London: Whurr.

Coles, R., & Eales, C. (1999). The aphasia self-help movement in Britain: A challenge and an opportunity. In R. Elman (Ed.), *Group treatment for neurogenic communication disorders: The expert clinician's approach* (pp. 107–114). Woburn, MA: Butterworth-Heinemann.

Csikszentmihalyi, M. (1990). *Flow: The psychology of optimal experience.* New York: HarperCollins.

Csikszentmihalyi, M. (1993). *The evolving self.* New York: HarperCollins.

Csikszentmihalyi, M. (1997). *Finding flow: The psychology of engagement with everyday life.* New York: HarperCollins.

Damico, J. S., Simmons-Mackie, N., & Schweitzer, L. A. (1995). Addressing the third law of gardening: Methodological alternatives in aphasiology. In M. L. Lemme (Ed.), *Clinical aphasiology* (Vol. 23, pp. 83–93). Austin, TX: Pro-Ed.

Darley, F. (1991). I think it begins with an A. In T. Prescott (Ed.), *Clinical aphasiology* (Vol. 20, pp. 9–20). Austin, TX: Pro-Ed.

Davis, A. (1986). Pragmatics and treatment. In R. Chapey (Ed.), *Language intervention strategies in adult aphasia* (pp. 251–265). Baltimore: Williams & Wilkins.

Davis, A., & Wilcox, J. (1985). *Adults' aphasia rehabilitation: Applied pragmatics.* San Diego: College Hill Press.

Davis, G., & Wilcox, J. (1981). Incorporating parameters of natural conversation in aphasia treatment. In R. Chapey (Ed.), *Language intervention strategies in adult aphasia.* Baltimore: Williams & Wilkins.

de Hann, R., Aaronson, N., Limburg, M., Langton Hewer, R., & van Crevel, H. (1993). Measuring quality of life in stroke. *Stroke, 24*, 320–327.

de Hann, R., Horn, J., Limburg, M., van der Meulen, J., & Bossuyt, P. (1993). A comparison of five stroke scales with measures of disability, handicap, and quality of life. *Stroke, 24*, 1179–1181.

Dickson, H. G. (1996). Problems with the ICIDH definition of impairment: Clinical commentary. *Disability and Rehabilitation, 18*, 52–54.

Disability Alliance (1995). *Disability rights handbook.* London: Disability Alliance Educational and Research Associations.

Doolittle, N. (1992). The experience of recovery following lacunar stroke. *Rehabilitation Nursing, 17*, 122–125.

Doolittle, N. (1994). A clinical ethnography of stroke recovery. In P. Benner (Ed.), *Interpretive phenomenology: Embodiment, caring and ethics in health and illness.* Thousand Oaks, CA: Sage.

Duchan, J. (1995). *Supporting language learning in everyday life.* San Diego: Singular.

Duchan, J. (1997). A situated pragmatics approach for supporting children with severe communication disorders. *Topics in Language Disorders, 17*, 1–18.

Duchan, J., Maxwell, M., & Kovarsky, D. (1999). Evaluating competence in the course of everyday interaction. In D. Kovarsky, J. Duchan, & M. Maxwell (Eds.), *Constructing (in)competence* (pp. 3–26). Mahwah, NJ: Lawrence Erlbaum.

Eldridge, M. (1968). *A history of the treatment of speech disorders.* Edinburgh: Livingstone.

Elman, R. (1995). Multimethod research: A search for understanding. *Clinical Aphasiology, 23*, 77–81.

Elman, R. (1998a). Diversity in aphasiology: Let us embrace it. *Aphasiology, 12*(6), 456–457.

Elman, R. (1998b). Memories of the 'plateau': Health-care changes provide an opportunity to redefine aphasia treatment and discharge. *Aphasiology, 12*, 227–231.

Elman, R. (Ed.). (1999). *Group treatment of neurogenic communication disorders.* Woburn, MA: Butterworth-Heinemann.

Elman, R., & Bernstein-Ellis, E. (1995). What is functional? *American Journal of Speech-Language Pathology, 4*, 115–117.

Elman, R., & Bernstein-Ellis, E. (1999a). The efficacy of group communication treatment in adults with chronic aphasia. *Journal of Speech, Language, and Hearing Research, 42*, 411–419.

Elman, R., & Bernstein-Ellis, E. (1999b). Psychosocial aspects of group communication treatment: Preliminary findings. *Seminars in Speech & Language, 20*(1), 65–72.

Enderby, P. (1997). *Therapy outcome measures: Speech-language pathology technical manual.* San Diego: Singular.

Evans, R. L., Dingus, C. M., & Haselkorn, J. K. (1993). Living with a disability: A synthesis and critique of the literature on quality of life, 1985–1989. *Psychological Reports, 72*, 771–777.

Ewing, S. (1999). Group process, group dynamics, and group techniques with neurogenic communication disorders. In R. Elman (Ed.), *Group treatment for neurogenic communication disorders: The expert clinician's approach* (pp. 9–16). Woburn, MA: Butterworth-Heinemann.

Ezrachi, O., Ben-Yishay, Y., Kay, T., Diller, L., & Rattock, J. (1991). Predicting employment in traumatic brain injury following neuropsychological rehabilitation. *Journal of Head Trauma Rehabilitation, 6*(3), 71–84.

Ferguson, A. (1994). The influence of aphasia, familiarity, and activity on conversational repair. *Aphasiology, 8*, 143–157.

Ferguson, A. (1996). Describing competence in aphasic/normal conversation. *Clinical Linguistics and Phonetics, 10*, 55–63.

Ferguson, D. (1994). Is communication really the point? Some thoughts on interventions and membership. *Mental Retardation, 32*, 7–18.

Finkelstein V. (1991). Disability: An administrative challenge. In M. Oliver (Ed.), *Social work, disabled people and disabling environments* (pp. 19–39). London: Jessica Kinglsey.

Flickinger, E. E., & Amato, S. C. (1994). School-age children's responses to parents with disabilities. *Rehabilitation Nursing, 19*, 403–406.

Florence, C. (1981). Methods of communication analysis used in family interaction therapy. In R. Brookshire (Ed.), *Clinical aphasiology: Conference proceedings* (pp. 204–211). Minneapolis, MN: BRK.

Flowers, C., & Peizer, E. (1984). Strategies for obtaining information from aphasic persons. In R. Brookshire (Ed.), *Clinical aphasiology: Conference proceedings* (pp. 106–113). Minneapolis, MN: BRK.

Fougeyrollas, P., Cloutier, R., Bergeron, H., Cote, J., Cote, M., & St. Michel, G. (1997). *Revision of the Quebec Classification: Handicap creation process.* Lac St-Charles, Quebec: International Network on the Handicap Creation Process.

Fox, L., & Fried-Oken, M. (1996). AAC Aphasiology: Partnership for future research. *Augmentative and Alternative Communication, 12*, 257–271.

Fraser, R., & Baarslag-Benson, R. (1994). Cross-disciplinary collaboration in the removal of work barriers after traumatic brain injury. *Topics in Language Disorders, 15*(1), 55–67.

Frattali, C. (1992). Functional assessment of communication: Merging public policy with clinical views. *Aphasiology, 6*, 63–85.

Frattali, C. (1993). Perspective on functional assessment: Its use for policy making. *Disability and Rehabilitation, 15*, 1–9.

Frattali, C. (1996). Measuring disability. *ASHA Special Interest Division 2 Newsletter-Neurophysiology and Neurogenic Speech and Language Disorders, 6*, 6–10.

Frattali, C. (1997). Clinical care in a changing health system. In N. Helm-Estabrooks & A. Holland (Eds.), *Approaches to the Treatment of Aphasia* (pp. 241–265). San Diego: Singular.

Frattali, C. (1998). Measuring modality-specific behaviors, functional abilities, and quality of life. In C. Frattali (Ed.), *Measuring outcomes in speech-language pathology* (pp. 55–88). New York: Thieme.

Frattali, C., & Sutherland, C. (1994). Improving quality in the context of managed care. *Managing Managed Care.* Rockville, MD: ASHA.

Frattali, C., Thomson, C., Holland, A., Wohl, C., & Ferketic, M. (1995). *The American Speech-Language-Hearing Association functional assessment of communication skills for adults (ASHA FACS).* Rockville, MD: ASHA.

French, S. (1993). What's so great about independence? In J. Swain, F. Finkelstein, S. French, & M. Oliver (Eds.), *Disabling barriers-enabling environments* (pp. 44–48). London: Sage.

French, S. (1994a). Dimensions of disability and impairment. In S. French (Ed.), *On equal terms: Working with disabled people* (pp. 17–34). Oxford: Butterworth Heinemann.

French, S. (1994b). The disabled role. In S. French (Ed.), *On equal terms: Working with disabled people* (pp. 47–60). Oxford: Butterworth Heinemann.

French, S. (1994c). Researching disability. In S. French (Ed.), *On equal terms: Working with disabled people* (pp. 136–147). Oxford: Butterworth Heinemann.

Fuhrer, M. J. (1994). Subjective well-being: Implications for medical rehabilitation outcomes and models of disablement. *American Journal of Physical Medicine and Rehabilitation, 73*, 358–364.

Gainotti, G. (Ed.). (1997). Emotional, psychological and psychosocial problems of aphasic patients [Special Issue]. *Aphasiology, 11*(7).

Garcia, L. J., Barrette, J., & Laroche, C. (in press). Perceptions of the obstacles to work reintegration for persons with aphasia. *Aphasiology.*

Garnes, H., & Olson, D. (1995). Parent-adolescent communication and the circumplex model. *Child Development, 56*, 438–447.

Garrett, K. (1996). Augmentative and alternative communication: Applications to the treatment of aphasia. In G. Wallace (Ed.), *Adult aphasia rehabilitation* (pp. 259–278). Boston: Butterworth-Heinemann.

Garrett, K. (1999). Measuring outcomes of group therapy. In R. Elman (Ed.), *Group treatment for neurogenic communication disorders: The expert clinician's approach* (pp. 17–30). Woburn, MA: Butterworth-Heinemann.

Garrett, K., & Beukelman, D. (1992). Augmentative communication approaches for persons with severe aphasia. In K. Yorkston (Ed.), *Augmentative communication in the medical setting* (pp. 245–338). Tucson, AZ: Communication Skill Builders.

Garrett, K., & Beukelman D. (1995). Changes in the interactive patterns of an individual with severe aphasia given three types of partner support. In M. Lemme (Ed.), *Clinical Aphasiology* (Vol. 23, pp. 237–251). Austin, TX: Pro-Ed.

Garrett, K., & Ellis, G. (1999). Group communication therapy for people with long-term aphasia: Scaffolded thematic discourse activities. In R. Elman (Ed.), *Group treatment for neurogenic communication disorders: The expert clinician's approach* (pp. 85–96). Woburn, MA: Butterworth-Heinemann.

Gerber, S., & Gurland, G. (1989). Applied pragmatics in the assessment of aphasia. *Seminars in Speech and Language, 10*, 263–281.

Goodwin, C. (1995). Co-constructing meaning in conversations with an aphasic man. In E. Jacoby & E. Ochs (Eds.), *Research on language and social interaction, 28*, 233–260.

Gordon, J. (1997). Measuring outcomes in aphasia: Bridging the gap between theory and practice . . . or burning our bridges. *Aphasiology, 11*, 845–854.

Graham, M. (1999). Aphasia group therapy in a subacute setting: Using the American Speech-Language-Hearing Association Functional Assessment of Communication Skills. In R. Elman (Ed.), *Group treatment for neurogenic communication disorders: The expert clinician's approach* (pp. 37–46). Woburn, MA: Butterworth-Heinemann.

Granger, C., Hamilton, B., Keith, R., Zielezny, M., & Sherwin, F. (1986). Advances in functional assessment for medical rehabilitation. *Topics in Geriatric Rehabilitation, 1*, 569–574.

Hales, G. (1996). *Beyond disability—Towards an enabling society.* London: Sage.

Hemsley, G., & Code, C. (1996). Interactions between recovery in aphasia, emotional and psychosocial factors in subjects with aphasia, their significant others and speech pathologists. *Disability and Rehabilitation, 18*, 567–584.

Hermann, M., & Code, C. (1996). Weightings of items on the Code-Müller protocols: The effects of clinical experience of aphasia therapy. *Disability and Rehabilitation, 18*, 509–514.

Hermann, M., & Wallesch, C. (1989). Psychosocial changes and psychosocial adjustments with chronic and severe nonfluent aphasia. *Aphasiology, 3*, 513–526.

Hermann, M., & Wallesch, C. (1990). Expectations of psychosocial adjustment in aphasia: A MAUT study with the Code-Müller scale of psychosocial adjustment. *Aphasiology, 4*, 527–538.

Hersh, D. (1998). Beyond the 'plateau': Discharge dilemmas in chronic aphasia. *Aphasiology, 12*, 207–218.

Hinckley, J. (1998). Investigating the predictors of lifestyle satisfaction among younger adults with chronic aphasia. *Aphasiology, 12*, 509–518.

Hinckley, J., Packard, M., & Bardach, L. (1995). Alternative family education programming for adults with chronic aphasia. *Topics in Stroke Rehabilitation, 2*, 53–63.

Hoen, R., Thelander, M., & Worsley, J. (1997). Improvement in psychological well-being of people with aphasia and their families: Evaluation of a community-based programme. *Aphasiology, 11*(7), 681–691.

Holland, A. (1977). Some practical considerations in the treatment of aphasic patients. In M. Sullivan & M. Kommers (Eds.), *Rationale for adult aphasia therapy* (pp. 167–180). Omaha, NE: University of Nebraska Press.

Holland, A. (1980). *Communicative abilities in daily living—CADL.* Austin TX: Pro-Ed.

Holland, A. (1982). Observing functional communication of aphasic adults. *Journal of Speech and Hearing Disorders, 47*, 50–56.

Holland, A. (1991). Pragmatic aspects of intervention in aphasia. *Journal of Neurolinguistics, 6*, 197–211.

Holland, A. (1992). Some thoughts of future needs and directions for research and treatment of aphasia. *NIDCD Monograph* (Vol. 2, pp. 147–152).

Holland, A. (1996). Pragmatic assessment and treatment for aphasia. In G. Wallace (Ed.), *Adult aphasia rehabilitation* (pp. 161–173). Boston: Butterworth-Heinemann.

Holland, A. (1998a). Some guidelines for bridging the research-practice gap in adult neurogenic communication disorders. *Topics in Language Disorders, 18*, 49–57.

Holland, A. (1998b). Why can't clinicians talk to aphasic adults? Clinical forum. *Aphasiology, 12*, 844–846.

Holland, A., & Beeson, P. (1999). Aphasia groups: The Arizona experience. In R. Elman (Ed.), *Group treatment for neurogenic communication disorders: The expert clinician's approach* (pp. 77–84). Woburn, MA: Butterworth-Heinemann.

Holland, A., Frattali, C., & Fromm, D. (1998). *Communicative abilities in daily living—CADL 2.* Austin TX: Pro-Ed.

Holland, A., Fromm, D., DeRuyter, F., & Stein, M. (1996). Treatment efficacy: Aphasia. *Journal of Speech and Hearing Research, 39*, 527–536.

Holland, A., & Ross, R. (1999). The power of aphasia groups. In R. Elman (Ed.), *Group treatment of neurogenic communication disorders* (pp. 115–117). Boston, MA: Butterworth-Heinemann.

Holland, A., & Thompson, C. (1998). Outcomes measurement in aphasia. In C. Frattali (Ed.), *Measuring outcomes in speech-language pathology* (pp. 245–266). New York: Thieme.

Howard, D., & Hatfield, F. (1987). *Aphasia therapy: Historical and contemporary issues.* Hillsdale, NJ: Lawrence Erlbaum.

Hughes, B., & Paterson, K. (1997). The social model of disability and the disappearing body: Toward a sociology of impairment. *Disability and Society, 12*, 325–340.

Hux, K., Beukelman, D., & Garrett, K. (1994). Augmentative and alternative communication for persons with aphasia. In R. Chapey (Ed.), *Language intervention strategies in adult aphasia* (3rd ed.) (pp. 338–357). Baltimore: Williams & Wilkins.

Ireland, C., & Wootton, G. (1993). *Time to talk: ADA counseling project, Department of health report.* London: Action for Dysphasic Adults.

Iskowitz, M. (1998). Preparing for managed care in long-term care. *Advance for Speech-Language Pathologists and Audiologists*, January 12th, 7–9.

Jennings, B., Callahan, D., & Caplan, A. (1988). *Ethical challenges of chronic illness.* Briarcliff Manor, NY: A Hastings Center Report.

Johnson, E. (1993). Open your doors to disabled workers. In M. Nagler (Ed.), *Perspectives on disability* (pp. 475–479). Palo Alto, CA: Health Markets Research.

Johnson, R. (1987) Return to work after severe head injury. *International Disability Studies, 9*, 49–54.

Jordan, L. (1998). 'Diversity in aphasiology': A social science perspective, *Aphasiology, 12*, 474–480.

Jordan, L., & Kaiser, W. (1996). *Aphasia—A social approach.* London: Chapman & Hall.

Kagan, A. (1995a). Family perspectives from three aphasia centers in Ontario, Canada. *Topics in Stroke Rehabilitation, 2*, 1–19.

Kagan, A. (1995b). Revealing the competence of aphasic adults through conversation: A challenge to health professionals. *Topics in Stroke Rehabilitation, 2*, 15–28.

Kagan, A. (1998). Supported conversation for adults with aphasia: Methods and resources for training conversation partners. *Aphasiology, 12*, 851–864.

Kagan, A., & Cohen-Schneider, R. (1999). Groups in the 'introductory program' at the Pat Arato Aphasia Centre. In R. Elman (Ed.), *Group treatment of neurogenic communication disorders* (pp. 97–106). Woburn, MA: Butterworth-Heinemann.

Kagan, A., & Gailey, G. (1993). Functional is not enough: Training conversation partners for aphasic adults. In A. Holland & M. Forbes (Eds.), *Aphasia treatment: World perspectives* (pp. 199–215). San Diego: Singular.

Kagan, A., & Kimelman, D. (1995). 'Informed' consent in aphasia research: Myth or reality? *Clinical Aphasiology, 23,* 65–75.

Kagan, A., Winckel, J., & Shumway E. (1996a). *Pictographic communication resources.* North York, Canada: Pat Arato Aphasia Centre.

Kagan, A., Winckel, J., & Shumway E. (1996b). *Supported conversation for aphasic adults: Increasing communicative access* (Video). North York, Ontario, Canada: Pat Arato Aphasia Centre.

Kaufman, S. (1988a). Illness, biography, and the interpretation of self, following a stroke. *Journal of Aging Studies, 2,* 217–227.

Kaufman, S. (1988b). Toward a phenomenology of boundaries in medicine: Chronic illness experience in the case of stroke. *Medical Anthropology Quarterly, 2,* 338–354.

Keatley, M. A., Miller, T. I., & Mann, A. (1995). Treatment planning using outcome data. *ASHA, 37*(2), 49–52.

King, R. B. (1996). Quality of life after stroke. *Stroke, 27,* 1467–1472.

Kovarsky, D., Duchan, J., & Maxwell, M. (Eds.). (1999). *Constructing (in)competence: Disabling evaluations in clinical and social interaction.* Hillsdale, NJ: Lawrence Erlbaum.

Kraat, A. (1990). Augmentative and alternative communication: Does it have a future in aphasia rehabilitation? *Aphasiology, 4,* 321–338.

Krefting, L. (1991). Rigor in qualitative research: The assessment of trustworthiness. *The American Journal of Occupational Therapy, 45*(3), 214–222.

Kwa, V., Limburg, M., & de Hann, R. J. (1996). The role of cognitive impairment in the quality of life after ischemic stroke. *Journal of Neurology, 243,* 599–604.

LaCoste, L. D., Ginter, E. J., & Whipple, G. (1987). Intrafamily communication and familial environment. *Psychological Reports, 61,* 115–118.

Lafond, D., Joanette, Y., Ponzio, J., Degiovani, R., & Sarno, M. (Eds.). (1993). *Living with aphasia: Psychosocial issues.* San Diego: Singular.

LaPointe, L. (1989). An ecological perspective on assessment and treatment of aphasia. *Clinical Aphasiology, 18,* 1–4.

LaPointe, L. (1996). On being a patient. *Journal of Medical Speech-Language Pathology, 4* (1).

LaPointe, L. (1997). Adaptation, accommodation, aristos. In L. LaPointe (Ed.), *Aphasia and related neurogenic disorders.* (2nd ed.) (pp. 265–287). New York: Thieme.

LeDorze, G., & Brassard, C. (1995). A description of the consequences of aphasia on aphasic persons and their relatives and friends, based on the WHO model of chronic diseases. *Aphasiology, 9,* 239–255.

LeDorze, G., Croteau, C., & Joanette Y. (1993). Perspectives on aphasia intervention in French-speaking Canada. In A. Holland & M. Forbes (Eds.), *Aphasia treatment, world perspectives* (pp. 87–114). San Diego: Singular.

Light, J. (1988). Interaction involving individuals using augmentative and alternative communication systems: State of the art and future directions. *Augmentative and Alternative Communication, 4,* 66–82.

Livneh, H. (1991). On the origins of negative attitudes toward people with disabilities. In R. Marinelli & A. Dell Orto (Eds.), *The psychological and social impact of disability* (pp. 181–196). New York: Springer.

Lomas, J., Pickard, L., Bester, S., Elbard, H., Finlayson, A., & Zoghaib, C. (1989). The communication effectiveness index: Development and psychometric evaluation of a functional communication measure for adult aphasia. *Journal of Speech and Hearing Disorders, 54,* 113–124.

Lomas, J., Pickard, L., & Mohide, A. (1987). Patient versus clinician item generation for quality-of-life measures: The case of language-disabled adults. *Medical Care, 25,* 764–769.

Lord, M. (1993). Away with barriers. In M. Nagler (Ed.), *Perspectives on disability* (pp. 471–474). Palo Alto, CA: Health Markets Research.

Lubinski, R. (1981). Environmental language intervention. In R. Chapey (Ed.), *Language intervention strategies in adult aphasia* (pp. 223–248). Baltimore: Williams & Wilkins.

Lubinski, R. (1986). Environmental systems approach to adult aphasia. In R. Chapey (Ed.), *Language intervention strategies in adult aphasia* (pp. 267–291). Philadelphia, PA: Williams & Wilkins.

Lubinski, R., Duchan, J., & Weitzner-Lin, B. (1980). Analysis of breakdowns and repairs in aphasic adult communication. In R. Brookshire (Ed.), *Clinical aphasiology conference proceedings.* Minneapolis, MN: BRK.

Lund, N., & Duchan, J. (1993). *Assessing children's language in naturalistic contexts* (3rd ed.). Englewood Cliffs, NJ: Prentice Hall.

Luterman, D. (1996). *Counseling persons with communication disorders and their families* (3rd ed.). Austin, TX: Pro-Ed.

Lyon, J. (1992). Communication use and participation in life for adults with aphasia in natural settings: The scope of the problem. *American Journal of Speech-Language Pathology, 1,* 7–14.

Lyon, J. (1995a). Drawing: Its value as a communication aid for adults with aphasia. *Aphasiology, 9*(1), 33–50.

Lyon, J. (1995b). Communicative drawing: An augmentative mode of interaction. *Aphasiology, 9*(1), 84–94.

Lyon, J. (1996a). Measurement of treatment effects in natural settings. *ASHA Special Interest Division 2 Newsletter-Neurophysiology and Neurogenic Speech and Language Disorders, 6,* 10–15.

Lyon, J. (1996b). Optimizing communication and participation in life for aphasic adults and their prime caregivers in natural settings: A use model for treatment. In G. Wallace (Ed.), *Adult aphasia rehabilitation* (pp. 137–160). Newton, MA: Butterworth Heinemann.

Lyon, J. (1997a). Treating real-life functionality in a couple coping with severe aphasia. In N. Helm-Estabrooks & A. Holland (Eds.), *Approaches to the treatment of aphasia* (pp. 203–239). San Diego: Singular.

Lyon, J. (1997b). Volunteers and partners: Moving intervention outside the treatment room. In B. Shadden & M. Toner (Eds.), *Communication and aging* (pp. 299–324). Austin, TX: Pro-Ed.

Lyon, J. (1998). *Coping with aphasia.* San Diego: Singular.

Lyon, J. (in press). Finding, defining, and refining functionality in real-life for people confronting aphasia. In L. Worrall & C. Frattali (Eds.), *Neurogenic communication disorders: A functional approach.* New York: Thieme.

Lyon, J. Cariski, D., Keisler, L., Rosenbek, J., Levine, R., Kumpula, J., et al. (1997). Communication partners: Enhancing participation in life and communication for adults with aphasia in natural settings. *Aphasiology, 11,* 693–708.

Lyon, J. G., & Sims, E. (1989). Drawing: Its use as a communicative aid with aphasic and normal adults. *Clinical Aphasiology, 18,* 339–356.

Markus, H., & Nurius, P. (1986). Possible selves. *American Psychologist, 41*(9), 954–969.

Marshall, R. (1993). Problem focused group therapy for mildly aphasic clients. *American Journal of Speech-Language Pathology, 2,* 31–37.

Marshall, R. (1999a). An introduction to supported conversation for adults with aphasia: Perspectives, problems and possibilities. *Aphasiology, 12,* 811–816.

Marshall, R. (1999b). *Introduction to group treatment for aphasia: Design and management.* Woburn, MA: Butterworth-Heinemann.

Marshall, R. (1999c). A problem-focused group treatment program for clients with mild aphasia. In R. Elman (Ed.), *Group treatment for neurogenic communication disorders: The expert clinician's approach* (pp. 57–65). Woburn, MA: Butterworth-Heinemann.

Marshall, R., Freed, D., & Phillips, D. (1997). Communicative efficiency in severe aphasia. *Aphasiology, 11,* 373–384.

McClenahan, R., Johnston, M., & Denham, Y. (1992). Factors influencing accuracy of estimation of comprehension problems in patients following cerebro-vascular accident by doctors, nurses and relatives. *European Journal of Disorders of Communication, 27,* 209–219.

Meeuwesen, L., Schaap, C., & Van der Staak, C. (1991). Verbal analysis of doctor-patient communication. *Social Science in Medicine, 32,* 1143–1150.

Milroy, L., & Perkins, L. (1992). Repair strategies in aphasic discourse: Towards a collaborative model. *Clinical Linguistics and Phonetics, 6,* 17–40.

Müller, D. (1984). Psychological adjustment to aphasia. Brief Research Report. *International Journal of Rehabilitation Research, 7,* 195–196.

Müller, D., & Code, C. (1983). Interpersonal perception of psychosocial adjustment to aphasia. In C. Code & D. J. Müller (Eds.), *Aphasia therapy* (pp. 101–112). London: Edward Arnold.

National Joint Committee for the Communicative Needs of Persons with Severe Disabilities (1992). Guidelines for meeting the communication needs of persons with severe disabilities. *ASHA, 34* (March, Suppl. 7), 1–8.

Nester, M. (1984). Employment testing for handicapped persons. *Public Personnel Management Journal, 13*(4), 417–434.

Nettleton, S. (1996). *The sociology of health and illness.* Cambridge, UK: Polity Press.

Newhoff, M., Tonkovich, J., Schwartz, S., & Burgess, E. (1985). Revision strategies in aphasia. *Journal of Neurological Communication Disorders, 2,* 2–7.

Nicholas, L., & Brookshire, R. (1993). A system for quantifying the informativeness and efficiency of the connected speech of adults with aphasia. *Journal of Speech and Hearing Research, 36,* 338–350.

Niemi, M., Laaksonen, R., Kotila, M., & Waltimo, O. (1988). Quality of life 4 years after stroke. *Stroke, 19,* 1101–1107.

Nisbet, J. (Ed.) (1992). *Natural supports in school, at work and in the community for people with severe disabilities.* Baltimore, MD: Paul H. Brookes.

Oelschlaeger, M., & Damico, J. (1998). Spontaneous verbal repetition: A social strategy in aphasic conversation. *Aphasiology, 12,* 971–988.

Oliver, M. (1996). *Understanding disability: From theory to practice.* London, UK: Macmillan.

Parr, S. (1994). Coping with aphasia: Conversations with 20 aphasic people. *Aphasiology, 8,* 457–466.

Parr, S. (1996a). The road more traveled: Whose right of way? *Aphasiology, 10,* 496–503.

Parr, S. (1996b). Everyday literacy in aphasia: Radical approaches to functional assessment and therapy. *Aphasiology, 10,* 469–479.

Parr, S., & Byng, S. (1998). Breaking new ground in familiar territory. Clinical forum. *Aphasiology, 12,* 839–844.

Parr, S., Byng, S., & Gilpin, S. (1997). *Talking about aphasia: Living with loss of language after stroke.* Buckingham, UK: Open University Press.

Patterson, J., & Garwick, A. (1992). The impact of chronic illness on families: A family systems perspective. *Annals of Behavioral Medicine, 16,* 131–142.

Patterson, R., Paul, M., Wells, A., Hoen, B., & Thelander, M. (1994). *Aphasia: A new life. Handbook for helping communities.* Stoufville, Ontario, Canada: York-Durham Aphasia Centre.

Peach, R. (1993). Clinical intervention for aphasia in the United States of America. In A. Holland & M. Forbes (Eds.), *Aphasia treatment: World perspectives* (pp. 335–369). San Diego: Singular.

Penn C. (1998). Clinician-researcher dilemmas: Comment on 'supported conversation for adults with aphasia.' Clinical forum. *Aphasiology, 12,* 839–844.

Pessar, L., Coad, M., Linn, R., & Willer, B. (1992). The effects of parental traumatic brain injury on the behavior of parents and children. *Brain Injury, 7,* 231–240.

Petheram, B., & Parr, S. (1998). Diversity in aphasiology: A crisis in practice or a problem of definition? *Aphasiology, 12,* 435–446.

Petheram, B., & Parr, S. (1998). Reply: Plenty of room in the wardrobe: A response to Bastianne, Edwards, Cappa, Elman, Ferguson, Gordon, and Jordan. *Aphasiology, 12,* 481–488.

Pound, C. (1996). New approaches to long term aphasia therapy and support. *Bulletin of the Royal College of Speech and Language Therapists, 12–13.*

Pound, C. (1998). Therapy for life: Finding new paths across the plateau. *Aphasiology, 12,* 222–227.

Prutting, C., & Kirchner, D. (1987). A clinical appraisal of the pragmatic aspects of language. *Journal of Speech and Hearing Disorders, 52,* 105–119.

Ramsburger, G. (1994). Functional perspective for assessment and rehabilitation of persons with severe aphasia. *Seminars in Speech and Language, 15,* 1–16.

Rao, P. (1997). Functional communication assessment and outcome. In B. Shadden & M. Toner (Eds.), *Aging and communication* (pp. 197–225). Austin, TX: Pro-Ed.

Rice, B., Paull, A., & Müller, D. (1987). An evaluation of a social support group for spouses of aphasic partners. *Aphasiology, 1,* 247–256.

Robey, R. (1998). A meta-analysis of clinical outcomes in the treatment of aphasia. *Journal of Speech, Language and Hearing Research, 421,* 172–187.

Robillard, A. (1994). Communication problems in the intensive care unit. *Qualitative Sociology, 17,* 383–395.

Rolland, J. S. (1994). In sickness and in health: The impact of illness on couples' relationships. *Journal of Marital and Family Therapy, 20,* 327–347.

Roter, D. L., & Hall, J. L. (1992). *Doctors talking with patients/patients talking with doctors: Improving communication in medical visits.* Westport, UK: Auburn House.

Ryan, E., Bourhis, R., & Knops, U. (1991). Evaluative perceptions of patronizing speech addressed to elders. *Psychology and Aging, 6,* 442–450.

Ryan, E., Meredith, S., MacLean, M., & Orange, J. (1995). Changing the way we talk with elders: Promoting health using the communication enhancement model. *International Journal of Aging and Human Development, 4,* 89–107.

Ryff, C. (1989a). Happiness is everything, or is it? Explorations on the meaning of psychological well-being. *Journal of Personality and Social Psychology, 57*(6), 1069–1081.

Ryff, C. (1989b). In the eye of the beholder: Views of psychological well-being among middle and old-aged adults. *Psychology and Aging, 4,* 195–210.

Ryff, C. (1989c). Scales of psychological well being (short form). *Journal of Personality and Social Psychology, 57,* 1069–1081.

Ryff, C., & Singer, B. (1998). The contours of positive human health. *Psychological Inquiry, 9*(1), 1–29.

Sacchett, C., & Marshall, J. (1992). Functional assessment of communication: Implications for the rehabilitation of aphasic people: Reply to Carol Frattali. *Aphasiology, 6,* 95–100.

Sacks, H., Schegloff, E., & Jefferson, G. (1974). A simplest systematics for the organization of turn-taking for conversation. *Language, 50,* 696–735.

Sandin, K. J., Cifu, D. X., & Noll, S. F. (1994). Stroke rehabilitation: Psychological and social implications. *Archives of Physical Medicine and Rehabilitation, 75,* S-52–S-55.

Sands, E., Sarno, M., & Shankweiler, D. (1969). Long term assessment of language function in aphasia. *Archives of Physical Medicine and Rehabilitation, 50,* 202–206.

Sarno, M. (1965). A measurement of functional communication in aphasia. *Archives of Physical Medicine and Rehabilitation, 46,* 101–107.

Sarno, M. (1969). *The functional communication profile: Manual of directions.* New York: Institute of Rehabilitation Medicine.

Sarno, M. (1993). Aphasia rehabilitation: Psychosocial and ethical considerations. *Aphasiology, 7,* 321–334.

Sarno, M. (1997). Quality of life in aphasia in the first post-stroke year. *Aphasiology, 11*(7), 665–678.

Sarno, M. T. (1991). The psychological and social sequelae of aphasia. In M. T. Sarno (Ed.), *Acquired aphasia* (2nd ed.) (pp. 521–582). San Diego: Academic Press.

Sarno, M. T. (1992). Preliminary findings in a study of age, linguistic evolution and quality of life in recovery from aphasia. *Scandinavian Journal of Rehabilitative Medicine,* Suppl. 26, 43–59.

Sarno, M. T., & Chambers, N. (1997). A horticultural therapy program for individuals with acquired aphasias. *Activities, Adaptation and Aging, 22,* 81–91.

Schuling, J., de Haan, R., Limburg, M., & Groenier, K. H. (1993). The Frenchay activities index. *Stroke, 24,* 1173–1177.

Sherman, S., & Anderson, N. (1982). *Ability testing of handicapped people: Dilemma for government, science and the public.* Washington, DC: National Academy Press.

Shewan, C. (1986). The history and efficacy of aphasia treatment. In R. Chapey (Ed.), *Language intervention strategies in adult aphasia.* (2nd ed.). Philadelphia, PA: Williams & Wilkins.

Shewan, C., & Bandur, D. (1986). Language-oriented treatment: A psycholinguistic approach to aphasia. In R. Chapey (Ed.), *Language intervention strategies in adult aphasia* (3rd ed.) (pp. 184–206). Philadelphia, PA: Williams & Wilkins.

Shontz, F. C. (1991). Six principles relating disability and psychological adjustment. In R. Marinelli & A. Dell Orto (Eds.), *The psychological and social impact of disability* (pp. 107–110). New York: Springer.

Simmons, N. (1986). Beyond standardized measures: Special tests, language in context, and discourse analysis. *Seminars in Speech and Language, 7,* 181–205.

Simmons, N., Kearns, K., & Potechin, G. (1987). Treatment of aphasia through family member training. In R. Brookshire (Ed.), *Clinical aphasiology: Conference proceedings* (Vol. 17, pp. 106–116). Minneapolis, MN: BRK.

Simmons-Mackie, N. (1998a). A solution to the discharge dilemma in aphasia: Social approaches to aphasia management. Clinical forum. *Aphasiology, 12,* 231–239.

Simmons-Mackie, N. (1998b). In support of supported communication for adults with aphasia: Clinical forum. *Aphasiology, 12,* 831–838.

Simmons-Mackie, N. (in press). Social approaches to the management of aphasia. In Worrall, L., & Frattali, C. (Eds.), *Neurogenic communication disorders: A functional approach.* New York: Thieme.

Simmons-Mackie, N., & Damico J. (1995). Communicative competence in aphasia: Evidence from compensatory strategies. *Clinical Aphasiology, 23,* 95–105.

Simmons-Mackie, N., & Damico J. (1996a). Accounting for handicaps in aphasia: Communicative assessment from an authentic social perspective. *Disability and Rehabilitation, 18,* 540–549.

Simmons-Mackie, N., & Damico J. (1996b). The contribution of discourse markers to communicative competence in aphasia. *American Journal of Speech Language Pathology, 5,* 37–43.

Simmons-Mackie, N., & Damico J. (1997). Reformulating the definition of compensatory strategies in aphasia. *Aphasiology, 8,* 761–781.

Simmons-Mackie, N., & Damico, J. (1999). Social role negotiation in aphasia therapy: Competence, incompetence and conflict. In D. Kovarsky, J. Duchan, & M. Maxwell (Eds.), *Constructing (in)competence: Disabling evaluations in clinical and social interaction* (pp. 313–341). Hillsdale, NJ: Lawrence Erlbaum.

Simmons-Mackie N., Damico, J., & Damico, H. (1999). A qualitative study of feedback in aphasia therapy. *American Journal of Speech-Language Pathology, 8,* 218–230.

Simmons-Mackie, N., & Kagan, A. (1999). Communication strategies used by 'good' versus 'poor' speaking partners of individuals with aphasia. *Aphasiology, 13,* 807–820.

Slansky, B., & McNeil, M. (1997). Resource allocation in auditory processing of emphatically stressed stimuli in aphasia. *Aphasiology, 11,* 461–472.

Spencer, K., Tompkins, C., Schulz, R., & Rau, M. (1995). The psychosocial outcomes of stroke: A longitudinal study of depression risk. *Clinical Aphasiology, 23,* 9–23.

Stainback, W., & Stainback, S. (Eds.) (1990). *Support networks for inclusive schooling.* Baltimore, MD: Paul H. Brookes.

Starkstein, S., & Robinson, R. (1988). Aphasia and depression. *Aphasiology, 2,* 1–20.

Stiell, D., & Gailey, G. (1995). Cotherapy with couples affected by aphasia. *Topics in Stroke Rehabilitation, 2,* 34–39.

Strauss Hough, M., & Pierce, R. (1994). Pragmatics and treatment. In R. Chapey (Ed.), *Language intervention strategies in adult aphasia*. Philadelphia, PA: Williams & Wilkins.

Sutherland, A. (1981). *Disabled we stand*. London, UK: Souvenir Press.

Swanson, K. (1993). Nursing as informed caring for the well-being of others. *Journal of Nursing Scholarship, 25*, 352–357.

Taylor, M. (1965). A measurement of functional communication in aphasia. *Archives of Physical Medicine and Rehabilitation, 46*, 101–107.

Thompson, C. (1989). Generalization research in aphasia: A review of the literature. *Clinical Aphasiology, 18*, 195–222.

Thompson, C. (1994). Treatment of nonfluent Broca's aphasia. In R. Chapey (Ed.), *Language intervention strategies in adult aphasia*. Baltimore, MD: Williams & Wilkins.

Tippett, D., & Sugarman, J. (1996). Discussing advance directives under the patient self determination act: A unique opportunity for speech-language pathologists to help persons with aphasia. *American Journal of Speech-Language Pathology, 5*, 31–54.

Verbrugge, L. M., & Jette, A. M. (1994). The disablement process. *Social Science and Medicine, 38*, 1–14.

Wahrborg, P. (1989). Aphasia and family therapy. *Aphasiology, 3*, 479–482.

Wahrborg, P. (1991). *Assessment and management of emotional and psychosocial reactions to brain damage and aphasia*. San Diego: Singular.

Wahrborg, P., & Borenstein, P. (1989). Family therapy in families with an aphasic member. *Aphasiology, 3*, 93–98.

Walker-Batson, D., Curtis, S., Smith, P., & Ford, J. (1999). An alternative model for the treatment of aphasia: The Lifelink© approach. In R. Elman (Ed.), *Group treatment for neurogenic communication disorders: The expert clinician's approach* (pp. 67–75). Woburn, MA: Butterworth-Heinemann.

Wang, C. (1993). Culture, meaning and disability: Injury prevention campaigns and the production of stigma. In M. Nagler (Ed.), *Perspectives on disability* (pp. 77–90). Palo Alto, CA: Health Markets Research.

Warren, R. (1996). Outcome measurement: Moving toward the patient. *ASHA Special Interest Divisions—Neurophysiology and Neurogenic Speech and Language Disorders, 6*, 5–6.

Webster, E., Dans, J., & Saunders, P. (1982). Descriptions of husband-wife communication pre and post aphasia. In R. Brookshire (Ed.), *Clinical aphasiology conference proceedings* (pp. 64–74). Minneapolis, MN: BRK.

Weisman, C. S. (1987). Communication between women and their health care providers: Research finding and unanswered questions. *Public Health Reports, 102*, 147–151.

Weniger, D., & Sarno M. (1990). The future of aphasia therapy: More than just new wine in old bottles? *Aphasiology 4*, 301–306.

Wertz, R. (1984). Language disorders in adults: State of the clinical art. In A. Holland (Ed.), *Language disorders in adults* (pp. 10–78). San Diego: College Hill Press.

West, J. (1993). "Ask me no questions": An analysis of queries and replies in physician-patient dialogues. In T. A. Dundas & S. Fosher (Eds.), *The social organization of doctor-patient communication* (pp. 127–157). Hillsdale, NJ: Ablex.

Whiteneck, G. G., Charlifue, S. W., Gerhart, K. A., Overholser, J. D., & Richardson, G. N. (1992). Quantifying handicap: A new measure of long-term rehabilitation outcomes. *Archives of Physical Medicine and Rehabilitation, 73*, 519–526.

Whurr, R., Lorch, M., & Nye, C. (1992). A meta-analysis of studies carried out between 1946 and 1988 concerned with the efficacy of speech and language therapy treatment for aphasic patients. *European Journal of Disorders of Communication, 27*, 1–17.

Wilcox, M. (1983). Aphasia: Pragmatic considerations. *Topics in Language Disorders, 3*(4), 35–48.

Wilcox, M., & Davis, G. (1977). Speech act analysis of aphasic communication in individual and group settings. In R. Brookshire (Ed.), *Clinical aphasiology conference proceedings* (pp. 166–174). Minneapolis, MN: BRK.

Wood, L., & Ryan, E. (1991). Talk to elders: Social structure attitudes and address. *Ageing and Society, 11*, 167–188.

World Health Organization (1980). *International classification of impairments, disabilities, and handicaps: A manual for classification relating to the consequences of disease*. Geneva, Switzerland: WHO.

World Health Organization (1997). *International classification of impairments, activities and participation. A manual of dimensions of disablement and functions. Beta-1 draft for field trials*. Geneva, Switzerland: WHO.

Worrall, L. (1992). Functional communication assessment: An Australian perspective. *Aphasiology, 6*, 105–110.

Yalom, I. (1985). *The theory and practice of group psychotherapy*. (3rd ed.). New York: Basic Books.

Zemba, N. (1999). Aphasia patients and their families: Wishes and limits. *Aphasiology, 13*, 219–224.

Zraik, R. I., & Boone, D. R. (1991). Spouse attitudes toward the person with aphasia. *Journal of Speech and Hearing Research, 34*, 123–128.

Chapter 11

Social Approaches to Aphasia Intervention

Nina Simmons-Mackie

OBJECTIVES

Major strides have been made in the past decade in the development of social approaches to aphasia (Byng & Duchan, 2005; Byng, Pound, & Parr, 2000; Elman, 2005; Elman & Bernstein-Ellis, 1999a, 1999b; Holland, 1999; Kagan, 1998; Kagan, Black, Duchan, Simmons-Mackie, & Square, 2001; LPAA Project Group, 2000; Lyon, 1992, 1996; Parr, 1996; Pound, Parr, Lindsay, & Woolf, 2000; Sarno, 1993a, 2004; Simmons-Mackie, 1993, 1994, 1998a, 1998b, 2000, 2004b; Worrall, 2000b). It is the objective of this chapter to explain the rationale, philosophy, and principles of socially motivated approaches to aphasia and to provide examples of assessment and intervention methods that fit into the social model philosophy.

This chapter will (1) introduce and define a social model of aphasia intervention; (2) describe social approaches and contrast social approaches with traditional restorative and functional approaches; (3) outline the principles of a social approach to intervention; (4) introduce assessment strategies appropriate to a social model of management; and (5) describe intervention objectives and examples that fit within a social approach.

RATIONALE FOR SOCIAL APPROACHES

The goal of a social approach is to promote membership in a communicating society and participation in personally relevant activities for those affected by aphasia. The ultimate aim of a social approach, enhancing the living of life with aphasia, is consistent with the philosophy of "Life-Participation Approaches to Aphasia" (see Chapter 10). The need for a social approach to aphasia management draws from several sources.

First, aphasia is a chronic disorder with long-term consequences beyond the acute disruption of communication. In spite of linguistic gains, many people with aphasia experience

residual communication problems that significantly impact their daily lives. Those affected by aphasia report social isolation, loneliness, loss of autonomy, restricted activities, role changes, and stigmatization (Herrmann, Johannsen-Horback, & Wallesch, 1993; LeDorze & Brassard, 1995; National Aphasia Association, 1988; Parr, 1994; Parr, Byng, Gilpin, & Ireland, 1997; Sarno, 1993a, 1997). In fact, "a frequent tale from people who live with aphasia is of being disengaged from life, excluded from involvement, or allowed in, but only on the periphery" (Pound, 2004, p. 50). Many of these long-term consequences are not addressed by traditional aphasia intervention. Such untreated psychological and social problems can increase disability, diminish community reintegration, and reduce response to rehabilitation (Sandin, Cifu, & Noll, 1994). The cycle of diminished participation in various aspects of life can take a drastic toll on self-confidence and personal identity (Shadden, 2005).

In addition, funding sources have pressed for more "functionally relevant" outcomes and evidence that our services make a difference in the lives of our clients (Frattali, 1996, 1998a; Johnson, 1999). Restructuring in health care has forced us to balance quality outcome with cost of care. Pressure from consumers, desire to improve outcomes, and changes in the health-care industry suggest an urgent need for creative approaches that increase the quality of communicative life for those affected by aphasia. A social model provides a philosophical framework for implementing interventions that fulfill these requirements.

EXPANDING THE MANAGEMENT FOCUS

In traditional aphasia therapy the emphasis has been on improving linguistic or cognitive processing. These restorative therapies have been effective in changing language performance. Such approaches tend to focus on the "impairment" of the individual with aphasia, and rely on formal tests and treatment probes to determine the level of deficit and degree of change after therapy. Certainly, restoration of communicative processes is an important goal for people with aphasia. However, gaps between changes on linguistic measures and "real-life" functional performance of people with aphasia have been noted (Holland, 1998a). Therefore, functional therapies have been developed to address performance of daily activities and communication "in use" (Frattali, 1998a; Holland, 1982, 1991; Worrall & Frattali, 2000). Functional-skills approaches often focus on the ability to utilize compensatory strategies and perform typical tasks such as using the telephone or making a grocery list. However, the personal experience of aphasia and individual life-style adjustments have rarely been addressed in restorative and skills approaches. For example, in spite of improved linguistic processing and success on "functional" tasks, clients and families continue to report social isolation, loss of confidence, decreased roles, and limited communication opportunities (Parr et. al., 1997). Therefore, expansion of functional approaches to encompass quality of life and social participation has been recommended (Frattali, 1998a; Kagan & Gailey, 1993; Worrall, 2000a). A social approach expands intervention to address the living of life with aphasia, including life-style changes and psychosocial issues.

CONTRASTING MEDICAL AND SOCIAL MODELS

The traditional health-care paradigm has been described as a "medical" or "biomedical" model with an explicit focus on management of "illness." Social models have arisen in an effort to shift the emphasis away from treating the illness to promoting health. The medical model has been the prevailing paradigm in aphasiology (Sarno, 1993b), and the influence of the medical model remains evident in our practices. For example, when the responsibility for "cure" and authority for decision-making is placed with the clinician (i.e., the "expert"), then clinicians tend to dictate goals and control treatment. While professional expertise is needed, the marked power differential can create a passive, dependent "patient" who learns to "take the cure" with little participation in life choices (Pyypponen, 1993). In a social model, clients take an active, participatory role in their own health-care decisions. The focus of rehabilitation shifts towards a "client-centered" perspective that involves maximizing opportunities for informed choices and taking full account of each person's preferences, needs, and social contexts (Cardol, De Jong, & Ward, 2002).

The medical model is also evident in our terminology. Thus, "patients receive treatment," as though treatment is a tonic that will cure aphasia (Pyypponen, 1993; Sarno, 1993a, 1993b). When complete recovery is not the result, individuals with residual aphasia face discharge from treatment with little attention to chronic affects (Hersh, 1998). By contrast, the social model requires a long-term view of aphasia. The focus shifts to optimally "living with" aphasia, with the emphasis on health rather than illness (LPAA, 2000; Lyon, 1992; Pound, 1998b).

In a medical model, "problems" tend to be located within the individual. A social model orients away from defining the problem as situated wholly within the individual. That is, problems result from an interaction between the individual's organic condition and his or her social and physical environment (World Health Organization, 2001). In a social model disability is a consequence of disabling attitudes and barriers imposed by society, not simply an impairment that resides within the individual. Thus, aphasia is not only a disorder, but also a situation in which opportunities and rights are not readily available. Both internal problems and external barriers must be addressed for optimal return of function and well-being.

ELEMENTS OF A SOCIAL MODEL

The "social" of social model refers to the broad concept that people are members of society and reside within a sociocultural context. As Goodwin (1995) describes, aphasia is more than a lesion within the skull; aphasia is also located outside of the person in dynamic relationships with others and in the social community. Thus, aphasia is addressed as an element of a social system and communication is viewed as a social act. Through communication we express and create our ideas, and also our personalities, our culture, and our life values. Communication fulfills a critical social goal when it allows us to reveal a healthy identity or "create a positive face" (Goffman, 1967). Because of the social significance of communication, disrupted communication entails social meanings and consequences; hence, the importance of a social model.

INTEGRATING PSYCHOSOCIAL AND COMMUNICATION INTERVENTION

When social systems do not support communicative access and participation, psychosocial well-being and quality of life are diminished (Cruice, Worrall, Hickson, & Murison, 2003; Doyle et al., 2004). Participation in various realms of life (e.g., leisure activities, social relationships) is closely tied to positive affective states and subjective well-being (Sveen, Thommessen, Bautz-Holter, Wyller, & Laake, 2004), yet participation in such activities is closely tied to the ability to communicate. Studies report relationships between communication disorders and quality of life or psychological well-being (Cruice et al., 2003; Doyle et al., 2004). For example, negative mood states, restricted social participation, and less life satisfaction are associated with communication disability (Doyle et al., 2004), while communication ability is associated with greater well-being and social functioning (Cruice et al., 2003).

While psychosocial issues associated with aphasia have long been recognized, they have remained on the outskirts of therapy. Traditionally, remediation of psychosocial problems has been divorced from the communication impairment and aphasia therapy. Typically, counseling and education are considered the approaches of choice for psychosocial issues. Yet these services are often unavailable or tangential to the "real" therapy. In addition, psychosocial problems such as depression and loneliness are sometimes accepted as a natural and expected consequence of aphasia. Finally, an aggressive research emphasis on the linguistic dimensions of aphasia has tended to overshadow psychosocial issues, resulting in neglect of "the person" (Byng et al., 2000; Sarno, 1993a, 1993b).

Attention to the psychosocial dimensions of aphasia is considered an integral part of communication in a social model (Bouchard-Lamothe et al., 1999; Brumfitt, 1993; Lafond, DeGiovani, Joanette, Ponzio, & Sarno, 1993; Müller, 1999; Müller & Code, 1989; Pound et al., 2000; Sarno, 1991; Simmons-Mackie, 1998b, 2000). Psychosocial issues are not separable from communication. Social affiliation and maintaining a healthy identity are major goals of human communication (Tannen, 1984). We craft our utterances and construct our interactions as a social and emotional endeavor. When communicative interactions are successful, we obtain emotional and social rewards. Through communication we obtain membership in a communicating society. This critical aspect of communication cannot be overlooked. Although often artificially separated in the literature, communication and psychosocial issues are woven together into the fabric of human existence. A social model recognizes that those affected by aphasia must fulfill psychosocial needs through communication. In fact, LaPointe (2002) has argued that psychosocial issues and neurolinguistic aspects should be integrated to create a "sociology" of aphasia.

DEFINING APHASIA IN A SOCIAL MODEL

The definition of aphasia is expanded within a social model to reflect more than linguistic or cognitive-processing deficits. Thus, aphasia is an impairment due to brain damage in the formulation and reception of language, often associated with diminished participation in life events and reduced fulfillment of desired social roles. Kagan (1995) defines aphasia as an impairment in communication that masks inherent competence. Byng and colleagues (2000, p. 53) define functional-communication goals in aphasia as "being able to communicate competently, through your own communication skills and those of others and feeling comfortable that you are representing who you are." By expanding the definition of aphasia we acknowledge that the meaning of aphasia to the person with aphasia and to those around him or her is greater than the linguistic deficit alone. Aphasia is a diagnosis, but also aphasia is a socially constructed way of being that is created through the experiences of the person with aphasia, those around the person, and society (Penn, 2004).

SOCIAL MODEL VERSUS SOCIAL APPROACHES

The phrase "social model" is used in this chapter to refer to a philosophy that guides and frames assessment and intervention. A social model is not a specific therapy approach or technique; rather, it is a value system adopted by clinicians, organizations or programs that deliver services within this philosophy. Social-model values call for aphasia intervention that promotes meaningful life changes and outcomes that are viewed relative to the individual's preferred roles and responsibilities within society. Furthermore, intervention is considered part of the individual's social context. Thus, the intervention experience and therapy interactions promote healthy identity and social integration. Social-model values invite people with aphasia and their families to share control and decision-making with clinicians, and treatment reflects client-centered values and practices (Byng & Duchan, 2005).

The "social model" has often been viewed as an alternative to impairment-focused treatment (Duchan, 2001). In fact, a social-model philosophy provides a framework within which any treatment approach might be employed. Intervention within a social model is determined more by the values and beliefs of therapists and organizations than by the actual "activities" carried out in therapy (Byng & Duchan, 2005). For example, conversational group therapy is touted as an approach that fits within social approaches to aphasia. However, an authoritarian clinician who sets all goals, controls therapy decisions, rations turns, and evaluates productions is not functioning within a social model philosophy.

While this chapter helps to define a social model, the specific methods and techniques described will constitute "social approaches" practiced within a social model philosophy. Social approaches focus specifically on social participation, psychosocial well-being, and life contexts. Social approaches to aphasia intervention have appeared under general labels such as social model approaches, consequences therapy (e.g., addressing the consequences of aphasia) (Holland, 2005, personal communication), life participation approaches (LPAA, 2000), or functional communication approaches (Worrall, 2000b). Within the general umbrella of social approaches are a wide range of therapies that address living life with aphasia.

PRINCIPLES OF A SOCIAL APPROACH

A social approach to aphasia management can best be conceptualized through a set of basic principles. Management is designed to (1) address both information exchange and social needs as dual goals of communication; (2) address communication within authentic, relevant, and natural contexts; (3) view communication as dynamic, flexible, and multidimensional; (4) focus on the collaborative nature of communication; (5) focus on natural interaction, particularly conversation; (6) focus on personal and social consequences of aphasia; (7) focus on adaptations to impairment; (8) embrace the perspective of those affected by aphasia; and (9) encourage qualitative as well as quantitative measures.

Dual Goals of Transaction and Interaction

Communication is designed to meet two primary goals: the exchange of information (transaction) and the fulfillment of social needs (interaction) (Simmons, 1993; Simmons-Mackie & Damico, 1995). In traditional aphasia therapy clinicians have focused on the transactional aspects of communication. For example, functional therapies have been designed to promote message exchange and to get ideas across in whatever way possible (Davis & Wilcox, 1985). Social goals of communication have been largely ignored. While certainly the exchange of messages is important, the social goals are equally, if not more, important. Through communication we not only exchange information, but also develop and maintain an identity and sense of self, fulfill emotional needs, provide connections with other people, and promote our membership in groups. Appreciation of the social goals of communication is critical to fully addressing the consequences of aphasia.

Address Communication within an Authentic Context

Communicative change must make a difference in personally relevant contexts of those affected by aphasia. Much traditional aphasia therapy and most formal aphasia tests are conducted in relatively controlled contexts and focus on decontextualized tasks and discrete elements of language (e.g., naming, sentence completion). By contrast, natural communication occurs in a complex, dynamic social context with shifting expectancies, social roles, and goals. When communication is stripped of its natural context, we get a skewed appreciation of a person's communicative life. A full appreciation of communication within natural, personally relevant contexts is imperative to ensuring effective therapy outcomes. "Authentic contexts" are at the forefront of decision-making, assessment, and intervention in a social approach.

Communication as Dynamic, Flexible, and Multidimensional

Aphasiologists have evaluated communication in terms of "idealized" normal language. We assess "deficits" based on expectations of how a standard speaker would perform. While this helps determine an objective skill level, it potentially deludes us into viewing communication as invariant and static. In reality, informal communication includes dysfluencies, word errors, revisions, and sentence fragments (Button & Lee, 1987; Shiffrin, 1987). The following is a transcription of a question asked to a presenter at an aphasia conference: "So is this like one of the uh uh one of those that we've seen before . . . at least I have . . . and how can we be sure to make the uh uh reee uh make the shift?" No one seemed disturbed by this question proffered by a well-respected aphasiologist; yet, according to traditional standards the production would not be considered normal. In fact, such deviations are typical of the informal discourse of standard speakers. It is important that clinicians fully appreciate the flexibility and creativity of language in use. Many devices that deviate from "idealized language norms" are used in natural conversation to meet communicative goals. Tannen (1984) examines the use of interruptions and joint talk in standard conversation as a means of achieving affiliation in certain cultural groups. Utterances such as "oh," "well," and "you know" are used to bracket information and manage the flow of discourse (Shiffrin, 1987; Simmons-Mackie & Damico, 1996b). Goodwin (1987) describes purposeful "forgetfulness" as a strategy used by couples to bring a spouse into a conversation. Thus, strategies are often used to serve a goal beyond the accurate and grammatical production of language. Perhaps in the practice of aphasia assessment and intervention, a more open-minded view of behavior and an appreciation of situated pragmatics are needed (Duchan, 1997; Simmons, 1993). Social approaches assume the flexibility and creativity of communication, and social goals are taken into account when assessing communication.

Communication Is Collaborative

In a social approach the focus is shifted away from the individual with aphasia and onto the collaborative nature of communication (Simmons, 1993). Conversation is a co-constructed activity in which participants negotiate important social actions and work to help each other understand with as little effort as possible (Clark & Wilkes-Gibbs, 1986; Milroy & Perkins, 1992). Research repeatedly affirms that communication is a collaborative achievement (Goodwin, 1995, 2003; Hengst, 2003; Hengst, Frame, Neuman-Stritzel, & Gannaway, 2005; Klippi, 1996; Oelschlaeger & Damico, 1998a, 1998b; Simmons-Mackie, Kingston & Schultz, 2005). Social roles are established and maintained through interactive cooperation (Brumfitt, 1993; Simmons-Mackie & Damico, 1999). Speaking style, content, discourse structure, and even opinions are modified to accommodate to speaking partners and context (Bell, 1984; Giles, Taylor, & Bourhis, 1973). A view of communication as a collaborative achievement requires expanding research and management efforts beyond the individual with aphasia to include the communicative skills of those "around" the person with aphasia and the dynamics of interaction.

Focus on Natural Interaction: Conversation

Conversation in its myriad forms has been labeled the primary site of human communication in our society (Clark & Wilkes-Gibbs, 1986). However, "functional communication" is often defined in terms of very goal-directed, transactional tasks such as cashing a check, asking for directions, or ordering in a restaurant. It is likely that the social chat that surrounds these activities is as important as the task itself.

Therefore, success in and enjoyment of conversational interactions is a potentially important objective in aphasia intervention. Until recently, research rarely focused on natural
conversation in aphasia, assessment rarely included a sample
of natural conversation, and few intervention approaches
directly targeted conversation. Fortunately, research on conversation and other communicative genres in aphasia has
grown considerably in the past decade, providing valuable
data to aid in focusing on natural interaction and conversation (Goodwin, 2003; Hengst et al., 2005; Oelschlaeger &
Damico, 1998a, 1998b).

Focus on Adaptations and Enablement Rather than Impairment and Disability

A social approach involves a positive stance towards life with
aphasia. While impairment tends to be the focus of traditional aphasia therapy, successful adaptations to aphasia and
ability (rather than disability) are primary in social
approaches (LaPointe, 2005). Attention to the prevalence of
adaptive strategies used by a person with aphasia can make a
difference in our predictions of functional outcomes.

In fact, an overemphasis on deficits might obscure appreciation of adaptive behavior. For example, when asked to describe a client's naming response—"uh uh pen"—clinicians
routinely described word-finding problems or processing
delays (Simmons-Mackie, 1993). However, the "uh uh"
behavior could also be described as a successful floor-hold-
ing strategy. When communication is disrupted, nonstandard compensations might be required to meet communicative goals. Successful adaptations are often contrary to what
are considered normal or preferred behaviors (Booth &
Perkins, 1999). For example, one client with chronic aphasia
often bombastically announced "I can't talk" when addressed by strangers. Analysis suggested that he preferred to
"powerfully" terminate the interaction rather than expose
his communicative "weakness." Thus, to meet his own identity needs, this man chose what some might consider a prag-
matically undesirable behavior. What is deemed "appropriate" is judged in terms of the goal of the behavior and
available alternatives.

In addition, the adaptive skills and attitudes of speaking
partners of people with aphasia will influence the success of
interactions. Therefore, emphasis expands beyond the
adaptation of the individual with aphasia, to adapting society to enable the person's participation. A considerable literature has arisen that describes characteristics of enabling
or disabling physical and social environments (Howe,
Worrall, & Hickson, 2004). Social approaches necessitate a
focus on aspects of the environment that enable the person
with aphasia. In a social approach the clinician focuses on
the adaptive purpose of behaviors, builds on existing adaptations, and takes into account social as well as linguistic
goals.

Focus on Personal and Social Consequences

As noted, a social model assumes that communication has a
critical sociocultural role. Impaired communication can be
associated with social consequences, potential social barriers, and resulting psychological issues. Thus, understanding
the impact of aphasia on a person's life is as important as
consideration of the disorder itself (Cardol et al., 2002).
Consequences are judged based on the personal experience
of the communication problem, which will undoubtedly
vary among those affected by aphasia. Thus, one individual
with mild aphasia might experience no life changes while
another individual with the same impairment might experience significant life changes and personal loss. Aphasia also
creates personal and social consequences for family and
friends, who might experience loneliness, stigma, embarrassment, energy depletion, and changed roles.

Consequences not only vary among individuals, but also
might vary from one context to another. Thus, using a picture board to convey food choices at home might be quite
different from using the aid in a restaurant with an unpre-
pared waitress. In part, the personal experience of aphasia
depends on cultural attitudes and knowledge regarding the
disability and expected life roles of those affected by aphasia.
Addressing the consequences for all those affected by aphasia will help to promote a healthy social system.

The Perspective of Those Affected by Aphasia

It is difficult to address consequences of aphasia without a
full appreciation of how those affected "perceive" these consequences. Consumer perspectives and consumer satisfaction are a priority. Rather than simply deciding what a client
"needs," intervention is based on consumer perceptions of
life changes, barriers to participation, and important life
goals. Research confirms that people with aphasia are able to
participate in interviews and ratings in order to share their
perspectives (Doyle, 2005; Hilari, Wiggins, Roy, Byng, &
Smith, 2003; Hoen, Thelander, & Worsley, 1997; Kagan,
1999; LeDorze & Brassard, 1995; Lyon, 1998b; Parr et al.,
1997; Simmons-Mackie & Damico, 2001). Personal choice
and autonomy are driving factors in management. The focus
is broadened from reducing impairment, to building meaning and purpose in life *as perceived by* those affected by aphasia. That is, in a social approach those confronting aphasia
chart the direction of intervention in concert with clinicians.

Qualitative as well as Quantitative Measures

In a social approach clinicians access the subjective experience of aphasia and describe outcomes relative to the rich
authentic context of daily communicative life. Subjective
experience and richly contextualized events call for qualitative as well as quantitative approaches to description.
Qualitative approaches such as ethnographic interviews,

personal narratives, and observational assessment provide important insights to drive management plans (Simmons-Mackie & Damico, 2001). Qualitative and descriptive methods are gaining attention as viable additions to research and assessment (Booth & Perkins, 1999; Damico, Simmons-Mackie, Oelschlaeger, Elman, & Armstrong, 1999; Fox, Poulsen, Bawden, & Packard, 2004; Perkins, Crisp, & Walshaw, 1999; Simmons-Mackie & Damico, 1996a, 1999; Sorin-Peters, 2004a).

EFFECTIVENESS OF SOCIAL APPROACHES

Although the social model is a relative newcomer to aphasiology and additional research is needed, a growing data base is accumulating to support the notion that social communication, communication opportunities, and well-being are amenable to intervention. For example, improvements in communication, relationships, and social participation have been documented after including communication partners in treatment (Boles, 1997; Hickey, Bourgeois, & Olswang, 2004; Hopper, Holland, & Rewega, 2002; Kagan et al., 2001; Lyon, 1998b; Lyon et al., 1997; Rayner & Marshall, 2003; Rogers, Alarcon, & Olswang, 1999; Simmons-Mackie, Kearns, & Potechin, 2005). Changes in adjustment, knowledge of aphasia, and functioning were reported among people with aphasia and their families after participating in brief intensive programs offering psychosocial support and education (Fox et al., 2004; Hinckley & Packard, 2001). Improvement in communicative success as well as qualitative changes in knowledge, confidence, and relationships were found by adapting principles of adult learning to working with couples on communicative skills and issues related to living with aphasia (Purdy & Hindenlang, 2005; Sorin-Peters, 2004b). Elman and Bernstein-Ellis (1999a, 1999b) report positive effects of social group therapy for patients with chronic aphasia on both linguistic and psychosocial measures. Integrating psychosocial support and access to social interaction into a community-based program has also been successful (Hoen et al., 1997; Ireland & Wotton, 1996; Kagan, 1999). Reports have begun to surface regarding intervention focusing specifically on enhancing participation in relevant life situations. For example, Lasker, LaPointe, and Kodras (2005) report successful ratings of job performance for a college professor with aphasia after intervention designed to facilitate teaching. The cost-effectiveness of social approaches has been reported since "meaningful" life and/or relationship changes have been effected with relatively few sessions (Lyon, 2004; Sorin- Peters, 2004b). There are also reports of positive effects of approaches that modify external barriers or facilitate participation in activities of choice (Garrett & Beukelman, 1995; Howe et al., 2004; Lyon et al., 1997; Rose, Worrall, & McKenna, 2003; Simmons-Mackie & Damico, 1996a, 2001; Simmons-Mackie et al., 2007). Indirect evidence of the potential

importance of socially oriented goals has come from research demonstrating associations between social relationships or participation and well-being, quality of life, and recovery (Cruice et al., 2003; Doyle, 2005; Hilari & Northcutt, 2006).

GOALS OF INTERVENTION IN A SOCIAL APPROACH

Socially motivated approaches conform to the ultimate goal of Life Participation Approaches to Aphasia—that is, to enhance the living of life with aphasia. To achieve the overall goal of living a satisfying life with aphasia, objectives might include (1) enhancing natural communication; (2) increasing successful participation in authentic events; (3) providing support systems within the speaker's community; (4) increasing communicative confidence and positive sense-of-self; and (5) promoting advocacy and social action. These objectives serve to guide intervention. Actual goals evolve out of a dialogue through which individuals with aphasia and clinicians negotiate specific outcome targets.

ASSESSMENT WITHIN A SOCIAL MODEL

Assessment in a social model encompasses a variety of tools that document accomplishment within the goal domains outlined above. Traditional measures such as standardized tests remain appropriate to determine the level and pattern of deficits. However, measures of outcome beyond linguistic or cognitive skills are needed to determine whether intervention is making a difference in the lives of those affected by aphasia (Frattali, 1998a, 1998b; Holland & Thompson, 1998). For people with aphasia, making a difference probably means returning to work, enjoying dinner with friends, sharing a good joke, or gossiping over coffee. Thus, assessment is designed to provide insight into well-being, personal consequences, and lifestyle affects of aphasia.

Situating Intervention within a Framework

Various frameworks and models are available to help organize assessment. For example, the World Health Organization (WHO) International Classification of Functioning, Disability and Health (ICF) (2001) emphasizes the multiple domains that comprise health, including body structure and function, activities and participation, and contextual factors. Kagan and colleagues (2005; in progress) have adapted and expanded the ICF framework and designed a simple schematic (Living with Aphasia: Framework for Outcome Measurement [A-FROM]) that serves as a guide to situate assessment and intervention. Figure 11–1 depicts the four key domains of life that dynamically interact and intersect to form one's "quality of life" at the center.

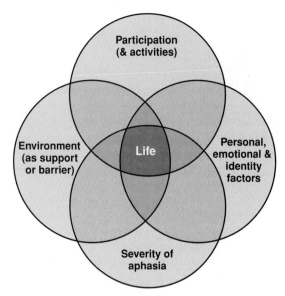

Figure 11–1. Living with Aphasia: Framework for Outcome Measurement (A-FROM) (adapted from Kagan et al., in press).

also can be divided into evaluation of capacity versus evaluation of actual performance (WHO, 2001). "Capacity" refers to a person's *ability* to perform a task in a clinical setting or test situation. "Performance" refers to what a person actually *does* in his or her daily life. For example, someone with aphasia might be able to make a phone call (capacity), but does not make phone calls during daily life (performance). Assessment approaches applicable to social intervention for aphasia are described below, and examples of tools are listed in Table 11–1. Measures of the linguistic or cognitive deficits are not included since this topic is covered in detail elsewhere.

Perspectives of Those Affected by Aphasia

A variety of tools assist the clinician in obtaining information from the perspective of those affected by aphasia relative to aphasia severity (the impairment), life participation, the communicative environment, and emotional factors.

Ethnographic Interviews

Ethnographic interviews have been recommended to determine the personal viewpoints of those affected by aphasia (Simmons-Mackie & Damico, 1996a, 2001). By analyzing interviews before, during, or after the intervention, general themes are identified that help focus intervention or document outcomes. Aspects of life participation, emotional adjustment, and environmental factors relevant to intervention and outcome can be accessed through interviews. Candidates for interviews include both the person with aphasia and others impacted by the aphasia. Ethnographic interviewing and analysis requires training and practice in order to access the authentic perspectives of informants. Readers are directed to Spradley (1979) and Westby (1990) for explanations of the methodology.

Communicative Profiling System (CPS)

An approach to assessment based on qualitative research methods is the Communicative Profiling System described by Simmons-Mackie and Damico (1996a, 2001). Interviews, personal journals, and observation are used to identify personally relevant behaviors, social relationships, emotions, and situational contexts of participation. Thus, the client and significant others catalog the behaviors that they consider significant to life with aphasia. A social-network diagram is devised to represent the people with whom the person with aphasia interacts on a regular basis, as shown in Figure 11–2. Description of relationships helps identify the quality of social networks. Psychosocial and affective issues are also catalogued. Finally, the contexts or activities that the person participates in on a regular basis are described. These layers of description help the clinician gain insight into communication patterns and motivations.

Assessment in the domain of *aphasia severity* entails documenting relevant linguistic or cognitive processes, either those targeted on traditional aphasia batteries or the impairment as viewed by the person with aphasia. The domain of *participation* includes a person's relevant life habits, roles, and situations, such as employment, relationships, social conversation, or leisure activities. This domain also includes activities that are components of life habits or situations such as activities of daily living or functional tasks. *Personal, emotional, and identity* factors refer to inherent characteristics of the person (e.g., age, gender) as well as to factors related to psychosocial well-being and identity (e.g., confidence, self-esteem). *Environment* refers to the physical or social environment in which a person functions. Aspects of these domains interact to create life with aphasia or *quality of life* at the center of the schematic. Assessment might target one or more of these domains. For example, changes might be documented in a person's self-esteem and confidence (personal domain) after intervention aimed at eliminating environmental barriers to communicative participation (environment domain).

In addition to different domains of assessment, measurements might accrue from different sources. These include the perspectives of the person with aphasia, clinician judgments (e.g., clinician ratings or observations), or proxy ratings or reports. The source of information should be clear since "insider" judgments (e.g., perspectives of the person with aphasia) often differ from "outsider" judgments (e.g., reports of others, clinician evaluation) (Cardol, de Haan, Van den Bos, & de Groot, 1999; Cruice, Worrall, Hickson, & Murison, 2005; Doyle, 2005; Parr et al. 1997). Assessment

TABLE 11-1

Examples of Assessment Tools for a Social Approach to Aphasia

Obtaining Perspectives of Those Affected by Aphasia

Ethnographic interviews (Simmons-Mackie and Damico 1996a; 2001; Spradley, 1979; Westby, 1990)
Communicative Profiling System (CPS) (Simmons-Mackie & Damico, 1996a, 2001)
Opinion or consumer-satisfaction surveys (Patterson & Wells, 1995)
Analysis of personal narratives (Frank, 1995; Greenhalgh & Hurwitz, 1999)

Functional Communication and Activities

Functional Assessment of Communication Skills for Adults (ASHA FACS) (Frattali et al., 1995)
Functional Communication Profile (Sarno, 1969)
Communication Profile (Payne, 1994)
CADL-2 (Holland, Frattali, & Fromm, 1999)
Conversational rating scales (Erlich & Barry, 1989; Garrett, 1999)
Interactive Communication Scales (Lyon, 1998b)
Discourse analysis
  • Content units (Yorkston & Beukelman, 1980)
  • Correct information units (Nicholas & Brookshire, 1993)
  • Lexical efficiency (Helm-Estabrooks & Albert, 1991)
  • Turns, initiations, time, and efficiency (Packard & Hinckley, 1997)
Functional scenario ratings (Lyon et al., 1997)
Communicative effectiveness/content/efficiency
Measure of Skill in Providing Supported Conversation for Adults with Aphasia (M-SCA) (Kagan et al., 2004)
Measure of Participation in Conversation by Adults with Aphasia (M-PCA) (Kagan et al., 2004)
Rating of transactional success in conversation (Ramsberger & Rende, 2002)
Communicative Effectiveness Ratings (Lyon et. al., 1997)
Communicative Effectiveness Index (Lomas et al., 1989)
Everyday Language Test (Blomert, Kean, Koster, & Schokker, 1994)
Pragmatic assessments (e.g. Penn, 1988)
Descriptive measures of number, success, and type of compensatory strategies
Conversation Analysis Profile for People with Aphasia (CAPPA) (Whitworth et al., 1997)

Participation

Adapted Activity Card Sort (Haley et al., 2005)
Frequency counts (e.g., number of social contacts, number of activities, hours of participation)
Community Integration Questionnaire (Corrigan, Smith-Knapp, & Granger, 1998)
Social-network analysis/contextual analysis (Simmons-Mackie & Damico, 1996a, 2001)
Personal goal-attainment scales (Schlosser, 2004)
Assessment of Life Habits (Life-H) (Noreau et al., 2004)

Personal, Emotional, and Psychosocial Factors

Affect Balance Scale (Bradburn, 1969)
Code-Müller Protocols (Code & Müller, 1992)
Psychosocial well-being index for aphasia (Lyon et al., 1997)
Visual Analogue Mood Scale (Stern et al., 1997)

(continued)

TABLE 11–1

Examples of Assessment Tools for a Social Approach to Aphasia (continued)

Environment
Observation and/or interview: Catalog barriers to and enablers of participation
Craig Hospital Inventory of Environmental Factors (CHIEF) (2001)

Quality of Life
ASHA Quality of Communicative Life Scales (Paul et al., 2004)
Burden of Stroke Scale (BOSS) (Doyle et al., 2004)
The Stroke and Aphasia Quality of Life Scale (SAQOL-39) (Hilari, 2003)
Life Satisfaction Index (Neugarten, Havighurst, & Tobin, 1961)
Satisfaction with Life Scale (Larsen, Diener, & Emmons, 1985)
Life Satisfaction Survey (Chubon, 1987)
Ryff scales (Ryff, 1989)
Present Life Survey (Records et al., 1992)

Professional Judgments

Assessment from the perspective of the professional is another source of measured outcomes. The speech-language pathologist evaluates performance as compared to defined target goals or expectations of "normal." In fact, most traditional assessment tools involve scoring or ratings completed by the professional to document aspects of communication.

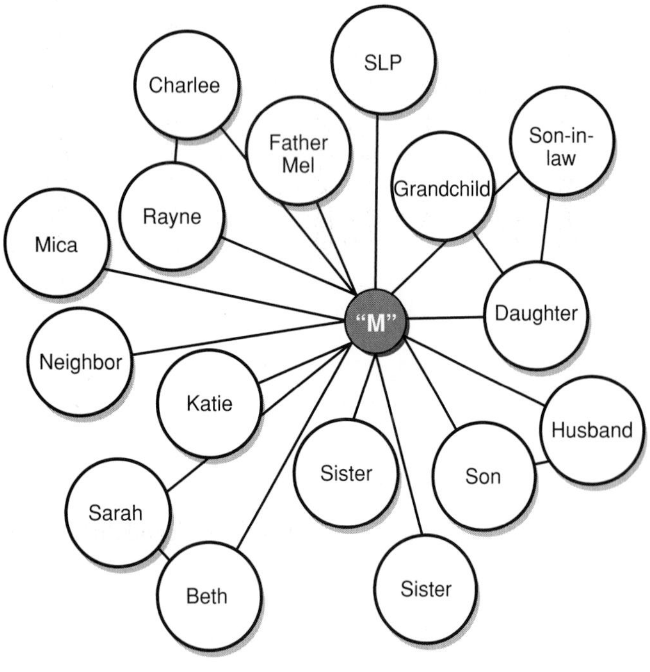

Figure 11–2. Example of a Social Network Analysis for "M," an Individual with Aphasia (Simmons-Mackie & Damico, 1996a, 2001).

Professional judgments or ratings are typical for measuring communicative effectiveness, performance of functional daily activities, and describing characteristics of conversation.

Activities and Participation

Functional Assessment and Activities of Daily Living

Using tests of functional communication clinicians assess or rate performance across a variety of categories or tasks typical of the daily activities of most people (Frattali, Thompson, Holland, Wohl, & Ferketic, 1995; Worrall, 1992). For example, the clinician rates observed or reported performance on "talking on the phone" or "reading the newspaper." In a social model, interpretation of such data must be balanced with information on the personal relevance of each task, since the importance of functional tasks varies from person to person (Davidson, Worrall, & Hickson, 1999; Payne, 1994; Smith, 1985). Talking on the phone might be deemed highly important to one person, yet minimally important to another, even when their lifestyles appear similar. In addition, it is important that clinicians are aware of *actual* function in daily life, not simply the ability to perform various functional tasks.

Communicative-Effectiveness Ratings and Conversation Analysis

Analyzing communicative interactions using communicative-effectiveness ratings is a prevalent approach to assessment. Aspects of an exchange, such as success of message transmission, efficiency, naturalness, or pragmatic appropriateness are rated for baseline or follow-up data. Barrier activities, "simulated" functional scenarios, or samples of

TABLE 11–2

Example of an Inventory of Key Life Activities Before the Onset of Aphasia, at Assessment (2 Years Post-Onset), and After Participation-Focused Intervention

Pre-Onset	Initial Assessment	Outcome Assessment
Teaching 1st grade		Preschool volunteer
Church on Sunday	Church on Sunday	Church on Sunday
Cook for church (Wednesday)		
Carnival club Secretary		Carnival club attendee
Walk 2 miles daily		Walk with friend daily
Prepare family dinner		Host family dinner
Baby sit grandchild	Baby sit grandchild	Baby sit grandchild
Garden club		
Gardening	Gardening (some)	Gardening (some)
Reading	Reading (news)	Reading (news)
	Television	Television

(Adapted from Simmons-Mackie, N., & Damico, J. (2001). Intervention outcomes: A clinical application of qualitative methods. *Topics Language Disorders, 22*(1), 21–36.)

natural conversation provide contexts for rating behaviors of interest (Lyon et al., 1997). The interaction, not simply the behavior of the client alone, is an important target of assessment (Leiwo, 1994). Kagan and colleagues (2004) report on two scales that provide insight into both the interactional and message-transmission skills of the person with aphasia and a communication partner. Ramsberger and Rende (2002) describe a method of analyzing "transactional" success in conversation. Communicative-effectiveness ratings need not come solely from the perspective of the professional. Clients or others (e.g., family, friend, employer) can rate their own perceptions of communicative effectiveness, as in the Communicative Effectiveness Index (Lomas et al., 1989). In addition, perceived conversational engagement or enjoyment during natural conversation might be a rating target.

Since performance on linguistic tasks does not necessarily predict how one performs in natural conversation (Beeke, Wilkinson, & Maxim, 2003; Horton, 2004; Wilkinson, 2004), analysis of conversation is an important component of assessment, particularly if intervention is to effect changes in natural social interactions. Conversation Analysis (CA) is a potential tool for documenting communicative interactions (Perkins et al., 1999). The Conversation Analysis Profile for People with Aphasia is based on principles of CA (Whitworth, Perkins, & Lesser, 1997).

Measures of Participation

While the preceding functional and communication measures provide useful information, documenting actual social participation is important for capturing meaningful life changes. There are a number of approaches to measuring participation. Simmons-Mackie & Damico (1996a, 2001) apply social-network analysis and contextual inventories to identify social contacts and activities performed on a regular basis as reported by people with aphasia and their significant others. Personally relevant changes in these inventories represent life-participation accomplishments. An activity inventory for a person with aphasia who entered therapy 2 years post-onset is presented in Table 11-2; it is clear from visual inspection that both the number and quality of activities increased after "activity-focused" intervention. Similarly, social-network maps (as in Fig. 11-2) can serve as visual evidence of increased social relationships (Simmons-Mackie & Damico, 1996a, 2001). Lyon (2000) lists "obligated" and "free-time" activities pre- and post-aphasia to provide data on lifestyle changes. Others (Haley et al., 2005) describe an adaptation of the Activity Card Sort (ACS) (Baum & Edwards, 2001) to obtain information from adults with aphasia regarding their current and prior life activities. Simple frequency counts also provide data. For example, if a goal involves increasing the number of social contacts per week or the variety of activities, then simple counts document increases over time. Similarly, hours of participation might serve as a "quick and dirty" measure of increased activity.

Participation can be judged from either an outsider perspective (e.g., ratings or counts by experts) or an insider perspective (e.g., reports or ratings by the person with aphasia). For example, clinicians, family members, or hospital staff might keep journals or observational diaries to document aspects of communication and participation of the person with aphasia. Observational data collected by the clinician in natural communication situations is valuable in documenting the presence and success of adaptations or compensations and changes over the course of treatment. Increasingly, however, assessment of social participation and functioning in society *as judged by those affected by aphasia* has been viewed as an essential element in rehabilitation (Cardol et al., 1999; Kagan et al., in press). In other words, people place different values on particular life situations, frequency of activities, or social contacts. It is difficult to judge the "success" of social participation without capturing whether or not the changes are meaningful to the person with aphasia and/or family.

Goal-Attainment Scales

Improvement over time in actual participation can be measured with scales designed to judge movement towards particular individually defined life-participation goals (Pound et al., 2000; Simmons-Mackie, 2000). For example, the individual who wishes to participate in an adult-education class works with the therapist to identify requirements to be achieved in order to meet this goal. Relevant scales can be developed to document achievement towards selected life goals. For example, return to work might be documented along an ordinal scale ranging from unemployed (rated as 1) to working full-time at full pay with adaptations (rated as 5). Within the goal scale, each rating is defined (e.g., a 3 = half-time, reduced salary/benefits). While results of such measures are not always comparable across patients and do not inherently indicate the significance of changes (Hesketh & Hopcutt, 1997), personal-goal-attainment scales are valuable in combination with other measures. Methods of developing goal-attainment scales and statistically analyzing results are available (Schlosser, 2004).

Communicative Environment

Interview and observation are the most widely used methods of documenting environmental barriers to and enablers of communicative or life participation for people with aphasia (e.g., Simmons-Mackie et al., in press). Clinicians might interview people with aphasia and their family members to identify barriers to participation, particularly in personally relevant environments (e.g., home, hospital, work). Observation of authentic events and situations also provides information on social, physical, attitudinal, temporal, and organizational factors that enable or disable participation. Such assessments are typically directed at improving participation of a particular individual with aphasia; however, a more broad-based assessment might be conducted to determine the "aphasia friendliness" of various settings, facilities, or organizations.

Quality of Life

Another approach to assessment includes gathering self-reports or ratings of life satisfaction or quality of life (QOL).

Numerous measures are grouped as quality-of-life tools (Engell, Hutter, Willmes, & Huber, 2003; Hilari et al., 2003; Paul et al., 2004; Records, Tomblin, & Freese, 1992; Ross, 2005; Ross & Wertz, 2003; Ryff, 1989; Worrall & Holland, 2003). Typically, the person with aphasia conducts a rating across one or more dimensions believed to represent aspects of well-being, satisfaction, or QOL. Since QOL is highly personal and subjective, those actually affected by aphasia should complete the ratings, and the dimensions rated must be meaningful and important to the person. Many quality-of-life tools include items reflecting various domains, including aspects related to the health condition itself (e.g., aphasia severity), psychological or emotional state (e.g., confidence, depression), and/or social activities and participation (e.g., leisure activities).

INTERVENTION WITHIN A SOCIAL MODEL

A social approach to intervention involves the ever-present and overt goal of enhancing overall QOL and participation in activities of choice. Individual goals explicitly address practical and personally relevant outcomes. Specific objectives to be discussed below include (1) enhancing communication; (2) increasing participation in events; (3) providing support systems; (4) increasing confidence and positive identity; and (5) promoting advocacy.

Enhancing Communication

To participate fully in life, one important goal of intervention is enhanced communicative interactions. Thus, increasing the communicative skill and confidence of the person with aphasia and/or potential communication partners might constitute a focus of therapy.

Expanding Skill and Confidence in Conversation

Skill and confidence in conversation is an appropriate objective of socially motivated intervention. Significant attention to natural conversation is only recently being addressed in the aphasia literature. As Leiwo (1994, p. 480) explains, "a genuine social interaction with meaningful discourse topics sets different goals for communication than the more or less artificial metalinguistic tasks, role-playing tasks or discussions that employ stimulus pictures and cards. Different goals evoke different discourse strategies." Research supports Leiwo's statement. For example, traditional therapy discourse includes a pervasive "teaching" discourse structure—the Request-Response-Evaluation (RRE) triad—in which the therapist "requests" the client to perform some task (e.g., What is this?), the client "responds" (e.g., pencil), and the therapist "evaluates" the response (e.g., "good job") (Simmons-Mackie & Damico, 1999; Simmons-Mackie, Damico, & Damico, 1999). This RRE structure is not typical of adult social conversation. Natural conversation—the everyday, ordinary talk that serves both social and transactional goals—involves varied discourse structures, creative discourse devices, varying social stances, and shifting social roles. This contrasts markedly with the relatively rigid structure of traditional therapy, in which therapist-patient roles tend to be maintained and discourse structures are relatively restricted (Ferguson & Armstrong, 2004; Silvast, 1991; Simmons-Mackie et al., 1999; Wilcox & Davis, 1977). Even conversation between therapist and client often conforms to interview patterns, with therapists asking questions and clients responding (Holland, 1998b; Simmons-Mackie & Damico, 1999). Restricted discourse structures and passive roles provide little occasion for practicing the myriad skills typical of natural conversation. In order for people with aphasia to practice strategies for engaging in conversation, then mediated and supported opportunities should be provided.

Conversation Therapy

One means of enhancing conversational interaction is direct conversation therapy (Simmons-Mackie, 2000). Conversation therapy refers to planned intervention that is explicitly designed to enhance conversational abilities. It does not necessarily involve "conversing" during therapy, although usually a conversational context is appropriate. Conversation therapy is goal-directed and individualized. It is not simply having a conversation. The goal of having a conversation is to exchange information and fulfill social needs. The goal of conversation therapy is to improve one's skill and confidence as a conversational participant. Conversation therapy focuses not only on message exchange, but also on social communication skills appropriate to specific communicative events. Thus, aspects of interaction such as power and control, variety of social roles, range of discourse structures, and issues of self-esteem gain equal importance to linguistic form and content. Improving skill in activities such as arguing, joke-telling, storytelling, and gossiping might be addressed, along with the usual speech act repertoire. Conversation therapy might also focus on exploiting the use of paralinguistic, nonlinguistic, and contextual cues to enhance conversation (Goodwin, 2003; Hengst et al., 2005; Simmons-Mackie et al., 2005). Finally, emphasis is placed on gaining confidence as well as building skill in participating in communicative interactions.

Enhanced Compensatory-Strategy Training

Improving natural interactions often requires the use of compensatory strategies. Traditionally, the individual with aphasia has been taught compensatory strategies designed to enhance message transmission across a variety of situations. For example, strategies such as gesture, writing, asking for repeats, and using augmentative aids are widely used to improve communication in the face of residual aphasia

(Simmons, 1993). Training in such message transmission strategies has not always generalized as well as we might expect (Kraat, 1990; Simmons, 1993; Thompson, 1989). One reason is probably related to the social appropriateness of strategies and the necessity for both parties to understand and use strategies. For example, Sachett, Byng, Marshall, and Pound (1999) demonstrated that communication partners must modify their own communication to accommodate strategy use by the person with aphasia. Simmons-Mackie (1998a) suggests that accommodation theory might explain this to some degree—that is, people in conversation tend to alter their manner of communication to be "like" the other person's style of communication (Bell, 1984; Giles et al., 1973). If a nonaphasic partner does not use writing, then it is less likely that the aphasic speaker will feel comfortable doing so. Furthermore, most compensatory strategies are trained independent of their natural use; thus, natural social contingencies are not present. Also, strategy training has not emphasized creativity and flexibility in generating novel applications during the rapid, dynamic flow of conversation. Therefore, an expanded approach to compensatory strategy training is suggested.

In enhanced compensatory strategy training, creativity, generativity, and interactivity are priorities. For example, rather than simply training a corpus of gestures or drawings, the client learns to generate ideas via vocalization, drawing, or gesture within a dynamic interchange. Examples include Lyon's (1995) interactive-drawing approach to training drawing as a collaborative effort between communication partners, and Demchuk's (1996) creative communication approach in which people with aphasia generate pantomime scenarios using principles drawn from dramatic enactment. In such approaches, creativity and spontaneity are reinforced. Clients are encouraged and supported in generating their own novel strategies, and existing strategies are reinforced and expanded. Therapy is conducted in a richly contextualized interaction. For example, drawing is practiced within a conversational exchange in which both the client and clinician augment verbal productions with drawings. The person with aphasia is considered a partner in identifying and elaborating a strategy repertoire.

Interactive as well as transactional strategies are included in enhanced compensatory strategy management. For example, strategies for shifting the communicative burden or encouraging the nonaphasic partner to continue talking might be important methods for a person with severe aphasia to stay in a conversation. A range of variables is considered in selecting strategies, such as the amount of "burden" placed on the partner (e.g., having to guess what a gesture means), stigma associated with the strategy (e.g., does it call attention), naturalness (e.g., performed relatively automatically versus requiring much conscious effort), time constraints (e.g., does it take too long), affect on the "flow" of interaction, and appropriateness in a specific context (e.g., attitudes, cultural norms) (Simmons-Mackie & Damico, 1997).

We as clinicians must maintain an open mind about potential strategies. That is, many strategies are not "normal" yet they constitute the best available alternative for a given person. For example, avoiding interaction is often considered a "problem" by speech-language pathologists who are anxious for their clients to use their residual communication skills to participate in society. However, if the client feels that participating is more "punishing" than sitting home alone, then the avoidance behavior serves a necessary social objective. In such a case it might be important to identify "supported" activities that are rewarding and work towards building contexts that satisfy the client's social needs, rather than eliminating a strategy without a viable alternative.

Conversational Coaching

Conversational coaching, introduced by Holland (1988; Hopper et al., 2002), provides for practice of communicative scenarios with the guidance of the speech-language pathologist, who serves as a "coach." The approach involves (1) identifying a goal or scenario to target in therapy; (2) planning what is needed; (3) developing a script and resources; (4) practicing with coaching as needed; (5) performing the scenario; and (6) evaluating the outcome. For example, one client wanted to "argue" with her dietitian about her unpalatable diet. Planning involved identifying the main ideas, how to begin, possible strategies, useful resources such as pictures and written words, and important details to convey. Together, the client and clinician developed a scripted scenario. Practice sessions revealed a number of potential weak spots and alternative strategies. In addition, manner of delivery was targeted to avoid angering the dietitian. In the process, the client identified strategies applicable to other situations and her confidence soared. Thus, a scripted scenario not only met a specific communicative need, but also served to build confidence and skill in general. In addition, the format of conversational coaching tends to "equalize" the roles of therapist (coach) and client (communication player), creating a more client-centered approach. Thus, an important element of coaching is the emphasis on symmetric discourse, the client's active role and attention to "face saving" as a priority (Leiwo, 1994). Another important element of conversational coaching is script-training. Scripts, prescribed or routinized courses of action or talk, pervade our daily lives. For example, favorite stories that are told and retold within families often have a relatively set structure and content. Routine activities often entail relatively habitual elements of communication (e.g., ordering from a catalog, calling a taxi). Various approaches to script- and text-training have been advocated for improving a range of discourse genres such as telling jokes or making introductions (Armstrong, 1993; Hinckley

& Carr, 2005; Youmans, Holland, Munoz, & Bourgeois, 2005).

Group Therapy

Group therapy is an effective context for improving communication and well-being in aphasia (Elman & Bernstein-Ellis, 1999a, 1999b). Moreover, groups provide an ideal context for conversation therapy. The key to addressing conversational skills within a group format is to focus on interaction rather than practicing didactic, discrete skills. Such groups foster a sense of joint purpose and emphasize meaningful communicative interactions (Graham & Avent, 2004). Overlaying a teaching style and traditional therapy tasks (e.g., naming, sentence formulation) onto a group is unlikely to fulfill the requirements of conversation therapy. Rather, promoting conversation within a group context requires considerable skill in facilitating participation, equalizing control, and promoting confidence. In addition to peer conversation, groups can build skill and confidence in a variety of natural communication genres such as telling stories, arguing, or complaining. Role-playing has been suggested as a mechanism for easing into difficult communication activities since groups can jointly problem-solve, enact roles, and evaluate performances. Texts and videos are now available with information and ideas for managing aphasia groups (Avent, 1997; Elman, 2007; Marshall, 1999; Pound et al., 2000).

Scaffolded and Supported Conversations

One method of promoting conversation that works well in a group or role-play context is to employ scaffolding techniques. In order to scaffold communication the clinician or other group members provide cues or facilitators within the natural flow of interaction. In other words, others mediate the participation of a person with aphasia. Damico (1992) proposes suggestions for scaffolding.

1. The clinician follows the communicative contributions of the client rather than controlling or directing the discourse. In other words, the clinician is available to expand and facilitate, but avoids "taking over" (e.g., asking all the questions, dictating topics, requesting performances).
2. Interaction emerges from a meaningful activity. For example, sharing vacation photos might elicit more interactive communication than asking someone to tell about a trip.
3. Responses are mediated or facilitated within the natural give-and-take of the interaction. For example, the clinician might use subtle gestural prompts or write key words to support a client during the interaction.
4. Feedback should be appropriate to the communication event. If the communication is understood, then the talk

proceeds; if not, then a request for clarification is in order. Thus, clients experience natural consequences for communicative success and failure, rather than evaluative feedback such as "good talking."

Contrast the following examples of communication. A group of people with aphasia have watched a short excerpt from an "I Love Lucy" show.

Example 1

Clinician: John, can you tell me about Lucy's job?
John: (Laughs) Eating.
Clinician: Well, (laughs) that is what she did, but what was her real job?
John: (Shrugs)
Clinician: George, what was her job supposed to be?
George: Candy.
Clinician: Good, she worked with candy. Claire, what was her job?
Claire: (gestures)
Clinician: Right, she was supposed to put the candy in the box.

Example 2

Clinician: (Laughing) Oh boy! Isn't that Lucy something?
Claire: (Laughing) (gestures shoving food into her mouth)
Clinician: (Laughs) (writes "eating" in large letters while Claire gestures)
John: Eating, eating (gestures).
Claire: Too much (laughing and gesturing).
Clinician: Eating candy! Not too much for me—I could eat it all.
George: Me too. Eat it all. Candy.
John: Mmm. I like candy.

The first example is a didactic, clinician-focused interaction in which the therapist attempts to elicit specific responses from the group members. The second example is a scaffolded conversation in which the content and direction flows with the group interaction. The clinician provides a written prompt ("eating") and models a verbal production ("I could eat it all") within the natural give-and-take of conversation. Although scaffolded conversation is the intent, it is appropriate for both the clinician and group members to occasionally "step outside" of the interaction to serve as "coaches" and make "meta" comments or suggest potentially useful strategies.

Duchan (1997) expands on the idea of scaffolding discourse to suggest that the therapist support multiple aspects of the interaction. She provides guidelines for interactive therapy with children that can be generalized to adults with aphasia. She suggests that the role of the clinician shifts from that of "interventionist imparting knowledge" to that of "facilitator supporting role change" (Duchan, 1997, p. 10). The supports provided include social (e.g., relating well, creating positive role identity), emotional (e.g., helping one another save face, feel empowered), functional (e.g., achieving communication goals), physical (e.g., providing accessible materials), discourse (e.g., scaffolding), and event support (e.g., providing contexts, letting participants know what to expect).

Partner Training

Another method of enhancing communication is through trained and knowledgeable communication partners. Partner-training is appropriate for family members, caregivers, friends, colleagues at work, and the community at large. Thus, interactions ranging from social conversation with poker buddies to discussion with one's attorney can be facilitated when speaking partners are knowledgeable and skilled. Training speaking partners actually improves the communication of the person with aphasia (Boles, 1997; Hickey et al., 2004; Hopper et al., 2002; Kagan et al., 2001; Lock et al., 2001; Lyon, 1997, 1998b; Lyon et al., 1997; Rogers et al., 1999; Simmons-Mackie et al., 2005). In fact, Kagan (1995, 1998; Kagan et al., 2001) reports that onlookers judge the aphasic speaker as more competent when they interact with a trained partner who provides "communication support." Thus, success of the interaction and judgments of competence depend not only on the person with aphasia, but also on the skills of the nonaphasic communication partner.

Partner training accomplishes several objectives. First, speaking partners learn concrete strategies to support communication when aphasia interferes. Second, trained speaking partners who use augmentative tools provide a context that encourages the partner with aphasia to use such modes. Third, partner training results in altered expectations and perceptions of speakers with aphasia. Once partners recognize that people with aphasia can be competent and interesting human beings, they are less likely to avoid interactions or feel bewildered by communicative failures. Finally, partner-training can expand opportunities for communication. By alleviating embarrassment, feelings of helplessness, and fear, it is more likely that partners will provide supportive opportunities to communicate.

Direct partner training and feedback are necessary for interactive patterns and techniques to be learned and incorporated into daily use (Simmons et al., 2005). Counseling or providing lists of do's and don'ts is insufficient. Moreover, communication partner training does not involve teaching partners to be "therapists" for the person with aphasia. In fact, such an approach often creates a teacher-student inter-active relationship that differs in structure and social dynamics from natural adult social interaction. Rather, a successful speaking partner requires an understanding of how to facilitate a satisfying conversation. This includes knowledge of potential strategies and insight into characteristics of interactive communication. Appendix 11-1 lists examples of compensatory strategies for speaking partners of people with aphasia. In addition to successful communication strategies, partners need to learn how to create an interaction that feels natural and reinforces the confidence and autonomy of the person with aphasia. Research suggests that an empowering attitude might be as important as use of a concrete strategy for speaking partners of people with aphasia (Simmons-Mackie & Kagan, 1999; Simmons-Mackie et al., 2005).

Improving the skills of the partner is only one part of the intervention: the person with aphasia is also responsible for promoting successful exchanges. Thus, intervention might be directed at people with aphasia along with their regular partners. Intervention aimed at the dyad often extends beyond didactic instruction in communicative skills. For example, programs have focused on various combinations of communicative-skills training, counseling, and education (Boles & Lewis, 2000; Fox et al., 2004; Hinckley & Packard, 2001; Purdy & Hindenlang, 2005; Sorin-Peters, 2004b).

Increasing Successful Participation in Authentic Communication Events

Without opportunities to communicate, improved language is a trivial accomplishment. For most of us, communication takes place in the context of life activities. For example, people converse while eating lunch with friends, attending art openings, or playing cards. In fact, research suggests that subjective well-being and involvement in social activity are positively associated (Cardol et al., 2002; Diener, 1984; Fuhrer, 1994; Fuhrer, Rintala, Hart, Clearman, & Young, 1992). Among individuals with physical disability "greater life satisfaction was reported by persons who were doing more to maintain customary social relationships . . . and spending more time in ways customary for their gender, age and culture" (Fuhrer, 1994, p. 362). In a social approach the speech-language pathologist is responsible for increasing opportunities for communication outside of the clinical environment and for addressing barriers beyond the individual's impairment.

One means of increasing participation in relevant communication events is to ensure that relevant life activities are accessible and successful (Lyon, 1996, 1997; Lyon et al., 1997; Simmons-Mackie, 1993, 1994, 2000). This might involve programs designed to provide supported-participation opportunities. Dedicated aphasia centers are now offering a variety of supported opportunities, such as leisure, exer-cise, and conversation groups for people with aphasia (e.g., www.aphasiacenter.org; www.aphasia.ca; www.ukconnect. org; www.ydac.on.ca). For example, the Aphasia Center of California provides a participation-based approach to improving reading skill and enjoyment. Book clubs are offered that involve guided reading assignments, adapted materials appropriate for various levels of aphasia, and facilitated group discussion (Bernstein-Ellis & Elman, 2006). Such participation provides a typical experience of everyday life with support. Moreover, anecdotal evidence suggests that guided participation may facilitate reading skill.

Other approaches focus specifically on enhancing participation in relevant life situations. (Lyon, 1996, 2000; Sarno & Chambers, 1997). Lyon (2004) describes individual intervention at the level of "life processes." His approach involves identifying what is important in someone's life, identifying barriers, and working with all concerned to facilitate participation in authentic life situations. Lyon warns that a good outcome of such intervention is a renewed sense of purpose and engagement in life, not necessarily "complete happiness" (since this is rarely achievable with or without aphasia). Similarly, activity-focused intervention involves identifying potential activities or life situations with the client and intervening to ensure successful participation (Simmons-Mackie, 2000). The activity need not be "communication-centered"; rather, the goal is to enhance life participation. Once an activity of choice is identified, then the clinician in collaboration with the person affected by aphasia determine characteristics of the activity that will be addressed to ensure success. This might involve working with the client to build specific skills or strategies and/or modifying the activity to accommodate the person with aphasia. It is particularly helpful for the clinician to participate in the identified activity in order to fully appreciate the requirements and identify an entry point that helps smooth the way for participation. Prior or existing pastimes as well as new activities are appropriate targets of intervention. It is not the intent to strive for a "pre-aphasia" lifestyle. Rather, a satisfying life with aphasia is the goal. The clinician, client, and others identify activity goals such as hobbies, interests, functional tasks, volunteer jobs, or employment in which the client would like to participate. Through interviews, prior interests and future aspirations can be gleaned. An interest survey can identify potential new activities. For example, clients might sort a large variety of activity pictures (e.g., grooming pets, cooking, gardening, painting, walking, etc.) into preference categories. In this way a rough inventory of preferences can serve as a starting point for identifying potential activities. It is important that choices are client-motivated and that participation is directly facilitated. Simply identifying an activity and encouraging participation is generally unsuccessful.

Case Example

Moderate Aphasia

TG, a woman with moderate aphasia, expressed interest in returning to her Bible class at church. In spite of improvements in communication and her expressed desire to return to class, she avoided doing so. A visit to the event with the clinician was initiated. During this visit TG and the clinician met privately with the bible-class teacher. At the suggestion of the teacher, TG agreed to pass out coffee and snacks, but insisted that she did not want to participate in the class discussion. The teacher suggested that TG and the clinician explain aphasia to the class. Since TG was visibly alarmed at this prospect, the clinician offered to present to the class. As TG greeted her old friends and served coffee her demeanor changed; the demands of serving did not require sophisticated conversation and allowed her a "soft" initiation back into the group. Interestingly, once the clinician began to talk to the class about aphasia TG "forgot" about her pledge to remain quiet and became absorbed in the discussion. During this discussion the therapist modeled various methods for facilitating interaction and made suggestions to the class members. Over the next few weeks, a variety of additional adaptations were identified. For example, the teacher provided TG with a written lesson-script that TG could use to follow the discussion and access difficult words. The class began using a flip chart to write key words during the discussions; all agreed that this facilitated their discussion as much as it helped TG. In effect, the teacher and other class members learned how to support TG's communication and facilitate her reentry into the class, and TG gained confidence in her ability to participate.

has been defined as a limitation of access to normal life due to physical or social barriers (French, 1993; Byng et al., 2000). Frameworks of health and disability have helped focus intervention on factors that affect participation (Kagan et al., in press; WHO, 2001). In such models both internal and external factors affect one's participation in life. Internal factors pertain to physical and psychological functions such as cognitive, linguistic, motor, or sensory integrity. These internal consequences, such as language-processing deficits, are often addressed in traditional rehabilitation. Environmental factors include the physical and social structures of the outside world. Physical barriers include architectural, visual, auditory, or temporal elements that disrupt communication or participation. For example, attempting to communicate in a noisy bank lobby or trying to conduct business when impatient people are waiting in line could be very difficult for a person with aphasia. Societal barriers to communication include attitudinal, political, governmental, economic, and educational factors. Barriers can be observable, such as complex written signs in buildings, or hidden, such as prejudice, negative attitudes, and ignorance. Garcia, Barrette, and Laroche (2000) suggest that sometimes a simple shift in viewpoint will reconfigure an impairment into a barrier that can be removed. For example, a person with aphasia who has difficulty talking on the telephone would be unable to perform a job that depends on phone use. Thus the "verbal impairment" of the individual prevents job performance. However, if the individual with aphasia could perform the same functions using electronic mail, then "phone use" can be considered a barrier that could be removed to help accommodate the disability. This shift in focus away from the problems of the individual and onto the external barriers is an important paradigm shift required in adopting a social approach (Garcia et al., 2000).

Providing Communicative Support Systems within the Speaker's Community

Related to measures designed to increase participation in relevant activities is the concept of providing an environment conducive to successful communication and participation. Participation in society is most likely to occur when environments are "aphasia-friendly" or communicatively accessible (Ghidella, Murray, Smart, McKenna, & Worrall, 2005; Kagan & LeBlanc, 2002; Simmons-Mackie et al., in press). A communicatively accessible environment provides ease of communication and access to information, systems, and choices (Howe et al., 2004). Thus, a goal of intervention is to create an environment that facilitates participation (Cardol et al., 2002). As noted above, this can be accomplished in part by identifying and modifying barriers within the environment. Similarly, it is important to identify methods of enabling participation, such as providing physical and

Activity-focused intervention shares similarities with traditional functional therapies that address performance of specific activities. However, many functional therapies focus on discrete tasks or generic skills such as writing a grocery list or ordering in a restaurant. Unfortunately, learning specific tasks does not ensure actual participation in the event. Functional approaches can be expanded to be more socially valid by ensuring that intervention is contextually situated and by modifying the environment as well as training the client. Thus, the functional task should be defined to address all parameters that will increase participation. Finally, a satisfying life is rarely limited to performing "chores"; therefore, it is important that an array of chosen life activities provide opportunities for socialization and fulfilling engagement.

In addition to intervention focusing directly on life habits, a related method of increasing participation is to identify and eliminate barriers to participation. Disability social accommodations. People with aphasia have a right to accessible communication and services even if this requires accommodations (ADA, 1990; ASHA, 1992). As Kagan and Gailey (1993) suggest, supported communication can be considered the "ramp" that enables people with aphasia to participate. A variety of environmental and social factors have been identified as potential barriers or facilitators for people with aphasia (Howe et al., 2004; Parr et al., 1997).

Skilled Partners and Prosthetic Communities

Partner-training (as discussed above) not only enhances communication, but also potentially expands opportunities for satisfying interactions. Thus, trained partners within an individual's community serve as communicative support systems and enable improved participation of the person with aphasia. In order to build expanded support systems, intervention might focus on training individuals within existing social networks. For example, a number of successful interventions with family members of the person with aphasia are reported in the literature (Boles, 1997; Hopper et al., 2002; Lyon, 1998b; Rogers et al., 1999; Simmons-Mackie et al., 2005). However, social life usually extends beyond our immediate family. Therefore, potential communication partners outside of the immediate family might be identified and trained. For example, a friend within the community (e.g., fellow club member, neighbor) might be willing to support community reentry.

In addition, the support system might be expanded to include new communication partners such as new acquaintances, aphasia-group members, volunteers, or peer mentors. Lyon (1992, 1997) has paired individuals with aphasia with a volunteer and worked on effective communication as a dyad. He also works with the dyad to identify an activity they can share as a means of facilitating life participation. Kagan (1998) and Hoen and colleagues (1997) describe community-based programs designed to provide opportunities for successful conversation between trained volunteers and people with aphasia. Peer mentors are another source of expanded social networks and supported communication. Peer mentors are individuals with aphasia who agree to visit, serve as social contacts, assist as advocates, help with counseling, or perform other needed services (Cohen-Schnieder, 1996; Ireland & Wotton, 1996). For example, two people with aphasia might be matched to fulfill some need such as providing a ride to an aphasia group or helping with a project. The helping relationship serves both individuals since helping others is often an important missing element after the onset of aphasia.

In addition to training specific individuals to interact with people with aphasia, community training is an important element of a social approach. Community education at religious institutions, community organizations, businesses, medical facilities, or educational institutions increases public knowledge and promotes positive attitudes. For example, Simmons-Mackie and colleagues (2007) describe a project designed to improve access to information and decision-making for people with aphasia within three health-care facilities. The project included staff training and on-site problem-solving to establish and support sustainable improvements in communicative access. Staff of the facilities reported changes, not only in their own ability to facilitate communicative access, but also in the culture of their programs and in the participation and well-being of clients with aphasia. Training people within the community in methods of supporting communication could have far-reaching consequences. Gradually the "community" of people trained to support communication with people with aphasia can be expanded, resulting in aphasia-friendly "prosthetic communities."

Resources as Supports

In addition to trained partners, a variety of resources such as pictures, paper and markers, remnant books, written aids, vocabulary notebooks, maps, or communication boards can support communication. The Pictographic Communication Resource Manual is a collection of thematically organized pictures developed specifically to support conversation with people with aphasia (Kagan, Winckel, & Shumway, 1996a, 1996b). In addition, pictographic resources aimed at particular groups (e.g., clergy, nurses, physical therapists) can enhance communicative interactions (Kagan & Shumway, 2003). Studies have demonstrated that graphic support or written key-word choices during conversation promote increased participation of the person with aphasia (Garrett & Beukelman, 1995; Garrett & Huth, 2002). Lasker and colleagues (2005) describe resources used to support a college professor with aphasia that included a computer-based communication system with synthesized voice output and "key word" PowerPoint slides. Others also report various computer aides designed to support communication in aphasia (Bruce, Edmundson, & Coleman, 2003). A variety of resources have been suggested to prevent institutionalized individuals with aphasia from remaining "anonymous" to caregivers. Communication plans that specify likes and dislikes and life-story notebooks that give a brief history with family photos, and key life events can provide a context for sharing information with caregivers (Genereux et al., 2004; LeDorze, 1997). Remnant books or memory albums also serve as resources to initiate topics and sustain conversation. Changes in physical environments can also support communication (e.g., a surface for writing, changing seating arrangements) (Lubinski, 2001). Finally, several reports describe the potential power of "aphasia-friendly" Web sites for linking people with aphasia to goods and information. Characteristics of accessible Web sites include a variety of modifications such as simplified text, reduced visual distractions, pictures to augment text, and large print (Egan, Worrall, & Oxenham, 2004; Elman, 2001; Elman, Parr, & Moss, 2003; Ghidella et al., 2005; Petheram, Parr, Moss, Byng, & Newbery, 2004; Rose et al., 2003; Singh, 2000).

Increasing Communicative Confidence and Positive Sense of Self

Human beings place great value on feeling important and successful. In fact, much of our communication is crafted to present a public identity or "face" (Goffman, 1967). Our view of ourselves is "reevaluated" constantly as we interact with others and obtain verification or contradiction of our perceived self-image and roles (Brumfitt, 1993). Communication and identity are entwined with the social roles we enact. Unfortunately, role change is a major consequence of aphasia. For example, unemployment after aphasia often results in the loss of a significant role and important part of one's "identity." Similarly, each communicative interaction has the potential to disrupt one's self-image as a competent person. The cycle of communication breakdown, changed social roles, and loss of identity can undermine the goals of aphasia therapy. Therefore, a positive outcome depends on the development of a healthy sense of self with aphasia (Brumfitt, 1993; Byng et al., 2000; Sarno, 1993a, 1993b, 1997). A robust identity not only contributes to improved quality of life but also directly relates to one's willingness to use residual communication skills. The person who lacks confidence is far less likely to risk participating in social situations. Development of productive new roles, robust identities, and healthy relationships often depends on support and external assistance or direction (Rolland, 1994). For example, research suggests that positive supportive relationships (i.e., those that foster autonomy while facilitating communication) strengthen self-esteem and confidence among people with aphasia, while patronizing, controlling, or negative interactions reduce confidence and motivation to participate (Andersson & Fridlund, 2002).

Modifying the Structure and Content of Services

In part, a healthy identity can be encouraged by attending to how our services promote or inhibit an empowered identity. Impairment-oriented therapy might actually undermine the development of a healthy identity with aphasia by emphasizing what is wrong and exposing failures (Byng et al., 2000; Ferguson & Armstrong, 2004; Simmons-Mackie & Damico, 1999). The social structure of traditional therapy could also devalue the person with aphasia by reinforcing the roles of "expert" therapist and "impaired" patient (Simmons-Mackie & Damico, 1999). Byng and colleagues (2000) caution that we must work on impairments with sensitivity, keeping in mind the potential effects on the developing sense of self of the person with aphasia. Perhaps by modifying the didactic

structure of therapy and moving towards a collaborative partnership approach, we might enhance the client's autonomy and sense of self. Furthermore, moving the emphasis away from the impairment and onto the interaction and external barriers reduces the emphasis on individual problems. Attention to the emotional impact of our services is as important as attention to the linguistic effects.

Case Example

Anomic Aphasia

RT, a 55-year-old man with anomic aphasia, contacted a university clinic seeking therapy. RT was 10 years post-onset and had functioned for the past 8 years independently. Although unemployed, he managed his own investments and enjoyed travel to visit friends. RT described his disability as "not too bad." His reasons for self-referral were to improve his ability to write letters and to converse in groups. RT attended the university clinic for an initial assessment that entailed administration of several standardized aphasia tests by a young female student-clinician. Later, the student-clinician and supervisor conducted a detailed counseling session to appraise RT of the test results. The assessment and subsequent conference were typical of a traditional evaluation. RT was visibly upset during the testing and conference. He remarked that he had no idea he was "so bad off" and appeared embarrassed to have "appeared the fool" in front of the "pretty girl." His usually outgoing personality gave way to depression as he faced his self-delusion regarding the extent of his disability.

This example raises an important ethical question: Was the exposure of residual deficits via standard testing in the best interest of this client? Standardized assessment did not allow RT to use many of his compensatory strategies to succeed. The assessment did provide a "window" into the pattern and severity of his language disorder; however, it also markedly impacted RT's self-confidence and sense of self. Traditionally, the importance of linguistic data might outweigh the negative psychosocial impact. However, a social model forces us to reconsider and weigh the overall impact of our practices on the person as a whole. This example is not an argument for eliminating standard tests; rather, it is an argument for carefully considering the client's stated goals and the potential impact of each procedure on communicative, social, and psychological well-being.

Modifying Our Own Language and Attitudes

Our language and attitudes can also empower or enable others. As specialists in language, aphasiologists undoubtedly know the power of words. Duchan (1997) describes "negative rhetoric" associated with medical approaches and more positive rhetoric often used in participation approaches. Shifting our usage to wording that avoids the biases of the medical model might help the client focus on living with aphasia over the long term. Thus, words such as "patient," "treatment," and "discharge" imply a "treatment and recovery" course similar to illness. Such terms reinforce the illness model and possibly allow us to shed some of our responsibility for long-term outcome. Substituting goals such as "reintegration" as opposed to "discharge" shifts the emphasis to the chronic nature of aphasia, and promotes a client-centered rather than service-delivery emphasis.

In addition, language can help those affected by aphasia learn that the person is not the disorder (Rolland, 1994). Too often the disability and the "self" become one (Goffman, 1963). Language can help externalize the disorder to reinforce the fact that the person is far more than the aphasia. For example, saying "you seem to be having trouble with your bridge club" places the burden on the person, while saying "the aphasia seems to be getting in the way of participating in your bridge club" places the onus on the aphasia. Thus, problems are the disorder, not the person. Attention to service-delivery styles and language use can help ensure that our practices promote a healthy identity as well as improved communication.

Counseling and Psychosocial Support

In addition to examining the structure of therapy and our own language, speech-language pathologists have a responsibility for aspects of counseling (Brumfitt, 1993; Cunningham, 1998; Holland, 1999; Luterman, 2001; Müller, 1999; Wahrborg, 1989). Those affected by aphasia need information and guidance in exploring the effects of aphasia on their lives. The speech-language pathologist is uniquely qualified to help other professionals understand the consequences of aphasia, to teach supported communication, and to ensure that counseling needs are met. In addition, counseling and communication intervention overlap. For example, disability powerfully affects relationships and role boundaries within families and couples (Rolland, 1994). Typically communication processes are critical for reestablishing a functional, balanced relationship. With aphasia the pre-onset modes of communication within relationships are altered. Focusing intervention at the level of the "couple" can assist both parties in identifying new ways of communicating (Boles, 1997; Boles & Lewis, 2000; Lyon, 1998b; Purdy & Hindenlang, 2005; Sorin-Peters, 2004b).

In fact, many aspects of aphasia therapy fall squarely within the realm of counseling. Counseling should be an integral part of therapy for aphasia since language is required for negotiating new identities and developing strategies for coping with life (Moss, Parr, Byng, & Pertheram, 2004). Clinicians can promote well-being by adopting an active "listening" role instead of an "instructing" role; that is, by sharing control with the person with aphasia and acknowledging his or her lived expertise in aphasia. Holland (in progress) advocates for applying principles of positive psychology to aphasia intervention. The values of a positive health approach can promote well-being, optimism, and hopefulness—elements important to living successfully with aphasia (Andersson & Fridlund, 2002; Sveen et al., 2004). In addition, LaPointe (2005) reminds us that an important aspect of coping involves finding the small things in life that make it worth living—"dressing up . . . soaking in a Jacuzzi . . . saving a manatee . . . helping others . . . renting a goofy movie . . . [or] listening to an audiotape" (p. 16).

Psychosocial support groups, caregiver support groups, and self-advocacy groups might serve to expand this counseling focus (Byng et al., 2000; Elman, 2007; Holland & Ross, 1999; Pound et al., 2000). The chance to "tell their stories" not only provides communication opportunities for people with aphasia and caregivers but, when appropriately validated, sharing stories is an important means of building a new sense of self with aphasia (Moss, Parr, Byng, & Pertheram, 2004; Pound, 2004). Groups provide a context for exploring topics related to living with aphasia such as identity, stress management, relationships, and emotions. Caregiver groups help those who experience aphasia as a family member or caregiver to address concrete issues, provide psychological support, and help build new identities. Self-help groups provide a mechanism for people confronting aphasia to define their own needs and assist each other in addressing these needs (Coles & Eales, 1999).

Adult-learning approaches that combine elements of education, counseling, and communication skills-training have been introduced for people with aphasia and their family members (Purdy & Hindenlang, 2005; Sorin-Peters, 2004b). Such methods approach the "learners" (people with aphasia and family members) as competent adults and collaborators in the learning process. Change evolves out of the learner's own experiences, reflective observations, and active experimentation. An important "counseling" element of such programs is the chance for participants to explore and validate the experience of living with aphasia. Reported outcomes include not only improved communicative skills but also changes in emotional well-being and relationships.

Self-Advocacy and Empowerment

Byng and colleagues (2000) propose self-advocacy as a means of (1) enhancing self-esteem, (2) developing skills and knowledge, and (3) promoting empowerment. Strategies for promoting self-advocacy include focusing on strengths, building social and political consciousness, promoting a group or community identity, gaining a role in community service, and ensuring that people with aphasia are partners in, rather than recipients of, services. Pound (1998a) described a self-advocacy project in which people with aphasia developed personal portfolios. Like pictorial vitae many of the portfolios depicted life before and after the onset of aphasia. Clients reported that this process of examining their lives resulted in significant insights into their own identity and appreciation for their accomplishments since the onset of aphasia.

Self-advocacy groups have addressed topics such as identity and life roles, attitudes towards disability, assertiveness, and development of support networks (Pound, 1998a; Byng et al., 2000). Individuals explore personal values and identify values that are inconsistent with a healthy self with aphasia (Fuhrer, 1994). For example, placing high value on being an expert storyteller might be contrary to achieving a satisfactory view of oneself. Instead of the "storyteller," the person with aphasia might need to identify other aspects of his or her self upon which to build self-worth (e.g., pet lover, father, spiritual person). Clients might explore new ways of expressing personalities. For example, Simmons-Mackie (2004a) offers suggestions for alternate methods of conveying humor. Clients can learn that methods of expressing oneself need not be traditional; painting, drawing, poetry, dramatics, and music also serve self-expression and release. Exploring such issues in a group with other people with aphasia can help with the reassessment of life values and objectives.

Caveats of a Social Approach

Communication provides a foundation for maintaining autonomy—the right to make our own decisions, freedom from control by others, and the ability to enforce our own values. Thus, a goal of aphasia intervention is to promote choice, freedom from control, and expression of personal values. However, any therapy approach carries with it the potential for invading rights and privacy. Therapists must avoid imposing their own values and choices in the name of treatment. Expanding and supporting participation is not to be construed as a license to "remake" peoples' lives according to our own prescriptions and values. Work must be conducted in complete collaboration with those affected by aphasia and with an understanding of their values and desires. Confidentiality and sensitivity to intrusion into personal situations and relationships are extremely important. If partners are to be recruited and trained, the clinician must ensure that the help is not invasive or embarrassing to those involved. Explanations of intervention procedures or contracts in simple written and pictograph form might ensure that clients fully understand the methods and objectives of intervention, and participate in the plan and implementation. Part of a successful outcome in aphasia intervention involves enforcing a sense of one's own autonomy and personal rights.

Promoting Advocacy and Social Action

The role of the speech-language pathologist includes not only intervention with those affected by aphasia but also development of social and political systems that support par-

ticipation for people with aphasia. Advocacy means that we "practice what we preach" relative to inclusion. For example, people with aphasia can serve as aphasia-group leaders or co-facilitate groups. People with aphasia can be "teacher-clients," rather than patients, in university clinics in recognition of their unique and valuable perspectives. People affected by aphasia are qualified to serve on our boards of advisors or as co-investigators in research. Aphasia-group members can offer services as a panel of experts to educate others such as allied-health students or community leaders. Byng and Duchan (2005) provide examples of how people with aphasia might be integrated into organizations at all levels. For example, board meetings with aphasic members are conducted in accessible language with aphasia-friendly supports. Through these expanded roles, accessibility strategies are modeled. Such partnerships offer many advantages, not the least of which is the bold affirmation of the expertise and value of people with aphasia.

Speech-language pathologists and those affected by aphasia have an important role in building public recognition of aphasia and promoting availability of accessible services. Aphasia is a relative "unknown." In fact, in a recent public survey only 5% of those surveyed knew the meaning of the term "aphasia" (Simmons-Mackie, Code, Armstrong, Stiegler, & Elman, 2002). Aphasia is mentioned in the public press with much lower frequency than other disorders with similar incidence rates (Elman, Ogar, & Elman, 2000). The impacts of poor public awareness include reduced funding for research and services, lack of understanding and acceptance by the public, and barriers inadvertently reinforced by political and public actions (Elman et al., 2000). Advocacy activities promote the development of a "group identity" for those affected by aphasia and increase public awareness. Advocacy efforts can also be integrated into aphasia management to provide a context for building a positive sense of self with aphasia while simultaneously educating the public.

Case Example

Identity Work

MC, a 62–year old woman with Broca's aphasia and apraxia of speech, had attended individual and group therapy for several years. According to her family, MC remained depressed and socially isolated and failed to participate in former activities. Within her aphasia group MC often complained about the "bad treatment" that she received in the community, particularly in medical encounters. For example, she described how nurses and doctors talked to her husband and ignored her "like she was a lump of nothing." She related stories of overhearing nurses talking about her as if she were not present, and described patronizing and incomprehensible interactions with health-care providers. After hearing these stories on several occasions, the clinician suggested that she and other group members "do something" to educate health-care providers. The result was an "expert panel" designed for people with aphasia to present their stories to classes in a local nursing program. Panel members worked with their therapists to create scripts and practice presentations with various communication supports. MC approached this experience with gusto—she felt that she must be an advocate for people with aphasia. Each semester the group described their prior feelings of helplessness and inadequacy in health-care encounters and offered insight into methods that the nursing students might use to facilitate communication and interactions. MC announced to her therapist that she felt like a "new me" and described recent encounters in health care—"now they listen to me." Friends and family noted a change in MC's demeanor and confidence. The panel experience not only provided MC with a communication opportunity; it also gave her life renewed meaning and enhanced her self-esteem and assertiveness.

Along with public recognition, inclusion of people with aphasia in existing community services is necessary. People with aphasia have a right to access information and services such as adult-education and leisure programs. Texts that provide information about coping with aphasia can be made available to those confronting aphasia (e.g., Lyon, 1998a). Manuals written in a style that is accessible to people with aphasia can outline available resources and benefits (e.g., Parr, Pound, Byng, & Long, 1999; Sarno & Peters, 2004). Aphasia-friendly Web sites can provide information as well as social connections to other people with aphasia (e.g., www.aphasiahelp.org; www.shrs.uq.edu.au/cdaru). Pictographic "consent forms" and documents promote access to health-care choices for people with severe aphasia (Kagan & Kimelman, 1995; Simmons-Mackie et al., 2007). Organizations such as the National Aphasia Association (United States) (www.aphasia.org), the Aphasia Hope Foundation (www.aphasiahope.org), and Speakability (United Kingdom) (www.speakability.org.uk) provide information and support. Public education can help inform others of methods that can be used to increase accessibility and participation (Appendix 11-2).

THE FUTURE OF SOCIAL APPROACHES: EXPANDING SERVICE-DELIVERY OPTIONS

With the advent of social models and changing health-care systems, alternative means of delivering services are being explored and advocated. For example, the prevailing practice of offering treatment for aphasia only during the acute stage

has been criticized (Elman, 1998; LPAA, 2000; Lyon, 1992; Simmons-Mackie, 1998b). Rather than shift from treatment to no treatment, a continuum of services should be available throughout the person's life with aphasia (Elman, 1998; Pound, 1998b; Simmons-Mackie, 1998b). Expanding our concept of services in aphasia requires that we recognize that aphasia is both an acute problem and a lifelong condition for those affected. As people learn to live with aphasia and as life situations change, the need for and type of services will change. Changed living arrangements, marriage, death of a loved one, or an opportunity for employment can create new goals and challenges. Ideally, those affected by aphasia should have access to support and professional expertise during such life changes. Services might constitute an array from which clients can select those appropriate to their current life goals (Elman, 1998). Thus, in addition to individual and group therapy, a range of services such as community-based programs, support groups, self-help programs, advocacy services, vocational programs, leisure programs, educational services, and counseling might be appropriate (Müller, 1999). An expanded service-delivery model will likely involve changes in our own services, as well as addition of services outside the domain of speech-language pathology. Expanding services beyond the health-care umbrella to include social or community agencies is a possibility. Adult day-centers and programs for the elderly might be re-engineered to accommodate those affected by aphasia. Adult-education programs such as basic computer and Internet training or art classes can be tailored to people with communication disabilities. Although not all of these services should or can be offered by speech-language pathologists, the speech-language pathologist is uniquely situated to ensure that the availability of varied services is adequately addressed. Thus, our roles, responsibilities, and payment sources are likely to shift as service delivery adjusts to changing demands.

As recently as 2004, Sarno listed the most compelling issues affecting intervention for aphasia, including: (1) limited access to services due to funding; (2) continued adherence to a medical model of recovery and rehabilitation; (3) views that aphasia intervention is exclusively a process of language repair; (4) ongoing stigmatization of aphasia associated with an uninformed and intolerant society; and (5) a lack of specialized services that include intervention aimed at the communicative, social, and psychological consequences of aphasia. Clearly, the future must address these barriers to holistic services for those affected by aphasia. A first step for clinicians and programs is to build a culture consonant with social model values.

CONCLUSION

Social approaches to intervention hold promise for promoting inclusion of people affected by aphasia in a communicating society. Creative and socially motivated approaches to management of aphasia are emerging around the world. Such approaches have arisen from the belief that communication is more than putting words together to get an idea across. Rather, communication is part of the foundation of social structure and human dignity. This philosophy drives efforts to establish effective and efficient methods for enhancing the living of life with aphasia. As Sarno has suggested, aphasia rehabilitation is a moral imperative in which "those who work with the communication-disabled are members of a moral community seeking to empower and restore individuals to a meaningful life experience" (Sarno, 2004, p. 28). The opportunity to retool aphasia management in keeping with this view is both an exciting and daunting prospect.

KEY POINTS

1. Adopting a social model requires a philosophical shift from traditional, medical-model approaches.
2. A social model is based on the belief that communication is a social act; through communication we create and express our ideas, our identities, and our life values, and ensure our membership in society.
3. In a social approach, communication and psychosocial functioning are considered inseparable.
4. A social approach focuses not only on communication and life participation of those affected by aphasia, but also on the communicative, physical, social, and emotional environment.
5. Long-term personal consequences of aphasia are the focus of intervention in a social approach.
6. Traditional clinician roles and service-delivery models are likely to expand and change with the adoption of social approaches.
7. The ultimate aim of a social approach is to enhance the living of life with aphasia.

ACTIVITIES FOR REFLECTION AND DISCUSSION

1. List all of the activities or events that you participated in over the past week. Consider the effects that aphasia might have on each of these activities or events. Choose one of the activities and consider methods for modifying the activity to support someone with moderate aphasia.
2. Discuss the differences between a medical model of aphasia intervention and a social model of aphasia intervention.
3. Explain the relationship between psychosocial adjustment and communication.

4. What are the principles of a social approach as defined in this chapter?
5. Listen to a "real" conversation (e.g., friends, coworkers). Identify examples of the following within the conversation:
   a. Behavior designed to "save face" or project an "identity"
   b. Evidence of "collaboration" in conversation
   c. Behavior that "deviates" from accurate, syntactically complete sentences
   d. Strategies that seem to help manage the interaction rather than add specific "information"
6. Garcia and colleagues (2000) provide an example of reconfiguring a functional disability (inability to use the phone) into an external barrier (lack of availability of electronic mail) as a means of identifying accommodations for people with aphasia. Think of two examples of "problems" in aphasia that might be "recast" as external barriers.
7. How does assessment in a social approach differ from traditional assessment (e.g., standardized aphasia tests, probes of language behaviors)?
8. How does traditional therapy discourse usually differ from natural, adult conversation?
9. What is "enhanced compensatory-strategy training"?
10. What are four possible benefits of training the communication partner of a person with aphasia?
11. What is an aphasia-friendly "prosthetic community"?
12. Describe one method of enhancing a positive sense of self with aphasia.

References

Americans with Disabilities Act (ADA) 1990, Public law 101-336(s.933); July 26, US Congressional Record, 36, 104 STAT, 327–379.

American Speech-Language-Hearing Association (1992). Communication and the ADA. *ASHA*, 62–65.

Andersson, S., & Fridlund, B. (2002). The aphasic person's views of the encounter with other people: A grounded theory analysis. *Journal of Psychiatric and Mental Health Nursing, 9*, 285–292.

Armstrong, E. (1993). Aphasia rehabilitation: A sociolinguistic perspective. In A. Holland (Ed.), *Aphasia treatment: World perspectives* (pp. 263–290). San Diego: Singular.

Avent, J. (1997). *Manual of cooperative group treatment for aphasia.* Boston: Butterworth-Heinemann.

Baum, C., & Edwards, D. (2001). *Activity Card Sort.* St. Louis: Washington University School of Medicine.

Beeke, S., Wilkinson, R., & Maxim, J. (2003). Exploring aphasic grammar 2: Do language testing and conversation tell a similar story? *Clinical Linguistics and Phonetics, 17*, 109–134.

Bell, A. (1984). Language style as audience design. *Language and Society, 13*, 145–204.

Bernstein-Ellis, E., & Elman, R. (2006). *The Book Connection™: A life participation book club for individuals with acquired reading impairment*. [Manual]. Oakland, CA: Aphasia Center of California. (available at www.aphasiacenter.org).

Blomert, L., Kean, M., Koster, C., & Schokker, J. (1994). Amsterdam-Nijmegen Everyday Language Test: Construction, reliability, and validity. *Aphasiology, 8*, 381–407.

Boles, L. (1997). Conversation analysis as a dependent measure in communication therapy with four individuals with aphasia. *Asia Pacific Journal of Speech, Language and Hearing, 2*, 43–61.

Boles, L., & Lewis, M. (2000). Solution-focused co-therapy for a couple with aphasia. *Asia Pacific Journal of Speech, Language and Hearing, 5*, 73–78.

Booth, S., & Perkins, L. (1999). The use of conversation analysis to guide individualized advice to careers and evaluate change in aphasia: A case study. *Aphasiology, 13*, 283–304.

Bouchard-Lamothe, D., Bourassa, S., Laflamme, B., Garcia, L., Gailey, G., & Stiell, K. (1999). Perceptions of three groups of interlocutors of the effects of aphasia on communication: An exploratory study. *Aphasiology, 13*, 839–856.

Bradburn, N. (1969). *The structure of well-being*. Chicago: Aldine.

Bruce, C., Edmundson, A., & Coleman, M. (2003). Writing with voice: An investigation of the use of a voice recognition system as a writing aid for a man with aphasia. *International Journal of Language and Communication Disorders, 38*, 131–148.

Brumfitt, S. (1993). Losing your sense of self: What aphasia can do. *Aphasiology, 7*, 569–591.

Button, J., & Lee, J. (Eds.). (1987). *Talk and social organization*. Clevedon, England: Multilingual Matters.

Byng, S., & Duchan, J. (2005). Social model philosophies and principles: Their applications to therapies for aphasia. *Aphasiology, 19*(10–11), 906–922.

Byng, S., Pound, C., & Parr, S. (2000). Living with aphasia: A framework for therapy interventions. In I. Papathanasiou (Ed.), *Acquired neurological communication disorders: A clinical perspective* (pp. 49–75). London: Whurr.

Cardol, M., de Haan, R., Van den Bos, G., & de Groot, I. (1999). The development of a handicap assessment questionnaire: The impact on participation and autonomy (IPA). *Clinical Rehabilitation, 13*, 411–419.

Cardol, M., De Jong, B., & Ward, C. (2002). On autonomy and participation in rehabilitation. *Disability and Rehabilitation, 24*(18), 970–974.

Chubon, R. A. (1987). Development of a quality-of-life rating scale for use in health care evaluation. *Evaluation and the Health Professions, 10*, 186–200.

Clark, H., & Wilkes-Gibbs, D. (1986). Referring as a collaborative process. *Cognition, 22*, 1–39.

Code, C., & Müller, D. (1992). The Code-Müller Protocols. London: Whurr.

Cohen-Schneider, R. (1996, November). *Peer support and leadership training program for aphasic adults*. Paper presented at the meeting of the American Speech-Language-Hearing Association, Seattle, WA.

Coles, R., & Eales, C. (1999). The aphasia self-help movement in Britain: A challenge and an opportunity. In R. Elman (Ed.), *Group treatment for neurogenic communication disorders: The expert clinician's approach* (pp. 107–114). Woburn, MA: Butterworth-Heinemann.

Corrigan, J., Smith-Knapp, K., & Granger, C. (1998). Outcomes in the first 5 years after traumatic brain injury. *Archives of Physical Medicine and Rehabilitation, 79*, 298–305.

Craig Hospital Inventory of Environmental Factors (CHIEF). (2001). Englewood, CO: Craig Hospital. Retrieved on August 12, 2004 from http://www.tbims.org/combi/chief/chiefprop.html

Cruice, M., Worrall, L., Hickson, L., & Murison, R. (2003). Finding a focus for quality of life in aphasia: Social and emotional health, and psychological well-being. *Aphasiology, 17*(4), 333–354.

Cruice, M., Worrall, L., Hickson, L., & Murison, R. (2005). Measuring quality of life: Comparing family members' and friends' ratings with those of their aphasic partners. *Aphasiology, 19*(2), 111–129.

Cunningham, R. (1998). Counseling someone with severe aphasia: An explorative case study. *Disability and Rehabilitation, 20*, 346–354.

Damico, J. (1992). *Whole language for special needs children*. Buffalo, NY: Educom Associates.

Damico, J., Simmons-Mackie, N., Oelschlaeger, M., Elman, R., & Armstrong, E. (1999). Qualitative methods in aphasia research: Basic issues. *Aphasiology, 13*, 651–666.

Davidson, B., Worrall, L., & Hickson, L. (1999, September). *Activity limitations in aphasia: Evidence from naturalistic observations*. Paper presented at the British Aphasiology Conference, London,

Davis, A., & Wilcox, J. (1985). *Adults aphasia rehabilitation: Applied pragmatics*. San Diego: College Hill Press.

Demchuk, M. (1996, November). *Creative communication in aphasia*. Paper presented at the meeting of the American Speech-Language-Hearing Association, Seattle, WA.

Diener, E. (1984). Subjective well-being. *Psychological Bulletin, 95*, 542–575.

Doyle, P. (2005). Advancing the development and understanding of patient-based outcomes in persons with aphasia. *Neurophysiology and Neurogenic Speech and Language Disorders, ASHA Special Interest Division 2, 15*(4), 7–9.

Doyle, P., Mikolic, J., Prieto, L., Hula, W., Lustig, A., Ross, K., et al. (2004). The Burden of Stroke Scale (BOSS) provided valid and reliable score estimates of functioning and well-being in stroke survivors with and without communication disorders. *Journal of Clinical Epidemiology, 57*, 997–1007.

Duchan, J. (1997). A situated pragmatics approach to supporting children with severe communication disorders. *Topics in Language Disorders, 17*, 1–18.

Duchan, J. (2001). Impairment and social views of speech-language pathology: Clinical practices re-examined. *Advances in Speech-Language Pathology, 3*(1), 37–45.

Egan, J., Worrall, L., & Oxenham, D. (2004). Accessible internet training package helps people with aphasia cross the digital divide. *Aphasiology, 18*, 265–280.

Elman, R. (1998). Memories of the 'plateau': Health-care changes provide an opportunity to redefine aphasia treatment and discharge. *Aphasiology, 12*, 227–231.

Elman, R. Editor. (2007). *Group treatment for neurogenic communication disorders: The expert clinician's approach*. (Second Edition). San Diego, CA: Plural Publishing.

Elman, R. (2000). *Working with groups: Neurogenic communication disorders* (Video). American Speech-Language-Hearing Association

(Producer) Rockville, MD: American Speech-Language-Hearing Association.

Elman, R. (2001). The internet and aphasia: Crossing the digital divide. *Aphasiology, 15,* 895–899.

Elman, R. (2005). Social and life participation approaches to aphasia intervention. In L. LaPointe (Ed.), *Aphasia and related neurogenic language disorders* (pp. 39–50). New York: Thieme.

Elman, R., & Bernstein-Ellis, E. (1999a). The efficacy of group communication treatment in adults with chronic aphasia. *Journal of Speech, Language, and Hearing Research, 42,* 411–419.

Elman, R., & Bernstein-Ellis, E. (1999b). Psychosocial aspects of group communication treatment: Preliminary findings. *Seminars in Speech & Language, 20*(1), 65–72.

Elman, R., Ogar, J., & Elman, S. (2000). Aphasia: Awareness, advocacy, and activism. *Aphasiology, 14,* 455–459.

Elman, R., Parr, S., & Moss, B. (2003). The internet and aphasia: Crossing the digital divide. In S. Parr, J. Duchan, & C. Pound (Eds), *Aphasia inside out* (pp. 103–116). Buckingham, UK: Open University Press.

Engell, B., Hutter, B., Willmes, K., & Huber, W. (2003). Quality of life in aphasia: Validation of a pictorial self-rating procedure. *Aphasiology, 17,* 383–396.

Erlich, J., & Barry, P. (1989). Rating communication behaviors in the head injured adult. *Brain Injury, 3,* 193–198.

Ferguson, A., & Armstrong, E. (2004). Reflections on speech-language therapists' talk: Implications for clinical practice and education. *International Journal of Language and Communication Disorders, 39*(4), 469–507.

Fox, L., Poulsen, S., Bawden, K., & Packard, D. (2004). Critical elements and outcomes of a residential family-based intervention for aphasia caregivers. *Aphasiology, 18*(12), 1177–1199.

Frank, A. (1995). *The wounded storyteller: Body, illness and ethics.* Chicago: University of Chicago Press.

Frattali, C. (1996). Clinical care in a changing health care system. In N. Helm-Estabrooks & A. Holland (Eds.), *Approaches to the treatment of aphasia* (pp. 241–265). San Diego: Singular.

Frattali, C. (1998a). Assessing functional outcomes: An overview. *Seminars in Speech and Language, 19,* 209–221.

Frattali, C. (1998b). Measuring modality-specific behaviors, functional abilities, and quality of life. In C. Frattali (Ed.), *Measuring outcomes in speech-language pathology* (pp. 55–88). New York: Thieme.

Frattali, C., Thompson, C., Holland, A., Wohl, C., & Ferketic, M. (1995). *The American Speech-Language-Hearing Association functional assessment of communication skills for adults (ASHA FACS).* Rockville, MD: ASHA.

French, S. (1993). What's so great about independence? In J. Swain, F. Finklestein, S. French, & M. Oliver (Eds.), *Disabling barriers—Enabling environments* (pp. 44–48). London: Sage.

Fuhrer, M. (1994). Subjective well-being: Implications for medical rehabilitation outcomes and models of disablement. *American Journal of Physical Medicine and Rehabilitation, 73,* 358–364.

Fuhrer, M., Rintala, D., Hart, K., Clearman, R., & Young, M. (1992). Relationship of life satisfaction to impairment, disability and handicap among persons with spinal cord injury living in the community. *Archives of Physical Medicine and Rehabilitation, 73,* 552–557.

Garcia, L., Barrette, J., & Laroche, C. (2000). Perceptions of the obstacles to work reintegration for persons with aphasia. *Aphasiology, 14,* 269–290.

Garrett, K. (1999). Measuring outcomes of group therapy. In R. Elman (Ed.), *Group treatment of neurogenic communication disorders: The expert clinician's approach* (pp. 17–30). Boston: Butterworth-Heinemann.

Garrett, K., & Beukelman, D. (1995). Changes in the interactive patterns of an individual with severe aphasia given three types of partner support. In M. Lemme (Ed.), *Clinical aphasiology,* (Vol. 23, pp. 237–251). Austin, TX: Pro-Ed.

Garrett, K., & Huth, C. (2002). The impact of graphic contextual information and instruction on the conversational behaviors of a person with severe aphasia. *Aphasiology, 16,* 523–536.

Genereux, S., Julien, M., Larfeuil, C., Lavoie, V., Soucy, O., & LeDorze, G. (2004). Using communication plans to facilitate interactions with communication-impaired persons residing in long-term care institutions. *Aphasiology, 18*(12), 1161–1175.

Ghidella C., Murray, S., Smart, M., McKenna, K., & Worrall, L. (2005). Aphasia websites: An examination of their quality and communicative accessibility. *Aphasiology, 19*(12).

Giles, H., Taylor, D., & Bourhis, R. (1973). Towards a theory of interpersonal accommodation through language: Some Canadian data. *Language in Society, 2,* 177–192.

Goffman, I. (1963). *Stigma: Notes on the management of spoiled identity.* New York: Touchstone.

Goffman, I. (1967). *Interaction ritual.* New York: Pantheon Books.

Goodwin, C. (1987). Forgetfulness as an interactive resource. *Social Psychology Quarterly, 50,* 115–131.

Goodwin, C. (1995). Co-constructing meaning in conversations with an aphasic man. *Research on Language and Social Interaction, 28,* 233–260.

Goodwin, C. (Ed.) (2003). *Conversation and brain damage.* New York; Oxford University Press.

Graham, M., & Avent, J. (2004). A discipline-wide approach to group treatment. *Topics in Language Disorders, 24,* 105–117.

Greenhalgh, T., & Hurwitz, B. (1999). Why study narrative? *British Medical Journal, 318,* 48–50.

Haley, K., Jenkins, K., Hadden, C., Womack, J., Hall, J., & Schweiker, C. (2005). Sorting pictures to assess participation in life activities. *Neurophysiology and Neurogenic Speech and Language Disorders: ASHA Special Interest Division 2, 15*(4), 11–15.

Helm-Estabrooks, N., & Albert, M. (1991). *Manual of aphasia therapy.* Austin, TX: Pro-Ed.

Hengst, J. (2003). Collaborative referencing between individuals with aphasia and routine communication partners. *Journal of Speech-Language-Hearing Research, 46*(4), 831–848.

Hengst, J., Frame, S., Neuman-Stritzel, T., & Gannaway, R. (2005). Using others' words: Conversational use of reported speech by individuals with aphasia and their communication partners. *Journal of Speech, Language and Hearing Research, 48,* 137–156.

Herrmann, M., Johannsen-Horback, H., & Wallesch, C. (1993). The psychosocial aspects of aphasia. In D. Lafond, R. DeGiovani, Y. Joannette, J. Ponzio, & M. Sarno (Eds.), *Living with aphasia: Psychosocial issues* (pp. 17–36). San Diego: Singular.

Hersh, D. (1998). Beyond the 'plateau': Discharge dilemmas in chronic aphasia. *Aphasiology, 12,* 207–218.

Hesketh, A., & Hopcutt, B. (1997). Outcome measures for aphasia therapy: It's not what you do, it's the way you measure it. *European Journal of Disorders of Communication, 32*, 189–202.

Hickey, E., Bourgeois, M., & Olswang, L. (2004). Effects of training volunteers to converse with nursing home residents with aphasia. *Aphasiology, 18*(5/6/7), 625–637.

Hilari K. (2003) The Stroke and Aphasia Quality of Life Scale- 39 item version. London: City University.

Hilari, K., & Northcutt, S. (2006). Social support in people with chronic aphasia. *Aphasiology, 20*, 17–36.

Hilari, K., Wiggins, R., Roy, P., Byng, S., & Smith, S. (2003). Predictors of health-related quality of life (HRQL) in people with chronic aphasia. *Aphasiology, 17*(4), 365–381.

Hinckley, J., & Carr, T. (2005). Comparing outcomes of intensive and non-intensive context-based aphasia treatment. *Aphasiology, 19*(10/11), 965–974.

Hinckley, J., & Packard, M. (2001). Family education seminars and social functioning in adults with chronic aphasia. *Journal of Communication Disorders, 34*, 241–254.

Hoen, B., Thelander, M., & Worsley, J. (1997). Improvement in psychological well-being of people with aphasia and their families: Evaluation of a community-based programme. *Aphasiology, 11*, 681–691.

Holland, A. (1982). Observing functional communication of aphasic adults. *Journal of Speech and Hearing Disorders, 47*, 50–56.

Holland, A. (1988). *Conversational coaching in aphasia.* Paper presented at the Deep South Conference on Communicative Disorders, Baton Rouge, LA.

Holland, A. (1991). Pragmatic aspects of intervention in aphasia. *Journal of Neurolinguistics, 6*, 197–211.

Holland, A. (1998a). Functional outcome assessment of aphasia following left hemisphere stroke. *Seminars in Speech and Language, 19*, 249–260.

Holland, A. (1998b). Why can't clinicians talk to aphasic adults? *Aphasiology, 12*, 844–846.

Holland, A. (1999). *Counseling adults with neurogenic communication disorders.* (Video). American Speech-Language-Hearing Association, Rockville, MD: ASHA.

Holland, A. (2007). *Counseling for communication disorders: A wellness perspective.* San Diego: Plural.

Holland, A., Frattali, C., & Fromm, D. (1999). *Communication Activities of Daily Living-2 (CADL-2).* Austin, TX: Pro-Ed.

Holland, A., & Ross, R. (1999). The power of aphasia groups. In R. Elman (Ed.), *Group treatment for neurogenic communication disorders: The expert clinician's approach* (pp. 115–120). Boston: Butterworth-Heinemann.

Holland, A., & Thompson, C. (1998). Outcomes measurement in aphasia. C. Frattali (Ed.), *Measuring outcomes in speech-language pathology* (pp. 245–266). New York: Thieme.

Hopper, T., Holland, A., & Rewega, M. (2002). Conversational coaching: Treatment outcomes and future directions. *Aphasiology, 16*, 745–762.

Horton, S. (2004). Critical reflection in speech and language therapy: Research and practice. *International Journal of Language and Communication Disorders, 39*(4), 486–490.

Howe, T., Worrall, L., & Hickson, L. (2004). What is an aphasia-friendly environment? *Aphasiology, 18*(11), 1015–1037.

Ireland, C., & Wotton, G. (1996). Time to talk: Counseling for people with dysphasia. *Disability and Rehabilitation, 18*(11), 585–591.

Johnson, A. (1999). Dealing with change in service reimbursement: Managing or caring? *Neurophysiology and Neurogenic Speech and Language Disorders; ASHA Special Interest Division 2, 9*(1), 6–8.

Kagan, A. (1995). Revealing the competence of aphasic adults through conversation: A challenge to health professionals. *Topics in Stroke Rehabilitation, 2*, 15–28.

Kagan, A. (1998). Supported conversation for adults with aphasia: Methods and resources for training conversation partners. *Aphasiology, 12*, 816–830.

Kagan, A. (1999) *Supported conversation for adults with aphasia: Methods and evaluation.* Unpublished thesis. Institute of Medical Science, University of Toronto.

Kagan, A., Black, S., Duchan, J., Simmons-Mackie, N., & Square, P. (2001). Training volunteers as conversation partners using "supported conversation for adults with aphasia" (SCA): A controlled trial. *Journal of Speech, Language and Hearing Research, 44*(3), 624–638.

Kagan, A., & Gailey, G. (1993). Functional is not enough: Training conversation partners for aphasic adults. In A. Holland & M. Forbes (Eds.), *Aphasia treatment: World perspectives* (pp. 199–215). San Diego: Singular.

Kagan, A., & Kimelman, M. (1995). Informed consent in aphasia research: Myth or reality? In M. Lemme (Ed.), *Clinical aphasiology* (Vol. 23, pp. 65–76). Austin, TX: Pro-Ed.

Kagan, A., & LeBlanc, K. (2002). Motivating for infrastructure change: Toward a communicative accessible, participation-based stroke care system for all those affected by aphasia. *Journal of Communication Disorders, 22*, 153–169.

Kagan, A., & Shumway, E. (2003). *Talking to your nurse: Help your nurse to help you (An interactive resource for people and their health practitioners).* Toronto, Canada: Aphasia Institute.

Kagan, A., Simmons-Mackie, N., Hicks, J., O'Neill, C., Shumway, E., McEwen, S., et al. (2005, November). *Living with Aphasia: Framework for Outcome Measurement (A-FROM).* Presentation at the American Speech-Language-Hearing Association Annual Conference, San Diego, CA.

Kagan, A., Simmons-Mackie, N., Hicks, J., O'Neill, C., Shumway, E., McEwen, S., et al. (in press). *Aphasiology.* Counting what counts: A framework for capturing real-life outcomes of aphasia intervention.

Kagan, A., Winckel, J., Black, S., Duchan, J., Simmons-Mackie, N., & Square, P. (2004). A set of observational measures for rating support and participation in conversation between adults with aphasia and their conversation partners. *Topics in Stroke Rehabilitation, 11*(1), 67–83.

Kagan, A., Winckel, J., & Shumway, E. (1996a). *Pictographic communication resources.* Toronto, Canada: Aphasia Institute.

Kagan, A., Winckel, J., & Shumway E. (1996b). *Supported Conversation for aphasic adults: Increasing communicative access* (Video). (available from Aphasia Institute. Toronto, Ontario, Canada).

Klippi, A. (1996). *Conversation as an achievement in aphasics.* Studia Fennica Linguistica 6. Helsinki: Finnish Literature Society.

Kraat, A. (1990). Augmentative and alternative communication: Does it have a future in aphasia rehabilitation? *Aphasiology, 4*, 321–338.

Lafond, D., DeGiovani, R., Joanette, Y., Ponzio, J., & Sarno, M.T. (eds.), (1993). *Living with aphasia.* San Diego: Singular.

LaPointe, L. (2002). The sociology of aphasia. *Journal of Medical Speech-Language Pathology, 10*, vii–viii.

LaPointe, L. (2005). Foundations: Adaptation, accommodation, aristos. In L. LaPointe (Ed.), *Aphasia and related neurogenic language disorders* (3rd ed.). (pp. 1–18). New York: Thieme.

Larsen, R., Diener, R., & Emmons, R. (1985). An evaluation of subjective well-being measures. *Social Indicators Research, 17,* 1–17.

Lasker, J., LaPointe, L., & Kodras, J. (2005). Helping a professor with aphasia resume teaching through multimodal approaches, *Aphasiology, 19*(3–5), 399–410.

LeDorze, G. (1997). *Towards understanding communication in communication disorders such as aphasia.* Paper presented at the Nontraditional Approaches to Aphasia Conference, Yountville, CA.

LeDorze, G., & Brassard, C. (1995). A description of the consequences of aphasia on aphasic persons and their relatives and friends based on the WHO model of chronic diseases. *Aphasiology, 9,* 239–255.

Leiwo, M. (1994). Aphasia and communicative speech therapy. *Aphasiology, 8,* 467–482.

Lock, S., Wilkinson, R., Bryan, K., Maxim, J., Edmundson, A., & Bruce, C., et al. (2001). Supporting Partners of People with Aphasia in Relationships and Conversation (SPPARC). *International Journal of Language and Communication Disorders, 36,* 25–30.

Lomas, J., Pickard, L., Bester, S., Elbard, H., Finlayson, A., & Zoghaib, C. (1989). The communication effectiveness index: Development and psychometric evaluation of a functional communication measure for adult aphasia. *Journal of Speech and Hearing Disorders, 54,* 113–124.

LPAA Project Group (2000). Life participation approaches to aphasia: A statement of values for the future. *ASHA Leader, 3,* 4–6.

Lubinski, R. (2001). Environmental systems approach to adult aphasia. In R. Chapey (Ed.), *Language intervention strategies in adult aphasia* (4th ed.) (pp. 269–296). Baltimore: Lippincott, Williams & Wilkins.

Luterman, D. (2001). *Counseling persons with communication disorders and their families* (4th ed.). Austin, TX: Pro-Ed.

Lyon, J. (1992). Communication use and participation in life for adults with aphasia in natural settings: The scope of the problem. *American Journal of Speech-Language Pathology, 1,* 7–14.

Lyon, J. (1995). Drawing: Its value as a communication aid for adults with aphasia. *Aphasiology, 9,* 33–50.

Lyon, J. (1996). Optimizing communication and participation in life for aphasic adults and their prime caregivers in natural settings: A use model for treatment. In G. Wallace (Ed.), *Adult aphasia rehabilitation* (pp. 137–160). Newton, MA: Butterworth Heinemann.

Lyon, J. (1997). Volunteers and partners: Moving intervention outside the treatment room. In B. Shadden & M.Toner (Eds.), *Communication and aging* (pp. 299–324). Austin, TX: Pro-Ed.

Lyon, J. (1998a). *Coping with aphasia.* San Diego: Thomsen Learning (formerly Singular Publishing).

Lyon, J. (1998b). Treating real-life functionality in a couple coping with severe aphasia. In N. Helm-Estabrooks & A. Holland (Eds.), *Approaches to the treatment of aphasia* (pp. 203–239). San Diego: Singular.

Lyon, J. (2000). Finding, defining, and refining functionality in real-life for people confronting aphasia. In L. Worrall & C.

Frattali (Eds.), *Neurogenic communication disorders: A functional approach.* (pp. 137–161). New York: Thieme.

Lyon, J. (2004). Evolving treatment methods for coping with aphasia: Approaches that make a difference in everyday life. In J. Duchan, & S. Byng (Eds.), *Challenging aphasia therapies* (pp. 54–82). Hove, East Sussex, UK: Psychology Press.

Lyon, J., Cariski, D., Keisler, L., Rosenbek, J., Levine, R., Kumpula, J., et al. (1997). Communication partners: Enhancing participation in life and communication for adults with aphasia in natural settings. *Aphasiology, 11,* 693–708.

Marshall, R. (1999). *Introduction to group treatment for aphasia: Design and management.* Woburn, MA: Butterworth-Heinemann.

Milroy, L., & Perkins, L. (1992). Repair strategies in aphasic discourse: Towards a collaborative model. *Clinical Linguistics and Phonetics, 6,* 17–40.

Moss, B., Parr, S., Byng, S., & Pertheram, B. (2004). 'Pick me up and not a down down, up up': How are the identities of people with aphasia represented in aphasia, stroke and disability websites? *Disability and Society, 19*(7), 753–768.

Müller, D. (1999). Managing psychosocial adjustment in aphasia. *Seminars in Speech and Language, 20,* 85–92.

Müller, D. J., & Code, C. (1989). Interpersonal perceptions of psychosocial adjustment to aphasia. In C. Code & D. Müller (Eds.), *Aphasia therapy* (2nd ed.) (pp. 101–112). London: Cole & Whurr.

National Aphasia Association (1988). *Impact of aphasia on patients and family: Results of a needs survey.* New York: NAA. Retrieved November 13, 1999 from http://www.aphasia.org/.

Neugarten, B., Havighurst, R., & Tobin, S. (1961). The measurment of life satisfaction. *Journal of Gerontology, 16,* 134–143.

Nicholas, L., & Brookshire, R. (1993). A system for quantifying the informativeness and efficiency of the connected speech of adults with aphasia. *Journal of Speech and Hearing Research, 36,* 338–350.

Noreau, L., Desrosiers, J., Robichaud, L., Fougeyrollas, P., Rochette, A., & Viscogliosi, C. (2004). Measuring social participation: Reliability of the LIFE-H in older adults with disabilities. *Disability and Rehabilitation, 26,* 346–352.

Oelschlaeger, M., & Damico, J. (1998a). Joint productions as a conversational strategy in aphasia. *Clinical Linguistics and Phonetics, 12,* 459–480.

Oelschlaeger, M., & Damico, J. (1998b). Spontaneous verbal repetition: A social strategy in aphasic conversation. *Aphasiology, 12,* 971–988.

Packard, M., & Hinckley, J. (1997). *Measuring conversational burden in adults with moderate and severe aphasia.* Paper presented at the American Speech-Language-Hearing Association Annual Convention, Boston.

Parr, S. (1994). Coping with aphasia: Conversations with 20 aphasic people, *Aphasiology, 8,* 457–466.

Parr, S. (1996). Everyday literacy in aphasia: Radical approaches to functional assessment and therapy. *Aphasiology, 10,* 469–479.

Parr, S., Byng, S., Gilpin, S., & Ireland, S. (1997). *Talking about aphasia: Living with loss of language after stroke.* Buckingham, UK: Open University Press.

Parr, S., Pound, C., Byng, S., & Long, B. (1999). *The aphasia handbook.* Leicestershire, UK: Ecodistribution.

Patterson, R., & Wells, A. (1995). Involving the family in planning for life with aphasia. *Topics in Stroke Rehabilitation, 2,* 39–46.

Paul, D., Frattali, C., Holland, A., Thompson, C., Caperton, C., & Slater, S. (2004). *Quality of Communicative Life Scale*. Rockville, MD: American Speech-Language-Hearing Association.

Payne, J. (1994). *Communication profile: A functional skills inventory*. San Antonio, TX: Communication Skill Builders.

Penn, C. (1988). The profiling of syntax and pragmatics in aphasia. *Clinical Linguistics and Phonetics, 6*, 11–25.

Penn, C. (2004). 'Festina lente': A case for making haste slowly in reflective practice. A response to Ferguson and Armstrong. *International Journal of Language and Communication Disorders, 39*(4), 490–497.

Perkins, L., Crisp, J., & Walshaw, D. (1999). Exploring conversation analysis as an assessment tool for aphasia: The issue of reliability. *Aphasiology, 13*, 259–282.

Petheram, B., Parr, S., Moss, B., Byng, S., & Newbery, J. (2004). *The internet for people with aphaisa: Their evaluation of an attempt at facilitation*. Paper Presented at the 11th International Aphasia Rehabilitation Conference, Milos, Greece.

Pound, C. (1998a). *Power, partnerships and perspectives: Social model approaches to long term aphasia therapy and support*. Paper presented at the 8th International Aphasia Rehabilitation Conference, S. Africa.

Pound, C. (1998b). Therapy for life: Finding new paths across the plateau. *Aphasiology, 12*, 222–227.

Pound, C. (2004). Dare to be different: The person and the practice. In J. Duchan & S. Byng, (Eds.), *Challenging aphasia therapies* (pp. 32–53). Hove, East Sussex, UK: Psychology Press.

Pound, C., Parr, S., Lindsay, J., & Woolf, C. (2000). *Beyond aphasia: Therapies for living with communication disability*. Bicester, UK: Speechmark.

Purdy, M., & Hindenlang, J. (2005). Educating and training caregivers of persons with aphasia. *Aphasiology, 19*(3/4/5), 377–385.

Pyypponen, V. (1993). The point of view of the clinician. *Aphasiology, 7*, 579–581.

Ramsberger, G., & Rende, B. (2002). Measuring transactional success in the conversation of people with aphasia. *Aphasiology, 16*, 337–354.

Rayner, H., & Marshall, J. (2003). Training volunteers as conversation partners for people with aphasia. *International Journal of Language and Communication Disorders, 38*(2), 149–164.

Records, N., Tomblin, J., & Freese, P. (1992). The quality of life of young adults with histories of specific language impairment. *American Journal of Speech-Language Pathology, 1*, 44–53.

Rogers, M., Alarcon, N., & Olswang, L. (1999). Aphasia management considered in the context of the WHO model of disablements. In I. R. Odderson & E. Halar (Eds.), *Physical medicine and rehabilitation clinics of North America on stroke* (pp. 907–923). Philadelphia: WB Saunders.

Rolland, J. S. (1994). In sickness and in health: The impact of illness on couples' relationships. *Journal of Marital and Family Therapy, 20*, 327–347.

Rose, T., Worrall, L., & McKenna, K. (2003). The effectiveness of aphasia-friendly principles for printed health education materials for people with aphasia following stroke, *Aphasiology, 17*, 947–963.

Ross, K. (2005). Assessing quality of life with aphasia: An annotated bibliography. *Neurophysiology and Neurogenic Speech and Language Disorders: ASHA Special Interest Division 2, 15*(4), 15–18.

Ross, K., & Wertz, T. (2003). Quality of life with and without aphasia. *Aphasiology, 17*(4), 335–364.

Ryff, C. (1989). Scales of psychological well being (short form). *Journal of Personality and Social Psychology, 57*, 1069–1081.

Sachett, C., Byng, S., Marshall, J., & Pound, C. (1999). Drawing together: Evaluation of a therapy programme for severe aphasia. *International Journal of Disorders of Language, 34*, 265–290.

Sandin, K., Cifu, D., & Noll, S. (1994). Stroke rehabilitation. Psychological and social implications. *Archives of Physical Medicine and Rehabilitation, 75*, S52–S55.

Sarno, M. T. (1969). *Functional Communication Profile*. New York: Institute for Rehabilitation Medicine, NYU Medical Center.

Sarno, M. T. (1991). The psychological and social sequelae of aphasia. In M.T. Sarno (Ed.), *Acquired aphasia* (2nd ed.) (pp. 521–582). San Diego: Academic Press.

Sarno, M.T. (1993a). Aphasia rehabilitation: Psychosocial and ethical considerations, *Aphasiology, 7*, 321–334.

Sarno, M. T. (1993b). Ethical-moral dilemmas in aphasia rehabilitation. In D. Lafond, R. DeGiovani, Y. Joannette, J. Ponzio, & M. Sarno (Eds.), *Living with aphasia: Psychosocial issues* (pp. 269–277). San Diego: Singular.

Sarno, M. T. (1997). Quality of life in aphasia in the first post-stroke year. *Aphasiology, 11*, 665–678.

Sarno, M. T. (2004). Aphasia therapies: Historical perspectives and moral imperatives. In J. Duchan, & S. Byng (Eds.), *Challenging aphasia therapies* (pp. 17–31). Hove, UK: Psychology Press.

Sarno, M. T., & Chambers, N. (1997). A horticultural therapy program for individuals with acquired aphasia. *Activities, Adaptation and Aging, 22*, 81–91.

Sarno, M. T., & Peters, J. E. (2004). *The aphasia handbook: A guide for stroke and brain injury survivors and their families*. New York: National Aphasia Association (NAA).

Schlosser, R. (2004). Goal attainment scaling as a clinical measurement technique in communication disorders: A critical review. *Journal of Communication Disorders, 37*, 217–239.

Shadden, B. (2005). Aphasia as identity theft: Theory and practice. *Aphasiology, 19*, 211–223.

Shiffrin, D. (1987). *Discourse markers*. Cambridge, UK: Cambridge University Press.

Silvast, M. (1991). Aphasia therapy dialogues. *Aphasiology, 5*, 383–390.

Simmons, N. (1993). *An ethnographic investigation of compensatory strategies in aphasia*. Ann Arbor, MI: University Microfilms International.

Simmons-Mackie, N. (1993). *Management of aphasia: Towards a social model*. Workshop presented at the Julie McGee Lambeth Conference, Denton, TX.

Simmons-Mackie, N. (1994). *Treatment of aphasia: Incorporating a social model of communication*. Workshop presented at the Aphasia Centre, North York, Toronto, Canada.

Simmons-Mackie, N. (1998a). In support of supported communication for adults with aphasia. *Aphasiology, 12*, 831–838.

Simmons-Mackie, N. (1998b). A solution to the discharge dilemma in aphasia: Social approaches to aphasia management. *Aphasiology, 12*, 231–239.

Simmons-Mackie, N. (2000). Social approaches to the management of aphasia. In L. Worrall, & C. Frattali (Eds.), *Neurogenic communication disorders: A functional approach* (pp. 162–187). New York: Thieme.

Simmons-Mackie, N. (2004a). Just kidding! Humor and therapy for aphasia. In J. Duchan & S. Byng (Eds.), *Challenging aphasia therapies* (pp. 101–117). Hove, East Sussex, UK: Psychology Press.

Simmons-Mackie, N. (2004b). *The role of social participation in intervention for aphasia*. Rockville, Maryland: American Speech-Language-Hearing Association.

Simmons-Mackie, N., Code, C., Armstrong, E., Stiegler, L., & Elman, R. (2002). What is aphasia? Results of an international survey. *Aphasiology, 16*, 837–848.

Simmons-Mackie, N., & Damico, J. (1995). Communicative competence in aphasia: Evidence from compensatory strategies. *Clinical aphasiology* (Vol. 23, pp. 95–105). Austin, TX: Pro-Ed.

Simmons-Mackie, N., & Damico, J. (1996a). Accounting for handicaps in aphasia: Communicative assessment from an authentic social perspective. *Disability and Rehabilitation, 18*, 540–549.

Simmons-Mackie, N., & Damico, J. (1996b). The contribution of discourse markers to communicative competence in aphasia. *American Journal of Speech-Language Pathology, 5*, 37–43.

Simmons-Mackie, N., & Damico, J. (1997). Reformulating the definition of compensatory strategies in aphasia. *Aphasiology, 8*, 761–781.

Simmons-Mackie, N., & Damico, J. (1999). Social role negotiation in aphasia therapy: Competence, incompetence and conflict. In D. Kovarsky, J. Duchan, & M. Maxwell (Eds.), *Constructing (in)competence: Disabling evaluations in clinical and social interaction*. Mahwah, NJ: Erlbaum.

Simmons-Mackie, N., & Damico, J. (2001). Intervention outcomes: A clinical application of qualitative methods. *Topics in Language Disorders, 22*(1), 21–36.

Simmons-Mackie, N., Damico, J., & Damico, H. (1999). A qualitative study of feedback in aphasia therapy. *American Journal of Speech-Language Pathology, 8*, 218–230.

Simmons-Mackie, N., & Kagan, A. (1999). Communication strategies used by 'good' versus 'poor' speaking partners of individuals with aphasia. *Aphasiology, 13*, 807–820.

Simmons-Mackie, N., Kagan, A., O'Neill Christie, C., Huijbregts, M., McEwen, S., & Willems, J. (2007). Communicative access and decision making for people with aphasia: Implementing sustainable health care systems change. *Aphasiology, 21*(1), 39–66.

Simmons-Mackie, N., Kearns, K., & Potechin, G. (2005/1987). CAC Classics: Treatment of aphasia through family member training. *Aphasiology, 19*, 583–593. (Originally published in 1987).

Simmons-Mackie, N., Kingston, D., & Schultz, M. (2005). "Speaking for another": The management of participation frames in aphasia. *American Journal of Speech-Language Pathology, 13*, 114–127.

Singh, S. (2000). Designing intelligent interfaces for users with memory and language limitations. *Aphasiology, 14*, 157–177.

Smith, L. (1985). Communicative activities of dysphasic adults: A survey. *British Journal of Disorders of Communication, 20*, 31–44.

Sorin-Peters, R. (2004a). The case for qualitative case study methodology in aphasia. *Aphasiology, 18*, 937–949.

Sorin-Peters, R. (2004b). The evaluation of learner-centered training programme for spouses of adults with aphasia. *Aphasiology, 18*, 951–975.

Spradley, J. (1979). *The ethnographic interview*. New York: Holt, Rinehart & Winston.

Stern, R., Arruda, J., Hooper, C., Wolfner, G., & Morey, C. (1997). Visual analogue mood scales to measure internal mood state in neurologically impaired patients: Description and initial validity evidence. *Aphasiology, 11*, 59–71.

Sveen, U., Thommessen, B., Bautz-Holter, E., Wyller, T., & Laake, K. (2004). Well-being and instrumental activities of daily living after stroke. *Clinical Rehabilitation, 18*, 267–274.

Tannen, D. (1984). *Conversational style: Analyzing talk among friends*. Norwood, NJ: Ablex.

Thompson, C. (1989). Generalization research in aphasia: A review of the literature. In T. Prescott (Ed.), *Clinical aphasiology* (Vol. 18, pp. 195–222). Boston: College-Hill Press.

Wahrborg, P. (1989). Aphasia and family therapy. *Aphasiology, 3*, 479–482.

Westby, C. (1990). Ethnographic interviewing: Asking the right questions to the right people in the right ways. *Journal of Childhood Communication Disorders, 13*, 101–112.

Whitworth, A., Perkins, L., & Lesser, R. (1997). *Conversation Analysis Profile for People with Aphasia*. London: Whurr.

Wilcox, J., & Davis, A. (1997). Speech act analysis of aphasic communication in individual and group settings. In R. Brookshire (Ed.), *Clinical aphasiology: Conference proceedings* (pp. 166–174). Minneapolis, MN: BRK.

Wilkinson, R. (2004). Reflecting on talk in speech and language therapy: Some contributions using conversation analysis. *International Journal of Language and Communication Disorders, 39* (4), 497–503.

World Health Organization (WHO) (2001). *International Classification of Functioning, Disability and Health (ICF)*. Geneva, Switzerland: World Health Organization. Retrieved on April 3, 2006 from http://www.who.int/classification/icf.

Worrall, L. (1992). Functional communication assessment: An Australian perspective. *Aphasiology, 6*, 105–111.

Worrall, L. (2000a). A conceptual framework for a functional approach to acquired neurogenic disorders of communication and swallowing. L. Worrall, & C. Frattali (Eds.), *Neurogenic communication disorders: A functional approach* (pp. 3–18). New York: Thieme.

Worrall, L. (2000b). The influence of professional values on the functional communication approach to aphasia. *Neurogenic communication disorders: A functional approach* (pp. 191–205). New York: Thieme.

Worrall, L., & Fratalli, C. (Eds.). (2000). *Neurogenic communication disorders: A functional approach*. New York: Thieme.

Worrall, L., & Holland, A. (2003). Quality of life in aphasia. *Aphasiology, 17*, 329–416.

Yorkston, K., & Beukelman, D. (1980). An analysis of connected speech samples of aphasic and normal speakers. *Journal of Speech and Hearing Disorders, 45*, 27–36.

Youmans, G., Holland, A., Munoz, M., & Bourgeois, M. (2005). Script training and automaticity in two individuals with aphasia. *Aphasiology, 19*, 435–350.

APPENDIX 11.1
Examples of Strategies for Communication-Partners of People with Aphasia

Slow the rate of speech

Chunk ideas with pauses between

Insert pauses between topics

Simplify sentence structure

Convey one idea at a time

Place key information at the end of the sentence

Repeat key words

Write key words as referents

Rephrase when not understood

Use direct instead of indirect referents ("Mary" vs. "she")

Use gestures, body lean, and gaze to shift topics

Use verbal terminators to end a topic ("so much for that")

Use verbal introductions to open topics ("Let's talk about . . .")

Use redundancy ("Where's Spot, the dog?" vs "Where's Spot?")

Use alerting phrases or gestures (touch, "uhh, John")

Emphasize key content with stress and intonation

Tolerate the other person's silence

Use gestures and pantomime to add information while talking

Backchannel to encourage the aphasic speaker ("mhm," "I see," "oh yes")

Paraphrase, summarize, or reinterpret to verify, elaborate, and sustain topic

Verify your understanding by paraphrasing, repeating, or questioning as needed

Use "thematic written support" (Garrett & Beukelman, 1995)

Use props (magazines, photo albums, pictures)

Subtly incorporate words that the person with aphasia "didn't get" into your own utterances

Get information from his or her body language—focus on more than the talk

Progress from the general to the specific in questioning

Provide and use paper and markers to support talk

Draw or write key ideas while talking

Use the augmentative strategies of the person with aphasia to model and establish equality

Use the environment (talk about a picture on the wall)

Establish shared experiences as topics (sports, gardening)

Focus on doing things together versus carrying out discussions

Avoid teaching comments such as "you said that right"

Reflect feelings communicated nonverbally ("Oh boy, that makes you angry")

Establish equality in relationship by following the aphasic individual's lead, acknowledge opinions, etc.

APPENDIX 11.2
Advocacy Strategies for Supporting Participation of the Person with Aphasia

Build public awareness and understanding of aphasia

Establish attitudes and behaviors that promote inclusion

Promote public knowledge of facilitating behaviors and accommodations

Provide communication aids and materials to support communication

Provide communication in an accessible format (e.g., alternatives such as pictures and written instructions, multiple-modality communication, large print)

Encourage environmental adaptations to promote communication (reduce noise, provide alerting systems, make speakers visible to the person with aphasia, alter signage)

Alter information complexity

Prepare for management of emergency or unexpected situations (e.g., written message for transport driver, police, or hospital staff)

Provide accessible information regarding services

(Adapted from American Speech-Language-Hearing Association (1992). Communication and the ADA. Fact Sheet. Rockville, MD: Author Retrieved on 10/1/07 at eric.ed.gov/ERIC-DOCS/data/ericdocs2sq1/comment_storage_01/0000019b/80/13/22/cd.pdf.)

Chapter 12

Environmental Approach to Adult Aphasia

Rosemary Lubinski

OBJECTIVES

The primary objective of this chapter is to introduce new and practicing clinicians to the concept that their clinical endeavors involving adults with aphasia will be enhanced if they consider the physical and social environment as part of their intervention. After reading and discussing this chapter, clinicians should be able to define the components of the physical and social environment, state their environmental philosophy regarding adult aphasia, identify physical and social factors in the environment that impede communication opportunities, and plan strategies to create a positive communication environment for the adult with aphasia, family members, and staff working in rehabilitation, long-term care, and home care.

The concept of **functional** dominated rehabilitation in the 1990s, and now **evidenced-based practice** emerges as the emphasis in the new century. Rehabilitation specialists are required by private and governmental health care insurers, and by consumers themselves, to demonstrate that therapy simultaneously emanates from scientifically proven methodology and makes a discernible difference in the everyday life of the patient. Numerous trends in health care have generated this focus, and the most potent of these is rapidly increasing financial cost, particularly to the escalating population of older adults. In 2004, Medicare and Medicaid, two of the primary health care insurers for the elderly, cost the U.S. population $308.9 billion and $276.9 billion, respectively (Hoffman, Klees, & Curtis, 2005). These expenses will swell as the first wave of baby boomers reaches age 65 in the next few years and as they enjoy a longer life span. Thus, payers want to reimburse for proven methodologies that result in real-life benefits for those receiving speech-language pathology services.

Speech-language pathologists have a particular challenge—providing intervention to adults with aphasia that meets the two criteria of scientific merit and functional relevance. Well-accepted models, such as those offered by the Quality Standards Subcommittee of the American Academy of Neurology (Miller et al., 1999) and a rating scale used in the Scottish Intercollegiate Guideline Network (n.d.), exist for determining the best scientific evidence. Graduate programs in speech-language pathology are introducing evidence-based practice in both academic coursework and clinical practicum. The American Speech-Language-Hearing Association (ASHA) has a focused initiative on evidence based practice and has published several documents, including a position statement (2005) on this topic.

Only a limited body of research currently meets the highest levels of scientific rigor for evidence-based practice yet addresses the unique needs that each adult with aphasia brings to the therapeutic context. Most importantly, we have few well-established models of what variables should be considered to be important functional outcomes; consequently, few standardized assessment tools exist for documenting changes in functional communication (e.g., Frattali, Thompson, Holland, Wohl, & Ferketic, 1995). Clinicians are well aware that their therapeutic efforts often extend beyond the individual with aphasia to the broader social and physical environment, and that these outcomes should be documented and provided as evidence for the value of speech-language intervention. For example, a growing literature on quality-of-life issues, both for adults with aphasia and for their caregivers, reveals a recognition that outcomes need not be limited to changes in receptive or expressive communication skills alone. (For in-depth discussions regarding quality of life for survivors of stroke, see, e.g., Brumfitt & Sheeran, 1999; Duncan et al., 1999; Paul-Brown, Frattali, Holland, Thompson, & Caperton, 2001; Ross & Wertz, 2003; Sarno, 1997; Sturm et al., 2002; Vickery, Gontkovsky, & Caroselli, 2005; Williams, Weinberger, Harris, & Biller, 1999. For in-depth discussions regarding quality of life for the family members of survivors of stroke, see, e.g., Evans, Connis, Bishop, Hendricks, & Haselkorn, 1994; Kalra et al., 2004; McCullagh, Brigstocke, Donaldson, & Kalra, 2005; Palmer & Glass, 2003; Visser-Meily, Post, Schepers, & Lindeman, 2005). A new generation of clinical research must be performed to

Specific communication skills	Effectiveness of communication	Caregiver effectiveness	Satisfaction with clinical services	Quality of life	Environment
Improves receptive access to expressive, community cognitive skills to maximum	Demonstrated personal communicative competence despite disorder(s)	Uses facilitating strategies to repair communication breakdowns	Extends treatment strategies outside the clinic	Participates in a variety and quantity of activities of choice	Provides physical and social home and thinking and communicating
Improves social and vision and hearing to maximum aphasia	Adapts proactively to communication changes	Copes with stress and burden associated with caregiving and communication breakdowns	Assumes independent problem solving for communication breakdowns	Has a sense of control and choice regarding communication partners and activities	Provides financial support for short and long term intervention
	Uses alternate means when needed				Increases public awareness of and its personal and societal effects

Client focused _____

Caregiver focused _____

Society focused _____

Figure 12–1. Array of intervention outcomes.

blend the science of the brain with the authentic needs of patients with aphasia and their caregivers.

One of the present needs we have as clinical aphasiologists is a model for conceptualizing the range of therapeutic outcomes we might achieve with our clients. Such a model should include specific receptive and expressive communication skills and extend to broader environmental outcomes for both the individual, significant others, and society. Figure 12–1 illustrates a continuum of intervention outcomes that begins with specific receptive and expressive communication skills that are identified and measured through formal traditional tests or trained observation of such skills in communicative interaction. Clinicians typically initiate intervention by improving these skills and concentrating on topics that are of everyday usefulness to the client. Clinicians assume that improvement in discrete skills within the context of isolated therapy will be reflected in everyday communicative interaction with a variety of communication partners.

The focus on using these skills in a variety of contexts moves us to another level of possible intervention outcomes, which are called "effectiveness skills." Effectiveness skills

allow the individual to demonstrate, to the degree possible, personal communicative competence regardless of the presence of communication difficulties. For some individuals with aphasia, skill development will be modest, yet their ability to communicate through a variety of communication channels and with skilled communication partners will result in effective communication. These are the individuals who "max out" on traditional aphasia tests but are able, to some extent, to understand and express themselves in real-life communicative contexts. They are often those persons with chronic aphasia who have been dismissed from therapy, want to participate in an intervention program, but may not demonstrate continued progress on traditional outcome measures. Effectiveness skills involve the individual's ability to adapt proactively to communicative changes. Some individuals might combine communication channels such as speaking and gesturing, use augmentative and assistive devices, or seek communicative support from communication partners when needed. Thus, regardless of his or her performance in terms of communicative skills, the individual is able to maintain an active communication role.

Because communication is a dyadic process, effective functional intervention must include primary and potential communication partners, particularly family members and other formal and informal caregivers. Two subtypes are possible for this third domain of outcomes. The first outcome is the ability of communication partners to use facilitating strategies to maintain communicative interaction with the individual who has aphasia. Thus, communication partners understand that they have a responsibility to become active and creative problem solvers when communication breakdowns occur with the individual having aphasia. A second outcome is to maximize caregiver ability to cope with the challenges of communicating on a daily basis with someone who has communication difficulties. Caregivers will not support therapeutic outcomes or use strategies if they feel burdened when communicating with an individual with aphasia. Outcomes that involve increasing the ability of caregivers to facilitate interaction and cope with the communicative challenges should be legitimate outcomes of speech-language pathology intervention.

A fourth type of outcome is assumed under the rubric of satisfaction with clinical services. This category is more than patients "liking" therapy or the clinician. Patients and caregivers are more likely to implement therapy strategies in their daily interaction if they perceive that the clinical services they are receiving reflect their communicative needs and genuinely benefit them on a daily basis. Clinicians have an obligation to seek frequent verbal and written feedback to document perceived satisfaction with the intervention program. An added benefit of seeking such input is that the client and caregiver assume more accountability for defining their needs and evaluating progress. Satisfaction can be measured in several ways, including use of the ASHA NOMS Measurement System that has a section devoted to patient satisfaction (ASHA, 1998). Most clinics design their own in-house tools to document patient satisfaction with clinical services, and some centers also might use large-scale health-care patient satisfaction instruments, such as those developed by the Rand Corporation (1994).

The very essence of what we do in therapy is ultimately intended to create a better quality of life for adults with aphasia and caregivers. Quality of life is a complex, multidimensional, and subjective category of outcomes that is based on respondent self-perceptions of numerous and often overlapping areas, including health, independence, socialization, and so forth (Ross, 2005). Outcomes can be documented with broad quality-of-life assessment tools, either those created for patients with aphasia or those designed for caregivers. Data from such instruments indicate that speech-language outcomes can embrace an extensive array of physical, health, social, psychological, and emotional needs of both the individual with aphasia and family members.

Finally, many clinicians realize inherently that therapeutic effectiveness is influenced by the dynamic physical and social environments in which our clients live and communicate. Two individuals with similar communication profiles might demonstrate their communicative competence differently because of how their physical and social environments create, support, or impede opportunities to communicate. Adults with aphasia and their environment create a single, inextricably interwoven unit that in turn affects the people, events, and relationships occurring around them. It may be efficient to isolate the communication sequelae of stroke from individuals and their environment, but the process results in a synthetic assessment of the individuals and their communication assets and difficulties. The stroke and its physical, cognitive, emotional, and communicative sequelae serve as active agents of change for individuals, their social networks, and the physical surroundings. Therefore, if communication therapy is to be functional and truly tailored to the individual's needs and resources, a broader perspective on the goals of therapy, the agents of change, and the evaluation of outcomes must be offered.

Further, environmental outcomes should also include changes in public awareness of aphasia and increased commitment to providing social and financial support for short- as well as long-term intervention. As therapeutic effectiveness across the continuum is documented, collated, and analyzed, this information must be shared with the general public and policy makers at local and national levels as well as with the professional community. A circular relationship exists between what the public perceives as important intervention endeavors, what the public supports both politically and financially, and what services are available (and for how long) to the individual and family.

ENVIRONMENT

Here, "environment" is defined as the spectrum of influences that impinge on and are influenced by an individual during his or her life cycle. These forces emanate from the external physical and social environment together with those that arise from the unique internal contributions of each individual. Note that these influences do not have a simple summative effect; rather, a change in any one can reverberate within the whole system. Each component has the potential to cross-fertilize the others. The combination of these external and internal stimuli forms a "total environment" for each person. Figure 12–2 presents a schematic diagram for the relationship of the individual to his or her total environment. Keep in mind that all environments contain a variety of individuals who in turn influence each other.

External Environment

The external environment is comprised of the physical world, the immediate social milieu in which an individual resides, and the social, political, and economic values,

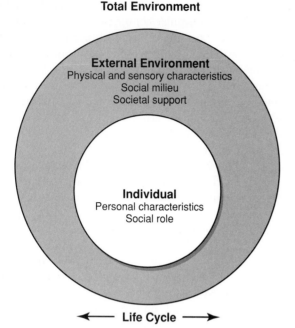

Figure 12–2. Relationship of a person to his or her total environment.

norms, and institutions of the larger society. These concurrent and interactive stimuli operate in tandem to help define how individuals will function in any setting.

Physical Environment

The physical stimuli in a person's external environment include the natural phenomena perceived through the senses, man-made contributions of buildings and artifacts (built environment), and the use of time and space. These stimuli create the physical context in which individuals function and help to determine both where and how they will live and the rules they will develop to maintain order within that landscape. Individuals assume control over their physical environment when possible to enhance their way of life.

The physical environment can create either access or barriers to communication for individuals who reside or function in a particular environment. If communication is to occur, individuals must perceive that they or their communication partners can function and move both safely and easily within that setting (Brawley, 1997). The environment must be structured so that communicating individuals can come within a reasonable and effective physical distance of each other. Distance is determined by one's sensory abilities and by sociocultural conventions. Effective communication also depends on having physical access to individuals and activities of choice that generate topics and desire to communicate. Persons must perceive that they have the option

to gain access either independently or with easily accessible personal or technological assistance.

Thus, the physical environment can either impede or support access to communication opportunities for those with aphasia. Keep in mind that in addition to the physical and communicative disabilities associated with stroke, many of these persons will also experience physical, sensory, and cognitive changes related to aging that interact powerfully with the built environment (e.g., arthritis, presbycusis, low vision, and dementia). Among the most important physical environmental impediments to communication is the reality—or the individual's perception—that the environment is unsafe or difficult to navigate. Some individuals are anchored to a limited number of physical environments because they or their communication partners cannot safely and independently traverse within or between settings. Such physical isolation is true for many adults with aphasia who reside in the community or in some level of institutional care. Other examples of barriers include confusing spatial design; lengthy hallways, stairways, or floor coverings that preclude independent navigation; inadequate and poorly controlled lighting, acoustical, and heating/cooling treatment; limited areas designed for group or private communicative interaction and activities that generate socialization; and furnishings that create physical obstacles to interaction.

Such physical environmental barriers become critical for individuals with aphasia for two reasons. First, there may be little or no awareness on the part of caregivers or individuals with aphasia that the physical environment affects access to communication opportunities. Other health, financial, and caregiving issues frequently take precedence over creating physical access to communication opportunities. It is not unusual that a person with aphasia is relegated to one location that is chosen by caregivers for reasons of safety and efficiency of care. Both in the home or in an institution, adults with aphasia are often placed in front of a television or near where meals are served. Physical placement is generally decided by a caregiver to facilitate delivery of care. Second, persons with aphasia have limited communication skills to verbally control their physical environment. For example, it may be difficult to communicate how the environment could be structured or modified to facilitate desired interaction and activities that stimulate conversations.

Immediate Social Milieu

Through social interaction, individuals learn their roles and the expectations of others in their environment. From infancy to old age, individuals assume a variety of roles that are influenced by the expectations of the sociocultural environment as well as by their own characteristics. Societies prescribe guidelines for how an individual should progress to and from various roles during the life cycle.

Formal social behavior is learned through direct, explicit communication (e.g., by the rules and laws of social organizations). In contrast, mores, or traditional customs, are acquired more subtly. These are learned through informal interaction within specific subsystems, such as family, work groups, and social activities (Ittelson, Proshansky, Rivlin, & Winkel, 1974). These two types of norms determine how much individual involvement, support, independence, personal growth, and expressiveness will be tolerated (Moos, 1976).

Each environment creates its own personality and provides individuals with a network of social capital. Social capital is created by the combined resources and values of all the social networks in which individuals function (Putnam, 1995). Hopefully, these social networks can be mobilized to provide adults with aphasia with social and physical support, meaningful opportunities to communicate, and assistance when communication difficulties create breakdowns in interaction. Social networks, such as the family as well as religious, work, and fraternal organizations, help individuals to realize their physical and emotional needs through both real and perceived support. A strong body of evidence suggests that social support is important in successful aging (e.g., Krause, 2001) and in coping with disability (e.g., Young & Olson, 1991).

Fundamental to the immediate social environment is the family. "Family" is broadly defined here as the network of individuals with whom the an individual with aphasia is closely involved on a daily basis. This can be an immediate system of spouse and/or children, or it can extend to other, multiple networks of relatives, friends, and informal or professional caregivers (Turnbull & Turnbull, 1991). An individual's family provides information about its broader culture and affords economic, socialization, daily care, and emotional support. The characteristics of the family, or of any of its components, will affect and be influenced by their relationships with larger social groups such as work, school, church, political, leisure, and medical/rehabilitation organizations.

Both individuals and their immediate and extended families are challenged when the individual incurs some type of disability, such as a stroke and ensuing aphasia. The roles and relationships that have been established may be imbalanced, and the family system must adapt if it is to remain integral and meet the needs of the individual family members (Maitz, 1991). Scholte op Reimer, de Haan, Rijnders, Limburg, and van den Bos (1998), in a study of 115 partners 3 years after a stroke, found that they perceived a high level of responsibility, uncertainty about patient needs, and restraints on their own socialization. Some partners also felt that the patient relied exclusively on them for care. In a meta-analysis of stroke caregiving, Han and Haley (1999) found that stroke caregivers exhibit high levels of depression at both the acute and chronic phases of stroke.

Some families are equipped to cope with such difficulties. For example, LeDorze (1995) found that some spouses believed aphasia united them with the individual having aphasia. Many families will face some degree of confusion or chaos unless they are provided with support. From the initial crisis through living with chronic aphasia, most families will experience an evolution in their reaction to the difficulties of coping with stroke and aphasia.

Family caregivers often assume added responsibilities regarding their loved one and the management of their home and daily life. These are in addition to changes in married life, family relationships, work, and social life. Besides the physical toll related to caregiving, the emotional impact includes increased irritability and anxiety, depression, loneliness, and fatigue (Michallet, LeDorze, & Tetreault, 2001; Michallet, Tetreault & LeDorze, 2003; Zemva, 1999). Michallet and colleagues (2003) state that communication difficulties are a "central source of stress . . . that combines with others sources of stress in lifestyle habits" (p. 853). Such reactions may result in increased burden and stress. Numerous studies indicate that increased depression in caregivers results in exacerbated depression in the adult with aphasia and in reduced rehabilitation outcomes (Han & Haley, 1999). This establishes a cycle of depression fueling depression.

Hemsley and Code (1996) caution us to remember that adults with aphasia and their caregivers have heterogeneous perceptions of recovery and adjustment to communication problems. For example, some studies show that families are not adjusted at 5 years poststroke (Holbrook, 1982), whereas others (e.g., Silliman, Fletcher, Earp, & Wagner, 1986) show that families improve over time. The need for individualized and qualitative assessment of family needs and conversational skills is echoed by LeDorze, Croteau, Brassard, and Michallet (1999).

Table 12–1 portrays a model for the stages through which individuals with aphasia and their families will evolve after the stroke. This model begins with the severe illness or crisis stage, and it evolves to subsequent stages of recuperation, rehabilitation, postrehabilitation, and institutionalization. This model is presented as a specific sequence of stages, but in reality, stages may be of varying lengths of time for individuals with aphasia and their families.

The family's initial concern after the stroke is coping with the sudden, life-threatening illness. The family, particularly the spouse, likely fears that the stroke will result in death or some disability. Not only is this fear directed toward the patient, but the family also feels anxiety about how their own lives will be changed by this crisis event. Numerous feelings, including obsessive concern, anxiety, helplessness, grief, and guilt, cloud this time. Few changes in family roles are likely to occur, however, because the family's energy is directed toward the immediate health crisis.

TABLE 12–1

Patient Stages, Possible Family Effects, and Potential Family Needs

Patient Stage	Possible Effects on Family	Potential Family Needs
Severe illness or crisis (acute)	Fear and shock Disequilibrium Anxiety Depression Guilt Helplessness Grief Obsessive concern Fatigue	Emotional support for entire family, particularly spouse and adult child caregiver, significant others
Recuperation	Sense of relief from acute stage Family works toward homeostasis Members assume needed roles and jobs Search for help begins Individuals try to maintain self-image	Continued emotional support Information about family demands, resources, concerns Informal education about stroke and its effects Family mobilized to work together Facilitative communication strategies modeled while communicating with adult who has aphasia
Rehabilitation	"Hope" that things will improve Expectation that patient will improve Want information about stroke, aphasia, depression, changes in personality, and other co-morbidities Solidification of new family roles Beginning of isolation from community Physical changes in home Possible logistical problems in attending therapy by patient and/or family members Possible financial problems Difficulties with travel and independence	Continued emotional support with more emphasis on self-reliance Information giving and counseling Problem-solving approach to communication difficulties Direct involvement in rehabilitation Discussion of family, individual, and clinician goals and expectations of therapy Definition of and access to community resources regarding financial aid, insurance, Medicare and Medicaid, etc. Peer support groups Counseling from social worker, occupational therapists, physical therapists, others Planning for postrehabilitation stage
Postrehabilitation	Frustration with daily communication Possible role overload for primary caregiver Possible health problems for primary caregiver Long-term changes in family roles Isolation of family from extended groups Possible reduction in intimacy between person with aphasia and spouse or significant other Over- or underexpectations for continued improvements	Participation in support groups Realization and support for caregiver personal needs Peer and extended group support Increase in normative features of home and person with aphasia Continued emotional support—referral to community counselors

TABLE 12–1

Patient Stages, Possible Family Effects, and Potential Family Needs (continued)

Patient Stage	Possible Effects on Family	Potential Family Needs
Institutionalization	Physical/psychological overload Lack of awareness of community alternatives Conflicting feelings of relief and guilt Further role changes Discomfort with setting Reduction in contact with institutionalized family member Preparation for family member's deterioration or death	Help in decision making Counseling regarding alternatives Support during decision making and entry Encouragement to visit; strategies for productive visits Information regarding impact of institutionalization on family member Modeling of facilitative communication strategies in this setting Work with facility staff to stress importance of communication with the individual who has aphasia Encouragement to develop new roles in this setting Encouragement to participate in activities with the patient both within and outside this setting Counseling regarding deterioration and death

Once the health of the patient who has had a stroke is stabilized, the patient and the family move into the recuperation stage. Initially, there is relief that the patient will live. The family tries to return to its pre-crisis state (homeostasis). In actuality, numerous changes are influenced by the normative stage of the family, its historical ability to cope with problems, the immediate tasks that need to be done and the resources for accomplishing them, and other demands on the family. For example, a mature family that has clear lines of communication, an established resource network of family and friends, and a history of successfully coping with problems may face a crisis differently than a family that is disengaged, interacts poorly, and has numerous conflicting demands on its members.

Stroke may occur in younger adults who are in the early stages of family development, but it is more likely to occur when the family is in the late life cycle. The elder spouse is likely to assume primary caregiving responsibility, although adult children play an increasingly important role in providing assistance to their parents. Further, children, particularly adult daughters, are likely to be employed outside the home and to be caught in the "sandwich" of caring for their own children and parents or for those of a spouse. The older family, however, comes to the stroke situation with both advantages and disadvantages. This family has many years of life resources and social capital that may assist in coping with stroke and aphasia (Rolland, 1990). The caregiving spouse, however, also may have health, physical, cognitive, or sensory problems that complicate his or her ability to provide optimum care.

During the recuperation stage, the family is likely to concentrate on activities of daily living, such as walking, feeding, dressing, and toileting. They also have a simultaneous awareness that communication is disrupted. The communication difficulties now evident between the individual with aphasia and family members confound both physical care and social relationships. Kinsella and Duffy (1979) found that difficulty in communication results in a loss of the intimacy and support found in most marriages.

Most families in which someone has had a stroke do not come as units untouched by other problems in life. Numerous concurrent demands have an impact on the family dealing with aphasia. For example, Jones and Lubinski (unpublished), in a family-systems study of nine poststroke families, found that all families contended with stresses faced by maturing families, such as those related to launching children, managing retirement, and coping with the needs of elderly parents. Kelly-Hayes et al. (1988) found that family and social factors were equal to medical factors in determining the final outcome of patients after a stroke.

When medical conditions have stabilized and physical recuperation appears to be possible, therapies are likely to begin. For many families, this will be their first encounter with therapy for aphasia. During this rehabilitation stage, the focus is on helping the individual with aphasia to improve his or her communication skills. The family system is also continuing its restructuring during this time. Role changes become more solidified so that even when individuals with aphasia return to their families, modifications in roles and routine are in place. Difficulties in communicating contribute significantly to the need for, yet also impede, the participation of the patient with aphasia in the restructuring of family roles. Unwittingly, the patient may become a marginal member of the family.

At some point, active rehabilitation will end as the individual with aphasia moves into the chronic stage post-rehabilitation. This is the beginning of a "new normal" set of roles and relationships for the individual and family (Allan, 2006). Some family caregivers may be overloaded by the demands of care and possible conflict with personal needs, and health problems are common among this group. Over time, family caregivers may realize that they need psychological support (Van den Heuvel et al., 2002)

Some individuals with aphasia may require relocation to long-term care if caregiving resources in the community are strained. This decision is generally difficult for the individual and family, and family members need information regarding their caregiving and residential options. Psychological support is important before and after making the decision.

The extended family of a person with aphasia is also affected by the stroke and the resulting communication problems. Friends and acquaintances may feel uncomfortable during interactions with the patient and may withdraw from former social interactions with the entire family unit or individual members within it. The family may lose some of its opportunities for social connectedness because one member cannot communicate. This results in disengagement of the family from the mainstream of the community.

Finally, the extended social system of the individual with aphasia is likely to include some new members, such as professional caregivers. Nurses and nursing assistants assume a prominent role in the lives of many patients with aphasia in the hospital, home, or long-term care settings. These individuals assume "quasi-family" roles, in that they perform intimate caregiving tasks and serve as primary communication partners for the individual with aphasia. They may or may not understand the nature of aphasia and how to reinforce gains made in therapy.

Broader Cultural Milieu

The broader social milieu is comprised of the social, political, and economic values of the culture that are translated to individuals through the social interaction they have with a variety of groups throughout their life. Basically, society is guided by the values that it deems as being important to pass on through the generations. Particularly relevant here is how society views disability.

How our broader society and individual cultures within it view disability in general and aphasia in particular also affects opportunities to communicate as well as financial and physical access to rehabilitation services. North American culture has a divided view on how it perceives disability. First, it views disability as a consequence of interaction between individual characteristics and the "natural, built, cultural and social environments" (National Institute on Disability and Rehabilitation Research, 1999, p. 68578). Sotnick and Jezewski (2005) state that acknowledgment of and outside intervention for disabilities are favored in mainstream American culture (p. 26). Second, Western societies also feel a need to "protect the less fortunate." Protection may lead to elimination of situations where the individual with aphasia (and, hence, society) might face communication frustration or failure. The individual with aphasia is now out of mainstream society and part of an unfamiliar and isolated minority group. Reintegration into society thus becomes more challenging.

Finally, when communication problems are evident, the individual has more difficulty demonstrating intelligence, social competence, and productive social roles—all qualities that are valued by Western industrialized societies. Safilios-Rothchild (1970) says that such societies do not tolerate "behavioral deviations [such as communication difficulties] that tend to disrupt the smooth functioning and easy flow of interpersonal relations" (p. 127). In general, contact with adults who have difficulty communicating arouses anxiety. The cultural norm is to mask such aversion, usually through avoidance.

Other cultures, even within North America, may have contrasting views of etiology, intervention options, and family involvement in rehabilitation. Thus, although there may be prevailing views on disability and rehabilitation within North America, the home culture of individuals with aphasia greatly influences how the client and family will perceive the problem and avail themselves of rehabilitation services. This is particularly important as the United States becomes an increasingly multicultural society. Note, too, that clinicians' cultural views of disability and rehabilitation may differ from those of the individuals with whom they work. This difference may affect the formation of goals and the inclusion of family or others in the therapeutic process.

Finally, the political and economic environment also influences the individual, the family, and the larger society. Society must constantly evaluate its economic resources against the multiple needs of various constituencies. The growing number of elderly, particularly the very old, stresses the balance between social needs and economic resources. The current emphasis on evidence-based practice demonstrates society's need to provide wisely for those with disabilities.

How health care and rehabilitation are approached is also influenced by the financial resources of those with aphasia and their social networks (Ingstad, 1990). The availability of personal financial resources or finances and of third-party insurance to cover prolonged rehabilitation may affect the person's willingness to participate in therapy. Speech-language pathologists are encouraged to be culturally sensitive, but they must also be "economically sensitive" to client and family concerns about the cost of therapy and the perceived cost/benefit ratio. Knowing that a family cannot afford extensive therapy or that the costs of therapy will deplete a family's savings may determine how and where therapy is done and how progress is evaluated. Individuals with aphasia and their families appreciate a speech-language pathologist who acknowledges the financial burden of therapy.

Internal Environment

The individual is at the core of the environmental approach presented in this chapter. By contributing personal characteristics to the environment, the individual becomes an active member of it. Basic characteristics include the total and evolving array of physical, sensory, psychological, cognitive, communicative, and emotional traits and needs. Human beings enrich their environment with these distinctive features yet must rely on other individuals and groups for information, support, and feedback. The individual generates social imperatives but must also respond to social conventions.

Ideally, pressure from the physical and sociocultural environment will never exceed the person's ability to respond competently. Individuals are expected to know their social roles and match them to their biologic, intellectual, and emotional abilities. The interplay between human beings and their environment is delicate and dynamic, creating challenges for our ability to adapt and survive. Person-environment congruence, or "fit," is defined as the similarity between what the individual can contribute and the demands of the environment (Kahana, Lovegreen, Kahana, & Kahana, 2003; Lawton, 1970).

Individuals with aphasia come to their environment with a constellation of characteristics, including their personal history, age-related changes, and stroke-related disabilities. Physical and health concerns may have priority over communication rehabilitation for the individual or caregivers. The loss of social roles for survivors of stroke is particularly devastating. Dowswell and colleagues (2000) concluded in their qualitative study of survivors of stroke that these patients "deeply felt their change in status from 'doers' to receivers, from active to passive. Particularly painful was the inability to help others" (p. 513). This study also documented the deterioration of social life for survivors of stroke, partly as a result of physical obstacles but also because of feelings of shame and perceived moral judgments.

From these findings, it is not surprising that many survivors of stroke incur depression, a potential co-morbidity (e.g., Starkstein & Robinson, 1988; Wahrborg, 1991). Depression may be related to biochemical changes resulting from site of lesion or as a reaction to the challenges of stroke

and aphasia. From 30% to 60% of patients with stroke exhibit depression following their insult, and this depression may be long term (e.g., Cullum & Bigler, 1991; Egelko et al., 1989; Robinson & Benson, 1981). Grief and anxiety are natural consequences of the physical and psychological losses associated with stroke. As family members cope with the demands of the stroke and with their own feelings of loss, they may provide few opportunities for communication with the adult who has aphasia. A vicious cycle ensues, as fewer opportunities result in diminished social roles that then generate depression for the individual and hence fewer opportunities to communicate.

The depressive symptoms that individuals with aphasia may show can be multiple, ranging from pervasive sadness, dependency, and indecisiveness to physical and cognitive problems. The most extreme symptom includes suicide (Jenike, 1988). Such depression symptomatology may be interpreted, however, by family or professionals as confusion or dementia. The individual with aphasia and depression is in double jeopardy because of his or her difficulty in verbally and therapeutically expressing feelings.

Depression is not the only affective disorder exhibited among individuals with aphasia. Affective changes can be any of a constellation of reactions, including frustration, anger, hostility, anxiety, aggression, withdrawal, denial, regression, boasting, and catastrophic reactions (Wahrborg, 1991). Further, individuals with aphasia may also incur other cognitive changes, such as dementia including Alzheimer's disease, multi-infarct dementia, and dementia related to Parkinson's disease. Again, these must be differentially diagnosed from the aphasia itself and from any other concomitant psychological problems, such as depression.

Of particular interest in this chapter are the communication abilities and disabilities that individuals with aphasia contribute to their environment. For successful communication to occur, the individual must have some degree of ability to send and receive messages. Language, speech, and hearing mechanisms must be minimally capable of sending and receiving signals. Visual acuity also contributes to effective communication, because one decodes many nonverbal cues through vision. Communication will be unsuccessful when the sender transmits an unintelligible message, when he or she misperceives the availability of the receiver, and/or when the content is ambiguous, inappropriate, or irrelevant. Communication also becomes ineffectual when the individual does not comprehend signals, receives a distorted signal, is distracted by extraneous stimuli, or loses interest.

The inability to communicate successfully may be the most significant problem for individuals with aphasia—and the greatest price they must pay for their illness. Some patients may be stigmatized by their communication problem (Goffman, 1964). Each time they attempt to communicate and fail, they strengthen their own or others' perception that they are incompetent communicators. At a time when communication is essential for adjustment and reintegration into the family and the community, their skill is impaired, and opportunities to interact are often seriously reduced.

Individuals with aphasia face a crisis each time they cannot quickly and efficiently express or comprehend the symbols of their environment. For example, each time individuals are bombarded by communication that comes too abundantly or quickly, they may reply unintelligibly or inaccurately, or they even may not respond at all. They find it difficult to fulfill their roles as adult communicators within their family and other social groups. Similarly, a crisis occurs each time individuals are isolated from communication opportunities by their voluntary withdrawal or by the retreat of significant communication partners. It may be easier to avoid communication and, thereby, lessen the frustration of failure.

ENVIRONMENTAL PHILOSOPHY

This chapter presents a model of assessment and intervention for adults with aphasia that derives from environmental and family systems theory and their application to aphasia rehabilitation. The philosophy discussed here is one that can be easily incorporated with other approaches presented in this text. Ideally, the environmental systems approach should complement and enhance other cognitive, linguistic, and communicative approaches while increasing their functionality for individuals with aphasia in their physical and social environment.

The environmental systems approach is based on the philosophy that effective and functional therapy emanates from a comprehensive rehabilitative management model that takes into consideration the interrelatedness of individuals, their communication abilities, the effectiveness of communication partners to facilitate communication, and the physical and social environment. Therapeutic goals should rightly focus on primary communication disorders, but the goals must also facilitate and strengthen those strategies that allow individuals with aphasia and their significant others to become effective communication problem solvers. If we acknowledge the principle that communication is a dyadic process, we realize that aphasia, by its very nature, creates problems for both members of that communication team. Although one individual incurs the stroke, each individual with whom that person communicates will face a predicament. The natural response by some communication partners is to talk for the individual with aphasia; for others, to anticipate every need; and for still others, to avoid communication because of potential problems. Each of these responses results in a loss of opportunity for the individual with aphasia to demonstrate intact or improving communication ability. Communicative avoidance also results in fewer opportunities for individuals with aphasia and their partners to initiate and evaluate productive communication problem-solving strategies. The diminution of communication

opportunities negatively affects the social relationships between those with aphasia and their communication partners, and it reverberates to larger social systems, including family, friends, and other social groups.

The philosophy underscoring this chapter is congruent with at least four models of disability and rehabilitation. First, Banja (1990) stated that rehabilitation should focus on "empowering a disabled person to achieve a personally fulfilling, socially meaningful and functionally effective interaction with the world" (p. 615). Speech-language pathologists who suspect that their therapy for aphasia is incomplete, artificial, and unfulfilling to the client, to significant others, or to themselves might find this approach to be a starting point for answering these questions. As Lyon (1992) states, "[S]ole preoccupation with the act of communicating has failed, so far, to deliver a solution to the problem of restoring optimal function (i.e., communication use and participation in life) in natural settings" (p. 9). The approach described here helps the speech-language pathologist to leave the cloister of the therapy office and enter the physical and social environment of the patients with aphasia.

Second, the environmental philosophy is compatible with the social model of disability that focuses on the relationship between individuals with impairments and society. Disability is viewed as the loss of ability to interact as a legitimate equal because of the barriers created by the physical, social, and economic environment (Burchardt, 2004). The significance of the environment in understanding disability is evident in this philosophy. For example, individuals with aphasia will communicate best in an environment that values and supports them regardless of their skill level. The World Health Organization (2001) framework that encompasses impairment, activity, and participation as well as the Life Participation Approach to Aphasia could both be assumed under the rubric of a social model of disability. In particular, a philosophy of communication rehabilitation emanating from England (e.g. Parr, Byng, Gilpin, & Ireland 1997; Parr, Duchan, & Pound, 2003) and Canada (Kagan, 2003) recognizes the impact of aphasia on a person's self-identity and the important role of the community in reintegrating this individual into society. MacKay (2003), himself an individual with aphasia, considers aphasia as "a social problem that is subject to social action" (p. 812).

A third, relatively new framework that supports an environmental approach to intervention is called the capabilities framework. Originally proposed by Sen (1980) and Nussbaum (2000), this model suggests that capabilities should be the object of value. Burchardt (2004) describes these as a combination of individual ability resources, practical means and knowledge to carry out a variety of functions of choice, and the social, physical, and economic environment to support the individual in these endeavors (p. 738). Applied to communication and the environmental model, the capabilities framework focuses on the ends (communication effectiveness, opportunities, and competence) rather than the means (specific skills).

The work of Hinckley (2001) on self-efficacy for aphasia and the philosophy of Shadden and Agan (2004) of renegotiation of identity in aphasia support groups complement both the social model of disabilities and the capabilities framework. In each, the active influence of the social environment is critical to the ability of individuals with aphasia to maximize their communicative competence.

OVERVIEW OF ENVIRONMENTAL INTERVENTION

The ultimate goal of environmental intervention is to create a positive communication environment. A positive communication environment is one in which individuals have plentiful access to communication opportunities of choice and are valued as meaningful communication partners. At the core of this intervention is the belief that, even in the face of severe communication disability, individuals with aphasia need and want to communicate and that the physical and social environment can be a catalyst to promote successful communication. Such an environment respects and supports individuals with aphasia and their significant partners. In addition, it eliminates or moderates physical barriers that impede the transmission and reception of messages and that preclude independent or assisted access to meaningful communication opportunities of choice within a variety of physical and social settings. A positive communication environment provides opportunities for socialization so that individuals with aphasia can demonstrate, to the extent possible, that they are socially and communicatively competent persons. Finally, keeping in mind that communication is a dyadic process, the environmental approach considers family members and other caregivers to be essential partners in the diagnostic and rehabilitation process.

Thus, twin benefits arise from adopting an environmental approach. First, individuals with aphasia achieve some degree of independent and successful communicative participation in their environment. Second, the physical and social environment becomes a stimulating and accepting milieu in which communicative interaction is likely to occur. Simply stated, the person with aphasia needs a stimulating and supportive physical and social environment that perceives communication as an important outcome of care. Accordingly, the therapeutic "client" consists of both the individual with aphasia *and* his or her environment.

Specifically, the environmental goals within the total rehabilitation program are:

1. To develop communication skills and those sensory and cognitive skills that underpin communication to the highest degree possible so that meaningful communication can occur.

2. To create a physical environment that promotes successful communicative interaction.

3. To create a positive communication environment that contains stimulating activities and a variety of interesting communication partners of choice.

4. To provide communication partners with techniques for facilitating and reinforcing communication through a variety of communication channels.

5. To develop self-actualization skills for individuals with aphasia and their significant others so that rehabilitation becomes a realistic and effective process.

6. To develop greater societal awareness of the nature and impact of aphasia and a philosophical and financial commitment to supporting communication intervention within the community.

IDENTIFICATION OF A COMMUNICATION-IMPAIRED ENVIRONMENT

The first step in the environmental rehabilitation program is to identify how the physical and social environment creates opportunities for, or barriers to, communicative interaction for adults with aphasia and their significant communication partners. A "communication-impaired environment," the antithesis of a positive communication environment, is one that limits communication opportunities through its physical and social characteristics. Such an environment exhibits the following characteristics:

1. Lack of sensitivity to the value of communication as a cornerstone of effective functioning.

2. The idea that communication is a by-product, not a goal, of care.

3. Restrictive stated or unstated rules that limit communicative interaction.

4. Few or no communication partners of choice.

5. Limited physical accessibility to activities and partners.

6. Few reasons to talk that emanate from meaningful activities and interaction.

7. Lack of private, easily accessible places to talk.

8. Sensory dimensions that confound communicative interaction.

9. Cognitively boring.

10. Limited or no support for communication partners.

Many clinicians will recognize a communication-impaired environment by its obvious inadequate quantity and quality of communicative interaction, but more formal tools are needed to document the nature of these deficiencies. A Communication Environment Inventory is presented in Table 12–2. This inventory provides clinicians with a broad and qualitative guideline for evaluating the communication opportunities and barriers that reduce interaction

TABLE 12–2

Communication Environment Inventory

Name_____ Date of Evaluation_____ Re-evaluation ____

Setting: Home___ Hospital ___ Rehabilitation ___ Community___

Long-Term Care _____

Communication Environment Inventory

Communication Factors	Frequency of Occurrence[1]		
	Frequently	Occasionally	Never

Physical Environment

1. Can the individual physically access communication opportunities in a variety of settings?
   a. Home
   b. Community
   c. Work
   d. Hospital/rehabilitation center
   e. Long-term care setting
   f. Other

2. Is personal or technologic assistance easily attainable within setting(s) to access communication opportunities?
   a. Caregiver assistance is readily available
   b. Assistive aids are available and feasible within the setting

3. Is environmental design conducive to communication?
   a. Adequate lighting
   b. Visual access to stimulation
   c. Noise control
   d. Proper ventilation and temperature control
   e. Physical layout
   f. Furniture design and placement

4. Are there objects and activities that stimulate thinking and interaction?
   a. Age appropriate
   b. Variety
   c. Easy access
   d. Appropriate to personal interests

5. Does the physical environment stimulate thinking and communication through use of:
   a. Color
   b. Sound
   c. Texture
   d. Smell
   e. Taste
   f. Movements and actions

6. Are private places clearly identifiable and accessible for personal conversations?

Social Environment

1. Does the individual participate in an activity of choice that stimulates conversation?
   a. Daily
   b. Weekly

TABLE 12–2

Communication Environment Inventory (continued)

Name_____ Date of Evaluation_____ Re-evaluation _____

Setting: Home___ Hospital ___ Rehabilitation ___ Community___

Long-Term Care _____

Communication Environment Inventory

Communication Factors	Frequency of Occurrence[1]		
	Frequently	Occasionally	Never
2. Do members of the environment encourage the individual to engage in interesting activities of choice?			
a. Spouse/family	_____	_____	_____
b. Roommate	_____	_____	_____
c. Medical staff/caregivers	_____	_____	_____
d. Friends, volunteers	_____	_____	_____
e. Others (specify)	_____	_____	_____
3. How available are communication partners of choice?			
a. Family or spouse	_____	_____	_____
b. Roommate	_____	_____	_____
c. Medical staff/caregivers	_____	_____	_____
d. Friends, volunteers	_____	_____	_____
e. Others (specify)	_____	_____	_____
4. Does the individual have at least one person of choice with whom to communicate personal thoughts?			
a. Spouse/family	_____	_____	_____
b. Roommate	_____	_____	_____
c. Medical staff/caregivers	_____	_____	_____
d. Friends, volunteers	_____	_____	_____
e. Others (specify)	_____	_____	_____
5. Does the individual have a variety of reasons to communicate? For example:			
a. Needs, wants, requests	_____	_____	_____
b. Safety and health	_____	_____	_____
c. Emotional release	_____	_____	_____
d. Personal history/interests	_____	_____	_____
e. Complaints	_____	_____	_____
f. Other (specify)	_____	_____	_____
6. What topics generate conversations for the individual?			
a. Personal history and interests	_____	_____	_____
b. Family	_____	_____	_____
c. Domestic/residential life	_____	_____	_____
d. Work	_____	_____	_____
e. Medical or physical needs	_____	_____	_____
f. Relationships with others	_____	_____	_____
g. Current events	_____	_____	_____
h. Other (specify)	_____	_____	_____
7. Do communication partners value the communication content and efforts of the individual?	_____	_____	_____

(continued)

TABLE 12–2

Communication Environment Inventory (continued)

Name_____ Date of Evaluation_____ Re-evaluation ____

Setting: Home___ Hospital ___ Rehabilitation ___ Community___

Long-Term Care _____

Communication Environment Inventory

Communication Factors	Frequency of Occurrence[1]		
	Frequently	Occasionally	Never
8. Are rules governing communication in the setting modified to encourage all communication attempts by the individual?	_____	_____	_____
9. Are communication partners skilled in the use of communication strategies to facilitate communication or repair breakdowns?			
a. Spouse/family	_____	_____	_____
b. Medical staff	_____	_____	_____
c. Other caregivers	_____	_____	_____
d. Friends, volunteers	_____	_____	_____
e. others	_____	_____	_____
10. Do communication partners have opportunities for physical and emotional wellness activities?	_____	_____	_____

[1] Frequency is subjectively defined for each individual.
Comments:
Plan of Action:
Environmental Goals:

---

of the person with aphasia. This tool can be used to assess the communication environment in the family home or some level of institutional care, from assisted-living settings to long-term care facilities. Although it is not standardized, the evaluation tool can form the basis for a structured observation and discussion with clients and caregivers. The individual items on the list are rated on a continuum from frequently, which signifies items conducive to a positive communication environment, to never, which portrays a communication-impaired environment. Frequency of occurrence may differ for individuals and should reflect client, caregiver, and clinician definitions. For example, some patients with aphasia and their family members may define "frequently" as every day, whereas others may define it as three times per week. Note, too, that perception of the adequacy of frequency may change as the person with aphasia tries to enter more communicative contexts and faces environmental barriers.

Those items rated on the negative end of the scale provide areas for possible environmental intervention. This type of assessment process should naturally complement other approaches to communication evaluation for clients and their caregivers. For example, more in-depth assessment of the individual's communication, sensory, and intellectual func-

tioning and evaluation of family or caregiver interaction with the client are essential and discussed elsewhere in this text.

The Communication Environment Inventory is divided into two major sections. The first section, Physical Environment, focuses on the built or structural environment. The second section, Social Environment, concentrates on social factors that may stimulate or decrease communicative interaction. Intervention focuses on strengthening those items that are frequently identified as encouraging communication and on reducing or eliminating those factors that create a more restrictive communication environment.

ENVIRONMENTAL INTERVENTION

Once the clinician has completed an environmental assessment, environmental concerns need to be prioritized through discussion with the client and caregivers. This discussion alone alerts the participants that effective intervention goes beyond development of communication skills. For therapy to be truly functional and successful, the participants need to become both sensitive to the environmental effects and environmental problem solvers. Keep in mind that goals must be identified that are reasonable and functional within

TABLE 12–3

Sample Goal Plans for Environmental Intervention

Environmental Concern	Environmental Goal
1. Client has restricted access to activities/partners of choice that stimulate conversation because of limited independent mobility.	1a. Family or staff will provide assistance to activities on a daily basis (e.g., personal aid, walker, cane, ramp) 1b. Client will communicate his or her preference for activities and partners of choice on a daily basis.
2. Hallway background noise masks communicative intelligibility of client.	2a. Staff will close door to hallway when communicating with client. 2b. Client will indicate through gesture that door should be closed during interaction.
3. Staff members ignore verbal attempts by the client.	3a. At least two staff members will have a one-on-one conversation with client on a daily basis. 3b. Client will verbally or nonverbally advocate the need for communication partners.
4. Spouse does not know what to do when client has word-finding problems and avoids communication to avoid further stress.	4. Spouse will learn several strategies that facilitate word recall and use them on a daily basis.

the guidelines of the setting and payment sources. Examples are shown in Table 12–3.

Goal 1: Improve Communication, Sensory, Cognitive, and Emotional Skills

Rehabilitation efforts focus primarily on empowering the person with aphasia to use communication to lead a meaningful social role in a variety of contexts. The most immediate need is to help the individual retain or achieve status as an active and viable communication partner. This is done by strengthening specific receptive and expressive skills whereby individuals can intelligibly and meaningfully contribute their personal ideas and have their needs appropriately met. Traditionally, this goal is achieved through individual and group speech-language therapy sessions using a variety of approaches.

In addition, it is critical that the individual with aphasia come to the intervention arena with adequate sensory, cognitive, and emotional skills. Patients may need to be referred for hearing and vision examinations and possible follow-up with assistive devices. Additional visual and acoustic environmental accommodations may be needed to supplement individual interventions.

Some individuals with aphasia may have co-existing dementia. Aphasic versus dementia-related language and cognitive changes must be differentiated. Identification of dementia as a co-morbidity may mitigate progress and influence prognosis. It may also change the content and nature of information provided to and counseling of both the patient and caregivers. For example, individuals with declining cognitive skills may benefit from engagement in a variety of cognitive stimulation programs, such as Montessori based group activities (Camp, 1999).

Finally, the speech-language pathologist must constantly be alert for symptoms of depression in the client with aphasia and in family caregivers. In some situations, referral to the family physician or a mental health specialist is appropriate. Several approaches to relieving symptoms of depression can be incorporated into daily therapy for aphasia. Tanner, Gerstenberger and Keller (1989) suggest that the speech-language pathologist incorporate frequent positive reinforcement into every session as a means of reducing depression. Other suggestions include encouraging the client to participate in activities of choice as well as peer-group therapeutic activities. Peer-group activities in particular are an excellent venue for peer counseling and discussion of coping strategies.

Perhaps the most important way to help cope with depression is to allow adults with aphasia time to talk. Ireland and Wotton (1996) provided 20 persons who had aphasia with 20 hours of counseling. Their descriptive study revealed that the participants valued being given time to talk in an attentive, noncritical, and private context. Outcomes included decreased depression, increased confidence, and better understanding of the emotional impact of aphasia and consequent life changes. One implication of this study is that speech-language pathologists may need to set aside specific therapeutic goals to allow individuals time to vent feelings in a therapeutic context.

Speech-language pathologists also need to consider long-term goals for the client with aphasia, including strengthening coping skills to deal with residual communication difficulties, achieving independence and socially fulfilling roles in the community, returning to employment, and for some, preparing for long-term care. Preserving the self after a stroke is essential. For example, Kvigne, Kirkevold, and Gjengedal (2004) found that female survivors of stroke were able to return to their social roles and reestablish their sense of self and a meaningful life when supported. Teamwork with other rehabilitation specialists provides the optimum vehicle for accomplishing these goals.

Goal 2: Create a Physical Environment that Promotes Communication

No matter the setting in which the person with aphasia lives, either a family home or an assisted-living or long-term care setting, the physical characteristics of that environment become an important backdrop for communicative interaction. The physical setting should be a source of information, stimulation, and access to communication activities and partners for the individual with aphasia. It may be impractical to redesign the hospital or family home, but some realistic modifications that facilitate communication are usually possible. The factors that can be manipulated in most environments include (a) lighting and visual cues, (b) acoustic treatment, (c) furniture arrangement, and (d) environmental props. For a more in-depth discussion of these topics, the reader is referred to Calkins (1988) and Lubinski (1995).

Lighting and Visual Cues

Adequate illumination contributes to the safety and independence of persons with aphasia and their communication partners while creating a visually stimulating environment. A high proportion of patients and their spouses will exhibit visual changes associated with stroke itself (e.g., hemianopsia), aging (e.g., presbyopia, dry eyes, and blepharitis), and age-related diseases (e.g., glaucoma, cataracts, diabetic retinopathy, and age-related macular degeneration). These visual changes result in loss of visual acuity, blindness, low or blurred vision, and changes in central or peripheral vision. Older persons with aphasia may also have difficulty with glare, perception of patterns, contrast differentiation, color perception, and adjusting to changes in levels of illumination (Brawley, 1997).

In general, older patients will require more light that is uniformly bright and does not create shadows. O'Keeffe (2006) suggests that seniors need 30% more light for general tasks and fivefold brighter light for reading and task completion. This is best presented through natural daylight and dimmable, high-quality fluorescent lamps (Aging Eye, 2006; Brawley, 1997). Areas of diagnostic and therapeutic activity should also have focused task lighting that can be moved as needed. Visual stimuli necessitate clear contrast, and font size should be larger than normal (18-point print in a clear font is recommended). Rooms that are filled with glare from shiny surfaces or poorly controlled lighting

reduce the individual's ability to comprehend nonverbal cues, take advantage of contextual information, and derive cognitive and social stimulation from the visual environment. Glare is reduced by the use of ambient indirect lighting, non-glare floor coverings or non-gloss waxed floors, semi-gloss paint on walls, and adjustable window treatments (Brawley, 1997).

When possible, the person with aphasia should have visual access to windows facing outdoors or to areas where everyday activities occur, such as the kitchen and living room at home or the nursing station and lounge areas in a nursing home. Visual access gives the person with aphasia a sense of connectedness and cognitive stimulation with the physical and social environment.

The use of color in the environment also plays an important role. O'Keeffe (2006) suggests that older individuals perceive colors at the warm end of the spectrum best but will have difficulty with blue tones, pastels, and low-contrast colors. Improving visual contrasts through color enhances information and aids in visual discrimination. For example, walls painted in primary colors with contrasting colors for floors and doors aid in the identification of one's own personal areas. Patterned wallpaper also provides stimulation and orientation cues. Nameplates or other identification should be printed in large-size white letters on a contrasting dark surface.

Other simple strategies that enhance visual access include adding texture to surfaces of walls, furniture, and bedding and using warm, medium-intensity colors to facilitate orientation. Because some individuals with aphasia will be seated in wheelchairs, placement of visual information such as clocks, televisions, book cases, and bulletin boards should be adjusted appropriately for a seated person. Visual access stimulates thinking and, in turn, orientation and conversations.

Clinicians may find that persons with aphasia and their family members do not attend evening support programs, particularly during the winter months. This may result from difficulties in night driving and concern about walking in dimly lit parking areas. Keep this in mind when scheduling programs. Alternate transportation may be needed as well as additional lighting in walkways.

Perhaps the simplest strategy to enhance visual access is to ensure that the individual with aphasia has the best vision possible through regular referral for ophthalmologic or optometric evaluations. Use of prescription lenses or other visual assistive devices should be easily accessible. Speech-language pathologists should check a patient's chart to note whether visual-field disturbances exist or if glasses are needed for evaluations and therapy. Use of large-print, high-contrast materials and access to handheld or stand magnifying glasses or magnifying sheets should be encouraged. Individuals who have aphasia and severe visual difficulties may benefit from "talking books," high-tech reading machines, pocket-sized telescopes, or specially adapted, closed-circuit televisions for the visually impaired (Orr, 1997). Finally, visual access is enhanced by coming face to face with the patient and asking what positioning facilitates visual access. Individuals with macular degeneration in particular may have better peripheral vision and be able to see when people or items are place in that area. It is prudent to check with the client and ask, "Can you see me here? Move the page so you can best see it."

Acoustic Treatment

The primary goal of enhancing the acoustic environment is to ensure that intact auditory information reaches the individual with aphasia. In addition to difficulties in auditory comprehension, the patient may have difficulties hearing related to the aging process (e.g., presbycusis) or previous life experiences (e.g., employment in noisy environments) and other physical disorders. Note that hearing loss is the third most prevalent chronic condition associated with aging and increases both with aging and with institutionalization. Listening to speech in background of noise is particularly difficult for older persons in general (Kricos, 2006).

The first step in enhancing the acoustic environment is to begin with a referral for a complete otologic and audiologic evaluation. Keep in mind that untreated hearing loss is linked to both depression and social isolation in seniors regardless of the presence of aphasia (American Academy of Audiology, 2006). Individuals with both aphasia and a hearing loss should be encouraged to use a personal hearing aid or other assistive listening device to receive auditory information more adequately. Face-to-face communication also will optimize the use of listening aids and the reception of nonverbal cues.

Ambient noise in the environment may reduce the patient's auditory attention and comprehension skills, particularly during conversation. Clinicians should be aware of the auditory characteristics where they provide therapy and where individuals with aphasia are likely to converse or participate in activities. Institutional environments, such as hospitals and rehabilitation centers, often contain hard surfaces, which increase reverberation, as well as a variety of peripheral noise sources. Even therapy provided in a client's home may be susceptible to unwanted background noise. When possible, therapy should be provided in areas that are acoustically treated with sound-absorbing materials (e.g., acoustic tiles or panels, carpeting, and draperies) to reduce ambient noise and reverberation. Areas to avoid include those near doors, windows, and high activity centers. Heating/cooling systems, vacuuming devices, and food service also contribute background noise. Other noise-control strategies include turning off the radio or television when talking or providing therapy as well as closing a door or window to reduce noise from other areas or corridors. Always seek permission from the client before adjusting lighting or noise-producing sources. Individuals with aphasia may take better advantage of visual cues during conversation if they have appropriate seating and adequate lighting. Each of these techniques is inexpensive. In addition, note that individuals with aphasia and a hearing loss may not understand information presented on public address systems. They may also benefit from telephones designed for those with motor or hearing impairments (e.g., remote speaker phones, cordless phones, voice print phones, and amplifiers) (Mann, 1997).

Clinicians and communication partners should consistently employ communication-enhancing techniques, including natural and clearly articulated speech with a slightly slower rate and a louder volume, eye contact, and appropriate pauses (Kricos, 2006). Communication that occurs within about a 3- to 4-foot radius from the person with aphasia is more likely to be heard than communication that occurs at greater distances.

Ideally, long-term care settings should have FM or other sound-reinforcement systems available, particularly in congregate areas, such as dining rooms and lounges (Crandell, Smaldino, & Flexer, 1995; Pichora-Fuller, 1997). Speech-language pathologists and consulting audiologists should define the acoustic needs of older patients with aphasia in long term care settings and provide suggestions for use of environmental assistive listening devices both in the design of new facilities and in the renovation of existing ones.

Individuals with aphasia and their caregivers who reside in the community should also use assistive listening devices that may be available in congregate settings such as senior centers, churches, theaters, and auditoria. Speech-language pathologists and audiologists should provide information about the types of environmental listening technology that are available and how to access them in community venues.

Noise control is important for adults who have aphasia with and without hearing loss. It does not, however, mean creating a sterile auditory environment. Everyday sounds are a source of stimulation, safety, and conversation. Stimulation from the myriad sounds of daily life, music, radios, and television can stimulate interaction with others in the environment. Auditory stimulation gives the individual with aphasia knowledge about his or her surroundings and a sense of belonging.

Furniture Arrangement

The arrangement of furniture determines where, when, and with whom the person with aphasia will talk. For example, the patient in a wheelchair may lack easy or independent access to favorite activities and social groups. Individuals with aphasia will be more likely to join a group if they feel they can enter with a minimum of inconvenience and disruption. Furniture, particularly chairs, should be movable to promote easy access, fit the person's size, and provide stable support while sitting or standing (Brawley, 1997). Circular furniture arrangement also facilitates eye contact and auditory reception with a variety of people. Small dining tables (four to six seats) encourage conversational interaction more than larger tables do. Wheelchair accessibility is a priority for many adults with aphasia, and again, it is critical that furniture be movable to accommodate wheelchair accessibility.

Furniture arrangement in long-term care facilities should encourage access and participation in both large group activities and in one-on-one private conversations. Key to the large groups is flexibility and mobility of furniture to meet programming needs. Opportunities for small group activities, in which intimate, informal conversations might occur in a relaxed and comfortable context, should also be available.

It is crucial that persons with aphasia retain control or autonomy over some personal space in their home or institutional environment (Barnes & the Design in Caring Environments Study Group, 2002). Morgan and Stewart (1998) found that privacy is a vitally important aspect of the environment for older people in general. Some residents of long-term care settings may prefer settings that enhance privacy rather than socialization. All individuals, however, require areas and objects that reflect their unique histories, personalities, and interests. Adults with aphasia must perceive a sense of choice and ownership in their environments.

Some individuals with aphasia may be satisfied to sit in one area for extended periods of time if that area provides good visual access to the outside (e.g., street, garden, and activities) or to areas where activities occur (e.g., kitchen, nurses' station, and lounge). Finally, furniture arrangement should provide opportunities for privacy and intimate talk with chosen partners. This is especially true in long-term care settings, where conversations can become the property of all interested listeners. Areas in which private conversations can occur should be both available and accessible. Clinicians should also keep in mind that therapy provided in public areas, such as the patient's room in an institutional setting, can be a source of interest and eavesdropping. The issue of privacy should be considered when therapy is provided in community homes as well.

Environmental Props

Physical props in the environment also stimulate the general orientation of the person with aphasia and are a source of topics for communication. Keep in mind that the environment provides much information that the individual can use to remain independent, safe, and active. For example, adults with aphasia in the community need easy access to spaces and objects that support activities of daily living and personal interests. Any assistive devices that promote physical independence (e.g., walkers, canes, and handrails) also provide access to activities of choice and, hence, communication.

For individuals with aphasia who have relocated to long-term care, personal items and furniture, mementos, and favorite pictures give them consistency with their family, home, and lifelong identity. Other props can promote comprehension and way-finding. For example, wall color and coverings, signage and visual stimuli, and bulletin boards serve as orientation devices. As much as possible, the physical "stuff" of the environment should reflect the person's history and interests while providing multi-sensory cues about time and place. Individuals with aphasia may need a variety of information sources to promote their way-finding.

Safety Issues

Safety should be a critical focus of communication intervention with adults who have aphasia. These adults may have impaired mobility related to hemiplegia and other health or sensory concerns. Both patients and their caregivers may limit opportunities for interaction if they perceive a potential threat to safety. Falls in particular are an important cause of injury and disability for older people and affect one in three adults aged 65 years and older (American Academy of Family Physicians, 2000). If adults with aphasia are to remain in the community, they need to be able to understand information that will keep them safe and secure. They also need to be able to communicate their safety needs both efficiently and effectively.

Safety topics for receptive therapy might focus on reading environmental signage related to medications, entrances and exits, hazardous materials, and instructions. For persons with aphasia who travel independently, reading transportation schedules and ticketing may be important. Similarly, expressive therapy might focus on verbal and nonverbal ways to communicate personal safety concerns on the telephone or in person. A variety of safety technologies may be suggested, including the telephone (e.g., cordless and voice activated), intercom systems, warning and signaling devices, and wearable lifeline devices) (Newton, 1997). Note, too, safety-focused therapy is also ideal for caregivers, who will better understand the patient's ability to function independently. Such a focus provides the family with a sense of security and comfort.

In addition, the environment needs to be designed to meet the safety needs of adults with aphasia. Although this chapter cannot discuss the topic in detail, major efforts should be made to assess the environment where these persons reside and delineate potential threats to safety. Examples include assessment of major living areas for design features and objects that might increase a potential for falls. A partial sample of suggestions includes creating clutter-free paths to the bathroom and telephone, providing adequate and non-glare illumination, using non-skid flooring, keeping assistive devices (e.g., walkers and canes) close, removing extension cords from pathways, and installing handrails in bathrooms and on both sides of steps (Family Caregivers Online, 2006).

Goal 3: Create a Positive Communication Environment with Stimulating Activities and Partners

The value of socialization for all persons, particularly older individuals, is undisputed. The recent MacArthur Study of Successful Aging investigated factors that contribute to healthy aging. Those investigators found that elders who participate in social activities or groups appear to gain the protective benefits associated with exercise. In particular, contact during conversation and exchange of friendship are key to optimizing the senior years (Rowe & Kahn, 1998; Seeman, 2000; Stern & Boyle, 2002).

Socialization is also an important factor in recovery following stroke. For example, in a meta-analysis of 39 quality-of-life studies of patients with stroke, limited socialization was one of the important factors related to reduced quality of life (Bays, 2001). Belanger, Bolduc, and Noel (1988) found a decrease in leisure and management of personal affairs 6 months poststroke. They also found that social contacts with family increase poststroke, but that a concomitant decrease occurs in contact with friends and others. Ellis-Hill and Horn (2000) found that even post-acute stage stroke respondents who received inpatient and outpatient rehabilitation reported a depressed sense of self, limited social activity, and psychological morbidity.

LeDorze and Brassard (1995) documented the perception of the consequences of aphasia held by patients, family members, and others. Both patients and family members noted reduction in interpersonal family relationships and intimacy as well as a restriction on activities. Helmsley and Code (1996) showed that social dysfunction remained an area of concern for both patients and their significant others at 9 months poststroke. Numerous other studies and reviews have also commented on the social isolation experienced following aphasia (e.g., Hermann & Wallesse, 1989; Lyon, 1992).

It is logical, therefore, that socialization is important for those with aphasia. Persons with aphasia may have to rely on family members for socialization activities because of both physical and communicative difficulties. Such reliance places the responsibility on family members to serve both as sources of stimulating activities and as communication partners.

Thus, one of the goals of communication intervention is to create a positive communication environment with stimulating activities and partners. In general, this goal will be accomplished indirectly through educating family and other caregivers and counseling the adult with aphasia regarding both the importance of and how to access socialization activities. Family and other caregivers need to learn the value of socialization and their role in maximizing access to a variety of meaningful social activities for the individual with aphasia. This may be accomplished in educational programs, informal discussion, and counseling. At a time when caregivers are absorbed in meeting the myriad needs of the survivor of stroke, socialization may not be a priority. In fact, family members' own socialization needs may be neglected.

Remember that a positive communication environment is one that values the communication contribution of its members. Key to being considered a viable communication partner is the understanding that, despite the presence of aphasia, the individual is respected as a valuable adult communication partner. Thus, caregivers and others need to provide real opportunities in which individuals with aphasia can offer their ideas through verbal and other means of communication.

Caregivers also need to realize their critical role in encouraging individuals with aphasia to reengage in old or new favored activities. Caregivers are also catalysts who encourage people outside the immediate family to interact with the person who has aphasia. They may need to model communication-facilitating strategies so that partners feel comfortable in communicating with the patient. Further, caregivers must understand the importance of activities of choice as the basis of communicative interaction. Speech-language pathologists may also use such activities as the foci of individual and group therapy to prepare the client for these interactions.

Caregivers will want to know which activities to suggest and what to talk about with patients. Encourage caregivers to follow the lead of the individual with aphasia. Such choices are likely to reflect prestroke interests and experiences, but they may also involve new activities and partners. The act of soliciting options from patients with aphasia is important socialization in itself. Topics generate from activities, but conversations that reflect reminiscing, philosophizing, and evaluating are also meaningful and adult-like. For example, opinions can be solicited with open-ended questions for those with aphasia and a high level of expressive skills: "What is your opinion on ___?" "What do you think about ___?" For those with more limited expressive skills, yes/no questions or those that contain options can be presented: "Do you think your property taxes are too high?" "Do you think Mr. Jones or Mrs. Wilson should run for mayor?"

Some individuals with aphasia may return to work or leisure activities, and these are natural sources of conversational topics. Others may participate in language stimulation groups at local aphasia centers. Such participation provides a supportive environment in which those with aphasia can demonstrate their communicative competence in a supportive environment. Many provide an array of adult-like activities that stimulate thinking and conversation. Involvement in other types of cognitive stimulation programs available in the community, college training programs, and long-term care settings also encourage interaction. These include reminiscence, remotivation, and cognitive stimulation programs. Many of these programs are geared for those with cognitive decline, but some may be appropriate for those with aphasia. Before suggesting such programs, however, the speech-language pathologist should try to observe the level of skill needed to participate and the cognitive level of the attendees.

Keep in mind that adults with aphasia should be encouraged, but not forced, to participate in programs. Some individuals with aphasia may be unsure of their ability to communicate in such contexts, and others may perceive some activities as demeaning. A good strategy is to provide information about an array of available activities and discuss those that the patient could attempt on a trial basis. Some individuals with aphasia may attend if they know that they can observe anonymously or participate with a caregiver. Finally, it is good to discuss the parameters of the activity, including length of the program, who attends, cost, transportation, and access to bathroom facilities. Role playing may help as a precursor to actually attending new activities.

Goal 4: Create Skilled and Empathic Communication Partners

Skilled clinicians know intuitively that support from family and other caregivers is critical to the success of speech-language intervention in patients with aphasia. Research on family intervention concretizes this clinical perception. Two studies by Hinckley and Packard (2001) investigated the effects of a family education program on adults with aphasia and their families. Both studies clearly demonstrated that family education improves knowledge, family adjustment, and functional activity level. Fox, Poulsen, Bawden, and Packard (2004) studied the outcomes of a 2-day residential family program held at a rustic camp. Participants identified five intervention outcomes: a sense of hope, a view of support from a social support network, an ability to monitor emotional and physical well-being, acceptance, and the creation of a new social support network.

The most typical approach to creating skilled and empathic communication family partners is to provide information in some type of education program. Avent and colleagues (2005), in focus group interviews of family members, found that they needed different information depending on the poststroke stage (acute initial rehabilitation or chronic phase). Michallet and colleagues (2001, p.734-5) found that spouses of patients with severe aphasia identified six needs: (1) need for information, (2) how to communicate more effectively, (3) how to have better interpersonal relations with their family and others, (4) need for a partnership relationship with professionals, (5) need for emotional and practical support, and (6) the need for respite. Thus, a one-time approach to counseling and education is not likely to meet the needs of most caregivers.

Stroke Education

When designing an education program for families, several things need to be kept in mind. First, the time or phase poststroke is critical to what information the family needs and how ready they are to participate meaningfully in the programming. Figure 12–2 illustrates the needs and ways to meet these needs by stages.

During the crisis and early recuperation stages, the focus is on providing family members with emotional support and beginning the process of engaging them as part of the therapeutic process. Support is generally provided through communication between the speech-language pathologist (or other professional) and the family. Emotional support involves letting the individuals know that someone in the unfamiliar world of the hospital knows who they are and understands the trauma they have experienced. Generally, this is a time when simple introductions, active listening, and comforting nonverbal communication are important. Such supportive counseling helps to establish an atmosphere of trust whereby individual family members can eventually express their feelings and concerns to the speech-language pathologist (Ziolko, 1991).

Emotional support may also be offered by other professionals, volunteers, peer visitors, and the family's own support network. Some families may be ready at this time for a limited amount of information regarding stroke and aphasia, but it is important not to overwhelm them. Stroke/aphasia packets or brochures may be provided that include easy-to-read information and clear directions to further resources. The American Stroke Association and the National Aphasia Association are good sources for such materials. Generally, families will want information about physical problems at this stage (Michallet et al., 2001).

The recuperation stage may be a time when the speech-language pathologist can model some simple communication facilitating strategies for the family members to use. Simple strategies include (a) alerting the patient with aphasia that conversation will begin, (b) maintaining eye contact during conversation, (c) using well-formed short utterances, (d) pausing frequently and using a slow to moderate speaking rate, and (e) including the individual with aphasia in conversation even if his or her responses are limited to single words, gestures, or eye gazes.

As the patient moves into the rehabilitation stage, more formal and extensive education may be provided to families. In fact, most family education will be done during this phase. This is the time to solidify the family as active members in the communication rehabilitation process. This involves soliciting their goals for therapy and enlisting them in the therapeutic process itself. The speech-language pathologist should discuss both goals and expectations and how these coincide with neurologic and communication diagnostic findings. The family can also be an excellent source of information regarding the strategies they have developed to facilitate interaction.

Families will also want specific information about a range of topics during this time. Evans and colleagues (1994) found that the most important constructs for families to understand are physical loss, cognitive and perceptual disorders, language impairment, and sexuality. Specifically, the nature of the communication problems, prognosis, how to facilitate communication, and how to make the transition to home and the postrehabilitation stage should be discussed in some depth. Family members should be encouraged to participate in therapy sessions and practice communication facilitating techniques with their family member. Encourage a problem-solving approach to repairing communication breakdowns with the patient. Practical issues, such as financial coverage of therapy and transportation needs, should be addressed. This is also the time to continue to provide emotional support as family members assume new responsibilities. Family members may be reluctant to discuss their feelings of stress and burden associated with caregiving. Many are grateful to express their emotions in a safe environment. This is a prime time to encourage participation in a support group.

It is not always easy to incorporate families in therapeutic activities or counseling programs because of limited time for therapy and the personal schedules of family members. To work effectively with the family during rehabilitation, we must be available during nontraditional times for therapy, such as evenings and weekends. Such availability demonstrates our commitment to helping family members maintain active participation in rehabilitation.

A smooth transition to the postrehabilitation stage is critical for the carryover of therapeutic techniques and family adjustment. The chronic stage presents long-term challenges for family members. This is a time when family members and the individual with aphasia no longer have the expectation that rehabilitation will result in improvement. Now, they must truly rely on their own internal and external resources. Michallet and colleagues (2001) found that if information needs were not met soon after the stroke, spouses experienced increased needs, worry, and difficulties in their interpersonal relationships with the patient and with others. Evans and colleagues (1988) found that families showed significantly less deterioration when they participated in a combination of education and counseling at 6 to 12 months poststroke. The results were sustained even after a year.

The individual with aphasia and the family members should not be surprised when therapy is terminated, and they should be well-prepared during the rehabilitation stage to assume their role as communication problem solvers. Avent and colleagues (2005) also suggest that this is a time to present information regarding long-term planning, travel and finances, living options, vocational retraining, volunteer opportunities, alternative therapies, and support groups. Referral to other rehabilitation counselors and support groups may be beneficial. With careful planning and guidance, the family should be able to reintegrate the individual with aphasia into the family and their extended social network in former or newly created roles.

Some individuals with aphasia may need to relocate to some level of long-term care, ranging from an assisted-living to a skilled nursing facility. The decision to relocate from the family home may be made during the recuperation stage or some time after the individual has returned to the community. This decision is difficult for everyone involved, because it will change the nature of the relationship between the person with aphasia and his or her family. The decision is usually made because family caregivers are unable to provide the extensive physical care needed by some persons with aphasia. For some families, acceptance of permanent institutionalization may instill feelings of guilt; for others, institutionalization may bring a sense of relief. In either case, families continue as an important source of cognitive and social stimulation for the individual with aphasia. Counseling for the family should concentrate on helping them to understand the meaning of institutionalization, their role in the communication life of their loved one, and strategies for communicating in that setting. Teamwork with the social worker and nursing staff can facilitate adjustment to the new setting. Finally, families should be encouraged to join support groups and participate in family-focused activities within the settings.

Aphasia Family Groups and Self-Help Groups

One of the best ways to provide long-term support to the family is through involvement of the family in group programming, including language stimulation programs, aphasia family support groups, and self-help groups. Language stimulation groups may be formed as part of formal communication therapy or as a post-therapeutic strategy. These groups help individuals with aphasia to practice communication skills in a realistic context. This is also an excellent opportunity to have family members serve as communication partners and reinforce their use of facilitating strategies.

A natural adjunct to the language stimulation group is the aphasia family support group. This group can be a combination of individuals with aphasia and family members, or it can be family members alone. Family members may appreciate having their own reference group, in which they can openly exchange ideas and feelings. Such groups may be organized by speech-language pathologists or other mental health personnel. Some groups are organized by family members themselves and become self-help groups. A "self-help group" is composed of peers who share a common problem and unite to form a collective identity.

Speech-language pathologists may be asked to present one or a series of talks on aphasia and related disorders to such family groups. McCormick and Williams (1976) organized a 17-week program that covered such topics as the etiology of stroke, rehabilitation services, physical and medical management, psychological/emotional changes, environmental barriers, diet, relaxation, and role changes. Pasquarello (1990) evaluated a similar type of program and found that family members specifically appreciated the opportunity to share feelings with others and find out how other families coped with a stroke. In another study on the effectiveness of support groups, Halm (1990) found that families perceived such groups as reducing anxiety and instilling hope. Support groups may assist families in locating available services and in advocating for services where they do not exist. Thus, topics chosen for such groups should be less didactic and include more open discussion and problem solving.

Another creative approach to supporting the family is family-to-family programs (Williams, 1991). Bissett, Haire, and Nelson (1978) designed a spouse advocate program, in which a family member of a person with aphasia assisted other individuals with aphasia and their families. By their unique kinship and empathy with the problem, these individuals can offer families special support. Such family-to-family programs are based on the premise that individuals with intimate knowledge of a problem can be excellent resources for other families while gaining a positive reward themselves from the helping experience. Such programs are not intended to replace professional counseling, but the families can help to relieve feelings of isolation and offer practical information about the logistics of obtaining funding and other assistive services. Williams (1991) states that family-to-family programs give families a "sense of control, predictability, and opportunity" (p. 305).

Family advocacy groups offer yet another dimension. Family members may wish to affiliate and become involved with local, state, and national family advocacy groups, such as the National Stroke Foundation and the National Head Injury Foundation. These groups serve important functions, such as affecting legislation on issues related to stroke and head injury and helping to change health-care and rehabilitation policies. Some families assume prominent roles in such organizations.

The speech-language pathologist should be available to these extended groups as a consultant, leader, counselor, or presenter. The goal in working with such groups is to provide strategies for facilitating communication with the individual with aphasia and informational resources regarding stroke and aphasia. Role playing and problem solving focused on difficult communicative interactions, rather than on didactic information regarding aphasia, are the most effective means of participation with family groups. Speech-language pathologists who feel competent in leading counseling sessions should also offer this service.

Respite and Wellness Programs

One of the most important programs to suggest to families of individuals with aphasia is a respite program. Known as the gift of time, "respite" is short-term, temporary care that allows families to take a break from the daily routine of caregiving. Respite care may extend from a few hours to overnight to a longer period of time. Respite helps family to attend to their own needs and take vacations while knowing their loved one is safe and comfortable. Use of respite programs may actually forestall institutionalization and prevent abuse or neglect. Some family members may perceive respite and wellness programs as an abrogation of their devotion to the person with aphasia when, in fact, use of these programs is a healthy approach to caregiving. Respite may be offered by other family members or by formal, paid caregivers. Such services may be offered in the family home, in long-term care settings on a temporary basis, or through adult day-care programs associated with senior centers or settings. Van den Heuvel and colleagues (2002) suggest that long-term family programs that focus on coping and providing information should be combined with respite programs for maximum effect. Good sources of information about the availability of respite programs in a community include senior citizens centers, discharge planners in health-care settings, self-help groups, and respite locators on the Internet (e.g., www.respitelocator.org). Families should check the credentials of the centers or personnel who provide respite services.

A second option to suggest to families falls under the rubric of "wellness" programs. Such programs encourage individuals to assume responsibility for their own physical and emotional health through self-education, active participation in a healthy lifestyle, disease management programs, and attention to preventive measures for reducing risks to health. Some wellness programs are comprehensive; others focus on special areas of concern, such as physical health, walking, emotional health, and nutrition. Such programs may be offered at senior citizens centers, workplaces, hospitals, YMCAs, and other community centers. Caregivers should check with their insurance plans for information on funding for participation.

Staff Inservice

Paid caregivers play an enormous role in the success of speech-language intervention. Such caregivers include medical staff (e.g., physicians, nurses, and nursing assistants), rehabilitation staff (e.g., occupational, physical, and recreational therapists), housekeeping and personal-care aides, social work staff, and others. The primary responsibility for therapy rests with the speech-language pathologist, but the staff, particularly in the hospital-rehabilitation-nursing home contexts, have intense daily contact with the patient. These are the folks who make therapy functional. Staff-patient communication can be therapeutic if it facilitates the communication skills of the individual with aphasia and serves to stimulate and reinforce his or her communicative attempts.

Staff education may be done in several contexts, including orientation programs, traditional lecture-type inservice programs, role-playing inservices, self-instructional written or computer packages, video demonstrations, discussions, and modeling by the speech-language pathologist. How and when education is provided to the staff depends on the setting. For example, some settings may have orientation modules on topics such as communication problems for new employees. Others may schedule periodic inservices that are attended on a voluntary basis. Keep in mind that informal modeling of communicative strategies during everyday interaction is a natural way to show the staff successful ways of facilitating communication with those who have aphasia.

Traditional didactic inservices tend to focus on three major topics: (1) the nature of speech, language, and comprehension problems of the patient with aphasia and any associated disorders, such as apraxia and dysarthria; (2) the concept of a positive communication environment for the patient and other patients/residents; and (3) strategies for understanding and speaking with the patient. Aphasia inservices traditionally have some content devoted to defining aphasia and its symptomatology. When conducting this portion of the inservice, it is important not to overwhelm the staff with technical detail and jargon but, rather, to focus quickly and primarily on those topics that will help the audience to communicate more effectively and create a positive communication environment.

Staff are specifically interested in how they can communicate more easily during the delivery of care. Some clinicians may choose to present a list of "do's and don't's" for communicating (e.g., speak slowly and clearly, talk about concrete topics, pause, check for comprehension, and ask questions that require forced choice responses). A more fruitful inservice technique, however, is to elicit facilitating techniques in role playing that focuses on solving communicative dilemmas. The clinician should role play various types of aphasia (e.g., predominantly expressive, receptive, and global) and have the staff role play themselves in these contexts. Following the role playing, the staff and clinician should discuss the scenario, which strategies were successful, and which strategies were not. Such an inservice fosters a problem-solving mentality in the staff and makes them active learners in the process. Two possible scenarios for role playing include:

Scenario 1 The staff member must convey to the patient with aphasia that he or she will be going to the podiatrist in 1 hour and must get ready.

Scenario 2 The staff member must respond to an unintelligible request by an individual with aphasia for something that is not obvious.

In addition, a second focus of an inservice should be on the importance of a rich, meaningful communication environment for all patients, including those with aphasia.

Staff-patient communication will be enhanced when staff members understand the value of successful communication and strategies for creating and maintaining a positive communication atmosphere. Examples of guidelines to suggest to staff include:

1. Staff should talk with the patient during medical and routine daily life care. Staff should talk about what they are doing during care, seek input from the patient regarding care, and solicit information about the individual's interests. In addition, staff members should offer some information about themselves. Persons who know something about each other are more likely to identify with each other and communicate more frequently.

2. Provide the patient with clear, specific information about his or her status, the routine for the day, and other information that helps the patient to understand his or her care and setting.

3. Encourage the patient to talk or communicate through any verbal or nonverbal means possible about his or her needs and ideas. Providing positive reinforcement to the patient for communicating will generate more frequent attempts.

4. Provide the patient with active listening or supportive attention. Encourage staff to maintain eye contact while communicating and reflect on the content and underlying meaning of the patient's communication. Other strategies include slowing or stopping an activity while talking, asking follow-up questions that demonstrate active listening, and reinforcing attempts at communication.

5. Encourage the individual with aphasia to participate in and talk about activities of interest.

6. Encourage other patients/residents to talk during the day with the patient who has aphasia. This may involve modeling communicative strategies and forming buddy/friendly visitor dyads.

7. Use positive humor during interactions. Humor can generate conversations and promote a positive atmosphere.

8. Value the communicative contribution of the patient. Remind staff that regardless of the communication difficulties that are present, the person with aphasia deserves adult-like respect.

9. Create a physical environment that promotes easy access to activities and persons of choice and facilitates hearing and vision while communicating.

10. Limit formal or informal rules that restrict communication attempts or topics.

Goal 5: Develop Self-Efficacy and Self-Actualization Skills for Client and Communication Partners

One of the goals of the environmental approach to therapy for aphasia is to develop self-efficacy and self-actualization skills in our clients and their communication partners. Self-efficacy is defined as what people believe they are capable of doing (Kricos, 2006). If therapy is to be successful, persons with aphasia and their communication partners must view themselves as capable communication problem solvers. It is unrealistic that communication intervention will meet all the long-term needs of adults with aphasia, particularly in a time of limited financial support for extended therapy. From the very first interactions in diagnostic and therapeutic contexts, the speech-language pathologist needs to cultivate the concept that the individual with aphasia and his or her communication partners must independently define their own communication needs and solve communication dilemmas. When they accept responsibility for self-evaluation and continued problem solving, they will be better able to resolve new communication problems. This attitude of "I think I can" leads to self-empowerment and an attitude of long-term self-therapy.

Similarly, communication intervention should help to maximize the client's self-actualization skills. Maslow (2006) states that self-actualizing people are realistic, accept themselves and others, act spontaneously and naturally, and have a mission in life. Clinicians have a responsibility to discuss how to access communication opportunities of choice. Other examples of self-actualization include asking for help when needed, discussing communication difficulties to relieve frustration, and self-advocating with policy makers for continued intervention.

Participation in community-based aphasia centers and in aphasia and family support groups are two long-term programs that promote opportunities for interaction, counseling, and continued communication problem solving (e.g., Kagan, 2003). They may also serve as a context for social programs as well as for political and social advocacy programs for those with aphasia. Families and patients with aphasia may unite to influence local and other governmental agencies about the needs of those with disabilities in the community. Such grass roots campaigns may influence social movements and promote social changes that reverberate across society.

As individuals with aphasia and their families move further away from direct rehabilitation, many will seek opportunities to reintegrate meaningfully into the community. Some may be able to return to work, and others may seek volunteer positions through their religious and community organizations, hospitals, and schools. One program that capitalizes on the unique knowledge of stroke is the Peer Visitor Program offered by the American Stroke Association.

Goal 6: Develop Greater Societal Awareness of Aphasia

The average person does not know what aphasia is or its short- and long-term impact on survivors of stroke and their caregivers (Code, Simmons-Mackie, Armstrong, & Armstrong, 2000). Unawareness leads to indifference and lack of support. Unless they have had a personal encounter with someone who has aphasia, most individuals are oblivious to the physical and social barriers that face such persons in the larger community. This is one reason why so many families, when faced with a stroke, are naïve regarding rehabilitation services and options. They may rely on their physicians and third-party payers for education and counseling, which may or may not be offered. Few persons with aphasia or their caregivers have a clear conception of what intervention is available at each stage of recovery, and most do not fully understand the difficulties that persons with aphasia will have in reintegrating meaningfully into their communities.

Third-party payers in particular have a vested interest in providing intervention at the least financial cost. Third-party payers such as Medicare and Medicaid are well aware of the increasing number of elderly, many of whom are at risk for stroke. These numbers translate to increased rehabilitation costs for the insurers, which want quality outcomes in the least amount of time and, hence, at the least cost. Long-term intervention is usually not an option with most insurance programs.

A number of efforts can be made to increase societal awareness of aphasia. It is essential that speech-language pathologists, both individually and through their professional organizations, accept responsibility for increasing social and political consciousness regarding this communication problem. Speech-language pathologists can articulate the dilemma of aphasia and argue for innovative programming to meet the needs of patients and their families. As stated previously, aphasia community groups have the potential to create social and political changes through the creation of organized lobby groups.

Research and Public Dissemination

The increased emphasis on functional and outcome-based research into aphasia should be made available to the public through local media, popular reading materials, and the Internet. Researchers and clinicians should take every opportunity to share their findings with the public and with colleagues. We cannot expect the public to search our literature or attend our conferences for information on innovative and effective approaches. We have the responsibility to share our knowledge base and, thus, educate the public on intervention options and outcomes.

Community Awareness Programs

Professional groups, rehabilitation programs, and individual professionals should participate in community awareness programs. This might involve programming during Aphasia Awareness Month. For example, rehabilitation programs might do special staff and family inservice programs or design bulletin boards or Microsoft PowerPoint programs devoted to aphasia. Interviews and articles in local newspapers and television programs that describe aphasia services will have a broad circulation. Local malls are often willing to provide display space for community-oriented projects. Other community centers that support such presentations include senior centers and public schools. Key to each of these options is a personal approach to which the audience can relate. The audience wants to know what aphasia is and how to talk to someone who has it. Many communities have local newspapers or senior citizen-focused circulars featuring periodic special inserts on health-related topics. An article on aphasia and programs for those with aphasia and their families in such publications would be highly visible to the public.

College and university programs need to build this type of awareness and responsibility into training speech-language pathologists at the pre-professional level. For example, a consortium of college programs in Boston organized graduate students to educate hotel staff and local merchants about aphasia before the Speaking Out! Conference in that city in 2006 (National Aphasia Association, 2006). Undergraduate and graduate student organizations or aphasia classes can also assume responsibility for educating some facet of their community.

Clinicians should take every opportunity to do presentations on aphasia to community groups, including professional physician, nursing, and pharmacy groups as well as political, third-party, and policy-maker groups and service and religious organizations. The word needs to go out!

The Internet provides a relatively new and increasingly popular medium for sharing information about aphasia. VanBiervliet and Edwards-Schafer (2004) found increasing reliance on the Internet across all age groups, demographic groups, and geographic regions. Internet use is growing the fastest among older persons. Such information is assumed under the rubric of consumer health informatics. Rehabilitation centers can highlight their specific programs, technologies, and outcomes and offer vignettes of success cases. Aphasia associations and support groups can also advertise programs and disseminate research findings in everyday language. It is important that clinical practitioners keep abreast of the nature of aphasia information on the Internet, because this is where older persons and their caregivers are now turning for information.

Aphasia Centers

An increasing number of aphasia centers have been established in Canada, England, and the United States. Kagan (2003), who started the Aphasia Institute of Toronto, states that these centers provide an aphasia-friendly community and reflect a life participation approach to long-term intervention. Interestingly, Kagan states that participants in her center prefer to be called "members" rather than "clients" or "patients." In England, the Connect program (www.ukconnect.org) has opened the community to those with aphasia. Such centers focus on creating a positive communication environment where individuals with aphasia can use their communication abilities in meaningful, adult-like interaction. Many also offer programs that help caregivers to communicate more effectively and understand the challenges of living with a survivor of stroke. In addition to innovative and traditional interventions, these centers often have outreach programs that provide education on how persons with aphasia can be integrated into the physical and social community.

Volunteer Programs

Survivors of stroke, including those with aphasia, and their caregivers may want to help others who have incurred a stroke. Benefits of formal volunteerism for seniors in general include decreased depression (Li and Ferraro, 2005), slower decline in self-reported health and functioning levels, and improved mortality rates (Lum & Lightfoot, 2005). One example of a volunteer program is the Peer Visitor Program (Insalaco, Sellers, & Lubinski, 2004). After a seven-session training program, survivors/caregivers visit survivors of stroke in acute and rehabilitation settings. Originally designed by the American Stroke Association, the program has been modified and trained more than 30 individuals who have provided hundreds of visits to survivors of stroke and their families in a hospital during the past 2 years. Initial visits are supervised by the training staff, but visitors soon become independent. Problem areas are discussed at quarterly meetings. Peer visitors frequently comment on the "transformative" benefits they receive, including having a new purpose in life. Many add that they wish they had had such a visit when they were in the early stages after a stroke. Several of the original peer visitors have assumed leadership positions within the volunteer program during the past 2 years. Even those who have aphasia are able to communicate effectively with patients and families. Another volunteer program is Speaking Out!, a 10-week functional communication program delivered by trained volunteers (Worral & Yiu 2000). Undoubtedly, numerous other volunteer programs exist in which adults with aphasia and their caregivers can participate. Major problems in establishing volunteer programs with older persons include the cost of formal training, finding optimum training times, and the attrition rate of volunteers over time.

FUTURE TRENDS

This chapter challenges us to think outside the traditional aphasia intervention box and toward the physical and social environment of the person with aphasia. This chapter encourages you to choose between a narrow, skill focus to your therapy and a broader ambition—one that includes the creation or reinforcement of a positive communication environment. The environmental philosophy presented in this chapter is perhaps the most holistic of those presented in this text in that it encompasses the individual with aphasia, the family and other caregivers, the physical and social milieu, and the broader sociopolitical community.

Fortunately, much has been done in the past 25 years that has implemented many of the ideas presented in the original environmental approach to aphasia (Lubinski, 1981). The World Health Organization framework for functioning, disability, and health has done much to focus on the relatedness of communication and participation for those with aphasia. The study of communication disability and quality of life continues to grow and creates an important database. Outcome measurement is becoming more inclusive of a variety of potential outcomes for both the person with aphasia and the caregivers. More documentation of environmental outcomes is needed. Innovative aphasia centers and community volunteer approaches offer a growing range of programming for persons with aphasia and their families. Increased finances to support the creation of such centers are needed. Political action groups that emanate from these programs are needed to influence governmental funding sources of the value of long-term, community-based communication programs. The challenge now is to sustain the momentum of creativity and promote greater societal understanding of, and support for, innovative aphasia programs across the community.

KEY POINTS

1. Clinicians must be aware that their therapeutic efforts often extend beyond the individual with aphasia to the broader social and physical environment and that these outcomes should be documented and provided as evidence of the value of speech-language intervention.
2. "Environment" is defined as the spectrum of influences that impinge on and are influenced by an individual during his or her life cycle. These forces emanate from the external physical and social environment together with those that arise from the unique internal contributions of each individual. The combination of these external and internal stimuli forms a "total environment" for each person.
3. The external environment is comprised of the physical world, the immediate social milieu in which an individual resides, and the social, political, and economic values, norms, and institutions of the larger

society. The internal environment created by the individual's own characteristics include the total and evolving array of physical, sensory, psychological, cognitive, communicative, and emotional traits and needs.
4. The environmental systems approach is based on the philosophy that effective and functional therapy emanates from a comprehensive rehabilitative management model that takes into consideration the interrelatedness of individuals, their communication abilities, the effectiveness of communication partners to facilitate communication, and the physical and social environment.
5. Communication is a dyadic process. Therefore, by its very nature, aphasia creates problems for both members of that communication team. Although one individual incurs a stroke, each individual with whom that person communicates will face a predicament that must be resolved if communication is to continue successfully.
6. The environmental philosophy complements current thinking on disability, including empowerment philosophy, social and capabilities models of disability, and self-efficacy.
7. A positive communication environment is one where individuals have plentiful access to communication opportunities of choice and are valued as meaningful communication partners. At the core of this intervention is the belief that, even in the face of severe communication disability, individuals with aphasia need and want to communicate and that the physical and social environment can be a catalyst to promote successful communicative interaction.
8. A communication impaired environment is characterized by:
   a. A lack of sensitivity to the value of communication as a cornerstone of effective functioning.
   b. The idea that communication is a by-product, not a goal, of care.
   c. Restrictive stated or unstated rules that limit communicative interaction.
   d. Few or no communication partners of choice.
   e. Limited physical accessibility to activities and partners.
   f. Few reasons to talk that emanate from meaningful activities and interaction.
   g. Lack of private places to talk that are easily accessible.
   h. Sensory dimensions that confound communicative interaction.
   i. Cognitively boring.
   j. Limited or no support for communication partners.

9. Environmental goals within a comprehensive therapy program include:
    a. Developing communication skills and those sensory and cognitive skills that underpin communication to the highest degree possible so that meaningful communication can occur.
    b. Creating a physical environment that promotes successful communicative interaction.
    c. Creating a positive communication environment that contains stimulating activities and a variety of interesting communication partners of choice.
    d. Providing communication partners with techniques for facilitating and reinforcing communication through a variety of communication channels.
    e. Developing self-actualization skills for individuals with aphasia and their significant others so that rehabilitation becomes a realistic and effective process.
    f. Developing greater societal awareness of the nature and impact of aphasia as well as a philosophical and financial commitment to supporting communication intervention within the community.
10. Central to enacting an environmental approach is working effectively with family and other caregivers. This may involve inservice education, working with support groups, creating aphasia community centers, and encouraging those with aphasia and their families to participate in community volunteer programs, particularly ones that enhance aphasia awareness.

ACTIVITIES FOR REFLECTION AND DISCUSSION

1. Third-party payers may be skeptical that environmental intervention will enhance the communication of an adult with aphasia. Provide an argument to justify an environmental approach as part of a comprehensive program of therapy for aphasia.
2. Make a visit to each of the following venues where therapy for aphasia might be done. How would you describe the way the physical and social environment either creates a positive communication environment or a communication-impaired environment?
    a. Medical rehabilitation unit in a hospital.
    b. Outpatient rehabilitation.
    c. Home health care (patient's own home).
    d. Long-term care.
3. After making the visit to each of the settings listed in the second activity, what physical and social characteristics need improvement? What would you do to create a more positive communication environment in each setting? What obstacles might you have in implementing your plans? What might you do to reduce or eliminate these obstacles?
4. Create an outline or a Microsoft PowerPoint presentation for nursing staff in a long-term care setting that discusses the topic "Creating a Positive Communication Environment." Present this to your peers, and ask for their feedback.
5. Working with families is an essential component to creating a positive communication environment. Consider the following questions regarding working with families:
    a. What resources do families bring that will facilitate success in therapy?
    b. What demands might family members have on them that might impede the success of therapy?
    c. What strategies might be used to incorporate productively family members in therapy and help them to create a positive communication environment?
6. An important issue in all therapies is outcome measurement. How would you document changes in the communication environment of your client with aphasia?
7. One of the key points in this chapter is the need for greater societal awareness regarding adult aphasia.
    a. Design a program for your agency that highlights Aphasia Awareness Month.
    b. How can you incorporate adults with aphasia and their family caregivers in efforts to improve community awareness of aphasia?
    c. Compare what can and should be done at the grass roots level versus the state and national levels to improve awareness of aphasia. Who should be involved, and what are the expected outcomes of such awareness programming?

References

Aging Eye. (2006). *Eye changes with aging*. Available at http://agingeye.net/visionbasics/theagingeye.php.

Allan, E. (2006). Personal communication.

American Academy of Audiology. (2006).*Untreated hearing loss linked to depression, social isolation in seniors*. Available at http://audiology.org/publications/documents/positions/aging/sendep.htm?PF+1.

American Academy of Family Physician. (2000). *Falls in the elderly*. Available at http://aafp.org/afp/20000401/2159.html.

American Speech-Language-Hearing Association. (1998). *National Outcomes Measurement Systems*. Rockville, Maryland: Author.

American Speech-Language-Hearing Association. (2005). *Evidence based practice in communication disorders* [Position Statement]. Available at http://www.asha.org/members/deskref/journals/.deskref/default.

Avent, J., Glista, S., Wallace, S., Jackson, J., Nishioka, J., & Wip, W. (2005). Family information needs about aphasia. *Aphasiology, 18,* 365–375.

Banja, S. (1990). Rehabilitation and empowerment. *Archives of Physical and Medical Rehabilitation, 71,* 614–615.

Barnes, S. (2002). The design of caring environments and the quality of life of older people *Aging and Society, 22.* 775–780.

Bays, C. (2001). Quality of life of stroke survivors: A research synthesis. *Journal of Neuroscience Nursing, 33,* 310–316.

Belanger, L., Bolduc, M., & Noel, M. (1988). Relative importance of after-effects, environment, and socio-economic factors on the social integration of stroke victims. *International Journal of Rehabilitation Research, 11,* 251–260.

Bissett, J., Haire, A., & Nelson, M. (1978). *Involving the aphasic's wife in the rehabilitation of other aphasics.* Poster session at the Annual Convention of the American Speech and Hearing Association, San Francisco, CA.

Brawley, E., (1997). *Designing for Alzheimer's disease.* New York: Wiley and Sons.

Brumfitt, S., & Sheeran, P. (1999). The development and validation of the Visual Analogue Self Esteem Scale (VASES). *British Journal of Clinical Psychology, 39.* 387–400.

Burchardt, T., (2004). Capabilities and disability: The capabilities framework and the social model of disability. *Disability and Society, 19,* 735–751.

Calkins, M. (1988). *Design for dementia: Planning environments for the elderly and confused.* Owing Mills, MD: National Health.

Camp, C. (1999). *Montessori-based activities for persons with dementia* (Vol. 1). Beechwood, Ohio: Menorah Park Center for Senior Living.

Code, C., Simmons-Mackie, N., Armstrong, J., & Armstrong, E. (2000). *Public awareness of aphasia.* Paper presented at the 9th International Aphasia Rehabilitation Conference Rotterdam, The Netherlands.

Crandell, C., Smaldino, J., & Flexer, C. (1995). Sound field FM amplification: Theory and practical applications. San Diego: Singular Press.

Cullum, C. M., & Bigler, E. (1991). Short- and long-term psychological status following stroke. *Journal of Nervous and Mental Diseases, 179,* 274–278.

Dowswell, G., Lawler, J., Dowswell, T., Young, J., Forster, A., & Hearn, J. (2000). Investigating recovery from stroke: A qualitative study. *Journal of Clinical Nursing, 9,* 507–535.

Duncan, P., Wallace, D., Lai, S., Johnson, D., Embretson, S., & Laster, L. (1999). The stroke impact scale version 2.0. Evaluation of reliability, validity, and sensitivity to change. *Stroke, 30,* 2131–2140.

Egelko, S., Simon, D., Riley, E., Gordon, W., Ruckdeschel-Hibbard, M., & Diller, L. (1989). First year after stroke: Tracking cognitive and affective deficits. *Archives of Physical and Medical Rehabilitation, 70,* 297–302.

Ellis-Hill, C., & Horn, S. (2000). Change in identity and self-concept: A new theoretical approach to recovery following stroke. *Clinical Rehabilitation, 14,* 279–287.

Evans, R., Connis, D., Bishop, R., Hendricks, R., & Haselkorn, J. (1994). Stroke: A family dilemma. *Disability and Rehabilitation, 16,* 110–118.

Evans, R., Matlock, A., Bishop, D., et al. (1988). Family intervention after stroke: Does counseling or education help? *Stroke, 19,* 1243–1249.

Family Caregivers Online. (2006). *Fall prevention.* Available at http://familycaregiversonline.com/module_6_fall-prevent. htm.

Fox, L., Poulsen, K., Bawden, K., & Packard, D. (2004). Critical elements and outcomes of a residential family-based intervention for aphasia caregivers. *Aphasiology, 18,* 1177–1199.

Frattali, C., Thompson, C., Holland, A., Wohl, C., & Ferketic, M. (1995). *American Speech-Language-Hearing Association Functional Assessment of Communication Skills for Adults.* Rockville, MD: ASHA.

Goffman, E. (1964). *Stigma.* Englewood Cliffs, NJ: Prentice-Hall.

Halm, M. (1990). Effects of support groups on anxiety of family members during critical illness. *Heart and Lung, 19,* 62–70.

Han, B., & Haley, W. (1999). Family caregiving for patients with stroke: Review and analysis. *Stroke, 30,* 1478–1485.

Hemsley, G., & Code, C. (1996). Interactions between recovery in aphasia, emotional and psychosocial factors in subjects with aphasia, their significant others and speech pathologists. *Disability and Rehabilitation, 18,* 567–584.

Hermann, M., & Wallesch, C. (1989). Psychosocial changes and psychosocial adjustment with severe aphasia. *Aphasiology, 13,* 513–526.

Hinckley, J. (2001). *Development and application of a measure of self-efficacy for aphasia.* Annual Convention of the American Speech-Language-Hearing Association, New Orleans.

Hinckley, J., & Packard, M. (2001). Family education seminars and social functioning of adults with chronic aphasia. *Journal of Communication Disorders, 34,* 241–254.

Hoffman, E., Klees, B., & Curtis, C. (2005). *Brief summaries of Medicare and Medicaid.* Washington, D. C.: Centers for Medicare and Medicaid Services.

Holbrook, M. (1982). Stroke: Social and emotional outcome. *Journal of the Royal College of Physicians of London, 16,* 100–104.

Ingstad, B. (1990). The disabled person in the community: Social and cultural aspects. *International Journal of Rehabilitation Research, 13,* 187–194.

Insalaco, D., Sellers, C., & Lubinski, R. (2004). Development of the Buffalo peer visitation program for stroke survivors. *Perspectives on Gerontology, 9,* 21–24.

Ireland, C., & Wotton, G. (1996). Time to talk: Counseling for people with dysphasia. *Disability and Rehabilitation, 18,* 585–591.

Ittelson, W., Proshansky, H., Rivlin, L., & Winkel, G. (1974). *An introduction to environmental psychology.* New York: Holt, Rinehart, & Winston.

Jenike, M. (1988). Depression and other psychiatric disorders. In M. Albert & M. Moss (Eds.), *Geriatric neuropsychology.* New York: Holt, Rinehart, & Winston.

Jones, K., & Lubinski, R. (unpublished manuscript). *Communication disorders research: Building scientific alliances in research for clinical relevance.*

Kagan., A. (2003). Aphasia centres and community: More than just a sum of parts. In S. Parr, J. Duchan, & C. Pound (Eds.), *Aphasia inside out.* (pp. 41–50). Berkshire, England: Open University Press.

Kahana, E., Lovegreen, L., Kahana, B., & Kahana, M. (2003). Person, environment, and person-environment fit as influences on residential satisfaction of elders. *Environment and Behavior, 33,* 434–453.

Kalra, L., Evans, A., Perez, I., et al. (2004). Training informal caregivers of patients, with stroke improved patient and caregiver quality of life and reduced costs. *British Medical Journal, 328*, 1099.

Kelly-Hayes, M., Warf, P., Kannel, W., Sytkowski, P., D'Agostino, R., & Gresham, G. (1988). Factors influencing survival and need for institutionalization following stroke: The Framingham study. *Archives of Physical and Medical Rehabilitation, 69*, 415–418.

Kinsella, G., & Duffy, R. (1979). Psychosocial readjustment in the spouses of aphasic patients. *Scandinavian Journal of Rehabilitation Medicine, 11*, 129–132.

Krause, N. (2001). Social support. In R. Binstock & L. George (Eds.). *Handbook of Aging and the Social Sciences* (pp. 273–294). San Diego: Academic Press.

Kricos, P. (2006). Audiologic management of older adults with hearing loss and compromised cognitive/psychoacoustic auditory processing capabilities. *Trends in Amplification, 10*, 1–27.

Kvigne, K., Kirkevold, M., & Gjengedal, E. (2004). Fighting back—Struggling to continue life and preserve the self following a stroke. *Health Care for Women International, 25*, 370–387.

Lawton, M. (1970). Assessment, integration and environments for older people. *Gerontology, 10*, 38–46.

LeDorze, G. (1995) *L'aphasie selon la perspectioe des personnes aphasiques et de leurs proches: Une analyze qualitative des consequences de l'aphasie.* Rapport de recherché subventionnee par le Programme National de Recherche en matiere de Sante. As cited Le Dorze, G., Croteau, C., Brassard, C., & Michallet, B. (1999). Research considerations guiding interventions for families affected by aphasia. *Aphasiology, 13*, 922–927.

LeDorze, G., & Brassard, C. (1995). A description of the consequences of aphasia on aphasic persons and relatives and friends, based on the WHO model of chronic diseases. *Aphasiology, 9*, 239–255.

LeDorze, G., Croteau, C., Brassard, C., & Michallet, B. (1999). Research considerations guiding interventions for families affected by aphasia. *Aphasiology, 13*, 922–927.

Li, Y., & Ferraro, K. (2005). Volunteering and depression in later life: Social benefit or selection processes? *Journal of Health and Social Behavior, 46*, 69–84.

Lubinski, R. (1981). Environmental language intervention. In R. Chapey (Ed.), *Language intervention strategies in adult aphasia.* Baltimore, MD: Williams & Wilkins.

Lubinski, R. (1995). Environmental considerations for elderly patients. In R. Lubinski (Ed.), *Dementia and communication.* San Diego: Singular.

Lum, T., & Lightfoot, E. (2005). The effects of volunteering on the physical and mental health of older people. *Research on Aging, 27*, 31–55.

Lyon, J. (1992). Communication use and participation in life for adults with aphasia in natural settings: The scope of the problem. *American Journal of Speech-Language Pathology, 1*, 7–14.

Mackay, R. (2003). 'Tell them who I was': The social construction of aphasia. *Disability and Society, 18*, 811–826.

Maitz, E., (1991) Family systems theory applied to head theory. In J. Williams & T. Kay (Eds.), *Head injury: A family matter* (pp. 81–100). Baltimore: Brookes.

Mann, W. (1997). An essential communication device: The telephone. In R. Lubinski & D. J. Higginbotham (Eds.), *Communication technologies for the elderly: Vision, hearing, and speech.* (pp. 323–340). San Diego: Singular.

Maslow, A. (2006). *Self-actualization.* Available at http://performance-unlimited.com/samain.htm.

McCormick, G., & Williams, P. (1976). The Midwestern Pennsylvania Stroke Club: Conclusions following the first year's operation of a family centered program. In R. Brookshire (Ed.), *Clinical aphasiology: Conference proceedings.* Minneapolis, MN: BRK.

McCullagh, E., Brigstocke, G., Donaldson, N., & Kalra, L. (2005). Determinants of caregiving burden and quality of life in caregivers of stroke patients. *Stroke, 36*, 2181.

Michallet, B., Le Dorze, G., & Tetreault, S. (2001). The needs of spouses caring for severely aphasic persons. *Aphasiology, 15*, 731–747.

Michallet, B., Tetreault, S., & Le Dorze, G. (2003). The consequences of severe aphasia on the spouses of aphasic people: A description of the adaptation process. *Aphasiology, 17*, 835–859.

Miller, R. G., Rosenberg, J. A., Gelinas, D. F., Mitsumoto, H., Newman, D., Sufit, R., et al. (1999). Practice parameter: The care of the patient with amyotrophic lateral sclerosis (an evidence based review). *Neurology, 52*, 1311–1325.

Moos, R. (1976). *The human contest.* New York: John Wiley & Sons.

Morgan, D., & Stewart, N. (1998). Multiple occupancy versus private rooms on dementia care units. *Environment and Behavior, 30*, 487–503.

National Aphasia Association. (2006). *News archives.* Available at http://aphasia.org/aphasianews4062006.php.

National Institute on Disability and Rehabilitation Research. (1999). Long-range plan for fiscal years 1999–2004. *Federal Register, 64*, 68576–69614.

Newton, M. (1997). Communication technology and safety of the elderly. In R. Lubinski & D. J. Higginbotham (Eds.), *Communication technologies for the elderly: Vision, hearing, and speech* (pp. 2295–2322). San Diego: Singular.

Nussbaum, M. (2000). *Women and human development.* Cambridge, England: Cambridge University Press.

O'Keefe, J., (2006). *Creating a senior friendly physical environment in our hospitals.* Available from the Regional Geriatric Assessment Program of Ottawa.

Orr, A. (1997). Assistive technologies for older persons who are visually impaired. In R. Lubinski & D. J. Higginbotham (Eds.), *Communication technologies for the elderly: Vision, hearing, and speech* (pp. 71–102). San Diego: Singular.

Palmer, S., & Glass, T. (2003). Family function and stroke recovery: A review. *Rehabilitation Psychology, 48*, 255–265.

Parr, S., Byng, S., Gilpin, S., & Ireland, C. (1977). *Talking about aphasia: Living with loss of language after stroke.* Buckingham, England: OUP.

Parr, S., Duchan, J., & Pound, C., (2003). *Aphasia inside out.* Berkshire, England: Open University Press.

Pasquarello, M. (1990). Developing, implementing, and evaluating a stroke recovery group. *Rehabilitation Nursing, 15*, 26–29.

Paul-Brown, D., Frattali, C., Holland, A., Thompson, C., & Caperton, C. J. (2001) *Quality of Communication Life Scale. Field test version.* Unpublished manuscript. Rockville, Maryland: American Speech-Language-Hearing Association.

Pichora-Fuller, M. K. (1997). Assistive listening devices for the elderly. In R. Lubinski & D. J. Higginbotham (Eds.), *Communication technologies for the elderly: Vision, hearing, and speech* (pp. 161–202). San Diego: Singular.

Putnam, R. (1995). Bowling alone: America's declining social capital. *Journal of Democracy, 6,* 65–78.

Rand Corporation. (1994). *The patient's view on health care.* Santa Monica, California: Author.

Robinson, R. G., & Benson, D. F. (1981). Depression in aphasia patients: Frequency, severity, and clinicopathological correlations. *Brain and Language, 14,* 282–291.

Rolland, J. (1990). Anticipatory loss: A family systems developmental framework. *Family Process, 29,* 229–243.

Ross, K. (2005). Assessing quality of life with aphasia: An annotated bibliography. *Perspectives on Neurophysiology and Neurogenic Speech and Language Disorders, 15,* 15–19.

Ross, K., & Wertz, R. (2003). Quality of life with and without aphasia. *Aphasiology, 17,* 355–364.

Rowe, J., & Kahn, R. (1998). *Successful aging: The MacArthur foundation study.* New York: Random House.

Safilios-Rothchild, C. (1970). *The sociology and social psychology of disability and rehabilitation.* New York: Random House.

Sarno, M. (1997). Quality of life in aphasia in the first post-stroke year. *Aphasiology, 11,* 665–679.

Scholte op Reimer, W., de Haan, R., Rijnders, P., Limburg, M, & van den Bos, G. (1998). Burden of caregiving in partners in long-term care survivors. *Stroke, 29,* 1605–1511.

Scottish Intercollegiate Guideline Network. [On line]. Available at http://www.sign.ac.uk.

Seeman, T. (2006). *Successful aging: Fact or fiction.* Available at http://aging.ucla.edu/successfulaging.html.

Sen, A. (1980). Equality of what. In S. McMurrin. (Ed.), *The Tanner lectures on human values.* Cambridge, England: Cambridge University Press.

Shadden, B., & Agan, J. (2004). Renegotiation of identity: The social context of aphasia support groups. *Topics in Language Disorders, 24,* 174–186.

Silliman, R., Fletcher, R., Earp, J., & Wagner, E. (1986). Families of elderly stroke patients: Effects of home care. *Journal of American Geriatric Society, 34,* 643–648.

Sotnick, P., & Jezewski, M. (2005). Culture and the disability services. In J. Stone (Ed.), *Culture and disability* (pp. 15–30). Thousand Oaks: Sage.

Starkstein, S., & Robinson, R. (1988). Aphasia and depression. *Aphasiology, 2,* 1–20.

Stern, S., & O'Boyle, R. (2002). *Successful aging: Optimizing life in the second half.* Available at http://ec-online.net/Knowledge/Articles/successfulaging.html.

Sturm, J., Osborne, R., Dewey, H., Donnan, G., Macdonell, R., & Thrift, A. (2002). Brief comprehensive quality of life assessment after stroke: The assessment of quality of life instrument in the north east Melbourne stroke incidence study. *Stroke, 33,* 2888–2894.

Tanner, D., Gerstenberger, D., & Keller, C. (1989). Guidelines for the treatment of chronic depression in the aphasia patient. *Rehabilitation Nursing, 14,* 77–80.

Turnbull, A., & Turnbull, H. R. (1991). Understanding families from a systems perspective. In J. Williams & T. Kay (Eds.), *Head injury: A family matter.* Baltimore, MD: Paul Brookes.

VanBiervliet, A., Edwards-Schaefer, P. (2004). Consumer health information on the web: Trends, issues, and strategies. *Dermatology Nursing, 16,* 519–523.

Van den Heuvel, E., de Witte, L., Stewart, R., Schure, L., Sanderman, R., & Meyboom-de Jong, B. (2002). Long-term effects of a group support program and an individual support program for informal caregivers of stroke patients: Which caregivers benefit the most? *Patient Education and Counseling, 47,* 291–299.

Vickery, C., Gontkovsky, S., & Caroselli, J. (2005). Self-concept and quality of life following acquired brain injury: A pilot investigation. *Brain Injury, 19,* 657–665.

Visser-Meily, A., Post, M., Schepers, V., & Lindeman, E. (2005). Spouses' quality of life one year after stroke: Prediction at the start of clinical rehabilitation. *Cerebrovascular Diseases, 20,* 443–448.

Wahrborg, P. (1991). *Assessment and management of emotional and psychological reactions to brain damage and aphasia.* San Diego: Singular.

Williams, J. (1991). Family reaction to head injury. In J. Williams & T. Kay (Eds.), *Head injury: A family matter.* Baltimore, MD: Paul Brookes.

Williams, L., Weinberger, M., Harris, L., & Biller, J. (1999). *Neurology, 53,* 1839.

World Health Organization. (2001). *International Classification of Functioning, Disability and Health.* Available at http://who.int/classification/icf.

Worrall, L., & Yiu, E. (2000). Effectiveness of functional communication therapy by volunteers for people with aphasia following stroke. *Aphasiology, 14,* 911–924.

Young, R., & Olson, E. (Eds.), (1991). *Health, illness, and disability in later life.* Newbury Park, California: Sage.

Zemva, N. (1999). Aphasic patients and their families: Wishes and expectations. *Aphasiology, 13,* 219–224.

Ziolko, M. (1991). Counseling parents of children with disabilities: A review of the literature and implications for practice. *Journal of Rehabilitation, 57,* 29–34.

Chapter 13

Focusing on the Consequences of Aphasia: Helping Individuals Get What They Need

Linda J. Garcia

OBJECTIVES

The objectives of this chapter are (1) to introduce the reader to fundamental principles of disability models, (2) to illustrate how these can be used to structure intervention programs focused on the consequences of aphasia, and (3) to review existing programs that can be incorporated into a life consequences approach to intervention. It is hoped that the reader will better understand better the complexities of a life consequences approach to intervention while, at the same time, adopt a concrete framework for organizing this information.

Approximately 1 million Americans live with the consequences of aphasia at any given time, with approximately 80,000 new cases every year (National Stroke Association, 2006). In addition, an estimated 4.5 million Americans have Alzheimer's disease (Alzheimer's Association, 2006), and 1.4 million sustain traumatic brain injury each year (National Center for Injury Prevention and Control, 2006). If one adds to these numbers those who live, work, and interact with the individual who has the disorder, the human impact of these conditions on everyday life can take on incredible proportions.

You may have wondered how you or someone you know might react to becoming aphasic or how this would affect your life. You might have wondered what your priorities for intervention would be. Likely, you would want to regain as much of your language as possible and do as many of the same life activities you did before your stroke, or, as some, you might see this as an opportunity to set different goals and develop other skills. Do you think your priorities would be different if you became aphasic at age 20 than if you became aphasic at age 75? How about if you worked as a speech-language pathologist or a lawyer versus a heavy machine operator? Do you think the impact of a language loss might be different? How about if you were living with a spouse and children, or just with your spouse, or living alone? Would the life priorities be different? What *would* be your priorities? In light of these questions, would you prioritize mobility, communication, pain management, or dealing with your incontinence? The point here is that even though two people might have exactly the same linguistic impairments, the impact on each of their lives could be completely different. Interventions focused on life consequences are preoccupied with exactly this impact.

THE NEED FOR A MODEL TO GUIDE INTERVENTION: A FRAMEWORK

No recipes exist for helping individuals return to their lives or redefine new ones following disease, disorder, or trauma. One solution may be adequate for one situation or one person but not for another. Likewise, one solution might work at one specific time in the person's life and not at another. Because aphasia is generally a chronic disorder, its impact may be felt differently at its onset as opposed to 10 years later. The only way to understand the interaction of these many factors is to use a framework that explains the relationships among the person and his or her abilities, environment, and life goals. Disability models can do this. Traditionally, our interventions have been guided by medical ideology. More modern models are based on social ideology (Byng & Duchan, 2005; Mackay, 2003).

To couch aphasia within the context of disability models is to accept that communication is only part of the story. To illustrate this point, let us use the analogy of the six blind men and the elephant (Saxe, 1963). This legend recounts the story of six blind men who, wondering what an elephant looked like, each touched a different part of the elephant's anatomy. The first touched its side and concluded that the elephant looked like a wall. The second touched its tusk and compared it to a spear. The third touched the trunk and decided it was a snake. The fourth touched the leg, which seemed to be a tree without leaves. The fifth found the ear and concluded the elephant looked like a fan, and the sixth touched the tail and imagined it to look like a rope. Each was convinced of the truth of his conclusions, yet each one of them was wrong.

How might this apply to our knowledge of the consequences of aphasia? Not unlike the six blind men, the foremothers of speech-language pathology relegated communication to the speech apparatus without necessarily considering the other aspects of communication (Duchan, 2006). With increasing scientific knowledge, we came to see communication as a complex system of interrelated abilities. We might use the analogy of the six blind men and the elephant to compare the phonetic system, phonology, syntax, semantics, pragmatics, and discourse as different parts of the elephant's anatomy, with the elephant itself representing the system of communication. No clinician or researcher today would argue against the fact that communication involves at least all of these elements. In terms of guiding intervention, for instance, we know that if we intervene on the syntactic aspects of language, we must be cognizant of the impact of the semantic system. We have theories as to how these elements function together and how we might use one aspect to facilitate the other during intervention.

Let us take the analogy one step further by considering communication as part of a cognitive system, with elements such as memory, attention, vision, and audition being the other components. Again, few would argue against the fact that all these elements are important to understand how one communicates. As in the first example, one might intervene and focus on the receptive aspects of communication while being cognizant of the impact of sensory systems, such as vision or audition, or other components, such as attention. We have conceptual frameworks with which to understand the interdependence of these elements so that we can better intervene on the communication aspects.

What happens if we use this same analogy yet again to understand and intervene on the impact of a communication disorder on an individual's life? Let us say that the elephant represents the person's integration into different aspects of his of her life (e.g., work integration and interpersonal relationships). In this context, communication is only one part of the elephant. The others might include culture, a supportive spouse, and disability laws. We would be foolish to consider looking at just one aspect of the elephant (e.g., communication) and assume that this is the only thing that influences a person's functioning. Disability models give us the framework from which to understand the interaction of these larger-scale elements (Byng & Duchan, 2005). Variations of international disability models have been around for more than 25 years and, as Ross and Wertz (2005) have pointed out, they are likely to stay. Although it can be argued that much work remains to be done, the basic philosophies behind these models provide a useful framework from which to understand the possible relationships among components of individual functioning that go beyond the communication patterns per se.

The ICF: Getting a Framework to Guide Intervention

Use disability models such as the International Classification of Functioning, Disability, and Health (World Health Organization, 2001), or ICF, to capture the impact of aphasia on everyday life is a growing trend (Simmons-Mackie, Kearns, & Potechin, 2005; Threats, 2006; Threats & Worrall, 2004). This framework has been widely diffused to both clinicians and researchers, and reference to this model is almost routine for those who are interested in psychosocial functioning.

Although an argument exists over whether the ICF can be used as part of an appraisal of aphasia (Ross & Wertz, 2005), the American Speech-Language-Hearing Association (2001), or ASHA, encourages the use of the ICF "to describe the role of speech-language pathologists in enhancing quality of life by optimizing human communication behavior, swallowing, or other upper aerodigestive functions regardless of setting." (p. I-22a-b). Travis Threats, a speech-language pathologist, is currently working with colleagues to develop a clinical manual to help prepare clinicians to use the ICF framework and classification (Reed et al., 2005). A better understanding of the historical development of the ICF may help the clinician to evaluate the relevance and importance of a framework such as the ICF in planning therapy.

The ICF is part of what the World Health Organization (WHO) considers to be a "family of classification systems." The intention is that these classification systems be used, as much as possible, in a complementary fashion. The International Classification of Diseases (WHO, 1999), or ICD, which is in the process of being updated, classifies health conditions. The ICF was developed to classify human functioning as a result of these health conditions. The impetus behind the ICF was to develop a common international language to describe the consequences of disease, trauma, and disorder. The WHO wished the classification to be used (1) for **scientific** reasons to look at the impact of health conditions, (2) for improving **services** by offering a framework for designing interventions and outcomes, (3) for helping individuals specify their **needs**, (4) for **economic** planning, and (5) for helping in the defense of the **rights** of individuals with functional limitations. The classification is not an evaluation system, nor is it meant to be a list of discipline-specific functions. Its aim is to capture an individual's level of functioning through use of a common language that includes a series of codes and categories.

Since its publication, researchers have offered preliminary applications of the ICF framework to the area of aphasia (Davidson & Worrall, 2000; Howe, Worrall, & Hickson,

2004; Threats, 2006; Threats & Worrall, 2004; Worrall, McCooey, Davidson, Larkins, & Hickson, 2002). As early as 1980, the WHO had already given us the International Classification of Impairments, Disabilities, and Handicaps (WHO, 1980), or ICIDH, and speech-language pathologists later applied these concepts to aphasia (LeDorze & Brassard, 1995). Today, however, neither the ICF nor the ICIDH has yet been proven to be useful in terms of its classification categories. In a pilot study, Garcia and colleagues (2003) used the categories from the ICF to describe the level of functioning of two individuals with aphasia. They found the classification to be incomplete in its ability to describe language functions as well as difficult to code in terms of environmental influence. Most uses still tend to focus on the philosophy rather than the classification per se.

The ICF was developed as an improvement over the original ICIDH, which was a linear model (Fig. 13–1). In the ICIDH, the model basically suggested that a disease or disorder (e.g., cerebrovascular accident [CVA]), would lead to impairments (e.g., a brain lesion), which in turn would lead to disabilities (e.g., aphasia), which in turn would lead to handicaps (e.g., not being able to work). Although the international community was pleased to see that we now considered the impact of "disabilities" such as aphasia, it was concerned about the linearity of the model. Individuals with functional limitations, clinicians, and disability researchers were dismayed that this model portrayed individuals with functional limitations as being "doomed" to have handicaps in the real world. The unidirectional impact (as suggested by the direction of the arrows in Fig. 13–1), indicated the likely effect on a handicap, suggesting that the disorder dictated the outcome. In this model, neither the physical environment nor society was held to be even partly accountable for creating obstacles to integration. It followed from this model, then, that if we worked on the impairments (e.g., brain lesion) and/or the disability (e.g., the aphasia itself), we would prevent the person from living with a handicap and from being "handicapped." The bottom line was that if the language impairment could be reduced, the consequences could also be reduced.

Newer models of disability encourage us to put these impairment-based therapies in a larger context. After many years of international consultation and the development of alpha and beta versions of the ICIDH-2, the WHO pro-

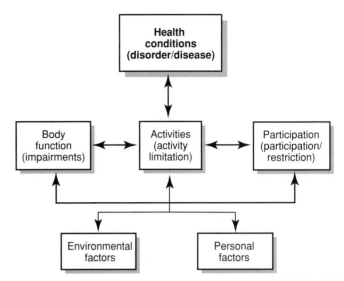

Figure 13–2. Model of the International Classification of Functioning, Disability and Health (ICF) (World Health Organization, 2001).

posed the newer ICF. One of the main differences between the ICF and the original ICIDH is the recognition that environmental factors (both physical and social) play a role in determining the level of functioning. Figure 13–2 provides a graphic representation of the ICF framework.

In this newer framework, the three key elements—Body function, Activities, and Participation (roughly the neutral versions of the three ICIDH domains)—are influenced by environmental factors and by personal factors. The premise here is that each of these three basic elements can be classified within an environmental context. Therefore, functioning can be interpreted in the context of a supportive spouse, a facilitative conversational partner, or access to an electronic communication board. Functioning can also be interpreted in the context of personal factors, such as age, sex, and cultural background.

The ICF has been criticized on many levels, including having a framework that remains more medically based than socially based (Fougeyrollas, 2006; Hilari, 2005; Whiteneck, 2006). Part of this criticism is that no clear distinction is made between the domains of Activities and Participation. As Worrall and Cruice (2005) clarify, the differences are more in relation to the levels of context. Activities refers more to what the person can do and Participation to what the individual actually does do in his or her real environments. Because the environmental factors interact with all elements in this model, however, the distinction between Activities and Participation remains nebulous. In fact, the list of Activities and Participation elements are actually all in one list in the ICF. It is understandable, therefore, that the clinician may have difficulty distinguishing the two. Nonetheless, the principles of the ICF help us to see all

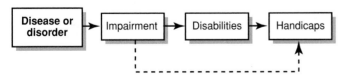

Figure 13–1. The International Classification of Impairments, Disabilities and Handicap (ICIDH) model (World Health Organization, 1980).

components of functioning. If we see ourselves as focusing on only one aspect of the model, we are back to the six blind men and the elephant.

An Alternative: The DCP Model

The current discussion surrounding these frameworks may appear to be academic to some, but it is important for the clinician to use some type of framework to guide consequence-based therapy. Interventions using a life consequences approach are not new, but clinicians might find it hard to understand how all the components fit together. For this reason, I would like to introduce an alternative model that might help clinicians to focus on an integrated approach—the Disability Creation Process model (Fougeyrollas, Cloutier, Bergeron, Côté, & St. Michel, 1998), or DCP. Both the ICF and the DCP models are closely related and use similar concepts. I find the DCP to be easier to interpret, however, and the reader is therefore encouraged to see the remainder of this chapter as a possible application of the ICF principles through use of the DCP conceptual model (1998).

Fougeyrollas and colleagues were very much involved in the ICIDH revision process and were instrumental in the inclusion of environmental factors in the WHO framework. The primary difference between the ICF and the DCP is the exclusivity of the components. In the DCP model, a clear distinction exists between the Activities, which is called Capabilities, and Participation, which is called Life Habits (Fig. 13–3). Capabilities do not include environmental factors, but participation necessarily includes the influ-ence of the environment. This is much more than an academic distinction and is extremely important, because it helps the clinician to distinguish what belongs to the person (personal factors) and what belongs to the environment (environmental factors). Hence, intervention strategies can be geared toward one, the other, or both. The model acknowledges that if the therapist chooses to work at the Capabilities level (e.g., working on the linguistic aspects of aphasia), improvement is likely to influence performance in life activities and roles. If the therapist chooses to work on the environmental factors (e.g., partners), however, reduction of environmental obstacles, in and of themselves, can impact participation.

Teasing out the environmental factors is important for advocacy, because it offers the opportunity to identify those factors that belong to the society and to the individual's milieu. Hence, comparisons across nations and health-care systems are more easily made. For instance, the impact of managed care versus universal health care in rehabilitation can be easily explained using these principles. CVAs or aphasia (personal factors in the DCP) can affect individuals in very similar ways across countries, because human bodies function, overall, in similar ways. The health-care system in one country can be a facilitator, and in another, an obstacle, when it comes to allowing people with aphasia to receive therapy. Environmental factors themselves constitute a sep-arate component and should be viewed as such by therapists. This concept allows us to identify society's responsibility and acknowledges the role that it plays in facilitating integration (Kagan & Leblanc, 2002).

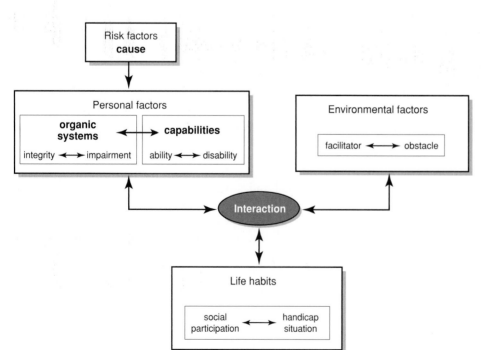

Figure 13–3. The Disability Creation Process (DCP) model. (From Fougeyrollas et al., 1998; with permission.)

Another important concept supported by the proponents of the DCP model is that the model applies to all human beings. The DCP model, in its historical development, was derived from anthropological theories of human development (Fougeyrollas being an anthropologist himself by profession). Hence, the proponents of this model stress that it can be applied to all individuals with or without perceived "disabilities." The premise is that all of us live with the consequences of some type of health disorder, disease, or trauma. Whether you struggle with relationships because of a lack of self esteem or you need reading glasses or you live with aphasia, you are at risk of living in a situation of handicap. A clinician who gives you reading glasses (an environmental factor) or a surgeon who performs corrective surgery (impacting on body structure) can remove this situation of handicap and allow you to function in your selected life activities or roles. Likewise, if you are the parent of a child with a health disorder or the adult child of an ailing parent, the model can be applied to your situation. Your own life activity or role (e.g., work) may be affected by someone else's (your child's or parent's) health condition. You are then the person who can be seen to live the consequences of your ailing parents', spouse's, or child's health condition. Take, for instance, the case of dementia. Informal caregivers who live with individuals who have dementia live the consequences of their loved one's disorder each and every day. Seeing the consequences through the disability model helps us to appreciate how the loved one's health condition (dementia) impacts the spouse's life activities. Helping the individual with dementia through programs such as respite care helps the caregiver to return, momentarily, to some of those life activities. This reasoning could and should be applied to aphasia as well.

Later in the chapter, you, the reader, will be asked to apply the model to yourself. Seeing yourself in a human developmental model will help you to recognize the impact of health conditions and, perhaps, better prepare you for understanding the possible consequences of aphasia.

Bottom line: Environment should be considered as an independent component capable of influencing integration and, therefore, as a potential focus of intervention, regardless of your preferred model.

Operational Definitions

The following section will help the clinician to understand conceptually the different elements of a disability model by way of the DCP definitions. The choice of the DCP model for this discussion is to help clinicians operationalize the concepts of Activities and Participation to guide intervention.

The Life Activities and Roles

The logical place to start is the Life Participation component—or "life habits" in the DCP model. A life habit is "a daily activity or a social role valued by the person or his socio-cultural context according to his characteristics (age, sex, socio-cultural identity, etc.) which ensures his survival and well-being in his society throughout his lifetime." (Fougeyrollas et al., 1998, p. 131). This can include anything from being involved in your personal self-care (physical and mental) to taking part in community activities or interpersonal relationships. A person's success in his or her life activity or role can be measured on a scale going from full social participation (meaning no problems at all with this activity or role) to a situation of handicap. A "situation" of handicap should be understood conceptually as something that might be temporary. It is influenced by the individual's abilities and by the support of his or her environment. Hence, the more the individual's abilities improve (i.e., less aphasia) and the more the environment becomes supportive, the less the individual lives with a situation of handicap, and the more his or her performance "slides" along the continuum toward social participation.

The key, then, clinically is to determine which daily activities or social roles are valued by the person at that point in time in his or her life. The activities or roles that appear to cause problems are not likely to be permanent. An individual can live a situation of handicap at some point in time and not at another, despite having the same functional limitation (e.g., same degree of aphasia). Because some situations can disappear (e.g., no longer need to return to work) and other situations can be created (e.g., planning more leisure activities), speech-language pathology services should be available throughout the life span. For instance, someone who wishes to reintegrate the workforce at age 45 following a stroke may be faced with a situation of handicap; however, at retirement, this may no longer be an issue. This person may also be experiencing situations of handicap in some leisure activities that may warrant different interventions from a speech-language pathologist. An approach to therapy based on life consequences would start by identifying the life activities and roles that are (1) important to the individual and/or to his or her culture or society and (2) done frequently by the individual at a certain point in time. Examples of creative ways for identifying these goals will be discussed later.

The Personal Factors

Assuming that the individual you are seeing is experiencing a situation of handicap with an activity and/or social role, the model suggests that this is the case because the person (1) has limitations related to personal factors (body structure or mental or physical capabilities) and/or (2) is subject to obstacles in the environment that prevent the achievement of higher participation levels. The next step to intervention will then be to identify these contributing factors.

Personal factors include a person's characteristics and capabilities. In addition to age, sex, culture, education, and the like, it includes how the body structures function and how limited or accomplished the individual is in terms of physical, sensory, mental, and cognitive abilities. The actual aphasia as well as motivation levels or attention are part of these personal factors. Some conceptualize these factors as "within the skin" (what the individual brings to the situation of handicap). If it was felt that the situation of handicap could be helped by intervening at the level of body structure, interventions that target body systems would be warranted (e.g., surgical procedures for aneurysms). If it was felt that the situations of handicap were caused by specific functional limitations in the individual's physical, sensory, mental, and/or cognitive capabilities, therapy for these capabilities would be warranted. A "capability" is defined as "the potential of a person to accomplish mental or physical activities" (Fougeyrollas et al., 1998, p. 69) without taking any environmental factors into account. Therapy focused on capabilities, when applied to aphasia, might involve linguistic or neuropsychologically based therapies as well as therapies aimed to improve other psychological components, such as motivational levels. Within a team context, it would also include other therapies, such as physical therapies or psychological therapies. It is important to note that the link is always made with participation levels in life activities and roles.

At the personal factors level, the clinician looks for what the person can do *without* environmental obstacles or environmental help. This gives the clinician a clearer perspective from which to identify the impact of environmental factors as an independent, equally important component.

Environmental Factors

The situation of handicap experienced by the individual is also likely to be the result of environmental barriers. An "environmental factor" is "a physical or social dimension that determines a society's organization and context" (Fougeyrollas et al., 1998, p. 111). It can create an obstacle to integration, or it can facilitate integration. These factors can include physical barriers, such as noise; social barriers, such as an unsupportive spouse; or organizational barriers, such as lack of services. The clinician's goal here is to help reduce the barriers and increase the number of facilitators. So, if it was felt that the environmental obstacles contributed to the situation of handicap, intervention at this level would be warranted. Examples of how to apply these strategies to aphasia are given later in this chapter.

Summary of Disability Models

In summary, disability models can be used to offer a framework for planning team interventions. Whether one impacts on personal or environmental factors or both, intervention has the potential to help achieve the ultimate outcome, which is to improve quality of life and integration into society. The premise is that an individual may have few functional limitations but face environmental factors that create enormous

obstacles to intervention. Likewise, a person may have very significant functional limitations yet, because of a facilitative environment, succeed in participating in his or her life activity or role. Hence, intervention on environmental factors can be just as important as focusing on language skills.

Applying a Disability Model to Your Own Functioning

If clinicians are to apply disability model concepts to help people with aphasia and their loved ones better integrate their lives, what better way to understand the philosophy than to apply these concepts to their own lives? As stated earlier, the concepts underlying disability models are meant, conceptually, to be universal. The following exercise is geared to helping the reader learn the concepts through personal applications. Similar questions will arise with those who seek our services.

First, pick a life activity or role that you feel you are not achieving to your fullest but that is important to you and/or your culture. Make sure this is something that you normally do or would like to do, and make sure it is something that you want to do frequently enough for it to be considered important to you. You might consider nutrition (e.g., diet), fitness (e.g., both mental and physical fitness), housing (e.g., finding lodging and/or decorating it), financial and family responsibilities, sexual activities, affective and social interpersonal relationships, community and spiritual involvement, education or employment, or leisure (e.g., sports or arts) activities. Just pick one life activity that impacts your quality of life.

Let us call this your "unfulfilled life activity," and for illustrative purposes, let us say that this activity falls into the Fitness category. You feel that you would like to take part in more physical activity so that you can keep in shape. To help you, we must identify the reasons why you are unable to take part in activities that keep you in shape. First, is there a body structure or system that prevents you from fulfilling your life activity? Perhaps a past knee injury prevents you from doing many of the physical activities you once did or would like to do. If so, is there anything you can do about this body structure or system? Would surgery help? Would medication help?

Next, take a quick inventory of your personal capabilities and see if any might limit your ability to take part in your unfulfilled life activity. These might include your intellectual capabilities (e.g., consciousness, memory, and thought), language capabilities, behavior capabilities (e.g., volition and affectivity), sensory and perceptual capabilities, motor activity capabilities (e.g., voluntary body part movements and manual activities), as well as capabilities related to breathing, digestion, excretion, reproduction, protection, and resistance (e.g., tolerance to sound and humidity as well as mental endurance).

We are basically looking for the contribution these capabilities might be having on your inability to fulfill your life activity. In the example given above, you might find that you are unable to perform your life activity of keeping in shape because of a lack of motivation on your part or, again, because of limited motor capabilities (e.g., perhaps because of a previous injury). Can something be done about these capabilities? Whereas intervention based on body structures might come in the form of knee surgery, one based on capabilities might come in the form of physiotherapy, for instance.

Your inquiry does not stop here. According to models such as the DCP, fulfillment of your life activity is the result of two elements: personal factors, and environmental factors. We examined your body structure as a possible cause for not keeping in shape. We looked at what you can or cannot do (capabilities) as a cause for the unfulfilled activity. We must also, however, look at the environmental factors. Consider again your specific situation. Does your physical environment, such as where you live or elements related to nature (e.g., too much snow or too much heat), contribute? Are these things preventing you from taking part in your activity or role? Also, think of social environments, such as family and friends and work colleagues, or yet again, you might look at organizational or governmental rules and regulations. For instance, in the example given above, there may not be many activities available to people in your age group or geographic area, thereby diminishing the chances you will be involved with these types of physical activities. To resolve your problem, you might think of finding a friend who can do a physical activity with you, starting a local activity yourself, or lobbying the municipal government to develop other activities for your age group.

In conclusion, to help you take part in your selected life activity or role, you might need to work on the body structure (e.g., knee surgery), work on the capability (e.g., improve movement through physiotherapy or work on your motivation), or get a facilitator (e.g., find a friend to join a physical activity program with you). The challenge is to find which of these parameters is most efficient over the short and long term in helping you to integrate your life activity or role. Basically, the disability models, whether you espouse to the DCP or the ICF, stress that the individual's functioning is not solely the result of a series of reduced functional limitations (e.g., aphasia + hemiplegia + lack of motivation) but, rather, interact with social and physical environments.

Bottom line: Current disability models are meant to use concepts that are applicable to all human beings. The number and level of severity of the situations of handicap will vary as a function of personal and environmental factors.

APPLYING THE FRAMEWORK TO APHASIA

The First Component: Identifying Disrupted Life Activities and Roles

As has been said, any clinician wishing to use a framework that takes into account the consequences of aphasia must identify the very consequences that might need intervention. The challenge in applying a life consequences approach is to identify the life activity or social role that the individual would like to address with the help of the therapeutic team. Whereas in more traditional approaches the therapist examines the results of the linguistic evaluation to determine the goals of therapy, the life consequences approach requires the therapist to obtain information from individuals regarding their involvement in life activities and roles as well as their perceptions of the successes they feel they are attaining.

A Question of Perspective

A key element in successful identification of life participation activities and roles is the perception of the individual with aphasia. The clinician should make every effort to include the individual with the disorder in identifying the perceived level of accomplishment of life activities and roles as well as the level of satisfaction. Not only should the individual be instrumental in choosing the goal, he or she should indicate the level of importance as well as the frequency with which the life activities are performed. This will influence the clinical decision to incorporate these activities as target goals for therapy. Only as a last result should a substitute decision maker be requested to help identify the life participation goals for the person with aphasia.

The aphasia literature contains considerable evidence that proxies are not good substitutes for respondents with aphasia. The paper by Byng and Duchan (2005) on the application of social model philosophies to therapy for aphasia stresses the importance of involving the person with aphasia in all decisions that concern therapeutic interventions. An excellent study by Cruice, Worrall, Hickson, and Murison (2005) compared patients' own ratings of quality of life to those of family and friends. These ratings were taken from (1) a global quality of life measure ("How would you rate your quality of life?"); (2) the Short Form 36 Health Survey, which is a scale of functional outcome; (3) a short, usable quality-of-life scale called the Dartmouth COOP Charts; and (4) the condensed Ryff Psychological Well-Being scale. The authors found that, overall, the perceptions of proxy respondents could not be assumed to be interchangeable with those of the individuals with aphasia. This, of course, depended on the nature of the questions being asked—the more subjective the category, the larger the discrepancy in ratings between the groups. Sometimes, it might be difficult to obtain this type of information from persons with aphasia, but Engell, Hütter, Willmes, and Huber (2003) found an effective way to evaluate quality of life in aphasia using a pictorial self-rating procedure. They, too, found differences in ratings between persons with aphasia and their relatives.

Using a more qualitative interview approach, Parr, Byng, and Gilpin (1997) interviewed 50 individuals with aphasia and reported on their experiences in living with aphasia. In a subsequent paper, Parr (2001) reflected on the importance of the perspective of these individuals with aphasia and highlighted how this might affect an "outsider's" view of the consequences of aphasia. She pointed out, for instance, that a person with aphasia may view the impact of aphasia on his or her inability to return to work as being much more invasive compared with the perceptions of the outsider clinician.

In conclusion, it is important to adopt a person-centered approach when identifying the primary areas of life participation that are most problematic. Doing so elevates our level of professionalism as clinicians.

Bottom line: Include the person with aphasia when identifying the goals based on life participation.

Getting Help from Formal Measures of Quality of Life

The therapist has several options, none of them ideal, for obtaining quality-of-life information. Options include generic or disease-specific quality of life measures, informal questionnaires and interviews, and participation=level assessment scales.

The WHO Quality of Life (WHOQOL) group (1998) defines "quality of life" as "individuals' perceptions of their position in life in the context of the culture and value systems in which they live and in relation to their goals, expectations, standards and concerns" (p. 551). This description of quality of life includes many components of what has been reviewed so far under life participation. Because aphasia can affect an individual's capacity to understand and/or express written or oral language, it is no small task to obtain this information using formal measures (Hilari & Byng, 2001).

In aphasia, many of our measures of functioning focus greatly on communication (Frattali, 1998), and when communication is impaired, we assume quality of life is also impaired. Hence, the measures we have of communication and conversational abilities become central to the measure of functional outcome. In her chapter on social approaches to aphasia intervention, Simmons-Mackie (2001) offers a comprehensive list of measures used to assess functional communication, either through scales such as the ASHA Functional Assessment of Communication Skills for Adults (Frattali, Thompson, Holland, Wohl, & Ferketic, 1995), or ASHA-FACS, or through judgment ratings such as the Communicative Effectiveness Index (Lomas et al., 1989), or CETI, in which, using a brief scale, families and friends rate how effectively the person with aphasia communicates in various daily communication activities. These are not meant to be quality-of-life scales, nor are they meant to be scales of overall functioning. Unfortunately, some clinicians interpret the results from these scales as outcome scales of overall functioning.

Simmons-Mackie, Threats, and Kagan (2005) surveyed speech-language pathologists on their practice of outcome assessment. In that study, the majority of respondents viewed outcomes as changes in therapy or intervention, with only a few viewing outcome as a change in life participation. In fact, only four respondents even referred explicitly to the term "participation" despite the increasing use of models such as the ICF in the literature. Close to half of the respondents stated that they used some model or theory to guide their choice of outcome assessment methods. The authors concluded, "There appeared to be no general consensus regarding how one measures or reports improvement after intervention or what constitutes improvement" (p. 12). If clinicians are not in agreement about what constitutes outcome despite half of them using some model of functioning, how can we hope to document and effect change on the life consequences of aphasia?

The ASHA guidelines (ASHA, 2001) stress that speech-language pathologists should have, as an outcome goal, the overall improvement of quality of life for the individuals in their care. Outcome cannot be limited to communication skills alone, and it does not appear to be the case that clinicians have access to a ready-made, universally accepted way of measuring perceived quality of life or participation of individuals with aphasia (Simmons-Mackie, Threats, & Kagan, 2005). This is where disability models can help. In disability terms, and for the purposes of the current chapter, the goal of intervention might be the outcome that improves the client's perceived quality of life by improving participation in life situations or decreasing the number of situations of handicap. As explained previously in this chapter, the focus might be on linguistic intervention, behavioral intervention, elimination of environmental obstacles, or adoption of new life goals. Whatever the approach, however, the outcome goals per se may not, in and of themselves, be communication goals.

In other words, whether one aims to improve cellular activity poststroke, improve naming ability, or facilitate conversations in real-world settings, agreement hopefully exists that our ultimate outcome is improved quality of life. Further, we can assume that quality of life encompasses much more than communication despite the important effect of communication on quality of life (Cruice, Worrall, & Hickson, 2003). Although quality of life is closely linked to participation in life activities and goals, they are not one and the same (Hirsh & Holland, 2000). From this perspective, functional communication assessments are not sufficient. Hirsh and Holland (2000) point out that although quality-of-life measures were originally used for economic reasons and to obtain population-level information regarding health status, most quality-of-life measures now include some assessment of the individual's perception of how he or she is getting along with his or her life. A recent DVD video developed by McWreath (2005) helps the public and others with aphasia understand, through words and pictures, the impact of aphasia.

Throughout the quality-of-life literature, much discussion is found about its measurement and whether scales (McDowell & Newell, 1996) are disease specific or generic. All can be useful, and the choice depends on the clinician's goals. This discussion extends beyond the scope of this chapter but is intrinsic to the clinician's understanding of participation, so a brief discussion is warranted. The proponents of disease-specific scales take the position that, as a group, the lived experiences of individuals with similar health conditions will also be similar. For instance, people with aphasia may find similar difficulties in the realization of their life activities that are not usually problematic for people with other types of health conditions. The underlying assumption is that the health condition is directly influencing the quality of life. These scales will be most sensitive to linguistic change following intervention, because the very design of the scale includes language-dependent items. In the area of aphasia, very few quality-of-life scales have been designed specifically for people with aphasia. The Stroke and Aphasia Quality of Life Scale–39 (Hilari, Byng, Lamping, & Smith, 2003), or SAQOL, is an adapted version of the Stroke-Specific Quality of Life Scale (Williams, Weinberger, Harris, Clark, & Biller, 1999), or SSQOL. The SSQOL includes 49 items within 12 domains (energy, family roles, language, mobility, mood, personality, self-care, social roles, thinking, upper extremity function, vision, and work/productivity), which must be self-evaluated on a five-point scale. The SAQOL includes four additional items specifically related to communication. Figure 13–4 gives a sample of the scoresheet used in the SAQOL; a more aphasia-friendly presenter's sheet is available with the test. Psychometric data on the use of the SAQOL with the stroke population at large will be available shortly. As with the SF-36 Health Survey (Ware, Kosinski, & Gandek, 2000), the scale evaluates functional limitations in the way of abilities as much as it does participation levels. The role of environmental factors, however, is not looked at specifically. Many of the domains that are included are actually "personal factors" (using DCP terminology). In fact, some items are actually perceptions of how well individuals feel they are doing on capabilities (e.g. "Do you have trouble seeing things off to one side?") rather than life activities or roles. Other scales, such as the Burden of Stroke Scale, or BOSS, by Doyle, McNeil, Hula, and Mikolic (2003) will offer an interesting tool for looking at the limitations stroke might have on different activities and psychological states. Once again, however, this scale mixes activity limitations with participation levels. This tool was also specifically designed for survivors of stroke. Both scales try to make links between the health condition (in this case, stroke) and success in various life activities.

Another point of view in assessing quality of life is that generic measures are preferable if one wants to bring about policy changes. Generic scales permit comparisons across diagnoses, whether across individuals with different diagnoses or within one individual who lives with the impact of several diagnoses (McDowell & Newell, 2006). Generic measures of quality of life may allow clinicians to discover other areas of life participation that might have been affected by the disorder but not been identified a priori as a potential area of difficulty. Likewise, they may discover that conditions other than the aphasia are contributing to the situation of handicap. The proponents of generic quality-of-life measures hold that the purpose of these measures is to look at the impact on overall functioning, not to obtain more information about the health condition itself. They believe that a ripple effect exists in terms of impact and that the health condition can affect other parameters of functioning not previously foreseen.

Generic quality-of-life measures allow us to compare the life consequences of aphasia to other conditions—for example, rhinitis, which has a much higher prevalence in the population but life consequences that may be very different. Such generic quality-of-life measures include the WHO-QOL (WHOQOL Group, 1998), which is quite comprehensive and evaluates many life domains. The WHOQOL comes in a long version (100 items) and an abbreviated version (26 items) and is available in 20 languages. It looks at six domains: (1) physical health (energy, pain, and sleep), (2) psychological (negative and positive feelings, self esteem, and thinking), (3) level of independence (mobility, activities of daily living, and work capacity), (4) social relations (including support), (5) environment (financial, home, leisure, and transport), and (6) spirituality (religion and spiritual beliefs). This scale is quite lengthy and, like many others, might be difficult to administer to people with aphasia. One of the attractive features of this tool is that it is standardized across many different countries and languages.

Other generic scales focus on life satisfaction. The Life Satisfaction Questionnaire (Carlsson & Hamrin, 2002) evaluates the level of functioning and the respondent's perceived satisfaction with life areas. For instance, it looks at the impact of various symptoms, such as tiredness, lack of fitness, loss of appetite, pain, how happy the respondent is with work, financial situation, health, where the respondent lives, level of activity, and relationships. The astute clinician might want to look at the relationship between the ratings from those with aphasia on certain of these items and (1) the severity of their aphasia and (2) the support they are receiving.

Two other scales based on disability models also merit consideration. The Craig Hospital Assessment and Reporting Technique (Whiteneck et al., 1988), or CHART, and the Life-H scale (Fougeyrollas et al., 1997; Noreau et al., 2004; Noreau, Fougeyrollas, & Vincent, 2002) were designed using disability models as a theoretical underpinning (the CHART from the original ICIDH and the Life-H from the DCP model). Participation scales rate the life

Item ID	During the past week: Did you (repeat before each item or as necessary)	Definitely yes	Mostly yes	Not sure	Mostly no	Definitely no	Physical	Commun-ication	Pyscho-social	Energy
T4	Have to write things down to remember them (*or ask somebody else to write things down for you to remember*)?	1	2	3	4	5				
T5	Find it hard to make decisions?	1	2	3	4	5				
P1	Feel irritable?	1	2	3	4	5				
P3	Feel that your personality has changed?	1	2	3	4	5				
MD2	Feel discouraged about the future?	1	2	3	4	5				
MD3	Have no interest in other people or activities?	1	2	3	4	5				
MD6	Feel withdrawn from other people?	1	2	3	4	5				
MD7	Have little confidence in yourself?	1	2	3	4	5				
E2	Feel tired most of the time?	1	2	3	4	5				
E3	Have to stop and rest often during the day?	1	2	3	4	5				
E4	Feel too tired to do what you wanted to do?	1	2	3	4	5				
FR7	Feel that you were a burden to your family?	1	2	3	4	5				
FR9	Feel that your language problems interfered with your family life?	1	2	3	4	5				
SR1	Go out less often than you would like?	1	2	3	4	5				
SR4	Do your hobbies and recreation less often than you would like?	1	2	3	4	5				
SR5	See your friends less than you would like?	1	2	3	4	5				
SR7	Feel that your physical condition interfered with your social life?	1	2	3	4	5				
SR8	Feel that your language problems interfered with your social life?	1	2	3	4	5				
	SAQOL- 39 mean score	Add all items and divide by 39								
	Physical score	(SC items + M items + W items + UE items + SR7) / 17								
	Communication score	(L items + FR7 + SR8) / 7								
	Psychosocial score	(T5 + P items + MD items + FR7 + SR1 + SR4 + SR5) / 11								
	Energy score	(T4 + E items) / 4								

Figure 13–4. Sample scoresheet from the Stroke and Aphasia Quality of Life Scale–39 (SAQOL-39). (From Hilari et al., 2003; with permission.)

activities and roles in which individuals participate and generally do not mix activity-level items with participation-level items, like some of the quality-of-life scales. The CHART asks respondents to indicate the number of hours they spend performing a specific activity (i.e., frequency). For instance, respondents note the frequency with which they got out of bed or the number of hours involved in active homemaking or working, hobbies, and so on. The Life-H scale (some items from the short form are shown in Fig. 13–5) is an assessment tool that includes 58 items based on the life habits section of the DCP classification. Respondents are required to score three aspects for each item: (1) level of accomplishment, (2) type of assistance needed, and (3) level of satisfaction. For example, an individual may no longer be able to do housework following a stroke; however, this individual might have hired help with this life activity (performed by substitution) and may be very satisfied with this arrangement. For level of accomplishment, the respondent

Answer the following 2 questions (check the appropriate boxes).

Question 1:
For each of the following life habits, indicate
A How the personal generally accomplishes it
and
B The type of assistance required to accomplish it

Question 2:
For each of the following life habits, indicate
the level of satisfaction with the way it is accomplished.
Note: Keep in mind that answers should reflect the person's usual way of carrying out the habits.

	Question 1		Question 2
	Level of accomplishment (check only 1)	Type of assistance (check all that apply)	Level of satisfaction (check only 1)

	No difficulty	With difficulty	Accomplished by a proxy	Not accomplished	Not applicable		No assistance	Assistance device	Adaptation	Human assistance		Very dissatisfied	Dissatisfied	More or less satisfied	Satisfied	Very satisfied	
Dressing and undressing the upper half of your body (clothing, accessories, including the choice of clothes)	☐	☐	☐	☐	☐		☐	☐	☐	☐		☐	☐	☐	☐	☐	3.3.1
Dressing and undressing the lower half of your body (clothing, accessories, including the choice of clothes)	☐	☐	☐	☐	☐		☐	☐	☐	☐		☐	☐	☐	☐	☐	3.3.2
Putting on, removing and maintaining your assistive devices (orthodontics, prosthetics, contact lenses, glasses, etc.)	☐	☐	☐	☐	☐		☐	☐	☐	☐		☐	☐	☐	☐	☐	3.3.3
Taking care of your health (first aid, medication, following treatment instructions, etc.)	☐	☐	☐	☐	☐		☐	☐	☐	☐		☐	☐	☐	☐	☐	3.4.1
Using services provided by a medical clinic, hospital or rehabilitation center.	☐	☐	☐	☐	☐		☐	☐	☐	☐		☐	☐	☐	☐	☐	3.4.2

Communication

Communication with another person at home or in the community (expressing needs, holding a conversation, etc.)	☐	☐	☐	☐	☐		☐	☐	☐	☐		☐	☐	☐	☐	☐	4.1.1
Communicating with a group of people at home or in the community (expressing needs, holding a conversation, etc.)	☐	☐	☐	☐	☐		☐	☐	☐	☐		☐	☐	☐	☐	☐	4.1.2
Written communication (writing a letter, message, etc.)	☐	☐	☐	☐	☐		☐	☐	☐	☐		☐	☐	☐	☐	☐	4.1.3
Reading and understanding written information (newspapers, books, letters, signs, etc.) Note: If you use glasses to read, check assistive devices	☐	☐	☐	☐	☐		☐	☐	☐	☐		☐	☐	☐	☐	☐	4.1.4
Using a phone at home or at work	☐	☐	☐	☐	☐		☐	☐	☐	☐		☐	☐	☐	☐	☐	4.3.1
Using a public or cell phone	☐	☐	☐	☐	☐		☐	☐	☐	☐		☐	☐	☐	☐	☐	4.3.2
Using a computer	☐	☐	☐	☐	☐		☐	☐	☐	☐		☐	☐	☐	☐	☐	4.3.3
Using a radio, television or sound system	☐	☐	☐	☐	☐		☐	☐	☐	☐		☐	☐	☐	☐	☐	4.3.4

Housing

Choosing a home that suits your needs (house, apartment, group home)	☐	☐	☐	☐	☐		☐	☐	☐	☐		☐	☐	☐	☐	☐	5.1

Figure 13–5. Items from the Life-H scale. (From Fougeyrollas et al., 1997; with permission.)

can score *No difficulty*, *Some difficulty*, *Realized by substitution* (meaning someone else is carrying out this activity for the respondent), *Not performed*, or *Not applicable*. For type of assistance to achieve the life habit, respondents can indicate *No assistance*, *Assistive device*, *Adaptation*, or *Human assistance*. This allows clinicians to identify what environmental help, human or otherwise, is helping the individual take part in his or her life activities. The last category is level of satisfaction, which can be rated on a five point scale from *Very dissatisfied* to *Very satisfied*. Taken as a whole, these participation rating scales allow the respondents to identify problematic areas of life participation.

The clear advantages of these tools are that they track the perception of the impact of environmental factors as well as level of satisfaction for each and every participation item and that they do not mix activity-level items. Unfortunately, they, too, may be difficult to apply to the area of aphasia. For instance, the visual presentation of the Life-H tool itself makes it difficult for individuals with aphasia to score the items themselves. The response forms may need to be adapted for use with this population. The Life-H scale was used in a pilot study comparing caregivers' responses to those of their loved ones with dementia (Wright, Garcia, Neault, & Fergus, 2002) as well as to those of individuals with traumatic brain injury in evaluating the environmental factors that contribute to workplace integration (Laroche et al., 1999). In both instances, the clinician asked the participant the questions.

In short, all of these scales can help the therapist identify how persons with aphasia perceive their level of functioning in daily life. No ideal tool is currently on the market that captures all the elements necessary for therapeutic planning using a life consequences approach, and the clinician will need to examine these clinical tools more closely. McDowell and Newell's book (2006) on measuring health is an interesting start.

In a pilot study using the DCP and ICF models to describe functioning in the area of aphasia, Garcia and colleagues (2003) preferred to use an interview format to identify the life participation areas. Questions were devised based on the participation domains found in the ICF and DCP. The questionnaire may be found in Appendix 13.1. Others also preferred to use tailor-made interviews and questionnaires with individuals with aphasia (Parr, Duchan, & Pound, 2003 Pound, Parr, Lindsay, & Woolf, 2000; Simmons-Mackie & Damico, 1995) to capture individuals' perceptions of the impact of their disorder on overall life participation.

Byng and Duchan (2005) give an excellent overview of how one can construct interventions based on life participation roles. Lyon and Shadden (2001) have also stressed the importance of looking at global life goals. In fact, successful participation in leisure activities has been shown to correlate most with quality of life and overall well-being poststroke (Bays 2001; Sveen, Thommessen, Bautz-Holter, Wyller,

& Laake, 2004). Level of linguistic functioning is not always the predictor of overall functioning (Ross & Wertz, 2002).

Bottom line: Whatever method is used by the clinician (quality-of-life scales, participation scales, or interviews), what is important is to identify those life participation areas that pose problems for the individual with aphasia.

The problematic life participation areas may or may not be reflected in explicit communication goals. In fact, it is very difficult, if not impossible, to tease out communication as a separate entity from life participation (Penn, 2005). Further, identifying areas of life participation as a goal for therapy may seem too global and unmanageable to some clinicians. In addition to using participation scales such as the Life-H and the CHART, or using informal questionnaires, those who are more systematic in their approach may choose a technique such as Goal Attainment Scaling (Schlosser, 2004) to evaluate progress in life participation. This technique (described in greater detail in the section entitled "Fitting it together: interprofessional strategies for rehabilitation, p. 366) involves assigning a numeric value to therapeutic goals as per the individual's priorities. A continuum of outcomes is identified pre-intervention using a five-point scale, and each goal is then defined in terms of this scaling. At the end of the intervention, together with the clinician, the person with aphasia can see which goals, if any, have been attained. Goal Attainment Scaling can be used with any therapeutic goal, including those based on life participation.

The Second Component: Intervention on the Personal Factors

Once the life activity or role has been identified in collaboration with the individual with aphasia but before a therapy plan can be designed, an inventory of the individual's capabilities must be made. These skills will normally be identified through discipline-specific evaluations. In speech-language pathology, this includes a comprehensive appraisal of the speech and language skills. Therapies designed for these skills are the subject of many chapters in this text. All of these techniques can impact the life participation of individuals with aphasia provided the links are made with life domains.

Although most, if not all, clinicians are concerned with the impact of language abilities on their clients' lives, the missing step is often the direct correlation of these abilities with improvements on subsequent life activities and roles that are important to the person with aphasia. Further, the clinician must not ignore the behavioral personal factors, such as level of motivation, and their correlation with life activities and roles. These correlations will allow the clinician to identify those life habits that likely are mildly affected, those that are compromised, and those that are at risk of being compromised (Castelein, Noots-Villers,

Buxant, & Spicher, 1994). For instance, a reading problem could mildly affect the life participation activity of preparing meals (i.e., reading recipe books) but would compromise the job of a lawyer and risk compromising leisure if the person reads for pleasure. Based on this information, the capabilities can be prioritized and incorporated into a cohesive therapeutic plan.

In identifying these capabilities, the clinician should pay specific attention to communication skills as an interactive process. Not only are the linguistic levels of phonology, syntax, and semantics important, but pragmatics becomes a central theme in intervention. Hence, the ability to express one's intention and/or understand others' intentions through language is fundamental to successful life participation. It is so fundamental, in fact, that we often define who we are through communicative interactions.

Verderber (1981) suggests that people communicate on three social levels: (1) For the sheer pleasure of interaction (in these cases, the topic is unimportant), (2) To demonstrate their ties with other people, and (3) to build and maintain relationships. In this sense, the goal of communication is to facilitate social interactions and not necessarily to transmit information. The therapist must remember that individuals may need to communicate with the intention to make relational ties and that this might demand different abilities from those needed to read a book. Luterman (1996) says, "The major means by which we alleviate our interpersonal loneliness is verbal communication, and when that is difficult, we become disturbed" (p. 22). Hence, an approach based on the life consequences cannot focus solely on the transactional aspects of communication (i.e., transmitting a message) (Simmons-Mackie & Damico, 1995). Aside from designing intervention strategies that focus on the linguistic aspects per se, as described in the various chapters of this text, the clinician can also focus on helping the individual with his or her communication skills to function as a social being. Functional communication techniques might include augmentative and alternative communication (McCall, Shelton, Weinrich, & Cox, 2000; Waller, Dennis, Brodie, & Cairns, 1998), drawing (Lyon, 1996; Ward-Lonergan & Nicholas, 1995), or PACE treatment (Carlomagno, Losanno, Emanuelli, & Casadio, 1991; Pulvermüller & Roth, 1991). Cunningham and Ward (2003) used videos to help functional communication by teaching repair strategies to conversational partners so that they become more efficient communicators. Another technique, called reciprocal scaffolding (Avent & Austerman, 2003), uses a reciprocal model of learning where the person with aphasia is in interaction with a student partner. In the reported case, the person with aphasia teaches a science lesson to 25 children. In this situation, the person with aphasia has the opportunity to improve not only in language but also in terms of life participation.

One of the more formal therapeutic interventions designed specifically for conversation is the method developed by Holland (1991) called conversational coaching. The conversational coaching technique is used to help the person with aphasia transfer the strategies learned in therapy to a more functional context. The first step in this process is to develop a predesigned script that the person with aphasia will practice with the clinician. This script can vary in difficulty depending on the amount of information that needs to be conveyed and on the level of improvisation left to the person with aphasia. The person with aphasia practices the script with the clinician as he or she guides the client in using the most efficient and effective conversational strategies. The person with aphasia will then practice the script with a familiar person, usually a family member, while being filmed on videotape. The therapist will coach both the person with aphasia and the family member in conversational strategies. Other, less familiar individuals can then be called in to make the task a little more difficult. The clinician and person with aphasia will then view the videotape together and discuss what worked and what did not.

Hopper, Holland, and Rewega (2002) looked at the efficacy, both pre- and post therapy, of using a videotaped story as a script. They looked at the number of concepts that were effectively communicated post-therapy and found this therapy to be effective. In another technique using script training, Youmans, Holland, Muñoz, and Bourgeois (2005) used a systematic technique to render scripted phrases more and more automatic in the conversational discourse of two individuals with aphasia. As the participants mastered the scripts, more and more information was added. The scripts were tested for robustness in a contextual conversation, and raters were then used to examine parameters such as speaking rate and naturalness of the conversations.

Any clinician wishing to use these techniques must remember some fundamental principles about communication. Normal speakers do not communicate all the necessary information to communicate their intention, and speakers may not reveal their intentions explicitly. This is important to remember when we engage in techniques that work on turn taking, topic shifting, or conversational repair. How close is the correlation between what is perceived as a breakdown in communication by the therapist (e.g., a breakdown in topic shifting) and the actual breakdown in the person's communicative intention? Which part of the message should be allocated to what is explicit, and which part should be deducted as a function of the context and the links with the speaker? Any approach that focuses on the life consequences must consider the intended goal of the communication event. It is not only about the clarity of the linguistic message. As a reaction to the paper by Ross and Wertz (2005) on the use of the ICF in the appraisal of aphasia, Penn (2005) remarked that communication, in and of itself, is not a life participation domain but, rather, transpires all domains. Nothing could be closer to the truth. What we see (or hear) is not always what is underlying the problem.

Sometimes, linguistic difficulties directly influence other domains, such as self-esteem.

How people feel about themselves and how they feel the disorder has affected them and their loved ones will impact whether individuals with aphasia can take part in life activities and roles. These are equally part of the personal factors of those with aphasia. Because communication affects the very fabric of interpersonal interactions, these feelings cannot be ignored by the therapist. In his book on counselling, Luterman (1996) stated that "the goal of counselling is not to make people feel better, but to separate feelings from non-productive behaviour. The feelings must always be acknowledged" (p. 47). To move ahead in therapy, Luterman suggested that we listen to clients. As with the identification of life participation events, clients can participate with the therapist to switch their focus from what they cannot do to what they may choose not to do. This is a very important distinction to make when one takes a life consequences approach. This perspective suggests that the therapists can use the individual's state of mind to help the person adopt new life roles by choosing to let go of past roles. The level of motivation and the sense of identity the person has can either facilitate or be an obstacle to full reintegration. Counselling on the other personal factors that interact with communication can be a very important step to recovery.

Assessment tools such as the Code-Müller Protocols (Code, Müller, Hogan, & Herrmann, 1999) or the Visual Analogue Self-Esteem Scale (Brumfitt & Sheeran, 1999), or VASES, are both designed to offer a standardized way of evaluating an individual's psychosocial adjustment. The VASES will offer the clinician an assessment of the individual's self-perception (e.g., optimist/pessimist, attractive/ unattractive, and so on), whereas the Code-Müller Protocols will evaluate the self-perceptions of individuals regarding how they are doing on items such as ability to work, ability to cope with depression, or ability to follow interests and hobbies. Sometimes, the best way to find out how people are doing is through informal and formal interviews or autobiographies (Parr, 2001; Pound, Parr, & Duchan, 2001). The clinician can use counselling techniques to probe issues of psychosocial adjustment as they relate to communication situations.

As mentioned previously, aphasia affects much more than one's ability to transmit a message. Kagan (1995) has spoken of aphasia as masking an individual's competence, whereas Shadden (2005) has written a paper describing how aphasia impacts one's perception of one's own identity. No matter how mild the aphasia may seem to the therapist, renegotiation of involvement in life events and roles will need to take place if the therapy is to be successful. Even with mild aphasia, those affected may see an impact on the fact that they can no longer be as witty or have deep conversations with a spouse. The demand placed on communication skills is far greater in real life than in a clinic situation. The individual must process multiple pieces of information—and process them quickly. Even with mild aphasia, the sequelae of the CVA might affect these subtle aspects, which in turn impact on the individual's ability to function as he or she did previously. The effect may be withdrawal from these events. As individuals are counselled into reconstructing this new identity with less efficient communication skills, they will need some external validation that they can once again become socially functioning human beings. Validation will come with help from the clinician as opportunities are offered in the form of successful communication situations. Some techniques, such as the conversational coaching technique described above, will help individuals attain success. Other activities, such as group therapy (Kearns & Elman, 2001) and techniques designed to help the conversational partner (see next section), will also help with the validation of a person's competence as a communicator. The therapist can help to unveil the mask of incompetence caused by aphasia (Kagan, 1995) and reveal who those affected were and may now choose to be (Mackay, 2003) by guiding their involvement in communication situations. The clinician must remember that the individual with aphasia has a premorbid life that comes with a premorbid personality and psychosocial situation. Ignoring these aspects is likely to doom the therapy to failure in terms of life participation.

Bottom line: Capabilities, as assessed by discipline specific evaluations, can be correlated with identified life participation goals.

The level of impairment will contribute to the realization of the life event. Therapy can then be prioritized into work on linguistic aspects and/or social conversational skills. It must not be forgotten that the psychological state of the individual will also play an important role in helping his or her return to past life activities and/or development of new life goals. Counselling will be necessary to guide the individual through these stages.

Improving linguistic, conversational, and psychological skills will most certainly help in improving quality of life (Cruice Worrall & Hickson, 2005); however, a life consequences approach demands that this be considered in the context of other environmental factors that impact real-life functioning. Opportunities for validation and inclusion will most easily occur if the therapist knows how to modify the environment, increasing the number of facilitators and decreasing the obstacles. The life participation goal is modified not only through work on personal factors but also through work on environmental factors. Therapy that focuses on both is more likely to be successful (Ross & Wertz, 2003).

The Third Component: Intervention on the Environmental Factors

To many people, the term "environmental factors" refers only to physical environments and includes such things as architectural designs, snow-covered sidewalks, or noisy environments. In the disability model approach, however, environment includes much more. It includes social environments, such as family members and colleague support, as well as sociopolitical systems and attitudes. Using the ICF model, Howe and colleagues (2004) offered an excellent review of environmental factors that can influence the life participation of individuals with aphasia, and Lubinski (2001) explained how environmental factors can be seen to interact at the individual, family, and systemic levels.

The most obvious environmental factor influencing the integration of individuals with communication deficits such as aphasia is the conversational partner. For as long as social scientists have studied conversational discourse, the role of the conversational partner has been instrumental in establishing coherent and cohesive interactions (Schegloff, 1987). A conversation cannot occur without a partner. Depending on the words used by conversational partners and their behaviors, this can negatively affect the functional communication levels of the person with aphasia. To reduce these effects, the therapist can use a number of the techniques mentioned previously to help turn negative-impact conversational partners into positive-impact conversational partners. For instance, volunteers were used to facilitate conversations using scripts in the "Speaking out" program of Worrall and Yiu (2000), and Hopper and colleagues (2002) explained how the conversational coaching technique not only benefits the individual with aphasia but also trains family members in how to coach for more fluid communication. Cunningham and Ward (2003) also used videotaping to train couples in conversational repair strategies, and Simmons-Mackie, Kearns, and Potechin (2005) showed evidence for generalization of family training techniques to better, fluid conversations in more naturalistic environments.

Conversational partners do more, however, than just help to construct coherent conversations. As mentioned in the previous section, conversational partners play an important role in validating the competence of the person with aphasia. Supported Conversation for Adults with Aphasia, or SCA, is one of the more formal approaches for training conversational partners. Designed by Kagan, Black, Duchan, Simmons-Mackie, and Square (2001), this program capitalizes on the inherent cognitive and social skills of the person with aphasia to facilitate communication. The program teaches conversational partners to see the person with aphasia as an equal conversationalist, and it encourages the partner to use whatever is at his or her disposal to engage the person with aphasia in a meaningful interaction. Tools that facilitate communication might include visual material (e.g., photographs), writing partial messages to clarify information, drawing, or natural "props" (e.g., newspaper clips). Partners are taught to offer feedback that is as natural and context dependent as possible and focus on the communicative intent rather than the clarity of the linguistic output.

By intervening at the environmental level, the therapist is making the world more accessible to the person with aphasia and helping others to facilitate rather than hinder integration. Nonetheless, environmental obstacles go beyond the individual conversational partner. Kagan and LeBlanc (2002) report on efforts to render health-care services more accessible to individuals with aphasia. Worrall and colleagues (2005) give further examples of how to render written environments more accessible. All environments with which the person interacts, including physical environments (Lubinski, 2001), attitudes (Parr, 2001), and work environments (Garcia, Barrette, & Laroche, 2000), or how health-care teams are structured and function (Golper, 2001), can be examined to see if they are perceived by individuals with aphasia as being obstacles or facilitators to integration.

Much more information is needed regarding the impact of these environmental factors on the life participation of individuals with aphasia. Parr (2001) correctly points out that identifying the exact impact of environmental factors on life participation is far from straightforward. Further, working on the environmental factors alone might be counterproductive. To focus only on the environmental factors minimizes the role of the personal factors (i.e., aphasia) on life participation (Parr, 2001). Just as the traditional medical model might be criticized for not acknowledging the role of environment, a purely environmental approach likewise does not do justice to the role of the impairment. The interaction must be symbiotic.

Lawton and Nahemow (1973) introduced the ecological model of aging (Fig. 13–6) to help articulate the role of personal and environmental factors. The concepts from this model are still relevant today, and they have been improved upon and incorporated into modern disability models. The level of competence of the individual is represented on the y-axis of this model. For our purposes, this would include personal factors, such as linguistic and behavioral capabilities. Following evaluation, this can be rated from a low level of competence to a high level of competence. The x-axis represents how demanding the environment can be toward the individual. This can be rated as very low in demand value to very high in demand value. The diagonal lines suggest a direct link between level of competence and demand from the environment. If a person has a high level of competence but is in an environment that demands little, the person will lose his or her ability to adapt and will develop negative affect and maladaptive behavior. The individual will not be working hard enough to stimulate development of his or her skills, because the environment demands very little. Conversely, if the person has lower competence skills for what the environment demands, he or she will also be unable to perform, because this individual will not have the skills to respond to the high demands of the environment. Hence, a relationship exists between the person's level of competence and what is asked by the environment to achieve maximal

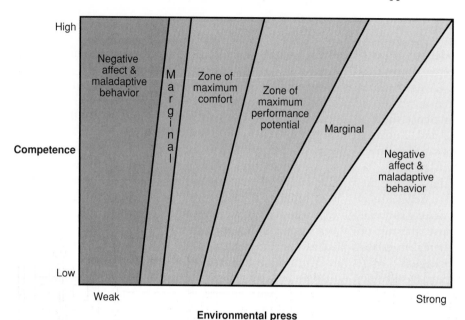

Figure 13–6. The ecological model of aging (Lawton & Nahemow, 1973).

performance. This is called "environmental press." The higher the level of competence, the more the environment can demand—up to a point. To use a concrete example, imagine an individual who can manage some stairs but who cannot manage a full staircase. If all stairs are removed from this person environment, he or she is likely to lose whatever is left of the competence to manage stairs. If this person must manage many stairs in the environment, he or she will likely be overwhelmed and unable to function.

These same principles can be applied to individuals with aphasia. A person with significant residual language must be in an environment that is sufficiently stimulating to reveal competence and enhance development but also not overwhelming enough to elicit discouragement, isolation, and demotivation. Therefore, in addition to stimulating linguistic aspects, the therapist has a role in shaping an environment that will be conducive to the "zone of maximum comfort," using the model of Lawton and Nahemow (1973).

The clinician's job, then, is to identify those environmental factors that are contributing to integration, either in a positive or a negative way, and help to impact on these factors. Using the environmental press model, this means that the individual with aphasia must come into contact with communication partners who are stimulating enough to encourage the use of communication strategies on the part of the individual with aphasia yet also facilitating enough not to be overwhelming. The Supported Conversation for Aphasia technique of Kagan et al. (2001) is precisely in line with the Lawton and Nahemow model of environmental press. Here, the clinician facilitates communication sufficiently enough to reveal the competence of the individual.

Two standardized tools may be useful to the clinician for identifying the frequency and impact of environmental factors. The Craig Hospital Inventory of Environmental Factors (Craig Hospital Research Department, 2001), or CHIEF, and the Measure of the Quality of the Environment (Fougeyrollas, Noreau, St-Michel, & Boschen, 1999), or MQE, are scales used measure environmental factors. The CHIEF helps the clinician identify barriers by asking the individual about the level of the barrier and the frequency with which he or she encounters it. Barriers include items such as the layout of built environments, natural environments, light, and noise, as well as more human barriers, such as human help, attitudes, and policies and rules. The MQE (Fig. 13–7) has similar items and asks the respondent to rate items on a scale going from +2 (very much a facilitator) to 0 (neutral impact) to −2 (very much an obstacle).

The Environmental Partner as an Object of Intervention

Until now, much of this chapter has focused on individuals with aphasia and their interactions with their environments. More and more writings, however, suggest that the clinician should also consider the individuals surrounding the person with aphasia as a focus of intervention. Bakas, Kroenke, Plue, Perkins, and Williams (2006) looked at family caregivers of individuals with aphasia and of individuals without aphasia following stroke. The impact of functioning with an individual who had aphasia was more demanding than with an individual who did not have aphasia.

Just as it is difficult for individuals with aphasia to communicate with their environment, it is difficult for the environment to communicate with an individual who has aphasia. Work on conversational discourse not only benefits the person with aphasia but also the conversational partner.

Measure the quality of the environment

	Influence scale						I do not know	Does not apply
While taking into consideration your abilities and personal limits, indicate on the scale to what extent the situations or factors generally influence your daily life.	Obstacle ←	No influence			→ Familiar			
	major	medium	minor		minor	medium	major		

Social network (support from people around you)	major	medium	minor		minor	medium	major	I do not know	Does not apply
• Your family situation (living alone, with a spouse, or with children).	-3	-2	-1	0	1	2	3	☐	☐
• Support from members of your family or close friends who take the place of family (presence, physical assistance, household assistance, encourgement).	-3	-2	-1	0	1	2	3	☐	☐
• Support from your friends.	-3	-2	-1	0	1	2	3	☐	☐
• Support from your neighbors.	-3	-2	-1	0	1	2	3	☐	☐
• Support from you colleages at work, school, or place of principal occupation.	-3	-2	-1	0	1	2	3	☐	☐

Attitudes of the people around you....	major	medium	minor		minor	medium	major	I do not know	Does not apply
• The attitudes of your family or close friends who take the place of family towards you.	-3	-2	-1	0	1	2	3	☐	☐
• The attitudes of your friends toward you.	-3	-2	-1	0	1	2	3	☐	☐
• The attitudes of your colleagues at work, school or place of principal occupation towards you.	-3	-2	-1	0	1	2	3	☐	☐
• The attitudes of your superiors (professors, supervisors, employees) towards you.	-3	-2	-1	0	1	2	3	☐	☐
• The attitudes of your neighbors towards you.	-3	-2	-1	0	1	2	3	☐	☐
• The attitudes of your service providoers (public service agents, salespeople, cashiers, etc.) toward you.	-3	-2	-1	0	1	2	3	☐	☐

Figure 13–7. Example of the Measure of the Quality of the Environment (MQE). (From Fougeyrollas et al., 1999; with permission.)

Shadden (2005) brings this point home in the area of personal identity by suggesting a specific burden associated with the impact of aphasia:

Using an identity perspective, it is clear that efforts must be made to understand how each significant other projects his or her identity both now (poststroke), and in the past (prestroke). There is a need to know relational dynamics, to go beyond questions such as "How does he communicate at home?" (p. 219).

In a life consequences perspective, the aphasia almost certainly affects the spouse's, the colleague's, or the friend's life participation. As with the individual who has aphasia, intervention on the aphasia itself or reduction of environmental barriers might help these partners. Sorin-Peters (2003) used an adult learning model to help couples deal with the consequences of aphasia. Her focus was not only on the communication aspects but also on the impact of the aphasia on the marital relationship. Other members in the person's entourage, such as health-care providers, can also be considered. Although Allan (2006) refers to health workers involved with individuals who have dementia, the same can be said about workers involved with individuals with aphasia:

A system which calls upon workers' humanity in the very delivery of the services it provides cannot simultaneously deny the needs of staff that arise in the course of the work that they do. (p. 191)

Bouchard-Lamothe and colleagues (1999) found that some physicians reported struggling when involved with individuals who have aphasia. Interventions at this level not only help the person with aphasia to obtain better care but also helps the health-care worker to do his or her job and offer better care to all individuals with communication disorders. Using disability models, the therapist can focus on the life participation of the health-care worker, family member, or colleague. This person, who does not have aphasia, has also been affected by it. His or her life habits (e.g., work, activities, and interpersonal relationships), not to mention his or her identity as a spouse or colleague, have likely been disrupted by the partner's aphasia. These are clearly life consequences of aphasia.

Bottom line: Environment is just as important a target of intervention as is linguistic capacity. Environment can include physical environment, social supports, and organizational structures. Those people in the individual's entourage can just as likely become a focus of intervention.

FITTING IT TOGETHER: INTERPROFESSIONAL STRATEGIES FOR REHABILITATION

For a speech-language pathologist to embark on a life consequences approach to intervention is quite challenging. Quickly, the clinician will realize the need for more information from other professionals to understand the full impact of the stroke on the patient's life activities and roles. The best way to facilitate this is to take an interprofessional approach in which the members of the team (including the person with aphasia) work toward common life participation goals. Each discipline can then work on disciplinary elements and keep informed through discussions with the team regarding the progress made on the patient-initiated life activities and roles. This will both save time and be more efficient. Simmons-Mackie, Threats, and Kagan (2005) reported that time constraints were the biggest obstacle to doing outcome measurement in clinic. Using a team approach allows clinicians to concentrate on life consequences goals in a more efficient and effective manner. For a team to be effective, its members must orient their efforts toward a clear, common objective (Golper, 2001), and a model such as the ESOPE (*Evaluation systémique des objectifs prioritaires en réadaptation* [Systemic Evaluation of Priority Goals in Rehabilitation]) will give them this opportunity.

The ESOPE model is one suggestion that might be useful as a guide for operationalizing this approach. It was developed by a Belgian team under the direction of Pierre Castelein and Patricia Noots-Villers (Castelein et al., 1994). These occupational therapists have proposed a model to guide the setting of team rehabilitation goals based on the DCP disability model. The ESOPE program (see Figure 13–8) uses a computer system to help an interprofessional team adopt a life consequences approach. The team first works from a common set

of life participation goals, which are identified based on the frequency with which the client engages in the life habit or role as well as the perceived importance by the client of this life habit or role. A correlation is made between the individual's capabilities and these life habits or roles based on formal or informal evaluation of the life habits and disciplinary evaluations. The clinical rehabilitation team, in collaboration with the individual with aphasia, will (1) target the capabilities that need to be prioritized as a function of life habits and roles, (2) suppress environmental obstacles that prevent integration or augment facilitators, and/or (3) work with the client to adopt new life habits. According to the ESOPE model of intervention, the individual will then be able to diminish situations of handicap and develop a more harmonious interaction with his or her social and physical environments.

To help persons with aphasia determine when they have attained some success in their goals, the therapeutic team can use the technique of Goal Attainment Scaling (Schlosser, 2004) discussed previously in this chapter. This technique offers a systematic way to determine progress on an individual goal. Here are the steps as outlined by Schlosser (p. 218):

1. **Specify a set of goals** In our case, these goals can be the life participation goals set by the team and the person with aphasia in the section entitled, "The First Component: Identifying Disrupted Life Activities and Roles (p. 355)" of this chapter.
2. **Assign a weight for each goal according to priority** The priority given to these goals will be influenced by the frequency and the importance of the goal to the person with aphasia.
3. **Specify a continuum of possible outcomes** Each goal is assigned a worst expected outcome (-2), a less than expected outcome (-1), an expected outcome (0), a more than expected outcome ($+1$), and a best expected outcome ($+2$). This is where the Goal Attaining Scaling is most useful; however, this is also the most difficult stage of the process. The team, always in conjunction with the client, will operationally define what each of the levels might be for each of the chosen goals.
4. **Specify the criteria for scoring at each level** The team will then clearly identify what is operationally needed to conclude that the goal has been attained.
5. **Determine current or initial performance** This could be determined through measurable evaluations of life participation or quality of life, environmental factors, and/or disciplinary clinical measures.
6. **Intervene for a specified period** As mentioned above, intervention might take the form of therapy aimed at (a) improving abilities, including linguistic and psychosocial adjustment abilities; (b) reducing environmental obstacles; or (c) helping define new life goals.
7. **Determine performance attained on each objective**
8. **Evaluate extent of attainment**

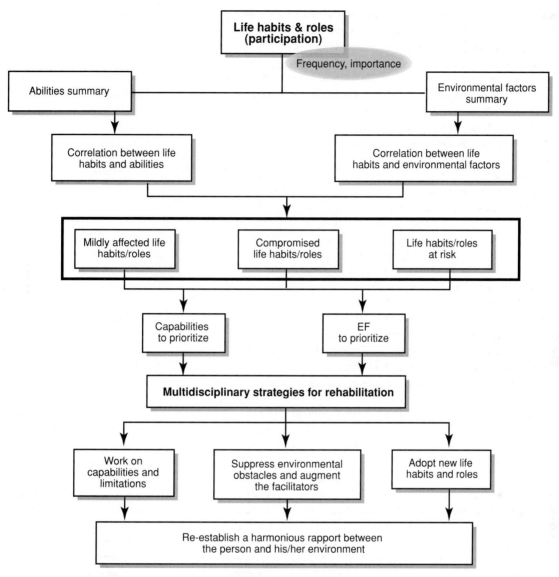

Figure 13–8. The ESOPE (*Évaluation systémique des objectifs prioritaires en réadaptation* [Systemic Evaluation of Priority Goals in Rehabilitation]). EF = environmental factors. (Adapted from Castelein et al., 1994; with permission.)

Regular meetings with the team will ensure that the overall life participation goal is being met and that each member is facilitating the person with aphasia's integration in the best possible way as defined by these goals. The professionals involved in the team will be able to focus their own therapeutic plans on the disciplinary items that offer a continued improvement of life participation goals. Like the elephant in the legend of the six blind men, the composite picture is more than the sum of its parts.

It is also important to remember that these goals will change over time (Parr, 2001; Shadden, 2005). As environmental factors change (e.g., the death of a spouse or the purchase of an electronic device) and personal factors improve (e.g., more motivation or improved language skills), the consequence on the life participation goal will also be affected. Further, as Shadden (2005) so eloquently states, the self-identity of the person will also change, and this will be influenced by his or her life experiences. Hence, the chronic condition of aphasia will have differing effects depending on this context. The clinician is therefore encouraged to continuously evaluate the extent of participation in life activities and roles as well as the extent to which the current personal skills and environmental factors are influencing the achievement of these goals.

TABLE 13–1

Applying The Philosophy

	Acute Care	Rehabilitation Settings	Long-Term Facilities	Community-Care Settings
Enhancement of life participation	• Unable to express needs/wants	• Return to work • Return to day living (shopping, cooking, homekeeping, driving, computer, telephone talking) • Return to social network	• Person with aphasia cannot communicate basic needs • Group/recreational activities (in-house and outside facility) • Using communication boards	• Participate in some community activity • Specific work goals Social participation
All those affected are entitled to service	• Nursing staff • Family • MDs • Rehabilitation team	• Medical staff • Family • Friends • Colleagues • Community workers • Lawyer, insurance personnel • Clergy	• Family • Friends • Caregivers	• Lack of funding for initiating/continuing support services • Family • Friends • Co-workers • Employers • MDs • Rehabilitation team
Measures of success include documented life enhancement changes	• Ongoing evaluation • Staff input/feedback • Improved communication on ward	• Anecdotal information • Family rating scale • Questionnaire • Formal assessment tool • Client interview	• Feedback from staff • Improvement in goals • Diagnostic measures • Documentation of room restorative programs • MDs • Nursing documentation	• Ability to return to work • Measures of self satisfaction • Ability to return to previous activities • Ability to learn new participation activities
Personal factors are targets	• Cognitive status • Motivation • Fatigue	• Cognitive status • Motivation • Client awareness/insight • Mental/physical/emotional status • Financial situation • Overall life style/behavior	• Feelings of isolation and depression • Premorbid level	• Age • Previous roles (e.g., managing finances) • Finances • Motivation • IADLs
Environmental factors are targets	• Other testing procedures • PT/OT • Family members • Noise • Roommates	• Living situation • Responsiveness of employer, community, family • Geographic isolation/location • Transportation	• Family attitudes • Privacy issues • Effects of psychotropic drugs • Noise • Lighting • Ventilation • Roommates • Lack of follow-through with strategic staff commitment and turnover • Language barrier • Cultural differences • Age factor	• Family situation • Transportation • Community involvement • Availability of support personnel

TABLE 13–1

Applying The Philosophy (continued)

	Acute Care	Rehabilitation Settings	Long-Term Facilities	Community-Care Settings
Availability of service	• Lack of SLP • Productivity issue • Lack of staff/MD knowledge	• Accessibility to service • Insurance • Transportation • Lack of/shortage of SLPs • Shortage of skilled clinicians • Poor communication of client to express needs/goals	• Insurance • Staffing issues • Time constraints	• Counselling services for adjustment • Aphasia groups
What would prevent SLPs from applying the philosophy?	• Priority given to vital life functions (swallowing, breathing)	• Medicare, availability • Time constraints • Ability • Lack of objective documentation • Lack of funding • Lack of employer support	• Time constraints • Excessive paperwork • Travel time	• Ongoing services (payment)

Key: IADLs = Instrumental Activities of Daily Living; PT/OT = Physiotherapy/Occupational Therapy; SLP = speech-language pathologist.
(Suggestions from participants at a New Jersey Speech and Hearing Conference.)

APPLYING THE PHILOSOPHY TO DIFFERENT CLINICAL CONTEXTS

Speech-language pathologists can deliver services in many different contexts, ranging from hospitals to rehabilitation centers to long-term care facilities to independent clinics to home care. The life consequences approach can be applied in all of these contexts and should not be relegated only to home care. Remember that the consequences of aphasia are felt the minute the person has survived the stroke; therefore, a life consequences approach can be just as appropriate in acute care as in home care.

To illustrate this, I will use the suggestions pooled from a conference I gave to the New Jersey Speech and Hearing Association in 2001 on the applications of the new disability models. The participants were asked to reflect on how the principles of the Life Participation Approach to Aphasia (LPAA Project Group, chapter 10, this book), which summarizes principles of practice using disability model notions, could be applied to the different clinical contexts. Table 13–1 summarizes their suggestions.

The Life Participation Approach to Aphasia guidelines mirror the approach taken in this chapter:

1. The explicit goal is enhancement of life participation.
2. All those affected by aphasia are entitled to service.

3. The measures of success include documented life enhancement changes.
4. Both personal and environmental factors are targets of intervention.
5. Emphasis is on availability of services as needed at all stages of aphasia.

The participants in the New Jersey Speech and Hearing Association conference offer clinicians a first look at targets that can be identified across health-care sectors. The life consequences approach to aphasia not only helps us in looking at the impact of aphasia on an individual's life but also has great promise in helping us understand the impact of aphasia as lived by individuals in different cultures. This can only be done through consideration of environmental factors. By helping individuals with aphasia and their loved ones get what they need to participate more fully in life at a certain point in their lives, we may contribute greatly to their sense of meaning and personal identity.

KEY POINTS

1. Disability model principles and frameworks, such as the International Classification of Functioning, Disability and Health (ICF) and the lesser-known

Disability Creation Process Model (DCP), provide a good starting point for understanding the relationship among all the factors that contribute to helping individuals reenter their lives following aphasia. They can help to identify whether the focus of therapy should be on (a) regaining language abilities, (b) diminishing environmental obstacles or encouraging environmental facilitators, (c) helping the individual to define new life goals, or (d) any combination of the first three.

2. Social and physical environments can facilitate integration or create obstacles to integration and, therefore, can be a focus for intervention just as capabilities can. The environment should be challenging enough to foster development yet facilitative enough to reduce frustration.

3. Goals of therapy should be identified in consultation with the person who has aphasia.

4. Problems in life participation should be seen as *situations* of handicap that change over time rather than as permanent states.

5. Current disability models are meant to use concepts that are applicable to all human beings.

6. Intervention aimed at the personal factors, such as capabilities, should also consider the psychological impact of the disorder on the individual.

7. The individual who interacts with the person who has aphasia also lives with the impact of aphasia. Hence, colleagues, spouses, children, and friends should be the focus of intervention when appropriate.

8. The most efficient way to keep life participation goals in focus is to work within an interprofessional team context.

ACTIVITIES FOR REFLECTION AND DISCUSSION

Use the following hypothetical case to help structure your answers to the following activities and thoughts.

S.H. is a 45 year-old woman who fell while skating on the canal (a 7-km skating surface) in Ottawa, Ontario, Canada. She was found to have had a left frontoparietal hemorrhage, leaving her with a hemiplegia and aphasia. She has no remarkable past medical history. She is married and has one adolescent child aged 15 years. She is the parent that is most involved with her daughter, and of late, she and her daughter have been experiencing some parenting conflicts surrounding her daughter's request for independence. S.H.'s husband is present but very involved with his work. When possible, they used to enjoy a variety of outdoor sports, such as skiing and skating. This has now become impossible since the

CVA. Before her CVA, S.H. worked as a policy analyst for the Canadian government.

Her language testing reveals the following:

A. Spontaneous language	6/20
B. Oral comprehension	
i. Questions	48/60
ii. Words	58/60
iii. Commands	41/80
C. Repetition	33/100
D. Lexical access	
i. Naming (Western Aphasia Battery)	6/60
ii. Naming (Boston Naming Test)	Unable
iii. Fluency	0/20
iv. Sentence completion	2/10
v. Responding to questions	1/10
E. Reading comprehension	
i. Sentences and paragraphs	28/40
ii. Commands	8/20
iii. Words	6/6 (×3)
F. Writing	
i. Name and address	6/6
ii. Spontaneous writing (paragraph)	Unable
iii. Dictation (sentences)	3/10
iv. Dictation (words)	7/10
G. Apraxia	46/60

1. Identify the personal factors, environmental factors, and life participation activities and roles in S.H.'s case.

2. How would you design your therapy for the personal factors, considering her participation levels?

3. Think about how you would design your therapeutic intervention if you wished to focus on:
   a. S.H.'s lexical access problem.
   b. S.H.'s language and communication skills as a whole.
   c. S.H.'s difficult relationship with her daughter and her (in)ability to return to work.
   Use the elephant analogy in the chapter to help you reflect on this. Use the disability models to help you identify the types of information you would need to plan your therapy. Look at the interview guidelines to see if you have enough information.

4. How are you going to monitor the changes in S.H.'s participation with her daughter and at work?

5. Now look at the daughter's perspective. How is her mother's new health condition affecting their relationship? What impact do you think the aphasia per se is having on their relationship? How much is unrelated or due to non-linguistic factors?

6. What kinds of things/people might be helpful in the environment? What might hinder integration?

7. Are there any other professionals you would like to include? If so, which ones? Design a therapeutic plan using the principles from the ESOPE model.

8. Think about the chronicity of neurologic language disorders such as aphasia, and evaluate how each of the service environments might impact on this chronicity (e.g., rehabilitation versus acute care). Fill out the categories in Table 1 using the hypothetical case above. Think about S.H.'s possible experiences as she takes part in the different levels of care.

9. Do you think your objectives match S.H.'s objectives?

10. Discuss the relevance of health-related quality of life measures and generic quality of life measures for capturing the impact of aphasia in life participation activities and roles.

11. Think about what motivated you to become a speech-language pathologist, and think about the changes you hoped or are hoping to bring about as a clinician. Does a therapy focused on the social consequences of aphasia respond to these aspirations?

▶ *Acknowledgment*—All of the animals except man know that the principle business of life is to enjoy it. (Anonymous)

▶ *Acknowledgment*—Above all, as clinicians and researchers, we need to recognize that our knowledge of aphasia provides, at best, a shallow representation of the reality in which our clients and their significant others live. (Shadden, 2005, p. 221)

▶ *Acknowledgment*—To Juliette, my mother, who became aphasic at the time I was writing this chapter.

References

Allan, K. (2006). Environmental and team approaches to communication in the dementias. In K. Bryan & J. Maxim (Eds.), *Communication disability in the dementias* (pp. 184–200). West Sussex: Whurr.

Alzheimer's Association. Retrieved September 25, 2006, from http://www.alz.org/overview.asp.

American Speech-Language-Hearing Association. (2001). *Scope of practice in speech-language pathology*. Rockville, MD.

Avent, J. R., & Austermann, S. (2003). Reciprocal scaffolding: A context for communication treatment in aphasia. *Aphasiology, 17*(4), 397–404.

Bakas, T., Kroenke, K., Plue, L. D., Perkins, S. M., & Williams, L. S. (2006). Outcomes among family caregivers of aphasic versus nonaphasic stroke survivors. *Rehabilitation Nursing, 31*(1), 33–42.

Bays, C. L. (2001). Quality of life of stroke survivors: A research synthesis. *Journal of Neuroscience Nursing, 33*(6), 310–316.

Bouchard-Lamothe, D., Bourassa, S., Laflamme, B., Garcia, L. J., Gailey, G., & Stiell, K. (1999). Perceptions of three groups of interlocutors of the effects of aphasia on communication: An exploratory study. *Aphasiology, 13*(9–11), 839–855.

Brumfitt, S. M., & Sheeran, P. (1999). The development and validation of the Visual Analogue Self-Esteem Scale (VASES). *British Journal of Clinical Psychology, 38*, 387–400.

Byng, S., & Duchan, J. F. (2005). Social model philosophies and principles: Their applications to therapies for aphasia. *Aphasiology, 19* (10/11), 906–922.

Carlomagno, S., Losanno, N., Emanuelli, S., & Casadio, P. (1991). Expressive language recovery or improved communicative skills: Effects of P. A. C. E. Therapy on aphasics' referential communication and story retelling. *Aphasiology, 5*(4/5), 419–424.

Carlsson, M., & Hamrin, E. (2002). Evaluation of the Life Satisfaction Questionnaire (LSQ) using Structural Equation Modelling (SEM). *Quality of Life Research, 11*, 415–425.

Castelein, P., Noots-Villers, P., Buxant, P., & Spicher, C. (1994). Creation and testing of a « tool » for systemic assessment of brain damaged patients. *ICIDH and Environmental Factors Network Journal, 7*, 7–26.

Code, C., Müller, D. J., Hogan, A., & Herrmann, M. (1999). Perceptions of psychosocial adjustment to acquired communication disorders: Applications of the Code-Müller protocols. *International Journal of Language and Communication Disorders, 34*(2), 193–207.

Craig Hospital Research Department (2001). *The Craig Hospital inventory of environmental factors* (Manual, Version 3.0). Englewood, CO: Craig Hospital.

Cruice, M., Worrall, L. E. & Hickson, L. (2005) Personal Factors, Communication and Vision Predict Social Participation in Older Adults. *Advances in Speech-Language Pathology, 7*(4), 220–232.

Cruice, M., Worrall, L, Hickson, L., & Murison, R. (2005). Measuring quality of life: Comparing family members' and friends' ratings with those of their aphasic partners. *Aphasiology, 19*(2), 111–129.

Cunningham, R., & Ward, C. D. (2003). Evaluation of a training programme to facilitate conversation between people with aphasia and their partners. *Aphasiology, 17*(8), 687–707.

Davidson, B. J., & Worrall, L. E. (2000). The assessment of activity limitation in functional communication: Challenges and choices. In L. E. Worrall & C. M. Frattali (Eds.), *Neurogenic communication disorders: A functional approach* (pp. 19–34). New York: Thieme.

Doyle, P. J., McNeil, M. R., Hula, W. D., & Mikolic, J. M. (2003). The Burden of Stroke Scale (BOSS): Validating patient-reported communication difficulty and associated psychological distress in stroke survivors. *Aphasiology, 17*, 291–304.

Duchan, J. (2006). *Getting here: A short history of speech pathology in America*. Last revised on February 12, 2006. http://www.acsu.buffalo.edu/~duchan/history.html

Engell, B., Hütter, B.- O., Willmes, K., & Huber, W. (2003). Quality of life in aphasia: Validation of a pictorial self-rating procedure. *Aphasiology, 17*(4), 383–396.

Fougeyrollas, P. (2006). *Convergences and differences between ICF and DCP: The issue of environmental factors' influence in the construction of human functioning and disability*. Paper presented at the 12th Annual North American Collaborating Center Conference on ICF, June 5–7, Vancouver, B.C.

Fougeyrollas, P., Cloutier, R., Bergeron, H., Côté, J., St Michel, G. (1998) *The Quebec classification: Disability creation process*. International Network on the Disability Creation Process, Lac St. Charles, Quebec.

Fougeyrollas, P., Noreau, L., Dion, S. A., Lepage, C., Sévigny, M., & St. Michel, G. (1997). *Life Habits (LIFE-H)*. International Network of the Disability Creation Process, Lac St. Charles, Québec.

Fougeyrollas, P., Noreau, L., St Michel, G., & Boschen, K. (1999). *Measure of the quality of the environment* (Version 2.0). International Network of the Disability Creation Process, Lac St. Charles, Québec.

Frattali, C. M. (Ed.). (1998). *Measuring utcomes in speech-language pathology*. New York: Thieme.

Frattali, C. M., Thompson, C. K., Holland, A. L., Wohl, C. B., & Ferketic, M. M. (1995). *Functional assessment of communication skills for adults*. Rockville, MD: ASHA.

Garcia, L. J., Barrette, J., & Laroche, C. (2000). Perceptions of the obstacles to work reintegration for persons with aphasia. *Aphasiology, 14*(3), 269–290.

Garcia, L. J., Eriks-Brophy, A., Daneault, C., Gravel, M., Séguin, M. J., & Rochette, M. C. (2003). Comparaison de deux méthodes pour décrire l'impact de l'aphasie sur le fonctionnement de deux individus—Étude pilote. (Comparison of two methods to describe the impact of aphasia on the global functioning of two individuals: A pilot study). *Développement Humain, Handicap et Changement Social. (Human Development, Handicap and Social Change), 12*(1), 31–49.

Golper, L. A. C. (2001). Teams and partnerships in aphasia intervention. In R. Chapey (Ed.), *Language intervention strategies in aphasia and related neurogenic communication disorders* (4th ed., pp. 194–207). Brooklyn: Lippincott Williams & Wilkins.

Hilari, K. (2005). Choosing relevant outcomes for aphasia: A commentary on Ross and Wertz, "Advancing appraisal: Aphasia and the WHO". *Aphasiology, 19*(1), 870–875.

Hilari, K., & Byng, S. (2001). Measuring quality of life in people with aphasia: The Stroke Specific Quality of Life Scale. *International Journal of Language and Communication Disorders, 36*(Suppl), 86–91.

Hilari, K., Byng, S., Lamping, D. L., & Smith, S. C. (2003) Stroke and Aphasia Quality of Life Scale-39 (SAQOL-39): Evaluation of acceptability, reliability, and validity. *Stroke, 34*, 1944–1950.

Hirsh, F. M., & Holland, A. L. (2000). Beyond activity: Measuring participation in society and quality of life. In L. E. Worrall & Frattali, C. M. (Eds.), *Neurogenic communication disorders: A functional approach* (pp. 35–54). New York: Thieme.

Holland, A. L. (1991). Pragmatic aspects of intervention in aphasia. *Journal of Neurolinguistics, 6*(2), 197–211.

Hopper, T., Holland, A., Rewega, M. (2002). Conversational coaching: Treatment outcomes and future directions. *Aphasiology, 16*(7), 745–761.

Howe, T. J., Worrall, L. E., & Hickson, L. (2004) What is an aphasia-friendly environment? *Aphasiology, 18*(11), 1015–1037.

Kagan, A. (1995). Revealing the competence of aphasic adults through conversation: A challenge to health professionals. *Top Stroke Rehabilitation, 2*(1), 15–28.

Kagan, A., Black, S. E., Duchan, J. F., Simmons-Mackie, N., & Square, P. (2001). Training volunteers as conversation partners using "Supported Conversation for Adults with Aphasia" (SCA): A controlled trial. *Journal of Speech, Language, and Hearing Research, 44*, 624–638.

Kagan, A., & LeBlanc, K. (2002). Motivating for infrastructure change: Toward a communicatively accessible, participation-based stroke care system for all those affected by aphasia. *Journal of Communication Disorders, 35*, 153–169.

Kearns, K. P., & Elman, R. J. (2001). Group therapy for aphasia: Theoretical and practical considerations. In R. Chapey (Ed.), *Language intervention strategies in aphasia and related neurogenic communication disorders* (4th Ed., pp. 316–337). Brooklyn: Lippincott Williams & Wilkins.

Laroche, C., Garcia, L. J., Barrette, J., Desjardins, M., Lefrançois, R., & Barbier, S. (1999). Revision process of the MQE for individuals with communication disorders within their work environment. *ICIDH and Environmental Factors Network Journal, 10*(1-2), 31–38.

Lawton, M. P., & Nahemow, L. (1973). Ecology and the aging process. In C. Eisdorfer, M. P. Lawton (Eds.), *The psychology of adult development and aging* (pp. 619–674). Washington, D.C. American Psychological Association.

LeDorze, G., & Brassard, C. (1995). A description of the consequences of aphasia on aphasic persons and their relatives and families, based on the WHO model of chronic diseases. *Aphasiology, 9*, 239–255.

Lomas, J., Pickard, L., Bester, S., Elbard, H., Finlayson, A., & Zoghaib, C. (1989). The communicative effectiveness index: Development and psychometric evaluation of a functional communication measure for adult aphasia. *Journal of Speech and Hearing Disorders, 54*, 113–124.

LPAA Project Group (Chapey, R., Duchan, J. F., Elman, R. J., Garcia, L. J., Kagan, A., Lyon, J. G., et al.) (2001). Life participation approach to aphasia: A statement of values for the future. In R. Chapey (Ed.), *Language intervention strategies in aphasia and related neurogenic communication disorders* (4th ed., pp. 235–245). Brooklyn: Lippincott Williams & Wilkins.

Lubinski, R. (2001). Environmental systems approach to adult aphasia. In R. Chapey (Ed.), *Language intervention strategies in aphasia and related neurogenic communication disorders* (4th ed., pp. 269–296). Brooklyn: Lippincott Williams & Wilkins.

Luterman, D. M. (1996). *Counseling persons with communication disorders and their families*. Austin: Pro-Ed.

Lyon, J. G. (1996). Optimizing communication and participation in life for aphasic adults and their prime caregivers in natural settings: A use model for treatment. In G. L. Wallace (Ed.), *Adult aphasia rehabilitation*. Boston: Butterworth-Heinemann.

Lyon, J. G., & Shadden, B. B. (2001). Treating life consequences of aphasia's chronicity. In R. Chapey (Ed.), *Language intervention strategies in aphasia and related neurogenic communication disorders* (4th ed., pp.297–315). Brooklyn: Lippincott Williams & Wilkins.

Mackay, R. (2003). 'Tell them who I was': The social construction of aphasia. *Disability and Society, 18*(6), 811–826.

McCall, D., Shelton, J. R., Weinrich, M., & Cox, D. (2000). The utility of computerized visual communication for improving natural language in chronic global aphasia: Implications for approaches to treatment in global aphasia. *Aphasiology, 14*(8), 795–826.

McDowell, I., & Newell, C. (1996). *Measuring health: A guide to rating scales and questionnaires*. New York: Oxford University Press.

McWreath, J. M. (2005). *Picturing aphasia*. Los Angeles (www.aphasia.tv), National Center for Injury Prevention and Control. http://www.cdc.gov/ncipc/tbi/TBI.htm, consulted on September 25, 2006.

National Stroke Association (2006). *Stroke facts*. Englewood: National Stroke Association.

Noreau, L., Desrosiers, J., Robichaud, L., Fougeyrollas, P., Rochette, A., & Viscogliosi, C. (2004). Measuring social participation: Reliability of the LIFE-H in older adults with disabilities. *Disability and Rehabilitation, 26*(6), 346–352.

Noreau, L., Fougeyrollas, P., & Vincent, C. (2002). The LIFE-H: Assessment of the quality of social participation. *Technology and Disability, 14*(3), 113–118.

Parr, S. (2001). Psychological aspects of aphasia: Whose Perspectives? *Folia Phoniatrica et Logopaedica, 53*, 266–288.

Parr, S., Byng, S., & Gilpin, S (1997). *Talking about aphasia: Living with loss of language after stroke*, Philadelphia: Open University Press.

Parr, S., Duchan, J., & Pound, C. (2003). *Aphasia inside out: Reflections on communication disability*. Berkshire, England: Open University Press.

Penn, C. (2005). Who's tired of the WHO? A commentary on Ross and Wertz, "Advancing appraisal: Aphasia and the WHO". *Aphasiology, 19*(9), 875–879.

Pound, C., Parr, S., & Duchan, J. (2001). Using partners' autobiographical reports to develop, deliver, and evaluate services in aphasia. *Aphasiology, 15*(5), 477–493.

Pound, C., Parr, S., Lindsay, J., & Woolf, C. (2000). *Beyond aphasia therapies for living with communication disability*. Oxford: Winslow Press.

Pulvermüller, F., & Roth, V. M. (1991). Communicative aphasia treatment as a further development of PACE therapy. *Aphasiology, 5*(1), 39–50.

Reed, G. M., Lux, J. B., Bufka, L. F., Petersen, D. B., Threats, T. T., & Trask, C. (2005). Operationalizing the international classification of functioning, disability and health in clinical settings. *Rehabilitation Psychology, 50*(2), 122–131.

Ross, K. B., & Wertz, R. T. (2002). Relationships between language-based disability and quality of life in chronically aphasic adults. *Aphasiology, 16*(8), 791–800.

Ross, K. B., & Wertz, R. T. (2003). Quality of life with and without aphasia. *Aphasiology, 17*(4), 355–364.

Ross, K. B., & Wertz, R. T. (2005). Advancing appraisal: Aphasia and the WHO. *Aphasiology, 19*(9), 860–900.

Saxe, J. G. (1963). *The blind men and the elephant; John Godfrey Saxe's version of the famous Indian legend. Pictures by Paul Galdone.* New York: Whittlesey House.

Schegloff, E. A. (1987). Analyzing single episodes of interaction: An exercise in conversation analysis. *Social Psychology Quarterly, 50*(2), 101–114.

Schlosser, R. W. (2004). Goal attainment scaling as a clinical measurement technique in communication disorders; A critical review. *Journal of Communication Disorders, 37*, 217–239.

Shadden, B. B. (2005). Aphasia as identity theft: Theory and practice. *Aphasiology, 19*(3/4/5), 211–223.

Simmons-Mackie, N. N. (2001). Social approaches to aphasia intervention. In R. Chapey (Ed.), *Language intervention strategies in aphasia and related neurogenic communication disorders* (4th ed., pp. 246–268). Brooklyn: Lippincott Williams & Wilkins.

Simmons-Mackie, N. N., & Damico, J. S. (1995). Communicative competence in aphasia: Evidence from compensatory strategies. *Clinical Aphasiology, 23*, 95–105.

Simmons-Mackie, N. N., Kearns, K. P., & Potechin, G. (2005). Treatment of aphasia through family member training. *Aphasiology, 19*(6), 583–593.

Simmons-Mackie, N. N., Threats, T. T., & Kagan, A. (2005). Outcome assessment in aphasia: A survey. *Journal of Communication Disorders, 38*, 1–27.

Sorin-Peters, R. (2003). Viewing couples living with aphasia as adult learners: Implications for promoting quality of life. *Aphasiology, 17*(4), 405–416.

Sveen, U., Thommessen, B., Bautz-Holter, E., Wyller, T. B., & Laake, K. (2004). Well-being and instrumental activities of daily living after stroke. *Clinical Rehabilitation, 18*, 267–274.

Threats, T. (2006). Towards an international framework for communication disorders: Use of the ICF. *Journal of Communication Disorders, 39*, 251–265.

Threats, T., & Worrall, L. (2004). Classifying communication disability using the ICF. *Advances in Speech-Language Pathology, 6*(1), 53–62.

Verderber, R. F. (1981). *Communicate!* Belmont, CA: Wadsworth.

Waller, A., Dennis, F., Brodie, J., & Cairns, A. Y. (1998). Evaluating the use of Talks Bac, a predictive communication device for nonfluent adults with aphasia. *International Journal of Communication Disorders, 33*(1), 45–70.

Ward-Lonergan, J. M., & Nicholas, M. (1995). Drawing to communicate: A case report of an adult with global aphasia. *European Journal of Disorders of Communication, 30*, 475–491.

Ware, J. E., Kosinski, M., & Gandek, B. (2000). *SF-36 Health survey: Manual and interpretation guide.* Lincoln, RI: Quality Metric Inc.

Whiteneck, G. (2006). Conceptual models of disability: Past, present, and future. In M. J. Field, A. M. Jette, & L. Martin (Eds.), *Workshop on disability in America: A new look (Appendix B)*. Washington, D. C.: The National Academies Press.

Whiteneck, G., Brooks, C., Charlifue, S., Gerhart, K., Mellick, D., Overholser, D., et al. (1988). *Guide for use of the CHART: Craig handicap assessment and reporting technique.* Englewood, CO: Craig Hospital.

The WHOQOL Group (1998). Development of the The World Health Organization WHOQOL-BREF quality of life assessment. *Psychological Medicine, 28*, 551–558.

Williams, L. S., Weinberger, M., Harris, L. E., Clark, D. O., & Biller, J. (1999). Development of a stroke-specific quality of life scale. *Stroke, 30*, 1362–1369.

World Health Organization (1980). *International Classification of Impairments, Disabilities, and Handicaps (ICIDH): A manual of classification relating to the consequences of disease.* Geneva: World Health Organization.

World Health Organization (1999). *International Classification of Diseases* (9th Revision). Geneva: World Health Organization.

World Health Organization (2001). *International Classification of Functioning, Disability and Health (ICF).* Geneva: World Health Organization.

Worrall, L. (2006). Professionalism and Functional Outcomes. *Journal of Communication Disorders, 39*, 320–327.

Worrall, L., & Cruice, M. (2005). Why the WHO ICF and QOL constructs do not lend themselves to programmatic appraisal for planning therapy for aphasia. A commentary on Ross and Wertz, "Advancing appraisal: Aphasia and the WHO". *Aphasiology, 19*(1), 885–893.

Worrall, L., McCooey, R., Davidson, B., Larkins, B., & Hickson, L. (2002). The validity of functional assessments of communication and the activity/participation components of the ICIDH-2: Do they reflect what really happens in real-life? *Journal of Communication Disorders, 35,* 107–137.

Worrall, L., Rose, T., Howe, T., Brennan, A., Egan, J., Oxenham, D., & McKenna, K. (2005). Access to written information for people with aphasia. *Aphasiology, 19*(10/11), 923–929.

Worrall, L., & Yiu, E. (2000). Effectiveness of functional communication therapy by volunteers for people with aphasia following stroke. *Aphasiology, 14*(9), 911–924.

Wright, M., Garcia, L. J., Neault, M. J., & Fergus, S. L. (2002). Use of the Disability Creation Process model in the evaluation of language in dementia. *Human development, Disability and Social Change, 11*(1), 36–54.

Youmans, G., Holland, A., Muñoz, M. L., & Bourgeois, M. (2005). Script training and automaticity in two individuals with aphasia. *Aphasiology, 19*(3/4/5), 435–450.

APPENDIX 13.1
Interview Guidelines for Looking at Functioning

Notes to Interviewer:

1. It is important to ask, in all areas, whether a person does not do the activity by choice.
2. Items indicated with bullets are suggested areas to explore.

Housing/Living at Home

Q1. Who do you live with?

Q2. Are you able to take care of your house/apartment? Any technologic help? Any human help?
  - Cleaning and laundry
  - Acquisition and adaptation of residence
  - Management of home and possessions (furnishings, animals, pets)
  - Paid home adaptation services?

Nutrition

Q3. Do you have any difficulty with your daily nutrition needs? Any meal providing services?
  - Getting food, buying food (restaurant, school cafeteria, store), preparing food (appliances, recipes)
  - Use of utensils? Feeding aids?
  - Do you eat well?

Personal Maintenance

Q4. How would you consider your physical and mental health?
  - Stress management and behavioral modification
  - Physical conditioning (relaxation, fitness, sleep)
  - Use of health-care services and resources
  - Health promotion (eating well, yoga, etc.)
  - Medication intake
  - Are services available to you?

Q4.1. Any problems handling different emotional situations?
  - Frustration
  - Anger
  - Sadness
  - Happiness

Q4.2. Does anybody help you with handling emotions?
  - Friends
  - Therapist
  - Family

Q5. Do you have issues related to your personal appearance and cleanliness?
  - Washing (self, teeth, clothes)
  - Dressing
  - Toileting
  - Technical or human aids?

Mobility

Q6. Can you get around your home and in your neighborhood for short walking distances?
  - Walking
  - Running
  - From sitting to standing
  - From standing to lying
  - Staying in one position
  - Balance

Q6.1. Do you have physical limitations that require modifications to your environment (accessibility, accommodations, distance to services)?

Q6.2. Do you require any type of special equipment, or services to help you move from one place to another (walker, wheelchair, special transportation services, etc.)?

Q6.3. How is your mobility when traveling long distances?
  - Using transportation (as a passenger, as a driver)

Communication/Exchange of Information

Q7. To what extent can you communicate with others? When do you encounter difficulties? What strategies do you use to overcome these difficulties?
- Spoken
- Written
- Sign language
- Nonverbal
- Body language
- Public symbols
- Drawings and photographs

Q7.1. Use of communication devices and technologies?

Q7.2. How do people react to you when you communicate?

Interpersonal Relationships

Q8. Describe your relationships with people. Do you have problems initiating and/or maintaining relationships?

Q8.1. Do you receive support or assistance (encouragement) from people?
- Spouse/intimate partners
- Children
- Friends
- Work colleagues
- Family
- Strangers
- Home-care providers
- Health professionals

Community Life

Q9. What is your involvement in all aspects of your community?
- Social life (activities organized by the community)
- Community associations or groups (scouts, self-help groups, political party, etc.)
- Spiritual life or organized religion

Work

Q10. To what extent can you participate in any type of work or employment?
- Work preparation (seeking employment)
- Self-employment
- Remunerative employment (full time, part-time)
- Nonremunerative work

Q10.1. Are you satisfied with your work and work environment?
- Colleague support and attitudes
- Physical environment at work (noise, lighting, number of colleagues, etc.)
- Organization of tasks (workload, change in duties, number of hours, etc.)

Q10.2. Do you need any special technical or human aid?

Education

Q11. How do you manage in school?
- Trouble understanding what's going on in class
- Friends at school
- Organization of class activities
- Problems with any subjects
- Taking notes
- Exams
- Extracurricular activities

Q11.1. Do you like school?

Q11.2. Do you need any special technical or human aid (adapted classroom, hearing aids, etc.)?
- When something is difficult to understand at school, are there things that the teacher can do to help you learn?

Leisure

Q12. Are you involved in any form of leisure activity?
- Sports
- Arts and culture (music)
- Cinema/theater
- Games
- Hobbies
- Travel (including preparing trips)
- Socializing

Responsibilities/Finances

Q13. Do you have problems managing your finances, your civil and family responsibilities? Have your social roles changed?
- Economic transactions and self-sufficiency (budget, going to the bank)
- Citizenship (social, political, and legal role of a citizen)
- Family (care and responsibility of others: parents, children, spouse)

Q13.1. What is your main source of income, and are you satisfied with it?

Q13.2. Do you receive any additional financial assistance from your family, governmental agencies, or private programs?

Q14. Any general comments about attitudes and support from people?

Q15. Are there things in your physical environment, at home, at work, or in other public places that you would like to change.

Q16. Are you satisfied with your quality of life? Is there anything that you would like to change? What would be your priorities?

Chapter 14

Group Therapy for Aphasia: Theoretic and Practical Considerations

Kevin P. Kearns and
Roberta J. Elman

OBJECTIVES

The need to synthesize the group treatment literature, describe current clinical practice, and develop specific treatment approaches that can be both clinically useful and experimentally validated continues to exist. Therefore, the purpose of this chapter is (a) to critically review and summarize the aphasia group therapy literature and (b) to present a perspective on group therapy for aphasia that is consistent with information in the literature on facilitating generalization. Suggestions will also be provided regarding the future role of speech-language pathologists in this area of rehabilitation.

The content and focus of group therapy for aphasia is predominantly a function of the skills and biases of the group leader (Elman, 1999, 2007; Marquardt, 1982; Marquardt, Tonkovich, & Devault, 1976). In general, however, most aphasia groups focus on one or more of the following parameters: psychosocial adjustment, speech-language treatment, and/or counseling (Eisenson, 1973; Fawcus, 1989). This clinical taxonomy is, of course, somewhat arbitrary, because communication and psychosocial factors are intricately related and improvement of one factor may affect the other (Marquardt et al., 1976). Therefore, the interrelatedness and complexity of therapeutic goals in group treatment of aphasia should be kept in mind during the following discussion of group treatment approaches.

Group therapy for aphasia evolved in the United States as a practical response to the large influx of head-injured veterans returning from World War II. At that time, relatively few professionals were specifically trained to provide clinical services for individuals with aphasia, and burgeoning caseloads necessitated group treatment. Group therapy has remained a common method of treating aphasia both in the United States and abroad (Fawcus, 1989; Pachalska, 1991a; Tsvetkova, 1980).

Ironically, changes in reimbursement and public policy (Frattali, 1992) as well as a renewed interest in psychosocial aspects of recovery from aphasia have stimulated a renewed interest in group treatment (Avent, 1997a, 1997b; Borenstein, Linell, & Wahrborg, 1987; Brindely, Copeland, Demain, & Martyn, 1989; Elman, 1999, 2005, 2007; Elman & Bernstein-Ellis, 1999a, 1999b; Marshall, 1999a, 1999b; Pachalska, 1991a, 1999b; Radonjic & Rakuscek, 1991). Lyon (1992) argued that clinical aphasiologists broaden their clinical perspective by incorporating psychological as well as functional communicative goals into the endeavors and should use treatment plans that facilitate or encourage "participation in life." The Life Participation Approach to Aphasia (LPAA Project Group, 2000) (see Chapter 10), further articulated this perspective. Similarly, Frattali has noted, "We must remember that human communication sciences and disorders is a discipline dedicated to improving the quality of life of persons with communication disorders" (p. 81). Psychosocial factors are classified in the World Health Organization (WHO) International Classification of Functioning, Disability, and Health, or ICF. The WHO framework seeks to integrate medical and social models of medicine using a biopsychosocial approach. The reader is referred to the WHO publication for a compete description of this framework (WHO, 2001).

Of course, interest in the broader aspects of recovery from aphasia are not new. Descriptive accounts of group therapy and its benefits abound in the aphasia literature (Agranowitz, Boone, Ruff, Seacat, & Terr, 1954; Aronson, Shatin, & Cook, 1956; Chenven, 1953; Gordon, 1976; Holland, 1970; Inskip & Burris, 1959; Nielson, Schultz, Corbin, & Crittsinger, 1948; Schlanger & Schlanger, 1970; Wepman, 1947). Advocates have claimed that group intervention results in widespread changes in speech and language skills as well as increased psychosocial adjustment to aphasia. Unfortunately, few objective studies have supported these claims, and the efficacy of group therapy for aphasia has more recently been established. Although the results of recent investigations indicate that group therapy is an effective form of aphasia management (Aten, Caligiuri, & Holland, 1982; Avent, 1997a; Brindely et al., 1989; Elman & Bernstein-Ellis, 1999a, 1999b; Radonjic & Rakuscek, 1991; Wertz et al., 1981), aphasiologists have only recently given attention to this important area of clinical investigation. Renewed interest in group therapy for aphasia is reflected in recent publications that specifically address clinical goals and procedures for group intervention (Avent, 1997b; Elman, 1999, 2007; Marshall, 1999a; Vickers, 1998). These texts are a welcome addition to the clinical armamentarium, because clinical aphasiology textbooks contain only brief descriptions of group treatment and minimal discussion of the procedures employed in group therapy (Brookshire, 1992; Darley, 1982, 1992; Eisenson, 1973; Jenkins, Jimenez-Pabon, Shaw, & Sefer, 1981; Sarno, 1981). Before the recent publication of texts that focus on group treatment, few critical summaries of the group treatment literature were available (Fawcus, 1989; Marquardt et al., 1976).

While recognizing the need for empirically based group treatment procedures, recent interest in broader rehabilitation goals has occurred within a conceptual and methodologic framework that heretofore had been lacking. From a conceptual perspective, clinical aphasiologists have begun to appreciate the complexities associated with facilitating generalized changes in people with aphasia (Van Harskamp & Visch-Brink, 1991). More important, an ecological perspective on intervention, which considers the complexity of environmental, personal, social, emotional, and communicative factors on treatment, is finally evolving into specific, testable treatment suggestions for both individual and group therapy (Aten et al., 1982; Davis & Wilcox, 1981; Elman & Bernstein-Ellis, 1999a, 1999b; LaPointe, 1989). Consistent with the trend toward a more ecological approach to intervention, a concomitant emphasis on methodologic issues may provide a procedural framework for group therapy. For example, calls for reliable and appropriate functional (Frattali, 1992), psychosocial (Lyon, 1992), and life participation assessment tools (LPAA Project Group, 2001), as well as the development of a generalization planning approach to intervention (Garrett & Pimentel, 2007; Kearns, 1989; Thompson, 1989), have direct relevance to group intervention for aphasia.

GROUP TREATMENT APPROACHES

Psychosocial Groups

Although psychotherapeutic and sociotherapeutic approaches to group management have been distinguished in the aphasia literature (Marquardt et al., 1976), these approaches share more similarities than differences. That is, despite differing descriptive labels, the purpose and procedures discussed in reports of sociotherapeutic and psychotherapeutic group

therapy are often indistinguishable. Psychosocial groups provide a supportive atmosphere in which individuals with aphasia can ventilate feelings and learn to cope with the psychological impact of aphasia. In addition, the goals and procedures of these groups emphasize interpersonal relationships while providing social contacts with other persons who are "in the same boat." The primary purpose of psychosocial aphasia groups is to foster the development of emotional and psychological bonds that help group members to cope with the consequences of aphasia (Ewing, 1999, 2007; Inskip & Burris, 1959; Luterman, 1996; Oradei & Waite, 1974; Redinger, Forster, Dolphin, Godduhn, & Wersinger, 1971; Yalom, 1995).

Earliest reports of psychosocial group treatment gave minimal attention to subject description, procedural specification, or evaluation of treatment results (Backus & Dunn, 1947, 1952; Blackman, 1950; Blackman & Tureen, 1948; Godfrey & Douglass, 1959). Aronson et al. (1956), however, provided a detailed description of a "social-psychotherapeutic" approach to group therapy and attempted to evaluate the effectiveness of such a program. They developed a task continuum in an attempt to facilitate group discussion, provide an emotional outlet, and allow patients to develop interpersonal relationships. Tasks in the hierarchy ranged from nonverbal (e.g., music rhythm group) to solely verbal (e.g., group discussion), and they included (a) using rhythmic musical instruments, (b) participating in group singing, (c) listening to short stories read by a group leader, (d) participating in various speech games and discussion of proverbs, (e) taping and replaying speech samples, and (f) taking part in group-centered discussion. Activities from the hierarchy were introduced as needed to maintain motivation and facilitate group interaction whenever adequate group discussion could not be elicited.

The effectiveness of this approach was evaluated for 21 chronic and acute patients who attended an average of 14 hourly treatment sessions. Results of interviews and clinical ratings revealed that the patients and staff reacted quite favorably to the treatment program. The group leaders also observed a reduction in anxiety, an increased level of intragroup, and a heightened ability for constructive self-criticism among group members. Another early report of psychosocial group therapy notable for its attempt to outline specific group treatment procedures was provided by Schlanger and Schlanger (1970). They recommended the use of role playing as a method for reducing anxiety about communication and establishing spontaneous, functional discourse in the group setting. Their primary purpose was to "try to 'get something across' both inter- and intra-personally" (p. 230) through the use of (a) gesture and pantomime, (b) role playing one's self in realistic situations, (c) role playing other individuals, and (d) psychodrama.

As Schlanger and Schlanger (1970), reported gestures and pantomime were employed to enhance the communication of chronic patients with aphasia who had severely limited verbal abilities. Gestural and pantomime training included the use of descriptive gestures to transmit information about pictorial referents, pantomiming daily activities such as mailing a letter, and using "universal" iconic gestures.

Following gesture and pantomime training, the patients participated in role-playing activities involving nonstressful and stressful situations. Nonstressful situations included activities such as shopping or attending a picnic. Role playing in stressful situations involved having patients interact with a clinician in a "Candid Camera"–like situation. Unexpected events were blended into everyday experiences so that the patient had to problem solve and communicate in a natural situation.

Another aspect of this approach involved having the individuals with aphasia role play other people during simulated situations. During this activity, patients used pantomime and verbal skills to depict people in contrived scenes from a bakery, a florist, and so on.

A final aspect of the group treatment program used psychodrama to act out the problems and frustrations of each group member. During this activity, patients assumed roles that allowed them to vent feelings and release hostility.

The aphasia group members gradually progressed through the four facets of training, and several benefits of the program were noted. Patients demonstrated an increased ability to cope with stressful situations, a reduction in anxiety concerning communication deficits, a feeling of accomplishment, a loss of emotional inhibition, and a better insight regarding feelings and problems. Schlanger and Schlanger (1970) concluded that role-playing activities provide an important means of adjusting to the psychosocial impact of aphasia.

More recent clinical reports have also targeted psychosocial goals within the aphasia group setting. Borenstein et al. (1987), for example, examined the psychological, linguistic, and neurologic effects of a 5-day, intensive residential treatment program for participants with aphasia and their relatives. Eleven participants with aphasia and seven family members attended the group. Sessions were conducted by a speech-language pathologist, a psychologist, and a neurologist. Formal assessments of the family members' psychological adjustment and of the participants with aphasia's language ability and neurologic status were conducted. The content of the intervention program included family-centered therapy, social excursions that encouraged functional communication, and group discussions of everyday problems and adjustment strategies. Reevaluations of the participants conducted 1 year after the intensive treatment period revealed some improvements in psychological and interpersonal adjustment but not in neurologic or communicative status. A 10-year follow-up study involving eight of the original participants (Wahrborg, Borenstein, Linell, Hedber-Borenstein, & Asking, 1997) found the improvements that had been achieved at the end of the course of treatment were diminished after 10 years. All but one of the participants showed a more severe aphasia at the 10-year follow-up; however, seven of the eight participants reported that their quality of life was improved at 10 years post-treatment as compared with the end of the psychosocial group.

Johannsen-Horbach, Wenz, Funfgeld, Hermann, & Wallesch (1993) reported on their aphasia groups that focused on aspects of coping with aphasia and its consequences. Two groups were described—one for younger participants (eight members, ages 26–51), and one for elderly participants (seven members, ages 60–80). Content of the group treatment included interactional and conversational exchange about psychosocial burden, communication strategies (e.g., PACE [Davis & Wilcox, 1985]), role playing, and tasks from a verbal/visual memory training program. The groups, which were led by a psychologist and a speech-language pathologist, met once a week for 2 hours. The younger group met a total of 22 times, and the elderly group met a total of 16 times. The authors reported that participants had higher degrees of self-esteem following participation in the group treatment and were able to use "new behavioral strategies." The authors stated that younger participants had more difficulty accepting their deficits as compared with the elderly clients and wanted to focus their efforts on communicative deficits. The authors concluded that their observations support the usefulness of psychosocial groups and reinforce their belief that separating participants by age is a useful clinical strategy.

Hoen, Thelander, & Worsley (1997) reported on psychosocial changes following participation in their community-based program offered to people with aphasia following stroke and head injury. Their study evaluated changes on a condensed form of psychological scales of well being (1989). Thirty-five clients with aphasia attended volunteer-run communication groups twice weekly for half-days. In addition, a social worker led caregiver support groups with 12 family members. Although improvement was measured over a 6-month period, treatment time in the program before enrollment in the study was not controlled. In addition, total treatment time for each subject was not reported. Results indicated that clients with aphasia showed positive changes on the scales, which measure autonomy, environmental mastery, personal growth, purpose in life, and self-acceptance. The scale designed to assess positive relations with others did not show significant change. The results for family members were also encouraging; family members showed significant change on all scales except for "environmental mastery." Despite these positive findings, the authors note that the design of this study is flawed and does not permit an objective assessment of the benefits of group intervention.

Penman and Pound developed a short-term, self-advocacy group for people with aphasia at the City Dysphasic Group at City University in London (Pound, 1998; Penman,

2007). The course ran for 10 weeks with 2-hour sessions. The focus of the group was twofold: (1) to identify disabling barriers in the environment, and (2) to develop a positive personal identity that was inclusive of aphasia and disability. Two people, a speech-language therapist and a person with aphasia, facilitated the groups. Eight individuals with chronic aphasia participated. Group discussion was used as the vehicle for working on many different issues, including communication, self-esteem, autonomy, leisure life, and financial status.

The outcomes of the therapy were evaluated by examining personal interviews and personal portfolios that had been developed by each group member. Post-treatment evaluations suggested that group members felt more confident, had improved self-esteem, and were more positive about living with aphasia. Participants also reported feeling an increased sense of social participation and "belonging."

Shadden (2007) described an ongoing monthly support group, the Stroke Support Group of Northwest Arkansas (NWA), originally established in 1982. She noted how the group has evolved into a community in which members exchange life stories, thereby renegotiating "self and identity." The NWA includes survivors of stroke, both with and without aphasia, as well as family members or others who are dealing with the impact of stroke. No formal agenda is followed; instead, group sessions start with a sharing time, followed by breakout sessions for survivors of stroke and significant others. Shadden listed 12 core values of the group: (1) respect for the concerns and competence of each member; (2) acceptance, (3) affirmation and validation, (4) actions speak louder than words, (5) feelings are okay, (6) reflection and problem solving are encouraged, (7) flexible goals, (8) a clean slate, (9) participant oriented, (10) focus on the story, (11) interaction oriented, and (12) celebration of change. The rules and routines that characterize the NWA include putting the survivors of stroke first, focusing on new members, and sharing updates and life stories.

Useful supplements to the specific psychosocial treatment programs outlined above are provided by Elman (2000), Ewing (1999, 2007), and Luterman (1996). These authors summarize information regarding group process, group dynamics, and other group considerations that speech-language pathologists must be aware of when facilitating treatment groups. Both authors emphasize group techniques that need adaptation when working with members who have neurogenic communication disorders.

Summary and Observations

The literature contains a general consensus that psychosocial group therapy provides psychological, emotional, and social benefits for individuals with aphasia. Specific benefits that have been reported include an opportunity for increased socialization; a supportive atmosphere in which individuals

with aphasia can express anger, hostility, and other emotions; and the development of skills that allow patients to cope with emotional and life-style changes resulting from aphasia (Aronson et al., 1956; Backus & Dunn, 1947; Blackman, 1950; Blackman & Tureen, 1948; Byng et al., 1998; Eisenson, 1973; Friedman, 1961; Godfrey & Douglass, 1959; Hoen et al., 1997; Inskip & Burris, 1959; Johannsen-Horbach et al., 1993; Marquardt et al., 1976; Oradei & Waite, 1974; Pound, 1998; Redinger et al., 1971; Schlanger & Schlanger, 1970; Shadden, 2007). Despite near-unanimous agreement regarding the benefits of psychosocial group treatment, it should be cautioned that the findings of most reports in this area are based on subjective assessment and anecdotal observations. Data-based studies are practically nonexistent in the psychosocial group literature, and those that have been reported have not been rigorous (Aronson et al., 1956; Godfrey & Douglass, 1959; Oradei & Waite, 1974). Although the psychometric difficulties involved in measuring psychological and social parameters are substantial, a pressing need exists to begin evaluating the psychosocial impact of group treatment for aphasia.

Prerequisite to the establishment of a solid database for this approach to aphasia management is the development of specific, replicable treatment procedures. Unfortunately, with few notable exceptions (Aronson et al., 1956; Schlanger & Schlanger, 1970), investigators have not delineated specific treatment principles or procedures for conducting psychosocial group therapy for aphasia. Descriptions in the literature do not provide the procedural detail necessary to translate them into clinical practice (e.g., Friedman, 1961; Oradei & Waite, 1974; Redinger et al., 1971), and psychosocial group therapy remains largely an undefined entity. Moreover, when attempts have been made to document the effectiveness of psychosocial treatment groups (e.g., Borenstein et al., 1987), failure to meet minimal psychometric standards limits the usefulness of these efforts.

Family Counseling and Support Groups

In addition to the psychosocial adjustment difficulties of individuals with aphasia, the emotional, psychological, and life-style changes for family members of individuals with aphasia have also been documented (Friedland & McColl, 1989; Johannsen-Horbach et al., 1993; Kinsella & Duffy, 1978, 1979; Lafond, Joanette, Ponzio, Degiovanni, & Sarno, 1993; Lyon, 1998; Malone, 1969; Parr et al., 1997; Rice, Paul, & Müller, 1987). More than 30 years ago, Malone (1969) observed that "in most cases the family as a closely knit unit no longer existed" (p. 147) once a family member was stricken by aphasia. He concluded that family counseling programs are needed to help spouses and family members learn about aphasia and cope with its devastating consequences. The group setting is frequently used for counseling and educating both patients with aphasia and their families.

Brookshire (1997) notes that the primary objective of family support or counseling groups is to educate patients with aphasia and their families about the nature of aphasia and to explore the impact of aphasia on family dynamics. Counseling groups provide a medium for discussing physical, psychological, and social consequences of brain damage. They also serve as a forum for expressing feelings and learning to adjust to newly acquired family roles and life-style changes. Brookshire observed that patient-family and spouse support groups also function as a social or recreational outlet for individuals with aphasia and their families.

Examples of family counseling groups abound in the aphasia literature (Davis, 1992; Derman & Manaster, 1967; Friedland & McColl, 1989; Gordon, 1976; Johannsen-Horbach et al., 1993; Kisley, 1973; Mogil, Bloom, Gray, & Lefkowitz, 1978; Newhoff & Davis, 1978; Porter & Dabul, 1977; Puts-Zwartes, 1973; Redinger et al., 1971). Turnblom and Myers (1952) provided one of the earliest examples of group counseling for families of individuals with aphasia. Following this early report, the area of rehabilitation was virtually neglected for approximately 20 years. Redinger et al. (1971) subsequently described a multidisciplinary discussion group for patients with severe aphasia and their spouses. The purpose of the group was to facilitate emotional adjustment and to help the group members work through family and social issues using problem-oriented discussions. The group, which met on a weekly basis for 1 year, consisted of several co-leaders (a speech-language pathologist, a psychiatric nurse, and a psychiatrist), six patients with aphasia, and four spouses. Participation of the spouses was viewed as a critical element in rehabilitation, because problems discussed in the group inevitably involved adjustment difficulties that were shared by the patients with aphasia and their spouses.

Redinger and colleagues (1971) observed that the group evolved through several stages during the course of therapy. Initially, a period of anxiety occurred, and group members experienced difficulty communicating with one another. During the second stage, the members expressed regrets about their condition and complained about various factors associated with rehabilitation. Finally, during the third stage, the group evolved into a friendly, understanding, and supportive unit. As the group evolved through these stages, participants gradually became better adjusted to home and social environments, and they developed a more realistic view of family problems. In addition to these benefits, the counseling group also provided a social outlet for patients and spouses.

Many reports of spouse counseling groups highlight the importance of planning treatment to meet the specific needs of individual patients with aphasia and their families. The spouse counseling group of Gordon (1976), for example,

developed in response to the needs expressed by wives of patients with aphasia. The group provided an atmosphere in which spouses acquired a better understanding of aphasia, felt free to express feelings and share their reactions, and worked through problems that occurred as a result of the aphasia. The ultimate goal of the group was to improve the interpersonal relationships of the individuals with aphasia and their spouses.

A speech-language pathologist and a psychiatric social worker acted as co-leaders for the group. Meetings were held on a weekly basis, and attendance ranged from 4 to 10 spouses per session. The duration of individual spouse participation in the group varied from several months to 3 years. The co-leaders adopted a nondirective counseling approach, in which wives increasingly assumed more responsibility for the content and direction of the group while the leaders provided information and guidance as needed. Psychosocial aspects of adjustment addressed by the social worker included feelings of resignation, guilt, and loneliness; shifts in family roles; and the need to maintain interests outside the home. The speech-language pathologist discussed the nature of aphasia, the prognosis for recovery of language skills, and strategies for improving communication with their partners who have aphasia. Wives were encouraged not to demand verbal responses from their husbands, to accept nonverbal communication, and to modify their input to their partners with aphasia.

Gordon (1976) concluded that wives' emotional problems hindered communication with their husbands who had aphasia before participation in the group. The group, however, helped to alleviate many of the wives' emotional problems, and formal psychotherapy was seldom required. Still, Gordon cautioned that multiple repetitions were often needed before the wives comprehended group-counseling information. Some redundancy may, therefore, be necessary for spouses to receive maximum benefit from group treatment.

Bernstein (1979) also described a multidisciplinary spouse group that evolved out of concern for the emotional needs of family members. He stressed that interpersonal problems between patients with aphasia and their wives may interfere with speech-language treatment. More important, Bernstein believed that the family unit itself may be endangered if we ignore the emotional and psychological trauma suffered by spouses and other family members. He stressed that we cannot meet the complex emotional needs of spouses simply by providing a list of "do's and don't's" and then discussing them. Bernstein also indicated that the team leaders benefited from the group as well; he stated, "We are all better clinicians for the experience" (p. 35).

Recognizing the scarcity of studies in the aphasia counseling area, Newhoff and Davis (1978) reported their attempt to objectively plan and implement a spouse intervention program. Four spouses, two male and two female, participated in this study. Spouses were individually interviewed to determine target areas for intervention, and a questionnaire was administered both before and at the termination of the study to evaluate the effectiveness of the program.

The questionnaire examined seven areas: (1) communication strategies, (2) changes in life style and social pursuits, (3) spouses' feelings regarding their partner's disability, (4) spouses' perceptions of how well they understood their partner's problems, (5) actual level of spouse understanding, (6) spouse-partner independence, and (7) advice sought by spouses. The items in the questionnaire were all "Do you . . ." questions. For example, one item asked, "Do you talk with your spouse as you did before the accident?" (Newhoff & Davis, 1978, p. 320). The spouses circled appropriate answers on a seven-point rating scale that ranged from "very often" to "never."

The spouse intervention group met for a 50-minute session once a week for a period of 7 weeks. A speech-language pathologist served as group leader, but the spouses provided the direction for the group. The leader served as a catalyst for discussions and provided information as needed. The purpose of the group was to accomplish the following "counseling functions": (a) provide information to the spouses, (b) receive information from spouses that might be useful during their partner's rehabilitation, (c) facilitate the spouses' acceptance of their own feelings and help them to accept and understand their partners with aphasia, and (d) effect change in the spouses' behavior.

After 7 weeks of group counseling, the questionnaire was readministered to evaluate the effectiveness of the intervention. A comparison of responses to pre- and post-study questionnaires revealed considerable variability in the spouses' responses, and no discernible pattern of change was apparent. However, Newhoff and Davis (1978) concluded that they had accomplished their primary counseling objectives. They also concluded that, although the measurement problems involved in evaluating group counseling are difficult, they are not insurmountable.

Rice et al. (1987) also described their social support group for the spouses of 10 patients with aphasia. The purpose of this 12-week group was to provide information and social support, enhance psychosocial adjustment, and facilitate communication between persons with aphasia and their spouses. The authors reported significant improvement on scales of psychological adjustment for those individuals who consistently attended the group. No significant differences were found in the post-treatment functional communication ability of patients with aphasia whose spouses regularly attended versus those whose spouses did not regularly attend. Although this report is noteworthy for its attempt to evaluate the psychosocial effects of the spouse counseling group, the results must be interpreted cautiously given the small number of participants in the evaluation and the lack of appropriate experimental control.

Friedland and McColl (1989) attempted to operationalize the definition of social support for their spouse program.

Their model conceptualizes social support as having three dimensions: (1) source of support, (2) types of support, and (3) how satisfied the patient is with the support received. Common sources of support may include personal, friend/ family, community, and professional resources. Relatedly, the type of support received may include emotional and informational support. Their parsing of social support has potential as a taxonomy for future studies of counseling and support groups.

A number of comprehensive aphasia programs offer caregiver and family support groups as part of their regular programming (Beeson & Holland, 2007; Bernstein-Ellis & Elman, 2007; Hersh, 2007; Kagan, Cohen-Schneider, Sherman, & Podolsky, 2007; Penman & Pound, 2007). Kagan and colleagues (2007) provided a detailed description of a 12-week program support and education program that included a "family and friends" group. The family and friends group consisted of 15 to 25 individuals. The primary goals of the group included the following: (1) sharing experiences of living with aphasia, (2) increasing understanding of aphasia as well as ways to overcome communication breakdowns, and (3) finding new ways to live and find hope for the future.

Summary and Observations

Patient and family counseling groups have been widely advocated in the aphasia literature. The primary purpose of patient-family and spouse groups has been to provide educational information regarding aphasia and to provide emotional support for individuals with aphasia and their families. At times, speech-language pathologists and psychologists have acted as group co-leaders for aphasia counseling groups. Their primary function has been to lead topic-oriented discussions that center on issues of communication and emotional adjustment. The emphasis in counseling groups for individuals with aphasia and their relatives has been on "working through" the communication, emotional, and life-style changes that affect family dynamics.

The devastating effects of aphasia on interpersonal relationships and the family unit are well documented, and the need for counseling persons with aphasia and their families is unassailable. Little documentation, however, exists regarding the best format for accomplishing counseling objectives in the group setting. Although not specifically mentioned in most reports of group counseling, topic-oriented discussions should be accompanied by printed counseling information and/or appropriate audiovisual materials. Bevington (1985), for example, described an educational program that included the use of videotaped educational materials, lectures, and printed materials. The National Aphasia Association is a nonprofit organization that promotes public education, research, rehabilitation, and support for people with aphasia and their families. The National Aphasia Association Web site (www.aphasia.org)

provides access to a variety of counseling and educational materials, including *The Aphasia Handbook* (Sarno & Peters, 2004), that can be used to support individual or group counseling efforts. Web sites for other professional organizations, such as the Aphasia Hope Foundation (www.aphasiahope.org), the National Stroke Association (www.stroke.org), and the American Stroke Association (www.strokeassociation.org), also provide an invaluable resource for the clinical management and counseling of persons with aphasia.

Information provided in the counseling packets can be supplemented with counseling films. Printed information provided in patient-family counseling can be supplemented with videotaped material, such as *Pathways: Moving Beyond Stroke and Aphasia* (Ewing & Pfalzgraf, 1991a) and *What Is Aphasia?* (Ewing & Pfalzgraf, 1991b).

Films and printed materials can be shared with individuals who have aphasia and/or with spouses before their participation in counseling and support groups. This common information base allows new members to immediately interact with the other group members if they wish to do so. Clinical experience indicates that this approach alleviates some of the anxiety that may be present before entering the group. Discussions generated from the counseling materials may also help clinicians to determine if a client or spouse might benefit from individual counseling. For example, spouses can be referred to a clinical psychologist for evaluation if they do not appear to be psychologically ready to share their feelings and emotions in the group setting. Similarly, spouses who discuss sensitive issues such as divorce or suicide may also be referred for individual counseling.

The invaluable contributions of professionals specifically trained in psychological assessment and counseling emphasize the importance of an interdisciplinary approach to family counseling for aphasia. Group counseling sessions are often very emotionally laden, and speech-language pathologists require specific training to manage the psychological and emotional impact of disability (Ewing, 1999, 2007; Kearns & Simmons, 1985; Luterman, 1996). Group counseling for aphasia may be best conducted within a multidisciplinary approach that recognizes and treats emotional and psychological difficulties arising from disordered communication (Friedland & McColl, 1989; Pachalska, 1991a; Radonjic & Rakuscek, 1991).

Speech-Language Treatment Groups

Speech-language treatment of patients with aphasia has been conducted in group settings for nearly half a century, yet despite this history, group therapy for aphasia remains a controversial area. Many authors have viewed group therapy as being an "adjunct" to, or a substitute for, individual therapy (Chenven, 1953; Eisenson, 1973; Makenzie, 1991; Marquardt et al., 1976; Schuell, Jenkins, & Jimenez-Pabon, 1964; Smith, 1972), rather than a substitute for it. Schuell

et al. (1964), for example, noted that "we are unable to have confidence in group therapy as a basic method of treatment for aphasia" (p. 343), because benefits derived from group treatment are likely to be emotional or social in nature. Similarly, although he acknowledges potential speech-language benefits, Eisenson (1973) states, "The first and most important [objective] is providing psychological support for individuals within the group" (p. 188). The prevalent attitude has been that group treatment methods may not facilitate speech-language recovery in aphasia but are not, at least, detrimental to recovery.

In opposition to the stance that group therapy for aphasia is merely palliative, a number of authors have indicated that group intervention is an effective means of treating speech-language deficits (Aten et al., 1981, 1982; Avent, 1997a; Beeson & Holland, 2007; Bloom, 1962; Elman, 2007; Elman & Bernstein-Ellis, 1999a, 1999b; Fawcus, 1989; Garrett & Ellis, 1999; Graham, 1999; Hersh, 2007; Makenzie, 1991; Marshall, 1993, 1999a, 1999b; Penman & Pound, 2007; Penn & Jones, 2007; Van der Gaag et al., 2005; Walker-Batson, Curtis, Smith, & Ford, 1999; Wertz et al., 1981; Worrall, Davidson, Howe, & Rose, 2007). Although the data are not yet available to conclude that individual and group therapy for aphasia are equally effective, recent data and opinions that support this conclusion are stimulating investigative interest in the group treatment approach. In the sections that follow, we will examine the speech-language treatment group literature and explore emerging trends in this area.

Advocacy Reports

For our purposes, the term "advocacy reports" is used to designate articles that advocate the use of group speech-language therapy for aphasia without clearly delineating treatment procedures or presenting data to support their position. Johnston and Pennypacker (1980) originally described an advocacy research style as one in which the experimenter's prejudices interfere with his or her objectivity. That is, the experimenter "has taken the role of an advocate who defends a cause, not a scientist who searches for understanding" (p. 424).

Advocacy reports may reflect, in part, a paucity of efficacy research, a strong clinical bias toward unproven techniques, and a genuine interest in sharing clinical ideas. Clinicians are often more influenced by teachers, colleagues, and nondata-based presentations than they are by clinical research. This has often been the case with clinical aphasiology, in which few data existed regarding the efficacy of group therapy approaches. Unfortunately, discussions of group therapy for aphasia continue to be based primarily on clinical experience and bias. Some descriptions of group therapy approaches have attempted to document change in psychosocial skills (Borenstein et al., 1987) and in communication skills (Radonjic & Rakuscek, 1991) following intervention. Few studies, however, have incorporated appropriate experimental controls, such as the use of control groups and reliable measurement techniques. These limitations may negate the contributions of such efforts, making them comparable to earlier advocacy reports.

The current emphasis on intensive, multidisciplinary, functional aphasia treatment groups is reminiscent of approaches that have been advocated for decades (Borenstein et al., 1987; Pachalska, 1991a; Repo, 1991). Sheehan (1946) was among the earliest advocates of group speech-language therapy for aphasia. Her initial writings described "group speech classes," in which small groups of patients with aphasia worked on everyday vocabulary. Five or six patients usually participated in the group at a given time. The specific content of "lessons" included greetings and farewells, personal identification information, money, calendar use, right-left orientation, and body part identification. As Sheehan noted, "The list is endless—a product of a little imagination and ingenuity and of observation of the things needed by the patients in their daily living" (p. 152). Sheehan (1948) was also an early advocate of establishing individualized goals for each patient with aphasia in treatment groups.

Wepman (1947) described a model program for inpatient rehabilitation of individuals with aphasia. This program was carried out by a multidisciplinary team that included speech-language pathologists, psychologists, occupational and physical therapists, social workers, and special education teachers. Both individual and group speech therapy sessions were included in the program. The speech-language pathologist directed speech-related groups, and special educators taught writing, spelling, reading, and arithmetic in a group setting. Wepman outlined an intensive program that included 6 to 8 hours of treatment per day, 5 days per week. He concluded that an intensive, multidisciplinary approach is necessary if patients with aphasia are to make maximum gains in therapy. A similar approach for patients with "motor aphasia" was outlined by Corbin (1951).

The earliest writers in this area emphasized the importance of functional communication therapy in the group setting, but the rationale for this approach was not fully developed for several years. Bloom (1962) was the first to clearly articulate a pragmatic philosophy of group therapy for aphasia. Her rationale for group treatment combined an awareness of contextual influences on communication and meaning with an appreciation for the power of operant training techniques.

Although several treatment groups were conducted in her setting, Bloom emphasized the feasibility of group treatment for patients with severe impairments. Individuals with aphasia who participated in her rehabilitation program attended one session of individual treatment, one session of auditory stimulation, and an hourly group session each day. The primary goal of group treatment was to improve functional communication abilities. All treatment activities were directed toward improving performance of activities of daily living. Unlike many of the previously reported group treatments, however, this approach did not segment sessions into classroom-like activities according to separate language modalities.

Bloom emphasized a situational group approach, one in which language stimulation was provided in meaningful contexts. Situations that occurred in daily experience were recreated in the naturalistic group environment; role playing and rote memorization of scripts were avoided. Verbal tasks were used to practice greetings, directions, ordering from a menu, and handling money. In addition, auditory stimulation was provided during group sessions.

Summary and Observations

To summarize, advocacy style treatment reports promoted the use of group therapy techniques as a primary method of intervention for aphasia. These reports described ongoing group treatment programs and presented a sampling of tasks employed in the group setting. A consensus existed that group speech-language treatment was efficacious, although data to support this claim were lacking.

Despite their shortcomings, advocacy reports of group treatment for aphasia were farsighted in several respects. They were, for example, ahead of their time in recommending a multidisciplinary treatment approach (Nielson et al., 1948; Sheehan, 1946; Wepman, 1947). Sheehan (1946) held regular team conferences that included speech-language pathologists, occupational therapists, and physical therapists. An effort was made to coordinate these services so that an overall plan of rehabilitation could be developed. Wepman (1947) also strongly advocated the multidisciplinary approach; he indicated that "only by this overall cooperative approach can the maximum recovery level for the brain injured aphasic adult be achieved" (p. 409). Advocacy reports laid the historical foundation for current group therapy approaches that incorporate a multidisciplinary format (Pachalska, 1991a; Radonjic & Rakuscek, 1991; Walker-Batson et al., 1999).

In addition to establishing a multidisciplinary approach to aphasia management, early advocates of group therapy were nearly unanimous in their call for an intensive therapeutic regimen (Corbin, 1951; Huber, 1946; Sheehan, 1948; Wepman, 1947). Wepman (1947) and his contemporaries suggested daily treatment, and many advocated several sessions per day. Huber (1946), for example, indicated that most patients with aphasia could participate in 3 to 6 hours of therapy daily if appropriate rest periods were scheduled. Perhaps the most impressive aspect of the early group treatment literature is the consistent emphasis on functional, real-life treatment activities (Agranowitz et al., 1954; Bloom, 1962; Corbin, 1951; Huber, 1946; Sheehan, 1946, 1948). During the embryonic stages of group therapy for aphasia, clinicians developed treatment tasks that were based on the patients' communicative needs in the living environment.

Treatment approaches included a consideration of contextual factors despite the lack of a supporting theoretic basis for "pragmatic" aspects of communication.

The previous examples of advocacy reports are primarily from the post–World War II era. Recent reports considered below, however, are also advocacy reports in nature (Borenstein et al., 1987; Friedland & McColl, 1989; Radonjic & Rakuscek, 1991; Rice et al., 1987). These authors present data obtained from uncontrolled group treatment studies to support the effectiveness of their approaches. Whereas earlier advocacy reports presented detailed clinical information and subjective clinical impressions, more recent descriptions of group therapy have included relatively less detailed information regarding clinical techniques and quasi-experimental results.

Taken together, early and more recent advocacy reports appear to have had a subtle and, perhaps, negative impact on the cumulative growth of objective information in this area. That is, the legacy of advocacy reports has been the tacit acceptance of the efficacy of group therapy for aphasia despite meager evidence to support this claim. Initial reports of group therapy provided convincing, albeit unsubstantiated, testimonials as to the effectiveness of this method of patient management, and more recent efforts have included clinical data that provide an appearance of scientific legitimacy. Acceptance of subjective reports and uncontrolled treatment data as evidence for the efficacy of group treatment, however, may have had the deleterious effect of retarding legitimate investigative efforts in this area. More than 20 years ago, Gilbert et al. (1977) stated that "repeated weakly controlled trials are likely to agree and build up an illusion of strong evidence because of a large count of favorable studies. Not only does this mislead us into adopting and maintaining an unproven therapy, but it may make proper studies more difficult to mount" (p. 687). It seems that advocacy reports of group therapy have seduced clinicians and researchers alike into uncritically accepting this approach, and the cumulative effect of this literature has been an "illusion of strong evidence." Recent data-based clinical efforts represent a legitimate initial effort to examine the effectiveness of treatment, but these efforts must be followed up with more rigorous studies of efficacy that examine specific treatment approaches for clearly defined groups of patients with aphasia.

In the section that follows, we will examine contributions to the group treatment literature and explore the current status of research in this area. Five types of aphasia treatment groups—direct, indirect, sociolinguistic, transition, and maintenance—will be considered.

Direct Language Treatment Groups

Davis (1992) has distinguished "direct" from "indirect" treatment approaches. He states:

Direct approaches focus the clinician-patient interaction on the exercising of specific language processes. They are referred to as stimulus-response training, in which the clinician elicits specific language responses from the patient. They are structured . . . so that the patient is using discrete functions such as auditory language comprehension or word retrieval. (p. 241)

Brookshire (2003) was apparently referring to "direct" speech-language training groups when he noted that many aphasia treatment groups are didactic, relatively structured, and clinician directed. Tasks that are chosen for direct treatment groups of 10 individuals mimic those used in individual treatment.

Holland (1970) provided an early example of the application of "stimulus-response training" in a direct group treatment program. She applied "shaping and reinforcement procedures to direct language work with aphasics in a group setting" (p. 385). Unlike previously discussed group treatment reports, she established specific treatment goals in an attempt to improve verbal categorization, naming, plurality, subject-verb agreement, and syntactic ordering abilities. Language tasks were arranged in hierarchies of difficulty so that patients with various levels of aphasia could participate in the same group. Although Holland did not report objective data to support her exploratory approach, she did indicate that she was able to arrange treatment so that individual patient needs were met.

Additional examples of direct language treatment groups are also available from studies of specific training techniques. Skelly, Schinsky, Smith, and Fust (1974), for example, combined group treatment with individual treatment in their study of the effects of American-Indian sign on patients' verbal production. They stated that the sign group was an integral part of their gestural program. Skelly and colleagues did not evaluate the contributions of group training to the acquisition of American-Indian signs. Relatedly, Sparks, Helm, and Albert (1974) used "less structured" Melodic Intonation Therapy (MIT) in direct group treatment of aphasia. Although not specifically evaluated in their study, group MIT therapy was suggested to possibly increase patients' ability to intone basic, purposeful utterances.

More often than not, group therapy is viewed as an adjunct to individual therapy (Davis, 2000). Makenzie (1991) examined the effectiveness of a combined regimen of direct individual and group intervention. The five subjects in this study had previously been dismissed from nonintensive speech therapy after having plateaued. All participants were at least 9 months post-onset of aphasia. The primary focus of this investigation was to examine the value of an intensive period of therapy.

The stated aim of the aphasia group was "information giving." All participants were encouraged to use an available modality to communicate effectively during discussions of daily topics. In addition, each individual participated in daily individual therapy in which two verbal goals were targeted for improvement. In total, subjects received approximately 85 hours of individual and group therapy during a 1-month period, and a 1-month period of no treatment followed the period of intensive therapy. A screening battery for aphasia, a test of verbal naming ability, and a test of functional communication were among the measures used to evaluate treatment gains. The results of this clinical report indicate that all five patients improved on at least one clinical measure. Some decrease in performance was found following a period of no treatment.

Indirect Language Treatment Groups

Indirect treatment approaches are unstructured and may consist of general conversation, social groups, role playing, and field trips (Davis, 1992). Despite the fact that they are largely undefined, many of these approaches are purported to have therapeutic merit for improving deficient language skills. Previously presented examples of psychosocial group therapy for aphasia, which used unspecified or poorly described techniques, differ from indirect treatment approaches primarily in the orientation and general goals of the group leaders. That is, whereas the general purpose of psychosocial groups has been to facilitate emotional and psychological adjustment to aphasia, the orientation of indirect language training groups has been to stimulate language recovery.

Despite the vague nature of indirect treatment groups, reason exists to believe that loosely defined language stimulation and group discussion are commonly applied treatment methods. In a survey of group therapy for aphasia in a Veterans Administration Medical Center, Kearns and Simmons (1985) asked clinicians to estimate the percentage of time spent on various clinical activities during a typical aphasia group treatment session. The respondents indicated that "general, topic oriented discussions" were the most prevalent (31%) activity during group treatment. Considerably less group time was spent on "structured tasks" (e.g., word retrieval [22%]).

As in all areas of group therapy for aphasia, few data are available regarding the effectiveness of indirect language treatment groups. The poorly defined nature of these treatment approaches severely limits the ability of investigators to examine the usefulness of such approaches. A Veterans Administration cooperative study on aphasia (Wertz et al., 1981), however, compared the effectiveness of individual treatment and indirect group treatment. A treatment protocol was developed to help ensure uniform training within both groups. Strict selection criteria were also used in this study, and only patients having a single, left-hemisphere, cerebrovascular accident were included.

Participants with aphasia in both treatment conditions received 8 hours of therapy per week for up to 44 weeks. Subjects in the group treatment condition received 4 hours of therapy in a social setting and 4 hours of recreational activities. Group treatment activities did not include direct manipulation of speech or language abilities; that is, no specific treatment tasks were presented to improve performance in verbal, auditory, visual, or graphic language modalities. Typical group tasks included participation in discussions of current events or other interesting topics. Subjects in the individual treatment condition received 4 hours of direct "stimulus-response" treatment of speech and language deficits. Specific tasks were presented for the various language modalities, and contingent feedback and reinforcement were provided by the clinician. In addition to individual treatment, subjects also received 4 hours per week of machine-assisted treatment.

The results of this study revealed that subjects in the individual treatment condition improved significantly more than subjects in the indirect treatment group conditions in terms of overall performance on the Porch Index of Communicative Ability (Porch, 1967), or PICA. No significant differences were, however, apparent on other language tests. Further, subjects in both the individual and group treatment conditions made significant gains in their language test scores beyond the recognized period of spontaneous recovery. Wertz and colleagues (1981) concluded that relatively few differences exists in the amount or type of improvement exhibited by subjects in the two treatment conditions. They surmised that "individual and group treatment are efficacious means for managing aphasia" (p. 593).

Sociolinguistic Treatment Groups

Sociolinguistic treatment groups have evolved as a reaction to the highly structured treatment techniques employed in direct treatment approaches. Proponents of sociolinguistic treatment approaches have pointed out that direct treatment approaches may limit the types of communicative exchanges that occur between the clinician and the patient. Wilcox and Davis (1977), for example, found that clinicians primarily produced "questions" and "requests" during direct treatment sessions and that patients responded to the clinicians with assertions. A similar pattern of restricted responding was evident in a social group setting. Clinicians and patients produced a restricted number of "speech acts" in both settings. Wilcox and Davis concluded that individual and group treatment should be less didactic and permit the exchange of a wider variety of communicative interactions, including advising, arguing, and congratulating.

Davis (1992) also advocates a sociolinguistic approach to group therapy for aphasia. Rather than drilling patients on specific treatment tasks that are adapted from individual treatment, he recommended that group sessions emphasize interaction among the patients while minimizing clinician directiveness. For example, principles of PACE therapy (Davis & Wilcox, 1981) can be incorporated into group treatment so that patients "take turns, convey new information, practice using multiple channels, and provide each other with feedback to overcome obstacles" (p. 263).

As a participant in the panel discussion of group therapy for aphasia conducted by Aten and colleagues (1981), they elaborated on Davis's principles of treatment. They defined the purpose of group treatment as an attempt to "maximize (the patients') communicative strengths in order to improve interpersonal communication" (Aten et al., 1981, p. 146). Her group treatment activities centered around a preplanned task or game, and PACE treatment principles were incorporated into the sessions. Aten et al. (1982) investigated a sociolinguistic treatment approach that was described as "group functional communication therapy." Seven patients with chronic aphasia participated in this study. All subjects had suffered a single, left-hemisphere, cerebrovascular accident at least 9 months before the initiation of treatment. The subjects participated in hourly group sessions twice weekly for a period of 12 weeks, and a total of 24 treatment sessions were administered.

The goal of treatment was to improve functional communication, and a variety of everyday communicative situations from the Communicative Activities of Daily Living (Holland, 1980), or CADL, were selected for training. The "real-life" training situations included (a) shopping, (b) giving and following directions, (c) greetings, (d) giving personal information, (e) reading signs, and (f) gestural expression of ideas. Therapeutic activities included role playing and use of menus, grocery lists, and other materials from the patients' living environment. The results of training were evaluated by examining pre- and post-study performance on the PICA (Porch, 1967) and the CADL. Pre- and post-treatment PICA scores revealed nonsignificant differences, but statistically significant differences were apparent for pre- and post-treatment CADL scores. The authors concluded that group functional communication treatment is efficacious and that functional measures, such as the CADL, should be included in our clinical assessments.

A partial replication of the study by Aten and colleagues was provided by Bollinger, Musson, and Holland (1993). In this study, group treatment was provided using a treatment/withdrawal design, with "structured" treatment followed by a period of no treatment. Ten individuals with chronic aphasia who were at least 18 months post-onset received 3 hours per week of group treatment for a total of 40 weeks. Treatment consisted of 10-week segments of "contemporary group treatment" and "structured television viewing group treatment" alternating with 10 weeks of no treatment. "Contemporary group treatment" consisted of greetings and socialization, a core activity focusing on a real-life activity, and specific communication-related activities, such as group repetition of words and naming activities. "Structured television viewing group treatment" consisted of subjects watching specific television programs with later group discussion of specific communicative elements by group members. Bollinger and colleagues found significant improvement on both the CADL and the PICA but not on the third measure of language, which tested auditory comprehension. Results did not demonstrate the superiority of either treatment.

Avent (1997a) described the use of cooperative learning methods with eight brain-injured individuals (seven post–cerebrovascular accident and one Traumatic Brain Injury). A single-subject, multiple baseline across behaviors design was used to evaluate the effectiveness of cooperative group treatment on narrative and procedural discourse of participants. Each participant was paired with another for a total of four dyads. The role of the speech-language pathologist was to provide guidance and structure to the treatment. Each participant with aphasia alternated in the role of "recaller" and "facilitator" of 10 narrative and 10 procedural stories having 100 to 120 words each. Initially, the therapist read the target story aloud, with participants listing 8 to 10 key words and/or phrases from the story. Then, the recaller retold the story. Each dyad's facilitator used the key words/phrases to cue his or her partner as needed. The therapist also prompted the facilitator to cue the reteller with the key words. Following a practice period, the reteller once again told the story, followed by feedback from both the facilitator and the therapist. Five procedural stories and five narrative stories were used in treatment, with the remaining stories used as generalization probes.

The outcome measure in this study was an analysis of content units (Nicholas & Brookshire, 1993). Results indicated that following 18 sessions of cooperative group treatment, three of the eight participants improved their narrative and procedural discourse in the treatment stories and the generalization probes. The remaining five participants, however, showed either slight improvement or no change in performance. Avent (1997a) concludes that participants who showed improvement were those with the mildest aphasia as measured pre-treatment by the Western Aphasia Battery and the content unit analysis (i.e., 20% or higher content units per minute).

Graham (1999) described the use of aphasia groups in subacute and skilled nursing facilities. Graham used the American Speech-Language-Hearing Association Functional Assessment of Communication Skills for Adults (1995), or ASHA FACS, as a framework for planning and evaluating treatment in these groups. Following evaluation to determine communicative strengths and weaknesses as well as the ability to use compensatory strategies, patients were enrolled into group treatment. (Group members could also be enrolled in individual treatment sessions.) Both individual and group treatment goals were selected from the ASHA FACS in combination with Hartley's (1995) functional communication goals. Treatment groups consisted of two to six members meeting 5 days per week for 45-minute sessions. Treatment tasks focused on functional and "survival" skills, and Graham described how she used videotape segments for viewing and discussion by group members.

Garrett and Ellis (1999) described a group language intervention program developed in 1994 at the University of Nebraska–Lincoln's Speech Language and Hearing Clinic. This program continued at Duquesne University (Garrett, Staltari, & Moir, 2007). The primary goal of this aphasia group program is to provide a vehicle for individuals with long-term aphasia to continue to improve their communication skills. In addition, the program provides learning opportunities for graduate students in speech-language pathology. The authors describe the Nebraska treatment program as combining principles of discourse, thematicity, contextual support, and functional use. A continuum of language activities, communication goals, and scaffolding strategies are incorporated into conversation, context building, language mediation, and discourse activities. The authors provide specific communication goals and explicit prompting information. Group sessions are 90 minutes in length, with 6 to 10 people participating in each group. Garrett and colleagues report that group members frequently indicated the groups helped them to become more competent communicators.

Additional data are needed to establish the validity of sociolinguistic group treatment for aphasia. For example, evaluation of the efficacy of discourse exercises (Osiejek, 1991) and other communication-based therapies in the group setting are warranted.

Transition Groups

In addition to the direct, indirect, and sociolinguistic treatment approaches described above, several authors have described transition or maintenance group treatment for aphasia. Brookshire (1997) indicates that transition groups "prepare patients for communication in daily life by giving them training and practice with strategies and problem-solving skills that are useful in daily life" (p. 286). Tasks employed in these groups, such as role playing, are usually selected to help individuals with aphasia adapt to communicative situations that occur in their living environment. Information may also be provided in transition groups regarding community services, such as adult day-care centers and home health services. Transition groups often meet one or more times weekly, and patients usually participate in these groups for a limited and specified period of time before discharge from treatment.

As a member of the group therapy panel conducted by Aten et al. (1981) she described her unique approach to transition groups. Three groups—a discharge-planning group, a community involvement group, and a "stroke club" group—were used to facilitate the transition between inpatient hospital services and release to the home environment. Patients in West's program participated in each of the groups in sequential order in an attempt to develop an increasing level of functional independence from the hospital staff.

The overall goals of the transition groups were (a) to help patients accept changes in physical and cognitive abilities, (b) to develop a realistic view of progress and altered ability, (c) to assist patients in finding an alternate life style within available family and community resources, (d) to reinforce gains made in individual therapy, and (e) to help patients with community placement.

In addition to these general goals, each group had a specific purpose. For example, the main purpose of the discharge-planning group was to prepare patients for life-style changes that would occur on dismissal from the hospital. Practical difficulties encountered during home visitations were also discussed in this group.

Once patients were discharged from the hospital, they participated in the community involvement group in an attempt to facilitate emotional and psychological adjustment to their new environment. The emphasis in this group was on helping patients to accept their new life styles and assist them in developing productive alternate life styles. The group also discussed emotional incidents that occurred in the home setting, and it provided an opportunity for emotional venting by the group members. The community involvement group attempted to "confront reality without destroying hope" (Aten et al., 1981, p. 150).

The final stage in West's transition group program was participation in a monthly "stroke club." This group provided emotional support and education, and it helped patients to maintain the level of communicative ability that had been reached following individual speech-language treatment. In general, West concluded that her three-group transition process was successful, because it reduced dependence on the hospital staff and integrated patients into existing family and community structures.

Maintenance Groups

In the final analysis, West's "stroke club" group appears to be similar in function to a maintenance group. Brookshire (1997) notes that maintenance groups provide regular stimulation so that patients' speech-language skills do not deteriorate once they are dismissed from intensive individual therapy. He indicates that maintenance group activities are frequently social in nature and may emphasize social interaction and communication in social contexts. Participation in maintenance groups may last from months to years, depending on the individual needs of the patient and his or her family. Brookshire observed that maintenance group meetings are seldom held more than once per week; in fact, they may be held only once per month. Maintenance groups continue to be a medium for encouraging retention of therapeutic gains made during aphasia rehabilitation (Springer, 1991).

Hunt (1976) described a language maintenance group that provided support, information, and language stimulation for patients who had been dismissed from individual treatment. From 8 to 12 patients participated in the groups, which met once per week for 2 hours. Family members were excluded from group participation.

The emphasis of this maintenance program was on stimulation of language in a social setting. Group activities were planned around the patients' interests and included movies, slide presentations, and guest speakers. These activities provided an opportunity for using residual language skills. Although specific language goals were not established, all attempts to communicate in the group setting were reinforced.

Hunt concluded that the social language group provided valuable language stimulation, practice of previously acquired abilities, social interaction, and entertainment. The maintenance group also acted as a source of information, support, and referral for the families of patients with aphasia, and it provided a valuable training experience for student clinicians.

Coles and Eales (1999) describe Action for Dysphasic Adults, an organization that provides self-help groups for individuals with aphasia in the United Kingdom. Speech-language therapists work for Action for Dysphasic Adults as regional development advisers. Each adviser supports a number of self-help groups and provides direction as each group is formed. The speech-language therapist also serves as the link to the national body. Ultimately, each group is run by its members, with the speech-language therapist providing assistance only when requested. Because different locales have varied interests and/or needs, each group identifies its relevant goals and sets its own rules, including the number of members permitted in the group.

Multipurpose Groups

Taxonomies of group treatment procedures for aphasia are inherently flawed, because clinicians often identify several purposes for their groups. The results of a survey by Kearns and Simmons (1985) of clinical practices indicate that 80% of the respondents listed multiple goals for their groups. As might be expected, language stimulation, often in combination with support or social goals, was the most frequent aim (84%) of aphasia groups. Following language stimulation, the next most frequently listed goals were emotional support (59%), carryover (47%), and socialization (45%). As previously indicated, attempts to classify types of aphasia group treatment approaches are generally for the sake of convenience alone, and they should not be construed as being a reflection of clinical reality. More often than not, group therapy is undertaken with several aims in mind—even when a primary focus is evident. Most recent reports of group therapy for aphasia reveal that programs are typically multipurpose in nature, often combining psychosocial and speech-language goals into treatment.

Kagan and colleagues (1990, 1999, 2001, 2004, 2007) described a unique, community-based group treatment approach, provided at the Aphasia Institute in Toronto, Canada, that is designed to facilitate functional communication, promote independence, and maintain gains resulting from individual therapy. An important aspect of the program is the use of community volunteers who are trained and supervised by speech-language pathologists to work, in a group setting, on communication goals with individuals who have with aphasia. A comparison of the results of pre- and post-testing for participants with chronic aphasia who participated in the community group versus a group of untreated, community-dwelling control subjects was reported (Kagan, 1990). Results revealed significant improvement in the post-treatment performance of the group participants on a test of communicative effectiveness (Lomas et al., 1989) (see Chapter 6), but not on traditional language testing. A significant between-group difference favoring the treated patients was also found on this measure.

A primary component of this aphasia community program is training agency volunteers and health-care professionals to use supported conversation techniques (Kagan, 1998). Kagan and colleagues (2001) investigated whether these techniques improve the conversational skills of volunteers and, if so, whether the improvements affect the communication of their conversation partners with aphasia. Twenty volunteers received training in supported conversation techniques, and 20 control volunteers were merely exposed to people with aphasia. Trained volunteers scored significantly higher than untrained volunteers on ratings of acknowledging competence and revealing competence of their partners with aphasia. The training also produced a positive change in ratings of social and message-exchange skills of individuals with aphasia, even though these individuals did not participate in the training. These results support the efficacy of supported conversation techniques.

Radonjic and Rakuscek (1991) described a multipurpose group that was established to decrease emotional tension; prevent social isolation; encourage the need for communication; encourage the ability to search for, develop, and use communication in social situations; and develop confidence and self-respect. The group was developed by a clinical psychologist and a speech-language pathologist, and it generally ranged in size from four to seven participants, with a maximum of 10 group members. Group activities included such varied activities as "learning about each other, relaxation techniques, games to strengthen psycholinguistic ability, drawing, pantomime, and therapeutic techniques involving music" (p. 451). A five-point scale of communication was administered at the beginning and end of each patient's participation in an attempt to examine the impact of intervention. A descriptive analysis of difference scores for 108 patients with aphasia revealed improvements on patients' post-treatment communication ratings as compared with pretreatment ratings. The authors concluded from their analysis that the best results were obtained for patients who participated in at least 10 treatment sessions in small groups (three to five members). Although intriguing, these clinical data must be replicated under more rigorous experimental conditions before they can be considered unassailable.

Pachalska (1991a) reviewed the group therapy literature and presented her treatment approach. Based on her literature review and clinical experience, she suggests making groups as homogeneous as possible in terms of patient type and level of language involvement. Pachalska also recommends that the size of aphasia groups should not exceed four or five members and that treatment sessions should last no more than an hour. A structured treatment approach is also advocated. Pachalska refers to a "holistic" method of treatment, which apparently refers to a multidisciplinary, multipurpose approach, such as her own Complex Aphasia Rehabilitation Model, or CARM. Citing publications in her native language (Polish), she asserts that the holistic approach is "the most effective approach" (p. 547) to group treatment. CARM is described as having both individual and group treatment components, and group therapy is seen primarily as an adjunct to individual treatment. Group sessions are run by a multidisciplinary team of clinicians who provide cognitive physiotherapy, physical therapy, speech therapy, psychotherapy, and sociotherapy. Tasks are directed toward facilitating natural conversation. Pachalska (1991b) also indicates that a goal of CARM is to stimulate transfer of information between the cerebral hemispheres. Consequently, both linguistic and nonlinguistic stimuli are employed in treatment, and special emphasis is placed on "language-oriented art therapy." Linguistic materials used in therapy include popular poems and word games. In addition to the language emphasis, other aspects of rehabilitation, such as physical therapy and group discussions with family members, are also included. Social activities, such as "car rallies," are considered to be part of the rehabilitation process as well. Pachalska (1991a) makes the broad claim that "all abilities which underwent training in the program significantly improved, and that the disturbances in the communicative, psychological and social domains were eliminated to a considerable degree; the reintegration was more complete" (p. 551).

The clinical forum that highlighted the work of Pachalska (1991a, 1991b) included commentaries by distinguished aphasiologists (Aten, 1991; Fawcus, 1991; Loverso, 1991; Repo, 1991; Springer, 1991). Fawcus (1991) emphasized that "the whole essence of group work is its flexibility and spontaneity" (p. 555) and cautioned against using overly structured approaches. Others agree that the mechanics of group therapy, such as group size and session length, cannot be dictated by prescription (Loverso, 1991; Springer, 1991). Our clinical experience is consistent with their suggestion that group sessions of longer than 1 hour are possible and that larger groups are manageable and, sometimes, desirable.

Larger, more heterogeneous groups may be particularly appropriate when the emphasis is not on direct communication or language training (Springer, 1991).

Another example of a multipurpose group is provided by Marshall's (1993, 1999b, 2007) description of problem-focused group therapy for patients with mild aphasia. The goals of this program are to provide a forum for discussing social, vocational, and recreational reintegration into society and assisting members in solving everyday communication problems. Examples of the problem-solving activities used during treatment include communicating in an emergency, meeting new people, and preparing for a physician's visit. Unique aspects of this program include the fact that it provides one of the few available descriptions of clinical management for patients with mild aphasia as well as a rationale for intervention that focuses on everyday problems and community reintegration. Clinical data are presented that show the range of post-treatment improvements on standardized language test scores of the 18 patients for whom pre- and post-treatment comparisons were available. Marshall recognizes the potential of functional communication assessments for evaluating progress in group therapy (Lomas et al., 1989), and he suggests that seldom-used formats, such as the client self-report, may also provide a measure of clinical accountability. This issue is further considered in the sections that follow.

Walker-Batson and colleagues (1999) describe the Texas Women's University transdisciplinary Aphasia Center Lifelink© program, which uses theme-based activities to prepare clients for community reentry. Lifelink© is a half-day, university-based program with graduate students in speech-language pathology, physical therapy, and occupational therapy in addition to rehabilitation professionals providing services. Clients are assessed on a battery of measures to evaluate speech and language skills, participation in leisure activities, affect/mood, and quality of life. Speech-language treatment is determined by placement of each client on the "recovery-compensation continuum" (Elman, 1994). Intensity of intervention is based on the client's severity level as measured by the Boston Diagnostic Aphasia Examination (Goodglass & Kaplan, 1983). The most severe clients receive individual as well as group treatment; those with less severe aphasia are discharged from individual treatment, with continuation in group therapy and community activities. The authors describe a "Visual Retrieval Language System" that provides theme-related vocabulary and structure for each client and is used in both individual and group treatment. Group size ranges from three to five members, and groups are 75 minutes in length. Group sessions often focus on themes developed by the clinician; however, higher-level groups can select their own topics.

Beeson and Holland (2007) describe the University of Arizona group treatment program. Treatment here is focused on facilitating successful communication using any modality in addition to client-specific communication strategies. Groups are 1 hour in length, include between five and seven members, and are facilitated by faculty and graduate students. Beeson and Holland suggest that the Arizona treatment groups serve many purposes including direct and indirect language treatment, modeling of communication strategies, psychosocial support, and continuing education for group members, their families, and the student-clinicians. (Separate groups are conducted for family members.) Holland and Beeson report the Western Aphasia Battery (WAB) scores, before and after group participation, for 40 individuals with chronic aphasia. All had participated in the aphasia group for at least 1 calendar year. More than one-third of the group members showed a positive change of at least five points on the WAB. A regression analysis suggests that individuals who are younger and closer to onset improve more than those who are older and further from stroke onset (Holland & Beeson, 1999; Beeson & Holland, 2007).

Elman & Bernstein-Ellis (1999a) investigated the efficacy of group communication treatment on linguistic and communicative performance for 24 participants with chronic aphasia. Their research design used random assignment to immediate-treatment and deferred-treatment groups, which were balanced for age, education level, and initial aphasia severity. In the treatment condition, all participants received 5 hours of group treatment per week, provided by a speech-language pathologist, for a total of 4 months. The focus of treatment was on increasing initiation of conversation and exchanging information using whatever means possible. Communicative topics were relatively unconstrained, with a wide variety of topics addressed, including psychosocial and poststroke issues. Specific clinical procedures and content are described in detail by Bernstein-Ellis and Elman (1999, 2007). While awaiting group communication treatment, participants in the deferred-treatment group engaged in activities such as support, performance, or movement groups to control for the effects of social contact.

Dependent measures included the Shortened PICA (Disimoni, Keith, & Darley, 1980), or SPICA; the WAB Aphasia Quotient (Kerstesz, 1982), or WAB AQ; and the Communicative Abilities in Daily Living (Holland, 1980), or CADL. All participants received these tests at entry, after 2 and 4 months of treatment, and after 4 to 6 weeks of no treatment. In addition, participants in the deferred-treatment group received an additional administration of the measures just before beginning treatment.

Results revealed that group communication treatment was efficacious. Participants receiving treatment had higher scores on the SPICA and WAB AQ compared with those participants not receiving treatment. In addition, those participants with moderate-to-severe aphasia who received treatment had higher scores on the CADL compared with those who did not receive treatment. Significant improvement was observed after both 2 months and 4 months of treatment. No significant decline was observed at the time of follow-up. This study was the first to demonstrate that group communication treatment and not social contact alone was responsible for treatment gains.

Elman and Bernstein-Ellis (1999b) also reported on results from participant and caregiver interviews collected during and after group communication treatment. Semistructured interviews were conducted, with questions focusing on the positive and negative aspects of participation in the communication treatment groups. Interview transcripts were transcribed verbatim, and a qualitative analysis (Miles & Huberman, 1994; Strauss & Corbin, 1990) was applied. In this analysis, both positive and negative aspects of group treatment were noted and then coded and grouped into common themes. Finally, all transcripts were reread multiple times to produce a limited number of themes that captured the information expressed in the interviews.

Interview data for 12 participants and their relatives/caregivers were reported by Elman and Bernstein-Ellis (1999b). The positive psychosocial aspects of group communication treatment reported by participants with aphasia included (a) like being with others, (b) like the support of others with aphasia, (c) like making friends, (d) like being able to help others, (e) like seeing others improve, and (f) feel more confident. The positive speech-language aspects included (a) enjoy conversations, (b) improvement in talking, and (c) improvement in reading/writing. The relatives/caregivers reported very similar positive psychosocial and speech-language aspects of their family member's or client's participation in group communication treatment. Psychosocial aspects included (a) more confident, (b) more social, (c) more independent, (d) more motivated, (e) like making friends, (f) happier, and (g) like helping others. Positive speech-language aspects included (a) improvement in talking and (b) improvement in reading/writing. Negative aspects were rarely reported. It is important to note that many of these psychosocial behaviors were not directly treated during group communication treatment. Elman and Bernstein-Ellis posited that many of these changes were a result of increased confidence and motivation that participants gained from attending the groups. They suggested that the group environment can be an extremely powerful one for producing change.

Van der Gaag and colleagues (2005) evaluated the impact of attending a community-based aphasia program on quality of life and communication skills for 28 people with chronic aphasia as well as 14 significant others. Individuals with aphasia attended group treatment either once or twice per week for an average of 1.7 hours a week. Caregivers received an average of 1.4 hours of therapy per week. Group activities included conversation groups, communication skill groups, and self-advocacy groups. Both qualitative and quantitative methods were used to assess the participants before and after 6 months of therapy. Participants were evaluated by semistructured interviews and two quantitative measures assessing quality of life, the CETI and a caregiver assessment. Results indicated statistically significant improvement in the CETI and one of the two quality-of-life measures but no statistically significant differences on the caregiver assessment. The qualitative interviews revealed similar results, with a majority of the participants reporting improved communication skills. It is not possible to determine which aspects of the therapeutic program contributed to these changes.

Inspired by the Aphasia Institute in Toronto, several independent, community-based aphasia centers were created in the 1990s. These included the Aphasia Center of California (Bernstein-Ellis & Elman, 1999, 2007; Elman, 1998), the Talkback groups in South Australia (Hersh, 2007), and Connect in London (Penman & Pound, 2007; Pound, Parr, Lindsay, & Woolf, 2000). In addition, various university-sponsored aphasia programs were developed (Penn & Jones, 2007; Walker-Batson et al., 1999; Worrall et al., 2007). These programs advocate a social approach to programming for individuals and family members affected by aphasia (Elman, 2005) (see chapter 11) and provide a variety of groups that emphasize successful communication strategies, rebuilding identity, and community reengagement. Several of these programs also provide specialized groups, including Internet training (Bernstein-Ellis & Elman, 2007; Egan, Worrall, & Oxenham, 2004; Worrall et al., 2007) and aphasia book clubs (Bernstein-Ellis & Elman, 2006).

Efficacy of Speech-Language and Multipurpose Treatment Groups

Examination of group treatment as a primary and independent form of patient management has only recently been undertaken (Aten et al., 1982; Avent, 1997a; Elman & Bernstein-Ellis, 1999a, 1999b; Radonjic and Rakuscek, 1991; Van de Gaag et al., 2005; Wertz et al., 1981). In addition, several studies have explored the value of combined individual and group treatment for aphasia (Chenven, 1953; Makenzie, 1991; Smith, 1972). Research evaluating the effectiveness of specific group speech-language treatment is growing, but the scientific basis of clinical aphasiology will not be sturdy unless this investigative effort continues.

Summary and Observations

Recent reports of group speech-language treatment for aphasia were reviewed and five group therapy approaches identified. These included (a) direct language treatment groups, (b) indirect language treatment groups, (c) sociolinguistic treatment groups, (d) transition groups, and (e) maintenance groups. Although each approach is unique, the common denominator is that their primary purpose is to facilitate recovery and/or maintenance of speech-language abilities. Considerable variability, however, exists among group treatment approaches. Speech-language treatment groups range from structured, so-called "stimulus-response" approaches to essentially undefined, indirect treatment approaches. Group treatment tasks also show considerable variability and include specific techniques, such as MIT (Sparks et al., 1974) as well as group discussions and recreational activities (Wertz et al., 1981). As previously noted, the variety of group treatment approaches probably reflects the training and biases of the clinicians who conduct group therapy (Elman, 1999, 2007; Marquardt et al., 1976).

Obvious parallels exist between speech-language treatment group therapy and individual therapy for aphasia. Direct language treatment groups, for example, often employ tasks similar to those used in individual treatment sessions. Similarly, clinicians conducting sociolinguistic group therapy often adopt recently developed functional treatment approaches, such as PACE therapy (Davis & Wilcox, 1981), to the group format. Given these parallels between individual and group treatment, Holland's (1975) inquiry about the differences between these two approaches is poignant. If a group leader sequentially treats each individual in a group and little interaction occurs other than individual exchanges between the clinician and a given patient, the result may be inefficient individual treatment in a group setting. To avoid this possibility, group leaders must be aware of the strengths and communicative needs of individual group members. Ideally, tasks should be structured so that all group members can participate (Holland, 1970), but interactive aspects of communication should not be sacrificed (Davis, 1992; Elman, 2000; Ewing, 1999). Moreover, the objectivity of direct approaches should be combined with the common-sense rationales for sociolinguistic group therapy. The development of data-based, pragmatic treatment approaches will be challenging, but clinical aphasiologists have recently demonstrated the feasibility of this approach to program development (Cochrane & Milton, 1984; Davis & Wilcox, 1981; Elman & Bernstein-Ellis, 1999a, 1999b; Kearns, 1986; Osiejek, 1991; Van der Gaag et al., 2005).

Clinicians should eschew indirect treatment approaches that have no explicit communication goals and serve as a social outlet for their patients with aphasia. Socialization can be a legitimate goal of group therapy for aphasia, but clinicians should be leery about letting group treatment deteriorate into totally unstructured activities that neither facilitate nor support identified communication aims. Like individual therapy for aphasia, group intervention should be based on sound clinical logic, and it should be goal directed without being overly rigid (Fawcus, 1991).

CLINICAL ACCOUNTABILITY

Measurement problems encountered in group therapy are significant but not insurmountable, and proper attention must be given to assessing speech-language treatment gains in the group setting. To date, few authors of group therapy reports have attempted to measure treatment gains, and those who have examined the success of treatment have, for the most part, relied on standardized tests of aphasia (Aten et al., 1982; Wertz et al., 1981). Although tools designed to measure functional communication ability (Holland, 1980; Lomas et al., 1989) may be of particular value, standardized aphasia tests do not measure interactive aspects of communication, and the development and use of reliable supplemental measurement tools, in addition to qualitative methods of investigation, are sorely needed (Elman & Bernstein-Ellis, 1999b; Garrett, 1999; Garrett & Pimentel, 2007).

The importance of measurement issues in group therapy for aphasia cannot be overestimated. Kearns and Simmons (1985) reported that 73% of survey respondents used periodic standardized testing to evaluate group members and that 33% employed standardized testing in combination with "behavioral ratings of task performance." Surprisingly, 20% of the clinicians indicated that patient performance was *not* routinely evaluated. A recurring problem for clinicians who run aphasia groups is the issue of clinical accountability; finding appropriate measures for assessing the effects of group therapy is problematic. As Aten (1991) pointed out in his commentary on Pachalska's work, treatment effectiveness will not be easily demonstrated until better assessments of psychosocial changes and conversational language are available. Similarly, Loverso (1991) addressed the need to develop and adopt tools that examine the roles of individuals within aphasia groups and the interaction of these roles during treatment. This novel suggestion is exemplified by the earlier work by Loverso et al. (1982), in which they demonstrated the reliability of a process evaluation form. Loverso, Young-Charles, and Tonkovich (1982) assessed the "roles" of individual group members and classified their interactions. They demonstrated that task (e.g., giving and receiving information), maintenance (e.g., encouraging following), and non-functional (e.g., disruptive) behaviors could be reliably rated in the small-group setting. Other novel, supplemental measures that may be employed in aphasia groups include the use of discourse analyses and interactive coding procedures (Cochrane & Milton, 1984; Garrett & Pimentel, 2007).

Given the nature of the abilities targeted for intervention in group settings, clinicians often must devise their own clinical probes or "mini-tests" to sample skills such as turn-taking ability, initiation of interactions, and other skills, because standard assessments are not routinely available. Garrett and Pimentel (2007) describe numerous outcome measures that clinicians can use to assess basic communication skills, functional communication, quality of life, customer satisfaction, and overall cost/benefit ratios. They state that most of these measures can be adapted for use in medical, outpatient, and/or community settings. Whatever the procedure or outcome measure that is chosen, it is important to evaluate

routinely the communicative abilities of aphasia group members.

GUIDING PRINCIPLES

Thus far, we have considered psychosocial, family counseling and support, and speech-language treatment groups for aphasia. Among the speech-language treatment reports, we distinguished early advocacy groups from more recent speech-language and multipurpose treatment groups. Our review of recent speech-language treatment group reports revealed a number of distinct approaches, including direct language treatment groups, indirect language treatment groups, sociolinguistic groups, transition groups, and maintenance groups. It should be apparent from this brief summary that no single therapeutic model can accommodate the variety of aphasia groups that have been reported in the literature. Recent trends in the generalization literature, however, may serve as a cornerstone for the development of eclectic, principled group treatment approaches.

The ultimate goal of therapy for aphasia is to develop maximum communication ability in non-training settings and situations. In essence, generalization of target behaviors across stimuli, settings, people, behavior, and time (i.e., maintenance) is the desired end product of therapy. Treatment effects are notoriously restrictive, and generalization is the exception rather than the rule in aphasia rehabilitation and other applied fields. A growing generalization literature, however, that provides suggestions regarding specific techniques that may facilitate carryover (Baer, 1981; Horner et al., 1988; Hughes, 1985; Kearns, 1989; McReynolds & Spradlin, 1989; Spradlin & Siegel, 1982; Warren & Rogers-Warren, 1985). A philosophy of group management that is geared toward facilitating generalization may provide an opportunity to empirically test our assumptions about generalization and allow us to examine the efficacy of group therapy for aphasia.

Reviews of the aphasia generalization literature also indicated that generalization of aphasia treatment effects is not an automatic by-product of intervention (Thompson, 1989). More often than not, clinical investigations of aphasia are what Stokes and Baer (1977) labeled "Train and Hope Studies." That is, investigators attempt to measure generalization of communicative improvements, but they seldom do anything to actively try and achieve generalized responding. Further, when generalization does not occur following intervention, no additional follow-up steps are taken to obtain carryover. If the ultimate goal of therapy for aphasia is to achieve maximum communicative functioning in settings and situations where patients live, work, and interact, we have an obligation to do everything in our power to achieve functional carryover. As Horner and colleagues (1986) note, "[T]here is an ethical obligation, if not a responsibility, to make sure that generalization programming is incorporated into every program that endeavors to make important social and life-style changes for clients" (p. 16).

Generalization Planning

Clinical practice in speech-language pathology often includes four discrete and relatively independent sequential phases: (a) assessment, (b) intervention, (c) generalization, and (d) maintenance. As is true of other clinical specialties in speech pathology, clinical aphasiologists have attended to the assessment and intervention phases of the clinical process while placing relatively little emphasis on the generalization and maintenance phases. In contrast to the traditional approach to treatment planning, a generalization planning approach to the clinical process is conceptualized as a means of integrating the known clinical phases into a continuous loop that incorporates specific procedures to maximize the possibility of promoting generalization (Baer, 1981; Horner et al., 1988; Hughes, 1985; Warren & Rogers-Warren, 1985).

Kearns (1989) notes the following differences between a generalization planning approach to intervention and the traditional, discrete-phase approach. First, separation of the clinical process into discrete phases encourages the establishment of clinical goals based on performance on clinical tasks within the treatment setting. Thus, within the traditional model, an aphasia test is given during the assessment phase, and the results of this testing are used to establish clinical goals. When these goals are met, clinicians may then begin to examine aspects of generalization and maintenance. By contrast, a generalization planning approach to clinical management assumes that carryover of improvements in functional communicative abilities is the primary goal of intervention, and as a result, assessment, goal setting, and intervention are all influenced by this assumption. The desire to facilitate generalization is foremost from the initial contact with the person with aphasia and his or her family. Within a generalization planning framework, carryover of functional abilities is the clinical glue that bonds all aspects of patient management into an integrated whole. Thus, all steps in the process are woven together for the express purpose of effecting change in a patient's ability to communicate in nonclinical settings as well as with people and in situations they experience in daily life. Whereas generalization and maintenance are too often a clinical afterthought with the discrete-phase model of clinical practice, their attainment is the driving force behind generalization planning.

The distinction between traditional treatment planning and generalization planning is far more than philosophical. After all, most clinical aphasiologists would contend that carryover is a primary goal of group therapy. From a practical viewpoint, however, a generalization training approach is procedurally more complex and, sometimes, more time-consuming than its traditional counterpart. For example,

whereas the discrete-phase approach to assessment of individuals with aphasia may include standard and nonstandard tests of language and functional communication, the generalization planning approach expands the evaluation process to include gathering information that is directly relevant to maximizing the chances of obtaining carryover of treatment effects. Expansion of the traditional assessment may include, for example, naturalistic observations, interviewing significant others to determine communicative needs, and recording and analyzing spontaneous interactions with familiar and unfamiliar partners. Baer (1981) suggests using every available means to make lists of all (communication) behaviors, settings, individuals, people, and actions of significant others that might affect generalization. These lists can then be narrowed down to a reasonable few, which are then prioritized for the purposes of deciding what combination of client behaviors and environmental factors need to be altered to maximize the probability of obtaining generalization.

The primary outcome of an expanded, more ecologically valid assessment is to choose generalization goals. That is, based on the information gathered, the clinician attempts to determine the most critical factors that should be targeted for intervention if improved communicative ability is likely to carry over to real-life settings and conditions. Importantly, the clinician also sets a criterion for evaluating whether a sufficient level of generalization occurs. The clinician is also charged with the task of determining how best to measure progress toward generalization goals. Because specific tests are rarely available to determine if generalization of specific target behaviors improves, clinicians must often develop their own means of assessing performance or adapt nontraditional measures (Garrett & Pimentel, 2007). These clinical probes (i.e., mini-tests) can be given periodically over time to evaluate progress toward generalization goals. This information can subsequently be graphed and used as a visual aid to monitor the effectiveness of treatment (Connell & McReynolds, 1988; Kearns, 1986a). In addition, ongoing assessment and visuographic data presentation also serve as a guide in making treatment decisions. For example, clinical probe data can be examined to determine if generalization occurs to targeted people, settings, and conditions, and appropriate modifications can then be made to intervention strategies as needed. Because generalization of aphasia treatment effects clearly does not automatically occur as a result of intervention, it is imperative that progress toward generalization goals be monitored so that appropriate clinical modifications can be initiated.

Kearns (1986a), Kearns and Scher (1988), Kearns and Yedor (1991), for example, reported a treatment approach, Response Elaboration Training (RET), which has been adopted clinically in group settings. The thrust of this approach is to use a forward-chaining technique to lengthen patient-initiated utterances and encourage response variety. Novel appropriate utterances are encouraged and reinforced.

That is, any patient-initiated response that was relevant for a given stimulus item is acceptable regardless of the form or content of that response. A unique aspect of this approach is that the patient directs the content of treatment. Once treatment stimuli are selected, the patient's spontaneous utterances are used as building blocks for developing more elaborate responses. The clinician combines successive patient responses, models them for repetition by the patient, and then prompts him or her to provide additional information. Each novel elaboration is subsequently added to the chain until the patient's spontaneous responses are lengthened to preselected levels. Throughout RET, an interactive, turn-taking format is maintained so that it can be readily adopted to group treatment. That is, each spontaneous conversational turn during group activities can serve as an opportunity for the clinician to prompt more elaborate verbal (and nonverbal) responses and reinforce the use of novel but appropriate utterances.

Although the RET format has not been tested experimentally in the group setting, a series of studies has examined the efficacy and generalization of this approach for individuals with aphasia. Results to date indicate that generalized increases in verbal response length and variety have occurred following RET (Kearns, 1986; Kearns & Scher, 1989; Kearns & Yedor, 1991). In addition, this approach has also successfully facilitated improvements in nonverbal means of communication (Gaddie-Cariola, Kearns, & Defoor-Hill, 1990) and communicative drawing (Kearns & Yedor, 1991).

Both RET and other "loose training" approaches to treatment are based, in part, on the rationale that loosening and diversifying treatment parameters may facilitate generalization (Baer, 1981; Horner et al., 1988; Hughes, 1985; Stokes & Baer, 1977; Stokes & Osnes, 1986). Attempts to target generalization directly, as a goal of therapy, by incorporating procedures that may facilitate carryover are an integral component of a generalization planning approach to intervention for aphasia. The group setting provides an environment for refining this clinical process, and it also provides a rich arena for future research and development of strategies that promote generalization.

By appropriately targeting generative responding in the group setting, we may increase the probability of obtaining carryover to the natural environment. Generalization training should, however, go beyond simply reinforcing selected responses when they occur. Task hierarchies should be developed to elicit responses under conditions that increasingly approximate the natural environment.

Summary

In summary, a generalization planning approach has been reviewed and related to group therapy for aphasia. It was suggested that group therapy for aphasia may provide a means of incorporating generalization prompting techniques. The group setting provides an important link between individualized treatment and the natural environment. Only future research can determine the most effective means of using group treatment to facilitate generalization.

FUTURE TRENDS

Group therapy for aphasia is at a crossroads. We can fall back on the worn path of investigative complacency, or we can continue along a newer path of rigorous research to add to the knowledge base regarding group therapy for aphasia (Elman & Bernstein-Ellis, 1999). Although the choice may seem to be obvious, the road to group therapy research will continue to be challenging. Group therapy for aphasia has become strongly entrenched in our clinical repertoire because of historical precedent and practical clinical exigencies. Very few experimental studies of group treatment methods, however, are available to guide our clinical practice. Intensive group treatment research will not be forthcoming unless we overcome the "illusion of strong evidence" (McPeek & Mostellar, 1977) that supports current clinical practices. The future direction of group therapy for aphasia depends on whether clinical aphasiologists will continue to research group treatment methods aggressively. The ultimate goal of research in this area should be to identify specific, replicable, and effective group treatment procedures. Ideally, it would be desirable to be able to predict with reasonable certainty which patients would benefit from which types of group treatment. Thus, future research should eventually compare the relative effectiveness of group treatment methods.

In addition to investigating treatment approaches, the future direction of group therapy for aphasia will bring an increased awareness regarding the training needs of group clinicians. It has been suggested that not all clinicians are appropriately trained to conduct group therapy (Eisenson, 1973; Elman, 1999, 2000, 2007; Ewing, 1999, 2007; Sarno, 1981; Simmons-Mackie, Elman, Holland, & Damico, submitted). We do not, however, have academic or training guidelines to evaluate the skill level of group leaders. Kearns and Simmons (1985) found that 74% of a large sample of clinicians who conduct group therapy for aphasia reported no additional training beyond their speech-language pathology coursework. Only 24% of the survey respondents indicated that they had taken coursework or training in group dynamics, counseling, or related areas. While it is not clear exactly what type of additional training is advisable for group clinicians, this issue must be addressed in the near future. Group therapy for aphasia presents additional challenges that are not encountered in individual sessions, and investigators and academicians alike need to consider clinical training factors relating to group intervention (Elman, 2000; Simmons-Mackie et al., submitted).

Along with research and training, the future direction of group treatment will also be shaped by technologic advances. The rapid development of computer technology, including the Internet, will no doubt have an impact on group treatment methods. Individualized treatment programs may be expanded to allow patients to interact with one another and jointly solve communication problems. Similarly, treatment approaches may be enhanced by expanding technology, and virtual communicative interactions may eventually replace static picture cards as the primary stimulus material used during group sessions.

In the final analysis, the future direction of group therapy for aphasia will depend on people rather than technology. If researchers are firmly committed to this area of investigation and clinicians are willing to challenge traditional assumptions about the effectiveness of group approaches, the benefits of group therapy for aphasia may eventually be fully realized.

KEY POINTS

Given the historical roots, it would be tempting to conclude that group therapy for aphasia is nothing more than "old wine in a new bottle." It should be emphasized, however, that group therapy for aphasia, while in existence since the post–World War II era, has taken on a new and more important role in clinical practice.

1. The advent of managed care and the resultant decrease in services for individuals with aphasia (Elman & Bernstein-Ellis, 1995; Frattali, 1998; Warren & Kearns, 2000) have forced clinicians and clinical researchers to reevaluate the efficiency and efficacy of their therapy techniques.
2. In the context of reductions in reimbursement for clinical services and less time to treat persons with aphasia, sound group therapy approaches clearly are playing an increasingly significant role in patient management.
3. General trends in rehabilitation, including the emphasis on treating individuals at the level of life participation or well-being rather on treating their impairments per se, also bode well for the future of group therapy for aphasia.
4. Multipurpose groups that attempt to address the needs of the "whole" patient are rapidly becoming the norm rather than the exception. Importantly, the resurgence of interest in group techniques is not simply a matter of necessity.
5. Clinical researchers have recently developed novel group treatment methods (Avent, 1997b; Bernstein-Ellis & Elman, 1999, 2007; Kagan et al., 1990, 2007) that incorporate clearly articulated treatment ratio-

nales, and long overdue interest has emerged regarding issues relating to the measurement of client progress in treatment (Garrett, 1999; Garrett & Pimentel, 2007).
6. Treatment efficacy is finally being put to the scientific test, and data are accumulating to support the use of group treatment for aphasia (Elman & Bernstein-Ellis, 1999a, 1999b; Marshall, 1993; Van der Gaag et al., 2005; Wertz et al., 1991).
7. Group therapy for aphasia should now be considered an essential component of our clinical armamentarium rather than a convenient supplement to individual treatment.

ACTIVITIES FOR REFLECTION AND DISCUSSION

Interested readers may wish to observe and compare individual and group therapy for aphasia. Attempt to categorize the group intervention into one of the types of therapy discussed in the chapter. What are the important similarities and differences observed between individual and group treatment?

References

Agranowitz, A., Boone, D., Ruff, M., Seacat, G., & Terr, A. (1954). Group therapy as a method of retraining aphasics. *Quarterly Journal of Speech, 40,* 17–182.

Aronson, M., Shatin, L., & Cook, J. C. (1956). Sociopsycho-therapeutic approach to the treatment of aphasic patients. *Journal of Speech and Hearing Disorders, 21,* 352–364.

Aten, J. (1991). Group therapy for aphasic patients: Let's show it works. *Aphasiology, 5,* 559–561.

Aten, J. L., Caligiuri, M. P., & Holland, A. (1982). The efficacy of functional communication therapy for chronic aphasic patients. *Journal of Speech and Hearing Disorders, 47,* 93–96.

Aten, J., Kushner-Vogel, D., Haire, A., West, J. F., O'Connor, S., & Bennett, L. (1981). Group treatment for aphasia panel discussion. In R.H. Brookshire (Ed.), *Clinical aphasiology conference proceedings* (pp. 141–154). Minneapolis, MN: BRK.

Avent, J. R. (1997a). Group treatment in aphasia using cooperative learning methods. *Journal of Medical Speech-Language Pathology, 5*(1), 9–26.

Avent, J. R. (1997b). *Manual of cooperative group treatment for aphasia.* Boston, MA: Butterworth-Heinemann.

Backus, O. & Dunn, H. (1947). Intensive group therapy in speech rehabilitation. *Journal of Speech and Hearing Disorders, 12,* 39–60.

Backus, O. & Dunn, H. (1952). The use of a group structure in speech therapy. *Journal of Speech and Hearing Disorders, 17,* 116–122.

Baer, D. M. (1981). *How to plan for generalization.* Austin, TX: Pro-Ed.

Barlow, D. H., Hayes, S. C., & Nelson, R. O. (1984). *The scientist practitioner: Research and accountability in clinical and educational settings.* New York: Pergamon Press.

Beeson, P. & Holland, A. (2007). Aphasia groups in a university setting. In R. Elman (Ed.), *Group treatment of neurogenic communication disorders: The expert clinician's approach*. Second Bernstein, J. (1979). A supportive group for spouses of stroke patients. *Aphasia Apraxia Agnosia, 11*, 30–35.

Bernstein-Ellis, E. & Elman, R. (1999). Group communication treatment of individuals with aphasia: The Aphasia Center of California approach. In R. Elman (Ed.), *Group treatment for neurogenic communication disorders: The expert clinician's approach* (pp. 47–56). Boston, MA: Butterworth-Heinemann.

Bernstein-Ellis, E., & Elman, R. (2006). *The Book Connection™: A life participation book club for individuals with acquired reading impairment, Manual*. Oakland, CA: Aphasia Center of California. Available at: www.aphasiacenter.org.

Bernstein-Ellis, E. & Elman, R (2007). Aphasia group communication treatment: The Aphasia Center of California approach. In R. Elman (Ed.), Group treatment of neurogenic communication disorders: The expert clinician's approach. Second edition. San Diego, CA: Plural Publishing. www.pluralpublishing.com.

Bevington, L. J. (1985). The effects of a structured educational programme on relatives' knowledge of communication with stroke. *Australian Journal of Communication Disorders, 13*, 117–121.

Blackman, N. (1950). Group psychotherapy with aphasics. *Journal of Nervous Mental Disorders, 111*, 154–163.

Blackman, N. & Tureen, L. (1948). Aphasia: A psychosomatic approach in rehabilitation. *Transactions of American Neurological Association, 73*, 1931–96.

Bloom, L. M. (1962). A rationale for group treatment of aphasic patients. *Journal of Speech and Hearing Disorders, 27*, 11–16.

Bollinger, R., Musson, N., & Holland, A. (1993). A study of group communication intervention with chronically aphasic persons. *Aphasiology, 7*, 301–313.

Borenstein, P., Linell, S., & Wahrborg, P. (1987). An innovative therapeutic program for aphasic patients and their relatives. *Scandinavian Journal of Rehabilitation Medicine, 19*, 51–56.

Brindely, P., Copeland, M., Demain, C., & Martyn, P. (1989). A comparison of the speech of ten chronic aphasics following intensive and no-intensive periods of therapy. *Aphasiology, 3*, 695–707.

Brookshire, R. H. (2003). *An introduction to neurogenic communication disorders* (5th ed.). Saint Louis, MO: Mosby Year Book.

Chenven, H. (1953). Effects of group therapy upon language recovery in predominantly expressive aphasic patients. Doctoral dissertation, New York University.

Cochrane, R. & Milton, S. B. (1984). Conversational prompting: A sentence building technique for severe aphasia. *Journal of Neurological Communication Disorders, 1*, 423.

Coelho, C. A. & Duffy, R. (1985). Communicative use of signs in aphasia: Is acquisition enough? *Clinical Aphasiology, 15*, 222–228.

Coles, R., & Eales, C. The aphasia self-help movement in Britain: A challenge and an opportunity. In R. Elman (Ed.), *Group treatment of neurogenic communication disorders: The expert clinician's approach* (pp. 107–114). Woburn, MA: Butterworth-Heinemann.

Connell, P. & McReynolds, L. V. (1988). A clinical science approach to treatment. In L. McReynolds, N. Lass, & D. Yoder (Eds.), *Handbook of speech-language pathology and audiology* (pp. 1058–1075). Toronto: BC Decker.

Corbin, M. L. (1951). Group speech therapy for motor aphasia and dysarthria. *Journal of Speech and Hearing Disorders, 16*, 21–34.

Darley, F. L. (1982). *Aphasia*. Philadelphia, PA: WB Saunders.

Davis, G. A. (2000). *Aphasiology disorders and clinical features*. Boston, MA: Allyn and Bacon.

Davis, G. A. (1992). *A survey of adult aphasia*. Englewood Cliffs, NJ: Prentice Hall.

Davis, G. A. & Wilcox, M. J. (1981). Incorporating parameters of natural conversation in aphasia treatment. In R. Chapey (Ed.), *Language intervention strategies in adult aphasia*. Baltimore, MD: Williams & Wilkins.

Derman, S. & Manaster, H. (1967). Family counseling with relatives of aphasic patients at Schwab Rehabilitation Hospital. *ASHA, 9*, 175–177.

Disimoni, R., Keith, R., & Darley, R. (1980). Prediction of PICA overall score by short version of the test. *Journal of Speech and Hearing Research, 23*, 511–516.

Egan, J., Worrall,, L., & Oxenham, D. (2004). Accessible Internet training package helps people with aphasia cross the digital divide. *Aphasiology, 18*(3), 265-280.

Eisenson, J. (1973). *Adult aphasia*. New York: Appleton-Century-Crofts.

Elman, R. J. (1994, October). Aphasia treatment planning in an outpatient medical rehabilitation center: Where do we go from here? In C. Coelho (Ed.), *Neurophysiology and neurogenic speech and language disorders special interest division 2 newsletter* (pp. 9–13). Rockville, MD: American Speech-Language-Hearing Association.

Elman, R. (Ed.), (1999). *Group treatment of neurogenic communication disorders: The expert clinician's approach*. Woburn, MA: Butterworth-Heinemann.

Elman, R. (1998). Memories of the 'plateau': Health care changes provide an opportunity to redefine aphasia treatment and discharge. *Aphasiology 12*(3), 227–231.

Elman, R. (2000). Working with groups: Neurogenic communication disorders and the managed care challenge. [Videotape.] Rockville, MD: American Speech-Language-Hearing Association.

Elman, R. (2005). Social and life participation approaches to aphasia intervention. In L. LaPointe (Ed.), *Aphasia and related neurogenic language disorders* (3rd edition, pp. 39-50). New York: Thieme Medical Publishers.

Elman, R. (2006). Evidence-based practice: What evidence is missing? *Aphasiology, 20*, 103–109.

Elman, R. (Ed.). (2007). *Group treatment of neurogenic communication disorders: The expert clinician's approach*. Second Edition. San Diego, CA: Plural Publishing. www.pluralpublishing.com.

Elman, R. & Bernstein-Ellis, E. (1995). What is functional? *American Journal of Speech and Language Pathology, 4*, 115–117.

Elman, R. & Bernstein-Ellis, E. (1999a). The efficacy of group communication treatment in adults with chronic aphasia. *Journal of Speech, Language, and Hearing Research, 42*, 411–419.

Elman, R. & Bernstein-Ellis, E. (1999b). Psychosocial aspects of group communication treatment: Preliminary findings. *Seminars in Speech & Language, 20*(1), 65–72.

Ewing, S. (1999). Group process, group dynamics, and group techniques with neurogenic communication disorders. In R. Elman (Ed.), *Group treatment for neurogenic communication disorders: The expert clinician's approach* (pp. 9–16). Boston, MA: Butterworth-Heinemann.

Ewing, S. (2007). Group process, group dynamics, and group techniques with neurogenic communication disorders. In R. Elman

(Ed.), *Group treatment of neurogenic communication disorders: The expert clinician's approach*. Second edition. San Diego, CA: Plural Publishing. www.pluralpublishing.com.

Ewing, S. & Pfalzgraf, B. (1991a). *Pathways: Moving beyond stroke and aphasia*. [videotape]. Novi, MI: Epcom Enterprises.

Ewing, S. & Pfalzgraf, B. (1991b). *What is aphasia?* [videotape]. Novi, MI: Epcom Enterprises.

Fawcus, M. (1989). Group therapy: A learning situation. In C. Code & D.J. Müller (Eds.), *Aphasia therapy* (2nd ed.). London: Cole & Whurr.

Fawcus, M. (l991). Managing group therapy: Further considerations. *Aphasiology*, 5–6, 55–557.

Frattali, C. M. (1998). *Measuring outcomes in speech-language pathology*. New York: Thieme.

Frattali, C. M. (1992). Functional assessment of communication: Merging public policy with clinical views. *Aphasiology*, 6–I, 630–683.

Frattali, C. M. Thompson C. K., Holland, A. L., Wohl, C. B., & Ferketic, M. M. (1995). The *American Speech-language Hearing Association functional assessment of communication skills for adults (ASHA FACS)*. Rockville, MD. ASHA.

Friedland, J. & McColl, M. (1989). Social support for stroke survivors: Development and evaluation of an intervention program. *Physical and Occupational Therapy in Geriatrics*, 7, 55–69.

Friedman, M. H. (1961). On the nature of regression in aphasia. *Archives of General Psychiatry*, 5, 60–64.

Gaddie, A., Keams, K., & Yedor, K. (1989). A qualitative analysis of response elaboration training effects. *Clinical Aphasiology*, 19, 171–184.

Gaddie-Cariola, A., Kearns, K., & Defoor-Hill, L. (1990). Response elaboration training: Treatment effects using a visual communication system. Paper presented at the annual meeting of the American Speech-Language-Hearing Association, Seattle, WA.

Garrett, K. (1999). Measuring outcomes of group therapy. In R. Elman (Ed.), *Group treatment of neurogenic communication disorders: The expert clinician's approach* (pp. 17–30). Woburn, MA: Butterworth-Heinemann.

Garrett, K. & Ellis, G. (1999). Group communication therapy for people with long-term aphasia: Scaffolded thematic discourse activities. In R. Elman (Ed.), *Group treatment of neurogenic communication disorders: The expert clinician's approach* (pp. 85–96). Woburn, MA: Butterworth-Heinemann.

Garrett, K., & Pimentel, J. (2007). Measuring outcomes of group therapy. In R. Elman (Ed.), *Group treatment of neurogenic communication disorders: The expert clinician's approach*. Second edition. San Diego, CA: Plural Publishing. www.pluralpublishing.com.

Garrett, K., Staltari, C., & Moir, L. (2007). Contextual group communication therapy for persons with aphasia: A scaffolded discourse approach. In R. Elman (Ed.), *Group treatment of neurogenic communication disorders: The expert clinician's approach*. Second edition. San Diego, CA: Plural Publishing. <www.pluralpublishing.com>.

Gilbert, T. P., Mcpeek, B., & Mosteller, F. (1977). Statistics and ethics in surgery and anesthesia. *Science*, 198, 684–699.

Godfrey, C. M. & Douglass, E. (1959). The recovery process in aphasia. *Canadian Medical Association Journal*, 80, 618–624.

Gordon, E. (1976). A bi-disciplinary approach to group therapy for wives of aphasics. Paper presented at the Annual Convention of the American Speech and Hearing Association, Houston, TX.

Goodglass, H. E. & Kaplan, E. (1983). *The assessment of aphasia and related disorders* (2nd ed.). Philadelphia, PA: Lea & Febiger.

Graham, M. (1999). Aphasia group therapy in a subacute setting: Using the American Speech-Language-Hearing Association Functional Assessment of Communication Skills. In R. Elman (Ed.), *Group treatment of neurogenic communication disorders: The expert clinician's approach* (pp. 37–46). Woburn, MA: Butterworth-Heinemann.

Hartley, L. (1995). *Cognitive-Communicative Abilities Following Brain Injury. A Functional Approach*. Singular, San Diego, CA.

Hersh, D. (2007). "From the ground up": The Talkback group program in South Australia. In R. Elman (Ed.), *Group treatment of neurogenic communication disorders: The expert clinician's approach*. Second edition. San Diego, CA: Plural Publishing. www.pluralpublishing.com.

Hoen, R., Thelander, M., & Worsley, J. (1997). Improvement in psychological well-being of people with aphasia and their families: Evaluation of a community-based programme. *Aphasiology*, 11(7), 681–691.

Holland, A. L. (1970). Case studies in aphasia rehabilitation using programmed instruction. *ASHA*, 35, 377–390.

Holland, A. L. (1975). The effectiveness of treatment in aphasia. In R.H. Brookshire (Ed.), *Clinical aphasiology conference proceedings*, 1972–1976 (pp. 145–159). Minneapolis. MN: BRK.

Holland, A. L. (1980). *Communicative abilities in daily living*. Baltimore, MD: University Park Press.

Holland, A. L. & Beeson, P. (1999). Aphasia groups: The Arizona experience. In R. Elman (Ed.), *Group treatment of neurogenic communication disorders: The expert clinician's approach* (pp. 77–84). Woburn, MA: Butterworth-Heinemann.

Horner, R. H., Dunlap, G., & Koegel, R. L. (1988). *Generalization and maintenance: Lifestyle changes in applied settings*. Baltimore, MD: Paul H. Brookes.

Horwitz, B. (1977). An open letter to the family of an adult patient with aphasia. *The National Easter Seal Society for Crippled Children and Adults*, 30, Reprint A-186.

Huber, M. (1946). Linguistic problems of brain-injured servicemen. *Journal of Speech Disorders*, II. 143–147.

Hughes, D. L. (1985). *Language treatment and generalization: A clinician's handbook*. San Diego, CA: College Hill Press.

Hunt, M. I. (1976). Language maintenance group for aphasics. Paper presented at the Annual Convention of the American Speech and Hearing Association, Houston, TX.

Inskip, W. M. & Burris, G. A. (1959). Coordinated treatment program for the patient with language disability. *American Archives of Rehabilitation Therapy*, 7, 27–35.

Jenkins, J. J., Jimenez-Pabon, E., Shaw, R. E., & Sefer, J. W. (1981). *Schuell's aphasia in adults: Diagnosis prognosis and treatment* (2nd ed.). Hagerstown, MD: Harper & Row.

Johannsen-Horbach, H., Wenz, C., Funfgeld, M., Herrmann, M., & Wallesch, C. (1993). Psychosocial aspects in the treatment of adult aphasics and their families: A group approach. In A. Holland & M. Forbes (Eds.), *Aphasia treatment: World perspectives*. San Diego, CA: Singular Publishing Group.

Johnston, J. M. & Pennypacker, H. S. (1980). *Strategies and tactics of human behavioral research*. Hillsdale, NJ: Lawrence Erlbaum.

Kagan, A. (1998). Supported conversation for adults with aphasia: Methods and resources for training conversation partners. *Aphasiology*, 12, 851–864.

Kagan, A., Cambell-Taylor, I., & Gailey, G. (1990). A unique community based programme for adults with chronic aphasia. Paper presented at the Fourth International Aphasia Rehabilitation Congress, Edinburgh.

Kagan, A. & Cohen-Schneider, R. (1999). Groups in the introductory program at the Pat Arato Aphasia Centre. In R. Elman (Ed.), *Group treatment of neurogenic communication disorders: The expert clinician's approach* (pp. 97–106). Woburn, MA: Butterworth-Heinemann.

Kagan, A., Black, S., Duchan , J., Simmons-Mackie, N., & Square, P. (2001). Training volunteers as conversation partners using "Supported Conversation for Adults with Aphasia" (SCA): a controlled trial. *JSLHR*, 44(3), 624-38.

Kagan, A., Winchel, J. Black, S., Duchan, J. Simmons-Mackie, N., & Square, P. (2004). A set of observational measures for rating support and participation in conversation between adults with aphasia and their conversation partners. *Topics in Stroke Rehabilitation*. 11(1), 67–83.

Kagan, A., Cohen-Schneider, R., Sherman, C., & Podolsky, L. (2007). Groups in the Aphasia Institute's Introductory Program: Preparing to live successfully with aphasia. In R. Elman (Ed.), *Group treatment of neurogenic communication disorders: The expert clinician's approach*. Second edition. San Diego, CA: Plural Publishing. <www.pluralpublishing.com>.

Kearns, K. P. (1986a). Flexibility of single-subject experimental designs II: Design selection and arrangement of experimental phases. *Journal of Speech and Hearing Disorders, 51*, 204–214.

Kearns, K. P. (1986b). Systematic programming of verbal elaboration skills in chronic Broca's aphasia. In R.C. Marshall (Ed.), *Case studies in aphasia rehabilitation* (pp. 225–244). Austin, TX: Pro-Ed.

Kearns, K. P. (1989). Methodologies for studying generalization. In L.V. McReynolds & J. Spradlin (Eds.), *Generalization strategies in the treatment of communication disorders* (pp. 13–30). Toronto: BC Decker.

Kearns, K. P. & Scher, G. (1988). The generalization of response elaboration training effects. *Clinical Aphasiology, 18*, 223–242.

Kearns, K. P. & Simmons, N. N. (1985). Group therapy for aphasia: A survey of Veterans Administration Medical Centers. In R. H. Brookshire (Ed.), *Clinical aphasiology conference proceedings* (pp. 176–183). Minneapolis, MN: BRK.

Kearns, K. P. & Yedor, K. (1991). An alternating treatments comparison of loose training and a convergent treatment strategy. *Clinical Aphasiology, 20*, 223–238.

Kearns, K. P. & Yedor, K. (1992). Artistic activation therapy: Drawing conclusions. Paper presented at the Clinical Aphasiology Conference, Durango, CO.

Kertesz, A. (1982). *Western Aphasia Battery*. New York: Grune & Stratton.

Kinsella, G. & Duffy, F. D. (1978). The spouse of the aphasic patient. In Y. Lebrun & R. Hoops (Eds.), *The management of aphasia*. Amsterdam: Swets-Zeitlinger.

Kinsella, G. & Duffy, F. D. (1979). Psycho-social readjustments in the spouses of aphasic patients. *Scandinavian Journal of Rehabilitation Medicine, 11*, 129–132.

Kisley, C. A. (1973). Striking back at stroke. *Hospitals, 47*, 4–72.

Lafond, D., Joanette, Y., Ponzio, J., Degiovani, R., & Sarno, M. (Eds.) (1993). *Living with aphasia: Psychosocial issues*. San Diego: Singular Publishing Group.

LaPointe, L. L. (1989). An ecological perspective on assessment and treatment of aphasia. *Clinical Aphasiology, 18*, 1–4.

Lomas, J., Pickard, L., Bester, S., Elbard, H., Finlayson, A., & Zoghab, C. (1989). The Communicative Effectiveness Index: Development and psychometric evaluation of a functional communication measure for adult aphasia. *Journal of Speech and Hearing Disorders, 54*, 113–124.

Loverso, F. L. (1991). Aphasia group treatment, a commentary. *Aphasiology, 5*, 567–569.

Loverso, F. L., Young-Charles, H., & Tonkovich, J. D. (1982). The application of a process evaluation form for aphasic individuals in a small group setting. In R.H. Brookshire (Ed.), *Clinical aphasiology conference proceedings* (pp. 1–17). Minneapolis, MN: BRK.

LLPA Project Group. (2000). Life participation approach to aphasia: A statement of values for the future. *ASHA Leader, 5*, 4–6. Retrieved June 27, 2006, from http://www. asha.org/public/speech/disorders/LPAA.htm

Luterman, D. (1996). *Counseling persons with communication disorders and their families* (3rd ed). Austin, TX: Pro-Ed.

Lyon, J. G. (1992). Communication use and participation in life for adults with aphasia in natural settings: The scope of the problem. *American Journal of Speech-Language Pathology, 1–3*, 7–14.

Lyon, J. (1997). *Coping with aphasia*. San Diego: CA: Singular.

Makenzie, C. (1991). Four weeks of intensive therapy followed by four weeks of no treatment. *Aphasiology, 5* (4–5), 435–437.

Malone, R. L. (1969). Expressed attitudes of families of aphasics. *Journal of Speech and Hearing Disorders, 34*, 146–151.

Marquardt, T. P. (1982). *Acquired neurogenic disorders*. Englewood Cliffs, NJ: Prentice-Hall.

Marquardt, T. P., Tonkovich, J. D., & Devault, S. M. (1976). Group therapy and stroke club programs for aphasic adults. *Journal of the Tennessee Speech-Hearing Association, 20*, 2–20.

Marshall, R. C. (1993). Problem focused group therapy for mildly aphasic clients. *American Journal of Speech-Language Pathology, 2(2)*, 31–37.

Marshall, R. C. (1999). *Introduction to group treatment for aphasia: Design and management*. Woburn, MA: Butterworth-Heinemann.

Marshall, R. C. (1999b). A problem-focused group treatment program for clients with mild aphasia. In R. Elman (Ed.), *Group treatment of neurogenic communication disorders: The expert clinician's approach* (pp. 57–65). Woburn, MA: Butterworth-Heinemann.

Marshall, R. C. (2007). A problem-focused group treatment program for clients with mild aphasia. In R. Elman (Ed.), *Group treatment of neurogenic communication disorders: The expert clinician's approach*. Second edition. San Diego, CA: Plural Publishing. <www.pluralpublishing.com>.

McReynolds, L. V. & Spradlin, J. (1989). *Generalization strategies in the treatment of communication disorders*. Toronto: BC Decker.

Miles, M. & Huberman, A. (1994). *Qualitative data analysis* (2nd ed.). Thousand Oaks, CA: Sage.

Mogil, S., Bloom, D., Gray, L., & Lefkowitz, N. (1978). A unique method for the follow-up of aphasic patients. In R. H. Brookshire (Ed.), *Clinical aphasiology conference proceedings* (pp. 314–317). Minneapolis, MN: BRK.

Newhoff, M. N. & Davis, G. A. (1978). A spouse intervention program: Planning, implementation and problems of evaluation. In R. H. Brooksbire (Ed.), *Clinical aphasiology conference proceedings* (pp. 318–326). Minneapolis, MN: BRK.

Nicholas, L. & Brookshire, R. (1993). A system for quantifying the informativeness and efficiency of the connected speech of adults with aphasia. *Journal of Speech and Hearing Research, 36*, 338–350.

Nielson, J. M., Schultz, D. A., Corbin, M. A., & Crittsinger, B. A. (1948). The treatment of traumatic aphasics of World War II at Birmingham. General Veterans Administration Hospital, Van Nuys, California. *Military Surgery, 102*, 351.

Oradei, D. M. & Waite, J. S. (1974). Group psychotherapy with stroke patients during the immediate recovery phase. *American Journal of Orthopsychiatry, 44*, 386–395.

Osiejek, E. (1991). Discourse exercises in aphasia therapy. *Aphasiology, 5*(45), 443.

Pachalska, M. (1991a). Group therapy for aphasia. *Aphasiology, 5*(6), 541–554.

Pachalska, M. (1991b). Group therapy: A way of integrating patients with aphasia. *Aphasiology, 5*(6), 573–577.

Parr, S., Byng, S., Glpin, S., & Ireland, C. (1997) *Talking about aphasia–Living with less of language after stroke*. Buckingham, UK: Open University Press.

Penman, T. (1999). Breaking down the barriers. *Bulletin of the College of Speech and Language Therapists*, August, 14–15.

Penman, R. & Pound, C. (2007). Making connections: Involving people with aphasia as group facilitators. In R. Elman (Ed.), *Group treatment of neurogenic communication disorders: The expert clinician's approach*. Second edition. San Diego, CA: Plural Publishing. <www.pluralpublishing.com>.

Penn, C., & Jones, D. (2007). "We all speak the same language…we all speak aphasia": The evolution of therapy groups within a changing sociopolitical context. In R. Elman (Ed.), *Group treatment of neurogenic communication disorders: The expert clinician's approach*. Second edition. San Diego, CA: Plural Publishing. www.pluralpublishing.com.

Porch, B. (1967). *The Porch Index of Communicative Ability*. Palo Alto, CA: Consulting Psychologists Press.

Porter, I. L. & Dabul, B. (1977). The application of transactional analysis to therapy with wives of adult aphasic patients. *ASHA, 19*, 24.

Pound, C. (1998). Power, partnerships and practicalities: Developing cost-effective support services for living with aphasia. Paper presented at the Clinical Aphasiology Conference, Asheville, NC.

Pound, C., Parr, S., Lindsay, J., & Woolf, C. (2000). *Beyond aphasia: Therapies for living with communication disability*. Oxon, UK: Winslow Press.

Puts-Zwartes, R. A. (1973). Group therapy for the husbands and wives of aphasics. *Logopaed, Fomiatr, 45*, 93–97.

Radonjic, V. & Rakuscek, N. (1991). Group therapy to encourage communication ability in aphasic patients. *Aphasiology, 5*(4–5), 451–455.

Rao, P. (1986). The use of Amer-Ind code with aphasic adults. In R. Chapey (Ed.), *Language intervention strategies in aphasia* (2nd ed.) (pp. 360–369). Baltimore, MD: Williams & Wilkins.

Redinger, R. A., Forster, S., Dolphin, M. K., Godduhn, J., & Wersinger, J. (1971). Group therapy in the rehabilitation of the severely aphasic and hemiplegic in later stages. *Scandinavian Journal of Rehabilitation Medicine, 3*, 89–91.

Repo, M. (1991). The holistic approach to rehabilitation: A commentary. *Aphasiology, 5*, 571–572.

Rice, B., Paul, A., & Müller, D. (1987). An evaluation of a social support group for spouses of aphasic partners. *Aphasiology, I*, 247–256.

Sarno, M. T. (1981). Recovery and rehabilitation in aphasia. In M. T. Sarno (Ed.), *Acquired aphasia*. New York: Academic Press.

Sarno, M. T. & Peters, J. (2004). *The aphasia handbook*. New York: National Aphasia Association.

Schlanger, P. H. & Schlanger, B. B. (1970). Adapting role-playing activities with aphasic patients. *Journal of Speech and Hearing Disorders, 35*, 229.

Schuell, H., Jenkins, J. J., & Jimenez-Pabon, E. (1964). *Aphasia in adults*. New York: Harper and Row.

Shadden, B. (2007). Rebuilding identity through stroke support groups: Embracing the person with aphasia and significant others. In R. Elman (Ed.), *Group treatment of neurogenic communication disorders: The expert clinician's approach*. Second edition. San Diego, CA: Plural Publishing. www.pluralpublishing.com.

Sheehan, V. M. (1946). Rehabilitation of aphasics in an army hospital. *Journal of Speech and Hearing Disorders, 2*, 149–157.

Sheehan, V. M. (1948). Techniques in the management of aphasics. *Journal of Speech and Hearing Disorders, 13*, 241–246.

Simmons-Mackie, N., Elman, R., Holland, A., & Damico, J. (2007). Management of discourse in group therapy for aphasia.

Skelly, M., Schinsky, L., Smith, R. W., & Fust, R. S. (1974). American Indian Sign (AMERIND) as a facilitator of verbalization for the oral verbal apraxic. *Journal of Speech and Hearing Disorders, 39*, 445.

Smith, A. (1972). *Diagnosis, intelligence, and rehabilitation of chronic aphasics: Final report*. Ann Arbor, MI: University of Michigan.

Sparks, R., Helm, N., & Albert, N. (1974). Aphasia rehabilitation resulting from melodic intonation therapy. *Corte, 10*, 303–316.

Spradlin, J. E. & Siegel, G. M. (1982): Language training in natural and clinician environments. *Journal of Speech and Hearing Disorders, 47*, 2.

Springer, L. (1991). Facilitating group rehabilitation. *Aphasiology, 6*, 563–565.

Stokes, T. F. & Baer, D. M. (1977). An implicit technology of generalization. *Journal of Applied Behavior Analysis, 10*, 349–367.

Stokes, T. & Osnes, P. P. (1986). Programming generalization of children's social behavior. In P. S. Strain, M. Guralnick, & H. Walker (Eds.), *Children's social behavior: Development, assessment, and modification* (pp. 407–443). Orlando, FL: Academic Press.

Strauss, A. & Corbin, J. (1990). *Basics of qualitative research: Grounded theory procedures and techniques*. Thousand Oaks, CA: Sage.

Thompson, C. K. (1989). Generalization in the treatment of aphasia. In L. V. McReynolds & J. Spradlin (Eds.), *Generalization strategies in the treatment of communication disorders* (pp. 82–115). Toronto: BC Decker.

Thompson, C. K. & Kearns, K. P. (1991). Analytical and technical directions in applied aphasia research: The Midas touch. *Clinical Aphasiology, 19*, 41–54.

Tsvetkova, L. S. (1980). Some ways of optimizing aphasic rehabilitation. *International Journal of Rehabilitation Research, 3*, 183–190.

Turnblom, M. & Myers, J. S. (1952). A group discussion program with the families of aphasic patients. *Journal of Speech and Hearing Disorders, 17*, 383–396.

Van der Gaag, A., Smith, L., Davies, S., Moss, B., Cornelius, V., Laing, S., et al. (2005). Therapy and support services for people with long term stroke and aphasia and their relatives: A six month follow up study. *Clinical Rehabilitation, 19*(4), 372–380.

Van Harskamp, F. & Visch-Brink, F. E. G. (1991). Goal recognition in aphasia therapy. *Aphasiology, 5–6*, 529–535.

Veterans Administration (1983). *A stroke: Recovering together.* St. Louis: V. A. Regional Learning Resources.

Vickers, C. (1998). *Communication recovery: Group conversation activities for adults.* San Antonio, TX: Communication Skill Builders.

Wahrborg, P., Borenstein, P., Linell, S., Hedber-Borenstein, E., & Asking, M. (1997). Ten-year follow-up of young aphasic participants in a 34-week course at Folk High School. *Aphasiology, 11*(7), 709–715.

Walker-Batson, D., Curtis, S., Smith, P., & Ford, J. (1999). An alternative model for the treatment of aphasia: The Lifelink© approach. In R. Elman (Ed.), *Group treatment of neurogenic communication disorders: The expert clinician's approach* (pp. 67–75). Woburn, MA: Butterworth-Heinemann.

Warren, R. L. & Kearns, K. P. (2000). The influence of capitation on rehabilitation and clinical aphasiology. Paper presented at the Clinical Aphasiology Conference, Waikola, HI.

Warren, S. F. & Rogers-Warren, A. K. (Eds.) (1985). *Teaching functional language.* Austin, TX: Pro-Ed.

Wepman, J. M. (1947). The organization of therapy for aphasia: 1. The inpatient treatment center. *Journal of Speech and Hearing Disorders, 12*, 405–409.

Wertz, R. T., Collins, M. H., Weiss, D., Kurtzke, J. F., Friden, T., Porch, B. E., West, J. A., Davis, L., Matovitch, V., Morley, G. K., & Resurreccion, E. (1981). Veterans Administration cooperative study on aphasia: A comparison of individual and group treatment. *Journal of Speech and Hearing Research, 24*, 580–594.

Wilcox, M. H. & Davis, G. (1977). Speech act analysis of aphasic communication in individual and group settings. In R. H. Brookshire (Ed.), *Clinical aphasiology conference proceedings* (pp. 166–174). Minneapolis, MN: BRK.

World Health Organization. (2001). *International classification of functioning, disability and health: ICF.* Geneva, Switzerland: Author.

Worrall, L., Davidson, B., Howe, T., & Rose, T. (2007). Clients as teachers: Two aphasia groups at The University of Queensland. In R. Elman (Ed.), *Group treatment of neurogenic communication disorders: The expert clinician's approach.* Second Edition. San Diego, CA: Plural Publishing. www.pluralpublishing.com.

Yalom, I. D. (1995). *The theory and practice of group psychotherapy* (4th ed.). New York: Basic Books.

Section IV

Traditional Approaches to Language Intervention

A. Stimulation Approaches

Chapter 15

Schuell's Stimulation Approach to Rehabilitation

Carl A. Coelho, Michele P. Sinotte, and
Joseph R. Duffy

OBJECTIVES

Hildred Schuell's stimulation approach to therapy for aphasia represents one of the main schools of thought in aphasia rehabilitation and has been one of the most widely used treatment approaches employed in this country. This chapter reviews Schuell's definition, theory, and classifications of aphasia as well as the principles, rationale, and specific goals associated with the stimulation approach.

This chapter deals with an approach to the treatment of aphasia that places its primary emphasis on the stimulation presented to the patient. Hildred Schuell was among the most lucid, scientifically minded, and insightful clinicians to propose and offer support for this approach. Because of her major role in its development, the approach described in this chapter is often referred to as "Schuell's therapy" or "Schuell's stimulation approach."

The bulk of Hildred Schuell's work in aphasiology spanned the 1960s and 1970s, and it included significant contributions in the areas of diagnostic testing, classification of patients with aphasia, and theory development regarding the underlying nature of the disorder. It was probably this sound foundation in theory, evaluation, and methods of observing and categorizing behavior that helped Schuell to develop the compelling rationale for the stimulation approach. This sound foundation also helps to explain why the stimulation approach represents one of the main schools of thought in therapy for aphasia and has been one of the most widely used treatment approaches employed in this country (Darley, 1975; Davis, 1993; Sarno, 1981). In this chapter, Schuell's definition, theory, and classifications of aphasia will be reviewed briefly as prerequisites for understanding the stimulation approach. The remainder of the chapter will emphasize the principles, rationale, and specific goals, procedures, and techniques associated with the stimulation approach to aphasia rehabilitation.

Before proceeding, it is necessary to delimit further the territory to be covered in this chapter. First, virtually all approaches used by speech-language pathologists for the treatment of aphasia must necessarily involve stimulation of some kind (Wepman, 1953); for that reason, the stimulation approach may be thought to encompass all approaches to aphasia rehabilitation. The presence of numerous other chapters in this book, however, makes it clear that this is not intended to be the case. The material presented here is conceptually related to Schuell's specific approach to treatment, and it is her name that signals the scope of this chapter and distinguishes it from other treatment approaches that use stimulation in more broadly, or more narrowly, defined ways.

The second point is intended to qualify the narrowed scope described in the previous paragraph. Although Schuell was a "prime mover" in the development of the stimulation approach, many other clinicians and investigators have contributed to the development or refinement of its rationale, principles, design, and techniques. Wepman's (1951) contribution, for example, is particularly noteworthy, because it was the first complete elaboration of the approach (Darley, 1972). Therefore, although all current approaches to the treatment of aphasia will not be discussed, attention will be given to the contributions of many individuals in addition to those of Hildred Schuell. Receiving special emphasis will be those investigations that continuously help to refine the approach by identifying stimulus factors influencing the adequacy of language performance in persons with aphasia.

PREREQUISITES TO UNDERSTANDING THE STIMULATION APPROACH
Definition and Primary Symptoms of Aphasia

Systematic observation and testing of more than a thousand patients with aphasia led Schuell and her colleagues to define aphasia as "a general language deficit that crosses all language modalities and may or may not be complicated by other sequelae of brain damage" (Schuell, Jenkins, &

Jiménez-Pabón, 1964, p. 113). The language modalities referred to in the definition include comprehension of spoken language, speech, reading, and writing. The "other sequelae"—that is, the nonaphasic disturbances—most often would include modality-specific perceptual disturbances, dysarthrias, and sensorimotor deficits (including apraxia of speech). Also, other complications and secondary symptoms, such as a reduction of communication generated by depression or an altered attitude toward communication, may occur as a reaction to the primary symptoms of aphasia (Jenkins, Jiménez-Pabón, Shaw, & Sefer, 1975).

Schuell consistently viewed a reduction of available vocabulary, linguistic rules, and verbal retention span, as well as impaired comprehension and production of messages, as being the primary characteristics of aphasia (Schuell, 1969, 1974a; Schuell & Jenkins, 1961a; Schuell et al., 1964). In addition, her observations indicate that the impaired ability to retrieve and use the language code not only crosses all modalities but also tends to be evident in all modalities in a similar manner. Finally, "the impairment is regular and orderly, and operates in a manner that is lawfully related to known language phenomena" (Schuell et al., 1964, p. 104). The occurrence of similar deficits across modalities within patients, as well as the predictable nature of those deficits, are important additional characteristics, and they figure strongly in the rationale and procedures used in the stimulation approach.

Underlying Nature of Aphasia

In most scientific clinical endeavors, it is preferable that the rationale for using a particular method precede the application of that method. This is particularly important in clinical aphasiology, because the efficacy of treatment continues to be debated and we cannot always confidently, though superficially, say, "I use this approach because it works!" Until the efficacy of any approach to the rehabilitation of a person with aphasia is unequivocally demonstrated, what we do must at least be defensible on theoretic grounds. Schuell (1974b) supported such a notion with her belief that "what you do about aphasia depends on what you think aphasia is" (p. 138). Therefore, it is important that our methods of treatment be linked to our beliefs about the organization of language in the brain and the nature of that language breakdown that occurs when the brain is damaged. The adoption of such beliefs, however, is complicated by an abundance of choices. In fact, the existence of numerous beliefs about the underlying nature of aphasia has led to the existence of numerous approaches to treatment. Because treatment is subject to such beliefs, it is essential that we have some understanding of the model of language and beliefs about the nature of aphasia that specifically underlie the stimulation approach. If such a model and beliefs are palatable, procedures and techniques become logical extensions of the underlying rationale.

Schuell's beliefs about the organization of language and the nature of the language breakdown in aphasia can be summarized as follows:

1. Language cannot be thought of as a simple sensorimotor dichotomy or a three-system cortical relay involving reception, transmission, and execution (Schuell et al., 1964). Such classical models ignore the complexity of perceptual and motor processes and view language as an activity bound to sensation and movement. They also allow aphasia to be thought of in terms of isolated, pure disorders reflecting disturbances at different stages of the dichotomy or relay system (e.g., receptive or Wernicke's aphasia, conduction aphasia, and expressive or Broca's aphasia). To many investigators, including Schuell, such notions do not correspond to modern concepts of neurophysiology and, more important, to the clinical behavior of most patients with aphasia.

2. Neurophysiologically, language is the result of the dynamic interaction of complex cerebral and subcortical activities. Such complex interactions preclude the existence of simply segregated sensory and motor divisions and, in effect, place the existence of isolated sensory or motor deficits outside the realm of aphasia. Likewise, the various elements of language cannot be separated neurophysiologically. For example, the relationship between the semantic and syntactic aspects of language is so strong that their separation at the physiological level is arbitrary at best (Schuell et al., 1964).

3. The language mechanism contains a system of stored, learned elements and rules, the use and maintenance of which require discrimination, organization, storage, comparison, retrieval, transmission, and feedback control. Like Wepman, Jones, Bock, and Van Pelt (1960), Schuell viewed language as an integrative activity that is linked, but not bound, to sensory and motor modalities. That is, the stored elements and rules are common (central) to all input and output modalities; speech, verbal comprehension, reading, and writing "involve the same referents and the same categorizations of individual and collective experience" (Schuell et al., 1964, p. 104). In the adult, therefore, language can exist unimpaired even in the presence of severe sensory and/or motor deficits, although it might be difficult to receive or express language through an impaired modality. Conversely, the language mechanism can be impaired in the absence of sensory or motor deficits. In such instances, however, the disturbance will be reflected in all modalities, because the same language system is used by (or linked to) all input and output modalities through which language is channeled. Consequently, aphasia is viewed as a multimodality disturbance that is unidimensional in nature. That is, not only do all

modalities tend to be impaired in aphasia, they also tend to be impaired in the same manner and to about the same degree.

4. It is important to recognize that Schuell's unidimensional, multimodality concept of aphasia does not require that patients with aphasia vary only along a severity continuum. Schuell and Jenkins (1961b) wrote that among patients with aphasia, "many dimensions of impairment resulting from language deficit are identifiable, and need to be studied, in addition to the common or general dimension of language deficit" (p. 299). They also stated, "[A]t a given level of language deficit, language tests may be arranged in subgroups which show systematic regularities in aphasic performance in various modalities as well as systematic differences in the performance of various segments of aphasic populations (p. 299)." The point here is that Schuell did not believe that all patients with aphasia were alike, but based on her clinical observations and objective analyses of data, she chose to emphasize the apparent universal feature of the disorder—a general disturbance of language that is reflected in a similar manner in all modalities.

5. In aphasia, the problems of most patients appear to be more related to performance factors than to competence factors (Schuell, 1969). That is, it appears that linguistic elements and rules are not lost or destroyed but that the language system either is working with reduced efficiency or is "swamped in noise, due to faulty connections, disturbed internal signal sources, defective speech analyzers, and the general asynchronous chaos of processes whose mass action can no longer be properly coordinated" (Jenkins et al., 1975, p. 59). Schuell's belief that language is not lost or destroyed in aphasia is an important factor in determining that the stimulation approach does not involve the "teaching" or "re-teaching" of language.

6. Although the language mechanism can exist separately from both input and output modalities, our primary language processes are acquired and organized through complex, interacting sensory systems and sensorimotor processes. Notably, auditory processes are at the apex of those interacting systems that aid in the acquisition, processing, and control of language (Schuell et al., 1964). The importance of auditory processes for language and in the stimulation approach to language remediation will be discussed in more detail later.

Classification of Aphasia

Schuell's classification system for aphasia is unique when compared to most other popular systems. Her view of aphasia as a multimodality, unidimensional impairment clearly precluded categorizing patients according to modality of impairment (e.g., expressive, receptive, agraphia, or alexia) or the element of language involved (e.g., semantic, syntactic, or anomic). Instead, her classification system aimed at descriptive and predictive utility by classifying patients according to the severity of language impairment, presence or absence of related sensory or motor deficits, and prognosis. Originally, Schuell's system contained five categories and two minor syndromes. Later (Jenkins et al., 1975), the minor syndromes were treated as major categories. The seven categories are summarized below.

These classifications are useful in planning treatment with the stimulation approach in two ways. First, the various categories indicate the severity of language impairment and, therefore, give some indication of the level at which stimulation should be directed. Second, the identification of associated non-aphasic deficits indicates those input avenues with the least intact access to the language system as well as those output avenues through which evidence of language processing is least likely to be valid or interpretable. Such input and output problems signal a possible need to modify stimuli or restructure response demands. They also identify non-linguistic disturbances that also may require remediation.

Simple Aphasia

"Simple aphasia" is considered to be relatively mild multimodality language impairment with no specific perceptual, sensorimotor, or dysarthric components. The prognosis for recovery is excellent.

Aphasia with Visual Involvement

"Aphasia with visual involvement" refers to mild aphasia complicated by central impairment of visual discrimination, recognition, and recall. The prognosis for language recovery is excellent, but reading and writing recover more slowly.

Aphasia with Persisting Dysfluency

"Aphasia with persisting dysfluency" is mild aphasia with associated verbal dysfluency as an apparent result of proprioceptive disturbance (Jenkins et al., 1975). The prognosis for recovery from aphasia is excellent, but continued conscious control over speech execution remains necessary.

Aphasia with Scattered Findings

"Aphasia with scattered findings" is considered to be moderate aphasia involving a variety of problems compatible with generalized brain injury (e.g., dysarthria, visual involvement, or emotional lability). Although the potential for functional language exists, the prognosis is limited by the concomitant physiological and psychological problems.

Aphasia with Sensorimotor Involvement

"Aphasia with sensorimotor involvement" is defined as severe language impairment with impaired perception and production of phonemic patterns. The prognosis is for limited but functional recovery of language with persisting signs of sensorimotor impairment.

Aphasia with Intermittent Auditory Imperception

"Aphasia with intermittent auditory imperception" is usually considered to be severe aphasic impairment with severe involvement of auditory processes. Recovery of some language may occur, but normalcy is not achieved.

Irreversible Aphasia Syndrome

"Irreversible aphasia syndrome" is nearly complete multimodality loss of functional language skills. The prognosis for recovery of functional language is poor.

APPROACH—GENERAL DESCRIPTION

Definition and Rationale

The stimulation approach can be defined as the approach to treatment that employs strong, controlled, and intensive auditory stimulation of the impaired symbol system as the primary tool to facilitate and maximize the patient's reorganization and recovery of language. It is an approach that recognizes the stimuli to which an intact language system can respond may be inadequate for eliciting responses from an impaired system. Because "sensory stimulation is the only method we have for making complex events happen in the brain" (Schuell et al., 1964, p. 338), the approach employs the manipulation and control of stimulus dimensions to aid the patient in making maximal responses.

Although numerous input modalities may be used, the auditory modality is at the foundation of the stimulation approach. The use of intensive, controlled auditory stimulation is supported by the following:

1. Sensory stimulation affects brain activity. For example, sensory input alters the electrical activity of the brain, increasing stimulus strength increases the frequency of firing of neurons and the number of fibers activated, and the threshold of response can be altered by repetitive stimulation (Eccles, 1973; Naeser, et. al, 2005; Thompson, 1967). In addition, repetitive stimulation can increase the firing of neurons in homologous right-hemisphere brain regions in individuals with left-hemisphere cortical and subcortical lesions (Calautti, Warburtion, & Baron, 2003, Hillis, 2002). Thus, at the neurophysiological level, stimulation can and does influence brain structure and function.

2. Many lines of research indicate that repeated sensory stimulation is essential for the acquisition, organization, storage, and retrieval of patterns in the brain. Language "patterns" appear to be no exception, because language proficiency is largely the result of linguistic stimulation

and experience. In addition, it is likely that language retrieval works through patterns of excitation laid down during original learning and that appropriate stimuli are required for adequate retrieval (Schuell et al., 1964).

3. The auditory system is of prime importance in the acquisition of language, and ongoing functional language is dependent on the auditory system for processed information and control through feedback loops (Schuell et al., 1964).

4. Numerous studies indicate that nearly all people with aphasia exhibit deficits in the auditory modality (Duffy and Ulrich, 1976; Schuell, 1953b; Schuell et al., 1964; Smith, 1971). It has been suggested that many of the multimodality impairments that patients with aphasia experience stem from these auditory deficits (Schuell, 1953b) and that recovery of auditory functions, for many patients, is a prerequisite to recovery of other speech and language abilities (Brookshire, 1976a; Holland and Sonderman, 1974). Finally, the clinical observations of Schuell and colleagues (1955, 1964) as well as of Schuell alone (1953a, 1969) suggest that the use of intensive, controlled auditory stimulation results in multimodality improvement greater than that when treatment focuses on movement patterns or on each modality separately. Schuell (1974c) considered the notion of intensive auditory stimulation to be "the most important clinical discovery that we ever made" (p. 112).

5. The use of intensive auditory stimulation is consistent with the definition of aphasia as a multimodality deficit that results from an underlying disturbance of language. That is, if the patient's problems in each modality are a reflection of a common underlying language disturbance, it makes sense to channel treatment through the auditory modality because of its crucial link to language processes. In doing so, we should expect that gains made through the auditory modality will extend to all other input and output language channels.

A caveat regarding the primacy of the auditory modality in treatment is in order. Experience tells us that for some patients, the auditory channel is not the most appropriate avenue for stimulation. For example, some patients with disproportionately severe impairment of auditory processes respond, on baseline testing, more favorably to written or gestural input. For such individuals, the primary stimulus channel in therapy may be visual instead of auditory. The use of intensive auditory stimulation in the stimulation approach should therefore be viewed as a rule for which important-to-recognize exceptions exist.

What the Stimulation Approach is Not

The stimulation approach can be further understood by identifying some things that it is not. Wepman (1953, 1968) argued that patients with aphasia do not recover because they are taught to speak. He indicated that the purpose of stimulation is not to convey new learning but, rather, to focus on "old learning" and stimulate the patient to produce new integrations for language. Schuell and colleagues (1955, 1964) emphasized that aphasia clinicians are not teachers; their role is to stimulate the adequate functioning of disrupted processes. Martin (1975), viewing the stimulation approach as being conceptually related to cognitive theories of learning, indicated that the approach is an attempt "to reorganize a system already reorganized by brain damage" (p. 73). He pointed out that, because the approach is based on a model which views aphasia as an interference with (not a loss of) language processes, therapy does not emphasize memory or the reproduction of stimuli as stimulus-response learning approaches do. Instead, the approach emphasizes the action that is elicited within the patient by the stimuli that are presented. Such an approach treats the patient as an active participant in the reorganization of language and adjusts stimulation to maximize the ability of the patient to participate in the process.

Finally, what Taylor (1964) has called nonspecific stimulation, or the spontaneous recovery approach, is not part of the approach being discussed here. Nonspecific stimulation would include merely talking to the patient as much as possible; working to establish rapport, socialization, or interest; and reducing anxiety. Clearly, such approaches to treatment should be distinguished from the more carefully planned and controlled approach that is the focus of this chapter.

Individuals for Whom the Approach is Appropriate

Relative to Severity

The rationale and general goals of the stimulation approach do not preclude its use with particular degrees of language impairment; however, the approach is not invariant along the severity continuum. The severity of aphasia should—and does—influence the nature of stimulation, the specific treatment goals and procedures, and the frequency and duration of treatment. For example, severe aphasia (Schuell's irreversible aphasia syndrome) may sharply limit use of the stimulation approach and reduce treatment to a short-term program aimed at improving comprehension, counseling of the patient and family, and preventing withdrawal and depression (Schuell, 1969). Variations of the approach as a function of severity will be discussed in more detail later.

Relative to Associated but Non-Aphasic Communicative Deficits

The stimulation approach attempts to improve language or reduce the functional handicap imposed by the disruption of language processes. It is not intended to remediate problems that often co-exist with aphasia, such as perceptual deficits,

apraxia of speech, or dysarthrias; such deficits may interfere with communication but do not disturb language per se. When present, they require treatment that differs significantly from the stimulation approach used therapy for the aphasia. The treatment of concomitant non-aphasic deficits may be secondary to, take precedence over, or coincide with therapy for aphasia. Although non-aphasic deficits often places limits on the application of the stimulation approach and the expected outcome of therapy for aphasia, their presence does not necessarily preclude use of the stimulation approach to treat the aphasia; nor does the presence of aphasia and use of the stimulation approach for its treatment necessarily preclude the use of other approaches to treat the non-aphasic deficits.

Philosophical Underpinnings

Before discussing the general principles and design of intervention, a brief summary of the general philosophy underlying the stimulation approach is in order. This philosophy should temper any desire on the part of the reader for a rigid, universal approach to treatment.

First, Schuell and colleagues (1964) stated, "We believe in a general philosophy of treatment, but not an arbitrary method. There is no room for rigidity in clinical practice . . . If the method leaves the patient behind, or if a patient outstrips the method, the method must be altered" (p. 332). Schuell believed that the main objective of treatment is to increase communication and that techniques merely assist in achieving that end. Therefore, methods should be flexible enough to be discarded if they are not working.

Second, diagnosis is a crucial part of the therapeutic process. That is, treatment must not proceed without some knowledge of the patient's assets and liabilities in each modality and some information about why performance breaks down when it does. Only with such information do we know what to work on and where to begin.

Third, treatment must be relevant. The neurologic, linguistic, and social needs and interests of the patient need to be considered and used (Schuell et al., 1964; Wepman, 1953, 1968). Not only do such considerations reflect the clinician's personal sensitivity, they also help to identify motivating material and pinpoint stimuli that may have very strong associational linkages in the patient's brain. Using stimuli and focusing treatment on skills that have functional relevance to the patient have been demonstrated to show greater gains in restoration of skills and/or increased use of compensatory strategies in individuals with aphasia (Pulvermüller et al., 2001).

Finally, as stated earlier, treatment should be logically related to beliefs about the nature of aphasia. The stimulation approach includes no material to be taught and no student to learn a lost language. Instead, the stimulation approach involves a person whose communication ability may be improved with appropriate stimulation. Such a philosophy significantly affects the principles and conduct of therapy.

GENERAL PRINCIPLES OF REMEDIATION

The design of intervention used in the stimulation approach is based on a number of general principles, many of which were articulated by Schuell and colleagues (1964). A number of additional, very practical principles that also apply to the stimulation approach have been presented by Brookshire (1997). It should be noted that several of these principles are indigenous to good clinical practice, regardless of the specific approach used. They are addressed here because they have grown out of observations of patients treated with a general stimulation approach. Information pertinent to the validity of the applied principles will be presented when the design of intervention is discussed. The general principles derived from those discussed by Schuell and/or Brookshire are as follows:

1. Intensive auditory stimulation should be used. As noted earlier, this is the framework of the stimulation approach and is based on the primacy of the auditory modality in language processes and the notion that the auditory modality represents a key area of deficit in aphasia. The auditory modality need not be used exclusively. One modality may be used to reinforce another, and combined auditory and visual stimulation may be especially appropriate.

2. The stimulus must be adequate—that is, it must get into the brain. Therefore, it needs to be controlled, perhaps along a number of dimensions. The application of this principle may be highly dependent on baseline data and may involve considerable individualized pretreatment planning. Brookshire (1997) states that the difficulty of tasks should match the level at which patients are working or be just below maximum performance level (i.e., approximately 60% to 80% prompt and correct responses, and task difficulty is increased when prompt correct responses exceed 90% to 95% accuracy).

3. Repetitive sensory stimulation should be used. Auditory material that is ineffective as a single stimulus may become effective after it is repeated a number of times.

4. Each stimulus should elicit a response. This is the only way we can assess the adequacy of stimulation, and it provides important feedback that both the patient and the clinician may use to modify future stimuli and responses.

5. Responses should be elicited, not forced or corrected. If a stimulus is adequate, there will be a response. If a response is not elicited, the stimulus was not adequate.

What the patient needs in such cases is more stimulation, not correction or information about why a response was inadequate.

6. A maximum number of responses should be elicited. A large number of adequate responses indicate that a large number of adequate stimuli have been presented. Numerous responses also provide frequent feedback and reinforcement of language and help to increase confidence and language attempts outside the treatment setting.

7. Feedback about response accuracy should be provided when such feedback appears to be beneficial, and such feedback should show patients their progress. The necessity for feedback may vary from patient to patient, but it is generally advisable. Showing patients their progress may be motivating, reinforcing, and extremely helpful in "proving" that progress is, in fact, taking place or that different approaches or termination of treatment should be considered.

8. The clinician should work systematically and intensively. Treatment requires a sequenced plan of action. It should be implemented often enough to meet the patient's needs, taking into account their overall condition and prognosis for recovery.

9. Sessions should begin with relatively easy, familiar tasks. This allows an adjustment and "warm-up" time, and it enables the patient to proceed to more difficult activities after experiencing success.

10. Abundant and varied materials (Schuell et al., 1955) that are simple and relevant to the patient's deficits should be used. Treatment does not involve the learning of vocabulary or rules, so content need not be limited to "items-to-be-learned." As Wepman (1953) indicated, the specific content of treatment is not as important as the manner in which the treatment is conducted. A variety of material also reduces the frustration often induced by drills on a small amount of material.

11. New materials and procedures should be extensions of familiar materials and procedures. This allows the patient to concentrate on language processing and minimizes the possible disruptive effects of new material and response demands.

DESIGN OF INTERVENTION

In this section, those factors that must be considered in developing a treatment program will be considered. Because the most important component of the stimulation approach is, by definition, the stimulation provided to the patient, those variables that are potentially most important to structuring stimulation will receive primary emphasis. Response demands, feedback, and the sequencing of treatment steps also will be discussed. The reader is cautioned, however, that the recommendations offered here for implementing the stimulation approach are based on rather broad generalizations derived from a potpourri of research and observation of heterogeneous groups and individual patients. Consequently, few, if any, of the recommendations can be assumed to apply effectively to all patients with aphasia.

Structure of Stimulation

A great deal of information has been acquired about stimulus variables that may affect the performance of patients with aphasia. Such data are largely the result of basic clinical and experimental research and are not primarily derived from specific treatment studies. Nonetheless, the data are invaluable to the clinician who must decide how to make stimulation adequate and effective during treatment. As Holland (1975) and Tikofsky (1968) have suggested, one strategy for designing treatment is to follow leads provided from research by turning the experimental techniques designed to isolate a particular problem into potential treatment tasks. Nowhere in the aphasiology literature are there so many "leads" as in the area related to stimulus variables that affect performance, and these leads have at least three practical applications to patient management. First, knowledge about stimulus manipulations that may maximize performance can be used to ensure that a patient is working at a level where "failure" is minimized. Second, and conversely, knowledge about stimulus manipulations can be applied in the opposite direction to challenge mildly impaired patients or those who respond without difficulty to tasks designed to maximize performance. Third, many of the factors to be discussed may be useful when counseling people in the patient's environment who need information about how best to communicate with the patient in everyday interactions.

The following discussion represents a review of the variables most relevant to the structuring of stimulation.

Auditory Perceptual Clarity (Volume and Noise)

Although Schuell and colleagues (1964) suggested that most patients prefer to hear speech at conversational levels, those authors indicated that an increase in volume (not shouting!) is sometimes desirable. Only a few controlled studies, however, have been conducted to evaluate the effects of increasing volume on auditory comprehension.

Glaser, Stoioff, and Weidner (1974) found that auditory comprehension of persons with aphasia under sound field conditions at the conversational level was superior to comprehension under earphones (binaurally and monaurally) at 25 dB above the conversational level. Because of the interaction between volume level and earphone/sound field methods of presentation, the results are difficult to interpret, but they do suggest that increasing volume above the normal levels does not facilitate comprehension.

McNeil, Darley, Rose, and Olsen (1979a) found no significant improvement in a group of 10 patients with aphasia on a word discrimination and word sequencing task or on portions of the Revised Token Test (McNeil and Prescott, 1978) when stimuli were presented under earphones at 75, 85, and 100 dB sound pressure level (SPL). Group data were representative of individual performance. The authors concluded that simple increases in stimulus intensity do not improve the auditory comprehension of patients with aphasia.

Although little evidence supports increasing the volume of auditory stimulation, reducing noise or increasing the signal/noise ratio does appear to be beneficial. Patients with aphasia often complain about the negative effects of noise on performance (Rolnick & Hoops, 1969; Skelly, 1975). Although Birch and Lee (1955) found that a binaural masking tone improved the naming and reading performance of patients with aphasia, other investigators have not concurred. Weinstein (1959), Wertz and Porch (1970), Schuell and colleagues (1964), and Siegenthaler and Goldstein (1967) found either no difference in performance accuracy in quiet versus noise or found noise to have a detrimental effect on performance on language tasks. Darley (1976) concluded from a review of such studies that "background noise apparently reduces the efficiency of the patient's performance" (p. 4).

These studies suggest that reducing noise or working in quiet generally facilitates language performance. Simply increasing loudness, on the other hand, does not appear to be useful, although such an increase may enhance performance in isolated cases. Many clinicians feel confident in advising patients' families that verbal comprehension is typically better in quiet than in the presence of a variety of distracting or competing auditory stimuli (e.g., television, radio, or background conversation).

Nonlinquistic Visuoperceptual Clarity (Dimensionality, Size, Color, Context, Ambiguity, and Operativity)

Visual materials are often used as an integral part of the stimuli to which patients are asked to respond. The importance of visual stimulation, in fact, led Eisenson (1973, p. 162) to call Schuell's stimulation approach to treatment a "visual-auditory" approach. Clinical observations suggest that the properties of visual stimuli may influence responses, and the importance of the visual modality to language behavior in general has led to the investigation of visual redundancy as a potential factor influencing linguistic processing in aphasia.

In a study of 21 patients with severe verbal comprehension deficits, Helm-Estabrooks (1981) compared performance on a single-word comprehension task in which stimulus conditions consisted of line drawings, each on individual cards arranged in rows; smaller line drawings of items, all on a single page; and real objects around the room. For the group as a whole, picture-pointing was superior to identification of objects around the room, but no differences were found between the two picture conditions. Not all patients followed the group pattern, however. Helm-Estabrooks concluded that auditory comprehension can be influenced by variables extrinsic to central auditory processing, such as visual search skills. The posteroinferior frontal gyrus has been demonstrated to be involved in the execution of visual search activities (Manjaly et al., 2005). Given that individuals with Broca's aphasia often present with lesions in this area, these findings support Schuell's notion that the properties of visual stimuli may influence responses during treatment.

Bisiach (1966) compared the naming performance of nine subjects with aphasia in response to pictures of realistically colored objects, line drawings of the same objects, and the same line drawings with superimposed curved or jagged lines. Although no differences were found among stimulus conditions for object recognition, subjects' naming of the realistically colored pictures was 15% to 18% more accurate than their naming of line drawings and of distorted line drawings. The visual redundancy of the realistically colored drawings was felt to facilitate naming.

Benton, Smith, and Lang (1972) examined the naming performance of 18 persons with aphasia in response to real objects, large line drawings, and small line drawings. Accuracy of real object naming was superior to that for small line drawings; accuracy for large line drawings fell between the two. The redundancy provided by three-dimensionality was felt to enhance the conceptual associations underlying word retrieval. Because of the relatively small differences between conditions, however, the authors questioned the clinical significance of their results. The possible insignificance of three-dimensionality was supported by Corlew and Nation (1975), who found no differences in the performance of 14 persons with aphasia when they named the 10 common, real objects used in the Porch Index of Communicative Ability (Porch, 1967), or PICA, than when they named reduced-size line drawings of the same objects.

In a theoretically interesting study, Whitehouse and Caramazza (1978) compared the ability of 10 persons with aphasia to identify line drawings of three objects (a cup, a bowl, and a glass) varying in physical features such as height and width. Stimuli consisted of prototypes (unambiguous representations) of the three objects as well as drawings in which the height-width dimensions were varied to make the perceptual distinction among the objects "fuzzy." In addition, some of the drawings had a handle, and some did not. Context (functional information) was also varied by presenting stimuli either alone or in context with a coffee pot, a cereal box, or a water pitcher. Subjects "named" the pictures by selecting from multiple-choice presentations of the names of the three objects. Results were not uniform across subjects. Those with a diagnosis of Broca's aphasia performed similarly to normal control subjects in their use of context and in their ability to deal with fuzzy perceptual boundaries. Patients with a diagnosis of anomic aphasia, however, had difficulty integrating and using perceptual and functional cues (dimension and context). These findings, along with those of Caramazza, Berndt, and Brownell (1982), have led to the conclusion that, for some patients, naming difficulty is related to an inability to organize adequately the concepts underlying word meaning in terms of functional and perceptual information, as opposed to difficulty with retrieval of an adequately perceived/conceived lexical item. Although the implications of these findings for clinical practice are neither clear-cut nor universal, it appears that the perceptual characteristics of visual stimuli should be as unambiguous as possible for all patients. Placing a target object in a redundant conceptual setting (e.g., pairing a cup with a coffee pot) may enhance word retrieval when the target is perceptually ambiguous. When pairing a target stimulus with other visual stimuli, however, the additional stimuli should never introduce ambiguity about the nature of the target.

The findings of Gardner (1973) suggest that the number of modalities in which associations may be evoked should be considered when selecting visual materials for treatment. He compared naming pictures of "operative" objects (discrete, firm to the touch, and available to several modalities [e.g., "rock"]) to "figurative" objects (not operative [e.g., "cloud"]), while accounting for the effects of picturability and word frequency. Most patients with aphasia performed more accurately in response to the operative items, and the effects of operativity were most pronounced for patients with difficulty initiating speech. Gardner argued that operative items were superior because they aroused associations in several modalities, whereas the figurative items were limited to visual associations. This perspective is supported by findings of Nickels and Howard (1995), who noted that operativity and imageability (i.e., how easy it is to create a visual or auditory image of the referent) were predictive of naming performance for some individuals with aphasia. The implication for treatment, therefore, is that visual stimuli which also may trigger auditory, tactile, kinesthetic, or olfactory associations are potentially more effective in aiding word retrieval than stimuli which trigger only visual associations.

To summarize, although some data suggest that some properties of visual stimuli are relatively unimportant to the performance of individuals with aphasia, the clarity and redundancy of visual stimuli do not seem to influence linguistic processing (Caramazza and Berndt, 1978). Darley (1976) recommends that we "play safe" and use the redundant and realistic stimuli in treatment. The most potent visual stimuli appear to be characterized by three-dimensionality, color, redundant physical properties, operativity, and a lack of ambiguity in perceptual characteristics and context.

Linguistic Visuoperceptual Clarity (Size and Form)

Few data suggest that the size or form of reading material affects comprehension, but some clinical observations are relevant. Rolnick and Hoops (1969) reported that patients with aphasia complain about small print for word and sentence stimuli and prefer large print—even when visual field deficits are not present. McDearmon and Potter (1975) observed varying preferences for upper-case, lower-case, or script stimuli. Schuell and colleagues (1955) recommended upper-case print for patients with visual impairments and felt that script should not be introduced until the patient's reading rate for printed material is normal.

Boone and Friedman (1976) examined single-word reading comprehension in response to cursive versus manuscript stimuli in 30 patients with aphasia, and Williams (1984) investigated the same factors' influence on the word and sentence comprehension of 20 patients. Neither study found significant differences between the two written forms. Williams, however, observed that two of her patients reliably responded better to manuscript than to cursive.

No compelling evidence suggests that the size and form of written input are powerful stimulus factors affecting reading comprehension. When providing reading material for patients, however, the clinician should be aware of a general preference for large print and potential idiosyncratic preferences for upper-case, lower-case, cursive, or manuscript format.

Method of Delivery of Auditory Stimulation

Many clinicians have speculated about ways to improve the delivery of auditory stimuli to patients. For example, are there better alternatives to live-voice, binaural, free-field stimulation?

The use of earphones is intuitively attractive because of its potential for reducing extraneous noise and focusing attention. Schuell and colleagues (1964), however, observed that patients usually prefer direct presentation to earphones, because they rely on more than auditory cues or, perhaps, because earphones produce distortions to which they are sensitive. The preference for free-field presentation is supported by the previously mentioned study of Glaser and colleagues (1974), who found that the comprehension under free-field conditions was superior to binaural as well as right- and left-ear monaural presentations through earphones. The superiority of the free-field condition was maintained even when the intensity of the earphone conditions was 25 dB greater than the intensity in the free-field.

It has been suggested that selective left-ear/right-hemisphere presentation of auditory stimuli may improve comprehension. Such speculation is based on the results of dichotic listening studies that have found a left-ear advantage for patients with aphasia (e.g., Johnson, Sommers, & Weidner, 1977; Sparks, Goodglass, & Nickel, 1970). LaPointe, Horner, and Lieberman (1977) examined the responses of patients with aphasia to portions of the Token Test (DeRenzi & Vignolo, 1962) when presented to the right ear, the left ear, or binaurally and found no significant differences among the three conditions. They concluded that selective monaural presentation of auditory stimuli is not a useful procedure. McNeil, Darley, Rose, and Olsen (1979b) examined the effects of selective binaural SPL variations in which stimuli were presented at 85 or 100 dB SPL to one ear while stimuli to the other ear were presented at 70 dB SPL. Although a trend toward better comprehension on some tasks was noted when the left ear was more intensely stimulated, their general conclusion was that the unilateral intensity increase is not a potent mechanism for improving auditory comprehension.

To date, the data indicate that response adequacy to free-field presentation is not exceeded when earphones are used and that selective stimulation of one ear/hemisphere does not surpass binaural stimulation. It should also be noted that the findings of Green and Boller (1974) and of Boller, Vrtunski, Patterson, and Kim (1979) suggest that live-voice presentation is superior to taped presentation of stimuli. Therefore, we have no compelling reason not to continue presenting auditory stimuli directly with live voice, binaurally, and in the free field.

Discriminability (Semantic, Auditory, Visual)

Verbal responses of patients with aphasia are often characterized by errors associated in meaning or experience. Such errors (e.g., "table" for "chair") are, in fact, the "best" errors a patient can make (Schuell and Jenkins, 1961a; Schuell et al., 1964). These characteristics suggest that response alternatives provided to patients should not promote semantic errors. This is particularly relevant for comprehension tasks, which require the patient to choose from among a set of alternatives (e.g., responding to a verbally and/or visually presented word or sentence by pointing to one of several choices). Assuring that response choices are unrelated semantically will often facilitate speed and accuracy of performance. Conversely, tasks can remain unchanged in nature but often can be made more difficult by introducing semantically related response choices (Duffy and Watkins, 1984; Pizzamiglio and Appicciafuoco, 1971).

Semantic discriminability among response choices is more important than visuoperceptual discriminability. This is illustrated by the findings of Chieffi, Carlomagno, Silveri, and Gainotti (1989). Their patients with aphasia made more errors on a single-word comprehension task when response choices were semantically related (e.g., banana, apple, and grapes) than when they were visually related (e.g., wheel, button, and lifebelt). Performance on a task in which response choices were both semantically and visually related (e.g., chair, bench, and stool) was poorer than in the semantically related condition, suggesting that semantic and perceptual effects may be cumulative, although the authors argued that the semantic demands of the combined semantic and visual task were more potent than the demands of the visual ones.

Difficulty discriminating between words with minimal phonemic differences (e.g., cake/take or horse/house) is an important aspect of auditory impairment in some patients (Schuell, 1973). In addition, patients with aphasia may confuse letters or words with similar visual configurations (e.g., E/F, p/b, or store/stone).

An investigation by Linebaugh (1986) sheds some light on the importance of semantic, auditory, and visual discriminability in single-word reading comprehension tasks. He presented a picture-to-written word matching task to 25 patients with aphasia under two conditions. In one, all three response foils (written words) were either semantically, auditorily, or visually related to the target response. In the other, the three foils consisted of one semantically, one auditorily, and one visually related word. When all foils were of the same type, the error rates were higher with visually than with auditorily related foils, with no differences among other foil comparisons. When foils contained one of each foil type, both semantic and visual errors were more frequent than auditory errors, with no differences between semantic and visual errors. Considerable variability was found among subjects in their patterns and degree of susceptibility to the semantic, visual, and auditory influences, with a minority of subjects making more than 50% of their errors in one category and only two subjects doing so in both experimental conditions. These findings suggest that semantic and visual discriminability, on average, are more potent than auditory discriminability in single-word reading tasks, but the power of each factor is seldom overwhelming in individual patients.

The discriminability factor apparently is also relevant to word retrieval tasks. The findings of Mills, Knox, Juola, and Salmon (1979), for example, have implications for the semantic distinctiveness of visual stimuli used in naming tasks. (They are also relevant to the information discussed under nonlinguistic visuoperceptual clarity.) These authors examined the effects of "uncertainty" on the naming performance of 10 patients with aphasia, with uncertainty being defined as "the number of equally probable binary choice decisions necessary to achieve a final name selection from one or several correct names available in the lexicon" (p. 75). For example, when shown a picture of a cup, most control subjects respond "cup"; few alternative responses are correct (i.e., little uncertainty). On the other hand, a picture of a country home in winter generates considerable uncertainty, because "winter . . . country," "cabin . . . house," and other

words would be reasonable responses, thus requiring a greater number of word retrieval decisions. The patients with aphasia made significantly more errors and had greater response latencies regarding high-uncertainty pictures than regarding low-uncertainty pictures, leading the authors to conclude that uncertainty affects naming performance in patients with aphasia. Their findings suggest that another way to simplify word retrieval on picture naming tasks is to select stimuli to which only a few alternative responses exist. Similarly, reducing the number of response alternatives reduces error probability on point-to comprehension tasks.

Finally, discriminability of task format is important to consider when evaluating a language deficit. To illustrate this point, Breese and Hillis (2004) examined the sensitivity of a word/picture verification task versus a word/picture identification task in identifying an auditory comprehension deficit in individuals with aphasia. For the word/picture verification task, subjects were asked if a picture corresponded to a spoken name—for example, a picture of knife with "Is this a fork?" For the word/picture identification task, subjects were asked to point to a named object in a set of four pictures. Results demonstrated that the word/picture verification task was more sensitive than the word/picture identification task for identifying impairments of auditory comprehension. Clinically, these findings suggest that greater discriminability of stimuli occur in verification tasks versus identification tasks when evaluating auditory comprehension deficits.

In summary, compelling data suggest that verbal comprehension tasks in which several response choices are offered can maximize performance if alternatives are semantically unrelated to the target response. The auditory and visuoperceptual "distinctiveness" of the target from response alternatives may also be important, with visual similarity generally being more important than auditory similarity on written-word comprehension tasks. Although considerable variability exists among patients in their responsiveness to these semantic, auditory, and visual influences, reducing the number of response choices on point-to tasks will usually lead to improved performance. In addition, picture verification tasks show greater sensitivity than point-to tasks in identifying auditory comprehension tasks.

Combining Sensory Modalities

Although the auditory modality is paramount in the stimulation approach, the use of several modalities in combination is often recommended. Schuell (1974b) indicated that various modalities should be used to reinforce one another and, in fact, felt that patients often do better when auditory and visual stimuli are combined. Schuell and Jenkins (1961a) reported that patients do better on single-word comprehension tasks when written and auditory stimuli are used instead of auditory stimuli alone.

Goodglass, Barton, and Kaplan (1968) examined the naming performance of 27 patients in response to auditory (characteristic sound associated with the target item), tactile, olfactory, and picture stimuli. They found a uniformity in performance across all modalities for the great majority of patients, although reaction times were fastest to visual stimuli. By extension, the work of Mills (1977) and Smithpeter (1976) suggest that combining some of those stimuli may enhance performance. Mills found that pairing an environmental sound (e.g., whinny) with a picture to be named (e.g., horse) facilitated naming performance over time, generalized to nondrilled words, and resulted in post-therapeutic improvement in naming without the auditory stimulus. Smithpeter reported that olfaction was effective in stimulating accurate language responses in some patients with aphasia when it preceded or accompanied other stimuli.

Caramazza and Berndt (1978) cite the work of North (1971), who found that the word recall of patients with aphasia improved when information was available through several sense modalities. North argued that various senses may contribute additively to word recall. The previously discussed findings of Gardner (1973) regarding operativity suggest that such additivity of multisensory stimulation need not be overt. That is, performance may be enhanced if visual stimuli, for example, are capable of "arousing" multisensory associations.

Combining the auditory and visual modalities is the most widely used form of multisensory stimulation, and a number of studies support the practice, although with some qualifications. Gardner and Brookshire (1972) found naming and single-word reading performance of eight patients with aphasia to be better during combined auditory and visual stimulation than during auditory or visual stimulation alone. By varying the order in which the stimulus conditions were presented, they also determined that combined stimulation facilitated performance during subsequent unisensory stimulus conditions. Analysis of single subject profiles indicated that combined stimulation may not be best for all patients, but these results generally supported the conclusion that combined stimulation is better than unisensory. They also suggest that combined auditory-visual stimulation should generally precede auditory or visual stimulation alone, at least during treatment tasks that require naming responses. Halpern (1965a, 1965b), reporting similar results, supported the concept of multisensory stimulation but noted that a multisensory approach sometimes can be distracting. Additional evidence related to multisensory stimulation may be derived from the study of electrophysiological activity in the brain during various stimulation activities. Moore (1996) investigated the hemispheric alpha asymmetries (through the use of electroencephalography) of normal male and female subjects and of male patients with aphasia during recall and recognition of high- and low-imagery words presented auditorily, visually, and in a multimodality (combined auditory and visual) condition. Results indicated that the subjects with aphasia demonstrated higher mean scores on the recall and recognition tasks during the multimodality condition than during either the visual or auditory condition alone. Further, for the subjects with aphasia, the multimodality stimulation appeared to activate the left hemisphere to a greater degree than either auditory or visual stimulation alone. Moore commented that "the multimodality stimulation appears to have facilitated the left hemisphere's participation in language processing, which may have contributed to increased language performance" (p. 683).

Auditory stimulation often involves some potentially useful visual input as well; for example, the patient's visual contact with the examiner may provide a number of facilitatory verbal or paralinguistic cues. Green and Boller (1974) found that the comprehension of severely impaired patients with aphasia was not as accurate or appropriate when stimuli were presented by tape or with the examiner behind the patient as when stimuli were presented face to face. Boller and colleagues (1979) confirmed the superiority of face-to-face presentation over the use of taped stimuli, and Lambrecht and Marshall (1983) showed that the comprehension of severely impaired patients was better when they looked and listened than when stimuli were simply heard. Whether the performance differences in these studies resulted from situational, extralinguistic, or additional visuoverbal input through lipreading is not clear. Such an interpretation is supported by recent studies of the contribution by visual sources of contextual information to speech perception. Records (1994) reported that, as auditory information became more ambiguous, individuals with aphasia and poor language comprehension made greater use of accompanying referential gestures to facilitate their understanding of verbal messages. Similarly, the successful application of therapy focused on auditory discrimination of minimal pairs at the phonemic level, using lipreading, has also been reported (Morris, Franklin, Ellis, Turner, & Bailey, 1996). Regardless, it seems that having the visual and auditory attention of the patient during the presentation of verbal material is important. Other combinations of sensory input have been noted to be facilitative as well. For example, Lott, Friedman, and Linebaugh (1994) successfully paired tactile-kinesthetic cues (i.e., tracing letters on the palm of the hand) with visual cues to improve the reading skills of an individual with aphasia and alexia.

Recent studies have investigated computer-administered auditory and visual stimulation for the treatment of anomia. The results of these studies are consistent and indicate that incorporating computers into stimulation treatments facilitate naming skills (Adrian, Gonzalez, & Buiza, 2003; Pedersen, Vinter, & Olsen, 2001). Other promising approaches have included combining verbal and gestural treatments (Rose & Douglas, 2001; Rose, Douglas, & Matyas, 2002).

To summarize, providing multimodality stimulation can improve response adequacy for many patients with aphasia, and combining auditory and visual stimulation may be the best and most practical way of doing so. Combined auditory and visual stimulation may facilitate responses to subsequent unisensory stimuli and, therefore, may be employed first when responses to unisensory stimulation are deficient to a significant degree. Other modalities, such as the tactile, or use of a computer may also be helpful. It seems that the effectiveness of multimodality stimulation stems from the redundancy of the information that it provides and the additional associations it might help to trigger. This appears to be desirable for many patients, although the clinician needs to be sure that such multiple inputs improve performance and do not, somehow, overload or exceed the capacity of the patient to use them effectively.

Stimulus Repetition

Repetitive sensory stimulation is a principle of treatment espoused by Schuell and colleagues (1964). They recommended, for example, that, on word recognition or repetition tasks, as many as 20 repetitions of a stimulus word might be appropriate or necessary before eliciting a response. Few studies, however, have directly examined the effects of repetitive stimulation on language comprehension or expression in patients with aphasia.

Helmick and Wipplinger (1975) examined naming behavior in one patient with aphasia under a no-treatment and two treatment conditions, with each condition containing different target words. In a minimal stimulus condition, six "stimulations" (including verbal identification, contextual cue, picture identification/discrimination, tracing, and copying) were provided before eliciting a naming response. In the maximum stimulus condition, the six stimulations were repeated four times for each word. Both conditions were more effective than the no-treatment condition, but no differences were found between the results obtained from minimum and maximum stimulation. The authors concluded that a relatively small amount of stimulation can be as effective as a great deal of stimulation.

LaPointe, Rothi, and Campanella (1978) evaluated the effects of two methods of repetition of Token Test commands on the auditory comprehension of 12 patients with aphasia. In one condition, stimulus repetitions of commands preceded responses; in the other, repetition occurred only following incorrect responses. When items were repeated following failure (to a ceiling of four repetitions of the original stimulus), significant improvement occurred in response to the first and second repetitions, and further but nonsignificant gains were noted for the third and fourth repetitions. In numeric terms, accuracy was 24% without repetition, which rose to 58% after repetition to ceiling level. Degree of language impairment was negatively correlated with gains from repetition. In contrast, when items were presented two or four times before a response, no significant

group gains over the no-repetition condition were noted. However, some individual subject differences were noted. One subject did "remarkably poorer" when commands were repeated before responses, and another apparently benefited from the preresponse repetition.

Contextual priming, a relatively new concept in treating word retrieval deficits, also incorporates stimulus repetition into its procedures. Contextual priming combines "massed repetition of picture names with context effects, by training pictures in small sets that are related in some way semantically or phonologically" (Martin, Fink, & Laine, 2004, p. 458). During treatment, blocks of stimuli are formed—for example, one group of stimuli that is semantically related, one group that is phonologically related, and one group that is unrelated. In a session, the subject is required to name each item in a block using a massed practice priniciple—that is, rapid and repetitive stimulation to one class of related pictures. Each block of related stimuli is presented in every session, and the accuracy of performance is recorded. Several recent studies examining the effectiveness of contextual priming have noted that not only was exposure to related stimuli beneficial in realizing treatment gains, the massed practice of each block of stimuli provided further substantial gains in naming skills (Cornelissen et al., 2003, Martin, Fink, & Laine, 2004; Martin, Fink, Laine, & Ayala, 2004; Martin & Laine, 2000, Renvall, Laine, Laakso, & Martin, 2003).

Another relatively new treatment approach that uses stimulus repetition is constraint-induced language treatment, the key principles of which include: (1) massed practice in an enriched, therapeutic, and communicatively relevant environment; (2) constraint of other communication modalities; and (3) forced use of spoken language through the application of visual barriers. Massed practice involves repetitive stimulation provided by the clinician, and the subject is required to practice a new or previously acquired language skill for several hours on a daily basis. During the period of massed practice on a variety of communication tasks, the subject is prevented from using either alternative modalities of communication, such as gesture, or other communicative compensatory strategies, such as circumlocution. Complementary studies have found that both constraining a language modality and requiring massed practice of a language behavior effected positive gains in language functions for individuals with chronic aphasia (Maher et al., 2003; Pulvermüller et al., 2001; Hinckley & Carr, 2005). Further research is required, however, to tease out the individual effects of massed practice and constraint during functionally relevant treatment.

As described above, recent research seems to support the use of numerous repetitions of stimulation as a general principle of therapy for aphasia. Earlier studies identified some individuals who responded differently to preresponse repetitive stimulation, with some benefiting and others deteriorating. In contrast, repetition of stimuli subsequent to errors generally does appear to increase adequate responses, with maximum benefits being derived from the first or second repetition.

Rate and Pause

It has been suggested that slowing speech rate may aid in auditory comprehension (Schuell et al., 1964) and that this is something experienced clinicians apparently are aware of subconsciously. Salvatore, Strait, and Brookshire (1978) reported that experienced clinicians give Token Test commands more slowly than their inexperienced colleagues by inserting more pause time within commands. They also found that experienced clinicians tend to slow their presentation rate when repeating commands that previously had generated error responses. Such clinician behavior obviously is not desirable during standardized diagnostic testing and some baseline procedures, but it does offer indirect support for the facilitating effect of rate reduction on verbal comprehension.

Gardner, Albert, and Weintraub (1975) examined sentence comprehension in 46 patients with aphasia and comprehension problems ranging from mild to severe. They reported improvement in comprehension—independent of the form of aphasia—when sentences were spoken at a rate of one word per second. They recommended that, when proceeding from single-word to sentence stimuli, words should initially be enunciated slowly."

Weidner and Lasky (1976) found improved performance in a group of 20 patients with aphasia on four measures of auditory comprehension when the presentation rate was reduced from 150 words per minute (wpm) to 110 wpm. Differences between the two rate conditions were greatest for patients scoring above the 50th percentile on the PICA. Similarly, Poeck and Pietron (1981) induced an 11% to 12% improvement in Token Test scores of a group of 42 patients with aphasia through electronically expanding the speech rate by 25%. Pashek and Brookshire (1982) extended these findings by showing that reducing the rate from 150 wpm to 120 wpm facilitated paragraph comprehension in a group of 20 patients; performance was facilitated in those with poor as well as those with good sentence-level comprehension.

The facilitative effect of reduced rate also has been demonstrated for a patient with aphasia and severe auditory imperception (Albert & Bear, 1974). The authors found that the patient's comprehension improved dramatically when rate was slowed to a third of the normal rate or less.

Liles and Brookshire (1975) examined the comprehension of 20 patients when 5-second pauses were inserted into various portions of Token Test commands. The insertion of pauses facilitated comprehension for many of their patients. Patterns of patient performance led the authors to hypothesize that the pauses aided in the processing of strings of lexical items but not in the processing of syntactic components. In contrast, Hageman and Lewis (1983) inserted 2-second pauses at major within-sentence breaks of the Revised Token Test and failed to find qualitative or quantitative performance differences compared to a no-pause condition. They suggested that a 2-second pause may not be long enough to facilitate performance.

Salvatore (1976) reported a facilitation of comprehension for a patient with aphasia when 4-second pauses were inserted into Token Test commands. By gradually fading the pause duration, it was also possible to maintain improved comprehension with 2-second and, sometimes, only 1-second pauses. Although no generalization to nonpause stimulation was found, the results do suggest that pause time can be faded, to some degree, while maintaining high levels of comprehension.

Are the effects of rate reduction and pause insertion cumulative? Lasky, Weidner, and Johnson (1976) examined the effects of rate reduction (120 wpm vs. 150 wpm) and the insertion of 1-second interphrase pauses on the sentence comprehension of 15 persons with aphasia. Comprehension improved when the rate was slowed or when the pauses were inserted, and the combination of reduced rate and interphrase pauses resulted in the best performance.

In an effort to examine how slowing rate facilitates comprehension, Blumstein, Katz, Goodglass, Shrier, and Dworetsky (1985) compared comprehension by patients with aphasia of sentences spoken at normal rates to (1) a vowel condition, in which vowel duration in each word was increased (140 wpm); (2) a word condition, in which silences were added between words (110 wpm); (3) a syntactic condition, in which silences were added at constituent phrase boundaries (90 wpm); and (4) a natural condition, in which sentences were read at a naturally slowed rate (110 wpm). In general, reducing rate had a relatively small facilitatory effect and was significant only for the syntactic condition and for patients with Wernicke's aphasia. The authors concluded that it may not be slowed rate per se that facilitated comprehension but, rather, the effect of a syntactically well-placed pause on the processing of preceding syntactic and semantic elements. Although this may be the case, the fact that the rate of the syntactic condition (90 wpm) was slower than any other slowed condition confounds the interpretation and leaves open the possibility that slowing rate to a comparable degree in other ways might also facilitate comprehension.

The positive effects of slowed rate may not be as robust for narrative discourse. Nicholas and Brookshire (1986a) examined narrative comprehension across two test sessions in patients with aphasia and relatively good and relatively poor comprehension; narratives were spoken at fast (190 wpm to 210 wpm) versus slow (110 wpm to 130 wpm) rates. Only the group with relatively poor comprehension benefited from rate reduction, and this held only for the first of the two test sessions. In addition, the facilitatory effect of slow rate was not present for all patients in the poor comprehension group. The authors concluded that the effect of slow rate was undependable and transitory, and they noted that variables with strong effects on comprehension at the sentence level may have only weak effects at the level of discourse.

To summarize, it appears that slowing rate and lengthening pauses at phrase boundaries can have a facilitatory effect on sentence comprehension. This effect is neither always present nor generally dramatic, and no consistent indications are found across studies that the ability to benefit from rate and pause modifications is tied to either type or severity of aphasia. The positive effects of slowing rate may be less consistent and pervasive at the level of discourse than at the sentence level. From the practical standpoint, however, it is reasonable to accept the advice of Nicholas and Brookshire (1986a) that "it seems reasonable to counsel those who speak with brain-damaged listeners to speak slowly, because slow speech rate does not affect most brain-damaged listeners negatively, and for some it may be beneficial, at least on some occasions" (p. 469).

Length and Redundancy

As previously stated, Schuell felt that reduced verbal retention span is a near-universal feature of aphasia. Although pervasive, she reported that retention deficits are highly reversible with the use of carefully controlled, intensive auditory stimulation characterized by gradual increases in stimulus length (Schuell, 1953a; Schuell et al., 1955).

The importance of stimulus length receives additional support from a number of sources, including patients themselves. Rolnick and Hoops (1969), interviewing several patients with mild aphasia, found numerous complaints about the processing and retention demands imposed by lengthy messages. Patients felt that reduced message length facilitated comprehension and retention.

In addition, numerous studies have demonstrated that, with other factors held constant, sentence comprehension tends to decrease as sentence length increases (e.g., Curtiss, Jackson, Kempler, Hanson, & Metter (1986); Shewan & Canter, 1971; Weidner & Lasky, 1976).

Although Goodglass, Gleason, and Hyde (1970) found that 52 patients with different classical forms of aphasia had varying degrees of success on a verbally presented retention span test, all patients were deficient to some degree. Albert (1976) examined the ability of 28 patients with aphasia on a short-term memory task in which they pointed to objects named serially by the examiner. The results of patients were inferior to those of control subjects and of patients with brain injury but without aphasia on total item retention and in retention of the accurate sequence of presentation. Response patterns indicated that sequencing problems increased as information load increased. Information load and sequencing deficits were both present regardless of the

clinical type of aphasia. The findings of Martin and Feher (1990) suggest that the degree of short-term memory limitation in aphasia affects semantic processing (i.e., sentences with a large number of content words) but is not strongly related to the processing of syntactic complexity. Finally, Gardner and colleagues (1975) found poorer comprehension when length increased from single words to nonredundant sentences containing the same single words.

Length appears to be an important factor in the visual as well as the auditory modality. Siegel's (1959) 31 patients with aphasia had more difficulty reading words of two or more syllables (six or more letters) than single-syllable words of less than five letters. Halpern (1965a, 1965b) compared verbal responses of 33 patients on tasks involving single-word repetition, reading single words, and reading single words with simultaneous auditory and visual stimulation. Stimuli in each task were either long (two or more syllables or six letters) or short (one syllable or less than four letters) and also varied as a function of abstraction level and part of speech. Results showed that long words resulted in more verbal errors—including preservation—compared with short words, regardless of the modality of presentation. Differences between errors on long and short words were greatest for the visual modality. On the basis of his findings, Halpern recommended that, for such tasks, auditory or auditory with visual stimulation should usually precede visual stimulation alone.

Going beyond the word level, Webb and Love (1983) examined the reading abilities of 35 patients with aphasia and found (1) more errors on sentence recognition than on letter or word recognition, (2) more errors on oral reading of sentences and paragraphs than of letters or words, and (3) more errors on paragraph comprehension than on sentence comprehension.

Friederici, Schoenle, and Goodglass (1981) have shown that word length also influences writing. In their group of 12 patients with aphasia, written accuracy was reduced by more than 50% as word length increased from one to three syllables. Increased word length (i.e., number of phonemes in the spoken word) has also been shown to negatively influence naming performance in some individuals with aphasia (Nickels & Howard, 1995).

Wepman and Jones (1961) found that verbal responses to words are easier than verbal responses to sentences whether stimuli are presented auditorily or visually. At the word level, verbal responses to written stimuli were better for one-syllable than for two-syllable words. On the other hand, verbal responses to auditorily presented words did not differ between one-syllable and two-syllable words. In contrast to the findings of Halpern (1965a, 1965b), these authors indicated that the length factor for sentence material is most pronounced for the auditory, not for the visual, modality. It is possible that the different results are caused by the fact that Halpern was dealing with variations of length within single words but Wepman and Jones were referring to differences between words and sentences. If so, this highlights the fact that differences in the processing and/or retention of words between modalities are not identical to differences in the processing and/or retention of sentences (and discourse) between modalities.

It is important to note that the detrimental effects of increasing message length may vary as a function of message redundancy. For example, the findings of Gardner and colleagues (1975) support the notion that patients with aphasia comprehend redundant sentences better than nonredundant sentences of equal length. Clark and Flowers (1987) demonstrated that increasing sentence redundancy facilitated comprehension even when redundant sentences were longer and syntactically more complex than nonredundant ones (e.g., sentences like "Which one is the book you read?" were easier than sentences like "Which one is the book?"). Also, the remarkable sensitivity of the Token Test to subtle deficits of comprehension is at least partially the result of the nonredundant properties of its verbal stimuli. Clearly, the potent effect of length strongly interacts with redundancy—the two factors can seldom, if ever, be considered separately. (Further discussion of this interaction can be found in the section on grammar and syntax.)

To summarize, there can be little doubt that controlling length at the word and the sentence levels is a potent stimulus factor for most or all patients with aphasia, and most clinicians discuss this factor when counseling families about their verbal input to the patient. Length is an influential factor regardless of whether stimuli are auditory, visual, or auditory and visual. In the visual modality, reducing length at both the word and the sentence levels can be expected to facilitate comprehension. For auditory input, length may be relatively unimportant at the word level, but it becomes highly important when proceeding from the word to the phrase to the sentence level. When controlling length, it seems that nonredundant components are the most crucial elements to control, because increases in message redundancy may limit or even overcome the generally negative effects of increases in message length. This may be particularly true at the levels of paragraph and narrative discourse (to be discussed in the section on context).

Cues, Prompts, and Prestimulation

It is well recognized that, under the right circumstances, the skillful clinician can employ a variety of techniques—often referred to as cues, prompts, or prestimulation—that will facilitate a patient's word retrieval or comprehension. Such techniques are often used following an inadequate response to a less powerful stimulus. When less powerful stimuli are consistently incapable of generating a high proportion of adequate responses, however, the cue (prompt or prestimulus) may become a distinct treatment condition to which

acceptable responses must be generated before proceeding to the less powerful stimuli. In this section, a number of potentially useful cues that have not been covered already under other headings will be discussed.

McDearmon and Potter (1975) offered a number of suggestions regarding representational prompts, which they defined as symbolic or realistic cues that directly suggest the concept being referred to in a response. Prompts are strongly related to the concepts of stimulus redundancy and multimodality stimulation; they suggest that more than one representation of the response be presented and that one representation (i.e., the prompt) gradually be faded. For example, on naming tasks, pictures and their written names may be presented with resultant adequate responses. The written prompts may then be faded gradually by blocking out increasing portions of the word until that word is entirely eliminated. Some other suggested prompts not already implied under other headings include (a) tracing letters to facilitate letter recognition, (b) writing words to aid word retrieval, (c) pantomime or American-Indian sign to facilitate word retrieval, and (d) using pictures in conjunction with corresponding written words to facilitate reading.

Barton, Maruszewski, and Urrea (1969) examined word retrieval of 36 patients under three conditions: (1) picture naming, (2) sentence completion (e.g., "You clean teeth with a _____."), and (3) object description. In order, the most powerful cues were sentence completion, picture naming, and object description. It is important to note, however, that 44% of the subjects in their study did not follow the group's ordering of responses to the three naming conditions. This highlights the importance of examining the individual patient's responsiveness to stimulus cues; a powerful cue for one patient may not be as powerful for another. Along these lines, Marshall and Tompkins (1982) as well as Golper and Rau (1983) point out that careful analysis of individual patient strategies may provide clues about the best cues for the clinician to provide during therapy. Such information may also be used to increase the patient's own use of successful cues.

Freed, Marshall, and Nippold (1995) examined two cueing techniques with 30 individuals having mild to moderate aphasia in associative learning tasks. Real English words were paired with black-and-white, abstract symbols, and subjects were required to label each symbol. During the task, subjects were given either their own previously elicited associations for the word-symbol pairs (personalized cues) or associations developed by the examiner (provided cues). Results indicated that both cueing techniques were equal in terms of yielding correct responses. The authors observed that subjects in the "provided cue" condition were given complete rationales for why the cues were used; thus, the provided cues may have inadvertently become similar to the personalized cues. Freed and colleagues concluded that both the provided and the personalized cues contained components that might be beneficial to include in a treatment protocol for word retrieval deficits.

Linebaugh and Lehner (1977) have described a cueing program for word retrieval that is based on two principles: (1) that recovery is best served by eliciting the desired response with a minimal cue, and (2) that when a cue is successful, continued elicitation of the appropriate response with less powerful cues is reinforcing and conducive to stimulating the processes underlying word retrieval. When a patient is unable to name a pictured object, the following cues, in order, are given until an adequate response is elicited: (1) directions to state the object's function, (2) statement of the function, (3) statement and demonstratation of the function, (4) sentence completion, (5) sentence completion plus the silently articulated first phoneme of the response, (6) sentence completion plus the vocalized first sound, (7) sentence completion plus the first two phonemes vocalized, and (8) word repetition. When an adequate response is elicited, the order of cues is reversed until the patient names the picture without a cue. Linebaugh and Lehner presented data for several patients that demonstrate improved word retrieval and generalization to nontreatment words. Importantly, they indicate that cueing hierarchies must be individually determined.

The effectiveness of personalized cues and self-cues in naming tasks has been investigated in two recent studies. In the first, the nature of information contained in personalized cues for naming of subordiante categories was examined. Personalized cues were elicited from 15 individuals without brain damage and 15 individuals with aphasia and evaluated to determine if the cues facilitated learning of unknown dog breeds. Five different types of cues were identified and evaluated for their faciliatory effect. Results revealed that cues containing semantic information led to greater accuracy of naming for the individuals with aphasia (Marshall, Karow, Freed, & Babcock, 2002). In a related study on treatment of naming deficits, individuals with chronic aphasia were required to generate self-cues characterized by either partial written word information or tactile cues. Results revealed improvements in naming of target items with generalization to performance on standardized language measures (DeDe, Parris, & Waters, 2003). The results of both studies support the value of personalized and self-generated cues in naming tasks.

A facilitatory effect of semantic cues also seems to exist for online tasks (i.e., tasks in which the cues are not necessarily obvious to the patient). Chenery, Ingram, and Murdock (1990) studied the ability of patients to recognize whether the second word in a pair of verbally presented words was real or nonsense when the first word was functionally related to the target (e.g., eat-knife), superordinally associated (e.g., cutlery-knife), unrelated (e.g., door-knife), or nonsense (e.g., lamiel-knife). Subjects were told to ignore the first word. All subjects with aphasia, including a subgroup with severe comprehension and naming deficits, more accurately identified words as being real in response to the functional and superordinate semantic

primes than in the other priming conditions. This led to a conclusion that information is preserved in semantic memory in patients with aphasia. (This online facilitation of semantic processing may partially explain why redundancy can facilitate sentence comprehension.) In a related study, Leonard and Baum (1997) noted faster responses to words preceded by primes that were both phonologically and orthographically related to the target word (i.e., words that shared both spelling and sound-syllable rhyme [e.g., "blood-flood"]) than those that were unrelated (e.g., "dish-room"). Phonologically related primes (i.e., word pairs that shared syllable rhymes but were orthographically unrelated [e.g., "seed-bead"]) alone did not facilitate reaction times, and responses were also slower relative to the primes that were orthographically, but not phonologically, related (i.e., word pairs that shared rhyme spelling but were pronounced differently [e.g., "tough-cough"]).

Podraza and Darley (1977) investigated the effects of three types of prestimulation on picture naming in five patients with aphasia. The prestimulus conditions (i.e., cues presented before picture presentation) included the first phoneme of the target word, an open-ended sentence (three words, one of which was the target word), and three semantically related words. Naming was generally facilitated by the phoneme, open-ended sentences, and three words containing the target word cues, whereas performance decrements occurred for the three semantically related word cues. The facilitative failure of the semantically related word cues is in disagreement with the findings of Weigl (1968) and of Blumstein, Milberg, and Shrier (1982) that such cues may serve a "deblocking function" and facilitate retrieval. Podraza and Darley suggest that their own patients may already have been operating in the appropriate "semantic field" (Goodglass and Baker, 1976, p. 361) and that additional stimuli in that field may have served to confuse the selection of an appropriate response. Similarly, patients with Wernicke's aphasia, who frequently make phonemic errors, benefit less from phonemic cues than patients with other types of aphasia (Kohn and Goodglass, 1985).

Breen and Warrington (1994) have also compared a variety of cues in an individual with severe anomia. Phonologic and semantic cues were noted to be far less facilitative, in a naming task, than were sentence frames (i.e., sentence completion). Further, neither picture frames, associated verbs, nor syntactically correct but semantically meaningless sentence frames were effective cues. The authors suggest that two modes of name retrieval may exist, one that uses a nominative system and one that employs an online language processor involved in propositional speech production. The latter system may account for the preservation of fluent speech in individuals with severe anomia. Similarly, sentence completion cues containing a semantically related word were noted to be more effective than semantically empty sentence frames (e.g., "This is a ____.") or semantic information alone (i.e., associated verbs) in facilitating naming performance in eight subjects with aphasia (McCall, Cox,

Shelton, & Weinrich, 1997). These findings were felt to support the notion that naming is enhanced most by a combination of syntactic and semantic variables.

Stimley and Noll (1991) examined naming accuracy in a group of patients with aphasia when pictures were accompanied by a semantic cue (e.g., "This is something you wear on your foot," for "sock") or a phonemic cue (e.g., "This is something that starts with /S/," for "sock"). Compared to a no-cue condition, the semantic and phonemic cues both facilitated naming, although the average effect was only on the order of 9% to 10%. The authors felt the small effect may have occurred because cues were presented for all items, not just following a failure to name without a cue. They also observed (as have others) that semantic errors were more frequent in the semantic cue condition and that phonemic errors were more frequent in the phonemic cue condition (Li & Canter, 1991, have made similar observations). Thus, although semantic and phonemic cues are generally facilitatory, they also tend to "move" errors toward the cueing category. Along similar lines Wambaugh and colleagues (2004) compared the effects of a phonological cueing treatment and a semantic cueing treatment. Results indicated that both treatments yielded positive increases in naming, with effects being similar across treatments. The authors concluded that both treatments have potential for facilitating action naming in aphasia.

Other recent investigations have examined the effects of only semantic cues on naming performance. Semantic feature analysis (SFA) is an elaborate cueing technique in which the client is encouraged to produce words semantically related to the target. For example, for the target word "pan," the cues might involve questions related to its use (cooking), its properties (metal, copper, and wooden handle), where it might be used (kitchen), what group it belongs to (cookware), and what might be associated with it (stove, spoons, ladles, and pots). SFA is thought to improve the retrieval of conceptual information by accessing semantic networks (Massaro & Tompkins, 1992). By activating the semantic network surrounding the target, the target itself should be activated above its "threshold" level, thus increasing the likelihood that its name can be retrieved. Results have consistently documented improved confrontational naming scores with the SFA technique for treated pictures as well as generalization to untreated pictures (Boyle & Coelho, 1995; Boyle, 2004; Coelho, McHugh, & Boyle, 2000; Lowell, Beeson, & Holland, 1995). Generalization to conversational speech, however, has either been quite modest (Coelho et al., 2000) or not observed at all (Boyle & Coelho, 1995). In a subsequent study, Conley and Coelho (2003) examined the effects of SFA in combination with Response Elaboration Training (RET) (Kearns, 1985) on word retrieval deficits for an individual with chronic Broca's aphasia. The combined SFA and RET treatment improved confrontation naming skills for the individual studied, but the results were equivocal in delineating the individual effects of each type of treatment.

Whether a semantic cue should be accompanied by the referent word has also been investigated (LeDorze, Boulay, Gadreau, & Brassard, 1994). Using a comprehension task format, two types of semantic cues were compared. In the first, the individuals with aphasia were to point to a picture (in a field of three pictures) of the referent word presented, then to match the written word to the corresponding picture, and then to answer a question about the referent word (e.g., "Does an organ have just one keyboard?" for the word "organ"). The other cueing procedure also involved three steps: The individuals with aphasia were to point to a picture of the referent word identified by a definition, then to match a written definition to the corresponding picture, and finally, to answer a yes/no question related to the referent word (e.g., "Does this mollusk have pincers?" for the word "lobster"). Results indicated that naming improved significantly when the semantic cues were accompanied by the referent word. The authors speculate that naming was facilitated because both word form and the word semantics were activated.

Some recent efforts have attempted to tailor the type of cue to the level at which naming tends to break down. Thompson, Raymer, and le Grand (1991) examined the effects of a phonemic cueing treatment program on two patients with Broca's aphasia whose naming deficits appeared to be related to phonologic breakdowns (e.g., they had naming difficulties despite being able to match spoken words to pictures and perform conceptual matching tasks; in other words, they appeared to have access to word meaning but not to the phonologic form of words). The program consisted primarily of providing a rhyming cue (e.g., "It sounds like mat" for the target "bat") or, if that failed, the first phoneme, whenever the patient failed to name without a cue. Both subjects improved in oral naming, and some generalization to untrained items and to oral reading tasks occurred. Li and Williams (1989) examined the effect of semantic and phonemic cues on noun and verb naming after failure to name on picture confrontation. Patients with Broca's and conduction aphasia responded better to phonemic than to semantic cues, and the opposite pattern occurred for patients with anomic aphasia. In general, phonemic cues were more effective than semantic cues for nouns, and the two cue types did not differ for verbs. This suggests that the effectiveness of cue type may vary both as a function of the source of naming failure (semantic vs. phonologic, presumably related to aphasia type) and of word category (nouns vs. verbs). (Li & Williams, 1990).

Are cues presented in combination more effective than single cues? The findings of Weidner and Jinks (1983) say yes. They examined the naming performance of 24 patients who were presented with single cues (e.g., sentence completion, written words, or first phoneme) or with cues in combination. Combined cues were more facilitative than single cues or single cues presented in succession. They suggest that if one cue fails, a combination of cues may help.

Finally, cueing also may facilitate sentence production. Roberts and Wertz (1986) used a contrastive task paradigm to facilitate sentence production in two patients with chronic aphasia. After demonstrating comprehension of sentence meaning, patients imitated the clinician production of a sentence (e.g., "The bed is made.") and then spontaneously produced a minimally contrasting sentence in response to a picture stimulus (e.g., "The bed is not made."). Imitation was then faded over additional steps to the point at which the patient had to produce on their own contrasting sentences in response to picture stimuli. The sentence production of both patients improved, and evidence of some carryover to spontaneous sentence production was found.

It is reasonable to conclude that a large number of cues, prompts, including computer-mediated approaches (Doesborgh, van de Sandt-Koenderman, Dippel, at al., 2004; Fink, Brecher, Sobel, et al., 2005) and preparatory stimuli exist that may facilitate language processing in patients with aphasia. Care must be taken to demonstrate the utility of cues in each case, because even the most widely used facilitators may not be effective for every patient. Careful analysis of the level at which language tends to break down (e.g., semantic vs. phonologic) and the types of successful cues that patients adopt spontaneously can help to identify the type of cueing that is likely to be most successful.

Frequency and Meaningfulness

It has been repeatedly established that the reduction of available vocabulary in patients with aphasia is related to the frequency of occurrence of words in the language. Schuell (1969, 1974d) also predicted a reduction of available linguistic rules and a hierarchy for their recovery, and Schuell speculated that the hierarchy is related to the frequency of occurrence of those structures in general or to individual language usage.

Schuell, Jenkins, and Landis (1961) tested the auditory comprehension of 48 patients with aphasia in response to four word lists varying in frequency of occurrence. Decrements in performance as a function of decreasing word frequency were found, supporting the conclusion that word frequency is an important factor in comprehension. They also reported that single-word comprehension improves in an orderly and predictable manner that is strongly related to word frequency. Relatedly, Gerratt and Jones (1987), in a reaction time task, have shown that individuals with aphasia, like individuals without aphasia, recognize words as real (vs. nonsense) more rapidly when they have multiple meanings and high frequency of occurrence than when they have few meanings and low frequency of occurrence. Finally, Hauk and Pulvermuller (2004) found lower evoked-response potential amplitudes for high-frequency versus low-frequency words, indicating physio-logical differences in the activation and processing of these different types of words.

Word frequency remains a factor at the sentence level. Shewan and Canter (1971) found that increasing vocabulary difficulty (reducing word frequency) reduced the accuracy and promptness of sentence comprehension in patients with aphasia. In addition, frequency of occurrence also applies to phrases and sentences when they occur as familiar units. For example, Van Lancker and Kempler (1987) have shown that patients with aphasia comprehend familiar phrases (idiomatic expressions, e.g., "While the cat's away, the mice will play.") more readily than novel sentences matched for word frequency, length, and structure.

Word frequency effects are also apparent in verbal output, reading, and writing. For example, Schuell and colleagues (1964), Gardner (1973), and Williams and Canter (1982) have reported negative correlations between errors on naming tests and frequency of occurrence. Siegel (1959) has found that less frequently occurring words were more difficult to read than frequently occurring words. Bricker, Schuell, and Jenkins (1964) reported that word frequency (and length) accounted for almost all aphasic spelling errors; and Santo Pietro and Rigrodsky (1982) found that verbal perseveration on naming and reading tasks increased as word frequency decreases.

In contrast to the notion that word frequency is an important factor in verbal expression, Nickels and Howard (1995) found small effects of word frequency on naming performance. Their series of experiments involved two groups of individuals having aphasia. The first group consisted of six fluent and six nonfluent individuals, and the second was made up of three nonfluent, two nonfluent with apraxia of speech, two with primarily apraxia of speech, and eight with fluent aphasia. The authors investigated the effect of eight variables on naming: (1) word age-of-acquisition, (2) operativity (i.e., figurative vs. operative), (3) frequency, (4) familiarity (i.e., based on a rating of how often one might see, hear, or use the referent word), (5) imageability (i.e., ease of creating visual or auditory image of referent), (6) concreteness (i.e., how accessible to sensory experience the subjects rated the referent word), (7) length (i.e., number phonemes in the spoken word), and (8) visual complexity (i.e., complex vs. simple, based on number of elements in stimulus picture). Results indicated a far less marked effect of frequency on naming when the effects of the other variables had been accounted for (i.e., by means of simultaneous multiple regression or discriminate analysis procedures). Further, because of intercorrelations between variables and the wide range of variables that have been found to affect naming performance in individuals with aphasia, these findings must be interpreted cautiously. The authors concluded that previously, the effects of frequency on naming have been overstated because of the confounding effect of other variables, such as length and imageability. Finally, the two groups of individuals with aphasia showed quite different patterns of predictor variables for naming performance, and the variables that affected an individual's performance was often different from those of the overall group, calling into question the applicability of conclusions drawn from group studies.

Although word frequency is certainly positively correlated among speakers of the language, we need to bear in mind that word frequency for individuals is determined by their unique experiences, needs, occupation, culture, and numerous other factors (e.g., the word "aphasia" is certainly more available to the speech-language pathologist than it is to the political scientist!). Although word lists such as that of Thorndike and Lorge (1944) are useful in selecting stimulus material, it is also important to identify verbal stimuli that are meaningful, relevant, and personally significant to the individual (Schuell, 1969; Schuell et al., 1955; Wepman, 1953).

The importance of this was demonstrated by Wallace and Canter (1985), who examined the responses of severely impaired patients with aphasia to personally relevant versus nonpersonal stimuli on verbal and reading comprehension tasks (e.g., "Is your birthday in _____" vs. "Is Christmas in February?"), repetition tasks (e.g., patient repeats their name vs. another name), and naming tasks (e.g., television vs. giraffe). Performance was better in response to personally relevant materials on all tasks, although the authors pointed out that personally relevant stimuli had a generally higher frequency of occurrence than nonpersonal material. Relatedly, Correia, Brookshire, and Nicholas (1989) asked if gender bias in pictures used to elicit narrative responses from male patients with aphasia affects what the patients say about them. After having subjects without aphasia identify picture stimuli as male or female biased (e.g., men working out in a gym vs. women in a beauty salon), these authors used the pictures to obtain narratives from aphasic and non-brain-damaged subjects. Subjects produced more words in response to male-biased stimuli, but no differences were found in measures of efficiency or amount of information conveyed. The authors concluded that gender bias in picture stimuli is not of great concern (at least for male subjects) unless the number of words in responses is important. Thus, some dimensions of personal relevance may or may not affect all dimensions of performance to the same, or to an important, degree.

The concept of meaningfulness is also tied to emotion and expectations. Reuterskiöld (1991) has demonstrated that patients with significant verbal comprehension deficits perform more adequately on single-word comprehension tasks when stimuli consist of objects and actions with emotional connotations (e.g., casket or kissing) than when they have no obvious emotional connotations (e.g., paper or typing). Graham, Holtzapple, and LaPointe (1987) examined the comprehension of patients with aphasia in response to contextually relevant commands (e.g., ring the bell), contextually neutral commands (e.g., touch the bell), and contextually inappropriate commands (e.g., roll the bell). Contextually related tasks were easier than neutral or inappropriate ones, leading the authors to state that "if we pair objects with actions that are most expected both in terms of meaning and structure, we facilitate comprehension" (p. 183). Finally, Deloche and Seron (1981) as well as Kudo (1984) have established that comprehension is better when sentence meaning does not violate our knowledge of the world (e.g., "The policeman arrests the thief.") than when the meaning is implausible or unlikely (e.g., "The thief arrests the policeman.").

Abstractness

It has been suggested that individuals with aphasia have more difficulty with abstract than with concrete words (Goldstein, 1948) and that these individuals categorize words in a relatively concrete emotional manner when compared to individuals without aphasia (Zurif, Caramazza, Myerson, & Calvin, 1974).

Two problems present themselves when the concept of abstractness arises. First, abstractness is strongly tied to—and difficult to separate from—frequency of occurrence (concrete words occur more frequently than abstract words). Spreen (1968), however, has pointed out that, even when frequency of occurrence is controlled, words scaled as abstract are not perceived or recalled as readily as words scaled as concrete. Halpern (1965a), controlling for frequency of occurrence, found that patients with aphasia made more verbal errors in response to written words of high or medium abstractness than in response to words of low abstractness. Abstractness did not, however, play a role in repetition of verbally presented stimuli.

The second problem is more relevant to stimulus selection and is related to the fact that "abstractness" is a difficult concept to define. Words, however, are scalable on an abstractness dimension (Darley, Sherman, & Siegal, 1959), and Spreen (1968) has suggested that the degree of abstractness can be related tangibly to sense experience (e.g., "book" is more concrete than "hope," because it presumably generates more multimodality associations).

The performance of patients with aphasia suggests that we should be aware of the abstractness factor when selecting and ordering stimulus material. Problems related to isolating and defining abstractness, however, present practical clinical problems. Fortunately, we probably account for most of the effects of abstractness when we account for the more easily defined concepts of word frequency and intersensory redundancy or operativity.

Part of Speech and Semantic Word Category

When word retrieval and comprehension abilities are examined or treated at the single-word level, a marked tendency exists for clinicians to focus on nouns, particularly object nouns. The evidence makes clear, however, that all parts of speech and word categories are typically affected in aphasia. This speaks against an object-noun orientation to treatment.

Kiran and Thompson (2003) investigated the role of semantic complexity in treating naming deficits in fluent individuals with aphasia. Subjects participated in a form of semantic feature treatment to improve naming of both typical and atypical exemplars within a semantic category. Training procedures were counterbalanced for whether typical versus atypical exemplars were trained first. Results revealed greater improvements in naming and generalization for those individuals who were trained on the atypical exemplars first versus the typical exemplars first.

Because different parts of speech (e.g., nouns vs. verbs) serve different linguistic functions, it seems possible that, for some patients or under some circumstances, they may present varying levels of difficulty. Consistent with this notion, recent research has demonstrated selective impairments in nouns versus verbs in some individuals with aphasia. For example, verb production has been noted to be more difficult than nouns for individuals with agrammatical aphasia, whereas nouns appear to be more problematic than verbs for some individuals with anomic aphasia (Marshall, Pring, & Chiat, 1988; Miceli, Silveri, Nocentini, & Caramaza, 1988; Miceli, Silveri, Villi, & Caramaza, 1984; Orpwood & Warrington, 1995; Saffran, Berndt, & Schwartz, 1989; Thompson, Shapiro, Li, & Schendel, 1994; Williams & Canter, 1987; Zingeser & Berndt, 1990). In addition, where a discrepancy exists between nouns and verbs on synonym-generating and sentence-generating tasks, the difference favors nouns over verbs (Kohn, Lorch, & Pearson, 1989). Finally, that the processing of nouns versus verbs can differ is also supported by the finding of Li and Canter (1991) that patients with aphasia responded better to phonemic than to semantic cues for noun naming, but that no difference existed between the cue types for verb naming. The authors felt that the greater concreteness, static nature, and imageability of nouns than verbs might explain some of the differences between them.

The observation that naming may be differentially impaired across semantic categories has led investigators to question whether verb production might also be differentially affected—that is, that certain types of verbs may be more difficult than others for some individuals. According to Thompson, Lange, Schneider, and Shapiro (1997), an important distinction among verbs pertains to their syntactic properties (i.e., the number and type of arguments or participant roles required by certain verbs). Like other classes of words, verbs are acquired and stored in memory on the basis of their phonologic form and lexical category. Verbs, however, are also represented in the lexicon by virtue of the sentence structures in which they occur. For example, the verb "wash" must always be followed by a noun phrase

and by a prepositional phrase. These rules of phrase structure are referred to as strict subcategorization and are related to, but separate from, argument structure. Argument structure pertains to meaning relations between the verb and constituents within a sentence (or the number of participant or thematic roles described by a verb). For example, the verb "wash" has two participant roles: an agent (someone doing the washing), and a theme (the thing being washed). The verb "put" has three roles: an agent (someone doing the putting), a theme (the thing that is put), and a location (the place where the thing is put). For certain verbs, all participant roles must be specified in sentence production for the sentence to be grammatical. Returning to the example of the verb "put," it is obligatory that all three of its arguments be represented when it is used, whereas for other verbs, some arguments are optional and do not need to be specified in the syntax. This is the case for the verb "eat", which can be produced with an agent only, as in "Tom ate," or with both its arguments, as in "Tom ate the corn." The critical issue is that the verb's lexical representation includes information about its argument structure and that the grammaticality of sentences and syntax is determined by these argument structures and their representation in the sentence (Thompson et al., 1997).

To investigate the type of verb deficits that occur in those with aphasia, Thompson and colleagues (1997) examined verb and verb argument structure production in 10 individuals with agrammatical aphasic and in 10 individuals without brain damage. Production of six types of verbs—obligatory one-place (verbs with only one external argument [e.g., "The boy smiles."]), obligatory two-place (verbs requiring both arguments [e.g., "The boy catches the ball."]), obligatory three-place (verbs that require three arguments [e.g., The girl gives the bone to the dog."]), optional two-place (verbs that require one external argument and a second optional argument [e.g., "The woman eats." and "The woman eats spaghetti."]), optional three-place (verbs that require an agent and theme but for which a third argument is optional [e.g., "The woman throws the stick." and "The woman throws the stick to the dog."]), and complement verbs (verbs that require external and internal arguments [e.g., "The girl knows the answer." and "The girl knows the cat is in the tree.")—were examined in confrontation and elicited labeling conditions. Results indicated that individuals with aphasia produced the obligatory one-place verbs correctly significantly more often than they did the three-place verbs. In addition, a consistent hierarchy of verb difficulty was found in both the confrontation and elicited conditions. Data indicated that argument structure properties of verbs are important dimensions of lexical organization and influence verb retrieval.

Differences may also exist for other word categories and tasks. Halpern (1965a) found that patients with aphasia made more errors when repeating or reading adjectives and verbs than they did with nouns. Siegel (1959) as well as Marshall and Newcombe (1966) reported similar findings for reading tasks. In contrast, Noll and Hoops (1967) did not find selective spelling difficulty among nouns, verbs, adjectives, and adverbs for a group of 25 patients, but they did find that pronouns, prepositions, and conjunctions were more difficult than other parts of speech. Finally, Goodglass and colleagues (1970) found different comprehension patterns among patients Broca's, Wernicke's, and anomic aphasia across measures of receptive vocabulary (nouns and verbs) and of comprehension of directional and grammatical prepositions.

It appears that the process of stimulus selection should consider possible differences among substantive word categories, such as nouns, verbs, and adjectives, with nouns likely to be easiest when word frequency is controlled. In general, the literature suggests that grammatical words, such as prepositions, conjunctions, and articles, are more difficult for patients with aphasia to comprehend than are substantive words (Lesser, 1978). The above findings suggest that both semantic categories and grammatical class are critical aspects of lexical organization. Such differences should be considered during stimulus selection.

The possibility that specific semantic word categories may be selectively impaired in aphasia is a matter of debate (Lesser, 1978, pp. 97–107), but some studies suggest that semantic word categories should be considered for some patients. For example, Goodglass, Klein, Carey, and Jones (1966) assessed the naming and comprehension of objects, actions, letters, numbers, and colors in patients with aphasia. Objects and actions were the easiest to comprehend and letters the most difficult, but objects were the most difficult to name and letters the easiest. This not only suggests differences among word categories but also implies that the difficulty of a particular category may vary between input and output tasks.

Although many investigators and clinicians argue convincingly against common or marked differences among semantic word categories, it does appear that stimuli restricted to a single semantic category (e.g., objects) occasionally may yield misleading diagnostic and treatment results. In addition, consideration of semantic category may lead to the identification of treatment stimuli with varying degrees of difficulty.

Grammar and Syntax

As noted earlier, Schuell hypothesized a hierarchically based reduction of available linguistic rules in aphasia. Her idea that such a hierarchy is based on the frequency of occurrence of grammatical structures in general language usage is untested and, perhaps, overly simplistic in light of current linguistic theory, but ample evidence suggests that grammatical complexity is an important factor in language activi-

ties. In other words, as for intact language users, a grammatical hierarchy of difficulty exists for patients with aphasia, with some grammatical structures being more difficult to comprehend and produce than others. Grammar and syntax therefore are important variables to consider when devising language stimuli. The following discussion is a sampling of the numerous studies that have examined the relationship between grammatical variations and performance in aphasia. (For more information on these factors, see Chapter 27 in this volume.)

The importance of grammar is illustrated by the fact that, even when lexical comprehension is quite good, sentence interpretation may be impaired because of grammatical processing deficits. Caramazza and Zurif (1976), for example, have shown that some patients have problems when sentence comprehension is dependent on syntax rather than on the logical relations expressed by individual semantic elements. To illustrate, the meaning of the semantically constrained sentence "The apple that the boy is eating is red" can be derived from an understanding of the meaning of its critical elements and the limited logical relationships among them. That is, our knowledge of the world tells us it must be the boy, not the apple, who is eating and it must be the apple that is red. On the other hand, consider the requirements for accurate comprehension of the reversible sentence "The girl that the boy is hitting is tall." Here, either the boy or the girl logically can do the hitting, and either can be tall. Correct interpretation requires the appropriate pairing of "boy" with "hitting" and of "girl" with "tall"—an interpretation arrived at only through adequate syntactic processing. Several studies have found that some patients have considerably more difficulty comprehending reversible sentences than semantically constrained ones, implying the presence of significant deficits in grammatical processing (Caramazza & Zurif, 1976; Kolk & Friederici, 1985; Sherman & Schweikert, 1989; Wulfeck, 1988).

Ample additional evidence indicates that sentences requiring structural-syntactic analysis are generally difficult for patients with aphasia (usually regardless of aphasia type) and that sentence comprehension is probably maximized when interpretation can be based on world knowledge and the understanding of critical individual elements (e.g., see Ansell & Flowers, 1982a, 1982b; Blumstein, Goodglass, Statlender, & Biber, 1983; Caplan & Evans, 1990; Curtiss et al., 1986; Friederici, 1983; Gallaher, 1981; Gallaher & Canter, 1982; Mack, 1982; Parisi & Pizzamiglio, 1970; Peach, Canter, & Gallaher, 1988). Constructing sentence stimuli with this in mind is of practical import for another reason. Gallaher and Canter (1982) suggest that the syntactic impact on comprehension in *real life* may be minimal, because much of what is said in everyday communication can be interpreted on the basis of real-world knowledge and comprehension of lexical items, with grammar and syntax providing largely redundant information.

Demands for processing of grammar and syntax should not—and cannot—be avoided entirely. A number of studies provide very useful information about the relative ease or difficulty of processing a variety of grammatical and syntactic devices for patients with aphasia. The following represent a sampling of these findings:

1. Present tense sentences are easier than past- or future tense sentences (Naeser et al., 1987; Parisi and Pizzamiglio, 1970; Pierce, 1981). When the tense changes, the use of an additional tense marker tends to facilitate tense comprehension (e.g., "The man has caught the ball" should be easier than "The man caught the ball"; "The man has already combed his hair" should be easier than "The man has combed his hair."). Words like "yesterday" and "tomorrow" also help to mark tense (Ansell and Flowers, 1982b; Pierce, 1981, 1982, 1983).

   The distinction discussed in the preceding paragraph is one example of what seems to be a fairly consistent hierarchy of syntactic difficulty that can affect comprehension. For example, gender, negative/affirmative, and singular/plural distinctions tend to be easier than past/present, subject/object, and past/future/present distinctions. Within distinctions, the marked features tend to be more difficult; for example, negative is more difficult than affirmative, plural more difficult than singular, and future and past tenses more difficult than present tense (Lesser, 1974; Naeser et al., 1987; Parisi and Pizzamiglio, 1970).

2. Other morphologic distinctions can also affect comprehension. For example, Goodglass and Hunt (1958) examined the ability of patients with aphasia to comprehend and express noun plurals and possessives that are represented by identical phonologic forms (e.g., "horses-horse's"). Expressively, patients made many more errors on possessive endings than on plurals. Receptively, the same pattern was noted, with the additional observation that third person singular verbs also generated more errors than plurals. Goodglass and Berko (1960) have reported similar error patterns, and Goodglass (1968) indicated that such patterns of deficit are independent of the form of aphasia (nonfluent vs. fluent) and, therefore, are not just specific to patients who are labeled "agrammatical." At the same time, it is important to keep in mind that syntactic deficits in aphasia are not an all-or-nothing phenomenon. In addition, the source of agrammatical production errors appears to be independent of comprehension errors (Goodglass, Christiansen, & Gallagher, 1993). The deficits typically encountered are relative, not absolute, and patients with aphasia (even "agrammatical" patients) are often able to process a good deal of syntactic information (Baum, 1989).

3. Patients with aphasia tend to use an active subject-verb-object (SVO) strategy for processing sentences and find active sentences easier to comprehend than other forms. In general, this means that sentences in which the order of mention reflects the agent-action-object relationship ("The mother kissed the baby.") are easier than sentences in which the word order does not reflect that relationship ("The policeman was punched by the robber.") (Ansell & Flowers, 1982b; Brookshire & Nicholas, 1980, 1981; Friederici & Graetz, 1987; Grossman & Haberman, 1982; Hickok & Avrutin, 1995; Hickok, Zurif, & Canseco-Gonzalez, 1993; Laskey et al., 1976; Pierce, 1983; Shewan & Canter, 1971). As mentioned above, SVO sentences that are nonreversible are easier to comprehend than reversible sentences.

4. Patients with aphasia tend to have more difficulty processing grammatically encoded (compact) sentences (e.g., "The man greeted by his wife was smoking a pipe" or "The woman was taller than the man.") than sentences that are simplified syntactically by expansion into a series of propositions (e.g., "The man was greeted by his wife and he was smoking a pipe" or "The woman was tall and the man was short.") (Goodglass et al., 1970; Nicholas and Brookshire, 1983). Similarly, individuals with aphasia have more difficulty processing object-gap relative clauses (e.g., "It was the farmer that the robber chased.") than subject-gap relative clauses (e.g., "It was the farmer that chased the robber.") (Hickok & Avrutin, 1995). These findings demonstrate that sentence comprehension is not simply a function of the amount of information and length, because compact and expanded sentences can contain the same amount of information and easier-to-comprehend sentences can be longer than compact ones. Results like these also highlight the complexity of the interactions among stimulus factors and show that maximizing the facilitatory effect of one factor may increase the difficulty imposed by another; for example, the generally desirable strategy of reducing sentence length may necessitate a generally undesirable increase in syntactic complexity. In addition, it has become evident that factors influencing sentence comprehension do not have the same effects on discourse comprehension and that performance on sentence-level material does not always predict discourse comprehension (Brookshire & Nicholas, 1984) (for further discussion, see the section on context).

5. Syntactic context, or the form in which sentence-level tasks are expressed, can influence response appropriateness, if not accuracy. For example, Green and Boller (1974) evaluated auditory comprehension in severe aphasia by testing differences in response to commands, yes/no questions, and information questions when such tasks were directly worded (e.g., "Point to the ceiling."), indirectly worded (e.g., "I would like you to point to the

ceiling."), or directly worded but preceded by an introductory sentence (e.g., "Here's something. Point to the ceiling."). Commands constituted the easiest task, followed by yes/no questions and information questions. The various syntactic contexts did not affect response accuracy, but directly worded items were associated with a greater number of appropriate (i.e., relevant but incorrect) responses than were indirectly worded items. Directly worded items preceded by an introductory sentence were easier than indirectly worded items.

6. As discussed in the previous section, verb argument structure properties are important influences of lexical organization for verb retrieval; however, these structures are also important factors in sentence production by individuals with agrammatical aphasia. Previous research has indicated that subjects with agrammatical aphasia do not produce all argument structures required by the verb in their sentence productions (Caplan & Hanna, 1996; Thompson et al., 1994; 1995). Thompson and colleagues (1997) have also investigated the effects of these structures on sentence production in those with agrammatical aphasia during narrative tasks. The subjects with aphasia were noted to produce fewer verbs than the normal subjects. In addition, the individuals with aphasia showed a preference for producing simple one- and two-place verbs (i.e., verbs with the fewest participant roles) and rarely produced three-place or complement verbs (i.e., the most complex verbs). When complex verbs were produced by the subjects with aphasia, they were produced in their simplest argument structure forms. These results indicated that sentence production was also influenced by the number of arguments or participant roles as well as by the type of arguments required by the verb. The complexity of the verb (i.e., the number of possible argument structure configurations) influenced sentence production, with simple verbs being produced correctly with their arguments more often than complex ones. Finally, obligatory arguments were produced correctly more often than optional ones, even when the production of optional arguments was requested.

Clearly, a number of syntactic and grammatical factors may influence comprehension, repetition, and verbal formulation performance. It also appears that the hierarchy of difficulty for a number of syntactic and grammatical tasks may be differentially influenced by the nature of the aphasia.

Recently, Thompson, Shapiro, and colleagues (Jacobs & Thompson, 2000; Mitchum, Greenwald, & Berndt, 2000; Rochon, Laird, Bose, & Scofield, 2005; Thompson & Shapiro, 2005; Thompson, Shapiro, Kiran, & Sobecks, 2003) have invesitgated the effectiveness of training more complex grammatical forms through a series of treatment studies. In each study, complexity of sentence structure was counterbalanced for each subject; that is, some were trained first on simpler sentence structures (who questions [e.g., "Who did the thief chase?"]) and others on more complex structures (object-relative clausal embedded sentences [e.g., "The man saw the artist who the thief chased."]. Across all studies, results revealed greater generalization to untrained structures when the more complex structures were trained first. Similar findings have also been reported for individuals with Fluent-aphasia profiles (Murray, Ballard, & Karcher, 2004) The authors have proposed a Complexity Account of Treatment Efficacy based on their results. This theory states that greater generalization of treatment effects may be realized by training more complex sentence structures first, because these sentences contain all the information necessary for linguistically related, simpler sentence structures plus additional information that may enhance learning.

A number of syntactic and grammatical factors clearly may influence comprehension, repetition, and verbal formulation performance. It also appears that the hierarchy of difficulty for a number of syntactic and grammatical tasks must be carefully considered in treatment planning. For example, Thompson, Shapiro, and colleagues have presented convincing data that support the notion of beginning treatment of grammatical structures with complex rather than, as previously believed, simple forms.

Context

In recent years, interest has surged in the discourse comprehension and expression, the factors that influence discourse comprehension and expression, and the relationship of discourse to word- and sentence-level abilities of patients with aphasia. Findings indicate that word and sentence comprehension do not predict the comprehension of discourse (Brookshire & Nicholas, 1984; Hough, 1990; Hough, Pierce, & Cannito, 1989; Pashek & Brookshire, 1982; Stachowiak, Huber, Poeck, & Kerschensteiner, 1977; Waller & Darley, 1978) very well and that discourse comprehension is often better than single sentence comprehension. Brookshire (1992) points out that, because communication in daily life usually occurs more in the form of connected speech than single sentences, it may be that measures of sentence comprehension underestimate daily life comprehension competence.

It appears that context, redundancy, predictability, and extralinguistic cues within discourse and conversation facilitate communication for patients with aphasia. The following summary represents a sampling of findings from studies regarding comprehension and expression of language in discourse or natural communicative contexts by patients with aphasia. These studies provide clues for the design of intervention tasks that, for some patients, may be easier than shorter and, apparently, simpler word- and single-sentence-level activities:

1. Comprehension of syntactically complex sentences (e.g., reversible passive sentences) is facilitated when these sentences are preceded or followed by contextually relevant sentences containing semantic or syntactic information that predicts the relationship expressed in the target sentence (Boyle & Canter, 1986; Cannito, Vogel, & Pierce, 1989; Pierce, 1988; Waller & Darley, 1978; Wright & Newhoff, 2004). (An example of a previous facilitative context task is "The girl is on the ground. The girl was tripped by the boy. Who was tripped?" An example of a subsequent facilitative context task is "The woman went to the library. She returned a book. Where did the woman go?" [Pierce, 1988]). Some studies also show that the context that precedes or follows a target sentence may not have to predict specific information as long as it facilitates processing of the target information by, for example, identifying the topic, setting, or theme (Cannito, Jarecki, & Pierce, 1986; Hough, Pierce, & Cannito, 1989). Nonpredictive context, however, has also been noted not to facilitate comprehension of target sentences (Cannito et al., 1989; Cannito, Hough, Vogel, & Pierce, 1996). Contextual facilitation for both types of paragraphs has been reported to increase as a positive function of stage of recovery from aphasia (Cannito et al., 1996). Individuals with aphasia who are in the early stage of recovery (<1 month) demonstrated no advantage for predictive or nonpredictive narratives, those in the intermediate stage (1–6 months) demonstrated an advantage only for predictive narratives, and those with chronic aphasia (>6 months) exhibited facilitative effects of both predictive and nonpredictive narrative contexts. Finally, extralinguistic context, in the form of a picture depicting target sentence information, also facilitates comprehension (Pierce & Beekman, 1985), although Waller and Darley (1978) found that the facilitatory effect of a contextual picture was less powerful than verbal context.

   Pierce (1991) has pointed out that these facilitatory effects are most apparent for patients with relatively poor comprehension. The benefits of this kind of contextual cue seem to derive from redundancy or the fact that certain events or relationships are made more plausible than others.

2. Predictability provided by discourse may explain why discourse is comprehended better than sentences. Armus, Brookshire, and Nicholas (1989) found that the knowledge of scripts by patients with mild to moderate aphasia is not significantly compromised (scripts are used to organize common situations [e.g., after repeatedly eating in restaurants, we "know" the events that usually occur]). Thus, if a patient has an internalized script for a discourse event, it may allow that person to predict what will happen next, infer what is not stated, and organize it for recall. The authors suggest that scripts may be used in treatment to facilitate comprehension, with fading of the degree to which discourse follows a script when comprehension improves.

3. Patients with aphasia comprehend implied meanings quite well, especially in situations aided by extralinguistic context. In fact, Foldi (1987) reported that those with aphasia, like those without brain injury, tend to prefer the pragmatic interpretation of indirect requests over the literal interpretation. Wilcox, Davis, and Leonard (1978) presented videotaped "natural" situations to patients in which the correct interpretation of an utterance was the meaning conveyed by the request in a particular context. For example, the literal interpretation of "Can you move the table?" simply requires a yes/no response, but the indirect, conveyed/contextual meaning is a request that the table be moved. Patients with aphasia generally performed similarly to normal control subjects in their ability to use extralinguistic cues to comprehend the intent conveyed in many indirect requests. These results suggest that the use of natural communicative contexts in treatment may raise communicative performance over and above that derived from more traditional, relatively pure linguistic tasks that often intentionally minimize extralinguistic cues.

   It also appears that linguistic information may help some patients to appreciate the meaning of extralinguistic information. For example, Tompkins (1991) found that increased semantic redundancy facilitated the interpretation of emotions that were conveyed linguistically or prosodically to patients with aphasia.

4. Patients with aphasia have been shown to comprehend the main ideas expressed in discourse—that is, the most salient information—better than the details, and information that is expressed directly better than information that must be inferred (Katsuki-Nakamura, Brookshire, & Nicholas, 1988; Nicholas & Brookshire, 1986a). Of interest, increasing directness and salience (through repetition or elaboration) seems to be a more reliable way than decreasing speech rate to improve discourse comprehension. Nicholas and Brookshire (1986b) have also shown that the advantage of directly expressed information over that requiring inference is maintained in multiple-sentence reading tests.

5. Context can facilitate performance in certain word retrieval tasks. This same effect has been demonstrated (Bendt et al., 2002; Hough & Pierce, 1989; Hough, 1989) for tasks requiring generation of words in ad hoc categories (categories that are constructed for use in specialized contexts [e.g., things not to eat on a diet]). Significantly, more items were generated when contextual vignettes preceded ad hoc category tasks (e.g., before listing things to take on a picnic, the patient heard "Sam wanted to spend time outdoors. It was a beautiful day so he packed up some items and went to a

nearby park.") than when they did not. The facilitative effect of context was not found for common categories (e.g., foods). Hough and Pierce suggest that ad hoc category tasks may be useful for patients with aphasia because they are more divergent in nature and allow reliance on experience and world knowledge to a greater extent than common category tasks.

6. Methods used to elicit narrative discourse from patients with aphasia have variable effects. For example, picture sequences representing stories generally lead to a greater number of words in narratives compared with single-pictured scenes, but the two types of stimuli generally do not affect other measures of production differently (Bottenberg, Lemme, & Hedberg, 1987). Gender bias of pictures (e.g., men in a gym vs. women in a beauty salon) may result in differences in the number of words and information but does not affect wpm or efficiency, at least in males (Correia, Brookshire, & Nicholas, 1990).

7. Main ideas are expressed to a proportionately greater degree than details when stories are retold (Ernest-Baron, Brookshire, & Nicholas, 1987). This may explain why patients get along reasonably well in daily life; it is usually main ideas that must be recalled rather than details.

8. Situational context may affect the manner in which patients with aphasia respond. Glosser, Wiener, and Kaplan (1988) reported that, despite their linguistic deficits, patients with aphasia showed appropriate and predictable changes in response to nonlinguistic social contextual variables (e.g., face-to-face conversation vs. telephone vs. conversation over video monitors). In contrast, Brenneise-Sarshad, Nicholas, and Brookshire (1991) found few meaningful differences in the verbal output of patients with aphasia when they narrated a sequenced picture story for a listener known to them who looked at the pictures as the story was being told versus a newly introduced person who could not see the picture stimuli. The authors felt that it may not be important to create treatment situations in which the patient believes the listener is naive to the information to obtain valid measures of communicative effectiveness.

In summary, the contextual information provided within discourse and natural communicative contexts can exert significant facilitative effects on language and communication for patients with aphasia. These effects occur not only for the processing of the main ideas and intents expressed in discourse but also extend "backward" to the comprehension and expression of semantic and syntactic relationships expressed within the context of discourse. Discourse tasks, particularly comprehension tasks, clearly need not await recovery of word and sentence comprehension ability to become a focus of treatment. In fact, in some instances, it appears that dis-course should precede word- and sentence-level tasks in the treatment hierarchy.

Stress

Despite some evidence that patients with aphasia may be deficient in their ability to derive meaning from information provided by vocal stress (Baum, Daniloff, Daniloff, & Lewis, 1982) or that stress representation may be selectively impaired after brain damage (Cappa, Nespor, Ielasi, & Mozzo, 1997), it appears that stress can influence response adequacy in a positive way. For example, Swinney, Zurif, and Cutler (1980) have shown that patients with aphasia respond more rapidly to stressed than to unstressed words. More important, Pashek and Brookshire (1982) as well as Kimelman and McNeil (1987) found improved paragraph comprehension when exaggerated stress on critical words was employed. Pashek and Brookshire (1982) observed that improved comprehension in response to exaggerated stress was independent of improvement induced by a slowed rate, suggesting that slowed rate and exaggerated stress may be additive facilitators of auditory comprehension. More recently, Kimelman and McNeil (1989) showed the comprehension of normally stressed target words in paragraphs by patients with aphasia is better when preceded by a stressed as opposed to a normally stressed context. The magnitude of the facilitatory effect was greater for the patients with more severe impairment (those individuals most likely to need extralinguistic cues for comprehension). Kimelman (1991) has presented data that suggest the facilitative effect of stressing target words may actually derive from changes in duration and fundamental frequency in the context preceding the target word. Finally, emphasizing rhythm may facilitate phrase repetition abilities of individuals with nonfluent aphasia (Boucher, Garcia, Fleurant, & Paradis, 2001). Thus, it may be contextual stress modifications that alert the listener to the salience of the target word.

Eliminating consideration of information strongly associated with Melodic Intonation Therapy (see Chapter 31), most representative study on stress and speech output in aphasia has been conducted by Goodglass, Fodor, and Schuloff (1967). They found that fluent and nonfluent patients omitted initial unstressed function words much more frequently than initial stressed words in a sentence repetition task. The omission of unstressed words occurred more frequently for nonfluent patients. They also found that the stress pattern "/-/" was easier to repeat than any other three-word pattern tested when a function word was in the first or second position. Moreover, the facilitating effect of this stress pattern seemed to override grammatical complexity. For example, the negative interrogative "Can't you swim?" (/-/) was easier to repeat than the grammatically simpler "Can you swim?" (-//). The authors felt that nonfluent (and, therefore, usually apraxic) patients, in particular, may depend on stress features to initiate and maintain a flow of speech. Goodglass (1968) interpreted these and similar findings as supporting the importance of "saliency" in the initiation of speech. That is, many patients need a salient word to initiate speech, with saliency being characterized by stress and phonologic prominence, as well as other factors already discussed, such as informational and personal significance.

The clinical implications of these findings are obvious. The selection of sentence and paragraph material for comprehension and repetition tasks should consider stress-saliency as a variable capable of affecting the verbal comprehension and verbal production of patients with aphasia.

Order of Difficulty

Within a given treatment task, stimuli probably should be ordered so that more difficult items are presented last. This recommendation is based on evidence suggesting that success tends to breed success—and failure to breed failure—for patients with aphasia.

Brookshire (1972) studied the effects of task difficulty on naming behavior in nine patients. A group of easy-to-name and a group of hard-to-name pictures were derived from baseline measures for each patient and then subsequently presented in different orders. When easy pictures preceded hard pictures, responses to hard pictures were better than predicted on the basis of baseline measures. When easy pictures followed hard pictures, performance on easy pictures was poorer than expected on the basis of baseline measures. Brookshire speculated that when a patient experiences a high proportion of failures, emotional responses may be generated that disrupt subsequent responses. Although such negative effects tended to decay over time, he suggested that treatment should keep error rates low and that easy items should precede difficult ones. Brookshire (1976b) subsequently demonstrated very similar task difficulty effects for a sentence comprehension task in a group of 22 patients. The results differed from the study on naming only in that easy items facilitated comprehension on subsequent hard items for only a small number of patients.

Support for an order effect can be found in several other studies. Gardner and Brookshire (1972) found that naming performance under unisensory conditions is often facilitated when preceded by a generally easier auditory-visual stimulus condition and that responses to auditory-visual stimuli are reduced when preceded by a generally more difficult visual stimulus condition. Similarly, Brookshire (1971b) found that forcing subjects to respond at rapid rates depresses performance on subsequent items in which they are given more time to respond. Finally, Brookshire and Lommel (1974) reported the disruptive effects of failure on the performance of patients with aphasia and subjects without on a nonverbal sequencing task.

Dumond, Hardy, and Van Demark (1978) questioned (or qualified) the significance of the order effect. They readministered the PICA to 20 patients in split-half form, with the 18 subtests rearranged in two orders of difficulty, one ascending and one descending. No performance differences were found between the two orders of difficulty. In contrasting their results with those of Brookshire (1972), who examined a single task containing items of varying difficulty, Dumond and colleagues (1978) examined differences across tasks containing items of equal difficulty. They also indicated that "the changes in difficulty level between subtests were apparently less extensive than the changes in difficulty level within Brookshire's experiment" (p. 358) and that this may have reduced subjects' perception of their performance adequacy. They concluded that presenting PICA-like tasks in order of increasing difficulty is not likely to adversely affect performance on nonevaluative tasks for which difficulty levels do not vary extensively.

The available data appear to warrant the following generalizations regarding order of presentation during treatment:

1. Error rates should be kept low.
2. Stimulus presentation should generally proceed from easiest to hardest (with the possible exception of grammatical structures; see previous discussion in the grammar and syntax section), particularly within a given task and on tasks in which the patient is likely to be most sensitive to performance inadequacies).
3. If error rates are kept low, potential across-task order effects should be minimized.

In line with these generalizations, Crosky and Adams (1969) present some practical procedures for selecting and ordering vocabulary stimulus materials for individual patients. It is also reasonable to follow the suggestion of Brookshire (2000) that sessions begin with familiar and easy tasks, proceed to less familiar and more difficult ones, and end with tasks that result in a great deal of success.

Psychological and Physical Factors

In addition to stimuli that are directly intended to stimulate language, factors that affect the psychological and physical "set" of patients can influence response adequacy.

Skelly's (1975) interviews with patients who have aphasia indicate that even relatively subtle signs of disinterest or impatience on the part of the clinician "bothers" patients. Stoicheff (1960) found that the overt attitudes expressed during instructions to patients can significantly affect responses. Using three groups of patients with aphasia, she examined the effects of encouraging, discouraging, and neutral instructions and comments during performance on naming, reading, and self-evaluation tasks. After 3 days of exposure to one of the conditions, the self-evaluation, naming, and reading performance of the group receiving the discouraging instructions was lower than the performance of the groups receiving neutral or encouraging instructions. No differences were found between the encouraging and neutral conditions. Obviously, the performance differences were attributed to the negative effects of discouraging instructions. Finally, the previously discussed findings of Brookshire and colleagues on the effects of order of stimulus difficulty suggest that failure—or stress induced by failure—may produce emotional responses that disrupt subsequent responses. It seems, therefore, that disruptive psychological effects may result from negative attitudes expressed by the clinician during instructions and performance or from the failures that patient may experience during the course of a treatment session.

The effects of physical fatigue on language performance have been examined by Marshall and King (1973). Subjects were given the PICA following a period of isokinetic exercise and, on another day, following rest. The PICA scores were significantly lower following exercise than following rest for verbal, graphic, and overall PICA measures. Fatigue had its most pronounced effect on speaking and writing tasks. The authors suggested that language therapy be scheduled before physical exertion, such as physical or occupational therapy. In another study that probably reflects the cumulative effects of fatigue over the course of a day, Marshall, Tompkins, and Phillips (1980) found that patients with aphasia did better on assessment measures administered in the morning compared with measures administered in the afternoon.

It seems that psychological and physical factors facilitate performance best when treatment is conducted in a positive, encouraging, success-producing milieu and at a time when the patient's physical status during the treatment day is optimal.

Pattern of Auditory Deficit

Auditory impairments are not uniform and may reflect a number of different underlying problems. As a result, to ignore differences in the auditory deficits of patients with aphasia is to ignore a factor that may bear on the way in which we structure auditory stimulation during treatment. Consideration of such differences may help to identify stimulus factors that are especially important for a given patient and, in some cases, may serve to qualify or alter the generalizations and recommendations that have been made about those factors thus far.

Brookshire (1974) summarized and discussed five kinds of auditory deficits, supported by a variety of subsequent studies (e.g., LaPointe, Horner, Lieberman, 1977; DiSimoni, Keith, Holt, & Darley, 1975; McNeil, Hageman, & Matthews, 2005), the characteristics of which may have an important bearing on treatment planning. These characteristics reflect the need to avoid considering auditory deficits in aphasia as a unitary problem. These deficits and implications for stimulus selection are:

Slow Rise Time

Patients whose auditory systems are characterized by a slow rise time tend to miss the initial portion of incoming messages. They may be able to repeat or comprehend only the last part of sentences, may miss short messages entirely, or may do better on the final items of a subtest or treatment activity than on the initial items. Brookshire (2000) suggests that the use of warning signals before presenting auditory stimuli may facilitate processing for these patients, and Loverso and Prescott (1981) provide some indirect support for this. They found response times of subjects with aphasia on a same/different visual judgment task to be reduced when the visual stimuli were preceded by a half-second warning tone; maximum benefit was derived when the tone preceded the stimulus by 1.5 seconds. Presenting items with gradually increasing intervals between successive items may also help the patient to keep his or her "processor" active over longer intervals or help to activate the processor more quickly.

Patients with a slow rise time illustrate the fact that generalizations about a number of stimulus factors do not always hold. For example, contrary to "average" performance, the patient with a slow rise time may respond better to redundant sentences than to single words or may respond more appropriately to directly worded input preceded by an introductory sentence than to a directly worded sentence alone.

Noise Buildup

Patients with noise buildup tend to respond more accurately to the initial portion of auditory messages than to the following portions. More complex material tends to produce noise more rapidly than less complex material. Such patients may not be able to repeat or comprehend the final portion of sentences, may make more errors on complex than on simple materials, and may deteriorate progressively across items on a particular task. Brookshire (2000) suggests that they may benefit from a program with messages of gradually increasing length and complexity, with gradually decreasing intervals of silence between successive items.

Retention Deficit

Patients with retention deficits also deteriorate as length increases, but they are not as susceptible to complexity factors as are those with noise buildup. Performance breakdown tends to occur at the same point in all messages regardless of complexity. The important treatment consideration here is to gradually increase message length.

Information Capacity Deficit

Patients with information capacity deficit do not seem able to receive and process information at the same time (see Wepman (1972) for a discussion of the "shutter principle"). In such cases, performance may be alternately good or poor within a message, good for information that is received and can be acted on and poor for information directed at the system while processing of previous stimuli is taking place. Such patients may, for example, be able to repeat the beginning and end, but not the middle elements, of a sequence of words. Brookshire (2000) suggests that these patients may benefit from the insertion of pauses within messages. Such pauses may initially be frequent and of relatively long duration, with fading of their frequency and duration as processing ability improves.

Intermittent Auditory Imperception

Patients with this problem constitute a separate category in Schuell's system of classification. Their auditory processing ability appears to fade in and out randomly, leading to sporadic and unpredictable performance. Because we do not understand the controlling factors in such a problem, Brookshire recommends that treatment be directed to other areas of deficit.

Brookshire points out that the above categories may be simplistic and incomplete, although the existence of several of them appears to have been verified by other investigators (McNeil & Hageman, 1979; Porch, 1967; Schuell et al., 1964). It is quite probable, however, that they exist in varying combinations within many patients, and are seen atypically in pure form. Regardless, the ability to recognize them when they occur has direct implications for the selection of potent stimulus factors when planning treatment.

Response Considerations

Although the emphasis of the stimulation approach is on input to the patient, the effectiveness of such stimulation can be assessed only if responses are elicited. Regardless of the form of response, three of the general principles of remediation stated earlier are relevant to response considerations:

1. There should be a response to each stimulus.
2. Responses should not be forced.
3. A maximum number of responses should be elicited.

To those, we can add one additional principle—response demands generally should proceed from short to long. Just as length is a potent stimulus factor, it is also a potent response factor for most patients, with short responses nearly always easier than long ones. In addition to these principles, certain other response considerations must be addressed when planning treatment.

Response Mode

Decisions regarding the mode of response are based on specific goals and baseline data. For example, if we wish to improve auditory comprehension or retention, we should place minimal demands on output and let baseline data aid us in selecting the most intact mode of response. If the goal

is to improve spoken language ability, the response mode has already been determined by the chosen goal.

Response adequacy in a particular modality can sometimes be facilitated by a simultaneous response in another modality. For example, Hanlon, Brown, and Gerstman (1990) found that patients with anterior lesions, hemiparesis, and Broca's aphasia named pictures more adequately when they simultaneously attempted to point to the picture with their hemiparetic right arm. (Note that this may represent facilitation of problems more related to apraxia of speech than to language per se.)

Output modes usually include pointing, nodding, object or picture manipulation, pantomime, other gestures, speech, and writing. Point-to tasks are frequently used when treatment focuses on auditory processes, because the motor control of simple pointing responses is usually unimpaired. However, Brookshire (1992) observes that such tasks can be relatively difficult for some patients. Such observations reinforce the need for letting the individual patient's abilities determine the mode of response.

Temporal Relationship

The temporal relationship between stimulus and response should be considered. Responses may be elicited in unison with a stimulus, immediately following a stimulus, or after a delay. Patients also may be asked to repeat a response consecutively.

Unison responses may be especially appropriate for severely impaired patients, because they give simultaneous auditory and visual feedback and are a step down the response hierarchy from repetition (Schuell et al., 1955; Wertz, 1978). Although immediate responses represent the most frequent and desirable temporal relationship, they may impose unreasonable demands on some patients; for some patients, requiring rapid responses may depress the adequacy of performance. In such cases, allowing a delay for processing may be very useful. Marshall (1976), for example, found that delay was the most effective response "strategy" employed by patients with aphasia for word retrieval.

How much delay? Schuell and colleagues (1964) suggested 60 seconds for some tasks. Brookshire (1971b) found that 30 seconds were better than 0, 5, or 10 seconds on an object naming task but also noted that, when patients were able to name objects, they usually did so within 10 seconds. Thus, it seems that delays allowed for processing to occur should rarely have to exceed 30 seconds, and probably should not, considering the principle that treatment should elicit a large number of responses.

On comprehension tasks, the effect of imposing delays between stimulus and response may not be predictable. Schulte (1986) examined the comprehension of 10 patients with aphasia on a Token Test type of task in which 0-, 5-, 10-, and 20-second delays were imposed before patients were allowed to look at response choices and respond. No consistent effects on comprehension were found among the delay conditions for the group as a whole. Performance within subjects varied by nearly 20% between some conditions, however, and a few of the more severely impaired patients benefited from brief delays in some conditions. Schulte suggested that, for some patients, an imposed delay may facilitate full processing before a response but may be detrimental for others because of poor rehearsal mechanisms or reduced retention capacity. It therefore appears that imposing a delay between stimulus presentation and response has no generally predictable influence on sentence comprehension accuracy but that it may be a useful response parameter if its effects are predictable for individual patients.

In addition to using delay as an aid to comprehension or formulation, imposing delays before allowing the patient to respond may be a useful strategy for improving retention span. Imposing a delay between a patient's response and the next stimulus may also be an effective strategy for reducing perseveration in some patients. Santo Pietro and Rigrodsky (1982) found that the frequency of perseveration on sentence completion, naming, and reading tasks decreased as the time between a response and subsequent stimulus increased from 1 to 10 seconds.

Delay sometimes can be used actively by patients to improve response adequacy (this point could also be considered under the section dealing with consequences/feedback). Berstein-Ellis, Wertz, and Shubitowski (1987) instructed a mildly impaired patient with aphasia and reduced conversational fluency (because of hesitation, revisions, and paraphasias) in the use of a pacing board (Helm, 1979) to slow the rate of speech. This reduced syntactic and paraphasic errors and permitted the same or more information to be conveyed with fewer verbalizations. Whitney and Goldstein (1989) used a different technique and achieved the same result for three patients with mild aphasia whose discourse was dysfluent because of revisions, repetitions, and audible pauses. After learning to recognize and identify their dysfluencies from audiorecorded samples of their speech, the patients were trained to monitor/identify their dysfluencies during picture description tasks. This resulted in reduced speech rate, a dramatic reduction of dysfluencies, and increased efficiency in the form of increased length of uninterrupted utterances.

Finally, some subtle uses of temporal relationships in stimulus presentation may influence processing demands and response adequacy. Brookshire and Nicholas (1980) have shown that patients with aphasia tend to use a find-and-compare strategy on sentence verification tasks in which the truth value of a sentence is based on a comparison with a simultaneously presented picture stimulus; in other words, instead of processing the full meaning of the sentence, they may simply match key words to elements in the picture. To force the patient to deal with the fuller meaning of the sentence, those authors suggest that the spoken sentence and the picture stimulus presentations be staggered (e.g., present the sentence and then the picture) rather than simultaneous. It is quite possible that this more challenging approach to stimulus presentation in a verification task would also apply to point-to comprehension tasks (i.e., present sentence and then present picture choices).

Response Characteristics

Although accuracy is certainly the most commonly expected response characteristic, it is not the only relevant one. Green and Boller (1974) found that severely impaired patients (i.e., unable to respond very accurately to auditory tasks) often are able to respond appropriately; that is, they show signs of rudimentary comprehension by, for example, looking around the room when asked to point to the door or nodding when asked yes/no questions. In such cases, appropriateness of response may be the most appropriate expectation for an initial response. At the other end of the continuum, when a patient can respond with a relatively high degree of accuracy, it may be appropriate to expect a reduction of self-corrections and of incomplete, delayed, or distorted responses. (Such response characteristics are reflected in Porch's multidimensional scoring scale and are discussed in Chapter 28.) The important point is that response expectations need not be geared solely toward accuracy. For some patients, a high degree of accuracy may not be possible, and expectations may have to be lowered. For others, a high proportion of accurate responses may still leave considerable room for response refinement along a number of other response dimensions.

Consequences (Feedback)

The stimulation approach presumes that the stimulus (i.e., the antecedent event) is that part of the treatment sequence which facilitates, or is largely responsible for, the ability of the patient to respond adequately. This is in contrast to operant approaches, in which increased adequacy of responses is attributed primarily to the controlling influence of consequences on subsequent behavior. Because antecedents are, theoretically, the crucial modifier of language processing in the stimulation approach, however, does not mean that we should not respond to patient behavior.

It has already been stated that feedback about response accuracy and appropriateness should be given when necessary. Boone (1967) suggests that any specific response-contingent feedback may be trivial or unnecessary when patients are motivated (as is usually the case), know the target response, and can assess their response in relation to the target. Support for this type of feedback comes from research on the concept of "errorless learning," in which treatment is structured to decrease the likelihood of a patient producing an inaccurate response. The notion behind this approach is that the brain is prevented from incorrect or inefficient processing to maximize accuracy of new learning (Fillingham, Hodgson, Sage, & Lambon Ralph, 2003). Additional support comes from the finding that mild to moderately impaired patients with aphasia modify their picture descriptions in response to failure in a referential communication task in the same way that speakers without aphasia do. In the relatively rare case when a patient is not motivated, response-contingent rewards or punishment may be necessary; but in general, reinforcement or punishment have little effect on speech and language performance in aphasia (Brookshire, 1977). When patients are motivated but give deficient responses, it may be most appropriate to confirm response adequacy or to give information about the closeness of a response to the target. Whether feedback is in the form of reward, punishment, confirmation, or information, Brookshire's (1971a) finding that patients with marked to severe impairment were sensitive to the effects of short delays between responses and their consequences on a nonlanguage learning task implies that feedback, when appropriate, should be immediate.

What information should be given to patients when their responses are inadequate? First, in most instances, such information should not be negative. The findings of Stoicheff (1960) suggest that discouraging comments during performance, such as "that's wrong," at least when combined with discouraging instructions, have a detrimental effect on performance. Second, Schuell and colleagues (1964) felt that one of the most common errors made by clinicians was overcorrection or overexplanation of errors and that the proper contingency for an inadequate response is usually more stimulation. In support of this, Holland and Sonderman (1974), in their evaluation of an auditory comprehension program, felt that explaining errors to patients confused, rather than aided, subsequent performance. The analysis by Brookshire and Nicholas (1978) of clinical interactions in treatment of aphasia indicated that patients tend to make errors following corrective explanations of previous errors. It seems that confirmation of adequate performance may be helpful and encouraging and, generally, represents good clinical practice. Explanation and correction, on the other hand, should be carefully controlled and concise, bearing in mind that such feedback may be of little value, waste time, and be counterproductive.

In addition to considering response-dependent feedback, general encouragement and reassurance during a treatment session is always desirable. Brookshire (1997) supports the value of showing patients their progress over time, with graphs often being an effective format for doing so. Such feedback—aside from being information the patient has a right to know about—has motivational and reinforcement functions, and it provides a framework for discussing and/or

supporting the continuation, alteration, or termination of certain treatment activities.

Sequencing Steps in the Treatment Program

Where to Start

Schuell and colleagues (1964) indicated that treatment should begin at the level where language breaks down and should proceed through gradually increasing levels of difficulty. Bollinger and Stout (1976), arguing for the critical importance of stimulation in treatment, suggested that treatment should progress from highly clinician-cued antecedent events to low-cued events in which the patient carries most of the processing load. Brookshire (1997) offers some more specific suggestions regarding starting points. which can be summarized as follows.

1. Treatment should begin at levels where slight deficiencies exist and never where performance is completely inadequate. This assures that patients are not pushed beyond their capacity but, instead, forces them to work near capacity.
2. Tasks for which 60% to 80% of responses are correct and immediate represent good starting points. That is, not more than 20% to 40% of responses should be self-corrected or delayed.
3. Tasks should not be too easy. Difficulty should be increased when 90% or more of responses are completely adequate in the dimensions that are the focus of treatment.

The selection of appropriate starting points should be based on adequate baseline data, because without such information, treatment begins without knowing if tasks or stimuli are appropriate. Baseline data may be established through standardized tests, systematic sampling of patients' responses to their environment (this is critical for the establishment of relevant, practical tasks and stimuli) or selected stimuli, or probing of variations in stimuli to see how changes influence speech and language behavior (Hendrick, Christman, & Augustine, 1973). For example, standardized testing may indicate that the ability to identify objects named from among 10 choices is very adequate (e.g., 90% immediate, accurate responses) but also that identifying object-by-function from among 10 choices is below the level at which treatment would be appropriate (e.g., 50% inaccurate responses). Subsequent assessment of responses to functional items might confirm standardized results, but probing might establish that identifying those same objects-by-function from among only four choices generates response characteristics at a level appropriate for treatment (e.g., 80% accurate, with 20% delayed or self-corrected responses). Such baseline data identify a starting point for stimulating auditory abilities, specify the stimulus conditions and response expectations to be employed during treatment, and give direction about the organization of succeeding steps. No less important is the fact that baseline data provide a pre-treatment measure of ability against which the results of treatment can be compared.

Criteria for Determining Success

Once tasks and stimuli have been established and target behaviors or response characteristics identified, we must determine the criterion for acceptable performance. When this criterion is reached, it is assumed that the specific task is no longer necessary and that the patient is ready to move on to tasks with greater demands. Experienced clinicians agree that a target behavior criterion of 90% is generally appropriate (Brookshire, 1992; LaPointe, 1977). LaPointe also suggests that the criterion be maintained for three consecutive sessions before terminating the task to ensure that the behavior is stable. When a patient's performance plateaus at a level below the criterion for a number of sessions, he suggests that the task be terminated or modified to make it slightly easier.

Compatibility of the Stimulation Approach and Programming

The discussion regarding the design of intervention has included information about stimulus and response considerations, contingencies, selection of starting points, and progression of activities. The acquisition of baseline data and the setting of criterion levels also have been highlighted. All these considerations can be strongly associated with programmed approaches to treatment. This may be somewhat surprising, because the appearance of information about the stimulation approach and the programmed approach to treatment in the same discussion has typically been in the form of contrast (e.g., see Darley (1975) and Sarno (1974)). Although operant-programmed approaches are dissimilar to the stimulation approach because of their emphasis on consequences as the primary modifiers of behavior, it is inappropriate to consider the stimulation approach and the application of general programming principles as being mutually exclusive treatment strategies (LaPointe, 1978b). A careful reading of Schuell's work shows that her principles and suggestions regarding treatment are compatible with the rigor and systematic nature of programming. Her admonitions to choose realistic goals, know where performance breaks down, elicit large numbers of responses, work systematically, and discard ineffective techniques are things with which a systematic, behavioral approach program is highly capable of assisting. It seems to be most appropriate, in this context, to consider programming as a tool for systematically implementing the stimulation approach. Programming is particularly desirable because of its commitment to accountability and its capacity for making treatment both replicable and

accessible to analysis (Holland, 1975; LaPointe, 1983). LaPointe's (1977) "Base-10 Programmed Stimulation" as well as Bollinger and Stout's (1976) "Response-Contingent Small-Step Treatment" are excellent, clinically applicable examples of the compatibility of the stimulation approach and structured behavioral methods.

EXAMPLES OF THERAPY TASKS

The preceding discussion regarding the design of intervention included numerous implied suggestions about tasks and techniques that may be appropriate for therapy. In this section, a number of specific tasks will be listed. They are offered as examples of activities that are considered to be appropriate for patients with aphasia and have enjoyed varying or undefined degrees of success. They are not offered as prescriptions or even as recommendations, because given our current state of knowledge, we have no way of predicting reliably which tasks and techniques work best with individual patients.

The focus of the examples here will be on tasks that emphasize auditory processes, because this is consistent with the stimulation approach. A number of examples of tasks requiring verbal output, many of which also involve auditory input, will be given as well. It should be understood that nearly all auditory and verbal tasks are readily adaptable to the reading and writing modes, but a few examples of tasks unique to reading and writing will be given.

The examples offered here cover a range of difficulty so as to include suggestions that are appropriate for patients with mild to severe impairment. The tasks are ordered from the anticipated easiest to hardest, but the reader is cautioned that the order provided is not empirically derived—and, probably, cannot be—because of patient variability. It is also important to note that difficulty level can be altered not only by switching tasks but also merely by altering certain stimulus factors or stimulus-response relationships associated with a given task. For example, increasing the number of response choices in a point-to auditory comprehension task may significantly increase task difficulty.

Many of the examples given below have been derived from suggestions offered in the following sources: Schuell and colleagues (1955, 1964); Schuell (1953a); Brookshire (1997); Kearns and Hubbard (1977); LaPointe (1978a); Darley (1982); and Rosenbek, LaPointe, and Wertz (1989). Many other examples are of such universal, long-standing use that they either defy or make accurate referencing trivial.

Tasks Emphasizing Auditory Abilities

Point-To Tasks

These activities involve the presentation of information auditorily and require a simple identification-by-pointing response. The ease of the motor response allows patients to focus primarily on the reception, processing, and retention of the auditory message. Difficulty level on these and many other auditory tasks can be altered by variations of many of the stimulus factors discussed earlier in the chapter (e.g., rate, pause, stress, similarity and number of response choices, visual cues, syntactic complexity). Many of these tasks can be employed as speech activities by requiring verbal instead of gestural responses. Some examples include:

1. Point to an item (picture or object) named.
2. Point to an item described by function ("Point to the one used for writing.").
3. Point to an item to complete a sentence ("Please pass the bread and _____.").
4. Point to an item in response to questions ("What do you find in the kitchen?"—points to a stove). A more complex but analogous task might involve responses to questions based on the preceding sentence or paragraph material.
5. Point to two (or more) items named ("Point to the book and point to the pen," or "Point to book-comb.").
6. Point to two (or more) items described by function.
7. Point to an item best described by a sentence ("Those people are very busy"—represented by people building a house).
8. Point to an item whose name is spelled.
9. Point to an item described by a varying number of descriptors ("Point to the large white circle," or "Point to the one that is long, silver, and sharp"—points to a knife).

Following Directions

These tasks allow greater flexibility and complexity in the auditory demands placed on the patient. For example:

1. Follow one-verb instructions ("Pick up the pen.").
2. Follow two-object location instructions ("Put the pencil in front of the cup.").
3. Follow two-verb instructions ("Point to the cup. Pick up the eraser.").
4. Follow two-verb instructions with time constraint ("Before touching the penny, pick up the spoon.").

Yes/No Questions and Sentence Verification

These formats also increase flexibility, can reduce the possible effects of visual deficits on performance, and often allow the extension of stimulus material beyond the immediate environment. Only a simple verbal or nonverbal response is required. For example:

1. Questions dealing with general information ("Was Kennedy President in 1861?").

2. Questions requiring phonemic discrimination ("Do people wear shoes and blocks on their feet?").
3. Questions requiring semantic discrimination ("Do you start a car with a tire?").
4. Questions about picture material ("Is the boy wailing?"—picture of boy running).
5. Questions involving verbal retention ("Are cows, horses, dogs, trees, and lions all animals?").
6. Questions about preceding sentences or paragraph material ("I like to swim, play tennis, and go to the ballpark. Did I say I like to play football?").
7. The above question examples may be converted to sentence or paragraph verifications tasks, in which the patient is asked to verify the truth of various statements ("Kennedy was President in 1861," or "Cows, horses, dogs, trees, and lions are all animals.").

Response Switching

These tasks require the patient to switch responses from item to item and, therefore, require close attention to the nature of the task on each trial. Such activities may simply combine the auditory tasks previously discussed or also may include items requiring speech, reading, or writing abilities. For example, a response switching activity might include the following successive items:

1. Point to the door.
2. Give me the cup.
3. Is the floor lower than the ceiling?
4. Spell your name.
5. How are you feeling today?
6. Have I asked you to give me the cup?
7. Read this, and do what it says to do.

Tasks Emphasizing Verbal and Auditory Abilities

Repetition Tasks

These require reception and retention of auditory information and the ability to repeat the information verbally. Auditory comprehension is not necessary, although it may facilitate performance. Minimal demands are placed on word retrieval. For example:

1. Repeat spoken words.
2. Repeat phrases ("in the house"; "on the beach"; "to the store"; "black and white"; "shoes and socks").
3. Repeat series of items ("book-table"; "penny-key-knife"; "long-under-baby-pencil").
4. Repeat stereotyped or functional phrases ("Where are you going?"; "What time is it?"; "Please pass the salt"; "How are you?")
5. Repeat sentences with or without corresponding picture stimuli ("The girl is chasing the boy"; "The cat is up in the tree.").

Sentence or Phrase Completion

These tasks typically place more demand on auditory comprehension and word retrieval processes and less demand on auditory retention compared with repetition tasks. For most patients, they are more difficult than single-word repetition tasks but less difficult than single-word recall tasks without auditory input. For example:

1. Complete sentences with nouns with varying degrees of predictability ("Please pass the salt and _____"; "Throw me the _____"; "Read a _____"; "Buy me some _____.").
2. Complete sentences with verbs ("I use a fork for _____"; "I use a paint brush for _____.").
3. Complete paired-associates ("black and _____"; "hot and _____"; "salt and _____").

Verbal Association

These tasks require verbal comprehension but minimal retention. Verbal retrieval processes are taxed. For example:

1. Oral opposites ("hot-cold"; "night-day"; "early-late").
2. Rhyming—clinician says word and patient rhymes ("hot—pot").
3. Word fluency/rapid word retrieval—clinician provides a letter of the alphabet, a common category (e.g., clothes, sports) or a concept (e.g., things to do on vacation, things that can roll), and the patient generates as many words, categories, or concepts as possible.
4. Synonyms—"think of a word that means the same as 'car.'"

Answering "Wh-" Questions

These tasks always place some demand on auditory comprehension and may require significant retention as well. Word retrieval and sentence formulation may be taxed to varying degrees. For example:

1. Answering questions after imitative cues and a question prompt (clinician—"Answer the phone"-patient imitates; clinician—"What should I do?", and patient—"Answer the phone").
2. Answering questions after a model (clinician— "The boy went to the movies. What did the boy do?").
3. Answer familiar conversational questions ("How old are you?"; "How do you feel?").
4. Answer questions about the preceding sentence or paragraph material (e.g., "John was on the ground. John was tripped by Mary."— "Who was on the ground?")
5. Answer general questions ("What do you do when you're hungry?"; "Who is the President of the U.S.A.?"; "How did you get here today?"). High-level patients may be asked questions requiring lengthy responses ("How do you change a flat tire?"; "Exactly how do you get from here to _____?").

Connected Utterances in Response to Single Words

Minimal demands are placed on auditory input processes. Maximal demands are placed on word retrieval and sentence formulation. For example:

1. Use selected words of varying parts of speech, word class, tense, and so on in sentences (put-how; television; red; running; bigger; given in a sentence).
2. Define words.
3. Use sentences beginning (or ending) with selected words or phrases (I eat; when; if, she).

Although these tasks are not listed in a hierarchy of difficulty, Thompson and colleagues (Thompson et al., 2003) have suggested that initiating treatment with stimuli that require a more complex response, such as using intransitive verbs in sentence formulation, may increase the generalization of this skill to less complex responses, such as using transitive verbs in sentence formulation.

Retelling

These tasks can place relatively heavy demands on comprehension and retention and always tax word retrieval and sentence formulation. For example:

1. Listen to paragraph material, and then retell it.
2. Listen to radio or television broadcast, and then retell it.
3. Retell a familiar story.

"Self-Initiated" or Conversational Verbal Tasks

These tasks are not dependent on preselected auditory input to the patient, with the exception of directions about the general nature of the task. Other stimuli may be used to focus content and aid retrieval, but the primary demands are placed on the patient's verbal retrieval and formulation abilities and, often, on the ability to follow naturally occurring auditory and situational cues. For example:

1. Name pictures.
2. Describe the function of objects.
3. Describe activities in pictures.
4. Tell everything possible about pictured objects or activities (urge patient to describe all possible uses of objects, objects' physical properties, associated situations, people, etc.).
5. Describe activity of the clinician (clinician points to two pictures—patient describes; clinician touches an object, places another object near it, and then places an object on top of another—patient describes the activity when completed).
6. General conversation about a selected topic with one or more individuals.
7. Open-ended conversation on unrestricted topics with one or more individuals.

Tasks Involving Reading and Writing Abilities

Reading

Nearly all of the tasks previously described involving auditory input can be adapted easily for reading tasks simply by using written input. The following are some additional tasks that are associated more uniquely with reading:

1. Match written words, phrases, or sentences to pictures (gradually reducing the stimulus exposure time may be employed in an effort to increase the reading rate).
2. Identify letters named by the clinician among a number of written choices.
3. Name letters.
4. Read in unison with the clinician, with a gradual increase in rate and/or fading of the clinician's input.
5. Fill in missing words in sentences from among written choices ("They went to the movies last (day, night, show, fight)"; "John is (to, went, going, come) in a little while.").
6. Read sentences or paragraphs silently, followed by questions about content.
7. Read aloud a paragraph or story, and then retell.

Writing

Most of the examples offered under the sections dealing with auditory and verbal activities also can be adapted readily to the writing mode merely by requiring written instead of gestural or verbal responses. The following are some additional tasks that are associated more uniquely with writing modality activities:

1. Copy forms, letters, and words.
2. Write letters to dictation.
3. Write words dictated letter-by-letter.
4. Write overlearned materials (e.g., name, the alphabet, and the numbers 1–10).
5. Fill-in missing letters or words in written stimuli, with or without associated picture stimuli ("He is reading a book _____"; "He is reading a _____ b-ok.").
6. The clinician reads paragraph material, and the patient writes down the essential facts. Have the patient rewrite the paragraph based on those notes.

RESOURCE ALLOCATION MODEL FOR APHASIA

Resource allocation models provide a useful format in searching for the underlying causes of impaired performance. Recently, McNeil and colleagues (McNeil & Kimelman, 1986; McNeil, Odell, & Tseng, 1990) have proposed a resource allocation model for aphasia. Essentially, what resource allocation models suggest is that all humans have a limited amount of cognitive resources for conducting mental or cognitive processes involved with perception, comprehension, memory, and response formulation. The mental energy, or fuel, required for carrying out these processes is referred to as "processing resources" and is contained in a central pool. With the activation of any process, resources must be transferred from the pool to the process. The number of cognitive processes that are called on simultaneously as well as the complexity of a given process determine how much fuel is drawn from the central resource pool. If the demands of the cognitive processes exceed the resources within the pool, the cognitive processes will not be provided with adequate resources, and performance will be negatively affected. If, on the other hand, the resource demands for a given process are low, the finite resources in the pool will not be exceeded, and performance will be normal. The issue of whether brain damage reduces the amount of resources within the central pool or hinders access to the pool is unclear. In either case, however, the allocation of suitable resources is insufficient for the task at hand; consequently, the performance of the individual with brain damage on a given task is at a level below that of the individual without brain damage. Performance will vary depending on the number and complexity of cognitive processes involved.

Resource allocation models have important implications for application of the stimulation approach to therapy for aphasia. If elements of treatment tasks are simplified, the demands on the resource pool will be decreased, thus improving the performance of the individual with aphasia performance. Brookshire (1997) provides an example that illustrates this notion. An individual with aphasia who has a visuoperceptual impairment is engaged in an auditory comprehension task involving pointing to black-and-white line drawings named by function ("Point to the one used for..."). After 10 trials, he has made eight errors. The patient comments that he cannot see what the pictures represent, so the clinician substitutes colored pictures for the line drawings. After 10 more trials, only three errors are noted. Although the targeted process was an aspect of auditory comprehension, this task required the individual to call on processes involved in visual perception that were impaired; consequently, the available resources were exceeded. By modifying the visual characteristics of the stimuli, the visuoperceptual demands of the task were decreased, freeing up cognitive resources, and performance on the auditory comprehension aspects of the task improved. As Brookshire notes, "[C]linicians can focus treatment on a targeted process by controlling the processing load associated with incidental task variables that are not related to the treatment objectives" (p. 217). The primary manner in which clinicians can manipulate the processing load is through manipulation of the task stimuli. Stimulus manipulations involve adjusting the factors that have been discussed throughout this chapter, such as visuoperceptual clarity, length and redundancy, frequency and meaningfulness, grammar and syntax, and so on, which get to the heart of the stimulation approach—that is, the stimulus must be adequate. In other words, it must get into the brain.

EFFICACY OF THE STIMULATION APPROACH

It is impossible to make a single, empirically based statement about the efficacy of the stimulation approach. Nor would it be appropriate or particularly enlightening, within the context of this chapter, to review all of the group and single-subject studies that might bear on the issue of treatment efficacy (the reader is referred to Fucetola, Tucker, Blank, & Corbetta, 2005; Holland, Fromm, DeRuyter, & Stein, 1996; Robey and Schultz, 1998; Robey, Schultz Crawford, & Sinner, 1999; and Wertz and Irwin, 2001, for comprehensive reviews of such studies and issues related to assessing the effectiveness of treatment). A number of general statements about the effectiveness of treatment, however, and particularly about the stimulation approach, may help to put the current state of the art in perspective.

No single study can conclusively "prove" the efficacy of treatment (Holland, 1975), but reviews and observations by well-respected, active clinical aphasiologists and some neurologists generally have yielded cautious to confident conclusions that therapy helps patients with aphasia (see, e.g., Albert, 2003; Benson, 1979; Darley, 1977, 1979, 1982; Helm-Estabrooks, 1984; Wertz, 1983, 1991). In addition, since 2001, the Academy of Neurologic Communication Disorders and Sciences (ANCDS) has been engaged in an objective, far-reaching project involving the development and dissemination of evidence-based practice guidelines for several neurogenic disorders of communication, including aphasia. The ANCDS committee developing the evidence-based practice guidelines for aphasia has been charged with the following: (1) conducting systematic and comprehensive literature reviews, (2) evaluating the levels of evidence against objective criteria, (3) formulating guidelines based exclusively on the reviews and assessments of levels of scientific evidence, (4) disseminating this information to practicing clinicians, and (5) delineating those areas in which additional research is needed (Frattali et al., 2003). To date, the review process has identified aphasia treatment studies categorized into seven groups by primary outcome variable, including (1) overall language performance, (2) lexical retrieval, (3) syntax, (4) speech production/fluency, (5) reading, (6) writing, and (7) alternative communication. Each of the studies has been evaluated in terms of study design (e.g., case-study, single subject, within-group, or between-group designs), strength of evidence, and phase of treatment (i.e., ranging from pre-efficacy to efficacy). The current tables of evidence are available online (www.u.arizona.edu/~pelagie/ancds/index.html). Although the review of aphasia treatment studies is still underway and the evidence-based guidelines have yet to be summarized, the evidence accumulated from several group and single-subject treatment studies,

including at least one well-designed randomized, controlled clinical trial (Wertz et al., 1986a), justifies, at the least, a general conclusion that "there is ample evidence that what we do for some aphasic patients does some good" (Wertz, 1991, p. 318).

Do we know something about the effectiveness of the stimulation approach that we do not know about therapy for aphasia in general? We do know that Schuell and her colleagues believed in and reported observations of the effectiveness of the stimulation approach, excluding patients with an irreversible (severe) aphasic syndrome. Many other users of the approach also report measurable progress (for more recent, relatively unambiguous examples of studies supporting the efficacy of the stimulation approach, see Basso et al., 1979; Marshall et al., 1989; Poeck, Huber, & Willmes, 1989; Shewan & Kertesz, 1984; Wertz et al., 1981, 1986b). Because of its widespread use, the stimulation approach has probably been studied more extensively than any other approach to treatment (although the interpretation of most efficacy studies requires this conclusion to be inferred, because treatment approaches have rarely been well specified). A final point pertains to the timelessness of Schuell's approach to the treatment of aphasia. Although underlying language processing models may differ according to each clinician's bias, the manner in which treatment is administered by these same clinicians is consistent and strikingly similar to that which Schuell described nearly 50 years ago. These tenets of therapy continue to be introduced in graduate aphasia courses across the country.

Therefore, conclusions that therapy is generally effective are based on studies that have used—or probably have used—a stimulation approach. More pessimistically, we can say that much of our inconclusive evidence about treatment efficacy is derived from studies of the stimulation approach. It is very possible, however, that such inconclusiveness results more to the study of the treatment than to the treatment itself. Taken as a whole, treatment studies employing the stimulation approach are more conclusive than inconclusive, and the conclusion they generate is that it has a significant positive effect on the communication ability of many patients with aphasia.

FUTURE TRENDS

What does the future hold for the stimulation approach? Answering this question is risky business, subject to the predictor's biases and misconceptions, new fads and fashions, major advances in other therapeutic approaches, altered availability of funding for continued investigation, and so on. With these pitfalls in mind, we can address three questions about the future:

1. Will we increase our understanding of the efficacy and dynamics of the stimulation approach?

2. Is the approach likely to change?
3. How will we understand and use it in relation to other therapy approaches?

Will we increase our understanding about the efficacy of the stimulation approach and the dynamics that explain its success? A number of reasons exist to anticipate that this will happen. First, clinical aphasiologists have made a commitment to accountability—that is, a commitment to providing "proof" of the effectiveness, or lack thereof, of therapy for aphasia. The development of evidence-based practice guidelines for aphasia initiated by the ANCDS is an example of such a commitment. Second, we have identified many of the flaws in our previous attempts, as well as those variables that must be accounted for in any study of treatment efficacy. Third, our measuring instruments have become more sensitive and reliable (e.g., the PICA). Fourth, we have begun to specify and study the dynamics of treatment more precisely (especially in single-subject studies) so that we know better what is effective and under what circumstances. Fifth, although we have acquired a substantial body of data regarding stimulus factors that affect the performance of patients with aphasia in nontreatment conditions, we know very little about the specific effects of using such stimulus manipulation in ongoing treatment. That is, the simple observation of improved performance under a certain stimulus condition in a single-trial, nontreatment study does not constitute proof that use of that stimulus factor in treatment will be responsible for short- or long-term language gains within or beyond the specific language task. This gap in our knowledge is true for many of the stimulus factors reviewed in this chapter, and it is close to the heart of questions about whether stimulation in general and/or specific stimulation is important to inducing language gains with the stimulation approach. We are in a position to test the effects of many stimulus factors in treatment, and this will likely be pursued in the future. Finally, the effect of stimulus factors and other variables that affect communication in discourse, conversation, and natural communicative settings are receiving increased attention. These efforts should help to identify the components of stimulation likely to have the greatest impact on communication in daily life and, thus, stimulus factors that are most meaningful to the patients we treat (i.e., social validation of the stimulation approach).

Is the stimulation approach likely to change? Probably not in any fundamental way. Major change is unlikely because the stimulation approach is an old and established one, the major principles and techniques of which have been reasonably well articulated and, in principle, consistently employed. Any major departures from the basic approach will likely be considered to be new approaches, given new names, and studied and employed separately. Several chapters in this volume reflect this trend and demonstrate divergence from the stimulation approach along many different lines.

The change that can be expected for the stimulation approach is refinement of our understanding of stimulus factors that do—and that do not—influence performance and, as mentioned previously, an increase in our ability to selectively and effectively employ that knowledge in treatment. Hopefully, these changes will be rapid and numerous and significantly improve overall treatment efficacy. Probably, they will be slow and painstakingly acquired. Certainly, they will require the efforts of many investigators who are interested in the increased understanding of the essence of aphasia as well as its effective management.

Finally, how will we understand and use the stimulation approach in relation to other therapeutic approaches? We have no way to answer this, because so little has been done to compare the effects of different treatment approaches. This is at least partly a result of the enormous past efforts expended to establish that treatment, in general, is effective (Albert, 2003) and to develop new approaches and preliminary efficacy data for them. Another reason, one that is really not to be confronted until more comparative studies are attempted, has been perceived by Sarno (1981). She said, "It is probably appropriate that there have been few studies comparing treatment methods in view of the seemingly insurmountable methodologic problems associated with such research and our present state of knowledge" (p. 512). Despite these past priorities and ever present methodologic challenges, it can be argued that, unless comparative studies are done, we will not learn what works best and with whom, and we will either become complacent in our use of a single "old and familiar" approach or, out of boredom, frustration, or fadism, will move randomly from one approach to another. Numerous comparative questions should be addressed, including:

1. How do various treatment approaches differ in terms of ultimate level of recovery, time demands, cost-effectiveness, professional and family requirements, and so on?
2. What is the best approach to use for patients with particular severity levels and forms of aphasia?
3. Are some approaches more effective early post-onset or late post-onset?
4. Is there a best sequence of approaches to use over the course of treatment?
5. Is language recovery enhanced if certain approaches are used in combination?
6. Do some approaches have to be used in isolation for them to be effective?

Finally, although Schuell's stimulation approach was developed for the treatment of aphasia, the utility of the approach for the treatment of cognitive deficits that often accompany aphasia is also worthy of study because of its sound clinical methodologies.

It is likely that some of the above questions will be addressed in the next 5 to 10 years. The number of approaches now in use make this increasingly necessary for rational, data-based clinical decision making. In addition, because more appears to be known about the efficacy of the stimulation approach compared with almost any other, it likely will frequently be among the approaches compared. In fact, we might anticipate that it will be the standard against which the effectiveness of other approaches will be measured.

1. The bulk of Hildred Schuell's work in aphasiology spanned the 1960s and 1970s and included significant contributions in the areas of diagnostic testing, classification of patients with aphasia, and theory development regarding the underlying nature of aphasia. It was probably this sound foundation in theory, evaluation, and methods of observing and categorizing behavior that helped to develop the compelling rationale for the stimulation approach. Schuell's beliefs about the organization of language and the nature of language breakdown in aphasia can be summarized as follows:

   a. Language cannot be thought of as a simple sensorimotor dichotomy or a three-system cortical relay involving reception, transmission, and execution.

   b. Neurophysiologically, language is the result of the dynamic interaction of complex cerebral and subcortical activities.

   c. The language mechanism contains a system of stored, learned elements and rules, the use and maintenance of which require discrimination, organization, storage, comparison, retrieval, transmission, and feedback control.

   d. Schuell's unidimensional, multimodality concept of aphasia does not require that patients vary only along a severity continuum. In aphasia, the problems of most patients appear to be more related to performance factors than to competence factors.

   e. Although the language mechanism can exist separately from input and output modalities, our primary language processes are acquired and organized through complex, interacting sensory systems and sensorimotor processes. Notably, auditory processes are at the apex of those interacting systems that aid in the acquisition, processing, and control of language.

2. Schuell's classification system for aphasia aimed at descriptive and predictive utility by classifying patients according to severity of language impairment, the presence or absence of related sensory or motor deficits, and prognosis. She identified seven categories: (a) simple aphasia, (b) aphasia with visual involvement, (c) aphasia with persisting dysfluency, (d) aphasia with scattered findings, (e) aphasia with sensorimotor involvement, (f) aphasia with intermittent auditory imperception, and (g) irreversible aphasia syndrome.

3. The stimulation approach can be defined as that approach to treatment that employs strong, controlled, and intensive auditory stimulation of the impaired symbol system as the primary tool to facilitate and maximize the patient's reorganization and recovery of language. Although numerous input modalities may be used, the auditory modality is at the foundation of the stimulation approach.

4. The design of intervention used in the stimulation approach is based on a number of general principles:

   a. Intensive auditory stimulation should be used.

   b. The stimulus must be adequate—that is, it must get into the brain. Therefore, it needs to be controlled, perhaps along a number of dimensions.

   c. Repetitive sensory stimulation should be used.

   d. Each stimulus should elicit a response.

   e. Responses should be elicited, not forced or corrected. If a stimulus is adequate, a response will occur.

   f. A maximum number of responses should be elicited.

   g. Feedback about response accuracy should be provided when such feedback appears to be beneficial and should show patients their progress.

   h. The clinician should work systematically and intensively.

   i. Sessions should begin with relatively easy, familiar tasks.

   j. Abundant and varied materials that are simple and relevant to the patient's deficits should be used.

   k. New materials and procedures should be extensions of familiar materials and procedures.

5. The following variables have been found to be most relevant to the structuring of stimulation:

   a. Auditory perceptual clarity.

   b. Nonlinguistic visuoperceptual clarity.

   c. Linguistic visuoperceptual clarity.

   d. Method of delivery of auditory stimulation.

   e. Discriminability.

   f. Combining sensory modalities.

   g. Stimulus repetition.

   h. Rate and pause.

   i. Length and redundancy.

   j. Cues, prompts, and prestimulation.

   k. Frequency and meaningfulness.

   l. Abstractness.

   m. Part of speech and semantic word category.

n. Grammar and syntax.

o. Context.

p. Stress.

q. Order of difficulty.

r. Psychological and physical factors.

s. Pattern of auditory deficit.

6. With regard to implementing the stimulation approach to treatment:

   a. Schuell indicated that treatment should begin at the level where language breaks down and should proceed through gradually increasing levels of difficulty.

   b. Once tasks and stimuli have been established and target behaviors or response characteristics identified, we must determine criterion for acceptable performance.

7. Conclusions that therapy for aphasia is generally effective are based on studies that have used—or probably have used—a stimulation approach. Treatment studies employing the stimulation approach are more conclusive than inconclusive, and the conclusion they generate is that it has a significant positive effect on the communication ability of many patients with aphasia.

ACTIVITIES FOR REFLECTION AND DISCUSSION

1. How is Schuell's definition of aphasia reflected in her aphasia classification system and the stimulation treatment approach?

2. Compare and contrast three treatment approaches for aphasia discussed in this text. How are they similar to and different that Schuell's approach?

3. Which of the stimulus variables described by Schuell would be most difficult to manipulate in the design of an individualized treatment task?

4. Design a treatment task for improving auditory comprehension of short sentences that could be used for an individual with severe aphasia. How could this task be modified for an individual with mild aphasia?

5. Design a treatment task for improving auditory comprehension of sentences by an individual with mild to moderate aphasia and significantly reduced visual acuity.

6. Design a 30-minute treatment session for an individual with moderate aphasia that targets naming of noun pictures.

7. Your client, a 60-year old man with mild to moderate aphasia, has just been authorized by his insurance company for 20 sessions of outpatient speech and language therapy. Design a treatment program that will maximize this treatment, and describe how you will demonstrate the effectiveness of your intervention.

References

Adrian, J. A., Gonzalez, M., & Buiza, J. J. (2003). The use of computer-assisted therapy in anomia rehabilitation: A single-case report. *Aphasiology, 17*(10), 981–1002.

Albert, M. (2003). Aphasia therapy works! (editorial). *Stroke, 34,* 992–993.

Albert, M. L. (1976). Short-term memory and aphasia. *Brain and Language, 3,* 28–33

Albert, M. L., & Bear, D. (1974). Time to understand: A case study of word deafness with reference to the role of time in auditory comprehension. *Brain, 97,* 373–384.

Ansell, B. J., & Flowers, C. R. (1982a). Aphasic adults' understanding of complex adverbial sentences. *Brain and Language, 15,* 82–91.

Ansell, B. J., & Flowers, C. R. (1982b). Aphasic adults' use of heuristic and structural linguistic cues for sentence analysis. *Brain and Language, 16,* 61–72.

Armus, S. R., Brookshire, R. H., & Nicholas, L. E. (1989). Aphasic and nonbrain-damaged adults' knowledge of scripts for common situations. *Brain and Language, 36,* 518–528.

Barton, M., Maruszewski, M., & Urrea, D. (1969). Variation of stimulus context and its effect on word finding ability in aphasics. *Cortex, 5,* 351–365.

Basso, A., Capitani, E., & Vignolo, L. A. (1979). Influence of rehabilitation on language skills in aphasic patients: A controlled study. *Archives of Neurology, 36,* 190–196.

Baum, S. R. (1989). On-line sensitivity to local and long-distance syntactic dependencies in Broca's aphasia. *Brain and Language, 37,* 327–338.

Baum, S. R., Daniloff, J. K., Daniloff, R., & Lewis, J. (1982). Sentence comprehension by Broca's aphasics: Effects of some suprasegmental variables. *Brain and Language, 17,* 261–271.

Benson, D. F. (1979). Aphasia rehabilitation (editorial). *Archives of Neurology, 36,* 187–189.

Benton, A. L., Smith, K. C., & Lang, M. (1972). Stimulus characteristics and object naming in aphasic patients. *Journal of Communication Disorders, 5,* 19–24.

Berndt, R. S., Burton, M. W., Haendiges, A. N., & Mitchum, C. C. (2002). Production of nouns and verbs in aphasia: Effects of elicitation context. *Aphasiology, 16,* 83–106.

Berstein-Ellis, E., Wertz, R. T., & Shubitowski, Y. (1987). More pace, less fillers: A verbal strategy for a high-level aphasic patient. In R. H. Brookshire (Ed.), *Clinical aphasiology* (Vol. 17, pp. 12–22). Minneapolis: BRK.

Birch, H. G., & Lee, M. (1955). Cortical inhibition in expressive aphasia. *A.M.A. Archives of Neurology and Psychiatry, 74,* 514–517.

Bisiach, E. (1966). Perceptual factors in the pathogenesis of anomia. *Cortex, 2,* 90–95.

Blumstein, S. E., Goodglass, H., Statlender, S., & Biber, C. (1983). Comprehension strategies determining reference in aphasia; A study of reflexivization. *Brain and Language, 18,* 115–127.

Blumstein, S. E., Katz, B., Goodglass, H., Shrier, R., & Dworetsky, B. (1985). The effects of slowed speech on auditory comprehension in aphasia. *Brain and Language, 24,* 246–265.

Blumstein, S. E., Milberg, W., & Shrier, R. (1982). Semantic processing in aphasia: evidence from an auditory lexical decision task. *Brain and Language, 17,* 301–315.

Boller, F., Vrtunski, B., Patterson, M., & Kim, Y. (1979). Paralinguistic aspects of auditory comprehension in aphasia. *Brain and Language, 7,* 164–174.

Bollinger, R. L., & Stout, C. E. (1976). Response-contingent small-step treatment: Performance-based communication intervention. *Journal of Speech and Hearing Disorders, 41,* 40–51.

Boone, D. R. (1967). A plan for the rehabilitation of aphasic patients. *Archives of Physical Medicine and Rehabilitation, 48,* 410–414.

Boone, D. R., & Friedman, H. M. (1976). Writing in aphasia rehabilitation: Cursive vs. manuscript. *Journal of Speech and Hearing Disorders, 41,* 523–529.

Bottenberg, D., Lemme, M., & Hedberg, N. (1987). Effect of story on narrative discourse of aphasic adults. In R. H. Brookshire (Ed.), *Clinical aphasiology* (Vol. 17, pp. 202–209). Minneapolis: BRK.

Boucher, V., Garcia, L. J., Fleruant, J., & Paradis, J. (2001). Variable efficacy of rhythm and tone in melody-based interventions: Implications for the assumption of a right-hemisphere facilitation in non-fluent aphasia. *Aphasiology, 15*(2), 131–149.

Boyle, M. (2004). Semantic feature analysis treatment for anomia in two fluent aphasia syndromes. *American Journal of Speech-Language Pathology, 13,* 236–249.

Boyle, M., & Canter, G. J. (1986). Verbal context and comprehension of difficult sentences by aphasic adults: A methodological problem. In R. H. Brookshire (Ed.), *Clinical aphasiology* (Vol. 16, pp. 38–44). Minneapolis: BRK.

Boyle, M., & Coelho, C. A. (1995). Application of semantic feature analysis as a treatment for aphasic dysnomia. *American Journal of Speech-Language Pathology, 4,* 94–98.

Breen, K., & Warrington, E. K. (1994). A study of anomia: Evidence for a distinction between nominal and propositional language. *Cortex, 30,* 231–245.

Breese, E. L., & Hillis, A. E. (2004). Auditory comprehension: Is multiple choice really good enough? *Brain and Language, 89,* 3–8.

Brenneise-Sarshad, R., Nicholas, L., & Brookshire, R. H. (1991). Effects of apparent listener knowledge and picture stimuli on aphasic and nonbrain-damaged speakers' narrative discourse. *Journal of Speech and Hearing Research, 34,* 168–176.

Bricker, A. L., Schuell, H., & Jenkins, J. J. (1964). Effect of word frequency and word length on aphasic spelling errors. *Journal of Speech and Hearing Research, 7,* 183–192.

Brookshire, R. H. (1971a). Effects of delay of reinforcemenet on probability learning by aphasic subjects. *Journal of Speech and Hearing Research, 14,* 92–105.

Brookshire, R. H. (1971b). Effects of trial time and inter-trial interval on naming by aphasic subjects. *Journal of Communication Disorders, 3,* 289–301.

Brookshire, R. H. (1972). Effects of task difficulty on the naming performance of aphasic subjects. *Journal of Speech and Hearing Research, 15,* 551–558.

Brookshire, R. H. (1974). Differences in responding to auditory materials among aphasic patients. *Acta Symbolica, 5,* 1–18.

Brookshire, R. H. (1976a). The role of auditory functions in rehabilitation of aphasic individuals. In R. T. Wertz & M. Collins (Eds.), *Clinical aphasiology: Conference proceedings,* 1972. Madison, WI: Clinical Aphasiology Conference.

Brookshire, R. H. (1976b). Effects of task difficulty on sentence comprehension performance of aphasic subjects. *Journal of Communication Disorders, 9,* 167–173.

Brookshire, R. H. (1977). A system for coding and recording events in patient-clinician interactions during aphasia treatment sessions. In M. Sullivan & M. S. Kommers (Eds.), *Rationale for adult aphasia therapy.* Omaha, University of Nebraska Medical Center.

Brookshire, R. H. (2005). *An introduction to neurogenic communication disorders* (6th ed.). St. Louis, MO: Mosby Year Book.

Brookshire, R. H., & Lommel, M. (1974). Perception of sequences of visual temporal and auditory spatial stimuli by aphasic, right hemisphere damaged, and non-brain-damaged subjects. *Journal of Communication Disorders, 7,* 155–169.

Brookshire, R. H., & Nicholas, L. S. (1978). Effects of clinician request and feedback behavior on responses of aphasic individuals in speech and language treatment sessions. In R. H. Brookshire (Ed.), *Clinical aphasiology: Conference proceedings.* Minneapolis: BRK.

Brookshire, R. H., & Nicholas, L. E. (1980). Sentence verification and language comprehension of aphasic persons. In R. H. Brookshire (Ed.), *Clinical aphasiology: Conference proceedings,* Minneapolis: BRK.

Brookshire, R. H., & Nicholas, L. E. (1981). Verification of active and passive sentences by aphasic and monoaphasic subjects. *Journal of Speech and Hearing Disorders, 23,* 878–893.

Brookshire, R. H., & Nicholas, L. E. (1984). Comprehension of directly and indirectly stated ideas and details in discourse by brain-damaged and non-brain-damaged listeners. *Brain and Language, 21,* 21–36.

Calautti, C., Warburton, E. A., & Baron, J.- C. (2003). Functional neuroimaging and recovery of function following brain damage in adults. In J. Grafman & I. H. Robertson (Eds.), *Handbook of neuropsychology* (2nd ed., Vol. 9). Amsterdam, Netherlands: Elsevier Science B. V.

Cannito, M. P., Hough, M., Vogel, D., & Pierce, R. S. (1996). Contextual influences on auditory comprehension of reversible passive sentences in aphasia. *Aphasiology, 10, 235*–252.

Cannito, M. P., Jarecki, J. M., & Pierce, R. S. (1986). Effects of thematic structure on syntactic comprehension in aphasia. *Brain and Language, 27,* 38–49.

Cannito, M. P., Vogel, D., & Pierce, R. S. (1989). Sentence comprehension in context: Influence of proper visual stimulation? In T. E. Prescott (Ed.), *Clinical aphasiology* (Vol. 18, pp. 433–446). Boston, MA: Little, Brown and Company.

Caplan, D., & Evans, K. L. (1990). The effects of syntactic structure on discourse comprehension in patients with parsing impairments. *Brain and Language, 39,* 206–234.

Caplan, D., & Hanna, J. E. (1996). Sentence production by aphasic patients in a constained task. *Brain and Language, 63,* 184–218.

Cappa, S. F., Nespor, M., Ielasi, W., & Miozza, A. (1997). The representation of stress: Evidence from an aphasic patient. *Cognition, 65,* 1–13.

Caramazza, A., & Berndt, R. S. (1978). Semantic and syntactic processes in aphasia: A review of the literature. *Psychological Review, 85,* 898–918.

Caramazza, A., Berndt, R. S., & Brownell, H. H. (1982). The semantic deficit hypothesis: Perceptual parsing and object classification by aphasic patients. *Brain and Language, 15,* 161–189.

Caramazza, A., & Zurif, E. B. (1976). Dissociation of algorithmic and heuristic processes in language comprehension: Evidence from ahpasia. *Brain and Language, 3,* 572–582.

Chenery, H. J., Ingram, J. C. L., & Murdoch, B. E. (1990). Automatic and volitional semantic processing in aphasia. *Brain and Language, 38,* 215–232.

Chieffi, S., Carlomagno, S., Silveri, M. C., & Gainotti, G. (1989). The influence of semantic and perceptual factors on lexical comprehension in aphasic and right brain-damaged patients. *Cortex, 25,* 592–598.

Clark, A. E., & Flowers, C. R. (1987). The effect of semantic redundancy on auditory comprehension in aphasia. In R. H. Brookshire (Ed.), *Clinical aphasiology* (Vol. 17, pp. 174–179). Minneapolis: BRK.

Coelho, C. A., McHugh, R. E., & Boyle, M. (2000). Semantic feature analysis as a treatment for aphasic dysnomia: A replication. *Aphasiology, 14*(2), 133–142.

Conley, A., & Coelho, C. A. (2003). Treatment of word retrieval impairment in chronic Broca's aphasia. *Aphasiology, 17*(3), 203–211.

Corlew, M. M., & Nation, J. E. (1975). Characteristics of visual stimuli and naming performance in aphasic adults. *Cortex, 11,* 186–191.

Cornelissen, K., Laine, M., Tarkiainen, A., Jarvensiuu, T., Martin, N., & Salmelin, R. (2003). Adult brain plasticity elicited by anomia treatment. *Journal of Cognitive Neuroscience, 15,* 444–461.

Correia, L., Brookshire, R. H., & Nicholas, L. E. (1989). The effects of picture content on descriptions by aphasic and non-brain-damaged speakers. In R. H. Brookshire (Ed.), *Clinical aphasiology* (Vol. 18, pp. 447–462). Boston, MA: Little, Brown and Company.

Correia, L., Brookshire, R. H., & Nicholas, L. E. (1990). Aphasic and nonbrain-damaged adults' descriptions of aphasia test pictures and genderbased pictures. *Journal of Speech and Hearing Disorders, 55,* 713–720.

Crosky, C. S., & Adams, M. R. (1969). A rationale and clinical methodology for selecting vocabulary stimulus material for individual aphasic patients. *Journal of Communication Disorders, 2,* 340–343.

Curtiss, S., Jackson, C. A., Kempler, D., Hanson, W. R., & Metter, E. J. (1986). Length vs. structural complexity in sentence comprehension in aphasia. In R. H. Brookshire (Ed.), *Clinical aphasiology* (Vol. 16, pp. 45–53). Minneapolis: BRK.

Darley, F. L. (1972). The efficacy of language rehabilitation in aphasia. *Journal of Speech and Hearing Disorders, 37,* 3–21.

Darley, F. L. (1975). Treatment of acquired aphasia. In W. J. Friedlander (Ed.), *Advances in neurology* (Vol. 7). New York: Raven Press.

Darley, F. L. (1976). Maximizing input to the aphasic patient. In R. H. Brookshire (Ed.), *Clinical aphasiology: Conference proceedings.* Minneapolis: BRK.

Darley, F. L. (1977). A retrospective view: Aphasia. *Journal of Speech and Hearing Disorders, 42,* 161–169.

Darley, F. L. (1979). Treat or neglect. *ASHA, 21,* 628–631.

Darley, F. L. (1982). *Aphasia.* Philadelphia: W.B. Saunders.

Darley, F. L., Sherman, D., & Siegal, G. M. (1959). Scaling of abstraction level of single words. *Journal of Speech and Hearing Disorders, 2,* 161–167.

Davis, G. A. (1993). *A survey of adult aphasia and related language disorders* (2nd ed.). Englewood Cliffs, NJ: Prentice-Hall.

DeDe, G., Parris, D., & Waters, G. (2003), Teaching self-cues: A treatment approach for verbal naming. *Aphasiology, 17*(5), 465–480.

Deloche, G., & Seron, X. (1981). Sentence understanding and knowledge of the world: Evidence from a sentence-picture matching task performed by aphasic patients. *Brain and Language, 14,* 57–69.

DeRenzi, E., & Vignolo, L. A. (1962). The Token Test: A sensitive test to detect receptive disturbances in aphasics. *Brain, 85,* 665–678.

Disimoni, F. G., Keith, R. L., Holt, B. L., & Barley, F. L., (1975). Practicality of shortening the porch Index of Communicative Ability. *Journal of Speech and Hearing Disorders, 41,* 110–119.

Doesborgh, S. J. C., van de Sandt-Koenderman, M. W. M. E., Dippel, D. W. J., van Harskamp, F., Koudstaal, P. J., & Visch-Brink, E. G. (2004). Cues on request: The efficacy of Multicue, a computer program for word finding therapy. *Aphasiology, 18*(3), 213–222.

Duffy, J. R., & Ulrich, S. R. (1976). A comparison of impairments in verbal comprehension, speech, reading, and writing in adult aphasics. *Journal of Speech and Hearing Disorders, 41,* 110–119.

Duffy, J. R., & Watkins, L. B. (1984). The effect of response choice relatedness on pantomime and verbal recognition ability in aphasic patients. *Brain and Language, 21,* 291–306.

Dumond, D. L., Hardy, J. C., & Van Demark, A. A. (1978). Presentation by order of difficulty of test tasks to persons with aphasia. *Journal of Speech and Hearing Research, 21,* 350–360.

Eccles, J. C. (1973). *The understanding of the brain.* New York: McGraw-Hill.

Eisenson, J. (1973). *Adult aphasia: Assessment and treatment.* Englewood Cliffs, NJ: Prentice-Hall.

Ernest-Baron, C. R., Brookshire, R. H., & Nicholas, L. E. (1987). Story structure and retelling of narratives by aphasic and non-brain-damaged adults. *Journal of Speech and Hearing Research, 30,* 44–49.

Fillingham, J. K., Hodgson, C., Sage, K., & Lambon Ralph, M. A. (2003). The application of errorless learning to aphasic disorders: A review of theory and practice. *Neuropsychological Rehabilitation, 13*(3), 337–363.

Fink, R. B., Brecher, A., Sobel, P., & Schwartz, M. F. (2005). Computer-assisted treatment of word retrieval deficits in aphasia. *Aphasiology, 19*(10/11), 943–954.

Foldi, N. S. (1987). Appreciation of pragmatic interpretations of indirect commands: Comparison of right and left hemisphere brain-damaged patients. *Brain and Language, 31,* 88–108.

Frattali, C., Bayles, K., Beeson, P., Kennedy, M. R. T., Wambaugh, J., & Yorkston, K. M. (2003). Development of evidence-based practice guidelines: Committee update. *Journal of Medical Speech-Language Pathology, 11,* ix–xviii.

Freed, D. B., Marshall, R. C., & Nippold, M. A. (1995). Comparison of personalized cueing on the facilitation of verbal labeling by aphasic subjects. *Journal of Speech and Hearing Research, 38,* 1081–1090.

Friederici, A. D. (1983). Aphasics' perception of words in sentential context: Some real time processing evidence. *Neuropsychologia, 21,* 351–358.

Friederici, A. D., & Graetz, P. A. M. (1987). Processing passive sentences in aphasia: Deficits and strategies. *Brain and Language, 30,* 93–105.

Friederici, A. D., Schoenle, P. W., & Goodglass, H. (1981). Mechanisms underlying writing and speech in aphasia. *Brain and Language, 13,* 212–222.

Fucetola, R., Tucker, F., Blank, K., & Corbetta, M. (2005). A process for translating evidence-based aphasia treatment into clinical practice. *Aphasiology*, *19*(3/4/5), 411–422.

Gallaher, A. J. (1981). Syntactic versus semantic performances of agrammatic Broca's aphasics on tests of constituent-element-ordering. *Journal of Speech and Hearing Research*, *2*, 217–223.

Gallaher, A. J., & Canter, G. J. (1982). Reading and lexical comprehension in Broca's apahsia: Lexical versus syntactical errors. *Brain and Language*, *17*, 183–192.

Gardner, B., & Brookshire, R. H. (1972). Effects of unisensory and multisensory presentation of stimuli upon naming by aphasic patients. *Language and Speech*, *15*, 342–357.

Gardner, H. (1973). The contribution of operativity to naming capacity in aphasic patients. *Neuropsychologia*, *11*, 213–220.

Gardner, H., Albert, M. L., & Weintraub, S. (1975). Comprehending a word: The influence of speed and redundance on auditory comprehension in aphasia. *Cortex*, *11*, 155–162.

Gerratt, B. R., & Jones, D. (1987). Aphasic performance on a lexical decision task: Multiple meanings and word frequency. *Brain and Language*, *30*, 106–115.

Glaser, R., Stoioff, M., & Weidner, W. E. (1974). The effect of controlled auditory stimulation on the auditory recognition of adult aphasic subjects. *Acta Symbolica*, *5*, 57–68.

Glosser, G., Wiener, M., & Kaplan, E. (1988). Variations in aphasic language behaviors. *Journal of Speech and Hearing Disorders*, *53*, 115–124.

Goldstein, K. (1948). *Language and language disturbances*. New York: Grune & Stratton.

Golper, L., & Rau, M. T. (1983). Systematic analysis of cuing strategies in aphasia: Taking your "cue" from the patient. In R. H. Brookshire (Ed.), *Clinical aphasiology: Conference proceedings*. Minneapolis: BRK.

Goodglass, H. (1968). Studies on the grammar of aphasics. In S. Rosenberg & J. Koplin (Eds.), *Developments in applied psycholinguistic research*. New York: Macmillan.

Goodglass, H., & Baker, E. (1976). Semantic field, naming, and auditory comprehension in aphasia. *Brain and Language*, *3*, 359–374.

Goodglass, H., Barton, M. I., & Kaplan, E. F. (1968). Sensory modality and object naming in aphasia. *Journal of Speech and Hearing Research*, *11*, 488–496.

Goodglass, H., & Berko, J. (1960). Agrammatism and inflectional morphology in English. *Journal of Speech and Hearing Research*, *3*, 257–267.

Goodglass, H., Christiansen, J. A., & Gallagher, R. (1993). Comparison of morphology and syntax in free narrative and structured tests: Fluent vs. nonfluent aphasics. *Cortex*, *29*, 377–407.

Goodglass, H., Fodor, I. G., & Schuloff, C. (1967). Prosodic factors in grammar: Evidence from aphasia. *Journal of Speech and Hearing Research*, *10*, 5–20.

Goodglass, H., Gleason, J. B., & Hyde, M. R. (1970). Some dimensions of auditory language comprehension in aphasia. *Journal of Speech and Hearing Research*, *13*, 595–606.

Goodglass, H., & Hunt, J. (1958). Grammatical complexity and aphasic speech. *Word*, *14*, 197–207.

Goodglass, H., Klein, B., Carey, P. W., & Jones, K. J. (1966). Specific semantic word categories in aphasia. *Cortex*, *2*, 74–89.

Graham, L. F., Holtzapple, P., & LaPointe, L. L. (1987). Does contextually related action facilitate auditory comprehension? Performance across three conditions by high and low comprehenders. In R. H. Brookshire (Ed.), *Clinical aphasiology* (Vol. 17, pp. 180–187). Minneapolis: BRK.

Green, E., & Boller, F. (1974). Features of auditory comprehension in severely impaired aphasics. *Cortex*, *10*, 133–145.

Grossman, M., & Haberman, S. (1982). Aphasics' selected deficits in appreciating grammatical agreements. *Brain and Language*, *16*, 109–120.

Hageman, C. F., & Lewis, D. L. (1983). The effects of intrastimulus pause on the quality of auditory comprehension in aphasia. In R. H. Brookshire (Ed.), *Clinical aphasiology: Conference proceedings*. Minneapolis: BRK.

Halpern, H. (1965a). Effect of stimulus variables on dysphasic verbal errors. *Perceptual and Motor Skills*, *21*, 291–298.

Halpern, H. (1965b). Effect of stimulus variables on verbal perseveration of dysphasic subjects. *Perceptual and Motor Skills*, *20*, 421–429.

Hanlon, R. E., Brown, J. W., & Gerstman, L. J. (1990). Enhancement of naming in nonfluent aphasia through gesture. *Brain and Language*, *38*, 298–314.

Hauk, O., & Pulvermuller, F. (2004). Effects of word length and frequency on the human event-related potential. *Clinical Neurophysiology*, *115*(5), 1090–1103.

Helm, N. (1979). Management of palilalia with a pacing board. *Journal of Speech & Hearing Disorders*, *44*, 350–353.

Helm-Estabrooks, N. (1981). "Show me the . . . whatever": Some variables affecting auditory comprehension scores of aphasic patients. In R. H. Brookshire (Ed.), *Clinical aphasiology: Conference proceedings*. Minneapolis: BRK.

Helm-Estabrooks, N. (1984). Treatment of the aphasias. *Seminars in Neurology*, *4*, 196–202.

Helmick, J. W., & Wipplinger, M. (1975). Effects of stimulus repetition on the naming behavior of an aphasic adult: A clinical report. *Journal of Communication Disorders*, *8*, 23–29.

Hendrick, D. L., Christman, M. A., & Augustine, L. (1973). Programming for the antecedent event in therapy. *Journal of Speech and Hearing Disorders*, *38*, 339–344.

Hickok, G., & Avrutin, S. (1995). Representation, referentiality, and processing in agrammatic comprehension: Two case studies. *Brain and Language*, *50*, 10–26.

Hickok, G., Zurif, E. B., & Canseco-Gonzalez, E. (1993). Traces in the explanation of comprehension of Broca's aphasia. *Brain and Language*, *45*, 371–395.

Hillis, A. E. (2002). Does the right make it right? Questions about recovery of language after stroke. *Annals of Neurology*, *51*(5), 537–538.

Hinckley, J. J., & Carr, T. H. (2005). Comparing the outcomes of intensive and non-intensive context-based aphasia treatment. *Aphasiology*, *19*(10/11), 965–974.

Holland, A. L. (1975). The effectiveness of treatment in aphasia. In R. H. Brookshire (Ed.), *Clinical aphasiology: Conference proceedings*. Minneapolis: BRK.

Holland, A. L., Fromm, D. S., DeRuyter, F., & Stein, M. (1996). Treatment efficacy: Aphasia. *Journal of Speech and Hearing Research*, *39*, S27–S36.

Holland, A. L., & Sonderman, J. C. (1974). Effects of a program based on the Token Test for teaching comprehension skills to aphasics. *Journal of Speech and Hearing Research*, *17*, 589–598.

Hough, M. S. (1989). Category concept generation in aphasia: The influence of context. *Aphasiology, 3*, 553–568.

Hough, M. S. (1990). Narrative comprehension in adults with right and left hemisphere brain-damage: Theme organization. *Brain and Language, 38*, 253–277.

Hough, M. S., & Pierce, R. S. (1989). Contextual influences on category concept generation in aphasia. In T. E. Prescott (Ed.), *Clinical aphasiology* (Vol. 18, pp. 507–519). Boston, MA: Little, Brown and Company.

Hough, M. S., Pierce, R. S., & Cannito, M. D. (1989). Contextual influences in aphasia: Effects of predictive versus nonpredictive narratives. *Brain and Language, 36*, 325–334.

Jacobs, B., & Thompson, C. K. (2000). Cross-modal generalisation effects of training non-canonical sentence comprehension and production in agrammatic aphasia. *Journal of Speech Language and Hearing Research, 43*, 5–20.

Jenkins, J., Jiménez-Pabón, E., Shaw, R., & Sefer, J. (1975). *Schuell's aphasia in adults* (2nd ed.). New York: Harper & Row.

Johnson, J., Sommers, R., & Weidner, W. (1977). Dichotic ear preference in aphasia. *Journal of Speech and Hearing Research, 20*, 116–129.

Katsuki-Nakamura, J., Brookshire, R. H., & Nicholas, L. E. (1988). Comprehension of monologues and dialogues by aphasic listeners. *Journal of Speech and Hearing Disorders, 53*, 408–415.

Kearns, K. P. (1985). Response Elaboration Training for patient initiated utterances. In R. H. Brookshire (ed.), *Clinical aphasiology.* (vol. 15) (pp. 196–204). Minneapolis: BRK

Kearns, K., & Hubbard, D. J. (1977). A comparison of auditory comprehension tasks in aphasia. In R. H. Brookshire (Ed.), *Clinical aphasiology: Conference proceedings.* Minneapolis: BRK.

Kimelman, M. D. Z. (1991). The role of target word stress in auditory comprehension by aphasic listeners. *Journal of Speech and Hearing Research, 34*, 334–339.

Kimelman, M. D. Z., & McNeil, M. R. (1987). Emphatic stress comprehension on adult aphasia: A successful constructive replication. *Journal of Speech & Hearing Research, 30*, 295–300.

Kimelman, M. D. Z., & McNeil, M. R. (1989). Contextual influences on the audio comprehension of normally stressed targets by aphasic listeners. In T. E. Prescott (Ed.), *Clinical aphasiology* (Vol. 18, pp. 407–420). Boston, MA: Little, Brown and Company.

Kiran, S., & Thompson, C. K. (2003). The role of semantic complexity in treatment of naming deficits: Training semantic categories in fluent aphasia by controlling exemplar typicality. *Journal of Speech, Language and Hearing Research, 46*, 773–787.

Kohn, S. E., & Goodglass, H. (1985). Picture-naming in aphasia. *Brain and Language, 24*, 266–283.

Kohn, S. E., Lorch, M. P., & Pearson, D. M. (1989). Verb finding in aphasia. *Cortex, 25*, 57–69.

Kolk, H. H. J., & Friederici, A. D. (1985). Strategy and impairment in sentence understanding by Broca's and Wernicke's aphasics. *Cortex, 21*, 47–67.

Kudo, T. (1984). The effect of semantic plausibility on sentence comprehension in aphasia. *Brain and Language, 21*, 208–218.

Lambrecht, K. J., & Marshall, R. C. (1983). Comprehension in severe aphasia: A second look. In R. H. Brookshire (Ed.), *Clinical aphasiology: Conference proceedings.* Minneapolis: BRK.

LaPointe, L. L. (1977). Base-10 programmed stimulation: Task specification, scoring, and plotting performance in aphasia therapy. *Journal of Speech and Hearing Disorders, 42*, 90–105.

LaPointe, L. L. (1978a). Aphasia therapy: Some principles and strategies for treatment. In D. F. Johns (Ed.), *Clinical management of neurogenic communicative disorders.* Boston, MA: Little, Brown.

LaPointe, L. L. (1978b). Multiple baseline designs. In R. H. Brookshire (Ed.), *Clinical aphasiology: Conference proceedings.* Minneapolis: BRK.

LaPointe, L. L. (1983). Aphasic intervention in adults: Historical, present, and future approaches. In J. Miller, D. E. Yoder, & R. Schiefelbusch (Eds.), *Contemporary issues in language intervention* (ASHA Reports, No. 12). Rockville, MD: American Speech-Language-Hearing Association.

LaPointe, L. L., Horner, J., & Lieberman, R. (1977). Effects of ear presentation and delayed response on the processing of Token Test commands. In R. H. Brookshire (Ed.), *Clinical aphasiology: Conference proceedings.* Minneapolis: BRK.

LaPointe, L. L., Rothi, L. J., & Campanella, D. J. (1978). The effects of repetition of Token Test commands on auditory comprehension. In R. H. Brookshire (Ed.), *Clinical aphasiology: Conference proceedings.* Minneapolis: BRK.

Lasky, E. Z., Weidner, W. E., & Johnson, J. P. (1976). Influence of linguistic complexity, rate of presentation, and interphrase pause time on auditory verbal comprehension of adult aphasic patients. *Brain and Language, 3*, 386–396.

LeDorze, G., Boulay, N., Gaudreau, & Brassard, C. (1994). The contrasting effects of a semantic versus formal-semantic technique for the facilitation of naming in a case of anomia. *Aphasiology, 8*, 127–142.

Leonard, C. L., & Baum, S. R. (1997). The influence of phonological and orthographic information on auditory lexical access in brain-damaged patients: A preliminary investigation. *Aphasiology, 11*, 1031–1042.

Lesser, R. (1974). Verbal comprehension in aphasia: An English version of three Italian tests. *Cortex, 10*, 247–263.

Lesser, R. (1978). *Linguistic investigations of aphasia.* New York: Elsevier.

Li, E. C., & Canter, G. J. (1991). Varieties of errors produced by aphasic patients in phonemic cueing. *Aphasiology, 5*, 51–61.

Li, E. C., & Williams, S. E. (1989). The efficacy of two types of cues in aphasic patients. *Aphasiology, 3*(7), 619–626.

Li, E. C., & Williams, S. E. (1990). The effects of grammatic class and cue type on cueing responsiveness in aphasia. *Brain and Language, 38*, 48–60.

Liles, B. Z., & Brookshire, R. H. (1975). The effects of pause time on auditory comprehension of aphasic subjects. *Journal of Communication Disorders, 8*, 221–235.

Linebaugh, C., & Lehner, L. (1977). Cueing hierarchies and word retrieval: A therapy program. In R. H. Brookshire (Ed.), *Clinical aphasiology: Conference proceedings.* Minneapolis: BRK.

Linebaugh, C. W. (1986). Variability of error patterns on two formats of picture-to-word matching. In R. H. Brookshire

(Ed.), *Clinical aphasiology* (Vol. 16, pp. 181–189). Minneapolis: BRK.

Lott, S. N., Friedman, R. B., & Linebaugh, G. W. (1994). Rationale and efficacy of a tactile-kinesthetic treatment for alexia. *Aphasiology, 8,* 181–196.

Loverso, F. L., & Prescott, T. E. (1981). The effect of alerting signals on left brain damaged (aphasic) and normal subjects' accuracy and response time to visual stimuli. In R. H. Brookshire (Ed.), *Clinical aphasiology: Conference proceedings.* Minneapolis: BRK.

Lowell, S., Beeson, P. M., & Holland, A. L. (1995). The efficacy of a semantic cueing procedure on naming performance of adults with aphasia. *American Journal of Speech-Language Pathology, 4,* 109–114.

Mack, J. L. (1982). The comprehension of locative prepositions in nonfluent and fluent aphasia. *Brain and Language, 14,* 18–92.

Maher, L. M., Kendall, D., Swearengin, J. A., Rodriguez, A., Leon, S., Pingel, K., et al. (2003). *Comparison of constraint induced language therapy and traditional therapy in rehabilitation of chronic aphasia: Preliminary findings.* Poster presentation at American Speech Language and Hearing National Convention, Chicago, IL.

Manjaly, Z. M., Marshall, J. C., Stephan, K. E., Gurd, J. M., Zilles, K., & Fink, G. R. (2005). Context-dependent interactions of left posterior inferior frontal gyrus in a local visual search task unrelated to language. *Cognitive Neuropsychology, 22*(3/4), 292–305.

Marshall, J., Pring, T., & Chiat, S. (1998). Verb retrieval and sentence production in aphasia. *Brain and Language, 63,* 159–183.

Marshall, J. C., & Newcombe, F. (1966). Syntactic and semantic errors in paralexia. *Neuropsychologia, 4,* 169–176.

Marshall, R. C. (1976). Word retrieval behavior of aphasic adults. *Journal of Speech and Hearing Disorders, 41,* 444–451.

Marshall, R. C., Karow, C. M., Freed, D. B., & Babcock, P. (2002). Effects of personalized cue form on the learning of subordinate category names by aphasic and non-brain-damaged subjects. *Aphasiology, 16*(7), 763–771.

Marshall, R. C., & King, P. S. (1973). Effects of fatigue produced by isokinetic exercise on the communication ability of aphasic adults. *Journal of Speech and Hearing Research, 16,* 222–230.

Marshall, R. C., & Tompkins, C. A. (1982). Verbal self-correction behaviors of fluent and nonfluent aphasic subjects. *Brain and Language, 15,* 292–306.

Marshall, R. C., Tompkins, C. A., & Phillips, D. S. (1980). Effects of scheduling on the communication assessment of aphasic patients. *Journal of Communication Disorders, 13,* 105–114.

Marshall, R. C., Wertz, R. T., Weiss, D. G., Aten, J. L., Brookshire, R. H. Garcia-Bunuel, L., Holland, W. L., et al. (1989). Home treatment for aphasia patients by trained nonprofessionals. *Journal of Speech and Hearing Disorders, 54,* 462–470.

Martin, A. D. (1975). A critical evaluation of therapeutic approaches to aphasia. In R. H. Brookshire (Ed.), *Clinical aphasiology: Conference proceedings.* Minneapolis: BRK.

Martin, N., & Laine, M. (2000) Effects of contextual priming on word retrieval in anomia *Aphasiology, 14,* 53–70.

Martin, N., Fink, R., & Laine, M. (2004). Treatment of word retrieval deficits with contextual priming. *Aphasiology, 18*(5/6/7), 457–471.

Martin, N., Fink, R., Laine, M., & Ayala, J. (2004). Immediate and short-term effects of contextual priming of word retrieval. *Aphasiology, 18*(10), 867–898.

Martin, R. C., & Feher, E. (1990). The consequences of reduced memory span for the comprehension of semantic versus syntactic information. *Brain and Language, 38,* 1–20.

Massaro, M. E., & Tompkins, C. A.(1992). Feature analysis for treatment of communication disorders in traumatically brain-injured patients: An efficacy study. *Clinical Aphasiology, 22,* 245–256.

McCall, D., Cox, D. M., Shelton, J. R., & Weinrich, M. (1997). The influence of syntactic and semantic information on picture-naming performance in aphasic patients. *Aphasiology, 11,* 581–600.

McDearmon, J. R., & Potter, R. E. (1975). The use of representational prompts in aphasia therapy. *Journal of Communication Disorders, 8,* 199–206.

McNeil, M., Darley, F. L., Rose D. E., & Olsen, W. O. (1979a, June). *Effects of diotic intensity increments on auditory processing deficits in aphasia.* Paper presented to the Ninth Annual Clinical Aphasiology Conference, Phoenix, AZ.

McNeil, M., Darley, F. L., Rose, D. E., & Olsen, W. O. (1979b, June). *Effects of selective binaural intensity variations on auditory processing in aphasia.* Paper presented to the Ninth Annual Clinical Aphasiology Conference, Phoenix, AZ.

McNeil, M., & Hageman, C. (1979). Prediction and pattern of auditory processing deficits on the Revised Token Test. In R. H. Brookshire (Ed.), *Clinical aphasiology: Conference proceedings.* Minneapolis: BRK.

McNeil, M. R., Hageman, C. F., & Matthews, C. T. (2005). Auditory processing deficits in aphasia evidenced on the Revised Token Test: Incidence and prediction of across subtest and across item within subtest patterns. *Aphasiology, 19*(2), 179–198.

McNeil, M. R., & Kimelman, M. D. Z. (1986). Toward an integrative information-processing structure of auditory comprehension and processing in adult aphasia. *Seminars in Speech and Language, 7,* 123–146.

McNeil, M. R., Odell, K., & Tseng, C. H. (1990). Toward the integration of resource allocation into a general model of aphasia. In T. Prescott (Ed.), *Clinical aphasiology* (Vol. 20, pp. 21–39). Austin, TX.

McNeil, M., & Prescott, T. E. (1978). *Revised Token Test.* Baltimore: University Park Press.

Miceli, G., Silveri, M. C., Nocentini, U., & Caramaza, A. (1988). Patterns of dissociation in comprehension and production of nouns and verbs. *Aphasiology, 2,* 207–220.

Miceli, G., Silveri, M. C., Villi, G., & Caramaza, A. (1984). On the basis for the agrammatic's difficulty in producing main verbs. *Cortex, 20,* 207–220.

Mills, R. (1977). The effects of environmental sound on the naming performance of aphasic subjects. In R. H. Brookshire (Ed.), *Clinical aphasiology: Conference proceedings.* Minneapolis: BRK.

Mills, R. H., Knox, A. W., Juola, J. F., & Salmon, S. J. (1979). Cognitive loci of impairments in picture naming by aphasic subjects. *Journal of Speech and Hearing Research, 22,* 73–87.

Mitchum, C. C., Greenwald, M. L., & Berndt, R. S. (2000). Cognitive treatments of sentence processing disorders: What have we learned? *Neuropsychological Rehabilitation, 10*(3), 311–336.

Moore, W. H. (1996). The effects of multimodality stimulation on hemispheric alpha asymmetries of aphasic and normal subjects. *Aphasiology, 10,* 671–686.

Morris, J., Franklin, S., Ellis, A. W., Turner, J. E., & Bailey, P. J. (1996). Remediating a speech perception deficit in an aphasic patient. *Aphasiology, 10,* 137–158.

Murray, L., Ballard, K., & Karcher, L. (2004). Linguistic specific treatment: Just for Broca's aphasia? *Aphasiology, 18*(9), 785–809.

Naeser, M. A., Martin, P. I., Nicholas, M., Baker, E. H., Seekins, H., Helm-Estabrooks, N., et al. (2005). Improved naming after TMS treatments in a chronic, global aphasia patient—Case report. *Neurocase, 11,* 182–193.

Naeser, M. A., Mazurskil, P., Goodglass, H., Peraino, M., Laughlin, S., & Leaper, W. C. (1987). Auditory syntactic comprehension in nine aphasia groups (with CT scans) and children: Differences in degree but not order of difficulty observed. *Cortex, 23,* 359–380.

Nicholas, L., & Brookshire, R. H. (1983). Syntactic simplification and context: Effects on sentence comprehension by aphasic adults. In R. H. Brookshire (Ed.), *Clinical aphasiology: Conference proceedings.* Minneapolis: BRK.

Nicholas, L. E., & Brookshire, R. H. (1986a). Consistency of the effects of rate of speech on brain-damaged adults' comprehension of narrative discourse. *Journal of Speech and Hearing Research, 29,* 462–470.

Nicholas, L. E., & Brookshire, R. H. (1986b). Types of errors in multiple sentence reading comprehension of aphasic adults. In R. H. Brookshire (Ed.), *Clinical aphasiology* (Vol. 16, pp. 190–195). Minneapolis: BRK.

Nickels, L., & Howard, D. (1995). Aphasic naming: What matters? *Neuropsychologia, 33,* 1281–1303.

Noll, J. D., & Hoops, H. R. (1967). Aphasic grammatical involvement as indicated by spelling ability. *Cortex, 3,* 419–432.

North, B. (1971). *Effects of stimulus redundancy on naming disorders in aphasia.* Unpublished doctoral dissertation, Boston University.

Orpwood, L., & Warrington, E. K. (1995). Word specific impairments in naming and spelling but not reading. *Cortex, 31,* 239–265.

Parisi, D., & Pizzamiglio, L. (1970). Syntactic comprehension in aphasia. *Cortex, 6,* 204–215.

Pashek, G. V., & Brookshire, R. H. (1982). Effect of rate and stress on auditory paragraph comprehension in aphasic individuals. *Journal of Speech and Hearing Research, 25,* 377–383.

Peach, R. K., Canter, G. J., & Gallaher, A. J. (1988). Comprehension of sentence structure in anomic and conduction aphasia. *Brain and Language, 35,* 119–137.

Pedersen, P. M., Vinter, K., & Olsen, R. S. (2001) Improvement of oral naming by unsupervised computerised rehabilitation. *Aphasiology, 15*(2), 151–169.

Pierce, R. S. (1981). Facilitating the comprehension of tense related sentences in aphasia. *Journal of Speech and Hearing Disorders, 46,* 364–368.

Pierce, R. S. (1982). Facilitating the comprehension of syntax in aphasia. *Journal of Speech and Hearing Research, 25,* 408–413.

Pierce, R. S. (1983). Decoding syntax during reading in aphasia. *Journal of Communication Disorders, 16,* 181–188.

Pierce, R. S. (1988). Influence of prior and subsequent context on comprehension in aphasia. *Aphasiology, 2,* 577–582.

Pierce, R. S. (1991). Short Report: Contextual influences during comprehension in aphasia. *Aphasiology, 5,* 379–381.

Pierce, R. S., & Beekman, L. A. (1985). Effects of linguistic and extralinguistic context on semantic and syntactic processing in aphasia. *Journal of Speech and Hearing Research, 28,* 250–254.

Pizzamiglio, L., & Appicciafuoco, A. (1971). Semantic comprehension in aphasia. *Journal of Communication Disorders, 3,* 280–288.

Podraza, B. L., & Darley, F. L. (1977). Effect of auditory prestimulation on naming in aphasia. *Journal of Speech and Hearing Research, 20,* 669–683.

Poeck, K., Huber, W., & Willmes, K. (1989). Outcome of intensive language treatment in aphasia. *Journal of Speech and Hearing Disorders, 54,* 471–479.

Poeck, K., & Pietron, H. (1981). The influence of stretched speech presentation on Token Test performance of aphasic and right brain damaged patients. *Neuropsychologia, 19,* 135–136.

Porch, B. E. (1967). *Porch index of communicative ability.* Palo Alto, CA: Consulting Psychologists Press.

Pulvermüller, F., Neininger, B., Elbert, T., Mohr, B., Rockstroh, B. Koebbel, P., et al. (2001). Constraint-induced therapy of chronic aphasia after stroke. *Stroke, 32,* 1621–1626.

Records, N. L. (1994). A measure of the contribution of a gesture to the perception of speech in listeners with aphasia. *Journal of Speech and Hearing Research, 37,* 1086–1099.

Renvall, K., Laine, M., Laakso, M., & Martin, N. (2003). Anomia rehabilitation with contextual priming: A case study. *Aphasiology, 17,* 305–308.

Reuterskiöld, C. (1991). The effects of emotionality on auditory comprehension in aphasia. *Cortex, 27,* 595–604.

Roberts, J. A., & Wertz, R. T. (1986). TACS: A contrastive-language treatment for aphasic adults. In R. H. Brookshire (Ed.), *Clinical aphasiology* (Vol, 16, pp. 207–212). Minneapolis: BRK.

Robey, R. R. (1998). A meta-analysis of clinical outcomes in the treatment of aphasia. *Journal of Speech, Language, & Hearing Research, 41,* 172–187.

Robey, R. R., & Schultz, M. C. (1998). A model for conducting clinical-outcome research: An adaptation of the standard protocol for use in aphasiology. *Aphasiology, 12,* 787–810.

Robey, R. R., Schultz, M. C., Crawford, A. B., & Sinner, C. A. (1999). Single-subject clinical-outcome research: Design, data, effect sizes, and analysis. *Aphasiology, 13*(6), 445–473.

Rochon, E., Laird, L., Bose, A., & Scofield, J. (2005). Mapping therapy for sentence production impairments in nonfluent aphasia. *Neuropsychological Rehabilitation, 15*(1), 1–36.

Rolnick, M., & Hoops, H. R. (1969). Aphasia as seen by the aphasic. *Journal of Speech and Hearing Disorders, 34,* 48–53.

Rose, M. L., & Douglas, J. M. (2001). The differential facilitatory effects of gesture and visualisation processes on object naming in aphasia. *Aphasiology, 15,* 977–990.

Rose, M. L., Douglas, J. M., & Matyas, T. A. (2002). The comparative effectiveness of gesture and verbal treatments for a specific phonological naming impairment. *Aphasiology, 16,* 1001–1030.

Rosenbek, J., LaPointe, L. L., & Wertz, R. T. (1989). *Aphasia: A clinical approach.* Boston, MA: College-Hill.

Saffran, E. M., Berndt, R. S., & Schwartz, M. F. (1989). The quantitative analysis of agrammatic production: Procedure and data. *Brain and Language, 37,* 440–479.

Salvatore, A. P. (1976). Training an aphasic adult to respond appropriately to spoken commands by fading pause duration within commands. In R. H. Brookshire (Ed.), *Clinical aphasiology: Conference proceedings.* Minneapolis: BRK.

Salvatore, A. P., Strait, M., & Brookshire, R. H. (1978). Effects of patient characteristics on delivery of Token Test commands by experienced and inexperienced examiners. *Journal of Communication Disorders, 11,* 325–333.

Santo Pietro, M. J., & Rigrodsky, S. (1982). The effects of temporal and semantic conditions of the occurrence of the error response of perseveration in adult aphasics. *Journal of Speech and Hearing Research, 25,* 184–192.

Sarno, M. T. (1974). Aphasia rehabilitation. In S. Dickson (Ed.), *Communication disorders: Remedial principles and practices.* Glenview, IL: Scott Foresman Co.

Sarno, M. T. (1981). Recovery and rehabilitation in aphasia. In M. T. Sarno (Ed.), *Acquired aphasia.* New York: Academic Press.

Schuell, H. (1953a). Auditory impairment in aphasia: Significance and retraining techniques. *Journal of Speech and Hearing Disorders, 18,* 14–21.

Schuell, H. (1953b). Aphasic difficulties understanding spoken language. *Neurology, 3,* 176–184.

Schuell, H. (1969). *Aphasia in adults.* (NINDS, Monograph No. 10). *Human communication and its disorders.* Washington, D.C.: Department of Health, Education and Welfare, National Institutes of Health.

Schuell, H. (1973). (Revised by J. W. Sefer). *Differential diagnosis of aphasia with the Minnesota test.* Minneapolis, MN: University of Minnesota Press.

Schuell, H. (1974a). Clinical symptoms of aphasia. In L. F. Sies (Ed.), *Aphasia theory and therapy: Selected lectures and papers of Hildred Schuell.* Baltimore: University Park Press.

Schuell, H. (1974b). The treatment of aphasia. In L. F. Sies (Ed.), *Aphasia theory and therapy: Selected lectures and papers of Hildred Schuell.* Baltimore: University Park Press.

Schuell, H. (1974c). The development of a research program in aphasia. In L. F. Sies (Ed.), *Aphasia theory and therapy: Selected lectures and papers of Hildred Schuell.* Baltimore: University Park Press.

Schuell, H. (1974d). A theoretical framework for aphasia. In L. F. Sies (Ed.), *Aphasia theory and therapy: Selected lectures and papers of Hildred Schuell.* Baltimore: University Park Press.

Schuell, H., Carroll, V., & Street, B. (1955). Clinical treatment of aphasia. *Journal of Speech and Hearing Disorders, 20,* 43–53.

Schuell, H., & Jenkins, J. J. (1961a). Reduction of vocabulary in aphasia. *Brain, 84,* 243–261.

Schuell, H., & Jenkins, J. J. (1961b). Comment on "dimensions of language performance in aphasia." *Journal of Speech and Hearing Research, 4,* 295–299.

Schuell, H., Jenkins, J. J., & Jiménez-Pabón, E. (1964). *Aphasia in adults.* New York: Harper & Row.

Schuell, H., Jenkins, J. J., & Landis, L. (1961). Relationship between auditory comprehension and word frequency in aphasia. *Journal of Speech and Hearing Research, 4,* 30–36.

Schulte, E. (1986). Effects of imposed delay of response and item complexity on auditory comprehension by aphasics. *Brain and Language, 29,* 358–371.

Sherman, J. C., & Schweickert, J. (1989). Syntactic and semantic contributions to sentence comprehension in agrammatism. *Brain and Language, 37,* 419–439.

Shewan, C. M., & Canter, G. J. (1971). Effects of vocabulary, syntax, and sentence length on auditory comprehension in aphasic adults. *Cortex, 7,* 209–226.

Shewan, C. M., & Kertesz, A. (1984). Effects of speech and language treatment on recovery from aphasia. *Brain and Language, 23,* 272–299.

Siegel, G. M. (1959). Dysphasic speech responses to visual word stimuli. *Journal of Speech and Hearing Research, 2,* 152–167.

Siegenthaler, B. M., & Goldstein, J. (1967). Auditory and visual figure-background perception by adult aphasics. *Journal of Communication Disorders, 1,* 152–158.

Skelly, M. (1975). Aphasic patients talk back. *American Journal of Nursing, 75,* 1140–1142.

Smith, A. (1971). Objective indices of severity of chronic aphasia in stroke patients. *Journal of Speech and Hearing Disorders, 36,* 167–207.

Smithpeter, J. V. (1976). A clinical study of responses to olfactory stimuli in aphasic adults. In R. H. Brookshire (Ed.), *Clinical aphasiology: Conference proceedings.* Minneapolis: BRK.

Sparks, R., Goodglass, H., & Nickel, D. (1970). Ipsilateral versus contralateral extinction in cichotic listening resulting from hemisphere lesions. *Cortex, 8,* 249–260.

Spreen, O. (1968). Psycholinguistic aspects of aphasia. *Journal of Speech and Hearing Research, 11,* 467–480.

Stachowiak, F. K., Huber, W., Poeck, K., & Kerschensteiner, M. (1977). Text comprehension in aphasia. *Brain and Language, 4,* 177–195.

Stimley, M. A., & Noll, J. D. (1991). The effects of semantic and phonemic prestimulation cues on picture naming in aphasia. *Brain and Language, 41,* 496–509.

Stoicheff, M. L. (1960). Motivating instructions and language performance of dysphasic subjects. *Journal of Speech and Hearing Research, 3,* 75–85.

Swinney, D. A., Zurif, E. B., & Cutler, A. (1980). Effects of sentential stress and word class upon comprehension in Broca's aphasics. *Brain and Language, 10,* 132–144.

Taylor, M. T. (1964). Language therapy. In H. G. Burr (Ed.), *The aphasic adult: Evaluation and rehabilitation.* Charlottesville, VA: Wayside Press.

Thompson, C. K., Lange, K. L., Schneider, S. L., & Shapiro, L. P. (1997). Agrammatic and non-brain-damaged subjects' verb and verb argument structure production. *Aphasiology, 11,* 473–490.

Thompson, C. K., Raymer, A., & le Grand, H. (1991). Effects of phonologically based treatment on aphasic naming deficits: A model-driven approach. In T. E. Prescott (Ed.), *Clinical aphasiology* (Vol. 20, pp. 239–261). Austin, TX: Pro-Ed.

Thompson, C. K., & Shapiro, L. P. (2005). Treating agrammatic aphasia within a linguistic framework: Treatment of Underlying Forms. *Aphasiology, 19*(10/11), 1021–1036.

Thompson, C. K., Shapiro, L. P., Kiran, S., & Sobecks, J. (2003). The role of syntactic complexity in treatment of sentence deficits in agrammatic aphasia: The complexity account of treatment efficacy (CATE). *Journal of Speech, Language and Hearing Research, 46*(3), 591–607.

Thompson, C. K., Shapiro, L. P., Li, L., & Schendel, L. (1994). Analysis of verbs and verb-argument structure: A method for quantification of aphasic language production. In P. Lemme (Ed.), *Clinical aphasiology* (Vol. 23, pp. 121–140). Austin, TX: Pro-Ed.

Thompson, C. K., Shapiro, L. P., Tait, M. E., Jacobs, B., Schneider, S., & Ballard, K. (1995). A system for the linguistic analysis of agrammatic language production (Abstract). *Brain and Language, 51*, 124–127.

Thompson, R. F. (1967). *Foundations of physiological psychology*. New York: Harper & Row.

Thorndike, E. L., & Lorge, I. (1944). *The teacher's word book of 30,000 words*. New York: Columbia University.

Tikofsky, R. (1968). Basic research in aphasic behavior: Could it and should it contribute to rehabilitation. In J. Black & E. Jancosek (Eds.), *Proceedings of the conference on language retraining for aphasics*. Washington, D.C.: Social and Rehabilitation Service, Department of Health, Education, and Welfare.

Tompkins, C. A. (1991). Redundancy enhances emotional inferencing by right- and left-hemisphere-damaged adults. *Journal of Speech and Hearing Research, 34*, 1142–1149.

Van Lancker, D. R., & Kempler, D. (1987). Comprehension of familiar phrases by left- but not by right-hemisphere damaged patients. *Brain and Language, 32*, 265–277.

Wallace, G. L., & Canter, G. J. (1985). Effects of personally relevant language materials on the performance of severely aphasic individuals. *Journal of Speech and Hearing Research, 50*, 385–390.

Waller, M. R., & Darley, F. L. (1978). The influence of context on the auditory comprehension of paragraphs by aphasic subjects. *Journal of Speech and Hearing Research, 21*, 732–745.

Wambaugh, J., Cameron, R., Kalinyak-Fliszar, M., Nessler, C., & Wright, S. (2004). Retrieval of action names in aphasia: Effects of two cueing treatments. *Aphasiology, 18*(11), 979–1004.

Webb, W. G., & Love, R. J. (1983). Reading problems in chronic aphasia. *Journal of Speech and Hearing Disorders, 48*, 164–171.

Weidner, W. E., & Jinks, A. F. G. (1983). The effects of single versus combined cue presentations on picture naming by aphasic adults. *Journal of Communication Disorders, 16*, 111–121.

Weidner, W. E., & Lasky, E. Z. (1976). The interaction of rate and complexity of stimulus on the performance of adult aphasic subjects. *Brain and Language, 3*, 34–40.

Weigl, E. (1968). On the problem of cortical syndromes: Experimental studies. In M. L. Simmel (Ed.), *The reach of the mind: Essays in memory of Kurt Goldstein*. New York: Springer.

Weinstein, S. (1959). Experimental analysis of an attempt to improve speech in cases of expressive aphasia. *Neurology, 9*, 632–635.

Wepman, J. M. (1951). *Recovery from aphasia*. New York: Ronald Press.

Wepman, J. M. (1953). A conceptual model for the process involved in recovery from aphasia. *Journal of Speech and Hearing Disorders, 18*, 4–13.

Wepman, J. M. (1968). Aphasia therapy: Some relative comments and some purely personal prejudices. In J. Black & E. Jancosek (Eds.), *Proceedings of the conference on language retraining for aphasics*. Washington, D.C.: Social and Rehabilitation Service, Department of Health, Education and Welfare.

Wepman, J. M. (1972). Aphasia therapy: A new look. *Journal of Speech and Hearing Disorders, 37*, 203–214.

Wepman, J. M., & Jones, L. V. (1961). *Studies in aphasia: An approach to testing*. Chicago: University of Chicago Education Industry Service.

Wepman, J. M., Jones, L. V., Bock, R. D., & Van Pelt, D. (1960). Studies in aphasia: Background and theoretical formulations. *Journal of Speech and Hearing Disorders, 25*, 323–332.

Wertz, R. T. (1978). Neuropathologies of speech and language: An introduction to patient management. In D. F. Johns (Ed.), *Clinical management of neurogenic communicative disorders*. Boston: Little, Brown.

Wertz, R. T. (1983). Language intervention context and setting for the aphasic adult: When? In J. Miller, D. E. Yoder, & R. Schiefelbusch (Eds.), *Contemporary issues in language intervention* (ASHA Reports, No. 12). Rockville, MD: American Speech-Language-Hearing Association.

Wertz, R. T. (1991). Keynote Paper: Aphasiology 1990: A view from the colonies. *Aphasiology, 5*, (311–322).

Wertz, R. T., Collins, M. J., Weiss, D., Kurtzke, J. F., Friden, T., Brookshire, R. H., et al. (1981). Veterans Administration cooperative study on aphasia: A comparison of individual and group treatment. *Journal of Speech and Hearing Research, 24*, 580–594.

Wertz, R. T., & Irwin, W. H. (2001). Darley and the efficacy of language rehabilitation in aphasia. *Aphasiology, 15*, 231–247.

Wertz, R. T., & Porch, B. E. (1970). Effects of masking noise on the verbal performance of adult aphasics. *Cortex, 6*, 399–409.

Wertz, R. T., Weiss, D. G., Aten, J. L., Brookshire, R. H., Garcia-Bunuel, L., Holland, A. L., et al. (1986). Comparison of clinic, home, and deferred language treatment for aphasia: A Veterans Administration cooperative study. *Archives of Neurology, 43*, 653–658.

Whitehouse, P., & Caramazza, A. (1978). Naming in aphasia: Interacting effects of form and function. *Brain and Language, 6*, 63–74.

Whitney, J. L., & Goldstein, H. (1989). Using self-monitoring to reduce dysfluencies in speakers with mild aphasia. *Journal of Speech and Hearing Disorders, 54*, 576–586.

Wilcox, J. M., Davis, G. A., & Leonard, L. B. (1978). Aphasics' comprehension of contextually conveyed meaning. *Brain and Language, 6*, 362–377.

Williams, S. E. (1984). Influence of written form on reading comprehension in aphasia. *Journal of Communication Disorders, 17*, 165–174.

Williams, S. E., & Canter, G. J. (1982). The influence of situational context on naming performance in aphasic syndromes. *Brain and Language, 17*, 92–106.

Williams, S. E., & Canter, G. J. (1987). Action-naming performance in four syndromes of aphasia. *Brain and Language, 32*, 124–136.

Wright, H. H., & Newhoff, M. (2004). Priming auditory comprehension in aphasia: Facilitation and interference effects. *Aphasiology, 18*(5/6/7), 555–565.

Wulfeck, B. B. (1988). Grammaticality judgments and sentence comprehension in agrammatic aphasia. *Journal of Speech and Hearing Research, 31*, 72–81.

Zingeser, L. B., & Berndt, R. S. (1990). Retrieval of nouns and verbs in agrammatism and anomia. *Brain and Language, 39*, 14–32.

Zurif, E. B., Caramazza, A., Myerson, R., & Calvin, J. (1974). Semantic feature representation for normal and aphasic language. *Brain and Language, 1*, 167–187.

Chapter 16

Thematic Language-Stimulation Therapy

Shirley Morganstein and Marilyn
Certner-Smith

OBJECTIVES

In this chapter, we provide a theoretic background for
Thematic Language Stimulation (TLS), an intervention technique for aphasia; explain the rationale for TLS and delineate its various components; provide suggestions for clinical
and functional communication analysis as a precursor to the
use of TLS; and provide a template for replication of TLS
modules and directives for implementation in aphasia
therapy.

In the previous chapter, the reader will find an excellent
description and discussion of the work of Hildred Schuell.
Despite evolving knowledge gained in neurologic substrates of speech and language function, Schuell's model of
aphasia rehabilitation remains relevant. Schuell posited a
neurobiologic change with controlled stimulation, and so
do today's researchers in "the community of brain repair."[1]
Jenkins and colleagues (1990) found expansion of distal
digit representation in monkey brains after sensory training,
suggesting that the brain can change with systematic motor
stimulation. Similarly, Kilgard and Merzenich (1998) reported
changes in the organization of monkey auditory cortex after
exposure to a combination of sound and chemical neurotransmitters.

Thematic Language Stimulation is firmly rooted in
Schuell's stimulation treatment model. Indeed, as a graduate
student in the 1960s, the senior author was privileged to
have studied with Schuell during her tenure at the
University of Minnesota and the Minneapolis VA Hospital.
Some approaches to management of aphasia are based on

abstract or theoretic models of language (Boyle & Coelho,
1995; Drew & Thompson, 1999) Schuell's approach was
conceived as a result of focused clinical observation and data
collection on large numbers of patients. This clinical
approach enabled her to see and record relevant behaviors,
postulate and evaluate the underlying mechanisms for that
behavior, and find ways into the wounded brain. Since the
1960s, many aphasia therapists have found an intelligent and
comfortable point of entry in Schuell's work. It was from
that place of comfort that TLS was born.

Since the original formulation of TLS in 1982, a variety
of different therapeutic approaches have developed in
response to changes in the way that we, as a profession, perceive aphasia, the concept of disability, and the therapeutic
milieu. Specifically, we are looking more closely at the *person
with aphasia*, rather than the *disorder of aphasia*, as did Schuell.
This is not to say that Schuell did not consider the interpersonal aspects of communication—quite the contrary. All of
her investigations and interventions sought to alleviate the
symptoms that interfered with normal communication. She
did speak to the devastating effect of impaired communication on the person with aphasia:

> Like anyone who, suddenly in the midst of the journey of his life
> has found himself alone in a dark wood where the straight way is
> lost, the aphasic patient knows despair. Surely anyone partially
> paralyzed and unable to communicate must feel himself in a dark
> wood, indeed, and surely the straight road he took for the natural
> way must seem lost to him." (Schuell, 1964, p. 321)

Schuell would have greatly appreciated the work of individuals currently involved in the social, environmental, and
life participation approaches. Today, many speech-language
pathologists may feel a pull away from traditional interventions and into the more person-centered ones. Without
question, we are learning from people with aphasia what the
form and content of our therapy can be. The disability
empowerment movement is having a strong, positive effect
on the work of the aphasia therapist, yet some new views
about how we can intervene in the workings of the brain in
the person with aphasia also have appeared. Constraint-
induced therapy, for example (Maher et al., 2003;
Pulvermuller et al., 2001), is based on the neurophysiological finding that "doing" actually changes structure within

---

[1]Leslie Gonzalez-Rothi, *Speaking Out! 2004*, Tampa, Florida.

the brain. Other recent studies are revisiting the notion that some specific drugs may have an enhancing effect on brain function for communication (Greener, Enderby, & Whurr, 2001).

Perhaps more to the point is an examination not of *which* intervention is appropriate but, perhaps, *at what point in the therapeutic process, in what order, and for which persons with aphasia* different intervention approaches may be useful. As we noted in our chapter in the fourth edition of this text, a significant body of research that might help us to reliably identify specific candidates and the most beneficial timing for these specific techniques continues to be absent.

The current version of TLS continues to reflect its original stimulation roots. We also have found it to be helpful in the metalinguistic exploration of symptoms and strategy training and in the education of other speech-language pathologists and caregivers. We view TLS as one technique in a growing professional armamentarium. None of these techniques is mutually exclusive; indeed, some actually may be enhanced by the inclusion of others at another point in time.

DEFINITION

"Thematic language stimulation" is a systematic method of therapy for aphasia that employs thematically related vocabulary in multimodality stimulation, targeting changes in language processing for functional communication. Specifically, it begins with a select group of words related in meaning, places them in particular linguistic contexts, uses them in tasks that employ both input and output modes, and targets improvement of underlying language processes to impact on conversational success. The TLS hypothesis is that you are changing the way the brain is working by "working the brain." It extends concepts originally presented by Schuell and colleagues (1964) and by Wepman (1953, 1972). In addition, the authors have been influenced by the work of Edith Kaplan (1989) and of Nancy Helm-Estabrooks and M. Albert (1991), who emphasize the process approach in evaluation and treatment—that is, understanding the *why* as well as the *what* about aphasia.

Like all stimulation approaches, TLS places the burden of success on therapists, because they provide a possible neurobiologic link between what the person with aphasia knows and what the person with aphasia can produce. Theoretically, restoration of language proficiency comes about by means of carefully controlled stimulation. Stimulation targets overall improved understanding, speaking, reading, and writing. Observation of the person's behavior during stimulation reveals information about underlying processes. Awareness of these processes has value in the development of strategies for success in conversation.

TLS THEORY

Organizing Content and Delivery

The organization of the language used for stimulation is central to TLS. This is accomplished in two ways: first, in establishing a relevant, thematic "core vocabulary," and second, in creating predictable, systematic linguistic stimuli for each presented task.

Thematic Content

Wepman (1972), in his *content-centered treatment approach*, believed that treatment should focus on ideas. He advocated stimulation of thought to enhance verbal production during conversation. In contrast, TLS requires more stringent control of content and its manipulation within the session. Content themes heighten the saliency of the therapy and provide a context for both the stimulation and the subsequent conversation. Meaningful content in natural contexts strengthens the therapeutic effect. Rather than creating new ones, the TLS structure capitalizes on the organizational systems already established within the brain.

Both Schuell (1964) and Wepman (1972) agreed that treatment content should be *personally relevant*. At the most basic level, people tend to have more to talk about when the subject is connected to them (Wallace & Canter, 1985). In addition, Marshall (1994) noted that, for those with fluent aphasia, personally relevant material is "comforting and helps to break the garbage in-garbage out cycle" (p. 444). Human beings are simply more at ease and better equipped to talk about topics that interest them most. Therefore, in choosing a TLS topic that is relevant for the person with aphasia, we establish a heightened "performance edge" for therapy as well as a shared referent for subsequent exchanges. In addition, choosing material of high personal relevance can reassure patients that we know more of who they are than they are able to tell us. In this way, we foster an atmosphere of respect that affirms the present value of the patient in a therapeutic partnership.

Thematic language stimulation themes may be fairly universal, such as "cooking" or "sports." Often, however, the authors create units based on the unique backgrounds and interests of the individuals with whom we work. For example, we once used a family interview and a few trade magazines to construct a TLS unit on the garbage industry for a particular client, and it proved to be a great success. In this way, we have learned a good deal about the world in which our clients live and work. It is frequently most interesting in and of itself, but it also has practical value, in that we can sometimes use this information again in TLS sessions with others.

A TLS unit usually consists of 8 to 10 vocabulary words, primarily nouns and verbs, that are highly related to a topic. From this pool of core vocabulary items, we develop, for language practice, a variety of activities, all linked to the theme. (See Appendix 16-1 for an example of one such unit.) Simultaneously, the functional communication segment uses extensions and elaborations on this theme. The reader will note that, with some exceptions, the exercises employed are highly familiar: repetition tasks, fill-ins, multiple-choice selection, and more. What is different about TLS is the way they are created, selected, ordered, delivered, extended, and enhanced.

Stimulation Delivery in TLS

Chapter 15 (Duffy and Coelho) provided a comprehensive discussion about the principles of Schuell's stimulation therapy. Several of these are very important in the development and execution of TLS and warrant further elaboration here:

1. **Stimulus Adequacy** The adequate stimulus, by definition, is one that has an intended result. Such stimuli must be sufficiently intense, focused, and redundant to create a neurobiologic effect—that is, a change in brain-mediated language performance. In TLS, stimuli can be made adequate in several ways. First, the high degree of relevant content ensures saliency. Second, redundancy, in the form of repeated semantic and syntactic elements, and the use of multiple input and output channels are programmed into stimulus/response tasks that literally bombard the patient with linguistic stimuli. Third, the hierarchical development of task sequences builds and extends stimuli in familiar but varied contexts.

2. **Maximal Patient Response** TLS supports this principle by providing many opportunities for the client to respond in all modalities. That is, between 10 and 15 different multimodality exercises are presented for each vocabulary item over the course of five to seven sessions. In addition, therapists are encouraged to repeat activities with minor adaptations from session to session. Task repetition, reordering, adaptation, and extension in meaningful context enable maximal response. Using a variety of tasks that can be rearranged and adapted for use over a period of several sessions, therapists can broaden the stimulation base without shifting out of the theme. In addition, language can be extended further by using environmental materials and objects, such as a real restaurant menu for a unit on dining out or a trade magazine on a specific chosen topic.

3. **Systematic and Intense Presentation** TLS activities are composed and delivered systematically to obtain the greatest number of accurate responses. The progression is from introductory topical conversational material to identification of theme vocabulary to manipulation of language in carefully adapted and sequenced multimodality tasks and a return to conversational format— all within one session. Within that structure, the order of presentation also is from those likely to result in the greatest degree of success to the more difficult. Here, "more difficult" is relative; the TLS philosophy employs an 80% to 90% success level for activities. Less success than that simply affirms failure to both the client and the therapist—that is, failure to achieve an adequate stimulus. Greater than 90% success suggests the activity is not truly stimulating the brain but, instead, is riding the wave of current capabilities—rather enjoyable at times but, perhaps, not therapeutic. The degree to which clients achieve high numbers of "correct" responses in therapy is dependent on the therapist's understanding of performance variables and how to influence them, the intensity of language stimulation delivered and for which there is a response, and the moment-to-moment adjustments made during sessions. This is probably more about what is frequently called "the art of aphasia therapy," for which we believe there is a definite learning process.

Functional Communication

The stimulation of language in clinical exercises is not the only benefit of TLS; it also can be of value in the transition from language used in structured activities to conversational exchanges in a shared topical context. The desire for *functional change* is a powerful one and is shared by the clinician, client, family members, and more recently, the sources of therapeutic funding.

Intervention in the functional domain has become central in several models of therapy for aphasia. These social and ecological models propose that the effectiveness of intervention be measured by functional communication success in natural environments and that therapeutic interventions employ analysis and problem solving in that milieu (Boles, 1998).

In many therapeutic models, treatment includes a problem-solving component, in which the clinician tries various combinations of cues and strategies to facilitate improved language function (Chapey, 1994a; Holland, 1998; Kaplan, 1989; Wepman, 1972). This process draws on the very essence of our practice as speech-language pathologists: the ability to observe symptoms and behavior and apply interventions that help. In TLS, because we are keeping the treatment structure consistent, the process itself becomes more of a focus. Freed of the necessity of constantly learning new directions and rules of therapy for new tasks, clients engage more easily in problem-solving activity and can concentrate more on their own performance issues. This consistent structure helps both the clinician and the client to develop insights that assist in facilitating functional communication behaviors.

We believe that TLS may provide a link from clinical to functional language stimulation by manipulation of the theme. The daily segue from clinical task to relevant, theme-based conversation moves the clinician and the person with aphasia back and forth between both environments. Capitalizing on what may be improved access primed in the stimulation mode, the therapist skillfully shifts the environment of practice to functional conversation. Once there, both clinician and client continue the problem-solving process, exploring successful strategies, heightening awareness, and developing insights.

Metalinguistic Dialogue

Metalinguistic dialogue is used in conjunction with TLS to strengthen the clinical to functional link. A metalinguistic act requires that an observation be made about the use of language. The observation could be about one's own language or about another's use of his or her language. Engaging in metalinguistic dialogue requires skill, but the speech-language pathologist has the ability to describe and codify the speech, language, and communication behaviors that affect conversation. From the personal and experiential perspective, the person with aphasia has valid observations to contribute, and both perspectives are complementary. Conversation strategies that are personalized and congruent with the individual's ideas of what works or fits that individual's life, however, are more likely to be the strategies that are actually used. Nina Simmons-Mackie (2001), in her description of "enhanced compensatory strategy training," notes that "the person with aphasia is considered a partner in identifying and elaborating a strategy repertoire" (p. 254).

The metalinguistic dialogue can happen at any point in the therapy session. We have found that it usually occurs quite naturally toward the end of the session, after the client and therapist have experienced the activities and the follow-up functional conversation. The typical flow is from baseline conversation to TLS activities to functional conversation and, then, to metalinguistic dialogue.

This metalinguistic dialogue often begins with the speech-language pathologist sharing examples of positive performance that are tied specifically to language and communication. Such observations or questions may assist those with aphasia to explore and reflect on their own performance. Beyond its usefulness to develop strategies, the exchange may serve to increase the patients' understanding about the nature of aphasia and how it operates with their present brain function. Once such dialogues are integrated into the session and the patients are "on board" with this component of treatment, the therapist offers more detailed observations about performance and asks the clients for their discoveries. The dyadic exchange could include comments about performance during transaction, interaction, and eventually, to domains beyond language (e.g., metacognition). Commenting and problem solving about the style of various conversation partners in the social network that either supports or exists as a barrier to conversational success may lead to productive solutions.

Metalinguistic dialogue reinforces the collaborative relationship in problem-solving treatment outcomes. Because it encourages the person with aphasia to take on more responsibility and independence in symptom and communication management, it is a helpful tool for discovering those strategies that are most likely to actually be used with confidence both inside and outside the treatment session. An example of a metalinguistic dialogue is as follows:

Therapist I noticed that when you had trouble saying some of the words just now, you seemed to pause and think about it more in your head. What did you notice?
Patient Yes, I try to see the word.
Therapist So you see the word written in your mind, and then you can say it easier?
Patient Yes, that's right
Therapist Is that easier than trying to write it?
Patient Yes, and it's faster.

ASSESSMENT FOR TLS

Regardless of the theoretic basis for provision of language treatment, clinicians need specific information about language function to develop a program. Schuell (cited in Byng, Kay, Edmundson, & Scott, 1990) proposed that treatment planning requires knowledge of which cerebral processes are impaired, the level at which performance breaks down in each modality, and the reason why performance breaks down when it does. For the present authors, this is a prescription for a process-oriented examination of both functional performance and behaviors more typically elicited in a formal test milieu. Whereas formal aphasia tests can provide some information, clinicians would do well to heed the warning inherent in Edith Kaplan's (1991) comment that "batteries are for cars, not for people".

Assessing aphasia is one of the most complex requirements of speech-language pathologists. Competent evaluation requires astute observation of language behavior combined with a thorough knowledge concerning the range of possible symptoms and how they influence communication. The speech-language pathologist also must have the knowledge and skill to manipulate the environment and explore all possible avenues of success. Thus, proper aphasia assessment bridges both domains of science and art. When the therapist has a thorough understanding of the patient's clinical and functional picture, the therapist can create an appropriate therapy program; specifically, the therapist can choose a particular approach or environment suited to the information provided by the evaluation. Moreover, end-point recommendations then are more individualized and helpful for communicative partners.

Establishing Baseline Functional Conversation

At the onset of treatment, a baseline of functional communication is obtained. Although we have used some formal instruments to measure functional communication in research or for other purposes (Taylor, 1969; Yorkston & Beukelman, 1980), our approach for TLS usually is more informal. That is, we believe that the experienced clinician usually can answer questions about functional communication after a relatively short period of interaction with the client.

How Well Do Patients Initiate and Sustain Conversation?

Assessment of the client's overall level of participation in a conversational exchange establishes a baseline for measuring progress and helps the clinician to develop initial ideas about intervention. Therefore, the relative burden of information exchange as well as the degree to which information must be inferred need to be determined.

How Well Do Patients Express Themselves Verbally and Nonverbally?

Assessment focuses on content. Observations address the patient's relative use of alternatives to speech when they appear in the natural course of an exchange. This information about preferred modes, and relative ease of success in any mode, will assist in decisions about TLS activity selection and order. It also will guide the way in which we introduce options for enhanced communication and how we train the communicative partner.

How Well Do Patients Follow Conversation and Directions? How Complex Can Auditory Demands Be Before Performance Breaks Down?

Information regarding comprehension informs decisions about task selection and presentation and about adjustments that need to be made in the therapist's verbal behavior when introducing tasks, counseling the client, and engaging in conversation. Skilled clinicians can derive a good deal of information during conversational exchange about the intermittency of auditory processing, regardless of whether patients are aware of a loss in understanding and how well they comprehend subtleties, humor, and/or sublinguistic information.

Assessing Clinical Performance on Tasks

Thematic language stimulation is strongly dependent on a process approach. Therefore, we continually ask "Why?" when symptoms are revealed. It is only by understanding the "why" that we can determine "what" can be done about it in treatment. Standard aphasia tests tell some of the "what" but none of the "why." In comparing the various standard aphasia instruments, a core group of subtests occur repeatedly: repetition, naming, answering yes/no to questions, and so on. The value of these subtests is that they assist the clinician in the differential diagnosis of aphasia. They do not, however, explain what to do once aphasia is confirmed. Therefore, the clinician must engage in further analysis, adding probes to explore cognition, behavior, and therapeutic style to determine both "what to do" and "where to begin" in therapy.

Formal Testing

1. **Repetition** Some people with aphasia can repeat well, and some cannot. Because TLS relies completely on the objective of "language in, language out," therapists must know whether repetition will be a primary stimulation task, one to avoid completely, or one that will need to be adapted but can still be used successfully. Any formal test of repetition can provide the level of breakdown with respect to length and complexity of units, but further observations are required to assist in therapeutic decision making. For example, if repetition is better than spontaneous speech, the clinician has discovered a key aural-oral connection to modify speech output; if it is worse, the clinician must look elsewhere, most likely to the visual modality, for primary input. In addition, for many individuals with aphasia, repetition is not a "can do/can't do" phenomenon. Many patients "can do" once some structural stimulation requirements are met, such as slowing the rate of presentation or providing face-to-face delivery (particularly for the patient with apraxia). Such observations are critical to TLS planning, and success that can be achieved using this approach.

2. **Sentence Construction** Most formal aphasia batteries assess the ability of the patient to create sentences given a one-, two- or three-word stimulus. Creation or expansion of verbal utterances that are substantive and grammatically correct is an objective of many treatment approaches. Clinicians learn more about how best to facilitate this for a particular patient when they know (a) the required length and grammatical composition of stimuli, (b) the effect of vocabulary complexity, and (c) how much and what type of verbal or visual cues are needed to facilitate performance.

3. **Automatic Language** For some people, automatic language is far more preserved than propositional language, and automatic language should be facilitated first if it will create a base of success. Knowing the ease with which automatic language can be facilitated will help with therapeutic task selection and sequencing. For example, fill-in tasks with multiple-choice response requirements are high in predictability and might be considered to be a natural extension of automatic language material.

4. **Picture Description** A pictorial cue can be powerful for some clients in eliciting a flow of ideas. When aural-oral

presentation and response is tenuous, a pictorial cue also can provide a starting point for therapy. In addition, the contrast between narrative and spontaneous expression can be explored with respect to the complexity of ideas and vocabulary generated as well as the degree of clinician-initiated cueing that is necessary for a response.

5. **Following Instructions** Although it is desirable to minimize task instructions to the patient at each session, it is important to determine each particular patient's need for such repetition of procedures. When we apply process parameters to listening, the logical questions to be asked are (a) how complex and lengthy can directions be, (b) will a visual cue be needed to support the verbal request, (c) how does the rate of presentation affect comprehension, and (d) is the auditory mode a strong or weak one for the individual?

6. **Yes/No Reliability** For the client with more severe aphasia, ability to respond readily and consistently in a yes/no question format is an essential skill. Indeed, it is a valuable task for auditory, verbal, and visual stimulation of all clients. In addition, before construction of a TLS unit, the parameters of length, complexity, ease, and facilitation requirements should be noted via descriptive comments.

7. **Reading Comprehension** For many individuals with aphasia, reading comprehension is a valid alternative to auditory comprehension. In this instance, treatment first emphasizes presentation of information via the visual modality rather than the more traditional auditory mode. The comparison of results on subtests that tap auditory processing of directions and commands with those that examine silent reading of sentences and paragraphs allows the clinician to decide on a preferred input mode. It also is important to compare scores obtained during testing as well as the overall ease of performance in both modalities, because this information sometimes provides a clue about a client's "hardwiring" for processing language. For example, if visuographic expression is more preserved and preferred to the aural-oral system, that will be the road that we follow. In addition, for some individuals, silent reading before verbal performance has a priming effect; only when a detailed process approach is applied to tasks are such important pieces of information learned. This information then can be applied not only to task and cue selection but also can be shared with those who have aphasia and with their communicative partners. Thus, treatment decisions are made based on a balancing of the patient's strengths and weaknesses (Holland, 1998).

8. **Oral Reading** Oral reading is another avenue that provides an opportunity to get language "in and out." Therefore, the clinician needs to know if oral reading is more preserved than speaking and whether the patient

can correct errors that occur in this format. For some clients, visual stimuli are more salient. In addition, when the patient and clinician share a visual reference in the same context, this may reveal specific symptoms and procedures for modification.

9. **Graphic Expression** Writing adds to the sources of linguistic bombardment necessary to reach a threshold for response. Integrated into the therapeutic program, it comes to be thought of as a welcome addition, adding to the patient's repertoire of success. For the person with milder aphasia, one needs to know how much and what kind of assistance is needed for the production of words, phrases, sentences, or narratives and whether a self-initiated written cue aids verbal performance. Therefore, clinical and functional graphic abilities are explored fully. The therapist investigates writing and drawing not only as an augmentative communication tool but also as a source of stimulation itself. By integrating writing at an early stage of treatment, the clinician stimulates the patient's language system in yet another way. Many individuals with global aphasia can copy neatly and accurately. In addition, after several such trials are combined with repetition, they may even produce the target word verbally without struggle.

These formal test probes, combined with observation of performance, comprise our "minimal data set" for evaluative exploration in both clinical and functional domains.

Cognitive and Behavioral Considerations

Several non-language behaviors have an impact on the treatment planning process. Additional knowledge about the person's cognitive and behavioral strengths and weaknesses will influence the treatment model or approach that is chosen. In the case of TLS, such an analysis is necessary to customize both the content and delivery of therapeutic materials. As in the language analysis, certain behaviors are observed, described, and noted for future reference.

Patient Involvement

For some, the purpose of therapy is obvious, and they "get with the program" immediately, respond well to the treatment materials, and provide clinicians with evidence that they are on the right track. For others, however, lack of insight is as much an obstacle to recovery as their symptoms. Naturally, TLS works best with insightful, motivated clients who "get it." Therefore, very early in the period of evaluation and during the initial phases of therapy, we note the patient's ability to connect with the disorder, comment on the patient's own internal processes or performance for such behavior on task, and consider other types of metalinguistic analyses. Because of the way TLS is structured, however, it also is a treatment approach that can facilitate improved insight and understanding about the therapeutic process. Even at the lowest level of function for this type of reflection, we offer many opportunities and indicate to the person that such concerns are not only worthwhile but also essential to recovery. We share our observations with the patient, and we encourage the patient to do the same. This process is important, because recovery does not happen via neurobiologic stimulation alone but, rather, via the insights that people with aphasia derive from their own process. Therefore, we continually ask "why" of our clients, and sometimes, they can give us an answer.

Specific Symptom Awareness

Clients are asked to modify their symptoms as part of the therapeutic process. Some modifications result from the clinician's direct intervention; others result from the person's own insight regarding a specific symptom and the patient's resultant, focused response to it. To us, clients with specific symptom awareness seem to achieve greater progress and do better overall. Indeed, such awareness has a significant impact on how we structure material in tasks and how we cue or strategize for success. We all have memories of such moments in our therapy sessions. For example, one author recalls a person with conduction aphasia who taught her clinician the value of graphomotor association by producing a dictionary of words beginning with target sounds and then using that list to aid pronunciation of words in general.

Task Orientation and Retention

When clients have good task orientation and retention of treatment set, directions need not be repeated from day to day. Subsequently, a natural flow occurs from one task to the next and from one day to the next. In addition, because of its organization, TLS can assist even the person with severe aphasia to prepare himself cognitively for the tasks at hand. In turn, this sometimes engenders feelings of competence in the "knowing" of what to do. Therefore, keeping structure constant and changing the items within it, rather than the constant shifting of exercises that sometimes is seen in more traditional language therapy, is valuable.

Perseveration

For some people with aphasia, perseveration is a highly problematic and unwelcome intrusion for communication. In our experience, the semantic relatedness of TLS can make perseveration even worse for these clients. Typically, this tendency is discovered once treatment is underway and the clinician observes that the client's responses, rather than demonstrating the advances in vocabulary retrieval and sentence use, contain recycled errors in word choice that are not evolving into something better. For such an individual, TLS is not an appropriate treatment approach.

Visual Perception

Because TLS relies heavily on multimodality stimulation, any visual problems that affect task presentation, such as the presence of hemianopsia or the need for altered print size, should be known in advance. For some, it may simply be a matter of modifying the aural-oral elements and adapting visual materials. For others with severe accompanying visual impairments, TLS may not be effective.

TREATMENT DELIVERY

After completing an assessment of conversational proficiency, language, and cognitive/behavioral status, the clinician is ready to incorporate this information into an organized treatment delivery plan. Before therapy can begin, however, one more set of questions needs to be answered:

1. **Is this person a good candidate for TLS?** Candidacy for TLS is best determined in one or two sessions of trial therapy; however, certain rules of thumb seem to be of help in deciding which clients have the potential for success. Good candidates generally are those with no marked perseveration or semantic confusion in task performance and with good ability to understand the purpose of therapy, stable emotional status, and some amount of visual language preservation. Level of severity may vary, but patients with moderate to severe difficulties appear to profit most. Although preliminary research findings suggest otherwise, we feel the technique is of value to people with either fluent or nonfluent aphasia.

2. **How should tasks be chosen and sequenced?** Our analysis during assessment has told us very specifically which modalities and tasks are the strongest and which are the weakest. Therefore, to adhere to the principle of stimulus adequacy, we begin there. In addition, because it will prime the session for all subsequent task presentations and adaptations, the first task should be one that provides a high probability of success. If it is known, for example, that the patient does not repeat well but that he can read words and phrases both silently and orally with good success, then the TLS exercises chosen first should require this patient to do just that. Because treatment is multimodal, the next task might begin to include aural-oral requirements, such as answering questions using the material just practiced visually. This might be followed by a writing task at a level compatible with demonstrated skills in this modality; for example, the client might be able to copy or write the target words as the clinician dictates them.

3. **What cues are most beneficial to achieve maximal success in treatment?** Because successful language stimulation should neither involve too much struggle nor be so "easy" that it does not provide a neurobiologic effect, an 80% to 90% success rate is targeted in TLS therapy. To achieve this level of success, considerable experimentation regarding facilitatory cueing takes

place; however, our assessment analysis has provided clues about the likelihood that they will or will not succeed. Therefore, the clinician answers questions such as the following: (a) Are visual cues more powerful than auditory ones? (b) How much spontaneous writing is possible with and without input from dictation? (c) When can I fade out a verbal, auditory, or visual cue and still maintain an accurate response?

When we determine cueing that works at baseline, we also determine the beginning of a cueing hierarchy. These hierarchies are individualized and will change over time as the client progresses and needs to be challenged further. Maintaining a high level of success throughout treatment, however, should be a constant goal.

4. **How do I select theme and vocabulary?** As mentioned earlier, theme selection is based on each client's interests; personal relevance generates ideas and themes that provide a shared reference point for all subsequent interaction. The inclusion of material based on client input reflects respect for the client's personal contribution to the decision about treatment needs. Themes that are more concrete—or even able to be pictured—are easier to conceptualize. It is entirely possible, however, to select complex themes and create vocabulary and tasks that can be modified to levels consistent with normal language complexity. A minimum of 6 and maximum of 10 words are recommended.

A closed set of core vocabulary permits manipulations that fulfill some of the content and delivery principles described earlier: redundancy, multimodality presentation, and predictable task inventory. The majority of words are nouns; however, an occasional verb or adjective also is desirable. For example, if the theme is "restaurant," appropriate vocabulary words might be *waitress, tip, table, menu, appetizer, water, check, chef,* and *order.*

The actual tasks that we have employed in our TLS work are familiar to any experienced aphasia clinician. What is different is the constancy of theme that connects them all and the systematic way in which they are employed. A complete TLS unit ("Books") is provided for your use in Appendix 16-1.

PRELIMINARY RESEARCH WITH TLS

According to Darley in 1972 (as cited in Howard, 1986, p. 89), "If speech pathologists are to have a role in the management of aphasic patients, it must depend not on wishful thinking, but on unequivocal demonstration of effectiveness in significantly altering, in a favorable way, the course of recovery." In the 1980s, this was referred to as "evaluating efficacy." In 2005, American Speech-Language-Hearing Association adopted the term "evidence-based practice" and created a position statement reinforcing the need for evidentiary support for clinical interventions. Although in the typical speech therapy clinical

milieu, single-subject design studies are accomplished more easily than group studies, therapists, according to Siegel (1987) as well as Siegel and Spradlin (1985), often find it difficult to integrate them into a typical service delivery model. In 1993, we completed one such clinically based, single-subject study with TLS.

Defining Success

In the early stages of our clinical work with TLS, we were relatively comfortable with clinical evidence that the approach was making language more available during the execution of tasks. As sessions progressed, performance seemed to improve during each session and from session to session. If TLS or, for that matter, any restorative technique is to be judged efficacious, however, it must be held to the ultimate standard—that is, improvement in conversational speech. We found immediate difficulties in selecting functional conversation as the improvement measure, because few quantifiable options from which to choose were available and those that were available seemed to be insensitive to discriminating what would undoubtedly be very small changes. For that reason, we declined to use the CADL (Communication Activities of Daily Living) (Holland, 1980), the CETI (Communicative Effectiveness Index) (Lomas et al., 1989), and the FCP (Functional Communication Profile) (Taylor, 1969). We found support, however, in our frustration:

Clinicians and investigators who wish to quantify changes in the informativeness of the connected speech of adults with aphasia in response to manipulation of experimental variables have been hampered by the scarcity of standard measures for characterizing this aspect of connected speech. (Nicholas & Brookshire, 1993, p. 338).

At the time we embarked on our study, the only published system for measuring small improvements in discourse appeared to be that proposed by Yorkston and Beukelman in 1980. In their system, the individual's response to the cookie theft picture from the *Boston Diagnostic Aphasia Examination* (Goodglass & Kaplan, 1983) is analyzed for the number of *content units* produced and for a measure of communicative efficiency, which is determined by the ratio of content units per minute of discourse. Content units, or groupings of information expressed by normal speakers in response to the cookie theft picture, are finite and offer a clear index of relative performance in response to this specific picture stimulus. Concerns regarding the differences between connected speech elicited in this manner and that elicited in a conversational exchange remained, but a content unit analysis seemed to be our best method of defining success—that is, communication of information in discourse.

Design Choice

In general, single-subject studies investigating the efficacy of a particular approach to aphasia intervention employ either a reversal/withdrawal or multiple-baseline design (Pring, 1986). Our desire was to determine whether TLS was more effective than a "traditional" approach, and we therefore chose a reversal design in which TLS and non-TLS modules would alternate with each other for 3 weeks after a baseline determination of communicative efficiency. Modules 1 and 2 (i.e., TLS and non-TLS, respectively) were ordered such that subjects would receive either one first for a 3-week period. This served to control for the number of times that each was received. The same content unit analysis obtained at baseline was performed between each of the modules.

The decision regarding the content of the non-TLS module was of great concern, because many differing approaches to therapy for aphasia are available. Our personal journey involved exploration of many of these approaches, and we would—and will—employ many of them therapeutically when we felt it to be an appropriate choice for a specific individual. Our choice of non-TLS therapy for Module 2, however, was derived from what seemed to be "the norm" for many speech-language pathologists—that is, a "general language stimulation" approach employing a variety of exercises for word retrieval, comprehension, reading, and writing but *without* controlled content and delivery around thematic structure and Schuellian principles.

Therefore, Module 2 employed activities from the many easily accessible aphasia workbooks frequently used by clinicians. These activities were administered by us subsequent to completion of the same evaluative procedures described above. In other words, we attempted to treat the patient with traditional speech and language tasks selected for the individual's level of performance in each modality but without regard to semantic uniformity across modalities. We did not hesitate to assist patients in achieving success on these tasks within the session, and we provided whatever degree of stimulation and support was required for specific activities. Even

so, we avoided any linking of materials with conversational topics. It may be argued that we did not provide the best possible non-TLS modules because of our bias; however, we are accustomed to delivering other kinds of therapy to those for whom TLS is not appropriate and attempted to do that for this study. Our hope is that, in future studies, we will be able to employ other therapists so as to eliminate any possible bias in this regard.

Subject Selection

The individuals who participated in the study completed a 3-week course of treatment while at an inpatient acute rehabilitation facility, and they were selected without regard to age, type of aphasia, etiology, duration of symptoms, or any other particular characteristic. All were screened for adequate vision and hearing, and all received traditional aphasia testing before inclusion in the study.

Procedures

Before beginning the first module, in between modules, and again at the end of the last module, the responses of each patient to the cookie theft picture were audiotaped and videotaped. Written transcripts of these descriptions were obtained and analyzed according to the procedure of Yorkston and Beukelman (1980). Each therapy session was videotaped as well. All subjects received 30-minute sessions of therapy 5 days per week for each of the three consecutive weeks.

Results

Pring (1986) offers some encouragement for the analysis of data in a visual rather than a statistical manner when changes are likely to be small. Thus, as can be seen in Figure 16–1, two

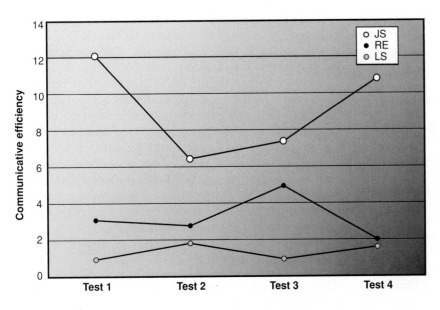

Figure 16–1. Treatment effects of thematic language stimulation. JS, RE, and LS refer to individual patients.

of the three subjects (both people with fluent aphasia) demonstrated treatment effects with TLS. That is, the communicative efficiency score (number of content units divided by rate) increased after TLS modules, and decreased after non-TLS modules, relative to baseline. No treatment effect was observed for patient JS; in fact, her scores appear to be poorer with both treatment approaches relative to baseline.

Discussion

Because of the very small number of subjects in our study, little about the efficacy of TLS can be confirmed. Certainly, we would need to test many more individuals before drawing any conclusions. What seems safe to assume, however, is that the use of a content unit analysis as a measure of discourse for revealing small, quantifiable changes in performance is a good idea. We found it interesting, however, that our best results were obtained when treating individuals with fluent, rather than nonfluent, aphasia given our clinical impression that people with nonfluent aphasia respond quite well. Even so, we observed that patient JS, the subject with nonfluent aphasia, lacked a sense of treatment purpose despite a good degree of cooperativeness regarding therapy. Our impression is that this person would have had difficulty with any intervention because of her inability to interact with the concept of treatment in general. Further exploration of TLS intervention is warranted with a greater number of subjects, individuals of varying aphasic syndromes, and consideration of the timing of implementation during the recovery phase.

FUTURE TRENDS

The World Health Organization's model for classification of functioning and disability differentiates deficit, activity, and participation as points of reference in the individual's health perspective. To treat individuals for their deficit or brain impairment in isolation is to ignore other critical features of their recovery. Improved language function that stays in the therapy room without application to functional activities and participation goals also reflects inadequate therapy. With a driving force to make life better for people with aphasia and those who matter most to them, our therapy needs to be authentic, flexible, and congruent at each of the various points in recovery. To meet these criteria, the speech-language pathologist needs to direct less, listen more, and support the direction described by patients and their chosen partners to assist in achieving a satisfactory recovery.

Our role as educators and trainers will continue to expand. If people are to be successful outside of the therapy room, they must be knowledgeable and empowered to problem solve and make choices. Similarly, families and others in the social network of those with aphasia need to be knowledgeable and comfortable with partnership to be supportive and effective.

Training aimed at understanding aphasia and how to be of help needs to be addressed early and frequently throughout the course of treatment. Although communicative partners generally cannot provide TLS therapy, they learn, by observing sessions and talking with us, about how those with aphasia organizes their language, employ appropriate strategies, and requires in the way of priming input or providing support to do their best. These lessons can be learned from many different approaches; because of its strong dependence on structure, TLS may simply be a more organized observational environment for shared insights and opportunities regarding problem solving.

Thematic Language Stimulation is an intervention that bridges treating the language deficit and facilitating function via the conversation focus. In recent years, addition of the metalinguistic component to complement the TLS format has reinforced the role of problem solving by the patient, family, and other supporters. Success in conversation often is a prerequisite to success in chosen activities and participation goals. Being skilled to problem solve and advocate for life's goals beyond the duration of the speech therapy intervention is of great value for the ultimate outcome.

Lastly, our training needs to involve the community. For the person with aphasia to participate successfully in chosen activities, we must assist the community with learning to recognize aphasia and to respond effectively. After all, the ultimate goal is for people with aphasia to succeed.

KEY POINTS

1. Thematic language stimulation is a neurobiologic approach to speech and language therapy, based on the theory of aphasia treatment first postulated by Hildred Schuell in the mid-twentieth century.
2. Success in implementation of TLS may depend on several factors, including the ability of the therapist to provide adequate stimulation and the abilities of the client to understand and respond to the aphasic symptoms.
3. Therapists who employ TLS must use the client's interests and talents to tap into the best possible subject matter for a successful outcome.
4. Thematic language stimulation extends out of the basic Stimulus-Response formats into the natural flow of speaking and listening in a conversation.
5. The ability of both therapist and client to examine language and cognitive abilities and make decisions about how to integrate treatment is key to the use of TLS.

1. Create your own "mini" TLS unit by following these steps:
   a. Select four vocabulary items on a topic of choice. Include nouns and verbs.
   b. Using the examples given in Appendix 16-1, place each vocabulary item:
      i. In a word-phrase-sentence format.
      ii. In an open-ended sentence for a fill-in.
      iii. In a multiple choice reading format.
      iv. In a question designed to elicit discussion.
   c. What other exercises NOT in Appendix 16-1 might be used with the same four vocabulary items?
2. Create a "cueing hierarchy" for someone who might not be able to succeed with item b.iii above. How would you adapt and change the presentation or task requirements to enable success?

References

American Speech-Language-Hearing Association. (2005). Evidence-based practice in communication disorders [Position statement].

Boles, L. (1998). Conducting conversation: A case study using the spouse in aphasia treatment. *Neurophysiology and Neurogenic Speech and Language Disorders, a publication of ASHA SID 2, 19*(3), 24–31.

Boyle, M., & Coelho, C. A. (1995). Application of semantic feature analysis as a treatment for aphasic dysnomia. *American Journal of Speech-Language Pathology, 4,* 94–98.

Byng, S., Kay, J., Edmundson, A., & Scott, C. (1990). Aphasia tests reconsidered. *Aphasiology, 4*(1), 24–31.

Chapey, R. (1994a). Cognitive intervention: Stimulation of cognition, memory, convergent thinking, divergent thinking, and evaluative thinking. In R. Chapey (Ed.), *Language intervention strategies in adult aphasia* (pp. 220–245). Baltimore, MD: Williams & Wilkins.

Chapey, R. (1994b). Introduction to language intervention strategies in adult aphasia. In R. Chapey (Ed.), *Language intervention strategies in adult aphasia* (pp. 2–26). Baltimore, MD: Williams & Wilkins.

Drew, R. L., & Thompson, C. K. (1999). Model-based semantic treatment for naming deficits in aphasia. *Journal of Speech and Hearing Research, 42,* 972–989.

Duffy, J. R., & Coelho, C. (2000). Schuell's stimulation approach to rehabilitation. In R. Chapey (Ed.), *Language intervention strategies in adult aphasia.* Baltimore, MD: Williams & Wilkins.

Goodglass, H., & Kaplan, E. (1983). *The Boston diagnostic aphasia examination.* Philadelphia, PA: Lea & Febiger.

Greener, J., Enderby, P., & Whurr, R. (2001) Pharmacological treatment for aphasia following stroke. *The Cochran Database of Systematic Reviews, 4.* Art. No.: CD000424.DOI:10.1002/14651858.CD000424.

Helm-Estabrooks, N., & Albert, M. L. (1991). *Manual of aphasia therapy.* Austin, TX: Pro-Ed.

Holland, A. (1980). *Communicative abilities in daily living.* Baltimore, MD: University Park Press.

Holland, A. (1998). A strategy for improving oral naming in an individual with a phonological access impairment. In N. Helm-Estabrooks & A. Holland (Eds.), *Approaches to the treatment of aphasia* (pp. 39–67). San Diego: Singular.

Howard, D (1986). *British Journal of Disorders of Communication, 21,* 89–102.

Jenkins, W. M., Merzenich, M. M., Ochs, M. T., Allard, T., & Guic-Robles, E. (1990, January). Functional reorganization of primary somatosensory cortex in adult owl monkeys after behaviorally controlled tactile stimulation. *Journal of Neurophysiology, 63*(1), 82–104.

Kaplan, E. (1989). A process approach to neuropsychological assessment. In T. Boll (Ed.), *Clinical neuropsychology and brain function: Research, measurement, and practice.* Washington, DC: APA.

Kaplan, E. (1991). *Neuropsychological assessment & language treatment: A process-based approach.* Seminar June 7–8 in Alexandria, VA, sponsored by Education Resources, Inc, Medfield MA and the Boston Neurobehavioral Institute, Boston, MA.

Kilgard, M. P., & Merzenich, M. M. (1998). Cortical map reorganization enabled by nucleus basalis activity. *Science, 270,* 1714–1718.

Lomas, J., Pickard, L., Bester, S., Elbard, H., Finlayson, A., & Zoghaib, C. (1989). The communicative effectiveness index: Development and psychometric evaluation of a functional communication measure for adult aphasia. *Journal of Speech and Hearing Disorders, 54,* 113–124.

Maher, L. M., Kendall, D., Swearengin, J. A., Pingle, K., Holland, A., & Rothi, L. J. G. (2003). Constraint-induced language therapy for chronic aphasia: Preliminary findings. *Journal of the International Neuropsychological Society, 9,* 192.

Marshall, R. C. (1994). Management of fluent aphasic clients. In R. Chapey (Ed.), *Language intervention strategies in adult aphasia* (pp. 389–406). Baltimore, MD: Williams & Wilkins.

Morganstein, S., & Certner-Smith, M. (1982). *Thematic language stimulation.* Tucson, AZ: Communication Skill Builders.

Morganstein, S., & Certner-Smith, M. (1993). Aphasia and right-hemisphere disorders. In W. Gordon (Ed.), *Advances in stroke rehabilitation* (pp. 103–133). Boston, MA: Andover Medical.

Nicholas, L. E., & Brookshire, R. H. (1993). A system for quantifying the informativeness and efficiency of the connected speech of adults with aphasia. *JSHR, 36,* 338–350.

Pring, T. R. (1986). Evaluating the effects of speech therapy for aphasics: Developing the single case methodology. *British Journal of Disorders of Communication, 21,* 103–115.

Pulvermuller, F., Neininger, B., Elbert, T., Mohr, B., Rockstrob, B., Koebbel, P., et al. (2001). Constraint-induced therapy of chronic aphasia after stroke, *Stroke, 32*(7), 1621–1626.

Schuell, H., Jenkins, J. J., & Jimenez-Pabon, E. (1964). *Aphasia in adults: Diagnosis, prognosis and treatment.* New York: Harper & Row.

Siegel, G. M. (1987). The limits of science in communication disorders. *Journal of Speech and Hearing Disorders, 52,* 306–312.

Siegel, G. M., & Spradlin, J. E. (1985). Therapy and research. *Journal of Speech and Hearing Disorders, 50,* 226–230.

Simmons-Mackie, N. (2001). Social approaches to aphasia intervention. In R. Chapey (Ed.), *Language intervention strategies in adult aphasia* (pp. 246–267). Baltimore, MD: Williams & Wilkins.

Taylor, M. L. (1969). *The functional communication profile*. New York: New York University Medical Center.

Wallace, G. L., & Canter, G. J. (1985). Effects of personally relevant language materials on the performance of severely aphasic individuals. *Journal of Speech and Hearing Disorders, 50,* 385–390.

Wepman, J. M. (1953). A conceptual model for the processes involved in recovery from aphasia. *Journal of Speech and Hearing Disorders, 18,* 4–13.

Wepman, J. M. (1972). Aphasia therapy: A new look. *Journal of Speech and Hearing Disorders, 37,* 201–214.

Wertz, R. T. (1986). Comparison of clinic, home, and deferred language treatment for aphasia. *Archives of Neurology, 43,* 653–658.

Yorkston, K. M., & Beukelman, D. R. (1980). An analysis of connected speech samples of aphasic and normal speakers. *Journal of Speech and Hearing Disorders, 45,* 27–36.

APPENDIX 16.1
Thematic Language Stimulation (TLS) Unit on Books with Instructions for Creating TLS Units.

How to Create a TLS Unit

Select between 8 and 10 words that have a close association to your chosen theme. These words will become your *core vocabulary*, which will be used in each exercise. Use nouns primarily, but verbs and adjectives are fine as well.

Twelve Exercises

Exercise 1: Repetition

This is controlled repetition practice, in which the stimuli gradually increase in length and complexity. Use each core vocabulary item, and create a phrase and sentence sequence for them in which the target word is in the final position, whenever reasonable.

Exercise 2: Speech Stimulation/Production

This is a grouping of three statements and one question, which evolves for each core vocabulary item from repetition to open-ended fill-ins to generation of novel utterances. Begin with a statement for the client to repeat in which the core vocabulary item is the last word. Create the next statement using the exact language of the first, but with the last word as a fill-in. Create a question requiring the target word as an answer. End with a question relevant to the content just practiced, but designed to elicit a novel response.

Exercise 3: Copying

Provide opportunity for the client to copy each target item at least three times, and attempt to write from memory.

Exercise 4: Categorization

This task is for identification of the core vocabulary in a list of words that vary in their semantic closeness to the target items.

First, randomize core vocabulary items in a list of roughly twice its size. Use foils (i.e., other words) that are varied in the degree to which they may be related, visually or semantically, to the targets. The semantic closeness of the foils will determine the difficulty of the task.

Exercise 5: Sentence Fill-Ins, Multiple Choice

These are fill-in sentences for which the target word is one of the choices. For each fill-in sentence, three choices are offered. Semantic closeness of the foils determines the complexity of the task.

Exercise 6: Yes/No Questions

Questions are formulated with target vocabulary, and the task is to provide a yes/no response.

Exercise 7: Answering Questions, Multiple Choice

Questions are developed for which correct answers are randomly ordered in a vocabulary grouping of four or five items. Place these choices above four or five questions. The client must choose and write the correct word.

Exercise 8: Sentence Arrangement

The client is provided with a scrambled sentence for each core vocabulary item. Create out-of-order sentences of varied complexity, but within the mild to moderate range for each vocabulary item.

Exercise 9: Sentence Construction

Pairs of words are provided with which to create sentences. Create two columns. On the left, list the core vocabulary first, followed by a verb. In the next column, list a noun phrase.

Exercise 10: Sentence Correction

The client is provided with sentences containing two errors of either word choice, grammar, or spelling, which the client must identify and correct.

Exercise 11: Paragraph Reading, Multiple Choice Questions

A paragraph is created in which all (or most) of the vocabulary has been used. The client must then answer some multiple-choice questions about the paragraph. When possible, use humor or idiomatic expressions to improve processing. Create three or four questions with multiple-choice answers for practice in processing factual and implied information.

Exercise 12: Conversational Questions

This is A list of questions on the topic designed to elicit conversation.

Vocabulary Unit: Books

Exercise 1: Repetition/Oral Reading

Directions: Repeat or read aloud these words, phrases, and sentence.

fiction	read
enjoy fiction	read my book
I always enjoy fiction.	Tonight I will read my book.
print	library
large print	at the library
The book comes in large print.	See you at the library.
glasses	characters
reading glasses	many characters
I've lost my reading glasses.	The novel has many characters.
writer	mystery
great writer	solve the mystery
She is a great writer.	Did you solve the mystery?

Exercise 2: Speech Stimulation/Production

Directions: Listen, fill in, and answer the questions.

1. I prefer to read fiction.

   I prefer to read _____.

   What do I prefer to read? _____

   What do you prefer to read?

2. The story is a mystery.

   The story is a _____.

   What is the story? _____

   Why are mysteries fun to read?

3. She is a famous writer.

   She is a famous _____.

   What is she? _____

   Name a famous writer.

4. The book comes in large print.

   The book comes in large _____.

   How is the book printed? _____

   How is large print helpful?

5. I wear reading glasses

   I wear reading _____.

   What do I wear? _____

   Where do you buy reading glasses?

6. I borrow books from the library.

   I borrow books from the _____.

   Where do I borrow books? _____

   How long can you borrow books?

7. The book has three main characters.

   The book has three main _____.

   What were there three of _____?

   How many characters are too many?

8. I've always liked to read.

   I've always liked to _____.

   What have I liked to do? _____.

   What kind of books do you read?

Exercise 3: Copying

Directions: Write each word three times. Then, cover it up, and try to write it from memory:

Name: _____

Date: _____

read

_____

_____

_____

print

_____

_____

_____

library

_____

_____

_____

glasses

_____

_____

_____

writer

_____

_____

_____

mystery

_____

_____

_____

fiction

_____

_____

_____

characters

_____

_____

_____

Exercise 4: Categorization

Directions: Circle the words that belong in the category "Books." If you prefer, you can cut these out, mix them up with another set of words from this book, and sort them into two categories.

fiction	butter
print	read
banana	salami
pill	rain
library	writer
spoil	weather
glasses	splash
inkling	characters
mystery	insult

Exercise 5: Sentence Fill-ins, Multiple Choice

Directions: Read the sentence, circle the correct word, and then write it.

night	print	perfect

1. The book is no longer in _____.

mystery	show	petal

2. A "whodunnit" is a _____.

ocean	travel	library

3. Borrow the books from the _____.

puppet	muffler	writer

4. Stephen King is a popular _____.

glasses	ears	advice

5. To read better, I need my _____.

filling	fiction	syrup

6. That type of book is _____.

wash	read	order

7. My cousin likes to _____.

characters	tumbles	services

8. The book has too many _____.

Exercise 6: Yes/No Questions

Directions: Read the question, and circle "yes" or "no."

1. Do you read only paperbacks?	Yes	No
2. Is fiction about real events?	Yes	No
3. Are all writers good?	Yes	No
4. Are most libraries quiet?	Yes	No
5. Are characters a key part of a book?	Yes	No
6. Do you wear glasses on your nose?	Yes	No
7. Does large print help some people?	Yes	No
8. Does a mystery keep you guessing?	Yes	No

Exercise 7: Answering Questions, Multiple Choice

Directions: Use each word to answer the questions that follow:

fiction	print	characters	writer

1. Who are the people in a novel? _____

2. What are the words on a page? _____

3. What is a story not based in fact? _____

4. Who creates a story? _____

read	library	glasses	mystery

5. Where can you borrow books? _____

6. What do you do with a book? _____

7. What do you wear to help you read? _____

8. What is a book about a crime? _____

Exercise 8: Sentence Arrangement

Directions: Rearrange these words to make a correct sentence. Write that sentence on the line.

1. I asked if the book: in   came   print   large

_____

2. Our library: new   has   a   wing

_____

3. My book: characters   many   has   too

_____

4. I bought a new: reading   pair   glasses   of

_____

5. Stephen King: writer is   a   popular

_____

6. The ending of the mystery: was total surprise   a

_____

7. I like: book to read reviews

_____

8. Her brother: fiction will   only   read

_____

Exercise 9: Sentence Construction

Directions: Create sentences with these word pairs.

1. fiction-prefer   fiction shelf
2. print-see   large print
3. library-borrow   new library
4. characters-admire   twelve characters
5. glasses-broke   reading glasses
6. writer-produced   well-known writer
7. mystery-confusing   clever mystery
8. read biography   never read

Exercise 10: Sentence Correction

Directions: There are two errors in each sentence below. Find the errors, circle them, and rewrite the sentence.

1. The print is two small for me to feed.

_____

2. Someone found my library cargo in them bathroom.

_____

3. She is famous for solvent the mystery before she funishes the book.

_____

4. Eye need a strongest prescription for my glasses.

_____

5. Do yous prefer function or nonfiction?

_____

6. I like to read the newspaper ever mourning.

_____

7. I cold easily identification with the lead character.

_____

8. The writer has writen nearly thirty books in his careen.

_____

Exercise 11: Paragraph Reading, Multiple-Choice Questions

Directions: Read the paragraph, and then answer the questions.

Once a month, Ellen goes to the public library to attend a book club. This month's selection was a mystery by Agatha Christie. Ellen asked her friend Laurie to read the book and try the club. At the meeting, Laurie was particularly annoying and negative. She had forgotten her glasses and could not read the print. She disliked the writer's style; said there were too many characters to keep straight, and she guessed the ending. When it was time to go, Laurie announced she would like to join the group, but insisted the next selection be contemporary fiction. Ellen reacted quickly and suggested another Agatha Christie book and that the group read only mysteries for the rest of the season.

1. The writer of book was:
   a. Stephen King
   b. Agatha Christie
   c. Ernest Hemmingway
   d. Angela Lansbury

2. Laurie didn't like the book because:
   a. too many characters
   b. too many pages
   c. it wasn't funny
   d. the print was in color

3. What did Laurie suggest that the club read next time?
   a. contemporary fiction
   b. another mystery
   c. a biography
   d. poetry

4. Ellen suggested they read more Agatha Christy because:
   a. she likes repetition
   b. she wants Laurie to drop out
   c. she wants Laurie to try harder
   d. she is a mystery buff

Exercise 12: Conversational Questions

Directions: Answer these conversational questions on the topic.

1. Why are books easier to read in large print for some people?
2. How has your library changed in the way you can borrow books?
3. Do you prefer fiction or nonfiction? Why?
4. What do you like or dislike about mysteries?
5. Why do drug stores now stock reading glasses?
6. Besides books, what else do you like to read?
7. What makes a character in a book memorable?
8. Why are the benefits of a writer holding a book signing?

Chapter 17

Cognitive Stimulation: Stimulation of Recognition/Comprehension, Memory, and Convergent, Divergent, and Evaluative Thinking

Roberta Chapey

OBJECTIVES

The objectives of this chapter are to define communication as a problem-solving, decision-making task; review the stimulation approaches to aphasia intervention; discuss the Guilford SOI model; define cognition, intelligence, language, problem solving, decision making, learning, information processing, and composite abilities within the context of the Guilford model; discuss assessment within a cognitive stimulation approach to aphasia management; explain the general and specific objectives of cognitive stimulation therapy and suggest possible tasks and materials for such therapy; and discuss the relationship between cognitive stimulation therapy and Wepman's Thought Process Therapy, Kearns' Response Elaboration Training, and the Life Participation Approach to Aphasia.

I served as a speech pathologist for a 6-week summer program in the NYC Board of Education that included a group of 5-year-old, nonverbal, language-impaired children. Each day, I used subsequent activities and lessons from the *Peabody Language Development Kit* (1965), based on the Guilford Structure-of-Intellect model—specifically, on divergent thinking, convergent thinking, and associative thinking. The results amazed me: The children gained a large amount of language in a very short time—so much so that they were not recommended for therapy that September. I became fascinated with the results, the kit, and the Guilford model, and the application of part of the model to adults with aphasia was the subject of my doctoral dissertation ("Divergent Semantic Behavior In Adult Aphasia"). The kit has subsequently been expanded to include multiple levels and is still used throughout the world.

COMMUNICATION: A PROBLEM-SOLVING/DECISION-MAKING TASK

Communication is a problem-solving/decision-making task. One possible model of problem solving and decision making may be the Guilford Structure-of-Intellect (SOI) model (Fig. 17-1). There are four reasons why this model may be appealing. First, it appears to have ecological and communicative validity. That is, communication usually involves deciding who can say what, to whom, in what way, where, and when (Prutting, 1979). It is a constant attempt to decide what is the message of best fit for this partner in this situation. It is the back and forth—the give and take—of ideas for a specific purpose or problem. During such communication, when we comprehend a literal or implied message (e.g., "What time is it?" perhaps meaning "You are late.") or that a problem exists, we use the mental operation of recognition/comprehension. When we comprehend a joke or double meaning of a word (e.g., "If the #2 pencil is the most popular, why is it still #2?" or "Why is the time of day with the slowest traffic called rush hour?"), we use recognition/comprehension of systems. When we remember what was said, we use memory; when we ask ourselves "What are all the possible reasons that I can use to explain the fact that I'm late?" we use divergent thinking. (Divergent thinking also is called brainstorming or creativity.) When we think of relevant contingent and/or adjacent utterances, we often use divergent thinking. When we decide between "My car broke down," "I overslept," and "The dog turned off my alarm clock," we use the mental operation of judgment.

When individuals have a communicative (or other) problem to solve or a decision to make, they make use of whatever *content* (figural, symbolic, semantic, and/or behavioral), *mental operation* (recognition/understanding, memory, convergent thinking, divergent thinking, and/or evaluative thinking), and/or *product* or *association* (units, classes, relations, systems, and transformations)—or some combination of these—is called for by the specific communication (or other) problem or decision at hand.

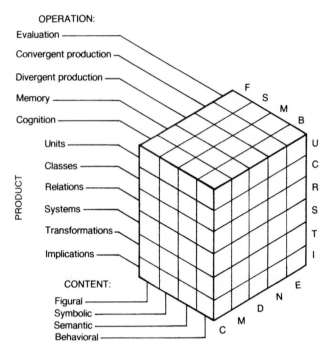

Figure 17–1. Guilford's Structure-of-Intellect model.

STIMULATION APPROACHES TO LANGUAGE INTERVENTION IN APHASIA

The stimulation approaches to therapy form the cornerstone of language intervention strategies used with adult patients who have aphasia (Chapey, 1981a). None of these approaches attempts to teach naming or other specific responses to particular stimuli. Rather, each emphasizes the reorganization of language through stimulation or increased cortical activity through problem solving (Duffy & Coelho, 2001). The stimulation approach first articulated and later developed and refined by Schuell and colleagues (1955, 1964) places its primary emphasis on the stimulation presented to the individual with aphasia. The stimulation approach is grounded in the observation that the patient has not lost linguistic elements or rules but, rather, that the language system is working with reduced efficiency. This approach, therefore, employs strong, controlled, and intensive auditory stimuli as the primary tool to facilitate and maximize the patient's reorganization and recovery of language. It emphasizes the action elicited within the patient by the stimuli presented, because "sensory stimulation is the only method we have for making complex events happen in the brain" (Schuell et al., 1964, p. 338). Some proponents of the stimulation approach encourage us to stimulate patient ability to solve problems (Jennings & Lubinski, 1981; Zachman et al., 1982), to predict outcomes and determine causes of events (Zachman et al., 1982), and to think (Chapey, 1977a, 1981b; Chapey & Lubinski, 1979; Chapey, Rigrodsky, & Morrison, 1976, 1977).

In light of the current emphasis on cognition, one might ask what types of cortical activity are increased through problem solving, predicting outcomes, and/or determining causes of events? What complex events happen in the brain when one stimulates a patient? What are cognition, intelligence, and information processing, and how do they relate to these complex events in the brain? Are problem solving and decision making unitary or composite abilities? What is the difference between cognitive processes and products? What language-based cognitive abilities elicit action within the patient and make complex events happen in the brain to stimulate the comprehension and production of language? Answers to these questions and operational definitions of these abilities are crucial if we are to develop a coherent and generative rationale for intervention, as opposed to the listing of tasks that should be presented to patients. We need a better understanding and specification of the processes we are stimulating in the brain as well as an operational definition of the action elicited within the patient and the complex events that happen in the brain. We need to concretize the cognitive processes and the processes involved in problem solving and decision making. Specification of the underlying targets of our stimulation therapy may increase the effectiveness of our intervention efforts.

The following discussion represents one possible way to answer the above questions.

DEFINITIONS OF COGNITION IN THE PSYCHOLOGY LITERATURE

The study of cognition represents the work of numerous psychologists with a variety of related approaches. Thus, no single comprehensive theory of cognition exists. Rather, cognitive psychologists are viewed as "information-processing" theorists who seek to determine what "functional mental events transpire while a person actually behaves" (Rosenthal & Zimmerman, 1978). Their focus is not on observable behavior but, rather, on examining the characteristics of internal, central brain processing or mental events, such as perception, recognition, reasoning, thinking, evaluation, concept formation, abstraction, generalization, decision making, and problem solving.

"Cognition," then, is a generic term for any process whereby an organism becomes aware of or obtains knowledge of an object (English & English, 1958). It "refers to all the processes by which sensory input is transformed, reduced, elaborated, stored, recovered, and used" (Neisser, 1967, p. 4). It is a group of processes by which we achieve knowledge and command of our world—that is, a method of processing information. It is "the activity of knowing; the acquisition, organization, and use of knowledge" (Neisser, 1967, p. 1)—knowledge that will, in turn, influence or instigate and guide subsequent and more overt behavior (Rosenthal & Zimmerman, 1978). It should be noted that cognitive psychologists do not interpret the above mental processes as occurring in stages or in isolation; rather, they are seen as dynamic and interacting variables.

HOW THE MIND WORKS

In his book *How the Mind Works*, Steven Pinker (1997) presents a computational theory of the mind and suggests that the mind is not the brain but, rather, is what the brain does. The brain's special status comes from what the brain does—information processing or computation. Thus, "beliefs and desires are *information*, incarnated as configurations of symbols" (p. 25). Computation "allows meaning to cause and be caused" (p. 25) by allowing patterns of connections and patterns of activity among the neurons (p. 25). The "content of brain activity lies in the patterns of connections and patterns of activity among the neurons" (p. 25). Also, "[o]nly when the program is run does the coherence become evident" (p. 25). Rather, it is the arrangement of neurons that matters. Programs are assemblies of simple information-processing units, which are functionally specialized and which must assemble themselves. "A program is an intricate recipe of logical and statistical operations directed by comparisons, tests, branches, loops, and subroutines embedded in subroutines" (p. 27).

According to Pinker, evolution equipped us with a neural computer that often supplies missing information and makes good guesses. It contains modules that are "defined by the special things they do with the information available to them, not necessarily by the kinds of information they have available" (p. 31). Pinker suggests we need ideas "that capture the ways a complex device can tune itself to unpredictable aspects of the world and take in the kinds of data it needs to function" (p. 33). Intelligence, Pinker says, "is the ability to attain goals in the face of obstacles by means of decisions based on rational (truth-obeying) rules" (p. 62).

INTELLIGENCE AS DEFINED IN THE PSYCHOLOGY LITERATURE

The most widely accepted definition of intelligence is that "intelligence is what the intelligence tests test." Another definition is the SOI model (Fig. 17-1), which was developed by J.P. Guilford (1967) during his 20 years as the director of the Aptitudes Research Project at the University of Southern California from 1949 to 1969. His project, funded by the Personnel and Training Branch of the Psychological Sciences Division of the U.S. Office of Naval Research, was designed to define various intellectual abilities to match the native skills of U.S. Navy personnel to specific job requirements. For example, Guildford sought to determine which subjects were best suited for officer status, for pilot training, and so on.

In an attempt to define the numerous intellectual abilities available to individuals and, thereby, achieve a taxonomy of intellectual functioning, Guilford (1967) as well as Guilford and Hoepfner (1971) developed numerous tests, each of which was thought to tap a specific intellectual ability. The validity of each test and ability was then assessed by performing numerous-factor analytic studies of responses to the tests and determining which of these tests loaded on specific statistical factors. Results of this research suggest that 120 factors exist in humans (Fig. 17-1). These 120 factors are divided into three parameters: (1) mental operations, (2) contents, and (3) products.

THE GUILFORD MODEL

The Guilford model has five mental operations, four content areas, and six products ($5 \times 4 \times 6 = 120$). An ability is a combination of one kind of operation, one kind of content, and one kind of product (e.g., convergent symbolic units or divergent semantic classes). Each operation is a computation.

Mental Operations

The five mental operations are cognition, memory, convergent thinking, divergent thinking, and evaluative thinking or judgment.

Cognition

The mental operation of cognition is basic to all other operations; hence, it is first. "If no cognition, no memory; if no memory, no production, for the things produced come largely from memory storage. If neither cognition nor production, then no evaluation" (Guilford, 1967, p. 63).

Cognition involves knowing, awareness, attention, immediate discovery (or rediscovery), and recognition of information in various forms (comprehension or understanding). Recognition involves acknowledgment that something has been seen or perceived previously. For example, cognition of semantic material might be tested by using a multiple-choice vocabulary test in which the correct alternative is a synonym of the word to be defined and the other alternatives are not. Tests of cognition determine how much the examinee knows or can readily discover on the basis of what is known. (The term "cognition" has been used to refer to all mental activity or operations by most cognitive psychologists; however, Guilford used the term to refer to one specific mental operation—recognition/comprehension—which can be confusing).

Memory

Memory is the power, act, or process of fixing newly gained information in storage. It involves the ability to insert new information into memory and to retain that new information. According to Guilford (1967), good memory tests require that subjects essentially have a full comprehension of the studied information. Therefore, test material is not difficult. Otherwise, tests may load on cognition, convergent thinking, and/or divergent thinking. The operation of memory, then, is the fixation and retention of new information.

Convergent Thinking

Convergent thinking is the generation of logical conclusions from given information, in which the emphasis is on achieving conventionally best outcomes. Usually, the information given fully determines the outcome, as in mathematics and logic. In accordance with the information given to them, examinees must converge on the one right answer (Guilford, 1967; Guilford & Hoepfner, 1971).

Convergent production is in the area of logical deductions or compelling inferences, and it involves the generation of logical necessities. An example of a convergent semantic test would be verbal analogies completion, in which subjects must supply their own answers, or picture group naming, in which subjects write a class name for each group of five pictured objects.

Divergent Thinking

Divergent production involves the generation of logical alternatives from given information, in which the emphasis is on variety, quantity, and relevance of output from the same source. It is concerned with the generation of logical possibilities, with the ready flow of ideas, and with the readiness to change the direction of one's responses (Guilford, 1967). It involves providing ideas in situations where a proliferation of ideas on a specific topic is required. Such behavior necessitates the use of a broad search of memory storage and the production of multiple possible solutions to a problem. It is the ability to extend previous experience and knowledge or to widen existing concepts (Cropley, 1967). Divergent behavior is directed toward new responses—new in the sense that the thinker was not aware of the response before beginning the particular line of thought (Gowan, Demos, & Torrance, 1967).

Divergent questions are open-ended and do not have a single correct answer. For example, the individual might be asked to list numerous things that are soft and fluffy, to think of problems that anyone might have when eating lunch, or to list what might happen if people no longer needed or wanted sleep. Responses can be grouped according to the number of ideas produced (fluency) and the variety of ideas suggested (flexibility). If an individual is asked to list objects that can roll and responds with "a baseball, a football, a basketball, a nickel, a dime, a quarter, a car, and a truck," this person would receive a fluency score of eight and a flexibility score of three (balls, money, and transportation). Guilford also uses originality and elaboration scores to measure divergent ability. "Originality" relates to the unusualness of the response, and "elaboration" is the ability

to specify numerous critical details in planning an event or making a decision. Responses also are evaluated for relevance. Answers that are not relevant to the specific questions are not scored. Thus, if the above individual had responded, "Isn't that an interesting question?" or "I like to eat lunch," these responses would not be scored, because they do not answer the question.

Evaluative Thinking or Judgment

According to Guilford (1967), judgment involves the ability of the individual to use knowledge to make appraisals or comparisons or to formulate evaluations in terms of known specifications or criteria, such as correctness, completeness, identity, relevance, adequacy, utility, safety, consistency, logical feasibility, practical feasibility, or social custom. Although judgment behavior is based on the individual's previous experience and knowledge of the subject involved, it is always an extension of what is known. It is an appraisal or evaluation based on knowledge.

Guilford (1967) developed a number of tests to study judgment or evaluation skills. These tests require that the individual keep specific criteria in mind and select one best answer or solution from among several alternatives. In one test, for example, the individual chooses the best word for the sentence "A sandwich always has (a) bread, (b) butter, (c) lettuce, (d) meat. Which one must it have in order to be a sandwich?" In another, the subject must judge whether a sentence expresses a complete thought—for example, "Is 'Milk comes from' a sentence?" In yet another test, the individual is given specific classifications and is asked to determine if new information can be assigned to the previously established class—for example, "Should the word 'chair' be put with the words 'cow' and 'horse' or with the words 'table' and 'lamp'?" Each judgment task has a predetermined best response or solution (Chapey & Lubinski, 1979).

Content

The human organism discriminates four broad, substantive, basic kinds (or areas) of information, material, or content: figural, symbolic, semantic, and behavioral.

Figural

Figural content pertains to "information in concrete form, as perceived or as recalled in the form of images." The term "figural" minimally implies figure-ground perceptual organization (Guilford & Hoepfner, 1971).

Symbolic

Symbolic content pertains to "information in the form of denotative signs having no significance in and of themselves, such as letters, numbers, musical notations [and] codes" (Guilford & Hoepfner, 1971).

Semantic

Semantic content pertains to "information in the form of conceptions or mental constructs to which words are often applied. Therefore, it involves thinking and verbal communication. However, it need not necessarily be dependent on words. For example, meaningful pictures also convey semantic information" (Guilford & Hoepfner, 1971).

Behavioral

Behavioral content pertains to psychological information—that is, to essentially nonfigural and nonverbal aspects of human interactions, in which the attitudes, needs, desires, moods, intentions, perceptions, and thoughts of others and ourselves are involved. Some of the cues that the human organism obtains about the attention, perception, thinking, feeling, emotions, and intentions of others come indirectly through nonverbal means, such as "body language." For example, this might involve matching two faces that are similar in terms of the mental state conveyed. Such ability enables us to remain aware of what behavior is going on and also to interpret it. It is important for coping with other individuals in face-to-face encounters, in solving interpersonal problems, in detecting and analyzing problems, and in generating information that is needed to derive solutions. This type of content sometimes is called social intelligence (Guilford & Hoepfner, 1971).

Products

The six types of products are units, classes, relations, systems, transformations, and implications. They represent the way that things are associated in the mind such that each level enters into the next level, producing a larger and larger number of associations between and among items of information. Thus, units enter into classes, classes into relations, relations into systems, and so on. Therefore, products represent a possible continuum from simple (units) to complex (implications) (Chapey, 1994).

Units

Units are things to which nouns often are applied. They are relatively segregated or circumscribed items or "chunks" of information having "thing" character (Guilford & Hoepfner, 1971) and often referring to one item, such as a cup or a chair. Units may be synonymous with the idea of "figure-on-ground" in Gestalt psychology. An example of a semantic units test might be a multiple-choice vocabulary test in which the correct alternative is a synonym of the word to be defined and the other alternatives are not. Semantic units are meanings, ideas, or thoughts in the form of a particular whole. Of the products, units are regarded as basic; hence, they appear at the top (Guilford, 1967).

Classes

Units enter into classes or "conceptions underlying sets of items of information grouped by virtue of their common properties" (Guilford & Hoepfner, 1971). They involve common properties within sets, such as dishes or furniture. Such semantic classes involve class ideas or concepts or choosing the class name that best describes a given set of words or objects.

Relations

Relations are meaningful connections between items of information based on variables or points of contact that apply to them (Guilford & Hoepfner, 1971). For example, a test of semantic relations can be the logical relations of a syllogism in which two premises and four alternative conclusions are presented, only one of which is correct. It also might involve an analogy task, in which case the individual must grasp the relations between the initial pair of words and apply it to the second (e.g., "soup is hot; ice cream is _____.").

Systems

Relations enter into systems or organized patterns or items of information; they are complexes of interrelated or interacting parts (Guilford & Hoepfner, 1971). For example, a semantic system can be a "sentence—a complex of relationships among ideas, an organized thought—a sequence of events, or a common situation" (Guilford & Hoepfner, 1971). It might involve double meanings, puns, homonyms, and redefinitions or shifts in meaning.

Transformations

Systems enter into transformations or changes of various kinds, such as redefinitions, shifts, transitions, or modifications in existing information.

Implications

Transformations enter into implications or circumstantial connections between items of information, such as connections by virtue of contiguity, or any condition that promotes "belongingness" (Guilford & Hoepfner, 1971). Implications involve information expected, anticipated, suggested, or predicted by other information. For example, a semantic implication can be sensitivity to problems such as stating two things seen wrong with a common appliance or those that might arise in the use of a given specific object.

Composite Abilities

According to Guilford and Hoepfner (1971):

It must not be supposed that, although the abilities are separate and distinct logically and they can be segregated by factor analysis, they function in isolation in mental activities of the individual. Two or more of the abilities are ordinarily involved in solving the same problem. The fact that they habitually operate together in various mixtures in ordinary mental functioning has been the reason for the difficulty of recognizing them by direct observation or even by ordinary laboratory procedures. (pp. 19–20)

Indeed, it was largely through the construction of special tests, each one aimed at a specific ability, and the sensitive and searching procedures of factor analysis that Guilford and colleagues clearly demonstrated the separateness of the various mental operations, contents, and products.

The following sections will explore the composite or unified notions of problem solving, decision making, and information processing.

PROBLEM SOLVING

According to Guilford and Hoepfner (1971), problem solving is a complex composite ability. A problem is presented whenever a situation calls for the individual doing anything novel to cope with something that is different from past behavior. Problem solving involves the use of all five mental operations, all types of content or information, and any kind of product, depending on the problem presented, the context in which the problem arises, and the kinds of products required to reach a solution.

Initially, the individual must become aware that a problem exists. This is a matter of cognition, often involving implications. Next, the problem must be analyzed or structured, which usually involves cognition of systems. After the problem is structured:

[The] individual generates a variety of alternative solutions, which is divergent production. If sufficient basis for a solution is cognized and then produced, there is convergent production. (Guilford & Hoepfner, 1971, p. 31)

At each stage in the problem-solving process, there is evaluation

in the form of accepting or rejecting cognitions of the problem and generated solutions. At any step what happens may become fixated and retained for possible later use, so that memory is involved. When evaluation leads to rejections, there may be new starts, with revised cognitions and productions. (Guilford & Hoepfner, 1971, p. 31)

Thus, problem solving can be said to have five steps: (1) preparation (recognition of a problem, cognition), (2) analysis (cognition), (3) production (divergent and convergent), (4) verification (evaluation), and (5) reapplication.

The problem-solving factors found by Guilford and his colleagues using factor analyses are as follows:

Cognition	CMU		
	CMC		
	CMR		
	CMS		Therefore, 8 factors are
	CMI[a]	Inductive	involved in reasoning
Divergent	DMU		(5 cognition, 3
	DMR		convergent)
	DMT		
Convergent	NMC		
	NMR	Deductive	
	MNI		
Evaluation	EMI		

[a]Sensitivity to problems = CMI, EMI.

DECISION MAKING

Decision making and planning ability both belong in the category of problem solving and usually entail all of the steps described above. Guilford (1967) notes that the more a problem, decision, or plan involves the generation of numerous responses or novelty, or the more creative the solution, then the more it involves divergent production abilities—especially divergent transformation abilities—or, possibly, all transformation abilities.

INFORMATION PROCESSING

The present writer suggests that Guilford's (1967) SOI model also can be viewed as an information-processing model (Fig. 17-2). Within this information-processing model, incoming sensory information is figural, symbolic, semantic, and/or behavioral. An attention mechanism selects a small portion of sensory information to be held for several seconds for further processing. This further processing takes place in the central processing unit. The processes of this central processing unit are cognition, memory, convergent thinking, divergent thinking, and evaluative thinking or judgment. It is suggested that these are the functional mental events that transpire while a person actually behaves. The mental events or processes by which sensory information is transformed, reduced, elaborated, stored, recovered, and used. This is the group of mental processes that are used to acquire, organize, store, and use knowledge—the processes whereby an organism becomes aware of or obtains knowledge of an object, event, or relationship.

Within this information-processing model, then, incoming figural, symbolic, semantic, and/or behavioral sensory information is attended to and processed in the central processing unit by one or more of the five SOI mental operations. If the information is immediately recognized, known, comprehended, or understood, the mental operation of cognition has occurred. When situations call for the individual to generate logical conclusions from given information, in which emphasis is on achieving conventionally best outcomes, then

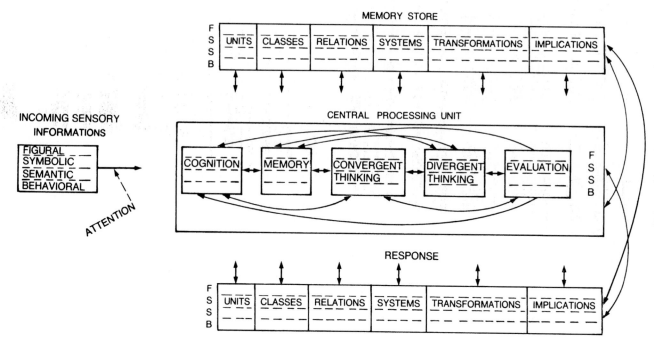

Figure 17–2. Human information processing model based on the Guilford Structure-of-Intellect model. (From Chapey, 1994; with permission.)

convergent thinking occurs. When a novel response is required, the divergent operation is generated. Inserting newly gained information into storage involves memory. Judging the appropriateness, acceptability, relevance, and/or correctness of information requires evaluation.

When the mental operations are used and new information or knowledge is produced, these new discriminations come about in the form of new products: units, classes, relations, systems, transformations, and implications. Products are the basic forms that figural, symbolic, semantic, and behavioral information take as a result of being processed by one or all of the organism's mental operations. These new associations usually are produced as responses and/or may be processed by the mental operation of memory and inserted into memory storage.

Memory

It is important to differentiate between memory as an operation, or short-term memory, and long-term memory, or memory storage. The operation of memory (or short-term memory) is the act or process of fixing newly gained information in storage. In contrast, long-term memory is a storage area that contains everything that is retained for more than a few minutes, such as all learned experience, including language and the rules of language. It retains the products generated by the various mental operations as they process or act on experience. Thus, each individual has his or her own summary of past experiences, or a memory structure of the

world in long-term memory. It has been shown that the capacity of this storage is not static or fixed; rather, it is dynamic. Indeed, "the more you know, the more you can know, the more you remember, the more you can remember" (Muma, 1978). This "theory of the world in our heads serves as the foundation for learning." Indeed, what we know makes our experience meaningful.

One of the characteristics of long-term memory is that what is recalled often is not simply what was seen or heard but, rather, is a modification of the original learning. That is, external stimuli cannot enter the organism. Instead, organisms do not react directly to representations of the world but, rather, to information that they themselves construct (Guilford, 1967). An individual's representation of reality as internal symbols and the interrelations among these symbols are what is called "information." When the amount of memory we need to process is large, the operation of memory is capable of collapsing (or "chunking") the data it receives in more efficient ways and treating it in groups, such as classes. Through chunking, we can deal successfully with larger amounts of information with only minimal difficulty in storage and retrieval. Chunking provides a way of representing information so that it conforms to one's conceptual organization (Muma, 1978)—that is, to one's previously stored associations or products.

When the individual is faced with a meaningful problem and uses all of the cognitive processes to solve a problem, the results of this information processing frequently are inserted into long-term memory. Rote memory, on the other hand, uses only one mental operation: memory. The use of more numerous operations during problem solving and the establishment of numerous associations, or products, during the process may be one reason why meaningful memory is longer lasting.

All of the mental operations depend on memory storage, because all operations retrieve information from this store (Fig. 17-2). That is, all of the mental operations search long-term memory to recall information that has been stored. Thus, there is cognitive retrieval, memory retrieval, convergent retrieval, divergent retrieval, and evaluative retrieval.

Perception/Attention

Where, one may ask, is perception in all this? In the literature, perception is defined as knowing and comprehending the nature of the stimulus (Muma, 1978). To perceive is to know. Attention is part of this process. Therefore, within this model, both perception and attention are viewed as part of cognition.

LEARNING

According to cognitive psychologists, learning is an active process of problem solving (Lazerson, 1975). A learning situation arises whenever our present cognitive structures prove to be inadequate for making sense of the world when something in our experience is unfamiliar or unpredictable (Smith, 1975). Thus, "learning" is an interaction between the world around us and the theory of the world in our heads. In this view, the learner is seen as a scientist who constructs theories or forms hypotheses about the world and then conducts experiments to test these hypotheses.

A distinguishing feature of the "cognitive" approach to learning is the assumption that what is learned are concepts or schema and conceptual associations about the relationships between and among objects, events, and relationships. This process of concept formation involves identifying common features and grouping together all things that have a common feature (i.e., forming classes). Concept learning involves the acquisition of a common response to dissimilar stimuli (Saltz, 1971). It is regarded as the process of making differentiations and discriminations, a process of recognizing similarities and differences or reorganizing material into new patterns or products. It involves the generation of lists of specific characteristics to differentiate membership into particular categories.

Concept formation enables us to transform the world of infinite appearances into finite essences (Saltz, 1971) and to organize past learning in such a way that it no longer is bound to the specific situation in which the learning occurred. Thus, instead of having to react to each object as something unique, we learn to make generalized responses to classes of objects. The generalized responses function as

principles or laws. When we learn something in this type of generic manner, we are able to benefit from analogy when we deal with a new problem. When this occurs, one of the major objectives of learning has been accomplished. We are able to adapt to our environment in more satisfactory ways, and we are saved from subsequent learning (Bruner, 1968).

According to Bruner (1968), all of a human being's interactions with the world involve classifying input in relation to classes or categories that he or she has already established. Bruner's contention is that to perceive is to categorize, to conceptualize is to categorize, to learn is to categorize, and to make decisions is to categorize.

In SOI theory, learning is "the acquisition of information which comes about in the form of new discriminations in terms of new products" (Guilford & Hoepfner, 1971, p. 30). Learning and concept formation employ the five operations of the SOI theory. According to Guilford and Hoepfner (1971):

[No] item of information has been learned until it has been cognized. That which is learned cannot have any future effects unless it is fixated and retained (memory). Items of information produced (divergent and convergent) in response to new cues may also be fixated and remembered. In attempting to learn, the individual makes errors and he must discriminate between errors and correct information. This involves evaluation. Evaluation is conceived as playing an important role in reinforcement. (p. 30)

Concept formations, the largest product of cognitive processing, are products of SOI operations and are called units, classes, relations, systems, transformations, and implications. Thus, the SOI model also is a model of learning.

Results of factor analyses led Guilford (1967) as well as Guilford and Hoepfner (1971) to redefine some of the terminology traditionally used in reference to learning. For example:

Serial learning is essentially dealing with systems, because learned order is a system.
Reasoning, redefined as relational thinking, involves mostly cognition and convergent production—but especially cognition of semantic systems.
Induction is thought to be in the area of cognition because of its discovery properties.
Deduction is primarily in the area of convergent production, because it has to do with drawing firm conclusions.
Classifying objects involves cognition of semantic classes.
Sensitivity to problems is primarily cognition of meaningful implications.
Analysis and synthesis are not coherent SOI factors.

Abstraction, generalization, and transfer

Abstraction occurs when the person selectively picks "abstract dimensions of the object" and reacts to those dimensions and no others. With transfer, "he is obviously adding some personal component to his original learning experience. Thus, more than the literal, external properties of stimuli guide the individual's behavior" (Rosenthal & Zimmerman, 1978). Abstraction is apparent during concept development: "Concepts are developed by abstracting the common stimulus elements in a series of stimulus objects" (Staats, 1968). After having experience with the common stimulus elements of the concept, the individual will be able to pick this common component from a new set containing the same element.

Abstraction and transfer are apparent during rule learning:

By a rule, we mean that two or more objects or events are related to one another in a systematic way. For example, we learn that a flashing red light signifies stopping before crossing an intersection. Later, we exhibit transfer of this rule by stopping when we unexpectedly see a flashing red light beside a stalled car on the highway. (Rosenthal & Zimmerman, 1978)

Abstraction and transfer are involved in a judgment of class inclusion. For example, a baby concludes that certain objects are movable. Understanding the "abstract dimension" of movability, the child transfers this by adding some personal component to his or her original learning experience: The child knows that one way of moving something is to pull it, another way is to kick it, and yet another is to get a parent to pull it (Boden, 1980). This is analogous to the child who knows that the class of beads includes the subclass of green beads (Boden, 1980).

The transfer of learning to new stimuli means that the individual will add quite dissimilar response elements that were not directly related to his or her original learning (Rosenthal & Zimmerman, 1978). Transfer is an additional concept used in problem solving; it is when an individual uses something he or she learned previously and transfers it to a new situation. Positive transfer is when what was learned for one situation helps to solve a problem in a new situation. Negative transfer is when what was learned for one situation makes it harder to solve a problem in a new situation. When an individual is continuously exposed to similar sorts of problems, he or she learns strategies for solving them. A skill that can be transferred to solve problems in new situations is termed a strategy. Harry Harlow (1949) calls this "learning to learn."

Strategies can be transferred from one situation to another. A strategy also can be divided into its components, and then the components can be recombined in new ways (transformations). A transfer in which the components are recombined to "suddenly" solve a problem is called an insight; it is when a problem is solved with the "Aha! Reaction" (Lazerson, 1975).

The intellectual ability to generalize is a significant component in the definition of "cognition." To incorporate specific knowledge and generalize it into everyday experiences is cognition that is well defined and developed (Scott, Osgood, & Peterson, 1979).

Why We Solve Problems or Learn

According to cognitive psychologists, the mind possesses an innate order-generating capacity—that is, a built-in drive to learn. We carry out that drive by acting on our environment. Thus, the individual must act on and interact with the physical, emotional, social, language, and thinking world for cognitive processing to occur. When something is unfamiliar or unpredictable, or when we do not understand, we are motivated to learn (Smith, 1975). According to Smith (1975):

We learn because we do not understand, cannot relate, cannot predict. Everything we know, then, is a consequence of all our previous attempts to make sense of the world. Our present knowledge arises out of a history of problem solving or of predicting the consequences of potential actions. (p. 161)

We learn by relating new information to previous information and by seeing relationships among various bits of information.

For cognitive psychologists, learning is an active process that is significantly influenced by motivation, especially intrinsic motivation (Bruner, 1968), and by curiosity (Yardley, 1974). Bruner (1968) explains this intrinsic motivation in terms of curiosity drive, a drive to achieve competence, and a need to work cooperatively with others, which he termed "reciprocity."

Leon Festinger (Lefrancois, 1982) conceived of cognitive dissonance—that is, the motivating effect of possessing simultaneously compatible items of information. "It is assumed that dissonance leads to behavior designed to reduce conflict" (Lefrancois, 1982, p. 71). An individual remembers more distinctly and for longer periods of time material that is somewhat different from what is already known. According to Ausubel (Lefrancois, 1982), if this material is completely new and unrelated to anything in the individual's cognitive structure, rote learning, rather than meaningful learning, will occur. If the material is too similar, it is rapidly forgotten.

Other variables that intervene between the stimuli and the response are the individual learner's purpose, aspirations, beliefs, and ideals (Marx, 1970). In addition, the learning potential of an individual includes the requisite intellectual capacities, the ideational context, and the existing store of knowledge as it is currently organized (Ausubel, 1965). On this basis, the potential meaningfulness of learning material varies with factors such as age, intelligence, occupation, and cultural membership.

Two people, therefore, are likely to respond differently to the very same stimuli because of what they have already learned, what they feel they are capable of achieving, differences in the ways their minds work, or other differences that distinguish one person from another (Dember & Jenkins, 1979). Smith (1975) observes two other crucial conditions for the individual to exercise a capacity to learn: the individual has the expectation that there is something to learn, and the learner must have some reasonable expectation of a positive outcome.

COGNITION

Cognition, then, can be operationally defined as the use of the five mental operations: (1) cognition (recognition/understanding/comprehension), (2) memory, (3) convergent thinking, (4) divergent thinking, and (5) evaluative thinking or judgment. These are the mental events or processes by which we learn or obtain knowledge about our world and by which we organize, store, recover, and use that knowledge. Knowledge is a product of cognition and is associated or organized into units, classes, relations, systems, transformations, and implications.

LANGUAGE DEFINED

Psycholinguistics is the study of the mental processes underlying the acquisition and use of language (Slobin, 1971). Within the context of the Guilford model, incoming information or language experience is semantic and behavioral (Fig. 17-3). This information is then processed by one or more of the five cognitive operations: cognition, memory, convergent thinking, divergent thinking, and evaluative thinking. These are the mental processes underlying the acquisition and use of language.

Language is something we know (Slobin, 1971). It is a body of knowledge represented in the brains of speakers of a language, the content of which is inferred from overt behavior (Slobin, 1971). According to Bloom and Lahey (1978),

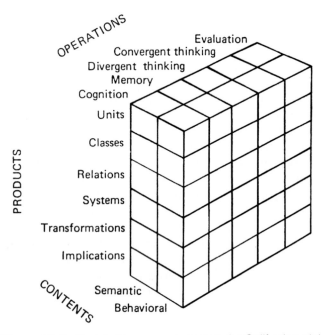

Figure 17–3. Model of language based on the Guilford model (From Chapey, 1994; with permission.)

language can be defined as "a knowledge of a code for representing ideas about the world through a conventional system of arbitrary signals for communication" (p. 23). Specifically, there are three types of language knowledge: content, form, and use. Thus, "language consists of some aspect of content or meaning that is coded or represented by linguistic form for some purpose or use in a particular context" (p. 23). These three types of language knowledge come together in both understanding and saying messages, and indeed, linguistic competence can be defined as the interaction of content, form, and use (Bloom & Lahey, 1978; Lahey, 1988).

Content: Language Represents Ideas About the World

Psycholinguistic research suggests that our

code or means of representing information can operate only in relation to what [we] the speaker and hearer of the language know about objects and events in the world. Speakers of a language need to know about objects and actions in order to know the names for objects and actions. [O]ne cannot know about sentences and the relations between the parts of a sentence unless one also knows about relations between persons and objects in different kinds of events . . . It is the knowledge that individuals have about objects, events and relations in the world that is coded by language—ideas about events are coded, not events themselves. (Bloom & Lahey, 1978, p. 5)

It is this knowledge, these ideas, that are the meaning, topic, or subject matter involved in conversation. For example, an individual might comment about a specific object, such as a pipe; a particular action, such as eating lunch; or a specific relation, such as that between Harry and his pipe. Or, meaning could relate to a content category, such as possession, or having or owning an object, quality, or ability; recurrence, or the reappearance of an object or event; and rejection, or the opposition to an action or object.

An individual learns to understand and use language in relation to the ideas or mental concepts that have been formed through experience (Bloom & Lahey, 1978). The experience of many different objects—some of which are more alike than others—is "an active process whereby persons perceive patterns of structure and invariance in the environment" (Bloom & Lahey, 1978, p. 7), such as similarities among different chairs and the mobility of certain objects but not others. The ability to perceive the similarities in repeated encounters with physical and social events involves the ability to process and analyze experience using the five cognitive processes. Words and categories represent regularities that the individual notes in his or her environment. Individuals learn new words and categories gradually, by testing hypotheses of what a word means in different situations in which they think one or another word might fit (Bloom & Lahey, 1978; Lahey, 1988). This results in the organization or association of information—or the formation of schema into units (or chunks of information having "thing" character; things to which words often are applied; meaning, ideas, or thoughts in the form of particular wholes [e.g., a cookie]); classes (or conceptions underlying sets of items [e.g., cookies]); relations (or meaningful connections between items of information [e.g., all desserts]); systems (or complexes of interrelated or interacting relationships among objects, ideas, and events; double meanings, puns, homonyms, and redefinitions or shifts in meaning [e.g., "This is what I call cheesecake."]); transformations (or various types of changes, such as redefinitions, shifts, transitions, or modifications in existing information [e.g., when baking a cake, if a recipe calls for two eggs and there is only one, a person might open one egg, put it into a measuring cup, and then double the volume by adding water or milk]); and implications (or the formation of hypotheses of what is expected, anticipated, suggested, or predicted by other information [e.g., "Desserts are sweet, fattening, and taste good; are sold in a bakery; are frequently chocolate; can often become stale or spoil," and so forth]).

New experiences may cause the brain to place the experience into an existing unit or class; to create a new concept; to reprocess existing information and reformulate the structure of individual units or to group units together into classes, systems, and/or relations; to transform the information; and/or to see the implications of such information.

Language content is developed and used within the context of the speech act. Communication, which is a problem-solving task, usually is initiated and/or maintained to convey meaning about certain topics or ideas or to convey an intent. For example, during communication, an individual may become aware that it is necessary to describe something (an intent) that he or she knows (cognition). The individual may sort through all the possible ways to express this intent (divergent thinking) and may make a judgment, based on past experience, that certain content would be inappropriate (evaluation) for his or her purpose, intent, or listener. The individual therefore comes to a logical conclusion about the conventionally best content for his or her intent (convergent thinking) and then conveys the content to the listener.

Form: Language Is a System

The rules of language specify how to arrange symbols to express ideas (McCormick & Schiefelbush, 1984). Specifically, a system of rules determines the "ways in which sounds combine to form words and words combine to form sentences for representing knowledge" (Bloom & Lahey, 1978, p. 7). For words, a limited number of rules specify which sounds can and cannot combine. For sentences, a limited number of rules specify how linguistic elements (words and morphemes) are combined to code meaning (Bloom & Lahey, 1978; Lahey, 1988). According to Slobin (1971), syntax is a device that relates sound and meaning. Thus, the form of language or system of rules "is the means for connecting sounds or signs with meaning" (Bloom & Lahey, 1978, p. 15).

Linguistic competence is a system of rules that relates semantic interpretations of a sentence to their acoustic phonetic representations (Slobin, 1971). It is a set or system of rules for processing utterances (Slobin, 1971).

Two rule systems in English are word order and markers. Word order tells us about the subject-object relationship. Markers can be divided into two types: function words (*the, a, with*) and suffixes (*-s, -ing*). The markers do such things as identify classes (e.g., *the* identifies a noun), specify relations (e.g., *with* relates *girl* to *eyes*), or signal meanings (e.g., *-ing* signals ongoing activity, and *-s* signals plurality), and so on (Slobin, 1971).

Chomsky (1957) postulated two basic sorts of rules or two levels of sentence interpretation. Phrase structure rules generate deep structures, which are directly related to the meaning of the sentence. The semantic component of grammar "relates deep structures to meanings" (Slobin, 1971, p. 19). Transformational rules convert deep structures into surface structures. The surface level of a sentence is directly related to the sentence as it is heard. The phonologic component of grammar "converts surface structures into sound patterns of spoken utterances" (Slobin, 1971, p. 19).

According to Chomsky (1972), the surface structure often is misleading and uninformative: "Our knowledge of language involves properties of a much more abstract nature, not directly in the surface structure" (p. 32). Because the meaning is not always directly expressed in the sounds we hear, we must have rich inner mental structures that make it possible to utter and comprehend sentences (Slobin, 1971). We cannot explain language learning on the basis of observable "stimuli" and "responses" alone, because all of the information for the processing of speech is not present in observable behavior" (Slobin, 1971, p. 19). Rather, the individual is biologically predisposed to learn a set or system of rules for processing utterances.

Grammar, then, is

a device for pairing phonetically represented signals [into a] system of abstract structures generated by the syntactic component. Thus, the syntactic component must provide for each sentence (actually for each interpretation of each sentence), a semantically interpretable deep structure and a phonetically interpretable surface structure, and in the event that these are distinct, a statement of the relation between these structures. (Chomsky, 1964, p. 52)

Abstract structural patterns underlie grammatical sentences. Understanding a sentence is based on knowledge of this structure. Indeed, "you can only make sense of the string of words you hear if you know . . . the grammar of your language" (Slobin, 1971). This syntactic knowledge or finite system of rules makes it possible for us to comprehend and generate an infinite number of sentences and connect sounds or signs with meaning.

These rules of language that allow us to process and/or generate utterances and connect sounds or signs with meaning are learned by "listening to the language of the environment and abstracting from it the rules that are used to generate it" (Naremore, 1980). Individuals do not learn language form and then apply it to meaning. Rather, they focus on what they see and hear and then "use their conceptual capacity for linguistic inductions" (Bloom & Lahey, 1978, p. 72) to develop a knowledge of language content, form, and use to communicate meaning. Meaning is the essence of language (Goodman, 1971).

Developing a language system is a problem-solving task. It involves, among other things, hypothesis formation, abstraction, transfer, judgment of class inclusion, and generalization. As individuals process and use semantic and behavioral information, they become aware that the system of rules they now possess is not adequate for expressing meaning or what they would like to say. Becoming aware that a problem exists is a matter of cognition, often involving implications. Next, the problem in the rule system is analyzed or structured, which usually involves cognition of systems. After the problem is structured, the individual generates a variety of possible ways to code what he or she wishes, which is divergent production. If sufficient basis for a solution to the rule system is cognized and then produced, there is convergent production. At each stage in the process, there is evaluation or judgment in the form of accepting or rejecting cognitions of the problem and the generated solutions. At any step, what happens may become fixated and retained for possible later use, so memory is involved. When evaluation leads to rejections, there may be new starts, with revised cognitions and productions.

Thus, we learn new forms of language when our present system of rules proves to be inadequate for expressing meaning. The acquisition of new rules comes about in the form of new discriminations in terms of new products. Individuals learn rules gradually, by testing hypotheses of what a form can express in different situations where they think the rule might be appropriate for the expression of meaning.

Use: Language Is Used for Communication

Communication is an assertive act of coping—an active problem-solving task. It is a constant attempt to vary the content, form, and acceptability of a message; to switch or shift sets of reference as topics change (Muma, 1975); and to be sensitive to the influence of one's communicative partner and the physical context in which communication occurs (Prutting & Kirchner, 1983) to achieve a message of best fit and, thus, effective and efficient communication (Muma, 1975).

Therefore, communicative competence implies knowledge of how to converse with different partners and in different contexts (Craig, 1983) as well as knowledge of the rights, obligations, and expectations underlying the maintenance of discourse (Ochs & Schieffelin, 1979). It is a knowledge of who can say what to whom, in what way, where, when, and by what means (Prutting, 1979).

Pragmatics involves the acquisition and use of such conversational knowledge and of the semantic rules necessary to communicate an intent to affect the hearer's attitudes, beliefs, or behaviors (Lucas, 1980). Such semantic knowledge develops and is "used within the context of a speech act, a theoretical unit of communication between a speaker and a hearer" (Lucas, 1980). According to Searle (1969), the speech act includes "what the speaker means, what the sentence (or other linguistic elements) uttered means, what the speaker intends, what the hearer intends, what the hearer understands, and what the rules governing linguistic utterances are" (p. 12). Speech acts include making promises, statements, requests, assertions, and so on (Table 17-1). In Searle's theory, the proposition is the words or sentences produced, and the elocutionary force of this proposition is the speaker's intent in producing the utterance.

Thus, pragmatics involves the interactional aspects of communication, including sensitivity to various aspects of social contexts (Prutting & Kirchner, 1983). It is an analysis of the use of language for communication. The emphasis is not on sentence structure but on how meaning is communicated—that is, how units of language function in discourse (Prutting & Kirchner, 1983).

Pragmatics is inextricably related to cognition, and indeed, the conversational knowledge or discourse structures that are derived by an individual are the products of one or all of the five SOI cognitive processes or operations. The incoming semantic and/or behavioral information is processed by cognition, memory, convergent thinking,

---

TABLE 17-1

Discourse Structures

1. Physical context variables
2. Communicative partner variables
3. Communication of intent

Label	Greeting	Attention
Response	Repeating	Protesting (Dore, 1974)
Request	Description	
Request	Order	Warn (Searle, 1969)
Assert	Argue	
Question	Advise	

4. Turn taking
   A. Initiation of speech act
   B. Maintenance of communication
      (i) Role switching/turn taking
      (ii) Sustaining a topic
         a. Contingent utterances
         b. Adjacent utterances
         c. Feedback to speaker
         d. Repair/revision
         e. Code switching

divergent thinking, and/or evaluative thinking to generate pragmatic (semantic and/or behavioral) units, classes, relations, systems, transformations, and implications. Communication (and, therefore, pragmatics or language use) is an active process of problem solving. We learn new pragmatic rules when our present pragmatic knowledge proves to be inadequate for a situation or when something in our experience is unfamiliar or unpredictable. The acquisition of new pragmatic information comes about in the form of new discourse structures as a result of the use of one or all of the five mental operations of the SOI model.

Discourse Structures

A number of cognitive/pragmatic products or discourse structures are discussed in the literature. These relate to physical context variables, communicative partner variables, communication of intent, and turn-taking rules (including topic selections, maintenance and change, code switching, and referential skills) (Table 17-1).

Physical Context Variables

A pragmatic view of language assumes that language will vary with each context, that contexts are dynamic, and that any language sample therefore will be the interactive product of contextual variables and the individual's structural linguistic knowledge (Gallagher, 1983). Various conversational settings may affect the number and variety of utterances produced by a speaker (Gallagher, 1983). For example, one may have a rule that says, "Don't talk in church"; one that says, "Don't talk loudly in an elegant restaurant"; and yet another that says, "Cheer loudly for your team at a football game."

As individuals encounter various contexts or settings, they categorize or classify these contexts and either simultaneously or subsequently develop rules for interacting in specific types of contexts. The individual tries to determine if he or she knows or recognizes the context; may, perhaps, try to think of all of the other possible responses or behaviors that might be appropriate to this context; may make judgments about certain variables within the context; may try to hypothesize what is expected, anticipated, or suggested for this or for analogous situations; and so on.

Communicative Partner Variables

Specific communicative partners may affect the length, complexity, redundancy, fluency, and responsiveness (e.g., elaborations of comments), semantic relatedness of comments, and amount of eye contact during an utterance (Gallagher, 1983). Indeed, partner characteristics, such as age, sex, familiarity, and status, frequently affect communication. Again, the individual categorizes and classifies partners and develops rules for interacting with specific partners, types of partners, and groups of partners.

When people first encounter a potential communicative partner, they may determine if they know or recognize the partner or type of partner. They may sort through all the possible topics or intents that would be appropriate for this partner and, subsequently, judge or evaluate the form, reference, and acceptability of various possible communications and the implications of such communication.

Communication of Intent

Language is used to communicate a variety of intentions. For example, Dore (1974) specified the following intents: to label, to respond, to request, to greet, to protest, to repeat, to describe, and to call attention to something. The intents specified by Searle (1969) are to request, to assert, to question, to order, to argue, to advise, and to warn.

Language intent may be communicated and comprehended through semantic-syntactic utterances and/or by previous or subsequent utterances. In addition, intent may be expressed (and comprehended) through facial expression or accompanying actions, gestures, or tone of voice. What is not said also may communicate intent. In addition, one can say one thing but mean another. Individuals frequently use their knowledge regarding the physical context variables and the communication partner to help them decipher between what is said and what is meant. Thus, the communication of intent involves the use of semantic content (what is said) as well as behavioral content, or the nonfigural and nonverbal information that communicates the attitudes, needs, desires, moods, intentions, perceptions, and thoughts of others and ourselves. It may even involve the use of symbolic content when symbolic gestures are used.

Individual intents are semantic and/or behavioral units—that is, items or "chunks" of information. These units are developed when the brain processes semantic and behavioral experiences using the five cognitive operations. New experiences may cause the brain to place the experience into an existing unit or class; to create a new concept; to reprocess existing information and reformulate the structure of individual units or to group units together into classes, systems, and/or relations; and/or to see implications of such information. The way in which the individual chooses to communicate an intent at any particular point will reflect his or her knowledge of physical context variables and his or her communicative partners. Thus, the individual evaluates group membership, ability of the listener to interpret the various levels of complexity, receptiveness to various intents, and so on. Comprehension of the intent will be based on the units, classes, systems, relations, transformations, and implications that the listener has already established as well as on the information, associations, or products that he or she has constructed with respect to this specific partner or class of partner, this type of context, and this type of topic. According to Haviland and Clark (1974), comprehension of an utterance in context also involves relating new information to assumed information. Thus, the individual makes a judgment based on past experience as to what is new information and what he or she can assume this particular partner knows.

Turn-Taking Rules

The reciprocal nature of communication involves a number of aspects, including the initiation of the speech act and the maintenance of communication. Initiation of the speech act (as speaker) includes topic selection and introduction and/or change of topic. Usually, the communicative act should contain new, relevant, and what is judged to be sincerely wanted information. It is important to evaluate the implicitly shared information aspect of the communication act. Thus, topical or referential identification involves searching one's long-term memory for information that is judged to be relevant to this partner, wanted by this partner, and perhaps, interesting.

Maintenance of communication involves a number of variables. First, role taking involves the establishment and variation of roles with respect to the speaker and the listener and the reciprocal roles of speaker-initiator and listener-respondent.

The listener's role is to comprehend the speaker's message, which involves cognition. The listener maintains this role with nonverbal (behavioral) responses that are "characterized by visual orientation rather than gaze avoidance" (Davis & Wilcox, 1981, p. 172), a nod of the head, or leaning forward. The listener also may respond with a short and, usually, affirmative verbal response, such as "Yes."

Feedback to the speaker is essential as well. This involves the listener's ability to monitor and evaluate the speaker's message and ability/willingness to indicate whether he or she believes it is effective and acceptable. Listener feedback will depend on the listener's previously established concepts of effectiveness and acceptability in general and his or her concepts that are relevant to this speaker and this context. Occasionally, the listener will assist the speaker in conveying the message, which involves cognition, judgment, and possibly, convergent and divergent thinking.

Role switching may occur as a result of the speaker's desire to relinquish the role. It can be communicated and/or comprehended semantically and/or behaviorally. In many instances, nonverbal (behavioral) cues are used by partners to signal a wish to maintain or change roles (Harrison, 1974; Rosenfeld, 1978). The speaker usually retains his or her role by gaze avoidance and a hand gesture that is not maintained or not returned to a resting state through a phonetic clause juncture (Rosenfeld, 1978). When a speaker wants a listener's reaction, he or she signals "with a pause between clauses" or "with a rising or falling pitch at the end of a phonemic clause" (Davis & Wilcox, 1981, p. 171). Thus, the listener needs to use knowledge of such cues as well as the cues themselves to formulate a judgment concerning the speaker's willingness to switch roles. When role switching occurs in the absence of the speaker's readiness to switch, however, it may be accompanied by overloudness and a shift of the head away from the speaker (Davis & Wilcox, 1981), which would be behavioral content.

Maintenance of communication also may involve a response that sustains a topic (the listener becomes the speaker)—one that involves a specific response to the speech act. For example, contingent utterances are utterances that share the same topic as the preceding utterance and that add information to the previous communication act. A contingent utterance is an elaboration of the speaker's topic. Production of contingent utterances usually involves semantic and behavioral cognition to understand or comprehend an utterance and its intent; convergent production, or a logical and sequentially ordered response; and divergent thinking, or an elaboration of a topic and judgment as to the relevance, accuracy, and appropriateness of a response in this context to this communicative partner.

Maintenance of communication also involves a sequential organization of topics. Thus, adjacent utterances are used as well. These are utterances that occur immediately after a partner's utterance but that are not related to the speaker's topic. Such utterances are considered to be logical or possible elaborations of communication and, therefore, involve convergent and divergent semantic thinking.

Repair and revision also are part of discourse maintenance and regulation. This involves the speaker's sensitivity to cues provided by the listener, which involves semantic and behavioral cognition and judgment and the ability to respond to such cues by repeating and/or modifying the message when necessary. It involves the speaker's use of convergent production, divergent production, and judgment. Moves by the speaker and the listener to repair sequences and respond to such regulatory devices as requests for clarification are essential to the maintenance of communication (Fey & Leonard, 1983).

Code switching is the degree to which the individual can produce stylistic variations in the form or frequency of specific acts to meet situational requirements (Fey & Leonard, 1983), such as the ability to role play. Judgment is essential.

In 1975, John Muma addressed the issue of role/code switching. In his article, he differentiated between two different variations in one's method of communication. One he called "dump," and the other he called "play." Dumping pertains to the issuance of a coded message. Play involves ascertaining needed changes for appropriate recoding of a message and making necessary adjustments to achieve the message of best fit. According to Muma, role-taking attitudes involve the active resolution of communicative obstacles of form, reference, and acceptability in an effort to achieve the message of best fit for a particular situation and listener. It is the ability to issue a "message in the most appropriate form for conveying intended meanings to a particular person for particular efforts" (p. 299). In role taking, "both speaker and listener are active participants in formulating, perceiving and revising messages until necessary adjustments are made in form, reference or psychological distance, and acceptability in order to convey intended meanings" (p. 299). The objective of true communication is aimed at ascertaining or judging which message is most suited to achieve effective and efficient communication.

Content, Form, and Use

Language learning and use, then, are problem-solving tasks. A problem is presented whenever a situation calls for the individual doing anything novel to cope with something that is different from his or her past behavior. A problem is a question or a proposition that necessitates consideration and a solution (Webster, 1977). Problem solving involves the use of all five mental operations, all types of content or information, and any kind of product, depending on the context in which the problem arises and the kinds of products that are required to reach a solution.

If the information is immediately recognized, known, comprehended, or understood, the mental operation of cognition has occurred. When situations call for the individual to generate logical conclusions from given information where emphasis is on achieving conventionally best outcomes, convergent thinking occurs. When a novel response is required, the divergent operation is generated. Inserting newly gained information into storage involves the operation of memory. Judging the appropriateness, acceptability, relevance, and/or correctness of information requires evaluation.

The three types of language knowledge that develop and are used (content, form, and use) are products of these five mental operations. Normal language functioning, then, requires the efficient action and interaction of all five cognitive processes for effective decoding (cognition and memory) and encoding (convergent thinking, divergent thinking, and evaluative thinking) to occur.

ASSESSMENT OF COGNITIVE OPERATIONS

Guilford and Hoepfner (1971) developed a number of tests to assess each of the five mental operations. A list of some of these tests follows.

Semantic Awareness/Recognition Tests

Verbal Comprehension Choose a word that means about the same as the given word.

Reading Comprehension Answer questions about a short passage.

Verbal Opposites Give a word that is opposite in meaning to the given word.

Sentence Synthesis Rearrange scrambled words to make a meaningful sentence.

Vocabulary Choose the alternative word that has the same meaning as a word that completes a sentence.

Semantic Memory Tests

Picture Memory Recall names of common objects pictured on a previously studied page.

Recalled Words Recall words presented on a study page.

Word Recognition Recognize whether given words were on a previously studied page.

Memory for Facts Answer questions regarding information previously given in two sentences.

Convergent Semantic Tests

Picture Group Naming Write a class name for each group of five pictured objects.

Associations Write a word that is associated with each of two given words.

Largest Class Form the largest class possible from a given list of words so that the remaining words also make a class.

Attribute Listing List attributes of objects needed to serve a specific function.

Divergent Semantic Tests

Common Situations List problems that are inherent in a common situation.

Brick Uses List many different uses for a common object.

Product Improvement Suggest ways to improve a particular object.

Consequences List the effect of a new and unusual event.

Object Naming List objects that belong to a broad class of objects.

Differences Suggest ways in which two objects are different.

Similarities Produce ways in which two objects are alike.

Word Fluency List words that contain a specified word or letter.

Planning Elaboration List many detailed steps needed to make a briefly outlined plan work.

Semantic Evaluation Tests

Word Checking Choose one of four words that fits a single criterion.

Double Descriptions Select the one object of four that best fits two given descriptions or adjectives.

Class Name Selection Select a class name that most precisely fits a group of four given words.

Commonsense Judgment Select the two best of five given reasons why a briefly described plan is faulty.

Behavioral Tests

Alternate Expressional Groups Group pictured expressions in different ways so that each group expresses a common thought, feeling, or intention.

Cartoon Predictions Choose one of three alternative cartoon frames that can be most reasonably predicted from the given frame.

Expression Grouping Choose one of four expressions that belongs with a given group by virtue of common psychological dispositions.

Expressions Choose one of four expressions that indicates the same psychological state as another given expression.

Other Assessment Techniques

Torrance (1966) adapted Guilford and Hoepfner's (1971) work on divergent thinking and developed the *Torrance Test of Creative Thinking* (Torrance, 1966). (Norms are available only for children.) Parts of this test, along with other tests from Guilford and Hoepfner (1971), have been used with patients who have aphasia, right brain damage, or closed-head injury as well as with elderly individuals (Braverman, 1990; Chapey, 1974, 1983; Chapey & Lubinski, 1979; Chapey et al., 1976, 1977; Diggs & Basili, 1987; Law & Newton, 1991; Schwartz-Crowley & Gruen, 1986) to assess abilities and impairments of specific mental operations in these groups. The *Test of Problem Solving* (Zachman et al., 1983), which was developed to measure reasoning abilities in children, also can be used with adults to assess specific cognitive semantic abilities, such as explaining inferences, determining causes, answering negative "wh-" questions, determining solutions, and avoiding problems.

Other techniques for assessing cognitive semantic abilities can be obtained through the Educational Testing Services' Test Collection Department, which has a number of unpublished research instruments measuring aptitude and cognition. Several of these measures target Guilford and Hoepfner's (1971) mental operations.

Clinicians who use the cognitive semantic approach to intervention also may evaluate the specific language assets and liabilities of each patient so that the therapeutic effort is individualized to fit the needs, interests, and abilities of each person who receives such therapy. For example, clinicians may want to explore the nature of each patient's language impairment, including performance on appropriate tasks, types(s) of errors made, and the manner in which each patient goes about tasks (Byng, Kay, Edmundson, & Scott, 1990).

In addition, clinicians may need to break tasks (e.g., comprehending sentences, reading aloud single words, gesturing, hailing a bus, filling in a check, and turn taking) down into their component processes and examine the functioning of each of those processes in detail (Byng et al., 1990) to derive hypotheses about the nature of the underlying processing problems in the language deficits in specific patients. A more in-depth discussion of assessment techniques can be found in Chapter 4.

INTERVENTION

The present writer agrees with Martin (1979) that:

1. **Normal functioning** is the "efficient action and interaction of the cognitive processes which support language behavior within and by the organism". The disorder is a "reduction of the efficiency of action and interaction of the cognitive processes which support language behavior".

2. **Therapy** is "the attempt to manipulate and to excite the action and interaction of the cognitive processes which support language behavior within and by the organism so as to maximize their effective usage . . . Therapy [is] directed toward the subsystems which process language" (pp. 157–158).

Within the context of the present chapter, the cognitive processes or subsystems that process language are cognition, memory, convergent thinking, divergent thinking, and evaluation. Aphasia is a reduction in the efficient action and interaction of these processes, and therapy is an attempt to manipulate and excite the action and interaction of these processes. We employ strong, controlled, and intensive figural, symbolic, semantic, and behavioral stimuli—most frequently, semantic stimuli—to elicit the action of cognition, memory, convergent thinking, divergent thinking, and evaluation. These are the cognitive processes or the complex events that happen in the brain.

What is happening between the stimulus and the response is that the individual is using one or all of his or her mental operations. Task input is defined as figural, symbolic, semantic, and/or behavioral stimuli. Processing occurs through the use of cognition, memory, convergent thinking, divergent thinking, and evaluative thinking. Output is generated in units, classes (or categories), relations, transformations, systems, and implications. This holds true for problem-solving, decision-making, learning, and language tasks.

Rationale

A cognitive approach to therapy is based on the belief that propositional language (H. Jackson; cited in Head, 1915) or functional communication is an active problem-solving task that necessitates the use of all five cognitive processes. These operations are the intervening, mediating variables or constructs responsible for language comprehension and production. Thus, cognitive semantic therapy advocates the stimulation of all five mental operations, because this type of processing is required for the comprehension and production of spontaneous language. Indeed, most definitions of language and communication have components that are highly suggestive of all five operations. For example, Hughy and Johnson (1975) state that language is used primarily for information getting and giving, problem solving, and persuasion. Another definition, that proposed by Muma (1975), notes that communication entails the ability to switch or shift sets of reference as topics change, to initiate such shifts, and to overcome obstacles to communication flow. Both definitions reflect the fact that language and communication require the use of all five cognitive processes.

The ability to produce functional communication or spontaneous speech also involves what Noam Chomsky (1957, 1964) refers to as deep structure and surface structure. Deep structure specifies the basic relationship being expressed—who did what to whom. It tells the meaning relationship. The surface structure is the actual sentences that are spoken and written. Meaning often is not audible or visible. Rather, the listener or reader must identify the relationships of the concepts to the events being communicated or described. Understanding a message depends on the memory structure of the people involved in the communication. The entire structure is not communicated if the receiver of the information can already be assumed to understand certain basic concepts. That is, some relations are assumed to be known or to be relatively easy to discover and, therefore, not necessary to mention.

According to Chomsky (1957, 1964), not everything we know about a sentence is revealed in the superficial string of words. That is, all information for processing speech is not present in observable behavior. Meaning is not directly expressed in the sounds we hear and the words we read. Our capacity to interpret sentences depends on our knowledge of deep structure. We do not learn a set of utterances (surface structures). Rather, we learn methods of processing utterances. We have rich cognitive structures that make it possible to utter and comprehend sentences.

In everyday communication, surface structure frequently is deficient, misleading, and uninformative. For example, there are extensive deletions, extensive use of pronouns, and ambiguous referents. Nevertheless, meaning structure may be communicated. Therefore, language is an aid to communication. Production of spontaneous, functional language, and therefore, deep and surface structure requires the use of all five mental operations. These are the methods for processing utterances, the rich cognitive structures that make it possible to comprehend and produce sentences. Cognitive therapy therefore targets all five mental operations for the production of meaningful ideas and the elaboration of those ideas.

A third rationale is based on the observation that patients with aphasia are unable to produce the highest-level central nervous system integrations (Wepman, 1951). Research by Bolwinick (1967) indicates that the highest-level cognitive integrations are thinking (e.g., convergent thinking, diver-

gent thinking, and evaluative thinking), problem solving (all five cognitive operations are viewed as essential components of problem solving), and creativity (divergent thinking is used as a synonym for creativity). Tasks using all five mental operations will focus on the essence of the aphasic impairment—that is, inability to produce the higher-level cognitive integrations.

Cognitive therapy also is rooted in the observation that aphasia is a problem in language retrieval (Schuell et al., 1964) or in the searching and scanning mechanism that selects among many possibilities. Schuell and colleagues (1964) noted that the search mechanism is controlled by instructions, directing it to go to a specific address and bring out information. They suggest that appropriate stimuli are required to activate or reactivate patterns. The information-processing model presented in this chapter hypothesizes that divergent production and evaluative production both involve the use of a broad search of memory storage, whereas cognition and convergent production involve a narrow search of long-term memory. Tasks that stimulate retrieval under a variety of cognitive operations appear to facilitate the patient's reorganization and retrieval of language. Specifically, the stimuli presented foster the action of a broad and narrow search of memory within the individual. The clinician attempts to manipulate the patient's retrieval strategy to aid the patient in making maximal responses.

Another appeal of the Guilford SOI model is that it is a model of learning (Chapey, 1994). Indeed, the acquisition and use of knowledge may involve the use of the five mental operations in the model: memory, recognition/comprehension, and convergent, divergent, and/or evaluative thinking (Chapey, 1994).

In addition, the Guilford SOI model has statistical validity. That is, the entire model has been proven to exist in "normal" individuals (Guilford, 1967; Guilford & Hoepfner, 1971), and the mental operations have been proven to exist in individuals with aphasia (Chapey, 1974, 1977a, 1983, 1988, 1992, 1994; Chapey & Lubinski, 1979).

The fourth appeal of the model is that some individuals may solve problems and make decisions more effectively and efficiently when they use a structured problem-solving, decision-making model.

Accountability

Despite the wide acceptance of the cognitive and pragmatic approaches to therapy in our literature, and the acceptance of the distinction between deep structure and surface structure, many intervention agencies and many government agencies mandate that each therapy session have an operationally written, behavioral goal. Many clinicians also use such goals. For example, the audience (American Speech-Language-Hearing Association–certified speech-language pathologists) at a workshop were asked to write short-term goals for a moderately language-impaired patient. More than half wrote goals such as "By the end of this session, X will say the name of five common objects."

Behavioral, operationally written objectives, however, are counterproductive to the development of language. They are unacceptable within both a cognitive model and a pragmatic model of intervention. Behavioral objectives target surface structures. Cognitive and pragmatic intervention focus on meaning or deep structure. In cognitive-pragmatic intervention, we attempt to increase the patient's viability as a communicative partner (Lubinski, 1986).

Behavioral, operationally written objectives are inappropriate, because they ignore the fact that meaning is the essence of language and that meaning is not an observable behavior. They ignore the fact that a conversation is like a game. It involves a series of moves by participants. Every conversation is altogether new for the participants. Therefore, we continually communicate creativity (Lindfors, 1980). (Lindfors' text concerns language intervention in children.)

Behavioral, operationally written objectives ignore the fact that content and form are developed and used within the context of a speech act. The individual develops communicative competence "through discerning rules underlying the diverse interaction contexts which she observes and in which she participates" (Lindfors, 1980, p. 311).

Behavioral, operationally written objectives ignore the fact that the speaker's intent in producing an utterance and a hearer's intent in hearing an utterance are the essence of communication and meaning. The intent of the message is the reason we communicate. The intent is the function that language serves. We use verbal utterances to express an intention or function. We use language to question, request, and inform. Our attention as speakers and listeners is on the meaning, the intention of what someone is trying to say (Cazden, 1976). Language forms are heard through the meaning that is intended (Cazden, 1976). Thus, communication is idea oriented, not word oriented. Language is rooted in meaning, not in surface structures. Language is used for communication. It is a tool, not an end in itself. Language is an aid to communication.

Clinical aphasiologists may wish to encourage regulating agencies to realize that language is facilitated by an environment that focuses on meaning rather than on form. Getting the message across is more important for individuals than the form they use to do so.

These agencies should realize that "language is not labeling or matching pictures to words or repeating what someone else said" (Holland, 1975, p. 518). (Holland's article concerns language intervention in children.) Instead, language is "an active, dynamic interpersonal interchange" (Holland, 1975, p. 518). If we focus on tasks like labeling, matching pictures to words, or repeating what someone else said, then "we run the risk of inadvertently teaching the

erroneous principle that language is a skill on the order of playing the piano. This helps the [individual] . . . miss the point of communicating" (Holland, 1975, p. 518). In fact:

Language training must be to some very significant extent concerned with helping [the individual] . . . discover his potential as a verbal communicator. Without this discovery, language will remain something akin to a well practiced talent, a recital, not a . . . part of him. (Holland, 1975, p. 519)

Verbalizations must not replace language. Drill is not language. According to Lindfors (1987), "there is no language apart from meaning" (p. 217). Language "is communicating—the back and forth, the give and take of ideas, not . . . the mindless parroting of rigid, fixed forms" (Lindfors, 1980, p. 218). Where in a language drill is the meaning that we know to be the very base of language (Lindfors, 1980)? Where is the creativity, the novel expression, that is the core of language? Where is the communicating—the interacting with someone, about something, for some reason (Lindfors, 1987)?

Drill is opposed to language in its meaninglessness, in its rigidity, and in its purposelessness (Lindfors, 1987). Drill may make clients very good at doing drills, but not at using language and communication. Indeed, according to Lindfors, drill may adversely affect language growth and retrieval. She maintains that problem solving, planning, discussing ideas, brainstorming, recording ideas, presenting ideas, and selecting the best ideas involve listening, speaking, reading, and writing with a purpose. The real question is, then, is the individual a more effective user of language after completing an exercise or drill? The answer is no. We become more effective communicators as a result of using language in communication with others. According to Lindfors (1980):

labeling syntactic (or semantic) items simply makes you a better "syntactic item labeler" (at least for a few days). Talking about forms doesn't help you express meaning more effectively. (p. 220)

Lindfors apparently believes that it is inappropriate to structure a simple-to-complex sequence of forms. Rather, the communication itself will determine the language forms that the individual uses and responds to. She believes that we need to focus on language use for effective communication. When we do so, our clients may then use the language forms that help them to accomplish effective communication.

Individuals, Lindfors (1987) claims, become effective interactants as they have more opportunities to interact. Language intervention should reflect the individual's interests, goals, activities, concerns, and life participation. Natural shaping of semantics and syntax happens not through sequenced curriculum but, rather, through feedback as to whether one has been understood and whether one has achieved the purpose of the communication.

New meanings find expression as individuals wonder, question, inform, argue, and reason through language in real-life situations rather than in contrived situations (Lindfors, 1987). Language lives in shared experience, in decision making, and in planning. Language is stimulated and facilitated by an environment that is rich in diverse verbal and nonverbal experiences. Language lives and grows in rich experiences.

As human beings, we develop a theory of the world in our head (Smith, 1975). Our theory shapes how we look at past experience (recall and interpret it) and how we look at new experience. We comprehend or interpret the world by relating new experience to the already known—that is, by placing new experiences in our existing cognitive structure or "theory" (Smith, 1975). To learn is to alter our existing cognitive structure when experience does not conform to our theory (Lindfors, 1987).

Language helps us to comprehend and learn—especially as language is used in questioning (curiosity and procedural or social-interactional questioning), focusing attention, making understandings more precise, making understandings more retrievable, reinterpreting past experience, and going beyond present personal experiences (Lindfors, 1987). Interaction is essential to both comprehension and learning. In real gut-level, meaningful learning, what is to be learned cannot be specified in advance. Such learning is characterized by curiosity, exploration, problem solving, planning, decision making, discussion of ideas, brainstorming, and evaluative thinking (Chapey, 1988, 1992; Guilford, 1967; Lindfors, 1980, 1987).

The present pressure to establish accountability has actively discouraged exploration, curiosity, and problem solving. Skills, drills, rules, and facts have become ends in themselves (Lindfors, 1987). We have packaged clinical programs with a renewed emphasis on memorizing words, defining words, and identifying parts of speech in sentences that no one ever said or ever will say, and all so that individuals can get higher standardized test scores and move on to the next-higher level of memorization, definition, and identification (Lindfors, 1987).

As a profession, we are first and foremost concerned that our clients become competent communicators (Frattali, 1992). Emphasis on learning rote skills and specified sets of behaviors means increased emphasis on the use of lower-level cognitive processes (Lindfors, 1987). Lower-level cognitive behavior means that clients can give back the same information they received (recalling, memorization), but to display higher-level cognitive behavior, they must go beyond the given information in some way—for example, relating it to something else, reorganizing it, inferring from it, and using it as a springboard for creatively solving new problems. It involves applying, analyzing, synthesizing, and evaluating. Questioning is the individual's most important tool for learning—especially curiosity questioning (Lindfors, 1987). Conversation should be the locus, process, and goal of language intervention (Warren & Rogers-Warren, 1985).

Content-centered discussion therapy and embellishment of ideas within a topic (Wepman, 1972, 1976) should be our focus.

OBJECTIVES OF THERAPY

The objective of a cognitive approach to rehabilitation is to stimulate the five cognitive processes—cognition (awareness/attention, immediate discovery, recognition, comprehension), memory, convergent thinking, divergent thinking, and evaluative thinking—to improve overall functional communication. Whenever possible, the focus should be on the stimulation of these abilities within the context of conversational discourse. That is, conventional discourse is seen as the procedural plan for intervention. Whenever possible, turn taking, cueing, modeling, and reinforcement are essential components of therapy.

General Objectives

The general objectives are:

1. To stimulate ability to recognize and comprehend language.
2. To stimulate ability to fix new information in memory to improve communication.
3. To stimulate ability to generate logical information or conclusions during communication.
4. To stimulate ability to generate logical alternatives to given information, produce a quantity and variety of responses during communication, and elaborate on ideas and plans during communication.
5. To stimulate ability to make judgments or appraisals or to formulate evaluations in terms of criteria such as correctness, completeness, identity, relevance, adequacy, utility, safety, consistency, feasibility, social custom, and so forth to communicate more effectively and efficiently.
6. To stimulate the integration of all cognitive operations through the use of problem-solving, decision-making, and planning tasks and through conversational discourse to communicate more effectively and efficiently.

This approach contains four levels of specific objectives. This model of therapy, however, suggests that, regardless of the level at which the patient is functioning, the initial stage of intervention should focus on language-related cognition: knowing, awareness, immediate discovery, recognition, comprehension, and understanding. This suggestion is based on the rationale that individuals with aphasia should be provided, over and over again, with opportunities to hear and grasp the language behavior of others. That is, auditory stimulation is seen as an essential component of language retrieval in patients with aphasia (Schuell et al., 1955). Thus, for example, the clinician might videotape a group of normal adults responding to a divergent task, such as "Can you think of a problem that anyone might have in eating lunch?" Concomitantly, the patient could be reinforced for all listening and attending behavior. Specifically, movements of the eye that result in a better visual stimulus for the patient or of the ear that result in a better auditory stimulus (Staats, 1968) of the videotape would be reinforced. Although no verbal responses would be required during this phase of therapy, all verbal responses that relate to the task at hand could be highly reinforced.

Exposure to the videotaped responses of others may prove to be a vicarious learning experience (Bandura & Walters, 1963; Harris & Evans, 1974) for the individual with aphasia. This suggestion appears to be in consonance with the finding by Cooper and Rigrodsky (1979) that persons with aphasia are able to model the verbal behavior of normal subjects and improve their explanations of the material presented. If modeling is to occur, however, it may be helpful to consider several facts. First, it may be beneficial if the subjects on the videotape are of comparable age and sex as the individual with aphasia; this way, the patient will identify with the person who is producing the divergent responses. Second, the clinician could attempt to choose tasks that are interesting and relevant to the particular subject. Third, considering that Pieres and Morgan (1973) empirically determined that a relaxed, receptive, and uncritical environment increased the divergent behavior of normal subjects, it may be important to provide this type of climate for persons with aphasia. This exposure to the divergent semantic behavior of others, perhaps filed in competitive "game show" style (Torrance, 1974), can continue to be a component of the intervention strategy throughout the process of therapy.

Principles

Intervention should be oriented toward the following traditional therapeutic principles:

1. Begin with the tangible (here and now), and move toward the representational.
2. Begin with the concrete, and move toward the abstract.
3. Begin with the simple, and move toward the complex.
4. Begin with the real, and move toward the complex.
5. Begin with actions on objects, and move toward verbalizations concerning these actions.
6. Begin with simple classifications, and move toward reclassifications and multiple classifications.
7. Begin with exaggerated sensory stimulation—for example, talking through a microphone or using a variety of inflectional patterns (McConnell, Love, & Smith, 1974)—and then gradually decrease this exaggeration.
8. Begin with short stimuli/responses, and move toward longer stimuli/responses.
9. Begin with continuous reinforcement, and move toward intermittent reinforcement (Grant, Hake, & Hornseth, 1951; Jensen & Cotton, 1960).
10. Begin with clinician reinforcement, and move toward self-reinforcement (Staats, 1968).

During the course of both diagnosis and therapy, the aphasiologist will attempt to isolate specific conditions under which language retrieval is maximized and to increase the number and variety of these conditions. That is, with whom and under what conditions does language behavior increase? The clinician may wish to manipulate some of the following variables and observe their effect on patient behavior: listener, referent, intent, situation, cueing devices, repetition and reauditorization, intonation, level of abstraction, cognitive complexity, linguistic complexity, length of stimuli, and frequency of occurrence of word stimuli. The conditions that augment semantic retrieval for each cognitive operation should become an integral component of all subsequent sessions. Examples of specific objectives at each of the four levels of therapy are presented below.

Level I: Specific Objectives

To stimulate ability

Cognition

To be aware of time/space/speech/emotional voice tone
To recognize stimulus equivalence, such as matching letters, matching objects to objects, matching objects to pictures, matching words to pictures, and matching words to objects
To recognize very high-frequency, concrete objects/events/relationships named
To recognize own name/family names
To follow one-part, simple commands
To understand simple greetings/requests/questions

Memory

To remember one to two letters/words/pictures
To remember one to two high-frequency, concrete objects/events named

Convergent Thinking

To repeat one-syllable, high-frequency objects/events/relationships
To produce automatic language
To complete high-probability closure tasks

Level II: Specific Objectives

To stimulate ability

Cognition

To recognize concrete, high-frequency, familiar objects/events/relationships

To recognize family names/body parts/community helper occupations

To recognize high-frequency objects given their function

To recognize high-frequency events described

To recognize concrete, brief ideas

To comprehend simple conversation with one person

To understand concrete, high-frequency statements about objects, such as existence, nonexistence, recurrence, rejection, denial, possession, food, clothing, and personal care objects

To understand concrete, high-frequency, brief statements about events, such as playing, eating, and activities of daily living

To comprehend concrete agent-action and action-object constructions

To comprehend concrete yes/no questions

To comprehend concrete active and negative phrases/sentences

To comprehend articles

To comprehend morphologic inflections, such as plural /s/, /z/, possessive /s/, /z/, and past /t/, /ed/

To comprehend concrete noun phrases and verb phrases

To recognize forms/letters/pictures

To recognize high-frequency printed words and pictures

To match high-frequency printed words to spoken words

To recognize printed letters

Memory

To remember one to three concrete, high-frequency objects/events/relationships, serially

To execute one- to two-step commands, serially

To remember one to four pictures, serially

To group items to facilitate ability to recall

Convergent Thinking

To produce automatic language

To complete high-probability phrases/closure tasks

To name high-frequency objects/events/relationships

To comment on objects noting their existence, nonexistence, recurrence, location, possession, and so forth

To talk about common objects, such as food, clothing, furniture, and transportation

To comment on events, such as cooking, eating, and activities of daily living

To produce agent-action and action-object constructions

To produce concrete speech acts, such as requesting, informing, greeting, and questioning

To name members of categories

To list many words that start with a specific letter

To generate numerous and varied objects within a class

To list numerous possible topics of conversation

Level III: Specific Objectives

To stimulate ability

Cognition

To recognize high- and low-frequency objects/events/relationships

To recognize high- and low-frequency objects/events/relationships described by function

To recognize letter/color/form/number names and rhyme words

To recognize phonetically similar words

To recognize categories

To comprehend concrete ideas/sentences

To understand relationships between words

To understand statements about objects, such as existence, nonexistence, recurrence, rejection, denial, possession, attribution, food, furniture, clothes, personal care objects, health, kitchen utensils, and family/other people/places/locations

To understand statements about events, such as play, entertainment, eating, activities of daily living, cooking, feelings, sports, school, work, travel, time, and news

To understand concrete speech acts, such as requesting, ordering, advising, warning, questioning, describing, greeting, repeating, and protesting

To hold the thread of discussion in mind, identifying main ideas

To distinguish between relevant and irrelevant information

To understand television/movies

To comprehend inferences

To comprehend short paragraphs

To recognize the existence of problems

To recognize own errors and errors of others

To comprehend simple, concrete analogies

To comprehend active and negative sentences

To comprehend pronouns, such as personal, reflexive, indefinite, demonstrative, interrogative, and negative

To comprehend adjectives, such as color, size, shape, length, height, width, age, taste, temperature, speed, distance, comparative, and superlative

To comprehend adverbs with "-ly"

To comprehend conjunctions

To comprehend prepositions, such as locative, temporal, and directional

To read concrete, high-frequency and low-frequency sentences

To read and comprehend sequences of material

To read and comprehend short paragraphs

To read and identify main ideas

To read and obtain facts
To read and locate answers
To read and draw conclusions
To read and grasp relationships
To read and grasp inferences
To read street signs
To read newspaper headlines/newspaper stories/newspaper ads

Memory

To identify one to five names serially
To follow one- to five-part directions and commands
To remember one to five ideas/facts just presented
To group items to facilitate recall
To remember meaning in sentences/short paragraphs/stories/songs

Convergent Thinking

To answer questions about self/family/everyday life
To name high- and low-frequency objects/events/relationships
To name categories
To name objects/events/relationships within categories
To describe objects/events/relationships
To tell the function of objects and the purpose of events
To define words
To judge the suitability of class inclusion
To judge the similarity of relationships
To judge the suitability of class properties
To identify absurdities
To evaluate implications
To express simple ideas with specificity
To sequentially order ideas or topics toward a purpose
To retell stories—both the literal (who, when, what, and where) details and the inferential implications
To describe procedures
To state the relationship between objects/events, such as similarities/differences
To predict possible outcomes
To make inferences and draw conclusions
To answer true/false, yes/no, and "wh-" questions
To write letters and numbers
To write own name and address
To write sentences with high-frequency, concrete words

Divergent Thinking

To produce numerous logical possibilities/perspectives/ideas where appropriate
To provide a variety of ideas where appropriate
To change the direction of one's responses
To generate categories of objects/events/relationships/ideas
To predict many different possible outcomes of situations

To generate many different solutions to problems
To list many different problems inherent in situations
To generate numerous steps in a plan
To elaborate on a topic

Evaluative Thinking

To judge the correctness, completeness, identity, relevance, adequacy, utility, safety, consistency, logical feasibility, and social acceptability of facts
To judge the suitability of words to a topic

Level IV: Specific Objectives

To stimulate ability

Cognition

To comprehend high- and low-frequency objects/events/relationships
To recognize concrete and more abstract classes/concepts
To understand relationships among objects/events/ideas
To comprehend analogies
To recognize problems
To recognize own errors and errors of others
To comprehend concrete and more abstract speech acts in conversation with one to five partners
To follow changes in the topic of conversation
To hold the thread of discussion in mind and identify main ideas
To understand changes in interpretation
To comprehend TV/movies
To comprehend more rapid, complex conversations
To comprehend longer sentences/directions/commands
To comprehend more complex/abstract relationships, such as comparative, possessive, spatial, temporal, inferential, familial, part-whole, object-action, action-object, cause-effect, sequential, degree, and antonym and synonym relationships
To comprehend negative, passive, and question transformations
To read both short and concrete as well as longer and more abstract sentences/paragraphs
To read and identify main ideas
To read and obtain facts
To read and locate answers
To read and draw conclusions
To read and grasp relationships
To read and draw inferences
To comprehend newspaper stories/ads
To comprehend catalog/mail-order forms
To comprehend a menu
To comprehend a table of contents/index
To use a dictionary/telephone directory

Memory

To remember one to nine high- and low-frequency objects/events/relationships/categories

To remember facts and commands of increasing length and complexity

To remember meaning in sentences and paragraphs

To use hierarchical organization to facilitate recall

To cluster information to facilitate recall

Convergent Thinking

To describe high- and low-frequency objects/events/relationships

To indicate the function of high- and low-frequency objects/events/relationships

To specify attributes of objects

To specify the defining attributes of concepts

To define words

To express ideas clearly and with variety

To use language to communicate specific ideas

To use language to elicit specific responses

To express relationships between and among objects/events/relationships and ideas, such as similarities and differences

To produce analogies

To sequentially order ideas toward a purpose

To use language to request, inform, explain, question, greet, advise, thank, order, and negotiate

To keep meaning going in conversation

To produce class names for groups of words/pictures

To logically deduce the most predictable outcome of a set of facts

To tell the literal (who, what, when, and where) details of a story

To make inferences and draw conclusions

To write high- and low-frequency words, sentences, and paragraphs

Divergent Thinking

To produce numerous logical possibilities and perspectives where appropriate

To provide a variety of ideas where appropriate

To change the direction of one's responses

To stimulate ability to generate many different uses for common and uncommon objects

To predict many possible outcomes of a situation

To list many different problems inherent in a common situation

To think of many different ways to initiate a conversation

To think of many different ways to maintain a conversation

To define many possible rules for communicative partners and communicative contexts

To think of many different ways to repair conversation

To elaborate on topics

To elaborate on or list many different steps needed to do a particular task

Evaluative Thinking

To make appraisals, comparisons, and formulate evaluations regarding correctness, completeness, relevance, adequacy, utility, safety, consistency, logical feasibility, and social acceptability

To judge the intent of messages

To judge the coherence of a conversation

To judge what can and cannot be said in different contexts and to different partners

To use context and partner variables to decipher between what is said and what is meant

To determine the meaning of proverbs

To judge a situation in which a proverb could be used

To select the word that best fits a single criterion

To select the best of given reasons why a briefly described plan is faulty

Integration of the Five Cognitive Processes

Within the present therapeutic approach, all five mental operations are integrated in therapy by requiring responses that involve composite abilities. Problem solving, planning, decision-making tasks, and conversational interaction are excellent for this purpose, because they are composite operations or processes depending on the content of the problem, decision, or conversation and on how the problem/decision/conversation is worded or phrased. Thus, whereas conversational interaction, such as the use of speech acts, sometimes is convergent in nature, it also often will involve the use of other mental operations and become problem solving, planning, and decision making in nature, depending on the listener, the context, and the intent. Individuals can be stimulated to use language to question, request, inform, wonder, argue, reason, and comprehend such speech acts.

In addition, formulating solutions to problems posed in the "Dear Abby" or "Dear Meg" column of the local newspaper can be used to stimulate all five cognitive operations. If carefully chosen, such tasks reflect "real-life" situations that patients face—or can allow patients to increase their self-concept, because their opinion is being sought and valued. The use of such tasks is conversational in nature and, frequently, allows reciprocal role reversal. These tasks therefore can be used to stimulate brainstorming, discussing, recording and presenting ideas, and selecting best outcomes. They also can be used to stimulate individuals to question (curiosity, procedural, and social-interactional), focus attention, make understanding more precise, reinterpret past experience, and go beyond present personal experience. In addition, conversational management, conversational turn taking, topic manipulation, and conversational repair management can be targeted using these tasks.

Thus, whenever possible, intervention should involve the stimulation of two or three (or more) mental operations. For example, the clinician might begin a session by asking the client, "Can you list all of the things that can be folded?" After the patient has produced some responses, the clinician summarizes these responses and asks, "Can you think of any more?" (Table 17-2). When the client has finished responding, the clinician then uses convergent techniques, such as those described by Aurelia (1974); Butfield and Zangwill (1946); Goldstein (1948); Keenan (1975); Sarno, Silverman, and Sands (1970); Schuell and colleagues (1955); Vignolo (1964); and Wepman (1953), to stimulate retrieval of appropriate and desired responses that the patient had not produced. Such techniques might involve confrontation naming, recognition naming, oral spelling, reading, categorizing similar responses, creating sentences with a word, and so forth (Table 17-2). In an attempt to develop each patient's ability to correct his or her own errors, the clinician may use cueing techniques, such as those suggested by Berman and Peelle (1967). For example, the initial letter of a word could be used as a cue technique. Alternative stimuli for self-cueing might include (a) the first phoneme of a word, (b) the association of a word with a gesture, or (c) the use of an incorrect associational response to cue the correct verbal response. Subsequently, the aphasiologist attempts to transfer the semantic material retrieved in the convergent context and integrate this information into a divergent one. For example, the clinician might ask another divergent question that would call for some of the responses that the patient has been able to retrieve, such as "Can you think of all of the things that we could pull over our heads?" (Table 17-2). Progress is evaluated by keeping a record of the number and variety of responses produced by the patient (Table 17-2).

Spontaneous language tasks that have divergent, convergent, and/or evaluative components also are used in therapy. For example, the clinician might present a picture description task, such as the cookie theft picture from the Boston Diagnostic Aphasia Examination (Goodglass & Kaplan, 1972), and encourage the client to produce as many responses as possible (see Yorkston & Beukelman, 1977). Clients also can be encouraged to produce functional spontaneous communication related to a specific theme (Wepman, 1976), such as food, nutrition, food service, restaurants, great parks, interesting sights, vacation destinations, health and diet, sexual issues, social security, legal and money issues, current events, and pharmaceutical issues (the American Association of Retired Persons' magazine, *Modern Maturity*, provides interesting and timely topics for the audience age 50 years or older). In each instance, the clinician records the number and variety of ideas produced by the client.

Levels III and IV: Specific Objectives to Stimulate Use of Composite Abilities

- To stimulate ability
- To use language to explain, request, correct information, report, advise, question, greet, thank, argue, and negotiate
- To comprehend speech acts produced by another
- To overcome obstacles in communication
- To keep meaning going in conversation
- To role play (especially to take the viewpoint of someone else) during communication
- To select, introduce, maintain, and change the topic of conversation
- To initiate and maintain conversation
- To use language to discuss objects, events, and relationships
- To use language to communicate specific ideas
- To use language to elicit specific responses
- To use language to verbalize a variety of possibilities and perspectives, such as the pros and cons of ideas and issues, the advantages and disadvantages of certain actions, and ideas
- To vary language depending on the context
- To vary language depending on the partner
- To comprehend various speech acts and intents in relationship to various partners and contexts
- To produce stylistic variations to meet situational requirements
- To overcome obstacles in communication
- To repair and revise communication
- To use cues as a signal to repeat or modify messages
- To provide feedback to the speaker, as listener, such as requesting message clarification/repetition/restatement, requesting that the message slow down, requesting the message in alternate form, and indicating agreement/disagreement with message
- To define the problems and solutions inherent in certain objects, events, and relationships
- To use a telephone
- To use a telephone directory, a dictionary, and a television schedule item
- To use street and store signs and maps

THERAPY TASKS AND MATERIALS

Guilford and Hoepfner (1971) developed a number of tasks for each of the five mental operations. Some of these tests have been listed previously under "Assessment." All of these tasks can be readily used to stimulate specific mental (cognitive) operations during therapy. Most traditional workbooks in the field of aphasia have presented tasks that stimulate cognition (recognition/comprehension) and convergent thinking. Within the last few years, however, a number of workbooks have been published that focus on the stimulation of divergent thinking, evaluative thinking, problem solving, and decision making.

TABLE 17–2

Sample Therapeutic Plan That Includes Both Divergent and Convergent Tasks

Objective	Tasks[a]	Cue	Evaluation
General—to stimulate the communication of ideas	Greeting *Divergent Tasks*		
Specific—to stimulate language related to a holiday, Christmas, through divergent and convergent thinking	1. We're coming close to Christmas. What are all of the things that you think of when you think of Christmas?	After 2 minutes, summarize responses given and ask, "Can you think of any more?"	1. (a) List responses _____ _____ Total fluency _____ (b) List categories _____ _____ Total flexibility _____
	2. Someone mentioned that Santa carries a sack. Can you think of all of the things that could fit into Santa's sack?	Same as above	2. Score as in question 1.

	3. What are all of the things we might get for Christmas that:
	    Could be folded?
	    Couldn't be folded?
	    Might break if they were dropped?
	    Wouldn't break if they were dropped?
	    We could wash?
	    Could be hauled in a truck?
	    We could pull over our head?
	    Might have buttons?
	    Could be worn in summer (winter)?
	    Could be made of paper?
	    Could come in a box?
	    Could be round (square)?
	    Are made of glass (plastic, rubber)?
	    Someone could drink?
	    Someone could eat?
	    Has handles?
	    Has a neck?
	    Moves?
		Same as above	3. Score as in question. 1.

	4. List all of the things that you could possibly use a Christmas box for (or bells, string, ribbon).	Same as above	4. Score as in question 1.
	5. How could you improve ___ so that it would be more useful (better, more fun)?	Same as above	5. Score as in question 1.
	6. If Santa didn't have a sack, he could use ___. If Santa lost his belt, he could use ___.	Same as above	6. Score as in question 1.

(continued)

TABLE 17–2

Sample Therapeutic Plan That Includes Both Divergent and Convergent Tasks (continued)

Objective	Tasks[a]	Cue	Evaluation
	7. Imagine you are in a department store (church, living room) at Christmas time. What are all of the things that you might possibly see?	Same as above	7. Score as in question 1.
	8. Let's make up a story about Christmas.	Same as above	8. Score as in question 1.
	9. The word *Christmas* begins with the sound "k." What other words can you think of that start with "k"? The word *bell* begins with the sound "b." What other words can you think of that start with "b"?	Same as above	9. Score as in question 1.
	10. What are all of the possible questions that you could ask about this Christmas picture?	Same as above	10. Score as in question 1.
	11. List all of the different parts of Santa's suit. How could we change each one to make it better?	Same as above	11. Score as in question 1.
	12. Suppose that we did not celebrate Christmas anymore. What do you think might happen? Can you guess?	Same as above	12. Score as in question 1.
	13. List all of the problems that someone might have in shopping for a Christmas present.	Same as above	13. Score as in question 1.
	14. Someone mentioned a cymbal and a drum. They make noise. Can you list all of the things that could be used to make noise?	Same as above	14. Score as in question 1.
	15. Santa's suit is red. What are all of the other things that could be red?	Same as above	15. Score as in question 1.
	16. Tomorrow we will have a Christmas party. What are all the different things we'll need to do before the party?	Same as above	16. Score as in question 1.
	Convergent Tasks Present responses given to question 1. Oral and/or visual representation of responses can be used. (Later, responses to question 2, then question 3, and so on, can be presented.)		
	Responses that might be appropriate to this question but that were not given by the patient are now presented.	Give first sound of a word	Use Porch's (1971) multidimensional scoring system to evaluate responses

TABLE 17–2

Sample Therapeutic Plan That Includes Both Divergent and Convergent Tasks (continued)

Objective	Tasks[a]	Cue	Evaluation
	Convergent techniques that might be used to stimulate retrieval of items not produced are: a) Confrontation naming b) Definition naming c) Closure naming d) Recognition naming e) Repetition naming f) Following oral and/or printed directions or commands g) Yes/no comprehension h) Word associations: antonyms, synonyms i) Rhyming j) Description k) Recognition spelling l) Oral spelling m) Analogies n) Recognition of categories o) Spontaneous generation of categories p) Concept learning q) Reading r) Writing s) Copying t) Creating sentences with words u) Creating sentences telling the function of an object v) Memory tasks w) Read a story, and ask questions x) Read a story, and retell a story y) Role play	Give first letter of a word Give semantic association	

[a]Turn taking, cueing, modeling, and reinforcement are essential components of therapy.

RELATIONSHIP OF COGNITIVE INTERVENTION TO WEPMAN THOUGHT PROCESS THERAPY

Wepman (1972) notes that the aphasic patient frequently substitutes a word that is associated with the word that he or she is attempting to produce, and that the remainder of the individual's communicative effort often relates to the approximated, rather than to the intended, word. In addition, the inaccurate verbal formulation of the person with aphasia may feed back an altered message to the thought process and, thereby, change the thought process so that it is in consonance with the utterance. For example, if the patient is trying to say "circle" and, instead, utters "square," his or concept of circle may change so that it agrees with the utterance, and the patient will begin to think of a circle as a square. Wepman suggested that aphasia may be a thought process disorder in which impairment of semantic expression is the result of an impairment of thought processes that "serve as the catalyst for verbal expression" (p. 207).

Individuals who cannot retrieve the most appropriate lexical symbol for a context are impaired in their ability to communicate a number and variety of specific propositional ideas. When the remainder of the person with aphasia's communication relates to the approximated rather than to the intended word, spontaneous language will be even more impaired, because in this instance, the patient becomes incapable of using the learned code to communicate his or her true feelings and thoughts.

For Wepman (1972, 1976), the first stage of therapy is content-centered, discussion therapy, in which the patient is stimulated to remain on a topic. Similarly, cognitive therapy is content centered and idea oriented; the individual is encouraged to generate functional communication and produce a variety of ideas related to topics.

During Wepman's (1972, 1976) second stage of therapy, individuals are encouraged to elaborate on various topics. The ability to elaborate on a topic is a divergent ability. Thus, Wepman's thought process therapy involves stimulating convergent, divergent, and evaluative thinking as well as recognition/comprehension and memory.

RELATIONSHIP OF COGNITIVE INTERVENTION TO RESPONSE ELABORATION TRAINING

Response elaboration training (RET) is a program developed by Kearns (1985, 1990; see also Gaddie, Kearns, & Yedor, 1991; Kearns & Potechin, 1988; Kearns & Yedor, 1991) to increase the length and information content of verbal responses of patients with nonfluent aphasia. RET is a "loose training" program that attempts to loosen control over stimuli and response during therapy by using client-initiated responses as the primary content of therapy. The emphasis is on shaping and chaining client-initiated responses. Patients are encouraged to elaborate (think divergently) on "whatever they are reminded of" when they are responding to picture stimuli of everyday activities and sports. Naming and describing are discouraged. Informational content rather than linguistic form is reinforced.

Specifically, according to Kearns (1990),

The basic RET sequence entails (1) eliciting spontaneous responses to minimally contextual picture stimuli, (2) modeling and reinforcing initial responses, (3) providing "wh-" cues to prompt clients to elaborate on their initial responses, (4) reinforcing attempted elaborations and then modeling sentences that combine initial and all subsequent responses to a given stimulus picture, (5) providing a second model of sentences that combine previous responses and then requesting a repetition of the sentence, (6) reinforcing repetitions of combined sentences and providing a final model of the sentence. Throughout this sequence clients' responses are not directly corrected by the clinician. Instead, naturalistic feedback is provided during the structured interactions through conversational modeling.

Progress during RET is measured by counting the number of content words per stimulus picture (fluency) and the variety of responses to the same stimulus picture (flexibility). Novel and varied responses are encouraged. Thus, RET stimulates fluency, flexibility, originality, and elaboration—or divergent semantic thinking as well as functional spontaneous speech, which necessitates all five mental operations.

Kearns' (1990) data demonstrate that RET procedures facilitate an increase in the amount of information (i.e., number of content words) generated by individuals with aphasia. Further, a moderate degree of generalization across stimuli, people, and settings was reported.

RELATIONSHIP OF COGNITIVE INTERVENTION TO LIFE PARTICIPATION APPROACH TO APHASIA

Communication creates and is created by life participation. Therefore, the Life Participation Approach to Aphasia (LPAA) model directs our choice of goals, priorities, activities, and strategies used in intervention to the purpose, direction, meaning, comfort, pleasure, needs, and life participation decisions and problems of each individual affected by aphasia. Such life participation necessitates the use of effective and efficient problem-solving and decision-making skills (Tables 17-3 and 17-4). In addition, various life-span theorists emphasize the importance of social integration and participation for the physical and emotional health and well-being of all individuals. Indeed, such participation in mundane yet meaningful, valued activities of everyday life provided the structure and meaning for living life (Duchan, 1999).

Case Study

P is a 67-year-old, mild to moderately impaired man with aphasia, 3 months poststroke, with a left cerebrovascular accident and right hemiplegia who lives with his wife, T. Before the stroke, both were active in the local church, but they had not returned since P's stroke. Both reported feeling isolated and cut off from life and wanted to go to an upcoming church-sponsored event—a trip to Atlantic City (famous for its gambling casinos, reasonable meals, beaches, and shopping). Both had reservations about how practical and advisable their involvement might be and about the reaction they might receive from others.

Goals

Life-enhanced participation governed management from day 1 (Tables 17-1 and 17-2). The main goal was to restore purpose, direction, meaning, comfort, and pleasure in the daily lives of P and T by facilitating their access to communication partners and events of their choice and to train caregivers, family, friends, and neighbors to communicate more effectively with both individuals. Therefore, the initial goals were:

- To determine the extent to which P and T and persons associated with them could partake in and achieve life participation goals
- To determine the extent to which P and T and persons associated with them were being hindered in the attainment of such goals

TABLE 17–3

Pre- and Post-Therapy Questionnaire for Life Participation/Communication: For the Person with Aphasia and Significant Others; Both Observational and Self-Reported—With and Without Support

Identity
Autonomy of life participation
  In social context
  In family
  In medical context
Degree of life participation
  In life events
  With other people
Relationships
  Value as participant
  Role
Count of number of people seen
  Of places
  Of activities
Environmental barriers (and changes)
Changes in social connection
Communication function (Simmons, 1993)
  Interactional (sharing ideas, thoughts, and opinions)
    Verbal, gestural, cued
  Transactional (transfer of information)
    Verbal, gestural, cued
Ability to communicate independently
Personal competence revealed
Impairment (and changes in)
Ability to cope with impairment
Degree of comfort
  Function
  Involvement
  Pleasure
  Success
  Quality of daily life
Feelings of self-esteem
Feeling of being in control of one's life
Level of flow in one's life
Analysis of specific life events (Duchan, 1999)
  Participants: Who is participating?
  Goal: Why are they participating?
  Type of interaction: What is the type of social interaction required?
  Part of activity: What part of the activity are they engaged in?
  Attitudes: What are the attitudes of the participants:
    Toward activity?
Toward their partners?
Toward goals?
Expectations (e.g., for social connection; general improvement in sense of well-being)
Perception of (and changes in perception)
Health-care worker
Family
Significant others

- To identify and increase personal and environmental factors facilitating harmony, comfort, purpose, and participation in life
- To identify and decrease personal and environmental obstacles disrupting harmony, comfort, purpose, and life participation
- To identify and facilitate attainment of the needs and goals of all individuals in the environment
- To increase/maximize P's ability to initiate and direct conversation/discussions, convey a number and variety of ideas across (with or without prompts, props, and cues), convey a message using whatever strategy might be useful (e.g., to encourage use of graphic and drawing representations, natural gesture, pictures, travel brochures, menus, and books), and practice conversational skills within the context of conversational exchanges
- To focus on conversation as a collaborative achievement, to provide communication/conversational support, and when appropriate and necessary, to train partners/communities in these techniques to use volunteers as conversational partners
- To provide and demonstrate a problem-solving, decision-making approach model for P and T and to encourage them to structure theme-oriented, problem-solving, decision-making, conversationally based interactions using the five mental operations.

Goals were constantly assessed, weighed, and prioritized to determine which personal and environmental factors should be targets of intervention and how best to provide freer, easier, and more autonomous access to activities and social connections. Every attempt was made to have consumer-based/self-generated rather than clinician-generated goals and activities and to provide autonomous choice whenever possible.

Methods

The upcoming trip to Atlantic City appeared to be an attractive initial target of intervention, both because it meant so much to P and T and because it focused on doing things that result in communication as participation rather than on communication itself. Therefore, intervention focused on developing strategies and skills to increase the possibility of success directly related to reengagement/participation in the upcoming event. Most therapeutic tasks were problem-solving, decision-making, role-playing tasks focused on the five mental operations. When appropriate, however, therapy also made use of Wepman's (1972, 1976) content-centered discussion therapy (see above), conversational prompting (Cochrane & Milton, 1984), conversational coaching (Holland, 1991), training of conversation partners (Kagan & Gailey, 1993), RET (Kearns, 1985) (see above as well as Chapters 1, and 14), PACE (Promoting Aphasic Communicative Effectiveness) therapeutic techniques (Davis &

TABLE 17–4

Reengagement, Enhancement/Inclusion Strategies to Facilitate Meaningful, Functional, Optimal Access to Participation in Life, Well-Being, Wellness, and Quality of Life: A Plan for Action

Goals	Outcomes
Foster optimal meaningful, purposeful life participation, autonomy, and choice of lifestyle and activities	Increased meaningful ties to others
Facilitate optimal inclusion in and meaningful, purposeful connection to social and community activities/life	
Encourage strong social connections with people who matter, such as spouse, caregiver, family, and close friends	
Facilitate the restoration of function, purpose, direction, pleasure, comfort, and sense of well-being in daily life	Mastery of environment
Encourage optimal mastery of daily life events	
Encourage and facilitate support from significant others to optimize meaningful, purposeful life participation	Purpose/direction
Encourage and facilitate support for significant others to optimize meaningful, purposeful life participation	Self-acceptance
Recognize and remove environmental, structural, attitudinal, and informational barriers that limit or prevent participation in normal social and community life	Harmony/well-being
Increase community resources that support life participation	Wellness
Work to build protected communities where individuals are valued participants	Quality of life
Enhance psychological adjustment, promote health and wellness, and foster a healthy sense of identity through life participation	Communication effectiveness
Reflect the fact that adaptation to the changes brought about by stroke is a complex, dynamic process that requires time and skill	Consumer satisfaction
Recognize and recalibrate the psychological effects that aphasia has on personal, social, and collective identities as well as on self-esteem, relationships, and role definitions	
Promote healthy psychological adjustment to grief and stress associated with the changes imposed by aphasia	
Facilitate the development of self-actualization, self-assertiveness, and self-advocacy skills	
Recognize and reduce negative internal barriers that decrease or prevent individuals from actively participating in life	
Reflect the curative factors in group work and the healing power of intimacy	
Increase feelings of harmony/well-being and quality of life	
Reflect that:	
Communication is a medium through which humans share life's experiences, happenings, and outcomes as well as ideas and feelings about them.	
Communication is inseparably bound to people, places, and purposes for its use.	
Communication creates and is created by participation in life.	
Communication is flexible and dynamic.	
Focus on conversation—and on conversation as a collaborative achievement	
Foster reasons to communicate	
Strive to enhance level of participation in conversation	
Promote abilities/opportunities:	
To communicate to maintain social relationships	
To communicate in natural, authentic contexts and social units or dyads	
To communicate to transmit information	
To communicate basic needs	
Empower individuals to demonstrate or reveal communicative competence and acknowledge such competence	
Work to increase ability to communicate independently	
Provide communication/conversational support, when appropriate and necessary, and train partners and communities in these techniques	
Work to reduce impairments while focusing on revealing competence/function	
Work to reduce impairments in the context of reducing barriers to life participation	
Relate functional communication to environmental factors as well as impairment	
Increase continuity and access to intervention[a]	

[a]*Intervention* is a consumer-driven, dynamic, assistive, advising, empowering, interactive, collaborative process that responds to the significant, immediate, and long-term consequences that aphasia imposes on the flow of daily living and recognizes both that communication is inseparably bound to people, places, and purposes for its use and that communication creates and is created by participation in life. All intervention goals reflect the complexity of aphasia and the multiple contexts that it affects. Such goals are established collaboratively and are constantly assessed, weighed, prioritized, and renegotiated to decrease the devastating negative consequences of aphasia, foster adaptation to change, and increase meaningful social participation, purpose, harmony, and well-being in the lives of all those who are affected by aphasia. It is a process that evolves and changes over time, increasingly empowering those who receive it to be responsible for their own care. Outcomes are measured qualitatively and quantitatively.

Wilcox, 1981), and for restorative, impairment-centered, skill-level work, both stimulation therapy (see Chapter 15) and thematic stimulation therapy (see Chapter 16).

Education

The church social committee, several participants of the upcoming trip, and the home care nurse attended two meetings in which they viewed the video *What Is aphasia?* and discussed the language, psychological, and social consequences of aphasia. Sample tasks under the five mental operations included:

- What are all the possible environmental barriers that will make functioning (including communication) in a bus difficult?
- What are all the possible things that we could change in the environment to make communication more successful?
- What are all the environmental factors that will make functioning (including communication) in the casino difficult?
- What are all the things that we can do to increase the chances of communication success in this environment?
- What are all the environmental barriers that make group communication more difficult than individual communication?
- What are all the things that we can do to decrease the level of this difficulty?
- What are all the things that we can do to increase our (our partner's) communication success/failure?
- What are all the things that communication partners can do to help someone be more successful in getting his or her ideas across?

In addition, the therapist led the group in a discussion and modeled strategies for facilitating communication, such as those suggested by Simmons-Mackie; interactive drawing (Lyon, 1994, 1995); alerting to topic initiation and change; cueing/retrieval feature analysis, as suggested by Boyle and Coelho (1995); and communication consequences, as developed by Norris and Hoffman (1990).

For example, the communication consequences discussed by Norris and Hoffman (1990) include (1) acknowledgments or confirming the truth value of an utterance, (2) using very specific language, (3) extensions or adding new ideas within the same topic, (4) nonverbal responses, (5) verbatim repetitions, (6) restating or rewording what was said, (7) summarizing and integrating, (8) negation or indicating how and why what was said is untrue or unclear, (9) self-talk, (10) parallel-talk, (11) semantically contingent remarks, (12) sharing personal reactions, (13) questions and comments, (14) predictions and projections, (15) requests for repair or clarification, (16) requests for repetition, and (17) concept formation.

Interaction with Patient and Spouse

During intervention, both partners discussed some of the same questions as above. In addition, other tasks, such as those discussed below, were used with the partners.

Comprehension and Memory

The POSSE strategy suggested by Englert and Mariage (1991) was used to facilitate comprehension of and memory for content for stories:

P = **PREDICT** what ideas may be in the story.
O = **ORGANIZE** your thoughts (What happens? Where is it? What does it look like? Main idea?).
S = **SEARCH the STRUCTURE** (draw the structure out schematically).
S = **SUMMARIZE** the main idea.
E = **EVALUATE**, compare, clarify, and predict.

For example, the patient and spouse were asked to predict what the article "Stay Busy, Live Longer, Experts Suggest" (*New York Times*, August 24, 1999, p. F8) might be about and what the author might possibly mean by the word "busy."

Later, the patient and spouse were asked to draw a picture of the information in the article by putting the main idea in the middle of the page (stay busy = live longer; sense of purpose = live longer) and other ideas around it (physical activity; social activity; productive activity: cooking, shopping, volunteering, gardening).

Questions relating to divergent thinking in relation to this article include:

- What are all the things that people can possibly do to live longer?
- What are all the ways that you could possibly apply this information to your everyday lives?
- What are all the personal and environmental factors that can increase (and decrease) life participation for individuals with aphasia, their families, and their communities?
- What are all the things that add purpose, direction, and meaning to our daily lives?
- What are all the things that can possibly lead to comfort and pleasure in our lives?
- What are all the things we can do to restore the purpose, direction, and meaning in the lives of P and T?
- What are all the ways that the trip to Atlantic City relates to this article?
- What other things can you think of that relate to this article?

Pre-Trip Questions

- Who are the possible participants in the group?
- What are all the things we could possibly think of to plan a trip to Atlantic City?
- What are all the things we could possibly need to consider in planning a bus trip?

- What are all the things you can think of about Atlantic City?
- What are all the things you can think of about the Jersey Shore?
- What are all the things you might possibly see in Atlantic City?
- What are all the possible things that someone might bring with him or her on a trip to Atlantic City?
- What are all the possible things that someone might do (participate in) in Atlantic City (e.g., go to the beach, nightclubs, restaurants, go shopping, walk on the boardwalk, swim, sightsee)?
- What are all the possible things we need to take care of before we go to Atlantic City (e.g., personal care, banking, and medical)?
- What are all the safety rules we might possibly follow on a trip (to Atlantic City)?
- What are all the topics someone could possibly talk about on a trip?
- What are all the possible ways that someone can be a good conversational partner?
- What are all the things a good citizen should do when he or she goes to a new place?
- What are all the things we could possibly change that could increase our ability to go on these trips?
- What are all of your strengths that will make this a successful trip?
- What are all the possible things that someone can do to make a trip successful?
- What are our weaknesses that could possibly hinder you from having a successful trip?
- What are all the possible community resources that someone could use in preparing for a trip?
- Who are all the possible people who might be able to help us make a trip more successful?
- What are all the things that could possibly restrict your access to a trip to Atlantic City?
- What are all the possible problems we might have in going to Atlantic City with a church group (e.g., getting to the bus, on the bus, in the casinos, in the restaurants, at the beach/boardwalk, in the shops, and on the way home)?
- What are all the possible environmental/structural, attitudinal, and informational obstacles that limit or prevent participation in a trip to Atlantic City?
- What are all the possible things we might be able to do to avoid these problems?
- What are all the possible ways we could solve each of these problems?
- What are all the possible ways to cope when we have a problem?
- What are all the things we can possibly eat in Atlantic City?
- What are all the possible foods that someone can eat in a restaurant?

- What are all the things we should eat to be healthy?
- What are all the things we should not eat to stay healthy?
- What are all the things that we can bring to Atlantic City that can be folded? Cannot be folded? That someone could drink? That someone could eat?
- What are all the ways that someone can get to Atlantic City?
- What are all the things that could fit into a bus?
- What are all the possible places that someone can go by bus?
- What are all the possible activities that we can attend through the church?

Post-Trip: Consumer Satisfaction Questionnaire

- What were all the possible benefits of going on the trip?
- What were all the possible benefits of being members of the group?
- What are all the feelings that you have about the trip?
- What are all the positive things that happened on the trip?
- What were all the problems that occurred that we did/did not anticipate?
- What are all the ways we could possibly have anticipated them?
- What are all the ways we could possibly have solved them or coped with them?
- What are all the ways that we (or others) could have been better conversational partners?
- What are all the things we did before the trip that made the trip more successful?
- What are all the things we did that gave us a feeling of connection with others? A feeling of comfort and harmony?
- What are all the things we could have done to have made the trip more successful?

Memory

To facilitate P's memory, several strategies were used. First, the scaffolding techniques or prompts suggested by Norris and Hoffman (1990) were used. These included various prompts to cue P for more information. They included:

- **Additive** (and . . .)
- **Temporal** (and then; first; after; next; and when; while . . .)
- **Causal** (because; so; since; so that's; in order to . . .)
- **Adversative** (but; except; however; except that . . .)
- **Conditional** (of; unless; if-then; in case; or . . .)
- **Spatial** (in; next to; until he got to; which was on . . .)
- **Contingent Queries** or "Wh-" questions to prompt for agents, actions, objects, locations, or relational information
- **Summarization** or **Evaluation** to give the individual a second opportunity to communicate
- **Binary Choices** to offer alternative utterances
- **Phonemic Cues** to offer the initial sound or syllable of a target word

In addition, the semantic feature analysis developed by Boyle and Coelho (1995) was used. This technique prompts the individual to identify the specific features of target pictures that they find hard to retrieve or name. For example, for "a quarter," P needed to identify the following:

- **GROUP:** money, coin
- **USE:** buy things
- **ACTION:** give, get, spend
- **PROPERTIES:** round, shiny, large
- **LOCATION:** in a pocket, at a bank, in the casino
- **ASSOCIATION:** spending, getting things

Cognition

Recognition/comprehension tasks included:

- Reading and following signs, directories, menus, travel brochures from the chamber of commerce, the casinos, and the AAA
- Comprehending the video *What Is Aphasia?*
- Comprehending the video *Casino*
- Comprehending other videotaped material
- Comprehending newspaper stories (e.g., "Ruling in California Crimps Indian Plans for a Casino Empire" [Todd Purdum, *New York Times*, August, 24, 1999, pp. A1 and A11]; "Little Tribe, Casino Threatened, Battles U.S." [*New York Times*, August 28, 1999, p. A7]; and "Stay Busy, Live Longer, Experts Suggest" [*New York Times*, August 24, 1999, p. F8])
- Reading short stories about gambling, Atlantic City, and the Jersey Shore

Skill-building, impairment-level recognition and understanding tasks included:

- **Matching Related Words** (e.g., draw a line from each word in the left-hand column to the related word in the right-hand column.)
- **Word Categorization Tasks** (circle the words that belong in the category "Atlantic City.")
- **Word Categorization Exclusion** (e.g., cross out the word on each line that does not belong)
- **Write in a New Word that Does Belong**
- **Yes/No Questions** (e.g., read each question, and mark "yes" or "no.")
- **Sentence Arrangement** of scrambled sentences for targeted core vocabulary items (e.g., Rearrange these words to form correct sentences: Atlantic City are we to going.)

Convergent Tasks

Answering "Wh-" question tasks include:

- What can I do when someone doesn't understand me?
- What can I do when I don't understand someone else?
- What can I do to get my partner to help me when I can't get my idea across?
- What can I do to help my partner to get his idea across when I can't understand him?

Other convergent tasks that might be useful are discussed below:

- **Using social greetings**
- **Object manipulation and description** (e.g., a slot machine).
- **Acting out and describing sequences with props** (e.g., using the slot machines or ordering lunch).
- **Picture description** (e.g., Describe this picture of "Taj Mahal Casino" or "Caesar's Palace Casino").
- **Event description** (e.g., Describe roulette).
- **Discussing** videotaped material
- **Structured answers** (e.g., What does the dealer deal? How many cards are in a deck?)
- **Identifying places and activities**
- **Answering questions** about reading material or videos
- **Barrier tasks**

Skill/impairment level convergent tasks included:

- **Repetition** of core vocabulary (e.g., Atlantic City—To Atlantic City—We're going to Atlantic City)
- **Closure tasks** (e.g., We're going to Atlantic City. We're going to _____.)
- **Naming tasks** (e.g., What do we swim in?)
- **Category naming**
- **Defining core vocabulary**
- **Using core vocabulary words**
- **Giving directions**
- **Creating sentences** for target core vocabulary items (e.g., create sentences for these words and phrases, such as game-play)
- **Multiple choice questions** relating to core vocabulary

Evaluative thinking or judgment tasks included:

- Which activity should we work on first? Atlantic City or the Garden Club lecture?
- Which trip means more to you: the trip to Atlantic City or the lecture on roses?
- Which game is easier to play: the slot machines or poker?
- Because the trip is in August, which would be more useful to have with us: a bathing suit or gloves? A beach towel or a coat? Suntan lotion or a lamp?
- I can't read the menu. Should I ask the waitress to tell me the choices or just point to anything?
- Which is more important for a pay phone call: a quarter or a five-dollar bill?
- Which is closer to New York: Atlantic City or Florida?
- Which is faster: a plane or a bus?
- I don't know how to play a game. Which should I do first: Watch others play, or start to play myself?
- The sign says "Wet floor." Should I walk across it or wait until it is dry?

Integrative tasks included:

- Conversation
- Procedural discourse

- Narrative discourse
- Unstructured discussions (e.g., the pros and cons of gambling, of a group trip, and of going to the beach)
- Role playing talking to fellow travelers on the bus
- Role playing being in the casino
- Role playing ordering in a restaurant
- Role playing shopping in a store
- Role playing being at the beach
- Watching video tapes about Atlantic City and discussing them
- Reading stories about the New Jersey shore and Atlantic City and discussing them

CONCLUSION

In summary, the model of problem solving and decision making presented here appears to be applicable to the LPAA approach because of its relevance to everyday life participation through its very specific structure or strategy for solving problems and the proven validity of the five mental operations both in "normal" individuals and in those with aphasia. It is hoped that use of this model, especially in conjunction with other models such as those cited in this chapter, will help those who use it to become more active, accurate, thorough, and effective problem solvers and decision makers, thus making it possible to achieve workable and effective solutions, resolutions, and adaptations to changing opportunities for participation in contexts that really matter and, thereby, facilitating optimum social, vocational, and recreational activity and reintegration.

Most of the literature on cognition, however, specifies what is learned, or the products of cognition. Similarly, the literature in language intervention specifies therapeutic objectives, or what is to be learned. Therapeutic objectives emphasize the types of tasks used. The goal of therapy is the appropriate accomplishment of these tasks. The criterion of success is based on the percentage of appropriate versus inappropriate responses.

Today, speech-language pathologists are shifting from an orientation of simplistic listing of tasks used in therapy, which define them as technicians, to a comprehensive understanding of the rationale behind the selection of these tasks and a description of why these tasks stimulate complex events to happen in the brain. This latter focus defines them as true clinicians.

An attempt to separate tasks into input, processing, and output components and, more important, the identification of the subsystems whose interaction is necessary for processing and specification of the complex events that happen in the brain may save us from performing therapeutic tasks backward. That is, we recognize that, during therapy, what we are attempting to stimulate is the patient's mental operations or processes, because these appear to be the complex events that happen in the brain. We also stimulate these mental operations because functional language requires the use of these

mental processes. Thus, language therapy must reflect the fact that language is communicating—that it is the give and take of ideas. It must reflect the belief that meaning is the essence of language; that communication is idea oriented, not word oriented; and that it is purpose/intent oriented. It must be recognized that the speech act involves creativity and novelty of expression. This is the core of language. Language is an aid to communication.

Applying the Guilford model to adult aphasia has several other advantages. Most importantly, it enables us to identify and operationally define the action elicited within the patient by the stimuli presented, the complex events that happen in the brain, and/or the cognitive processes that are used in generating language products, such as words, classes, rules of languages, and semantic implications. It enables us to make use of an empirical statistically documented model or taxonomy of behaviors to give the concepts of cognition, information processing, and problem solving a firm, comprehensive, and systematic theoretic and yet operationally defined foundation. Guilford supported the separate and distinct existence of each of the 120 abilities in normal individuals through the use of repeated research studies using factor analysis. Some of these abilities, such as memory, divergent thinking, convergent thinking, evaluative thinking or judgment, and semantic and behavioral content, also have been documented in persons with adult aphasia, right brain damage, and closed-head injuries and in elderly individuals (Braverman, 1990; Chapey, 1977b; Chapey & Lubinski, 1979; Chapey et al., 1976; Diggs & Basili, 1987; Law & Newton, 1991; Lubinski & Chapey, 1978; Schwartz-Crowley & Gruen, 1986). In addition, this model provides a set of tests whose validity and reliability have been established. These tests can be used in therapy to stimulate specific parameters of the model and to assess, evaluate, and describe patient behavior. Use of these tests may help us to someday make a statement about the efficacy of treatment based on this model.

FUTURE TRENDS IN COGNITIVE SEMANTIC INTERVENTION

Recovery today is very documentation oriented—very focused on cost containment. This orientation generates a "pricing by activity" mentality in which governmental and insurance agencies emphasize unimportant but measurable goals, activities, and abilities. Many of these do not help the patient to regain as much functional, meaningful propositional language as possible or increase his or her ability to become better adept at the back and forth—the give and take of ideas.

The current emphasis on measurable, operationally written behavioral goals should be reconsidered. In the future, we need therapeutic goals and procedures based on rich and shared experiences that encourage individuals to apply, analyze, synthesize, and evaluate such real-life experience; relate it to something else; reorganize it; infer from it; and use it as a springboard to solve new problems creatively. A cognitive approach to recovery appears to meet this need. In addition, it has the added advantage that stimulating thinking and cognitive processing may facilitate the individual with aphasia' natural acquisition ability—that is, the ability to acquire language independently.

A cognitive approach also may stimulate generalization. Therefore, a strong need exists to develop additional therapeutic materials appropriate for this approach. A strong need also exists to develop assessment protocols that will measure these cognitive-semantic processes separately and within the context of functional, meaningful communication. Such a measure may help clinicians to assess progress in therapy and generalization and, therefore, sharpen our quality-assurance systems.

KEY POINTS

1. The Guilford SOI model contains four types of content, five mental operations, and six types of products or associations.
2. Intelligence can be defined within this model in terms of 120 abilities (content × operation × product). Therefore, we can assess the individual's intelligence for each ability.
3. Cognition can be operationally defined by the use of one or more of the five mental operations in the Guilford model: recognition/understanding, memory, convergent thinking, divergent thinking, and evaluative thinking.
4. Communication is a problem-solving, decision-making task that usually involves the back and forth, give and take of ideas between partners in a specific context. This usually involves the use of one or all five mental operations or cognitive processes.
5. Language involves the use of three types of knowledge: content, form, and use or function. Each of these can be defined within the context of the Guilford model as semantic and behavioral information processed by one or more of the five mental processes and resulting in one or more associations or products.
6. Spontaneous speech, communication, problem solving, decision making, learning, and information processing are composite abilities, often requiring several abilities to function together to achieve a desired goal.
7. The objective of cognitive stimulation therapy is to stimulate the five mental operations at various levels of complexity and in composite abilities, such as spontaneous speech, to increase ability to participate in meaningful and personally relevant activities and life goals.

ACTIVITIES FOR REFLECTION AND DISCUSSION

1. Write a definition of language based on the five mental operations in the Guilford model. How would aphasia be defined within this definition?
2. Create an interactive exercise for clients to practice the use of divergent thinking using two of the following topics: gardening, travel, dining out, food shopping, meeting a stranger, and World War II. List vocabulary that you would consider to be important to this exercise.
3. Compare and contrast Chapey's cognitive definition of aphasia with those of:
   - Wepman
   - Schuell
   - Goldstein

   How are they the same, and how are they different?
4. List 10 questions that you would include on an assessment protocol for each of the following models of aphasia:
   a. Chapey's cognitive definition
   b. Wepman's definition
   c. Schuell's definition
   d. Goldstein's definition

References

Aurelia, J. (1974). *Aphasia therapy manual.* Danville, IL: Interstate.

Ausubel, D. (1965). Introduction. In R. Anderson & D. Ausubel (Eds.), *Readings in the psychology of cognition.* New York: Holt, Rinehart & Winston.

Bandura, A., & Walters, R. (1963). *Social learning and personality development.* New York: Holt, Rinehart & Winston.

Berman, M., & Peelle, L. (1967). Self-generated cues: A method for aiding aphasic and apractic patients. *Journal of Speech and Hearing Disorders, 32,* 372–376.

Bloom, L., & Lahey, M. (1978). *Language development and language disorders.* New York: John Wiley & Sons.

Boden, M. (1980). *Jean Piaget.* New York: Viking Press.

Bolwinick, J. (1967). *Cognitive processes in maturity and old age.* New York: Springer.

Boyle, M., & Coelho, C. (1995). Application of semantic feature analysis as a treatment for aphasic dysnomia. *American Journal of Speech-Language Pathology, 4*(4), 94–98.

Braverman, K. M. (1990). *Divergent semantic and behavioral production skills in aphasia and right-hemisphere communication impairment.* Unpublished doctoral dissertation. University of Cincinnati, Cincinnati, OH.

Bruner, J. (1968). *Processes of cognitive growth: Infancy.* Worcester, MA: Clark University Press.

Butfield, E., & Zangwill, O. (1946). Reeducation in aphasia: A review of 70 cases. *Journal of Neurology, Neurosurgery and Psychiatry, 9,* 75–79.

Byng, S., Kay, J., Edmundson, A., & Scott, C. (1990). Aphasia tests reconsidered. *Aphasiology, 4*(1), 67–92.

Cazden, C. B. (1976). How knowledge about language helps the classroom teacher–Or does it? A personal account. *Urban Review, 9*, 74–91.

Chapey, R. (1974). *Divergent semantic behavior in aphasia*. Unpublished doctoral dissertation. Columbia University, New York.

Chapey, R. (1977a). A divergent semantic model of intervention in adult aphasia. In R. Brookshire (Ed.), *Clinical aphasiology: Conference proceedings*. Minneapolis: BRK.

Chapey, R. (1977b). The relationship between divergent and convergent semantic behavior in adult aphasia. *Archives of Physical Medicine and Rehabilitation, 58*, 357–362.

Chapey, R. (Ed.). (1981a). *Language intervention strategies in adult aphasia*. Baltimore, MD: Williams & Wilkins.

Chapey, R. (1981b). Divergent semantic intervention. In R. Chapey (Ed.), *Language intervention strategies in adult aphasia*. Baltimore, MD: Williams & Wilkins.

Chapey, R. (1983). Language-based cognitive abilities in adult aphasia: Rationale for intervention. *Journal of Communication Disorders, 16*, 405–424.

Chapey, R. (1988). Aphasia therapy: Why do we say one thing and do another? In S. Gerber & G. Mencher (Eds.), *International perspectives on communication disorders*. Washington, DC: Gallaudet University.

Chapey, R. (1992). Functional communication assessment and intervention: Some thoughts on the state of the art. *Aphasiology, 6*(1), 85–93.

Chapey, R. (1994). Cognitive intervention. In R. Chapey (Ed.), *Language intervention strategies in adult aphasia*. Baltimore, MD: Williams & Wilkins.

Chapey, R., & Lubinski, R. (1979). Semantic judgment ability in adult aphasia. *Cortex, 14*, 247–255.

Chapey, R., Rigrodsky, S., & Morrison, E. (1976). The measurement of divergent semantic behavior in aphasia. *Journal of Speech and Hearing Research, 19*, 664–677.

Chapey, R., Rigrodsky, S., & Morrison, E. (1977). Aphasia: A divergent semantic interpretation. *Journal of Speech and Hearing Disorders, 42*, 287–295.

Chomsky, N. (1957). *Syntactic structures*. The Hague: Mouton.

Chomsky, N. (1964). *Current issues in linguistic theory*. The Hague: Mouton.

Chomsky, N. (1972). *Language and mind*. New York: Harcourt, Brace & Jovanovich.

Cochrane, R., & Milton, S. (1984). Conversational prompting: A sentence building technique for severe aphasia. *Journal of Neurological Communication Disorders, 1*, 4–23.

Cooper, L., & Rigrodsky, S. (1979). Verbal training to improve explanations of conservation with aphasic adults. *Journal of Speech and Hearing Research, 33*, 818–828.

Craig, H. (1983). Application of pragmatic language models for intervention. In T. M. Gallagher & C. A. Prutting (Eds.), *Pragmatic assessment and intervention issues in language*. San Diego: College Hill Press.

Cropley, A. (1967). *Creativity*. London: Longman.

Davis, G. A., & Wilcox, M. J. (1981). Incorporating parameters of natural conversation in aphasia treatment. In R. Chapey (Ed.), *Language intervention strategies in adult aphasia*. Baltimore, MD: Williams & Wilkins.

Dember, W., & Jenkins, J. (1979). *General psychology: Modeling behavior and experience*. Englewood Cliffs, NJ: Prentice-Hall.

Diggs, C., & Basili, A. (1987). Verbal expression of right cerebrovascular accident patients: Convergent and divergent language. *Brain and Language, 30*, 130–146.

Dore, J. (1974). A pragmatic description of early language development. *Journal of Psycholinguistic Research, 3*, 343–350.

Duchan, J. (April, 1999). Personal communication on LPAA.

Duffy, J. R., & Coelho, C. (2001). Schuell's stimulation approach to rehabilitation. In R. Chapey (Ed.), *Language intervention strategies in adult aphasia*. Baltimore, MD: Lippincott Williams & Wilkins.

Englert, C. S., & Mariage, T. V. (1991). Making student partners in the comprehension process: Organizing the reading 'POSSE.' *Learning Disability Quarterly, 14*, 129.

English, H. B., & English, A. C. (1958). *A comprehensive dictionary of psychological and psychoanalytic terms*. New York: McKay.

Fey, M., & Leonard, L. B. (1983). Pragmatic skills of children with specific language impairments. In T. Gallagher & C. A. Prutting (Eds.), *Pragmatic assessment and intervention issues in language*. San Diego: College Hill Press.

Frattali, C. (1992). Functional assessment of communication: Merging public policy with clinical view. *Aphasiology, 6*(1), 63–85.

Gaddie, A., Kearns, K., & Yedor, K. (1991). A qualitative analysis of response elaboration training effects. In T. Prescott (Ed.), *Clinical aphasiology: Conference proceedings, 21*, 171–184.

Gallagher, T. (1983). Pre-assessment: A procedure for accommodating language use variability. In T. Gallagher & C. A. Prutting (Eds.), *Pragmatic assessment and intervention issues in language*. San Diego: College Hill Press.

Goldstein, K. (1948). *Language and language disturbances*. New York: Grune & Stratton.

Goodglass, H., & Kaplan, E. (1972). *The assessment of aphasia and related disorders*. Philadelphia, PA: Lea & Febiger.

Goodman, P. (1971). *Speaking and language: Defense of poetry*. New York: Random House.

Gowan, J., Demos, G., & Torrance, E. (1967). *Creativity: Its educational implications*. New York: John Wiley & Sons.

Grant, D., Hake, H., & Hornseth, J. (1951). Acquisition and extinction of verbally conditioned response with different percentages of reinforcement. *Journal of Experimental Psychology, 42*, 1–5.

Guilford, J. P. (1967). *The nature of human intelligence*. New York: McGraw-Hill.

Guilford, J. P., & Hoepfner, R. (1971). *The analysis of intelligence*. New York: McGraw-Hill.

Harlow, H. (1949). The formation of learning sets. *Psychological Review, 56*, 51–56.

Harris, M., & Evans, R. (1974). The effects of modeling and instruction on creative responses. *Journal of Psychology, 86*, 123–130.

Harrison, R. P. (1974). *Beyond words: An introduction to nonverbal communication*. Englewood Cliffs, NJ: Prentice-Hall.

Haviland, S. E., & Clark, H. H. (1974). What's new? Acquiring new information as a process in comprehension. *Journal of Verbal Learning and Verbal Behavior, 13*, 512–521.

Head, H. (1915). Hughlings Jackson on aphasia and kindred affections of speech. *Brain, 38*, 1–7.

Holland, A. (1975). Language therapy for children: Some thoughts on context and content. *Journal of Speech and Hearing Disorders, 40*, 514–523.

Holland, A. (1991). Pragmatic aspects of interaction in aphasia. *Journal of Neurolinguistics, 6,* 197–211.

Hughy, J., & Johnson, A. (1975). *Speech communication: Foundations and challenges.* New York: Macmillan.

Jennings, E., & Lubinski, R. (1981). Strategies for improving productive thinking in the language impaired adult. *Journal of Communication Disorders, 14,* 255–271.

Jensen, G., & Cotton,, J. (1960). Successive acquisitions and extinctions as related to differing percentages of reinforcement. *Journal of Experimental Psychology, 60,* 41–49.

Kagan, A., & Gailey, G. (1993). Functional is not enough: Training conversation partners for aphasic adults. In A. Holland & M. Forbes (Eds.), *Aphasia treatment: World perspectives.* San Diego: Singular.

Kearns, K. (1985). Response elaboration training for patient initiated utterances. *Clinical Aphasiology, 15,* 196–204.

Kearns, K. P. (1985). Response elaboration training for patient initiated utterances. In R. Brookshire (Ed.), *Clinical aphasiology: Conference proceedings* (pp. 196–204). Minneapolis: BRK.

Kearns, K. P. (1990). Broca's aphasia. In L. LaPointe (Ed.), *Aphasia and related neurogenic language disorders.* New York: Thieme.

Kearns, K. P., & Potechin, G. (1988). The generalization of response elaboration training effects. In T. Prescott (Ed.), *Clinical aphasiology.* Boston, MA: College Hill Press.

Kearns, K., & Yedor, K. (1991). An alternating treatments comparison of loose training and a convergent treatment strategy. In T. Prescott (Ed.), *Clinical aphasiology, 20,* 223–238.

Keenan, J. A. (1975). *A procedure manual in speech pathology with brain-damaged adults.* Danville, IL: Interstate.

Lahey, M. (1988). *Language disorders and language development.* New York: Macmillan.

Law, P., & Newton, M. (1991). *Divergent semantic behavior in aged persons.* Atlanta, GA: American Speech-Language-Hearing Association Convention.

Lazerson, A. (Ed.). (1975). *Psychology today.* New York: Random House.

Lefrancois, G. (1982). *Psychological theories of human learning* (2nd ed.). Belmont, CA: Brooks-Cole.

Lindfors, J. W. (1980; rev. 1987). *Children's language and learning.* Englewood Cliffs, NJ: Prentice-Hall.

Lubinski, R. (1986). A social communication approach to treatment in aphasia in an institutional setting. In R. Marshall (Ed.), *Case studies in aphasia rehabilitation.* Austin, TX: Pro-Ed.

Lubinski, R., & Chapey, R. (1978). Constructive recall strategies in adult aphasia. In R. Brookshire (Ed.), *Clinical aphasiology: Conference proceedings.* Minneapolis: BRK.

Lucas, E. (1980). *Semantic and pragmatic language disorders: Assessment and remediation.* Rockville, MD: Aspen.

Lyon, J. (1994). Drawing: Its value as an aid for adults with aphasia. *Aphasiology, 8.*

Lyon, J. (1995). Drawing: Its value as a communication aid for adults with aphasia. *Aphasiology, 9*(1), 33–94.

Martin, A. D. (1979). A critical evaluation of therapeutic approaches to aphasia. In R. Brookshire (Ed.), *Clinical aphasiology: Conference proceedings.* Minneapolis: BRK.

Marx, M. (1970). *Learning theories.* London: Macmillan.

McConnell, F., Love, R., & Smith, B. (1974). Language remediation in children. In S. Dickson (Ed.), *Communication disorders: Remedial principles and practices.* Glenview, IL: Scott Foresman.

McCormick, L., & Schiefelbush, R. (1984). *Early language intervention: An introduction.* Columbus, OH: Charles E. Merrill.

Muma, J. (1975). The communication game: Dump and play. *Journal of Speech and Hearing Disorders, 40,* 296.

Muma, J. R. (1978). *Language handbook: Concepts, assessment and intervention.* Englewood Cliffs, NJ: Prentice-Hall.

Naremore, R. (1980). Language disorders in children. In T. Hixon, L. Shriberg, & J. Saxman (Eds.), *Introduction to communication disorders.* Englewood Cliffs, NJ: Prentice-Hall.

Neisser, U. (1967). *Cognitive psychology.* New York: Appleton-Century-Crofts.

Norris, J., & Hoffman, P. (1990). Language intervention within naturalistic environments. *Language, Speech and Hearing Services in the Schools, 21,* 72–84.

Ochs, E., & Schieffelin, B. (Eds.). (1979). *Developmental pragmatics.* New York: Academic Press.

Peabody Language Development Kit. Level One. (1965). Circle Pines, MN: American Guidance Service.

Pieres, E., & Morgan, F. (1973). Effects of free associative training on children's ideational fluency. *Journal of Personality, 41,* 42–49.

Porch, B. (1971). Multidimensional scoring in aphasia testing. *Journal of Speech and Hearing Research, 14,* 776–792.

Prutting, C. (1979). Process/pra/ses/n: The action of moving forward progressively from one point to another on the way to completion. *Journal of Speech and Hearing Disorders, 44,* 3–10.

Prutting, C., & Kirchner, D. (1983). Applied pragmatics. In R. M. Gallagher & C. A. Prutting (Eds.), *Pragmatic assessment and intervention issues in language.* San Diego: College Hill Press.

Rosenfeld, N. M. (1978). Conversational control function of nonverbal behavior. In A. W. Siegman & S. Felstein (Eds.), *Nonverbal behavior and communication.* Hillsdale, NJ: Lawrence Erlbaum.

Rosenthal, T., & Zimmerman, B. (1978). *Social learning and cognition.* New York: Academic Press.

Saltz, E. (1971). *The cognitive bases of human learning.* Homewood, IL: Dorsey Press.

Sarno, M., Silverman, M., & Sands, E. (1970). Speech therapy and language recovery in severe aphasia. *Journal of Speech and Hearing Research, 13,* 607–623.

Schuell, H., Carroll, V., & Street, B. (1955). Clinical treatment of aphasia. *Journal of Speech and Hearing Disorders, 20,* 43–53.

Schuell, H., Jenkins, J., & Jiminez-Pabon, E. (1964). *Aphasia in adults.* New York: Harper & Row.

Schwartz-Crowley, R., & Gruen, A. (1986). Rehabilitation assessment of communicative, cognitive-linguistic, and swallowing functions. *Trauma Quarterly, 3*(1), 63–65.

Scott, W., Osgood, W., & Peterson, C. (1979). *Cognitive structure, theory and measurement of individual differences.* New York: Halstead Press.

Searle, J. (1969). *Speech acts.* London: Cambridge University Press.

Simmons, N. (1993). *An ethnographic investigation of compensatory strategies in aphasia.* Dissertation. Louisiana State University and Agricultural and Mechanical College.

Slobin, D. (1971). *Psycholinguistics.* Glenview, IL: Scott Foresman.

Smith, F. (1975). *Comprehension and learning.* New York: Holt, Rinehart & Winston.

Staats, A. (1968). *Learning, language and cognition.* New York: Holt, Rinehart & Winston.

Torrance, E. P. (1966). *Torrance Test of creative thinking.* Princeton, NJ: Personnel Press.

Torrance, E. P. (1974). Interscholastic brainstorming and creative problem solving competition for creatively gifted. *Gifted Child Quarterly, 18*, 3–7.

Vignolo, L. (1964). Evolution of aphasia and language rehabilitation: Retrospective exploratory study. *Cortex, 1*, 344–367.

Warren, S., & Rogers-Warren, A. K. (Eds.). (1985). *Teaching functional language.* Austin, TX: Pro-Ed.

Webster's new collegiate dictionary (1977). Springfield, MA: G. & C. Merriam.

Wepman, J. (1951). *Recovery from aphasia.* New York: Ronald Press.

Wepman, J. (1953). A conceptual model for the processes involved in recovery from aphasia. *Journal of Speech and Hearing Disorders, 18*, 4–13.

Wepman, J. (1972). Aphasia therapy: A new look. *Journal of Speech and Hearing Disorders, 37*, 203–214.

Wepman, J. (1976). Aphasia: Language without thought or thought without language. *ASHA, 18*, 131–136.

Yardley, A. (1974). *Structure in early learning.* New York: Citation Press.

Yorkston, K., & Beukelman, D. (1977). A system for quantifying verbal output of high level aphasia patients. In R. Brookshire (Ed.), *Clinical aphasiology: Conference proceedings.* Minneapolis: BRK.

Chapter 18

Early Management of Wernicke's Aphasia: A Context-Based Approach

Robert C. Marshall

OBJECTIVES

The early post-onset period encompasses the first 1 to 3 months after a stroke causing aphasia. This is a time when persons with aphasia and their families struggle with the uncertainties of the future and with day-to-day communication (Lyon, 1998; Marshall, 1997). Many patients with aphasia do not talk at this time, or they talk very little. Those with Wernicke's aphasia are an exception. These patients talk, but their aphasia interferes with communication in other ways. A different approach to clinical management therefore is required for these patients compared with that used for patients with other types of aphasia.

This chapter provides information on a context-based approach to management for patients with Wernicke's aphasia. This approach blends science, art, and common sense. Science comes from knowing and applying judiciously to treatment what research tells us about people with aphasia. The art is associated with knowing when to do what and with good clinical decision making. The common sense involves using therapy to improve communication skills relevant to the patient's daily life communication contexts. The material herein focuses on management during the early post-onset period, because this is when the patient's aphasia is most severe, when therapy occurs, and when the patient needs help the most. The chapter's objectives are (1) to provide a rationale for using the context-based with patients with Wernicke's aphasia, (2) to describe how context-based treatment is used to improve comprehension and information exchange in communication contexts, and (3) to increase clinicians' confidence and willingness to apply this unique approach to patient management.

WERNICKE'S APHASIA

Lesions responsible for Wernicke's aphasia occur posterior to the fissure of Rolando (Benson, 1967), leaving the patient with few, if any, associated deficits. Some patients may have a right visual field deficit, but usually, no sensory loss or paralysis occurs (Kirshner, 2002). Often, Wernicke's aphasia results from blockages in the smaller, posterior branches of the left middle cerebral artery. These damage the primary auditory cortex (Brodmann areas 41 and 42), Wernicke's area (Brodmann area 22), and portions of the second temporal and angular gyri (Brodmann areas 39 and 40), sometimes with white matter extension (Bachman & Albert, 1990).

Damage to Wernicke's area may produce severe loss of speech understanding, even though the patient may hear nonverbal sounds and music normally (Boatman, 2002). Some patients' comprehension deficits appear to be related to attention difficulties and inability to effectively ignore distracting stimuli (LaPointe & Erickson, 1991; Wiener, Connor, & Obler, 2004). Classic descriptions of Wernicke's aphasia indicate these patients have disproportionately impaired auditory comprehension in relationship to their fluent speech (Goodglass & Kaplan, 1983; Kertesz, 1979). Often, speech is perceived as rapid, with preserved rhythm, melodic line, and articulatory agility (Geschwind, 1970; Goodglass & Kaplan, 1983), but disrupted in other ways. Verbal output may be (1) devoid of content or empty (e.g., "Before the one, my son took another of them over to the one there."), (2) full of circumlocutory phrases (e.g., "The one you eat soup with") and indefinite words (e.g., "thing") rather than specific words (e.g., "spoon"), and (3) contaminated by paraphasia (unintended word substitutions not caused by motor difficulties). The paraphasias may be verbal (e.g., "tiger" for "knife"), semantic (e.g., "knife" for "spoon"), or phonemic ("spoot" for "spoon"), and if they contain several unrelated sounds, even neologistic ("veehall" for "trailer").

Unlike the halting, agrammatical speech of patients with nonfluent aphasia, the speech of the patient with Wernicke's aphasia contains a variety of grammatical forms. Some patients, however, make para-grammatical errors in which the substitution of one small word for another (e.g., "him" for "her" or "she" for "he") disrupts communication markedly. Self-correction effort and successful repair occur less often in Wernicke's aphasia (Marshall & Tompkins, 1982), and patients with severe cases of Wernicke's aphasia may be mistakenly diagnosed as being confused or mentally ill. Because Wernicke's area is the crossroads for all incoming meaningful sound patterns, these patients also have severe deficits in repetition, reading, and writing (Goodglass & Kaplan, 1983; Kirshner, Casey, Henson, & Heinrich, 1989).

Some writers have suggested patients with Wernicke's aphasia have a poorer prognosis for improvement compared with patients having other types of aphasia (Brookshire, 2003; Nicholas, Helm-Estabrooks, Ward-Lonergan, & Morgan, 1993). Research indicates that Wernicke's area and adjacent regions of the posterior language zones are vital to language processing and that extensive damage to these areas results in severe aphasia (Boatman, 2002; Metter et al., 1990). Lasting comprehension deficits and persistent aphasia usually are associated with larger lesions and, in some cases, complete destruction of Wernicke's area (Goldenberg & Spatt, 1994; Naeser, Helm-Estabrooks, Haas, Auerbach, & Srinivasan 1987; Selnes, Niccum, Knopman, & Rubens, 1984). Conversely, improvement in Wernicke's aphasia is associated with restored metabolic activity in the temporoparietal cortex (Metter, Hanson, Kempler, & Jackson, 1992) and the ability of this region of the brain to reperfuse

(Hillis & Heidler, 2002). It generally is believed that patients who improve their comprehension evolve to anomic aphasia (Goodglass, 1981; Kirshner, 2002; Pashek & Holland, 1988; Rosenbek, LaPointe, & Wertz, 1989).

RATIONALE FOR CONTEXT-BASED TREATMENT

An early question from the spouse of the person with aphasia is "when is my husband or wife going to talk again?" The field of clinical aphasiology has a long-standing practice of emphasizing what the person with aphasia produces (Doyle, Goda, & Spencer, 1995). Conversation is probably the biggest loss for many persons with aphasia, because it is via conversation that we illustrate our knowledge and capabilities as well as establish and maintain our human connections (Kagan, 1995). For the patient with Wernicke's aphasia, *talking* is a strong point—as long as the individual is talking in a conversational context rather than a noncontextual situation. Examples of the differences in noncontextual and contextual communication for three patients with Wernicke's aphasia—Glen, Marie, and Vern—are shown in Table 18-1.

TABLE 18–1

Differences in How Patients with Wernicke's Aphasia Communicated in Noncontextual and Contextual Situations

Patient: Glen, a 52-year-old man with severe Wernicke's aphasia

Noncontextual: I tested Glen with the Minnesota Test for Differential Diagnosis of Aphasia (MTDDA) (Schuell, 1965). He talked a blue streak but performed poorly on the easiest subtests of the MTDDA: repetition, matching, copying, and naming. To my chagrin, he often conveyed to me that the assessment was "stupid" and showed little appreciation for the help I was trying to give him. After an hour, I was frustrated, because Glen did all the talking and all I had to show for my efforts was a blank test form.

Contextual: As I pondered what to put in my report, I realized Glen had actually communicated a lot of information about his aphasia. It just did not relate to what the MTDDA tested. For example, when I asked him to name pictures, he informed me he hated this task and every time his wife asked him "What's this?" became angry. When I asked him to repeat short phrases, he was able to convey that he had no earthly idea why his doctors kept asking him to say "No if's, and's, or but's." He was unable to repeat single words accurately, but when I asked him to say the word "screw," he responded enthusiastically "I'd sure like to" and made an inappropriate gesture.

Patient: Marie, a 90-year-old woman with moderate Wernicke's aphasia

Noncontextual: I gave Marie the Porch Index of Communicative Ability (PICA; Porch, 1967) in the nursing home. Her overall score placed her at the 29th percentile in a large, random sample of adults with aphasia. Her only relevant performance during testing was on the matching and reading subtests. Marie lived alone, did not drive, and aside from her aphasia, was perfectly healthy. However, her physician felt that her communication deficits were so severe that she would be unable to live independently.

Contextual: When therapy began, all Marie would talk about was going home. She clearly understood the discharge plan and argued that she could, indeed, go home because she was essentially a recluse and had few communication needs. She asked that I talk to her neighbors about helping out in an emergency. She told me how she did her shopping and that her major responsibility was her cat. Marie was able to convince us all that she should go home, and the result was positive.

Patient: Vern, a 63-year-old man with moderate Wernicke's aphasia

Noncontextual: Vern could not name any of the common objects on the PICA accurately. Usually, he responded "No way" or "Can't get that today" after several aborted attempts to produce a specific verbal response.

Contextual: One day I asked Vern how things were going at home. He said, "Not so good." I asked, "Why?" Vern was able to convey he had been having trouble with insects (earwigs) and that the bugs were winning. He did this by (1) pointing to his ear and (2) then pointing to his bald head and saying, "I don't have any, so I need one up here." From this, I put together the word "earwig."

Context: A Common Denominator

Glen, Marie, and Vern had obvious aphasic deficits, but when communicating in a context about something relevant to them, they were remarkably successful, even though they appeared to be totally impaired when tested with the Minnesota Test for Differential Diagnosis of Aphasia, or MTDDA, or with the Porch Index of Communicative Ability, or PICA. Context was the common denominator that allowed them to communicate successfully despite pervasive aphasic deficits. The context-based approach exploits the differences in noncontextual and contextual communication with patients like Glen, Marie, and Vern.

A communicative context allows the participants to make inferences and derive interpretations about what transpires in a conversation (Paradis, 1998). When adults share knowledge about people, topics, events, and the world in general, the shared information guides the generation of appropriate requests for information.

Context is a multifaceted concept. It relates to the physical and social situations of the conversational participants as well as to their points of view (Winograd, 1977). Linguistic context refers to verbal behavior that occurs before and after a given utterance (Davis & Wilcox, 1985). Paralinguistic context refers to the "trappings" of utterances (e.g., intonation, prosody, facial expression, vocal quality, and rate of speech) that help us to convey affective information, highlight new information, and govern our behavior in communicative interactions. Research has shown that manipulation of linguistic and paralinguistic context enhances the comprehension of persons with aphasia (Freiderici, 1983; Hough, Pierce, & Cannito, 1988; Pierce, 1988; Pierce & Beekman, 1985; Pierce and DeStafano, 1987; Waller & Darley, 1978) and improves information exchange in general.

Of course, communicative contexts also vary in terms of where people live, whom they live with, what they do, where they go, and other factors. One thing is certain, however. Real-life communication always takes place in a context, and real-life communication is what persons with aphasia, especially Wernicke's aphasia, need to be prepared to do.

Rapid Discharges

One reason for using a context-based approach is that patients with Wernicke's aphasia are put into situations where effective communication is needed shortly after their stroke. This is because they rarely have major associated deficits (e.g., right-side weakness or paralysis) and do not require the same rehabilitation services as do other survivors of stroke. Frequently, they are sent home instead of to the rehabilitation center. The early transition from the hospital gives the patient no time to adjust to the residuals of the aphasia in the relatively "safe" environment of the rehabili-

tation center. Once home, the patient is thrust into decision-making situations where he or she needs to be able to communicate effectively. The context-based approach is well-suited for coping with this sudden transition. It forms the scaffolding for the clinician to provide the needed partner training, education, and counseling to help the patient cope, adjust to, and compensate for the residuals of the aphasia.

The Therapeutic Window

Context-based treatment is preferable when treatment time is limited (Hinckley & Carr, 2005). For patients with Wernicke's aphasia, individual speech-and-language therapy may not extend beyond the early post-onset period. For example, it the patient is funded for 20 speech-and-language treatments and is seen once a day, the funds for therapy will be exhausted in 4 or 5 weeks. Unless alternative monies are available or the patient should be fortunate enough to qualify for services elsewhere, the patient and the family will be left to their own devices approximately a month after the stroke. The context-based approach is a better way to prepare them for this possibility, because it focuses on communication situations that come up in real life.

Personalizing Treatment

The aphasia research indicates that persons with aphasia perform better when personally relevant materials are used as stimuli (Gray, Hoyt, Mogil, & Lefkowitz, 1977; Van Lancker & Klein, 1990; Van Lancker & Nicklay, 1992; Wallace & Canter, 1985). Most clinicians have experienced this firsthand in their practices. For example, the patient who might not be able to point to the "cigarette" on subtest 10 of the PICA might respond readily to "Have you got a cigarette?" or "Don't you know smoking is bad for you?" The context-based approach is all about personalizing treatment. This is congruent with life participation approaches to aphasia treatment (Byng & Duchan, 2005).

Clinician as a Communicator

Another advantage of the context-based approach is that it is naturalistic. That is, it stresses speaker-listener interactions to fulfill the language facilitation function. It keeps the focus of therapy on communication, and it inhibits the tendency to engage in forced production drills, convergent tasks, or pseudo-communication exchanges. Because the clinician takes the role of participant-communicator rather than director of operations, the patient and the clinician are both stakeholders in therapy. This also makes the clinician-patient relationship horizontal rather than vertical, thus reducing the performance pressure that typically is placed on the patient to come up with specific words and responses.

Improved Outcomes

Outcomes reflect the results of interventions (Fratalli, 1998). The chapters in this book indicate many routes are available for achieving favorable outcomes with persons who have aphasia. I believe, however, that outcomes may be better for patients with Wernicke's aphasia when a context-based approach is used. The context-based approach increases their "degrees of freedom" to communicate. This allows patients to increase problem-solving efforts to communicate about something important to them rather than searching for specific words. The belief that these patients have poorer prognoses may come from the fact that treatment success often is measured with standardized tests (e.g., PICA, MTDDA, and Wostein Aphasia Battery (WAB)) rather than with a conversational measure. When treatment outcomes are based on the ability to converse and/or communicate information relevant to day-to-day functioning, the prognoses of patients with Wernicke's aphasia may be as good as—or, perhaps, even better than—those of other patients.

ASSESSMENT

Early assessment of the patient with Wernicke's aphasia usually takes place in the acute-care hospital. All patients need to be evaluated before they are discharged. Those with severe language deficits need immediate attention from the speech-language pathologist, because their incomprehensible speech and faulty comprehension can result in a misdiagnosis (e.g., confusion, agitation, or psychiatric disease) and get them into trouble. For example, Leroy developed severe Wernicke's aphasia while having a beer with friends after work. He became upset when he could not be understood because of his garbled speech. The police were called and took Leroy to jail before it was discovered he had had a stroke and was taken to the hospital.

Individuals with less severe aphasia also are vulnerable. Joe's mild Wernicke's aphasia quickly evolved to an anomic aphasia during his brief hospitalization. Assuming he would soon be back to normal, the physician discharged Joe before he could be evaluated and counseled by the speech-language pathologist. After he got home, Joe became so frustrated with his anomic deficits that he contemplated selling his thriving garage business. His wife insisted Joe come back to the hospital for a speech-and-language evaluation. This evaluation revealed that Joe's anomic deficits, although still obvious, would not interfere with his ability to work on cars. Joe returned to work successfully and made good progress as an outpatient.

Some patients with Wernicke's aphasia can be given a standardized aphasia test during the early post-onset period. Many, however, perform poorly on any type of formal test. Moreover, the results provide little information to help guide treatment during the early post-onset period. Several strategies, however, are available to the clinician for obtaining information to identify the patient's strengths and weaknesses, answer the physician consult, and plan early intervention. Early assessment is all about (1) doing the necessary homework to personalize the assessment and (2) using this information in an interview to engage the patient in the process so you can learn as much as possible.

Obtaining Patient-Relevant Information

Knowing as much as possible about the patient before the interview and the beginning of treatment aids the clinician in providing the perceptual support for the conversations that drive the context-based approach. Patient-relevant information comes from (1) the medical chart, (2) observation, (3) learning about the patient's premorbid communication habits, (4) biographies, and (5) staff observations. This information helps clinicians to ask questions with a reasonable expectations as to what a given patient's answers should be. This also allows clinicians to compare what they already know with the patient's actual performance and eliminates some of guesswork from the assessment process.

Medical Chart

The medical chart contains identifying (date of birth), demographic (work history), medical (previous illnesses), and other information. Suppose the clinician learns from reviewing the chart that the patient is a Harvard graduate. In the interview, the clinician could make an open-ended comment, such as "I understand you went to school in the East" and see if the patient comes up with relevant information about Harvard. This might be followed with a statement such as "I understand Ivy League schools are expensive," which would be expected to evoke a response from the patient such as "Wow, they sure are." This one simple fact from the medical chart could set the scene for an entire conversation.

Observation

Because patients with Wernicke's aphasia have few associated deficits, they often move about the hospital rather than remain in their rooms. It may be possible to observe how or if the patient communicates in other situations (e.g., day room, cafeteria, or nurse's station) and with other people (e.g., family, friends, physicians, or staff) and if the patient attempts to resume normal communication activities (e.g., phone calls, reading the paper, writing, or watching television). Holland (1982) has commented on the importance of observing communication of the patient in other situations; in her early paper on observation of persons with aphasia, she provides a convenient form for this purpose.

Premorbid Communication Skills

Knowledge of the patient's premorbid communication habits should be collected before the interview. For example, if the clinician knew a patient was a quiet person who rarely initiated communication or elaborated on what was said, the clinician would have different expectations from the interview than if the patient was a highly verbal individual. Swindell, Pashek, and Holland (1982) have developed a form that can be filled out by the spouse to obtain information about a patient's communication style, and Green (1984) has published a checklist of factors that the clinician should consider in determining the patient's premorbid communication habits.

Biography

Family members should be included in the assessment process. One way get them involved is to ask a family member to write a short biography that gives information about the patient's work, friends, hobbies, interests, likes, dislikes, accomplishments, and related factors. Some family members may choose to include photos, artifacts (items of personal interest to the patient [e.g., sculptures, paintings, or woodwork]), and related materials. The clinician needs to tell the volunteer biographer that (1) the information is confidential, (2) the task is not a writing exercise and need not be perfect, and (3) how the information will be used in treatment.

Staff Observations

Staff (e.g., physical therapists, occupational therapists, and nurses) also can participate in assessment and treatment. One way to facilitate this is to give staff members a brief synopsis about the patient's background. For example:

John Marks is a 54-year-old college graduate who worked as an architect for Pitney-Wilson before his stroke on 10-7-06. He's married (Camilla), and his wife teaches math at St. Joseph High School. His daughter, Jocelyn, age 20, is a junior majoring in international business at Duke. His older child, Brian, is a professional baseball player in the Mets organization and currently plays third base for a farm team. John (nickname Duke because of his height and resemblance to John Wayne) is a 4-handicap golfer and longtime member of the Olympic Club. His daughter is getting married in the summer following her graduation in 07.

Staff can be trained to use this information to probe comprehension and expression in their interactions with the patient. With respect to John, the physical therapist might say, "Show me with your fingers, the position your son plays in baseball" to probe comprehension of directions. As an expression probe, she might ask John to tell her where his daughter is attending college. Successes and failures can be noted in the patient's chart. This is a way to include all staff in the effort to improve communication and provide the patient with more communication opportunities.

The Interview

During the early post-onset period, the interview forms the basis of the clinician's assessment of the patient with Wernicke's aphasia. The patient should be prepared for the interview with an advanced visit from the clinician. At this visit, the clinician should tell the patient that he or she is setting up a time to "find out a little more" about the patient's communication. It may be helpful to leave the patient a note to remind him or her about the time of the appointment. The interview should take place in a quiet, distraction-free space. What the clinician does in the interview itself largely depends on the patient's status. The suggestions for conducting the interview that follow are not prescriptive and constitute only a few of the things that might be accomplished.

Para-Standardized Testing

Para-standardized testing procedures are well-suited to assess the patient with Wernicke's aphasia. Para-standardized guidelines published by Sparks (1978), with some modifications of my own, are shown in Table 18-2. As shown in the table, the guidelines cover four broad content areas—therapeutic set, pragmatics, auditory comprehension, and verbal expression—within which specific behaviors (e.g., following conversational rules) are examined with respect to their presence or absence and positive or negative impact on communication. Para-standardized testing procedures are certainly applicable, but not necessarily to patients with Wernicke's aphasia. Most importantly, the guidelines are flexible and permit the clinician to obtain information regarding what aids and disrupts comprehension and expression. This gives the clinician information that is immediately useful for planning early treatment and counseling the patient and the family. For example, the para-standardized format allows the clinician to determine the variables that can be manipulated to aid comprehension and enhance information exchange by testing certain hypotheses (e.g., Will the patient comprehend better if I reduce his talking?). Videotaping the examination or developing a form for recording observations may aid in writing the consult and in counseling the patient and family at a later time.

Bedside Items

Holland and Fridriksson (2001) suggest that early assessment of the patient with aphasia center on activities relevant to the hospital stay. They suggest that clinicians make use of items in the patient's room when carrying out an initial assessment. Representative examples include reading get-well cards, selecting foods from the menu, choosing television programs, naming objects in the room, testing memory for the therapist's name, and writing the names of one's children.

TABLE 18–2

Modified Para-Standardized Examination Guidelines

Feature 1. Therapeutic Set

Area of Concern	*Negative Signs/Behaviors*	*Positive Signs/Behaviors*
Ease or difficulty establishing and maintaining a therapeutic set	Hostility toward examiner; distractibility because of ambient noise	Accepts the therapist in the situation; displays a realistic appraisal of situation; acknowledges clinician is there to help
Presence of rigidity or perseveration	Continuing to produce a response without regard to change in stimulus; difficulty switching tasks	Recognizing task switches; awareness of errors and effort to correct them
Behavioral rigidity	Ego-minded responses (e.g., when asked "What do you wear on your head?" says "I don't ever wear hats.")	Ability to role play and pretend

Feature 2. Pragmatics

Area of Concern	*Negative Signs/Behaviors*	*Positive Signs/Behaviors*
Follows conversation rules	Limited turn taking; not aware when to terminate a conversation; violates social conventions	Obeys conversational conventions
Realizes the reasons for language processing deficit	Blames problems on outside forces (e.g., missing dentures, people talking too fast, no glasses)	Understands a stroke has occurred
Initiate communication	Initiates few communication interactions; only responds when asked to	Initiates communication to make needs known
Persistence in face of failure	Gives up when communication snag occurs	Persists until thought has been communicated

Feature 3. Auditory Comprehension

Area of Concern	*Negative Signs/Behaviors*	*Positive Signs/Behaviors*
Peripheral hearing loss	Asks for repeats; phonetic confusions (e.g. rake-lake); history of working in noise	Examiner judges hearing acuity to be within normal limits
Understanding a conversation	Looking confused or perplexed; difficulty following conversation containing personally relevant material	Responds more enthusiastically to conversation about personal interests (e.g., sports, family, work)
Comprehension in structured auditory comprehension tasks	Difficulty pointing to objects, body parts, following simple commands	Once oriented to task, points to objects and body parts and follows simple commands
Responses to different methods of presentation	Not helped by slower rate, alerting phrases, shorter and simplified messages, orientation to topic	Comprehension of conversation and structured material when clinician uses different methods of presenting material
Comprehension when verbal output is restricted	Examiner is unable to halt "press of speech" or patient's comprehension does not improve when speech is restricted	Comprehension in conversation and on structured tasks improves when patient is asked to "listen" rather than talk
Intrapersonal monitoring	Does not ask for repeats or verify what has been said	Asks for repetitions; verifies what has been said
Comprehension when treatment materials are thematically organized	Comprehension does not improve when questions flow from mutually known topic (e.g., family)	Comprehension improves when task is organized (e.g., "I want to know about your family. Are you married? Do you have any children? Are the children still at home?")
Effect of visual supplementation	No improvement when provided a visual cue (e.g., written word "Military")	Comprehension improves with visual cue in form of written word (e.g., "Were you in the service? What branch of the military were you in?")
Self-criticism	No awareness of errors in speech output	Aware of errors and possibly upset by them

TABLE 18–2

Modified Para-Standardized Examination Guidelines (continued)

Feature 4. Verbal Expression

Area of Concern	Negative Signs/Behaviors	Positive Signs/Behaviors
Accuracy and use of substantive words	Not aware when correct target has been produced; empty speech; rejects target word when it is provided; errors do not resemble target word	Aware that speech lacks content words; recognizes target word when provided; errors are variable and sometimes approximate the target word
Quantity of speech	Unrestricted verbal output with no awareness of its content	Fluent speech that sometimes becomes less fluent as the patient evidences concern for his errors
Grammatical structure	High number of para-grammatical errors (e.g., he/she, from/for, they/we) and lack of awareness of them	Speech reflects full range of grammatical constructions with few para-grammatical errors
Degree to which paraphasic errors approximate target word	Errors bear no resemblance to target word (e.g., for "pillow": "grabbitz, rafunta")	Errors contain some of the constituents of the target word (e.g., pister/pillar) and may "in the ball park"
Self-correction accuracy and effort	No awareness of errors; makes no effort to correct errors; overcorrects a response when its meaning has been conveyed	Recognizes most errors; makes efforts to correct errors and sometimes succeeds
Stimulability	No improvement when errors are pointed out and model provided; response does not improve with semantic or phonetic cue	May improve production when model provided; responds to semantic or phonetic cues
Response to restriction in verbal output	Brief responses continue to be in error	Verbal expression is improved when shorter responses are elicited
Verbal compensations	Unable to find alternative means of verbal expression to convey intended word (zebra)	Conveys meaning of target word through description (e.g., "black-and-white horse thing") or other means
Compensations in other modalities	Uses only speech to express thoughts	Uses alternative modalities (e.g., writing, gesturing)

Author's modifications based on Sparks (1978).

Everyday Language Test

The Everyday Language Test is a verbal test that elicits responses to specific questions and/or situations (Blomert, Kean, Koster, & Schokker, 1994). For example, for one of the test items, the clinician says, "You are at the florist. You want a bouquet of flowers delivered to a friend. I am the salesperson. What do you say?" Responses are scored on a 0-to-4 scale for understandability (content) and intelligibility (perception of the message regardless of the content or meaning). A complete listing of items on the test can be found in the article by Blomert and colleagues (1994). Because the Everyday Language Test is not readily available in the United States, clinicians may want to make up their own version.

Inpatient Functional Communication Interview

The Inpatient Functional Communication Interview, or IFCI, is a measure of functional communication to be used in

an acute hospital setting (O'Halloran, Worrall, Toffolo, Code, & Hickson, 2004). Specifically, the IFCI measures the patient's ability to communicate during everyday tasks, actions, and situations that might occur in a hospital. The test is administered in four steps. Step 1 consists of documenting information about the patient from the medical chart. Step 2 involves a structured bedside interview using the IFCI. The clinician first establishes a communication context so as to evaluate the patient's performance in 15 situations that are relevant to the hospital environment. For example, one situation seeks information about whether the patient can give relevant information concerning their pre-admission history. Based on the amount and quality of the information provided, the patient receives a score of 2 (successful communication), 1 (partially successful communication), or 0 (unsuccessful communication). Step 3 consists of discussing the necessary information with the staff, and step 4 involves writing a report of the findings. The IFCI comes with a test manual, instructions, and recording and scoring forms.

TREATMENT

During the early post-onset period, many patients with Wernicke's aphasia will have severe communication problems. Their communication status often changes from day-to-day as well, because spontaneous recovery is ongoing. Some patients may begin early treatment with obvious "press of speech," nonstop talking, and pay little or no attention to their errors. Once a therapeutic set has been established and comprehension improves, however, patients may try to correct themselves, and their speech will become less fluent. With these patients, the clinician functions as a "behavioral engineer"—keeping the train (patient) on the track; changing speeds and routes; and heeding the signals regarding what the clinician should—and should not—do. The clinician's job is to steer the patient, family, and staff through the early post-onset period and make the trip as smooth as possible. The goals of treatment are to improve the patient's comprehension and ability to exchange information in contextual situations.

Therapeutic Set

The term "therapeutic set" describes the patient's attitude toward therapy and its environment and to being helped in general (Sparks, 1978). It is important that the patient understand the clinician is there to help and that he or she needs help. This may be difficult with patients who are improving so rapidly that they feel treatment is unnecessary. At the very least, the clinician should try to explain to the patient and family what aphasia is and leave the door open for later evaluation and treatment.

Establishing a therapeutic set for patients who are not improving also is difficult. These patients may be unaware or unwilling to admit that anything is wrong. The useful cues and prompts that help patients with nonfluent aphasia to produce accurate verbal responses (e.g., counting, sentence completion, and repetition) rarely help and/or sometimes are confusing to them. To show these patients that help is available and establish a therapeutic set, I have found it beneficial to identify something important that the patient needs to communicate to the staff, physician, or family and work to help the patient with that. Often, this is a problem the patient wants to solve, and it is a time-consuming process of trial and error that delays evaluation and treatment. It can pay dividends, however, as it did with Wes, a 47 year-old man with severe Wernicke's aphasia. I knew that Wes wanted to tell me something important. I wanted to evaluate him, but it seemed prudent to try and figure out what he wanted to tell me instead. Using yes/no questions, writing, and a lot of guessing, I learned that Wes was worried about his dog. He lived alone, and no one was around to take care of the animal. I dealt successfully with the situation, and that succeeded in establishing a therapeutic set for Wes.

Establishing a Communication Context

The clinician establishes a communication context to prepare the patient for a conversation. In the conversation, the clinician and the patient function as receivers and senders of messages. During the early post-onset period, the patient will be most interested in talking about personal issues (e.g., going home, returning to work, the family, health, and finances). Discussing these concerns requires the clinician to have some personal knowledge about the patient's situation. Should the clinician not have the necessary information to communicate with the patient about these issues, other, less personal topics *shared* by the clinician and the patient can be used to establish a conversational context. For example, how could anyone living in or around Boston not be able to converse about the Red Sox, the Patriots, or the "Big Dig?" Certainly, I would be hard-pressed to find a patient in Lexington that would not be able to talk about Kentucky basketball. Also, communicative contexts do not always need to be pre-established. An enterprising clinician can establish a communicative context on the "spur of the moment" by using humor, emotion, or absurdity. Further, different perceptual props and items in the patient's room (e.g., maps, pictures, newspapers, pictures of family, and books) can be used to establish contexts for communication. In a pinch, general topics (e.g., the weather, upcoming holiday, or quality of hospital food) also can be used to create a communicative context. Table 18-3 provides several examples of communication contexts and what type of information stimulated their creation.

Improving Comprehension

Auditory processing involves comprehension of spoken messages and their retention in memory. Most would agree that disorders of auditory processing in persons with aphasia reflect difficulties understanding spoken messages that are not attributable to sensory, (hearing loss), cognitive, or attention deficits (Boller, Kim, & Mack, 1977). Clinical diagnosis of Wernicke's aphasia is based on the patient's performance on receptive language tests of standardized aphasia test batteries (Boatman, 2002). Two models of auditory processing have received widespread attention in the aphasia literature. The bottom-up model suggests that understanding a message is the cumulative result of analyzing the sounds of an utterance (phonemes), combining the sounds into word representations, retrieving the meanings of the words, and constructing a mental representation for the meaning of the message (Brookshire, 2003). The top-down model has more to do with how listeners comprehend messages in naturalistic conversations. Here, the starting point is the knowledge shared by listeners in the communication situation. This shared knowledge leads to the development of inferences and expectations. The result is that participants interpret what they hear in the conversation on the basis of what they know.

TABLE 18–3

Establishing Communication Contexts

Strategy	Stimulus	Clinician Comment	Patient Response
Shared knowledge	Clinician learns from chart review that she and the patient share the same birthday	"I learned that you were born on the same day as I was."	"Oh wow, October 7 too."
Bedside prop	Picture of patient's family on the bedside table	"You have beautiful children."	"Right." [looks at picture] "Three of them."
Emotion/humor	Clinician notices patient is not eating a rather unappetizing meal	"Are you really going to eat that crap?" "I bet you would prefer a steak."	"Oh yeah. I gotta." "Right rare." [gestures thickness of steak]
Spur of the moment	Sees the patient is wearing a ring from Stanford	"Good-looking ring on your finger. Does Stanford have a good team this year?"	"I think all the way."

During the early post-onset period, the patient's comprehension deficits are relatively severe. For some patients, it is difficult—if not impossible—to work on comprehension with structured tasks, particularly at the single-word and sentence level. Working to improve comprehension in conversational contexts is a better approach to use at this time. With the context-based approach, this involves (1) identifying and manipulating linguistic and temporal variables to improve comprehension in conversations, (2) encouraging the patient to take responsibility for comprehension, and (3) training caregivers how to talk to the patient using demonstration and modeling.

Linguistic Variables

The aphasia literature indicates that linguistic variables can be manipulated to improve comprehension of spoken messages. Normal speakers do this naturally in relation to whom they are speaking. For example, when talking with my 99-year-old father, I do things that the aphasia literature shows improve the auditory comprehension of persons with aphasia. I use short, syntactically simple, plausible sentences that do not contain unfamiliar or "big" words. The aphasia literature on auditory comprehension, as reviewed by several writers (Boller et al., 1977; Marshall, 2002), suggests these tactics facilitate auditory comprehension for persons with aphasia (Marshall, 2002). Comprehension is improved in other ways as well. Some of these include:

- Highlighting the main ideas of what is being talked about in relationship to less important details (Brookshire & Nicholas, 1982, 1984, 1993; Wegner, Brookshire, & Nicholas, 1984).

- Giving added prosodic stress to the important words of the message so that they stand out (Kimelman & McNeil, 1987; Pashek & Brookshire, 1982; Swinney, Zurif, & Cutler, 1980).

- Stating information directly (e.g., "Time to eat. It's six o'clock.") rather than indirectly (e.g., "Now it's time for dinner, and we better go in to eat.") so that the patient does not have to make inferences about implied information (Katsuki-Nakamura, Brookshire, & Nicholas, 1988; Nicholas & Brookshire, 1995).

- Using repetition and appropriate synonyms to create lexical ties to link the information of a message together (e.g., "Susan and Andy got out of the car. Susan wore a blue dress. Andy wore a black tuxedo.") (Brookshire, 2003; Halliday & Hasan, 1976).

- Using repetition, paraphrasing, and expansion to increase message redundancy (Gardner, Albert, & Weintraub, 1975; Graville & LaPointe, 1983; West & Kaufman, 1972).

Temporal Variables

People with aphasia like to talk to clinicians. This may be because clinicians adjust certain temporal variables to help the patient understand what is said. This was seen in a novel experiment (Salvatore, Strait, & Brookshire, 1975) that compared speech rates of experienced and inexperienced clinicians giving Token Test commands to patients with severe and mild aphasia. The experienced clinicians intuitively slowed their rate of speech when giving the commands to the severe, but not the mild, patients; the inexperienced clinicians did not make these differential adjustments. Similar to what it tells us about manipulating linguistic components of messages, the aphasia literature provides information about the effects of temporal manipulations on auditory comprehension of persons with aphasia:

- Patients benefit when spoken to at slightly slower, but not unnatural, rates of speech (Cermak & Moreines, 1976; Lasky, Weidner, & Johnson, 1976; Pashek & Brookshire, 1982; Weidner & Lasky, 1976).
- Rate slowing is best achieved by inserting brief pauses at syntactic boundaries within sentences (Fehst & Brookshire, 1980; Salvatore, 1979). This serves to group information into meaningful "chunks," and it permits the patient to catch up to facilitate storage and processing of the message.
- Attention deficits may cause the patient to miss the initial portions of message and/or not pick up shifts in topic, a problem referred to as "slow rise time" (Brookshire, 1974). These deficits can be compensated for by alerting the patient to an incoming message. This helps the patient to reallocate his or her attention and may improve comprehension (Campbell & McNeil, 1983; Loverso & Prescott, 1981; Marshall & Thistlethwaite, 1977).

Finding the Hole in the Screen

To understand how the clinician might manipulate linguistic and temporal variables in a conversational context to maximize comprehension, imagine you are looking at a screen at which someone has thrown mud. You probably would see that some of the squares were plugged with mud but that others were open. Consider that the message sender, in this case the clinician, is on one side of the screen and that the patient with Wernicke's aphasia, Pete, is on the other. For Pete to understand the clinician's message, it needs to be sent through an "open square." If the message hits a "plugged square," Pete will not comprehend it. The clinician's challenge is to manipulate linguistic and temporal variables so as to get the message through an "open hole" so that the patient will comprehend it. This is shown in the following example of a conversation with a patient with Wernicke's aphasia centering on the patient's family. In the example, the bolded information provides a rationale for what the clinician is attempting to accomplish:

Clinician: I would like to talk to you about your family. **(Establish context)**
Patient: Oh boy.
Clinician: I know you have a *large* family [presents written word "FAMILY"]. **(Stress; visual supplement)**
Patient: Oh, my family, well it's a big one.
Clinician: I understand you have quite a few children. How many do you have? **(Increased redundancy)**
Patient: Let me see, Tony, Markee, Martee, Muckee—Oh no.
Clinician: That's a hard word to say, but I'm interested in HOW MANY [stresses this word]: four, five, six [gestures higher]. **(Redirect to topic; stress; gesture supplement)**

Patient: No more than that [holds up 10 fingers].
Clinician: Wow, 10 kids. That must keep you busy. All boys? **(Humor; syntactic simplification)**
Patient: No way, no way. Lots of girls [holds up seven fingers].
Clinician: Seven girls. That means you have three boys [holds up three fingers]. **(Verify, gesture supplementation)**
Patient: Yep, three of them.
Clinician: I understand one of your *boys* is quite *famous*. **(Stress key words; put words at the end of the sentence)**
Patient: Huh? [looking quizzical] What did you say?
Clinician: I'm glad you asked me to repeat that question. Any time. I was asking about your FAMOUS son. **(Reinforce for asking for repeat; stress word famous; redundancy)**
Patient: Oh, you mean Buddig, Bodie, Booby.
Clinician: Right, Buddy. I understand he's a rather good football player? [Buddy is really a baseball player.] **(Give false information to help patient integrate and consolidate response)**
Patient: Not that one, the other one.
Clinician: Sorry, wrong sport. You mean golf? **(Humor; again give information to integrate and consolidate response)**
Patient: Nope.
Clinician: Tennis? **(Humor; continue to consolidate and integrate)**
Patient: Get out of here.
Clinician: Baseball? **(Syntactic simplification; one word; salient word)**
Patient: That would be the one. He's a [gestures pitching motion] you know.
Clinician: A pitcher? Wow. Is he right or left handed? **(Emotion and facial expression; redundancy)**
Patient: One of these [gestures with his left hand].

In the example provided, the clinician established the context by telling the patient that the conversation would be about his family. Once the patient understood this, the clinician selectively manipulated linguistic and timing variables (see bolded text) to work on comprehension. Because the objective was to improve the patient's comprehension, the clinician paid little attention to the production errors, and only short verbal responses were required. The clinician noted those manipulations that were helpful in getting messages "through the open holes of the screen" and made adjustments accordingly. For patients with Wernicke's aphasia and severe comprehension deficits, many holes of the screen will be plugged at first, but as comprehension improves, more squares in the screen will open. During the early post-onset period, much of the work done to maximize comprehension for the patient with Wernicke's aphasia is a trial-and-error process. As treatment progresses, the tactics that aid—and hinder—comprehension become clearer, and some strategies are abandoned and others retained and expanded on.

Taking Responsibility for Comprehension

Patients with Wernicke's aphasia look and move perfectly normally. Sometimes, they pretend to understand so that the listener will not know they have aphasia. Signs of pretending to understand include vigorous bobbing of the head "yes" and lots of "uh-huh's." A necessary part of improving the patient's comprehension integral to the context-based approach involves encouraging the patient to take responsibility for comprehending what is said. At first, clinician need to demonstrate what they want the patient to do. Thus, the clinician might (1) ask for a repetition (e.g., "Could you run that by me again?"), (2) give the patient a quizzical look to indicate the patient has not been understood, (3) verify what the patient says by paraphrasing the message (e.g., "You said your wife is coming at three o'clock? It's almost here."), or (4) ask a rhetorical question (e.g., "When is your wife coming?"). The clinician also promotes the patient taking responsibility for comprehension by liberally reinforcing the patient's requests for repetitions and use of verification strategies. There also may be times when the patient cannot listen anymore, because his or her auditory system is overloaded. In such cases, the patient needs to withdraw from the competitive listening situation and take a break. The clinician needs to reassure that patient that it's all right to take a break from listening and that this may help in the long run.

Training Caregivers

The patient with Wernicke's aphasia will have more conversations with family, friends, and other people than with the speech-language pathologist. To improve the patient's comprehension in conversations outside the therapy room, these individuals need to be trained how to talk to the patient. Specifically, this involves the clinician teaching them how to do what the aphasia literature tells us to do that helps in comprehension.

It will not help to tell these communication partners that the "test results" suggest the patient has comprehension problems. A study by Czvik (1977) found that family members tended to disagree with the speech-language pathologist's test results documenting the patient's comprehension deficits and viewed aphasia as an expressive problem only. It is necessary for clinicians to show, though demonstration and modeling, what they want family, staff, and friends to do. This is powerful therapy, and it is apparent that good coaching helps.

Several recent studies have provided empirical evidence that a variety of conversational partners can be trained how to talk to people with aphasia and that training improves the information transaction of persons with aphasia (Hickey, Bourgeios, & Olswang, 2004; Hopper, Holland, & Rewenga, 2002; Kagan, Black, Duchan, Simmons-Mackie, & Square, 2001; Legg, Young, & Bryer, 2005; Lyon et al., 1997; Purdy & Hindenlang, 2005; Simmons-Mackie, Kearns, & Potechin, 2005). When the training involves professional staff, clinicians may want to refer to a recent paper by Marshall and English (2004) that provides functional strategies physical therapists can use to enhance the auditory comprehension of persons with aphasia in the physical therapy gym. This is practical information that can easily be posted in the clinic and used in providing in-service training for staff.

Improving Information Exchange

Speech output of patients with Wernicke's aphasia may be unchecked. Excessive speech flow is associated with a "rambling" style of communication, which seems to occur when the patient's comprehension deficits are severe and talking is less punitive than listening (Marshall, 1983). If the patient's speech output is markedly defective, a situation is created in which the "defective utterances" are fed back to an impaired auditory system, a condition I have referred to in the past as "the garbage-out/garbage-in cycle" (Marshall, 1994). Information exchange also can be impeded by (1) perseverations, (2) pervasive word-finding difficulties, (3) lack of or excessive self-correction, and (4) prolonged circumlocution.

Breaking the Cycle

A "stop" strategy can be used to break up the garbage-out/garbage-in cycle. This involves directing patients to listen to themselves, stop when they make an error, and try to correct themselves. At first, the clinician may need to signal the patient to stop and say, "What do you need to do now?" Ultimately, the goal is to have the patient identify and correct his or her errors, first in treatment and then outside the clinic. At times, merely stopping the patient from talking so much, encouraging shorter replies, and framing questions so that answers are within his or her capabilities will suffice.

Some patients, however, are not able to benefit from the stop strategy, because their comprehension and self-monitoring skills are too impaired. Martin (1981a) offers an alternative. He suggests that, rather than stopping patients and having them try to correct an error, the clinician should translate a patient's defective utterance as best possible. (This often is easy to do, because the clinician is working in a context.) The clinician's translation and ensuing paraphrasing or modeling of the defective utterance in a correct form gives the patient some positive feedback for communicative adequacy (getting the message across) and breaks the garbage-out/garbage-in cycle. For example:

Patient [waving an issue of the *American Kennel Club* Magazine]: Here's the one smasher, master boy, oh nuts! It's there, where is it? My caster, the ones out there where I live. I know it. What's wrong with me? [Pause]. Smash. M-A-T-T-E-R. Matteree. Oh, God.

Clinician: I understand you are a dog breeder. What types of dogs do you raise?

Patient [opening the magazine]: Well they're not in here but they are big and mean. [Opens the page to show Bulldogs.] Almost like this, but bigger. Smasbees, masters, mastees, on nuts. Why can't I say it? [now frustrated]

Clinician Do you mean Bull Mastiffs? They are big fellows?

Patient Bull Mastiffs, Bull Mastiffs, that's it. You got it. Those are my boys. [now enthusiastic]

Clinician: Very protective animals?

Patient: Oh you bet, they'll bite your head off if you mess with me.

In the above example, the *American Kennel Club* magazine was the prompt that established the communicative context. The clinician's knowledge of the situation and the patient's interests in dogs allowed him to interpret the patient's defective utterances and break the cycle.

Perseveration

Perseveration is the repetition of a response when a new response is called for. For example, I asked Jim to tell me about his work. He replied, "I own a flower shop." Then, I asked, "Do you have a family?" and he said "Yes, I have a flower shop." Wepman (1972) believed that perseveration was the result of not taking enough time to consolidate and integrate a response. He suggested that the mind operates like a camera shutter. When the shutter is open, stimulation is possible. If the shutter is closed, however, new information cannot be processed, and calling for a new response will result in perseveration. He suggested that clinicians take time to consolidate and integrate the patient's accurate response before calling for a new response to reduce perseveration. With Jim, I could have done this by following up his correct response with questions such as "How's business?" and "What's your busy time of the year?" Helm-Estabrooks, Emery, and Albert (1987) also have proposed a mechanism for treating perseveration errors in aphasia that highlights the fact that a new response is called for.

Anomic Difficulties

Anomic difficulties are a hallmark of patients with Wernicke's aphasia in conversation and whenever a specific word is needed. Anomic struggle takes place at both the pre- and post-lexical levels. The latter suggests that the patient is having problems accessing word meanings and/or forms. For example, if the target word is "Wal-Mart," the patient might produce a semantic error ("Rite Aid"), a description ("Where we buy medicine cheap"), a phonemic approximation ("Swallmart—that's almost it."), or an indefinite word ("the place"). Post-lexical anomic difficulties are reflected in a variety of behaviors that suggest the patient has accessed the word's meaning and form but cannot map the phonologic shapes of the word onto the lexical entries for outputting. For example, if the patient is having problems coming up with the word "pillow," he or she might make several near-attempts to produce it, write the word or a portion of it, or point to the pillow on the bed. Finally, some patients simply choose to talk around the anomic difficulty (circumlocution) or simply say, "I don't know." Anomic difficulties of the patient with Wernicke's aphasia can be dealt with indirectly (by teaching compensations) and directly.

Indirect Approaches

Indirect approaches minimize the impact of anomic struggle by keeping the focus on communication. The clinician or trained communication partner makes "on the spot" decisions as to how best to keep communication or track—or get it back on track—when anomic difficulties threaten to interfere. Golper and Rau (1983) have described this as "taking your cue from the patient."

The first example in Table 18-4 shows that the clinician has determined the patient's struggle will not result in successful production of the word "cigarette." The clinician has elected to *fill in* the blank, terminate Joanne's 3-minute effort, and move on. In the second example shown in Table 18-4, the clinician sensed that the patient was close to producing the target word. This clinician's decision was that it

---

TABLE 18–4

Examples of Anomic Struggle in Conversations that Require a Clinician Decision as How Best to Keep Communication on Track (Target Word in Parenthesis)

(Cigarette) Patient PJ:	"You smoke a cig, a sigg, oh what is it? I want one now. Smittring, ciggerthing, almost, what is it called? You put in your mouth and smuch it. Smucher, smuch, smukker, chitter, No." [clinician fills in]
(Alaska) Patient HB:	"I always wanted to go to Alasta, where its cold, Alasta, Alaskan, Alasker." [pause; clinician signals to go on] "Alaska."
(Coffee) Patient BB:	"Well since my heart went bad, my doctor said no more cokkee, I mean coffee. It's not good for my blood pressure." [clinician lets it go]

was better to let the patient work through the difficulty. The clinician gave the patient an *encouraging gesture* that signaled him to keep going. Encouragement could be verbal (e.g., "You're almost there."). The last example in Table 18-4 shows that the clinician has decided the patient has successfully communicated that "he does not drink coffee because of a heart condition." This clinician deduced that the patient communicated successfully what he wanted to say and elected to *let it go*. Thus, the clinician said, "Oh, yes, I drink too much coffee myself" to give him feedback that he had communicated his message adequately. It also has been shown that information provided by patients with aphasia as they search for specific words (self-cues) could be used to make decisions to fill in the missing word, encourage the patient to keep trying to produce the target word, or accept what has been produced and move on (Tompkins & Marshall, 1982; Tompkins, Scharp, & Marshall, 2006).

Wepman's content-centered therapy also puts communication at the forefront (Martin, 1981b; Wepman, 1972). In this approach, the clinician and the patient discuss topics of prestroke interest to the patient. Wepman recommends ignoring the patient's struggles to find specific words and keeping the discussion on track by reflecting back the individual's intended thoughts and paraphrasing when anomic difficulties occur. His rationale for this unique, but empirically untested, approach is that speech should be the "handmaiden of thought" and not visa versa (Wepman, 1976).

Compensations

Using alternative modalities of communication (e.g., drawing, gesture, writing, and pointing) is highly recommended for individuals with nonfluent aphasia, primarily because these patients generate little speech. It is also helpful, however, for the patient with Wernicke's aphasia to be able to communicate using other modalities if talking fails. Some studies show that these patients make little use of alternative modalities (Marshall, Freed, & Phillips, 1997), but reports also show that patients with Wernicke's aphasia can use gestures (Simmons & Zorthian, 1979) and body movements (Ahlsen, 1991) to aid communication. In treating many patients with Wernicke's aphasia, I have seen individuals compensate for what they could not immediately communicate in several ways. Some examples include going through things in a series (e.g., numbers, days of the week, months, or names of family members) to come up with specific words, writing, gesturing, and pointing. I remember that Paul used to write words that were important to him on small scraps of paper. Then, when he needed one of these words during therapy, he would pull all the scraps from his jacket pocket and search through them diligently. This worked for Paul and suggests that the best guide to using compensations for patients with Wernicke's aphasia is whether the compensatory efforts aid or hinder communication.

Direct Approaches

Numerous direct approaches to the treatment of anomia have been described in the aphasia literature (Nickels, 2002). Three specific methods—circumlocution-induced naming, personalized cueing, and semantic feature analysis—are presented here. These do not necessarily fit within the context-based treatment approach. Many patients with Wernicke's aphasia are concerned about their naming errors, however, and the end-point for most of them is anomic aphasia. Thus, some specific methods for treatment of naming may be useful in therapy for Wernicke's aphasia, especially as the early post-onset period comes to an end and the patient is able to be treated directly.

Circumlocution-induced naming is a novel approach to the treatment of anomia. A recent report described its use in treatment of a patient with pervasive anomia (Francis, Clark, & Humphreys, 2002). When the patient could not supply the name of a picture, she was encouraged to "talk around" the topic to try and access the specific name. When she had trouble, the therapist joined in the conversation and reinforced the information provided by the patient, but the therapist did not provide the name. During therapy, the therapist did not provide the name. Results of the study revealed improved naming from pre- to posttest assessments.

Personalized cueing is a procedure for treating anomia that has been used successfully with patients having a variety of types of aphasia (Freed, Celery, & Marshall, 2004; Freed & Marshall, 1995; Marshall & Freed, 2006). When using this method, the clinician and patient work together to create a personally relevant associational cue to help the patient remember an important word. For example, in one study (Freed et al., 2004), a patient created the cue "old red one" to help her remember the word "bathrobe." In therapy, the cue and the target word are repeatedly paired. The success of personalized cueing is assessed with naming probes administered at later points in time when the cues are not provided. Several studies have shown that the benefits of this training are highly durable and result in improved naming of target words as long as 6 months after the end of treatment.

Semantic feature analysis is a procedure for treating anomic deficits that has widespread popularity. The patient is presented with a picture that is difficult to name (e.g., a giraffe) and is asked to respond to questions about its semantic features, such as location (Africa), actions (eats leaves), color (brown and yellowish), and characteristics (tall, long neck). Several studies have shown that semantic feature analysis (Boyle, 2004; Boyle & Coelho, 1995, Coelho, McHugh, & Boyle, 2000) and other semantic treatments (Davis, Harrington, & Baynes, 2006; Drew & Thompson, 1999) improve naming and that the benefits of this treatment generalize to untrained words and other speech tasks, such as connected speech. It has been argued that these improvements result from possible repair of a damaged semantic system, increased the specificity of semantic representations, and increased activation of the semantic network surrounding the target word, all of which elevate the word's threshold for being retrieved (Boyle & Coelho, 1995; Hillis, 1998).

Promoting Self-Correction

Wepman (1958) suggested a continuum of self-correction exists for patients with aphasia and that the patient's location on the continuum was predictive of recovery from the disorder. At the lower end are those patients who fail to recognize or attempt to correct their production errors. In the middle are those who make the effort and sometimes succeed. At the upper end are those patients who always make the effort and who usually are successful. Research has shown that patients with Wernicke's aphasia rank last in terms of their frequency and success of verbal self-correction among various aphasia classifications (Marshall & Tompkins, 1982). In a larger sense, self-correction relates to intra- and interpersonal monitoring (Martin, 1981a).

Intrapersonal monitoring involves attention to language structure and usage, such as selection of a word or determination of word order. Interpersonal monitoring refers to the act of attending to signals from the environment and from the communication partner that are important to sustaining communication. These signal indicate when it is appropriate to change roles or follow certain conventions (e.g., be quiet, move closer, or lower one's voice).

Within the context-based approach, the clinician reinforces the patient for appropriate self-monitoring. For example, after a successful self-correction, the clinician might say, "That's great that you changed to a different word." After a successful struggle to produce a specific word, the patient's persistence should be acknowledged (e.g., "I like the way you stuck with that."). If the patient attempts to self-correct but fails, encouragement remains important (e.g., "That word was tough today."). Also important to the promotion of self-monitoring is to acknowledge and ease the patient's concerns about day-to-day variability in performance. For example, George called his wife "Mildred" on one day and addressed her as "Bernice" (his ex-wife's name) on the next. This upset the him, and he said "Mildred, Mildred, Mildred—stupid. I said it yesterday, why not today?" In this case, the clinician needs to help George understand day-to-day fluctuations in word retrieval efforts are a product of the stroke will get better with time.

Other Individual and Group Approaches

Other individual and group treatment approaches also can be used within the context-based approach with the patient who has Wernicke's aphasia. Most of the therapeutic approaches that follow are not exclusive to patients with Wernicke's aphasia. All are applicable to context-based treatment, however, because they emphasize communication and give the patient options to reflect his or her communicative competence.

Promoting Aphasic Communicative Effectiveness

Promoting Aphasic Communicative Effectiveness (Davis, 2005; Davis and Wilcox, 1985), or PACE, was developed to make treatment situations more like natural conversations. The PACE principles include (1) the use of new information, (2) equal participation by patient and clinician as sender and receiver of messages, (3) freedom of communication channel selection (e.g., patient can gesture, write, draw, point, or speak), and (4) giving feedback based on communicative adequacy rather than on production accuracy. In the traditional PACE format, the clinician and patient take turns describing pictures unknown to each other following the PACE principles. Several studies have shown that PACE improves the communicative effectiveness of persons with aphasia (Glindemann, Willmes, Huber, & Springer, 1991; Li, Kitselman, Dusatko, & Spinelli, 1988; Springer, Glindemann, Huber, & Willmes, 1991). This body of research has not focused on patients with Wernicke's aphasia, but PACE could be used with these patients inasmuch as their verbalizations do not always conveying their intended messages (Ahlsen, 1991; Marshall et al., 1997). Also, since PACE was developed, other researchers (Carlomagno, Losanno, Emanuelli, & Casadio, 1991; Pulvermuller & Roth, 1991) have expanded it to incorporate other speech acts (e.g., bargaining, requesting, and arguing) and tasks (e.g., describing pictures, cartoon sequences, and talking about famous people) that fit within context-based approach.

Response Elaboration Training

Response elaboration training (Kearns, 1985, 1986), or RET, is a loose-training procedure based on the premise that highly structured and constrained-task therapies will restrict the patient's use of creative language (Stokes & Baer, 1977). In using RET, the clinician elaborates on the patient's novel utterances with the goal of increasing the length and content of those utterances. Several studies by Kearns and colleagues (Gaddie, Kearns, & Yedor, 1991; Kearns, 1985, 1986; Kearns & Scher, 1989; Kearns & Yedor, 1991; Yedor, Conlon, & Kearns, 1993) have shown that RET increases the verbal productions of speakers with aphasia. A recent study indicated that a modification of RET successfully increased the number of content information units produced in response to picture stimuli by three speakers with chronic apraxia-aphasia (Wambaugh & Martinez, 2000). Although RET has been used sparingly with the patient who has aphasia and is talking, its goal is to facilitate generalized improvement of the patient's ability to elaborate on

TABLE 18–5

How the Game of Blackjack Could Be Used to Work on Improving Word Retrieval and Other Skills

Materials: Cards, betting tokens (e.g., chips, pennies, beans) allocated to clinician (dealer) and client (player).

Representative skills and abilities needed: 1 = attention; 2 = decision making; 3 = simple computation; 4 = auditory comprehension (following simple command); 5 = differential responding verbally or gesturally (e.g., signaling for "hit" or "stay"), 6 = turn taking; 7 = correcting erroneous information

Using the Game of Blackjack as a Treatment Module: Examples of Clinician and Patient Actions

Clinician Actions	Patient Responses	Skills and Abilities
Mixes cards; gives cards to player to cut	Cuts cards; signals he does not want to cut the cards	1, 2
Place your bet	Puts out chips or tokens	1, 2, 4
Deals king and six to patient; shows an ace for dealer	Signals for "hit" or "stay"	1, 2, 3, 5
After "hit" signal, deals a queen to the patient	Turns up cards to show "busted"; pushes money to dealer	2, 3, 5
Deals eight and two to patient; dealer shows queen	Signals for hit and receives an ace; signals he's "just right"	1, 2, 3, 5
Dealer pays patient too much money	Corrects error and gives money back to clinician (dealer)	2, 7
Deals king and ace to patient; dealer shows a four	Turns up cards and smiles; says, "Oh boy."	3, 5
Dealer pays even money instead of the blackjack rate	Patient corrects error	7

conversational topics and share communicative burden. Thus, it seems ideal for use with certain clients with Wernicke's aphasia.

Games

Games provide an excellent resource for working on communication in a context. These might include blackjack, poker, checkers, Monopoly, and other similar games. McDonald and Pearce (1995) have described how the "dice" game can be used to assess pragmatic language skills in patients with closed-head injuries. With their appropriate pragmatic and turn-taking skills, patients with Wernicke's aphasia can work on communicating in a context using such games. An added advantage is that some games provide the opportunity to work on cognitive and executive function skills that support language, such as attention, decision making, and planning. Table 18-5 provides relevant examples of the skills that would be worked on in the game of blackjack.

Reminiscence

Reminiscence therapy (Harris, 1997) capitalizes on the patient's ability to recall and converse about events, people, and places from earlier times. Usually, these are salient events deeply imbedded in one's episodic memories, such as buying a first car, how you met your wife, and what you were doing when the World Trade Center was destroyed. Reminiscence therapy can be used in a group or individual setting.

Problem-Focused Treatment

Problem-solving activities also are suitable for use with the context-based approach to treatment. Marshall (1993) describes a problem-focused group treatment approach that could easily be used to treat, support, and guide patients with less severe Wernicke's aphasia in managing day-to-day communication difficulties. During treatment sessions, group members discuss problems that arise in their daily lives. Members work together to come up with solutions, alternatives, and plans to solve problems. For example, Roy was upset that it now took him more time disassemble and reassemble his furnace than before he had his stroke. His group came up with several organizational strategies to improve his speed. Credit card woes caused another group member (Cecile) to develop hypertension. She failed to read the information on interest when presented with several credit card offers and went over her credit limit. The problem was discussed in the group and resulted in her (1) seeking individual treatment to learn how interest worked, (2) meeting with a consumer credit counselor to develop a plan to pay off the debt, and (3) tearing up her credit cards.

DEVELOPING CONFIDENCE IN THE CONTEXT-BASED APPROACH

Eisenson (1964) defined "language therapy" as a relationship between the clinician and patient in which both recognize and understand that improvement of communication is the purpose and the goal. His view of therapy captures what the context-based approach is designed to do—specifically, to improve communication. To use the context-based approach with confidence, however, clinicians need (1) to select the appropriate measure or measures to document treatment outcomes and (2) to increase their cognitive flexibility as therapists.

Measurement

Many direct and indirect measures are available to document treatment outcomes (Fratalli, 1992, 1998; Marshall, 2000). Direct measures, such as the Amsterdam Nijmegan Everyday Language Test (ANELT) and IFCI (reviewed earlier), require the patient to respond in some way, and the examiner scores those responses. Indirect measures, such as the Functional Independence Measure (1993), or FIM, require the clinician to rate the patient's ability to do certain tasks based on what is known about the patient, but they do not require the patient to do anything.

Regardless of whether the clinician measures treatment outcomes directly on indirectly, the documentation measure must be representative of the treatment given (Marshall, 2000). For the context-based approach, this should be a measure related to conversational success. Using a standardized test, such as the PICA, with a patient who has Wernicke's aphasia and is being treated with the context-based approach would be ill-advised, because success on the PICA is integrally linked to retrieving the labels of 10 common objects that make up the core of the test. Some representative measures of transactional success that can be used to document the effects of context-based treatment follow.

Message Exchange Task

The message exchange task was used in a study of information transfer with four patients with articulatory apraxia (Fawcus & Fawcus, 1990). For this task, the patient is given a message to convey to a partner. The patient is allowed to convey the message in any way that he or she chooses. The patient and the partner interact until consensus is reached. The partner rates the efficiency and speed of message exchange and records how each of the critical elements of the message were conveyed (e.g., pointing, gesture, speech, writing, or drawing). Table 18-6 provides an example.

Interaction Competence Scale

Table 18-7 provides another scale, the interaction competence scale (Garrett & Sittner, 1995), that can easily be used to rate the communication success of the patient with Wernicke's aphasia in a conversational interaction.

TABLE 18–6

Example of Message Exchange Task

Message: I am canceling therapy next week because I have to go to Chicago for my sister's wedding

Step 1. Patient conveys message to partner.

Step 2. Partner translates and notes elements of the message conveyed by speech (S), writing (W), drawing (D), gesture (G), or pointing (P).

Canceling (G) therapy (S) next week (P); wedding (S) in Chicago (P)

Step 3. Partner rates efficiency of message exchange: 4 = highly efficient; 3 = efficient; 2 = somewhat efficient; 1 = inefficient; 0 = no basis for understanding.

Step 4. Partner rates speed of message exchange: 4 = prompt, within normal limits; 3 = delayed, but not noticeable; 2 = markedly delayed; 1 = delay made listener uncomfortable; 0 = message not delivered.

Transactional Success

Ramsberger and Rende (2002) have recently developed a way to measure what has been understood and exchanged at the end of a conversation between persons with aphasia and their conversational partners. Those authors did this by examining the conversations of 14 adults with aphasia about a series of *I Love Lucy* episodes. The participants with aphasia had to relay information about each of the episodes to four different partners. Transactional success was measured by examining the amount and type of information the partners could convey after having a conversation with the patient with aphasia.

Increasing Cognitive Flexibility

Clinicians who like order, control, and certainty may have difficulty working with individuals who have Wernicke's aphasia. In particular, this could be the case during the early post-onset period, when the patient's deficits are most pronounced. Clinicians seeped in the use of structured treatment approaches will not be comfortable with the context-based approach, because it is a treatment demanding flexibility and a willingness to experiment. Flexibility connotes a willingness to switch, to deviate from a plan, and to make on-the-spot decisions to enhance communication. Experimentation involves balancing the science and the art—and having the common sense to focus on what is important to the patient. Importantly, clinicians who choose to use a context-based approach need to free themselves of the guilt associated with conversing with the patient and not evoking a specific number of preselected responses.

TABLE 18–7	

Scale of Interaction Competence

1. How much did the communicator participate in the interaction?

1	2	3	4	5	6	7
none			some			a lot

2. How much of the time was Communicator X able to get his or her message across?

1	2	3	4	5	6	7
none			some			a lot

3. How much of the time did Communicator X take an active role in the interaction by asking questions, generating unsolicited comments, or expressing opinions?

1	2	3	4	5	6	7
none			some			a lot

4. How frequently did Communicator X use different ways of communicating when trying to get his or her message across (e.g., speaking, writing, or Augmentative Alternative Communication (AAC) system)?

1	2	3	4	5	6	7
didn't use methods		used some different methods				used many methods

5. How flexible and strategic was Communicator X when trying to convey messages that were not understood by others?

1	2	3	4	5	6	7
not flexible			some flexibility			very flexible

6. How many communication functions (e.g., asking questions, arguing, giving advice, greeting, or commenting) did the communicator use when conveying messages?

1	2	3	4	5	6	7
none			some			a lot

7. On a scale of 1 to 5, how would you rate Communicator X's total communication ability?

1	2	3	4	5	6	7
poor ability			some ability			good

Cognitive flexibility refers to the ability to shift cognitive set, thought, or attention so as to respond in different and, hopefully, successful ways (Rende, 2000). Cognitive flexibility can be reactive and involve altering one's behavior in response to a situation; it also can be spontaneous and involve considering alternatives and formulating ideas on one's own. Successful communication by persons with aphasia is associated with a greater degree of cognitive flexibility (Chapey, Rigrodsky, & Morrison, 1977; Keil & Kaszniak, 2002; Purdy & Koch, 2005; Wepman, 1972). Patients manifesting this trait recognize their errors, come up with solutions to correct them, and to do what is needed to communicate successfully despite the aphasia. This is what clinicians want them to do.

Cognitive flexibility is important to the patient's success, but clinicians also need to increase their own cognitive flexibility. Patients with aphasia do not use compensatory strategies unless they see the clinician doing the same thing (Simmons-Mackie & Damico, 1997). The patient learns to compensate from the modeling and the demonstrations of the clinician who uses the context-based approach. Using a context-based approach is hard work, because this approach has no script or set of steps to follow. What clinician do, they do based on antecedent events, and this requires continuous decision making. This underscores that using a context-based approach is more than just talking to the patient but, rather, is something that requires a great deal of skill and experience.

FUTURE TRENDS

Before the fourth edition of *Language Intervention Strategies in Adult Aphasia and Related Disorders* was published in 2001, Holland (1995) noted that the crystal ball looked "cloudy" for specialists in neurogenic communication disorders, because the rising costs of health care and the growth of managed care threatened to reduce funding for treatment of aphasia. Holland's fears have been realized. In slightly more than a decade, the crystal ball is no longer just cloudy—the crystal ball is black. Most old-guard clinical aphasiologists remember that, not long ago, aphasia clinicians were under fire from the medical profession, because they lacked empirical data to support the efficacy of aphasia therapy (Darley, 1972). That time has long past. Today, a plethora of group, single-subject design, case reports, and qualitative research demonstrate the benefits of therapy for aphasia (Holland, Fromm, DeRuyter, & Stein, 1996; Robey, 1994, 1998; Robey, Schultz, & Crawford, 1999; Wertz & Irwin, 2001). Nevertheless, funding for therapy remains scarce, prompting Rogers, Alarcon, and Olswang (1999) to describe the present-day situation as ironic.

It is obvious what the future does not hold. This is hope for the U.S. Congress to drop a boatload of money into the hands of service providers to pay for more treatment of persons with aphasia. It is only possible to speculate what could be done in the future to improve things. Three possibilities are discussed here: (1) increasing advocacy for aphasia treatment, (2) directing more research effort at people with acute rather than chronic aphasia, and (3) training future aphasia clinicians for what their jobs will be instead of what those jobs used to be.

Advocacy

People get terribly frustrated with aphasia, but they do not die from it (Marshall, 1997). Regrettably, an international survey of public awareness of aphasia indicated most individuals have little knowledge of what aphasia is (Simmons-Mackie, Code, Armstrong, Stiegler, & Elman, 2002). Another study examined the frequency with which the word "aphasia" occurred in newspapers in comparison to other chronic conditions (Elman, Olgar, & Elman, 2000). Results indicated that "aphasia" was found far less often than references to less frequently occurring conditions, such as Parkinson's disease and muscular dystrophy. So perhaps, as recommended by Elman and colleagues (2000), something that we will see in the future will be greater unification and effort from those affected by aphasia (e.g., patient, families, friends, and professionals) to "energize and pressure politicians and insurance companies" (p. 459) to increase funding for aphasia treatment.

Research

More aphasia research has not increased funding for treatment of the disorder. In fact, things are worse now than when Holland looked into the crystal ball in 1995 and the Balanced Budget Act was passed in 1997. Perhaps aphasia research has had little effect on funding because it has not, for several years, focused on the patient and the family during the early post-onset period, when concern is greatest about the impact of aphasia on the future, but has focused instead on those living with chronic aphasia who may have adjusted to the condition. It appears that the only clinicians who are able to see patients with chronic aphasia work in universities, VA hospitals, or socialized medical-care systems; these are the people doing most of the research on aphasia. This research, however, is being carried out with very chronic patients. Of course, this research is valuable. Rarely, however, front-line clinicians are able to treat patients with aphasia much past the early post-onset period (1–3 months), because no money is available to pay for it. Ongoing research is studying people with aphasia who are being provided pharmacological and other medical treatments shortly after the onset of aphasia to minimize the impact of brain injury (Hillis & Heider, 2002; Hillis et al., 2002; Shisler, Baylis, & Frank, 2000; Walker-Batson et al., 2001). Thus, the future may see more aphasia treatment research being done closer to the time of the patient's stroke, and perhaps, the results of that research will impact funding decisions.

Training

Hopefully, the future will see graduate students being trained for the jobs they will have rather than for the jobs of the past. This might involve the following:

1. Introducing students to contemporary measures of assessment that capture how treatment impacts the patient's day-to-day life and psychosocial functioning.
2. Teaching students how to talk to physicians to help them understand that communication is as important as swallowing.
3. Educating students about and providing them with experiences in group treatment.
4. Including information about social approaches to treatment of aphasia in the graduate curriculum.
5. Promoting altruistic behavior in students to stimulate the initiation of support groups and involvement in groups such as the National Aphasia Association.
6. Developing mechanisms to keep abreast of the aphasia literature, which continues to grow exponentially.

1. Neurological damage in Wernicke's aphasia affects the posterior language zones, causing aphasia, but spares the primary motor cortex. Clients with Wernicke's aphasia therefore do not suffer motor deficits, seldom need physical and/or occupational therapy, and are discharged early from the hospital.

2. Clients with Wernicke's aphasia reflect marked differences in terms of auditory comprehension in situations with and without contextual support. Most clients will perform far better in a conversational situation than on an aphasia test.

3. Individuals with Wernicke's aphasia have been regarded as having poorer prognoses for improvement following language therapy compared with patients who have nonfluent aphasias. Largely, this is because improvement following treatment of aphasia is dependent on changes in test scores on standardized aphasia tests that may not capture improvements made by clients with Wernicke's aphasia.

4. Treatment outcome research and treatment programs for persons with aphasia rarely address clients with Wernicke's aphasia. This may result from the fact that "talking aphasic people" are able to get by in most communicative situations and do not seek further treatment beyond the basic coverage provided by most health-care programs.

5. Training of students and successful use of a context-based approach with clients who have Wernicke's aphasia requires knowledge of personal biographical information about the client that can be used to create client-relevant assessment and treatment procedures.

6. Successful therapy for the client with Wernicke's aphasia is highly dependent on the flexibility of the clinician and on his or her the willingness to try different approaches rather than any single treatment or combination of treatments.

7. Group treatment is appropriate for clients with Wernicke's aphasia and may offer a long-term solution to the management of this condition.

1. Describe how you would convince a client with Wernicke's aphasia about to be discharged home 2 days after a stroke that it was vital to return to the hospital for an outpatient evaluation of his communication deficits.

2. Prepare an interactive in-service for the rehabilitation staff on how to maximize auditory comprehension for a specific client with Wernicke's aphasia.

3. Create verbatim transcriptions for descriptions of the cookie-theft picture from clients with moderate Wernicke's and Broca's aphasia. Describe how these two transcriptions differ in terms of phonologic, semantic, and syntactical features.

4. Prepare a list of home assignments for a client with Wernicke's aphasia that would supplement your treatment goals and improve generalization.

5. Describe how you would carry out a program of conversational coaching that would improve communication between clients with Wernicke's aphasia and their spouses.

6. Mr. Jones, a man with Wernicke's aphasia now a year post-onset, loves to play poker every week with his friends. They stopped inviting him to their games after his stroke. Develop a plan of action for facilitating Mr. Jones returning to this formerly enjoyed activity.

7. Describe the types of responses on a naming test would you expect from a patient with Wernicke's aphasia that would be reflective of semantic, phonologic, and post-lexical errors.

8. Prepare a series of tasks that you could use to measure improvement in receptive and expressive functions for a client with Wernicke's aphasia, and describe how these will be used to measure therapeutic outcomes.

References

Ahlsen, E. (1991). Body communication as compensation for speech in a Wernicke's aphasic—A longitudinal study. *Journal of Communication Disorders, 24*, 1–12.

Author (1993). *Functional Independence Measure.* Buffalo, NY: State University of New York at Buffalo Research Foundation.

Bachman, D. L., & Albert, M. A. (1990). Auditory comprehension in aphasia. In H. Goodglass (Ed.), *Handbook of neuropsychology* (pp. 281–306). New York: Elsevier.

Benson, D. F. (1967). Fluency in aphasia: Correlation with radioactive scan localization. *Cortex, 1*, 373–392.

Blomert, L., Kean, M. L., Koster, C., & Schokker, J. (1994). Amsterdam-Nijmengen Everyday Language Test: Construction, reliability, and validity. *Aphasiology, 8*, 381–397.

Boatman, D. (2002). Diagnosis and treatment of auditory disorders. In A. E. Hollis (Ed.), *Handbook of adult language disorders* (pp. 281–295). London: Psychology Press.

Boller, F., Kim, Y., & Mack, J. (1977). Auditory comprehension in aphasia. In H. Whitaker & H. Whitaker (Eds.), *Studies in neurolinguistics* (pp. 1–64). New York: Academic Press.

Boyle, M. (2004) Semantic feature analysis treatment for anomia in two fluent aphasia syndromes. *American Journal of Speech Language Pathology, 13*, 236–249.

Boyle, M., & Coelho, C. (1995). Application of semantic feature analysis as a treatment for aphasic dysnomia. *American Journal of Speech Language Pathology, 4*, 94–98.

Brookshire, R. (2003). *Introduction to neurogenic communication disorders.* St. Louis, MO: Mosby.

Brookshire, R. H. (1974). Differences in responding to auditory-verbal materials among aphasic patients. *Acta Symbolica, 1,* 1–18.

Brookshire, R. H., & Nicholas, L. E. (1982). Comprehension of directly and indirectly picture verbs by aphasic and nonaphasic listeners. In R. H. Brookshire (Ed.), *Clinical aphasiology: Conference proceedings* (pp. 200–206). Minneapolis: BRK.

Brookshire, R. H., & Nicholas, L. E. (1984). Comprehension of directly and indirectly stated main ideas and details in the discourse of brain-damaged and non-brain-damaged listeners. *Brain and Language, 21,* 21–36.

Brookshire, R. H., & Nicholas, L. E. (1993). *The Discourse Comprehension Test.* Minneapolis: BRK.

Byng, S., & Duchan, J. F. (2005). Social model philosophies and principles: Their applications to therapies for aphasia. *Aphasiology, 19,* 906–922.

Campbell, T. F., & McNeil, M. R. (1983). Effects of presentation rate and divided attention on auditory comprehension in acquired childhood aphasia. Abstract. In R. H. Brookshire (Ed.), *Clinical aphasiology: Conference proceedings* (pp. 193–194). Minneapolis: BRK.

Carlomagno, S., Losanno. N., Emanuelli, S., & Casadio, P. (1991). Expressive language recovery or improved communication skills: Effects of PACE therapy on aphasics' referential communication and story telling. *Aphasiology, 5,* 419–424.

Cermak, L., & Moreines, J. (1976). Verbal retention deficits in aphasic and amnesic patients. *Brain and Language, 3,* 16–27.

Chapey, R., Rigrodsky, S., & Morrison, E. M. (1977). Aphasia: A divergent semantic interpretation. *Journal of Speech and Hearing Disorders, 42,* 287–295.

Coelho, C., McHugh, R. E., & Boyle, M. (2000). Semantic feature analysis as a treatment for aphasic dysnomia: A replication. *Aphasiology, 14,* 133–142.

Czvik, P. (1977). Assessment of family attitudes towards aphasic patients with severe auditory processing disorders. In R. Brookshire (Ed.), *Clinical aphasiology: Conference proceedings* (pp. 160–164). Minneapolis: BRK.

Darley, F. L. (1972). The efficacy of language rehabilitation in aphasia. *Journal of Speech and Hearing Disorders, 37,* 3–21.

Davis, A. G. (2005). Pace revisited. *Aphasiology, 19,* 21–38.

Davis, A. G., & Wilcox, M. J. (1985). *Adult aphasia: Applied pragmatics.* San Diego: College Hill Press.

Davis, C., Harrington, G., & Baynes, K. (2006). Intensive semantic treatment in fluent aphasia: A pilot study with fMRI. *Aphasiology, 20,* 59–83.

Doyle, P. J., Goda, A. J., & Spencer, K. A. (1995). The communicative informativeness and efficiency of connected discourse by adults with aphasia under structured and conversational sampling conditions. *American Journal of Speech Language Pathology, 4,* 130–134.

Drew, R., & Thompson, C. K. (1999). Model-based semantic treatment for naming deficits in aphasia. *Journal of Speech, Language, and Hearing Research, 42,* 972–989.

Eisenson, J. (1964). Aphasia: A point of view as to the disorder and the factors that determine prognosis for recovery. *International Journal of Neurology, 4,* 287–295.

Elman, R. J., Olgar, J., & Elman, S. H. (2000). Aphasia: Awareness, advocacy, and activism. *Aphasiology, 14,* 455–460.

Fawcus, M., & Fawcus R. (1990). Information transfer in four cases of articulatory apraxia. *Aphasiology, 4,* 207–211.

Fehst, C. A., & Brookshire, R. H. (1980). Aphasic subjects' use of within-sentence pause time. In R. Brookshire (Ed.), *Clinical aphasiology: Conference proceedings* (pp. 67–75). Minneapolis: BRK.

Francis, D. R., Clark, N., & Humphreys, G. W. (2002). Circumlocution-induced naming: A treatment for effecting generalization in anomia? *Aphasiology, 16,* 243–260.

Fratalli, C. M. (1992). Functional assessment of communication: Merging public policy with clinical views. *Aphasiology, 6,* 63–82.

Fratalli, C. M. (1998). *Measuring clinical outcomes in speech-language pathology.* New York: Thieme.

Freed, D. B., Celery, K., & Marshall, R. C. (2004). Effectiveness of personalized and phonological cueing on long-term naming performance by aphasic subjects: A clinical investigation. *Aphasiology, 18,* 743–757.

Freed, D. B., & Marshall, R. C. (1995). The effects of personalized cueing on the long-term naming of realistic visual stimuli. *American Journal of Speech Language Pathology, 4,* 105–108.

Friederici, A. (1983). Aphasics' perception of words in sentential context: Some real-time processing evidence. *Neuropsychologia, 21,* 351–358.

Gaddie, A., Kearns, K. P., & Yedor, K. (1991). A qualitative analysis of response elaboration training effects. *Clinical Aphasiology, 19,* 171–183.

Gardner, H., Albert, M. L., & Weintraub, S. (1975). Comprehending a word: The influence of speed and redundancy on auditory comprehension in aphasia. *Cortex, 11,* 155–162.

Garrett, K., & Sittner, M. (1995). *Perceptions of interactional competence of persons with aphasia.* Paper presented at the annual convention of the American Speech-Language-Hearing Association, Orlando, FL, November.

Geschwind, N. (1970). The organization of language and the brain. *Science, 170,* 940–944.

Glindemann, R., Willmes, K., Huber, W., & Springer, L. (1991). The efficacy of modeling in PACE-therapy. *Aphasiology, 5,* 425–429.

Goldenberg, G., & Spatt, J. (1994). Influence of size and site of cerebral lesions on spontaneous recovery of aphasia and success of language therapy. *Brain and Language, 47,* 684–698.

Golper, L., & Rau, M. T. (1983). Systematic analysis of cueing strategies in aphasia: Taking your cue from the patient. In R. H. Brookshire (Ed.), *Clinical aphasiology: Conference proceedings* (pp. 52–61). Minneapolis: BRK.

Goodglass, H. (1981). The syndromes of aphasia: Similarities and differences in neurolinguistic features. *Topics in Language Disorders, 1,* 1–14.

Goodglass, H., & Kaplan, E. (1983). *The Assessment of aphasia and related disorders* (2nd ed.). Philadelphia: Lea & Febiger.

Gravel, J., & LaPointe, L. L. (1983). Length and redundancy in health care providers' speech during interaction with aphasic and nonaphasic listeners. In R. Brookshire (Ed.), *Clinical aphasiology: Conference proceedings* (pp. 211–217). Minneapolis: BRK.

Gray, L., Hoyt, P., Mogil, S., & Lefkowitz, N. (1977). A comparison of clinical tests of yes/no questions in aphasia. In R. H. Brookshire (Ed.), *Clinical aphasiology: Conference proceedings* (pp. 265–268). Minneapolis: BRK.

Green, G. (1984). Communication in aphasia therapy. Some of the procedures and issues involved. *British Journal of Disorders of Communication, 19,* 35–46.

Halliday, M., & Hasan, R. (1976) *Cohesion in English.* New York: Longman.

Harris, J. L. (1997). Reminiscence: A culturally and developmentally appropriate language intervention for older adults. *American Journal of Speech-Language Pathology, 6,* 19–26.

Helm-Estabrooks, N, Emery, P., & Albert, M. (1987) Treatment of aphasic perseveration (TAP) program. *Archives of Neurology, 44,* 1253–1255.

Hickey, E. M., Bourgeois, M. S., & Olswang, L. B. (2004). Effects of training volunteers to converse with nursing home residents with aphasia. *Aphasiology, 18,* 625–637.

Hillis, A. E. (1998). Treatment of naming disorders: New issues regarding old therapies. *Journal of the International Neuropsychological Society, 4,* 648–680.

Hillis, A. E., & Heidler, J. (2002). Mechanisms of early aphasia recovery. *Aphasiology, 16,* 885–896.

Hillis, A. E., Kane, A., Tuffiash, E., Ulatowski, J. A., Barker, P., Beauchamp, N., et al. (2002). Reperfusion of specific brain regions by raising blood pressure restores selective language functions in subacute stroke. *Brain and Language, 79,* 495–510.

Hinckley, J. J., & Carr, T. H. (2005). Comparing the outcomes of intensive and non-intensive context-based aphasia treatment. *Aphasiology, 19,* 965–974.

Holland, A. L. (1982). Observing functional communication in aphasic adults. *Journal of Speech and Hearing Disorders, 47,* 50–56.

Holland, A. L. (1995). A look into a cloudy crystal ball for specialists in neurogenic language disorders. *American Journal of Speech-Language Pathology, 3,* 34–36.

Holland, A. L., & Fridriksson, J. (2001). Aphasia management in the early phases of recovery following stroke. *American Journal of Speech-Language Pathology, 10,* 19–28.

Holland, A. L., Fromm, D., DeRuyter, F., & Stein, M. (1996). Treatment efficacy: Aphasia. *Journal of Speech and Hearing Research, 40,* 27–36.

Hopper, T., Holland, A. L., & Rewenga, M. (2002). Conversational coaching: Treatment outcomes and future directions. *Aphasiology, 16,* 745–761.

Hough, M., Pierce, R., & Cannito, M. (1988). Contextual influences in aphasia: Effects of predictive versus non-predictive narratives. *Brain and Language, 38,* 252–277.

Kagan, A. (1995). Revealing the competence of aphasic adults through conversation: A challenge for health care professionals. *Topics in Stroke Rehabilitation, 2,* 15–28.

Kagan, A., Black, S. E., Duchan, J. F., Simmons-Mackie, N., & Square, P. (2001). Training volunteers as conversational partners using "Supported Conversation for Adults with Aphasia" (SCA): A controlled trial. *Journal of Speech, Language Hearing Research, 44,* 624–628.

Katsuki-Nakamura, J., Brookshire, R. H., & Nicholas, L. E. (1988). Comprehension of monologues and dialogues by aphasic listeners. *Journal of Speech and Hearing Research, 53,* 408–415.

Kearns, K. P. (1985). Response elaboration training for patient initiated utterances. In R. H. Brookshire (Ed.), *Clinical aphasiology: Conference proceedings* (pp. 196–204). Minneapolis: BRK.

Kearns, K. P. (1986). Systematic programming of verbal elaboration skills in chronic Broca's aphasia. In R. C. Marshall (Ed.), *Case studies in aphasia rehabilitation* (pp. 225–244). Austin, TX: Pro-Ed.

Kearns, K. P., & Scher, G. P. (1989). The generalization of response elaboration training effects. *Clinical Aphasiology, 18,* 223–242.

Kearns, K. P., & Yedor, K. (1991). Alternating treatments comparison of loose training and a convergent treatment strategy. *Clinical Aphasiology, 20,* 223–238.

Keil, K., & Kaszniak, A. W. (2002). Examining executive function in individuals with brain injury: A review. *Aphasiology, 16,* 305–336.

Kertesz, A. (1979). *Aphasia and associated disorders.* New York: Grune & Stratton.

Kimelman, M. Z., & McNeil, M. R. (1987). An investigation of emphatic stress comprehension in aphasia: A replication. *Journal of Speech and Hearing Research, 30,* 295–300.

Kirshner, H. (2002). *Behavioral neurology* (2nd ed.). Boston: Butterworth-Heinemann.

Kirshner, H. S., Casey, P. F., Henson, H, & Heinrich, J. J. (1989). Behavioral features and lesion localization in Wernicke's aphasia. *Aphasiology, 3,* 169–177.

LaPointe, L. L. & Erickson, R. J. (1991). Auditory vigilance during divided task attention in aphasia. *Aphasiology, 5,* 511–520.

Lasky, E. Z., Weidner, W. E., & Johnson, J. P. (1976). Influence of linguistic complexity, rate of presentation, and interphrase pause time on auditory-verbal comprehension of adult aphasic patients. *Brain and Language, 3,* 386–395.

Li, E. C., Kitselman, K., Dusatko, D., & Spinelli, C. (1988). The efficacy of PACE in the remediation of naming deficits. *Journal of Communication Disorders, 21,* 491–503.

Legg, C., Young, L., & Bryer, A. (2005). Training sixth-year medical students in obtaining case-history information from adults with aphasia. *Aphasiology, 19,* 559–575.

Loverso, F. L., & Prescott, T. E. (1981) The effects of alerting signals on left brain damaged (aphasic) and normal subjects' accuracy and response time to visual stimuli. In R. H. Brookshire (Ed.), *Clinical aphasiology: Conference proceedings* (pp. 55–67). Minneapolis: BRK.

Lyon, J. (1998). *Coping with aphasia.* San Diego: Singular.

Lyon, J., Cariski, D., Keisler, L, Rosenbek, J., Levine, R., & Kumpula, J. et al. (1997). Communication partners: Enhancing participation in life and communication for adults with aphasia in natural settings. *Aphasiology, 11,* 693–708.

Marshall, R. C. (1983). Communication styles of fluent aphasic clients. In H. Winitz (Ed.), *Treating language disorders* (pp. 163–180). Baltimore: University Park Press.

Marshall, R. C. (1993). Problem-focused group treatment for clients with mild aphasia. *American Journal of Speech-Language Pathology, 2,* 31–37.

Marshall, R. C. (1994). Management of fluent aphasic clients. In R. Chapey (Ed.), *Language intervention strategies for adult aphasia* (pp. 390–406). Baltimore: Williams & Wilkins.

Marshall, R. C. (1997). Aphasia treatment in the early post onset period: Managing our resources effectively. *American Journal of Speech-Language Pathology, 6,* 5–12.

Marshall, R. C. (2000). Documentation in medical speech-language pathology: Some clinician-friendly suggestions to keep the tail from wagging the dog. *Journal of Medical Speech-Language Pathology, 8,* 37–53.

Marshall, R. C. (2002). *The Marshall auditory comprehension training program (MACTP)*. Missoula, MT: Lexicon Press.

Marshall, R. C., & English, L. (2004). Functional strategies to enhance auditory comprehension of persons with aphasia for neurologic physical therapists. *Journal of Neurological Physical Therapy, 28*, 138–144.

Marshall, R. C., & Freed, D. B. (2006). The personalized cueing method: From the laboratory to the clinic. *American Journal of Speech Language Pathology, 15*, 103–111.

Marshall, R. C., Freed, D. B., & Phillips, D. S. (1997). Communicative efficiency in severe aphasia. *Aphasiology, 11*, 373–384.

Marshall, R. C., & Thistlethwaite, N. (1977). *Verbal and nonverbal alerters: Effects on auditory comprehension of aphasic subjects.* (Unpublished manuscript).

Marshall, R. C., & Tompkins, C. A. (1982). Verbal self-correction behaviors of fluent and non-fluent aphasic subjects. *Brain and Language, 15*, 292–306.

Martin, A. D. (1981a). Therapy with the jargonaphasic. In J. Brown (Ed.), *Jargonaphasia* (pp. 305–326). New York: Academic Press.

Martin A. D. (1981b). An examination of Wepman's thought centered therapy. In R. Chapey (Ed.), *Language intervention strategies in adult aphasia* (pp. 141–154). Baltimore, MD: Williams and Wilkins.

McDonald, S., & Pearce, S. (1995). The 'dice' game: A new test of pragmatic language skills after closed head injury. *Brain Injury, 9*, 255–271.

Metter, E. J., Hanson, W. R., Jackson, C. A., Kempler, D., van Lancker, D., Mazziotta, J. C., et al. (1990). Temporoparietal cortex in aphasia—Evidence from positron emission tomography. *Archives of Neurology, 47*, 1235–1238.

Metter, E. J., Jackson, C. A., Kempler, D., & Hanson, W. R. (1992). Temporoparietal cortex and the recovery of language comprehension in aphasia. *Aphasiology, 6*, 349–358.

Naeser, M. A., Helm-Estabrook, N. A., Haas, G., Auerbach, S., & Srinivasan, M. (1987). Relationship between lesion extent in "Wernicke's area" on computed tomographic scan and predicting recovery of comprehension in Wernicke's aphasia. *Archives of Neurology, 44*, 73–82.

Nicholas, L. E., & Brookshire, R. H. (1995). Comprehension of spoken narrative discourse by adults with aphasia, right hemisphere brain damage, or traumatic brain injury. *American Journal of Speech-Language Pathology, 4*, 69–81.

Nicholas, M. I., Helm-Estabrooks, N. A., Ward-Lonergan, J., & Morgan, A. R. (1993). Evolution of severe aphasia in the first two years post onset. *Archives of Physical Medicine and Rehabilitation, 74*, 830–834.

Nickels, L. (2002). Therapy for naming disorders: Revisiting, revising, and reviewing. *Aphasiology, 16*, 935–979.

O'Halloran, C., Worrall, L., Toffolo, R., Code, C., & Hickson, M. (2004). *Inpatient Functional Communication Interview* (IFCI). Oxon, UK: Speechmark.

Paradis, M. (1998). *Pragmatics in neurogenic communication disorders.* New York: Elsevier.

Pashek, G. V., & Brookshire, R. H. (1982). Effects of rate of speech and linguistic stress on auditory paragraph comprehension of aphasic individuals. *Journal of Speech and Hearing Research, 25*, 377–383.

Paskek, G. V., & Holland, A. L. (1988). Evolution of aphasia in the first year post-onset. *Cortex, 24*, 411–423.

Pierce, R. S. (1988). The influence of prior and subsequent context on comprehension in aphasia. *Aphasiology, 2*, 577–582.

Pierce, R. S., & Beekman, L. (1985). Effects of linguistic and extralinguistic context on semantic and syntactic processing in aphasia. *Journal of Speech and Hearing Research, 28*, 250–254.

Pierce, R. S., & DeStefano, C. (1987). The interactive nature of auditory comprehension in aphasia. *Journal of Communication Disorders, 20*, 15–24.

Porch, B. E. (1967). *Porch index of communicative ability.* Palo Alto, CA: Consulting Psychologists.

Pulvermuller, F., & Roth, V. M. (1991). Communicative aphasia treatment as an further development of PACE therapy. *Aphasiology, 5*, 39–50.

Purdy, M., & Hindenlang, J. (2005). Educating and training caregivers of persons with aphasia. *Aphasiology, 19*, 377–388.

Purdy, M., & Koch, A. (2005). Prediction of strategy usage by adults with aphasia. *Aphasiology, 20*, 337–348.

Ramsberger, G., & Rende, B. (2002). Measuring transactional success in the conversation of people with aphasia. *Aphasiology, 16*, 337–354.

Rende, B. (2000). Cognitive flexibility: Theory, assessment, and treatment. *Seminars in Speech and Language, 21*, 121–133.

Robey, R. R. (1994). The efficacy of treatment for aphasic persons: A meta-analysis. *Brain and Language, 47*, 582–608.

Robey, R. R. (1998). A meta-analysis of clinical outcomes in the treatment of aphasia. *Journal of Speech, Language, and Hearing Research, 41*, 172–187.

Robey, R. R., Schultz, R., & Crawford, A. B. (1999). Single-subject clinical outcome research: Designs, data, effect sizes, and analyses. *Aphasiology, 13*, 445–473.

Rogers, M. A., Alarcon, N. B., & Olswang, L. B. (1999). Aphasia management considered in the context of the World Health Organization model of disablements. *Physical Medicine and Rehabilitation Clinics of North America, 10*, 907–923.

Rosenbek, J., LaPointe, L. L., & Wertz, R. T. (1989). *Aphasia: A clinical approach.* San Diego: Singular.

Salvatore, A. (1979). Clinical treatment of auditory comprehension deficits in acute and chronic aphasic adults: An experimental analysis of within-message pause duration. In R. H. Brookshire (Ed.), *Clinical aphasiology: Conference proceedings* (pp. 203–212). Minneapolis: BRK.

Salvatore, A., Strait, M., & Brookshire, R. H. (1975). Effects of patient characteristics on the delivery of Token Test commands by experienced and inexperienced examiners. In R. H. Brookshire (Ed.), *Clinical aphasiology: Conference proceedings* (pp. 103–112). Minneapolis: BRK.

Schuell, H. (1965). *The Minnesota Test for Differential Diagnosis of Aphasia.* Minneapolis, MN: University of Minnesota Press.

Selnes, O. A., Niccum, N., Knopman, D. S., & Rubens, A. B. (1984). Recovery of single word comprehension: CT-scan correlates. *Brain and Language, 21*, 72–84.

Shisler, R. J., Baylis, G. C., & Frank, E. M. (2000). Pharmacological approaches to the treatment and prevention of aphasia. *Aphasiology, 14*, 1163–1186.

Simmons-Mackie, N. Code, C., Armstrong, E., Stiegler, L., & Elman, R. J. (2002). What is aphasia? Results of an international survey. *Aphasiology, 16*, 837–848.

Simmons-Mackie, N., & Damico, J. (1997). Reformulating the definition of compensatory strategies in aphasia. *Aphasiology, 8,* 761–781.

Simmons, N., & Zorthian A. (1979). Use of symbolic gestures in a case of fluent aphasia. In R. H. Brookshire (Ed.), *Clinical aphasiology: Conference proceedings* (pp. 278–285), Minneapolis: BRK.

Simmons-Mackie, N. N., Kearns, K. P., Potecin, G. (2005). Treatment of aphasia through family member training. *Aphasiology, 19,* 583–593.

Sparks, R. (1978). Parastandardized examination guidelines for adult aphasia. *British Journal of Disorders of Communication, 13,* 135–146.

Springer, L., Glindemann, R., Huber, W., & Willmes, K. (1991). How efficacious is PACE-therapy when 'Language Systematic Training' is incorporated? *Aphasiology, 5,* 391–399.

Stokes, T., & Baer, D. M. (`1977) An implicit technology of generalization. *Journal of Applied Behavior Analysis, 22,* 157–170.

Swindell, C., Pashek, G., & Holland, A. (1982). A questionnaire for surveying persons and communicative style. In R. H. Brookshire (Ed.), *Clinical aphasiology: Conference proceedings* (pp. 50–63). Minneapolis: BRK.

Swinney, D., Zurif, E. B., & Cutler, A. (1980) Effects of sentential stress and word class upon comprehension in Broca's aphasics. *Brain and Language, 10,* 132–144.

Tompkins, C. A., & Marshall, R. C. (1982). Communicative value of self-cues in aphasia. In R. H. Brookshire (Ed.) *Clinical Aphasiology: Conference proceedings* (pp. 77–82), Minneapolis: BRK.

Tompkins, C. A., Scharp, V. L., & Marshall, R. C. (2006). Communicative value of self-cues in aphasia: A re-evaluation. *Aphasiology, 20,* 684–704.

Van Lancker, D., & Klein, K. (1990). Preserved recognition of familiar personal names in global aphasia. *Brain and Language, 39,* 511–529.

Van Lancker, D., & Nicklay, C. K. (1992). Comprehension of personally relevant (PERL) versus novel language in two globally aphasic patients. *Aphasiology, 6,* 37–62.

Walker-Batson, D., Curtis, S., Natarajan, R., Ford, J., Dronkers, N., et al. (2001). A double-blind, placebo-controlled study of the use of amphetamine in the treatment of aphasia. *Stroke, 32,* 2093–2098.

Wallace, G. J., & Canter, G. (1985). Effects of personally relevant language materials on the performance of severely aphasic individuals. *Journal of Speech and Hearing Disorders, 50,* 385–390.

Waller, M., & Darley, F. L. (1978). The influence of context on the auditory comprehension of paragraphs by aphasic subjects. *Journal of Speech and Hearing Research, 21,* 732–745.

Wambaugh, J., & Martinez, A. (2000). Effects of modified response elaboration training with apraxic and aphasic speakers. *Aphasiology, 14,* 603–618.

Wegner, M. L., Brookshire, R. H., & Nicholas, L. E. (1984) Comprehension of main ideas and details in coherent and noncoherent discourse by aphasic and nonaphasic listeners. *Brain and Language, 21,* 37–51.

Weidner, W. E., & Lasky, E. Z. (1976). The interaction of rate and complexity of stimulus on the performance of adult aphasic subjects. *Brain and Language, 3,* 34–40.

Weiner, D. A., Connor, L. T., & Obler, L. K. (2004). Inhibition and auditory comprehension in Wernicke's aphasia. *Aphasiology, 18,* 599–609.

Wepman, J. M. (1958). The relationship between self-correction and recovery from aphasia. *Journal of Speech and Hearing Disorders, 23,* 302–305.

Wepman, J. M. (1972). Aphasia therapy: A new look. *Journal of Speech and Hearing Disorders, 37,* 203–214.

Wertz, R. T., Collins, M. J., Weiss, D., Kurtzke, J. F., Friden, T., Brookshire, R. H., et al. (1981). Veterans Administration cooperative study on aphasia: A comparison of individual and group treatment. *Journal of Speech and Hearing Research, 21,* 580–594.

Wertz, R. T., & Irwin, W. H. (2001). Darley and the efficacy of language rehabilitation in aphasia. *Aphasiology, 15,* 231–248.

West, J. F., & Kaufman, M. (1972). *Some effects of redundancy on the auditory comprehension of adult aphasics.* Paper presented at the annual convention of the American Speech-Language-Hearing Association, San Francisco (November).

Winograd, T. (1977). A framework for understanding discourse. In M. Just & P. Carpenter (Eds.), *Cognitive processes in comprehension.* Hillsdale, NJ: Erlbaum.

Yedor, K., Conlon C. P., & Kearns, K. P. (1993). Measurements predictive of generalization of response elaboration training. *Clinical Aphasiology, 21,* 213–223.

Chapter 19

Rehabilitation of Subcortical Aphasia

Stephen E. Nadeau and
Leslie J. Gonzalez Rothi

OBJECTIVES

The objectives of this chapter are to elucidate features and mechanisms of thalamic and nonthalamic subcortical aphasias, to analyze these aphasias in terms of the impairments they reflect in the neural networks supporting language function, and to review behavioral consequences of subcortical lesions associated with aphasia that may seriously interfere with the rehabilitation process.

Subcortical aphasia is defined as a language disorder associated with damage to subcortical brain structures, such as the basal ganglia, the thalamus, or the white matter pathways in the general vicinity of these structures. Usually, it is caused by ischemic strokes, and less often by intracerebral hemorrhages. When these disorders were first described, the aphasia was assumed to be a direct consequence of the damage to subcortical structures that was revealed by structural imaging studies, such as computed tomography and magnetic resonance imaging. Further research has shown this assumption to be substantially incorrect (Nadeau & Crosson, 1997). Aphasia is actually an indirect consequence of subcortical lesions. In the case of subcortical aphasias stemming from thalamic lesions, the language disorders appear to stem from the impact of thalamic dysfunction on cerebral cortical function (i.e., a disorders of neural systems). In the case of subcortical aphasias stemming from lesions outside the thalamus, the language disorders reflect either invisible cortical damage or dysfunction associated with the vascular event that caused the visible subcortical lesion, or they reflect the impact of the subcortical lesion on pathways between the thalamus and language cortex.

We will begin this chapter by describing the neural mechanisms underlying thalamic aphasias and the pathogenesis of nonthalamic subcortical aphasias. We also will review the linguistic features of these disorders, with a particular emphasis on the dysfunction of the underlying neural systems that these disorders reflect. We know of no adequately controlled scientific studies regarding the efficacy of therapy for subcortical aphasias. For the time being, therefore, we assume that therapy for specific deficits commonly associated with cortical lesions (e.g., word-retrieval impairment) will show similar efficacy when the lesion is subcortical. Clearly, this idea requires testing. We will conclude with a consideration of nonlinguistic behavioral disorders that frequently are present in patients with subcortical aphasia and that may have a major impact on prognosis.

Thalamic Aphasias

The thalamus is located at the center of the cerebrum at its junction with the midbrain (Figs. 19–1 through 19–3). Although its function is by no means simple, the thalamus is far simpler and better understood than that of any other cerebral structure. In essence, it functions as a *relay device*. Specific groups of neurons within the thalamus (nuclei) relay sensory information from more peripheral neural waystations to the cerebral cortex. For example, visual information is transmitted from the retinas via the lateral geniculate bodies to the primary visual cortex (calcarine cortex) in the occipital lobes. Auditory information is relayed through a chain of nuclei within the brain stem to the medial geniculate bodies, from which it is transmitted to primary auditory cortex (Heschl's gyrus) on the dorsal surface of the temporal lobe deep within the sylvian fissure. Somatosensory information is relayed by two major pathways within the spinal cord and brain stem to two specific thalamic nuclei, the ventral posteromedial (subserving the face) and ventral posterolateral (subserving the body) (Table 19–1), from which it is then relayed to somatosensory cortex on the surface of the cerebral hemispheres. Thus, these three pairs of nuclei relay information derived from sensory organs outside the brain to the cerebral cortex. The remainder of the thalamic nuclei relay information from one part of the brain to another. For example, neural transmission from motor areas of the cerebrum to the cerebellum and the putamen is relayed back to separate portions of the ventrolateral nucleus of the thalamus,

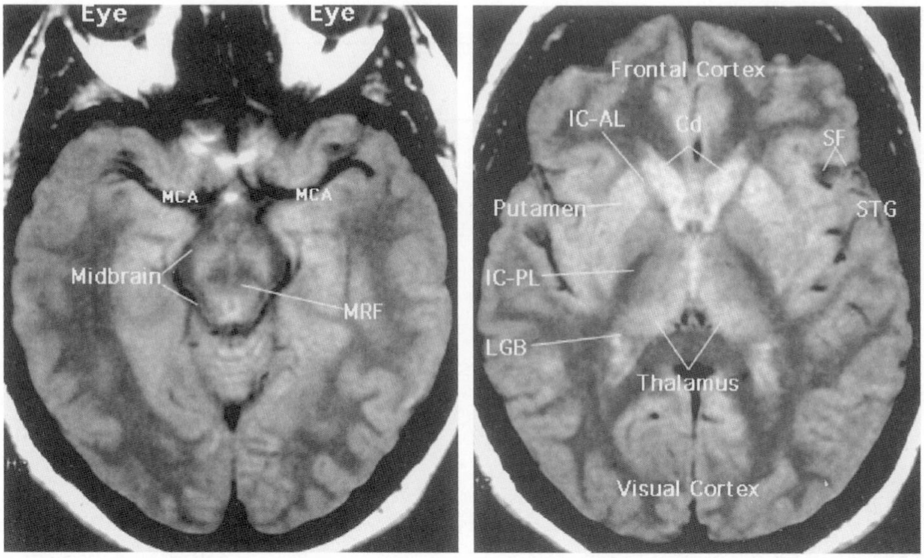

Figure 19–1. Major cerebral structures and landmarks relevant to the problem of subcortical aphasia (thalamus, caudate, and putamen), anterior limb of the internal capsule (IC_{AL}), posterior limb of the internal capsule (IC_{PL}), midbrain reticular formation (MRF), visual cortex, lateral geniculate body (LGB), and primary auditory cortex.

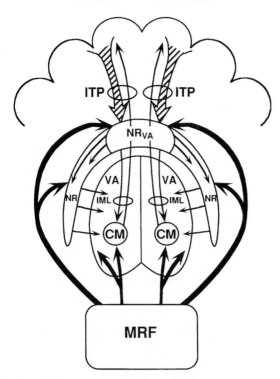

FRONTAL CORTEX

Figure 19–2. Schematic diagram of essential relationships involved in regulation of the thalamic gating mechanism. See text for details. ITP = inferior thalamic peduncle; NR = nucleus reticularis; NR_{VA} = the portion of the NR immediately anterior to ventral anterior nucleus that receives input both from the midbrain reticular formation (MRF) and the prefrontal cortex via the ITP; CM = center median nucleus; IML = internal medullary lamina, the white matter fascicle separating the medial from the lateral thalamus and containing the connections between prefrontal cortex and CM. (From Nadeau & Crosson, 1997; with permission.)

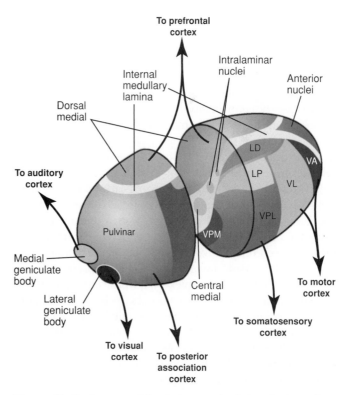

Figure 19–3. Cartoon of the thalamus, depicting the loci of the major nuclei. Center median (Cm) is labeled "central medial" in this figure, and parafascicularis (Pf), located anterior, ventral, and medial to Cm, is not depicted. From Nadeau et al,.2004. Medical Neuroscience. (Philadelphia: Saunders (imprint of Elsevier)).

TABLE 19–1

Abbreviations

Cd_H	Head of the caudate nucleus
GABA	γ-Aminobutyric acid
IC_{AL}	Internal capsule, anterior limb
ITP	Inferior thalamic peduncle
MCA	Middle cerebral artery
MRF	Midbrain reticular formation
PCA	Posterior cerebral artery
Thalamus	
CmPf	Center-median parafascicularis nuclear complex
DM	Dorsomedial nucleus
IML	Internal medullary lamina
LP	Lateral posterior nucleus
MTT	Mammillothalamic tract
NR	Nucleus reticularis
NR_{VA}	Portion of NR over anterior pole of VA, interfacing with ITP
VA	Ventral anterior nucleus
VLa	Ventrolateral nucleus, anterior portion
VPL	Ventroposteromedial nucleus
VPM	Ventroposterolateral nucleus

and from there back to motor areas of the cortex. For all these nuclei—as, indeed, for every nuclear group in the thalamus—the cortical projections to the thalamus are at least as extensive as the projections from the thalamus to the cortex. This two-way connectivity is entirely consistent with our emerging understanding of the neural network basis of brain function (Nadeau, 2001).

Of particular interest with respect to language and language-related processes are two other nuclear groups, the dorsomedial nucleus (DM) and the pulvinar-lateroposterior (LP) complex. These nuclear groups resemble the ventrolateral nucleus, in that they relay information originally derived from the cerebral cortex back to the cerebral cortex. The DM, however, relays information from the prefrontal cortex and several subcortical structures back to the prefrontal cortex. The pulvinar-LP complex relays projections from the frontal, temporal, and parietal cortices (including those portions of the dominant hemisphere directly implicated in language function) as well as from some subcortical structures back to these same cortices. As we shall see below, there appears to be a logical relationship between dysfunction in these two nuclear groups and particular features of thalamic aphasias.

It is more accurate to characterize the thalamus as a regulated or gated-relay device. This gating feature helps to address two questions. First, what could conceivably be the purpose of long connections descending from, for example, the temporoparietal cortex to the pulvinar-LP complex only

to be sent right back to the very same cortex? One product of passing cortical information through the thalamus may be that this information—and, by implication, the originating cortex—is subjected to the regulatory mechanism provided by the thalamic gate. Second, considering that ischemic strokes involving either the DM or pulvinar-LP complex (the thalamic regions being linked most directly to the language cortex) are extremely rare, how do we explain thalamic aphasia in terms of dysfunction of these two regions? To do so, we must look for a cause of dysfunction other than direct damage. It appears that thalamic strokes sparing these nuclear groups produce aphasia by damaging key components of the thalamic gating mechanism. At this point, we must address four questions: (1) how does the thalamic gating mechanism work, (2) how do strokes impair its function, (3) what purpose could such a gating mechanism serve, and (4) what is likely to be the specific impact of disorders of the gating mechanism on cortices supporting higher neural function, most specifically language function? The neuroscientific data needed to answer these questions are limited, so our answers necessarily involve considerable inference and speculation.

How Does the Thalamic Gating Mechanism Work?

Nearly the entire thalamus is enveloped by a paper-thin layer of cells comprising the thalamic reticular nucleus (NR; Fig. 19–3). The cells of this nucleus, unlike those in the remainder of the thalamus, send their projections back into the thalamus, where they synapse both on thalamic relay neurons and on inhibitory thalamic interneurons. They employ an inhibitor neurotransmitter (γ-aminobutyric acid [GABA]). Thus, they are admirably suited to regulating thalamic transmission to the cortex, either by directly inhibiting thalamic relay neurons or by indirectly potentiating their activity through inhibiting the inhibitory interneurons within the thalamus.

The neurons of the NR are regulated by a host of brain systems. Two systems appear to be particularly important. The first is the midbrain reticular formation (MRF), a complex network of neurons within the core of the midbrain immediately below the thalamus. The MRF defines the level of wakefulness or arousal. With high levels of arousal, the MRF inhibits the NR at the same time that it excites thalamic relay neurons, thereby allowing all neural transmission to pass readily through the thalamus. Thalamic relay neurons fire at a rate that is a linear function of input, thereby functioning to relay the input to their cortical projection targets faithfully. With low levels of arousal, as in deep sleep or coma, because of low input from the MRF, the NR neurons exert maximally inhibitory effects on thalamic relay neurons at the same time that these relay neurons receive little excitatory input from the MRF. In this state, relay neurons fire in intermittent, high-frequency bursts that convey little information about temporal fluctuations in their input amplitude. Cortical relay of thalamic input is effectively blocked. In this way, the impact of the MRF on thalamic transmission is global and nonselective.

The second major regulatory system is provided by projections from the entire cerebral cortex to the NR. Two subsystems can be defined within this set of projections: a *direct* system, involving modality-specific cortical projections to individual thalamic nuclei that largely reciprocate thalamocortical projections and synapse on NR neurons as they pass through the NR; and an *indirect* system, involving projections from the prefrontal cortex to the NR via the inferior thalamic peduncle (ITP), providing a potential basis for multimodal regulation of thalamic transmission. Both systems provide a mechanism by which thalamic transmission from specific regions of specific nuclei can be selectively gated to the cortex.

The mechanisms underlying selective NR regulation of thalamocortical transmission are currently the subject of intense study and much debate, and the last 10 years have seen a surge of interest in the role of NR in attentional processes (Bezdudnaya et al., 2006; Crabtree & Isaac, 2002; McAlonan, Cavanaugh, & Wurtz, 2006; Pinault, 2004; Sherman, 2005). This work has focused almost exclusively on the direct corticothalamic system. Corticothalamic neurons synapsing on the NR and thalamic relay neurons are glutamatergic and, therefore, excitatory. Because this excitatory input to NR neurons inhibits thalamocortical transmission (NR neurons are GABAergic and, therefore, inhibitory), it is difficult to understand how this mechanism could serve to selectively release thalamic transmission to cortex.

Two possible explanations have emerged. First, a given NR neuron may project to neurons in several specific regions of the thalamus, and NR neurons have extensive dendrodendritic contacts with one another. This anatomy provides a mechanism by which a given region of the cerebral cortex could shape thalamocortical transmission from one or more nuclei both spatially and temporally. Evidence also has emerged that NR neurons not only have ion channel–linked glutamate receptors (uniformly excitatory) but also metabotropic (non-ion channel) glutamate receptors, some of which may exert inhibitory effects (Cox & Sherman, 1999). Second, although in our previous discussion of MRF effects on NR activity we linked the intermittent burst mode of thalamic relay neuron activity to low arousal states and closing of the thalamic gate, evidence in multiple species, including humans, now suggests that brief epochs of intermittent bursting can be observed in the awake state. Because these bursts are associated with a particularly high signal to noise ratio, they could effectively break through ongoing cortical activity to signal the need for a change in focus of attention or function. They are associated with onsets of stimulus change and occur either when the subject is awake but not attentive or when the subject is attending to a stimulus in one modality and a salient stimulus is presented in another. It has been suggested that this mechanism may serve to give the cortex a "wake-up call," either during drowsiness or during attention to another stimulus, that will lead the organism to focus on a stimulus that, by virtue of its sudden appearance, may be particularly important (Sherman, 2005). In this way, the thalamic intermittent burst mode could serve as one mechanism underlying reactive attention—that is, attention elicited by the intrinsic properties of the stimulus (Nadeau & Heilman, 1991).

The indirect corticothalamic regulatory system, involving a pathway from the prefrontal cortex to the NR via the ITP, provides a mechanism by which thalamic transmission to specific regions of the cortex might be regulated volitionally. Because language largely is produced volitionally, it would seem logical that, to the extent the thalamus is involved in language, dysfunction of this system would lead to aphasia. Empirical studies bear this out (see below). Unfortunately, little neuroscientific study of this system has occurred since our last review (Nadeau & Crosson, 1997).

How Do Strokes Impair the Function of the Thalamic gate?

The projections from both the MRF and the prefrontal cortex to the NR terminate in a dense neural complex near the anterior pole of the thalamus (NR_{VA}), which is immediately adjacent to the ventral anterior (VA) nucleus of the thalamus (Fig. 19-3). This NR_{VA} neural complex appears to play a role in regulating the entirety of the NR. The mechanism by which the prefrontal cortex regulates the thalamic gate also appears to require the participation of the center-median parafascicularis (CmPf), a nuclear complex buried deep within the posterior portions of the thalamus (Figs. 19-2 and 19-3). Fibers from the prefrontal cortex to and from the CmPf pass within the thalamus in a neural fascicle, the internal medullary lamina (IML), which also envelopes the CmPf. Immediately in front of the thalamus, these fibers pass through the ITP, which is continuous with the anterior limb of the internal capsule and the deep white matter of the frontal lobe (Figs. 19-1 and 19-3). Although the means we use to localize strokes within the thalamus are prone to error, all the thalamic strokes that have been reported to result in aphasia appear to have involved either VA at the nexus of the connections between the prefrontal cortex (the ITP), the MRF, and the NR_{VA}; the IML carrying connections from the prefrontal cortex to CmPf; or the CmPf itself. Thus, it appears that all ischemic strokes causing thalamic aphasia disrupt the regulatory system for the thalamic gate for the entire hemithalamus by damaging either the prefrontal-NR_{VA} junction or the prefrontal-NR_{VA}-IML-CmPf axis. This disruption would implicate transmission from all thalamic nuclei, including the pulvinar-LP complex, which is heavily connected to language cortices. Thalamic strokes that are not associated with aphasia appear to spare these structures and pathways. Disorders of executive function also often occur with lesions of the prefrontal-NR$_{VA}$-IML-CmPf axis (Van der Werf et al., 2003), perhaps because of associated dysfunction of the DM, which is heavily interconnected with prefrontal cortex. Hemorrhages, which do not respect vascular territories, may directly damage the pulvinar-LP or DM.

What Purpose Could Such a Gating Mechanism Serve?

The brain contains approximately 100 billion neurons organized into hundreds of systems, each of which is nearly infinitely malleable. It appears logical that there should be, given this situation, that some systems function simultaneously to maintain order and to optimize the resources that are brought to bear on a particular problem—that is, systems that allocate processing demands either among the multitude of different neural networks or within parts of particular networks. Several lines of research have begun to delineate executive systems that serve this purpose.

More than 20 years ago, Moran and Desimone (1985) performed a clever experiment that provides particular insight into the fundamental nature of one of these allocation processes. Scientists were recording the activity of single neurons in the inferotemporal cortex (visual-association cortex) of macaque monkeys. In one study, they identified a neuron that was sensitive only to red light. If the monkey had been trained to pull a lever to be rewarded with of a squirt of apple juice whenever a red light came on, this neuron fired vigorously in response to the red light. If the monkey had been trained to expect reward for a pulling a lever in response to a green light, however, this neuron failed to fire in response to a red light. In other words, this neuron required two inputs to fire, one from visual cortex signaling the presence of red and one from elsewhere in the brain, almost certainly the frontal lobes, signaling that red was behaviorally important, because it indicated an opportunity to get a reward. During the red-light rewarded condition, input from the frontal lobes preferentially sensitized red-sensitive neural systems; that is, it recruited red-sensitive neurons to working memory. This corresponded to particular attention by the monkey to red lights. The process exhibited by the monkeys in the experiment of Moran and Desimone can be termed "intentional attention," because it subserves attentional behavior and constitutes a deliberate, volitional allocation of sensory (visual) resources to achieve a particular end (get a juice reward).

Recently, Minamimoto and Kimura (2002) reported an experiment that sheds light on the potential role of the prefrontal-NR$_{VA}$-IML-CmPf axis in intentional attention.

They trained macaque monkeys in the Posner paradigm.[1] When CmPf was inactivated by injection of the GABA$_A$-agonist muscimol, the validity effect was abolished—that is, correct cues to the side on which the stimulus would appear no longer produced a reduction in reaction time. No other aspect of task performance was affected. Thus, inactivation of the CmPf produced a selective deficit of intentional attention. An earlier experiment by Weese, Phillips, & Brown (1999) showed that a cellular lesion at a different locus along this pathway, the NR, had the same effect.

Attention also may be reactive (Nadeau & Heilman, 1991). For example, we orient to a brilliant flash of light or a sudden movement in our environment because of the intrinsic value the brain assigns to these types of stimuli. A precise but flexible balance must be maintained between intentional (volitional) and reactive attentional systems. For example, a rat must engage intentional attention to search for edible material but also, simultaneously, must maintain reactive attention to detect approaching predators.

The attentional phenomena we have been discussing so far involve the selection of particular neural networks or components of networks in cerebral association cortices in the service of focusing sensory systems on some particular locus in the environment (i.e., orienting). Abundant reason now exists to believe that precisely analogous processes occur in polymodal or supramodal cerebral cortices, such as those supporting language function, that correspond to thinking and the formulation of behaviors other than orienting. These processes have been the focus of considerable study over the past 20 years (Fuster, 1991; Goldman-Rakic, 1990). The term "working memory" often is used to refer to the information maintained by activation of a selected neural network (e.g., memory that the color red is important, as in the experiment of Moran and Desimone, 1985), although we prefer the more neutral term "selective engagement." In this conceptualization, attentional processes represent the subtype of selective engagement involved in allocating components of neural networks located in sensory association cortices in the service of attentional behavior.

The thalamus also appears to support selective engagement processes. Nonhuman primate research, however,

---

[1]In the Posner paradigm (Posner, Walker, Friedrich, & Rafal, 1987), the subject begins by focusing on cross-hairs at the center of a computer screen. A cue subsequently appears on either the right or left of the screen that indicates to the subject on which side a subsequent stimulus is likely to appear (with 80% accuracy). As soon as the stimulus actually appears, the subject makes a response. The experimental measure is the reaction time. The cue will lead the subject to volitionally direct attention to the side of the cue, providing the basis for a reaction time advantage if the stimulus actually appears on that side (the validity effect). On those 20% of trials when the cue is misleading, the stimulus engages reactive attentional mechanisms, which ultimately lead the subject to make an orienting response, but with a somewhat longer reaction time.

suggests that, at this stage in the evolution of the brain, very little of this regulation involves thalamic projection to primary sensory cortices. The thalamus appears to be only minimally involved in *ongoing* gated relay to primary sensory cortices of visual or auditory information, but it may be involved to some extent in regulating the relay of somatosensory information. That is, attentional mechanisms (selective engagement) involving visual and auditory modalities have been subsumed by the cerebral cortex.[2] For thalamic nuclei such as the DM and pulvinar-LP complex that have evolved in tandem with the burgeoning of cerebral cortex in higher primates, indirect evidence suggests that their role in ongoing selective engagement has not been superceded. In nonhuman primates, ongoing attentional modulation of neural activity in the pulvinar occurs in parallel with modulation of neural activity in visual and polymodal association cortices, though to what extent the pulvinar modulation is responsible for cortical modulation cannot be determined from this experiment (Bender & Youakim, 2001). Even so, neglect, extinction, and delayed reorienting of attention have been induced by injection of the GABA-agonist muscimol into the pulvinar (Desimone, Wessinger, Thomas, & Schneider, 1990; Petersen, Robinson, & Morris, 1987). These studies, coupled with evidence of cortical dysfunction after thalamic lesions in human subjects, suggest that the thalamus is responsible for at least certain aspects of selective engagement of cortex. Thus, in humans, thalamic gating mechanisms appear to be most important in regulating selective engagement of *association* cortices (unimodal and polymodal) as well as supramodal association cortices supporting higher neural functions, such as language.

Recent studies have further elucidated this process. Wester, Irvine, & Hugdahl (2001) reported that in consonant-vowel dichotic listening tasks (in which processing likely takes place in the auditory association cortex, Brodmann's area 22, and frontal operculum [Nadeau, 2001]), patients with subacute and chronic thalamic hemorrhages exhibit a strong ipsilesional ear advantage, which they cannot overcome even when told to direct their attention to the contralesional ear. These findings suggest a disorder of selective engagement affecting reactive attention (hence the ipsilesional ear advantage) and intentional (volitional) attention (hence the inability to overcome the contralesional ear disadvantage). Kubat-Silman, Dagenbach, & Absher (2002) reported impairment on letter, object location, and object

shape N-back task performance[3] in six subjects with old thalamic infarcts (five right-sided and one left-sided). The N-back tasks are widely accepted as probes of working memory—a function that depends on selective engagement, as discussed previously. Of note, even though both hemispheres likely are engaged by these tasks, unilateral thalamic lesions were disruptive, and no clear differences were found in performance between the patient with the left-side lesion and the five patients with right-sided lesions. In this same study, forward digit span was normal in all subjects, even when articulation was suppressed by the requirement that subjects repeatedly say the word "the" during task performance. This finding is consistent with the evidence that thalamic aphasia relatively spares repetition and, thus, relatively spares the procedural knowledge domain underlying phonologic processing that is engaged in repetition and digit span performance (Nadeau, 2001) (see next section).

What Is Likely To Be the Specific Impact of Disorders of the Thalamic Gating Mechanism on Function of the Cerebral Cortex (Most Specifically the Language Cortex)?

The neuroscience of thalamocortical interaction has not advanced to the point of providing a precise picture of how disorders of thalamic gating impact higher cortical function, and we are dependent primarily on human data in the inferences that we draw regarding this subject. Thalamic aphasia is characterized classically by anomia in spontaneous language (at times severe), some impairment in naming to confrontation, apparently normal grammar, normal articulation, and usually flawless repetition. Naming deficits disproportionately affect low-frequency words (Raymer, Moberg, Crosson, Nadeau, & Gonzalez-Rothi, 1997). In the worst cases, modest impairment in comprehension may be noted. Some patients make semantic paraphasic errors, and rare patients, primarily those with thalamic hemorrhages, transiently produce neologisms. Can we relate this pattern of deficits to any fundamental functional attributes of the cerebral cortices involved? We have proposed that linguistic deficits wrought of thalamic dysfunction reflect selective functional impairment of cortices supporting declarative memories, with sparing of cortices supporting procedural memories (Nadeau & Crosson, 1997).

Declarative or explicit memory consists of knowledge regarding facts and events and ordinarily is available to

---

[2]Note that we stress *ongoing* gated relay. As noted in an earlier section (see the section *How Does the Thalamic Gating Mechanism Work?*), the thalamic burst mode state may provide a mechanism to give the cortex a brief "wake-up call" that will result in shifting thalamic relay neurons into a linear transmission mode, thereby opening thalamic transmission to the cortex in a fashion that no longer is regulated at the thalamic level.

[3]In N-back tasks, the subject hears or sees a steady stream of stimuli (e.g., letters) presented one at a time at a fixed rate. The subjects has to respond when the current stimulus matches the immediately preceding stimulus (i.e., the N=1 N-back task); the current stimulus matches the stimulus that occurred before the immediately preceding stimulus (i.e., the N=2 N-back task), and so on.

conscious recollection. It is represented in association cortices throughout the brain. New declarative memories are encoded by a system comprised of the hippocampus; cortices overlying the hippocampus; several structures in the limbic system, which presumably help to define which facts are worth remembering; and the DM and the anterior nuclear group of the thalamus (Squire, 1987, 1992).

Nondeclarative memory consists of a heterogeneous collection of abilities (including skills and habits), implicit memory, and some forms of classical conditioning. Nondeclarative memory is reflected only in behavioral change, as when one's tennis game improves with practice or an experimental subject demonstrates an autonomic response or a correct decision when reexposed to a stimulus previously presented too briefly to provide even a sense of familiarity, let alone a basis for conscious recognition. Skills, habits, and some forms of classical conditioning are represented in the motor and premotor cortex, the cerebellum, and possibly, the basal ganglia. Unlike declarative memory, nondeclarative memory does not appear to require a special auxiliary processing mechanism like the hippocampal system to be instantiated. Patients with impaired declarative memory generally have preserved nondeclarative memory.

The principal linguistic deficit exhibited by patients with thalamic aphasia is in lexical-semantic access (Nadeau & Crosson, 1997), a process that clearly depends on declarative memories. In contrast, linguistic processes involving phonologic processing and grammar generally are spared. Although we have declarative knowledge of the spelling of words, we rely on entirely automatic processes not available to conscious recollection in the actual production of spoken words. Although we have declarative knowledge of the concepts about which we plan to speak, the process of translating concepts into clause sequences and appropriate phrase structures also largely is an automatic one and largely unavailable to conscious recollection (except to the extent that we deliberately modify grammar to meet situational demands). Thus, the preponderance of data regarding phonologic and grammatical processes in thalamic aphasia appears to indicate substantial sparing of procedural memory systems.

Unfortunately, this tidy picture cannot be reconciled completely with available data regarding phonologic and grammatical function in patients with thalamic lesions. First, patients with thalamic hemorrhages often have been reported to produce phonemic paraphasic errors and neologisms. This phenomenon also occasionally can be seen in patients with ischemic lesions (Ebert, Vinz, Görtler, Wallesch, & Herrmann, 1999; Raymer et al., 1997). Because it appears to represent dysfunction involving phonologic sequence knowledge, which would seem to be procedural in nature (Nadeau, 2001; Nadeau & Gonzalez-Rothi, 1993) (see Chapter 26), this finding is not easily reconciled with a concept that the thalamus is mechanistically involved only in declarative processes. The disproportionate occurrence of neologisms

with acute hemorrhage raises the question of some kind of pathologic excitatory phenomenon. Whether hemorrhage or ischemic lesion, however, we are still left without an explanation for the occasional occurrence of neologisms, but we have offered two possibilities (Nadeau & Crosson, 1997):

1. The process of becoming literate serves to additionally define phonemes, inflectional grammatical morphemes, derivational morphemes, and syllables as lexical elements in their own right, which are consciously retrievable like any item in declarative memory and, therefore, are susceptible to errors of selection, as whole words are (Bertelson & De Gelder, 1989; Semenza, Butterworth, Panzeri, & Ferreri, 1990). This "sublexicalization" may create susceptibility to the production of sublexical paraphasias manifesting as phonologic errors and neologisms in the presence of thalamic injury.

2. Thalamic lesions may sufficiently disrupt mutually inhibitory relationships within cortices supporting semantics that competing semantic entrees can vie simultaneously for translation into a phonologic sequence, with the ultimate outcome being a word blend that constitutes a neologism.

An important recent paper has provided compelling evidence of syntactic simplification and, possibly, agrammatism in a patient with bilateral paramedian thalamic infarcts (De Witte, Wilssens, Engelborghs, De Deyn, & Mariën, 2006). How might this be explained? A concept representation, corresponding to a noun phrase, can be represented in neural network terms as a specific pattern of activation of the neurons in association cortices representing the various features of that concept (see Chapter 26). Production of a sentence invariably involves modification of that distributed concept representation, and it usually involves generation and reciprocal modification of two or more distributed concept representations and the binding of these representations into a superdistributed representation. For example, the sentence "the old man shot the burglar" involves simultaneously generating two distributed concept representations, one corresponding to an old man and one corresponding to a burglar. It also requires reciprocal modification of these representations to yield a new representation corresponding to "shooter old man" that now is linked to another new representation corresponding to "shot burglar." The use of verbs mandating three arguments would correspond to the simultaneous maintenance and reciprocal modification of three distributed concept representations, and addition of embedded clauses will demand still further active distributed concept representations.

The production of normal syntax requires both the ability to generate and maintain multiple distributed concept representations (i.e., selective engagement/working memory) and skill in the modification of these various representations.

Broca's aphasia occurs with lesions that damage the frontal apparatus that is apparently required to modify distributed concept representations and is certainly required to reciprocally modify multiple distributed concept representations (and, hence, simplification of syntax, among other things). It may be that selective engagement mechanisms supporting needed working memory are integral to this apparatus or that frontal networks involved in this selective engagement are, to some degree, anatomically separate. The report of De Witte and colleagues (2006) suggests that disorders of selective engagement caused by thalamic lesions could produce a pattern of language abnormality having some similarities to that of Broca's aphasia. Even some abnormalities of grammatical morphology might be explained in terms of working memory deficits, even though we suspect that in Broca's aphasia, the loss of phonologic sequence knowledge involving words, their affixes, and short phrases (caused by the perisylvian component of the lesions) makes a major contribution to agrammatism (see Chapter 26). For example, the use of articles is particularly dependent on sustained working memory of what has just been said to determine whether the reference should be definite or indefinite. Absent working memory of what has been said, the lack of a concept of definiteness or indefiniteness may result in a failure to produce the article, as in the case described by De Witte and colleagues.

The notion that thalamic lesions can lead to disorders of endogenous generation of distributed concept representations invites comparison with adynamic aphasia (Gold et al., 1997). In adynamic aphasia, subjects appear to be incapable of endogenous generation of any distributed concept representations, hence their extreme nonfluency. When distributed concept representations are generated from without, however, as in a picture description task, subjects with adynamic aphasia perform relatively normally. The report of De Witte and colleagues suggests that, at least with certain uncommon thalamic lesions, distributed concept representations can be generated endogenously to the degree that the patient can translate them into words but that these representations cannot be sustained in the manner necessary for them to be related to each other and modified in the well-practiced ways that instantiate the rules of syntax (see Chapter 26). Thus, we might employ the term "paradynamic" to describe the patient of De Witte and colleagues to indicate that the fundamental problem involves endogenous selective engagement but also that, rather than a complete failure of endogenous engagement, as in adynamic aphasia, it constitutes disjointed, excessively brief, and substantially dysfunctional engagement.

Intimations of the problem observed by De Witte and colleagues can be found in the older thalamic aphasia literature. Goldenberg, Wimmer, & Maly (1983) noted disproportionately impaired ability to elaborate in the spontaneous description of remote memories—a problem reminiscent of adynamic aphasia. Lhermitte (1984) observed evidence of problems with conceptual delineation and sequencing in patients with thalamic lesions. He noted that "narration is no longer chronologic . . . a passage from one story slides into another story. . . the patient cannot control the order of his ideas" (p. 106). He also noted that disorders of this type are seen in patients with left frontal lesions. Nevertheless, De Witte and colleagues appear to be the first to provide such detailed evidence of syntax simplification and at least some evidence of agrammatism in thalamic aphasia. Does this merely reflect the thoroughness of their investigation, or might it reflect something unusual about their patient's lesion? The lesion in their case might, in fact, have been somewhat unusual. In particular, the lesion was bilateral (as in the case of many paramedian artery distribution infarcts), and it likely involved the prefrontal-NR$_{VA}$-IML-CmPf axis bilaterally, thus producing bilateral disorders in thalamic engagement involving the pulvinar-LP and DM. It also extended relatively anterior and deep, potentially destroying prefrontal-to-DM pathways that run beneath the thalamus before curving upward to extend into the DM (Nadeau & Crosson, 1997; Steriade, Parent, & Hada, 1984). In contrast, Raymer and colleagues (1997) noted normal syntax in a patient with a very large left paramedian artery distribution infarct, verbal amnesia, severe anomia, and major disruption of prefrontal function.

In summary, if these ideas find support in future investigations of syntactic disorders and agrammatism in subjects with thalamic aphasia, it may still be possible to account for thalamic aphasia as a disorder of declarative knowledge processing.

NONTHALAMIC SUBCORTICAL APHASIA

Whereas the development of aphasia after thalamic lesions is a natural consequence of the disrupted function of neural systems implicated in language processing, the development of aphasia after nonthalamic subcortical lesions appears to be largely a consequence of direct damage to language cortices that is not visible on imaging studies, reflecting mechanisms of stroke pathogenesis. That is, nonthalamic subcortical aphasias are not fundamentally different in character or pathogenesis from cortical aphasias.

At first, the problem of nonthalamic subcortical aphasia seems formidable, given the enormous variety in size and location of lesions as well as the spectrum of linguistic disorders observed. In our approach to this problem, we chose to simplify by focusing on one type of subcortical lesion producing aphasia, the striatocapsular infarct (Nadeau & Crosson, 1997). We did so for two reasons. First, this is a relatively common lesion that is typically fairly stereotyped in size and configuration. Second, because this infarct apparently is confined to structures that appear to have nothing to do with language (i.e., the head of the caudate nucleus, the putamen, and the interleaved anterior limb of the internal capsule) (Fig. 19-1), the very existence of aphasia in patients

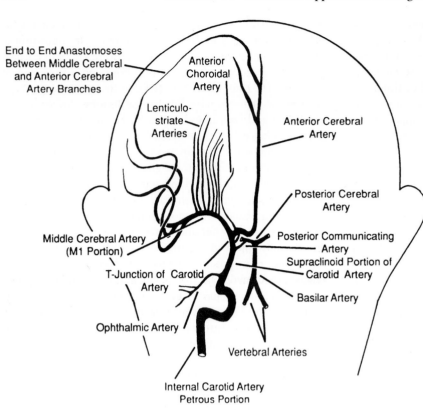

End to End Anastomoses Between Middle Cerebral and Anterior Cerebral Artery Branches

Anterior Choroidal Artery

Lenticulo-striate Arteries

Anterior Cerebral Artery

Posterior Cerebral Artery

Middle Cerebral Artery (M1 Portion)

Posterior Communicating Artery

Supraclinoid Portion of Carotid Artery

T-Junction of Carotid Artery

Basilar Artery

Ophthalmic Artery

Vertebral Arteries

Internal Carotid Artery Petrous Portion

Figure 19–4. Anteroposterior view of cerebral vascular anatomy relevant to the problem of nonthalamic subcortical aphasia. (From Nadeau et al., 2004; with permission.)

with this lesion provides compelling evidence of either an unrecognized neural mechanism or a completely non-neural mechanism. In fact, the latter proved to be the case.

The striatocapsular infarct is caused by the propagation of thrombus or the embolization of blood clot into the proximal (M1) portion of the middle cerebral artery (Fig. 19–4). There, the clot occludes the lenticulostriate arteries supplying the head of the caudate nucleus, the anterior limb of the internal capsule, and much of the putamen, causing essentially complete infarction (death) of these structures. It should be noted, however, that this same clot also severely reduces the flow of blood to the middle cerebral artery branches supplying the overlying cerebral cortex. This cortex becomes entirely dependent on blood flowing backward into the middle cerebral artery branches from their connections (anastomoses) with branches of the anterior cerebral artery and the posterior cerebral artery. If these anastomoses are abundant and large, the cortex will be relatively spared; if they are sparse and small, a massive stroke will occur. One might object that if ischemia exists sufficient to cause aphasia, the damaged tissue should be apparent on imaging studies, but this clearly is not the case. Even newer and more sensitive magnetic resonance imaging techniques, such as diffusion-weighted imaging (DWI), may fail to demonstrate any cortical abnormalities, at least within the first 24 hours (Hillis et al., 2002). Studies of cerebral blood flow in patients

with acute striatocapsular infarcts and otherwise normal structural images (including DWI), however, have shown dramatic reductions in cortical blood flow in precisely the regions that would be expected from the character of the aphasia (e.g., hypoperfusion in the posterior perisylvian temporal region in patients with features of Wernicke's aphasia); conversely, patients with subcortical lesions who exhibit no reductions in cortical blood flow do not have aphasia (Hillis et al., 2002, 2004; Nadeau & Crosson, 1997). Functional imaging studies in patients with chronic nonthalamic subcortical aphasia also demonstrate reduced blood flow or metabolism in cortical regions precisely corresponding to the pattern of the language impairment observed (Nadeau & Crosson, 1997). Furthermore, although a year later no focal abnormalities are observed on anatomic imaging studies of the cortex in these chronic patients, the studies demonstrate hemispheric cortical atrophy—unequivocal evidence of earlier cortical damage involving neurons or their connections (Weiller et al., 1993).

This hypothesis regarding the mechanism of nonthalamic subcortical aphasia predicts that cortical damage could occur anywhere within the cortex supplied by the middle cerebral artery, delimited only by the pattern and adequacy of arterial anastomoses. One would then expect aphasias of all types—or even no aphasia at all—with striatocapsular infarcts or any other subcortical infarct reflecting proximal middle cerebral artery occlusion. In fact, this turns out to be the case. In addition, some subcortical infarcts, as well as hemorrhages into the putamen, disrupt the connections between language cortex and the thalamus. Thus, they likely add features of thalamic aphasia to whatever language disorder results directly from the cortical damage. Striatocapsular infarcts also may disrupt frontothalamic projections traversing the anterior limb of the internal capsule, disrupting thalamic function as well (Tatemichi et al., 1992). Hemorrhages into the putamen can produce pressure on overlying cortex with associated ischemic damage.

One can immediately conclude from this discussion that nonthalamic subcortical aphasias likely are not fundamentally different from cortical aphasias, either in character or pathogenesis, and that they should be treated in the same way. Furthermore, unlike aphasias resulting from thalamic lesions, which appear to be intrinsically limited to impairment in declarative memory systems, cortical aphasias may implicate both declarative and procedural systems. Indeed, nonthalamic subcortical aphasias are as varied as cortical aphasias, and they commonly include impairment in grammatical and phonologic function as well as lexical-semantic function.

NONLINGUISTIC BEHAVIORAL DISORDERS RELEVANT TO THE REHABILITATION PROCESS

During the last 20 years, our estimates regarding the fundamental plasticity of the adult cerebrum have increased 100-fold. In principle, it seems that any type of cerebral dysfunction might be susceptible to rehabilitation. The function of several fundamental cerebral systems, however, appears to be critical to the very conduct of the rehabilitation process. We suggest that, when these systems are substantially impaired, any rehabilitation, but particularly rehabilitation at the level of sophistication and refinement of speech/language therapy, may be problematic and the prognosis for meaningful advances in therapy relatively poor. These functional systems include arousal, attention, and frontal systems. Faced as we are with overwhelming pressures to optimize the use of our treatment resources, it is important to identify these types of deficits ahead of time.

Arousal

Impairment in arousal typically reflects dysfunction of the MRF. A host of disorders commonly produce transient dysfunction of the MRF (e.g., metabolic disorders, drugs, infections, and intracerebral masses). Most often, however, patients develop *persistent* dysfunction because of embolism to the top of the basilar artery, which occludes small vessels supplying the MRF, as well as one or both posterior cerebral arteries (hence abnormalities in vision [e.g., hemianopia or cortical blindness]). Infarcts of the midline thalamus, some

of which produce aphasia, often extend caudally into the MRF. These patients often experience lethargy that, although most severe initially (to the point of coma), often persists for months or years. No treatment has been shown to be effective in mitigating this lethargy. Because these patients behave as if they are constantly half-asleep, they are unable to engage fruitfully in rehabilitation efforts, and their long-term prognosis for an active, interactive life is poor.

Attention

Arousal is a necessary substrate for attention, so patients with impaired arousal will have impaired attention. Patients with frontal system dysfunction also often will have a disorder of intentional or volitional attention, even though their level of arousal is normal. Thus, they are limited in their ability to sustain focused attention, and they tend to be very distractible. This behavior may substantially undermine any rehabilitation program. This type of impairment most often is seen with lesions implicating the dorsolateral frontal lobes bilaterally, but it also may be a feature of patients with midline thalamic lesions.

Patients with nondominant hemisphere dysfunction, most often caused by parietal lobe lesions (cortical or nonthalamic subcortical) and, occasionally, by thalamic lesions, often will exhibit a hemispatial disorder of attention known as hemispatial neglect, in which patients fail to attend or respond to any stimuli presented in the left hemispace. This same disorder sometimes is seen with dominant hemisphere lesions but, characteristically, is much less severe. Nevertheless, even patients with dominant hemisphere lesions (cortical, subcortical, or thalamic) without apparent right hemispatial neglect may benefit from presentation of stimuli in the left hemispace for reasons that are still poorly understood and controversial (Coslett, Schwartz, Goldberg, Haas, & Perkins, 1993; Crosson et al., 2005; Nadeau, Crosson, Schwartz, & Heilman, 1997; Nadeau & Heilman, 1991).

Frontal Systems Dysfunction

Frontal systems dysfunction may impede therapy in other ways. The precise impact depends on the locus of the predominant pathology. Patients with midline frontal systems dysfunction tend to be akinetic in their general behavior and nonfluent in their language. Typically, they are poorly motivated, cannot carry out multi-step commands, and may actively resist any type of intervention by caretakers. Patients with orbitofrontal system dysfunction may appear superficially to be normal, but they tend to be irresponsible, cannot be relied on to sustain goal-oriented activity, and tend to be socially inappropriate. Both of these types of patients pose major challenges for any type of rehabilitation program. Patients with dorsolateral frontal system dysfunction may retain strong motivation and exhibit excellent cooperation in rehabilitation programs. The side of the lesion often assumes major importance. Patients with dominant hemisphere lesions, such as patients with Broca's or global aphasia, often are excellent candidates for speech therapy. Patients with nondominant hemisphere lesions (seldom seen for aphasia rehabilitation), however, often exhibit anosognosia (denial of illness) or anosodiaphoria (lack of concern for illness). These patients are poorly motivated to participate in any rehabilitation program, because, put simply, they either do not recognize the problem or do not care about it.

Frontal systems disorders manifested in these ways rarely are a significant problem in patients with nonthalamic subcortical aphasia unless bilateral lesions exist. Midline thalamic lesions, however, are almost uniformly associated with prominent frontal systems dysfunction. When not lethargic, these patients often appear superficially to be quite normal in their general demeanor. Often, however, they exhibit the most profound lack of motivation, even to the point of perpetually placing obstacles in the way of any rehabilitation efforts (e.g., "I'm too tired;" "I have another appointment in two hours;" "I'm too busy;" "I think I've already done enough of that this week"). Thus, they reflect some blend of midline and orbitofrontal systems dysfunction.

Concept Formation

Spoken language depends on the translation of concepts into the articulatory motor sequences that will produce sounds that are intelligible to others. Concepts can be generated in two fundamentally different ways. First, if we look at something, a concept is automatically elicited as the visual input automatically generates a distributed representation in cerebral association cortices corresponding to that concept. Second, we have the power to intentionally generate a distributed representation corresponding to a concept from within—a fragment of a process we refer to as thinking. Some rare patients, usually with bilateral lesions, may exhibit impairment in their ability to automatically generate distributed concept representations in response to specific types of sensory input. They will be unable to name or describe the properties or use of objects they are observing. This disorder, most often seen after lesions of visual pathways, is termed "agnosia." Other patients exhibit selective impairment in their ability to generate distributed concept representations from within. These patients typically appear to be profoundly nonfluent in spontaneous language, tending either not to respond or to respond with single words or short phrases. When asked, however, to describe a complex picture (in which case distributed concept representations are automatically generated from without), they typically perform almost normally. This disorder is termed "adynamic aphasia" (Gold et al., 1997). It characteristically is

seen with frontal lobe lesions, most often affecting the dominant frontal lobe or being bilateral in location. It may be seen with nonthalamic subcortical infarcts. In addition, patients with thalamic infarcts associated with aphasia may exhibit some features of adynamic aphasia, although rarely in these cases is the fullest form of this disorder seen. Effective speech therapy is not absolutely precluded in such patients, but spontaneous language is unlikely to become fluent because of the more fundamental underlying deficit (Huntley & Rothi, 1988). For similar reasons, we suspect that patients with paradynamic aphasia (see the section *What Is Likely To Be the Specific Impact of Disorders of the Thalamic Gating Mechanism on Function of the Cerebral Cortex [Most Specifically the Language Cortex]?*) also likely are poor candidates for rehabilitation.

KEY POINTS

Subcortical aphasia is logically divided into thalamic and nonthalamic types. Aphasia caused by thalamic lesions appears to reflect dysfunction of cortical systems involved in language as a result of damage to the thalamic mechanisms for selectively engaging cortical neuronal networks. It is characterized almost exclusively by lexical-semantic dysfunction. Aphasia caused by nonthalamic subcortical lesions predominantly reflects acute hypoperfusion of the cortex or chronic damage to the cortex that is not apparent on structural imaging studies, caused in turn by ischemia in the distal territory of the middle cerebral artery, the proximal occlusion of which is directly responsible for the visible subcortical lesion. Nonthalamic subcortical infarcts therefore may be associated with any type of aphasia, and nonthalamic subcortical aphasia is not fundamentally different from cortical aphasia.

Disorders of brain systems supporting arousal, attention, and frontal systems function and causing lethargy, inattention, or poor motivation, which often are seen with thalamic strokes, as well as lesions impacting frontal systems function (frontal or thalamic) and causing adynamic or paradynamic aphasia, disorders of endogenous concept formation, may limit the effectiveness of speech therapy.

FUTURE TRENDS

The proposed mechanisms of thalamic aphasia discussed in this chapter, although both cogent and supported by human lesion studies as well as animal research, have not been adequately tested empirically. Whether our application of the declarative/procedural dichotomy to language processes in general, and to thalamic subcortical aphasias in particular, made in the hopes of clarifying fundamental mechanisms, ultimately will be vindicated also remains to be seen.

KEY POINTS

1. Aphasia caused by thalamic lesions (hemorrhages or infarcts) appears to reflect dysfunction of cortical systems involved in language as a result of damage to thalamic mechanisms for selectively engaging cortical networks. It is characterized predominantly by lexical-semantic dysfunction.

2. Aphasia caused by nonthalamic subcortical hemorrhages or infarcts stems mainly from acute hypoperfusion of the cortex or chronic damage to the cortex that is not apparent on structural imaging studies. It may be characterized by any of the linguistic disorders seen with aphasia caused by cortical lesions. A good correlation exists between the type of aphasia observed and the pattern of cerebral blood flow or metabolism seen on functional imaging studies.

3. Lesions causing thalamic aphasia also may cause lethargy, inattention, and poor motivation, all of which are behaviors that may limit the effectiveness of speech therapy. This is particularly seen with midline thalamic lesions.

4. The thalamus is best understood as a gated relay device. The pulvinar-LP complex of the thalamus relays cortico-cortical transmission from portions of the frontal, temporal, and parietal lobes involved in language function, and dysfunction of this nucleus in thalamic aphasia appears to impair the engagement or spoken word forms by concept representations. The DM relays cortico-cortical transmission from the frontal lobes, and dysfunction of this nucleus in thalamic aphasia appears to cause disorders of endogenous concept formation.

5. The thalamic gate can be opened or closed nonselectively by brain-stem structures, including the MRF responsible for maintaining our level of arousal. The thalamic gate can be opened or closed selectively and volitionally by the frontal lobes acting through a complex system that involves the thalamic NR, which envelopes the thalamus, and the CmPf deep with the thalamus. Thalamic aphasia occasionally is caused by hemorrhage into the thalamic nuclei most directly involved in language, the pulvinar-LP complex and the DM. In most cases, however, thalamic aphasia appears to be caused by disruption of the frontally controlled selective gating mechanism for one entire half of the thalamus.

6. The thalamus is a key component of one of the many mechanisms in the brain that enable selective engagement of cortical systems—that is, the bringing online of particular cortical neural networks needed at any given time to process a particular stimulus and generate an appropriate response.

7. Portions of the thalamus implicated in language function appear to be involved in processes involving declarative knowledge. The predominant deficit observed with thalamic lesions—namely, lexical-semantic dysfunction—is consistent with this idea. The rare subjects with thalamic lesions who produce neologisms or exhibit disorders of grammar appear to challenge this concept. Production of neologisms and grammatical dysfunction may be understandable, however, as disorders involving declarative knowledge.

ACTIVITIES FOR REFLECTION AND DISCUSSION

1. Why does the brain need selective engagement mechanisms? Discuss these mechanisms in relation to attention and language.

2. Discuss the differences between declarative and procedural memory in terms of the types of knowledge involved, the manner in which the brain acquires these types of knowledge, and the brain systems supporting knowledge acquisition.

3. Lexical-semantic function can be readily understood in terms of factual knowledge—that is, declarative memories. Consider how certain aspects of phonologic and grammatical function also might involve declarative knowledge and, thus, be susceptible to occasional disruption in subjects with thalamic aphasia.

4. Subjects with nonthalamic subcortical aphasia may exhibit nearly any pattern of language impairment. Consider how this can be explained in terms of the aberrations in blood flow to the brain that commonly occur with stroke.

5. Are thalamic and nonthalamic subcortical aphasias best viewed in terms of loss of language knowledge or in terms of loss of access to language knowledge? Why?

References

Bender, D. B., & Youakim, M. (2001). Effect of attentive fixation inmacaque thalamus and cortex. *Journal of Neurophysiology, 85,* 219–234.

Bertelson, P., & De Gelder, B. (1989). Learning about reading from illiterates. In A. M. Galaburda (Ed.), *From reading to neurons* (pp. 1–25). Cambridge: MIT Press.

Bezdudnaya, T., Cano, M., Bereshpolova, Y., Stoelzel, C. R., Alonso, J.- M., & Swadlow, H. A. (2006). Thalamic burst mode and inattention in the awake LGNd. *Neuron, 49,* 421–432.

Coslett, H. B., Schwartz, M. F., Goldberg, G., Haas, D., & Perkins, J. (1993). Multi-modal hemispatial deficits after left hemisphere stroke. *Brain, 116,* 527–554.

Cox, C. L., & Sherman, S. M. (1999). Glutamate inhibits thalamic reticular neurons. *Journal of Neuroscience, 19,* 6694–6699.

Crabtree, J. W., & Isaac, J. T. R. (2002). New intrathalamic pathways allowing modality-related and cross-modality switching in the dorsal thalamus. *Journal of Neuroscience, 22,* 8754–8761.

Crosson, B., Moore, A. B., Gopinath, K. S., White, K. D., Wierenga, C. E., Gaiefsky, M. E., et al. (2005). Role of the right and left hemispheres in recovery of function during treatment of intention in aphasia. *Journal of Cognitive Neuroscience, 17,* 392–406.

Desimone, R., Wessinger, M., Thomas, L., & Schneider, W. (1990). Attentional control of visual perception: Cortical and subcortical mechanisms. *Cold Spring Harbor Symposium on Quantative Biology, 55,* 963–971.

De Witte, L., Wilssens, I., Engelborghs, S., De Deyn, P. P., & Mariën, P. (2006). Impairment of syntax and lexical semantics in a patient with bilateral paramedian thalamic infarction. *Brain and Language, 96,* 69–77.

Ebert, A. D., Vinz, B., Görtler, M., Wallesch, C.- W., & Herrmann, M. (1999). Is there a syndrome of tuberothalamic artery infarction? A case report and critical review. *Journal of Clinical and Experimental Neuropsychology, 21,* 397–411.

Fuster, J. M. (1991). The prefrontal cortex and its relation to behavior. *Progress in Brain Research, 87,* 201–211.

Gold, M., Nadeau, S. E., Jacobs, D. H., Adair, J. C., Gonzalez-Rothi, L. J., & Heilman, K. M. (1997). Adynamic aphasia: A transcortical motor aphasia with defective semantic strategy formation. *Brain and Language, 57,* 374–393.

Goldenberg, G., Wimmer, A., & Maly, J. (1983). Amnesic syndrome with a unilateral thalamic lesion: A case report. *J Neurol, 229,* 79–86.

Goldman-Rakic, P. S. (1990). Cellular and circuit basis of working memory in prefrontal cortex of nonhuman primates. *Progress in Brain Research, 85,* 325–336.

Hillis, A. E., Wityk, R. J., Barker, P. B., Beauchamp, N. J., Gailloud, P., Murphy, K., et al. (2002). Subcortical aphasia and neglect in acute stroke: The role of cortical hypoperfusion. *Brain, 125,* 1094–1104.

Hillis, A. E., Work, M., Barker, P. B., Jacobs, M. A., Breese, E. L., & Maurer, K. (2004). Re-examining the brain regions crucial for orchestrating speech articulation. *Brain, 127,* 1479–1487.

Huntley, R. A., & Rothi, L. J. (1988). Treatment of verbal akinesia in a case of transcortical motor aphasia. *Aphasiology, 2,* 55–66.

Kubat-Silman, A. K., Dagenbach, D., & Absher, J. R. (2002). Patterns of impaired verbal, spatial, and object working memory after thalamic lesions. *Brain and Cognition, 50,* 178–193.

Lhermitte, F. (1984). Language disorders and their relationship to thalamic lesions. *Advances in Neurology, 42,* 99–113.

McAlonan, K., Cavanaugh, J., & Wurtz, R. H. (2006). Attentional modulation of thalamic reticular neurons. *Journal of Neuroscience, 26,* 4444–4450.

Minamimoto, T., & Kimura, M. (2002). Participation of the thalamic Cm-Pf complex in attentional orienting. *Journal of Neurophysiology, 87,* 3090–3101.

Moran, J., & Desimone, R. (1985). Selective attention gates visual processing in extrastriate cortex. *Science, 229,* 782–784.

Nadeau, S. E. (2001). Phonology: A review and proposals from a connectionist perspective. *Brain and Language, 79,* 511–579.

Nadeau, S. E., & Crosson, B. (1997). Subcortical aphasia. *Brain and Language, 58,* 355–402, 436–458.

Nadeau, S. E., Crosson, B., Schwartz, R. L., & Heilman, K. M. (1997). Gaze-related enhancement of hemispheric blood flow in a stroke patient. *Journal of Neurology, Neurosurgery, and Psychiatry, 62,* 538–540.

Nadeau, S. E., Ferguson, T. S., Valenstein, E. Vierck, C. S., Getraska, J. C., Streit W. J., Ritz, L. A. (2004). Medical Neuroscience. Philadelphia Saunders/Elsevier.

Nadeau, S. E., & Gonzalez-Rothi, L. J. (1993). Morphologic agrammatism following a right hemisphere stroke in a dextral patient. *Brain and Language, 43,* 642–667.

Nadeau, S. E., & Heilman, K. M. (1991). Gaze-dependent hemianopia without hemispatial neglect. *Neurology, 41,* 1244–1250.

Petersen, S. E., Robinson, D. L., & Morris, J. D. (1987). Contributions of the pulvinar to visual spatial attention. *Neuropsychologia, 25,* 97–105.

Pinault, D. (2004). The thalamic reticular nucleus: Structure, function and concept. *Brain Research Reviews, 46,* 1–31.

Posner, M. I., Walker, J. A., Friedrich, F. A., & Rafal, R. D. (1987). How do the parietal lobes direct covert attention? *Neuropsychologia, 25,* 135–145.

Raymer, A. M., Moberg, P., Crosson, B., Nadeau, S., & Gonzalez Rothi, L. J. (1997). Lexical-semantic deficits in two patients with dominant thalamic infarction. *Neuropsychologia, 35,* 211–219.

Semenza, C., Butterworth, B., Panzeri, M., & Ferreri, T. (1990). Word formation: New evidence from aphasia. *Neuropsychologia, 28,* 499–502.

Sherman, S. M. (2005). Thalamic relays and cortical functioning. *Progress in Brain Research, 149,* 107–126.

Squire, L. R. (1987). *Memory and the brain.* New York: Oxford University Press.

Squire, L. R. (1992). Declarative and non-declarative memory: Multiple brain systems supporting learning and memory. *Journal of Cognitive Neuroscience, 4,* 232–243.

Steriade, M., Parent, A., & Hada, J. (1984). Thalamic projections of nucleus reticularis thalami of cat: A study using retrograde transport of horseradish peroxidase and fluorescent tracers. *Journal of Comparative Neurology, 229,* 531–547.

Tatemichi, T. K., Desmond, D. W., Prohovnik, I., Cross, D. T., Gropen, T. I., Mohr, J. P., et al. (1992). Confusion and memory loss from capsular genu infarction: A thalamocortical disconnection syndrome? *Neurology, 42,* 1966–1979.

Van der Werf, Y. D., Scheltens, P., Lindeboom, J., Witter, M. P., Uylings, H. B. M., & Jolles, J. (2003). Deficits of memory, executive functioning and attention following infarction in the thalamus; A study of 22 cases with localised lesions. *Neuropsychologia, 41,* 1330–1344.

Weese, G. D., Phillips, J. M., & Brown, V. J. (1999). Attentional orienting is impaired by unilateral lesions of the thalamic reticular nucleus in the rat. *Journal of Neuroscience, 19,* 10135–10139.

Weiller, C., Willmes, K., Reiche, W., Thron, A., Insensee, C., Buell, U., et al. (1993). The case of aphasia or neglect after striatocapsular infarction. *Brain, 116,* 1509–1525.

Wester, K., Irvine, D. R. F., & Hugdahl, K. (2001). Auditory laterality and attentional deficits after thalamic haemorrhage. *Journal of Neurology, 248,* 676–683.

Chapter 20

Primary Progressive Aphasia and Apraxia of Speech

Joseph R. Duffy and
Malcolm R. McNeil

OBJECTIVES

In this chapter, primary progressive aphasia (PPA) and primary progressive apraxia of speech (AOS) will be defined; the criteria for their diagnoses reviewed; their common presenting histories and basic demographics discussed; the characteristics of the aphasia, AOS, and associated motor speech impairments summarized; common neuroimaging findings and the variety of possible underlying autopsy-based pathologic diagnoses reviewed; and theoretic and philosophical aspects of management as well as the meager treatment efficacy data summarized and discussed. Because considerably more is known about PPA than primary progressive AOS, the primary emphasis of this chapter will be on PPA.

Because aphasia and apraxia of speech (AOS) are most commonly caused by stroke, what we understand about their nature, assessment, diagnosis, prognosis, and management is overwhelmingly based on data derived from people in whom these conditions were stroke-induced. Despite this, clinicians recognize that the conditions of closed-head and penetrating head injuries, tumors, surgical complications, and infection can cause aphasia and AOS. All of these etiologies usually are acute or subacute in onset, and their natural (i.e., untreated) course usually is considered to be one of sudden or subacute onset, with severity being greatest early post-onset, followed by decelerating physiological improvement, ultimately to a point at which the disorder is considered to be resolved, or improving minimally without intervention and, thus, considered to be in its chronic state.

Twenty-five years ago, most speech-language pathologists and neurologists would have considered aphasia to be incompatible with a diagnosis of degenerative central nervous system (CNS) disease. The generally accepted principle was that degenerative neurologic diseases (e.g., Alzheimer's disease [AD]) impair cognitive functions diffusely and only rarely (or never) in a focal or selective way. Thus, any aphasic-like difficulties in individuals with degenerative CNS disease presumably were embedded within a constellation of cognitive difficulties that might include, but always extended beyond, the language domain.

It now is commonly recognized that aphasia can announce the presence of degenerative neurologic disease and that it may be the only manifestation of CNS disease for a substantial period of time—or perpetually. When this happens, the condition is commonly referred to as "primary progressive aphasia" (PPA). Less well recognized is the fact that AOS can present in the same way, often with aphasia and/or dysarthria but sometimes as the only communication impairment. In such cases, "primary progressive AOS" (PPAOS) is an appropriate diagnostic label.

PRIMARY PROGRESSIVE APHASIA

Basic Definition and Terminology

We reserve the term "aphasia" for language processing deficits that cross levels or domains of language (e.g., semantics, syntax, morphology, and phonology) as well as language modalities (e.g., listening, reading, writing, talking, and gesturing). These deficits are not attributable to sensory or motor deficits or to a loss of the representations or rules of language. They result from deficits of the cognitive apparatus used to buffer, activate, and inhibit, in precisely timed patterns, the rules and representations of language.

Aphasia, in the absence of other CNS deficits, is caused by relatively focal damage to the language-dominant hemisphere (usually the left) and is most often (but not in the case of PPA) of sudden onset. When, however, language or communication deficits are embedded within a constellation of other cognitive deficits (e.g., those seen in persons with dementia or traumatic brain injury), particularly (but not only) at its onset, it is *not* considered to be aphasia. The reasons for these inclusion and exclusion criteria are both theoretic and clinical, having implications for epidemiologic and other forms of research on prognosis, assessment, and intervention. It is beyond the scope of this chapter to discuss aphasia definitions and their inclusionary and exclusionary criteria in detail; such discussions can be found in Darley (1982), McNeil (1988), McNeil and Pratt (2001), and Mesulam (1987). To use the term "aphasia," however, modified by its onset and time-course, evidence is required that other cognitive deficits that cross non-linguistic domains of knowledge, such as procedural memory deficits, altered personality, visuoperceptual impairments, altered personal, temporal or spatial orientation, or psychiatric illness, are not present or are not accounted for by a single or common etiology.

Primary progressive aphasia can be defined as aphasia of insidious onset, gradual progression, and prolonged course, without evidence of non-language computational impairments that are shared by a common etiology to the aphasia, and caused by a degenerative condition that, presumably and predominantly, involves the left (language-dominant) perisylvian region of the brain (modified from Duffy, 1987). Because concomitant non-language processing and computational impairments probably become evident very often during later stages of the disorder, the term PPA is used only when the concomitant impairments are not manifest. At the point in time when non-language cognitive impairments become detectable during formal assessment and are functionally meaningful, the criteria for a different diagnosis are met (e.g., dementia), and the diagnosis changes from one of PPA to one of aphasia plus the other disorder or the other disorder alone. In addition, because aphasia is a behavioral manifestation of neurologic disease, it is important to remember that PPA is a clinical syndrome and not necessarily a reflection of a single, underlying brain pathology. This principle will become evident when the underlying histopathology associated with PPA is addressed.

Similar to many clinical disorders, particularly early in the history of their recognition, definition, and study, PPA has had a number of aliases, some of which can be considered as synonymous with PPA and others of which—under careful scrutiny—probably represent other diagnostic entities. The terms "slowly progressive aphasia" (e.g., Duffy, 1987; Kempler et al., 1990; Kushner, 1990; Poeck & Luzzatti, 1988) and "progressive aphasia without dementia" (e.g., Heath, Kennedy, & Kapur, 1983; Mesulam, 1982; Scheltens, Hazenberg, Lindeboom, Valk, & Wolters, 1990) probably refer to the same clinical entity as PPA; they seem

to have succumbed to PPA as the preferred diagnostic label.[1] In contrast, terms such as "aphasic (or dysphasic) dementia," "nonfamilial dysphasic dementia," "familial aphasia," and "hereditary dysphasic dementia" (e.g., Cole, Wright, & Banker, 1979; Kobayashi, Kurachi, Gyoubu, Imao, & Nakamura, 1990; Mehler, 1988; Morris, Cole, Branker, & Wright, 1984) may or may not be synonymous with PPA as defined here; at least some of the cases in reports using those labels had evidence of widespread impairment of cognition early in their course. It bears repeating that PPA does not include patients in whom language impairment or aphasia is just a prominent manifestation of dementia.[2]

Historical Perspective

Although modern interest in PPA was sparked by Mesulam in 1982, isolated or relatively isolated progressive language impairment in association with degenerative neurologic disease has been recognized since the late 1800s. For example, Pick published a paper in 1892 titled "On the relation between aphasia and senile atrophy of the brain" (translated by Girling & Berrios, 1994). In 1914, Mingazzini published a paper titled "On aphasia due to atrophy of the cerebral convolutions." Ironically, Maurice Ravel (1872–1937), whose *Bolero* musically chronicles a slow progression to a climactic conclusion, developed a relatively focal progressive neurologic disease at 52 years of age, with prominent aphasia, apraxia, agraphia, alexia, and loss of musical creativity (Henson, 1988). In a review article, Poeck and Luzzatti (1988) identified 19 cases in the literature before 1950 that, today, might be labeled PPA.

There is no doubt, however, that Mesulam's 1982 summary of six cases with slowly progressive aphasia without other cognitive deficits is the modern seminal work on the topic. It generated interest in PPA in particular, but also in the general concept that a variety of focal cognitive deficits

---

[1]We adhere to the term "primary" modifying the progressive nature of the aphasia with acknowledgement that it is philosophically inconsistent with our criteria for the syndrome's identification. We adhere to this term to avoid advancing yet another term to describe the emerging literature on this etiologically based category of aphasia. We believe it is important to recognize that the term does not, in our definition, imply that the aphasic signs and symptoms are simply the most obvious, prevalent, or severe deficit that is accompanied by deficits in other cognitive domains. If other such deficits are validly and reliably identifiable and are attributable to a common etiology, then the diagnosis of PPA probably is not appropriate.

[2]We *do* believe it is reasonable to include within the scope of the definition of PPA people in whom neuropsychological examination raises questions about impairment of cognitive functions beyond the language domain, but in whom there is no such evidence during basic clinical examination and no complaint of such impairment either by the patient or by those who know the patient well.

can be associated with degenerative neurologic disease. Since then, hundreds of cases have been reported, and subsequent reviews of their cumulative meaning have appeared (e.g., Duffy & Petersen, 1992; Mesulam, 2001, 2003; Mesulam & Weintraub, 1992; Rogers & Alarcon, 1999; Westbury & Bub, 1997). Mesulam (2001) has suggested that "PPA may well be the fifth most common form of degenerative dementia, following in prevalence AD, FLD [frontal lobe dementia], Parkinson-related dementia, and dementia with Lewy bodies" (p.431).

Because in recent years PPA frequently has been tied to more specific neurologic diagnoses, sometimes as a disease subtype (e.g., frontotemporal dementia [FTD]) and sometimes as one of the possible signs of a disease (e.g., corticobasal degeneration [CBD] and progressive supranuclear palsy [PSP]), its demographic features have become intermingled with those of the associated conditions. For that reason, the data reviewed in the basic demographics section of this chapter (and summarized in Table 20–1) rely heavily on reviews that have focused exclusively on PPA (Duffy &

TABLE 20–1

Demography/Epidemiology of Primary Progressive Aphasia

	Mean	Range	Standard Deviation
Age of onset (years)	Late 50s[1,2]	40–70[ab]	
Fluent aphasia	56.8[c]	40–69[c]	7.1[c]
Nonfluent aphasia	62[c]	40–81[c]	8.5[c]
"Undetermined" aphasia	62.6[c]	17–81[c]	13.2[c]
Average	60.5[c]	17–81	9.6[3\c]
Gender ratio (M:F)	~2:1[ab]		
Duration of isolated language signs & symptoms to onset of cognitive impairment or death (years)			
Fluent aphasia	5.6[c]	2–20[c]	3.9[c]
Nonfluent aphasia	4.8[c]	1.5–14[c]	2.5[c]
"Undetermined" aphasia	4.8[c]	1.5–11[c]	3.0[c]
Average	5.1[c]	1.5–20[c]	3.1[c]
Duration of isolated language signs & symptoms to onset of cognitive impairment (years)	5.3[a]	1–15[a]	
Fluent aphasia	6.6[c]	6–9[c]	
Nonfluent aphasia	4.3[c]	1.5–14[c]	
"Undetermined" aphasia	3.7[c]	1.5–11[c]	
Average (across reports)	5.0	1–15	
Percentage progressing to non-aphasic cognitive impairment	50[a]		
Fluent aphasia	27[c]		
Nonfluent aphasia	37[c]		
"Undetermined" aphasia	73[c]		
Average (across reports)	46.8		
Average time from symptom onset to death (years)[d]			
Fluent aphasia	8.8[c]	4–17[c]	
Nonfluent aphasia	6.8[c]	3–13[c]	
"Undetermined" aphasia	6.5[c]	3–12[c]	
Average	7.4[c]	3–17[c]	
Average age at death (years)			
Fluent aphasia	65.1[c]	62–67[c]	2.0[c]
Nonfluent aphasia	68.4[c]	48–84[c]	9.9[c]
"Undetermined" aphasia	69.0[c]	58–84[c]	11.0[c]
Average	67.4[c]	48–84[c]	7.6[c]

[a] Duffy & Petersen (1992).
[b] Westbury & Bub (1997).
[c] Rogers & Alarcon (1999).
[d] These data were computed from those presented by Rogers & Alarcon (1999). These data include those individuals who remained aphasic only and those that progressed to a diagnosis of dementia. The reader should interpret these and the other data reported here cautiously, because they are based on a retrospective analysis of published reports and on small subject samples.

Petersen, 1992; Mesulam & Weintraub, 1992; Rogers & Alarcon, 1999; Westbury & Bub, 1997), supplemented when possible by more recent data that can be linked unambiguously to PPA.

Considerable variability exists in the degree to which published case studies have met current criteria for the diagnosis of PPA. The large number of such cases, however, as well as the commonalities among them are now sufficient to establish that PPA, although representing an uncommon clinical phenomenon, is not an extremely rare one. Today, case presentations with the sole intent of supporting the existence of PPA are no longer of special interest. Of importance now are studies that improve and refine our understanding of its typical and atypical language manifestations, associated non-language clinical characteristics, clinical course, neuroimaging and other laboratory correlates, histopathology and biochemistry, and responses to behavioral and medical interventions.

Diagnostic Criteria

The criteria for establishing the diagnosis of PPA, originally suggested and subsequently slightly modified by Mesulam and colleagues (Mesulam, 2001, 2003; Weintraub, Rubin, & Mesulam, 1990) seem to be generally accepted at this time. They include:

1. A 2-year history of insidious onset and gradual decline in language ability (e.g., word finding, object naming, syntax, and word comprehension).
2. Relative preservation of other mental functions (e.g., patients with prominent language deficits in the first 2 years but who also have apathy, disinhibition, memory, attention or visuospatial or visual recognition deficits, or sensorimotor impairments, would not meet the criteria).
3. Any major limitations in activities of daily living (ADLs) attributable to the language impairment during the first 2 years.
4. Acalculia, ideomotor apraxia, difficulty copying simple drawings, or perseveration, if present in the first 2 years, that do not significantly limit ADLs.
5. A full neurologic workup that excludes other causes of aphasia (e.g., stroke, tumor, infection, or metabolic disturbances).
6. Comprehensive speech-language and neuropsychological evaluation yields results consistent with the complaint and clinical neurologic examination.

Mesulam (2001, 2003) suggests that non-language cognitive functions can be impaired after the first 2 years, but that language must remain the most impaired function and deteriorate faster than other cognitive functions for the diagnosis of PPA to be maintained.

Some of the above diagnostic criteria are worthy of discussion. Of particular importance is the required 2-year history

before a diagnosis of PPA can be established. This criterion presumably has been set to reduce the number of false-positive diagnoses of PPA (or false-negative diagnoses of dementia). The assumption is that an isolated deficit in the domain of language that has endured for a minimum of 2 years will increase the likelihood that the behaviors are not the initial signs of a more general cognitive deficit. In fact, however, not all investigators have required a 2-year history (Neary, Snowden, & Mann, 1993), and more important, the epidemiological research to support this assumption has not been conducted. Thus, no evidence indicates that this criterion helps to better define the PPA population (Knibb, Xuereb, Patterson, & Hodges, 2006). In addition, a 2-year hiatus in the diagnosis can delay aphasia management and general life planning. It seems that the diagnosis of PPA can and should be made without regard to the duration of its existence, recognizing that the diagnosis should be altered or discarded at such time that other criteria for PPA are no longer met.

A second assumption embedded within the diagnostic criteria is that the language deficit is disproportional to any other non-linguistic deficits. Again, the degree to which non-linguistic functions are or are not relatively spared would be the degree to which they meet the criteria for the diagnosis of aphasia of any etiology or type. It is important to remember that the only difference between the definition of aphasia, in general, and the definition of PPA, as provided here, is in the meaning of the adjectival modifiers "primary" and "progressive."

The third assumption of preserved ADLs is included to help exclude those persons with cognitive deficits outside of the language domain, such as personality, memory, or attention. Persons with aphasia certainly can have deficits of ADLs that involve language and communication. In addition, some individuals' reactions to their aphasia can affect ADLs outside of the language and communication domains. For example, reactive depression can impair ADLs, and embarrassment or frustration with failed communicative interactions can lead to social withdrawal. If a reduction in ADLs is taken at face value as a criterion for rejecting the diagnosis of PPA, it could lead to a decrease in the legitimate diagnosis of PPA and an increase in the false-positive diagnosis of dementia. It thus seems appropriate to modify this criterion to permit inclusion of persons with reduced ADL abilities that are a direct or indirect consequence of the aphasia.

A fourth assumption is that the diagnosis of PPA requires a relatively focal or asymmetric degenerative process, one that is progressive and is of unknown etiology. It is based on the assumption of an etiology that excludes stroke, tumor, infection, and metabolic disturbances. Stroke is focal, of known etiology, and non-progressive. Tumor is focal, of known etiology, and progressive. Infection and metabolic disorders may or may not be focally localized, are of known etiology, and are non-progressive when they are appropriately treated. Table 20–2 summarizes these distinctions.

TABLE 20–2

Aphasia Etiology by Symptom Distribution, Lesion Distribution, Etiology, Disease Course, and Medical Treatment

Etiology	Symptom Distribution	Lesion Distribution	Etiology	Typical Long-term Course	Medical Treatment
Primary progressive aphasia	Language only	Focal	Unknown	Progressive	Untreatable
Vascular	Can be language only	Focal	Known	Chronic	Some early post onset treatment
Infectious (bacterial)	Typically more than aphasia	Focal or diffuse	Known	Progressive until treated	Treatable
Infectious (viral)	Typically more than aphasia	Focal or diffuse	Known	Progressive	Largely untreatable
Metabolic	Typically more than aphasia	Diffuse > focal	Known	Progressive until treated	Treatable
Neoplastic	Can be language only	Focal or multifocal	Known	Progressive	Treatable
Traumatic	Typically more than aphasia	Focal, multifocal, or diffuse	Known	Chronic	Some early post onset treatment

It has been argued that PPA often is a precursor to generalized dementia or AD, and that it is simply a variant of degenerative diseases that typically present with a broader spectrum of deficits (e.g., Gordon & Selnes, 1984; Poeck & Luzzatti, 1988). Today, however, evidence suggests that PPA is only infrequently associated with AD pathology (Mesulam, 2003), which supports its separate diagnostic status. Regardless of the ultimate outcome in a given person, the early prominence of aphasia and its relative isolation for long periods of time justify its distinction from typical, common dementing illnesses. People with PPA must cope for an extended period of time with a different set of problems than do those with generalized dementia. In addition, the prognosis and the underlying pathology may be different, and management approaches may vary considerably (Duffy & Petersen, 1992).

Issues of Classification and Nomenclature

When PPA was considered solely as an independent clinical entity, as it was for the first decade or so after Mesulam brought attention to it, issues of classification generally were tied to subdividing the aphasia into fluent and nonfluent types or into more specific "classical" categories (e.g., Broca's, Wernicke's, or anomic). In the broad context of neurodegenerative diseases, however, it has become evident that PPA also can be thought of as one of several possible manifestations of a general category of disturbances known as asymmetric cortical degeneration syndromes (Caselli & Jack, 1992; Caselli, Jack, Petersen, Wahner, & Yanagihara, 1992) or focal cortical atrophy syndromes (Black, 1996). These generic labels emerged with the recognition of a vari-

ety of isolated cognitive deficits, such as visual agnosia (e.g., DeRenzi, 1986), prosopagnosia (e.g., Tyrrell, Warrington, Frackowiak, & Rosser, 1990), and limb apraxia (e.g., Azouvi et al., 1993; Dick, Snowden, Northen, Goulding, & Neary, 1989; Piccirilli, D'Alessandro, & Ferroni, 1990), that can be associated with degenerative neurologic disease, of which PPA may be the most common. Caselli (1995) argues for the term "asymmetric" as opposed to "focal," because although these cases may present with a progressing focal neurologic syndrome, more diffuse abnormalities often can eventually be demonstrated both clinically and histopathologically.

More recently, the classification of PPA has become intermingled with complex, diverse, and often confusing nomenclature and approaches to the classification of degenerative neurocognitive diseases (Boeve, 2003; Petersen, 2001). This complexity and diversity is fed by "a rapidly expanding body of information on the clinical, neuroimaging, neuropathological, and genetic fronts" (Petersen, 2001, p. 422) but in the absence of a unifying clinical, imaging, histopathological,[3] or biochemical basis for classification (Petersen, 2003). The next few paragraphs will provide some

---

[3] Petersen (2001) observes that histopathology does not solve problems of classification, because it is not necessarily distinctively associated with specific clinical diagnoses. For example, people with clinical diagnoses of PPA, FTD, semantic dementia (SD), and so on can have AD as their underlying pathology (although not typically). In addition, some labels have clinical and pathologic criteria that do not always correspond with one another (e.g., not all people with a clinical diagnosis of AD have AD pathology on autopsy).

examples of how PPA currently is being classified neurologically and of its relationship to broad classifications of degenerative neurocognitive diseases. Their content will not resolve the confusion, but it will identify some of the nomenclature in which information about PPA has become embedded within the neurology literature.

At the simplest level, PPA is now classified among many behavioral neurologists as progressive nonfluent aphasia (PNFA) or SD. Others seem to consider PNFA to be the only type of PPA and view SD as a separate entity, although one involving language (e.g., Hodges et al., 2004; Kertesz, McMonagle, Blair, Davidson, & Munoz, 2005; Neary, Snowden, & Mann, 1993). For those who consider SD to be a subtype of PPA, the term seems to have replaced fluent aphasia (e.g., Neary et al., 1998), which essentially means that SD and fluent aphasia can be considered to be synonymous. For others, fluent aphasia remains a major subcategory of PPA, with SD being a subtype of fluent aphasia (e.g., Grossman & Ash, 2004).

For those who consider SD to be a distinct entity (i.e., not synonymous with fluent PPA), the disorder is characterized by a "loss of word meaning"—affected individuals seem no longer able to associate a word with its meaning, stating, for example, that they do not recognize that the spoken word "fork" represents its eating utensil referent—in the presence of preserved grammar and syntax and preserved verbal comprehension that does not rely on understanding words whose meaning has been lost (e.g., Mesulam, 2001; Neary et al., 1998). This difficulty stands in contrast to that of many people with fluent PPA and anomia who recognize target words they have been unable to name when they are provided to them. Strictly speaking, the diagnosis of SD also should be associated with impaired recognition (visual agnosia) of faces (prosopagnosia) or object identity (associative agnosia) (e.g., Mesulam, 2001; Neary et al., 1998). As a result, Mesulam (2003) has argued that the presence of prominent prosopagnosia and visual associative agnosia during the initial 2 years is incompatible with his definition of PPA, although he recognizes that, in clinical practice, SD often is a diagnosis given to patients with fluent aphasia but without visual agnosia. He feels that such patients without visual agnosia should be labeled as having PPA, not SD. Obviously, this diversity in the use of the term "semantic dementia" is a considerable source of confusion that, at the least, requires careful definition in clinical and research communications.

Going beyond subclassifications of PPA, PPA itself now often is considered to be a subtype of FTD, a degenerative dementia that is second in prevalence only to AD, accounting for 10% to 15% of untreatable dementias (Boeve, 2003). Pathologic substrates of FTD include Pick's disease, CBD, and dementia lacking distinctive histology. Clinically, FTD is characterized by personality-behavioral changes, PPA, or both (Boeve, 2003). Patients with early prominent personality-behavioral changes are considered to represent the frontal phenotype of FTD, whereas those with early prominent language changes (PPA and, for some, SD) are considered to represent the temporal phenotype.

In a similar conceptual approach, PPA is considered to be one (or two) of three distinct manifestations of a broad category of disorders known as frontotemporal lobar degeneration (FTLD) (Neary et al., 1998). Included under this broad heading are (1) FTD, which is characterized by behavioral/personality changes (e.g., disinhibition, impulsivity, poor insight, perseveration, and inflexibility); (2) SD, which is characterized by loss of word or object meaning with preservation of language fluency and syntax; and (3) PNFA, characterized by "labored speech," anomia, and/or agrammatism. It has been suggested that PPA accounts for approximately 10% of FTLDs, and SD accounts for about 15% (Snowden, Neary, & Mann, 2002). Thus, in this scheme, PPA is not considered to be a subtype of FTD but, rather, a subtype of FTLD. Within this approach, patients with SD and PNFA could meet the criteria for a diagnosis of PPA (ignoring the issue of whether SD would capture all patients with fluent PPA).

Finally, Kertesz and Munoz (1997) have argued that several disorders, including PPA, FTD, Pick's disease, and CBD, should be classified as part of "Pick complex" because of shared histopathologic features (discussed later). At this point, however, imaging, neuropathology, genetics, and biochemistry have not provided an absolute answer to the problem of classification (Petersen, 2001). It may be that PPA is linked to multiple diseases sharing a common anatomic locus (i.e., the left hemisphere perisylvian language area). An alternative explanation is that it results from an as-yet-incompletely understood unitary disease (e.g., Pick complex, lobar atrophy-Pick's disease-tauopathy, or frontotemporal degeneration) that includes a spectrum of anatomically and behaviorally distinct degenerative brain disorders. This latter explanation receives some support from genetic analyses of so-called FTLD syndromes that include PPA and FTD (Mesulam, 2001; Mesulam, Grossman, Hillis, Kertesz, & Weintraub, 2003). Petersen (2001) points out that "it is incumbent on the clinician to classify persons with these disorders as accurately as possible to allow for diagnostic, treatment, counseling and prognostic advice for patients and families. In the final analysis there may be no gold standard" (p. 422) on which all of these disorders can be uniquely characterized.

Clinical Presentation

How do people with PPA present clinically? What is their history, and how do they behave? Initial diagnosis hinges strongly on the answers to these questions, so it is important to recognize typical presenting features.

People with PPA often present clinically many months or even a year or more after the onset of language difficulty.

Occasionally, they associate the onset with a specific event, giving the onset a superficially acute appearance; in such cases, more often than not, the event was one with significant language demands or psychological stress (e.g., a public speech). Most frequently, however, the onset is insidious, and the patient and family often are vague or even disagree about when symptoms first appeared. Unlike people with AD, however, those with PPA often are aware of the problem before their family, friends, or work colleagues.

Presenting speech and language complaints can be strikingly similar to those of people with stroke-induced aphasia. The classic refrain of the person with aphasia that "I know what I want to say but I can't find the words!" is commonly heard. Word finding difficulty seems to be the most frequent presenting complaint among people with PPA (Westbury & Bub, 1997).[4]

People with PPA rarely deny their deficits. In fact, they, rather than their families, usually initiate the search for diagnosis and treatment. They do not complain of memory disturbances outside the verbal domain, and they are not disoriented. They and their significant others do not report significant personality changes, although expressions or frank evidence of frustration and reactive depression are common. If work demands are not language-based, job performance can be unchanged. Daily routine activities (e.g., grooming, driving, shopping, and exercising) typically are unaffected. Conversely, if language demands for job performance or daily routine activities (e.g., reading, writing, and calculations for record keeping) are high, especially those involving rapid or large-capacity language processing and extemporaneous production and comprehension, then difficulty with job performance or routine daily activities can be the initial situations that reveal early signs or symptoms.

To summarize, the initial clinical presentation of people with PPA can be strikingly different from those of people with AD or other degenerative diseases that induce diffuse impairments of memory, thinking, organization, self-awareness, personality, and ability to succeed in routine social, self-care, and work activities. Conversely, they can be strikingly similar to stroke-induced and other static etiologies for aphasia.

Character of the Aphasia

It appears that any type of aphasia (as it traditionally has been classified) is possible. The types reported in the not-so-recent literature include fluent and nonfluent, Broca's,

Wernicke's, anomic, and transcortical (e.g., Karbe, Kertesz, & Polk, 1993; Kertesz, Davidson, & McCabe, 1998; Turner, Kenyon, Trojanowski, Gonatas, & Grossman, 1996); even pure word deafness has been reported (Mesulam, 1982; Otsuki, Soma, Sato, Homma, & Tsuji, 1998; Philbrick, Rummans, Duffy, Kokmen, & Jack, 1994).

Because of changing trends in the classification of PPA (see previous discussion), the recent neurologic literature tends to classify patients as having nonfluent or fluent PPA, or SD. Some investigators have also described a logopenic form, in which significant word finding difficulty is present, there is a slowing and decrease of verbal output, but syntax, phonology, and motor speech production are relatively preserved (e.g., Gorno-Tempini, Dronkers et al., 2004; Kertesz, Davidson, & McCabe, 2003; Weintraub et al., 1990).

It is important to note that the subclassification of PPA along a "fluency" dimension is not without problems, and that these problems are similar to those associated with classifying aphasia resulting from stroke or other acute-onset causes (Darley, 1982; McNeil, 1988; Schwartz, 1984). Specifically, the problem with using fluency or nonfluency as valid adjectives for aphasia is that they (1) are without theoretic motivation as a descriptor of language pathology, (2) are not assigned by a set of uniform criteria across users or standardized tests and are unreliably assigned to patients (Trupe, 1984), and (3) as typically applied, are more likely the result of concomitant sensorimotor speech pathologies (dysarthria or AOS) than of a language-specific impairment.[5]

With the above caveats, PPA with nonfluent verbal output characteristics (i.e., Broca's aphasia, agrammatism or telegraphic speech, brief and unelaborated verbal expression, and hesitant and/or dysprosodic speech) deserves some special comment, because it generally is unexpected during the earlier stages of probable AD. It thus contributes to neurologic differential diagnosis. In addition, its demographics, localization, etiology, prognosis, and responsiveness to medical and behavioral management may differ from those PPA without nonfluent language characteristics, which by default are usually termed "fluent" (see the subsequent discussion of neuroimaging correlates and histopathology). In fact, several studies and reviews support the distinction among several PPA subtypes (and SD) on behavioral, anatomical, or pathologic grounds (e.g., Gorno-Tempini, Dronkers et al., 2004; Grossman & Ash, 2004; Josephs et al., 2006a; Kertesz et al., 2003). Operational definitions for PPA types and the reliability of placement of patients into each type, however, are not reported in many studies. It is essential that the characterization of PPA be made on the basis of careful definitions and

---

[4]This complaint alone may not assist differential diagnosis, however, because it also is a common presenting complaint in patients with probable AD.

[5]See the case report of McNeil, Small, Masterson, & Fossett (1995) for a clinical example and discussion of the importance of accurate differential diagnosis of the speech production impairments that often are used to classify the "nonfluency."

descriptions of what constitutes fluent, nonfluent, and other types of aphasia, and with the recognition that many patients may not fit neatly into any single category. As will be discussed in following sections, it also is important to distinguish among aphasia, AOS, and dysarthria in studies of PPA. Only when large series of patients are reported, using strict diagnostic criteria, will the true characterization and distribution of the "type" of aphasia in PPA be clearly understood.

Basic Demographics

Gender Ratio and Age of Onset

Table 20-1 summarizes reviews by Duffy and Petersen (1992), Westbury and Bub (1997), and Rogers and Alarcon (1999). Although these reviews suggest that more men than women are affected, with an approximately 2:1 male:female ratio (Duffy & Petersen, 1992; Westbury & Bub, 1997), it should be noted that recent series of 30 or more patients have not found significant gender differences (e.g., Gorno-Tempini, Dronkers et al., 2004; Kertesz et al., 2003), or they have found male predominance in patients with fluent PPA and female predominance in those with nonfluent PPA (Clark, Charuvastra, Miller, Shapira, & Mendez, 2005). The age of onset is quite variable, covering nearly all adult decades, but onset most often is between 40 and 75 years, with average age of onset across reviews converging on 60.5 years (Duffy & Petersen, 1992; Rogers & Alarcon, 1999; Westbury & Bub, 1997). On average, therefore, PPA develops in the presenium (before age 65).

Time until Onset of Other Cognitive Deficits

Among the cases reported in the literature, the duration from onset of aphasia to the emergence of more widespread impairment of cognitive functions, when they emerge, has varied from 1 to more than 15 years,[6] with an average duration across reviews of about 5 years. Duffy and Petersen's (1992) review found that approximately 50% of persons with PPA eventually developed nonaphasic cognitive impairments. Rogers and Alarcon's (1999) review reported that an overall average of 45.7% (46.8% averaged across reviews) progressed to nonaphasic cognitive impairments. Sentiment is growing, however, that, although many patients have isolated language symptoms for an average of about 5 years

---

[6] Cases with a duration of less than 2 years would not meet Mesulam and colleagues' criteria for a diagnosis of PPA and, if embraced, might be labeled on initial evaluation as having "possible PPA." As stated, however, the diagnosis of PPA is best made on the coherence of both inclusionary criteria for aphasia of any type and exclusionary criteria for the disorders with which it is most likely to be confused (e.g., dementia and conversion disorder).

after onset and for as long as 15 years, the great majority eventually will experience symptoms in areas such as memory, personality, or mood (Green, Morris, Sandson, McKeel, & Miller, 1990; Krefft, Graff-Radford, Dickson, Baker, & Castellani, 2003; Thompson, 1997). Many of the exceptions, especially when onset is later in life, may be those who succumb to unrelated, acute, or more rapidly progressive conditions (e.g., heart attack, carcinoma, and stroke) before the PPA advances to affect other cognitive functions.

Life Expectancy

Although relatively few cases have been reported, the evidence summarized by Rogers and Alarcon (1999) suggests that the average age of death for persons with PPA is 67.4 years, with a 7.6-year standard deviation and a range from 48 to 84 years; the average duration from PPA symptom onset to death was 7.4 years, with a range of 3 to 17 years. These figures are in rough agreement with data from more recent studies of small to relatively large groups of patients with PPA (e.g., Josephs et al., 2005, 2006a,b; Kertesz et al., 2003; Knibb et al., 2006; Krefft et al., 2003). The difference between the number of years of isolated language deficits preceding the onset of non-linguistic cognitive deficits and the average time from symptom onset to death (i.e., the average time from onset of general cognitive deficits to death) was 2.4 years in the Rogers and Alarcon (1999) review; however, this duration spans the considerable range of 1 to 17 years.

Accompanying Deficits

Other neurologic signs and symptoms can accompany PPA. Dysarthria, dysphagia, right-central facial weakness, AOS, nonverbal oral apraxia, limb apraxia, right-extremity weakness or clumsiness, and extrapyramidal deficits (e.g., rigidity) have been reported (e.g., Duffy & Petersen, 1992; Fuh, Liao, Wang, & Lin, 1994; Krefft et al., 2003; McNeil, 1998).

Mesulam et al. (2003) consider dysarthria, ideomotor apraxia, dyscalculia, construction deficits, impaired executive functions, visual recognition deficits, extrapyramidal deficits, and decreased learning of word lists to be "boundary features" of PPA that usually arise later in the disease course and are less prominent than the aphasia. They also note that some patients with PPA develop personality changes characteristic of frontal lobe dementia, extrapyramidal deficits characteristic of CBD (typically characterized by cortical and extrapyramidal signs, including asymmetric limb rigidity and apraxia), or signs of motor neuron disease after 2 years. They suggest that such patients can be said to have a "PPA-plus" syndrome or, alternatively, frontal lobe dementia with aphasia, CBD with aphasia, and so on. It is well-documented that aphasia can be the initial sign (or a prominent early sign) of CBD (Frattali, Grafman, Patronas, Makhlouf, & Litvan, 2000; Gorno-Tempini, Murray et al.,

2004; Kertesz et al., 2003; Lehman Blake, Duffy, Boeve, Ahlskog, & Maraganore, 2003); aphasia was present in more than 50% of patients with CBD who were carefully studied by Frattali et al. (2000) and by Lehman Blake et al. (2003). In addition, PPA has been associated with atypical PSP (Boeve et al., 2003; Josephs et al., 2005) and, rarely, with dementia with Lewy bodies (Caselli, Beach, & Sue, 2002). These interrelationships support the contention that these conditions may belong to a common family of focal diseases and that the individual clinical syndromes reflect a different anatomy of disease onset and progression.

Neuroimaging Correlates

The results of neuroimaging studies that are conducted as part of clinical workups for suspected PPA sometimes are normal, supporting conclusions that the disorder does not stem from stroke, tumor, or other nondegenerative causes of focal lesions. In other cases, neuroimaging identifies abnormalities that contribute to understanding the anatomical bases of the aphasia. The methods most frequently reported include electroencephalography (EEG), magnetic resonance imaging (MRI), positron-emission tomography (PET; measuring glucose use), single-photon-emission computed tomography (SPECT; measuring blood flow), and voxel-based morphometry (VBM; an MRI-based measure of regional brain atrophy using voxel-based comparisons of gray matter volumes between groups of subjects). Abnormalities in blood flow (SPECT) and metabolism (PET) may emerge before evidence of atrophy (MRI and VBM) (Mesulam, 2001).

In a general summary of neuroimaging in PPA, Mesulam (2003) indicated that many patients with PPA have atrophy, EEG slowing, decreased blood flow, and decreased glucose use in left hemisphere language areas. The right hemisphere may be normal, especially early in the course of disease; when right-hemisphere abnormalities are present, they generally are less pronounced than abnormalities in the left hemisphere (Kertesz et al., 2003). Those with nonfluent PPA tend to have metabolic dysfunction and atrophy in the left inferior frontal cortex, whereas those who are fluent and have comprehension deficits have abnormalities in the left temporal lobe. Mesulam's generalizations are supported by previous literature reviews (Duffy & Petersen, 1992; Westbury & Bub, 1997). For example, Westbury and Bub (1997) found that 56% of patients with abnormalities on MRI had left hemisphere abnormalities only, with the remainder having bilateral abnormalities; the left hemisphere abnormalities most often were in the region of the sylvian fissure or temporal lobe. They also found that 97% of patients with PPA who underwent PET or SPECT had abnormalities and that 69% of the abnormalities were in the left hemisphere only (the remaining 31% were bilateral). Most of the left hemisphere abnormalities were in the temporal and/or frontal lobe.

More recent neuroimaging studies generally have identified left perisylvian and anterior temporal and inferior parietal lobe atrophy, without regard to PPA type. Some have found significant overlap and nonsignificant differences in the distribution of anatomic abnormalities between patients with fluent and nonfluent PPA (Clark et al., 2005; Sonty et al., 2003). In general, however, studies of patients classified as nonfluent find evidence of left frontal and perisylvian atrophy (e.g., Abe, Ukita, & Yanagihara, 1997; Josephs et al., 2006a), sometimes more narrowly localized to the left inferior frontal and insular areas (Gorno-Tempini, Dronkers et al., 2004; Nestor et al., 2003). In contrast, studies of fluent PPA or SD find more posterior abnormalities, such as left anterior temporal and inferior parietal lobe atrophy (Gorno-Tempini, Dronkers et al., 2004; Mummery et al., 1999) or superior, middle, and inferior temporal gyri, hippocampal, and parahippocampal gyrus atrophy (Abe et al., 1997); patients with SD tend to have bilateral abnormalities (e.g., Mummery et al., 1999). Findings on VBM of patients classified as logopenic have been localized to the inferior parietal lobe (Gorno-Tempini, Dronkers et al., 2004).

In summary, when patients with PPA have abnormal neuroimaging findings, they tend to show left hemisphere or more left than right hemisphere abnormalities. The fact that some patients with PPA have bilateral abnormalities suggests that their underlying disease is not confined to the left hemisphere, even if their current clinical syndrome is. This supports the contention that PPA and related syndromes may best be thought of as asymmetric rather than focal diseases. It will be important in future research to determine whether patients with PPA and neuroimaging evidence of bilateral disease progress more rapidly to diffuse cognitive deficits than those with neuroimaging evidence of left hemisphere disease only.

Histologic Pathology

Autopsy results for people with PPA are few, but increasing. In general, the pathologic changes in PPA (and SD, when analyzed separately) tend to be consistent with neuroimaging findings regarding the location of the brunt of pathologic changes. That is, they are more pronounced in the frontal lobes, perisylvian regions, and frontal and temporal lobes, in contrast to changes in AD, which typically are most pronounced in hippocampal areas (Davies et al., 2005; Mesulam, 2003).

Histopathologic findings identify a variety of pathologic diagnoses. In a sense, this is not surprising, because anatomical localization, not histopathology, determines the clinical manifestations of neuropathologic processes. The pathologic heterogeneity associated with PPA suggests that it can be caused by several entities whose initial or prominent effects happen to be, for unexplained reasons, located in those areas of the brain that, when affected, result in deficits of language processing consistent with those of aphasia.

Perhaps the most frequent autopsy findings in PPA are of cellular changes that do not correspond to well-known specific clinical or pathologic conditions. It is estimated that about 60% of patients with PPA have microscopic findings commonly called "dementia lacking distinctive histopathology" or "nonspecific focal atrophy," in which there is focal neuronal loss, gliosis, and mild spongioform changes in superficial cortical layers (Krefft et al., 2003; Mesulam, 2001, 2003; Mesulam et al., 2003),

In addition, PPA has been associated with the histopathology of Pick's disease (e.g., Craenhals, Raison-Van Ruymbeke, Rectem, Seron, & Laterre, 1990; Fukui, Sugita, Kawamura, Shiota, & Nakano, 1996; Graff-Radford et al., 1990; Holland, Mcburney, Moossy, & Reinmuth, 1985), which typically manifests clinically as significant cognitive, memory, or personality disturbances. It has been estimated that about 20% of patients with PPA have Pick's disease pathology (i.e., Pick bodies or tau-positive spherical neuronal inclusions) (e.g., Krefft et al., 2003; Mesulam, 2003; Mesulam et al., 2003).

In people with autopsy-confirmed pathologic diagnoses of AD, PPA can occur as well (e.g., Engel & Fleming, 1997; Green, Patterson, Xuereb, & Hodges, 1996; Kempler et al., 1990), but this is not the pathology in a majority of autopsied cases. Some have found AD pathology in about one-third of patients with PPA (split about evenly between those with PNFA and those with SD), although often with an atypical anatomic distribution (Knibb et al., 2006); however, some suggest that pathologic features of AD may not emerge until long after the onset of disease (Mesulam, 2003; Mesulam et al., 2003). Others estimate that less than 20% of people with PPA have AD pathology (e.g., Krefft et al., 2003; Mesulam, 2001, 2003; Mesulam et al., 2003; Mesulam, Johnson, Grujic, & Weintraub, 1997; Westbury & Bub, 1997). Mesulam (2001) points out that none of the genetically caused forms of AD leads to early or prominent language deficits, an observation that supports the distinction between PPA and AD.

Of interest, PPA also has been associated with autopsy-confirmed pathologic diagnoses of CBD, PSP, amyotrophic lateral sclerosis (ALS), Creutzfeldt-Jakob (CJD) disease,[7] and even motor neuron disease[8] (e.g., Arima et al., 1994;

Josephs et al., 2005, 2006b; Mandell, Alexander, & Carpenter, 1989; Sakurai et al., 1996; Shuttleworth, Yates, & Paltan-Ortiz, 1985; Yamanouchi, Budka, & Vass, 1986), the common clinical characteristics of which all include motor disturbances. For example, PSP and CBD pathology accounted for nearly 70% of the pathologic findings in 13 patients with nonfluent PPA studied by Josephs et al. (2006a). In general, although the descriptions of the speech-and-language characteristics of these cases are quite variable, patients with nonfluent verbal output characteristics and/or AOS seem to be over-repesented. In some instances, the aphasia or AOS was the first symptom of disease. For example, the first symptom for all four of the patients with pathologically "atypical PSP" described by Josephs et al. (2005) was speech or language difficulty that, on initial examination, reflected AOS (4/4 patients) and aphasia (3/4 patients).

It may be that this plethora of pathologies share histologic or biochemical features that unite many of them and, in fact, tie PPA to other neurodegenerative diseases. As noted previously, this suggests that PPA and FTLD/FTD may represent anatomically distinct manifestations of a unitary histologic process (Josephs et al., 2006b; Mesulam, 2003; Mesulam et al., 2003; Snowden, Neary, & Mann, 2002), possibly captured by the concept of the Pick complex (Kertesz, 1997; Kertesz, Hudson, MacKenzie, & Munoz, 1994; Kertesz & Munoz, 1997). This generic concept includes several neurodegenerative diseases associated with focal cortical degeneration, such as PPA, FTD, Pick's disease, and CBD. Support for this is exemplified in a recent clinicopathologic study of 60 patients with FTD/Pick complex, 22 of whom had PPA (Kertesz et al., 2005). Findings revealed clinical and pathologic overlap between FTD and PPA and suggested that patients clinically described as having CBD belong within the entity of Pick complex. The study found that patients within the Pick complex had a range of underlying pathologies that, on immunohistochemical analysis, primarily divided between tau-negative and tau-positive (often called "tauopathy"[9]) biochemistry, as well as differences in the cortical and subcortical distribution of lesions. Both PPA and CBD presented more frequently with tau-positive pathology, whereas the behavioral variety of FTD more frequently was tau-negative and associated with motor neuron disease pathology or dementia lacking distinctive histopathology. Kertesz et al. (2005) acknowledged that there may be many exceptions to this dichotomy, and that it may be premature to split the Pick

---

[7] Because most patients with CJD die within 2 years, they would not meet the Mesulam and Weintraub (1992) criteria for PPA diagnosis. Regardless, it is important to recognize that a progressive aphasia can announce the presence of CJD.

[8] A recent study (Davies et al., 2005) examined 18 consecutive cases with SD pathologically. "Motor neuron inclusion dementia" (motor neuron disease–type inclusions) was the most common pathology (13/18 patients); three cases had Pick's disease and two AD. It is noteworthy that only one patient had evidence of motor neuron disease during life, an observation that highlights the fact that clinical diagnosis does not always correspond to histopathologic diagnosis.

[9] Tauopathies are non-Alzheimer's dementias that are associated with abnormal accumulations of hypophosphorylated tau (a protein) in neurons or glia. Mutations in the tau gene (chromosome 17) can be associated with dementia and parkinsonism (Mesulam, 2000).

complex either clinically or pathologically. The tauopathy-nontauopathy distinction, however, seems to be a useful one. Among patients with PPA, it appears that tauopathy (tau-positive) is overrepresented in patients classified as nonfluent (Josephs et al., 2006a; Knibb et al., 2006) and that tau-negative findings are more common in those classified as fluent (Knibb et al., 2006). It thus appears that histopathologic/biochemical support is emerging for the distinction between fluent and nonfluent PPA (although the distinction may have more to do with the presence or absence of AOS than with differences in the aphasia).

What is known about the possible genetic basis of or risk factors for PPA? Very little at this time, although Neary et al. (1993) found that 42% of their patients with PPA had a first-degree relative with a "similar condition" (Neary et al., 1993). Apolipoprotein E genotyping (the E4 allele is a risk factor for AD) found that the pattern of allele distribution for 12 patients with PPA was similar to that of controls and different than of patients with a clinical diagnosis of probable AD or a histologic diagnosis of AD (Mesulam et al., 1997). This provides support for distinguishing between PPA and probable AD clinically, and it is in agreement with evidence that most patients with PPA do not have the histopathology of AD. Finally, Mesulam (2001) notes that frontal lobe dementia, PPA, lobar atrophy without distinctive histopathology, and Pick-like inclusions can result from mutations within chromosome 17, some of which have been traced to the tau gene. Within a kindred, some patients may develop prominent aphasia and others display a frontal lobe dementia; this suggests that chromosome 17 mutations are prone to marked phenotypic divergence. These observations also raise the possibility that sporadic FTDs (presenting as PPA or frontal lobe dementia) may have a unitary pathogenesis, perhaps related to tauopathy or to impairment of some other function of chromosome 17 (Mesulam, 2001).

PRIMARY PROGRESSIVE APRAXIA OF SPEECH

Because AOS very often is a component of the syndrome of Broca's (or nonfluent) aphasia (McNeil & Kent, 1990), it is reasonable to ask if its presence in PPA is important to variables such as emergence of non-language cognitive impairments, survival, etiology, or management. In addition, AOS is of interest because progressive AOS, in the absence of aphasia and nonaphasic cognitive impairment, has been reported in the literature and encountered by us frequently enough to tentatively label such occurrences as PPAOS.

Similar to PPA, PPAOS may herald more specific neurologic diseases but likely not any single neurologic disease. It has been our observation that when it is prominent and accompanied by dysarthria, it tends to progress in a direction that leads to clinical diagnoses with prominent motor

manifestations (e.g., PSP, CBD, and ALS). Whether these clinical diagnoses reliably predict ultimate histologic diagnosis remains to be determined, although emerging evidence suggests that it may have predictive value in this regard (Josephs et al., 2006a).

The distinction between PPAOS and PPA may be relevant to prognosis and, possibly, medical management, especially if it is found to have predictive value relative to underlying histopathology. That is, decisions about medical/pharmacological management often depend on predictions about the ultimate clinical or pathologic diagnosis. As a result, for example, existing or future pharmacologic treatments for probable AD likely will be different than those for PSP, ALS, and other degenerative sensorimotor disorders. The degree to which PPA and PPAOS eventually may be linked to different specific clinical neurologic diagnoses or to underlying histopathology may mean that they will be treated in medically as well as behaviorally different ways.

Basic Definition and Terminology

Primary progressive AOS can be defined as AOS of insidious onset, gradual progression, and prolonged course, in the absence of non-language cognitive impairments and, sometimes, in the absence of aphasia, for a substantial period of time or perpetually resulting from a degenerative condition that, presumably, involves the left hemisphere's apparatus for translating the phonologic aspects of language into the learned kinematic parameters necessary for their expression through speech.[10] When AOS occurs with PPA, its presence should be explicitly recognized (e.g., "PPA with AOS"). When the AOS is more prominent than the aphasia, the appropriate diagnostic label in our opinion should be "PPAOS with aphasia." When observed in the absence of aphasia, it should be labeled as PPAOS.

Historical Perspective

The existence of AOS as a problem distinct from aphasia often is neglected in the neurology literature, and when its characteristics are recognized, they tend to be subsumed under diagnoses of aphasia or dysarthria. This almost certainly has been the case within the literature on PPA. It is very likely that many patients said to have PPA, particularly PNFA, have had AOS, and it is very possible that some unknown percentage of them have had AOS and little or no

---

[10] The reader is referred to McNeil, Doyle, and Wambaugh (2000) or to McNeil, Robin, and Schmidt (1997) for a detailed definition and discussion of the nature of AOS.

aphasia. If true, this is unfortunate, because it will have distorted our understanding of PPA and limited our understanding of degenerative AOS.

The literature on neurodegenerative disease—and on PPA in particular—has begun to recognize problems of speech motor planning or programming as a problem separable from aphasia and, sometimes, as *the* predominant or only communication problem. During the last 10 to 15 years, a small but increasing number of case reports or relatively small case series have documented progressive AOS, sometimes in the absence of any aphasia and often as the predominant communication disorder (e.g., Broussolle et al., 1996; Chapman, Rosenberg, Weiner, & Shobe, 1997; Cohen, Benoit, Van Eekhout, Ducarne, & Brunet, 1993; Fukui et al., 1996; Hart, Beach, & Taylor, 1997; Josephs et al., 2005, 2006a; Tyrrell, Kartsounis, Frackowiak, Findley, & Rosser, 1991). Others have explicitly included AOS as a component of PPA, although not necessarily as the predominant communication disorder (e.g., Craenahls et al., 1990; Gorno-Tempini, Dronkers, et al., 2004; Hart et al., 1997). In general, the presence or possible influence of AOS in patients diagnosed as having PPA is increasingly recognized. For example, Clark and colleagues (2005), discussing findings for their subjects with PNFA, wondered if "the nonfluency of PPA results more from articulatory disturbances, such as apraxia of speech..." (p. 58). Kertesz and colleagues (2003) recently noted an "aphemic variety" of PPA. Mesulam et al. (2003) recommend that PPA be distinguished from "pure progressive dysarthria or phonological disintegration," a designation that probably is equivalent to AOS.

Recently, Duffy (2006) summarized data for 80 patients with progressive AOS that represented either the only or the most prominent communication disorder associated with degenerative neurologic disease. The findings support a conclusion that AOS can be the first and/or most prominent manifestation of neurodegenerative disease, and they highlight several reasons for distinguishing between progressive AOS and PPA. The data from this study will be relied on heavily in subsequent description of progressive AOS and PPAOS.

Diagnostic Criteria and Character of the AOS

The defining characteristics of AOS associated with degenerative neurologic disease appear to be very similar to those associated with AOS in general. The most common deviant perceptual features among the 80 patients with AOS associated with degenerative neurologic disease described by Duffy (2006) included slow rate (79%), distorted substitutions (78%), syllable segmentation and/or excess and equal stress (75%), poorly sequenced sequential motion rates (i.e., rapid repetition of "puhtuhkuh") (66%), increased off-target errors with increased utterance length (62%), and sound

sequencing errors (50%).[11] A minority of patients also exhibited false starts/restarts, distorted sound additions, reduced words per breath group despite adequate maximum vowel duration, effortful orofacial movements during speech, sound repetitions, inaccurate speech alternating motion rates (i.e., rapid repetition of "puhpuhpuh," "tuhtuhtuh," or "kuhkuhkuh"), and sound prolongations. Many of these features correspond to those felt to be consistent with a diagnosis of AOS in general (Duffy, 2006; McNeil et al., 1997, 2000). The finding of reduced words per breath group despite adequate maximum vowel duration in 26% of the sample is noteworthy, because it is not typically reported in AOS from non-degenerative causes and is not usually associated with dysarthria. Duffy (2006) suggests that it may turn out to be a distinguishing feature of degenerative AOS (i.e., distinctive relative to features of AOS resulting from nondegenerative causes).

Issues of Classification and Nomenclature

The heart of the issue here is the distinction between AOS and aphasia. As already noted, within the literature, progressive AOS often is embedded with the designation of PPA or PNFA, but often without recognizing its distinctiveness from aphasia. This appears to be changing, although slowly. For example, Grossman and Ash (2004) suggest that some findings in studies of PNFA suggest that, fundamentally, it is a modality-specific disorder of speech and articulation, known by some as "dysarthria." If so, the problem would not meet our definition of aphasia but could meet the definition of AOS. Others explicitly recognize that patients with PNFA caused by FTD can have AOS as part of the syndrome (Boeve, 2003). Nestor and colleagues (2003) have suggested that the breakdown of "fluency" in patients with PNFA "is due to a motor articulatory planning deficit (speech apraxia) combined with a variable degree of agrammatism" (p. 2406). Gorno-Tempini, Dronkers and colleagues (2004) noted that 9/11 subjects in their PNFA group had AOS. And, as already noted, Kertesz and colleagues (2003) have recognized an "aphemic" variety of PPA, with "predominantly phonological, articulatory errors and stuttering or verbal apraxia" (p. 715). In our opinion, PPAOS (i.e., in the absence of aphasia or when the AOS is the predominant

---

[11] We recognize that poorly sequenced sequential motion rates and sound sequencing errors, although clearly helpful in distinguishing aphasia and AOS from dysarthria, may not be helpful in distinguishing aphasic phonemic errors from AOS and, arguably, are more consistent with aphasia than with AOS (e.g., McNeil et al., 1997, 2000). Thus, the sequencing errors in these affected individuals may have reflected the influence of aphasia on their speech output. Nonetheless, the other prominent characteristics in the group are not expected in aphasia and are consistent with the diagnosis of AOS.

problem) should not be considered as a subcategory of PPA, because, simply, AOS is not aphasia.

In the larger picture of neurodegenerative diseases, PPAOS could be considered as another variant of the asymmetric cortical degeneration syndromes (Broussolle et al., 1996) and, possibly, as a member of disorders within the Pick complex.

Clinical Presentation

The clinical presentation of PPAOS is very similar to that of PPA in many respects (see previous discussion for a summary of what typically is *not* part of the presentation). The differences lie in the specifics of the complaints that are offered. In the absence of any aphasia, the person with PPAOS will deny difficulties with listening or reading comprehension and with writing. Instead of complaining about word retrieval problems or semantic or grammatical errors, they complain that "the right words don't come out the right way" and, often, that lengthy or complex words create more problems that simpler ones.

Basic Demographics

Gender Ratio and Age of Onset

Duffy (2006) provides the most comprehensive data to date. Sixty-one percent of his patients were men. Average age at onset was about 67 years, with a range of 36 to 86 years. The data on gender should be interpreted cautiously, however, because single-case reports and smaller case series reported in the literature (Broussolle et al., 1996; Chapman et al., 1997; Cohen et al., 1993; Didic, Ceccaldi, & Poncet, 1998; Fukui et al., 1996; Hart et al., 1997; Josephs et al., 2005, 1996; Sakurai et al., 1998), in which degenerative AOS has been explicitly identified, have reported more women than men. The average age at onset in those reports is a few years younger (about 63 years) than those reported by Duffy.

Time until Onset of Other Deficits

Data regarding this are limited. Fifty-six percent of the 75 patients reported by Duffy (2006), for whom data on nonlanguage cognitive functioning were available, had no evidence of nonaphasic cognitive impairment at the time of initial assessment (on average, about 2.5 years post-onset); only 3% of them complained of such deficits. Only 9% had nonspeech motor complaints as an initial symptom. In general, many patients eventually develop nonspeech motor deficits, but often not until several years after the AOS has emerged.

Life Expectancy Following Onset of PPAOS

The seven patients reported by Josephs et al. (2006a) who had a progressive AOS as their sole or predominant commu-

nication disorder died an average of 8.7 years after initial symptom onset (range, 4–16 years). Three of the patients with AOS reported by Broussolle et al. (1996) died at 6, 6, and 10 years post-onset. Other cases in the literature that were followed to death seem to fall within this distribution of survival duration.

Accompanying Deficits

Other neurologic symptoms and signs can accompany progressive AOS and PPAOS. Among the 80 patients with progressive AOS summarized by Duffy (2006), aphasia was unequivocally present in 49% and most often was nonfluent or Broca-like in character. Fifty percent of the cases were dysarthric, most often spastic and/or hypokinetic in type. Eleven percent of the cases had neither aphasia nor dysarthria.

Deficits beyond the speech and language domain can include dystonia, limb apraxia, nonverbal oral apraxia, and alien limb phenomena (Duffy, 2006; Gorno-Tempini, Murray et al., 2004). A majority of Duffy's patients with AOS for whom information about nonaphasic cognitive impairment was available did not have such impairment; in those who did, the cognitive deficits were never clearly worse than the AOS.

Deficits beyond the speech-language domain can lead to more specific clinical diagnoses. Twenty-nine percent of Duffy's patients received neurologic diagnoses tied to prominent motor signs, most frequently including CBD or PSP (16%) and ALS (7–9%). The association between AOS and CBD and PSP is now well-established. For example, in each of two separate studies, one that described 13 patients with autopsy-confirmed CBD (Lehman Blake et al., 2003) and the other 14 patients with a clinical diagnosis of CBD (Frattali & Sonies, 2000), 38% had AOS; in those studies as well as a case reported by Gorno-Tempini, Murray et al. (2004), AOS (and, often, aphasia) preceded the emergence of other signs that permitted the diagnosis of CBD in several instances. In addition, in a recent autopsy study, Josephs et al. (2006a) found that PSP was the pathologic diagnosis for five of seven patients whose predominant speech-language disorder was AOS (one had CBD, and one had Pick's disease). An additional three patients who had PPA and AOS that were of comparable severity had pathologic diagnoses of CBD.

Neuroimaging Correlates

Neuroimaging abnormalities are similar to those documented for PPA. Duffy (2006) concluded that neuroimaging can be normal but that, when abnormal, left or left-greater-than-right hemisphere abnormalities are common. SPECT was more sensitive to abnormalities than EEG, CT, or MRI, with 14% of patients having abnormalities confined to the left hemisphere and 48% having left-greater-than-right hemisphere abnormalities. Other studies, mostly focused on PNFA (but in which at least some subjects were identified as "aphemic" or having AOS), generally concur and add some anatomical specificity. They generally point to the left perisylvian region, most often in the frontal lobe and usually in the region of the inferior frontal lobe/frontal operculum and anterior insula (Gorno-Tempini, Dronkers et al., 2004; Kertesz et al., 2003; Nestor et al., 2003)

Histologic Pathology

Recently, Josephs et al. (2006a) studied 17 patients with degenerative aphasia or AOS for whom pathologic diagnoses were available. Seven patients were classified as "AOS" (those in whom AOS was more prominent than any aphasia, if present), and three patients were classified as "PNFA-AOS" (those with PNFA and AOS in which neither aphasia nor AOS clearly predominated). Among the seven patients classified as AOS, the pathologic diagnoses were PSP (five patients), CBD (one patient), and Pick's disease (one patient). The three patients classified as PNFA-AOS had pathologic diagnoses of CBD. The pathologic diagnosis for the remaining seven patients in the study (in whom aphasia could not be classified as SD or PNFA and in whom AOS or dysarthria, if present, nonetheless was dominated by the aphasia) was classified as "frontotemporal lobar degeneration with ubiquitin-only-immunoreactive changes" in five patients, PSP in one patient, and CBD in one patient. In addition, within the 11 cases that had evidence of AOS, all had underlying tau biochemistry. Among them, the pathologic diagnoses were PSP (six patients), CBD (four patients), and Pick's disease (one patient). Thus, a clinical diagnosis of predominant AOS was strongly predictive of tauopathy histochemistry and a pathologic diagnosis of PSP. When PNFA and AOS were roughly equivalent, tauopathy also was predicted, but with a predominance of CBD pathology. Less prominent or absent AOS suggested non-tauopathy. Although these results require replication, they highlight the potential value of distinguishing between AOS and aphasia. Not only are AOS and aphasia managed differently from a behavioral standpoint, it appears that the distinction may be helpful in predicting pathologic diagnosis and specific biochemical findings. Thus, the identification of AOS (and its predominance relative to aphasia) seems to have implications for clinical, histological, and biochemical levels of inquiry.

The results of the Josephs et al. (2006a) study are supported by other pathologic findings, if it can be assumed that many patients classified as PNFA also had AOS. Thus, for example, Knibb et al. (2006) characterized, both clinically and pathologically, 38 patients with PPA, 23 of whom had PNFA. Seventy-four percent of their patients with PNFA were said to have "phonetic paraphasia," and 26% had "dysprosody"—features that might reflect AOS. The most frequent pathology in the PNFA group was non-Alzheimer's tauopathy (10/23 patients). In their 15 cases with fluent PPA, FTLD with ubiquitin-positive, tau-negative inclusions was the most frequent pathology (8/15 patients). They concluded that tauopathies were over-represented in their PNFA group and that their findings provide pathologic support for the existence of two distinct PPA syndromes. Obviously, one might argue that the two syndromes do not really reflect fluent and nonfluent aphasia but, rather, aphasia and AOS, or fluent aphasia versus nonfluent aphasia and AOS.

MANAGEMENT OF PPA AND PROGRESSIVE AOS

As with all interventions for aphasia, the consideration of therapy for PPA and progressive AOS requires both philosophical and scientific inspection. This inspection has taken the form of a number of frequently asked questions. Duffy (1987) asked:

1. Should persons with PPA or progressive AOS receive speech-language services at all?
2. If the answer to the first question is affirmative, under what conditions should treatment be given?
3. What should be the nature of the management efforts?
4. What are the criteria for success?

To these queries, we might ask what about PPA or progressive AOS is similar to or different from other forms of therapy for aphasia or AOS and what about it would require different criteria for intervention initiation, treatment type, and expected or acceptable consequences to the treatment.

Once the theoretic/philosophical definitions of what aphasia and AOS are and are not have been answered, we can begin to address the questions raised above that make the progressive form different from a static or non-progressive form of aphasia or AOS. If the fundamental definitions of aphasia and AOS are the same (as we have argued that they must be, or the diagnosis is incorrect), then it is only the progressive nature of the disorder that demands our differential consideration for treatment implementation. That is, does the progressive nature of the disorder obviate the consideration of treatment? If so, this would be a rare exception among progressive disorders of speech and language that is not considered for intervention simply because of its degenerative nature. Likewise, the life expectancy of the individual has been raised as an issue in the decision to initiate treatment, especially for degenerative disorders. It seems to us that a decision to initiate or withhold treatment based only on the duration of life expectancy is ethically indefensible. On these bases alone, the question of whether PPA or PPAOS should be exempt from treatment consideration can be dismissed. Therefore, the question becomes whether the patient under consideration has the motivation, financial and other (e.g., transportation) resources, level of linguistic and other cognitive resources (e.g., attention and memory), and the potential for language or motor and communication learning and maintenance necessary to support a recommended treatment. When these determinations have been made, secondary questions can be asked about the potential to benefit from specific intervention procedures.

To our knowledge, the treatment data (administered under experimental conditions that allow the examination of its efficacy) for only three patients with PPA have been published (McNeil et al., 1995; Rapp, Glucroft & Urrutia, 2005; Schneider, Thompson & Luring, 1996).[12] One other uncontrolled case study (Murray, 1998) describes a sequence of treatments administered to one person with PPA, and a book chapter (Rogers, King, & Alarcon, 2000) describes the rationale and a detailed plan for the treatment of persons with PPA. The experimental data are, of course, too limited to provide guidance for the treatment of subsequent patients. What has become apparent from these experiments and from the treatment pundits, however, is that the same array of treatment options remains available to persons with PPA as to those persons with non-progressive aphasia. To the degree that this is true, it also is apparent that these options are governed, in large measure, by the same clinical and theoretic considerations and biases. That is, whether treatment potential is determined by an assessment of the patient's activity limitations and restrictions in social participatory roles alone or is based on the evaluation of the presumed underlying mechanisms for the communication disorder (impairment-level assessment) represents a major clinical/theoretic bias. Likewise, the type of intervention selected is determined, in great measure, by this bias. Other issues involve the commitment to treat areas of deficit to improve them temporarily or maintain them as long as possible, or, alternatively, to direct intervention toward the expected decline in abilities with augmentative/alternative communication as the goal and the method. Each of these considerations and biases can be found among the publications reviewed below.

McNeil et al. (1995) published the first experimental attempt to assess the efficacy of treatment for a person with PPA. They evaluated the effects of treatment directed to

dysnomia, the primary sign and symptom in a patient with PPA of recent onset. The patient presented with very mild spastic dysarthria, nonverbal oral apraxia, aphasia that crossed all modalities and levels of language, and no AOS. In the context of a single-subject, multiple-baseline design, data were derived that demonstrated improved word finding ability when that was the focus of treatment (Lexical-Semantic Activation Inhibition Treatment [L-SAIT]), declines in language abilities that were not treated, and stable non-language cognitive performance. The most effective treatment for the patient was a combination of behavioral treatment plus dextroamphetamine. Although this particular patient's course of degeneration was atypically short and was dominated toward its end by severe spastic dysarthria and dysphagia, the impairment-focused treatment was efficacious and bolstered the patient's interpersonal and intrapersonal communication for some time. Generalization to untreated and progressively deteriorating areas of language performance was evidenced to some degree, but secondary benefits of treatment were observed. During the periods in which the patient was receiving treatment, he had an additional purpose and goal for his life and his otherwise unfilled time. Although of no obvious consequence to his life expectancy, his demonstrated improvements in language and communication gave him a sense of control that was not available to him in other areas of his life. This benefit was acquired with full knowledge that his treatment would not retard progression of the underlying disease. Augmentative communication was not an acceptable modality to this patient, and other potential forms of treatment became unreasonable because of the rapid progression of his underlying disease.

Also in the context of a single-subject, experimental multiple-baseline design, Schneider and colleagues (1996) presented data for a person with PPA demonstrating that oral and oral plus gestural training of verb tense was learned and generalized to untreated verbs within tense, but not across tenses. This impairment-directed treatment for agrammatism using gestural plus oral responding resulted in higher levels of correct oral sentence production than verbal responding alone. Although generalization to untreated areas of language and communication was not robust, the gestural responding generalized and was maintained for a 3-month period following the withdrawal of treatment. This maintenance was achieved in the context of declines in other language functions.

Murray (1998) presented a detailed case study (without experimental control) describing a series of treatments administered to a single subject with nonfluent PPA. The patient presented 1 year post-onset of self-described "stuttering," with the complaint of increased "slurring" of speech and word finding difficulties. Although impaired across all modalities, the patient's progressing deficits during the course of treatment were characterized by agrammatism,

---

[12] A small number of studies have reported the results of treatment for "naming" or "forgotten" vocabulary in individuals with SD (Graham, Patterson, Pratt, & Hodges, 2001; Jokel, Rochon, & Leonard, 2002; Snowden & Neary, 2002). We have elected not to review them here because of our uncertainty about whether the study participants would meet the criteria for the diagnosis of aphasia aspresented in this chapter.

anomia, phonemic paraphasia, AOS, and auditory comprehension deficits. Treatment was first administered over an 11-month period and was directed at her auditory and reading comprehension. It was described as consisting of "traditional stimulus-response activities which were designed to stimulate and facilitate . . ."(p. 658). The second treatment involved 24 one-hour sessions over a 4-month period and used the "back to the drawing board" program (Morgan & Helm-Estabrooks, 1987), a treatment that involves drawing pictures for communicative purposes and claims to be both an alternative communication method and a deblocker of speaking and writing. The third treatment involved both individual and aphasia support group therapy. Individual treatment in this phase "focused on improving communication interactions between D.D. and her spouse" and involved identifying turn-taking and repair skills. The patient also was trained and appeared to use an augmentative communication device (Dyna Vox), although with poor situational generalization.

Although the lack of experimental control in this case study obviates the attribution of any change to the treatments that were administered, it clearly describes the change of treatment focus and technique as the patient's signs and symptoms changed over the course of her decline. This changing sequence of treatment goals and methods may represent the most common practice in the treatment of aphasia of any etiology. For this to represent a generalizable model for best practice in the planning and implementation of intervention for PPA, it will require the same level of evidence as for the treatment of aphasia of any etiology. It does, however, illustrate the apparent frequently used and perhaps necessary adaptations of treatment goals and methods that follow careful observation of patient change that accompanies any efficacious treatment.

In the context of a single-subject, multiple-baseline design (with a single averaged data point reported for each baseline, treatment, and follow-up for each trained and untrained list of stimuli), Rapp and colleagues (2005) reported positive acquisition effects of a writing intervention focused on spelling to dictation. This 63-year-old individual had an 8-year history from first-noticed dysgraphic symptoms to treatment. She was diagnosed with fluent PPA 4 months before the initiation of the experimental treatment. During the 4-month course of therapy, the individual demonstrated normal and stable performance on a number of non-linguistic tasks (e.g., Rey Figures, delayed verbal recall, and verbal recognition memory) while demonstrating a substantive decline in language (Rey auditory verbal learning; word fluency for the letters F, A, and S; spoken picture naming). In addition, a systematic and substantive decline in the untrained spelling lists occurred over the course of the treatment and at the 6- and 12-month post-treatment evaluations.

The treatment involved having the participant spell each word to dictation, study the word, and then attempt to spell it again if it had been spelled incorrectly. This sequence was repeated as many as three times or until the stimulus word was spelled correctly. A control condition also was administered whereby a matched list of stimuli were presented but without feedback regarding accuracy. A list of words also was given as homework and self-assessed at home. Finally, as mentioned above, a list of control words was presented only at the pre- and post-tests. Treatment effects were determined by the number of correct letters divided by the number of target letters. Repeated and treated lists were identical at pre-treatment (about 68% correct). The treated list improved to 76%, however, and the repeated list dropped to 67% accuracy. The untreated control list dropped from 65% pre-treatment to 60% post-treatment and then to about 52% at 6-month follow-up. Interestingly, the repeated words and the homework remained relatively stable during the treatment period but dropped substantially during the 6-month follow-up, as did the treated spelling list. The treated list, however, remained higher than either untreated list at this 6-month maintenance phase. Only the treated list improved, and with the withdrawal of treatment, performance on all spelling lists diminished to roughly equivalent levels.

This study adds to findings that intervention can provide short-term, positive consequences for communicative function in PPA and intermediate-term, protective consequences as well. They also underscore the important conclusion that behavioral treatment does not reverse or prevent progression of the underlying disease; however, it can provide meaningful relief to the burden of the unrelenting march of the disease and the limitation it imposes on communicative functions.

In an uncontrolled case study, Koenig-Bruhin, Studer-Eichenberger, Donati, Zwahlen, and Hohl (2005) reported improvement on the sentence repetition subtest of the Aachen Aphasia Test over a 5-month, once-per-week regimen in areas targeted for treatment (phonologic aspects of repetition and short-term memory). The other subtests of this test remained unchanged over this time period. These changes cannot be attributed to the intervention, but the targets of treatment chosen for this individual reflect the predominant impairment-based approach to remediation of PPA.

Impairment-based treatment is not, however, the only approach advocated for the treatment of PPA. Rogers and colleagues (2000) presented a detailed description of proactive management for PPA that they believe will minimize activity limitations and participation restrictions as well as maximize communication competence as speech and language decline. This is accomplished by "early intervention focused on the development and training of augmentative and alternative communication (AAC)" (p. 306). In addition to the early training in AAC, patient and family education and family/partner intervention is advocated, with particular attention being paid to activity and participation limitations in both patient assessment and treatment planning and implementation. It is the inherent assumption of this approach that AAC is both an efficacious method of therapy for aphasia and the inevitable treatment modality in persons with PPA. In terms of evidence-based practice, neither of these assumptions stands on firm ground. Treatment efficacy and effectiveness data for aphasia are essentially nonexistent concerning AAC. In addition, compliance data for patients with aphasia, an issue in AAC training for all communication disorders, is in need of verification and, perhaps, improvement.

It seems clear to us that the call by Rogers and colleagues (2000) for assessment of PPA that deemphasizes the understanding of the nature of the impairment (for treatment planning purposes) and shifts it toward the individual's communication needs, partners, and environments, and that prescribes the early initiation of AAC as the target of treatment, is potentially problematic—or at the least premature. One problem is that it may be destined for nonacceptance from a substantial segment of the PPA patient population. A second problem is that this approach neglects the potential to improve and/or maintain specific language processing functions that underlie both the interpersonal and intrapersonal communication deficits (and, consequently, communicative and other activities and participatory limitations) for a meaningful period of time. That is, it neglects the fact that many, if not most, patients with PPA decline at a rate and a level sufficient to support and maintain independent language and communication skills, supporting communicative activity and social participation for many years. It may be that planning for AAC is on firmer ground when the progressive disorder is motor in nature (e.g., PPAOS or dysarthria) or when PPA is accompanied by progressive motor speech impairment. It seems to us that a much more rational and palatable approach, depending on the rate of decline and the impairment level of the patient, is to direct treatment at the hypothesized deficits, at compensatory strategies, at psychosocial concomitants of the disorder, at environmental influences (e.g., significant others and caregivers), and when communicatively appropriate, accepted by the patient, and trained before their use is necessary, at AAC systems. One difference in the treatment of persons with PPA compared to treatment of those of aphasia and a more static course is the need for clear patient and family education and counseling that emphasizes the progressive nature of this disorder. As with other etiologies, counseling that spans the course of the treatment as well as the accompanying patient and family changes is essential.

Similar to these treatment recommendations, Thompson (1997) provided the following useful guidelines for the treatment of PPA:

1. Early speech-language-cognitive evaluation is important, as are frequent follow-ups to establish the pattern of decline.

2. Early treatment may focus on impaired functions but should be adjusted as decline occurs.
3. AAC should be introduced early, when it is most easily learned, so that it can be used as the need arises.
4. Family members/significant others must be involved to enhance awareness of successful strategies and to practice with patient.
5. Treatment will not reverse progression of the disease but may enhance communication ability.

In the absence of reported and documented attempts to treat PPAOS, it is seems altogether reasonable that the same principles for structuring intervention for PPA would apply. The single addition to these general treatment strategies would be to reiterate the potential for AAC intervention in persons with PPAOS over that of individuals whose access to language is impaired.

In summary, no a priori theoretic or philosophical reason exists to withhold language and communication treatment from persons with PPA or PPAOS if the usual criteria for treatment candidacy are met. It is, however, too early in the accumulation of evidence to determine whether treatment for persons with PPA or PPAOS is predictably efficacious and whether it will follow the same principles of management as aphasia and AOS resulting from other etiologies and of other natural courses. It has been demonstrated that persons with PPA can improve on language and communication tasks with impairment-directed treatments that are typical of and efficacious for persons with static aphasia. It is reasonable to assume that—but currently untested whether—persons with PPA can learn, will use if learned, and will benefit from AAC devices. Patient and family counseling and communication training are likely to be integral parts to any successful aphasia or AOS regimen.

KEY POINTS

1. Aphasia of insidious onset, gradual progression, and prolonged course, without evidence of non-language computational impairments, and resulting from a degenerative condition that, presumably and predominantly, involves the language-dominant perisylvian region of the brain, is known as PPA. The criteria for the diagnosis of aphasia of any etiology or type are the same as those required for establishing the diagnosis of PPA. The disorder does not include patients in whom language impairment is just a prominent manifestation of dementia. PPA is a clinical syndrome, not a reflection of particular underlying brain pathology.
2. Currently applied criteria for the diagnosis of PPA include (a) a minimum of a 2-year history of language decline; (b) prominent language deficits, with relative

preservation of other mental functions; (c) independence in ADLs; (d) a full neurologic workup that has excluded other causes of aphasia; and (e) a comprehensive speech-language and neuropsychological evaluation that yields results consistent with the complaint and clinical neurologic examination. It should be noted that the 2-year history criterion is somewhat arbitrary—a working diagnosis of PPA may be justified without regard to duration of the aphasia. In addition, reduced ADLs that can be explained by the aphasia should not preclude a diagnosis of PPA.

3. The initial clinical presentation of people with PPA can be very different from that of people with AD or other degenerative diseases that induce diffuse cognitive impairments. It can be strikingly similar to stroke-induced and other static etiologies for aphasia, with the exception of its temporal course.

4. More men than women have PPA. Age of onset is highly variable but averages about 60 years. The duration from onset of aphasia symptoms to the emergence of more widespread impairment of cognitive functions also is highly variable but averages about 5 years. About 45% of reported cases have eventually developed non-aphasic cognitive impairments, but an emerging general consensus is that the great majority eventually experience symptoms in areas such as memory, personality, or mood, if they live long enough.

5. Apraxia of speech, nonverbal oral apraxia, dysarthria, dysphagia, right-central facial droop or weakness, right-extremity weakness or clumsiness, rigidity, agnosia, and depression have been reported in persons with PPA.

6. MRI and SPECT are commonly used for the neuroradiologic evaluation of people with PPA. When abnormal, these modalities tend to show left hemisphere abnormalities or left-greater-than-right hemisphere abnormalities.

7. PPA can be associated with a variety of specific histopathologic diagnoses, including AD, corticobasal degeneration, PSP, motor neuron disease, and CBD. The most frequent autopsy findings are perhaps, however, of cellular changes that do not correspond to well-known, specific clinical or pathologic conditions (e.g., nonspecific focal degeneration with spongiform changes and gliosis, nonspecific cortical degeneration). Most patients with PPA will not have a histologic diagnosis of AD.

8. Apraxia of speech (AOS) may be the initial, only, or prominent manifestation of degenerative neurologic disease. Similar to PPA, it may herald more specific neurologic diseases and is unlikely to represent a single neurologic disease. Distinguishing between a progressive AOS and PPA may be relevant to prognosis, management, and perhaps, underlying histopathology.

9. Efficacy and outcome data regarding management of PPA and progressive AOS are very limited, but no a priori theoretic or philosophical reasons exist to withhold language, speech, or communication treatment from persons with either disorder if the usual criteria for treatment candidacy are met.

10. It is premature to draw conclusions about whether treatment of persons with PPA or PPAOS is generally effective, but it has been demonstrated that some affected persons with PPA can improve on language and communication tasks with impairment-directed treatments that are typical of, and efficacious for, persons with static aphasia. It is reasonable to assume that—but is currently untested whether—persons with PPA or progressive AOS can learn, will use if learned, or will benefit from AAC devices and strategies.

11. For persons with PPA or PPAOS and their families, a need exists for education and counseling that emphasizes the progressive nature of the disorder and that behavioral treatment to maximize communication ability cannot be expected to retard or reverse progression of the disease.

12. In general, it appears that the most rational approach to management of PPA or PPAOS is to gauge the rate of decline and the level of impairment, and then to direct treatment at the hypothesized deficits, at compensatory strategies, at psychosocial concomitants of the disorder, and at environmental influences (e.g., significant others and caregivers). When communicatively appropriate, accepted by the patient, and trained before their use is necessary, AAC systems may be used, particularly if substantive motor speech deficits accompany the PPA or if PPAOS is substantially greater in severity than aphasia.

ACTIVITIES FOR **REFLECTION AND DISCUSSION**

1. Discuss the unique features of PPA, other than its slow onset, that differentiate it from non-progressive courses of aphasia.
2. Discuss the criteria for diagnosing PPA.
3. List the neurogenic language disorders with which PPA is most likely to be confused or misdiagnosed, and identify the diagnostic features that differentiate each from PPA.
4. Discuss the evidence for and against the classification of PPA as a subtype of FTD.
5. What percentage of individuals with PPA can be expected to develop non-aphasic cognitive impairment?

6. What are the theoretic objections and clinical implications of classifying all persons with adult-onset language disorders as "aphasic"?

7. Discuss the neurologic degenerative diseases in which progressive AOS can be an accompanying or presenting sign or symptom.

8. Discuss the demographic and etiologic similarities and differences between PPA and PPAOS.

9. What are the two most significant theoretic biases governing the selection and implementation of treatment for progressive aphasia and AOS?

10. Discuss the amount and quality of the evidence supporting each theoretic bias governing the selection and implementation of treatment for progressive aphasia and AOS.

References

Abe, K., Ukita, H., & Yanagihara, T. (1997). Imaging in primary progressive aphasia. *Neuroradiology, 39*(8), 556–559.

Arima, K., Uesugi, H., Fujita, I., Sakurai, Y., Oyanagi, S., Andoh, S., et al. (1994). Corticonigral degeneration with neuronal achromasia presenting with primary progressive aphasia; Ultrastructural and immunocytochemical studies. *Journal of the Neurological Sciences, 127*(2), 186–197.

Azouvi, P., Bergego, C., Robel, L., Marlier, N., Durand, I., Held, J. P., et al. (1993). Slowly progressive apraxia: Two case studies. *Journal of Neurology, 240,* 347–350.

Black, S. E. (1996). Focal cortical atrophy syndromes. *Brain & Cognition, 31*(2), 188–229.

Boeve, B. F. (2003). Diagnosis and management of the non-Alzheimer dementias. In J. H. Noseworthy (Ed.), *Neurological therapeutics: Principles and practice* (pp. 2826–2854). New York: Martin Dunitz.

Boeve, B. F., Dickson, D., Duffy, J. R., Bartleson, J. D., Trennery, M., & Petersen, R. (2003). Progressive nonfluent aphasia and subsequent aphasic dementia associated with atypical progressive supranuclear palsy pathology. *European Neurology, 49,* 72–78.

Broussolle, E., Bakchine, S., Tommasi, M., Laurent, B., Bazin, B., Cinotti, L., et al. (1996). Slowly progressive anarthria with late anterior opercular syndrome: A variant form of frontal cortical atrophy syndromes. *Journal of Neurological Sciences, 144*(1–2), 44–58.

Caselli, R. J. (1995). Focal and asymmetric cortical degeneration syndromes. *The Neurologist, 1*(1), 1–19.

Caselli, R. J., Beach, T. G., & Sue, L. I. (2002). Progressive aphasia with Lewy bodies. *Dementia & Geriatric Cognitive Disorders, 14,* 55–58.

Caselli, R. J., & Jack, C. R., Jr. (1992). Asymmetric cortical degenerative syndromes: A proposed clinical classification. *Archives of Neurology, 49,* 770–780.

Caselli, R. J., Jack, C. R., Jr., Petersen, R. C., Wahner, H. W., & Yanagihara, T. (1992). Asymmetric cortical degenerative syndromes: Clinical and radiologic correlations. *Neurology, 42,* 1462–1468.

Chapman, S. B., Rosenberg, R. N., Weiner, M. F., & Shobe, A. (1997). Autosomal dominant progressive syndrome of motor-speech loss without dementia. *Neurology, 49*(5), 1298–1306.

Clark, D. G., Charuvastra, A., Miller, B. L., Shapira, J. S., & Mendez, M. F. (2005). Fluent versus nonfluent primary progressive aphasia: A comparison of clinical and functional neuroimaging features. *Brain & Language, 94,* 54–60.

Cohen, L., Benoit, N., Van Eekhout, P., Ducarne, B., & Brunet, P. (1993). Pure progressive aphemia. *Journal of Neurology, Neurosurgery, & Psychiatry, 56*(8), 923–924.

Cole, M., Wright, D., & Banker, B. Q. (1979). Familial aphasia due to Pick's disease. *Annals of Neurology, 6,* 158.

Craenhals, A., Raison-Van Ruymbeke, A. M., Rectem, D., Seron, X., & Laterre, E. C. (1990). Is slowly progressive aphasia actually a new clinical entity? *Aphasiology, 4*(5), 485–509.

Darley, F. L. (1982). *Aphasia.* Philadelphia: W.B. Saunders.

Davies, R. R., Hodges, J. R., Kril, J. J., Patterson, K., Halliday, G. M., & Xuereb, J. H. (2005). The pathological basis of semantic dementia. *Brain, 128,* 1984–1995.

DeRenzi, E. (1986). Slowly progressive visual agnosia or apraxia without dementia. *Cortex, 22,* 171–180.

Dick, J. P., Snowden, J. S., Northen, B., Goulding, P. J., & Neary, D. (1989). Slowly progressive apraxia. *Behavioral Neurology, 2,* 101–114.

Didic, M., Ceccaldi, M., & Poncet, M. (1998). Progressive loss of speech: A neuropsychological profile of premotor dysfunction. *European Neurology, 39,* 90–96.

Duffy, J. R. (1987). Slowly progressive aphasia. *Clinical Aphasiology, 16* 349–356.

Duffy, J. R. (2006). Apraxia of speech in degenerative neurologic disease. *Aphasiology, 20*(6), 511–527.

Duffy, J. R., & Petersen, R. C. (1992). Primary progressive aphasia. *Aphasiology, 6*(1), 1–15.

Engel, P. A., & Fleming, P. D. (1997). Primary progressive aphasia, left anterior atrophy, and neurofibrillary hippocampal pathology: Observations in an unusual case. *Neuropsychiatry, Neuropsychology, & Behavioral Neurology, 10*(3), 213–218.

Frattali, C. M., Grafman, J., Patronas, N., Makhlouf, M. S., & Litvan, I. (2000). Language disturbance in corticobasal degeneration. *Neurology, 54,* 990–992.

Frattali, C. M., & Sonies, B. C. (2000). Speech and swallowing disturbances in corticobasal degeneration. In I. Litvan, C. G. Goetz, & A. E. Lanf (Eds.), *Corticobasal degeneration. Advances in neurology* (Vol. 82). Philadelphia: Lippincott Williams & Wilkins.

Fuh, J. L., Liao, K. K., Wang, S. J., & Lin, K. N. (1994). Swallowing difficulty in primary progressive aphasia: A case report. *Cortex, 30*(4), 701–705.

Fukui, T., Sugita, K., Kawamura, M., Shiota, J., & Nakano, I. (1996). Primary progressive apraxia in Pick's disease: A clinico-pathologic study. *Neurology, 47,* 467–473.

Girling, D. M., & Berrios, G. E. (1994). On the relationship between senile cerebral atrophy and aphasia. *History of Psychiatry, 5,* 542–547.

Gordon, B., & Selnes, O. (1984). Progressive aphasia without dementia: Evidence of more widespread involvement. *Neurology, 34,* 102.

Gorno-Tempini, M. L., Dronkers, N. F., Rankin, K. P., Ogar, J. M., Phengrasamy, L., Rosen, H. J., et al. (2004). Cognition and anatomy in three variants of primary progressive aphasia. *Annals of Neurology, 55,* 335–346.

Gorno-Tempini, M. L., Murray, R. C., Rankin, K. P., Weiner, M. W., & Miller, B. L. (2004). Clinical, cognitive, and anatomical evolution from nonfluent progressive aphasia to corticobasal syndrome: A case report, *Neurocase, 10,* 426–436.

Graff-Radford, N. R., Damasio, A. R., Hyman, B. T., et al. (1990). Progressive aphasia in a patient with Pick's disease: A neuropsychological, radiologic, and anatomic study. *Neurology, 40,* 620–626.

Graham, K. S., Patterson, K., Pratt, K. H., & Hodges, J. R. (2001). Can repeated exposure to "forgotten" vocabulary help alleviate word-finding difficulties in semantic dementia? An illustrative case study. *Neuropsychological Rehabilitation, 11,* 429–454.

Green, J., Morris, J. C., Sandson, J., McKeel, D. W., & Miller, J. W. (1990). Progressive aphasia: A precursor of global dementia. *Neurology, 40,* 423–429.

Green, J. D., Patterson, K., Xuereb, J., & Hodges, J. R. (1996). Alzheimer disease and nonfluent progressive aphasia. *Archives of Neurology, 53*(10), 1072–1078.

Grossman, M., & Ash, S. (2004). Primary progressive aphasia: A review. *Neurocase, 10,* 3–18.

Hart, R. P., Beach, W. A., & Taylor, J. R. (1997). A case of progressive apraxia of speech and non-fluent aphasia. *Aphasiology, 11*(1), 73–82.

Heath, P. D., Kennedy, P., & Kapur, N. (1983). Slowly progressive aphasia without generalized dementia. *Annals of Neurology, 13,* 687–688.

Henson, R. A. (1988). Maurice Ravel's illness: A tragedy of lost creativity. *British Medical Journal, 296,* 1885–1588.

Hodges, J. R., Davies, R. R., Xuereb, J. H., Casey, B., Broe, M., Bak, T. H., et al. (2004). Clinicopathological correlates of frontotemporal dementia. *Annals of Neurology, 56,* 399–406.

Holland, A. L., McBurney, D. H., Moossy, J., & Reinmuth, O. M. (1985). The dissolution of language in Pick's disease with neurofibrillary tangles: A case study. *Brain and Language, 24,* 36–58.

Jokel, R., Rochon, E., & Leonard, C. (2002). Therapy for anomia in semantic dementia. *Brain & Cognition, 49,* 241–244.

Josephs, K. A., Boeve, B. F., Duffy, J. R., Smith G. E., Knopman D. S., Parisi J. E., et al. (2005). Atypical progressive supranuclear palsy underlying progressive apraxia of speech and nonfluent aphasia. *Neurocase, 11*(4), 283–296.

Josephs, K. A., Duffy, J. R., Strand, E. A., Whitwell, J. L., Layton, K. F., Parisi, J. E., et al. (2006a). Clinicopathological and imaging correlates of progressive aphasia and apraxia of speech. *Brain, 129,* 1385–1398.

Josephs, K. A., Petersen, R. C., Knopman, D. S., Boeve, B. F., Whitwell, J. L., Duffy, J. R., et al. (2006b). Clinicopathologic analysis of frontotemporal and corticobasal degenerations and PSP. *Neurology, 66,* 41–48.

Karbe, H., Kertesz, A., & Polk, M. (1993). Profiles of language impairment in primary progressive aphasia. *Archives of Neurology, 50*(2), 193–201.

Kempler, D., Metter, E. J., Riege, W. H., Jackson, C. A., Benson, D. F., & Hanson, W. R. (1990). Slowly progressive aphasia: Three cases with language, memory, CT and PET data. *Journal of Neurology, Neurosurgery, and Psychiatry, 53*(11), 987–993.

Kertesz, A. (1997). Frontotemporal dementia, Pick disease, and corticobasal degeneration: One entity or 3? *Archives of Neurology, 54,* 1427–1429.

Kertesz, A., Davidson, W., & McCabe, P. (1998). Primary progressive semantic aphasia: A case study. *Journal of the International Neuropsychological Society, 4*(4), 388–398.

Kertesz, A., Davidson, W., McCabe, P., & Takagi, K. (2003). Primary progressive aphasia: Diagnosis, varieties, evolution. *Journal of the International Neuropsychological Society, 9,* 710–719.

Kertesz, A., Hudson, L., MacKenzie, I. R. A., & Munoz, D. G. (1994). The pathology and nosology of primary progressive aphasia. *Neurology, 44,* 2065–2072.

Kertesz, A., McMonagle, P., Blair, M., Davidson, W., & Munoz, D. G. (2005). The evolution and pathology of frontotemporal dementia. *Brain, 128,* 1996–2005.

Kertesz, A., & Munoz, D. G. (1997). Primary progressive aphasia. *Clinical Neuroscience, 4*(2), 95–102.

Knibb, J. A., Xuereb, J. H., Patterson, K., & Hodges, J. R. (2006). Clinical and pathological characterization of progressive aphasia. *Annals of Neurology, 59,* 156–165.

Kobayashi, K., Kurachi, M., Gyoubu, T., Imao, G., & Nakamura, J. (1990). Progressive dysphasic dementia with localized cerebral atrophy: Report of an autopsy. *Clinical Neuropathology, 9*(5), 254–261.

Koenig-Bruhin, M., Studer-Eichenberger, F., Donati, F., Zwahlen, J., & Hohl, B. (2005). Language therapy in fluent primary progressive aphasia—A single case study. *Brain and Language, 95,* 135–136.

Krefft, T. A., Graff-Radford, N. R., Dickson, D. W., Baker, M., & Castellani, R. J. (2003). Familial primary progressive aphasia. *Alzheimer Disease and Associated Disorders, 17,* 106–112.

Kushner, M. (1990). MRI and ^{123}I-iodoamphetamine SPECT imaging of a patient with slowly progressive aphasia. *Functional Neuroimaging, 2*(4), 17–19.

Lehman Blake, M., Duffy J.R., Boeve, B.F., Ahlskog, J.E., and Maraganore, D.M. (2003). Speech and language disorders associated with corticobasal degeneration. *Journal of Medical Speech-Language Pathology, 11,* 131–146.

Mandell, A. M., Alexander, M. P., & Carpenter, S. (1989). Creutzfeldt-Jakob disease presenting as isolated aphasia. *Neurology, 39,* 55–58.

McNeil, M. R. (1988). Aphasia in the adult. In N. J. Lass, L. V. McReynolds, J. Northern, & D. E. Yoder (Eds.), *Handbook of speech-language pathology and audiology* (pp. 738–786). Toronto: B. C. Decker.

McNeil, M. R. (1998). The case of the lawyer's lugubrious language: Dysarthria plus primary progressive aphasia or dysarthria plus dementia? *Seminars in speech and language, 19*(1), 49–57.

McNeil, M. R., Doyle, P. J., & Wambaugh, J. (2000). Apraxia of speech: A treatable disorder of motor planning and programming. In S. E. Nadeau, L. J. Gonzalez Rothi, & B. Crosson (Eds.), *Aphasia and language: Theory to practice* (pp. 221–266). New York: Guilford Press.

McNeil, M. R., & Kent, R. D. (1990). Motoric characteristics of adult apraxic and aphasic speakers. In G. R. Hammond (Ed.), *Cerebral control of speech and limb movements* (pp. 349–386). New York: North Holland.

McNeil, M. R., & Pratt, S. R. (2001). A standard definition of aphasia: Toward a general theory of aphasia. *Aphasiology*, *15*(10/11), 901–911.

McNeil, M. R., Robin, D. A., & Schmidt, R. A. (1997). Apraxia of speech: Definition, differentiation, and treatment. In M. R. McNeil (Ed.), *Clinical management of sensorimotor speech disorders* (pp. 311–344). New York: Thieme.

McNeil, M. R., Small, S. L., Masterson, R. J., & Fossett, T. R. D. (1995). Behavioral and pharmacological treatment of lexical-semantic deficits in a single patient with primary progressive aphasia. *American Journal of Speech-Language Pathology*, *4*, 76–87.

Mehler, M. F. (1988). Mixed transcortical aphasia in nonfamilial dysphasic dementia. *Cortex*, *24*, 545–554.

Mesulam, M. M. (1982). Slowly progressive aphasia without dementia. *Annals of Neurology*, *11*, 592–598.

Mesulam, M. M. (1987). Primary progressive aphasia. Differentiation from Alzheimer's disease. *Annals of Neurology*, *22*, 533–534.

Mesulam, M. M. (2000). *Principles of behavioral and cognitive neurology*. New York: Oxford University Press.

Mesulam, M. M. (2001). Primary progressive aphasia. *Annals of Neurology*, *49*, 425–432.

Mesulam, M. M. (2003). Primary progressive aphasia—A language-based dementia. *New England Journal of Medicine*, *349*, 1535–1542.

Mesulam, M. M., Grossman, M., Hillis, A., Kertesz, A., & Weintraub, S. (2003). The core and halo of primary progressive aphasia and semantic dementia. *Annals of Neurology*, *54*(suppl 5), S11–S14.

Mesulam, M. M., Johnson, N., Grujic, Z., & Weintraub, S. (1997). Apolipoprotein E genotypes in primary progressive aphasia. *Neurology*, *49*, 51–55.

Mesulam, M. M., & Weintraub, S. (1992). Spectrum of primary progressive aphasia. In M. N. Rossor (Ed.), *Bailliere's clinical neurology. Unusual Dementias.* (Vol. 1, pp. 583–609). London: Bailliere Tindall.

Mingazzini, G. (1914). On aphasia due to atrophy of the cerebral convolutions. *Brain*, *36*, 493–524.

Morgan, A., & Helm-Estabrooks, N. (1987). Back to the drawing board: A treatment program for nonverbal aphasic patients. *Clinical Aphasiology*, *16*, 34–39.

Morris, J. C., Cole, M., Branker, B., & Wright, D. (1984). Hereditary dysphasic dementia and the Pick-Alzheimer spectrum. *Annals of Neurology*, *16*, 455–466.

Mummery, C. J., Patterson, K., Wise, R. J. S., Vandenbergh, R., Price, C. J., & Hodges, J. R. (1999). Disrupted temporal lobe connections in semantic dementia. *Brain*, *122*, 61–73.

Murray, L. L. (1998). Longitudinal treatment of primary progressive aphasia: A case study. *Aphasiology*, *12*(7/8), 651–672.

Neary, D., Snowden, J. S., Gustafson, L., Passant, U., Stuss, D., Black, S., et al. (1998). Frontotemporal lobar degeneration: A consensus on clinical diagnostic criteria. *Neurology*, *51*, 1546–1554.

Neary, D., Snowden, J. S., & Mann, D. M. (1993). The clinical pathological correlates of lobar atrophy. *Dementia*, *4*, 154–159.

Nestor, P. J., Graham, N. L., Fryer, T. D., Williams, G. B., Patterson, K., & Hodges, J. R. (2003). Progressive nonfluent aphasia is associated with hypometabolism centered on the left insula. *Brain*, *126*, 2406–2418.

Otsuki, M., Soma, Y., Sato, M., Homma, A., & Tsuji, S. (1998). Slowly progressive pure word deafness. *European Neurology*, *39*(3), 135–140.

Petersen, R. C. (2001). Focal dementia syndromes: In search of the gold standard (editorial). *Annals of Neurology*, *49*, 421–422.

Philbrick, K. L., Rummans, T. A., Duffy, J. R., Kokmen, E., & Jack, C. R. (1994). Primary progressive aphasia: An uncommon masquerader of psychiatric disorders. *Psychosomatics*, *35*(2), 138–141.

Piccirilli, M., D'Alessandro, P., & Ferroni, A. (1990). Slowly progressive apraxia without dementia. *Dementia*, *1*, 222–224.

Pick, A. (1892). Über die Beziehungen der senilen Hirnatrophie zur Aphasie. *Prager Medizinische Wochenschrift*, *17*, 165–167.

Poeck, K., & Luzzatti, C. (1988). Slowly progressive aphasia in three patients. *Brain*, *111*, 151–168.

Rapp, B., Glucroft, B., & Urrutia, J. (2005). The protective effects of behavioral intervention in a case of primary progressive aphasia. *Brain and Language*, *95*, 18–19.

Rogers, M. A., & Alarcon, N. B. (1999). Characteristics and management of primary progressive aphasia. *ASHA Special Interest Division Neurophysiology and Neurogenic Speech and Language Disorders*, *9*(4), 12–26.

Rogers, M. A., King, J. M., & Alarcon, N. B. (2000). Proactive management of primary progressive aphasia. In D. R. Beukelman, K. Yorkston, & J. Reichle (Eds.), *Augmentative communication for adults with neurogenic and neuromuscular disabilities* (pp. 325–338). Baltimore, MD: Brookes.

Sakurai, Y., Hashida, H., Uesugi, H., Murayama, S., Bando, M., Iwata, M., et al. (1996). A clinical profile of corticobasal degeneration presenting as primary progressive aphasia. *European Neurology*, *36*(3), 134–137.

Scheltens, P. H., Hazenberg, G. J., Lindeboom, J., Valk, J., & Wolters, E. C. (1990). A case of progressive aphasia without dementia: "Temporal" Pick's disease? *Journal of Neurology, Neurosurgery, and Psychiatry*, *53*, 79–80.

Schneider, S. L., Thompson, C. K., & Luring, B. (1996). Effects of verbal plus gestural matrix training on sentence production in a patient with primary progressive aphasia. *Aphasiology*, *10*(3), 297–317.

Schwartz, M. F. (1984). What the classical aphasia categories can't do for us, and why. *Brain and Language*, *21*, 3–8.

Shuttleworth, E. C., Yates, A. J., & Paltan-Ortiz, J. (1985). Creutzfeldt-Jakob disease presenting as progressive aphasia. *Journal of the National Medical Association*, *77*, 649–656.

Snowden, J. S., Mann, D. M. A., & Neary D. (1996). *Fronto-temporal lobar degeneration: Fronto-temporal dementia, progressive aphasia, semantic dementia*. New York: Churchill Livingstone.

Snowden, J. S., & Neary, D. (2002). Relearning of verbal labels in semantic dementia. *Neuropsychologia*, *40*, 1715–1728.

Snowden, J. S., Neary, D., & Mann, D. M. A. (2002). Frontotemporal dementia. *British Journal of Psychiatry*, *180*, 140–143.

Sonty, S. P., Mesulam, M. M., Thompson, C. K., Johnson, N. A., Weintraub, S., Parrish, T. B., et al. (2003). Primary progressive aphasia: PPA and the language network. *Annals of Neurology*, *53*, 35–49.

Thompson, C. K. (1997). *Primary Progressive Aphasia Newsletter—Readers Section*, *2*, 1–6.

Trupe, E. H. (1984). Reliability of rating spontaneous speech in the Western Aphasia Battery: Implications for classification. *Clinical Aphasiology*, *13*, 55–69.

Turner, R. S., Kenyon, L. C., Trojanowski, J. Q., Gonatas, N., & Grossman, M. (1996). Clinical, neuroimaging, and pathologic features of progressive nonfluent aphasia. *Annals of Neurology, 39*(2), 166–173.

Tyrrell, P. J., Kartsounis, L. D., Frackowiak, R. S. J., Findley, L. J., & Rosser, M. N. (1991). Progressive loss of speech output and orofacial dyspraxia associated with frontal lobe hypometabolism. *Journal of Neurology, Neurosurgery, and Psychiatry, 54*, 351–357.

Tyrrell, P. J., Warrington, E. K., Frackowiak, R. S. J., & Rosser, M. N. (1990). Progressive degeneration of the right temporal lobe studied with positron emission tomography. *Journal of Neurology, Neurosurgery, and Psychiatry, 53*, 1046–1050.

Weintraub, S., Rubin, N. P., & Mesulam, M. M. (1990). Primary progressive aphasia: Longitudinal course, neurological profile, and language features. *Archives of Neurology, 47*(12), 1329–1335.

Westbury, C., & Bub, D. (1997). Primary progressive aphasia: A review of 112 cases. *Brain and Language, 60*(3), 381–406.

Yamanouchi, H., Budka, H., & Vass, K. (1986). Unilateral Creutzfeldt-Jakob disease. *Cortex, 24*, 545–554.

APPENDIX 20.1
Information Resources

- The Association for Frontotemporal Dementias (AFTD). This nonprofit organization that promotes research into frontotemporal dementias, educates health professionals, and provides information, education, and support for affected individuals and their families.
  The Association for Frontotemporal Dementias
  P.O. Box 7191
  St. David's, PA 19087-7191
  www.FTD-Picks.org

- National Aphasia Association. The Association's Web site contains information about PPA.
  National Aphasia Association
  156 Fifth Avenue, Suite 707
  New York, NY 10010
  1-800-922-4622
  www.aphasia.org/NAAppa.html

- Primary Progressive Aphasia Newsletter. This newsletter about PPA is published through:
  The Cognitive Neurology and Alzheimer's Disease Center
  320 East Superior Street
  Searle 11-450
  Chicago, IL 60611-3008
  312-908-9339 (phone); 312-908-8789 (fax)
  www.brain.nwu.edu/core/ppal.htm

- Rare Dementia Registry. This registry is made up of individuals who have been diagnosed with a rare dementing illness and their primary caregivers. PPA is one of several rare dementias listed. The registry functions as a telephone support group. The database is confidential; names are shared with other registered families only. The service is provided by the:
  Alzheimer's Association, Greater Phoenix Chapter
  1028 East McDowell Road
  Phoenix, AZ 85006-2622
  602-528-0550; 1-800-392-0550
  www.alzaz.org

Chapter 21

Global Aphasia: Identification and Management

Richard K. Peach

OBJECTIVES

Following the completion of this chapter, the reader will be able to identify the features of global aphasia, its etiology, the patterns of evolution and outcome in global aphasia, and some factors that are related to recovery from this syndrome. The reader also will be able to provide a rationale for early intervention with these patients, describe contemporary goals for assessment, and develop treatment plans that exploit the residual language capacity and/or other functional abilities of patients with global aphasia. Finally, the reader will be able to identify current testing measures and both impairment-based and socially oriented treatment programs that emphasize improved language and functional communication and are appropriate for assessing and treating patients with global aphasia.

Positive developments regarding the rehabilitation of persons with global aphasia have continued to appear in the literature since publication of the last version of this chapter. Clinicians and families therefore have reasons to be guardedly optimistic concerning the communication outcomes from this condition. Among these developments are an improved understanding of the cerebral mechanisms underlying recovery of auditory comprehension following global aphasia (Zahn et al., 2004); novel approaches to treating naming, including phonologic treatment (Biedermann, Blancken, & Nickels, 2002) and transcranial magnetic stimulation (Naeser et al., 2005); and extended application of computer-based communication systems to produce sentences of varying syntactic complexity (Koul, Corwin, & Hayes, 2005; McCall, Shelton, Weinrich, & Cox, 2000). The emergence of social approaches for language and communication treatment, some of which have demonstrated efficacy, also provides an important dimension to rehabilitation for global aphasia (Kagan, Black, Duchan, Simmons-

Mackie, & Square, 2001). The prognosis for recovery of premorbid speech-language abilities is, indeed, poor following global aphasia, but these individuals do make significant improvements in communication skills with treatment during the first year post-onset (Nicholas, Helm-Estabrooks, Ward-Lonergan, & Morgan, 1993) and beyond (Naeser et al., 2005). Those improvements also occasionally exceed the outcomes observed in patients with other types of aphasia (i.e., Broca's and Wernicke's aphasia) that are associated with better prognoses for improvement (Basso & Farabola, 1997; Kertesz & McCabe, 1977). Identification of new treatments yielding limited but nonetheless positive communication benefits for these individuals is therefore an important advance, particularly when considered in the context of the historically pessimistic views associated with this clinical group.

The central questions regarding outcomes following global aphasia concern discovering the patient characteristics that can be associated with various prognoses and applying these in treatment planning (Peach, 1992). Some recent studies have attempted to do this by examining outcomes with regard to the patterns of lesion sites producing global aphasia (Basso & Farabola, 1997; Kumar, Masih, & Pardo, 1996; Naeser, 1994; Okuda, Tanaka, Tachibana, Kawabata, & Sugita, 1994). Others have investigated the role of an accompanying hemiplegia (Keyserlingk, Naujokat, Niemann, Huber, & Thron, 1997; Nagaratnam, Barnes, & Nagaratnam, 1996). Still others have employed positron-emission tomography to identify predictors that might account for the large amount of variability observed in recovery from aphasia generally and from global aphasia specifically (Heiss, Kessler, Karbe, Fink, & Pawlik, 1993; Okuda et al., 1994).

These developments are encouraging especially, because the largest percentage of patients with aphasia referred for speech-language services is composed of those presenting with global aphasia (Sarno & Levita, 1981). Despite the poor prognosis for recovery of oral language skills following global aphasia, clinicians now have more tools than ever to make informed decisions regarding both whether and how to treat individuals with global aphasia and the impact that this treatment will have on the patients' communication skills.

FEATURES

Incidence

Global aphasia may be one of the most frequently occurring types of aphasia. Previously, incidence rates of between 10% and 40.6% have been reported for global aphasia (Basso, Della Sala, & Farabola, 1987; Brust, Shafer, Richter, & Bruun, 1976; Collins, 1986; De Renzi, Faglioni, & Ferrari, 1980; Eslinger & Damasio, 1981; Kertesz, 1979; Kertesz & Sheppard, 1981). Some recent reports, however, suggest that the incidence rate during the acute stage may be even higher. Scarpa, Colombo, Sorgato, and De Renzi (1987) reported an incidence of 55.1% in an acute sample. All of the 108 patients with aphasia included in the study by Scarpa and colleagues (1987) were assessed between 15 and 30 days post-onset and were right-handed with a single, left hemisphere lesion. When these data are combined, they provide evidence indicating that patients with global aphasia are prominent among patients with aphasia as a whole. As a result, they constitute a significant demand on the resources of clinical aphasiologists from the acute stages of illness through the time of maximal recovery.

Characteristics

Age and Sex

Discrepancies appear in the literature with regard to age and global aphasia. Some studies suggest no effect of age on global aphasia (Habib, Ali-Cherif, Poncet, & Salamon, 1987; Scarpa et al., 1987; Sorgato, Colombo, Scarpa, & Faglioni, 1990), whereas others report differences only with patients demonstrating Broca's aphasia (i.e., patients with Broca's aphasia tend to be significantly younger than those with global aphasia). This difference appears to hold true not only for Western patients with stroke but also for Indian patients with stroke (Bhatnagar et al., 2002). The older patients in the sample of Sorgato and colleagues (1990), however, did tend to show atypical aphasias, including global aphasia from brain damage that was restricted to either anterior or posterior areas.

With regard to sex, there appears to be no observable difference in the distribution of global aphasia (Habib et al., 1987). Davis (1983) suggested a general bias toward males in the data generated among the VA Medical Centers because of the nature of the population seen at these hospitals. Further studies, including more representative patient distributions, may be necessary for reliable data regarding the influence of sex on global aphasia. Nonetheless, age and sex may not be considered to have a differential effect on the incidence of global aphasia.

Site of Lesion

Cerebrovascular lesions producing global aphasia have been described as involving Broca's (posterofrontal) and Wernicke's (superotemporal) areas (Kertesz, 1979) or, alternatively, both the prerolandic and postrolandic speech zones (Goodglass & Kaplan, 1983). The subjects with global aphasia described by Murdoch, Afford, Ling, and Ganguley (1986) exhibited large lesions extending from the cortical surface inferiorly to subcortical areas, including the basal ganglia, internal capsule, and thalamus. Basso and Farabola's (1997) subject with global aphasia had damage to the left frontal operculum, Wernicke's area, the premotor area, the supramarginal gyrus, inferior and superior parietal lobules, angular gyrus, and Heschl's gyri. All of these global aphasia–producing lesions involved the cortex and were extensive, dominating the left hemisphere. Numerous exceptions have been reported in the literature, however, suggesting that such an extensive lesion may not be necessary to produce a global aphasia.

Mazzocchi and Vignolo (1979) found global aphasia in 3 of 11 cases following lesions that were confined to anterior regions. In four additional cases, the lesions were deep and confined to the insula, the lenticular nucleus, and the internal capsule. Varying lesion effects also were described by Cappa and Vignolo (1983). Basso, Lecours, Moraschini, and Vanier (1985) observed global aphasia following discrete lesions confined to anterior (sparing of postrolandic centers) or posterior cortical sites. Alexander (2000) suggests that the comprehension deficit in patients with lesions limited to the frontal lobe may be the result of inattention, underactivation, unconcern, poor problem solving, or perseveration interacting with modest phonologic and/or semantic deficits to produce more profound functional comprehension deficits. Lüders and colleagues (1991) produced global aphasia during electrical stimulation of the basal temporal region. This region has its white matter in contact with the white matter deep to Wernicke's area, thereby favoring close interaction between these two areas. Sugiu, Katsumata, Ono, Tamiya, and Ohmoto (2003) observed global aphasia in a patient with a subarachnoid hemorrhage of the interhemispheric fissure identified by computed tomography (CT) and a small ischemic lesion in the territory of the distal left anterior cerebral artery identified by magnetic resonance imaging (MRI). Angiography demonstrated an anterior communicating artery aneurysm and severe vasospasm of the A1 segment of the anterior cerebral artery, the M1 segment of the middle cerebral artery, and the distal internal carotid artery. Conversely, Basso and colleagues (1985) reported other forms of aphasia following lesions that would have been suggestive of global aphasia.

Global aphasia also has been described in patients with lesions restricted to subcortical regions. Alexander, Naeser, and Palumbo (1987) found global aphasia in association with one lesion or with a series of primarily subcortical lesions that collectively damaged the striatum-anterior limb of the internal capsule; the anterior, superior, anterosuperior, and extraanterior periventricular white matter; and the temporal isthmus. Yang, Yang, Pan, Lai, and Yang (1989) also identified global aphasia in patients with lesions involving the internal capsule, basal ganglia, thalamus, and anteroposterior periventricular white matter. Okuda and colleagues (1994) described four patients with global aphasia who had lesions in the putamen, posterointernal capsule, temporal isthmus, and periventricular white matter of the left hemisphere. Kumar and colleagues (1996) observed global aphasia in their patient following a left thalamic hemorrhage.

Ferro (1992) as well as Basso and Farabola (1997) investigated the influence of lesion site on recovery from global aphasia. Ferro initially examined 54 subjects during either the first month (34 subjects), third month (7 subjects), or sixth month post onset (13 subjects). He then followed-up each patient at 3, 6, and 12 months and then yearly thereafter when possible. The lesions in his group of subjects with global aphasia were grouped into five types with differing outcomes. Type 1 included patients with large pre- and postrolandic middle cerebral artery infarcts; these patients had a very poor prognosis. The remaining four groups were classified as follows: type 2 = prerolandic; type 3 = subcortical; type 4 = parietal, and type 5 = double frontal and parietal lesion. Patients in these latter groups demonstrated variable outcomes, improving generally to Broca's or transcortical aphasia. Complete recovery was observed in some cases with type 2 and type 3 infarcts. In contrast to these findings, Basso and Farabola investigated recovery in three cases of aphasia based on the patients' lesion patterns. One patient had global aphasia from a large lesion involving both the anterior and posterior language areas, whereas two other patients had Broca's and Wernicke's aphasia from lesions restricted to either the anterior or posterior language areas, respectively. The patient with global aphasia was found to recover better than his two aphasic counterparts, but his overall outcome was considered to be outstanding. Based on these observations, Basso and Farrabola concluded that group recovery patterns based on aphasia severity and site of lesion may not be able to account for the improvement that occasionally is observed in individual patients.

Language

The hallmark of global aphasia is impaired language comprehension (up to the 30th percentile on the Boston Diagnostic Aphasia Examination [Alexander, 2000]) with concomitant deficits in expressive abilities (Damasio, 1991; Davis, 1983; Kertesz, 1979) in the context of almost universal buccofacial and limb apraxia (Alexander, 2000). Wallace and Stapleton (1991) suggested that, traditionally, the linguistic deficit in global aphasia has been interpreted as a loss of language competency (i.e., the knowledge of linguistic rules and operations). According to these authors as well as others (Rosenbek, LaPointe, & Wertz, 1989), the recent clinical evidence demonstrating preserved areas of language

functioning in global aphasia suggests that the loss for these patients may be viewed more appropriately as a variable mix of competence and performance deficits.

Comprehension

Patients with global aphasia may have considerable single-word comprehension (Alexander, 2000). Several isolated areas of relatively preserved comprehension following global aphasia also have been identified in the literature. These include recognition of specific word categories (McKenna & Warrington, 1978; Wapner & Gardner, 1979), familiar environmental sounds (Spinnler & Vignolo, 1966), and famous personal names (Van Lancker & Klein, 1990; Yasuda & Ono, 1998; but see also Forde & Humphreys, 1995, for a report of relatively impaired access to personal names following global aphasia). In the case of famous personal names, Yasuda and Ono (1998) found a distinct advantage for comprehending these items when reading versus listening. They attributed this finding to the nonsemantic, referential nature of personal names and to the probable processing of these stimuli in the patients' intact right hemispheres. Subjects with global aphasia also show relatively better comprehension for personally relevant information (Wallace & Canter, 1985; Van Lancker & Nicklay, 1992).

Wallace and Stapleton (1991) analyzed the responses of subjects with global aphasia on the auditory comprehension portion of the Boston Diagnostic Aphasia Examination (Goodglass & Kaplan, 1983), or BDAE, to identify patterns of preserved and impaired performance. Their results generally supported previous claims that distinct patterns of preserved components are absent in global aphasia; nonetheless, two or three of their subjects did show evidence of differential performance both within and across tasks. Interestingly, the scores for each of these subjects were collected during the acute stage of their recovery. The authors speculate that differential auditory comprehension performance during acute aphasia may be a useful prognostic indicator.

Expression

It has been suggested that patients with global aphasia may be most severely impaired in their expressive abilities. This may be a result of the greater contributions of the right hemisphere for comprehension than for expressive behaviors (Collins, 1986). The verbal output of many patients with global aphasia primarily consists of stereotypic recurring utterances or speech automatisms (Kertesz, 1979). Some authors have concluded that stereotypic recurring utterances are unique to global aphasia (Poeck, De Bleser, & Keyserlingk, 1984). Because of this and complementary evidence, Selnes and Hillis (2000) speculate that Tan, a patient with Broca's aphasia whose speech was limited to repetitions of the syllable "tan," actually may have presented with an atypical global aphasia rather than the historically accepted diagnosis of Broca's aphasia.

Stereotypes have been described as being either nondictionary verbal forms (unrecognizable) or dictionary forms (word or sentence) (Alajouanine, 1956). Blanken, Wallesch, and Papagno (1990) examined 26 patients demonstrating the nondictionary forms of speech automatisms. Of these cases, 24 were classified as having global aphasia. The other patients demonstrated signs more closely associated with Broca's and Wernicke's aphasia. Although speech automatisms frequently were associated with comprehension disturbances, the observed variability in language comprehension among these patients suggests that speech automatisms cannot be used to infer the presence of severe comprehension deficits. Blanken and colleagues (1990) proposed that speech automatisms relate only to speech output and do not necessarily indicate the presence of severe comprehension deficits.

Cognition

The cognitive abilities of patients with brain damage often are assessed by administration of the Raven's Colored Progressive Matrices (Raven, 1965), or RCPM, a nonverbal test of analogical reasoning. Conflicting results have been reported regarding the performance of subjects with aphasia relative to that of patients with left brain damage but without aphasia. Some studies have found that subjects with aphasia perform at lower levels (Basso, Capitani, Luzzati, & Spinnler, 1981; Basso, De Renzi, Faglioni, Scotti, & Spinnler, 1973; Colonna & Faglioni, 1966), but others have failed to show any significant difference between these two groups (Arrigoni & De Renzi, 1964; Piercy & Smith, 1962). Collins (1986) has reported significant positive correlations between the language ability of subjects with global aphasia and their performance on the RCPM. The subjects in the Collins study were in the early stages of recovery, and eventually, these subjects achieved RCPM scores similar to those of subjects with less severe aphasia.

Using a modified version of the RCPM to minimize the potential effect of unilateral spatial neglect, Gainotti, D'Erme, Villa, and Caltagirone (1986) compared acute and chronic subjects with varying types of aphasia to normal controls, subjects with right hemisphere damage, and subjects with left hemisphere damage but without aphasia. In this study, the subjects with aphasia performed worse than the subjects in the other groups. Further, the patients with global aphasia and with Wernicke's aphasia scored the poorest in comparison to those in the other aphasic groups (anomic, Broca's, and conduction). These results were similar to those obtained by Kertesz and McCabe (1975). Gainotti and colleagues (1986) did not obtain differences relative to the severity of aphasia, but they did link poor performance on the RCPM to the presence of receptive semantic-lexical disturbances. Gainotti colleagues conclude that "a

specific relationship exists in aphasia between cognitive non-verbal impairment and breakdown of the semantic-lexical level of integration of language" (p. 48).

Rossor, Warrington, and Cipolotti (1995) demonstrated relatively preserved calculation skills in a patient with global aphasia secondary to progressive atrophy of the left temporal lobe. Together with previous reports of selective impairment of calculation in patients with intact language skills, the authors posited that this double dissociation reflects a functional independence between the two domains of behavior (i.e., that calculation skills are not dependent on the language processing system). Because selective impairment of calculation skills has been associated with left parietal lesions, the authors also suggested that lesions producing language disturbances that spare the parietal lobe may be associated with preserved calculation skills.

Communication

Recurring utterances among individuals with global aphasia was addressed previously. Those who exhibit only recurring consonant-vowel syllables (e.g., "do-do-do" or "ma-ma-ma") often give the impression of somewhat preserved communicative abilities in that they may make use of the suprasegmental aspects of speech (Collins, 1986). The use of suprasegmentals in conversational turn taking may appear to indicate that the patient with aphasia is producing utterances with some communicative intent. deBlesser and Poeck (1984) studied a group of patients with global aphasia and found that they did not exhibit prosodic variability to the extent necessary for conveying communicative intent. The utterances used for analysis, however, were limited to those elicited during formal testing, and they may not have reflected the spontaneous use of inflection to convey intent (Collins, 1986). deBlesser and Poeck (1985) subsequently analyzed the spontaneous utterances of a group of subjects with global aphasia and output limited to consonant-vowel recurrences. Utterances were sampled during interviews in which the examiner asked a series of open-ended questions, and the length of the utterances and their pitch contours were analyzed for variability. The authors concluded that both length and pitch appeared to be stereotypic and that the prosody of these patients did not seem to reflect communicative intent. The appropriateness of these consonant-vowel recurring utterances with regard to turn taking remains questionable. These findings highlight the marked discrepancy that exists between research outcomes and clinical reports. deBlesser and Poeck (1985) suggest that the contributions to conversation for which these patients are credited may, in fact, be the result of the communicative partner's need for informative communication rather than the patient's use of prosodic elements to convey intent.

In a study by Herrmann, Koch, Johannsen-Horbach, and Wallesch (1989), a group of patients with chronic and severe nonfluent aphasia were described in terms of their communication strategies and communicative efficiency. The patients presented with either severe Broca's or global aphasia (50%). The results showed that the efficiency of the patients' communication depended on the type of question to which they were asked to respond. As might be expected, superior performance was observed for responses to yes/no questions (e.g., "Did your illness occur suddenly?") when compared to interrogative pronoun questions (e.g., "How long have you had language problems now?") and narrative requests (e.g., "Tell me what happened to you after you took ill."). Herrmann and colleagues (1989) reported that the patients used mostly gesture in their responses to the yes/no questions. The other types of questioning require increased verbal output and, thus, created the need for more complex communicative responses from the patients.

In examining the communication strategies utilized, Herrmann and colleagues (1989) found that patients rarely took the initiative or expanded on topics. The most frequent strategies reported by these authors were those enabling the patients to secure comprehension (e.g., indicating comprehension problems or requesting support for establishing comprehension). Herrmann and colleagues concluded that patients with global aphasia rely most heavily on nonverbal communication.

Marshall and colleagues (1997) also investigated the efficiency of different communication strategies used by three patients with severe aphasia: A patient with Broca's aphasia communicated primarily through writing and drawing; a patient with Wernicke's aphasia communicated primarily through speaking; and a patient with global aphasia and apraxia of speech communicated primarily through gesturing with a few single words. Marshall and colleagues assessed each patient's communicative efficiency and the degree of communicative burden assumed by a partner during a declarative message exchange task that was evaluated using a visual analogue scale. The investigators also analyzed the effects of context and shared knowledge on efficiency in communicative interactions by varying the extent of the raters' awareness of the message contents (e.g., no knowledge or partial or full knowledge). Their results demonstrated that the efficiency of communication by the patient with global aphasia approximated that of the most efficient patient (i.e., the patient with Broca's aphasia). Also, the burden imposed by his gestural strategy was nearly as low as the writing and drawing of the patient with Broca's aphasia. These findings support the effectiveness of the nonverbal strategies used by patients with global aphasia and further reinforce their training as a target of rehabilitation.

Affect

Depression following aphasia has been "underrecognized and undertreated" (Masand & Chaudhary, 1994). Masand and Chaudhary suggest this might be the result of heavy reliance on verbal responses for establishing a diagnosis of depression. Also, patients with global aphasia tend to be excluded from treatment studies because of their severe comprehension deficits. In a case report of a patient with chronic global aphasia hospitalized for deteriorating mental status, these authors describe positive benefits from administration of the psychostimulant methylphenidate for treatment of his major depression. From a pre-treatment state characterized by drowsiness and lethargy, sad affect, and an inability to participate in his care, the patient improved within 72 hours of achieving a therapeutic dose (15 mg/day) to become more alert, smiling, attentive, and actively involved in his care. These changes resulted in his improved candidacy for rehabilitation, and on referral, he reportedly made significant gains in speech-language treatment that included producing single words, following simple commands, and imitating gestures. Discontinuation of his medications, including the methylphenidate, secondary to two generalized tonic-clonic seizures resulted in a return to his previous apathetic state within a week.

ETIOLOGY

As described, the majority of lesions producing global aphasia are extensive and involve both pre- and postrolandic areas. The blood supply for these areas is via the middle cerebral artery, which is the largest branch of the internal carotid artery, branching at the point of the sylvian fissure. Because of the extent of the lesion, global aphasia most commonly results from a cerebrovascular event, the locus of which is in the middle cerebral artery at a level inferior to the point of branching. When accompanied by hemiplegia, the event causing global aphasia tends to be thrombotic more than embolic (Collins, 1986). The stroke mechanism causing global aphasia without hemiparesis, however, is heterogeneous (Bang et al., 2004; Hanlon, Lux, & Dromerick, 1999). Greater late recovery may be associated with large hemorrhages (Alexander, 2000).

Not all occurrences of global aphasia are the result of a cerebrovascular event in the middle cerebral artery. Interestingly, Wells, Labar, and Solomon (1992) reported a temporary case of global aphasia because of simple partial status epilepticus. The aphasia lasted during a period in which periodic lateralized epileptiform discharges occur. Wells and colleagues reported that the patient's language returned to near normal during the 24 hours following the seizures. A case of rapidly developing global aphasia and personality change in a young woman secondary to demyelinating disease also is described in the case records of the Massachusetts General Hospital (Anonymous, 1996). An MRI scan of the brain with gadolinium showed multiple enhancing white matter lesions predominating in the subcortical and periventricular white matter, the posterior limb of the left internal capsule, and the corona radiata and centrum semiovale bilaterally. Treatment with corticosteroids resulted in minimal improvements; administration of cyclophosphamide, an anti-inflammatory/immunologic agent, produced steady improvement. No other information was provided regarding her speech-language outcome. Katz, Shetty, Gobin, and Segal (2003) reported a case of transient global aphasia resulting from a giant dural arteriovenous fistula of the superior sagittal sinus that resolved after fistula embolization. Global aphasia also was reported following a ruptured anterior communicating artery aneurysm and vasospasm (Sugiu, Katsumata, Ono, Tamiya, & Ohmoto, 2003). His symptoms improved following endovascular treatment of the aneurysm.

RECOVERY

The outlook for recovery from global aphasia tends to be bleak. For this reason, the term "global aphasia" may be more prognostic than descriptive (Peach, 2004). Kertesz and McCabe (1977) reported that the group of subjects with global aphasia in their study generally demonstrated limited language recovery, a pattern similar to that reported by Wapner and Gardner (1979). When assessing the language recovery that does occur, better improvement is demonstrated in comprehension than in expression (Lomas & Kertesz, 1978; Prins, Snow, & Wagenaar, 1978). With regard to recovery of nonverbal cognitive abilities, Kertesz and McCabe (1975) found a precipitous and parallel rate of improvement for RCPM and language performance during the first 3 months post-onset. During the next 3 months, performance on the RCPM continued to increase substantially, surpassing language performance that was only mildly improved from levels attained at the end of the first 3 months. Patients appeared to reach a plateau in both RCPM and language performance during the period between 6 and 12 month post-onset. Overall, performance on the RCPM by the patients with global aphasia did not exceed approximately 50% of the maximum attainable score.

In relation to the recovery observed in other types of aphasia, Kertesz and McCabe (1977) described patients with global aphasia as having the lowest recovery rate. With regard to the temporal aspects of recovery in global aphasia, differences have been reported depending on whether the subjects were receiving speech and language treatment. For patients with global aphasia not receiving treatment, improvement appears to be greatest during the first months post-onset (Kertesz & McCabe, 1977; Pashek & Holland, 1988). Siirtola and Siirtola (1984) observed the greatest improvement in their untreated subjects during the first 6 months post onset.

Patients with global aphasia receiving treatment, however, demonstrate substantial improvements during the first 3 to 6 months but also continued improvement during the period between 6 and 12 months or more post-onset (Kertesz & McCabe, 1977; Nicholas et al., 1993; Sarno & Levita, 1979, 1981). In the study by Kertesz and McCabe (1977), significantly greater improvement was noted in treated versus untreated patients with global aphasia during this period, although the authors attributed this gain at least partially to subject heterogeneity. In the studies by Sarno and Levita (1979, 1981), improvement was most accelerated between 6 and 12 months poststroke. Nicholas and colleagues (1993) found different patterns of recovery for language and non-language skills following longitudinal administration of the Boston Assessment of Severe Aphasia (Helm-Estabrooks, Ramsberger, Morgan, & Nicholas, 1989), or BASA, an instrument developed specifically to evaluate communication performance in patients with severe aphasia. Substantial improvements in praxis and oral-gestural expression were noted only during the first 6 months post-onset, whereas similar improvements in auditory and reading comprehension were observed only between 6 and 12 months post-onset. Based on these findings, the authors stressed the need for analyzing subsets of communication skills rather than overall scores to evaluate recovery from global aphasia.

Evolution

The majority of patients with global aphasia will not recover to less severe forms of the disorder. Some patients, however, will improve to the extent that they evolve into other aphasic syndromes. A number of studies have documented these changes using a variety of assessment instruments and testing schedules.

Six studies used the Western Aphasia Battery (Kertesz, 1982), or WAB, to assess language performance during the acute period of recovery and at regular intervals for up to 1 year (or more) post-onset. Kertesz and McCabe (1977) tested 93 subjects with aphasia between 0 and 6 weeks post-onset and found that 5 of their 22 subjects with global aphasia progressed to other syndromes, including Broca's, transcortical motor, conduction, and anomic aphasia after 1 year or more. Siirtola and Siirtola (1984) classified subjects with aphasia within the first 2 weeks after hospitalization. At 1 year post-onset, 6 from among 14 subjects with global aphasia had evolved to other syndromes, including Broca's, conduction, anomic, and Wernicke's aphasia, or, in the case of one subject, had recovered completely. For 1 year, Holland, Swindell, and Forbes (1985) followed 15 patients who had been classified as having global aphasia immediately after stroke. In this study, classifications were based on results obtained from the WAB as well as from clinical impressions. Several patterns were observed at the end of the first year: Two patients (in their 30s) returned to normal language functioning, two (in their 40s) evolved to Broca's aphasia, two (59 and 61 years of age) evolved to anomic aphasia, two (in their 70s) evolved to Wernicke's aphasia, and two (in their 80s) remained global aphasic. The five remaining subjects died during the course of the study. Pashek and Holland (1988) described the evolution of 11 subjects with global aphasia from among a larger group of 32 subjects who were followed for at least 6 months. Language performance was assessed by repeated administration of the WAB, these subjects with aphasia were classified on the basis of descriptive criteria rather than WAB typology. All subjects were evaluated within the first 5 days after stroke. Four of these patients evolved to less severe syndromes, including Broca's, Wernicke's, and anomic aphasia. Two patients evolved to a less severe but unclassifiable aphasic syndrome. One subject recovered normal language, and two subjects demonstrated symptoms of dementia. Mark, Thomas, and Berndt (1992) reported the 1-year outcomes of 13 patients initially classified as having global aphasia at 7 to 10 days post-onset. One patient was no longer aphasic, whereas seven patients recovered to a less severe form of aphasia. Among the latter, two patients recovered to Wernicke's aphasia, two recovered to conduction aphasia, and three recovered to anomic, Broca's, and transcortical motor aphasias, respectively. Finally, 9 of 13 patients with global aphasia followed by McDermott, Horner, and DeLong (1996) evolved to other forms of aphasia. Seven of these patients evolved to Broca's aphasia, and two evolved to Wernicke's aphasia.

Nicholas and colleagues (1993) assessed 17 patients with global aphasia as well as seven other patients with severe aphasia for 2 years after the onset of their aphasia to describe the patterns of recovery. Patients were scheduled for testing with the BASA at 1 to 2 months after the onset of their aphasia and at every 6-month anniversary of their strokes thereafter up to 24 months. Of the patients with global aphasia initially, four changed classification during this period, and the remaining 13 continued to be classified as having global aphasia. For the patients who did evolve, one changed to a mild Wernicke's aphasia and changed to mixed nonfluent aphasia.

Sarno and Levita (1979) investigated recovery from global aphasia using selected subtests of the Neurosensory Center Comprehensive Examination for Aphasia (Spreen & Benton, 1977) and the Functional Communication Profile (Sarno, 1969), or FCP. Classification of aphasia was based on clinical impressions as well as language test scores. In the study by Sarno and Levita (1979), the earliest language observations were collected at 4-weeks post-onset, with a variation of no greater than plus or minus 1 week. Repeated testing was continued until 1 year after the stroke. In contrast to the above studies, none of these 14 subjects with global aphasia evolved to another type of aphasia by the end of the year. Similar results were observed in a follow-up study of seven subjects with global aphasia (Sarno & Levita, 1981).

Laska, Hellblom, Murray, Kahan, and Von Arbin (2001) studied the natural course of aphasia during the acute phase and at 3, 6, and 18 months after stroke onset in 119 consecutive, unselected patients. The median time for acute testing was 5 days (range, 0–30 days); 90% of all patients were tested within 11 days. Clinical tests included the "Grunntest for aphasi" (Reinvang, 1985, as cited in Laska et al., 2001), a test that the authors described as being similar to the WAB; the Amsterdam-Nijmegen-Everyday-Language-Test, or ANELT, which is a measure of functional verbal communication; and the Token Test. A subjective ranking of aphasia severity also was obtained. Recovery was determined by the degree of change in ANELT scores. A vast majority of the patients had either global, Wernicke's, or conduction aphasia. Improvements were observed in all types of aphasia, including global aphasia. A positive correlation was found for initial severity and degree of recovery. Of six patients who were diagnosed initially with global aphasia and were available at least three times during 18 months, four evolved to mixed nonfluent aphasia, one to conduction aphasia, and one to mixed fluent aphasia (the category of mixed aphasias on the Reinvang test includes the presence of two or more aphasic syndromes).

One apparent explanation for the discrepancies among these studies might be the greater instability of language scores and, therefore, aphasia classifications obtained during the first 4 weeks after stroke versus those obtained after the first month post-onset. McDermott and colleagues (1996) found greater magnitude-of-change scores and frequencies of aphasia type evolution in subjects tested during the first 30 days post-onset versus those tested during the second 30 days post-onset. Aphasia tends to be more severe during the acute stage, giving observers an initial impression of global aphasia. This symptomatology may be fleeting, however, and result in a seemingly greater potential for patients to evolve to a less severe aphasic syndrome following this early period (Table 21–1).

Holland and colleagues (1985) as well as Pashek and Holland (1988), however, found that patients with global aphasia who do progress to some other form of aphasia demonstrate changes that extend into the first months post-onset. In some cases, the global aphasia may not begin to evolve until after the first month has passed. In addition, Reinvang and Engvik (1980) initially assessed their subjects with aphasia between 2 and 5 months after their injuries (mean, 3 months) and found that four of the seven subjects with global aphasia had evolved to a less severe Broca's, conduction, or unclassifiable syndrome at retesting. The retesting was completed no sooner than 1 month after initial testing, with a mean time of 7.5 months after injury and a range of 3 to 30 months. Based on these findings, the discrepancies in recovery from global aphasia reported in these studies do not appear to be the result simply of the time at which the initial language observations were recorded. Apparently,

TABLE 21–1

Proportion of Subjects with Global Aphasia Evolving to Less Severe Aphasic Syndromes or Normal Language with Time of Initial Testing after Cerebral Injury

Study	Subjects (*n*)	Initial Testing	% Evolved[a]
Holland, Swindell, & Forbes (1985)	10	Immediately	80
Pashek & Holland (1988)	11	0–5 days	64
Laska, Hellblom, Murray, Kahan, &Von Arbin (2001)	6	0–30 days	100
Mark, Thomas, & Berndt (1992)	13	7–10 days	62
Siirtola & Siirtola (1984)	14	0–2 weeks	43
Kertesz & McCabe (1977)	22	0–6 weeks	23
McDermott, Horner, & DeLong (1996)	13	0–6 weeks	69
Sarno & Levita (1979)	11	4 weeks	0
Sarno & Levita (1981)	7	4 weeks	0
Nicholas, Helm-Estabrooks, Ward-Lonergan, & Morgan (1993)	17	1–2 months	24
Reinvang & Engvik (1980)	7	2–5 months	57

[a]End-stage assessments were completed between 6 to 12 months post-injury in all studies except Kertesz & McCabe (1977), Reinvang & Engvik (1980), Nicholas et al. (1993), McDermott and colleagues (1996), and Laska and colleagues (2001). Only 10 of the subjects with global aphasia studied by Kertesz and McCabe (1977) were assessed at 1 year or more post-onset. Specific data for the subjects with global aphasia of Reinvang & Engvik (1980) were not reported; the mean time post-onset for the end-stage observations of all subjects with aphasia in their study was 7.5 months, with a minimum time of 3 months post-onset. Fifteen of the 17 subjects with global aphasia followed by Nicholas and colleagues (1993) were assessed at 24 months post-onset; final testing for the remaining two subjects was completed at 18 months post-onset. Re-evaluation for the 13 subjects with global aphasia tested by McDermott and colleagues (1996) occurred approximately between 1 and 6 months post-onset, with a minimum intervening period of at least 30 days. The patients of Laska and colleagues (2001) received follow-up at 18 months post-onset of their aphasia.

evolution from global aphasia is the result of a complex interaction among a number of heretofore incompletely understood factors.

Prognostic Factors

Age

Following global aphasia, a patient's age appears to have an impact on recovery: The younger the patient, the better the prognosis (Holland et al., 1985; Pashek & Holland, 1988). Age also may relate to the type of aphasia at 1 year post-stroke. For example, in the study reported by Holland and colleagues (1985), younger patients with global aphasia evolved to a nonfluent Broca's aphasia, whereas older patients evolved to increasingly severe fluent aphasias with advancing age. The oldest patients remained global aphasic (see above).

Whether age can be considered a prognostic indicator has yielded differing conclusions. Advanced age has been found to have a negative influence on recovery (Holland & Bartlett, 1985; Holland, Greenhouse, Fromm, & Swindell, 1989; Marshall & Phillips, 1971; Sasanuma, 1988) and to be an insignificant predictor of recovery (Hartman, 1981; Kertesz & McCabe, 1977; Sarno, 1981; Sarno & Levita, 1971). Pashek and Holland (1988) noted specifically that age appeared to predict a poor prognosis for change in global aphasia but also identified a number of exceptions to this rule. Thus, age cannot be considered an absolute predictor.

The variability in evolution patterns and age effects identified by these authors is intriguing and suggests the need for further large-scale research studies in this area.

Hemiplegia

Occasionally, global aphasia occurs without an accompanying hemiparesis (Bogousslavsky, 1988; Ferro, 1983; Van Horn & Hawes, 1982). Motor abilities may be preserved following dual discrete lesions occurring in the frontal and temporoparietal regions, a single frontotemporoparietal lesion, or a single temporoparietal lesion. Absence of a hemiparesis in global aphasia may be a positive indicator for recovery (Legatt, Rubin, Kaplan, Healton, & Brust, 1987; Tranel, Biller, Damasio, Adams, & Cornell, 1987). Tranel and colleagues (1987) described patients with global aphasia with dual discrete lesions (anterior and posterior cerebral) that spared the primary motor area. The global aphasia of these patients aphasia improved significantly within the first 10 months post-onset. Deleval, Leonard, Mavroudakis, and Rodesch (1989) reported two cases of global aphasia without hemiparesis following discrete prerolandic lesions. Although both of these patients exhibited mild right arm weakness initially, this motor disturbance cleared within 48 hours of onset. The patients reported by Deleval and colleagues (1989) showed rapid recovery yet continued to exhibit what the authors referred to as a residual motor aphasia. The patient described by Basso and Farabola (1997) experienced global aphasia and a right hemiparesis that cleared within a few days following a single, left frontotemporal lesion. Although severely aphasic at the initiation of treatment 40 days post-onset, the patient's language outcome 2.5 years later was described as "outstanding." Nagaratnam and colleagues (1996) examined language recovery at 3 months poststroke in 12 patients diagnosed with global aphasia without hemiparesis 4 to 8 days post-onset. Eight patients with single lesions in either anterior language cortex or posterior language cortex recovered to no more than mild levels of impairment. Four patients with lesions in both anterior and posterior language areas continued to have severe language impairments.

Global aphasia without hemiparesis does not necessarily result in extensive language recovery. Keyserlingk and colleagues (1997) found that chronic patients with global aphasia and no history of hemiparesis secondary to a single, large lesion of the left perisylvian region did not fare any better with regard to language outcome than did their counterparts with global aphasia and hemiparesis from the time of onset. The critical difference between the two groups for motor, but not language, function depended on the degree to which the patients' lesions extended into the subcortical white matter and nuclei. Eight of the 11 patients studied by Bang and colleagues (2004) showed minimal improvement 8 weeks after stroke onset. Three patients demonstrated the classical pattern of dual lesions in the left inferior frontal gyrus and the superior temporal gyrus, five patients exhibited single lesions of either the left inferior frontal gyrus or the superior temporal gyrus, and three patients had a subcortical or cortical lesion outside the perisylvian area. Language recovery could not be predicted by lesion location.

Hanlon, Brown, and Gerstman (1999) found three distinct subtypes of global aphasia in 10 patients without hemiparesis. The subtypes were associated with different patterns of language outcome 10 to 12 weeks after their strokes. The auditory-verbal subtest scores and the aphasia quotient (AQ) from the WAB were entered into a cluster analysis to define the groups. Lesion patterns also were identified. Four patients with a mean AQ of 2.3 comprised cluster 1; these were the most severely impaired patients and were characterized by dense, nonfluent speech with severe initiation deficits, marked comprehension impairment, no repetition, and grossly defective naming. Their lesions primarily involved the left superior temporal gyrus. Patients in this cluster showed minimal or no change in language scores at follow-up and remained globally aphasic. Cluster 2 consisted of two patients with a mean AQ of 34.9 who were characterized by dense, nonfluent spontaneous speech; moderate comprehension impairment; minimal capacity for naming monosyllabic, high-frequency nouns; and limited repetition. The left inferior frontal gyrus and adjacent subcortical white matter, primarily involving the territory of the precentral, central, lenticulostriate, and insular branches of the middle cerebral artery, were lesioned. These patients recovered to a pattern most like transcortical motor aphasia, with relative preservation of repetition and improved comprehension and naming. Cluster 3 included four patients with a mean AQ of 13.9. These patients demonstrated low-level, dysfluent speech; marked comprehension impairment; minimal or no repetition; and severely defective naming characterized by perseverative monosyllabic utterances. Lesioning of the left pre- and postcentral gyri involving the central and posterior parietal vascular territories was found. At follow-up, increased speech fluency and improved comprehension were observed, accompanied by inconsistent changes in repetition and naming. All members of this group evolved to a pattern of Wernicke's aphasia. Degree of recovery was related to group subtype.

Neuroimaging Patterns

Both CT and functional MRI (fMRI) have been used to estimate outcome from global aphasia. In a two-part study, Pieniadz, Naeser, Koff, and Levine (1983) investigated the relationship between hemispheric asymmetries and recovery from aphasia. The first part of the study involved the analysis of hemispheric asymmetry in a large group of subjects with aphasia and in a group of control subjects without aphasia. The results demonstrated significant similarity and consistency in hemispheric asymmetry for both groups. The most frequent asymmetry involved left-greater-than-right occipital width. Frontal width was greater in the right hemisphere than in the left hemisphere. Length also was greater in the left occipital region. For frontal length, the hemispheres were typically equal.

In the second part of the study by Pieniadz and colleagues (1983), recovery patterns were examined in a group of subjects with global aphasia. These researchers found larger right occipital widths and lengths on CT scans for subjects demonstrating superior recovery of single-word comprehension, repetition, and naming. Pieniadz and colleagues suggested that these atypical asymmetries may indicate right hemisphere dominance for language. Evaluation of hemispheric asymmetries may be used, therefore, to predict recovery of single-word functions, with atypical patterns suggesting superior long-term gains.

Naeser, Gaddie, Palumbo, and Stiassny-Eder (1990) used CT to compare lesion location and language recovery in a group of subjects with global aphasia. The primary foci in their study were recovery of comprehension abilities and differentiation between temporal lobe lesions involving Wernicke's area and those restricted to the subcortical temporal isthmus. The subjects had either frontal, parietal, and temporal lobe lesions or lesions involving the frontal and parietal lobes with temporal lobe lesions restricted to the subcortical temporal isthmus. The results of this study showed significantly better recovery of auditory comprehension for the group without damage to Wernicke's area (lesions limited to subcortical temporal isthmus). Over the course of 1 to 2 years, the majority of these subjects reportedly obtained auditory comprehension scores on the BDAE (Goodglass & Kaplan, 1983) that were consistent with only mild to moderate comprehension deficits (Naeser et al., 1990). None of the subjects in this study made significant gains in speech output.

A group of patients with severe global aphasia and extreme loss of both verbal and nonverbal communication (including comprehension) was studied by De Renzi, Colombo, and Scarpa (1991). These authors found a variety of lesion patterns, only 35% of which involved the entire language area. Attempts to correlate specific types of lesions with some recovery of language abilities were unsuccessful. For the patients who showed some comprehension improvement, no common lesion pattern was found.

Mark and colleagues (1992) evaluated CT scans of patients with global aphasia in a routine acute-care setting to assess their viability of such scans for predicting language performance at 1-year post-onset. The scans were measured for lesion volume, total occipital asymmetry, and the cerebral volume occupied by the lateral ventricles and correlated with WAB (Kertesz, 1982) AQ and auditory comprehension scores. No clear relationship was found between acute imaging of the patients' lesions and their aphasia outcomes.

Zahn and colleagues (2004) used fMRI to investigate the underlying mechanism for recovery of auditory comprehension following global aphasia. Seven patients with large lesions following left middle cerebral artery infarction were identified using the Aachen Aphasia Test or the Aachen Aphasia Bedside Test during the acute or subacute stages of their illnesses. Different degrees of auditory comprehension recovery were demonstrated among these patients at follow-up 6 to 12 months later. A functional activation paradigm was used that allowed differentiation of anatomical patterns associated with processing of auditory word form versus meaning. When compared to normal subjects, no differences were observed in the patients having global aphasia with regard to the lateralization or the general regions of activations. The left extrasylvian temporal cortex and right posterior parietal cortex were the most consistently activated regions. The extrasylvian temporal activations were thought to represent correlates of recovery of lexical-semantic processing. The authors concluded that comprehension recovery occurs via functional compensation by spared parts of the partially damaged semantic word processing system (redundancy recovery). The results did not support other mechanisms for recovery that have been proposed, such as reactivation of functionally connected areas, substitution of previously nonactive areas, or transfer of function to right hemisphere homologues. Right hemisphere contributions, however, may be substantial for lexical-semantic processing of words presented visually, particularly when phonologic processing is severely impaired (Gold & Kertesz, 2000).

Language Scores

Collins (1986) has used scores obtained from patients with global aphasia on the Porch Index of Communicative Ability (Porch, 1981), or PICA, to predict recovery. According to Collins (1986), patients with global aphasia invariably obtain scores below the 25th percentile. High intra- and intersubtest variability, however, suggest at least the potential for recovery. Variability in this instance is defined as the difference between the mean score for a PICA subtest and the highest score within that subtest. A total variability score is derived by adding the variability scores for all PICA subtests. Variability scores of greater than 400 suggest excellent potential for recovery, whereas scores of less than 200 suggest poor potential for recovery.

Using medical and PICA data, Collins (1986) suggests that patients with global aphasia demonstrating some variability within subtests and variability scores of around 100, but relatively flat scores across all modalities, have a poor prognosis for recovery. Imitation, copying, and matching may be better than other test behaviors. Patients with variability scores of much greater than 100 and with greater divergence among modality scores have a fair prognosis for recovery. Performance generally is characterized by mostly correct object matching, good copying skills, the ability to name one or two of the objects, and production of some differentiated responses on the verbal subtests. Significant increases in overall variability relative to the previous two categories and occasionally higher scores (seven or above) on auditory comprehension, reading, and naming subtests are consistent with a good prognosis for recovery. One patient described by Collins (1986) achieved a variability score of greater than 400 while still performing at the 9th percentile.

The recommendations of Collins should be tempered by subsequent work. Wertz, Dronkers, and Hume (1993) tested the influence of PICA intrasubtest variability on prognosis for improvement in aphasia. Negative and nonsignificant correlations were obtained between variability scores at 1 month post-onset and improvement in PICA overall performance at 6 and 12 months post-onset. In addition, no significant differences in improvement were found at 6 and 12 months post-onset between two groups with high variability (score greater than 350) and low variability (score less than 300) at 1 month post-onset. Wertz and colleagues concluded that intrasubtest variability has no influence on prognosis. For other measures of aphasia, it generally appears that a lack of variability between auditory comprehension scores and other language scores may be viewed as a negative indicator. The more performance differs among tasks, the better the outlook. Further, higher test scores (i.e., less severe impairment) are consistent with a better prognosis. Within auditory comprehension scores, patients with global aphasia who provide yes/no responses to simple questions, regardless of their accuracy, seem to have a better outcome at 1 year post-onset compared with those who cannot grasp the yes/no format (Mark et al., 1992).

INTERVENTION

Before discussing clinical intervention for global aphasia, a few introductory remarks are provided in support of the management strategies that follow. The issues addressed here include some influences regarding the timing of intervention for global aphasia, the nature of the language assessment, and the behavioral targets of treatment.

Influences Regarding the Timing of Intervention

As described previously, the prognosis for recovery from global aphasia generally is poor (Kertesz & McCabe, 1977). Nonetheless, approximately one-fourth to three-fourths or more of these patients with global aphasia will recover to a less severe aphasia or even to a normal condition by the end of the first year after their stroke. Do these findings argue against early intervention for global aphasia? Should practitioners withhold assessment and treatment for these patients until a stable language profile is achieved? Clinicians have opposed withholding early treatment (Collins, 1986; Peach, 2001), and a number of reasons exist to continue to do so.

Prognostic Limitations

Primary among the reasons for advocating early intervention is the inability to identify accurately those patients with global aphasia who will evolve to less severe syndromes and those who will not. Even if it could be established that withholding early treatment from patients who have a high or low probability for good recovery is an acceptable clinical practice, current methodologies prevent clinicians from accurately identifying the recovery potential for these patients to make such decisions. Global aphasia cannot be reliably discriminated in the early stage (Wallesch, Bak, & Schulte-Monting, 1992), and any general conclusions about recovery in individual patients are "premature" (Basso & Farabola, 1997). Conflicting findings with regard to many of the factors identified above continue to present problems for estimating clinical prognosis.

Information derived from technologic applications may assist with this problem. In one study, the potential for recovery of auditory comprehension following global aphasia was estimated by examining the lesion site patterns on CT scans for these patients. As described earlier, better recovery was predicted at 1 to 2 years post-onset in patients whose temporal lesions spared Wernicke's area and involved only the subcortical temporal isthmus. Patients with temporal lesions that included more than half of Wernicke's cortical area, however, were expected to demonstrate moderate to severe comprehension deficits at 1 to 2 years after their injuries

(Naeser et al., 1990). Recent evidence derived from fMRI studies of patients initially diagnosed with global aphasia has demonstrated that activation of regions associated with lexical-semantic processing in normal subjects (left extratemporal and right posterior parietal cortex) is associated with good recovery of auditory comprehension at 6 months or greater following global aphasia (Zahn et al., 2004).

Recovery of spontaneous speech in severely nonfluent patients with stroke and left middle cerebral artery infarction can be estimated from the extent of lesion in two subcortical white matter areas: the medial subcallosal fasciculus (initiation of spontaneous speech), and the middle third of the periventricular white matter (motor/sensory aspects of spontaneous speech) (Naeser, Palumbo, Helm-Estabrooks, Stiassny-Eder, & Albert, 1989). For patients with lesions outside the left middle cerebral artery, Naeserand colleagues (1989) suggest examining other specific structures as well (e.g., supplementary motor area and cingulate gyrus).

These findings provide a promising approach to prognosis for global aphasia, but their application appears to warrant discretion on several accounts when making decisions regarding early intervention for global aphasia. For example, the findings of Naeser and colleagues (1989) are limited, because many of the patients in their most severe subject groups were not global aphasic. In addition, exceptions to expected patterns of recovery exist even in patients who meet the suggested neuroanatomical profiles (Naeser et al., 1989). Finally, the lack of clear patterns on CT scans that could be associated with recovery from global aphasia in other studies (De Renzi et al., 1991; Mark et al., 1992) suggests that these approaches are in need of further data before they can be applied rigorously.

Besides CT, a patient's levels of alertness or attention at the outset of global aphasia also might be assessed to predict superior recovery. Patients who initially are more alert or have better attention appear to show greater recovery from their global aphasia (Kertesz & McCabe 1977; Sarno & Levita, 1981). Because the evidence for these latter findings is primarily anecdotal, however, its application as a clinical guideline is tenuous until additional information becomes available. These observations, along with differing profiles in the evolution of global aphasia, underscore the fact that patients with global aphasia are a heterogeneous group. It is evident that research is needed to identify the particular factors and the way that they interact to account for better recovery. Clinicians might then more accurately identify the subgroups of patients with global aphasia who will demonstrate substantial language recovery and those who will not. This information can then be applied in management decisions regarding treatment (Ferro, 1992; Sarno, Silverman & Sands, 1970).

In the absence of accurate techniques for predicting recovery from global aphasia, the most powerful reasons for providing early treatment are (1) the latent recovery observed in those patients who receive acute speech and language treatment and (2) the greater effects generally observed in patients with aphasia when treated during the acute period of recovery. As a group, patients with global aphasia receiving early treatment show continued language improvement during the period between 6 and 12 months post-onset (Kertesz & McCabe, 1977; Nicholas et al., 1993; Sarno & Levita, 1979, 1981) that is not observed in untreated patients (Pashek & Holland, 1988; Siirtola & Siirtola, 1984). In addition, meta-analyses of the aphasia treatment literature have provided convincing evidence that outcomes for patients with severe aphasia are much greater when treatment is begun immediately after onset rather than during the post-acute period (Robey, 1998). Until more is known about the individual patient with global aphasia, these data suggest that clinicians should continue to intervene at the earliest opportunity to assist these patients at a time when such treatments may be most crucial to long-term recovery.

Treatment Objectives

A second reason for early intervention in global aphasia concerns the purpose of treatment. In deliberating this issue, consider a scenario in which the clinical limitations described above no longer applied in predicting recovery from global aphasia. With full awareness of whether a patient will experience a good versus a minimal recovery, which outcome would suggest the need for early treatment? For patients who are expected to evolve to a less severe aphasia, might treatment be deferred to obtain the more stable language profile that might subserve a more effective long-term management plan, or might treatment be initiated immediately to accelerate the patient's anticipated recovery? For patients who are not expected to demonstrate substantial recovery, might treatment be withheld because of the poor prognosis to allocate clinical and financial resources more effectively, or might these patients become primary candidates for treatment to develop a functional communication system from the outset of their aphasia that will provide the primary means through which they subsequently will communicate? When considering the purpose of treatment in either case, the arguments for early intervention with patients who have global aphasia, no matter their outcome, are more compelling than otherwise. The recovery patterns per se following global aphasia therefore do not provide an adequate rationale for postponing treatment of aphasia for these patients.

Global aphasia will be greatest during the acute phase of recovery. Often, as alluded to above, treatment during this phase focuses on the remediation of language deficits via stimulation of disrupted cognitive processes. Depending on the degree to which the condition renders the patient unable to communicate even the most basic of needs, however, the first goals of treatment also focus on establishing some means of communication, no matter how simple. Some methods to accomplish this would include establishing reliable yes/no responding or a basic vocabulary of functional items through oral or gestural means, such as head nodding, eye blinking, and pointing to pictures or specific icons. Interestingly, the activities associated with establishing these communication systems may, in and of themselves, be considered stimulatory for language. Clinicians also provide information to family, friends, and health-care staff during this phase regarding the patient's particular language profile (i.e., preserved versus deficient areas), prognosis, and suitable ways to improve communication with the patient. Early intervention in global aphasia therefore has the multiple purposes of language stimulation directed toward cerebral reorganization and recovery, identification of successful communication strategies, and patient, family, and staff counseling. None of these activities can—or should—be deferred until a stable language profile is achieved.

Goal Revisions

Patients with global aphasia do demonstrate varying improvements in linguistic, extralinguistic, and nonverbal communicative functioning (Kenin & Swisher, 1972; Mohr, Sidman, Stoddard, Leicester, & Rosenberger, 1973; Prins, Snow, & Wagenaar, 1978; Sarno & Levita, 1979, 1981; Wapner & Gardner, 1979). As discussed, these improvements may result in recovery to a less severe form of aphasia in some cases, whereas in others, the changes may be insufficient even at 1 year post-onset to suggest reclassification to another form of aphasia (Sarno & Levita, 1979, 1981). For this latter group, improvement can be anticipated in at least one of these categories, especially that of functional communication.

Most, if not all, clinical aphasiologists recognize the dynamic nature of aphasia. Early testing therefore is viewed only as a measure of the patient's language functioning at a single point in time that will be used to establish a baseline for intervention during the acute period. Because of recovery, frequent probes for improvement in treated and untreated behaviors during this early period as well as re-evaluation using formal instruments is not only encouraged, it is expected.

Withholding early treatment while awaiting more stable language profiles to improve treatment planning does not acknowledge that establishing and revising short-term treatment goals are inherent principles of aphasia rehabilitation. Whether treatment is provided before or after the first month post-onset, this process will be repeated regularly throughout the term of the patient's rehabilitation, regardless of the type of aphasia. There is little sense, therefore, in declaring this process to be less valid in global aphasia when treatment is initiated before the first month after injury.

Clinicians have much to offer patients with global aphasia and their families during the acute period of recovery. When patients improve, the treatment objectives reflect this change; when they fail to change, concerted rehabilitative efforts continue in the areas of the patients' greatest functional communicative needs.

Nature of the Assessment

Assessment of individuals with aphasia encompasses more than simple diagnosis. Ideally, assessment provides a profile not only of the patient's areas of weakness but also of his or her strengths. Reasonable treatment plans require both types of data. Formal tests provide one method for gathering such data and, in addition, facilitate discussion of patient findings among colleagues. To that end, Collins (1986, p. 62) provides a summary of the severity ratings for a number of these tests that are suggestive of global aphasia. Sometimes, however, formal tests may be inadequate for treatment planning (Rosenbek et al., 1989), especially in the case of severely impaired patients, such as those with global aphasia. Little can be gained about patients' preserved areas of communicative functioning from scores that are consistently near the floor for a given test. For these patients, information regarding their residual communicative capacities may be more readily available from a variety of informal (i.e., nonstandardized) measures. Such measures consist of patient observation to determine functional communication and the diverse methods for cueing behaviors that, when logically varied, allow a practical test of approaches that result in the most favorable responses. Methods that are successful in eliciting target behaviors are incorporated into treatment and provide an initial approach for developing subsequent behaviors.

Contemporary approaches include both formal and informal measures of assessment to establish a communication profile for the patient with global aphasia. From a practical point of view, initial contact with the patient should be preceded by a review of medical records and interviews with knowledgeable others to glean information about the patient's communicative status. To the degree possible, a formal language assessment should be completed using a standardized aphasia battery, sampling behaviors across tasks at least minimally in each language domain (i.e., speaking, listening, reading, and writing), and describing the patient's responses to each item. Given this baseline, assessment continues through what might be viewed as diagnostic treatment to identify the conditions that further promote successful language performance. Included here would be an analysis of patient responses during interviews focusing on familiar topics or in selected situations and the evaluation of hierarchical cues within language tasks.

In this "qualitative" approach, as described by Helm-Estabrooks (1986), neither type of language assessment (for-

mal or informal) is seen as simply augmenting the other. For the patient with global aphasia, both types are deemed mandatory for adequately describing communication functioning. A host of procedures are available to accomplish these objectives. These will be reviewed in the following sections.

Behavioral Targets for Treatment

Because the impairment in aphasia is, first and foremost, a linguistic one, the primary target for treatment traditionally has been that of language performance. As a result, the success of intervention most often has been evaluated by the extent of changes occurring exclusively in the patient with aphasia's grammatical and lexical behaviors. In such an approach, the potential for these changes is diminished with increases in the initial severity of the language impairment. Too often, this approach has resulted in underestimation of what has been accomplished regarding recovery of communication skills.

Nowhere might this problem be more prevalent than in the case of the patient with global aphasia. From the time that Sarno and colleagues (1970) suggested that patients with stroke and severe aphasia do not benefit from speech and language treatment, many health-care providers have taken a rather pessimistic view with regard to rehabilitation outcomes in this group of patients. The conclusions of Sarno and colleagues, however, and of others like them, were based solely on statistical comparisons of pre- and post-treatment language scores and failed to account for positive changes that may have occurred in other communication behaviors. In a subsequent study involving patients with global aphasia, Sarno and Levita (1981) examined the changes occurring not only in language scores but also in communication performance as assessed by the FCP. Clinically significant improvements in the patients' language scores were observed that, nonetheless, were insufficient to warrant reclassification to another aphasic syndrome. Inspection of nonverbal communication abilities revealed recovery of alternate skills (e.g., gesture, pantomime, and other extralinguistic behaviors) that exceeded the reported language changes. According to Sarno and Levita (1981), these improvements resulted in limited but effective communication by the end of the first year after stroke. Nicholas and colleagues (1993) also found significant improvements in the communication skills of their patients with global aphasia during the first year poststroke, even though the majority of those patients did not change classification.

These findings have given way in many instances to social approaches that exploit the residual language capacity and/or other functional abilities of these patients as well as the skills of conversation partners to improve communication and the patient's quality of life. Clinicians no longer attend exclusively to improving propositional speech in patients with global aphasia during or after the acute period of recovery. Such an emphasis is apparent in many of the treatment methods that have been developed recently for such patients.

ASSESSMENT

Assessment of communication functioning in patients with global aphasia is best achieved using both formal and informal measures. These measures are summarized in Table 21–2.

Formal Test Measures

General Language

The language features of global aphasia were described in a previous section. Some standardized aphasia test batteries that specifically address global aphasia in their classification schemes include Aphasia Diagnostic Profiles (Helm-Estabrooks, 1992), the BDAE (Goodglass, Kaplan, & Barresi, 2001), the Language Modalities Test for Aphasia (Wepman & Jones, 1961), the Minnesota Test for Differential Diagnosis of Aphasia (irreversible aphasia syndrome) (Schuell, 1974), the Sklar Aphasia Scale (Sklar, 1983), and the WAB (Kertesz, 1982). Additional batteries that comprehensively assess language performance to provide the clinical data for establishing a diagnosis of global aphasia include the Aphasia Language Performance Scales (Keenan & Brassell, 1975), Examining for Aphasia–Third Edition (Eisenson, 1994), the Neurosensory Center Comprehensive Examination for Aphasia (Spreen & Benton, 1977), the PICA (Porch, 1981), and Psycholinguistic Assessments of Language Processing in Aphasia (Kay, Lesser, & Coltheart, 1992). For Spanish speakers, the Multilingual Aphasia Examination-Spanish (Rey, Sivan, & Benton, 1991) can be used. The performance pattern for patients with global aphasia on any of the tests identified above generally is one of severe impairment in all language abilities.

Some modality-specific assessment instruments also might be appropriate in the evaluation of patients with global aphasia. These tests include the following: for auditory comprehension, the Token Test (De Renzi & Vignolo, 1962), the Auditory Comprehension Test for Sentences (Shewan, 1979; Shewan & Canter, 1971), the Revised Token Test (McNeil & Prescott, 1978), and the Functional Auditory Comprehension Task (LaPointe & Horner, 1978; LaPointe, Holtzapple, & Graham, 1985); for reading comprehension, the Reading Comprehension Battery for Aphasia-Second Edition (LaPointe & Horner, 1998) and the Gray Oral Reading Tests-Fourth Edition (Wiederholt & Bryant, 2001); and for naming, the Boston Naming Test (Kaplan, Goodglass, & Weintraub, 2001), the Object and

TABLE 21–2

Formal and Informal Measures for Assessment of Global Aphasia

Formal Assessment

General Language
Aphasia Diagnostic Profiles
Aphasia Language Performance Scales
Boston Assessment of Severe Aphasia
Boston Diagnostic Aphasia Examination
Examining for Aphasia–Third Edition
Language Modalities Test for Aphasia
Minnesota Test for Differential Diagnosis of Aphasia
Neurosensory Center Comprehensive Examination
  for Aphasia
Porch Index of Communicative Ability
Sklar Aphasia Scale-Revised
Western Aphasia Battery

Modality-Specific
Auditory Comprehension Test for Sentences
Boston Naming Test
Functional Auditory Comprehension Test
Gray Oral Reading Tests–Fourth Edition
Object and Action Naming Battery
Psycholinguistic Assessments of Language Processing
  in Aphasia
Reading Comprehension Battery for Aphasia–Second Edition
Test of Adolescent/Adult Word Finding
Token Test
Revised Token Test

Functional Communication
ASHA Functional Assessment of Communications Skills
  for Adults
Assessment of Language-Related Functional Activities
Communication Activities of Daily Living–Second Edition
Functional Communication Profile

Informal Measures

General Language
Auditory Comprehension Assessment (Edelman, 1984)
Behavioral Assessment (Salvatore & Thompson, 1986)

Functional Communication
Assessment of Communicative Effectiveness in Severe Aphasia
  (Cunningham et al., 1995)
Communicative Effectiveness Index (Lomas et al., 1989)
Functional Rating Scale (Collins, 1986)
Natural Communication (Holland, 1982)

Key: ASHA = American Speech-Language-Hearing Association.

Action Naming Battery (Druks & Masterson, 2000), and the Test of Adolescent/Adult Word Finding (German, 1990).

Unlike the foregoing instruments, the BASA (Helm-Estabrooks, Ramsberger, Morgan, & Nicholas, 1989) was developed "for the specific purpose of identifying and quantifying preserved abilities that might form the beginning steps of rehabilitation programs for severely aphasic patients" (p. 1). The BASA assesses performance on 61 items in 15 areas: social greetings and simple conversation; personally relevant yes/no question pairs; orientation to time and place; buccofacial praxis; sustained phonation and singing; repetition; limb praxis; comprehension of number symbols; object naming; action picture items; comprehension of coin names; famous faces; emotional words, phrases, and symbols; visuospatial items; and signature. Responses are scored for response modality (verbal, gestural, or both), communicative quality (fully communicative, partially communicative, noncommunicative, unintelligible, irrelevant, incorrect, unreliable, or task refused or rejected), affective quality, and perseveration. Raw scores are summed according to seven clusters of items: auditory comprehension, praxis, oral-gestural expression, reading comprehension, gesture recognition, writing, and visuospatial tasks. Norms are provided to convert the total raw score and item cluster raw scores to standard scores and percentile ranks. "Because an important goal of the BASA is to help determine whether a severe case of aphasia may be classified as global," (p. 42) two separate sets of norms are provided, one for cases of severe aphasia and one for global aphasia.

Functional Communication

Measures for the formal assessment of functional communication include the FCP (Sarno, 1969); Communication Activities of Daily Living–Second Edition (Holland, Fratalli, & Fromm, 1998), or CADL-2; the American Speech-Language-Hearing Association Functional Assessment of Communication Skills for Adults (Fratalli, Holland, & Thompson, 1995), or ASHA FACS; and the Assessment of Language-Related Functional Activities (Baines, Martin, & Heeringa, 1999), or ALFA. The FCP assesses 45 communication behaviors in a conversational situation that are considered to be common functions of everyday life. Behaviors are rated as normal, good, fair, or poor and are transformed to raw scores within five dimensions: movement, speaking, understanding, reading, and other behaviors. The raw scores are converted to a percentage and a weighted score representing the patient's performance relative to normal behavior for that dimension. An overall score is obtained by summing the weighted scores to represent the patient's percentage of normal communication.

The CADL-2 includes 50 items that assess communication skills in structured, simulated daily activities. It includes a series of context-dependent items that evoke a variety of speech acts and verbal interchanges as well as other items that assess functional reading, writing, and math. Responses can be communicated by a variety of verbal and nonverbal means and are scored as correct, adequate, or wrong. The CADL-2 has high inter- and intrarater reliability and includes standard scores and performance norms.

The ASHA FACS contains 43 items that assess functional communication in four areas: social communication; communication of basic needs; reading, writing, and number concepts; and daily planning. A seven-point quantitative scale rates the frequency of behaviors. A five-point qualitative scale rates the adequacy, appropriateness, and promptness of an individual's responses as well as the relative sharing of communication burden with the partner. The ASHA FACS has been found to be reliable and valid for use with adult aphasia resulting from left hemisphere stroke and adult cognitive communication disorders resulting from traumatic brain injury. It is available in both a paper-and-pencil version and a computerized version.

The ALFA consists of 10 subtests, including telling time, counting money, addressing an envelope, solving daily math problems, writing a check/balancing a checkbook, understanding medicine labels, using a calendar, reading instructions, using the telephone, and writing a phone message. The subtests probe auditory comprehension, verbal expression, reading and writing, as well as cognitive and motor skills. The test yields a raw score for each subtest that is associated with a rating of independent functioning levels for two populations (below and above 65 years of age). The ALFA was standardized on 495 patients between the ages of 20 and 96 years with neurological histories as well as a group of 150 normal adults.

Informal Measures

General Language

As described previously, informal measures of language assessment are conducted following formal assessment with a standardized battery to identify the conditions that further promote successful language performance. Such measures aim to identify isolated areas of preserved performance, such as those listed above as features of comprehension. Hierarchical cues are used to evaluate such residual areas within language tasks.

Salvatore and Thompson (1986) provide an example of informal assessment procedures designed to assess verbal and nonverbal communication systems in patients with global aphasia. The model used in their approach employs one stimulus to evoke a variety of responses. When stimuli are presented to evoke all levels of responding, stimulus-response relations that are preserved and those that are impaired are identifiable. For example, patients may be asked to provide several responses to a pictured stimulus, including matching it to an identical picture and both writing and saying its name. Responses are analyzed in different modes, including gesturing, drawing, reading, writing, and verbalizing. A matrix is developed to categorize the various relations that are tested. The results of the assessment provide important information that provides a basis for treatment.

Edelman (1984) provides an outline for the assessment of comprehension in global aphasia that specifically takes into account research findings identifying areas of residual function in global aphasia and factors that facilitate understanding. The suggested framework permits a systematic evaluation of understanding, both contextually and acontextually, while manipulating variables found to be facilitative. Performance is assessed using commands and questions at simple linguistic levels. Commands are divided into two sections. Those relating to the self involve whole-body movements, limb movements, and orofacial movements, and those relating to objects in the environment are divided into object recognition and object manipulation. These tasks are assessed respectively in a natural verbal context (e.g., "Have you any water?"; "Can you pass the tissues?") and acontextually (e.g., "Show me the comb"; "Pick up the comb"). Questions require affirmation or negation only, and they include those relating to self as well as those of less personal saliency. Responses are accepted when communicated either verbally or nonverbally. In addition, hierarchical cueing, consisting of repetition, utterance expansion, and gestural accompaniment, is incorporated and scored using a modified PICA system.

Functional Communication

A number of informal procedures that can be used to systematically evaluate the functional communication of patients with global aphasia also have appeared in the literature. Holland (1982) developed a procedure to score observations of natural communication in normal family interactions. The categories of behaviors included verbal and nonverbal output, reading, writing, math, and other communicative behaviors, such as talking on the phone and singing. The verbal behaviors were further subcategorized to capture the form, style, conversational dominance, correctional strategies, and metalinguistics of the production. Holland's procedure is "primarily concerned with the frequency and form of successful and failed verbal and nonverbal communicative acts" (p. 52).

Lomas and colleagues (1989) constructed the Communicative Effectiveness Index, or CETI, using communicative situations provided by patients with aphasia and their families that were thought to be important in day-to-day life. The CETI quantitatively assesses the performance of those with aphasia over time in 16 situations using judgments provided by spouses or significant others. Performance is rated relative to the person with aphasia's premorbid abilities using a visual analogue scale. The situations range from getting somebody's attention to describing or discussing something in depth. The index was found to be internally consistent, to have acceptable test-retest and interrater reliability, and to be a valid measure of functional communication when compared with other measures. The authors conclude that the CETI is an instrument that is capable of measuring the functional changes occurring during the recovery of patients with aphasia that have been difficult to measure previously.

Cunningham, Farrow, Davies, and Lincoln (1995) developed the Assessment of Communicative Effectiveness in Severe Aphasia, or ACESA. It consists of two sections: a structured conversation, and an assessment of the patient's ability to convey information about objects and pictures. Gesture, facial expression, speech, symbolic noise, and intonation are accepted ways for conveying information. Communicative effectiveness is rated using separate scales of recognizability for verbal and nonverbal responses. In an initial study to test the reliability of the instrument, test-retest reliability and intrarater reliability were found to be good. The authors therefore suggested that the tool can be useful for assessing change in communicative effectiveness when it is scored by the same person. Low interrater reliability, however, suggested that the tool needs further modifications before it can be used confidently for other clinical and/or research purposes.

Finally, a less systematic—but often effective—assessment of functional communication can be derived from patient interviews or questionnaires completed by individuals who are familiar with the patient who has global aphasia. Collins (1986) reviews several of these questionnaires and provides one such example, an adaptation of the FCP called the Functional Rating Scale.

TREATMENT

Given the generally poor outcome in chronic global aphasia (Kertesz & McCabe, 1977; Sarno & Levita, 1981) and the negative results that have been reported for treatment programs aimed specifically at remediating verbal skills (Sarno et al., 1970), treatment for these patients may emphasize functional and/or social approaches that attempt to improve participation in communication activities as well as impairment-based approaches that attempt to reduce the severity of the language impairment (Peach, 1993). Functional (patient-oriented) and social (partner-oriented) approaches use strategies that exploit the patient's residual linguistic and non-linguistic cognitive skills to increase successful communication (Herbert, Best, Hickin, Howard, & Osborne, 2003). Impairment-based approaches use structured methods that are carefully controlled for levels of difficulty to provide a context that will facilitate successful language responses and shape succeeding language behaviors of increasing complexity. Functional and social approaches tend to predominate during the chronic phase of the condition, but all approaches may—and should—be used during the course of recovery from global aphasia (Peach, 2001). Table 21–3 provides a summary of these approaches.

TABLE 21–3

Treatment Approaches for Global Aphasia

Impairment-Based Approaches
Auditory Comprehension
Matching pictures
Eliciting appropriate responses
Playing cards
Verbal Expression
Associating meaning with speech movements
Conversational prompting
Voluntary control of involuntary utterances
Phonologic treatment for naming
Transcranial magnetic stimulation for naming
Functional (Patient-Oriented) Approaches
Gestural Programs
Amer-Ind Code
Visual action therapy
Pantomime
Limited manual sign systems
Non-Speech Communication Aids
Non-electronic
    Preparatory training
    Communication boards
    Blissymbols
    Drawing
Electronic
    Computer-aided visual communication
    Lingraphica
    Gus multimedia speech system
    Promoting Aphasics' Communicative Effectiveness
Social (Partner-Oriented) Approaches
Supported Conversation for Adults with Aphasia
Conversational coaching
Partner training
Reciprocal scaffolding

Key: Amer-Ind = American-Indian.

Impairment-Based Approaches

Auditory Comprehension

Collins (1986, 1997) suggests that a realistic goal for treatment with the patient who has global aphasia consists of improving auditory comprehension, supplemented with contextual cues, to permit consistent comprehension of one-step commands in well-controlled situations. For the most severe comprehension deficits, picture matching, accompanied by the clinician's production of the name of the items to be matched, may provide the most basic level of auditory stimulation. Even in those cases when the patient has no understanding of the auditory stimulus accompanying the pictures, the response elicited by the matching task is assumed to evokes auditory representations of the visual stimuli that

may underlie subsequent association of meaning with the name of the pictures (Peach, 1993). Complexity may be increased within this task by (a) increasing the size of the response field; (b) moving from pairing real objects to realistic pictures of objects to line drawings of the objects; (c) matching objects to pictures and pictures to objects, a technique incorporated in Visual Action Therapy (Helm-Estabrooks, Fitzpatrick, & Barresi, 1982); and (d) using sets of pictures that represent nouns with decreasing frequency of occurrence in language usage. As performance improves, these tasks may be followed by word recognition for objects, pictures, or body parts and responding to simple questions.

Marshall (1986) provides an approach to treating auditory comprehension in patients with global aphasia that is presented in four phases: (a) eliciting responses, (b) eliciting differentiated responses, (c) eliciting appropriate responses, and (d) eliciting accurate responses. In the first phase, clinicians focus on attending, pointing, and yes/no responding; at a minimum, the clinician should help patients to express themselves through head nods, smiles, or frowns. Patients who cannot respond to spoken messages may engage in visual matching or orientation tasks. They also may be provided spoken messages accompanied by gestures. Questions and statements about personally relevant topics may comprise one of the best ways to elicit responses during this phase. In the second phase, the materials and techniques to elicit responses are not unlike those used in the first phase. At this time, however, the clinician accepts and reinforces any response that is different from the previous response given for those stimuli (e.g., varied facial expressions, head nods, gestures, and stereotypic utterances). To do this, the clinician records the patient's responses to a standard set of simple questions, looking for a variety of responses both between stimuli and from session to session. With progress, patients will move into the third phase, demonstrating appropriate responses with occasional accurate responses, such as pointing to a calendar when asked to show the date, saying "yes" instead of "no," and shrugging the shoulders when asked how they are feeling. Other appropriate responses consist of performing one command for another or production of jargon in response to a question or request for information. Marshall suggests that, for some patients, appropriate responses may represent their best performance and, therefore, should be encouraged by clinicians and others in the patient's environment. Finally, in the fourth phase, clinicians seek accurate responses to such tasks as object and picture identification, following commands, and responding to yes/no and "wh-" questions. Nonverbal responses may be facilitated with accompanying props, including pages with words and numbers written on them; a clock with movable hands; a calendar; a road atlas; lists of families, relatives, and friends; and a communication notebook.

Collins (1986, 1997) has designed a program to treat auditory comprehension using playing cards. This approach is based on the observation that patients with global aphasia often can recognize names that contain two salient features (e.g., "queen of hearts"), differentiate cards by suit, and place cards in a sequence when they are unable to perform similarly with other stimuli. Although not all patients achieve the highest levels of performance, Collins suggests that portions of the program are useful at some stage for most patients.

Verbal Expression

Despite conclusions that traditional treatment focused on verbal communication skills may be ineffective for global aphasia (Salvatore & Thompson, 1986; Sarno & Levita, 1981), short-term attempts to establish or expand verbal expression in patients with global aphasia may be a legitimate therapeutic activity during both the acute and chronic phases of recovery (Rosenbek et al., 1989). Rosenbek and colleagues (1989) do this by first attempting to associate meaning with speech movements. To do this, patients use available methods (e.g., showing fingers, pointing, gesturing, writing, matching, and selecting objects) to confirm the meaning of any successfully elicited verbalizations. Included among these may be serial productions, imitated words and phrases, or automatic, meaningful responses to conversations relating to a variety of topics. As described previously, conversational topics that are personally relevant will improve performance (Van Lancker & Klein, 1990; Van Lancker & Nicklay, 1992; Wallace & Canter, 1985). Patients who succeed in these tasks are taught to produce at least a small repertoire of useful spoken or spoken plus gestured responses. They suggest that these items include at least one greeting, the words "yes" and "no," a few proper names, single words that express important needs, and perhaps, one or more phrases, especially if they appear in the patient's spontaneous verbal productions. Imitation, either alone or supplemented by gestures and reading, is used to establish these responses (for a detailed approach to establishing an unequivocal yes/no response, see Collins, 1986, 1997). Imitated responses are then practiced in more functional contexts using questions or practical situations to facilitate response generalization.

Conversational prompting, a method reported by Cochran and Milton (1984), uses modeling, expansion, and feedback to develop the verbal responses of patients with severe aphasia in conversational contexts. Props and written cues are provided to facilitate verbal expression. Ten conversational levels are identified, ranging from concrete, structured contexts (e.g., manipulating objects or acting out and describing sequences) to more open contexts (e.g., structured interview or structured discussion). A cueing hierarchy is described to promote language retrieval. With its emphasis on conversational interaction, this technique may be particularly useful in developing contextually appropriate

communication for patients with global aphasia. It also may provide a suitable means for overcoming some of the problems traditionally associated with the generalization of trained responses to conversational contexts.

The verbal output of many patients with global aphasia consists primarily of stereotypic recurring utterances or speech automatisms. For many of these patients, productive usage of single words or phrases may not be a realistic goal. The treatment program Voluntary Control of Involuntary Utterances (Helm & Barresi, 1980; Helm-Estabrooks & Albert, 2004), or VCIU, can be used with these patients to bring these stereotypies into more productive usage. In this program, words that are involuntarily and inappropriately produced in the contexts of testing and treatment are identified and used as later targets in treatment. The words are trained in a sequence of activities, including oral reading, confrontation naming, and finally, conversational usage, until a vocabulary of between 200 and 300 words is established.

Two studies have investigated treatments for improving naming ability in patients with global aphasia. To test theories regarding the psycholinguistic representation of homophones as well as the effectiveness and generalization of phonologic treatment, Biedermann and colleagues (2002) treated naming to confrontation using phonologic cues in a 59-year-old man with global aphasia 13 years poststroke. The cuing hierarchy consisted of (a) an initial cue (consonant + schwa or vowel), (b) tapping the syllable number of the word, and (c) repetition. The design included four conditions: homophones, semantically related words, phonologically related words, and unrelated words. Item-specific, short-term improvements were observed for treated items; no generalization to untreated items, except for homophones, occurred. These results were consistent with previous studies of aphasia that have found poor generalization to untreated items following phonologic treatment.

Naeser and colleagues (2005) used transcranial magnetic stimulation (TMS) to treat the naming abilities of a 51-year-old woman with severe nonfluent/global aphasia who was 6.5 poststroke. TMS is a noninvasive procedure that uses magnetic fields to generate electrical currents over discrete brain regions. These lead to neuronal depolarization that can excite or inhibit the cortex. Functional imaging studies have suggested an anomalous right frontal response in patients with left frontal damage that is thought to interfere with language recovery. Naeser and colleagues therefore applied repetitive TMS (rTMS) to reduce the cortical excitability of right pars triangularis in this patient and effect improvements in language functioning. She received ten 20-minute, 1-Hz rTMS treatments 5 days a week for 2 weeks. Language testing at 2 and 8 months post-treatment demonstrated modest improvements in naming on the Boston Naming Test and the BDAE. Improvements at 1 year post-treatment were considered to be substantial enough to warrant referral for further speech-language treatment. This patient continued to improve, especially in auditory comprehension and in the voluntary use of words and phrases appropriate to her environment.

Functional (Patient-Oriented) Approaches

Gestural Programs

American-Indian Code

Gestural programs constitute a sizeable portion of the functional treatment approaches for global aphasia. Probably the best known of the gestural programs is American-Indian (Amer-Ind) Code (Rao, 2001; Skelly, 1979). Amer-Ind Code is adapted from Amer-Ind sign, a gestural system based on the concepts underlying words rather than on the word themselves (Skelly, Schinsky, Smith, Donaldson & Griffin, 1975). According to Rao and Horner (1980), Amer-Ind Code is concrete, pictographic, highly transmissible, easily learned, agrammatical, and generative. The system can be applied in aphasia rehabilitation as an alternative means of communication, as a facilitator of verbalization, and as a deblocker of other language modalities (Rao, 2001). A few reports have demonstrated the usefulness of Amer-Ind Code as an alternative means of communication (Rao 1995; Rao et al., 1980; Tonkovich & Loverso, 1982). The approach also might be combined with other nonverbal means of communication (e.g., drawing) (see below) to increase a severely affected patient's communicative effectiveness (Rao, 1995). The greatest utility of the technique, however, appears to be as a facilitator of verbalization, though reports of its effectiveness vary (Hanlon et al., 1990; Hoodin & Thompson, 1983; Kearns, Simmons, & Sisterhen, 1982; Rao & Horner, 1978; Raymer & Thompson, 1991; Skelly, Schinsky, Smith, Donaldson, & Griffin, 1974). Rosenbek and colleagues (1989) describe a treatment program for gestural reorganization that uses Amer-Ind Code as the primary system of gestures and has, as its end goal, verbalization without gestural accompaniment.

Visual Action Therapy

Visual Action Therapy (Helm-Estabrooks & Albert, 2004; Helm-Estabrooks et al., 1982; Helm-Estabrooks, Ramsberger, Brownell, & Albert, 1989; Ramsberger & Helm-Estabrooks, 1989), or VAT, uses gestures to reduce apraxia and improve the patient's verbal expression or ability to use symbolic gestures as a means of communication. Three programs constitute the approach: proximal limb, distal limb, and buccofacial VAT. A hierarchical procedure is used in each program to "move the patient along a performance continuum from the basic task of matching pictures and objects to the communicative task of representing hidden items with self-initiated gestures" (Helm-Estabrooks & Albert, 2004, p. 255). The authors suggest that the method produces improvements not only in the area of pantomime, as indicated by formal assessments, but also in the areas of auditory and reading comprehension, verbal repetition, and graphic copying.

Conlon and McNeil (1991) proposed that the efficacy of VAT has not been established because of experimental limitations in the original work of Helm-Estabrooks and colleagues (1982). Therefore, they investigated the effects of VAT on the communication abilities of two patients with global aphasia. Using a modified program for experimental purposes, positive treatment effects were observed on most steps of the program for their first subject and on about half the steps for their second subject. These results generally were consistent with those of Helm-Estabrooks and colleagues (1982), but generalization of these effects to untreated items was not observed. This lack of generalization suggested that the learned behaviors did not influence performance on untreated but similar behaviors. Conlon and McNeil (1991) determined that VAT is not effective in achieving the program's stated purpose of establishing "symbolic representation" as defined by Helm-Estabrooks and colleagues (1982). Conlon and McNeil concluded that further research is needed before VAT can be confidently recommended for the treatment of patients with global aphasia.

Some other gestural programs include pantomime; limited manual sign systems for hospitals and nursing homes, such as manual shorthand, manual self-care signals, or a hand-talking chart; gestures for "yes" and "no"; eye-blink encoding; and pointing (Silverman, 1989). Silverman (1989) offers a number of suggestions for the selective use of each of these approaches. For example, pantomime may be appropriate for the patient with aphasia who cannot use Amer-Ind Code. Limited manual sign systems may be used initially, on an interim basis, until other communication systems can be developed, but ultimately, these limited systems may provide the only means of communication in the most severely impaired patients (see, e.g., Coelho, 1990, 1991). Pointing is desirable for the patient who is going to use a communication board.

Non-Speech Communication Aids

Non-speech aids include those that assist communication by both non-electronic and electronic means. Strategies using non-electronic assistance include transmission of messages by communication boards, manipulation of symbol sequences, and drawing. One of the most prominent strategies in the rehabilitation of patients with global aphasia using electronic means is computer-aided visual communication (C-ViC) (Weinrich, Steele, Carlson, et al., 1989).

Preparatory Training

Alexander and Loverso (1993) developed a specific program for the treatment of global aphasia that supports the capacity to make categorical and associational semantic discriminations while being sufficiently easy to allow an understanding of the nature and purpose of the tasks. Those authors contend that therapy of this sort establishes a necessary precondition for subsequent treatment with communication programs using iconic/substitutional language (e.g., communication boards or C-ViC). Twenty-four common everyday objects, realistic pictures of those objects, and realistic pictures of the locations in which those objects would be found were used as treatment stimuli. The stimuli were described as being representationally similar to those adopted for communication boards or C-ViC. Eight hierarchically-arranged treatment levels were identified, beginning with object-to-object matching in a field of one and increasing to picture sorting into locatively related groups. Two of five patients with global aphasia who were studied reached the proposed goal of treatment—namely, demonstration of semantic capacity across categorical and associational boundaries. The remaining patients with global aphasia were unable to recognize the nature of the response required at more complex levels. The authors concluded that, even if only 40% of the cases respond successfully to the program, these patients constitute the appropriate group for substituted language systems.

Salvatore and Nelson (1995) described a training model for establishing equivalence relationships among visual stimuli that may have potential for use with gestural-assisted programs like those described below. In their study, four subjects with severe aphasia learned novel symbolic relationships and generalized these to untrained relationships. The authors suggested that demonstrations of such generalization may be used as an indicator of the patient's ability to benefit from further treatment efforts.

Communication Boards

Communication boards vary in type and complexity. For severely impaired patients, a typical board will contain personally relevant words and pictures, numbers, and the alphabet. Specific treatment is required for effective use of the board. Collins (1986, 1997) suggests a training procedure in which target items are identified in isolation, then after an imposed delay, and finally, from among increasing numbers of foils until a temporary ceiling is obtained for the number of items contained on one board. Alternative boards containing pictures within only one domain (e.g., family or familiar objects) may be used to increase the number of items available to the patient.

Bellaire, Georges, and Thompson (1991) investigated the acquisition, generalization, and maintenance effects of picture communication board training. Although their two subjects did not have global aphasia, their findings have potential application to the treatment of this population.

Treatment and acquisition probes were administered in a traditional treatment room, whereas generalization probes

and training occurred during a coffee hour in a nursing home care unit. Pictures were divided into three sets for communicating social responses, requests for food and other items, and personal information. Stimulus presentations were followed by a 5-second response interval. If an accurate response was not observed, cues consisting of a verbal cue, a model, and a physical assist were provided. Subjects received response-contingent verbal feedback. Generalization training was conducted using a role-playing procedure in the treatment room with a script employed during the coffee-hour probes or within the coffee-hour setting. Maintenance data were collected for up to 6 months.

Following treatment, requesting and personal information responses were acquired, but not social responses. No response generalization to untrained responses was observed, nor was generalization of board use seen during the coffee hour. Of the two procedures for training generalization, only training within the actual coffee-hour setting resulted in generalized use of all responses except for social responses. Based on these results, the authors recommended that (a) communication boards include primarily pictures that communicate specific content items and (b) treatment for the use of picture communication boards take place in the natural environments where the board is to be used.

Ho, Weiss, Garrett, and Lloyd (2005) speculated that the failure of symbol use to generalize to functional communication following global aphasia might be a result of (a) the difficulty individuals with global aphasia have extracting meaning from symbols referring to abstract concepts, (b) a correlation between the severity of the language impairment and the ability to use symbols, and (c) the absence of the cognitive ability to initiate symbol use without the support of conversational partners. To overcome these challenges, they suggested using remnants (actual objects or photographs depicting recent or past events) that have personalized value in conversational interactions with persons who have global aphasia. In a study using a combination ABA and alternating treatment single-subject design with two patients who had global aphasia, the authors demonstrated that the participants initiated more topics and had fewer unrepaired communication breakdowns during conversation when either remnants or pictographs were used versus when no symbols were available. Participants demonstrated more pointing behavior, however, with remnants than with pictographic symbols. The subjective evaluations of the communication partners also favored the remnants over the pictographs. The authors concluded that their results support the use of communication books with individuals who have aphasia.

Blissymbols

Johannsen-Horbach, Cegla, Mager, Schempp, and Wallesch (1985) assessed the benefits of treating four patients with global aphasia using Blissymbols, a visual symbol system of pictograms and ideograms. All patients had previously received at least 6 months of traditional therapy for aphasia without significant improvement in expressive language. For the procedures using Blissymbols, patients received individual treatment twice per week for a period of at least 2 months. The program was designed (a) to provide a basic lexicon of nouns, verbs, adverbs, and function words; (b) teach the production and comprehension of simple sentence in the symbol language; and (c) acquaint relatives with the symbol system to use in communicating with the patients. Symbols were introduced verbally along with simultaneous presentation of pictures or objects or the pantomime of the therapist. Training consisted of associating symbols and pictures for nouns, verbs, and function words in multiple-choice arrays and, subsequently, incorporating these items into Blissymbol sentences.

All patients acquired a symbol lexicon; three patients produced Blissyntactically correct sentences in response to pictures. Two of the patients successfully used the symbols in their communication with their relatives. In an important related finding, three patients evidenced the ability to articulate the correct words while pointing to the corresponding symbols, and one patient articulated grammatical sentences. Variable outcomes with regard to continued use of the symbols by these four patients were reported.

The success of some patients with severe aphasia in communicating using novel visual symbol systems has been interpreted as evidence for the superiority of such systems relative to the surface forms of natural language. To test this assumption, Funnell and Allport (1989) investigated the ability of two patients with severe aphasia (neither of whom appeared to have global aphasia) to use Blissymbols to communicate in conversational situations. By performing detailed analyses of the patients' abilities to process isolated words during listening, speaking, reading, and writing, the authors were able to compare the patients' use of Blissymbols to their processing of similar forms in natural language. Funnell and Allport found that the performance of the patients with aphasia using Blissymbols was entirely consistent with their processing of spoken and written words, and that the use of Blissymbols did not provide a channel for communication that was independent of natural language processes. Further inquiry will be necessary to determine whether these findings can be applied to patients with global aphasia who have more severely impaired natural language abilities than those of the subjects participating in the study by Funnell and Allport.

Drawing

Drawing has received considerable attention both as a communicative medium and as a means to deblock verbal and written communication. Morgan and Helm-Estabrooks (1987; see also Helm-Estabrooks & Albert, 2004) designed a program entitled Back to the Drawing Board (BDB) to teach patients to communicate messages through sequential drawings. Patients are trained to draw cartoons from memory using verbal instruction, demonstration, and practice through copying. The cartoons range from one to three panels. Criterion performance consists of reproducing a recognizable drawing that contains the critical details relevant to the humorous aspects of the cartoon. Treatment outcome is evaluated by increased accuracy in the patients' drawings of nine "accidents of living." Morgan and Helm-Estabrooks (1987) provide an operational definition of accuracy to facilitate comparison and interpretation of the drawings. Their post-treatment results for two patients indicated an improved ability to convey information through the use of drawing alone.

Lyon and Sims (1989) undertook a study to determine the degree to which patients with severe aphasia can communicate through drawing and to evaluate the effectiveness of a treatment program emphasizing drawing-aided communication. Eight patients with aphasia and eight comparable, normal adults participated in the study. The eight subjects with aphasia were enrolled in a treatment program focused on refining primary drawing skills (form, visual organization, detail, and perspective) within defined communicative contexts. Verbal and graphic cueing and requests for enlargement of distorted parts were used to improve the recognizability of the drawings. The drawings were then placed in a communicative interaction between the patient and a trained interactant who used specific strategies to optimize communicative effectiveness.

Communicative effectiveness was assessed using a 40-item drawing outcome measure to evaluate pre- and post-treatment performance both with and without the use of drawings. A scale of communicative effectiveness was designed to rate performance on the outcome measure, and a second scale was designed to rate the recognition of drawings. Pre- and post-treatment performance on the PICA also was used to measure communicative effectiveness.

Following drawing treatment, substantial gains were observed in the communicative effectiveness of subjects with aphasia compared to their pretreatment levels. Performance further improved following treatment to 88% of the communicative effectiveness score attained by the normal adults. The subjects with aphasia also improved in the recognizability of their drawings following treatment, achieving 65% of the normal adults' scaled value. Based on these data, the authors concluded that drawing serves as an important facilitator of communication by providing to patients with aphasia a fixed representation of a concept that is readily available for subsequent modification.

Kearns and Yedor (1992) have pointed out that specific programming may be needed in some cases to establish spontaneous use of drawing for communicative purposes. Ward-Lonergan and Nicholas (1995) described such a program for their patient with global aphasia. The program began with BDB (Morgan & Helm-Estabrooks, 1987), progressed to the less structured conversational framework employed in Promoting Aphasics' Conversational Effectiveness (Davis & Wilcox, 1981) (see below), and concluded with an unstructured, interactive approach they identified as Functional Drawing Training. The patient made substantial progress during the course of the program, and although spontaneous initiation of communicative drawing was still lacking at the end of the treatment, the patient was able to communicate effectively through drawing when given limited encouragement.

Computer-Aided Visual Communication

Computer-aided visual communication (Steele, Kleczewska, Carlson, & Weinrich, 1992; Steele, Weinrich, Kleczewska, Carlson, & Wertz, 1987; Steele, Weinrich, Wertz, Kleczewska, & Carlson, 1989; Weinrich, Steele, Kleczewska, et al., 1989) provides another approach to establishing alternative communication in severely impaired patients. Using procedures similar to those of visual communication (Gardner, Zurif, Berry, & Baker, 1976) but in a microcomputer environment, C-ViC is an iconographic system in which patients construct communications by selecting symbols from six "card decks" and arranging them according to certain syntactic conventions. The card decks contain interjections, animate nouns, verbs, prepositions, modifiers, and common nouns. The program has been used successfully to train comprehension of a variety of lexical categories (e.g., verbs and prepositions), although generalization to oral production of these items has been limited (Weinrich, Steele, Kleczewska et al., 1989, Weinrich et al., 1993). Formal procedures have been developed that extend training from introductory phases which teach the patient to follow simple commands to later phases designed to transfer C-ViC communication skills to use in a home setting (Baker & Nicholas, 1992). One patient with global aphasia was able to accurately select the lexical items for a message as well as apply simple syntactic rules to produce basic constructions (subject-verb, irreversible and reversible subject-verb-object) (McCall et al., 2000). This patient demonstrated great difficulty in multi-sentence production, however, and positive gains that were observed over the protracted period required for this training did not generalize to standardized assessment measures.

Naeser and colleagues (1998) investigated the lesion site patterns for 17 patients with severe aphasia who had undergone C-ViC training to determine whether these patterns were predictive of communication outcomes following C-ViC treatment. Although some of their patients did not have global aphasia, all of the patients did present with little or no spontaneous speech and impaired auditory comprehension. Before treatment, all patients were tested with the BASA (Helm-Estabrooks, Ramsberger, Morgan, & Nicholas, 1989) and underwent non–contrast enhanced CT at 3 months or later poststroke. The C-ViC training was initiated no earlier than 3 months after aphasia onset and was continued twice weekly for 6 months to 1 year. Outcomes were based on a rating scale that was developed to assess the quality of C-ViC–generated sentences.

The findings from this study suggested that the lesion site pattern associated with the best response (i.e., initiates communication) using C-ViC spares large portions of either posterior systems that include Wernicke's area and the temporal isthmus or anterior systems that include the supplementary motor area and the cingulate gyrus. Moderate responses (i.e., responds to questions but does not initiate interactions) were found following lesions that spared posterior systems but involved anterior systems. Patients who demonstrated no response to the program had bilateral lesions that included variable lesions in either left posterior or posterior and anterior systems. The authors also found, however, that prediction of outcome was optimized when these lesion site patterns were combined with behavioral results obtained from pre-treatment testing with the BASA (Naeser et al., 1998).

Similar to that reported with gestural strategies, verbal facilitation has been noted (personal observation) during C-ViC training that produces successful naming that is not seen in these same patients in other communicative contexts (e.g., conversation or formal testing). The ultimate goal of C-ViC is not verbalization without computer assistance (as might be the case with some of the foregoing gestural strategies), but these observations suggest that C-ViC is a powerful verbal reorganizer that may enhance the language production of patients using this tool.

Lingraphica

The Lingraphica is a speech-generating device combining images, animation, text, and spoken words to provide computer-based communication. It contains a large number of words represented by icons and can be customized with a user's special words and pictures. The user selects icons to express a thought or need, which the device then turns into audible words or sentences. The Lingraphica also is loaded with a wide range of practice materials that can be used in the clinic under the direction of a speech-language pathologist or independently at home.

Three studies have demonstrated positive effects for chronic patients with a wide range of types and severities of aphasia following treatment using the Lingraphica System. Aftonomos, Steele, and Wertz (1997) studied the responses to computer-based treatment of 23 patients with aphasia who were 6 months to more than 15 years post-onset and who had been discharged from previous courses of speech-language treatment. All patients received 1-hour treatment sessions with a speech-language pathologist using the Lingraphica System and, with the exception of one patient, used the system at home for practice between clinical treatment sessions. Comparison of pre- and post-treatment scores on a variety of formal language instruments demonstrated significantly improved performance in multiple modalities.

Aftonomos, Appelbaum, and Steele (1999) extended the previous work by assessing the outcomes of computer-based treatment on functional communication as well as formal language tests. Sixty subjects, consisting of 14 patients less than 6 months post-onset and 46 patients more than 6 months post-onset, were administered the WAB and CETI before the initiation of treatment. Treatment consisted of 1-hour sessions using the Lingraphica clinical exercises but with a focus on improving the patients' functional communication outside the clinic. The number of treatment sessions ranged from 10 to 132. Post-treatment group results demonstrated significant improvements for all subtests of the WAB and for the CETI. The acute and chronic aphasic groups each made significant improvements on both of the test measures, and all of the patients grouped by aphasia category, except for patients with Wernicke's and transcortical motor aphasia, made significant improvements. Eleven patients with global aphasia included in this group had a mean AQ improvement of 6.2 points.

Finally, Aftonomous, Steele, Applebaum, and Harris (2001) reported outcome data for both the impairment and functional levels following treatment with the Lingraphica System. Fifty patients, including six with global aphasia, completed at least 1 month of treatment, after which pre- and post-treatment scores on all items of the WAB and CETI were compared. Participants were found to have improved significantly on all language subtests of the WAB, on the WAB AQ, and for all items of the CETI following treatment. Patients with global aphasia made the second least gains (behind patients with anomic aphasia) at the impairment level and the third least gains in functional communication. When analyzed by patient severity, those with the most and least severe aphasias made the smallest, although still statistically significant, gains at the impairment level, whereas those with the most severe aphasias made the greatest gains in functional communication. The authors attributed the latter outcome to commonly observed "ceiling effects" in less impaired patients following treatment.

Gus Multimedia Speech System

Gus is a computer-based graphic symbol communication system that offers graphic and orthographic symbols along with synthetic speech output (Koul et al., 2005). The program presents symbols in a dynamic display format that allow the symbols to be presented across screens logically (e.g., superordinate categories in a first screen that explode into subordinate categories in a second screen, followed by specific items in that category in a third screen). The patient's cognitive, linguistic, motor, and visuoperceptual skills determine the number of symbols that are displayed in each screen, and each symbol can be programmed to produce a spoken message.

Koul and colleagues (2005) investigated the effect of Gus intervention on the production and generalization of graphic symbol sentences of varying grammatical complexity in 10 patients with severe aphasia, 2 of whom had global aphasia. The motivation for the study was to evaluate the extent to which patients with severe aphasia can use electronic communication aids to support or replace spoken language. The first patient with global aphasia was unable to produce even the most syntactically simple sentences (two word agent + action or action + object constructions). The second patient was able to achieve criterion for two out of six Level I constructions and one Level II construction (morphologic inflections [e.g., boy reading]); he did not achieve the criteria for any of the more complex constructions. No generalization was observed for any of the sentences that were probed. That even one of the two patients with global aphasia was able to use the computer-based system to produce sentences of varying syntactic complexity was viewed by the authors as evidence for the effectiveness of this approach following global aphasia when compared to the patients' natural language.

Promoting Aphasics' Communicative Effectiveness

The last functional approach to be considered here is Promoting Aphasics' Communicative Effectiveness, or PACE, treatment (Davis, 1980, 1986, 2005; Davis & Wilcox, 1981, 1985; Wilcox & Davis, 1978). Despite having attributes such as direct language stimulation and real-life conversation (Davis, 2005), its inclusion here (as in previous versions of this chapter) is based on the limited language of persons with global aphasia and the potential for using this procedure as a means to promote nonverbal, functional options for communication.

Because PACE procedures allow patients to freely choose the channels through which they will communicate, the technique provides opportunities for patients to use either a verbal strategy or any of the nonverbal strategies described above, with or without verbal accompaniment, to convey messages. In this way, the approach emulates natural conversation by allowing participants to exchange information through multiple modalities.

In addition to free selection, some of the other characteristics of natural conversation that provide guiding principles for PACE treatment include the following: (a) Clinician and patient participate equally as senders and receivers of messages, (b) the interaction incorporates the exchange of new information between clinician and patient, and (c) the clinician's feedback is based on the patient's success in communicating a message (Davis & Wilcox, 1985). PACE treatment also uses a multidimensional scoring system to better capture the full range of behaviors that may be observed in this interactive approach. Generalization of language gains observed following PACE treatment has been demonstrated on formal language assessment instruments. Given its emphasis on the pragmatic aspects of language, PACE is well suited as a means to incorporate compensatory strategies into communication treatment. An additional strength of the approach, however, lies in its use as a framework for incorporating traditional language stimulation techniques into a communicatively dynamic context.

Social (Partner-Oriented) Approaches

Social approaches (covered in greater detail elsewhere in this volume) target communication partners or other ways to reduce communication barriers in addition to improving language or compensatory functional language (LPAA Project Group, 2001; Simmons-Mackie, 2001). As such, they may be particularly appropriate for individuals with global aphasia, given their poor prognosis for language recovery. One particularly good example of this approach is Supported Conversation for Adults with Aphasia (Kagan, 1998; Kagan et al., 2001), or SCA. Others have included conversational coaching (Hopper, Holland & Rowega, 2002), reciprocal scaffolding (Avent & Austermann, 2003), partner training (Simmons-Mackie, 2004), and the use of autobiographical reports (Pound, Parr, & Duchan, 2001).

The SCA program teaches techniques to conversation partners that will help them better reveal the competence of people with aphasia (Kagan, 1998). It builds on the assumption that many adults with aphasia can capitalize on preserved cognitive and social abilities to participate in conversation. The SCA program involves training conversation partners to acknowledge the competence of individuals with aphasia and help them reveal what they think, know, and feel.

Kagan and colleagues (2001) investigated the efficacy of SCA in a single-blind, randomized, controlled, pre-post design study. Forty dyads consisting of a volunteer conversation partner and an adult with moderate to severe aphasia were divided evenly between a control and an experimental group. Fifteen percent of the participants with aphasia were diagnosed with global aphasia. The groups participated in videotaped semistructured interviews with or without SCA training. The SCA training focused on acknowledging and revealing the competence of adults with aphasia through supported conversation. For example, the topics for acknowledging competence included keeping talk as natural as possible, avoiding patronization, and explicitly indicating that competence of the person with aphasia is not in question; those for revealing competence included ensuring the person with aphasia understands what is being communicated and is given the opportunity to express what he or she knows, thinks, or feels and verifying that the conversation is on track from perspective of person with aphasia. The techniques

included gesture, writing key words, and drawing accompanied by pictographic resources. Two rating scales were developed to measure the amount of support provided by the conversation partner and the level of participation by the adult with aphasia. Trained volunteers scored significantly higher than untrained volunteers on ratings of acknowledging and revealing competence in their partners with aphasia. The adults with aphasia in the experimental group also performed significantly higher than their counterparts in the control group on measures of social and message exchange skills, even though they had not participated in the training. These results were interpreted as support for the efficacy of this particular approach to aphasia rehabilitation.

FUTURE TRENDS

Clearly, future clinical research must better identify the conditions under which treatment for global aphasia is maximally effective. To do so, several issues must receive further exploration. One of these concerns outcome from global aphasia and includes (a) identifying the factors that differentially account for evolution in some patients with global aphasia to less severe aphasic syndromes, (b) establishing or refining prognostic indicators or profiles that can reliably predict outcome in global aphasia, and (c) specifying the relationships between site and extent of lesion for outcome in global aphasia. A second issue concerns how this outcome information can be better applied to management decisions for patients with global aphasia. Naeser (1994) provides one example of the use of outcome information obtained during the acute phase of recovery for these purposes. This approach must be further developed to improve specificity and accuracy. Third, clinicians must continue to identify specific assessment and treatment approaches that are sensitive to the capabilities of patients with global aphasia and produce reasonable outcomes in functional communication relative to the time and effort expended during the rehabilitation process. Finally, greater emphasis will be placed on improving not just communication, but the overall quality of life of the patient with global aphasia. Rehabilitation programs will incorporate increasingly sensitive measures to evaluate the psychosocial outcomes of treatment. Common practice will extend the continuum of care for these patients to support groups and other community organizations following the completion of formal speech and language treatment.

KEY POINTS

1. Global aphasia may be one of the most frequently occurring types of aphasia; age and sex do not appear to have a differential effect on the incidence of global aphasia.

2. Global aphasia may result from extensive cortical lesions of the dominant hemisphere, lesions confined to either the anterior or posterior cortex, or lesions restricted to subcortical regions. Patients with global aphasia and large pre- and postrolandic middle cerebral artery infarcts generally have a poor recovery, but some individual patients with this lesion pattern may demonstrate outstanding outcomes.

3. Patients with global aphasia have several isolated areas of relatively preserved comprehension, including specific word categories, familiar environmental sounds, famous personal names, and personally relevant information. The verbal output of these patients consists primarily of stereotypic recurring utterances or speech automatisms.

4. Nonverbal cognitive impairment is correlated with the degree of language impairment in global aphasia.

5. Patients with global aphasia rely most heavily on nonverbal communication that may be nearly as effective as the communication strategies employed by patients with other types of aphasia.

6. Global aphasia most often results from middle cerebral artery occlusion below the point of branching, but cases have occurred from illnesses such as epilepsy and demyelinating disease.

7. Patients with global aphasia who are receiving treatment demonstrate substantial improvements during the first 3 to 6 months post-onset as well as continued improvement during the period between 6 and 12 months or more post-onset. Different patterns of recovery for language and non-language skills may be found during these periods.

8. Evolution from global aphasia is not simply the result of the time at which language is observed initially but, rather, is the result of a complex interaction of incompletely understood factors.

9. Younger patients with global aphasia and those without accompanying hemiparesis tend to have better prognoses for language recovery.

10. Greater right hemisphere asymmetries are associated with superior recovery of single-word language functions. Temporal lobe lesions that are limited to the subcortical temporal isthmus and spare Wernicke's area are associated with significantly better recovery of auditory comprehension following global aphasia.

11. Higher language test scores with greater variability among auditory comprehension and other language scores are consistent with a better prognosis. Patients with global aphasia who respond to yes/no questions, regardless of accuracy, may have a better outcome than those who cannot grasp the yes/no question format.

12. In the absence of accurate techniques for predicting recovery from global aphasia, the most powerful reasons for providing early treatment are the latent recovery observed in patients who receive acute speech and language treatment and the greater effects that are observed for patients with aphasia in general when treated during the acute period of recovery.

13. Early intervention in global aphasia has the multiple purposes of language stimulation directed toward cerebral reorganization and recovery, identification of successful communication strategies, and patient, family, and staff counseling.

14. Contemporary approaches to assessment include both formal and informal measures to establish a communication profile that documents not only the patient's areas of weakness but also the patient's strengths.

15. Treatment for global aphasia exploits the residual language capacity and/or other functional abilities of these patients to improve communication and the patient's quality of life.

References

Aftonomos, L. B., Appelbaum, J. S., & Steele, R. D. (1999). Improving outcomes for persons with aphasia in advanced community-based treatment programs. *Stroke, 30*, 1370–1379.

Aftonomous, L. B., Steele, R. D., Applebaum, J. S., & Harris, V. M. (2001). Relationships between impairment-level assessments and functional-level assessments in aphasia: Findings from LCC treatment programmes. *Aphasiology, 15*(10/11), 951–964.

Aftonomos, L. B., Steele, R. D., & Wertz, R. T. (1997). Promoting recovery in chronic aphasia with an interactive technology. *Archives of Physical Medicine & Rehabilitation, 78*, 841–846.

Alajouanine, M.S. (1956). Verbal realization in aphasia. *Brain, 79*, 1–28.

Alexander, M. P. (2000). Aphasia I: Clinical and anatomic issues. In M. J. Farah & T. E. Feinberg (Eds.), *Patient-based approaches to cognitive neuroscience* (pp. 165–181). Cambridge, MA: The MIT Press.

Alexander, M. P., & Loverso, F. L. (1993). A specific treatment for global aphasia. *Clinical Aphasiology, 21*, 277–289.

Alexander, M. P, Naeser, M. A., & Palumbo, C. L. (1987). Correlations of subcortical CT lesion sites and aphasia profiles. *Brain, 110*, 961–991.

Anonymous (1996). Weekly clinicopathological exercises: Case 8–1996: A 28 year old woman with the rapid development of a major personality change and global aphasia [Case records of the Massachusetts General Hospital]. *New England Journal of Medicine, 334*, 715–720.

Arrigoni, G., & De Renzi, E. (1964). Constructional apraxia and hemispheric locus of lesion. *Cortex, 1*, 170–197.

Avent, J. R., & Austermann, S. (2003). Reciprocal scaffolding: A context for communication treatment in aphasia. *Aphasiology, 17*(4), 397–404.

Baines, K. A., Martin, A. W., & Heeringa, H. M. (1999). *Assessment of language-related functional activities*. Austin, TX: Pro-Ed.

Baker, E., & Nicholas, M. (1992). *C-ViC training manual*. Unpublished manuscript.

Bang, O. Y., Heo, K. G., Kwak, Y. T., Lee, P. H., Joo, I. S., & Huh, K. (2004). Global aphasia without hemiparesis: Lesion analysis and its mechanism in 11 Korean patients. *Journal of the Neurological Sciences, 217*, 101–106.

Basso, A., Capitani, E., Luzzati, C., & Spinnler, H. (1981). Intelligence and left hemisphere disease: The role of aphasia, apraxia and size of lesion. *Brain, 104*, 721–734.

Basso, A., Della Sala, S., & Farabola, M. (1987). Aphasia arising from purely deep lesions. *Cortex, 23*, 29–44.

Basso, A., De Renzi, E., Faglioni, P., Scotti, G., & Spinnler, H. (1973). Neuropsychological evidence for the existence of cerebral areas critical to the performance of intelligence tasks. *Brain, 96*, 715–728.

Basso, A., & Farabola, M. (1997). Comparison of improvement of aphasia in three patients with lesions in anterior, posterior, and antero-posterior language areas. *Neuropsychological Rehabilitation, 7*, 215–230.

Basso, A., Lecours, A. R., Moraschini, S., & Vanier, M. (1985). Anatomoclinical correlations of the aphasias as defined through computerized tomography: Exceptions. *Brain and Language, 26*, 201–229.

Bellaire, K. J., Georges, J. B., & Thompson, C. K. (1991). Establishing functional communication board use for nonverbal aphasic subjects. *Clinical Aphasiology, 19*, 219–227.

Bhatnagar, S. C., Jain, S. K., Bihari, M., Bansal, N. K., Pauranik, A., Jain, D. C., et al. (2002). Aphasia type and aging in Hindi-speaking stroke patients. *Brain and Language, 83*, 353–361.

Biedermann, B., Blanken, G., & Nickels, L. (2002). The representation of homophones: Evidence from remediation. *Aphasiology, 16*(10/11), 1115–1136.

Blanken, G., Wallesch, C. W., & Papagno, C. (1990). Dissociations of language functions in aphasics with speech automatisms (recurring utterances). *Cortex, 26*, 41–63.

Bogousslavsky, J. (1988). Global aphasia without other lateralizing signs. *Archives of Neurology, 45*, 143.

Brust, J. C., Shafer, S. Q., Richter, R. W., & Bruun, B. (1976). Aphasia in acute stroke. *Stroke, 7*, 167–174.

Cappa, S. F., & Vignolo, L. A. (1983). CT scan studies of aphasia. *Human Neurobiology, 2*, 129–134.

Cochran, R. M., & Milton, S. B. (1984). Conversational prompting: A sentence building technique for severe aphasia. *Journal of Neurological Communication Disorders, 1*, 4–23.

Coelho, C. A. (1990). Acquisition and generalization of simple manual sign grammars by aphasic subjects. *Journal of Communication Disorders, 23*, 383–400.

Coelho, C. A. (1991). Manual sign acquisition and use in two aphasic subjects. *Clinical Aphasiology, 19*, 209–218.

Collins, M. (1986). *Diagnosis and treatment of global aphasia*. San Diego: College-Hill.

Collins, M. J. (1997). Global aphasia. In L. L. LaPointe (Ed.), *Aphasia and related neurogenic language disorders* (2nd ed., pp. 133–150). New York: Thieme.

Colonna, A., & Faglioni, P. (1966). The performance of hemisphere-damaged patients on spatial intelligence tests. *Cortex, 2*, 293–307.

Conlon, C. P., & McNeil, M. R. (1991). The efficacy of treatment for two globally aphasic adults using Visual Action Therapy. *Clinical Aphasiology, 19*, 185–195.

Cunningham, R., Farrow, V., Davies, C., & Lincoln, N. (1995). Reliability of the assessment of communicative effectiveness in severe aphasia. *European Journal of Disorders of Communication, 30*, 1–16.

Damasio, A. (1991). Signs of aphasia. In M. T. Sarno (Ed.), *Acquired aphasia* (2nd ed., pp. 27–43). San Diego: Academic Press.

Davis, G. A. (1980). A critical look at PACE therapy. *Clinical Aphasiology, 10*, 248–257.

Davis, G. A. (1983). *A survey of adult aphasia*. Englewood Cliffs, NJ: Prentice-Hall.

Davis, G. A. (1986). Pragmatics and treatment. In R. Chapey (Ed.), *Language intervention strategies in adult aphasia* (2nd ed., pp. 251–265). Baltimore: Williams & Wilkins.

Davis, G. A. (2005). PACE revisited. *Aphasiology, 19*(1), 21–38.

Davis, G. A., & Wilcox, J. (1981). Incorporating parameters of natural conversation in aphasia. In R. Chapey (Ed.), *Language intervention strategies in adult aphasia* (pp. 169–194). Baltimore: Williams & Wilkins.

Davis, G. A., & Wilcox, M. J. (1985). *Adult aphasia rehabilitation: Applied pragmatics*. San Diego: College-Hill.

deBlesser, R., & Poeck, K. (1984). Aphasia with exclusively consonant-vowel recurring utterances: Tan-Tan revisited. In F. C. Rose (Ed.), *Advances in neurology: Progress in aphasiology* (Vol. 42, pp. 51–57). New York: Raven Press.

deBlesser, R., & Poeck, K. (1985). Analysis of prosody in the spontaneous speech of patients with CV-recurring utterances. *Cortex, 21*, 405–416.

Deleval, J., Leonard, A., Mavroudakis, N., & Rodesch, G. (1989). Global aphasia without hemiparesis following prerolandic infarction. *Neurology, 39*, 1532–1535.

De Renzi, E., Colombo, A., & Scarpa, M. (1991). The aphasic isolate: A clinical-CT scan study of a particularly severe subgroup of global aphasics. *Brain, 114*, 1719–1730.

De Renzi, E., Faglioni, P., & Ferrari, P. (1980). The influence of sex and age on the incidence and type of aphasia. *Cortex, 16*, 627–630.

De Renzi, E., & Vignolo, L. A. (1962). The Token Test: A sensitive test to detect receptive disturbances in aphasics. *Brain, 85*, 665–678.

Druks, J., & Masterson, J. (2001). *An object and action naming battery*. Philadelphia: Psychology Press.

Edelman, G. M. (1984). Assessment of understanding in global aphasia. In F. C. Rose (Ed.), *Advances in neurology: Progress in aphasiology* (Vol. 42, pp. 277–289). New York: Raven.

Eisenson, J. (1994). *Examining for aphasia* (3rd ed.). Austin, TX: Pro-Ed.

Eslinger, P. J., & Damasio, A. R. (1981). Age and type of aphasia in patients with stroke. *Journal of Neurology, Neurosurgery and Psychiatry, 44*, 377–381.

Ferro, J. M. (1983). Global aphasia without hemiparesis. *Neurology, 33*, 1106.

Ferro, J. M. (1992). The influence of infarct location on recovery from global aphasia. *Aphasiology, 6*, 415–430.

Forde, E., & Humphreys, G. W. (1995). Refractory semantics in global aphasia: On semantic organization and the access-storage distinction in neuropsychology. *Memory, 3*, 265–307.

Frattali, C., Holland, A. L., & Thompson, C. K. (1995). *Functional assessment of communication skills for adults.* Rockville, MD: American Speech-Language-Hearing Association.

Funnell, E., & Allport, A. (1989). Symbolically speaking: Communicating with Blissymbols in aphasia. *Aphasiology, 3,* 279–300.

Gainotti, G., D'Erme, P., Villa, G., & Caltagirone, C. (1986). Focal brain lesions and intelligence: A study with a new version of Raven's colored matrices. *Journal of Clinical and Experimental Neuropsychology, 8,* 37–50.

Gardner, H., Zurif, E. B., Berry, T., & Baker, E. (1976). Visual communication in aphasia. *Neuropsychologia, 14,* 275–292.

German, D. J. (1990). *Test of adolescent/adult word finding.* Austin, TX: Pro-Ed.

Gold, B. T., & Kertesz, A. (2000). Preserved visual lexicosemantics in global aphasia: A right-hemisphere contribution? *Brain and Language, 75,* 359–375.

Goodglass, H., Kaplan, E., (1983). *The assessment of aphasia and related disorders* (2nd ed.). Philadelphia: Lea & Febiger.

Habib, M., Ali-Cherif, A., Poncet, M., & Salamon, G. (1987). Age-related changes in aphasia type and stroke localization. *Brain and Language, 31,* 245–251.

Hanlon, R. E., Brown, J. W., & Gerstman, L. J. (1990). Enhancement of naming in nonfluent aphasia through gesture. *Brain and Language, 38,* 298–314.

Hanlon, R. E., Lux, W. E., & Dromerick, A. W. (1999). Global aphasia without hemiparesis: Language profiles and lesion distribution. *Journal of Neurology, Neurosurgery, and Psychiatry, 66,* 365–369.

Hartman, J. (1981). Measurement of early spontaneous recovery from aphasia with stroke. *Annals of Neurology, 9,* 89–91.

Heiss, W. D., Kessler, J., Karbe, H., Fink, G. R., Pawlik, G. (1993). Cerebral glucose metabolism as a predictor of recovery from aphasia in ischemic stroke. *Archives of Neurology, 50,* 958–964.

Helm, N. A., & Barresi, B. (1980). Voluntary control of involuntary utterances: A treatment approach for severe aphasia. *Clinical Aphasiology, 10,* 308–315.

Helm-Estabrooks, N. (1986). Severe aphasia. In J. M. Costello & A. L. Holland (Eds.), *Handbook of speech and language disorders* (pp. 917–934). San Diego: College-Hill.

Helm-Estabrooks, N. (1992). *Aphasia diagnostic profiles.* Austin, TX: Pro-Ed.

Helm-Estabrooks, N., & Albert, M. L. (2004). *Manual of aphasia and aphasia therapy* (2nd ed.). Austin, TX: Pro-Ed.

Helm-Estabrooks, N., Fitzpatrick, P. M., & Barresi, B. (1982). Visual action therapy for global aphasia. *Journal of Speech and Hearing Disorders, 47,* 385–389.

Helm-Estabrooks, N., Ramsberger, G., Brownell, H., & Albert, M. (1989). Distal versus proximal movement in limb apraxia. *Journal of Clinical and Experimental Neuropsychology, 7,* 608.

Helm-Estabrooks, N., Ramsberger, G., Morgan, A. R., & Nicholas, M. (1989). *Boston assessment of severe aphasia.* Chicago: Riverside Press.

Herbert, R., Best, W., Hickin, J., Howard, D., & Osborne, F. (2003). Combining lexical and interactional approaches to therapy for word finding deficits in aphasia. *Aphasiology, 17*(12), 1163–1186.

Herrmann, M., Koch, U., Johannsen-Horbach, H., & Wallesch, C. W. (1989). Communicative skills in chronic and severe nonfluent aphasia. *Brain and Language, 37,* 339–352.

Ho, K. M., Weiss, S. J., Garrett, K. L., & Lloyd, L. L. (2005). The effect of remnant and pictographic books on the communicative interaction of individuals with global aphasia. *Augmentative and Alternative Communication, 21*(3), 218–232.

Holland, A. L. (1982). Observing functional communication of aphasic adults. *Journal of Speech and Hearing Disorders, 47,* 50–56.

Holland, A. L., & Bartlett, C. L. (1985). Some differential effects of age on stroke-produced aphasia. In H. K. Ulatowska (Ed.), *The aging brain: Communication in the elderly* (pp. 141–155). San Diego: College-Hill.

Holland, A. L., Fratalli, C. M., & Fromm, D. (1998). *Communication activities of daily living* (2nd ed.). Austin, TX: Pro-Ed.

Holland, A. L., Greenhouse, J. B., Fromm, D., & Swindell, C. S. (1989). Predictors of language restitution following stroke: A multivariate analysis. *Journal of Speech and Hearing Research, 32,* 232–238.

Holland, A. L., Swindell, C. S., & Forbes, M. M. (1985). The evolution of initial global aphasia: Implications for prognosis. *Clinical Aphasiology, 15,* 169–175.

Hoodin, R. B., & Thompson, C. K. (1983). Facilitation of verbal labeling in adult aphasia by gestural, verbal or verbal plus gestural training. *Clinical Aphasiology, 13,* 62–64.

Hopper, T., Holland, A., & Rewega, M. (2002). Conversational coaching: Treatment outcomes and future directions. *Aphasiology, 16*(7), 745–761.

Johannsen-Horbach, H., Cegla, B., Mager, U., Schempp, B., & Wallesch, C. W. (1985). Treatment of global aphasia with a nonverbal communication system. *Brain and Language, 24,* 74–82.

Kagan, A. (1998). Supported conversation for adults with aphasia: Methods and resources for training conversation partners. *Aphasiology, 12*(9), 816–830.

Kagan, A., Black, S. E., Duchan, J. F., Simmons-Mackie, N., & Square, P. (2001). Training volunteers as conversation partners using "Supported Conversation for Adults with Aphasia" (SCA): A controlled trial. *Journal of Speech, Language, and Hearing Research, 44,* 624–638.

Kaplan, E., Goodglass, H., & Weintraub, S. (2001). *The Boston naming test* (2nd ed.). Philadelphia: Lippincott Williams & Wilkins.

Katz, J. M., Shetty, T., Gobin, P., & Segal, A. Z. (2003). Transient aphasia and reversible major depression due to a giant sagittal sinus dural AV fistula. *Neurology, 61,* 557–558.

Kay, J., Lesser, R., & Coltheart, M. (1992). *Psycholinguistic assessments of language processing in aphasia.* East Sussex, UK: Psychology Press.

Kearns, K., Simmons, N. N., & Sisterhen, C. (1982). Gestural sign (Amer-Ind) as a facilitator of verbalization in patients with aphasia. *Clinical Aphasiology, 12,* 183–191.

Kearns, K. P., & Yedor, K. (1992, June). *Artistic activation therapy: Drawing conclusions.* Paper presented at the Clinical Aphasiology Conference, Durango, CO.

Keenan, J. S., & Brassell, E. G. (1975). *Aphasia language performance scales.* Murphreesboro, TN: Pinnacle Press.

Kenin, M., & Swisher, L. P. (1972). A study of patterns of recovery in aphasia. *Cortex, 8,* 56–68.

Kertesz, A. (1979). *Aphasia and associated disorders: Taxonomy, localization, and recovery.* Orlando: Grune & Stratton.

Kertesz, A. (1982). *Western Aphasia Battery.* New York: Grune & Stratton.

Kertesz, A., & McCabe, P. (1975). Intelligence and aphasia: Performance of aphasics on Raven's Coloured Progressive Matrices (RCPM). *Brain and Language, 2,* 387–395.

Kertesz, A., & McCabe, P. (1977). Recovery patterns and prognosis in aphasia. *Brain, 100,* 1–18.

Kertesz, A., & Sheppard, A. (1981). The epidemiology of aphasia and cognitive impairment in stroke. *Brain, 104,* 117–128.

Keyserlingk, A. G., Naujokat, C., Niemann, K., Huber, W., & Thron, A. (1997). Global aphasia—With and without hemiparesis. *European Neurology, 38,* 259–267.

Koul, R., Corwin, M., & Hayes, S. (2005). Production of graphic symbol sentences by individuals with aphasia: Efficacy of a computer-based augmentative and alternative communication intervention. *Brain and Language, 92,* 58–77.

Kumar, R., Masih, A. K., & Pardo, J. (1996). Global aphasia due to thalamic hemorrhage: A case report and review of the literature. *Archives of Physical Medicine and Rehabilitation, 77,* 1312–1315.

LaPointe, L. L., Holtzapple, P., & Graham, L. F. (1985). The relationships among two measures of auditory comprehension and daily living communicative skills. *Clinical Aphasiology, 15,* 38–46.

LaPointe, L. L., & Horner, J. (1978, Spring). The Functional Auditory Comprehension Task (FACT): Protocol and test format. *FLASHA Journal,* pp. 27–33.

LaPointe, L. L., & Horner, J. (1998). *Reading comprehension battery for aphasia* (2nd ed.). Austin, TX: Pro-Ed.

Laska, A. C., Hellblom, A., Murray, V., Kahan, T., & Von Arbin, M. (2001). Aphasia in acute stroke and relation to outcome. *Journal of Internal Medicine, 249,* 413–422.

Legatt, A. D., Rubin, M. J., Kaplan, L. R., Healton, E. B., & Brust, J. C. M. (1987). Global aphasia without hemiparesis: Multiple etiologies. *Neurology, 37,* 201–205.

Lomas, J., & Kertesz, A. (1978). Patterns of spontaneous recovery in aphasic groups: A study of adult stroke patients. *Brain and Language, 6,* 388–401.

Lomas, J., Pickard, L., Bester, S., Elbard, H., Finlayson, A., & Zoghaib, C. (1989). The communicative effectiveness index: Development and psychometric evaluation of a functional communication measure for adult aphasia. *Journal of Speech and Hearing Disorders, 54,* 113–124.

LPAA Project Group (2001). Life participation approach to aphasia: A statement of values for the future. In R. Chapey (Ed.), *Language intervention strategies for aphasia and related neurogenic communication disorders* (4th ed., pp. 235–245). Philadelphia: Lippincott Williams & Wilkins.

Lüders, H., Lesser, R. P., Hahn, J., Dinner, D. S., Morris, H. H., Wyllie, E., et al. (1991). Basal temporal language area. *Brain, 114,* 743–754.

Lyon, J. G., & Sims, E. (1989). Drawing: Its use as a communicative aid with aphasic and normal adults. *Clinical Aphasiology, 18,* 339–355.

Mark, V. W., Thomas, B. E., & Berndt, R. S. (1992). Factors associated with improvement in global aphasia. *Aphasiology, 6,* 121–134.

Marshall, R. C. (1986). Treatment of auditory comprehensive deficits. In R. Chapey (Ed.), *Language intervetion strategies in adult aphasia* (2nd ed., pp. 370–393). Baltimore: Williams & Wilkins.

Marshall, R. C., Feed, D. B., & Phillips, D. S. (1997). Communicative efficiency in severe aphasia. *Aphasiology, 11,* 373–384.

Marshall, R. C., & Phillips, D. S. (1971). Prognosis for improved verbal communication in aphasic stroke patients. *Archives of Physical Medicine and Rehabilitation, 64,* 597–600.

Masand, P., & Chaudhary, P. (1994). Methylphenidate treatment of poststroke depression in a patient with global aphasia. *Annals of Clinical Psychiatry, 6,* 271–274.

Mazzocchi, F., & Vignolo, L. A. (1979). Localization of lesions in aphasia: Clinical CT scan correlations in stroke patients. *Cortex, 15,* 627–654.

McCall, D., Shelton, J. R., Weinrich, M., & Cox, D. (2000). The utility of computerized visual communication for improving natural language in chronic global aphasia: Implications for approaches to treatment in global aphasia. *Aphasiology, 14*(8), 795–826.

McDermott, F. B., Horner, J., & DeLong, E. R. (1996). Evolution of acute aphasia as measured by the Western Aphasia Battery. *Clinical Aphasiology, 24,* 159–172.

McKenna, P., & Warrington, E. K. (1978). Category-specific naming preservation: A single case study. *Journal of Neurology, Neurosurgery, and Psychiatry, 41,* 571–574.

McNeil, M. R., & Prescott, T. E. (1978). *Revised Token Test.* Baltimore: University Park Press.

Mohr, J. P., Sidman, M., Stoddard, L. T., Leicester, J., & Rosenberger, P. B. (1973). Evolution of the deficit in total aphasia. *Neurology, 23,* 1302–1312.

Morgan, A. L. R., & Helm-Estabrooks, N. (1987). Back to the drawing board: A treatment program for nonverbal aphasic patients. *Clinical Aphasiology, 17,* 64–72.

Murdoch, B. E., Afford, R. J., Ling, A. R., & Ganguley, B. (1986). Acute computerized tomographic scans: Their value in the localization of lesions and as prognostic indicators in aphasia. *Journal of Communication Disorders, 19,* 311–345.

Naeser, M. A. (1994). Neuroimaging and recovery of auditory comprehension and spontaneous speech in aphasia with some implications for treatment in severe aphasia. In A. Kertesz (Ed.), *Localization and neuroimaging in neuropsychology* (pp. 245–295). San Diego: Academic Press.

Naeser, M. A., Baker, E. H., Palumbo, C. L., Nicholas, M., Alexander, M. P., Samaraweera, R., et al. (1998). Lesion site patterns in severe, nonverbal aphasia to predict outcome with a computer-assisted treatment program. *Archives of Neurology, 55,* 1438–1448.

Naeser, M. A., Gaddie, A., Palumbo, C. L., & Stiassny-Eder, D. (1990). Late recovery of auditory comprehension in global aphasia: Improved recovery observed with subcortical temporal isthmus lesion vs Wernicke's cortical area lesion. *Archives of Neurology, 47,* 425–432.

Naeser, M. A., Martin, P. I., Nicholas, M., Baker, E. H., Seekins, H., Helm-Estabrooks, N. et al. (2005). Improved naming after TMS treatments in a chronic, global aphasia patient—Case report. *Neurocase, 11,* 182–193.

Naeser, M. A., Palumbo, C. L., Helm-Estabrooks, N., Stiassny-Eder, D., & Albert, M. L. (1989). Severe non-fluency in aphasia: Role of the medial subcallosal fasciculus plus other white matter pathways in recovery of spontaneous speech. *Brain, 112,* 1–38.

Nagaratnam, N., Barnes, R., & Nagaratnam, S. (1996). Speech recovery following global aphasia without hemiparesis. *Journal of Neurologic Rehabilitation, 10,* 115–119.

Nicholas, M. L., Helm-Estabrooks, N., Ward-Lonergan, J., & Morgan, A. R. (1993). Evolution of severe aphasia in the first two years post onset. *Archives of Physical Medicine and Rehabilitation, 74,* 830–836.

Okuda, B., Tanaka, H., Tachibana, H., Kawabata, K., Sugita, M. (1994). Cerebral blood flow in subcortical global aphasia: Perisylvian cortical hypoperfusion as a crucial role. *Stroke, 25,* 1495–1499.

Pashek, G. V., & Holland, A. L. (1988). Evolution of aphasia in the first year post-onset. *Cortex, 24,* 411–423.

Peach, R. K. (1992). Efficacy of aphasia treatment: What are the real issues? *Clinics in Communication Disorders, 1,* 7–10.

Peach, R. K. (1993). Clinical intervention for aphasia in the Unites States of America. In A. Holland & M. Forbes (Eds.), *Aphasia therapy: World perspectives* (pp. 335–369). San Diego: Singular.

Peach, R. K. (2001). Further thoughts regarding management of acute aphasia following stroke. *American Journal of Speech-Language Pathology, 10,* 29–36.

Peach, R. K. (2004). Aphasia (global). In R. D. Kent (Ed.), *The MIT encyclopedia of communication disorders* (pp. 243–245). Cambridge, MA: The MIT Press.

Pieniadz, J. M., Naeser, M. A., Koff, E., & Levine, H. L. (1983). CT scan cerebral hemispheric asymmetry measurements in stroke cases with global aphasia: Atypical asymmetries associated with improved recovery. *Cortex, 19,* 371–391.

Piercy, M., & Smith, V. O. G. (1962). Right hemisphere dominance for certain non-verbal intellectual skills. *Brain, 85,* 775–790.

Poeck, K., De Bleser R., & Keyserlingk, D. F. (1984). Neurolinguistic status and localization of lesion in aphasic patients with exclusively consonant-vowel recurring utterances. *Brain, 107,* 199–217.

Porch, B. E. (1981). *Porch index of communicative ability* (3ʳᵈ ed.). Palo Alto, CA: Consulting Psychologists Press.

Pound, C., Parr, S., & Duchan, J. (2001). Using partners' autobiographical reports to develop, deliver, and evaluate services in aphasia. *Aphasiology, 15*(5), 477–493.

Prins, R. S., Snow, E., & Wagenaar, E. (1978). Recovery from aphasia: Spontaneous speech versus language comprehension. *Brain and Language, 6,* 192–211.

Ramsberger, G., & Helm-Estabrooks, N. (1989). Visual Action Therapy for bucco-facial apraxia. *Clinical Aphasiology, 18,* 395–406.

Rao, P. R. (1995). Drawing and gesture as communication options in a person with severe aphasia. *Topics in Stroke Rehabilitation, 2,* 49–56.

Rao, P. R. (2001). Use of Amer-Ind code by persons with severe aphasia. In R. Chapey (Ed.), *Language intervention strategies in aphasia and related neurogenic communication disorders* (4th ed., pp. 688–702). Philadelphia: Lippincott Williams & Wilkins.

Rao, P. R., Basili, A. G., Koller, J., Fullerton, B., Diener, S., & Burton, P. (1980). The use of Amer-Ind code by severe aphasic adults. In M. S. Burns & J. R. Andrews (Eds.), *Neuropathologies of speech and language: Diagnosis and treatment* (pp. 18–35). Evanston, IL: Institute for Continuing Professional Education.

Rao, P. R., & Horner, J. (1978). Gesture as a deblocking modality in a severe aphasic patient. *Clinical Aphasiology, 8,* 180–187.

Rao, P. R., & Horner, J. (1980). Nonverbal strategies for functional communication in aphasic persons. In M. S. Burns & J. R. Andrews (Eds.), *Neuropathologies of speech and language: Diagnosis and treatment* (pp. 108–133). Evanston, IL: Institute for Continuing Professional Education.

Raven, J. C. (1965). *Guide to using the Coloured Progressive Matrices.* London: H.K. Lewis.

Raymer, A. M., & Thompson, C. K. (1991). Effects of verbal plus gestural treatment in a patient with aphasia and severe apraxia of speech. *Clinical Aphasiology, 20,* 285–295.

Reinvang, I., & Engvik, H. (1980). Language recovery in aphasia from 3 to 6 months after stroke. In M. T. Sarno & O. Hook (Eds.), *Aphasia: Assessment and treatment* (pp. 79–88). New York: Masson.

Rey, G. J., Sivan, A. B., & Benton, A. L. (1991). *Examen de afasia multilingue (Multilingual Aphasia Examination-Spanish).* Iowa City, IA: AJA.

Robey, R. R. (1998). A meta-analysis of clinical outcomes in the treatment of aphasia. *Journal of Speech, Language, and Hearing Research, 41,* 172–187.

Rosenbek, J. C., LaPointe, L. L., & Wertz, R. T. (1989). *Aphasia: A clinical approach.* Austin, TX: Pro-Ed.

Rossor, M. N., Warrington, E. K., & Cipolotti, L. (1995). The isolation of calculation skills. *Journal of Neurology, 242,* 78–81.

Salvatore, A. P., & Nelson, T. R. (1995). Training novel language systems in severely aphasic individuals: How novel is it? *Clinical Aphasiology, 23,* 267–278.

Salvatore, A. P., & Thompson, C. K. (1986). Intervention for global aphasia. In R. Chapey (Ed.), *Language intervention strategies in adult aphasia* (2ⁿᵈ ed., pp. 403–418). Baltimore: Williams & Wilkins.

Sarno, M. R., & Levita, E. (1971). Natural course of recovery in severe aphasia. *Archives of Physical Medicine and Rehabilitation, 52,* 175–178.

Sarno, M. R., & Levita, E. (1979). Recovery in treated aphasia during the first year post-stroke. *Stroke, 10,* 663–670.

Sarno, M. T. (1969). *The functional communication profile: Manual of directions* (Rehabilitation Monograph 42). New York: New York University Medical Center, Institute of Rehabilitation Medicine.

Sarno, M. T. (1981). Recovery and rehabilitation in aphasia. In M. R. Sarno (Ed.), *Acquired aphasia* (pp. 485–529). New York: Academic Press.

Sarno, M. T., & Levita, E. (1981). Some observations on the nature of recovery in global aphasia after stroke. *Brain and Language, 13,* 1–12.

Sarno, M. T., Silverman, M. G., & Sands, E. S. (1970). Speech therapy and language recovery in severe aphasia. *Journal of Speech and Hearing Research, 13,* 607–623.

Sasanuma, S. (1988). Studies in dementia: In search of the linguistic/cognitive interaction underlying communication. *Aphasiology, 2,* 191–193.

Scarpa, M., Colombo, A., Sorgato, P., & De Renzi, E. (1987). The incidence of aphasia and global aphasia in left brain-damaged patients. *Cortex, 23,* 331–336.

Schuell, H. M. (1974). *The Minnesota test for differential diagnosis of aphasia* (revised edition). Minneapolis: University of Minnesota Press.

Selnes, O. A., & Hillis, A. (2000). Patient Tan revisited: A case of atypical global aphasia? *Journal of the History of the Neurosciences, 9*(3), 233–237.

Sugiu, K., Katsumata, A., Ono, Y., Tamiya, T., & Ohmoto, T. (2003). Angioplasty and coiling of ruptured aneurysm with symptomatic vasospasm: Technical case report. *Surgical Neurology, 59,* 413–417.

Shewan, C. M. (1979). *Auditory Comprehension Test for Sentences.* Chicago: Biolinguistics Clinical Institutes.

Shewan, C. M., & Canter, G. J. (1971). Effects of vocabulary, syntax, and sentence length on auditory comprehension in aphasic patients. *Cortex, 7,* 209–226.

Siirtola, T., & Siirtola, M. (1984). Evolution of aphasia. *Acta Neurologica Scandinavica, 69*(Suppl. 98), 403–404.

Silverman, F. H. (1989). *Communication for the speechless* (2nd ed.). Englewood Cliffs, NJ: Prentice Hall.

Simmons-Mackie, N. (2001). Social approaches to aphasia intervention. In R. Chapey (Ed.), *Language intervention strategies for aphasia and related neurogenic communication disorders* (4th ed., pp. 246–268). Philadelphia: Lippincott Williams & Wilkins.

Simmons-Mackie, N., Kingston, D., & Schultz, M. (2004). "Speaking for another": The management of participant frames in aphasia. *American Journal of Speech-Language Pathology, 13(2),* 128–141.

Skelly, M. (1979). *Amer-Ind gestural code based on universal American Indian hand talk.* New York: Elsevier.

Skelly, M., Schinsky, L., Smith, R., Donaldson, R., & Griffin, P. (1974). American Indian Sign (Amer-Ind) as a facilitator of verbalization for the oral-verbal apraxic. *Journal of Speech and Hearing Disorders, 39,* 445–456.

Skelly, M., Schinsky, L., Smith, R., Donaldson, R., & Griffin, P. (1975). American Indian Sign: Gestural communication for the speechless. *Archives of Physical Medicine and Rehabilitation, 56,* 156–160.

Sklar, M. (1983). *Sklar Aphasia Scale* (revised). Los Angeles: Western Psychological Services.

Sorgato, P., Colombo, A., Scarpa, M., & Faglioni, P. (1990). Age, sex, and lesion site in aphasic stroke patients with single focal damage. *Neuropsychology, 4,* 165–173.

Spinnler, H., & Vignolo, L. (1966). Impaired recognition of meaningful sounds in aphasia. *Cortex, 2,* 337–348.

Spreen, O., & Benton, A. L. (1977). *Neurosensory center comprehensive examination for aphasia* (revised edition). Victoria, B.C.: University of Victoria.

Steele, R. D., Kleczewska, M. K., Carlson, G. S., & Weinrich, M. (1992). Computers in the rehabilitation of chronic, severe aphasia: C-VIC 2.0 cross-modal studies. *Aphasiology, 6,* 185–194.

Steele, R. D., Weinrich, M., Kleczewska, M. K., Carlson, G. S., & Wertz, R. T. (1987). Evaluating performance of severely aphasic patients on a computer-aided visual communication system. *Clinical Aphasiology, 17,* 46–54.

Steele, R. D., Weinrich, M., Wertz, R. T., Kleczewska, M. K., & Carlson, G. S. (1989). Computer-based visual communication in aphasia. *Neuropsychologia, 27,* 409–426.

Sugiu, K., Katsumata, A., Ono, Y., Tamiya, T., & Ohmoto, T. (2003). Angioplasty and coiling of ruptured aneurysm with symptomatic vasospasm: Technical case report. *Surgical Neurology, 59,* 413–417.

Tonkovich, J. D., & Loverso, F. L. (1982). A training matrix approach for gestural acquisition by the agrammatic patient. *Clinical Aphasiology, 12,* 283–288.

Tranel, D., Biller, J., Damasio, H., Adams, H. P., & Cornell, S. H. (1987). Global aphasia without hemiparesis. *Archives of Neurology, 44,* 304–308.

Van Horn, G., & Hawes, A. (1982). Global aphasia without hemiparesis: A sign of embolic encephalopathy. *Neurology, 32,* 403–406.

Van Lancker, D., & Klein, K. (1990). Preserved recognition of familiar personal names in global aphasia. *Brain and Language, 39,* 511–529.

Van Lancker, D., & Nicklay, C. K. H. (1992). Comprehension of personnaly relevant (PERL) versus novel language in two globally aphasic patients. *Aphasiology, 6,* 37–61.

Wallace, G. L., & Canter, G. J. (1985). Effects of personally relevant language materials on the performance of severely aphasic individuals. *Journal of Speech and Hearing Disorders, 50,* 385–390.

Wallace, G. L., & Stapleton, J. H. (1991). Analysis of auditory comprehension performance in individuals with severe aphasia. *Archives of Physical Medicine and Rehabilitation, 72,* 674–678.

Wallesch, C. W., Bak, T., & Schulte-Monting, J. (1992). Acute aphasia—Patterns and prognosis. *Aphasiology, 6,* 373–385.

Wapner, W., & Gardner, H. (1979). A note on patterns of comprehension and recovery in global aphasia. *Journal of Speech and Hearing Research, 29,* 765–772.

Ward-Lonergan, J., & Nicholas, M. (1995). Drawing to communicate: A case report of an adult with global aphasia. *European Journal of Disorders of Communication, 30,* 475–491.

Weinrich, M., Steele, R., Carlson, G. S., Kleczewska, M., Wertz, R. T., & Baker, E. H. (1989). Processing of visual syntax in a globally aphasic patient. *Brain and Language, 36,* 391–405.

Weinrich, M., Steele, R., Kleczewska, M., Carlson, G. S., Baker, E. H., & Wertz, R. T. (1989). Representation of "verbs" in a computerized visual communication system. *Aphasiology, 3,* 501–512.

Weinrich, M., McCall, D., Shoosmith, L., Thomas, K., Catzenberger, K., & Weber, C. (1993). Locative prepositional phrases in severe aphasia. *Brain and Language, 45,* 21–45.

Wells, C. R., Labar, D. R., & Solomon, G. E. (1992). Aphasia as the sole manifestation of simple partial status epilepticus. *Epilepsia, 33,* 84–87.

Wepman, J. M., & Jones, L. V. (1961). *The Language Modalities Test for Aphasia.* Chicago: Education-Industry Service.

Wertz, R. T., Dronkers, N. F., & Hume, J. L. (1993). PICA intrasubtest variability and prognosis for improvement in aphasia. *Clinical Aphasiology, 21,* 207–211.

Wiederholt, J. L., & Bryant, B. R. (2001). *The Gray Oral Reading Tests* (4th ed.). Austin, TX: Pro-Ed.

Wilcox, M. J., & Davis, G. A. (1978, November). *Procedures for promoting communicative effectiveness in an aphasic adult.* Symposium conducted at the annual meeting of the American Speech and Hearing Association, San Francisco, CA.

Yang, B. J., Yang, T. C., Pan, H. C., Lai, S. J., & Yang, F. (1989). Three variant forms of subcortical aphasia in Chinese stroke patients. *Brain and Language, 37,* 145–162.

Yasuda, K., & Ono, Y. (1998). Comprehension of famous personal and geographical names in global aphasic subjects. *Brain and Language, 61,* 274–287.

Zahn, R., Drews, E., Specht, K., Kemeny, S., Reith, W., Willmes, K., et al. (2004). Recovery of semantic word processing in global aphasia: A functional MRI study. *Cognitive Brain Research, 18,* 322–336.

B. Cognitive Neuropsychological Approaches to Treatment of Language Disorders

Chapter 22

Cognitive Neuropsychological Approaches to Treatment of Language Disorders: Introduction

Argye E. Hillis and Melissa Newhart

OBJECTIVES

The purposes of this chapter are to (1) describe an approach to assessment and treatment of individuals with aphasia that begins with identifying, in each patient, the cognitive mechanisms that are impaired and those that are intact, within a cognitive neuropsychological model of the affected language task; (2) provide examples of this general approach that have resulted in functional gains in communication abilities; (3) delineate the uses and limitations of this approach to clinical management of persons with aphasia; and (4) speculate on the future trends in the areas of cognitive science and language rehabilitation. To set the stage, we first describe the main goals of cognitive neuropsychology and how this model characterizes the normal cognitive mechanisms (mental representations and processes) necessary to accomplish a given language task, such as naming or reading, on the basis of patterns of impaired performance due to brain damage. More recently, clinicians have used cognitive neuropsychological models of normal language to characterize impaired and spared cognitive processes important for focusing treatment of individuals with aphasia.

DEFINITION

This section provides illustrations of a general approach to the assessment and treatment of specific language tasks that makes use of cognitive analyses and models developed within the discipline of cognitive neuropsychology—a branch of psychology that seeks to understand normal human cognitive mechanisms through evidence from how cognitive mechanisms are modified by brain damage. This approach begins, for each patient, with identifying which cognitive processes and representations underlying the language task are impaired and which are intact. Treatment then focuses either on remediation of the impaired cognitive processes, compensation via the intact cognitive processes, or both. This framework involves consideration of the patient's performance of the task in light of a model of the cognitive processes and representations that underlie normal performance of the task. It should be emphasized that the treatment procedures themselves are not usually based on models from cognitive neuropsychology, although some computational models have been used to guide selection of treatment stimuli (Kiran & Thompson, 2003) or even treatment strategies (Martin, Lane, & Harley, 2003). However, most therapies are based on principles of learning, clinical experience with the sorts of input that successfully elicit better performance, and the clinician's other skills, talents, and knowledge—just like other therapy strategies in speech-language pathology. In fact, the selection of the chapter contributors reflects the fact that this approach has its foundations in the integration and cooperation across the professions of cognitive neuropsychology, speech-language pathology, behavioral neurology, and other professions within the discipline of cognitive science. Related areas include cognitive psychology (a branch of psychology devoted to the study of normal cognitive processing), psycholinguistics (a branch of psychology devoted to the study of rules and representations that underlie normal language comprehension and production), and linguistics (a profession devoted to investigation of the structure and computation of language). No one profession can lay claim to the sort of rehabilitation described in this section, although clinicians in each profession can engage in it equally.

PRINCIPLES AND PROCEDURES OF THE "COGNITIVE NEUROPSYCHOLOGICAL" APPROACH

The goal of cognitive neuropsychological research is to develop models of normal language processes, in the form of the cognitive architecture of specific language tasks. A model of this type specifies the mechanisms for solving the necessary computational problems of a particular task, such as naming, as a set of representations (i.e., stored visual, orthographic, semantic, or phonologic information) and the processes required to compute or activate each representation from earlier ones. So, for example, we might propose that picture-naming involves, at the very least, the following: discrimination of the lines, edges, and shadings of the picture to develop a representation of the visual image; matching the computed visual representation to a stored representation of the physical structure of the object (i.e., accessing the "structural/visual description"); accessing stored information about the set of instances with a particular name (i.e., accessing a "semantic representation"); accessing the stored pronunciation (the "phonologic representation") of the word to which it corresponds; and activating representations of the motor programs involved in articulating the word.

One such processing model of the lexical system is schematically depicted in Figure 22–1. This figure depicts some of the principal cognitive processes underlying reading, spelling, and naming, understood as a series of transformations of mental representations. Many models include

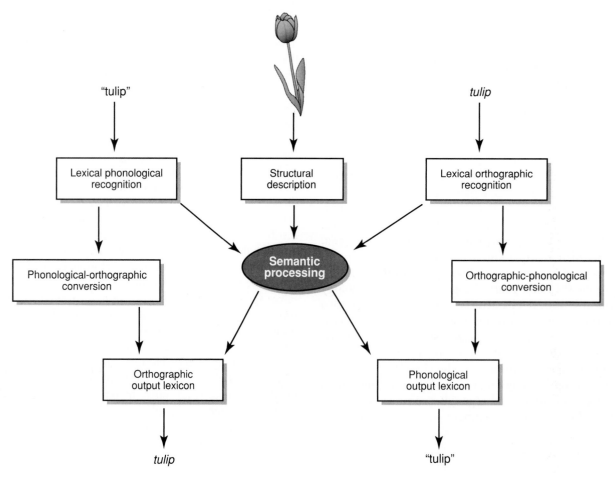

Figure 22–1. Schematic representation of the components of lexical processing.

additional levels of processing, such as a "lemma," a modality-independent syntactic representation that specifies the word class (and mass/count and gender in some languages), prior to accessing a phonologic or orthographic lexical representation. It is important to note that although each component is dedicated to a particular aspect of lexical processing, some of the components are involved in more than one lexical task. For example, both reading and naming involve computing the phonologic representation of a word for output from a semantic representation. Hence, if computation of the phonologic representation were to be disrupted by brain damage, it should be manifest as impairment in both reading and naming, although the consequences for output may be somewhat different in the two tasks. In the case of reading, additional information about the pronunciation of the name is available from the printed word. Therefore, if the patient is unable to compute "chair" from the semantic representation of CHAIR, he or she will be unable to name the pictured chair but may yet be able to correctly read *chair* on the basis of orthographic-to-phonologic conversion mechanisms (i.e., by "sounding out" the word). Of note, some models of naming are more explicitly computational in that they simulate the process of a limited number of neurons like units that represent features or even whole words. Some of these models also simulate learning or re-learning.

Motivation for proposing specific representations and processes comes from considering the computational requirements of the cognitive task, and the proposals are supported by empirical evidence from studies of normal subjects and from patterns of impaired performance by brain-damaged subjects. To illustrate, evidence for proposing separate mechanisms for computing phonologic and orthographic representations of words from a semantic representation comes from patients who show good comprehension of printed and spoken words (indicating adequate access to the semantic representation) and are able to write the corresponding written word (in dictation or picture-naming tasks), but are not able to access the pronunciation of the same word. Such a pattern of performance (Caramazza & Hillis, 1990; Ellis, Miller, & Sin, 1983; Hier & Mohr, 1977) is inconsistent with an alternative proposal that computation of the orthographic representation first requires computation of the phonologic representation. Thus, such models are constrained by patterns of performance of brain-damaged patients that cannot be otherwise explained by proposing specific loci of damage to the existing model. The subsequent chapters will cite cases that provide evidence for proposing those components of lexical processing that are involved in naming (Raymer & Gonzalez Rothi, Chapter 23, this volume; see also Fink, Brecher, Sobel, & Schwartz, 2005; Hillis, 1994), reading and writing (Beeson & Henry, Chapter 25, this volume; see also Beeson, 1999; Beeson & Hirsch, 1998; Beeson, Rewega, Vail, & Rapcsak, 2000; Coltheart, Patterson, & Marshall, 1980; Ellis, 1982; Friedman & Lott, 1996; Friedman & Lott, 2002; Friedman, Lott, & Sample, 1998; Friedman, Sample, & Lott, 2000; Goodman & Caramazza, 1986; Hillis & Heidler, 2005; Patterson, Coltheart, & Marshall, 1985; Rapp, 2005), and sentence processing (Mitchum & Berndt, Chapter 24, this volume; see also Garrett, 1980; Thompson & Shapiro, 1995; Thompson & Shapiro, 2005; Thompson, Shapiro, Ballard, Jacobs, & Tait, 1997; Thompson, Shapiro, Tait, Jacobs, & Schneider, 1996).

In turn, the models guide our understanding of performance patterns by individuals with aphasia. That is, language disorders resulting from brain damage (which disrupts previously normal language) can be characterized by proposing deformations of one or more of the constituent mental representations or processes underlying language tasks. For example, imagine a patient who understands spoken and written words and writes the names of pictures adequately but is unable to say the correct names, despite unimpaired motor skills for articulating the correct name. We might propose in this case that the patient is unable to retrieve the accurate pronunciation of the word from among the stored pronunciations of all words he or she knows ("the phonologic output lexicon"). Therefore, a pattern of performance that indicates a proposed locus of disruption in the lexical system at the level of the phonologic output lexicon would include (1) demonstrated access to the semantic system from printed and spoken words (i.e., intact reading and auditory comprehension) and from pictures, and (2) access to printed words from semantics (i.e., intact written expression of names and of self-generated ideas), but (3) failure to access the phonologic representation from pictures or objects (impaired oral naming) or from written words (impaired oral reading). This example illustrates that the data crucial to proposing a specific locus of damage include the patient's performance profile across lexical tasks in all modalities. To understand a patient's writing, for example, we need to know about his or her reading, comprehension, and speech, as well as performance on various spelling tasks. In addition, an analysis of the types of errors made in the affected task(s) and the stimulus parameters that influence performance (e.g., word frequency, part of speech, word length, and so on) may be required, as illustrated in several cases in the following chapters. Recent studies indicate that disruption of separate components of the lexical process are caused by distinct site of brain dysfunction (DeLeon et al., 2007).

Basic Assumptions

There are a few basic assumptions of cognitive neuropsychological research, which if proved to be incorrect would undermine the usefulness of this approach for understanding normal language processing. First, the universality assumption states that everyone has essentially "the same" cognitive processes. Certainly, there may be different modes of learning and thinking that reflect variable reliance on one type of processing relative to another, but presumably we all develop the same types of mental representations and processes.

Second, the "transparency assumption" states that brain-damaged patients also have basically the same cognitive processes, except for a focal modification at some level(s) of representation or processing, "transparently" revealed by the performance pattern in various tasks. In other words, brain damage does not result in new types of mental representations or operations, although it may change *which* of our normal components we rely on to accomplish a task. For example, referring to Figure 22–1, normal oral reading of a word such as "yacht" is accomplished by accessing a representation in the phonologic output lexicon (the repository of stored "pronunciations" of familiar words). However, when there is damage to the phonologic output lexicon a patient may now read aloud via letter-to-sound conversion mechanisms. This local modification in the system is transparently revealed by pronunciation of the word yacht as "yached" (/jætSt/, rhyming with thatched). Normally, oral reading of English is likely to be accomplished by an interaction of the two mechanisms (access to the phonologic output lexicon from semantics and letter-to-sound conversion mechanisms (Hillis & Caramazza, 1991, 1995), although some readers may rely more on one or the other, at least in learning to read.

Different Types of Cognitive Models

The classical cognitive neuropsychological model is the so-called "serial" or "box and arrow" schematic representation of the cognitive representations and their interactions that underlie a given task, such as reading, spelling, naming, or sentence production. These representations and processes do not necessarily correspond to locations in the brain. Rather, they represent distinct functional components of a cognitive operation. Several models of this type are illustrated in the following chapters, and a "serial" model of the lexical system is shown in Figure 22–1. The basis for proposing each level of representation comes from patients whose performance of the task, and pattern of performance across tasks, can be understood by proposing selective damage to that cognitive component and dependence on the other spared components. Such schema are described as serial because it was initially assumed that processing at each level of representation was completed before processing at the next level was started. In serial models, feedback from one level of representation to a prior level, and integration of the various components, were not considered. However, several cognitive mechanisms may interact to select or "access" a specific lexical representation at a subsequent level (Hillis & Caramazza, 1991, 1995; Patterson, Graham, & Hodges, 1994), and that information may "cascade" from one level to the next, such that several representations are simultaneously active and contributing to the final output (Humphreys, Riddoch, & Quinlan, 1988).

The concepts of integration and feedback are best seen in more recent, computational models of specific language tasks. This type of model is a computer simulation of the cognitive representations and procedures that underlie the task, utilizing several levels of "nodes" with feedback and feedforward connections between each level. In some of these models, the strength of the connections between nodes is not "programmed in," but is learned through many repeated simulations (Plaut & Shallice, 1993; Seidenberg & McClelland, 1989). Evidence for postulating specific characteristics of each model comes from patients whose pattern of performance can be simulated by "damaging" the simulation in some way (e.g., by reducing the connection strength between two levels of nodes). It is likely that each of these types of serial and computational models captures some of the characteristics of normal language processing. It is plausible that there are both feedback and feedforward interactions between at least some levels. (Dell, 1986; Dell, Burger, & Svec, 1997; Rapp & Goldrick, 2004). It is also likely that lexical and semantic representations consist of activation distributed across component units, some of which are shared by other, related representations (Plaut & Shallice, 1993; Seidenberg & McClelland, 1989).

Application of Models to Treatment

Focusing Treatment

The clinician's primary goal in understanding the patient's deficit is to focus treatment on just those levels of processing that are impaired or to identify methods that will allow the patient to process language successfully by "getting around" the deficit. Thus, the predominant usefulness of cognitive models is in identifying the level(s) of processing that are impaired in each patient, so that therapy can be directed toward remediation of that component and/or strategies to compensate for the loss of that component. Among the first illustrations of this application was a study by Byng and Coltheart (1986) showing that selective damage to particular components of the reading system in their patient could be treated successfully by focusing treatment on the impaired component (see Beeson & Henry, Chapter 25, this volume). Additional notable examples of studies in which cognitive analyses have been used to focus intervention are described in the subsequent chapters in this section. In each case, a model of the normal processes underlying the treated task served to pinpoint the patient's deficit and thereby focus intervention. For example, patient JJ (reported in Hillis & Caramazza, 1991), whose pattern of performance across lexical tasks indicated a disruption at the level of the semantic system, showed more improvement in naming performance when treatment tasks explicitly required semantic processing (printed word/picture matching) than when treatment tasks did not overtly require semantic processing (oral reading with phonologic cues). In contrast, patient HW, whose naming impairment could be localized to the phonologic output lexicon, showed greater improvement in naming performance as a consequence of the facilitated oral-reading treatment than as a consequence of treatment using printed word/picture matching to enhance semantic processing (see Hillis & Caramazza, 1994, for details and discussion). Raymer, Thompson, Jacobs, and LeGrand (1993) (see also McNeil et al., 1999; Thompson, Raymer, & LeGrand, 1991) also reported that phonologic strategies to facilitate naming (e.g., using rhyming word cues) improved naming performance of patients whose impairment was localized to the phonologic output lexicon. Additional reports of treatment focused on specific components of the naming process are reported by Raymer and Gonzalez Rothi in Chapter 23 (this volume). However, many types of naming treatment described in the literature, including those that directly facilitate production of the name in response to the picture, might improve naming at either the level of the semantic system or the level of the phonologic output lexicon or both (Hillis, 1989; Howard, Patterson, Franklin, Orchard-Lisle, & Morton, 1985; Linebaugh, 1983; Thompson & Kearns, 1981).

Another use of cognitive neuropsychological models has been in the prediction of patterns of generalization across tasks and across items. For example, in Chapter 25 of this volume, Beeson and Henry describe a patient, HG, whose performance across lexical tasks could be explained by assuming that she had partial damage to semantic representations of words and profound damage to the phonologic output lexicon (Hillis, 1990, 1994). In various tasks, such as written and spoken naming, repetition, written word/picture matching, and spoken word/picture matching, HG made semantic errors, such as "tulip" named or understood as "rose." However, her errors were inconsistent. Tulip might be named on one occasion as "rose" and on another occasion as "daisy." Furthermore, when shown a picture of a tulip she would accept the name "rose," "daisy," "tulip," or any other flower as the name of the picture. This pattern can be explained by assuming that HG accessed underspecified semantic representations, or meanings, of words. In this case, she might have had a semantic representation of "tulip" that consisted of a partial set of features that define tulip. While the normal semantic representation of "tulip" might include all of the features that jointly define a tulip and allow it to be distinguished from all other flowers, such as <flower>, <bulb>, <upright petals>, <slender, upright leaves>, <spring blooming>, <dutch>; HG's semantic representation might include only <flower> and <spring blooming>. Therefore, she would accept any word that corresponded to these features in word/picture verification. Furthermore, her underspecified semantic representation would access all phonologic representations and orthographic representations that correspond to these features, so that a picture of tulip might be named as any one of many spring flowers. In addition, HG mispronounced nearly every word in all tasks with spoken output (repetition, oral reading, spoken naming). This aspect of HG's performance was attributed to an additional deficit in accessing phono-

logic representations for output. Initially, treatment focused on her semantic impairment (see Chapter 25, this volume), by teaching her the features that distinguish semantically related words, for certain categories of words, such as foods and clothing. Based on the model in Figure 25–1, it was predicted that treatment (teaching/improving specific semantic representations) should improve her performance of all tasks that involve the semantic component—for example, spoken and written naming, and spoken and written word comprehension. And, indeed, although treatment engaged the task of written naming only, her reduction in semantic errors generalized to tasks of spoken naming and spoken and written word comprehension. However, the treatment was expected to be specific to the trained categories of words. That is, teaching her features that distinguish various types of clothing should not reduce her semantic errors in naming or understanding of furniture. And, consistent with this prediction, her gains generalized to untrained items within the trained categories, but not to untrained categories. Furthermore, the treatment of semantic representations utilizing the task of written naming was not expected to improve her pronunciation of words in spoken output, and it did not. Subsequent therapy directed toward teaching her accurate pronunciations by reestablishing phonologic representations (or access to them) in the task of oral reading did result in more accurate pronunciations in not only oral reading, but also in oral naming and repetition. In this case, treatment was item-specific, as expected, since reteaching a phonologic representation of "tulip" would only improve pronunciation of tulip. Behrmann and Lieberthal (1989) reported comparable generalization results—improvement in categorization of *untreated items* within *treated categories*— of a therapy strategy that also focused on teaching semantic distinctions among related items. Their patient, like HG, showed a pattern of performance consistent with damage to the semantic system, as indicated in particular by his category-specific impairment in comprehension (but unlike HG he showed some improvement of items in one of the untrained categories). Additional reports in the literature of item-specific treatment include treating reading of function words using association with visually/phonologically similar content words (Hatfield, 1983) and improving printed-word recognition by reinforcing correct word/nonword, semantic, and phonologic decisions about the "treated" set of words (Hillis, 1993). These reports are consistent with the hypothesis that if treatment influences specific representations (or access to them), performance involving the target representations (treated stimuli) should improve across tasks, but performance would not be expected to improve for other representations (of untreated words).

A different type of generalization concerns changes in performance across treated and untreated stimuli. Here, we would expect that if treatment influences a general processing mechanism (say, holding representations in a short-term memory system), processing should improve across all stimuli that are subject to that mechanism (Rapp, 2005). Many examples of therapy that influenced both treated and untreated stimuli have been reported, such as improving reading speed by reinforcing rapid semantic decisions about printed words ("gestalt processing") (Gonzalez Rothi & Moss, 1989), improving comprehension of sentences (Byng & Coltheart, 1986), improving use of a self-correction strategy in spelling (Hillis & Caramazza, 1987), and improving use of sublexical letter-to-sound conversion mechanisms or "phonologic assembly" to improve oral reading (Berndt & Mitchum, 1994; de Partz, 1986; Hillis, 1993) or sound-to-letter conversion mechanisms to improve spelling (Carlomagno, Iavarone, & Colombo, 1994; Hillis Trupe, 1986). Generalization to untrained items might be increased by starting of more complex or less protypical examples (Kiran & Thompson, 2003). The problem in making predictions as to whether or not to expect improvement across stimuli is that we have no way of knowing, a priori, how treatment affects processing. Indeed, we might instead use treatment results to propose whether a general mechanism or specific representations were affected by our treatment (see Goodman-Schulman, Sokol, Aliminosa, & McCloskey, 1990, for discussion and illustration).

Finally, we always work toward ensuring that treatment effects generalize to other tasks and settings outside the therapy session. For example, patient HG (above) showed dramatically improved use of trained words not only during therapy, but also in the job setting (documented by her job coach), at home (documented by her mother), and in restaurants (observed by her therapist). Hinckley, Patterson, & Carr (1999) also reported that treatment that focused on specific cognitive skills—"the cognitive neuropsychological approach"—resulted in better generalization of improvements to untrained tasks, such as the Communicative Abilities in Daily Living (CADL; Holland, 1980), than treatment that focused on a particular functional activity.

Limitations

Several authors have argued that cognitive neuropsychological models are simply models of cognitive tasks, not models of rehabilitation. That is, most current models of cognitive processing provide no direct motivation for specific treatment strategies. For example, knowing the patient's level of disruption in the naming process does not guide the clinician as to how to treat the problem (see Caramazza, 1989; Caramazza & Hillis, 1991; Wilson & Patterson, 1990 for discussion). In fact, such knowledge does not even guide the clinician as to what to treat. Should we treat the damaged component of processing, or should we try to exploit the preserved components in the hopes for more functional, but not normal, language processing? The models alone do not help us in this regard, because they do not specify which components are

subject to remediation, nor how the system might be reorganized following damage to circumscribed parts. Hence, choices of treatment must rely (as usual) on the clinician's intuitions about what might help, the goals of the person seeking therapy, and ongoing evaluation of treatment effects. Empirical reports of improvement in functioning associated with specific treatment approaches in well-described cases of damage to selective components of language processing might give the clinician hope that a particular component is treatable. However, valid predictions about improvement in a different case of damage to the same component would also require evidence regarding the patient characteristics that influence outcome and the nature of damage to the impaired component (see Hillis, 1993; Hillis & Caramazza, 1994, for detailed discussion). In fact, even patients who have the "same" deficit with respect to the level of representation in some cognitive task do not consistently respond to the same treatment. It is not clear, from considering the model, whether the differential response to treatment is due to different forms of damage to the same component or due to different overall learning abilities, motivation, or other patient characteristics. However, some authors have described how patients with different deficits (within a computational model of lexical processing) have responded to different therapies, as shown by many studies cited in the chapters in this section.

Another limitation in applying these sorts of models to treatment is that the analyses required to determine the patient's level of damage are often extremely time-consuming and may not be cost-effective (Schwartz, 1998). That is, with the recent limitations on the number of reimbursable therapy visits, and requirements to document improvement at each visit, it is often impractical to spend hours of time testing a patient to pinpoint precisely which components of each task are impaired. However, in other cases, such extensive evaluation may be justifiable. For instance, in the case of HG, whose deficits were quite complicated, it was difficult to know where to even begin treatment until damage to specific components of lexical processing were identified. She had undergone years of unfocused therapy for "cortical deafness" and other inaccurate psychiatric and language diagnoses, with virtually no improvement in language or communication, prior to careful analysis of her impairments. She made useful, albeit slow, gains after delineating her deficits. Furthermore, it is often possible to identify with some precision the impaired cognitive process(es) with relatively brief testing using carefully selected tasks and stimuli.

It has also been argued that treatment based on cognitive neuropsychological models fails to generalize across items or categories (for evidence for and against this claim, see Schwartz, 1998 and chapters in this section). Although this failure of generalization to untrained items or categories is far from ideal, item-specific gains are better than no gains. Recall HG, a patient described earlier in this chapter as having a semantic impairment, demonstrated by identical rates and types of semantic errors in all lexical tasks (oral naming, written naming, auditory word/picture matching, written word/picture matching, and writing to dictation). HG's improvements in oral production were item-specific, and her improvements in semantic processing generalized only to items that were semantically related to trained items (see also Hillis, 1998). Nevertheless, as mentioned above, HG's gains served a significant function. She gradually regained a functional vocabulary for daily activities (such as dining out and riding public transportation) and a vocabulary specific to the job for which she was training (as a stock clerk in a fabric store). Her item-specific gains, which generalized well across tasks and settings, thus permitted HG to obtain and maintain a job and independence in activities of daily living. At the time of this writing HG, who was globally aphasic for more than 6 years, remains gainfully employed.

Similarly, the "phonologic" therapy with a patient HW (see above and Chapter 25, this volume) that involved cued oral reading treatment seemed to result in improved access to specific phonologic representations in the output lexicon, irrespective of the setting. Like patient HG, patient HW produced mostly fluent speech with few content words before this item-specific therapy was initiated more than 5 years post-stroke. Her impairment was localized to the phonologic output lexicon (Fig. 22–1), because (1) she showed flawless performance in auditory word/picture and written word/picture matching tasks and was able to define both words and pictures she could not name, indicating that her processing of words and pictures was unimpaired through the level of the semantic system; (2) she produced accurate or recognizable written names of 100% of pictures, even though she could not produce the spoken name, indicating that semantics and access to the orthographic output lexicon were intact; and (3) she had perfect fluency, articulation, and repetition of words she could not name, ruling out a motor-speech deficit as the basis for her impaired spoken naming. HW's improvements in producing a trained set of words using the phonologic therapy were sufficiently rapid that she was able to receive treatment for many sets of words she selected. She was also observed to use trained words in conversation at home, in restaurants, and over the telephone in follow-up calls. In describing the "Cookie Theft" picture from the Boston Diagnostic Aphasia Examination (Goodglass & Kaplan, 1972), HW improved in the number of accurate content-units produced, from five before the phonologic treatment to 12 after treatment (c.f. Yorkston & Beukelman, 1980, for description of content-units). Furthermore, not only were her gains maintained more than a year after treatment, but additional gains were achieved: She later produced 15 content-units in describing the picture. The further progress was probably achieved in part through HW's oral-reading practice with her husband providing cues (which probably provided "treatment" of thousands of words).

Thus, item-specific gains that generalize across tasks and settings can lead to dramatic functional improvement resulting from therapy for naming and other oral production tasks. Gains that generalize across tasks but not always to other settings have also been reported for sentence production/comprehension therapies (see Mitchum & Berndt, Chapter 24, this volume). Several authors have reported not only generalization of improvements from comprehension to production (or vice versa) for the same items, but also generalization across trained and untrained sentence types (Ballard & Thompson, 1999). And, as previously discussed, improvements in many model-based treatments do show generalization to untrained stimuli as well as untrained tasks, if treatment addresses a process common to many stimuli or compensatory strategy that will result in improved access to a variety of stimuli.

An important limitation of conclusions reached about the results of a given treatment for an individual patient is that it is not possible to determine, a priori, which other patients will respond to the same treatment in the same way. Ideally, we would like to be able to conclude that treatment of a specific component of cognitive processing would help all patients with damage to that component. Unfortunately, such conclusions are not possible in light of our current levels of theory. As noted previously, we have no way of knowing how any specific mechanisms are actually modified by our interventions (see Baddeley, 1993 and Hillis, 2005 for discussion). Thus, the observation that a "semantic" approach was associated with improved naming in a patient with a semantic deficit does not directly imply that all patients with semantic deficits will show improved naming with that treatment. Earlier studies have shown that sometimes patients with putatively "the same" locus of impairment do not respond to the same treatment approach, but different approaches have been beneficial for individuals, and sometimes patients with different loci of damage in the lexical system respond to the same treatment (Fridrikson et al., 2005; Hillis, 1993; Hillis & Caramazza, 1994; Rapp, 2005). This finding is not unexpected, since the characteristics of the patient and the form of impairment at any given level of processing that may influence treatment outcomes have yet to be precisely defined. Although studies have identified recovery as a function of a variety of individual factors, these studies have not been integrated with (a) the specific cognitive mechanisms that are impaired in the patient, and (b) the cognitive mechanisms that might be influenced by the treatment.

This inability to predict whether a particular patient will benefit from a given treatment strategy is certainly not specific to the approach described in this chapter, which relies on a cognitive analysis of patient performance, but applies equally to other "schools" of treatment.

In summary, cognitive neuropsychological models of specific language tasks are useful for understanding the nature of impairment consequent to brain damage in individual patients but do not constitute a theory of language rehabilitation. The latter would require motivated hypotheses about how mental representations or transformations are modified, how particular interventions bring about these modifications, and how particular patient characteristics influence response to treatment. Moreover, a theory of rehabilitation would need to specify the interactions among these variables, in order to make predictions about results of a given treatment approach. Nevertheless, the following chapters illustrate how cognitive neuropsychological models can be useful in planning and designing individualized therapy, selecting stimuli, and predicting patterns of generalization across tasks or stimulus types.

INTRODUCTION TO THE CHAPTERS IN THIS SECTION

Scope of the Section

There has been no attempt to cover every domain of cognition in this section, nor even every domain of language. Instead, we have chosen to include chapters on those domains that have received the most attention in the cognitive neuropsychological literature. Therefore, there are chapters on spoken-word comprehension and naming, written-word comprehension and production (reading and writing), and sentence comprehension and production. Perhaps as a consequence of the number of studies in these areas, the models in these domains are the most clearly articulated and most widely (although not universally) accepted. Although each chapter will discuss models of tasks limited to that domain (e.g., a model of the cognitive processes underlying reading), it is important to understand that there is a great deal of overlap in the cognitive representations and processes that underlie reading, writing, naming, and word and sentence comprehension and production. For example, as discussed in the case of HG, it is likely that a single set of phonologic representations (a phonologic output lexicon) is accessed in the course of all tasks that have spoken-word output: oral reading, oral naming, repetition, oral sentence production, and spoken conversation. Similarly, a single semantic system is engaged in a variety of tasks that involve comprehension and/or production of words. Therefore, identifying the patient's problem in oral naming may require assessment of oral reading, comprehension, written naming, and so on. It is probably never possible to be sure of the level of damage by assessing performance on only one task.

It is also crucial to note that other cognitive abilities, such as attention and memory, are engaged in every language task. Impairments of sustained attention, selective attention, spatial attention, and/or short- or long-term memory can affect performance on any given language task. Although there are models and theories of each of these areas, we have not addressed them, since the focus of this book is on language intervention. Other important domains that have received much attention in the psychological literature are procedural and episodic memory, and the so-called "executive functions" such as planning, judgment, organization (sequencing, switching and maintaining tasks, etc.). Investigations in these domains have not yielded the types of models of specific component cognitive representations of the type we are considering in these chapters. Nevertheless, awareness of deficits in these areas is often helpful in understanding patients' responses or failure of response to particular treatment strategies.

Content of the Chapters

In Chapter 23, Anastasia Raymer and Leslie Gonzalez Rothi describe clinical diagnosis and treatment of spoken-word comprehension and production. They identify impairments at different levels of cognitive processing that result in poor auditory word comprehension and/or poor oral naming. The authors further report rehabilitation strategies that rely on this type of diagnosis, made in view of a cognitive neuropsychological model of word comprehension and naming. In Chapter 24, Charlotte Mitchum and Rita Berndt discuss evaluation and rehabilitation of sentence comprehension and production based on cognitive neuropsychological models of sentence processing. They focus on issues of the relationship between theory and therapy and issues of generalization. Finally, in Chapter 25, Pelagie Beeson and Maya Henry describe how to identify an individual patient's underlying deficit in comprehension or production of written words. This chapter focuses on assessment and treatment of reading and spelling at the single-word level, and shows how treatment can generalize to improved reading and spelling in untrained tasks.

FUTURE TRENDS

This section illustrates the integration of speech-language pathology with cognitive neuropsychology and behavioral neurology (the three disciplines represented by the chapter authors). The authors have been involved in integrative research centers in Gainesville, Tucson, and Baltimore. Other excellent interdisciplinary centers for aphasia research and rehabilitation exist in Philadelphia, Ann Arbor, and Pittsburgh in the United States, and in Belgium (the Brussels Neuropsychological Rehabilitation Unit), the United Kingdom, Italy, the Netherlands, France, Germany, and Australia (see Appendix 22-1 for contact person and names of several such centers). Many centers are also collaborating with other disciplines in the field of cognitive science, such as artificial intelligence, linguistics, and neuroscience. For example, interdisciplinary collaboration at Moss Rehabilitation, Temple University, Carnegie Mellon, and elsewhere have led to the development of computational models of naming that have been useful in understanding various forms of naming impairment (e.g., Dell et al., 1997b). It is expected that such collaborations are only a hint of what may come. Several authors have predicted that computational models of language may become important in directing rehabilitation as well (Plaut, 1996). Certainly, computational models are helping us to understand learning and recovery, two crucial aspects of rehabilitation. Functional imaging techniques (such as functional magnetic resonance imaging [fMRI], positron emission tomography [PET], magnetic resonance perfusion, and spectroscopy) have been used in many studies to shed light on physiologic aspects of learning and recovery. Perhaps more importantly, anticipated advances in cognitive neuroscience in understanding how the brain recovers through reorganization of neural representations (Hillis, 2005; Jenkins & Merzenich, 1987; Jenkins, Merzenich, & Recanzone, 1990), and how the brain changes with learning, through changes in neural synaptic strength and genetic expression (Kandel, Schwartz, & Jessell, 1995), will surely contribute to developing an interdisciplinary theory of aphasia rehabilitation.

▶ *Acknowledgments*—This work was supported in part by NIH grant RO1 DC05375. The author is grateful to Pelagie Beeson, Charlotte Mitchum, Roberta Chapey, Anastasia Raymer, and Leslie Gonzalez Rothi for helpful comments on an earlier draft.

KEY POINTS

Chapters 23 to 25 will illustrate how therapy for a particular patient with aphasia can be guided by pinpointing his or her impairment to one more components of a model of the cognitive processes underlying the specific language task to be treated. This approach to intervention has its foundations in the fields of cognitive neuropsychology, speech-language pathology, and behavioral neurology.

1. Most strategies utilized are not truly model-based interventions, since the strategies themselves rely more on clinical intuitions and experience than on the model of the language task to be treated.
2. Reference to a model of the task being treated often allows the therapist to understand when, how, and why a particular therapy procedure is likely to have an effect on performance.
3. Models can also sometimes help us to understand why therapy "works" for some individuals with aphasia and not for others.
4. Future developments through cooperative efforts in these fields, as well as in other areas of cognitive neuroscience, may further guide our models and our therapies.

References

Baddeley, A. (1993). A theory of rehabilitation without a model of learning is a vehicle without an engine: A comment on Caramazza and Hillis. *Neuropsychological Rehabilitation, 3*, 235–244.

Ballard, K. J., & Thompson, C. K. (1999). Treatment and generalization of complex sentence production in agrammatism. *Journal of Speech, Language, and Hearing Research, 42*, 690–707.

Beeson, P. M. (1999). Treating acquired writing impairment. *Aphasiology, 13*, 367–386.

Beeson, P. M., & Hirsch, F. M. (1998). *Writing treatment for severe aphasia.* Presentation at the Annual Convention of the American Speech-Language-Hearing Association. San Antonio, TX: November.

Beeson, P. M., Rewega, M., Vail, S., & Rapcsak, S. Z. (2000). Problem-solving approach to agraphia treatment: Interactive use of lexical and sublexical spelling routes. *Aphasiology, 14*, 551–565.

Behrmann, M., & Lieberthal, T. (1989). Category-specific treatment of a lexical-semantic deficit: A single case study of global aphasia. *British Journal of Communication Disorders, 24*, 281–299.

Berndt, R., & Mitchum, C. (1994). Approaches to the rehabilitation of "phonological assembly": Elaborating the model of non-lexical reading. In G. W. Humphreys & M. J. Riddoch (Eds.), *Cognitive neuropsychology and cognitive rehabilitation* (pp. 503–526).

Byng, S., & Coltheart, M. (1986). Aphasia therapy research: Methodological requirements and illustrative results. In E. Hjelmquist & L.-G. Nilsson (Eds.), *Communication handicap: Aspects of psychological compensation and technical aids.* (pp.191–213). North-Holland: Elsevier Science Publishers B.V.

Caramazza, A. (1989). Cognitive neuropsychology and rehabilitation: An unfulfilled promise? In T. Seron & G. DeLoche (Eds.), *Cognitive approaches in rehabilitation* (pp. 383–398). Hillsdale, NJ: LEA.

Caramazza, A., & Hillis, A. E. (1990). Where do semantic errors come from? *Cortex, 26*, 95–122.

Caramazza, A., & Hillis, A. E. (1991). For a theory of remediation of cognitive deficits. *Neuropsychological Rehabilitation, 3*, 217–234.

Carlomagno, S., Iavarone, A., & Colombo, A. (1994). Cognitive approaches to writing rehabilitation. In M. J. Riddoch & G. Humphreys (Eds.), *Cognitive neuropsychology and cognitive rehabilitation* (pp. 485–502). London: Lawrence Erlbaum Associates.

Coltheart, M., Patterson, K., & Marshall, J. C. (1980). *Deep dyslexia.* London: Routeledge and Kegan Paul.

DeLeon, J., Gottesman, R. F., Kleinman, J. T., Neunart, M., Davis, C., Lee, A., Hillis, A. E. (2007) Neural regions essential for distinct cognitive processes underlying picture naming. *Brain, 130*, 1408–22.

Dell, G. S., Burger, L. K., Svec, W. R. (1997a). Language production and serial order: A functional analysis and a model. *Psychological Review, 104*(1), 123–147.

Dell, G. S, Schwartz, M. E., Martin, N., Saffran, E. M., & Gagnon, D. A. (1997b). Lexical access in aphasic and nonaphasic speakers. *Psychological Review, 104*, 801–838.

de Partz, M. P. (1986). Re-education of a deep dyslexic patient: Rationale of the method and results. *Cognitive Neuropsychology, 3*, 149–177.

Ellis, A. W. (1982). Spelling and writing (and reading and speaking). In A. W. Ellis (Ed.), *Normality and pathology in cognitive functions* (pp. 113–146). London: Academic Press.

Ellis, A. W., Miller, D., & Sin G. (1983). Wernicke's aphasia and normal language processing: A case study in cognitive neuropsychology. *Cognition, 15,* 111–114.

Fink, R. B., Brecher, A., Sobel, P., Schwartz, M. (2005). Computer-assisted treatment of word retrieval deficits in aphasia. *Aphasiology, 19*(10/11), 943–954.

Fridriksson, J., Holland, A. L., Coull, B., Plante, E., Trouard, T., & Beeson, P. (2005). Spaced retrieval treatment of anomia. *Aphasiology, 19*(2), 99–109.

Friedman, R. B., & Lott, S. N. (1996). Phonologic treatment for deep dyslexia using bigraphs instead of graphemes. *Brain and Language, 72*(3), 219–237.

Friedman, R. B., & Lott, S. N. (2002). Successful blending in a phonologic reading treatment for deep dyslexia. *Aphasiology, 16*(3), 355–372.

Friedman, R. B., Lott, S. N., & Sample, D. M. (1998). A reorganization approach to treating phonological alexia. *Brain and Language, 65,* 196–198.

Friedman, R. B., Sample, D. M., & Lott, S. N. (2000). The role of level of representation in the use of paired associate learning for rehabilitation of alexia. *Neuropsychologia, 40,* 223–234.

Garrett, M. F. (1980). Levels of processing in sentence production. In B. Butterworth (Ed.), *Language production* (Vol. 1). New York: Academic Press.

Gonzalez-Rothi, L., & Moss, S. (October, 1989). *Alexia without agraphia: A model-driven therapy.* Paper presented at Academy of Aphasia, Santa Fe, NM.

Goodglass, H., & Kaplan, E. (1972). *The Boston Diagnostic Aphasia Examination.* Philadelphia, PA: Lea & Febiger.

Goodman, R. A., & Caramazza, A. (1986). Phonologically plausible errors: Implications for a model of the phoneme-grapheme conversion mechanism in the spelling process. In G. Augst (Ed.), *Proceedings of the international colloquium on graphemics and orthography* (pp. 300–325). New York: Walter de Gruyter.

Goodman-Schulman, R. A., Sokol, S., Aliminosa, D., & McCloskey, M. (October, 1990). *Remediation of acquired dysgraphia as a technique for evaluating models of spelling.* Paper presented at the Academy of Aphasia, Baltimore, MD.

Hatfield, M. F. (1983). Aspects of acquired dysgraphia and implications for re-education. In C. Code & D. J. Muller (Eds.), *Aphasia therapy* (pp. 157–169). London: Edward Arnold.

Hier, D. B., & Mohr, J. P. (1977). Incongruous oral and written naming. *Brain and Language, 4,* 115–126.

Hillis, A., & Caramazza, A. (1992). The reading process and its disorders. In D. I. Margolin (Ed.), *Cognitive neuropsychology in clinical practice* (pp. 229–261). Oxford: University Press.

Hillis, A. E. (1989). Efficacy and generalization of treatment for aphasic naming errors. *Archives of Physical Medicine and Rehabilitation, 70,* 632–636.

Hillis, A. E. (1990). Effects of a separate treatments for distinct impairments within the naming process. In T. Prescott (Ed.), *Clinical aphasiology* (Vol. 19, pp. 255–265). Austin, TX: Pro-Ed.

Hillis, A. E. (1993). The role of models of language processing in rehabilitation of language impairments. *Aphasiology, 7,* 5–26.

Hillis, A. E. (1994). Contributions from cognitive analyses. In R. Chapey (Ed.), *Language intervention strategies in adult aphasia* (3rd ed., pp. 207–219). Baltimore: Williams and Wilkins.

Hillis, A. E. (1998). Treatment of naming disorders: New issues regarding old therapies. *Journal of the International Neuropsychological Society, 4,* 648–660.

Hillis, A. E. (2005). For a theory of cognitive rehabilitation: Progress in the decade of the brain. In P. W. Halligan & D. T. Wade (Eds.), *Effectiveness of rehabilitation for cognitive deficits* (1st ed., pp. 271–279). Oxford: Oxford Press.

Hillis, A. E., & Caramazza, A. (1987). Model-driven treatment of dysgraphia. In R. H. Brookshire (Ed.), *Clinical aphasiology, 1987* (pp. 84–105). Minneapolis: BRK.

Hillis, A. E., & Caramazza, A. (1994). Theories of lexical processing and theories of rehabilitation. In M. J. Riddoch & G. Humphreys (Eds.), *Cognitive neuropsychology and cognitive rehabilitation* (pp. 449–484). Hove: LEA.

Hillis, A. E., & Caramazza, A. (1995). Converging evidence for the interaction of semantic and phonological information in accessing lexical information for spoken output. *Cognitive Neuropsychology, 12,* 187–227.

Hillis, A. E., & Heidler, J. (2005). Contributions and limitations of the cognitive neuropsychological approach to treatment: Illustrations from studies of reading and spelling therapy. *Aphasiology, 19*(10/11), 985–993.

Hillis Trupe, A. E. (1986). Effectiveness of retraining phoneme to grapheme conversion. In R. H. Brookshire (Ed.), *Clinical aphasiology, 1986* (pp. 163–171). Minneapolis: BRK.

Hinckley, J. J., Patterson, J., & Carr, T. H. (1999, June). *Differential effects of context- and skill-based treatment approaches: Preliminary findings.* Paper presented at Clinical Aphasiology Conference, Key West, FL.

Holland, A. (1980). *Communicative Abilities in Daily Living (CADL).* Baltimore, MD: University Park Press.

Howard, D., Patterson, K., Franklin, S., Orchard-Lisle, V., & Morton, J. (1985). The facilitation of picture naming in aphasia. *Cognitive Neuropsychology, 2,* 42–80.

Humphreys, G. W., Riddoch, M. J., & Quinlan, P. T. (1988). Cascade processes in picture identification. *Cognitive Neuropsychology, 5,* 67–104.

Jenkins, W. M., & Merzenich, M. M. (1987). Reorganization of neocortical representations after brain injury: A neurophysiological model of the bases of recovery from stroke. In F. J. Seil & B. M. Carlson (Eds.), *Progress in brain research, 71* (pp. 249–266).

Jenkins, W. M., Merzenich, M. M., & Recanzone, G. (1990). Neocortical representational dynamics in adult primates: Implications for neuropsychology. *Neuropsychologia, 28,* 573–584.

Kandel, E. R., Schwartz, J. H., & Jessell, T. M. (1995). *Essentials of neural science and behavior.* Stamford, CT: Appleton and Lange.

Kiran, S., & Thompson, C. K. (2002). Typicality of category exemplars in aphasia: Evidence from reaction time and treatment data. *Brain and Language, 79,* 27–31.

Kiran, S., & Thompson, C. K. (2003). The role of semantic complexity in treatment of naming: Training semantic categories in fluent aphasia by controlling exemplar typicality. *Journal of Speech, Language and Hearing Research, 46,* 773–787.

Linebaugh, C. (1983). Treatment of anomic aphasia. In C. Perkins (Ed.), *Current therapies for communication disorders: Language handicaps in adults.* (pp. 181–189). New York: Thieme-Stratton.

Martin, N., Lane, M., & Harley, T. A. (2003). How can connectionist cognitive models of language inform models of language rehabilitation? In A. E. Hillis (Ed.), *Handbook of adult language disorders: Integrating cognitive neuropsychology, neurology, and rehabilitation* (pp. 375–396). Philadelphia: Psychology Press.

McNeil, M. R., Matunis, M., Just, M., Carpenter, P., Haarman, H., Rosenblatt, H., et al. (1999, June). Paper presented at Clinical Aphasiology Conference, Key West, FL.

Patterson, K., Graham, M., & Hodges, J. (1994). The impact of semantic memory loss on phonological representations. *Journal of Cognitive Neuroscience, 6,* 57–69.

Patterson, K. E., Coltheart, M., & Marshall, J. C. (1985). *Surface dyslexia.* London: LEA.

Plaut, D. (1996). Relearning after damage in connectionist networks: Toward a theory of rehabilitation. Brain and Language, 52, 25–82.

Plaut, D., & Shallice, T. (1993). Deep dyslexia: A case study of connectionist neuropsychology. *Cognitive Neuropsychology, 10,* 377–500.

Rapp, B. (2005). The relationship between treatment outcomes and the underlying cognitive deficit: Evidence from the remediation of aquired dysgraphia. Aphasiology, *19*(10/11), 994–1008.

Rapp, B., & Goldrick, M. (2004). Feedback by any other name is still interactivity: A reply to Roelofs. *Psychological Review, 111*(2), 573–578.

Raymer, A. M., Thompson, C. K., Jacobs, B., & LeGrand, H. R. (1993). Phonological treatment of naming deficits in aphasia: Model-based generalization analysis. *Aphasiology, 7,* 27–53.

Schwartz, M. (1998, October). *Psycholinguistic theory and aphasia rehabilitation: When worlds collide.* Paper presented at Academy of Aphasia, Santa Fe, NM.

Seidenberg, M & McClelland, J. L. (1989). A distributed, developmental model of visual word recognition and naming. *Psychological Review, 96*(4), 523–568.

Thompson, C., & Kearns, K. (1981). Experimental analysis of acquisititon and generalization of naming behaviors in a patient with anomia. In R. H. Brookshire (Ed.), *Clinical aphasiology: Conference* (Vol. 10, pp. 35–45).

Thompson, C. K., Raymer, A., & le Grand, H. (1991). Effects of phonologically based treatment on aphasic naming deficits: A model-driven approach. In T. Prescott (Ed.), *Clinical aphasiology,* Vol. 20, pp. 239–259). Austin, TX: Pro-Ed.

Thompson, C. K., & Shapiro, L. P. (1995). Training sentence production in agrammatism: Implications for normal and disordered language. *Brain and Language, 50,* 201–224.

Thompson, C. K., & Shapiro, L. P. (2005). Treating agrammatic aphasia within a linguistic framework: Treatment of underlying forms. *Aphasiology, 19*(10/11), 1021–1036.

Thompson, C. K., Shapiro, L. P., Ballard, K. J., Jacobs, B. J., & Tait, M. E. (1997). Training and generalized production of wh- and NP-movement structures in agrammatic aphasia. *Journal of Speech, Language, and Hearing Research, 40,* 228–244.

Thompson, C. K., Shapiro, L. P., Tait, M. E., Jacobs, B. J., Schneider, S. L. (1996). Training wh-question production in agrammatic aphasia: Analysis of argument and adjunct movement. *Brain and Language, 52*(1), 175–228.

Wilson, B. A., & Patterson, K. E. (1990). Rehabilitation and cognitive neuropsychology. *Applied Cognitive Psychology, 4,* 247–260.

Yorkston, K., & Beukelman, D. (1980). An analysis of connected speech samples of aphasic and normal speakers. *Journal of Speech and Hearing Disorders, 45,* 27–36.

APPENDIX 22.1
Selected Interdisciplinary Centers for Aphasia Research and Rehabilitation

Name and Location	Contact Person, Telephone, e-mail Address
Aphasia Research Center Boston VA Medical Center Boston University Medical School 150 South Huntington Ave. Boston, MA 02130 USA	Martin L. Albert, M.D. (617) 232-9500 malbert@bu.edu
The Aphasia Research Center Moss Rehabilitation Hospital 1200 W. Tabor Road Philadelphia, PA 19141 USA	Myrna Schwartz, Ph.D. Ruth Fink, Ph.D. (215) 456-9605 mschwar@vm.temple.edu

Birkbeck College
Department of Psychology
University of London
Malet Street
London WC1E 7HX
UK

Wendy Best, Ph.D.
w.best@psych.bbk.ac.uk

Clinical Communication Studies
City University
Northampton Square
London EC1V 0HB
UK

Sally Byng, Ph.D.
0171-477-8000
s.c.byng@city.ac.uk

Georgetown Institute for Cognitive and
    Computational Sciences

Georgetown University Medical Center
3970 Reservoir Rd. NW
Washington, DC 20007
USA

Rhoda Friedman, Ph.D.
(202) 784-4134
rfried01@medlib.georgetown.edu

Instituto di Scienze Neurologiche
Universita Degli Studi di Napoli
I Facolta Di Medicina E Chirurgia
80131 Napoli
Via Pansini 5
Italy

Sergio Carlomagno, Ph.D.

National Center for Neurogenic
    Communication Disorders
University of Arizona
Tuscon, AZ 85721-0071
USA

Audrey Holland, Ph.D.
Pelagie Beeson, Ph.D.
(520) 621-9878
Pelagie@u.arizona.edu

School of Behavioural Sciences
Macquaire University
Sydney, New South Wales 2109
Australia

Max Coltheart, Ph.D.
Lyndsey Nickels, Ph.D.
612-9850-8448
lyndsey@frogmouth.bhs.mq.edu.au

VA RR&D Brain Rehabilitation
    Research Center-151A
Gainesville VA Medical Center
Gainesville, FL 32608
USA

Leslie Gonzalez Rothi, Ph.D.
(904) 376-1611
Gonazlj@medicine.ufl.edu

APPENDIX 22.2
Glossary

Behavioral neurology—branch of neurology devoted to understanding the neural mechanisms of behavior and cognition.

Cognitive neuropsychology—branch of psychology devoted to understanding normal cognitive processes through the study of people who have sustained brain damage.

Computational model—computer simulation of a particular task.

Lexical processing—mental representations and processes involved in comprehension and production of single words in various modalities.

Orthographic representation—stored spelling of a word.

Phonological representation—stored "sound" of a word.

Semantic representation—stored meaning of a word.

Chapter 23

Impairments of Word Comprehension and Production

Anastasia M. Raymer and
Leslie J. Gonzalez Rothi

OBJECTIVES

The objectives of this chapter are to describe a model of lexical processing that represents the mechanisms involved in word comprehension and production; delineate impairments in lexical comprehension and production with respect to breakdown of the mechanisms of lexical processing; review evidence for clinical application of this model for assessment, recovery, and treatment of lexical impairments; and consider the limitations and future trends in the use of lexical models in the clinical setting.

DEFINITION

Impairments of word comprehension and, in particular, word retrieval, are pervasive among patients with acquired aphasia (Goodglass, Kaplan, & Barresi, 2001). The nature of the lexical impairments, most often tested in constrained picture-recognition and naming paradigms, vary among patients in terms of their cognitive and neural bases. Traditional methods of aphasia-syndrome classification are usually insufficient to distinguish the mechanisms of lexical failure that occur among patients with aphasia—differences that may influence treatment decisions for those patients (Nickels, 2002; Raymer, Rothi, & Greenwald, 1995). An alternative approach to characterize the diverse lexical impairments that patients may display has its foundation in cognitive neuropsychology (CN) (Coltheart, 2001; Hillis, 2001), the study of brain-impaired individuals to provide evidence for theories of cognitive processing, including language. In the past two decades, much research has transpired using the CN approach as a backdrop to clinical

assessment and treatment of impairments related to lexical comprehension and production.

MODEL OF LEXICAL PROCESSING

Figure 23–1 depicts a model of lexical processing that forms the basis for this discussion of lexical impairments for spoken words. Recent years have seen an evolution in the structure and functioning of lexical models toward a more computational approach, such as that described by Nadeau and Rothi (see Chapter 19). Nonetheless, cognitive neuropsychological models, as shown in Figure 23–1, have served as a backdrop to a large clinical literature examining lexical impairments in aphasia, and will form the basis for this discussion of assessment and treatment of lexical impairments. Although the details vary to some extent across versions of such models, the fundamental components are similar (e.g., Goldrick & Rapp, 2007; Hillis, 2001; Lambon Ralph, Moriarty, & Sage, 2002; Nickels, 2001). The model includes a complex system of distributed and interconnected modules that allow for processing of different types of lexical information in cascade fashion (Chialant, Costa, & Caramazza, 2002). The activation of peripheral sensory structures with some form of sensory input, such as spoken or written words or viewed objects, triggers cognitive mechanisms in the central nervous system to recognize, conceptualize, and respond to that input. Subsequently, peripheral motor processes allow for planning and executing a response to the stimulus in the form of speech, writing, or gesture. The focus of this chapter is on the mechanisms involved in processing spoken words, so the description will center on the central mechanisms critical for lexical phonologic processing. In addition, because lexical tasks often incorporate visual stimuli, we will also briefly consider the mechanism responsible for object recognition.

To acquire skill in any behavior implies that the person is more efficient in the production of that behavior than in the production of less-skilled behaviors. The central nervous system can increase efficiency by storing memories based on previous exposure to a stimulus such that subsequent pro-

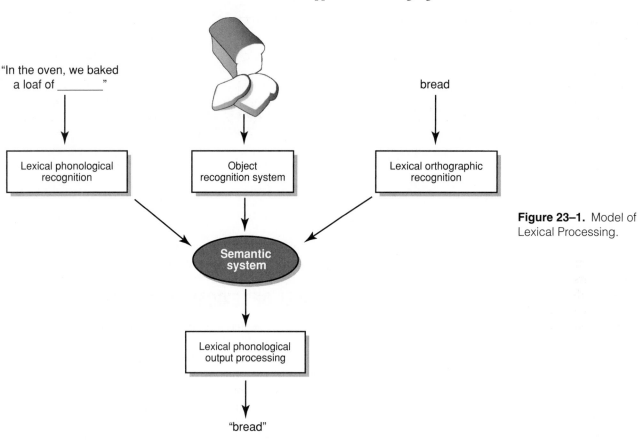

Figure 23–1. Model of Lexical Processing.

cessing experiences with that information can be expedited (Rothi, Raymer, Maher, Greenwald, & Morris, 1991). The model of lexical processing shown in Figure 23-1 indicates that lexical abilities are dependent upon the integrity of a number of different types of stored representations. We will review the mechanisms that make up this complex system and the types of impairments that we might observe associated with dysfunction of these mechanisms. Finally, we will mention the neurologic site of lesion often associated with dysfunction of the lexical mechanisms to suggest neural regions that mediate aspects of lexical processing.

Recognition Level Mechanisms

Following early sensory processing, stimulus-recognition processes allow for activation of representations that closely correspond to the input stimulus. Recognition represents the point at which a stimulus is identified as familiar compared to other physically similar stimuli (Tyler, 1987). It allows the individual to say "yes" when asked whether a stimulus is a familiar object or word. It does not yet allow the individual to state what that object or word means. Recognition processes provide a processing advantage that allows us to react quickly to whatever form the stimulus exemplar may take. For example, if the word is spoken with

an accent or written in an unusual font, or if an object is viewed from an unusual orientation, stimulus-recognition mechanisms allow for the quick realization that the stimulus is familiar in spite of input perturbations.

A number of lines of evidence support the notion that recognition-level processes are modality specific (Hillis, 2001), that is, that separate components represent knowledge for different types of familiar sensory stimuli (Fig. 23-1). The phonologic and orthographic lexical recognition stages represent stores of familiar spoken and written words, respectively. The object-recognition system stores memories of familiar objects. Other mechanisms for processing in other sensory modalities, such as visual gestures, touch, or smell, also may exist.

Visual Object Recognition

Impairments related to visual object representations will affect performance in lexical tasks that require the patient also to process viewed objects. For example, on clinical examination, patients may be impaired in picture-naming, and they may have difficulty in word-to-picture matching tasks that test comprehension. In contrast, the same patient may be able to name in response to other sensory inputs, such as spoken definitions, or to demonstrate comprehension with printed word-to-word matching tasks. That is, difficulty may occur only when visual stimuli are incorporated in the task.

Impairments may take different forms depending upon which stage of object processing is affected (Farah, 1990; Riddoch & Humphreys, 2001). "Agnosia" is the term used for failure (as a result of brain damage) to recognize a sensory stimulus, such failure not being attributable to dysfunction of peripheral sensory mechanisms. Dysfunction of early visual processes involved in developing a percept for the viewed object, prior to activation of visual object representations, may lead to apperceptive or integrative forms of visual agnosia (Lissauer, 1890/1988; Riddoch & Humphreys, 2001; Warrington & Taylor, 1978). These patients, who have adequate visual acuity, may be unable to copy a line drawing or even to match simple drawings. However, their stored object knowledge appears to be intact as they may be able to answer questions about the visual characteristics of named objects in visual imagery tasks. Patients with impairment of visual object representations have a form of visual associative agnosia (Riddoch & Humphreys, 2001), in which they can perform tasks dependent upon early visual processes such as matching line drawings or copying figures. Errors in naming may include visual misperceptions (e.g., "pen" for "dart"), or failures to respond ('I don't know') (Farah, 1990). Patients may be impaired in tasks requiring knowledge of the structure of a visual stimulus, such as distinguishing familiar from nonsense objects (visual object decision), drawing from memory, or answering questions about the visual characteristics of objects.

A phenomenon often discussed in the realm of visual object agnosia is optic aphasia, in which patients also experience naming failure restricted to the visual modality (modality-specific). They may, however, be able to describe the function of viewed objects, sort objects into categories, or gesture the appropriate use for the objects they are unable to name, arguing against visual agnosia in which meaning for viewed objects is not appreciated. One interpretation of optic aphasia is that it represents a visual-to-semantic access impairment in which visual object representations are unable to activate full semantic representations corresponding to the viewed objects (Hillis & Caramazza, 1995a, 1995b; Marsh & Hillis, 2005; Riddoch & Humphreys, 1987d). Thereby, some semantic information is available regarding a picture for the patient to sort by category or to provide an appropriate gesture, but the full semantic representation must be activated for accurate picture-naming to occur.

Several papers that have analyzed lesions in patients with visual agnosia and optic aphasia suggest brain regions critical for the neural representation of object knowledge (Iorio, Falanga, Fragassi, & Grossi, 1992; James, Culham, Humphrey, Milner, & Goodale, 2003; Marsh & Hillis, 2005; Schnider, Benson, & Scharre, 1994). Although bilateral-

posterior cerebral cortex lesions were commonly reported, researchers have also described visual associative agnosia in patients with unilateral left-posterior mesial cortex infarctions. Schnider and colleagues proposed that patients with visual agnosia tend to have less damage to the splenium of the corpus callosum, and apparently access and employ the impaired left-posterior hemisphere, which is a critical region for object recognition. Patients with optic aphasia, in contrast, have more extensive splenial lesions, preventing access to the damaged left hemisphere, and presumably must rely on the right hemisphere's contribution to visual and semantic processing (Coslett & Saffran, 1989, 1992; Raymer, Greenwald, Richardson, Rothi, & Heilman, 1997).

Phonologic Recognition

Damage affecting phonologic lexical recognition (Fig. 23-1) leads to impairments in any tasks that require patients to process spoken words, such as auditory word-to-picture matching tasks, naming to spoken definitions, or gesturing to verbal commands. Some general parallels may be seen between the impairments of object processing and phonologic lexical processing as represented in patients with pure word deafness (Boatman, 2002; Franklin, 1989; Polster & Rose, 1998; Vignolo, 1982). Some patients seem to have a pre-lexical impairment that affects processing of phonemic and other types of acoustic stimuli (Buchman, Garron, Trost-Cardmone, Wichter, & Schwartz, 1986; Buchtel & Stewart, 1989), similar to apperceptive visual impairments. In contrast, some patients reported with Wernicke's aphasia seem to have impairments of the phonologic lexicon as represented by modality-specific auditory comprehension impairment (Ellis, Miller, & Sin, 1983; Hillis, Boatman, Hart, & Gordon, 1999; Semenza, Cipolotti, & Denes, 1992). Because the reported patients had retained comprehension for written material, semantic processing was judged to be intact and the auditory comprehension impairment presumably related to presemantic, phonologic lexical processing. Some early theories had proposed that the processing of the orthographic word forms occurred subsequent to phonologic activation (Caplan, 1993), a dependency that leads to the prediction that patients with phonologic recognition dysfunction should also have impaired reading comprehension. Thereby, patients with selective impairment for phonologic input in the face of intact reading comprehension provide evidence for distinct input mechanisms for orthographic and phonologic lexical processing.

The phonologic correlate of optic aphasia may be represented in some patients with word-meaning deafness (Francis, Riddoch, & Humphreys, 2001; Kohn & Friedman, 1986). For example, one report described a patient who could process the phonologic components of words as indicated by preserved ability to discriminate and repeat words, and to perform auditory lexical decision, which presumably depends upon the integrity of phonologic input representations (Franklin, Turner, Ralph, Morris, & Bailey, 1996). Although the patient demonstrated intact reading comprehension, he had difficulty in auditory-comprehension tasks, particularly for abstract, low-frequency words. Franklin and colleagues attributed the failure to an impairment in activating the full semantic specification for spoken words, an argument similar to that proposed for optic aphasia.

Some studies have described the neural correlates of phonologic lexical recognition impairments. Individuals with pure word deafness typically have bilateral temporal or subcortical left-hemisphere lesions affecting input to Wernicke's area (Polster & Rose, 1998), suggesting that these regions are important for prelexical stages of phonologic processing. Cases of Wernicke's aphasia associated with left-posterior perisylvian lesions, including Wernicke's area, (Kertesz, Lau, & Polk., 1993; Weiller et al., 1995) may be characterized by an impairment of phonologic recognition. Therefore, it appears that the posterior portion of the left superior temporal cortex is a critical neural region subserving phonologic lexical knowledge.

Semantic Processing

Once a recognition-level representation achieves sufficient activation, it initiates activity in the semantic system (Fig. 23-1). Semantic representations contain stored knowledge shared by speakers of a language, including meanings for words, objects, or actions. The lexical model incorporates a unitary semantic system that can be accessed from any input modality and can access any output mode as appropriate. Semantic representations presumably involve a network of information about words, objects, and ideas that includes superordinate, coordinate, associated, and subordinate relationships. Discussion in cognitive neuropsychology continues regarding the structure of the semantic system (Funnell, 2000). Some proposals view semantic representations as modality-independent in that a single unitary semantic system provides meaning for a stimulus, regardless of input modality or output mode (Chialant et al., 2002; Hillis, Rapp, Romani, & Caramazza, 1990; Shelton & Caramazza, 2001). A contrasting view holds that the semantic system is structured into subsystems for different sensory information and knowledge systems, such as verbal semantics and visual semantics (Allport, 1985; Paivio, 1986; Saffran, 1997; Shallice, 1988).

A patient with a semantic impairment will have difficulty performing any tasks that require semantic mediation, including comprehension of spoken and written words, interpreting the meanings of objects and gestures, and spoken and written picture-naming. Performance in oral word-reading and writing to dictation may also be affected if alternative sublexical letter-sound conversion mechanisms are unavailable for decoding or encoding written words. If the unitary semantics system proposal is correct, the performance of individuals with semantic system impairment should demonstrate quantitatively and qualitatively similar impairments across lexical tasks. Researchers have described this association of impairments in some patients with vascular lesions (Hillis et al., 1990; Howard & Orchard-Lisle, 1984) and progressive neurologic impairments (Chertkow, Bub, & Seidenberg, 1989; Hodges & Patterson, 1996; Lambon Ralph, Ellis, & Franklin, 1995; Raymer & Berndt, 1996).

Researchers have also described individuals with aphasia whose naming and comprehension impairments fractionate, demonstrating selective preservation or impairment for specific semantic categories. Patients have demonstrated impairments for categories such as living and non-living things (Laiacona, Capitani, & Caramazza, 2003; Rosazza, Imbornone, Zorzi, Farina, Chiavari, & Cappa, 2003; Silveri, Gainotti, Perani, Cappelletti, Carbone, & Faxio, 1997; Warrington & McCarthy, 1983); fruits and vegetables (Farah & Wallace, 1992; Hart, Berndt, & Caramazza, 1985); tools (Ochipa, Rothi, & Heilman, 1989); and animals (Caramazza & Shelton, 1998; Ferreira, Giusiano, & Poncet, 1997; Hart & Gordon, 1992; Hillis & Caramazza, 1991). At first, one might use these unusual dissociations to infer that the semantic system is structured in a fashion that represents these specific categories of knowledge. Warrington and her colleagues (Warrington & McCarthy, 1983, 1987, 1994; Warrington & Shallice, 1984) attributed semantic category dissociations to the type of semantic information that is a defining characteristic for that category. They propose that category-specific deficits arise because the semantic system is structured along lines of sensory modalities and output modes in a complex network of subsystems (Allport, 1985; Saffran, 1997). Disruption of selective subsystems leads to impairments that affect semantic categories for which that subsystem contributes critical semantic information. For example, because visual semantic information may be critical for distinguishing exemplars within the category of animals, impairment of the visual semantic subsystem results in category-specific impairment for animals (Warrington & Shallice, 1984).

In contrast, Caramazza and colleagues (Caramazza, Hillis, Leek, & Miozzo, 1994; Caramazza & Shelton, 1998; Laiacona et al., 2003) have argued for a unitary semantics account of category-specific impairments. Rather, Caramazza and Shelton (1998) proposed that category-specific impairments arise because of texturing in the interconnections of properties comprising semantic representations for members of a category of objects. If critical shared properties happen to be localized in a neural region that is damaged by neurologic disease, any concepts that include those properties in their semantic representations will be affected. In particular, items within certain natural categories such as plants or animals may have a number of highly interconnected properties, making all exemplars of the category vulnerable upon neurologic injury and leading to category-specific deficits.

Regarding neural correlates of semantic-system impairments, lesion analyses in patients with semantic dysfunction provide clues as to the neural instantiation of semantic knowledge. In particular, left-hemisphere posterolateral cortical regions appear to play a critical role, as these regions are implicated in individuals with degenerative dementias leading to semantic dysfunction (Graham, Patterson, & Hodges, 1998; Hodges, Patterson, Oxbury, & Funnell, 1992; Kertesz, Davidson, & McCabe, 1998). Left posterior temporal regions also are compromised in patients with acute vascular lesions (Foundas, Daniels, & Vasterling, 1998; Hart & Gordon, 1990; Hillis et al., 2001; Hillis, Chaudhry, Davis, Kleinman, Newhart, & Heidler-Gary, 2006; Raymer, Foundas et al., 1997). In addition, the left thalamus also seems to be implicated in the complex semantic network. Transcortical sensory aphasia, a syndrome associated with semantic dysfunction, is observed in many individuals with vascular lesions affecting the left thalamic nuclei (Crosson, 1992; Raymer, Moberg, Crosson, Nadeau, & Rothi, 1997).

Neural regions associated with category-specific impairments also suggest critical regions representing specific aspects of semantic knowledge. Viral encephalitis, which has a predilection for damaging the inferior and mesial temporal cortex, has been associated with impairments for the category of living items (Warrington & Shallice, 1984). Damasio, Grabowski, Tranel, Hichwa, and Damasio (1996) investigated the location of lesions associated with impairments for three different semantic categories: (1) persons: left temporal pole lesions; (2) animals: left inferotemporal lesions; (3) tools: left temporoparietal-occipital lesions. Finally, Crosson, Moberg, Boone, Rothi, and Raymer (1997) reported a category-specific naming impairment for medical terminology associated with a left-thalamic hemorrhage. Findings from these lesion studies provide further support that damage to left-posterior temporoparietal-occipital and thalamic regions may lead to disruption of semantic processing.

Lexical Phonologic Output

Once recognition of a word or object has occurred and meaning has been activated, a response is initiated with activation of lexical representations in the output lexicons (Fig. 23-1). Evidence suggests that the output lexicons are modality-specific as there are separate stores for familiar spoken and written words as well as for gestures (Rothi, Ochipa, & Heilman, 1997). In this discussion, we focus on the mechanism for spoken words: lexical phonologic output processing. There is some indication that words are stored in phonologically similar groupings and that root morphemes are separated from affixes (e.g., "walk+" "-ed", "-ing," "-s") (Badecker &

Caramazza, 1991; De Bleser & Cholewa, 1998; Miceli & Caramazza, 1988). Word class distinctions (e.g., nouns and verbs) also appear to be represented at the level of the output lexicon (Caramazza & Miozzo, 1997; Chialant et al., 2002; Hillis, 2001). Factors such as age of acquisition and word frequency seem to exert their influence at this stage of processing (Goldrick & Rapp, 2007).

Dysfunction of lexical phonologic output processing leads to impairment in all verbal tasks that depend on the integrity of the stored phonologic representations. Patients will have difficulty in all oral naming tasks (e.g., picture-naming, name to definitions), and in oral reading, particularly for exception words (e.g., "choir," "yacht"), as sublexical grapheme-phoneme assembly processes are insufficient to derive accurate pronunciations for those words. Production errors may take a variety of forms, including semantic and phonemic paraphasias, no responses, or neologisms (Hillis, 2001), depending on the nature and severity of lexical phonologic dysfunction. Some individuals may have greater difficulty activating the output representations (Caramazza & Hillis, 1991; Le Dorze & Nespoulous, 1989; Miceli, Giustollisi, & Caramazza, 1991), leading to semantic or no-response errors. Others may have a disturbance affecting the internal structure of representations, resulting in neologistic responses (Kohn, Smith, & Alexander, 1996) or phonemic paraphasias (Ellis, Kay, & Franklin, 1992).

Researchers have inferred key features of the structure of the lexical system from observed lexical dissociations among brain-damaged patients. For example, some patients demonstrate retained auditory comprehension for words they are unable to pronounce (Kay & Ellis, 1987; Maher, Rothi, & Heilman, 1994; Nickels & Howard, 1995), a dissociation providing evidence for the input/output distinction for lexical phonologic processing. Some patients have selective impairments for phonologic production in the context of retained performance in written word spelling (Bub & Kertesz, 1982; Caramazza & Hillis, 1990), a dissociation that supports the distinction between phonologic and orthographic output stores, the latter remaining intact in some patients with phonologic output impairments. Nevertheless, it is often the case that neurologic injury affects multiple lexical mechanisms, so patients may be impaired in a variety of lexical tasks (e.g., impairments of both verbal and written output, Caramazza, Berndt, & Basili, 1983; Miceli et al., 1991; impairments of both phonologic input and output, Ellis et al., 1983, Kohn et al., 1996).

Whereas many studies of lexical retrieval impairments have focused largely on noun retrieval, other studies have also described disturbances of verb retrieval in some patients (Damasio & Tranel, 1993; Miceli, Silveri, Villa, & Caramazza, 1984; Shapiro & Caramazza, 2003; Zingeser & Berndt, 1990). Several patients have now been described who have more difficulty with nouns than verbs or with verbs than nouns, but within only one output modality, spoken or written production (Caramazza & Hillis, 1991; Hillis & Caramazza, 1995c; Hillis, Tuffiash, & Caramazza, 2002). These patterns of dissociation provide evidence that the grammatical class distinction observed only within a specific mode of output is represented at the level of the output lexical representations.

Distinct neural regions appear to be associated with impairments affecting lexical phonologic output. In particular, researchers typically have described noun-retrieval impairments in patients with fluent aphasia and left-posterior perisylvian cortex lesions, often including temporal regions (Damasio & Tranel, 1993; Miozzo, Soardi, & Cappa, 1994). In particular, area 37 at the inferior temporal/occipital junction has been associated with impairments of phonologic lexical retrieval (Antonucci & Beeson, 2004; Hillis et al., 2001, 2006; Raymer, Foundas et al., 1997). In contrast, impairments are worse for verb retrieval than noun retrieval in association with nonfluent aphasia and left-inferior frontal lesions (Caramazza & Hillis, 1991; Damasio & Tranel, 1993; Shapiro & Caramazza, 2003; Zingeser & Berndt, 1990).

In summary, studies examining impairments of lexical processing in a variety of patients with aphasia have provided evidence for a complex, distributed system of lexical processing as depicted in Figure 23-1. Overall, it is the left hemisphere that plays the key role in representing lexical knowledge, although the right hemisphere may contribute to certain aspects of lexical-semantic processing (Joanette & Goulet, 1998). Controversies persist regarding details of processing and representation in the lexical system; for example, whether there is an intervening amodal lexical representation stage (e.g., lemma level) between semantic and lexical phonologic output processing. Nevertheless, this general model provides a rational theoretical basis for guiding this discussion of clinical management for patients with lexical impairments.

CLINICAL APPLICATIONS OF THE LEXICAL MODEL

The model of lexical processing provides a framework for exploring the implications of the cognitive neuropsychological (CN) approach as applied within the clinical process. The CN framework may influence the form that lexical assessment takes. In addition, researchers have applied this approach to analyses of treatment of lexical impairments in patients with aphasia. The CN approach also has direct implications for predictions regarding generalization of treatment effects.

Assessment

The goal of assessment within cognitive neuropsychology is to characterize a patient's language impairments with respect to a cognitive model. The model of lexical processing shown in Figure 23-1 provides a basis for discussion of impairments specifically related to spoken word comprehension and production. Raymer and colleagues (1995) illustrated how a CN analysis played a significant role in distinguishing the lexical impairments of two patients whose standardized aphasia assessments acutely indicated anomic aphasia. When clinicians evaluated the profound word-retrieval impairments in greater detail, it became clear that the two patients differed considerably in the cognitive mechanisms for their word-retrieval impairments. One patient had an impairment affecting semantic activation of the lexical output mechanisms (Raymer, Foundas et al., 1997). The other had impairments affecting at least two stages of lexical processing: visual object activation of the semantic system, and semantic activation of lexical output (Raymer, Greenwald et al., 1997). Assessment results then had consequences for treatment for the word-retrieval impairment in the second patient (Greenwald, Raymer, Richardson, & Rothi, 1995). The challenge to clinicians is to tailor assessments to evaluate the integrity of the lexical mechanisms.

Mode/Modality Comparisons

A key concept in an assessment geared to identifying impairments in the lexical system is mode/modality comparisons. The lexical assessment should include a variety of single-word processing tasks in which the clinician systematically varies input modalities and output modes, and analyzes patterns of performance for tasks sharing modalities/modes of processing. Table 23–1 lists a number of lexical tasks that result when combining input modalities (auditory verbal, written, viewed objects) and output modes (speech, writing, gesture). The lexical assessment typically includes key tasks such as oral picture-naming, written picture-naming, naming to spoken definition, oral word reading, writing to dictation, auditory word comprehension, and written word comprehension, among others. Published psycholinguistic tests are available that allow systematic assessment of lexical processing (e.g., Psycholinguistic Assessments of Language Processing in Aphasia, Kay, Lesser, & Coltheart, 1992), and several research groups also have developed experimental batteries (Hillis et al., 1990; Raymer et al., 1990; Roach, Schwartz, Maratin, Grewel, & Brecher, 1996; Zingeser & Berndt, 1990).

Lexical Stimuli

A second important consideration in lexical assessment is the selection of appropriate stimulus materials. As tasks contrast modalities/modes of processing, it is important, to the extent possible, to employ the same set of stimuli across tasks. For example, in the Florida Semantics Battery (Raymer et al., 1990), we incorporated the same set of 120 nouns across tasks. (See Appendix 23-1 for the full set of 120

TABLE 23–1

Lexical Tasks to Include in Assessment

Output Tasks	Input Tasks
*Oral picture-naming	*Auditory word-to-picture matching
*Written picture-naming	*Written word-to-picture matching
*Oral naming to spoken definitions	Auditory word-picture verification
Written naming to spoken definitions	Written word-picture verification
*Oral word-reading	*Semantic-associates matching
*Writing to dictation	Auditory lexical decision
Name to tactile-object presentation	Written lexical decision
Name to environmental sounds	Category sorting
Gesture to command	
Gesture to viewed objects	

*Indicates key tasks in the general lexical assessment.

nouns.) Patients complete blocks of stimuli systematically across experimental tasks to control for effects of repeated exposure to the same stimuli. In this way, the clinician can attribute differences observed across tasks to the modality of processing and not to differences in stimulus variables.

On the other hand, there will be times when the clinician wants to evaluate performance for contrasting sets of materials, for example, when contrasting performance for nouns versus verbs, or for different semantic categories. In many studies examining factors influencing word retrieval in patients with aphasia, investigators often have discussed the effect of word frequency, as higher-frequency words are named better than lower-frequency words (Capitani & Laiacona, 2004; Raymer, Foundas et al., 1997; Zingeser & Berndt, 1988). However, carefully controlled studies have demonstrated that word frequency has a less potent effect on lexical processing than factors such as imageability, length, familiarity, and, especially, age of acquisition (Bell, Davies, Hermann, & Walters, 2000; Colombo & Burani, 2002; Cuetos, Monsalve, & Perez, 2005; Hirsh & Ellis, 1994; Kremin et al., 2001; Nickels & Howard, 1994, 1995) (Table 23–2). Words learned early in life are particularly resilient. Therefore, the clinician should evaluate the effect such variables have on their patient's performance, as certain factors may have implications for which materials are chosen for use in treatment. Several online resources are available for determining the psycholinguistic attributes of stimuli (e.g., MRC data base, Center for Research in Language data base).

Comprehension Tasks

In tasks that assess comprehension of single words, it can be difficult at times to detect an impairment, as the patient often can provide a correct response, sometimes by guessing. In word-to-picture matching tasks, individuals may respond correctly to an item on the basis of only basic semantic information if a target picture (e.g., "apple") and the distractor pictures are unrelated (e.g., "apple," "chair," "hammer," "dress") (Raymer & Berndt, 1996). For this reason it is important to evaluate comprehension performance in the context of semantically related distractors (e.g., "apple," "orange," "banana," "grapes"), which will require subjects to activate more specified semantic information to derive the correct answer.

An alternative task to assess comprehension is picture-word verification, in which the patient sees a picture and must decide (yes-no) whether a given word is the correct label. To be credited with a correct response, the patient must verify (yes) the correct name and reject foil names (no) that are semantically or phonologically related to the target

TABLE 23–2

Linguistic Factors That May Affect Performance for Items Within Lexical Tasks, with Selected Normative References

Word frequency (Francis & Kucera, 1982)
Grammatical category (noun, verb, functor)
Semantic category (living items, fruits, animals)
Lexicality (word, nonword)
Regularity (Berndt, Reggia, & Mitchum, 1987; regular spelling-"mat," exceptional spelling-"yacht")
Age of acquisition (Gilhooly & Logie, 1980)
Imageability (Coltheart, 1981; Gilhooly & Logie, 1980)
Operativity (Coltheart, 1981; tools and objects tools act upon)
Length (syllable length, phoneme length)
Familiarity (Snodgrass & Vanderwart, 1980)

word. Breese and Hillis (2004) compared performance in word-picture matching and word-picture verification tasks in a large sample of participants with left-hemisphere stroke. With 78% of participants performing more poorly in verification than matching, and only 8% showing the opposite pattern, the verification task was much more sensitive for identifying subtle deficits in word recognition. Semantic foils were more problematic than phonologic foils, suggesting the types of foils that might be more sensitive to mild comprehension impairments.

Error Patterns across Lexical Tasks

Another key concept to consider in the lexical assessment is the pattern of errors produced across tasks. Table 23–3 provides a list of some typical errors observed for verbal responses in lexical tasks (Mitchum, Ritgert, Sandson, & Berndt, 1990). The types of errors may provide clues as to the mechanism of a patient's lexical impairment. The same quantitative and qualitative pattern of errors should be observed in all tasks that engage the impaired mechanism.

TABLE 23–3

Types of Production Errors Commonly Observed in Lexical Tasks

Error Type	Description
Visual	In object-naming, names of objects sharing visual characteristics, e.g., "pencil" for "screwdriver"; in oral reading, words that share orthography, e.g., "chain" for "choir"
Semantic	
Superordinate	Semantic category name for the viewed object or word
Coordinate	Name of alternative item within the semantic category, e.g., "apple" for "pear"
Associate	Words bearing some relationship (e.g., function, location, attribute) to the target picture or word, e.g., "pound" for "hammer"
Circumlocution	Description of the semantic attributes of the object or word
Phonemic	Response sharing phonemic attributes of target; at times is a real word, e.g., "trick" for "truck," or nonword, e.g., "trut" for "truck"
Unrelated	Responses bearing no relationship to target, e.g., "cow" for "lamp"
No response	Refusal or inability to retrieve response, e.g., "I don't know"

For example, a deficit of semantic processing will affect performance in all comprehension and naming tasks (Hillis et al., 1990). Dysfunction of lexical phonologic output will result in parallel patterns of impairment in all verbal production tasks (e.g., oral naming of pictures and oral reading of single words with exceptional spellings) (Caramazza & Hillis, 1990).

Examination of the type of error itself within one lexical task is not sufficient to distinguish the level of lexical impairment responsible for the error. Semantic errors in picture naming are a case in point (Hillis, 2001). For example, for the target picture of a carrot, semantic-naming errors may include responses such as "vegetable" (superordinate), "celery" (coordinate), or "rabbit" (associated). On the surface, one might assume that these errors represent semantic-system dysfunction (see Fig. 23-1). Indeed, in some patients, semantic errors may represent semantic-system impairment (Hillis et al., 1990; Howard & Orchard-Lisle, 1984). Caramazza and Hillis (1990) describe a patient who produced semantic errors only for oral picture naming and oral word reading, but none in written picture naming and writing to dictation, suggesting that the semantic errors arose from a disturbance of the phonologic lexicon. In contrast, patients with optic aphasia often produce large numbers of semantic errors in picture-naming tasks (oral and written), but no semantic errors in naming to definition (Hillis & Caramazza, 1995a; Raymer, Greenwald et al., 1997), a pattern that may represent an impairment of visual object activation of the semantic system. These observations underscore the need to analyze error patterns across lexical tasks to develop an accurate hypothesis regarding the source of the lexical error (Raymer & Rothi, 2000).

Stage-Specific Analyses

Many lexical tasks involve processing at multiple stages in the lexical system. It is necessary to contrast performances across tasks sharing processing at one stage to develop a precise hypothesis about the nature of the impairment affecting performance at that stage. In this section we will review tasks that the clinician may administer to assess performance at each stage of lexical processing.

Visual Object Representation Tasks

Tasks that require processing of familiar pictures will depend on the integrity of visual object representations. Therefore, general tasks such as object naming and word-to-picture matching provide an initial screening for this mechanism. Object-recognition impairment is suspected if performance improves for contrasting tasks that don't require picture or object processing (e.g., name to definitions, word-to-word matching), or when patient responses in picture naming represent visually similar objects (e.g., "pencil" for "screwdriver"). Tasks that more directly target processing by visual object representations require subjects to determine the familiarity of objects or to use knowledge of the visual form of objects. Object decision, which requires a patient to decide whether a viewed stimulus is a familiar object, presumably depends on an intact visual object representation. Similarly, drawing from memory or answering questions about visual attributes of objects (i.e., visual imagery) also may tap this object-recognition process. Because impairments of object recognition may take a number of forms, tasks such as copying and matching line drawings may be necessary to distinguish early object-processing impairments from impairments affecting visual object representations themselves. The key feature is that impairment will be specific to the visual modality.

Lexical Phonologic Recognition Tasks

Any tasks that present stimuli through the auditory verbal channel will require activation of lexical phonologic recognition. Testing will include tasks that are part of the general lexical assessment, such as auditory word-picture verification (especially in the presence of semantic distractors), naming to spoken definitions, and gestures to verbal command. As in visual object representations, stage-specific phonologic tasks require patients to process auditory aspects of familiar phonologic stimuli. Auditory lexical decision, in which patients decide whether a given stimulus is a real or nonsense word, is such a task. Additional phonologic tasks such as phoneme discrimination, repetition, or identification of familiar environmental sounds may be useful to determine whether the impairment for phonologic lexical information relates to pre-lexical auditory impairments. A modality-specific dysfunction is suspected if performance improves when stimuli are presented through other nonphonologic modalities, such as written or viewed object input, and when responses to phonologic stimuli suggest misperception or confusion with phonologically related words.

Semantic-System Tasks

All lexical comprehension and production tasks presumably depend upon adequate processing by the lexical-semantic system, regardless of input modality and output mode. However, performance for oral reading and writing to dictation of regularly spelled words may be spared in the face of semantic impairments if sublexical print-sound conversion processes remain intact. In practice, it may be possible for a brain lesion to cause extensive damage to lexical input and output stages simultaneously, leading to mode/modality-consistent impairments that mimic semantic dysfunction. It can therefore be useful to administer additional semantic tasks that require more specific processing of the semantic attributes of stimuli or that avoid the use of lexical stimuli. Sorting objects by category, systematically manipulating the distance between categories, may

help detect semantic impairment. Asking patients to provide definitions for words also taxes semantic processing. A semantic-associates task, such as the Pyramids and Palm Trees test (Howard & Patterson, 1992), may be useful to detect semantic impairments. In the semantic-associates task, participants match a target item (e.g., "carrot") to a semantically associated item from several choices (e.g., associate-"rabbit"; distractors-"squirrel, cake"). This test can be sensitive to subtle impairments in semantic activation (Raymer, Greenwald et al., 1997).

Because semantic impairments can fractionate along the lines of specific semantic categories, it is useful to include tasks that are structured according to this dimension. Some experimental batteries incorporate the semantic category distinction (e.g., Florida Semantics Battery, see Appendix 23-1). Within standard aphasia tests, an astute examiner may notice either impaired or spared performance related to selective categories by noting errors and then exploring category distinctions with additional testing with relevant materials (e.g., animals, tools). It is also helpful to ask patients whether they notice problems for specific categories. During an extended hospitalization, one patient complained of experiencing great difficulty with medical words. Careful examination substantiated his complaint of a selective impairment for medical terminology (Crosson et al., 1997).

Clinicians may find it useful to develop informal sets of stimuli that include items from a variety of semantic categories that stress different types of semantic content. For example, visual information is purportedly an important characteristic of living categories such as animals, fruits, and vegetables; action output/operativity is relevant to categories of garage tools, kitchen implements, and office supplies. The results of testing that identifies selective categories of difficulty for a patient may allow the clinician to streamline efforts in rehabilitation.

Lexical Phonologic Output Tasks

On the general lexical assessment, tasks requiring verbal production of familiar words will require activation of lexical phonologic representations. Impairment in oral naming, oral word reading, or repetition tasks in the presence of good performance in auditory and reading comprehension, written naming, and writing to dictation leads one to suspect impairment of lexical phonologic output (Caramazza & Hillis, 1990). However, this dissociation may arise with subsequent post-lexical dysfunction (e.g., apraxia of speech). Furthermore, differences between nouns and verbs in word-retrieval tasks may indicate impairments of lexical phonologic output. It may be necessary to administer additional tasks to evaluate further the integrity of lexical phonologic representations. One such task is rhyme verification for picture pairs, in which the patient views two pictures and must determine whether their names rhyme (e.g., "whale-nail").

The rhyming task will prove difficult for individuals who fail to activate a full phonologic lexical representation for the pictures (Hillis, 2002). Word-nonword repetition is another task that may help determine whether an impairment stems from lexical phonologic output or beyond. Patients with post-lexical impairments often have greater difficulty for nonword stimuli (Kahn, Stannard, & Skinner, 1998), whereas patients with lexical impairments may have greater difficulty with word stimuli (Hillis et al., 2001).

Summary of Assessment

Overall, the CN approach to assessment of lexical function is distinguished by its systematic examination of patterns of performance across modalities of input and modes of output. Rather than employing a specific assessment protocol, assessment will be individualized on the basis of deficits identified in preliminary testing. Additional testing will proceed as the clinician develops hypotheses regarding suspected levels of impairment.

The CN assessment approach has a number of advantages (Raymer et al., 1995). Many patients with extensive neurologic lesions have dysfunction affecting multiple levels in the lexical system. An in-depth assessment will frequently suggest not only what mechanisms in lexical processing are impaired, but also what mechanisms are spared. In addition, the clinician may identify specific linguistic factors that affect performance across tasks. These types of information may be beneficial as the clinician turns toward devising treatments for each patient.

Some clinicians may argue that in these days of limited resources, it is unrealistic to promote such a lengthy assessment. Clinicians may adapt these methods using a more circumscribed set of available materials (e.g., Breese & Hillis, 2004). For example, it might be possible to select 10 stimuli representing a variety of semantic categories and to vary mode/modality of processing for key lexical processing tasks listed in Table 23-1. A systematic assessment may indeed be more cost-effective as clinicians understand their patients' impairments and direct treatments in the most expeditious manner.

RECOVERY OF LEXICAL IMPAIRMENTS

Researchers have described diverse lexical impairments in individuals with a variety of neurologic disorders. In general, the etiology of the brain disorder and the size and extent of the brain lesion will have the greatest influence on the prognosis for recovery of lexical impairment (Rothi, 1997). Recently, investigators have described more detailed analyses of language recovery in order to identify lexical factors predictive of recovery from aphasia. Recovery analyses described by Kohn and colleagues (1996) and Laiacona, Capitani, and Barbarotto (1997) provide information to help clinicians pre-

dict which patients are likely to recover from lexical impairment. Kohn and colleagues examined recovery of neologistic verbal output in four subjects with lexical impairment related to lexical phonologic output processing; only two demonstrated substantial improvement after 6 months. The distinguishing characteristic in the nonrecovering subjects was a perseverative phonemic pattern in their neologisms at onset. The authors proposed that the patients who recovered had an impairment that affected retrieval of phonologic representations, whereas the two with no recovery had substantial loss of lexical phonologic representations.

Laiacona and colleagues (1997) described recovery of lexical abilities in two patients with category-specific lexical impairments for living items as compared to nonliving items. One patient was initially less impaired than the other and had normal performance for nonliving items across tasks. One year later, that patient had improved to normal levels of performance for living items as well. In contrast, the second patient was initially severely impaired across categories, with an advantage for items in the nonliving category. After 2 years, performance had improved significantly only for the category of nonliving items; living items remained severely impaired. The authors proposed that distinct mechanisms of word-retrieval failure led to different resolution of the category-specific impairments in the two patients. Like the argument of Kohn and colleagues (1996), an impairment characterized by loss of semantic representations was associated with more limited recovery than an impairment that affected semantic-system access to intact lexical output representations.

Recovery analyses may serve to distinguish hypotheses generated to account for lexical impairments in individuals with similar patterns of impairments. Raymer, Foundas and colleagues (1997) described a patient with impaired word retrieval in oral and written naming tasks and intact performance in comprehension tasks. They proposed that the impairment arose at a late stage in semantic processing as semantic representations activate subsequent lexical output mechanisms. When Raymer and colleagues (Raymer, Maher, Foundas, Rothi, & Heilman, 2000) assessed the pattern of recovery for their patient, parallel patterns of improvement, qualitatively and quantitatively, were evident for both oral and written naming, as might be predicted if the impairment arose at a common stage in lexical processing. These parallel recovery patterns across output modes further substantiate the original proposal that the lexical impairment for speech and writing is related to a common stage in lexical-output processing.

Although fewer studies have assessed recovery from a CN perspective, those to date have demonstrated the implications of such analyses. Recovery analyses may allow researchers to confirm and contrast interpretations made regarding lexical impairments observed early after a neurologic lesion. Over time, clinicians may use the knowledge derived from recovery analyses to direct clinical efforts toward lexical processes that are predicted to recover. And finally, recovery analyses may ultimately provide additional evidence to validate proposed models of lexical processing (Martin, 1996).

TREATMENT

A number of clinical researchers have voiced optimism that CN models may provide a sound theoretical foundation on which to develop rational treatments for patients with aphasia (Riddoch & Humphreys, 1994; Seron & Deloche, 1989). Of course, cognitive models are not the sole determinant of decisions made in treatment for patients with aphasia (Caramazza & Hillis, 1993; Hillis, 1993). Clinicians also weigh a number of other medical, neurologic, and social factors as they develop a treatment plan for a given patient to optimize success.

Cognitive models of lexical processing lend themselves well toward a distinction in the kind of treatment to be attempted, restitutive or substitutive (Rothi, 1995). Restitutive treatments target semantic or lexical phonologic processes that clinicians have identified as impaired following the systematic lexical assessment. Substitutive treatments incorporate cognitive processes that remain intact and might be used to circumvent or facilitate processing by the impaired lexical mechanism. Clinical researchers have applied the CN approach in a number of lexical studies, some of which used a restorative approach, and others which used a substitutive approach.

Treatments for Comprehension Impairments

The process of word comprehension, in which meaning is applied to a lexical referent, involves activation of both lexical phonologic recognition and semantic processing. Restitutive treatments for auditory comprehension might target those mechanisms, whereas substitutive treatments would use alternative processes to accomplish word comprehension. A small number of studies have applied a CN approach in the treatment of auditory-comprehension impairments.

Restitutive Comprehension Treatments

Morris and colleagues (Morris, Franklin, Ellis, Turner, & Bailey, 1996) described a phonologic treatment for a patient with impairments of auditory comprehension arising at a prelexical phonologic stage of processing. In their treatment, the patient participated in a series of tasks engaging phonemic processing, including phoneme-grapheme matching, phoneme discrimination, auditory-word to picture and auditory-word to written-word matching and verification, and nonsense CV syllable discrimination. As needed, the

clinician provided additional lip-reading cues and hand signals (substitutive strategies) to embellish the phonemic input. Following 6 weeks of twice-weekly treatment, the patient demonstrated significant improvements in a variety of phonologic tasks, but no improvement in written word-comprehension and picture-naming tasks that do not involve phonologic recognition, indicating that the effect was modality-specific and not due to spontaneous recovery.

Grayson, Hilton, and Franklin (1997) implemented a semantic treatment for a patient with severe deficits of lexical comprehension related to dysfunction at both phonologic and semantic processing stages. They chose first to target the semantic impairment by having the patient execute a number of lexical tasks requiring semantic processing: auditory word- and written word-to-picture matching in which they systematically increased the number and relatedness of distractors; category-sorting for pictures and written words of increasing semantic relatedness; and matching associated written words. After 4 weeks of treatment, the patient improved in other word-picture matching tasks, but not in a phoneme-discrimination task. Subsequently, the clinicians added a phonologic component to their semantic treatment as they asked the patient to perform a word-picture matching task using all rhyming word foils. After an additional 4 weeks of treatment, improvement was seen in auditory word-picture matching tasks as well as a nonword phoneme-discrimination task, suggesting that repeated exposure to the treatment tasks affected both phonologic and semantic processing.

Raymer, Kohen, and Saffell (2006) used a similar semantic training paradigm to address the auditory comprehension and naming impairments in two patients with semantic dysfunction. The patients completed spoken word- and written word-to-picture matching tasks in the context of semantic distractors administered via a computer. They also rehearsed the spoken production of words, adding a phonologic component to the training. Both improved their comprehension of words rehearsed in training, and one improved for untrained word comprehension as well.

Behrmann and Lieberthal (1989) applied a semantic treatment in a patient with category-specific comprehension impairments that were particularly severe for the categories of body parts, furniture, and transportation. Clinicians trained the patient on superordinate and specific semantic details about the three targeted categories and then had the patient perform visual and verbal matching tasks applying the semantic information. Following treatment, their patient demonstrated improved categorization of items in the trained categories as well as one untrained category. Little improvement was noted in other semantic processing tasks.

Substitutive Comprehension Treatments

Substitutive treatments for auditory-comprehension impairments may take a number of forms. Some researchers have advocated the use of a lip-reading strategy to provide additional visual information during the course of phonologic processing (Ellis et al., 1983; Morris et al., 1996). Shindo, Kaga, and Tanaka (1991) demonstrated an advantage in processing spoken words when given lip-reading cues in four patients with impairments of phonologic recognition. Maneta, Marshall, and Lindsay (2001), however, reported that lip-reading was less effective than teaching a spouse to use communicative strategies to promote comprehension in a patient with word deafness. Thus, lip-reading may be useful to support auditory comprehension in some patients with intact semantic processing in the presence of phonologic processing impairments.

The orthographic recognition system is another modality for use in patients with phonologic processing impairments. Francis and colleagues (2001) reported their treatment of auditory-comprehension problems in a patient with word-meaning deafness, presumably due to disruption of access from phonologic recognition to semantic processing. They compared outcomes of two different treatments, a substitutive one in which the patient was presented all words only in written form, and a second one in which written words were paired with spoken presentation of stimuli. Both treatments led to improved comprehension of trained words, but the second treatment had more lasting effects, presumably acting more directly to restore phonologic processing.

In summary, having patients complete tasks that require some form of phonologic or semantic processing has the potential to improve future processing abilities for spoken input. It appears that these improvements relate to changes in phonologic recognition and semantic stages of lexical processing, as improvements were less evident in control conditions. Other nonverbal strategies also may be helpful to circumvent or support impaired comprehension abilities.

Treatment for Naming Impairments

Researchers have reported many studies applying the CN approach in the treatment of word-retrieval impairments in patients with aphasia. Word retrieval requires both semantic and phonologic output stages of lexical processing. Thereby, a number of studies have examined the usefulness of restitutive treatments incorporating various semantic and phonologic tasks, either independently or in combination, as shown in Table 23–4. Substitutive treatments, in contrast, have incorporated alternative modes of output to either circumvent an impairment or to vicariatively encourage word retrieval through alternative means.

Restitutive Word-Retrieval Treatments

Semantic Treatments

Recognizing the common role the semantic system plays in both word comprehension and retrieval, a number of studies

---

TABLE 23–4

Semantic and Phonologic Treatments Used to Improve Word Retrieval

Semantic Treatments

Semantic comprehension tasks (e.g., auditory word or picture matching; written word or picture matching; yes/no verification)

Contextual priming (e.g., word or picture matching and rehearsal of related sets of words)

Semantic features descriptions (e.g., distinguishing features between similar objects)

Semantic matrix training (e.g., category, function, attribute, associates)

Phonologic Treatments

Phonologic questions tasks (e.g., rhyming comprehension, syllable-number verification, initial-phoneme verification)

Oral word reading

Word repetition

Phonologic cueing hierarchy (e.g., rhyming word, initial phoneme, repetition)

Phonologic choice tasks (e.g., choose from correct and incorrect phonemic cues)

---

have implemented *comprehension treatments* in an attempt to facilitate word retrieval. Over several sessions, patients complete semantic processing tasks such as picture categorization with related categories (e.g., fruits vs. vegetables), spoken and written word-to-picture matching in the presence of semantic distractors (e.g., target-"corn," distractors-"beans, tomato, squash"), and answering yes/no questions about semantic attributes of target words (e.g., "Does corn grow on a tree?"). At times, the patients also say the word during the performance of the comprehension tasks, adding a phonologic component to the treatment (Byng, Kay, Edmundson, & Scott, 1990; Davis & Pring, 1991; Kiran & Thompson, 2002; Marshall, Pound, White-Thomson, & Pring, 1990; Nickels & Best, 1996). Following semantic comprehension treatments, a variety of individuals with word-retrieval impairments related to either semantic or phonologic dysfunction have demonstrated significant improvement in word-retrieval abilities, largely limited to words incorporated in training (Nickels, 2002).

Subsequent studies contrasted treatments in which semantic comprehension tasks were performed with and without phonologic production of target words to determine what role the phonologic-production component played in the treatment (Drew & Thompson, 1999; Le Dorze, Boulay, Gaudreau, & Brassard, 1994). Drew and Thompson (1999) showed that participants benefited maximally when training combined semantic comprehension tasks with phonologic rehearsal of target words compared to semantic comprehension tasks alone, a finding compatible with the interactive nature of semantic and phonologic lexical processing mechanisms.

One study used a word-retrieval training protocol in which semantic comprehension tasks were administered via the MossTalk computer program (word-picture matching with semantic distractors) along with spoken rehearsal of training words (Raymer, Kohen, & Saffell, 2006). All participants improved their production of trained words, with greater improvement in the three participants with phonologically based retrieval impairments than in the two with severe semantic impairments.

Earlier studies of semantic comprehension training targeted noun-retrieval abilities. Recent studies have examined effects for verb retrieval as well (Raymer & Ellsworth, 2002; Raymer et al., 2007; Rodriguez, Raymer, & Rothi, 2006; Webster, Morris, & Franklin, 2005). Improvements were evident in retrieval of trained verbs, with little generalization to untrained verbs. Some generalized improvements were reported in measures of communicative effectiveness and sentence production using trained words, presumably because of the important role verbs play in sentence generation. Gains were greater in patients whose verb-retrieval impairments stemmed from phonologic as compared to semantic dysfunction.

A modified version of semantic comprehension treatment is seen in studies of *contextual priming* (Martin, Fink, & Laine, 2004, Martin, Fink, Renvall, & Laine, 2006; Renvall, Laine, & Martin, 2005). Participants view a set of several pictures that are related either semantically (e.g., animals), phonologically (e.g., words beginning with "r"), or not at all. They then match spoken word to picture and repeat the name several times. Martin and colleagues reported that, although patients sometimes experience considerable interference from word to word during training, patients ultimately improved production of trained words. Improvements are less potent in patients with semantically based naming dysfunction (Martin et al., 2006).

In another modification of semantic treatment, Wambaugh and colleagues (1999, 2001, 2002, 2003) have examined effects of *semantic cueing treatment* (SCT) for word retrieval in patients with aphasia. In SCT, patients perform a spoken description-to-picture matching task, followed immediately by attempts to name the target picture. If unable to name the picture, patients are given a series of semantically loaded cues to elicit the target word, ending with repetition of the word, if necessary. Across studies, treatment was effective for improving retrieval of trained nouns and verbs in several patients whose word-retrieval impairment arose from semantic, phonologic, and mixed semantic plus phonologic dysfunction.

Some patients with semantic dysfunction seem to lack specific details of semantic knowledge, and thereby produce many semantic errors. Following a lexical assessment that indicated a word-retrieval impairment related to underspecified semantic representations, Hillis (1998) devised a semantic treatment for her patient in which she provided *semantic information* about target pictures the patient was unable to name, and contrasted those features with the semantic features of a closely related object. Ochipa, Maher, and Raymer (1998) used a similar semantic treatment with their patient with word-retrieval impairment stemming from semantic dysfunction. Patients in both studies demonstrated significant improvements in naming trained pictures as well as generalization to untrained pictures and untrained lexical tasks incorporating semantic processing (written-word production). Hillis also reported that this semantic-features treatment was more effective than a traditional cueing hierarchy treatment in her patient.

In another type of semantic treatment, developed on the basis of cognitive theories of how semantic representations are structured, clinicians attempt to improve word retrieval using *semantic-feature matrix training* (Haarbauer-Krupa, Smith, Sullivan, & Szekeres, 1985). Clinicians teach subjects to use a viewed matrix of printed cue words (e.g., function, properties, category, etc.) to assist in retrieving semantic information about a target picture along with its name. After training with a semantic-feature matrix, participants demonstrated improved naming of trained pictures as well as generalization of the strategy to some untrained pictures and conversational measures (Boyle, 2004; Boyle & Coelho, 1995; Conley & Coelho, 2003; Lowell, Beeson, & Holland, 1995). The psycholinguistic basis for word-retrieval impairment among patients was not well characterized in these studies, however.

Phonologic Treatments

Other studies have used treatment protocols presumably engaging lexical phonologic stages of word retrieval. A shared phonologic output representation may be activated in oral reading, word repetition, and oral picture-naming. Capitalizing on this relationship, Miceli and colleagues had their patient repeatedly *read aloud* or *repeat* target words (Miceli, Amitrano, Capasso, & Caramazza, 1996). Both procedures resulted in improved picture-naming for trained words in one subject with phonologically based word-retrieval failure. Mitchum and Berndt (1994) used a similar phonologic rehearsal treatment (incorporating repetition practice) in their patient with a selective verb-retrieval impairment. Following training, their subject demonstrated improvements in verb retrieval, but little improvement in the formulation of complete sentences using the trained verbs.

Other studies have incorporated treatments using a *phonologic cueing hierarchy* to assist patients in retrieving target words. Subjects who were repeatedly exposed to a hierarchy of initial phoneme, rhyme, and word-repetition cues demonstrated improvements in word retrieval for trained words (Greenwald et al., 1995; Hillis, 1993, 1998; Raymer & Ellsworth, 2002; Raymer, Thompson, Jacobs, & le Grand, 1993). Among these studies, treatment was effective for subjects with either semantic or phonologic word-retrieval dysfunction, although improvements were more limited in patients with semantic impairment (Raymer et al., 1993). Studies that systematically examined the impact on word retrieval of word repetition alone demonstrated improvements that were not as potent or lasting as when repetition was paired with other phonologic or semantic processing tasks, however (Greenwald et al., 1995; Raymer & Ellsworth, 2002).

Another treatment paradigm that presumably focuses on lexical phonologic stages of processing incorporated yes/no questions about the *phonologic characteristics* of target words (Howard, Patterson, Franklin, Orchard-Lisle, & Morton, 1985; Robson, Marshall, Pring, & Chiat, 1998). In these studies, patients completed tasks in which they made judgments about words, such as the number of syllables, the initial phoneme of words, or whether the words rhymed. Participants demonstrated improvement in retrieving words trained with this strategy, with some showing generalization of the process to naming of untrained pictures (Robson et al., 1998).

Some studies that contrasted semantic and phonologic training protocols seem to indicate that semantic treatments have longer-lasting effects than phonologic treatments (Howard et al., 1985). Hickin and colleagues reasoned that the difference in semantic treatments compared to phonologic treatments is the need to make a choice, which perhaps promotes deeper processing of the linguistic stimuli (Hickin, Best, Herbert, Howard, & Osborne, 2002). In their phonologic treatment protocol, therefore, participants attempted to name target words when given a *choice of two phonemic cues*, starting with initial phonemes and increasing to syllables and the full word if needed. Significantly improved naming was evident in five of seven participants trained.

In summary, the findings of a number of studies indicate that different types of restitutive semantic and phonologic treatments are effective in improving word retrieval for trained words. One observation is that there is little direct correlation between type of word-retrieval impairment (semantic or phonologic) and the most effective type of treatment (Hillis, 1993; Nickels, 2002). Either semantic or phonologic treatment seems to improve word retrieval in individuals with either semantic or phonologic impairments. In fact, the best restitutive treatments appear to be those that combine semantic and phonologic information during the course of training, to encourage the process of word retrieval in a manner compatible with the typical process (Drew & Thompson, 1999; Le Dorze et al., 1994). Patients with severe semantic dysfunction often show a more limited response to treatments than those with phonologic retrieval bases of impairment (Nickels, 2002).

Substitutive Word-Retrieval Treatments

An alternative approach to rehabilitation of word-retrieval impairments is to devise treatments that either circumvent the impaired lexical mechanism or develop an alternative means to vicariatively mediate word retrieval using other cognitive mechanisms. For example, the use of semantic circumlocution to describe a concept when a word-retrieval failure occurs would be a substitutive semantic strategy to circumvent failure at the subsequent stage of phonologic lexical retrieval. Some treatment studies have evaluated the effects of methods to vicariatively activate word retrieval.

Orthographic Mechanisms

Some patients with word-retrieval impairments stemming from failure to access lexical phonologic representations nevertheless may be able to access some knowledge about the word's spelling. In turn, using print-to-sound conversion processes, it may be possible to self-cue and generate the appropriate spoken form of the word. Patients with some retained spelling knowledge for words they were unable to produce were successfully taught either to type the letters into a computer, which in turn generated the initial phoneme of the word (Bruce & Howard, 1987), or to write the letters and self-cue the spoken production of the words (Bastiaanse, Bosje, & Fraansen, 1996). Some patients may need to be trained in print-to-sound conversion, however, before written self-cueing is useful to promote spoken naming (Nickels, 1992).

Hickin and colleagues (2002) used a task in which patients chose between two written-letter cues to promote production of target words. In a subsequent study they compared the effects of multiple written cues versus only one cue and showed that both techniques led to improvements in picture-naming (Hickin, Greenwood, Grassly, Herbert, Howard, & Best, 2005). Because repetition was used as a final step in training, it is likely that this training engaged both orthographic and phonologic stages of lexical processing. DeDe, Parris, and Waters (2003) used a similar rationale in their training study in which their patient practiced writing target words, given a choice of written cues from one letter to several letters as necessary. In addition, the patient rehearsed the use of tactile cues (e.g., hand-pointing to neck for "k"), corresponding to the word's initial letter, and phonemic cues to produce target words. Positive treatment effects were reported for spoken-naming, which may be a result of changes in orthographic or phonologic stages of lexical processing. Finally, Laganaro, Di Pietro, and Schnider (2006) used a computer-training protocol in which participants practiced written spellings of words. When spelling errors occurred, the participant was provided with more and more information about the spelling until the word was correctly spelled. Apparently, participants never said the words aloud during training, constraining the training paradigm largely to the orthographic modality. Nonetheless, their participants improved markedly in spoken-naming of words they had practiced spelling.

Some studies, in contrast, have used oral-reading treatments to promote spoken-naming abilities. Hillis (1998) described a remarkable patient who spontaneously used retained print-to-sound conversion abilities to support her impaired word retrieval. This patient often mispronounced words using regularized pronunciations (e.g., "/brid/" for "bread") when a word-retrieval failure occurred. Listeners who were familiar with her maladaptive technique could often perform a reverse translation and figure out the word the patient was attempting to say. To circumvent this awkward strategy, Hillis taught her patient to read aloud regularized spellings of common words with exceptional spellings (e.g., "kwire" for "choir"). Improvements in oral reading also were evident in oral naming of the same words. Similarly, Kiran, Thompson, and Hashimoto (2001) demonstrated in their patients with phonologic dysfunction that practice in oral reading of words led to improvements in spoken-naming of the same words.

Gesture

An alternative method that researchers have applied to mediate word retrieval is the use of the gestural-processing mechanisms through pantomime. Cognitive models of lexical and praxis processing recognize the interactive nature of the two systems (Rose, Douglas, & Matyas, 2002; Rothi et al., 1997), suggesting that gesture may be useful to mediate activation of lexical retrieval. Arbib (2005) has argued for a close relationship between gesture and language processing, making gesture particularly appropriate for use as a language-treatment modality. A desirable consequence of gestural facilitation with pantomimes is that, should verbal processes not improve with training, the patient may increase the use of gesture as an alternative communication mode. A number of single-participant studies have demonstrated that gestural training paired with spoken production of words improved word retrieval in individuals with aphasia (Pashek, 1997; Raymer & Thompson, 1991). For example, Rose and colleagues (2002) showed that treatment with iconic gestures was as effective as use of phonologic-orthographic cues in improving word retrieval in one individual with phonologic-retrieval dysfunction. Similarly, Rodriguez and colleagues (2006) reported that gestural training was as effective as semantic-phonologic training in one individual with phonologic-retrieval impairment for verbs. Three other participants with semantic impairments did not improve spoken verb-naming abilities during either treatment, although two demonstrated dramatic increases in the use of gestures corresponding to verbs.

Druks (2001) noted a close relationship between networks engaged in verb and gesture knowledge, suggesting that gestural treatment may be especially effective for verb retrieval as compared to noun retrieval. One participant described by Pashek (1998) improved retrieval of both nouns and verbs following gestural training, though improvement was greater for verbs than for nouns. In a larger study, Raymer and colleagues (2006) reported that gestural training led to improved word retrieval for both nouns and verbs in five of nine participants in the study, with no difference between noun and verb outcomes. Improvements in word retrieval were greater in individuals with phonologic-retrieval impairments and mild to moderate semantic impairments than in those with severe semantic impairments.

One problem with earlier gesture studies is that the integrity of the action mechanisms (limb apraxia) was often not well documented in the subjects with aphasia. Patients with severe limb apraxia may not be able to use pantomime as a viable communication mode, as their gestures are often unrecognizable. However, the studies by Raymer and colleagues (Raymer et al., 2006; Rodriguez et al., 2006) showed that patients with severe limb apraxia can improve their ability to produce recognizable gestures, even when word retrieval does not improve.

Summary of Treatment Research

Studies have demonstrated that restitutive treatments are effective for improving performance in individuals with impairments of either lexical comprehension or production. Other studies have shown that substitutive treatments also can benefit word comprehension and retrieval in some patients. One observation noted across treatment studies is that, whereas patients may present with impairments that implicate either semantic or phonologic stages of lexical processing, there is no direct relationship between type of impairment and type of treatment that seems to be most effective for naming recovery (Hillis, 1993). Some patients with semantic impairments benefit from treatment that focuses on phonologic output, and vice versa. In general, recovery of word-retrieval functions is more limited in patients with severe semantic dysfunction. Although simple rehearsal of spoken words can help a person improve word retrieval, the most effective treatments were those that engaged either semantic, phonologic, and, in particular, semantic plus phonologic processing within one treatment protocol. That is, treatments that attempted to facilitate the multistage process of word retrieval were often most effective.

GENERALIZATION

The CN approach has specific implications for analyzing the generalization of treatment effects for lexical impairments (Hillis, 1993; Raymer, Rothi, & Heilman, 1995).

First, if treatment facilitates processing in a particular lexical mechanism, improvements should be evident in all tasks that require processing by that mechanism. Hereafter, this type of generalization will be referred to as "generalization across tasks." Second, as treatment strengthens targeted lexical representations, other semantically or phonologically related lexical representations may benefit from the treatment as well. This type of generalization will be referred to as "generalization to untrained stimuli."

Generalization across Tasks

A number of studies have examined the effects of word-retrieval treatment on other untrained lexical tasks that draw upon semantic or phonologic mechanisms presumably impacted by treatment. Hillis (1998) examined generalization across untreated lexical tasks following her semantic-features treatment for word retrieval. Benefits of semantic treatments should be evident in all tasks involving semantic activation, including oral- and written-naming, comprehension, and possibly oral-reading and writing to dictation. Although semantic treatment focused solely on written-naming, improvements were also evident in all other lexical tasks, as predicted. Likewise, Ochipa and colleagues (1998) reported improvement in written-naming following semantic-features treatment targeting oral-naming. Similarly, benefits of phonologic treatments should be evident in oral-naming and oral-reading, and less likely in written-naming and comprehension. So, for example, when Hillis (1998) trained her patient to pronounce regularized spellings of words with exceptional spellings, her patient improved pronunciation of the same words in picture-naming and word repetition as well, but not in written-naming.

There are times, however, when treatment effects observed in additional lexical tasks extend beyond those predicted. For example, Raymer and colleagues (1993) used a phonologic cueing hierarchy to train oral picture-naming, and observed generalized improvements in oral word-reading as well as written picture-naming in one patient. Although one might expect that the phonologic training largely impacted on phonologic stages of word retrieval, semantic aspects of processing also may have been strengthened, leading to improvements in written-naming as well. In contrast, Greenwald and colleagues (1995) reported improvements in oral picture-naming following visual-semantic training, but no improvement in a visual picture-associate matching task that they predicted would also improve following training. These patterns of generalization that are contrary to the predicted patterns suggest that the complexity of the lexical mechanisms and the types of processing that occur among mechanisms also influence treatment in important, but as yet unspecified, ways.

Finally, the results of the CN assessment may assist the clinical researcher in selection of tasks to demonstrate that the effects of treatment indeed result from treatment and not from spontaneous recovery (Raymer et al., 1995). The clinician can identify other independent areas of cognitive/linguistic impairment that should not be affected by treatment and probe performance over time. The clinician demonstrates internal validity when treatment improves performance in the targeted task but not in the untreated task.

Generalization to Untrained Stimuli

Generalization to untrained stimuli may occur in two ways. Some treatments affect a lexical process, teaching patients to use this process or strategy to improve performance for a set of trained stimuli. If the patient learns this strategy or improves functioning in this process, performance should be affected when applying that process for all stimuli, trained or untrained. An example of such a process that may affect word-retrieval abilities is semantic-feature matrix training, in which clinicians train patients to use a matrix of cue words to encourage the recall of semantic information for a target word and ultimately word retrieval. Boyle and Coelho (1995; Boyle, 2004) and Lowell and colleagues (1995) reported that their patients who responded to semantic-feature matrix training also demonstrated some improvements in naming untrained pictures. It may be that the patients learned to self-generate semantic information whenever a word-retrieval failure occurred, thereby leading to activation of lexical responses for untrained words as well.

A second way in which generalization to untrained stimuli might occur is at the level of lexical representations. If word-retrieval training somehow restores features of representations to a more optimal state, then all items sharing those features should be affected. Therefore, generalization may be evident in predictable ways to items that share semantic or phonologic features. It may be this type of effect that can account for generalization to semantically related items found after semantic-feature training (Hillis, 1998; Ochipa et al., 1998) and after contextual priming with semantically related words (Martin et al., 2004).

Some studies have evaluated generalization of word-retrieval training effects that target specific semantic categories. Behrmann and Lieberthal (1989) evaluated generalization of category-specific semantic-comprehension treatment to naming of untrained items within trained and untrained categories. They observed generalization to untrained items within one trained category, as might be predicted. But they also noted improved naming in one untrained category, which cannot be completely explained on the basis of restoration of semantic features. Kiran and Thompson (2002d) provided word-retrieval training for subsets of words within a semantic category (e.g., birds, vegetables) and compared the effects when trained words were more typical exemplars of a category in that they have the characteristic features common to that category (e.g., robin, carrot), versus atypical exemplars that have unique features that differ from other exemplars in the category (e.g., peacock, olive). In keeping with computational simulations (Plaut, 1996), Kiran and Thompson found that training with atypical exemplars led to greater generalized improvements when naming untrained typical exemplars of the category than when training typical exemplars in four patients with semantically based anomia. Stanczak, Waters, and Caplan (2006) replicated the typicality findings in word-retrieval training for one patient with a semantic plus phonologic dysfunction, but the pattern of generalization was not seen in a second patient with a phonologic naming dysfunction. They proposed that training with atypical exemplars has a more global influence on semantic networks than does training with typical exemplars. Patients with semantic dysfunction may benefit more than those with phonologic dysfunction from training with atypical category exemplars.

More often than not, improvements in trained lexical tasks seem to be item-specific, and limited improvements are evident for untrained words. For example, Raymer and colleagues (1993) systematically assessed generalization of the effects of a phonologic cueing hierarchy to items that were either semantically or phonologically related to trained pictures. They observed no clear patterns of response generalization among the patients. It is interesting that studies showing more positive generalization to untrained items typically incorporated semantic treatments. However, not all semantic treatments led to response generalization (Pring et al., 1993). Because there is no indisputable reason to predict generalization to untrained items, it would be sensible to select treatment words that respect the functional needs of each individual patient. For example, Hillis (1998) used a cueing hierarchy to train her patient to retrieve the names of different types of fabrics after the patient took a job at a fabric store.

LIMITATIONS OF THE COGNITIVE NEUROPSYCHOLOGICAL APPROACH

While this discussion has focused largely on the positive ramifications of the CN approach for the clinical rehabilitation process, the CN approach has some recognized shortcomings. The systematic, in-depth assessment of lexical abilities advocated in this approach proves tremendously difficult to accomplish in many clinical settings. However, clinicians may find it possible to use this approach in a more condensed format to accumulate the information necessary to make informed treatment decisions. Clinicians may be able to complete a series of lexical tasks with a circumscribed set of materials in the course of diagnostic treatment in an attempt to characterize lexical abilities more specifically. It may prove helpful for clinicians to characterize impairments accurately, but, in addition, to identify retained lexical abilities, as the clinician may capitalize upon those retained abilities to devise appropriate substitutive treatments for lexical impairments. Furthermore, observations of overall patterns of impairments may eventually allow clinicians to develop better prognoses for impairments they observe in their patients. For example, disturbed oral-naming in the presence of preserved oral word-reading skills seemed to be predictive of best response to word-retrieval treatments (Raymer et al., 1993; Pring et al., 1990).

Although one of the initial goals of the CN approach was to identify more rational treatments that target identified impairments in the lexical system (e.g., semantic treatments for semantic impairments, and so forth), the findings to date do not support this notion. But the considerable body of research certainly has suggested a more favorable course to follow when attempting restorative treatments with patients with aphasia. Treatments that encourage activation of multiple stages in the lexical process (see Fig. 23-1) in the course of one treatment protocol appear to be most effective. Although the lexical mechanisms are distinct and distributed, they are highly interactive in the course of lexical processing.

Some clinicians have argued that the CN approach, which emphasizes impairment-oriented treatments, has few consequences for overcoming the disabling conditions posed by aphasia (Wilson, 1999). Because earlier treatment studies often neglected to report the functional aftermath of lexical treatments, this argument may have some merit. Substitutive treatments that researchers have generated on the basis of lexical theories definitely encourage progress in functional communication in a variety of patients. Recent studies have attempted to improve methods to document the substantial impact that impairment-oriented treatments have for patients and their families.

Hillis (1993) noted that although an assessment may help the clinician to characterize the nature of the patient's impairment, it does not help determine what specific strategy will be most effective—that is, how to treat the impairment. A number of additional neurologic, cognitive, and social factors also must play a role in the treatment decision. As researchers accrue a greater body of knowledge about treatment effects across patients, clinicians may be better at making predictions about who, what, and how to treat.

FUTURE TRENDS

A review of the limitations of the CN approach to lexical treatment suggests a number of areas for future research. Much of the treatment literature has reported the effects of one type of treatment, so that clinicians are unable to judge whether that treatment was as effective as other possible treatment options. Some recent studies have implemented crossover designs (e.g., Rodriguez et al., 2006) to add to the body of knowledge of what clinicians know are the most beneficial treatments. Future studies need to implement prospective randomized trials to solidify the evidence-base for treatments founded on the cognitive neuropsychological approach.

Also, the impairment-oriented approach to aphasia treatment has received much criticism and skepticism. Therefore, future studies must incorporate methods to evaluate the functional consequences of treatments for daily communication situations (Herbert, Best, Hickin, Howard, & Osborne, 2003). Finally, imaging studies are beginning to document the neural changes associated with successful behavioral treatments. Continued research in each of these areas will advance the effectiveness and efficiency of clinical practice for our patients with aphasia.

KEY POINTS

1. The lexical system is a complex, distributed system of modules that store information in sensory modality-specific and output mode-specific mechanisms that interact by way of a semantic system.
2. Lexical impairments take many forms depending on which component of the lexical system is affected.
3. Assessment focuses on mode/modality comparisons across lexical tasks. Patterns of performance, quantitatively and qualitatively, help the clinician develop an informed hypothesis about the nature of lexical impairments.
4. Recovery analyses may assist clinicians in predicting which patients will recover and in which direction, and may serve to confirm hypotheses generated on initial assessment.
5. Restitutive treatments target impaired lexical mechanisms. Treatments that are putatively semantic in nature, and others that focus on phonologic aspects of lexical information, have induced changes in auditory comprehension and word retrieval in a variety of patients. However, contrary to early predictions about the CN approach, there is not a direct correspondence between types of impairments and most effective treatments. Treatments that incorporate multiple stages of the lexical process seem most beneficial.
6. Substitutive treatments capitalize on retained aspects of lexical processing to either circumvent an impairment at some stage in lexical processing or to vicariatively mediate activation of the impaired mechanism.
7. Generalization of treatment effects is observed across all tasks for which the mechanism facilitated by treatment plays a necessary role in accurate performance. Generalization of treatment effects to untrained stimuli has been more limited, although there are indications that semantic treatments incite greater generalization to untrained semantically related words.
8. Less research has been focused on the functional outcomes of these impairment-oriented treatments.

ACTIVITIES FOR REFLECTION AND DISCUSSION

1. What is modality-specificity as it relates to the model of lexical processing?
2. What is the difference between lexical phonologic recognition, lexical semantics, and lexical phonologic output?
3. A dysfunction of the phonologic-recognition mechanism will result in a pattern of impairment in which lexical tasks and preserved performance for what other lexical tasks?
4. What is the pattern of lexical performance seen in patients with optic aphasia?
5. What is a category-specific impairment? For what semantic categories might we observe category-specific impairments?
6. What is the purpose of mode/modality comparisons in the cognitive neuropsychological assessment?
7. The presence of semantic errors in naming may represent dysfunction at which three stages of lexical processing?
8. Describe one stage-specific assessment task to target processing in each of the following: object recognition, lexical semantics, and lexical phonologic output.
9. How are analyses of lexical recovery useful in clinical practice?
10. Describe restitutive and substitutive treatments that may be useful to improve functioning in an individual with phonologic recognition impairment.
11. Why are semantic comprehension tasks useful as a restitutive treatment for word-retrieval impairments?
12. What are three different tasks a patient may practice to encourage restoration of functioning in the lexical-phonologic output stage of word retrieval?
13. How can the graphemic system be used in a substitutive strategy for word-retrieval impairments?
14. How do models of lexical processing assist in predicting generalization effects to untrained tasks?

References

Allport, D. A. (1985). Distributed memory, modular subsystems and dysphasia. In S. Newman & R. Epstein (Eds.), *Current perspectives in dysphasia* (pp. 32–60). Edinburgh: Churchill Livingstone.

Antonucci, S. M., & Beeson, P. M. (2004). Anomia in patients with left inferior temporal lobe lesions. *Aphasiology, 18,* 543–554.

Arbib, M. A. (2005). From monkey-like action recognition to human language: An evolutionary framework for neurolinguistics. *Behavioral and Brain Sciences, 28,* 105–167.

Badecker, W., & Caramazza, A. (1991). Morphological composition in the lexical output system. *Cognitive Neuropsychology, 8,* 335–367.

Bastiaanse, R., Bosje, M., & Fraansen, M. (1996). Deficit orented treatment of word finding problems: Another replication. *Aphasiology, 10,* 363–383.

Behrmann, M., & Lieberthal, T. (1989). Category-specific treatment of a lexical-semantic deficit: A single case study of global aphasia. *British Journal of Disorders of Communication, 24,* 281–299.

Bell, B. D., Davies, K. G., Hermann, B. P., & Walters, G. (2000). Confrontation naming after anterior temporal lobectomy is related to age of acquisition of the object names. *Neuropsychologia, 38,* 83–92.

Berndt, R. S., Reggia, J. A., & Mitchum, C. C. (1987). Empirically derived probabilities for grapheme-to-phoneme correspondences in English. *Behavior Research Methods, Instruments, and Computers, 19,* 1–9.

Boatman, D. (2002). Diagnosis and treatment of auditory disorders. In A. E. Hillis (Ed.), *The handbook of adult language disorders* (pp. 269–280). New York: Psychology Press.

Boyle, M. (2004). Semantic feature analysis treatment for anomia in two fluent aphasia syndromes. *American Journal of Speech-Language Pathology, 13,* 236–249.

Boyle, M., & Coelho, C. A. (1995). Application of semantic feature analysis as a treatment for aphasic dysnomia. *American Journal of Speech-Language Pathology, 4,* 94–98.

Breese, E. L., & Hillis, A. E. (2004). Auditory comprehension: Is multiple choice really good enough? *Brain and Language, 89,* 3–8.

Bruce, C., & Howard, D. (1987). Computer-generated phonemic cues: An effective aid for naming in aphasia. *British Journal of Disorders of Communication, 22,* 191–201.

Bub, D., & Kertesz, A. (1982). Evidence for lexicographic processing in a patient with preserved written over oral single word naming. *Brain, 105,* 697–717.

Buchman, A. S., Garron, D. C., Trost-Cardmone, J. E., Wichter, M. D., & Schwartz, M. (1986). Word deafness: One hundred years later. *Journal of Neurology, Neurosurgery, & Psychiatry, 49,* 489–499.

Buchtel, H. A., & Stewart, J. D. (1989). Auditory agnosia: Apperceptive or associative disorder? *Brain and Language, 37,* 12–25.

Byng, S., Kay, J., Edmundson, A., & Scott, C. (1990). Aphasia tests reconsidered. *Aphasiology, 4,* 67–91.

Capitani, E., & Laiacona, M. (2004). A method for studying the evolution of naming error types in the recovery of acute aphasia: A single-patient and single-stimulus approach. *Neuropsychologia, 42,* 613–623.

Caplan, D. (1993). *Language: Structure, processing and disorders.* Cambridge, MA: MIT Press.

Caramazza, A., Berndt, R. S., & Basili, A. G. (1983). The selective impairment of phonological processing: A case study. *Brain and Language, 18,* 128–174.

Caramazza, A., & Hillis, A. E. (1990). Where do semantic errors come from? *Cortex, 26,* 5–122.

Caramazza, A., & Hillis, A. (1993). For a theory of remediation of cognitive deficits. *Neuropsychological Rehabilitation, 3,* 217–234.

Caramazza, A., & Hillis, A. E. (1991). Lexical organization of nouns and verbs in the brain. *Nature, 349,* 788–790.

Caramazza, A., Hillis, A. E., Leek, E. C., & Miozzo, M. (1994). The organization of lexical knowledge in the brain: Evidence from category- and modality-specific deficits. In L. Hirschfeld & S. Gelman (Eds.), *Mapping the mind: Domain specificity in cognition and culture* (pp. 68–84). New York: Cambridge University Press.

Caramazza, A., & Miozzo, M. (1997). The relation between syntactic and phonological knowledge in lexical access: evidence from the 'tip-of-the-tongue' phenomenon. *Cognition, 64,* 309–343.

Caramazza, A., & Shelton, J. R. (1998). Domain-specific knowledge systems in the brain: The animate-inanimate distinction. *Journal of Cognitive Neuroscience, 10,* 1–34.

Chertkow, H., Bub, D., & Seidenberg, M. (1989). Priming and semantic memory loss in Alzheimer's disease. *Brain and Language, 36,* 420–446.

Chialant, D., Costa, A., & Caramazza, A. (2002). Models of naming. In A. E. Hillis (Ed.), *The handbook of adult language disorders* (pp. 123–142). New York: Psychology Press.

Colombo, L., & Burani, C. (2002). The influence of age of acquisition, root frequency, and context availability in processing nouns and verbs. *Brain and Language, 81,* 398–411.

Coltheart, M. (1981). The MRC psycholinguistic database. *Quarterly Journal of Experimental Psychology, 33A,* 497–505.

Coltheart, M. (2001). Assumptions and methods in cognitive neuropsychology. In B. Rapp (Ed.), *The handbook of cognitive neuropsychology* (pp. 3–21). Philadelphia: Psychology Press.

Conley, A., & Coelho, C. A. (2003). Treatment of word retrieval impairment in chronic Broca's aplasia. *Aphasiology, 17,* 203–211.

Coslett, H. B., & Saffran, E. M. (1989). Preserved object recognition and reading comprehension in optic aphasia. *Brain, 112,* 1091–1110.

Coslett, H. B., & Saffran, E. M. (1992). Optic aphasia and the right hemisphere: A replication and extension. *Brain and Language 43,* 148–161.

Crosson, B. (1992). *Subcortical functions in language and memory.* New York: Oxford University Press.

Crosson, B., Moberg, P. J., Boone, J. R., Rothi, L. J. G., & Raymer, A. M. (1997). Category-specific naming deficit for medical terms after dominant thalamic/capsular hemorrhage. *Brain and Language, 60,* 407–440.

Cuetos, F., Monsalve, A., & Perez, A. (2005). Determinants of lexical access in pure anomia. *Journal of Neurolinguistics, 18,* 383–399.

Damasio, A. R., & Tranel, D. (1993). Nouns and verbs are retrieved with differently distributed neural systems. *Proceedings of the National Academy of Sciences, USA, 90,* 4957–4960.

Damasio, H., Grabowski, T. J., Tranel, D., Hichwa, R. D., & Damasio, A. R. (1996). A neural basis for lexical retrieval. *Nature, 380,* 499–505.

Davis, A., & Pring, T. (1991). Therapy for word-finding deficits: More on the effects of semantic and phonological approaches to treatment with dysphasic patients. *Neuropsychological Rehabilitation, 1,* 135–145.

De Bleser, R., & Cholewa, J. (1998). Dissociations between inflection, derivation, and compounding: Neurolinguistic evidence for morphological fractionations within the lexical system. In

E. G. Visch-Brink & R. Bastiaanse (Eds.), *Linguistic levels in aphasiology* (pp. 231–243). San Diego: Singular.

DeDe, G., Parris, D., & Waters, G. (2003). Teaching self-cues: Atreatment approach for verbal naming. *Aphasiology, 17,* 465–480.

Drew, R. L., & Thompson, C. K. (1999). Model-based semantic treatment for naming deficits in aphasia. *Journal of Speech, Language, & Hearing Research, 42,* 972–989.

Druks, J. (2001). Verbs and nouns—A review of the literature. *Journal of Neurolinguistics, 15,* 289–315.

Ellis, A. W., Kay, J., & Franklin, S. (1992). Anomia: Differentiating between semantic and phonological deficits. In D. I. Margolin (Ed.), *Cognitive neuropsychology in clinical practice* (pp. 207–227). New York: Oxford University Press.

Ellis, A. W., Miller, D., & Sin, G. (1983). Wernicke's aphasia and normal language processing: A case study in cognitive neuropsychology. *Cognition, 15,* 111–144.

Farah, M. J. (1990). *Visual agnosia.* Cambridge, MA: MIT Press.

Farah, M. J., & Wallace (1992). Semantically-bounded anomia: Implications for the neural implementation of naming. *Neuropsychologia, 30,* 609–621.

Ferreira, C. T., Giusiano, B., & Poncet, M. (1997). Category-specific anomia: Implication of different neural networks in naming. *Neuroreport, 6,* 1595–1602.

Foundas, A. L., Daniels, S. K., & Vasterling, J. J. (1998). Anomia: Case studies with lesion localization. *Neurocase, 4,* 35–43.

Francis, D. R., Riddoch, M. J., & Humphreys, G. W. (2001). Cognitive rehabilitation of word meaning deafness. *Aphasiology, 15,* 749–766.

Francis, W. N., & Kucera, H. 1982. *Frequency analysis of English usage: Lexicon and grammar.* Boston: Houghton Mifflin.

Franklin, S. (1989). Dissociations in auditory word comprehension; Evidence from nine fluent aphasic patients. *Aphasiology, 3,* 189–207.

Franklin, S., Turner, J., Ralph, M., Morris, J., & Bailey, P. (1996). A distinctive case of word meaning deafness. *Cognitive Neuropsychology, 13,* 1139–1162.

Funnell, E. (2000). Models of semantic memory. In W. Best, K. Bryan, & J. Maxim (Eds.), *Semantic processing: Theory and practice* (pp. 1–27). Philadelphia: Whurr.

Gilhooly, K. J., & Logie, R. H. (1980). Age-of-acquisition, imagery, concreteness, familiarity and ambiguity measures of 1944 words. *Behavioral Research Methods and Instrumentation, 12,* 395–427.

Goldrick, M., & Rapp, B. (in press, 2006). Lexical and post-lexical phonological representations in spoken production. *Cognition.*

Goodglass, H., Kaplan, E., & Barresi, B. (2001). *Boston Diagnostic Aphasia Examination* (3rd ed.). Hagerstown, MD: Lippincott, Williams & Wilkins.

Graham, K., Patterson, K., & Hodges, J. R. (1998). Semantic dementia and pure anomia: Two varieties of progressive fluent aphasia. In E. G. Visch-Brink & R. Bastiaanse (Eds.), *Linguistic levels in aphasiology* (pp. 49–68). San Diego: Singular.

Grayson, E., Hilton, R., & Franklin, S. (1997). Early intervention in a case of jargon aphasia: Efficacy of language comprehension therapy. *European Journal of Disorders of Communication, 32,* 257–276.

Greenwald, M. L., Raymer, A. M., Richardson, M. E., & Rothi, L. J. G. (1995). Contrasting treatments for severe impairments of picture naming. *Neuropsychological Rehabilitation, 5,* 17–49.

Haarbauer-Krupa, J., Moser, L., Smith, G., Sullivan, D. M., & Szekeres, S. F. (1985). Cognitive rehabilitation therapy: Middle stages of recovery. In M. Ylvisaker (Ed.), *Head injury rehabilitation: Children and adolescents* (pp. 287–310). San Diego: College Hill Press.

Hart, J., Berndt, R. S., & Caramazza, A. (1985). Category specific naming deficit following cerebral infarction. *Nature, 316,* 439–440.

Hart, J., & Gordon, B. (1990). Delineation of single-word semantic comprehension deficits in aphasia, with anatomical correlation. *Annals of Neurology, 27,* 226–231.

Hart, J., & Gordon, B. (1992). Neural subsystems for object knowledge. *Nature, 359,* 60–64.

Herbert, R., Best, W., Hickin, J., Howard, D., & Osborne, F. (2003). Combining lexical and interactional approaches to therapy for word finding deficits in aphasia. *Aphasiology, 17,* 1163–1186.

Hickin, J., Best, W., Herbert, R., Howard, D., & Osborne, F. (2002). Phonological therapy for word-finding difficulties: A re-evaluation. *Aphasiology, 16,* 981–999.

Hickin, J., Greenwood, A., Grassly, J., Herbert, R., Howard, D., & Best, W. (2005, May). *Therapy for word finding difficulties using phonological and orthographic cues: A clinical application in progress.* Presentation at the annual Clinical Aphasiology Conference, Sanibel Island, Florida.

Hillis, A. E. (1993). The role of models of language processing in rehabilitation of language impairments. *Aphasiology, 7,* 5–26.

Hillis, A. E. (1998). Treatment of naming disorders: new issues regarding old therapies. *Journal of the International Neuropsychological Society, 4,* 648–660.

Hillis, A. E. (2001). The organization of the lexical system. In B. Rapp (Ed.), *The handbook of cognitive neuropsychology* (pp. 185–210). Philadelphia: Psychology Press.

Hillis, A. E. (2002). The organization of the lexical system. In B. Rapp (Ed.), *The handbook of cognitive neuropsychology* (pp. 185–210). Philadelphia: Psychology Press.

Hillis, A. E., Boatman, D., Hart, J., & Gordon, B. (1999). Making sense out of jargon: A neurolinguistic and computational account of jargon aphasia. *Neurology, 53,* 1813–1824.

Hillis, A. E., & Caramazza, A. (1991). Category-specific naming and comprehension impairment: A double dissociation. *Brain, 114,* 2081–2094.

Hillis, A. E., & Caramazza, A. (1995a). Cognitive and neural mechanisms underlying visual and semantic processing: Implications from "optic aphasia". *Journal of Cognitive Neuroscience, 7,* 457–478.

Hillis, A. E., & Caramazza, A. (1995b). The compositionality of lexical semantic representations: Clues from semantic errors in object naming. *Memory, 3,* 333–358.

Hillis, A. E., & Caramazza, A. (1995c). Representation of grammatical categories of words in the brain. *Journal of Cognitive Neuroscience, 7,* 396–407.

Hillis, A. E., Chaudhry, P., Davis, C., Kleinman, J., Newhart, M., & Heidler-Gary, J. (2006). Where (in the brain) do semantic errors come from? *Brain and Language, 99,* 84–85.

Hillis, A. E., Kane, A., Tuffiash, E., Ulatowski, J. A., Barker, P. D., Beauchamp, N. J., et al. (2001). Reperfusion of specific brain regions by raising blood pressure restores selective language functions in subacute stroke. *Brain & Language, 79,* 495–510.

Hillis, A. E., Rapp, B., Romani, C., & Caramazza, A. (1990). Selective impairment of semantics in lexical processing. *Cognitive Neuropsychology, 7,* 191–243.

Hillis, A. E., Tuffiash, E., & Caramazza, A. (2002). Modality-specific deterioration in naming verbs in nonfluent primary progressive aphasia. *Journal of Cognitive Neuroscience, 14,* 1099–1108.

Hirsh, K. W., & Ellis, A. W. (1994). Age of acquisition and lexical processing in aphasia: A case study. *Cognitive Neuropsychology, 11,* 435–458.

Hodges, J. R., & Patterson, K. (1996). Nonfluent progressive aphasia and semantic dementia: A comparative neuropsychological study. *Journal of the International Neuropsychological Society, 2,* 511–524.

Hodges, J. R., Patterson, K., Oxbury, S., & Funnell, E. (1992). Semantic dementia: Progressive fluent aphasia with temporal lobe atrophy. *Brain, 115,* 1783–1806.

Howard, D., & Orchard-Lisle, V. (1984). On the origin of semantic errors in naming: Evidence from the case of a global aphasic. *Cognitive Neuropsychology, 1,* 163–190.

Howard, D., & Patterson, K. (1992). *Pyramids and palm trees.* Bury St. Edmunds: Thames Valley.

Howard, D., Patterson, K., Franklin, S., Orchard-Lisle, V., & Morton, J. (1985). Treatment of word retrieval deficits in aphasia. *Brain, 108,* 817–829.

Iorio, L., Falanga, A., Fragassi, N. A., & Grossi, D. (1992). Visual associative agnosia and optic aphasia. A single case study and a review of the syndromes. *Cortex, 28,* 23–37.

James, T. W., Culham, J., Humphrey, G. K., Milner, A. D., & Goodale, M. A. (2003). Ventral occipital lesions impair object recognition but not object-directed grasping: An fMRI study. *Brain, 126,* 2463–2475.

Joanette, Y., & Goulet, P. (1998). Right hemisphere and the semantic processing of words: Is the contribution specific or not? In E. G. Visch-Brink & R. Bastiaanse (Eds.), *Linguistic levels in aphasiology* (pp. 19–34). San Diego: Singular.

Kahn, H. J., Stannard, T., & Skinner, J. (1998). The use of words versus nonwords in the treatment of apraxia of speech: A case study. *ASHA Special Interest Division 2: Neurophysiology and Neurogenic Speech and Language Disorders, 8*(3), 5–10.

Kay, J., & Ellis, A. (1987). A cognitive neuropsychological case study of anomia: Implications for psychological models of word retrieval. *Brain, 110,* 613–629.

Kay, J., Lesser, R., & Coltheart, M. (1992). *PALPA: Psycholinguistic assessments of language processing in aphasia.* East Sussex, England: Lawrence Erlbaum.

Kertesz, A., Davidson, W., & McCabe, P. (1998). Primary progressive semantic apahsia: A case study. *Journal of the International Neuropsychological Society, 4,* 388–398.

Kertesz, A., Lau, W. K., & Polk, M. (1993). The structural determinants of recovery in Wernicke's aphasia. *Brain and Language, 44,* 153–164.

Kiran, S., & Thompson, C. K. (2002). The role of semantic complexity in treatment of naming deficits: Training semantic categories in fluent aphasia by controlling exemplar typicality. *Journal of Speech-Language-Hearing Research, 46,* 608–622.

Kiran, S., Thompson, C. K., & Hashimoto, N. (2001). Training grapheme to phoneme conversation in patients with oral reading and naming deficits: A model-based approach. *Aphasiology, 15,* 855–876.

Kohn, S. E., & Friedman, R. (1986). Word meaning deafness: A phonological-semantic dissociation. *Cognitive Neuropsychology, 3,* 291–308.

Kohn, S. E., Smith, K. L., & Alexander, M. P. (1996). Differential recovery from impairment to the phonological lexicon. *Brain and Language, 52,* 129–149.

Kremin, H., Perrier, D., De Wilde, M., Dordain, M., Le Bayon, A., Gatignol, P., et al. (2001). Factors predicting success in picture naming in Alzheimer's disease and primary progressive aphasia. *Brain and Cognition, 46,* 180–183.

Laganaro, M., Di Pietro, M., & Schnider, A. (2006). What does recovery from anomia tell us about the underlying impairment: The case of similar anomia patterns and different recovery. *Neuropsychologia, 44,* 534–545.

Laiacona, M., Capitani, E., & Barbarotto, R. (1997). Semantic category dissociations: A longitudinal study of two cases. *Cortex, 33,* 441–461.

Laiacona, M., Capitani, E., & Caramazza, A. (2003). Category-specific semantic deficits do not reflect the sensory/functional organization of the brain. *Neurocase, 9,* 221–231.

Lambon Ralph, M. A., Ellis, A. W., & Franklin, S. (1995). Semantic loss without surface dyslexia. *Neurocase, 1,* 363–369.

Lambon Ralph, M. A., Moriarty, L., & Sage, K. (2002). Anomia is simply a reflection of semantic and phonological impairments: Evidence from a case-series study. *Aphasiology, 16,* 56–82.

Le Dorze, G., Boulay, N., Gaudreau, J., & Brassard, C. (1994). The contrasting effects of a semantic versus a formal-semantic technique for the facilitation of naming in a case of anomia. *Aphasiology, 8,* 127–141.

Le Dorze, G., & Nespoulous, J.-L. (1989). Anomia in moderate aphasia: Problems in accessing the lexical representation. *Brain and Language, 37,* 381–400.

Lissauer, H. (1890/1988). A case of visual agnosia with a contribution to theory. *Cognitive Neuropsychology, 5,* 153–192.

Lowell, S., Beeson, P. M., & Holland, A. L. (1995). The efficacy of a semantic cueing procedure on naming performance of adults with aphasia. *American Journal of Speech-Language Pathology, 4,* 109–114.

Maher, L. M., Rothi, L. J. G., & Heilman, K. M. (1994). Lack of error awareness in an aphasic patient with relatively preserved auditory comprehension. *Brain and Language, 46,* 402–418.

Maneta, A., Marshall, J., & Lindsay, J. (2001). Direct and indirect therapy for word sound deafness. *International Journal of Language and Communication Disorders, 36,* 91–106.

Marsh, E. B., & Hillis, A. E. (2005). Cognitive and neural mechanisms underlying reading and naming: Evidence from letter-by-letter reading and optic aphasia. *Neurocase, 11,* 325–337.

Marshall, J., Pound, C., White-Thomson, M., & Pring, T. (1990). The use of picture/word matching tasks to assist word retrieval in aphasic patients. *Aphasiology, 4,* 167–184.

Martin, N. (1996). Cognitive approaches to recovery and rehabilitation in aphasia. *Brain and Language, 52,* 3–6.

Martin, N., Fink, R., & Laine, M. (2004). Treatment of word retrieval deficits with contextual priming. *Aphasiology, 18,* 457–471.

Martin, N., Fink, R. B., Renvall, K., & Laine, M. (2006). Effectiveness of contextual repetition priming treatments for anomia depends on intact access to semantics. *Journal of the International Neuropsychological Society, 12,* 853–866.

Miceli, G., Amitrano, A., Capasso, R., & Caramazza, A. (1996). The treatment of anomia resulting from output lexical damage: Analysis of two cases. *Brain and Language, 52*, 150–174.

Miceli, G., & Caramazza, A. (1988). Dissociations of inflectional and derivational morphology. *Brain and Language, 35*, 24–65.

Miceli, G., Giustollisi, L., & Caramazza, A. (1991). The interaction of lexical and non-lexical processing mechanisms: Evidence from anomia. *Cortex, 27*, 57–80.

Miceli, G., Silveri, M. C., Villa, G., & Caramazza, A. (1984). On the basis for the agrammatic's difficulty in producing main verbs. *Cortex, 20*, 207–220.

Miozzo, A., Soardi, M., & Cappa, S. F. (1994). Pure anomia with spared action naming due to a left temporal lesion. *Neuropsychologia, 32*, 1101–1109.

Mitchum, C., & Berndt, R. S. (1994). Verb retrieval and sentence construction: Effects of targeted intervention. In M. J. Riddoch & G. Humphreys (Eds.), *Cognitive neuropsychology and cognitive rehabilitation* (pp. 317–348). Hove: Erlbaum.

Mitchum, C. C., Ritgert, B. A., Sandson, J., & Berndt, R. S. (1990). The use of response analysis in confrontation naming. *Aphasiology, 4*, 261–280.

Morris, J., Franklin, S., Ellis, A. W., Turner, J. E., & Bailey, P. J. (1996). Remediating a speech perception deficit in an aphasic patient. *Aphasiology, 10*, 137–158.

Nadeau, S. E., & Rothi, L. J. G. (2007). Rehabilitation of subcortical aphasia. In R. Chapey (Ed.), *Language intervention strategies in aphasia and related neurogenic disorders*. Baltimore: Williams & Wilkins.

Nickels, L. (1992). The autocue? Self-generated phonemic cues in the treatment of a disorder of reading and naming. *Cognitive Neuropsychology, 9*, 155–182.

Nickels, L. (2001). Spoken word production. In B. Rapp (Ed.), *The handbook of cognitive neuropsychology* (pp. 291–320). Philadelphia: Psychology Press.

Nickels, L. (2002). Therapy for naming disorders: Revisiting, revising, and reviewing. *Aphasiology, 16*, 935–979.

Nickels, L., & Best, W. (1996). Therapy for naming disorders (Part II): Specifics, surprises, and suggestions. *Aphasiology, 10*, 109–136.

Nickels, L., & Howard, D. (1994). A frequent occurrence: Factors affecting the production of semantic errors in aphasic naming. *Cognitive Neuropsychology, 11*, 289–320.

Nickels, L., & Howard, D. (1995). Aphasic naming: What matters? *Neuropsychologia, 33*, 1281–1303.

Ochipa, C., Maher, L. M., & Raymer, A. M. (1998). One approach to the treatment of anomia. *ASHA Special Interest Division 2: Neurophysiology and Neurogenic Speech and Language Disorders, 15*(3), 18–23.

Ochipa, C., Rothi, L. J. G., & Heilman, K. M. (1989). Ideational apraxia: A deficit in tool selection and use. *Annals of Neurology, 25*, 190–193.

Paivio, A. (1986). Mental comparisons involving abstract attributes. *Memory & Cognition, 2*, 199–208.

Pashek, G. V. (1997). A case study of gesturally cued naming in aphasia: Dominant versus nondominant hand training. *Journal of Communication Disorders, 30*, 349–366.

Pashek, G. V. (1998). Gestural facilitation of noun and verb retrieval in aphasia: A case study. *Brain and Language, 65*, 177–180.

Plaut, D. C. (1996). Relearning after damage in connectionist networks: Toward a theory of rehabilitation. *Brain and Language, 52*, 25–82.

Polster, M. R., & Rose, S. B. (1998). Disorders of auditory processing: Evidence for modularity in audition. *Cortex, 34*, 47–65.

Pring, T., Hamilton A., Harwood, A., & Macbride, L. (1993). Generalization of naming after picture/word matching tasks. *Aphasiology, 7*, 383–394.

Pring, T., White-Thomson, M. Pound, C., Marshall, J., & Davis, A. (1990). Picture/word matching tasks and word retrieval. *Aphasiology, 4*, 479–483.

Raymer, A. M., & Berndt, R. S. (1996). Reading lexically without semantics: Evidence from patients with probable Alzheimer's disease. *Journal of the International Neuropsychological Society, 2*, 340–349.

Raymer, A. M., Ciampitti, M., Holliway, B., Singletary, F., Blonder, L. X., Ketterson, T., et al. (2007). Semantic-phonologic treatment for noun and verb retrieval impairments in aphasia. *Neuropsychological Rehabilitation., 17*, 244–270.

Raymer, A. M., & Ellsworth, T. A. (2002). Response to contrasting verb retrieval treatments. *Aphasiology, 16*, 1031–1045.

Raymer, A. M., Foundas, A. L., Maher, L. M., Greenwald, M. L., Morris, M., Rothi, L. J. G., et al. (1997). Cognitive neuropsychological analysis and neuroanatomic correlates in a case of acute anomia. *Brain and Language, 58*, 137–156.

Raymer, A. M., Greenwald, M. L., Richardson, M. E., Rothi, L. J. G., & Heilman, K. M. (1997). Optic aphasia and optic apraxia: Case analysis and theoretical implications. *Neurocase, 3*, 173–183.

Raymer, A. M., Kohen, F. P., & Saffell, D. (2006). Computerised training for impairments of word comprehension and retrieval in aphasia. *Aphasiology, 20*, 257–268.

Raymer, A. M., Maher, L. M., Foundas, A. L., Rothi, L. J. G., & Heilman, K. M. (2000). Analysis of lexical recovery in an individual with acute anomia. *Aphasiology, 14*, 901–910.

Raymer, A. M., Maher, L. M., Greenwald, M. L., Morris, M., Rothi, L. J. G., & Heilman, K. M. (1990). *The Florida Semantics Battery*. Unpublished. (see Appendix 23-1).

Raymer, A. M., Moberg, P., Crosson, B., Nadeau, S.E., & Rothi, L. J. G. (1997). Lexical-semantic deficits in two patients with dominant thalamic infarction. *Neuropsychologia, 35*, 211–219.

Raymer, A. M., & Rothi, L. J. G. (2000). Semantic system. In L. J. G. Rothi, B. Crosson, & S. Nadeau (Eds.), *Aphasia and language: Theory to practice* (pp. 108–132). New York: Guilford Press.

Raymer, A. M., Rothi, L. J. G., & Greenwald, M. L. (1995). The role of cognitive models in language rehabilitation. *NeuroRehabilitation, 5*, 183–193.

Raymer, A. M., Rothi, L. J. G., & Heilman, K. M. (1995). Nonsemantic activation of lexical and praxis output systems in Alzheimer's subjects. *Journal of the International Neuropsychological Society, 1*, 147 (abstract).

Raymer, A. M., Singletary, F., Rodriguez, A., Ciampitti, M., Heilman, K. M., & Rothi, L. J. G. (2006). Gesture training effects for noun and verb retrieval in aphasia. *Journal of the International Neuropsychological Society, 12*, 867–882.

Raymer, A. M., & Thompson, C. K. (1991). Effects of verbal plus gestural treatment in a patient with aphasia and severe apraxia of speech. In T. E. Prescott (Ed.), *Clinical aphasiology* (Vol. 12, pp. 285–297). Austin, TX: Pro-Ed.

Raymer, A. M., Thompson, C. K., Jacobs, B., & le Grand, H. R. (1993). Phonologic treatment of naming deficits in aphasia: Model-based generalization analysis. *Aphasiology, 7,* 27–53.

Renvall, K., Laine, M., & Martin, N. (2005). Contextual priming in semantic anomia: A case study. *Brain and Language, 95,* 327–341.

Riddoch, M. J., & Humphreys, G. W. (1987). Visual object processing in optic aphasia: A case of semantic access agnosia. *Cognitive Neuropsychology, 4,* 131–185.

Riddoch, M. J., & Humphreys, G. W. (1994). Cognitive neuropsychology and cognitive rehabilitation: A marriage of equal partners? In M. J. Riddoch & G. W. Humphreys (Eds.), *Cognitive neuropsychology and cognitive rehabilitation* (pp. 1–15). London: Erlbaum.

Riddoch, M. J., & Humphreys, G. W. (2001). Object recognition. In B. Rapp (Ed.), *The handbook of cognitive neuropsychology* (pp. 45–74). Philadelphia: Psychology Press.

Roach, A., Schwartz, M. F., Martin, N., Grewal., R., & Brecher, A. (1996). The Philadelphia Naming Test: Scoring and rationale. *Clinical Aphasiology, 24,* 121–134.

Robson, J., Marshall, J., Pring, T., & Chiat, S. (1998). Phonologic naming therapy in jargon aphasia: Positive but paradoxical effects. *Journal of the International Neuropsychological Society, 4,* 675–686.

Rodriguez, A., Raymer, A. M., & Rothi, L. J. G. (2006). Effects of gesture and semantic-phonological treatments for verb retrieval. *Aphasiology, 20,* 286–297.

Rosazza, C., Imbornone, E., Zorzi, M., Farina, E., Chiavari, L., & Cappa, S. F. (2003). The heterogeneity of category-specific semantic disorders: Evidence from a new case. *Neurocase, 9,* 198–202.

Rose, M., Douglas, J., & Matyas, T. (2002). The comparative effectiveness of gesture and verbal treatments for a specific phonologic naming impairment. *Aphasiology, 16,* 1001–1030.

Rothi, L. J. G. (1995). Behavioral compensation in the case of treatment of acquired language disorders resulting from brain damage. In R. A. Dixon & L. Mackman (Eds.), *Compensating for psychological deficits and declines: Managing losses and promoting gains* (pp. 219–230). Mahwah, NJ: Lawrence Erlbaum.

Rothi, L. J. G. (1997). Transcortical motor, sensory, and mixed aphasia. In L. L. LaPointe (Ed.), *Aphasia and related neurogenic language disorders* (2nd ed., pp. 91–111). New York: Thieme Medical.

Rothi, L. J. G., Ochipa, C., & Heilman, K. M. (1997). A cognitive neuropsychological model of limb praxis and apraxia. In L. J. G. Rothi & K. M. Heilman (Eds.), *Apraxia: The neuropsychology of action* (pp. 29–49). East Sussex, UK: Psychology Press.

Rothi, L. J. G., Raymer, A. M., Maher, L. M., Greenwald, M., & Morris, M. (1991). Assessment of naming failures in neurological communication disorders. *Clinics in Communication Disorders, 1,* 7–20.

Saffran, E. M. (1997). Aphasia: Cognitive neuropsychological aspects. In T. E. Feinberg & M. J. Farah (Eds.), *Behavioral neurology and neuropsychology* (pp. 151–165). New York: McGraw-Hill.

Schnider, A., Benson, D. F., & Scharre, D. W. (1994). Visual agnosia and optic aphasia: Are they anatomically distinct? *Cortex, 30,* 445–457.

Semenza, C., Cipolotti, L., & Denes, G. (1992). Reading aloud in jargonaphasia: An unusual dissociation in speech output. *Journal of Neurology, Neurosurgery, & Psychiatry, 55,* 205–208.

Seron, X., & Deloche, G. (Eds.). (1989). *Cognitive approaches in neuropsychological rehabilitation.* Hillsdale, NJ: Erlbaum.

Shallice, T. (1988). *From neuropsychology to mental structure.* Cambridge: Cambridge University Press.

Shapiro, K., & Caramazza, A. (2003). Grammatical processing of nouns and verbs in left frontal cortex? *Neuropsychologia, 41,* 1189–1198.

Shelton, J. R., & Caramazza, A. (2001). The organization of semantic memory. In B. Rapp (Ed.), *The handbook of cognitive neuropsychology* (pp. 423–443). Philadelphia: Psychology Press.

Shindo, M., Kaga, K., & Tanaka, Y. (1991). Speech discrimination and lip reading in patients with word deafness or auditory agnosia. *Brain and Language, 40,* 153–161.

Silveri, M. C., Gainotti, G., Perani, D., Cappelletti, J. Y., Carbone, G., & Faxio, F. (1997). Naming deficits for non-living items: Neuropsychological and PET study. *Neuropsychologia, 35,* 359–367.

Snodgrass, J. G., & Vanderwart, M. (1980). A standardised set of 260 pictures: Norms for name agreement, image agreement, familiarity and visual complexity. *Journal of Experimental Psychology: Human Perception and Performance, 6,* 174–215.

Stanczak, L., Waters, G., & Caplan, D. (2006). Typicality-based learning and generalization in aphasia: Two case studies of anomia treatment. *Aphasiology, 20,* 374–383.

Tyler, L. K. (1987). Spoken language comprehension in aphasia: A real-time processing perspective. In M. Coltheart, G. Sartori, & R. Job (Eds.), *The cognitive neuropsychology of language* (pp. 145–162). London: Lawrence Erlbaum.

Vignolo, L. A. (1982). Auditory agnosia. *Philosophical Transactions of the Royal Society (London), 298,* 49–57.

Wambaugh, J. L. (2003). A comparison of the relative effects of phonologic and semantic cueing treatments. *Aphasiology, 17,* 433–441.

Wambaugh, J. L., Doyle, P. J., Linebaugh, C. W., Spencer, K. A., & Kalinyak-Fliszar, M. (1999). Effects of deficit-oriented treatments on lexical retrieval in a patient with semantic and phonological deficits. *Brain and Language, 69,* 466–450.

Wambaugh, J. L., Doyle, P. J., Martinez, A. L., & Kalinyak-Fliszar, M. (2002). Effects of two lexical retrieval cueing treatments on action naming in aphasia. *Journal of Rehabilitation Research & Development, 39,* 455–466.

Wambaugh, J. L., Linebaugh, C. W., Doyle, P. J., Martinez, A. L., Kalinyak-Fliszar, M., & Spencer, K. A. (2001). Effects of two cueing treatments on lexical retrieval in aphasic speakers with different levels of deficit. *Aphasiology, 15,* 933–950.

Warrington, E. K., & McCarthy, R. A. (1983). Category-specific access dysphasia. *Brain, 100,* 1273–1296.

Warrington, E. K., & McCarthy, R. A. (1987). Categories of knowledge: Further fractionation and an attempted integration. *Brain, 110,* 1273–1296.

Warrington, E. K., & McCarthy, R. A. (1994). Multiple meaning systems in the brain: A case for visual semantics. *Neuropsychologia, 32,* 1465–1473.

Warrington, E., & Shallice, T. (1984). Category specific semantic impairments. *Brain, 107,* 829–854.

Warrington, E., & Taylor, (1978). Two categorical stages of object recognition. *Perception, 7,* 695-705.

Webster, J., Morris, J., & Franklin, S. (2005). Effects of therapy targeted at verb retrieval and the realization of the predicate argument structure: A case study. *Aphasiology, 19,* 748–764.

Weiller, C., Isensee, C., Rijntjes, M., Huber, W., Muller, S., Bier, D., et al. (1995). Recovery from Wernicke's aphasia: A positron emission tomographic study. *Annals of Neurology, 37,* 723–732.

Wilson, B. A. (1999). *Case studies in neuropsychological rehabilitation.* New York: Oxford University Press.

Zingeser, L. B., & Berndt, R. S. (1988). Grammatical class and context effects in a case of pure anomia: Implications for models of language production. *Cognitive Neuropsychology, 5,* 473–516.

Zingeser, L. B., & Berndt, R. S. (1990). Retrieval of nouns and verbs in agrammatism and anomia. *Brain and Language, 39,* 14–32.

APPENDIX 23.1
Stimuli from the Florida Semantics Battery*

Key: HF = 40 highest frequency words, range 26–242;
MF = 40 middle frequency words, range 9–25;
LF = 40 lowest frequency words, range 0–8.

Body Parts	Frequency	Transportation	Frequency	Vegetables	Frequency	Fruits	Frequency
ankle	15 MF	airplane	21 MF	broccoli	1 LF	apple	15 MF
elbow	17 MF	jeep	16 MF	celery	4 LF	cherry	6 LF
wrist	16 MF	van	22 MF	lettuce	1 LF	lemon	4 LF
ear	67 HF	bus	42 HF	peas	24 MF	peach	4 LF
nose	65 HF	truck	80 HF	potato	30 HF	pineapple	9 MF
chin	25 MF	canoe	8 LF	carrot	5 LF	banana	4 LF
thumb	14 MF	sailboat	4 LF	corn	38 HF	grapes	10 MF
arm	217 HF	boat	123 HF	onion	19 MF	orange	15 MF
leg	126 HF	train	86 HF	pepper	13 MF	pear	8 LF
teeth	102 HF	wagon	72 HF	pumpkin	2 LF	raisin	1 LF

Kitchen Utensils	Frequency	Clothing	Frequency	Animals	Frequency	Personal Items	Frequency
fork	20 MF	mitten	2 LF	deer	13 MF	brush	36 HF
pan	16 MF	robe	10 MF	mouse	20 MF	mirror	27 MF
spoon	6 LF	sweater	18 MF	turtle	9 MF	razor	15 MF
cup	58 HF	dress	63 HF	cow	46 HF	toothbrush	6 LF
knife	86 HF	shoe	58 HF	fish	281 HF	towel	17 MF
jar	19 MF	pants	9 MF	frog	2 LF	comb	6 LF
skillet	2 LF	scarf	4 LF	pig	14 MF	perfume	11 MF
bottle	90 LF	coat	52 HF	cat	42 HF	soap	25 MF
glass	128 HF	hat	71 HF	dog	147 HF	toothpaste	2 LF
plate	44 HF	suit	64 HF	horse	203 HF	tissue	54 H

Furniture	Frequency	Office Items	Frequency	Tools	Frequency	Musical Instruments	Frequency
crib	8 LF	book	100 HF	axe	19 MF	accordian	1 LF
shelf	20 MF	newspaper	43 HF	hammer	6 LF	drum	20 MF
stool	8 LF	phone	46 HF	pliers	1 LF	guitar	10 MF
bench	42 HF	scissors	1 LF	saw	8 LF	harp	1 LF
desk	69 HF	tape	39 HF	shovel	8 LF	trumpet	5 LF
hammock	5 LF	clip	6 LF	clamp	2 LF	bell	17 MF
sofa	9 MF	pen	13 MF	hoe	1 LF	flute	3 LF
bed	139 HF	ruler	13 MF	rake	8 LF	harmonica	0 LF
chair	89 HF	stamp	8 LF	screwdriver	1 LF	piano	32 HF
table	242 HF	pencil	38 HF	wrench	1 LF	violin	9 M

*Includes 120 nouns from 12 different semantic categories.
†Frequencies based on Francis, W. N., & Kucera, H. (1982). *Frequency analysis of English usage: Lexicon and grammar.* Boston: Houghton Mifflin.)
(From Raymer, A. M., Maher, L. M., Greenwald, M. L., Morris, M., Rothi, L. J. G., & Heilman, K. M. (1990). The Florida Semantics Battery. Unpublished.)

APPENDIX 23.2
Glossary

Category-Specific Semantic Impairments—Disturbances in comprehension or production for selective semantic categories, with preserved performance for other categories.

Lexical Decision—Task in which the patient decides whether a given stimulus is a familiar real word or object, or a nonsense word or object.

Lexical Phonologic Output Processing—Mechanism of representations for familiar spoken words that have previously been produced.

Lexical Phonologic Recognition—Mechanism of representations for familiar spoken words that have previously been heard.

Lexical System—Complex, distributed set of mechanisms storing representations for familiar words, objects, and actions, as well as processes for decoding and encoding unfamiliar stimuli.

Optic Aphasia—Visual modality-specific impairment in naming viewed objects in the presence of basic semantic processing indicated through circumlocutions or gestures associated with the unnamed object.

Pure Word Deafness—Auditory modality–specific impairment in processing spoken input.

Recognition—The point in stimulus-processing at which a stimulus is distinguished and found to be familiar and previously experienced.

Restitutive Treatments—Strategies that encourage restoration of functioning in a manner compatible with normal language processing.

Semantic System—The lexical mechanism responsible for storing meaning representations for familiar words, objects, and actions.

Substitutive Treatments—Strategies that attempt to circumvent a dysfunctional language mechanism using other intact language and cognitive processes.

Visual Agnosia—The failure, as a result of brain damage, to recognize a viewed stimulus that is not due to a peripheral sensory visual disorder.

Visual Object Representation—The mechanism storing memories for familiar objects that have previously been seen.

Word-Meaning Deafness—Impairment in the ability to apply meaning to heard words despite intact phonologic processing.

Chapter 24

Comprehension and Production of Sentences

Charlotte C. Mitchum and
Rita Sloan Berndt

OBJECTIVES

In this chapter we illustrate how cognitive neuropsychology has been applied to assessment and intervention of sentence-processing disorders in aphasia. This approach differs from traditional assessment measures that classify subtypes of aphasia; it does not seek to establish a clinical label based on measures of contrasting symptoms (e.g., Broca's aphasia vs. Wernicke's aphasia), or to obtain a general measure of relative severity. Rather, specific symptoms are contrasted with normal sentence processing, with the goal being to identify how brain damage has altered normal functions.

Using a model of normal sentence processing is somewhat hampered by the lack of a complete understanding of all the details involved in sentence production and comprehension. There is no theoretic model that can fully account for normal sentence processing, nor can a model account for the myriad of problems observed in aphasic language (Berndt, 2001). Treatment can be guided by hypotheses about what needs to be restored or bypassed, but the mechanisms of change established with therapy remain poorly understood. Nonetheless, we illustrate how reference to a theoretic framework has provided a valuable mechanism for sorting out the array of symptoms associated with aphasic sentence processing, and has inspired new and effective approaches to the treatment of sentence-processing disorders.

SENTENCE-LEVEL DEFICITS IN APHASIA

Interest in aphasic symptoms that are specific to sentences has a long history in neurology (Luria, 1947; Pick, 1913) and linguistics (Jacobson, 1956); these symptoms have been interpreted primarily as grammatical disturbances. An important contrast is the one between "agrammatism,"

which typically occurs in the context of nonfluent (especially Broca's) aphasia, and "paragrammatism," which occurs in sentences produced by more fluent speakers (especially those with Wernicke's aphasia). The difference between these manifestations of grammatical disturbance has been widely described as involving distinct problems with grammatical morphemes (both bound and free), with agrammatism characterized primarily by omission of these elements and paragrammatism by their misuse (Goodglass, 1993). The following speech samples illustrate the differences between a typical Broca's pattern and the type of disordered sentences often produced by more fluent speakers (pauses > 1 sec are noted):

Pattern Associated with Broca's Aphasia

Cinderella (4s) poor and (4s) poor meaning not to be (3s) fire and all thing but (2s) stepsister two (4s) rich (2s) powerful man and (3s) well that after (6s) slim chance (3s) me and cleaning the house and serving the (2s) meals and rich man (3s) well the prince is (2s) going to (4s) east (2s) feast

Pattern Associated with (Mild) Wernicke's Aphasia

the Cinderella was his his father and his father but he's . . . passed away so she's his his mother-in-law was the really little bit angry and everything . . . and the Cinderella in the cellar . . . she also had the sisters-in-law two sisters and they have all they have all the sisters was old . . . nose and teeth and awful

Although these types of speech patterns sound markedly different to the listener, considerable overlap exists in the types of errors that can be noted. Analyses of such speech samples from patients demonstrating both of these patterns reveal omission and substitution of grammatical morphemes (Butterworth & Howard, 1987). In some cases, grammatical disturbances are primarily structural in nature, with relatively preserved use of grammatical morphology but an inability to produce a normally structured and elaborated sentence (Saffran, Berndt, & Schwartz, 1989; Tissot, Mounin, & Lhermitte, 1973). Although many different accounts of grammatical morpheme omissions in agrammatism have been offered (see Berndt, 1998 for review), it is important to note that impaired use of grammatical morphology is only one of many structural impairments observed in the

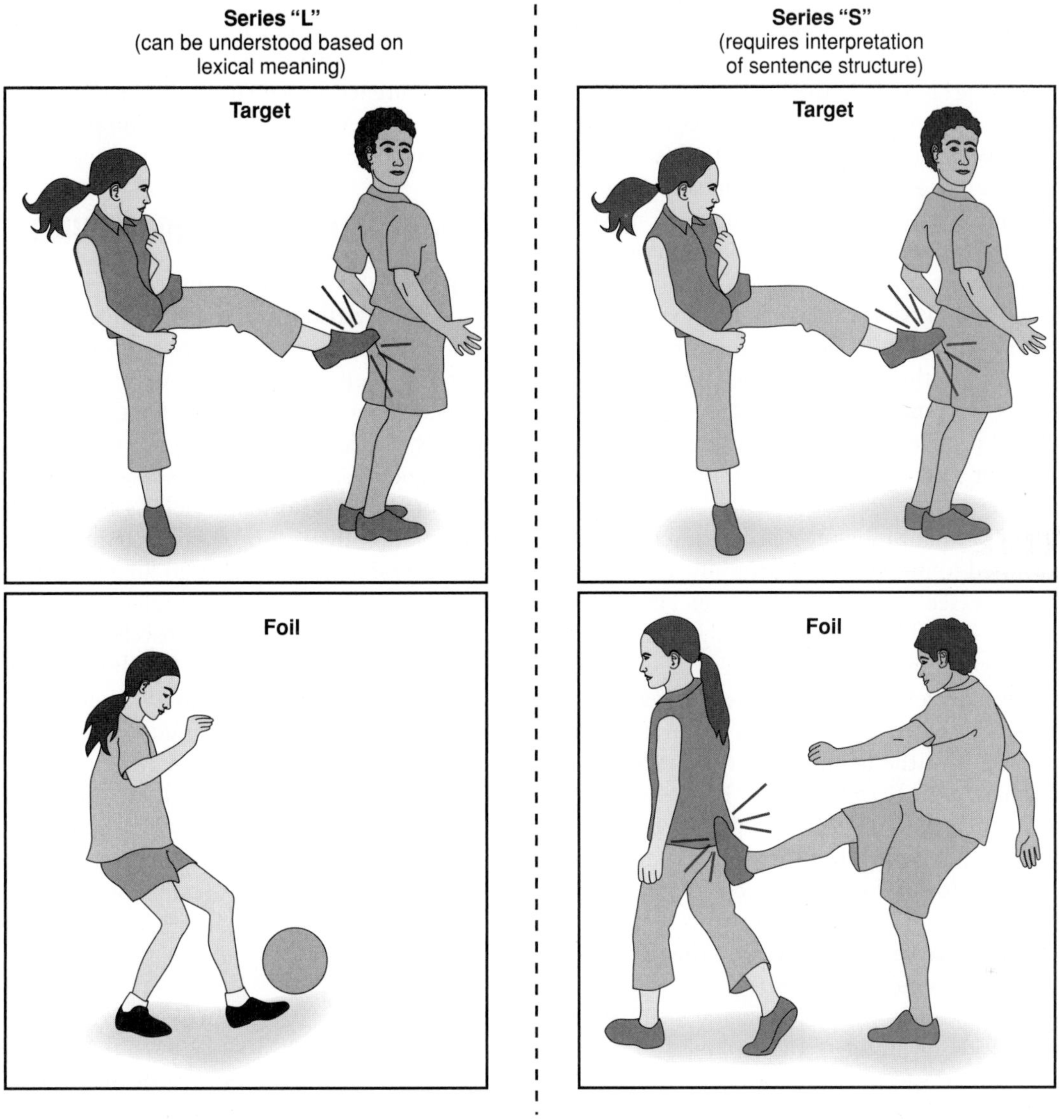

Series "L"
(can be understood based on
lexical meaning)

Target

Foil

Series "S"
(requires interpretation
of sentence structure)

Target

Foil

Figure 24–1. Examples of Stimuli Used to Assess Comprehension of Sentences Based on Lexical ("L") or Structural ("S") Cues to Meaning.

sentences of speakers with aphasia. It is also now widely recognized that symptoms associated with agrammatism do not always co-occur and are not unique to Broca's-type aphasia.

Agrammatism was long believed to be a uniquely "expressive" impairment, since patients with Broca's aphasia (by definition) demonstrate good comprehension on clinical testing. However, a set of studies in the late 1970s showed that agrammatic patients often failed to understand sentences correctly when the stimuli were constructed to require interpretation of grammatical features (Caramazza & Zurif, 1976; Schwartz, Saffran, & Marin, 1980). These studies revealed a pattern of impaired comprehension associated with Broca's aphasia that suggested that interpretation

of sentences was frequently based on semantic cues such as noun animacy, or on heuristics based on word order, rather than on sentence structure.

This type of sentence-comprehension disorder emerged only in tests that systematically eliminated the possibility of using non-syntactic cues to meaning. For example, sentence-picture matching tasks present a spoken sentence with two pictures showing a pair of actors performing the same action, but with the noun roles reversed. Other items in the test assure that patients' understanding of the individual words in the sentence is intact. As shown in Figure 24–1, it is possible to identify the depiction of "the girl kicking the boy" (vs. "the girl kicking the ball") simply by knowing the difference between the meaning of the words "boy" and "ball." That is, an interpretation based on single-word meaning may give the impression that the sentence has been fully comprehended. In the pair of pictures on the right, the same target sentence "the girl is kicking the boy" cannot be interpreted using the meaning of individual words because "boy," "kick," and "girl" are shown in both pictures. In this arrangement, the grammatical cues to the sentence meaning—word order, verb inflection, i.e., the syntactic structure—must be interpreted in order to identify which of the two nouns is *doing the kicking*. To test for a "first noun is agent" word-order strategy, active and passive versions of the same sentence are presented with pictures showing the correct depiction and a reversal of the thematic roles stated in the stimulus sentences. Patients cannot perform correctly on both the active and passive versions of the sentence if they assume that the first noun mentioned is the agent of the action.

Variants of these "semantically reversible" sentences have been very widely used to investigate structurally based comprehension disorders (see Berndt, Mitchum, & Haendiges, 1996 for review). In addition, tasks designed to test reversible sentence *production* reveal similar errors involving difficulty matching correct word order to sentence structure. This is observed when patients are "constrained" to begin their response with the noun that is not the agent of the action (Caramazza & Berndt, 1985). For example, if forced to start a sentence to describe the picture shown in Figure 24–1 (top) with the word "boy," it is difficult for some speakers with aphasia to produce a passive sentences (e.g., "the boy is kicked by the girl"). A typical error is to produce a sentence in the active voice and thus violate the sentence's meaning (e.g., "the boy is kicking the girl").

The finding that speakers with agrammatic aphasia frequently had difficulty interpreting structural cues to meaning in comprehension generated enormous interest in Broca's aphasia because it suggested that such patients suffered from a "central" syntactic deficit affecting all elements of language use. Agrammatism was viewed as a constellation of inseparable symptoms associated with the halting, telegraphic speech of Broca's aphasia. The characteristics of agrammatism were generally believed to include the following symptoms: (1) "closed class" word errors, especially the omission of free and bound grammatical morphemes; (2) "open class" word production, which mostly spared concrete nouns; (3) simplified syntactic complexity and reduced phrase length; and (4) poor comprehension of semantically reversible sentences (Berndt & Caramazza, 1980).

Although some researchers who still maintain some elements of this "syntactic deficit hypothesis," including the view that "Broca's area" of the brain is specialized for aspects of syntactic processing (Grodzinsky, 2000), there is strong evidence from many studies that these symptoms can dissociate from one another (see Berndt, 1991; Martin, 2006, for reviews). Current approaches to the study of sentence production and comprehension in aphasia do not assume that these symptoms will always occur together. Rather, recent work more often seeks to explain how a particular symptom contributes to the sentence-processing pattern observed in individual cases, or in groups of individuals who share (at least) a symptom of interest (Berndt, 1998; Berndt et al., 1996).

NORMAL SENTENCE PROCESSING

Normal speakers produce and comprehend sentences with little apparent effort, yet the cognitive operations that support the creation and interpretation of sentences must be remarkably complex. To utter or understand even a single sentence requires, at the very least, the integration of the products of lexical retrieval, syntactic formulation, phonologic encoding, and articulation. Exactly how the interplay of these components normally yields a final product is not well understood. Theories of normal sentence processing draw upon several sources of data in an attempt to describe the inner structure of language, including analyses of normal "slips of the tongue," results of psycholinguistic experiments, and computational modeling. The theories that result can be very useful for the speech-language clinician interested in understanding how aphasic language deviates from language that is unimpaired (Hillis, 1993; Mitchum & Berndt, 1995). In the sections to follow, we will identify subcomponents of sentence production and comprehension, within the context of what we know about normal language, and in light of evidence from cognitive neuropsychological studies.

Sentence Production

Operations necessary for sentence production range from the creation of an intended message to its ultimate articulation. Even in the absence of a formal theory, it would seem likely that sentences evolve through a series of fairly independent stages. Thoughts form a rough, preverbal idea of what one wants to say. Although thoughts may be candidates for verbal expression, they are not lexically specified or grammatically well-formed; many thoughts never become phonologically encoded. For selected thoughts, however, we seem to readily convert the unspecified message into an ordered utterance that contains both lexical (open-class) content and grammatical (closed-class) structure. The utterance is made known using an articulatory code common to both speaker and listener. However, this informal description tells us little about how these events are coordinated. That is, how do we construct a verbal sentence from thought? Importantly, for the speech-language pathologist, how do we determine what can go wrong in aphasic sentence production?

The production model proposed by Garrett (1975, 1982, 1988) characterizes the processes involved in creating a series of distinct sets of representations that transform ideas into speech. Figure 24–2 is a schematic of normal sentence

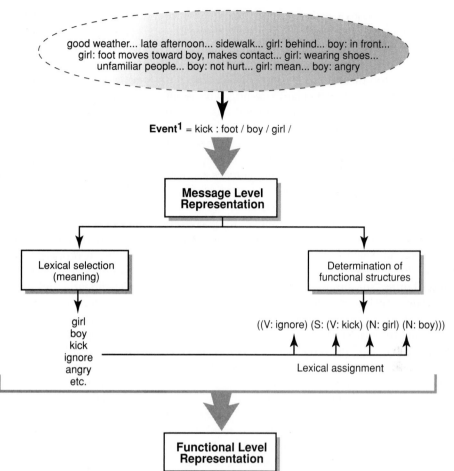

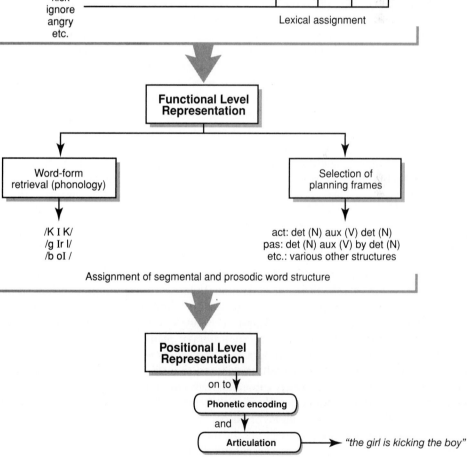

Figure 24–2. A Model of Normal Sentence Production Based on Garrett (1988).

production adapted from Garrett (1988), which we have elaborated to illustrate how the model conceives of the elements needed to produce a sentence. In this example, the message to be conveyed is that a girl is kicking a boy. We focus here on the top three levels of the model and do not consider the requirements of articulatory coding. This is not to diminish the importance of these operations, but to emphasize the issues that have been the primary focus of research on sentence processing in aphasia. It is important to keep in mind that this model describes only the representations that are constructed serially during sentence production. What are not detailed are the processes through which the speaker moves from one level to the next.

The three distinct levels within the model to be considered here consist of the following: A <u>Message Representation</u> may derive from a variety of verbal and nonverbal sources, and may be thought of as the conceptualization of some proposition that the speaker wants to convey. A <u>Functional Representation</u> encodes the conceptual proposition into abstract lexical entries representing word meanings and their functional (thematic) roles. Structural order is established at the <u>Positional Level</u> as phonologically specified lexical items are inserted into a surface structure based on their grammatical roles (e.g., subject, verb, object).

These levels of representation are motivated primarily by evidence from errors produced by normal speakers. For example, the postulation that word retrieval requires two steps (one semantic, one phonologic), as well as the details about what information these levels encode, is supported by regularities in the types of errors that occur in normal speech. Word-exchange errors demonstrate distinct characteristics from sound exchanges (exchanged portion italicized; all examples from Garrett, 1982):

a. " Well you can cut *rain* in the *trees*"
   "Why was that *horn* blowing its *train*?"
b. " No . . . it's . . . Bria*th* Kee*n*" (Brian Keith)
   "And this is the *l*arietal *p*obe" (parietal lobe)

Word-exchange errors (as in a.) tend to involve words in different phrases that are in the same grammatical category, whereas sound exchanges (b.) tend to occur within a phrase and to involve words of different grammatical classes. These distinctions lead to the postulation of a multiphrasal planning level in which the identity and phrasal role of words is important (i.e., the Functional Level), in addition to a single-phrase planning level at which (phonologic) form and serial order are represented (the Positional Level). The hypothesis is that word-exchange errors occur in the creation of Functional-Level structures from the message level, whereas sound exchanges arise in the construction of the Positional Level from Functional-Level structures.

One important characteristic of word- and sound-exchange errors is that they almost always involve words from major lexical categories (nouns, verbs, adjectives, and adverbs) rather than grammatical words (pronouns, auxiliary verbs, prepositions), suggesting that these two types of words are generated by different processes. This distinction is supported by another type of exchange error that generally occurs within phrases:

c. "that's why they sell the *cheap*s *drink*" (drinks cheap) "she *write*s her *slant*ing" (slants her writing)

These errors typically involve the "stranding" of inflections in their proper positions even though their stems are exchanged, suggesting that the construction of the Positional Level involves the insertion of phonologically specified major lexical items into a planning frame with inflectional elements and grammatical words already specified.

Many variants of this framework with relevance to aphasia have been proposed over the years, including an argument that bound and free grammatical morphemes are generated independently in the construction of phrasal frames (Lapointe, 1985), suggestions that there must be feedback from Positional to Functional Level to account for "mixed" (phonologic/semantic) speech errors (Dell & Reich, 1981), and debate about the level at which grammatical class information is encoded (Caramazza, 1997). Nonetheless, there is widespread agreement on the major distinctions expressed by the model, and it has been used frequently as a starting point for analyses of aphasic sentence production (Saffran, 1982; Schneider & Thompson, 2003; Schwartz, 1987).

Sentence Comprehension

It is likely that sentence comprehension shares many of the more abstract components that Garrett identifies for sentence production (e.g., at the Message and Functional Levels), whereas the details of the phonetic representations (acoustic/articulatory) for input and output must be quite different. Because Message- and Functional-Level representations are assumed to be shared for production and comprehension (Levelt, 1989; Levelt, Roelofs, & Meyer, 1999; Vigliocco & Hartsuiker, 2002), it is sometimes argued that if comprehension of Message and Functional elements is intact, then the source of a patient's production impairment must arise at a later point (Caramazza & Hillis, 1989). For this reason, and in the absence of a suitably detailed model of sentence comprehension, it is useful to consider a schematic of the components of the production model working in reverse as they decode the acoustic signal (see also Jacobs & Thompson, 2000).

Saffran (2001) presents a framework for sentence comprehension that corresponds to the Functional/Positional level distinguished by Garrett. As depicted in Figure 24–3, the listener interprets the acoustic signal by segmenting the phonetic sequence into recognizable spoken word forms and matches them to lexical entries. As each word is recovered, it is held in temporary storage as the syntactic structure of the

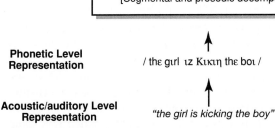

Conceptual Representation

Functional Level Representation

[Identification of functional structures]

(S: (V: kick) (N: girl/actor) (N: boy/recipient))

[Retrieval of word meaning]

"young female, young male, action with foot, surprise, anger, etc."

Positional Level Representation

Decoding of phonological word forms

Identification of structural components

/kick/
/girl/
/boy/

[S]

[NP]   [VP]

det /N/ aux /V/ det /N/

[Segmental and prosodic decomposition]

Phonetic Level Representation

/ ðə gɪrl ɪz Kɪkɪη the boɪ /

Acoustic/auditory Level Representation

"the girl is kicking the boy"

Figure 24–3. A Model of Normal Sentence Comprehension Based on Levels of Representation Similar to Those Proposed for Sentence Production.

sentence is assigned at the Positional Level. As the "structural components" (grammatical roles such as subject or object) of the words become available, they are linked to their thematic counterparts (agent, theme/patient) at the Functional Level. As sentence meaning unfolds, a concept is formed and the sentence is interpreted.

Normal sentence interpretation is based on access to, and memory for, a wide range of intermediate elements that the listener must immediately coordinate and integrate across several different levels of information (Saffran, 2001). Any

number of possible points of interruption could undermine sentence comprehension in aphasia. Some of these seem clearly to implicate the point of integration between syntactic structure (at the Positional Level) and sentence meaning (at the Functional Level).

Translating between Levels of Representation

The models described above were conceptualized as serial, feed-forward operations that specify how information is represented for processing. This type of framework is increasingly being challenged by production models that postulate two-way interaction among levels of representation; some of these studies support their assertions with computational implementations (Dell, 1986; Dell, Chang, & Griffin, 1999; Harley, 1995). These models have focused attention on the mechanisms by which information flows between the types of representational levels identified by Garrett.

Details of inter-level interaction is of great importance to considerations of aphasic language, in which it seems likely that perturbations in the timing and coordination of elements across levels could create much difficulty. Even for normal speakers, errors occur with the slightest aberrations in the normal flow of language, such as minor blocks to word-finding, or a change in thought, motivating a modification of the sentence under construction (Garrett, 1982; Levelt et al., 1999). Such aberrations in the normal flow of information are likely considerably greater for the speaker with aphasia, creating challenges for the comparison of aphasic speech to normal speech.

Several hypotheses have been put forth that implicate limitations of memory or other processing resources as critical causes of some types of sentence-processing failure. For example, Kolk (2005) attributes the fragmentary and poorly structured speech produced by many persons with aphasia to interruptions in the normal flow of information, caused either by delay in the activation of the relevant representations or by abnormally fast decay of such information, or by both. These deficiencies then cause strategic adaptations in which patients simplify or truncate structures, or rely on comprehension heuristics.

The lack of detail regarding how information is normally conveyed between levels, and about the memory and other resources necessary to support these processes, makes it difficult to identify a point of disruption in normal processing, since aphasic language problems clearly can involve both degraded representations and limitations on their translation between different forms (or levels).

IDENTIFYING THE SOURCE(S) OF APHASIC SYMPTOMS

Despite these challenges and limitations, considerable evidence suggests that reference to the normal model is an important and useful tool—one that can help to identify the sources of the overt symptoms of aphasia.

Message-Level Impairment

As noted previously, Message-Level representations are conceptual, nonverbal ideas about people, things, their attributes, and their relationships that might be expressible as language or understood from language. Although the types of "messages" that trigger sentence production are likely to differ somewhat from those that arise as sentences are understood, there is little evidence that these differences are either substantial or measurable. If this is the case, Message-Level impairments, when they occur, should be manifested in both production and comprehension.

Several studies of aphasic sentence processing that implicate a Message-Level impairment have identified an inability to construct "event representations" that establish a basis for sentence production (Dean & Black, 2005; Marshall, Pring, & Chiat, 1993; Nickels, Byng, & Black, 1991). These studies focus on difficulty with the extraction of linguistically relevant information from a concept of some action-based scenario (i.e., a "motion event"). Failure to construct event representations results in poor expression of noun/verb role relations—that is, of *who is doing what to whom*. This may be evident in aphasic production when what the patient says demonstrates no relational link between nouns and verbs; in other words, when it fails to establish a predicate-argument structure. This might be manifested as a preponderance of unlinked nouns in an utterance that does not appear to reflect solely impaired verb retrieval (Dean & Black, 2005). In the following excerpt, the speaker with aphasia is unable to express how two nouns in a pictured event (shown in Figure 24–4) relate to one another, although the speaker clearly perceives the independent activity of each noun:

Pt.: "the girl is in the sand . . . the boy is motionless."
Ex: "tell me about how they are interacting" (points to boy and girl)
Pt.: "the girl in the sand . . . the man . . . the girl is in the sand . . ." (points in the picture to where the sand is being poured) ". . . the girl is in the sand . . . pouring the woman . . . man . . . two separate . . . equal but . . . the girl is in the sand."

The use of copular constructions appears to reflect an inability to describe the interaction of the boy and girl depicted in the scene. Although her difficulty may involve impaired verb retrieval, note that she is unable to link a relevant verb "pour" to its correct noun arguments when she does eventually produce it. Thus, it is possible that at least part of the problem is a failure to appreciate the interactional nature of the event.

Another characteristic of aphasia that may reflect impaired event perception is the production of nouns that

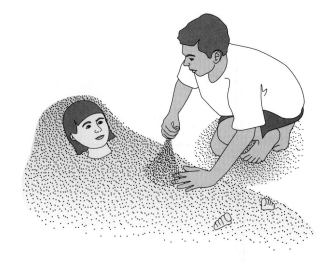

Figure 24–4. Stimulus Drawn to Elicit a Sentence (such as "The boy is burying the girl (in the sand)").

may express some part of a concept, but have no relevance to description of the *event*. Dipper, Black, and Bryan (2005) suggest that the lack of propositional thinking yields the type of noun-listing pattern of production associated with severe nonfluent aphasia, as is evident in the following speech sample in which a speaker with aphasia is retelling the story of Cinderella (from Marshall et al., 1993, p. 180):

crying . . . yes nice . . . (writes '12' on a pad) eleven o'clock yes . . . er dance . . . . er wine . . . cherio . . . er horses . . . horses . . . er twelve . . . finish . . . . shoe . . . . no no no (gestures towards her feet) ah . . . . ball . . . shoe . . . shoes . . . no no no big ones.

Although such a sample shows no evidence of propositional thinking, it is also possible that the symptoms arise from poor verb retrieval. Both Message-Level and verb-retrieval impairments could contribute to poor performance when the evidence is limited to verbal tasks such as storytelling. To address these concerns, nonverbal tests of conceptual-event processing have been developed that eliminate the lexical retrieval component of production and allow a clearer understanding of patients' Message-Level representations. Nickels and colleagues (1991) assessed event understanding in individuals with aphasia using a sorting task with pictures that portrayed an action event (a car being driven) or a "non-event" (a street scene without action). Successful sorting of the event pictures at baseline was associated with a more successful outcome following a sentence-production therapy that assumed intact ability to utilize message representations.

Several tasks designed to assess the ability to understand events have been reported in experimental studies (Dean & Black, 2005; Marshall & Cairns, 2005; Marshall et al., 1993), and a few have been published for clinical use. The Event Perception Test (Marshall et al., 1993; Nickels et al., 1991) assesses the ability to recognize fine distinctions in verb meaning that engage conceptual/semantic features of verbs (e.g., "pour" vs. "drip"). Performance on this measure is often assessed in conjunction with the Role Video Test (Marshall, 1995; Marshall & Cairns, 2005), in which the person with aphasia is asked to match a video scene to a photo showing the outcome of the event. For example, a video scene showing a woman burning a newspaper is matched to one of three photos: the target (burned paper) and two related distractors (torn paper; burned box). A different version of the task shows reversible scenarios that require knowledge of thematic role assignment (who is doing the action) to interpret the outcome of the event. The ability to interpret the nonreversible events is assumed to require broad decisions about cause and effect, as well as intact ability to interpret complex scenes. Understanding of the reversible scenarios requires the ability to extract role relations from events.

The assessment of patients' understanding of events and of other aspects of complex concepts is relatively unexplored in aphasia assessment. Yet it seems clear that it is critically important to understanding the nature of aphasic impairments, since difficulties at this level would be expected to have wide-ranging effects on sentence production and comprehension. Treatments that focus solely on specifically linguistic aspects of patients' performance are unlikely to succeed if patients do not have a secure understanding of concepts such as causality, agency, and temporal order within events.

Functional-Level Impairments

A major feature of the Functional-Level representation is the retrieval and interpretation of abstract lexical representations in accordance with the message (for production) or as dictated by the surface structure (in comprehension). Also created at this level is a representation of the thematic relations among selected lexical elements. By many accounts, a critical element at this level is the selection or interpretation of the verb. It is assumed in many models of normal sentence processing that the verb represents various types of information that contribute to the structure and meaning of a sentence. The choice of verb expresses the semantic concept of the action component of the event, and it determines the predicate-argument structure that will express the thematic relations between the verb and noun(s) involved in the event (c.f., Bresnan & Kaplan, 1982). For example, in describing an event showing a transaction between two people in a store, the speaker can use one of several different verbs (e.g., buy, sell) to express the event, and the choice of verb will influence the assignment of thematic (and grammatical) roles to the nouns. In comprehension, the listener matches the meaning of the verb to the thematic roles of its noun arguments.

Verbs are often classified into types based on their inherent features, such as the manner of motion (run/walk), or how they effect a change of state (melt/burn). Kemmerer (2000), based on Pinker (1989), proposed that grammatically relevant features of verbs are those that determine their syntactic argument structure, whereas features that enable verbs to encode more conceptual information, such as manner of motion or changes of state, are grammatically irrelevant. This finding is supported by evidence that speakers with aphasia can make very subtle perceptual and conceptual judgments about verbs, yet fail when making structure-relevant judgments about the same verbs. For example, Kemmerer (2000) showed that some patients could distinguish between the verbs "drip," "pour," and "spray" in tests of verb meaning, and yet were unable to judge the grammatical integrity of sentences using the same verbs, accepting as correct items such as "Sam is dripping the paper with water."

These findings suggest that different aspects of verb meaning may be differentially subject to disruption in aphasia, with different consequences for sentence processing. This semantic/syntactic distinction within verbs may not be quite so clear as the above results suggest, however. Berndt and Mitchum (1998) reported a pattern of response to sentence-comprehension therapy that indicated sensitivity to conceptual features of verbs that affect the ease of the assignment of thematic roles, independent of the sentence's argument structure. The relative complexity among types of verbs was indexed by such factors as the extent of relative motion of the event participants, and of degree of change of state experienced by the entity undergoing the action, that were encoded in the verbs' meanings. Verbs whose meanings implied an asymmetric distribution of motion and degree of affectedness across the sentence's nouns (e.g., "kick") were easier to understand following reversible sentence-comprehension therapy than were those with more symmetric distribution of such features (e.g., "chase") (Jones, 1984; Saffran, Schwartz, & Marin, 1980).

A hierarchy of verb difficulty based on these meaning components was generally supported in a larger study that demonstrated their effects on thematic role assignments in normal and aphasic participants listening to reversible active- and passive-voice sentences (Berndt, Mitchum, Burton, & Haendiges, 2004). The verb hierarchy also predicted response to treatment of reversible sentence comprehension, with more "symmetric" verbs responding more poorly to treatment than verbs with less inherent symmetry (Mitchum, Haendiges, & Berndt, 2004).

An impairment occurring at the Functional Level could give rise to a number of symptoms involving lexical selection and thematic role assignment, but as noted earlier it is often difficult to ascertain that Message-Level representations were sufficient to motivate the correct structures, on the one hand, and that later Positional structures were ultimately available to support correct productions, on the other hand. Although much testing typically must be carried out before a Functional-Level impairment can be confidently identified, occasionally such a deficit is relatively clear even from limited data. One speaker with aphasia showed an unusual pattern of excellent sentence production in connected speech, with good control over grammatical morphology and a wide range of complex structures. However, she had great difficulty understanding semantically reversible sentences, scoring at chance on numerous administrations of sentence/picture-matching tasks probing active- and passive-voice sentences. In contrast, her ability to detect grammatical violations in spoken sentences was intact. This speaker's great difficulty interpreting thematic roles in comprehension is difficult to reconcile with her excellent sentence production: if comprehension and production share Functional-Level representations, comprehension problems arising at the Functional Level should be mirrored by problems expressing thematic roles. The only way to make this problem evident is with production tasks that require expression of thematic roles. The following sample demonstrates that this is indeed the case when the production task is designed specifically to assess expression of thematic relations. The example also demonstrates how poor expression of thematic roles can occur despite excellent control over grammatical morphemes and a clear ability to obtain a relevant "message" from the picture stimulus shown in Figure 24–5.

Target response: The girl is leading the sheep (with a leash).

Instruction: "Describe this picture by telling me a sentence that starts with 'the girl'."

Response: "the little girl is being pulled along by the sheep. That's not good."

[repeats the sentence twice more, then studies the picture]

Instruction: "Try again."

Response: "the little girl is being pulled forward by the sheep . . . but that's wrong because the sheep is actually

behind . . . . the little girl is following the sheep on a leash . . . . the little girl is taking the sheep on a walk."

In this case, despite retained ability to produce sentences in the passive voice, and despite obvious appreciation of the event depicted, the speaker had difficulty integrating the order of the nouns with the verb she accurately chose to describe the picture. Note that the final sentence, though clearly correct, relied on a "light" verb construction that did not encode the *direction* of the action. This example clearly indicates that the problem of expressing thematic role relations is not limited to agrammatic speakers or to production of non-canonical structures in which the agent of the action is not the subject of the sentence (as in passive voice).

The impaired sentence production of some speakers with aphasia suggests an inability to assign nouns to the thematic roles dictated by the verb. As noted above, picture-description tasks (in which the target is known to the listener) sometimes elicit sentences with noun order that violates thematic role assignment. Role-reversal errors are infrequent in spontaneous aphasic speech (Menn & Obler, 1990), but can be elicited with carefully constructed tests (Schwartz, Fink, & Saffran, 1995). Production tasks (such as described above) are designed to elicit specific sentence structures and to assess the patient's ability to detect his or her own word-order errors (Caramazza & Berndt, 1985). Such impairments, although clearly implicating some problem with understanding of the thematic relations encoded by verbs, also seem to involve other problems with full expression of the sentence's structural frame at the Positional Level.

Positional-Level Impairment

Realization of a Positional-Level representation is a critical step of grammatical encoding. Although this aspect of sentence production appears especially vulnerable in aphasia, it is not easy to predict how a deficit specific to this level of processing would manifest itself. One problem is the difficulty in distinguishing between a deficit located at this level and one that emerges from failure to elaborate the information that feeds into this level (i.e., from the Message and Functional levels).

Caramazza and Hillis (1989) argued that an impairment arising from the Positional Level would be evident when the structural difficulties with sentence production co-occur with intact single-word retrieval and normal comprehension of reversible sentences (on the assumption that Functional-Level representations are also used in comprehension). This profile suggests that Functional-Level operations (word-meaning retrieval and thematic role assignment) are fully operational, thus localizing the symptom to a point at which the grammatical elements of the sentence are realized for production. Below we describe such a case in which a person with aphasia demonstrated excellent comprehension of active and passive reversible sentences, but was unable to

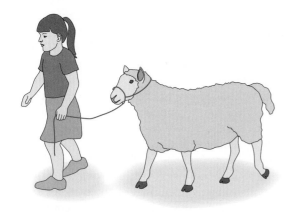

Figure 24–5. Stimulus Drawn to Elicit a Sentence (such as "The girl is leading the sheep (with a leash)").

produce passive-voice sentences. However, the functional locus of impaired sentence processing in this case was interpreted quite differently (see also Mitchum, Greenwald, & Berndt, 2000).

Exactly how the grammatical elements are derived at the Positional Level is left largely unspecified in Garrett's (1982, 1988) model of normal sentence production. Some patterns of production (as in the examples above) clearly indicate that the speaker has the ability to retrieve grammatical function words, but does not seem to know where to place them to form a structural sentence frame (Berndt, Haendiges, Mitchum, & Sandson, 1997). Further support that a variety of grammatical frame structures are available, but underutilized, comes from investigations using structural sentence "priming." Several studies have shown that some speakers with aphasia are significantly more likely to produce a specific structure immediately after hearing a different, but structurally similar, sentence that serves as a model or "prime" (Saffran & Martin, 1997), even for particularly difficult structures such as passive voice. In normal speakers, there is evidence that structural priming effects are sustained for a remarkably long time, measuring as many as 10 intervening sentences between the auditory prime and production of the primed sentence structure (Bock & Griffin, 2000).

Hartsuiker and Kolk (1998) obtained experimental evidence that the syntactic priming effect was diminished when participants with aphasia were explicitly told to model the priming sentence. When the same task was given without instruction to use the model, the effect of priming for agrammatic speakers was robust for both active and passive sentence types. This finding implies that the construction of a Positional-Level representation may be undermined by conscious effort in aphasic production, perhaps because the resources required to use the provided structure causes the patients to divide their attention from the content of the target sentence to its structure. Interestingly, the inverse was observed for control subjects: priming was facilitated when normal speakers were explicitly asked to match the structure of the model sentence.

USING THE MODEL TO MOTIVATE THERAPY: VERB PRODUCTION

The results of the studies described above can inspire novel approaches to aphasia therapy, and may be helpful in interpreting the effects of more traditional approaches. While there are diagnostic advantages of attempting to isolate a hypothetical component of normal sentence processing, therapies driven by the diagnostic findings tend to be more closely aligned to the symptom. This is due, in part, to underspecification of how representational levels are formed (as noted above) and to the possible interactive nature of subcomponent processes of production (Dell et al., 1999; Harley, 1995). Most therapies guided by normal models target a specific

symptom of sentence-processing impairment, then attempt to restore function by improving the integrity of the degraded representation, and/or access to it. Here we focus on the symptom of poor verb retrieval, especially with regard to its effect on the processes that support sentence production.

The effect of poor lexical access to verbs has been well studied in aphasia. Careful observation and analysis of spoken production can reveal patterns of verb omission, or strategic avoidance of lexical verbs in sentences, as described above. Although poor verb retrieval is highly correlated with structurally impaired sentence production, the correlation with clinical aphasia is imperfect (Berndt, Haendiges, et al., 1997; Berndt, Mitchum, Haendiges, & Sandson, 1997; Caramazza & Hillis, 1989). In the preceding section, the importance of the verb in many aspects of sentence processing was highlighted; yet it cannot simply be assumed that verb difficulties actually cause the grammatical disturbance. The nature of the relationship between verb retrieval and sentence production has been explored using experimental paradigms that improve access to lexical verbs by speakers with aphasia who have difficulty producing verbs in sentences. Tasks of "cued production," in which the phonologic form of an uninflected verb is provided to the speaker with aphasia to use in a sentence, have yielded mixed results (Berndt, Haendiges et al., 1997; Berndt, Haendiges, & Wozniak, 1997; Faroqi-Shah & Thompson, 2003; Marshall, Pring, & Chiat, 1998). Such variability underscores the complexity of the relationship between poor verb retrieval and impaired sentence production.

One of the problems in elucidating the role of the verb in aphasic sentence production has already been described: difficulties associated with verbs may arise at a number of levels within the normal stream of sentence formation and production, making it difficult to pinpoint the source(s) of disruption within a single person with aphasia. Moreover, problems arising at a specific point may give rise to different symptoms in different speakers with aphasia, depending on such things as the unique combination of associated problems and the indication that the strategies to overcome (even mask) the impairment. In addition, it is essentially impossible to avoid some engagement of several levels of processing with the clinical treatment tasks. For all of these reasons, it is more accurate to say that model-driven therapies "highlight" (rather than "isolate") specific representations or processing operations.

Message-Level (Event) Treatments

As suggested above, poor expression of propositional speech may be attributed in some cases to difficulty extracting relevant information from the Message. A few studies have specified therapy that directly targets the ability to understand events. Jane Marshall (1999) has pioneered these efforts using a variety of nonlinguistic and language tasks. One approach to therapy at this level is to place conscious effort on "unpacking" the elements of an observed or imagined event. Marshall (1999) encouraged one speaker with aphasia, with apparent difficulty conceptualizing events, to extract propositional information from events using imagery and gesture (p. 124):

Examiner: "Imagine yourself with the dog. There he is at your feet (points to door). You go and get some string and make a lead (gestures holding leash). You set off . . ."
Response: (copies the gesture and moves it away from her body) "Take . . . yes take . . . take the dog to the house."

The imagery and gesture therapy was used along with an attempt to help this woman focus on the aspect of a complex event that could be described with a simple proposition. The goal was to "promote the formation of highly focused concepts at the Message Level, which would place minimal demands on her language system." To encourage this, Marshall employed a variety of exercises to "alter (Bock & Levelt, 1994) conceptual preparations for language" (p. 124).

To simplify things, a set of "light" verbs was established for verbal descriptions, each being matched to a broad conceptual category (established earlier in therapy). These included verbs such as "go"/"come" (movement), "give"/"get" (change of possession), "put"/"take" (removal and location), and so on. The use of gesture, a natural tendency observed in this particular speaker, was encouraged to compliment the imagery exercises and to promote focus on the action component of scenarios. Post-therapy results showed improved production of verbs with specific arguments in storytelling tasks (i.e., narrative speech). Communicative effectiveness was also measurably improved as determined by both trained and naïve judges.

Marshall (1999) interpreted the results as indicative of improved conceptual preparation and attention to linguistically relevant components of events. As anticipated, Marshall's patient had learned to extract verb-relevant information that could be used in simple propositions. Of interest was that the use of light verbs as a substitute for lexical verbs was not considered an effective goal of therapy. Marshall found that such verbs were helpful in learning to isolate verb-relevant information from events, but that their use at later stages (i.e., as a substitute for lexical verbs) was actually a limiting factor.

Other therapies have been designed to help individuals with aphasia identify relevant conceptual information, addressing skills that have been described as "thinking for speaking" (Slobin, 1996). Such therapies attempt to filter, or "pare down" complex events to a single (expressible) proposition, and methodically increase event complexity as determined by the number of events and their variety of potential perspectives (Marshall & Cairns, 2005). In some cases, changes to the way events are interpreted can be guided to match the propositional structures available to the speaker with aphasia. For example, Marshall (1999) describes a treatment that uses complex video scenes presented with a systematic cueing hierarchy. The speaker was guided through the event by focusing on a serial description of the smaller sequences (e.g., the clinician says: "now he's at the door . . . what does he do next? Just the first thing." Response: mimes action; "put the bag on the ground") (p.124). A broader-ranging therapy described by Peach and Wong (2004) used written feedback to refine the conceptual content of spoken sentences, and to repair grammatical errors. This approach exercised a range of production levels to address the link from conceptual to Positional-Level representations.

Message-to-Functional Level Treatments

Verb-retrieval therapies that link the verb to possible noun arguments (sometimes described as "semantic" therapy) have been shown to improve the number of arguments produced (in sentences) in association with verbs. In some cases, the treatment must focus first on establishing that the patient understands the conceptual distinctions among different types of verbs. Marshall (1999) encouraged patient E.M. to recognize the intrinsic *manner* of verbs based on their motion ("spin"/"drive"), change of state ("melt"/"cook"), movement ("spray"/"splatter"), change of possession ("buy"/"learn"), or relative non-action ("bore"/"pity"). Queries enforced the fundamental verb concept (e.g., "When you *spray* paint on a wall, what moves? The wall or the paint?"). The therapy task also engaged conversation about the conceptual distinctions among the verb types.

Other therapies assume that the conceptual information is already available (i.e., that the problem is not in establishing a message), yet there is some difficulty identifying the correct verb at the Functional Level. Several studies describe treatment of sentence production using tasks that focus only on single-verb semantics. Marshall, Pring, and Chiat (1998), Raymer and Ellsworth (2002), and Schneider and Thompson (2003) describe therapy studies with different participants with aphasia that limited treatment to single words and used a semantic therapy, either in conjunction with, or contrasted with, other (nonsemantic) forms of single-word therapy. A common principle of these therapies is to allow the speakers with aphasia to appreciate a range of factors associated with a verb's meaning *and* its relation to other sentence elements (primarily nouns). These therapies collectively suggest that single-word therapies can provide a basis for generalization to sentence production for some speakers with aphasia. However, it may prove critical that noun/verb role relations are highlighted in such therapies to obtain generalization to sentence-level production. That is, such generalization may rely on a realization of how the verb and its (noun) arguments relate to one another at the sentence level, even though the therapy tasks involve only single words.

Some studies explicitly address the production of specific types of predicate-argument structures (PAS). Sentence-ordering tasks can be used to assess understanding of verb-argument structure by having participants arrange written anagram phrases (verbs plus arguments) into meaningful sentences (Jacobs & Thompson, 2000; Marshall, Chiat, & Pring, 1997; Marshall et al., 1993; Mitchum et al., 2000; Murray, Ballard, & Karcher, 2004). Schneider and Thompson (2003) compared the effects of semantic tasks (addressing verb properties such as direction of motion or change of state) with the effects of argument-structure tasks that highlighted the number and place of verb arguments. For example, a depiction of the three-argument verb "fill" was accompanied by the following information: "This picture shows fill. It shows 'the girl is filling the pitcher with water.' The girl is the person doing the filling; the water is the thing doing the filling; and the pitcher is the thing being filled." An attempt at production followed this instruction. Both forms of treatment (i.e., based either on semantics or PAS) yielded improved verb retrieval and sentence production. Webster, Morris, and Franklin (2005) describe a treatment study designed to target verbs' PAS production using therapy tasks to improve verb retrieval, establish thematic role relations between verbs and nouns, and practice sentence generation. Post-therapy sentence production contained more verbs and nouns as obligatory arguments and a greater variety of argument structures in connected speech.

As these results indicate, there is actually little distinction among tasks that are said to address construction of the PAS, to improve lexical-verb production, and/or to improve semantic processing of nouns and/or verbs. All of these approaches potentially serve to link verb/noun role relations and contribute to the formation of a Functional-Level representation. These tasks can also be difficult to distinguish from tasks that target event-role interpretation (as discussed above), which are presumed to occur earlier at the conceptual/message level. It is likely that tasks that involve multiple levels of processing, or therapies that involve a variety of different exercises, engage a wider range of sentence-processing components. The assumption behind this therapy approach is that treatment should target a broad range of functions to improve the potential for effective results. The disadvantage of providing a range of therapy tasks is the lack of specificity regarding exactly which elements of the therapy effected a positive outcome in a particular case.

In general, verb-based therapies that integrate noun/verb role relations, even without working at the sentence level, appear to be effective with many patients with aphasia. Demonstration therapies have yielded robust results with regard to production of canonical (i.e., active voice) sentences, often with multiple arguments. There is no indication, however, that lexically based single-word therapies generalize to production of non-canonical structures, an effect we elaborate on below with regard to treatments targeting the Positional-Level representation.

Functional-to-Positional Level Treatments

Verb Retrieval: Word Form

Therapies that practice simple stimulation of action words either with repetition/rehearsal (Raymer & Ellsworth, 2002) or with picture naming (Fink, Schwartz, & Myers, 1998; Mitchum & Berndt, 1994; Mitchum, Haendiges, & Berndt, 1993) may address only a part of the verb's lexical representation. If the therapy task stimulates only production of the phonologic word form from pictured meaning (devoid of thematic requirements), it may address problems of retrieval at the Positional Level (i.e., word forms), while leaving the earlier (Functional and Message level) representations of the sentence production process "untouched" by intervention. If a speaker with aphasia has additional impairments involving the Functional-Level representation (which may be indicated if reversible sentence comprehension is poor), the treatment predictably would not improve sentence production.

Mitchum and colleagues (1993, 1994) studied the relationship between verb-retrieval therapy and sentence production in two speakers with chronic aphasia (7 to 8 years post-onset). In terms of superficial symptoms of aphasia, both were clinically quite different. One was fluent, yet showed all the features associated with agrammatic production: reduced phrase structure, use of simple sentence structures, poor verb retrieval in sentence production, and impaired use of verb-related grammatical morphemes. Both patients were poor at comprehending reversible sentences. The other person was severely nonfluent. Although he could not produce sentences verbally, his attempts at written sentence production revealed the same pattern of response elicited verbally from the other person.

Following extensive diagnostics, it was hypothesized that, for both participants, facile availability of verbs would improve sentence production if, in fact, the unavailability of verb word forms was a source of the sentence-production impairment. The same technique was used with both patients although responses were elicited verbally for one participant and in writing for the other. Several picture exemplars of action verbs were repeatedly presented to elicit a set of verbs that "name the action." As criterion performance was reached for each targeted verb (correct response initiated within 3 seconds), a new verb was added until the treatment successfully established facile retrieval of eight verbs (an effect that was sustained for at least 1 month following therapy) (Mitchum & Berndt, 1994; Mitchum et al., 1993).

Despite significantly improved ability to retrieve specific lexical verbs, neither participant demonstrated an ability to *use* the newly acquired verbs in sentences. This result helps to clarify why traditional "naming therapies" that practice picture-naming (devoid of any attachment to morphologic

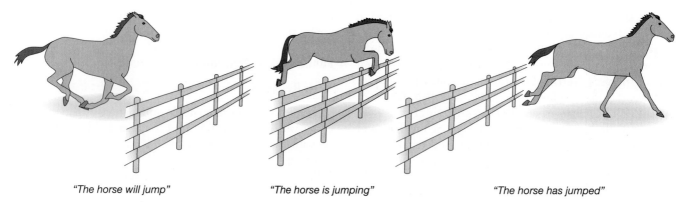

"The horse will jump"   *"The horse is jumping"*   *"The horse has jumped"*

Figure 24–6. Sequential Picture Stimuli Used to Elicit Time-Marking Grammatical Morphemes (Future, Present, and Past Tense). (Target responses reflect the temporal order of an action event.)

elements or semantic relations) often have a limited effect on production beyond the single-word level. Berndt and colleagues (1997) argued that only a small percentage of cases involving impaired verb production may be attributed to a localized impairment involving access to verbs' word forms. This argument was based on results showing that verb-cued retrieval (i.e., providing an uninflected verb form for patients to use in a sentence) usually fails to improve sentence production.

Verb Retrieval: Verb Morphology

The sentence production patterns of speakers with aphasia with poor production of verb inflections vary considerably (Faroqui-Shah & Thompson, 2003). Druks and Carroll (2005) concluded that the unavailability of verb-tense information was the basis for the poor production of the speaker with aphasia in their study. DOR used few verbs in narrative speech, and benefited from cued retrieval only when provided with verbs inflected in the present-progressive form (-ing); past tense (-ed) did not cue sentence production. In action picture-naming, DOR produced some verbs, but often substituted a noun for a verb. He also tended to inflect nouns as if they were verbs (e.g., "afternoon maybe it's *computering* or going out"; "today is *hoovering* and dusting" (c.f. classic examples in Saffran et al., 1980). Druks and Carroll (2005, p. 11) suggest that "verbs unmarked for tense, in contexts where tense is obligatory, are no longer grammatical units that participate in sentence construction; instead they are labels of actions." Further testing indicated that DOR appreciated the concept of tense (i.e., he was able to arrange sequential pictures into their temporal order), but suffered from a fundamental morphosyntactic problem marking and interpreting verb tense.

For many speakers with aphasia, verb morphology is available, but poorly used. In some cases, production is improved when inflected verbs are provided as cues (Faroqui-Shah & Thompson, 2003). For example, dependence on the present-progressive verb inflection (-ing) is often observed in aphasic speech, either as a natural tendency of production (Goodglass, 1993; Mitchum & Berndt, 1994; Mitchum et al., 1993), in response to cued verb retrieval (Faroqui-Shah & Thompson, 2003), or as a post-therapy characteristic (Raymer & Ellsworth, 2002). This does not demonstrate use of this inflection as a morphologic element, but indicates only knowledge that an inflection (of some sort) is expected.

Mitchum and colleagues (1993, 1994) interpreted the lack of generalization to sentence production from the uninflected verb-form treatments (described above) as an indication that the grammatical frame of the sentence was unavailable, evidenced by the patients' over-reliance on the present progressive in all contexts. A second intervention carried out with the same two patients linked the production of verb-tense markers (auxiliary "will," bound morphemes -ing, -ed) to the expression of temporal information using sequential pictures (Fig. 24–6). In a series of steps, therapy systematically diminished cues needed to elicit structurally well-formed sentences to express a future-, present-, or past-tense sentence to describe each picture. The intervention was successful in establishing verb retrieval for trained and untrained lexical verbs, including irregular past-tense verbs (Table 24–1). In addition, the generalization to untrained verbs suggested a robust effect of therapy that tapped intact lexical-verb representations, and was not dependent on the elicitation conditions used in therapy. Significant improvement was also noted in a sentence-generation task in which the patient was asked to construct a sentence using a specific noun or verb. However, there was no generalization to untrained sentence types; in particular, the past-tense verb morphology, once available, was not produced as the superficially similar past participle to support passive structures.

TABLE 24–1

Proportion of Sentences Containing the Target Verb Morphology Needed to Describe Sequential-Action Picture Stimuli (shown in Fig. 24–6)*

M.L. (spoken)	"will" + verb	"is" + verb + "ing"	"has" + verb + "ed"
before therapy	0.25	0.75	0.00
after therapy	1.00	1.00	1.00
E.A. (written)	**"will" + verb**	**"is" + verb + "ing"**	**"has" + verb + "ed"**
before therapy	0.00	0.00	0.00
after therapy	0.75	0.88	0.38

*n = 8 per type; elicited before and after therapy to improve grammatical sentence production. Pictures were not presented in sequential order for these assessments.

Two studies expanded upon the verb-tense training paradigm reported by Mitchum and Berndt (1994). Weinrich, Shelton, Cox, and McCall (1997) attempted to isolate the effects of verb-tense training to the Functional Level using a computerized iconic symbol system that focused therapy on the insertion of lexical terms (object/action icons) into a grammatical frame. Future-, present-, and past-tense morphology was trained using sequential pictures. All three participants (speakers with severe aphasia) showed marked improvement in verbal production and comprehension of sentences with tense-marked verbs following training; generalization to untrained verbs was also noted (Rochon & Reichman, 2003; Weinrich, Boser, & McCall, 1999). These studies observed no generalization to untrained sentence types.

Verb Retrieval: Non-Canonical Sentence Structures

The attention to grammatical frames focusing on verb tense exploits the structural information encoded in verb representations and draws attention to the need for structure in sentences. This points out to the speaker with aphasia that sentence meaning can be modified with grammatical elements. Verb-centered therapies have been generally successful in establishing improved sentence production as measured by increased use of lexical verbs (often within the trained verb class or semantic field), and of a greater number of verb arguments. However, there is considerable evidence that verb-centered therapy does not readily affect the production of non-canonical structures (Mitchum et al., 2000; Rochon & Reichman, 2003). Rather, improved production of non-canonical sentences requires explicit retraining.

Rochon and Reichman (2003) describe a phase of therapy in which their participant (DH) was trained to produce

non-canonical sentences using therapy tasks that demonstrated lexical insertion of nouns and verbs into passive sentence frames marked for tense with sequential pictures (future, present, past). In response to this therapy, DH learned to use passive sentences in narrative production and other untrained conditions, but at some expense to his ability to use active sentences.

Another example of therapy focused on non-canonical sentence production involved an unusual case of isolated impairment of passive-voice production. A.L. (described in Mitchum & Berndt, 2001; Mitchum et al., 2000) was a fluent speaker with intact comprehension of semantically reversible sentences and flawless repetition of active and passive sentences, all in conjunction with an inability to produce passive sentences in a constrained production task. As shown in Table 24–2, A.L. produced well-formed active-voice sentences without difficulty. However, when constrained to start his sentence with a non-agentive noun his responses were clearly impaired. The few responses that contained a passive structure were anomalous in meaning; presumably he was aware that walls cannot paint girls (see response to stimulus #1). Many attempts revealed either strategic avoidance of the target passive (as in stimulus #2), a lack of integration between the actor/object (stimuli #3 to #5), or some otherwise inadequate sentence (stimuli #6 to #8).

Following a demonstration that extensive sentence-repetition training was not effective in improving his passive sentence production (presumably because the source of impairment was at an earlier level), an intervention was designed to establish a link between active and passive sentence meanings at the pre-phonologic level. Using a written anagram version of a sentence-order task, A.L. learned to produce passive sentences by linking the change in word order and verb inflection of the passive to its counterpart active structure. After

TABLE 24–2

Sample of A.L.'s Responses in a Task of Picture Description*

Stimulus	Constrained Active Response	Constrained Passive Response
(1) girl painting wall	"The <u>girl</u> is painting the wall."	"The <u>wall</u> is painting the girl."
(2) girl kicking a boy	"The <u>girl</u> is kicking the boy."	"The <u>boy</u> is perturbed because the girl is kicking the boy."
(3) man drinking tea	"The <u>man</u> is drinking from the cup."	"The <u>tea</u> is hot."
(4) boy eating an apple	"The <u>boy</u> is eating the apple."	"The <u>apple</u> . . . is paramount."
(5) girl riding bike	"The <u>girl</u> is riding a bike."	"The <u>bike</u> is . . . not very pretty."
(6) man cutting a rope	"The <u>man</u> is cutting the rope."	"The <u>rope</u> is . . . . piecemeal."
(7) boy pushing a box	"The <u>boy</u> is fixing the boxes."	"The <u>box</u> . . ."
(8) horse jumping a fence	"The <u>horse</u> is jumping."	"The <u>fence</u> . . ."

* Responses are constrained by the requirement that each sentence start with the agent noun (for active targets) or the non-agent noun (for passive targets), underlined in the examples. The same picture is used in separate test sessions to elicit each type of sentence.

12 sessions, therapy proved successful. Unlike the result obtained with D.L. by Rochon and Reichmann (2003), there was no decline in the production of active sentences following passive-sentence training. One factor in the different outcomes may have been A.L.'s intact comprehension of both active and passive sentences at the start of intervention, whereas D.L. required additional training in sentence comprehension.

A therapy procedure described by Jacobs and Thompson (2000) similarly linked canonical and noncanonical structures (passives and object clefts) to the same underlying meaning. Anagram words were used to build sentences, and to demonstrate the moved content words and changes in the grammatical frame for noncanonical sentences. The treatment was preceded by attention to the central action (verb) and its thematic role relations. Production treatment required oral reading of the final sentence; comprehension required pointing to constituents (in pictures) with no verbal response. The treatment was effective with all (four) participants and generalized to untrained exemplars, but not to (theoretically) unrelated sentence types. This study further supports the necessity of direct training of noncanonical sentence structures and of motivating them by attention to sentence meaning.

INTERPRETING THE EFFECTS OF TREATMENT

While many model-driven therapies attempt to target specific functional components, others consider how therapy can "exercise" integration of the various subprocesses that support production. Successful therapies do not need to pinpoint the locus of treatment effects to be clinically relevant (e.g., Peach & Wong, 2004). However, attempts to interpret the effects of aphasia treatments have led to better understanding of what might have occurred in therapy; that is, of which cognitive mechanisms were used to accomplish the

treatment task. An understanding of how therapy affects cognitive function will inevitably lead to a better understanding of which treatment approach is most appropriate, and has the potential to offer the most widely applicable results. Therapy studies designed and executed in the context of a normal production model have provided a basis for interpreting sentence-processing therapy effects.

The Mapping-Deficit Hypothesis

As noted above, early analyses of agrammatism (the "syntactic-deficit hypothesis") attributed both comprehension and production impairments associated with agrammatism to an inability to establish a full syntactic representation (at the Positional Level) either because of difficultly producing and interpreting grammatical morphemes (Kean, 1979) or because of a more general inability to elaborate a syntactic structure (Berndt & Caramazza, 1980). However, a series of studies demonstrated spared sensitivity to syntactic structure in grammaticality judgment tasks in patients with poor sentence comprehension and production of reversible sentences (Linebarger, 1990; Linebarger, Schwartz, & Saffran, 1983; Saffran, Schwartz, & Linebarger, 1998; Schwartz, Linebarger, Saffran, & Pate, 1987). These findings indicated that the patients' difficulties did not arise from poor representation of syntactic information, but rather from an inability to coordinate the representations of syntactic functions (e.g., subject/object) and thematic roles (e.g., agent/object). This is, in effect, an inability to relate surface-structure cues to the underlying sentence meaning, as expressed by thematic role assignment (for comprehension) or to express thematic roles appropriately in a sentence structure (for production). In Garrett's (1988) model this indicated an inability to map between the Functional- and Positional-Level representations. This failure has been termed the "Mapping-Deficit Hypothesis" (MDH) (Saffran

Canonical sentence order:

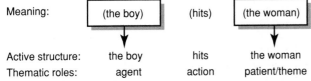

Noncanonical sentence order:

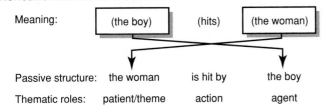

Figure 24–7. Illustration of Canonical vs. Noncanonical Sentence Structure. (The arrows characterize the shift in word order for two sentence types with shared meaning.)

& Schwartz, 1988), and provides a clear example of the importance of considering the transfer of information from one level of the model to the next.

Identifying a Thematic Mapping Impairment

Impaired thematic/syntactic mapping has been attributed to two potential sources. The "lexical" variant arises from poor access to verb-specific mapping rules, in other words, the syntactic and grammatical information that is inherently part of the lexical-verb representation. According to Saffran and Schwartz (1988), this type of problem could explain poor interpretation of simple, canonical sentences with a transparent mapping between grammatical roles (subject, object) and thematic roles (agent, patient) (Fig. 24–7). For more complex sentences in which the mapping is not transparent (such as in passive-voice sentences in which the subject noun does not map to the thematic role of agent), Saffran and Schwartz and colleagues (1987, 1988) proposed a "procedural" variant of the MDH, implicating the processes that move noun arguments out of their canonical (deep-structure) positions.

Therapies Designed to Improve Thematic Mapping

The hypothesis that failure to produce and/or comprehend sentences in aphasia could arise from a failure to link two levels of intact representation has significant implications for therapy (for reviews of "mapping" therapies, see Fink, 2001; Marshall, 1995; Mitchum et al., 2000). Despite their different formats, many sentence-comprehension treatment studies shared the goal of linking sentence structure (Positional-Level representation) to semantic/thematic

structure (Functional-Level representation). Initially, the objective of these experimental studies was not so much to test the efficacy of the therapy procedure but to test the hypothesis that poor mapping ability (either lexical or procedural) was an underlying cause of impaired sentence processing. Extensive pre/post-therapy measures were provided from each study to interpret what, if any, changes were established, and how they may have occurred.

Mapping therapies have been generally quite successful in improving sentence comprehension for *trained* reversible sentences, but often reveal wide variability in patterns of generalization (or lack thereof) among the participants (Marshall, 1995; Nickels et al., 1991; Schwartz, Saffran, Fink, Myers, & Martin, 1994). Few speakers with aphasia have shown improvement on all post-therapy measures, and most demonstrate persistent sentence-processing impairment.

Extensive post-therapy analyses indicate that therapies designed to improve thematic mapping between the Functional and Positional levels cannot assume that each representational level is intact. The small number of highly successful results observed with mapping therapies have likely addressed a relatively pure mapping impairment in these particular participants (Byng, 1988; Rochon, Laird, Bose, & Scofield, 2005; Schwartz et al., 1994), or the cases in which treatment also addressed the additional impairments. Most of the mapping-therapy outcomes have revealed far more limited effects of therapy, and they implicate a different, and perhaps more extensive, source of impairment in the patients who participated (Fink, 2001; Marshall, 1995; Mitchum & Berndt, 2001; Mitchum et al., 2000; Nickels et al., 1991).

The collective outcome of mapping therapies leads us to a conclusion that parallels the direction of other research in cognitive neuropsychology. Therapies cannot be based on the assumption that grammatically based symptoms of production and comprehension represent a homogenous entity. Rather, it appears far more promising to look at the relative symptom in individual cases that seems to give rise to the grammatical-processing impairment. The question(s) of interest have become more specific. Model-based treatment studies are motivated by assessment of what the speaker (or listener) fails to establish at the various representational levels, and whether or not information is communicated between levels.

Studying the Generalization of Treatment Effects

Cognitive-neuropsychological treatment studies typically assess aphasic participants' ability to acquire trained and untrained exemplars of the treatment material, and to generalize what is learned to other (related and/or unrelated) materials and conditions. Studies of how sentence-level treatments generalize across input/output modalities indicate that therapy tasks that address structural cues to sentence meaning effectively improve sentence *comprehension*, but tend to remain specific to comprehension (Berndt & Mitchum, 1998; Haendiges, Berndt, & Mitchum, 1996; Mitchum, Haendiges, & Berndt, 1995). Sentence-comprehension therapies that explicitly point out verb-centered thematic role relations and retrieval of predicate-argument structures have some effect on sentence production, particularly with regard to increased use of lexical verbs and an increased number of noun arguments (Byng, 1988; Fink et al., 1998; Jacobs & Thompson, 2000; Marshall, 1995). In contrast, sentence-production therapy has been shown to have little transfer to sentence comprehension (Jacobs & Thompson, 2000; Mitchum & Berndt, 1994; Mitchum et al., 1993; Murray et al., 2004; Rochon et al., 2005; Rochon & Reichman, 2003, 2004).

Research findings regarding cross-modal generalization are both theoretically and clinically important: patterns of generalization suggest how certain aspects of sentence processing are shared across modalities, and they may point to the most efficient approaches to therapy. Although considerable insights have been gained in recent years with regard to generalization of treatment effects, it remains important to recognize that our current impressions are influenced by a number of complicating variables, including variations in the techniques used in therapy, symptomatic differences among participants, and the methods used to measure generalization.

Interpreting Strategies Induced by Aphasia

The cognitive-neuropsychological approach has offered a framework for the identification and interpretation of strategies used by individuals with aphasia. The detailed attention to response patterns and subtle manipulations of stimuli inherent in model-based assessments can reveal much about a person's ability to process specific sentence types, and to use strategies when needed. It was a long-standing assumption that strategies were used in aphasia only when processing failed. More recently, research suggests that individuals with aphasic language may regularly avoid aspects of sentence processing, becoming overly dependent on normally influential cues such as word order (Caplan, 1992), verb-specific mapping information (Berndt & Mitchum, 1998), or primitive spatial strategies (Chatterjee, Maher, Gonzalez-Rothi, & Heilman, 1995). Linebarger (1995) suggests that the use of strategies is not compensatory, but rather reflects "normal mechanisms which have come to play an abnormally visible role" (p. 83). This interpretation is supported by evidence that even normal listeners use shallow processing for comprehension that is usually "good enough" to support a correct interpretation (see also Chatterjee, Southwood, & Basilico, 1999; Ferreira, 2003; Ferreira, Bailey, & Ferraro, 2002; Saffran, 2001).

In some cases, strategies are detected in post-therapy assessments. For example, apparent generalization to comprehension of passive sentences has been shown to hinge on the superficial detection of the "by" phrase in the surface structure (Berndt & Mitchum, 1998; Haendiges et al., 1996). This was revealed only when truncated versions of passive sentences (i.e., passives without the "by" phrase such as "the boy was hit") were not interpreted at the same level as full passive structures. Mitchum and colleagues (2004) demonstrated the clinical utility of identifying response biases in tests of sentence comprehension. Two individuals with aphasia responded to interventions that took their strategic tendencies into account. Of interest was the finding that the person who demonstrated a more superficial strategy was more responsive to intervention, presumably because the strategy represented a "good enough" approach that was easily displaced.

Strategies are also frequently observed in aphasic attempts at verbal sentence production. The use of "light" verbs, or simplified structures, implicates an attempt to produce a syntactically structured proposition in spite of the linguistic limitations imposed by aphasia (Marshall, 1999; Mitchum & Berndt, 1994). One well-developed theory of agrammatic sentence production emphasizes patients' ability to revert to simplified (but normal) elliptical structures when their processing resources become taxed (Kolk, 2005; Kolk & VanGrunsven, 1985). Kolk stresses that these elliptical structures are a type of speech register that may be used by normal speakers in some conditions, such as when talking to a foreign speaker.

A program of production therapy has been devised based on Kolk's hypothesis. Springer and colleagues describe good results for German speakers with aphasia using Reduced Syntax Therapy (REST) (Springer, Huber, Schlenk, & Schlenk, 2000). This intervention is based on the view that severe agrammatism is a compensatory response to the loss of syntactic ability that arises from the nondominant hemisphere (Springer et al., 2000). Like other linguistic approaches, treatment encourages activation of Functional-Level information and the mapping between thematic roles and (simple) syntactic structures. However, the production of morphosyntactic elements is actively *dis*couraged in favor of expanding the lexical content of telegraphic-style utterances. The authors suggest that their compensatory approach "frees up capacities for other aspects of the production process, like message planning, word activation and motor speech planning" (Springer et al., 2000).

The consistent use of response strategies by individuals with aphasia should be considered in diagnostic testing to avoid misinterpreting the nature of their language impairment. Such identification typically requires testing the patient with a variety of tasks using different response formats. It is equally important to identify the extent to which changes established with therapy reflect shifts in strategy, or whether they represent a fundamental change in cognitive processing. Although any positive change is a welcomed outcome, a better understanding of how therapy affects cognitive processing leads to a more efficient basis for matching the treatment candidate to the most effective intervention.

FUTURE TRENDS

Cognitive-neuropsychological studies have contributed to a better understanding of sentence-processing impairments in patients with aphasia. In this chapter, we illustrated how even a single symptom (e.g., impaired verb retrieval) can arise from multiple sources in the sentence-production process, and how such a symptom may be embedded within the unique combination of spared and impaired function of each individual with aphasia. In this respect, cognitive neuropsychology has served to reveal the complexity of the aphasic condition. At the same time, a cognitive-neuropsychological analysis offers a structured means of accounting for the differences in function that may be imposed by brain damage, and it provides a basis for therapy that seeks either to restore normal function, or to find new or compensatory ways to communicate around the impairment.

As models of normal cognition improve, there will be a better account of the flow of information within and across levels of representation. A more detailed understanding of normal cognition will provide a much-needed basis to develop a theory of the therapy process itself. Future research should be directed at refining the basis for selecting a therapy approach, with studies of how treatment effects generalize within and across cognitive domains. A less-developed area that is beginning to receive more attention is how certain cognitive domains (such as memory and perception), traditionally viewed as nonlinguistic functions, serve to support language in various ways and at multiple points in processing.

Increased interest in individual therapy outcomes dictates an individualized approach to therapy. Cognitive-neuropsychological studies of aphasia continue to offer a framework for addressing this challenge by approaching the problem in terms of the difference between normal and aphasic language, and not as an effort to classify individuals under diagnostic "labels" that reiterate the symptoms of impairment.

KEY POINTS

1. Models of normal cognitive function, such as sentence processing, can be used to guide diagnosis and intervention in aphasia. Even underspecified models are useful in this regard. As models are further developed, and theories of normal sentence processing are advanced, the extent to which models of normal cognition can be applied to clinical intervention will improve.

2. The set of symptoms traditionally associated with agrammatism do not always occur together, making it clear that agrammatism does not constitute a clearly defined syndrome. Current approaches to the study of sentence production and comprehension in aphasia seek to explain how a particular symptom (such as poor verb retrieval) contributes to the sentence-processing pattern observed in individual cases, or in groups of individuals who share (at least) the symptom of interest.

3. Treatment studies based on a cognitive-neuropsychological interpretation of aphasic sentence processing are largely conducted as a research endeavor. However, the recent emphasis on evidence-based therapy has forged a more direct and urgent link between research and clinical intervention. Although many of the treatment approaches described here have direct clinical relevance, the goal of such studies is generally not intended to test the efficacy of a particular therapy. Rather, such studies illustrate an *approach* to diagnosis and intervention that evolves from an understanding of the differences between normal and aphasic language.

4. Although the studies cited here describe experimental therapies, some general clinical implications have emerged. An important finding is that the most effective therapies for improving sentence production are those that integrate the full production process. Treatments that isolate later levels of lexical representation (such as traditional "picture-naming" therapies that practice repeated access to phonologic word forms) are effective only in a small percentage of cases. More often, the best outcomes are obtained from therapy that directs attention to the link between conceptual information about an event and the elements that allow for linguistic encoding of the event, such as meaning and thematic relations.

5. An understanding of noun/verb role relations is a critical element of sentence production that can be retrained effectively in aphasia. Therapy that targets this element of production can be limited to single words, with the expectation that therapy may generalize to sentences and narrative contexts (assuming that there are no additional impairments). Such effects are likely, however, to be limited to the production of canonical structures. Improved production of noncanonical structures (passive, object-relative clause), which give production improved flexibility, appears to require specific retraining of those sentence structures.

6. Studies of the manner in which treatment effects generalize within and among cognitive domains have

important implications for aphasia therapy. At the sentence level, recent studies indicate that generalization between production and comprehension of sentences is not equally bi-directional. Rather, current studies indicate that therapy directed at comprehension tends to generalize to production, whereas production therapy has a minimal effect on sentence comprehension. These findings remain preliminary, and are subject to further refinement through research. One of the least-developed aspects of this area of research is with regard to isolating the elements of production and comprehension that are employed *during* intervention.

7. A deficiency of this approach (noted several times in this review) is a lack of specificity about the details of information transmission among levels, and of the temporal and storage requirements that this transmission entails. Current research using implemented computational models of word production are beginning to contribute importantly to our understanding of these issues, and have great potential to "scale up" to incorporate elements that are specific to sentence processing.

ACTIVITIES FOR REFLECTION AND DISCUSSION

1. What is the cognitive-neuropsychological approach to assessment and intervention of aphasia? How do the goals of cognitive-neuropsychological assessment differ from more traditional approaches that classify subtypes of aphasia?

2. Use the model of normal sentence production (Fig. 24–2) to describe, in your own words, the major sequence of processing events that leads to the production of a single, well-formed sentence. Use Garrett's terms to describe each level of representation that is achieved during production (i.e., Message Level, Functional Level, Positional Level, etc.). Use the following example in your description: *The dog is chasing the cat.*

3. Explain the difference between canonical and noncanonical sentence structures (see Figs. 24–1 and 24–7). Why does a "word-order" strategy for sentence processing result in better performance with canonical, and poorer performance with noncanonical, stimuli?

4. Describe how Garrett and other researchers used the errors of normal speakers to develop a model of normal sentence production?

5. How can sequential pictures be used to assess the ability to produce and comprehend grammatical morphemes? (*Hint:* see Fig. 24–6.) Can you think of any other ways to assess the ability to process grammatical morphemes in sentences?

6. What is the ability to construct an "event representation" at the Message Level? How would an impaired ability to construct an event representation result in difficulty producing sentences? (Refer to the aphasic speech samples in the chapter, or try to create your own example.)

7. A major feature of the Functional-Level representation is the selection of a verb to describe the action in the event. How does the choice of verb influence the content and structure of the sentence? Consider different responses that describe the event shown in Figure 24–4. What responses would be produced for the following verbs: (1) burying; (2) pouring; (3) covered; (4) playing. Note what changes occur in the sentence structure based on the choice of verb. Do the thematic roles of the nouns change or remain constant with different verbs? Is it necessary to name the instrument (e.g., "sand") in some sentences, but not in others? Repeat the exercise with other pictures or stimuli that are used to elicit sentences.

8. Describe the effect of structural priming at the Positional Level of sentence production. How does structural priming differ in normal speakers as opposed to speakers with aphasia, according to the study by Hartsuiker & Kolk (1998)?

9. Why is it difficult to pinpoint the exact location of impaired sentence processing within the model of normal sentence processing?

10. Explain why the following two statements are false: (1) A verb-based approach to therapy is indicated only for speakers with aphasia who show poor verb retrieval in naming action pictures. (2) A verb-based approach to therapy is indicated only for speakers with aphasia who fail to produce any verbs. Consider the following points in your response: Does picture naming have the same task requirements as sentence production? Is it possible to produce some verbs (e.g., have/got, go/went, come) despite having an impaired ability to retrieve lexical verbs? Use some of the speech samples in this chapter to support your response.

11. Upon viewing a picture of a girl kicking a boy in the shin, a speaker with aphasia says "She really got 'em on the leg." Describe what the speaker does and does not convey in the response. Did he or she correctly express the thematic roles of the actors (nouns) in the picture? Was a semantically meaningful verb used? Does the speaker seem to use grammatical morphemes effectively? Repeat the exercise with the following responses:
    - "She pushed him right on there" (points to the boy's leg).

- "He got kicked by the other one."
- "The girl is . . . doing . . . something to the boy."
- "Oh, boy got hurt. Ouch!" (speaker grabs his or her own shin).
- "The boy" (gestures kicking) . . . "strike the girl" . . . "the foot, no shin."
- "The girl is the kick is shin."

12. Why is it important to be able to produce well-formed sentences? Is improved sentence production a reasonable goal of therapy for some speakers with aphasia?

▶ *Acknowledgement:* The preparation of this paper, and the conduct of much of the research reviewed here, were supported by grant R01-DC00262 from the National Institute on Deafness and Other Communication Disorders to the University of Maryland School of Medicine. Many people have contributed in various and substantial ways to the research that continues to shape our view of sentence-processing disorders in aphasia. They include our long-time collaborator Anne N. Haendiges, M.S., as well as Sarah Wayland, Ph.D, Margaret Greenwald, Ph.D., and Jennifer Sandson, Ph.D. Of course, our most important contributions are from the individuals with aphasia who tirelessly support our research efforts with their dedicated participation.

References

Berndt, R. S. (1991). Sentence processing in aphasia. In M. Sarno (Ed.), *Acquired aphasia* (2nd ed., pp. 223–270). San Diego: Academic Press.

Berndt, R. S. (1998). Sentence processing in aphasia. In M. Sarno (Ed.), *Acquired aphasia* (3rd ed., pp. 229–262). New York: Academic Press.

Berndt, R. S. (2001). More than just words: Sentence production in aphasia. In R. Berndt (Ed.), *Handbook of neuropsychology* (2nd ed., Vol. 3, pp. 173–187). Amsterdam: Elsevier.

Berndt, R. S., & Caramazza, A. (1980). A redefinition of the syndrome of Broca's aphasia: Implications for a neuropsychological model of language. *Applied Psycholinguistics, 1*, 225–278.

Berndt, R. S., Haendiges, A., Mitchum, C., & Sandson, J. (1997). Verb retrieval in aphasia: 2. Relationship to sentence processing. *Brain and Language, 56*, 107–137.

Berndt, R. S., Haendiges, A. N., & Wozniak, M. A. (1997). Verb retrieval and sentence processing: Dissociation of an established symptom association. *Cortex, 33*, 99–114.

Berndt, R. S., & Mitchum, C. C. (1998). An experimental treatment of sentence comprehension. In N. Helm-Estabrooks & A. L. Holland (Eds.), *Approaches to the treatment of aphasia*. San Diego: Singular.

Berndt, R. S., Mitchum, C. C., Burton, M. W., & Haendiges, A. N. (2004). Comprehension of reversible sentences in aphasia: The effects of verb meaning. *Cognitive Neuropsychology, 21*, 229–245.

Berndt, R. S., Mitchum, C. C., Haendiges, A. N., & Sandson, J. (1997) Verb retrieval in aphasia: 1. Characterizing single word impairments. *Brain and Language, 56*, 68–106.

Berndt, R. S., Mitchum, C. C., & Haendiges, A. N. (1996). Comprehension of reversible sentences in "agrammatism": A meta-analysis. *Cognition, 58*, 289–308.

Bock, J., & Levelt, W. (1994). Language production: Grammatical encoding. In M. A. Gernsbacher (Ed.), *Handbook of Psycholinguistics*. San Diego: Academic Press.

Bock, J. K., & Griffin, Z. M. (2000). The persistence of structural priming: Transient activation or implicit learning? *Journal of Experimental Psychology: General, 129*, 177–192.

Bresnan, J., & Kaplan, R. M. (1982). Grammars as mental representations of language. In J. Bresnan (Ed.), *The mental representation of grammatical relations*. Cambridge: MIT Press.

Butterworth, B., & Howard, D. (1987). Paragrammatisms. *Cognition, 26*, 1–37.

Byng, S. (1988). Sentence processing deficits: Theory and therapy. *Cognitive Neuropsychology, 5*, 629–676.

Caplan, D. (1992). *Language: Structure, processing and disorders*. Cambridge: The MIT Press.

Caramazza, A. (1997). How many levels of processing are there in lexical access? *Cognitive Neuropsychology, 14*, 177–208.

Caramazza, A., & Berndt, R. S. (1985). A multicomponent deficit view of agrammatic Broca's aphasia. In M. L. Kean (Ed.), *Agrammatism*. New York: Academic Press.

Caramazza, A., & Hillis, A. E. (1989). The disruption of sentence production: Some dissociations. *Brain and Language, 36*, 625–650.

Caramazza, A., & Zurif, E. B. (1976). Dissociation of algorithmic and heuristic processes in language comprehension: Evidence from aphasia. *Brain and Language, 3*, 572–582.

Chatterjee, A., Maher, L. M., Gonzalez-Rothi, L. J., & Heilman, K. M. (1995). Asyntactic thematic role assignment: The use of a temporal-spatial strategy. *Brain and Language, 49*, 125–139.

Chatterjee, A., Southwood, M. H., & Basilico, D. (1999). Verbs, events and spatial representations. *Neurpsychologia, 37*, 395–402.

Dean, M. P., & Black, M. (2005). Exploring event processing and description in people with aphasia. *Aphasiology, 19*(6), 521–544.

Dell, G. S. (1986). A spreading activation theory of retrieval in sentence production. *Psychological Review, 93*, 283–321.

Dell, G. S., Chang, F., & Griffin, Z. M. (1999). Connectionist models of language production: Lexical access and grammatical encoding. *Cognitive Science, 23*(4), 517–542.

Dell, G. S., & Reich, P. A. (1981). Stages in sentence production: An analysis of speech error data. *Journal of Verbal Learning and Verbal Behavior, 20*, 611–629.

Dipper, L. T., Black, M., & Bryan, K. L. (2005). Thinking for speaking and thinking for listening: The interaction of thought and language in typical and non-fluent comprehension and production. *Language and Cognitive Processes, 20*(3), 417–441.

Druks, J., & Carroll, E. (2005). The crucial role of tense for verb production. *Brain and Language, 94*(1), 1–18.

Faroqui-Shah, Y., & Thompson, C. K. (2003). Effect of lexical cues on the production of active and passive sentences in Broca's and Wernicke's aphasia. *Brain and Language, 85*, 409–426.

Ferreira, F. (2003). The misinterpretation of non-canonical sentences. *Cognitive Psychology, 47*, 164–203.

Ferreira, F., Bailey, K. G. D., & Ferraro, V. (2002). Good-enough representations in language comprehension. *Current Directions in Psychological Science, 11*, 11–15.

Fink, R. B. (2001). Mapping treatment: An approach to treating sentence level impairments in agrammatism. *Special Interest Division, 2*(11), 83–87.

Fink, R. B., Schwartz, M. F., & Myers, J. L. (1998). Investigations of the sentence query approach to mapping therapy. *Brain and Language, 65*, 203–207.

Garrett, M. F. (1975). The analysis of sentence production. In G. Bower (Ed.), *The psychology of learning and motivation* (pp. 133–177). London: Academic Press.

Garrett, M. F. (1982). Production of speech: Observations from normal and pathological language use. In A. Ellis (Ed.), *Normality and pathology in cognitive functions* (pp. 19–76). London: Academic Press.

Garrett, M. F. (1988). Processes in language production. In F. J. Newmeyer (Ed.), *Linguistics: The Cambridge Survey: 111. Language: Psychological and biolgical aspects*. Cambridge: Cambridge University Press.

Goodglass, H. (1993). *Understanding aphasia*. San Diego: Academic Press.

Grodzinsky, Y. (2000). The neurology of syntax: Language use without Broca's area. *Behavioral and Brain Sciences, 23*, 1–21.

Haendiges, A. N., Berndt, R. S., & Mitchum, C. C. (1996). Assessing the elements contributing to a "mapping" deficit: A targeted treatment study. *Brain and Language, 52*, 276–302.

Harley, T. A. (1995). *The psychology of language: From data to theory*. Hove: Psychology Press.

Hartsuiker, R. J., & Kolk, H. (1998). Syntactic facilitation in agrammatic sentence production. *Brain and Language, 62*, 221–254.

Hillis, A. E. (1993). The role of models of language processing in rehabilitation of language impairments. *Aphasiology, 7*, 5–26.

Jacobs, B. J., & Thompson, C. K. (2000). Cross-modal training effects of training noncanonical sentence comprehension and production in agrammatic aphasia. *Journal of Speech, Language and Hearing Research, 43*, 5–20.

Jacobson, R. (1956). Two aspects of language and two types of aphasic disturbances. In R. Jacobson & M. Halle (Eds.), *Fundamentals of language*. The Hague: Mouton.

Jones, E. V. (1984). Word order processing in aphasia: Effect of verb semantics. In F. C. Rose (Ed.), *Advances in neurology (progress in aphasiology)* (Vol. 42). New York: Raven.

Kean, M. L. (1979). *Agrammatism*. New York: Academic Press.

Kemmerer, D. (2000). Grammatically relevant and grammatically irrelevant features of verb meaning can be independently impaired. *Aphasiology, 14*(10), 997–1020.

Kolk, H. (2005). How language adapts to the brain: An analysis of agrammatic aphasia. In L. Progovac (Ed.), *The syntax of nonsententials: Multi-disciplinary perspectives*. London: John Benjamins.

Kolk, H., & VanGrunsven, M. F. (1985). Agrammatism as a variable phenomenon. *Cognitive Neuropsychology, 2*, 347–384.

Lapointe, S. (1985). A theory of verb form use in the speech of agrammatic aphasics. *Brain and Language, 24*, 100–155.

Levelt, W. J. M. (1989). *Speaking: From intention to articulation*. Cambridge: MIT Press.

Levelt, W. J. M., Roelofs, A., & Meyer, A. S. (1999). A theory of lexical access in speech production. *Behavioral and Brain Sciences, 22*, 1–75.

Linebarger, M. C. (1990). Neuropsychology of sentence processing. In A. Caramazza (Ed.), *Cognitive neuropsychology and neurolinguistics* (pp. 55–117). Hillsdale: Lawrence Erlbaum.

Linebarger, M. C. (1995). Agrammatism as evidence about grammar. *Brain and Language, 50*, 52–91.

Linebarger, M. C., Schwartz, M. F., & Saffran, E. M. (1983). Sensitivity to grammatical structure in so-called agrammatic aphasics. *Cognition, 13*, 361–392.

Luria, A. (1947). *Traumatic aphasia*. The Hague: Mouton.

Marshall, J. (1995). The mapping hypothesis and aphasia therapy. *Aphasiology, 9*(6), 517–539.

Marshall, J. (1999). Doing something about a verb impairment: Two therapy approaches. In S. Byng, Swinburn, K., & Pound, C. (Ed.), *Aphasiology*. Hove: Psychology Press.

Marshall, J., & Cairns, D. (2005). Therapy for sentence processing problems in aphasia: Working on thinking for speaking. *Aphasiology, 19*(10/11), 1009–1021.

Marshall, J., Chiat, S., & Pring, T. (1997). An impairment in processing verbs' thematic roles: A therapy study. *Aphasiology, 11*, 855–876.

Marshall, J., Pring, T., & Chiat, S. (1993). Sentence processing therapy: Working at the level of the event. *Aphasiology, 7*(2), 177–199.

Marshall, J., Pring, T., & Chiat, S. (1998). Verb retrieval and sentence production in aphasia. *Brain and Language, 63*, 159–183.

Martin, R. C. (2006). The neuropsychology of sentence processing: Where do we stand? *Cognitive Neuropsychology, 23*(1), 74–95.

Menn, L., & Obler, L. (1990). Cross-language data and theories of agrammatism. In L. Menn & L. Obler (Eds.), *Agrammatic aphasia* (Vol. 2, pp. 1369–1389). Amsterdam: John Benjamins.

Mitchum, C. C., & Berndt, R. S. (1994). Verb retrieval and sentence construction: Effects of targeted intervention. In J. Riddoch & G. Humphreys (Eds.), *Cognitive neuropsychology and cognitive rehabilitation*. London: Lawrence Erlbaum.

Mitchum, C. C., & Berndt, R. S. (1995). The cognitive neuropsychological approach to treatment of language disorders. *Neuropsychological Rehabilitation, 5*, 1–16.

Mitchum, C. C., & Berndt, R. S. (2001). Cognitive neuropsychological approaches to diagnosing and treating language disorders: Production and comprehension of sentences. In R. Chapey (Ed.), *Language intervention strategies in adult aphasia* (4th Ed.). Baltimore: Lippincott, Williams & Wilkins.

Mitchum, C. C., Greenwald, M. L., & Berndt, R. S. (2000). Cognitive treatments of sentence processing disorders: What have we learned? *Neuropsychological Rehabilitation, 10*(3), 311–336.

Mitchum, C. C., Haendiges, A., & Berndt, R. S. (1993). Model-guided treatment to improve written sentene production: A case study. *Aphasiology, 7*, 71–109.

Mitchum, C. C., Haendiges, A., & Berndt, R. S. (1995). Treatment of thematic mapping in sentence comprehension: Implications for normal processing. *Cognitive Neuropsychology, 12*, 503–547.

Mitchum, C. C., Haendiges, A., & Berndt, R. S. (2004). Response strategies in aphasic sentence comprehension: An analysis of two cases. *Aphasiology, 18*(8), 675–692.

Murray, L. L., Ballard, K., & Karcher, L. (2004). Linguistic specific treatment: Just for Broca's aphasia? *Aphasiology, 18*(9), 785–809.

Nickels, L., Byng, S., & Black, M. (1991). Sentence processing deficits: A replication of treatment. *British Journal of Disorders of Communication, 26*, 175–199.

Peach, R. K., & Wong, P. C. M. (2004). Integrating the message level into treatment for agrammatism using story retelling. *Aphasiology, 18*(5/6/7), 429–441.

Pick, A. (1913). *Die agrammatischen sprachstonungen.* Berlin: Springer-Verlag.

Pinker, S. (1989). *Learnability and cognition.* Cambridge: MIT Press.

Raymer, A. M., & Ellsworth, T. A. (2002). Response to contrasting verb retrieval treatments: A case study. *Aphasiology, 16*(10/11), 1031–1045.

Rochon, E., Laird, L., Bose, A., & Scofield, J. (2005). Mapping therapy for sentence production impairments in nonfluent aphasia. *Neurpsychological Rehabilitation, 15*(1), 1–36.

Rochon, E., & Reichman, S. (2003). A modular treatment for sentence processing impairments in aphasia: Sentence production. *Journal of speech-language pathology and audiology, 27*(4), 202–210.

Rochon, E., & Reichman, S. (2004). A modular treatment for sentence processing impairments in aphasia: Sentence comprehension. *Journal of speech-language pathology and audiology, 28*(1), 25–33.

Saffran, E. M. (1982). Neuropsychological approaches to the study of language. *British Journal of Psychology, 73,* 317–337.

Saffran, E. M. (2001). Effects of language impairment on sentence comprehension. In R. S. Berndt (Ed.), *Handbook of neuropsychology* (2nd ed., Vol. 3). Amsterdam: Elsevier.

Saffran, E. M., Berndt, R. S., & Schwartz, M. F. (1989). The quantitative analysis of agrammatic production: Procedure and data. *Brain and Language, 37,* 440–479.

Saffran, E. M., & Martin, N. (1997). Effects of structural priming on sentence production in aphasia. *Language and Cognitive Processes, 12,* 877–888.

Saffran, E. M., & Schwartz, M. F. (1988). 'Agrammatic' comprehension it's not: Alternatives and implications. *Aphasiology, 2,* 389–394.

Saffran, E. M., Schwartz, M. F., & Linebarger, M. (1998). Semantic influences on thematic role assignment: Evidence from normals and aphasics. *Brain and Language, 62,* 85–113.

Saffran, E. M., Schwartz, M. F., & Marin, O. S. M. (1980). Evidence from aphasia: Isolating the components of a production model. In B. Butterworth (Ed.), *Language production* (Vol. 1). London: Academic Press.

Schneider, S. L., & Thompson, C. K. (2003). Verb production in agrammatic aphasia: The influence of sematnic class and argument structure properties on generalisation. *Aphasiology, 17*(3), 213–241.

Schwartz, M. F. (1987). Patterns of speech production deficit within and across aphasia syndromes: Application of a psycholinguistic model. In M. Coltheart, G. Sartori, & R. Job (Eds.), *The Cognitive neuropsychology of language* (pp. 163–199). New Jersey: Lawrence Erlbaum.

Schwartz, M. F., Fink, R. B., & Saffran, E. M. (1995). The modular treatment of agrammatism. *Neuropsychological Rehabilitation, 5,* 93–127.

Schwartz, M. F., Linebarger, M. C., Saffran, E. M., & Pate, D. S. (1987). Syntactic transparency and sentence interpretation in aphasia. *Language and Cognitive Processes, 2,* 85–113.

Schwartz, M. F., Saffran, E. M., Fink, R. B., Myers, J. L., & Martin, N. (1994). Mapping therapy: A treatment programme for agrammatism. *Aphasiology, 8,* 9–54.

Schwartz, M. F., Saffran, E. M., & Marin, O. S. M. (1980). The word order problem in agrammatism: Comprehension. *Brain and Language, 10,* 249–262.

Slobin, D. (1996). From "thought and language" to "thinking for speaking". In J. L. Gumperz, S. (Ed.), *Rethinking linguistic relativity.* Cambridge: Cambridge University Press.

Springer, L., Huber, W., Schlenk, K.-J., & Schlenk, C. (2000). Agrammatism: Deficit or compensation: Consequences for aphasia therapy. *Neuropsychological Rehabilitation, 10,* 279–309.

Tissot, R. J., Mounin, G., & Lhermitte, F. (1973). *L'agrammatisme.* Brussels: Dessart.

Vigliocco, G., & Hartsuiker, R. J. (2002). The interplay of meaning sound and syntax in sentence production. *Psychological Bulletin, 128*(3), 442–472.

Webster, J., Morris, J., & Franklin, S. (2005). Effects of therapy targeted at verb retrieval and the realisation of the predicate argument structure: A case study. *Aphasiology, 19*(8), 748–764.

Weinrich, M., Boser, K. I., & McCall, D. (1999). Representation of linguistic rules in the brain: Evidence from training an aphasic patient to produce past tense verb morphology. *Brain and Language, 70,* 144–158.

Weinrich, M., Shelton, J. R., Cox, D. M., & McCall, D. (1997). Remediating production of tense morphology improves verb retrieval in chronic aphasia. *Brain and Language, 58,* 23–45.

Chapter 25

Comprehension and Production of Written Words

Pélagie M. Beeson and
Maya L. Henry

OBJECTIVES

The purpose of this chapter is:

1. To delineate the processes necessary for reading and spelling familiar and unfamiliar words.
2. To describe assessment procedures for the comprehension and production of written words, with particular emphasis on single-word processing.
3. To describe the nature of acquired impairments of reading and spelling.
4. To provide a description of treatment procedures for specific alexia and agraphia profiles.

Despite the fact that most individuals with aphasia have impaired comprehension and production of written words, treatment directed toward the improvement of reading and spelling abilities is often limited. This may reflect the prominence of spoken communication in our daily lives. In today's society, however, face-to-face communication is increasingly replaced by written communication in forms such as electronic mail; automated machines for banking, postage, and airline check-in; and Internet sites for chatting, news and entertainment, managing finances, and purchasing merchandise. Thus, the functional consequences of reading and writing impairments can be quite significant.

The limited attention given to reading and writing rehabilitation may also reflect, in part, limited knowledge of treatment approaches for acquired alexia and agraphia in comparison to the treatment of spoken language. Thus, the purpose of this chapter is to describe numerous approaches that have been shown to be effective for reading and spelling impairments. Our approach to treatment begins with an effort to understand the nature of a patient's impairment by determining what processes and representations necessary for reading and writing are impaired, and what skills are spared. Therefore, in this chapter, we begin with a review of the component processes that support reading and writing, and then describe how impairments to specified representations and processes result in reading and writing disturbances. We will not review the neural substrates for written language processing, but refer the interested reader to reviews by Hillis and Tuffash (2002) and Rapcsak and Beeson (2002). The major focus of this chapter is the review of evidence-based treatments for acquired alexia and agraphia. These impairment-based approaches constitute a central component of treatment plans that have as their ultimate goal the facilitation of meaningful, functional changes in patients' lives.

READING

Reading of familiar words is typically accomplished with relative ease as we recognize a string of letters as a word and comprehend its meaning. Despite the myriad of possible writing styles, we are able to recognize the letter identities that comprise a written word. The word "apple," for example, is activated by any of the following font styles: apple = *apple* = *apple* = apple = *apple*. In each case, the letter combination is recognized as the spelling for a word that we know. Our vocabulary of written words is variously referred to as the *visual input lexicon, graphemic input lexicon,* or *orthographic input lexicon* (the term that we will use here, as shown in Fig. 25–1). The orthographic input lexicon is the mental store of letter strings that we recognize as familiar words. In the figures in this chapter, we have depicted the cognitive processes that support reading and spelling with distinct input and output lexicons. We acknowledge, however, that reading and spelling may rely on shared lexical representations (see review in Tainturier & Rapp, 2001).

Under normal circumstances, orthographic representations activate the appropriate word meaning in the semantic system, allowing us to comprehend the words we read. When reading aloud (and often when reading silently), we access the stored representations for word pronunciations in the *phonological output lexicon*. In turn, this activated representation accesses the component phonemes of the word, which are

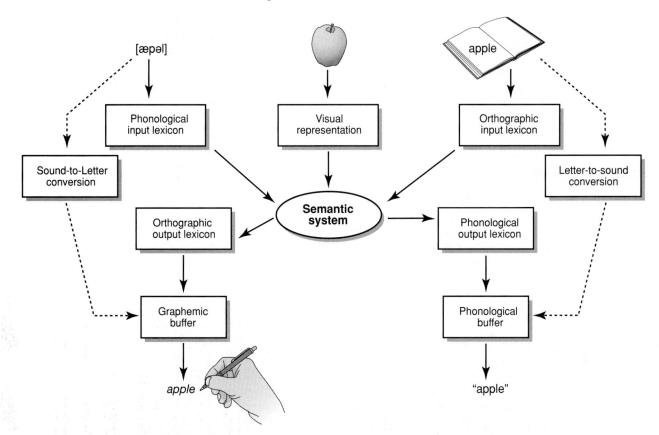

Figure 25–1. Schematic depiction of the component representations and processes for single-word reading and spelling. The solid lines depict lexical-semantic routes and the dashed lines indicate sublexical routes.

held in a short-term storage mechanism referred to as the *phonological buffer*, while we plan the appropriate articulatory movements. This cascade of events is referred to as reading via the *lexical semantic route*, because we derive semantic meaning by activation of words in the lexicon. In Figure 25-1, this is shown as follows: written word (*apple*) → orthographic input lexicon → semantic system → phonological output lexicon → phonological buffer → spoken word ("apple").

Although reading typically activates semantic knowledge, it is possible to read without accessing meaning. We can all recall occasions when we are reading aloud without processing the meaning of the words. In that case, the orthographic input lexicon directly addresses the phonological output lexicon, and meaning is bypassed. This is a lexical route because whole words are processed, but it is a *nonsemantic route* because word meanings are not activated. Reading without meaning is a rare occurrence for healthy adults, but is characteristic of some brain-damaged individuals, particularly those with dementia (Greenwald & Berndt, 1998; Schwartz, Saffran, & Marin, 1987).

When we attempt to read unfamiliar words, there is no corresponding representation to access in our orthographic

input lexicon, so we may take advantage of our knowledge of relatively predictable relations between letters and sounds. Letters or letter clusters that correspond to a single phoneme are referred to as *graphemes*; for example, *f* and *ph* are both graphemes for the sound /f/. In this way, we convert letters (or clusters of letters) to the appropriate sounds and assemble them to produce plausible attempts at their pronunciation. This approach is depicted in Figure 25-1 (with dashed lines) as the *letter-to-sound conversion route*; it is also referred to as *grapheme-to-phoneme conversion*, *orthography-to-phonology conversion*, or simply the *phonological reading route*. This reading process is considered a *sublexical*, or *nonlexical*, *reading route* because it does not depend on activation of words in our lexicon. Although we typically use this sublexical route to read unfamiliar words, it can be used if we are asked to read pronounceable nonwords or pseudowords, like "flig" or "merber." When brain damage causes reading failure via the lexical-semantic route, patients may rely on this sublexical approach for reading both words and nonwords. An obvious feature of the phonological approach is that it only works well if the letter-to-sound correspondences are predictable. Because there are a large number of irregularly spelled words in English, the sublexical route is susceptible to error. For example, the word "sword" might be mispronounced because of failure to appreciate the silent "w." Proper names, like the first names of the authors of this chapter, also present a challenge because the sound-to-letter correspondences may be difficult to predict:

Pelagie = [pe₁lɑ₁ʒiˈ]; Maya = /maɪˈyə/.

Impairments of Reading

Neurologic damage can disturb the processes necessary for reading in a variety of ways. In order to isolate the source of the reading impairment, it is helpful to examine performance on tasks that are dependent upon specified representations and processes, such as processing of single words presented variously in spoken, written, and pictured forms with spoken, written, or nonverbal (pointing) responses. Some processing components are specific to reading (e.g., visual analysis of letter strings, orthographic input lexicon, and letter-to-sound conversion), whereas other components are shared with other lexical processing tasks. For example, semantic processing is necessary for auditory comprehension tasks, writing, and oral naming, as well as reading. Similarly, the phonologic output lexicon is accessed for both oral naming and oral reading tasks. By contrasting performance for single-word comprehension and production in written and spoken modalities, the hypothesized locus (or loci) of impairment may be isolated.

In addition to examining performance across language modalities, it is also informative to determine the influence of various lexical features on reading accuracy (and reading speed, in some cases). Clues regarding the location of damage can be obtained by examining what types of words pose the greatest problem for reading. Carefully constructed word lists that control for lexical features such as word length, part of speech, frequency of use, and concreteness (or imagery) are useful to discern the nature of the impairment, as shown in Table 25–1. Controlled word lists are available in the *Psycholinguistic Assessments of Language Processing in Aphasia* (PALPA; Kay, Lesser, & Coltheart, 1992), the Battery of Adult Reading Function (Rothi, Coslett, & Heilman, 1986), and the Johns Hopkins University (JHU) Dyslexia and Dysgraphia Battery (Goodman & Caramazza, 1986), which is included in Appendix 25-1. The word lists provide contrasts of lexical features that allow examination of various processes for reading single words. The information gained from performance on these controlled word lists will be discussed further in the context of specific reading impairments.

When possible, reading should also be assessed at sentence and paragraph levels. Sentence and paragraph reading can be screened using subtests from standardized aphasia

---

TABLE 25–1

Summary of the Primary Features of Various Acquired Alexia Profiles

		Clinical Features						
Locus of Damage	Example Syndrome	Word Length Short > Long	Spelling Regularity Reg > Irreg	Frequency HF > LF	Imageability/ Concreteness HI > LI	Word Class N > F	Inability to Read Nonwords	Semantic Errors
Access to orthographic input lexicon	Letter-by-letter reading	√						
Orthographic input lexicon	Surface alexia		√	√				
Sublexical (letter-to-sound) procedures	Phonological alexia			√	√	√	√	
Semantics and letter-to-sound conversion	Deep alexia			√	√	√	√	√
Access to phonological output lexicon	Surface alexia		√	√				

Key: √ = significant disturbance; Reg = regular spelling; Irreg = irregular/exceptional spelling; HF = high frequency; LF = low frequency; HI = high imagery; LI = low imagery; N = nouns; F = functors.

tests including the *Western Aphasia Battery-R* (WAB-R; Kertesz, 2006) and the *Boston Diagnostic Aphasia Examination, Third Edition* (*BDAE-3*; Goodglass, Kaplan, & Barresi, 2000). The PALPA (Kay et al., 1992) also provides some sentence-comprehension subtests, and the Reading Comprehension Battery for Aphasia-2 (RCBA-2; LaPointe & Horner, 1998) samples reading for single words, sentences, and paragraphs. In the absence of a comprehensive assessment tool for reading at the paragraph level, some of the tests designed for the examination of developmental reading disorders are useful for examining acquired alexia. For example, the *Gray Oral Reading Test, Fourth Edition* (*GORT*-4; Wiederholt & Bryant, 2001) provides short essays of graded difficulty that can be used to assess reading rate and accuracy, as well as comprehension. The GORT-4 is particularly useful in that alternate forms (A and B) are available.

The pattern of impaired and preserved reading processes will differ among individuals, but there are discernible patterns of impairment that have been recognized as various acquired alexia syndromes (Ellis, 1993; Hillis & Caramazza, 1992; Margolin & Goodman-Schulman, 1992; Rapcsak & Beeson, 2002). Several patterns of acquired reading impairment will be reviewed here, and evidence-based treatment approaches are reported for each of the various patterns. We will show how the hypothesized nature of the impairment can help to guide the treatment approach. Reading impairments will be reviewed in an order that starts at the processing of visual input and ends with impairments in the spoken production of written language.

Impaired Access to the Orthographic Input Lexicon: Pure Alexia

In some cases of neurologic damage, patients fail to recognize strings of letters as familiar words, even though the individual letters are perceived. In its pure form, this disorder is specific to reading, while writing ability remains preserved, so it is referred to as *pure alexia* or *alexia without agraphia*. Many individuals with pure alexia are able to perceive and name the letters of words that they fail to recognize, and if they spell the word letter-by-letter it often helps them identify the word (see papers in Colheart, 1998). For example, a patient may fail to recognize the word *apple* but after spelling it aloud (or subvocally) quickly acknowledges, "oh, apple."

A schematic depiction of the impaired access to the orthographic input lexicon is shown in Figure 25–2 with *letter-by-letter reading* shown as a compensatory strategy. As indicated, the orthographic input lexicon is not impaired, and letter naming may provide an alternative means of activating the orthographic representations. The deficit is specific to the visual modality, so in most cases, individuals with pure alexia are able to quickly recognize words that are spelled aloud to them. Once a word is properly identified, its meaning is easily accessed because there is no impairment of the semantic system. There is also no difficulty in saying the word aloud once it has been recognized.

In pure alexia, access to the orthographic input lexicon is disrupted for all types of words, and reading accuracy typically is not strongly affected by features such as word frequency, concreteness (or imageability), grammatical class, or regularity of spelling, as shown in Table 25-1. When words are decoded letter-by-letter, however, there is a marked word-length effect and thus, long words take more time to read and are more prone to errors than short words. In fact, there is often a linear increase in reading time as a function of the number of letters. In some cases, there is also difficulty with letter identification, which limits the effectiveness of letter-by-letter reading even further.

Treatment for Pure Alexia

Several treatment approaches have been shown to improve access to the orthographic input lexicon or to provide compensatory strategies to support reading. The treatments vary with regard to the complexity of the stimuli used for treatment: text, single words, or single letters. The first approach, multiple oral rereading, is thought to strengthen access to the orthographic input lexicon either in a direct manner or via the compensatory letter-naming route. A different treatment approach is appropriate for patients who show impaired letter identification.

Multiple Oral Rereading. Multiple oral rereading (MOR) entails the use of repeated reading aloud of a given text as a means of facilitating whole-word, rather than letter-by-letter, reading. Several researchers have shown this procedure to be effective as a means to increase reading rate in letter-by-letter readers (Beeson, 1998; Beeson, Magloire, & Robey, 2005; Moyer, 1979; Tuomainen & Laine, 1991). It was hypothesized that repeated reading of the same text facilitates a shift from letter-by-letter reading to whole-word reading because of the support provided by sentence context and familiarity with the text. This approach is thought to improve or re-establish access to the orthographic input lexicon so that letter-by-letter reading can decrease. The procedures for implementing MOR are described in Table 25-2. Essentially, the treatment involves structured homework in which selected text is read aloud repeatedly so that reading rate improves and reading errors decrease. When successful, the improved reading for practiced text is accompanied by improvement in reading of novel (i.e., previously unread) text that more closely approximates normal adult oral reading rates, which range from 150 to 200 wpm (Rayner & Pollatsek, 1989).

The text used for MOR treatment should be controlled for length and complexity. In particular, the average word

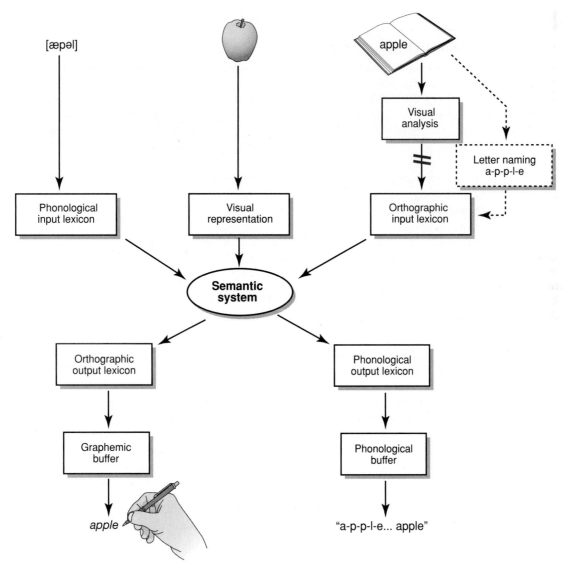

Figure 25–2. Schematic representation of impaired access to the orthographic input lexicon with strategic compensation in the form of letter-by-letter reading. Bold black hash marks indicate disrupted process.

length will affect reading performance. Treatment studies implementing MOR have used standardized text, such as passages from the Reading Laboratory by Scientific Research Associates (SRA; Parker & Scannell, 1998) because it has graded levels of difficulty. Reading material can also be selected from readily available sources including books, magazines, and the Internet. If the text is in electronic format, the difficulty level can be appraised using readability indices, such as the Flesch-Kincaid grade level (Kincaid, Fishbourne, Rogers, & Chissom, 1975). To do so using Microsoft® Office Word 2003, use the pull-down menu to select tools → options → spelling and grammar, and check the box for "show readability statistics." Then run the "spelling and grammar" check on the "tools" menu. At the completion of the spelling and grammar check, a reading grade level (from 1 to 12) according to Flesch-Kincaid is returned.

Although no studies document the ideal intensity and duration of MOR needed to be effective, therapeutic effects have been documented with a homework schedule of at least 30 minutes a day. A criterion rate of 100 words per minute for the practiced text has been used with even the slowest of letter-by-letter readers (10 seconds per word; Beeson, 1998). Once achieved, new passages are introduced for repeated oral reading as homework. To test whether MOR results in generalized improvements, reading rates and accuracy for previously unread passages are sampled during weekly therapy sessions. The expected outcome is a steady improvement in

TABLE 25–2

Steps for Implementing Multiple Oral Rereading (MOR) Treatment Approach*

A. Initial treatment session(s)
Step 1. Determine reading rate and accuracy for text-level material.
  a. Select a passage of appropriate difficulty, e.g., 100-word segment, to be used as practice text.
  b. Ask the patient to read the text aloud allowing for letter-by-letter decoding as needed.
  c. Calculate reading rate in words per minute and score reading errors in terms of number of deviations from print (self-corrected errors may be tallied separately).
Step 2. Establish multiple oral rereading procedures.
  a. Have the patient reread the text, providing assistance as needed to guide correction of reading errors. Multiple repetitions during therapy sessions provide an opportunity to increase familiarity with text, and should result in increased accuracy.
  b. Establish homework activity.
    1) Provide a copy of the written text for homework.
    2) Agree upon daily homework schedule, e.g., 30 minutes of repeated oral reading of specific text once or twice daily.
    3) Establish a log for recording completion of homework. Patients may time themselves and record the time taken to read the passage, or simply note completion of homework on a daily basis.
B. Subsequent therapy sessions
Step 1. Review patient's log to confirm consistency in completing MOR homework.
Step 2. Determine rate and accuracy of reading for practiced text.
  a. Have the patient read practiced text aloud.
  b. Keep a graphic plot of reading rate and accuracy.
Step 3. Determine target rate for practiced text, e.g., to achieve 50 wpm or 100 wpm. When target rate is attained (with acceptable accuracy) for practiced text, provide a new passage for MOR homework.
Step 4. Determine reading rate and accuracy for new (previously unread) text.
  a. Provide a new passage (about 100 words) for oral reading to determine whether reading rate or accuracy for new material improves.
  b. Calculate and record reading rate and accuracy during each session to determine effectiveness of MOR treatment.

*Rationale: Multiple oral reading is thought to improve access to the orthographic input lexicon, so that reliance on letter-by-letter reading decreases and whole-word recognition improves.
(After Beeson, P. M. (1998). Treatment for letter-by-letter reading: A case study. In N. Helm-Estabrooks & A. L. Holland (Eds.), *Approaches to the treatment of aphasia* (pp. 153–157). San Diego: Singular Press.

reading rate for new text while maintaining (or improving) the level of accuracy. Slow readers have shown improvement that is two, three, and four times their pre-treatment reading rates.

The MOR protocol can be implemented with relatively infrequent treatment sessions because it is heavily dependent upon the patient's accomplishment of reading homework. Weekly or even biweekly sessions may be adequate. Variations in the protocol might include adjustment of the criterion reading rate for practiced text from 100 wpm to a slower rate, such as 50 wpm, when deemed necessary.

Brief Orthographic Exposure. A different approach to treatment for impaired access to the orthographic input lexicon involves the presentation of written words for brief exposures so that letter-by-letter reading is not possible. The motivation for this treatment came from the observation that some individuals with pure alexia retain an ability to derive some meaning from words that they cannot explicitly name (Coslett & Saffran, 1989; 1994).

Rothi and Moss (1992) proposed that individuals with pure alexia might be stimulated to use this implicit knowledge gained from brief whole-word "reading" to facilitate comprehension and possibly to regain access to the orthographic input lexicon. They used a paradigm in which single words were presented on a computer screen for brief exposures (e.g., 500 msec), and the patient was asked to make a decision about the word, such as, "Is it an animal?" Although the patient often indicated that he had not actually read the word, he was encouraged to guess. Response accuracy was above chance, indicating some ability to apprehend the whole word at an implicit level. This brief exposure procedure resulted in improved reading rate (following 20 treatment sessions) in Rothi and Moss's patient, suggesting that it facilitated recovery of whole-word reading. However, Rothi and colleagues reported failure of this treatment approach with two other patients (Maher, Clayton, Barrett, Schober-Peterson, & Rothi, 1998; Rothi, Greenwald, Maher, & Ochipa, 1998), suggesting that it may be useful for a subset of people with pure alexia.

An adaptation of the brief exposure procedure could be implemented using written words presented on cards and shown for a brief duration rather than by computer presentation. Another variation involves contrasting real words with plausible nonwords for a lexical decision task in response to the question, "Is this a word?" These variations share the common goal of promoting whole-word apprehension rather than letter-by-letter reading.

Cross-Modality Cueing to Enhance Letter Identification. Letter-by-letter reading cannot be accomplished effectively if a significant number of letter identification errors are made. In some patients, letter identification is facilitated when information regarding the letter shape is provided via another modality. For example, some patients perceive a letter when it is traced on their palm, or when they trace the letter themselves (Seki, Yajima, & Sugishita, 1995). Tracing the component letters of a word with one's finger, or copying the written word, are compensatory strategies that can be used by the patient without assistance. It is assumed that the kinesthetic information about spelling provides access to the orthographic input lexicon, which substitutes for activation of the lexicon via visual input. Thus, the procedure has been referred to as cross-modality cueing.

A positive response to cross-modality cueing was reported by Maher and colleagues (1998) for a patient with pure alexia who had difficulty naming letters, so letter-by-letter decoding of words was not possible. This patient was able to identify letters in a word only after she traced each letter with her finger. Maher documented that treatment using this motor cross-cueing strategy resulted in improved word recognition and increased reading rate. With practice, letter recognition improved, such that simply tracing the first letter or two of a word was adequate to cue word identification.

Reading with Overreliance on Letter-to-Sound Conversion: Surface Alexia

Reading is disrupted when component processes of the lexical-semantic reading route are damaged. This can include impaired representations in the orthographic input lexicon (or impaired access to orthographic representations), as well as damage to the semantic system or the phonologic output lexicon. In the case of orthographic impairment, it appears as though the individual's vocabulary of written words has eroded, and thus, visually perceived words that were once familiar now appear unfamiliar and their meaning cannot be derived. If the ability to "sound out" words is retained, reading may be accomplished by means of the letter-to-sound conversion procedure (i.e., via the sublexical route), as shown in Figure 25–3. This procedure works well for words that have good letter-to-sound correspondences (i.e., regular words, such as *flake*), but words that have uncommon letter-to-sound correspondences (i.e., irregular words, such as

yacht) pose a problem and are often misread. For example, the word "blood" might be pronounced such that it rhymes with "mood." Thus, when reading is accomplished via the sublexical rather than the lexical route, performance is characterized by greater difficulty reading irregularly spelled words when compared to regularly spelled words, as indicated in Table 25-1. This reading profile has been referred to as *surface alexia* because reading is accomplished via phonology rather than meaning, so that it might be thought of as reading "on the surface" (see papers in Patterson, Marshall, & Coltheart, 1985). Because reading is accomplished by sounding-out, regularly spelled words and nonwords are read with at least fair accuracy, and phonologically plausible errors for irregularly spelled words are common. A consequence of overreliance on the sublexical route while reading is confusion of words that sound the same but are spelled differently (i.e., homophones, such as "dear" and "deer"), because access to semantics is gained from the oral reading response. Additionally, words that are spelled the same but pronounced differently (i.e., homographs) may be mispronounced for a given context; for example, "lead" might be (incorrectly) pronounced the same in the phrases "the lead pipe" and "I will lead the way." Typically, individuals with surface alexia also use a phonological strategy for spelling, and phonologically plausible errors are common when spelling irregular words, reflecting a concomitant syndrome referred to as *surface agraphia* (or lexical agraphia) that is discussed below.

In surface alexia, there are no strong effects of lexical-semantic features such as imageability or word class, because reading "bypasses" the semantic system. However, the impairment at the level of the orthographic input lexicon should be more notable on low frequency words compared to high frequency words (see Table 25-1), because high frequency words are thought to be more resistant to damage. Word length may have a negative effect on reading accuracy, because longer words provide more opportunities for errors in letter-to-sound conversion, and it may also take longer to sound out a long word rather than a short word; however, a word-length effect is not an essential feature associated with impaired representations in the orthographic input lexicon.

Lexical Treatment for Surface Alexia

Because surface alexia typically occurs with surface agraphia, treatment for the reading impairment may be addressed in the context of spelling treatment. A lexical approach to treatment involves retraining orthographic knowledge for specific words. Lexical treatment may focus on words that are prone to error, such as homophones and homographs. Hillis (1993) demonstrated successful treatment to increase reliance on lexical-semantic processing for reading and spelling in the context of retraining homographic and homophonic pairs. Each target word was presented in print with its written definition, which was read aloud by the

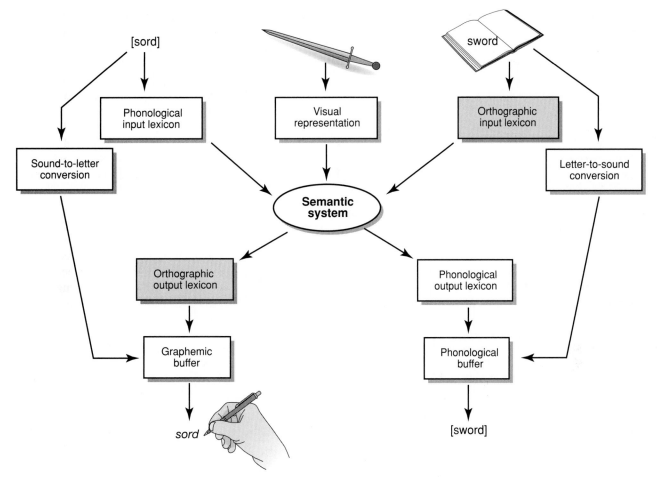

Figure 25–3. Schematic representation of damage to the orthographic input lexicon (shaded), and reliance on letter-to-sound conversion to decode written words (heavy black lines), resulting in phonologically plausible reading errors typical of surface alexia (on the right side of figure). Surface agraphia is depicted on the left side of the figure.

clinician. The patient was asked to write the target word in a sentence, and corrective feedback was provided. Treatment resulted in improved oral reading, spelling, and comprehension (as assessed by use of the word in sentence contexts) for trained words, as well as improved oral reading for the untrained members of the word pairs. Therefore, the pairing of specific orthographic representations with semantics served to strengthen the patient's ability to read via the lexical-semantic route, allowing him to disambiguate homophones and homographs.

Another approach to enhance reading via the lexical semantic route (and to reduce overreliance on a phonological strategy) involves the presentation of written words for brief exposures in a manner similar to that described by Rothi and colleagues in the case of pure alexia. Rapid visual presentation can force a lexical strategy for word recognition. Hillis (1993) showed that brief exposure to written words with corrective feedback during oral reading resulted in item-

specific learning for trained items. Because there may be limited generalization with this approach, it is important to select words of functional value for the patient.

Reading with Impaired Letter-to-Sound Conversion: Phonologic Alexia and Deep Alexia

When phonological abilities are impaired due to brain damage, patients have difficulty with letter-to-sound conversion, as depicted in Figure 25–4. Reading is accomplished via a lexical-semantic strategy, such that representations in the orthographic input lexicon should activate the semantic system. Impairments of the nonlexical route are clearly evident when the patient is asked to read unfamiliar words or phonologically plausible nonwords that do not have a lexical representation (e.g., "dusp"). The profile of impaired nonword reading relative to real word reading is referred to as *phonological alexia*. It reflects an inability to use sublexical

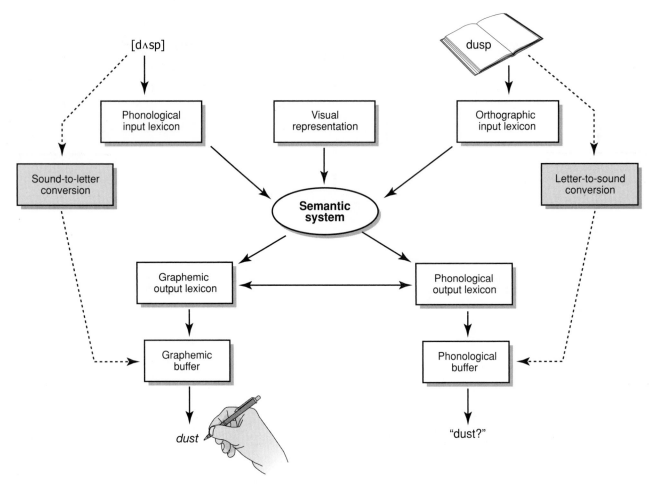

Figure 25–4. Schematic representation of impairment to letter-to-sound conversion procedures resulting in lexicalization error on nonword reading ("dust" for "dusp"), reflecting phonological alexia (on the right side of figure). Phonological agraphia is depicted on the left side of the figure.

processes to derive the appropriate sound for a given letter. A range of severity is observed in phonological alexia, with mild cases showing relatively preserved reading of real words but difficulty with nonwords. In more severe cases it is evident that the lexical-semantic route is vulnerable to error when deprived of phonological input. In most cases, the weakened lexical-semantic route typically results in a frequency effect, in that high frequency words are read better than low frequency words. There is also a concreteness (or imageability) effect, such that concrete words such as "apple" are read better than abstract words such as "pride." This profile may reflect the fact that concrete, high frequency nouns have stronger semantic representations and therefore are most resistant to damage. Abstract, low frequency words and grammatical functors have the weakest semantic representations, or have semantic representations that have a great deal of overlap with other words and are thus easily confused. For example, the meaning of "belief" is

difficult to define and overlaps considerably with the meaning of many other words: confidence, conviction, credence, creed, notion, thought, concept, faith, religion, hope, idea, presumption, principle, trust, and so on. In contrast, the meanings of concrete nouns like "fork" do not overlap as much with other meanings. A part-of-speech (or grammatical class) effect is also common in phonological alexia, in that nouns are read better than adjectives and verbs, which are read better than functors.

Because phonology provides little assistance, there is typically no difference in the reading accuracy of regularly spelled words compared to irregular words in phonological and deep alexia. That is, there is no regularity effect as seen in surface alexia. The overreliance on the lexical route often draws patients to misread nonwords as real words (e.g., "dusp" → "dust"), which is referred to as "lexicalization."

When damage to the sublexical route is accompanied by dysfunction of the lexical-semantic reading route, semantic

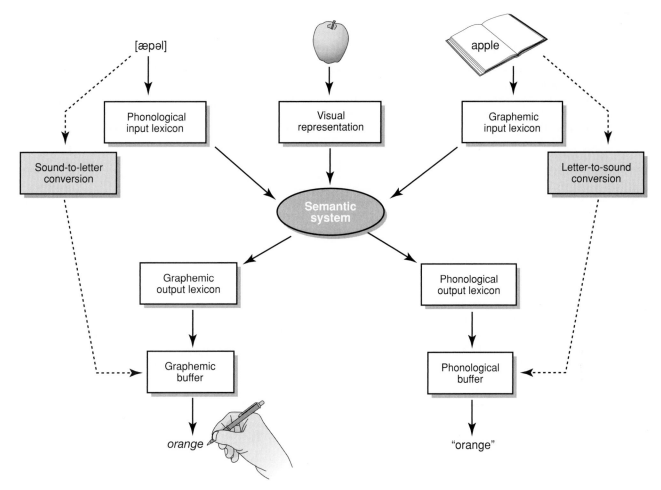

Figure 25–5. Schematic representation of impairments to the semantic system and letter-to-sound conversion resulting in a semantic error ("orange" for "apple"), reflecting deep alexia (on the right side of the figure). Deep agraphia is depicted on the left side of the figure.

errors are prevalent, such as reading *woman* as *girl*, or *apple* as *orange*, as shown in Figure 25–5. The presence of semantic errors is the hallmark feature of the acquired alexia syndrome referred to as *deep alexia*, or more commonly, *deep dyslexia* (Coltheart, Patterson, & Marshall, 1987; Newcombe & Marshall, 1984). Although phonological and deep alexia initially were considered to be distinct syndromes, they are currently viewed as points on a continuum, reflecting quantitative rather than qualitative differences (Glosser & Friedman, 1990; Rapcsak & Beeson, 2002). Deep alexia is usually associated with extensive left hemisphere lesions, suggesting that reading in these patients may be mediated by the right hemisphere (Coltheart et al., 1987; Patterson, Vargha-Khadem, & Polkey, 1989).

Treatment for Phonological and Deep Alexia

Treatments for phonological and deep alexia may be directed toward sublexical or lexical reading processes, or both.

Phonological treatments may serve to strengthen letter-to-sound correspondences that supplement lexical reading procedures. Lexical reading treatments typically include spoken production of target words or text-level material, so there is simultaneous stimulation of written and spoken language processes that ideally improves both language modalities. It is worth mentioning again that reading treatment is an inherent component of treatments for spelling, and thus, clinicians may find it efficient to combine the treatments described for phonological/deep alexia with those described for phonological/deep agraphia.

Strengthening Letter-to-Sound Conversion. The training of letter-to-sound correspondences has the potential to be an effective strategy for reading many words (rather than a specific set of words), so it is worthwhile to determine whether a given patient can relearn letter-sound associations. A number of treatment reports have documented

TABLE 25–3

Establishing Key Words That Are Associated with Specific Graphemes

A. Initial treatment sessions
  Step 1. Determine what grapheme-phoneme pairs will be targeted for training.
    a. Select consonants first because they have more consistent letter-to-sound correspondences than vowels.
    b. Select frequently occurring consonants (see Appendix 25-2); proceed to less frequent consonants and vowels as appropriate for a given patient. For example, train consonants in sets of five at a time:
      Set 1. r, t, n, s, l
      Set 2. k, d, m, p, f
      Set 3. b, sh, v, g, z
  Step 2. For each target grapheme, assist the patient in identifying a key word that begins with the grapheme.
    a. If possible, find key words that the patient can consistently say correctly, such as, "Ron" for r.
    b. If the patient does not have a key word available for a given grapheme, a word should be agreed upon and trained for consistency of production.
    c. Construct stimulus cards that have a grapheme on one side (e.g., R-r) and the associated key word on the other side (e.g., Ron).
B. Establish homework procedures
    a. Using stimulus cards, the patient should look at the grapheme and say the name of the key word. (Look at key word on the back of the card only as necessary for cueing.)
    b. Optional: Make a videotape of clinician showing the grapheme and asking for production of the key word (with model provided by clinician after a pause so that the patient can evaluate response relative to the model).
    c. Establish frequency of homework (e.g., daily practice).
C. Subsequent therapy sessions
    a. Review the patient's ability to retrieve the key word for each targeted grapheme.
    b. Target additional graphemes as appropriate.
D. Subsequent treatment
    a. Select (or develop) a subsequent protocol to take advantage of key words for deriving phonology from written words (for reading) or deriving graphemes from phonology (for writing).

*Rationale: to develop a corpus of key words that can be used to assist the patient in retrieving phonology from written words.

success in re-establishing links between orthography and phonology (e.g., de Partz, 1986; Nickels, 1992). A "key word" approach is often used, such as that described in Table 25-3. The training involves establishing at least one key word for each grapheme-phoneme pair targeted for treatment. As indicated in Table 25–3, key words are used to assist a patient in self-cueing the phonology for a given grapheme. The items selected as key words should be ones that the patient can consistently produce. In other words, it is typical that the list of key words is different for each individual, capitalizing on their success with specific words. Key words are typically nouns, and can include proper names that the patient can easily retrieve. Treatment typically begins with higher frequency phonemes, so it is useful to consider frequency of occurrence in English words to guide the choice of targets (see Appendix 25-2; Berndt, Reggia, & Mitchum, 1987; Hanna, Hanna, Hodges, & Rudorf, 1966). Because the predictability of letter-to-sound correspondences is stronger for consonants than vowels, it is most effective to establish key words for consonants first. For some patients, it may be too effortful to train the vowels at all. Although the time required to re-establish the letter-to-sound associations may be considerable, much of the work can be accomplished by self-drill outside of the therapy session. Videotaped homework is particularly useful to provide articulatory models for practicing letter-to-sound correspondences.

After key words are established, treatment proceeds to phonemic self-cueing, so that the patient can derive the appropriate phoneme from a grapheme. This training may be accomplished by having the patient say the key word with the first sound prolonged, and then say only the first phoneme in isolation (for example, "Sue . . . . . SSSSSue . . . . . . SSSS . . . [s]"). Thus, the key word provides the means to cue placement of the articulators for a given letter. The patient is then trained to produce only the first sound of the key word in response to its associated letter. In many instances, phonological information obtained via letter-to-sound conversion may be adequate to reduce or block phonological and semantic errors in oral reading and to initiate correct production of a word (de Partz, 1986). Training can also proceed to reading three- or four-letter monosyllabic words and nonwords by deriving the component sounds and blending them to produce a word (or nonword). In some patients, mastery of regular letter-to-sound associations provides the necessary additional information to support the impaired lexical-semantic reading route, such that treatment addressing the nuances of irregular spellings is not necessary.

Treatment for Impaired Semantics. Individuals with impairment of the letter-to-sound conversion mechanism and concomitant damage to semantics may also benefit from treatment to strengthen semantics. Such treatment may include written word-to-picture matching tasks that reinforce the links between word forms and their meanings. Hillis demonstrated the value of this approach with a patient who exhibited impaired semantics affecting his reading as well as written and spoken naming (patient JJ in Hillis & Caramazza; 1991a, 1991b, 1994). The semantic treatment entailed matching written words and their corresponding pictures, with error responses corrected and missed items re-presented after intervening items until a correct response was achieved. Treatment resulted in rapid improvement of oral reading and comprehension of the trained words.

Oral Reading Treatments. In some patients, semantic errors do not reflect a central impairment of semantic knowledge, but rather a failure to activate correct phonological representations. Hillis demonstrated that a cueing hierarchy to elicit correct oral reading of target words was an appropriate intervention approach (patient HW described by Hillis, 1993; Hillis & Caramazza, 1994). In effect, this cued oral reading treatment served to improve access to spoken word forms in an item-specific manner. To do so, written words were presented for oral reading, and phonemic cueing and repetition were provided as needed to elicit correct production. This treatment resulted in item-specific improvement of oral naming and oral reading of targeted items, which confirmed the hypothesized locus of damage to be the phonological output lexicon that is common to both tasks. The success of this procedure is best explained as a lowering of the activation threshold in the phonological output lexicon as a consequence of the increased frequency of production in the training context. This stimulation effect is a familiar result of effective hierarchical cueing and mass-practice effects. Despite the lack of generalization to other words, there can be considerable functional benefit from item-specific improvement of single-word reading and naming.

Oral reading treatments have also been implemented at the text level, with positive treatment outcomes. Cherney, Merbitz, and Grip (1986) documented the value of an approach referred to as Oral Reading for Language in Aphasia (ORLA), which involves oral reading in unison with the clinician. The protocol includes corrective feedback and modeling by the clinician to facilitate accurate oral reading of text-level stimuli. The nature of the reading impairment in the participants was not described from a cognitive perspective; however, spoken language impairment in these individuals suggested impairment to lexical and sublexical

procedures, typical of phonological and deep alexia. Administration of ORLA was associated with improved reading comprehension, as well as improved comprehension and production of spoken language. An adaptation of ORLA, referred to simply as Oral Reading Treatment, demonstrated similar benefits for spoken and written language performance in an individual with aphasia and phonological alexia (Orjada & Beeson, 2005). The outcomes from these studies suggest that reading treatments may stimulate interactive processing of orthography and phonology with benefits to both reading and spoken language in individuals with aphasia.

There is evidence to suggest that oral reading of text can also serve to strengthen access to grammatical words in individuals with relatively mild language impairment. This was demonstrated by Beeson and Insalaco (1998), who showed that the multiple oral rereading (MOR) approach can also benefit individuals who do not fit the classic profile of pure alexia but who appeared to have relatively mild phonological alexia. MOR was implemented with two individuals with anomic aphasia who reported slow reading rate as their primary complaint. Both showed a word-length effect for oral reading, slower reading rate for functors in comparison to nouns, and impaired reading of nonwords. Using the MOR approach, both patients were able to more than double their reading rate for new text to about 100 words per minute, an increase that was adequate to support pleasure reading. An examination of their reading rate and accuracy for single words before and after treatment showed the greatest improvement in reading rate for functors, suggesting that for some individuals MOR may be particularly beneficial for improving recognition of function words. These results suggested that the syntactic constraints offered by sentence contexts help to facilitate access to functors, and that repeated oral reading had a durable therapeutic effect.

Unspecified Alexia Profiles

In this chapter, we have taken a cognitive approach to describing the nature and treatment of written language processing. We acknowledge, however, that some treatment studies have shown positive responses to reading treatments for individuals with aphasia and acquired alexia that was unspecified with regard to the specific nature of the impairment. For example, Katz and Wertz (1997) demonstrated significant improvement on standardized aphasia tests in response to a hierarchical reading treatment presented via computer. The treatment provided structured reading tasks from single letters to words to sentences, with corrective feedback and performance-based advancement through the protocol hierarchy. Significant improvement was documented following the computerized reading treatment on measures of overall language performance when compared to conditions with nonlinguistic computer stimulation or no treatment. These outcomes support the notion that written-language treatments may engage and strengthen spoken-language processes.

Summary of Treatments for Acquired Reading Impairments

Reading disturbances may reflect impairments to the component processes necessary for comprehension and production of written words. Degraded representations (or impaired access to representations) may occur at the level of orthography, semantics, or phonology. Similarly, the sublexical reading route that enables sounding out words may be impaired. These impairments may occur in isolation or in various combinations. Numerous treatment approaches have been shown to be effective in strengthening lexical-semantic representations and processes, and improving letter-to-sound conversion abilities, as well as developing alternative strategies to support reading. Even when reading processes are not fully restored, item-specific improvements and the retrieval of partial information can serve to improve functional reading skills. It is also worth noting that several treatment approaches might be implemented in sequence, so that improved skills are incorporated in successive treatment stages. For example, initial treatment efforts may focus on lexical-semantic processes, whereas a later stage of treatment may include strengthening the sublexical route. In this way, progressive approximation of normal reading processes is achieved, and appropriate strategic compensations are established.

SPELLING

The act of expressing our ideas in writing involves clarifying our thoughts, formulating sentences, and sequentially translating each word to its written form according to the spelling conventions for the language. Writing calls upon a multitude of cognitive, linguistic, and perceptual-motor processes. We will focus here primarily on the processes that are specific to single-word spelling. Under normal circumstances, our semantic representation activates a written word in our mental dictionary. This collection of spellings that we know is referred to as the *orthographic output lexicon* (Fig. 25-1); or it may also be referred to as the *graphemic output lexicon* or the *visual output lexicon* (Ellis, 1993). As we write a word, it is held in short-term storage in the *graphemic output buffer*, which may simply be called the *graphemic buffer*. The information is held in the graphemic buffer as a series of graphemes, which are generic, abstract letter representations (as opposed to specific upper or lowercase exemplars in particular writing styles). The representation in the graphemic buffer allows realization of spelling in several forms—handwriting, typing, or oral spelling. Written spelling requires implementation of peripheral processes whereby

the specific letter forms (referred to as *allographs*) are selected and motor movements are planned and executed. The selection of a particular letter form is referred to as the *allographic conversion process*. Finally, graphic motor programs are implemented to write the component letters of a word.

The motivation to write a word most often reflects self-activation of a semantic concept; but in clinical situations, we may ask a patient to write a word that we dictate (i.e., in response to auditory input), write the name of a pictured item, or even copy a printed word. As is the case with reading, spelling may be accomplished via the lexical-semantic route, but it can also rely on sublexical knowledge of sound-to-letter correspondences, as shown in Figure 25-1. For an unfamiliar word (or a nonword), spelling can be derived by sounding out the word and converting sounds to letters, a process that is also referred to as *phoneme-to-grapheme conversion*. This sound-to-letter conversion is considered a non-lexical or sublexical process, because spellings are assembled rather than retrieved as whole words. Assembled spellings are likely to reflect regular spelling rules, such that irregularly spelled words might be regularized; for example, "cough" might be spelled as *coff*. This sublexical route can provide an important compensatory spelling strategy when the lexical-semantic spelling route is impaired.

Impairments of Spelling

The processes necessary to spell words can be disrupted by damage to central linguistic processes as well as more peripheral components involved in writing (Ellis, 1993; Rapcsak & Beeson, 2000; Tainturier & Rapp, 2001). A comprehensive assessment of writing includes examination of spontaneous writing, written naming, writing to dictation, and copying. A sample of spontaneous writing may be obtained by asking a patient to compose a short narrative; however, it may be preferable to request a written description of a standard picture, such as the picnic scene from the *WAB-R* (Kertesz, 2006) or the cookie-theft picture from the *BDAE-3* (Goodglass et al., 2000). The use of a standard stimulus allows for comparison over time and also provides referent information that may be helpful in discerning the intended content and spellings. Written narratives allow for examination of semantic organization, syntactic structure, word choice, and single-word spelling.

There are several sources of standardized stimuli that can be used to assess single-word spelling. Standardized aphasia tests, such as the *WAB-R* and *BDAE*-3, offer a small set of items for initial screening of writing. A comprehensive assessment of single-word writing requires the use of controlled word lists, such as those included in the *PALPA* (Kay et al., 1992) or the JHU Battery (Goodman & Caramazza, 1986; Appendix 25-1). Assessment of oral spelling, typing, spelling with anagram letters, and copying may be needed to

TABLE 25–4

Summary of the Primary Features of Various Acquired Agraphias

Locus of Damage	Example Syndrome	Clinical Features						
		Word Length Short > Long	Spelling Regularity Reg > Irreg	Frequency HF > LF	Imageability/Concreteness HI > LI	Word Class N > F	Inability to Read Nonwords	Semantic Errors
Sublexical (sound-to-letter) procedures	Phonological agraphia			√	√	√	√	
Semantics and sound-to-letter conversion	Deep agraphia			√	√	√	√	√
Orthographic output lexicon	Surface (lexical) agraphia		√	√				
Graphemic buffer	Graphemic buffer agraphia	√						

Key: √ = significant disturbance; Reg = regular spelling; Irreg = irregular/exceptional spelling; HF = high frequency; LF = low frequency; HI = high imagery; LI = low imagery; N = nouns; F = functors.

discern whether central or peripheral spelling processes are impaired. Given that clinical evaluations are typically constrained by time and financial considerations, it is important to select writing subtests that serve to test hypotheses regarding the locus of damage to the spelling system, in order to ensure that an appropriate treatment approach is selected.

As with acquired alexia, characteristic patterns of acquired agraphia may result when certain component processes are disturbed (Table 25-4). In this section of the chapter, several patterns of acquired spelling impairments will be described, with greatest attention given to the central (or linguistically based) writing impairments that often accompany aphasia. Treatment approaches directed toward particular components of the writing process are described, with reference to representative studies.

Spelling with Impaired Sound-to-Letter Conversion: Phonological Agraphia and Deep Agraphia

Selective impairment of sublexical spelling, or sound-to-letter conversion, has been referred to as *phonological agraphia* (Shallice, 1981). The defining feature of phonological agraphia is a disproportionate impairment of sound-to-letter conversion, with relative sparing of lexical-semantic procedures (see Fig. 25-4). Accordingly, individuals with phonological agraphia have a pronounced nonword spelling deficit and show little effect of spelling regularity. A pure form of phonological agraphia is relatively uncommon, and

would only affect spelling of unfamiliar words and nonwords (Alexander, Friedman, Loverso, & Fischer, 1992). In actuality, most individuals with impaired sublexical spelling also have some degree of concomitant lexical-semantic spelling impairment, suggesting that phonological processes are critical for both nonword and real word spelling (Henry, Beeson, Stark, & Rapcsak, 2007). Because spelling in these individuals is mediated by the lexical-semantic route, performance tends to be affected by lexical variables such as word frequency (high > low), imageability (high > low), and grammatical class (nouns > functors) (see Table 25-4). Spelling errors are typically not phonologically plausible, and often bear some visual or orthographic similarity to the target (e.g., *flewen* for *flower*). Morphological errors (e.g., *walking* for *walked*) and functor substitutions (e.g., *since* for *about*) are also prevalent.

In some individuals, impaired sound-to-letter conversion is accompanied by deficits at the semantic level. Written semantic errors occur when semantic representations are damaged or in some way underspecified, resulting in the retrieval of the incorrect orthographic representation. For example, a fully elaborated semantic representation of *apple* might include <fruit>, <round>, <red>, <juicy>, <sweet>. If the semantic representation included <fruit>, <round>, <juicy>, <sweet>, but failed to include <red>, then it might activate *orange* as shown in Figure 25-5. Such semantic errors are observed in spelling, but also may be evident in other output modalities, such as spoken production. The combined profile of written semantic errors and poor sound-to-letter conversion ability has been called *deep dysgraphia*, or *deep agraphia*, which is the analog of deep dyslexia. As with phonological/deep alexia, phonological and deep agraphia were initially considered distinct syndromes but have more recently been described as points along a continuum of increasingly severe phonological and lexical-semantic impairment (Rapcsak & Beeson, 2002). As shown in Table 25–4, these impairments result in spelling that is influenced by the same lexical features that affect performance in phonological agraphia (concreteness/imageability, word class, and frequency). As with phonological agraphia, there is little influence of spelling regularity, and nonword spelling is poor. Patients typically produce error types consistent with those seen in phonological agraphia (morphological errors, functor substitutions, and visually/orthographically similar misspellings) and also produce semantic errors (e.g., *apple* for *orange*) (Rapcsak, Beeson, & Rubens, 1991).

Treatment for Phonological and Deep Agraphia

As with phonological/deep alexia, treatment for individuals with phonological and deep agraphia may be directed toward sublexical and/or lexical processes. Phonological treatment may serve to strengthen sound-letter correspondences so that spellings can be derived phonologically. For individuals with concomitant damage to the lexical-semantic route, treatment may address damage to semantic representations or may focus on rebuilding specific spellings in the orthographic output lexicon.

Strengthening Sound-to-Letter Conversion. If a patient has impairment of sound-to-letter conversion, but has the ability to say words, it may be worthwhile to provide treatment to retrain sublexical spelling procedures (Cardell & Chenery, 1999; Hillis & Caramazza, 1994; Hillis Trupe, 1986). This treatment can be implemented using the same key word approach as used in reading treatment, with the potential for both modalities to be trained simultaneously (see Table 25-3). Once key words are established, training should be implemented to facilitate retrieval of phoneme-grapheme correspondences for spelling, as illustrated in Table 25–5. Hillis described clinical cases in which information derived from the sublexical route in combination with a partially damaged lexical-semantic system provided improved access to single words for written communication (Hillis Trupe, 1986; Hillis & Caramazza, 1994).

In individuals with deep agraphia, strengthening sound-to-letter conversion skills may provide access to initial graphemes, serving to block semantic errors or support activation of the orthographic output lexicon (Bub & Kertesz, 1982). In other words, semantic errors in writing might be avoided or self-corrected if a patient has at least some ability to translate the initial sounds of a word into the correspond-

ing graphemes. For example, if the intended target word is *movie*, but the patient incorrectly writes *TV*, the error might be self-corrected if the initial phoneme /m/ is converted to the grapheme *m*. While retraining sound-to-letter conversion skills may improve spelling in patients with deep agraphia, others require treatment directed toward the semantic system itself.

Treatment for Impaired Semantics. Effective remediation of semantic impairments may result in improved responses on oral naming and repetition tasks, as well as in written naming. For example, in cases where semantic errors suggest an underspecification of the features necessary to distinguish among items in the same semantic category, semantic treatment may be directed toward clarifying the semantic distinctions among written words as they are matched to corresponding pictures (Hillis, 1991). When errors are made, corrective feedback is offered that highlights distinctive features of the target in contrast to other members of the semantic category. For example, if *shirt* is written incorrectly as *pants*, then gestures, pointing, and simple verbal explanation highlight the distinction of *shirt* as clothing for the upper body and *pants* as clothing for the legs. This type of treatment has been shown to be effective in remediation of written naming within trained categories, even for untrained items. This pattern of improvement indicates the development of richer semantic representations, allowing for more accurate distinctions among items in treated categories. Semantic spelling treatment has also resulted in generalized improvement in other modalities, including oral naming and comprehension, again suggesting an improvement at the level of the semantic system (Hillis, 1991).

Lexical Spelling Treatments. As mentioned above, many individuals with damage to sublexical spelling procedures also have damage to the lexical-semantic spelling route. For individuals whose orthographic representations are damaged or unavailable and for whom a sublexical strategy is not feasible, treatment may be administered with the goal of rebuilding specific representations in the orthographic output lexicon. Because many of these individuals also have significant aphasia, item-specific lexical spelling treatment may be used to develop a functional written vocabulary that can augment, or substitute for, spoken language (Beeson, 1999; Clausen & Beeson, 2003; Robson, Marshall, Chiat, & Pring, 2001).

Several effective treatment protocols have been reported that include the task of arranging anagram letters to spell target words (Beeson, 1999; Beeson, Hirsch, & Rewega, 2002; Hillis, 1989). This lexical approach, called Anagram and Copy Treatment (ACT), is depicted in Figure 25–6. The treatment procedure consists of a task hierarchy to elicit correct spelling of the target words through the arrangement

---

TABLE 25–5

Cueing Hierarchy for Teaching Phoneme-to-Grapheme Conversion

A. Initial treatment sessions
  Step 1. Select target graphemes to be trained; for example, four sets of five graphemes (see Appendix 25-2).
  Step 2. Establish one key word that the patient can write for each grapheme (see procedures in Table 25-3).
B. Implement cueing hierarchy to train targeted graphemes
  Note that Step 1 is the most difficult task. If the patient cannot respond correctly, proceed to Step 2, then subsequent steps as needed. Follow the instructions to ascend the hierarchy when correct responses are achieved.
  Step 1. "Write the letter that makes the sound /phoneme/."
    a. If correct, move on to the next target phoneme.
    b. If in error, proceed to Step 2.

  Step 2. Provide an array of letters (five or more) including the correct target and say, "Point to the letter that makes the sound /phoneme/."
    a. If correct, remove array of letters and go to Step 1.
    b. If incorrect, proceed to Step 3.

  Step 3. "Think of a word that starts with /phoneme/." or "Think of your key word for /phoneme/."
    "Now point to the first letter of your key word" (from array of letters).
    a. If correct, say, "Yes, a word that starts with /phoneme/ is [key word]. [Key word] starts with the letter [target letter]." For example, "Yes, a word that starts with /b/ is baby. Baby starts with the letter B."
    Rearrange the letters in the array and go to back to Step 2.
    b. If incorrect, go to Step 4.

  Step 4. "A word that starts with /phoneme/ is [key word]. Point to the letter that makes the first sound of [key word]."
    a. If correct, rearrange the array of letters and go back to Step 2.
    b. If incorrect, go to Step 5.

  Step 5. "Write your key word for /b/. Write [key word]."
    "Now point to the letter that makes the first sound of [key word]."
    a. If correct, rearrange letters in the array and go back to Step 2.
    b. If incorrect, go to Step 6.

  Step 6. Clinician writes the key word for the target sound /phoneme/, and says, for example, "The letter B makes the first sound of *baby*. /b/ is the first sound of *baby*. B makes the sound /b/. Point to the letter B. Now copy the letter B." Return to Step 2.
C. Repeat the probe and cueing hierarchy for all targeted letters. Record responses only to initial trials of Step 1 to determine progress. Probe each letter at least three to five times per session.
D. Once single letters are reliably written in response to their associated phoneme, provide spoken words and ask the patient to write the first letter of the word.
  For example, "Write the first letter for the word 'basketball.'"
E. Determine next appropriate protocol to develop and take advantage of phoneme-to-grapheme conversion abilities.

*Rationale: to train patients the ability to derive graphemes from their associated phonemes.
(After Hillis Trupe, A. E. (1986). Effectiveness of retraining phoneme to grapheme conversion. In R. H. Brookshire (Ed.), *Clinical aphasiology* (pp. 163–171). Minneapolis: BRK.

---

of anagram letters, followed by repeated copying of the word. The goal is to strengthen the orthographic representations of specific words. After correct anagram arrangement and copying of the word, recall trials require repeated correct spelling from memory. The ACT approach relies heavily on the completion of homework (at least 30 minutes per day) that involves repeated copying of sets of target words presented with line drawings or photographs.

Another homework-based lexical spelling treatment is Copy and Recall Treatment (CART; Beeson, 1999; Beeson et al., 2002; Beeson, Rising, & Volk, 2003; Clausen & Beeson, 2003). For this treatment, individuals repeatedly copy target words, then test their memory by covering up the written example and attempting to recall the spelling. During the treatment sessions, patients are trained to appropriately implement CART homework and check the accuracy of their responses. Typically, five words are targeted for treatment at one time, with additional sets of words added sequentially as criterion is met. For individuals who can repeat spoken words, CART can also be implemented with

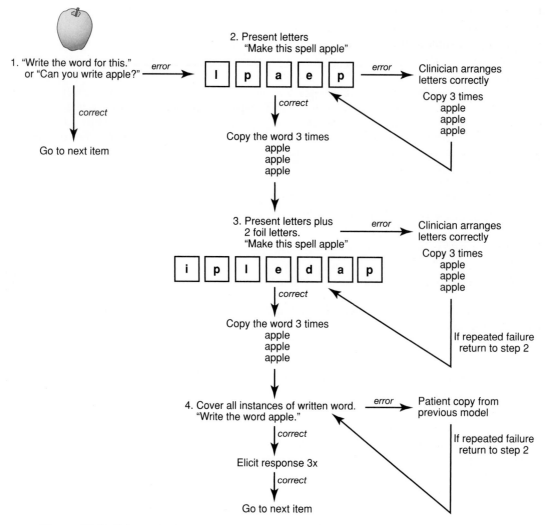

Figure 25–6. Schematic depiction of Anagram and Copy Treatment (ACT).

verbal repetition of target words in order to improve both written and spoken naming (Beeson & Egnor, 2006). The model for spoken repetition can be provided on videotape, or using a photo album with an audio-recording feature, or one of various augmentative communication devices. Patients are trained to produce both spoken and written responses for each target during their daily homework. This CART plus repetition treatment resulted in positive gains in both written and spoken modalities for two individuals with moderate aphasia and severe spelling impairment (Beeson & Egnor, 2006).

Improvements made using ACT and CART tend to be item-specific but can be highly functional when target words are individually selected and personally relevant. For example, written targets may be proper names, including those of family, friends, and favorite restaurants, allowing for specific, meaningful exchange of information. CART has proven beneficial in individuals with severe aphasia, even those with minimal pre-treatment spelling skills

(Beeson et al., 2003). Words practiced using the CART protocol may also be trained in the context of group-treatment sessions, wherein each individual is given opportunities to communicate using practiced written words (Clausen & Beeson, 2003). This type of treatment has resulted in increased use of written targets in structured group settings and also in the context of conversation with unfamiliar partners.

Spelling with Overreliance on Sound-to-Letter Conversion: Surface (Lexical) Agraphia

In many cases of acquired agraphia, patients appear to have lost the orthographic representations for words, or have degraded representations, such that they show partial knowledge of word forms that they once knew. Low frequency words are typically more vulnerable to impairment than high frequency words. If sound-to-letter conversion abilities are spared, as shown in Figure 25-3, spelling may be accomplished using the knowledge of sound-to-letter correspondences. This provides a useful strategic compensation; however, overreliance on the sublexical spelling route results in errors on words that have irregular spellings (for example, *knight* and *yacht* might be spelled as *nite* and *yot*). This spelling pattern is referred to as *surface agraphia*, in reference to the pattern of "writing how it sounds" (i.e., "on the surface"); it is also referred to as *lexical agraphia*, in reference to the damaged lexicon for writing (see Table 25-4). Because of patients' reliance on a sounding-out procedure for spelling, surface agraphia is characterized by poor spelling of homophones (e.g., *suite* and *sweet*) and relative sparing of nonword spelling.

Lexical Spelling Treatment for Surface Agraphia

Several studies have documented the utility of item-specific training for strengthening representations in the orthographic output lexicon. This type of treatment has been used to teach correct spellings for irregularly spelled words (Hillis & Caramazza, 1987) and homophones (Behrmann, 1987) in patients with surface agraphia. Hillis and Caramazza (1987) showed that repeated, corrected practice served to improve spelling of targeted words. Behrmann (1987) used a task that involved matching pictures and written words followed by written naming of the picture. This treatment also used homework that required selection of the appropriate homophone to complete printed sentences. The treatment was successful in improving spelling of homophones and some untreated irregularly spelled words, but did not generalize to untreated items.

The aforementioned lexical spelling treatments, ACT and CART, may be appropriate for individuals with damage to orthographic representations in order to retrain spellings for specific lexical items. In addition, individuals with lexical agraphia, who have relatively spared sublexical spelling, may be trained to take advantage of sound-letter conversion abilities in conjunction with residual lexical knowledge, as described below.

Training a Problem-Solving Approach to Spelling. Individuals with damage to the lexical-semantic route may demonstrate an overreliance on the sublexical spelling route, resulting in errors on irregularly spelled words and homophones. In some cases, plausible misspellings derived by sound-to-letter conversion may provide written cues that help patients resolve their own spelling errors. A problem-solving approach to spelling is appropriate for individuals who are capable of generating plausible or partial spellings. In this type of treatment, individuals learn to self-correct spelling errors by evaluating their written attempts relative to their lexical knowledge (Beeson, Rewega, Vail, & Rapcsak, 2000). Problem-solving treatment also includes training in the use of an electronic speller that accepts plausible misspellings to help resolve spelling difficulties. For example, an individual might use a sublexical strategy to generate an initial spelling (e.g., *sepost* for "supposed"), then evaluate this spelling relative to residual lexical knowledge for the target (resulting in a closer approximation, such as *suposed*). Finally, the individual is instructed to use the electronic speller to check their spelling or to correct it further, resulting in an accurate spelling of the target. Problem-solving strategies have proven useful for self-correction of spelling errors, and it has been documented that, following the implementation of homework-based writing treatment employing the problem-solving approach, individuals may show generalized improvement in spelling abilities (Beeson et al., 2000).

Impairment of the Graphemic Buffer

The orthographic representation that is derived either from the orthographic output lexicon or via the sublexical sound-to-letter conversion process is held in short-term storage while letter forms are selected and writing is initiated. It has been documented that some patients have an impairment of this graphemic buffer, such that information decays at an abnormally rapid rate (Hillis & Caramazza, 1995; Miceli, Silveri, & Caramazza, 1985). As shown in Figure 25–7, the graphemic buffer receives output from both lexical-semantic and sublexical routes. Therefore, an impairment of the graphemic buffer will affect all writing tasks, including spontaneous writing, written naming, writing to dictation, and delayed copying. Damage to the graphemic buffer affects spelling of all word types, and thus, there are no effects of frequency, imagery, grammatical class, or regularity of spelling (see Table 25-4). In contrast, word length has a significant effect on performance, with a tendency for short words to be more accurately spelled than long words, due to the increased demand on storage capacity for longer words. Damage to the graphemic buffer also tends to result in loss of information about the identity and serial ordering of letters, resulting in spelling errors such as letter omissions (e.g., sweater → *sweatr*), substitutions (e.g., peanut → *peanul*), transpositions (e.g., painter → *painetr*), and additions (e.g., flower → *flowaer*). In the case of left hemisphere brain damage, the initial letters of the word are most likely to be correct, with errors occurring in the middle or toward the end of words (Caramazza, Miceli, Villa, & Romani, 1987; Hillis & Caramazza, 1989, 1995; Katz, 1991).

Treatment for Impairment of the Graphemic Buffer

In cases of selective impairment to the graphemic output buffer, the spared cognitive processes for spelling may provide a means to compensate (or self-correct) for spelling errors. For instance, individuals with some degree of preservation of sublexical and lexical-semantic spelling processes

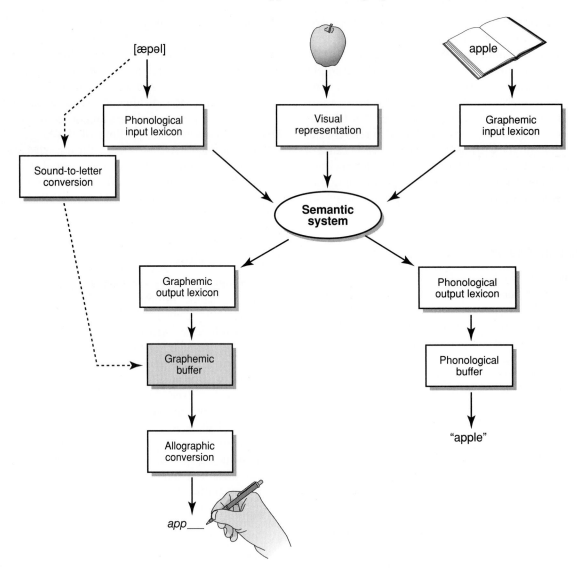

Figure 25–7. Schematic representation of impairment to the graphemic output buffer, resulting in loss of information for the rightmost part of the word.

may be trained to use strategies for self-correction of spellings (Hillis & Caramazza, 1987). Such strategies may include examining spellings to evaluate their accuracy (i.e., comparing to representations in the orthographic lexicon) and also sounding out each word as it is written (to call attention to phonologically implausible misspellings).

Spelling treatments targeting impaired lexical spelling procedures have resulted in improvement for individuals with deficits at the level of the orthographic output lexicon as well as the graphemic buffer, indicating that a single treatment approach may prove beneficial to more than one component of the spelling process. Raymer, Cudworth, and Haley (2003) used a modified version of CART to address a spelling impairment involving both the orthographic output

lexicon and the graphemic buffer, and they documented improvements at both levels of processing in a single patient. Rapp and Kane (2002) used a delayed copy treatment with two individuals, one with a deficit at the level of the orthographic output lexicon and the other with a graphemic buffer impairment. Both individuals demonstrated positive treatment effects for trained items, with the latter showing generalization to untrained items.

Impairment of Allographic Conversion

Writing requires the conversion of each grapheme (i.e., abstract letter identity) into a particular letter shape, or allograph, in order to form the string of letters for a word.

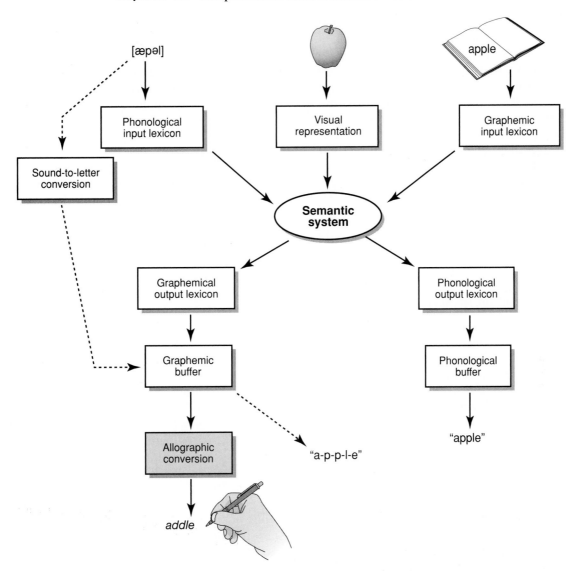

Figure 25–8. Schematic representation of impairment to the allographic conversion mechanism, resulting in errors of letter selection in writing. Preserved ability to perform oral naming is indicated.

There are many ways to write a given grapheme, including upper or lowercase, print or cursive, and individual variations in writing style. Therefore, each time a word is written, the appropriate letter shape must be selected for that instance. This stage of writing, the allographic conversion process, is specific to written spelling, and is not required for oral spelling (Fig. 25–8). Some patients show a selective impairment of the allographic conversion process. These patients can spell aloud but are impaired in the selection and generation of the correct letter shapes in handwriting (Margolin, 1984; Ramage, Beeson, & Rapcsak, 1998). This impairment may be specific to letter case (upper or lowercase; De Bastiani & Barry, 1986; Kartsounis, 1992) or style (print vs. cursive; Hanley & Peters, 1996). The characteristic features include incorrect letter selection, resulting in

well-formed but incorrect letters, and also in disturbed letter formation. In either case, the writing errors are accompanied by preserved oral spelling.

When examining allographic conversion processes, it is useful to ask patients to transcode printed words from lower to uppercase and vice versa (see Appendix 25-1). Performance on this task may be compared to direct copy of single words. If graphomotor skills appear preserved for copy, but performance on the transcoding task is impaired, the profile is suggestive of impairment at the level of allographic conversion.

Treatment for Allographic-Conversion Impairment

It makes sense that treatment for individuals with impaired allographic conversion processes should attempt to take advantage of superior oral spelling abilities. Self-dictation procedures have proven beneficial in improving spelling in individuals with preserved oral relative to written spelling (Pound, 1996; Ramage et al., 1998). Pound (1996) instructed a patient with impaired allographic conversion to engage in the following steps during treatment: orally spell each target word before attempting to write it; self-dictate each letter while writing one letter at a time; examine the written word one letter at a time while orally spelling the word again; self-correct any noted errors, using an alphabet card if a model is needed; finally, inspect the entire word to check it against the orthographic representation for the word. While spelling accuracy was not perfect post-treatment, this procedure proved successful in improving the patient's written spelling to a level commensurate with performance in oral spelling.

Summary of Treatment for Spelling Impairments

Spelling impairments can result from damage to one or more of the critical components of the cognitive processes that support written spelling. Treatment studies demonstrate that therapy directed toward lexical-semantic and sublexical spelling processes can improve spelling abilities of individuals with acquired writing impairments. In some cases, treatments serve to strengthen damaged or degraded representations, including semantic knowledge or orthographic word forms (i.e., spellings), as well as access to those representations. In other cases, the sublexical sound-to-letter conversion processes are strengthened. Finally, other treatments improve the operation of the graphemic buffer or allographic conversion processes that ultimately initiate the graphic motor plans for writing. The more peripheral sensorimotor impairments of writing (such as those resulting from cerebellar damage, subcortical lesions, and disorders of praxis) were not discussed here because they are less likely to accompany aphasia, but these disorders are reviewed elsewhere (Rapcsak & Beeson, 2000).

CLOSING COMMENTS

In this chapter, we sought to provide a framework for assessing reading and spelling and using the assessment findings to select or design treatments. The treatment approaches focused on those components of the reading or spelling process that are impaired or can be used more efficiently to compensate for damaged components. The illustrative evaluation and therapy methods we have described surely do not exhaust the possibilities for improving processing at each level. However, the general approach to identifying, in each patient, which processes are impaired and which processes are spared in the tasks of reading or spelling should provide a springboard for designing other focused treatments. In practice, sequential treatment approaches may be warranted

to develop and take full advantage of improved skills and compensatory strategies in a given individual. We caution that it is essential to monitor a patient's progress carefully so that only effective interventions are pursued. Additionally, specific treatment approaches should be tailored appropriately to meet the functional needs of the patient.

FUTURE TRENDS

We expect that advances in our understanding of the cognitive processes and neural substrates that support reading and spelling will continue to influence treatment approaches for acquired alexia and agraphia. In the past decade, a number of interdisciplinary efforts have contributed to the knowledge base, and reflect complementary perspectives from speech-language pathology, neuropsychology, behavioral neurology, cognitive science, and psycholingistics (e.g., Funnell, 2000; Hillis, 2002; Nadeau, Gonzalez Rothi, & Crosson, 2000; Rapp, 2001). We expect knowledge gained from behavioral research to be complemented by research using functional neuroimaging and computational modeling of normal and disordered language processes. Functional neuroimaging has the potential to clarify the neural substrates of recovery and the response to behavioral interventions (see, for example, Crosson et al., 2005; Marsh & Hillis, 2005). Computational modeling can be implemented to simulate the effects of brain damage and test different treatment approaches (see, for example, Houghton & Zorzi, 2003; Plaut, 1996). Advances in these endeavors may provide insights that improve our understanding of the nature of reading and spelling impairments, as well as maximize the effectiveness and efficiency of behavioral treatments.

Finally, the increased attention to evidence-based practice in speech-language pathology has promoted increased rigor in the experimental designs used to examine treatment outcomes. In particular, the quantification of treatment outcomes using standardized effect sizes should facilitate a better understanding of the therapeutic effects of different treatments (see, for example, Beeson & Robey, 2006). Ideally, treatment research should serve to clarify who are the ideal candidates for particular treatment approaches, and provide an estimate of treatment effect size for such individuals. This information can serve to guide clinicians as they select treatment for a particular individual.

▶ *Acknowledgment*—This work was supported in part by DC007646 and DC008286 from the National Institute on Deafness and Other Communication Disorders. The authors wish to thank Argye E. Hillis, M.D. for her significant contributions to the previous edition of this chapter. We also thank Roberta Goodman-Schulman and Alfonso Caramazza for generously sharing the Johns Hopkins Dyslexia and Dysgraphia Batteries.

1. Neurologic damage can disturb the processes necessary for reading and writing in a variety of ways. Careful examination of the component processes for reading and writing can serve to isolate the locus (or loci) of impairment and thus guide the treatment approaches.

2. Treatment for acquired reading and writing impairments include approaches that strengthen weakened processes and representations, as well as those that encourage the development and use of strategies to compensate for impaired processes.

3. Reading impairments can result from impairment to any or all of the following processes or representations: visual processing of written words, the orthographic input lexicon (the store of known written words), the semantic system, the phonological processes necessary for speech production (for oral reading), and the processes necessary to convert letters to the corresponding sounds.

4. Treatment for acquired reading impairments may be directed toward lexical-semantic processes, so that the links between written words and their meanings are strengthened. Conversely, treatment may be directed toward strengthening the sublexical route for reading, whereby letters are converted to their associated sounds and word pronunciations are assembled.

5. Writing impairments can result from impairment to any or all of the following processes or representations: the semantic system, the orthographic output lexicon (the store of spellings), the graphemic buffer that temporarily holds graphemic information for writing, the conversion processes necessary to select and form specific letters, and the graphic motor processes necessary for the implementation of writing.

6. Similar to reading, treatment for writing impairments may be directed toward lexical-semantic processes, sublexical spelling processes, or both.

7. Some treatment approaches result in item-specific improvements, whereas other approaches result in the development of strategies that are of general benefit. Both approaches are valid.

1. What are the components of the lexical-semantic route for reading?

2. Why do you always read "apple" as "apple," regardless of the style of the font?

3. Why is letter-by-letter reading a successful strategy for pure alexia, but not a useful strategy for surface or deep alexia?

4. When might you work on reading at the text level in a patient who has trouble reading single words?

5. What is the benefit of training a "key word" approach for alexia or agraphia?

6. Individuals with surface agraphia nearly always demonstrate surface alexia, but it is not uncommon to observe surface agraphia without surface alexia. Discuss why that is the case.

7. Describe an example of a lexical treatment for spelling.

8. What alexia syndrome is characterized by a word-length effect?

9. What agraphia syndrome is characterized by a word-length effect?

10. What is meant by an interactive, problem-solving approach to spelling treatment?

11. Deep alexia and deep agraphia are characterized by what hallmark feature?

12. What is meant by the statement that phonological and deep alexia/agraphia represent the ends of a severity continuum?

13. How might you combine treatment for spoken and written language at the same time? Give an example in the context of reading treatment, and an example in the context of spelling treatment.

References

Alexander, M. P., Friedman, R. B., Loverso F., & Fischer, R. S. (1992). Lesion localization in phonological agraphia. *Brain and Language, 43*, 83–95.

Beeson, P. M. (1998). Treatment for letter-by-letter reading: A case study. In N. Helm-Estabrooks & A. L. Holland (Eds.), *Approaches to the treatment of aphasia* (pp. 153–177). San Diego: Singular Press.

Beeson, P. M. (1999). Treating acquired writing impairment. *Aphasiology, 13*, 367–386.

Beeson, P. M., & Egnor, H. (2006). Combining treatment for written and spoken naming. *Journal of the International Neuropsychological Society, 12*, 816–827.

Beeson, P. M., Hirsch, F. M., & Rewega, M. A. (2002). Successful single-word writing treatment: Experimental analyses of four cases. *Aphasiology, 16*, 473–491.

Beeson, P. M., & Insalaco, D. (1998). Acquired alexia: Lessons from successful treatment. *Journal of the International Neuropsychology, 4*, 621–635.

Beeson, P. M., Magloire, J., & Robey, R. R. (2005). Letter-by-letter reading: Natural recovery and response to treatment. *Behavioural Neurology, 16*, 191–202.

Beeson, P. M., Rewega, M., Vail, S., & Rapcsak (2000). Problem-solving approach to agraphia treatment: Interactive use of lexical and sublexical spelling routes. *Aphasiology, 14*(5–6), 551–565.

Beeson, P., Rising, K., & Volk, J. (2003). Writing treatment for severe aphasia: Who benefits? *Journal of Speech and Hearing Research, 46,* 1038–1060.

Beeson, P. M., & Robey, R. R. (2006). Evaluating single-subject treatment research: Lessons learned from the aphasia literature. *Neuropsychology Review,16*(4), 161–169.

Behrmann, M. (1987). The rites of righting writing: Homophone remediation in acquired dysgraphia. *Cognitive Neuropsychology, 4,* 365–384.

Berndt, R. S., Reggia, J. A., & Mitchum, C. C. (1987). Empirically derived probabilities for grapheme-to-phoneme correspondences in English. *Behavior Research Methods, Instruments, & Computers, 19,* 1–9.

Bub, D., & Kertesz, A. (1982). Deep agraphia. *Brain & Language, 17,* 146–165.

Caramazza, A., Miceli, G., Villa, G., & Romani, C. (1987). The role of the graphemic buffer in spelling: Evidence from a case of acquired dysgraphia. *Cognition, 26,* 59–85.

Cardell, E. A., & Chenery, H. J. (1999). A cognitive neuropsychological approach to the assessment and remediation of acquired dysgraphia. *Language Testing, 16,* 353–388.

Cherney, L. R., Merbitz, C. T., & Grip, J. C. (1986). Efficacy of oral reading in aphasia treatment outcome. *Rehabilitation Literature, 47,* 112–117.

Clausen, N. S., & Beeson, P. M. (2003). Conversational use of writing in severe aphasia: A group treatment approach. *Aphasiology, 17,* 625–644.

Coltheart, M., (Ed.). (1998). *Pure alexia: Letter-by-letter reading.* Hove, East Sussex: Psychology Press.

Coltheart, M., Patterson, K., & Marshall, J. C., (Eds.). (1987). *Deep dyslexia* (2nd ed.). London: Routledge & Kegan Paul.

Coslett, H. B., & Saffran, E. M. (1989). Evidence for preserved reading in pure alexia. *Brain, 112,* 327–259.

Coslett, H. B., & Saffran, E. M. (1994). Mechanisms of implicit reading in alexia. In M. J. Farrah & G. Ratcliff (Eds.), *The neuropsychology of high-level vision* (pp. 299–330). Hillsdale, NJ: Lawrence Erlbaum.

De Bastiani, P., & Barry, C. (1986). After the graphemic buffer: Disorders of peripheral aspects of writing in Italian patients. *Cognitive Neuropsychology, 6,* 1–23.

de Partz, M. P. (1986). Re-education of a deep dyslexic patient: Rationale of the method and results. *Cognitive Neuropsychology, 3,* 147–177.

Ellis, A. W. (1993). *Reading, writing and dyslexia: A cognitive analysis.* Hillsdale, NJ: Lawrence Erlbaum.

Funnel, E. (2000). *Case studies in the neuropsychology of reading.* East Sussex, UK: Psychology Press.

Glosser, G., & Friedman, R. B. (1990). The continuum of deep/phonological alexia. *Cortex, 26,* 343–359.

Goodglass, H., Kaplan, E., & Barresi, B. (2000). *Boston Diagnostic Aphasia Examination* (3rd ed.), Psychological Assessment Resources.

Goodman, R. A., & Caramazza, A. (1986, unpublished). *The Johns Hopkins University Dyslexia and Dysgraphia Batteries.*

Greenwald, M. L., & Berndt, R. (1998). Letter-by-letter access without semantics or specialized letter name phonology (abstract). *Brain and Language, 65,* 149–152.

Hanley, J. R., & Peters, S. (1996). A dissociation between the ability to print and write cursively in lower-case letters. *Cortex, 32,* 737–745.

Hanna, P. R., Hanna, J. S., Hodges, R. E., & Rudorf, E. H. (1966). *Phoneme-grapheme correspondences as cues to spelling improvement.* Washington, DC, US Department of Health, Education, and Welfare.

Henry, M. L., Beeson, P. M., Stark, A. J., & Rapcsak, S. Z. (2007). The role of left perisylvian cortical regions in spelling. *Brain and Language, 100*(1), 44–52.

Hillis, A. E. (1989). Efficacy and generalization of treatment for aphasic naming errors. *Archives of Physical Medicine and Rehabilitation, 70,* 632–636.

Hillis, A. E. (1991). Effects of a separate treatments for distinct impairments within the naming process. In T. Prescott (Ed.), *Clinical aphasiology, 19,* 255–265.

Hillis, A. E. (1993). The role of models of language processing in rehabilitation of language impairments. *Aphasiology, 7,* 5–26.

Hillis, A. E. (Ed.). (2002). *Handbook of adult language disorders: Integrating cognitive neuropsychology, neurology, and rehabilitation.* Philadelphia: Psychology Press.

Hillis, A. E., Caramazza, A. (1987). Model-driven treatment of dysgraphia. In R. H. Brookshire (Ed.), *Clinical aphasiology* (pp. 84–105). Minneapolis: BRK.

Hillis, A. E., & Caramazza, A. (1989). The graphemic buffer and attentional mechanisms. *Brain and Language, 36,* 208–235.

Hillis, A. E., & Caramazza, A. (1991a). Mechanisms for accessing lexical representations for output: Evidence from a category-specific semantic deficit. *Brain and Language, 40,* 106–144.

Hillis, A. E., & Caramazza, A. (1991b). Category-specific naming and comprehension impairment: Theoretical and clinical implication. In T. Prescott (Ed.), *Clinical aphasiology* (Vol. 20, pp. 191–200). Austin, TX: Pro-Ed.

Hillis, A. E., & Caramazza, A. (1992). The reading process and its disorders. D. I. Margolin, (Ed.), *Cognitive neuropsychology in clinical practice.* New York: Oxford University Press.

Hillis, A. E., & Caramazza A. (1994). Theories of lexical processing and rehabilitation of lexical deficits. In M. J. Riddoch & G. W. Humphreys (Eds.), *Cognitive neuropsychology and cognitive rehabilitation.* Hillsdale, NJ: Lawrence Erlbaum.

Hillis, A. E., & Caramazza, A. (1995). Spatially-specific deficits in processing graphemic representations in reading and writing. *Brain and Language, 48,* 263–308.

Hillis Trupe, A. E. (1986). Effectiveness of retraining phoneme to grapheme conversion. In R. H. Brookshire (Ed.), *Clinical aphasiology* (pp. 163–171). Minneapolis: BRK.

Hillis, A. E., & Tuffash, E. (2002). Neuroanatomical aspects of reading. In A. E. Hillis (Ed.). *Handbook on adult language disorders: Integrating cognitive neuropsychology, neurology, and rehabilitation* (pp. 3–26). Philadelphia: Psychology Press.

Houghton, G., & Zorzi, M. (2003). Normal and impaired spelling in a connectionist dual route architecture. *Cognitive Neuropsychology, 20,* 115–162.

Kartsounis, L. D. (1992). Selective lower-case letter ideational dygraphia. *Cortex, 28,* 145–150.

Katz, R. B. (1991). Limited retention of information in the graphemic buffer. *Cortex, 27,* 111–119.

Katz, R. C., & Wertz, R. T. (1997). The efficacy of computer-provided reading treatment for chronic aphasic adults. *Journal of Speech, Language, and Hearing Research, 40*, 493–507.

Kay, J., Lesser, R., & Coltheart, M. (1992). *Psycholinguistic assessments of language processing in aphasia (PALPA).* East Sussex, England: Lawrence Erlbaum.

Kertesz, A. (2006). *Western Aphasia Battery—Revised.* New York: Grune & Stratton.

Kincaid, J. P., Fishbourne, R. P., Rogers, R. L., & Chissom, B. S. (1975). Derivation of new readability formulas (Automated Readability Index, Fog Count and Flesch Reading Ease Formula for Navy enlisted personnel). *CNTECHTRA Research Branch Report*, 8–75.

LaPointe, L. L., & Horner, J. (1998). *Reading Comprehension Battery for Aphasia* (2nd ed.), Austin, TX: Pro-Ed.

Maher, L. M., Clayton, M. C., Barrett, A. M., Schober-Peterson, D., & Rothi, L. J. G. (1998). Rehabilitation of a case of pure alexia: Exploiting residual abilities. *Journal of the International Neuropsychological Society, 4*, 636–647.

Margolin, D. I. (1984). The neuropsychology of writing and spelling: Semantic, phonological, motor and perceptual processes. *Quarterly Journal of Experimental Psychology, 36A*, 459–489.

Margolin, D. I., & Goodman-Schulman, R. (1992). Oral and written spelling impairments. In D. I. Margolin (Ed.), *Cognitive neuropsychology in clinical practice.* New York: Oxford University Press.

Miceli, G., Silveri, M. C., & Caramazza, A. (1985). Cognitive analysis of a case of pure dysgraphia. *Brain and Language, 25*, 187–212.

Moyer, S. B. (1979). Rehabilitation of alexia: A case study. *Cortex, 15*, 139–144.

Nadeau, S. E., Gonzalez Rothi, L. J., & Crosson, B. (Eds.), (2000). *Aphasia and language: Theory to practice.* New York: Guilford Press.

Newcombe, F., & Marshall, J. C. (1984). Task and modality—Specific aphasias. In F. C. Rose (Ed.), *Advances in neurology: Progress in aphasiology.* (Vol. 42). New York: Raven Press.

Nickels, L. (1992). The autocue? Self-generated phonemic cues in the treatment of a disorder of reading and naming. *Cognitive Neuropsychology, 9*, 155–182.

Orjada, S., & Beeson, P. M. (2005). Concurrent treatment for reading and spelling in aphasia. *Aphasiology, 19*, 341–351.

Parker, D. H., & Scannell, G. (1998). *Scientific Research Associates Reading Laboratory 1C.* Columbus, OH: McGraw-Hill.

Patterson, K. (1992). Reading, writing, and rehabilitation: A reckoning. In M. J. Riddoch & G. W. Humphries (Eds.), *Cognitive neuropsychology and cognitive rehabilitation* (pp. 425–448). Hillsdale, NJ: Lawrence Erlbaum.

Patterson, K. E., Marshall, J. C., & Colheart, M. (1985). *Surface dyslexia.* London, England: Lawrence Erlbaum.

Patterson, K., Vargha-Khadem, F., & Polkey, C. E. (1989). Reading with one hemisphere. *Brain, 112*, 510–530.

Plaut, D. C. (1996). Relearning after damage in connectionist networks: Toward a theory of rehabilitation. *Brain and Language, 52*, 25–82.

Pound, C. (1996). Writing remediation using preserved oral spelling: A case for separate output buffers. *Aphasiology, 10*, 283–296.

Ramage, A., Beeson, P. M., & Rapcsak, S. Z. (June, 1998). Dissociation between oral and written spelling: Clinical characteristics and possible mechanisms. *Clinical Aphasiology Conference.*

Rapcsak, S. Z., & Beeson, P. M. (2000). Agraphia. In L. J. G. Rothi, B. Crosson, and S. Nadeau (Eds.), *Aphasia and language: Theory and practice* (pp. 184–220). New York: Guilford.

Rapcsak, S. Z., & Beeson, P. M. (2002). Neuroanatomical correlates of spelling and writing. In A. E. Hillis (Ed.), *Handbook on adult language disorders: Integrating cognitive neuropsychology, neurology, and rehabilitation* (pp. 71–99). Philadelphia: Psychology Press.

Rapcsak, S. Z., Beeson, P. M., & Rubens, A. B. (1991). Writing with the right hemisphere. *Brain and Language, 41*, 510–530.

Rapp, B. (Ed.), (2001). *The handbook of cognitive neuropsychology: What deficits reveal about the human mind.* Philadelphia: Psychology Press.

Rapp, B., & Kane, A. (2002). Remediation of deficits affecting different components of the spelling process. *Aphasiology, 16*, 439–454.

Raymer, A. M., Cudworth, C., & Haley, M. A. (2003). Spelling treatment for an individual with dysgraphia: Analysis of generalization to untrained words. *Aphasiology, 17*, 607–624.

Rayner, K., & Pollatsek, A. (1989). *The psychology of reading.* Hillsdale, New Jersey: Lawrence Erlbaum.

Robson, J., Marshall, J., Chiat, S., & Pring, T. (2001). Enhancing communication in jargon aphasia: A small group study of writing therapy. *International Journal of Communication Disorders, 36*, 471–488.

Rothi, L. J. G., Coslett, H. B., & Heilman, K. M. (1986, unpublished test). *Battery of Adult Reading Function, Experimental Edition.*

Rothi, L. J. G., Greenwald, M., Maher, L. M., & Ochipa, C. (1998). Alexia without agraphia: Lessons from a treatment failure. In N. Helm-Estabrooks & A. L. Holland (Eds.), *Approaches to the treatment of aphasia* (pp. 179–202). San Diego: Singular.

Rothi, L. J. G., & Moss, S. (1992). Alexia without agraphia: Potential for model assisted therapy. *Clinical Communication Disorders, 2*, 11–18.

Schwartz, M. F., Saffran, E. M., & Marin, O. S. M. (1987). Fractionating the reading process in dementia: Evidence for word-specific print-to-sound associations. In M. Coltheart, K. Patterson, & J. C. Marshal (Eds.), *Deep dyslexia.* (2nd ed., pp. 259–269). New York: Routledge & Kegan Paul.

Seki, K., Yajima, M., & Sugishita, M. (1995). The efficacy of kinesthetic reading treatment for pure alexia. *Neuropsychologia, 33*, 595–609.

Shallice, T. (1981). Phonological agraphia and the lexical route in writing. *Brain, 104*, 413–429.

Tainturier, M.-J., & Rapp, B. (2001). The spelling process. In B. Rapp (Ed.), *The handbook of cognitive neuropsychology* (pp. 263–290). Philadelphia: Psychology Press.

Tuomainen, J., & Laine, M. (1991). Multiple oral rereading technique on rehabilitation of pure alexia. *Aphasiology, 5*, 401–409.

Wiederholt, J. L., & Bryant, B. R. (2001). *Gray Oral Reading Tests* (4th ed.). (GORT-4). Austin, Texas: Pro-Ed.

APPENDIX 25.1
Johns Hopkins University Dyslexia and Dysgraphia Batteries

The following word lists are controlled for lexical features including grammatical word class, frequency of occurrence in written English, concreteness, regularity of spelling based on sound-to-letter correspondences, and word length. Nonwords are also provided that are pseudohomophones (i.e., nonword spellings that are homophones with real words) and nonhomophones (i.e., pronounceble nonwords derived by altering real words by one grapheme). The words are grouped on the basis of their relevant features, so that the contrasts are apparent; however, items within a given list should be presented in random order during test administration. In many cases, the same word lists can be used to assess reading and writing, but as indicated below, some lists are specific to the dyslexia or dysgraphia batteries.

The dyslexia battery consists of oral reading of words and nonwords. The dysgraphia battery includes writing to dictation, written naming of pictures, transcoding by letter case (e.g., upper to lowercase), and copying of single words. Writing to dictation is accomplished by presenting a word or nonword auditorily and asking the patient to first repeat the stimulus aloud and then write it.

1. Grammatical Word Class
   List composition: 104 words (28 nouns, 28 adjectives, 28 verbs, 20 functors)
   a. Dyslexia Battery
      Task: oral reading
   b. Dysgraphia Battery
      Task: writing to dictation

Word	Class	Frequency	# Letters	Word	Class	Frequency	# Letters
body	noun	HF	4	jury	noun	LF	4
child	noun	HF	5	bugle	noun	LF	5
music	noun	HF	5	digit	noun	LF	5
noise	noun	HF	5	faith	noun	LF	5
ocean	noun	HF	5	glove	noun	LF	5
space	noun	HF	5	grief	noun	LF	5
bottom	noun	HF	6	motel	noun	LF	5
church	noun	HF	6	career	noun	LF	6
column	noun	HF	6	pillow	noun	LF	6
friend	noun	HF	6	priest	noun	LF	6
length	noun	HF	6	sleeve	noun	LF	6
member	noun	HF	6	stripe	noun	LF	6
nature	noun	HF	6	threat	noun	LF	6
street	noun	HF	6	lobster	noun	LF	7
loud	adj	HF	4	brisk	adj	LF	5
tiny	adj	HF	4	cheap	adj	LF	5
angry	adj	HF	5	crisp	adj	LF	5
broad	adj	HF	5	loyal	adj	LF	5
fresh	adj	HF	5	rigid	adj	LF	5
happy	adj	HF	5	sleek	adj	LF	5
short	adj	HF	5	vivid	adj	LF	5
afraid	adj	HF	6	absent	adj	LF	6
bright	adj	HF	6	decent	adj	LF	6
common	adj	HF	6	fierce	adj	LF	6
hungry	adj	HF	6	quaint	adj	LF	6
strong	adj	HF	6	severe	adj	LF	6
certain	adj	HF	7	strict	adj	LF	6
strange	adj	HF	8	vulgar	adj	LF	6

begin	verb	HF	5	deny	verb	LF	4
bring	verb	HF	5	adopt	verb	LF	5
carry	verb	HF	5	annoy	verb	LF	5
hurry	verb	HF	5	greet	verb	LF	5
learn	verb	HF	5	argue	verb	LF	5
solve	verb	HF	5	merge	verb	LF	5
speak	verb	HF	5	spoil	verb	LF	5
spend	verb	HF	5	borrow	verb	LF	6
become	verb	HF	6	pierce	verb	LF	6
bought	verb	HF	6	preach	verb	LF	6
caught	verb	HF	6	reveal	verb	LF	6
decide	verb	HF	6	sought	verb	LF	6
happen	verb	HF	6	starve	verb	LF	6
listen	verb	HF	6	conquer	verb	LF	7
both	functor	HF	4	since	functor	HF	5
into	functor	HF	4	these	functor	HF	5
only	functor	HF	4	those	functor	HF	5
what	functor	HF	4	under	functor	HF	5
about	functor	HF	5	while	functor	HF	5
above	functor	HF	5	before	functor	HF	6
after	functor	HF	5	enough	functor	HF	6
could	functor	HF	5	rather	functor	HF	6
often	functor	HF	5	should	functor	HF	6
shall	functor	HF	5	though	functor	HF	6

2. Word Concreteness List

List composition: 42 nouns (21 concrete, 21 abstract)

a. Dyslexia Battery

Task: oral reading

b. Dysgraphia Battery

Task: writing to dictation

Word	Feature	Frequency	# Letters	Word	Feature	Frequency	# Letters
cabin	concrete	HF	5	beauty	abstract	HF	6
cattle	concrete	HF	6	danger	abstract	HF	6
engine	concrete	HF	6	method	abstract	HF	6
valley	concrete	HF	6	moment	abstract	HF	6
window	concrete	HF	6	sister	abstract	HF	6
kitchen	concrete	HF	7	system	abstract	HF	6
village	concrete	HF	7	science	abstract	HF	7
college	concrete	MF	6	basis	abstract	MF	5
dollar	concrete	MF	6	advice	abstract	MF	6
insect	concrete	MF	6	degree	abstract	MF	6
palace	concrete	MF	6	effort	abstract	MF	6
planet	concrete	MF	6	theory	abstract	MF	6
spider	concrete	MF	6	courage	abstract	MF	7
turkey	concrete	MF	6	success	abstract	MF	7
salad	concrete	LF	5	mercy	abstract	LF	5
bullet	concrete	LF	6	belief	abstract	LF	6
fabric	concrete	LF	6	horror	abstract	LF	6
oyster	concrete	LF	6	status	abstract	LF	6
parent	concrete	LF	6	talent	abstract	LF	6
journal	concrete	LF	7	offense	abstract	LF	7
sparrow	concrete	LF	7	pursuit	abstract	LF	7

3. Word Frequency
   List composition: Use responses from any or all of the following lists
       Grammatical Class List (nouns, adjectives, verbs only) = 42 HF and 42 LF
       Word Concreteness List (concrete and abstract) = 14 HF, 14 MF, and 14 LF
       Word Length List = 35 HF and 35 LF
   a. Dyslexia Battery
      Task: oral reading
   b. Dysgraphia Battery
      Task: writing to dictation

4. Nonwords
   a. Dyslexia Battery
      Task: oral reading
      List composition: 34 pseudohomophones and 34 nonhomophones
   b. Dysgraphia Battery
      Task: writing to dictation
      List composition: 34 nonhomophones (* indicates 20 nonwords to be used for oral spelling task with real words in list 7)

Reading Only

Nonword	Type	# Letters
berd	pseudohomophone	4
bole	pseudohomophone	4
groe	pseudohomophone	4
hert	pseudohomophone	4
lern	pseudohomophone	4
meen	pseudohomophone	4
noys	pseudohomophone	4
rewt	pseudohomophone	4
snoe	pseudohomophone	4
sune	pseudohomophone	4
breth	pseudohomophone	5
ghurl	pseudohomophone	5
kroud	pseudohomophone	5
kwene	pseudohomophone	5
lytes	pseudohomophone	5
phait	pseudohomophone	5
reech	pseudohomophone	5
skurt	pseudohomophone	5
cherch	pseudohomophone	6
hunnee	pseudohomophone	6
kattul	pseudohomophone	6
lemmun	pseudohomophone	6
merder	pseudohomophone	6
mursee	pseudohomophone	6
phlore	pseudohomophone	6
sircle	pseudohomophone	6
windoe	pseudohomophone	6
wissel	pseudohomophone	6
consept	pseudohomophone	7
haytrid	pseudohomophone	7
kuntree	pseudohomophone	7
sertain	pseudohomophone	7
teybull	pseudohomophone	7
mushrume	pseudohomophone	8

Reading and Writing

Nonword	Type	# Letters
berk	nonhomophone	4
boke*	nonhomophone	4
troe	nonhomophone	4
herm*	nonhomophone	4
lorn*	nonhomophone	4
feen*	nonhomophone	4
foys	nonhomophone	6
dewt*	nonhomophone	4
snoy	nonhomophone	4
sume	nonhomophone	4
bruth	nonhomophone	5
ghurb	nonhomophone	5
kroid	nonhomophone	5
kwine*	nonhomophone	5
pytes	nonhomophone	6
phoit*	nonhomophone	5
reesh*	nonhomophone	5
skart*	nonhomophone	5
chench*	nonhomophone	6
hannee*	nonhomophone	6
kittul	nonhomophone	6
remmun*	nonhomophone	6
merber*	nonhomophone	6
murnee*	nonhomophone	6
phloke	nonhomophone	6
sarcle*	nonhomophone	6
wundoe	nonhomophone	6
wessel	nonhomophone	6
donsept*	nonhomophone	7
haygrid*	nonhomophone	7
kantree*	nonhomophone	7
sortain	nonhomophone	7
teabull*	nonhomophone	7
mushrame*	nonhomophone	8

5. Regularity of Spelling
   a. Dyslexia Battery—Letter-to-Sound Regularity
      Task: oral reading
      List composition: 60 words with regular spelling and 30 words with irregular spelling

Reading Only

Word	Regularity	Frequency	# Letters
but	regular	HF	3
base	regular	HF	4
bone	regular	HF	4
cook	regular	HF	4
cool	regular	HF	4
cord	regular	HF	4
corn	regular	HF	4
days	regular	HF	4
face	regular	HF	4
feed	regular	HF	4
feel	regular	HF	4
five	regular	HF	4
grow	regular	HF	4
home	regular	HF	4
life	regular	HF	4
lift	regular	HF	4
list	regular	HF	4
main	regular	HF	4
meat	regular	HF	4
nine	regular	HF	4
paid	regular	HF	4
race	regular	HF	4
sand	regular	HF	4
save	regular	HF	4
seen	regular	HF	4
thin	regular	HF	4
wake	regular	HF	4
shell	regular	HF	5
still	regular	HF	5
these	regular	HF	5
gut	regular	LF	3
boot	regular	LF	4
dare	regular	LF	4
dean	regular	LF	4
dock	regular	LF	4
dome	regular	LF	4
fern	regular	LF	4
fowl	regular	LF	4
gull	regular	LF	4
hike	regular	LF	4
jays	regular	LF	4
math	regular	LF	4
mode	regular	LF	4
mush	regular	LF	4
peat	regular	LF	4
pest	regular	LF	4
pill	regular	LF	4
pose	regular	LF	4
rave	regular	LF	4

Reading Only

Word	Regularity	Frequency	# Letters
eye	exception	HF	3
two	exception	HF	3
once	exception	HF	4
sign	exception	HF	4
view	exception	HF	4
earth	exception	HF	5
front	exception	HF	5
ghost	exception	HF	5
knife	exception	HF	5
laugh	exception	HF	5
piece	exception	HF	5
sword	exception	HF	5
friend	exception	HF	6
school	exception	HF	6
tongue	exception	HF	6
axe	exception	LF	3
heir	exception	LF	4
limb	exception	LF	4
quay	exception	LF	4
tsar	exception	LF	4
aisle	exception	LF	5
choir	exception	LF	5
chute	exception	LF	5
corps	exception	LF	5
fraud	exception	LF	5
gauge	exception	LF	5
seize	exception	LF	5
sieve	exception	LF	5
weird	exception	LF	5
brooch	exception	LF	6

rust	regular	LF	4
sock	regular	LF	4
teak	regular	LF	4
tile	regular	LF	4
wail	regular	LF	4
weld	regular	LF	4
greed	regular	LF	5
moose	regular	LF	5
pouch	regular	LF	5
stink	regular	LF	5
stint	regular	LF	5

b. Dysgraphia Battery—Sound-to-Letter Probability
   Task: writing to dictation
   List composition: 30 words with high probability spelling and 80 words with low probability spelling (probability based on likely phoneme-grapheme conversion)

Writing Only

Word	Probability	Frequency	# Letters
best	HIGH	HF	4
dust	HIGH	HF	4
fact	HIGH	HF	4
flat	HIGH	HF	4
hard	HIGH	HF	4
land	HIGH	HF	4
soft	HIGH	HF	4
spot	HIGH	HF	4
stop	HIGH	HF	4
cloud	HIGH	HF	5
count	HIGH	HF	5
drive	HIGH	HF	5
point	HIGH	HF	5
round	HIGH	HF	5
trade	HIGH	HF	5
grab	HIGH	LF	4
mend	HIGH	LF	4
plot	HIGH	LF	4
rent	HIGH	LF	4
twin	HIGH	LF	4
wept	HIGH	LF	4
blame	HIGH	LF	5
bribe	HIGH	LF	5
broom	HIGH	LF	5
chant	HIGH	LF	5
crime	HIGH	LF	5
grave	HIGH	LF	5
hound	HIGH	LF	5
trout	HIGH	LF	5

Writing Only

Word	Probability	Frequency	# Letters
book	LOW	HF	4
dead	LOW	HF	4
free	LOW	HF	4
give	LOW	HF	4
gone	LOW	HF	4
grew	LOW	HF	4
head	LOW	HF	4
keep	LOW	HF	4
love	LOW	HF	4
move	LOW	HF	4
snow	LOW	HF	4
stay	LOW	HF	4
talk	LOW	HF	4
true	LOW	HF	4
type	LOW	HF	4
shoe	LOW	HF	4
skin	LOW	HF	4
tree	LOW	HF	4
want	LOW	HF	4
blood	LOW	HF	5
check	LOW	HF	5
chief	LOW	HF	5
cross	LOW	HF	5
dance	LOW	HF	5
fence	LOW	HF	5
field	LOW	HF	5
fight	LOW	HF	5
floor	LOW	HF	5
fruit	LOW	HF	5
group	LOW	HF	5
knife	LOW	HF	5

learn	LOW	HF	5
leave	LOW	HF	5
noise	LOW	HF	5
share	LOW	HF	5
sheep	LOW	HF	5
speak	LOW	HF	5
voice	LOW	HF	5
breath	LOW	HF	6
bright	LOW	HF	6
beak	LOW	LF	4
crow	LOW	LF	4
debt	LOW	LF	4
dumb	LOW	LF	4
germ	LOW	LF	4
jeep	LOW	LF	4
jerk	LOW	LF	4
junk	LOW	LF	4
kiss	LOW	LF	4
lamb	LOW	LF	4
loaf	LOW	LF	4
myth	LOW	LF	4
skip	LOW	LF	4
toss	LOW	LF	4
urge	LOW	LF	4
worm	LOW	LF	4
yawn	LOW	LF	4
budge	LOW	LF	5
cheer	LOW	LF	5
cloak	LOW	LF	5
crawl	LOW	LF	5
glove	LOW	LF	5
gross	LOW	LF	5
knock	LOW	LF	5
ledge	LOW	LF	5
lodge	LOW	LF	5
moose	LOW	LF	5
phase	LOW	LF	5
pulse	LOW	LF	5
rinse	LOW	LF	5
sauce	LOW	LF	5
shack	LOW	LF	5
shove	LOW	LF	5
skull	LOW	LF	5
thief	LOW	LF	5
tread	LOW	LF	5
vague	LOW	LF	5
weave	LOW	LF	5
sketch	LOW	LF	6
sneeze	LOW	LF	6

6. Word Length
   a. Dyslexia Battery
      Task: oral reading
      List composition: 70 words (14 each of 4-letter, 5-letter, 6-letter, 7-letter, and 8-letter words, balanced for frequency)
   b. Dysgraphia Battery
      Task: writing to dictation
      List composition: 70 words (14 each of 4-letter, 5-letter, 6-letter, 7-letter, and 8-letter words, balanced for frequency)

Word	# Letters	Frequency	Word	# Letters	Frequency
baby	4	HF	edit	4	LF
copy	4	HF	evil	4	LF
iron	4	HF	jury	4	LF
lady	4	HF	odor	4	LF
open	4	HF	pity	4	LF
poem	4	HF	riot	4	LF
unit	4	HF	ruin	4	LF
color	5	HF	avert	5	LF
party	5	HF	cable	5	LF
power	5	HF	drama	5	LF
ready	5	HF	elbow	5	LF
seven	5	HF	fluid	5	LF
solid	5	HF	igloo	5	LF
value	5	HF	urban	5	LF
center	6	HF	excess	6	LF
future	6	HF	fumble	6	LF
letter	6	HF	pigeon	6	LF
pretty	6	HF	pirate	6	LF
reason	6	HF	shower	6	LF
region	6	HF	tragic	6	LF
travel	6	HF	vision	6	LF
brother	7	HF	absence	7	LF
machine	7	HF	curtain	7	LF
million	7	HF	cushion	7	LF
problem	7	HF	leopard	7	LF
provide	7	HF	rooster	7	LF
special	7	HF	sincere	7	LF
trouble	7	HF	suspend	7	LF
complete	8	HF	chipmunk	8	LF
language	8	HF	frequent	8	LF
mountain	8	HF	instinct	8	LF
pressure	8	HF	nuisance	8	LF
question	8	HF	province	8	LF
surprise	8	HF	schedule	8	LF
thousand	8	HF	scramble	8	LF

7. Oral Spelling and Copy Tasks—Dysgraphia Battery Only
   Task composition: 42 words (21 HF and 21 LF including nouns, adjectives, verbs, functors)
   a. Oral spelling—ask the patient to spell the word aloud
   b. Copy
      1) Cross-case transcoding—present written words in uppercase and ask patient to copy in lowercase
      2) Direct copy—present written words in lowercase and ask patient to copy in lowercase

Word	Class	Frequency	# Letters	Word	Class	Frequency	# Letters
poem	noun	HF	4	faith	noun	LF	5
length	noun	HF	6	glove	noun	LF	5
moment	noun	HF	6	grief	noun	LF	5
street	noun	HF	6	fabric	noun	LF	6
window	noun	HF	6	talent	noun	LF	6
fresh	adj	HF	5	pursuit	noun	LF	7
happy	adj	HF	5	brisk	adj	LF	5
afraid	adj	HF	6	crisp	adj	LF	5
bright	adj	HF	6	rigid	adj	LF	5
hungry	adj	HF	6	absent	adj	LF	6
bring	verb	HF	5	quaint	adj	LF	6
carry	verb	HF	5	severe	adj	LF	6
since	verb	HF	5	strict	adj	LF	6
speak	verb	HF	5	argue	verb	LF	5
listen	verb	HF	6	bring	verb	LF	5
provide	verb	HF	7	greet	verb	LF	5
what	functor	HF	4	spoil	verb	LF	5
under	functor	HF	5	borrow	verb	LF	6
enough	functor	HF	6	pierce	verb	LF	6
rather	functor	HF	6	starve	verb	LF	6
though	functor	HF	6	suspend	verb	LF	7

8. Written Naming—Dysgraphia Battery Only
   Line drawings of the following 52 items are presented for written naming

Word	Frequency	# Letters	Word	Frequency	# Letters	Word	Frequency	# Letters
car	HF	3	tie	MF	3	cane	LF	4
bear	HF	4	flag	MF	4	comb	LF	4
bell	HF	4	pipe	MF	4	drum	LF	4
fish	HF	4	shoe	MF	4	lamb	LF	4
foot	HF	4	lamp	MF	4	broom	LF	5
iron	HF	4	tent	MF	4	glass	LF	5
rope	HF	4	brush	MF	5	glove	LF	5
glass	HF	5	canoe	MF	5	nurse	LF	5
money	HF	5	pilot	MF	5	razor	LF	5
plant	HF	5	shirt	MF	5	onion	LF	5
table	HF	5	thumb	MF	5	skirt	LF	5
train	HF	5	basket	MF	6	snail	LF	5
watch	HF	5	castle	MF	6	spoon	LF	5
bottle	HF	6	cheese	MF	6	tiger	LF	5
church	HF	6	orange	MF	6	witch	LF	5
doctor	HF	6	rocket	MF	6	anchor	LF	6
island	HF	6	thread	MF	6	carrot	LF	6
						guitar	LF	6

9. Nonwords—Additional list for dyslexia battery

Nonword	Type	# Letters	Nonword	Type	# Letters
ded	pseudohomophone	3	ner	nonhomophone	3
dert	pseudohomophone	4	buke	nonhomophone	4
gard	pseudohomophone	4	cest	nonhomophone	4
gerl	pseudohomophone	4	dree	nonhomophone	4
groe	pseudohomophone	4	feve	nonhomophone	4
hert	pseudohomophone	4	fute	nonhomophone	4
lern	pseudohomophone	4	gand	nonhomophone	4
meen	pseudohomophone	4	gree	nonhomophone	4
rufe	pseudohomophone	4	leng	nonhomophone	4
snoe	pseudohomophone	4	nuck	nonhomophone	4
sune	pseudohomophone	4	pesh	nonhomophone	4
turm	pseudohomophone	4	plen	nonhomophone	4
werd	pseudohomophone	4	tink	nonhomophone	4
werk	pseudohomophone	4	trin	nonhomophone	4
wite	pseudohomophone	4	vece	nonhomophone	4
breth	pseudohomophone	5	plent	nonhomophone	5
munny	pseudohomophone	5	sheem	nonhomophone	5
reech	pseudohomophone	5	taght	nonhomophone	5
shure	pseudohomophone	5	thalk	nonhomophone	5
whall	pseudohomophone	5	thell	nonhomophone	5
whife	pseudohomophone	5	tuddy	nonhomophone	5
merder	pseudohomophone	6	jenior	nonhomophone	6
sircle	pseudohomophone	6	sloser	nonhomophone	6
consept	pseudohomophone	7	resords	nonhomophone	7
sertain	pseudohomophone	7	sountry	nonhomophone	7

(From Goodman, R. A., & Caramazza, A. (1986, unpublished). *The Johns Hopkins University Dyslexia and Dysgraphia Batteries.*)

APPENDIX 25.2
Rank Order of Phoneme Occurrences in Word Corpus and the Common Associated Graphemic Representations

Rank of Occurrence[1]	International Phonetic Alphabet	Compatible Representation	Keyboard Probable Grapheme[2]	Example
1	/r/	r	r	rat
2	/t/	t	t	tea
3	/n/	n	n	no
4	/s/	s	s	sun
5	/ɪ/	ih	i	pill
6	/ə/	uh-	o, a	button, about
7	/l/	l	l	lake
8	/k/	k	k, c	key, cat
9	/i/	ee	ee, ea	bee, eat
10	/æ/	ae	a	apple
11	/ɛ/	eh	e	egg
12	/d/	d	d	dog
13	/m/	m	m	man
14	/p/	p	p	pen
15	/ɚ/	er	er	mother
16	/o/	o	oa, o	boat, open
17	/b/	b	b	book
18	/e/	ay	a-e	ape
19	/a/	ah	a	father
20	/f/	f	f	fan
21	/ʃ/	sh	sh	shoe
22	/v/	v	v	van
23	/ai/	ai	i, i-e	find, ice
24	/ʌ/	uh+	u	up
25	/g/	g	g	goat
26	/z/	z	z	zebra
27	/dʒ/	dj	j	joke
28	/ɔ/	aw	aw, o	saw, soft
29	/h/	h	h	hat
30	/w/	w	w	window
31	/ŋ/	ng	ng	ring
32	/tʃ/	tch	ch	chin
33	/u/	oo	oo	food
34	/ð/	th-	th	then
35	/aʊ/	au	ou, ow	house, owl
36	/ʊ/	u	oo	book
37	/ɔi/	oy	oy	boy
38	/θ/	th+	th	thin
39	/j/	y	y	yellow
40	/ʒ/	zh	g	rouge

[1] Rank of occurrence was calculated from a corpus of 17,310 English words by Hanna, Hanna, Hodges, & Rudorf (1966) with modifications made by Berndt, Reggia, & Mitchum (1987).

[2] Phoneme-to-grapheme correspondences were taken from Berndt, et al. (1987) who used the Hanna, et al. (1966) data to calculate probability estimates for pronunciation of particular graphemes. The graphemes presented here reflect only the most probable spellings (see Berndt, et al. for a complete listing of graphemes for each phoneme).

APPENDIX 25.3
Glossary

Alexia without agraphia—An acquired reading impairment that is not accompanied by an impairment of writing; also called pure alexia. It is often characterized by a letter-by-letter reading approach.

Allographic conversion—The process whereby an abstract orthographic representation is converted to a specific physical manifestation of a given grapheme.

Allographs—The different forms that a grapheme can take, that is, the various ways one can write a given letter by varying, for example, font, case, script, and handwriting styles.

Deep agraphia (Deep dysgraphia)—An acquired writing impairment that is characterized by the presence of written semantic errors, as well as effects of word frequency (high better than low), imagery (high better than low), and grammatical class (nouns better than functors).

Deep alexia (Deep dyslexia)—An acquired reading impairment that is characterized by the presence of semantic errors in reading, as well as reading performance that is better for high-frequency, concrete nouns in comparison to low-frequency, abstract words.

Global agraphia—An acquired impairment of writing that disrupts lexical and sublexical spelling processes to such an extent that few words are spelled correctly and it is difficult to detect lexical influences on spelling accuracy.

Grapheme—The abstract representation of a letter's identity, e.g., *F* and *f* are letters that both represent the grapheme *f*. A grapheme is a letter or letter cluster (like sh) that corresponds to a single phoneme.

Grapheme-to-phoneme conversion mechanism—A mental process whereby a written word is sounded out by associating each letter identity with its corresponding sound.

Graphemic input lexicon—The corpus of written words that one recognizes.

Graphemic output buffer—The short-term storage mechanism for holding graphemes as one selects the specific allographs (letter form and style) and implements graphic motor programs.

Graphemic output lexicon—The corpus of words that one knows how to spell.

Homographs—Words that are spelled the same but pronounced differently; for example, the adjective *lead* as in "a lead pipe" and the verb *lead* as in "lead the group."

Letter-by-letter reading—An approach to reading whereby letters are identified in serial order; typically observed as a compensatory reading approach in individuals with pure alexia.

Letter-to-sound conversion—The process of reading aloud by converting a letter (or letter cluster) to the corresponding sound.

Lexical agraphia (Surface agraphia)—An acquired writing impairment that is characterized by an overreliance on sound-to-letter conversion processes; typical errors include regularization of irregularly spelled words (e.g., *yot* for *yacht*).

Lexical-semantic route—A means of processing information whereby lexical entries for words are activated along with their corresponding meanings.

Nonlexical route—A means of information processing that does not rely on activation of lexical representations; for example, non-lexical reading can be accomplished by converting letters to their corresponding sounds and nonlexical writing can be accomplished by converting sounds to their corresponding letters.

Orthographic input lexicon—The collection of mental representations for written words that one recognizes; also called the visual-input lexicon or the graphemic-input lexicon.

Orthographic output lexicon—The collection of mental representations for spellings that one knows; also called the graphemic-output lexicon.

Orthography-to-phonology conversion—The process of reading aloud by converting a letter (or letter cluster) to the corresponding sound; also referred to as letter-to-sound conversion.

Phoneme-to-Grapheme Conversion—The process of writing by means of deriving spelling based on knowledge of sound-to-letter correspondences.

Phonological agraphia—An acquired impairment of spelling that is characterized by the inability to write nonwords due to impairment of the sublexical sound-to-letter conversion processes.

Phonological alexia—An acquired impairment of reading that is characterized by an inability to read nonwords due to impairment to the sublexical letter-to-sound conversion processes.

Phonological buffer—The short-term storage mechanism whereby phonemes are held while articulatory planning for speech production is accomplished.

Phonological output lexicon—The collection of phonologic representations for words that one can produce.

Pure alexia—An acquired reading impairment that is not accompanied by an impairment of writing. It results from a disruption of visual input from the appropriate abstract word-form representation, so that words are visually perceived, but not recognized.

Semantic paralexias—Reading errors that are semantic in nature; for example, reading *bus* as "car."

Sublexical route—A means of information processing that does not rely on activation of lexical representations; for example, reading that is accomplished by converting letters to their corresponding sounds or writing that is accomplished by converting sounds to their corresponding letters.

Surface agraphia (Lexical agraphia)—An acquired writing impairment that is characterized by an overreliance on sound-to-letter conversion processes; typical errors include regularization of irregularly spelled words (e.g., *yot* for *yacht*).

Surface alexia (Surface dyslexia)—An acquired reading impairment characterized by reading according to letter-to-sound correspondence rules so that irregularly spelled words (such as *yacht*) tend to be mispronounced.

Visual input lexicon—The collection of mental representations for written words that one recognizes; also called orthographic-input lexicon or graphemic input lexicon.

Visual output lexicon—The collection of mental representations for spellings that one knows; also called orthographic output lexicon or graphemic output lexicon.

C. Cognitive Neurolinguistic Approaches to the Treatment of Language Disorders

Chapter 26

Language Rehabilitation from a Neural Perspective

Stephen E. Nadeau, Leslie J. Gonzalez Rothi, and Jay Rosenbek

OBJECTIVES

The objectives of this chapter are to detail a neural network model of language function that incorporates phonologic, semantic, lexical-semantic, and grammatical function; to discuss cerebral memory mechanisms in relation to the acquisition of knowledge and skills during language therapy; to define mechanisms by which knowledge and skills gained during therapy might generalize in ways that will enhance daily communicative function; to consider the implications of education psychology research for the structure, context, and temporal spacing of therapy, the nature of stimuli presented in therapy, and the nature of feedback delivered during therapy; and to review several specific therapies (including phonologic, semantic, and grammatical therapies; constraint-induced language therapy, and errorless learning) to illustrate the applications of neural principles to treatment and the potential opportunities for generalization.

Rehabilitation after brain injury depends on two processes: (1) the endogenous responses of neural tissues (reactive plasticity), which include reactive neurogenesis, neural migration, axonal sprouting and extension to target structures, and synaptogenesis (Kolb, 2004; Kolb & Cioe, 2004); and (2) the replacement of knowledge lost as a result of injury through behavioral therapy. Although we are at the scientific threshold of manipulating reactive plasticity

to therapeutic advantage, the clinical data so far are inconclusive and do not yet bear on rehabilitation of language processes. Therefore, the principal focus of this chapter will be on behavioral therapies.

The efficacy of behavioral therapies for language impairment has been demonstrated in a large number of studies, some providing level I evidence. These are reviewed at length in this text. In this chapter, we focus on the treatment of aphasia not from the perspective of clinical trials but, rather, from the perspective of neural science. We will begin with a very brief review of relevant aspects of neuroscience (see also Nadeau et al., 2004).

The brain contains 100 billion neurons. Half of these are located in the cerebrum. Any given neuron sends output, through its axon, to thousands or tens of thousands of other neurons, and any given neuron receives synaptic contacts providing input from up to tens of thousands of neurons. Neurons, through their connections, are organized into networks. These networks provide the basis for the representation of knowledge and for transforming knowledge in one domain (e.g., written language) into another domain (e.g., spoken language). For these reasons, neural networks (as opposed to neurons) have been identified as the essential unit of brain function (Buonomano & Merzenich, 1998). The brain is best viewed as webs of connected neural processes, including axons and dendrites, in which the neurons themselves serve mainly to provide metabolic support, structural maintenance, and the currency of neural processing (firing rates), and the knowledge is represented in synaptic connection strengths.

The state of the brain at any given moment (the substrate for conscious awareness) largely is defined by the pattern of neural activity in all its neural networks. Because active perceptions, thoughts, and plans correspond to patterns of spatially disseminated neural activity, we refer to their neural representations as being distributed.[1] When an excitatory neuron fires, it elicits firing in many of the neurons to which it is connected. In this way, neural activity can spread from a few neurons to many neurons within a network and from one network to another.

Information is not sent from one part of the brain to another (this is a digital computer concept); rather, a sustained pattern of neural firing in one network eventually elicits a sustained pattern of firing in another network. Most neural efferent (output) projections are reciprocated by returning (afferent) projections from the target networks. Thus, the transmission of information in the brain corresponds to an ongoing, two-way dialogue between a sending network and a receiving network in which the two networks ultimately settle into a steady state. The time to settle largely defines behavioral response latency. This dynamic additionally provides the neural basis for bottom-up/top-down processing effects. In practice, information transmission typically involves a large number of connected networks, each contributing its particular knowledge and expertise to the final steady-state pattern. In this way, the brain is able to meet multiple different constraints simultaneously—an emergent property of connected neural networks referred to as "parallel constraint satisfaction." Nowhere is parallel constraint satisfaction better illustrated than in the case of language, in which what we ultimately say reflects perceptual input (e.g., auditory); knowledge latent in our semantic networks; processing by neural networks supporting grammar, the translation of concepts into phonologic sequences, implicit rules governing phonologic sequences, and implicit rules governing modifications of phonologic sequences as language is produced (phonetic modifications); and constraints imposed by neural networks driving respiratory and pharyngeal musculature in actually producing sound.

A given neural network supports knowledge (long-term memory, represented in neural connection strengths), working memory (the pattern of neural activity in the network at any given time), and processing (the transformation of input patterns into output patterns). Learning corresponds to changes in connection strengths in the network. Knowledge includes facts and skills. Acquisition of declarative knowledge (fact memory) requires the participation of a unique ancillary processor (the hippocampal system). The acquisition of nondeclarative knowledge (e.g., procedural or skill memory) can be achieved through the incremental adjustment of neural connection strengths that may occur during neural network processing activities. Rules can be learned explicitly (e.g., "i" before "e" except after "c"). In general, however, such rules are best viewed as metamemory, and in the extremely rapid online processing that underlies language comprehension and production, rules are reflected as implicit knowledge of regularities in a network's experience.

There has been a long-standing debate in the linguistic and neuropsychological literatures as to whether deficits observed after brain damage reflect loss of knowledge or loss of access to knowledge. The fact that even subjects with severe impairment may demonstrate residual knowledge often is cited as support for the loss-of-access theory (e.g., subjects with agrammatical aphasia often display considerable ability in make judgments regarding grammar; semantic paraphasic errors tend to be near-misses, and phonemic paraphasic errors typically bear a semantic and/or phonologic relationship to the target). The neural network understanding of brain operations that we have achieved (summarized above) leads us to more nuanced conclusions. Because knowledge is distributed as connection strengths throughout a neural network, damage to a network may lead to a substantial probability of output error, but it does not eliminate all knowledge unless the network is completely destroyed, a phenomenon referred to as "graceful degradation." Thus, evidence of residual knowledge is perfectly consistent with partial loss of knowledge as a result of network damage. On the other hand, certain types of brain damage, particularly those involving major white matter pathways, may destroy connections between networks, leading to cognitive dysfunction that truly reflects loss of access to intact knowledge representations—that is, true disconnection syndromes (Geschwind, 1965). For example, following transection of the corpus callosum to treat refractory generalized epilepsy, the right hemisphere generally cannot express itself verbally, because it has no access to left hemisphere language networks and the left hemisphere cannot speak about right hemisphere perceptions, thoughts, and plans because it has no way of accessing these representations. Subjects with posterior cerebral infarcts that destroy the left occipital cortex and the splenium of the corpus callosum cannot read, because even though the right occipital cortex can see the printed words, it cannot relay this orthographic information to the left hemisphere for linguistic processing. In the final analysis, most aberrant behavior observed after brain damage likely reflects a mix of loss of knowledge as a result of destruction of neural networks and loss of access to knowledge as a result of damage to white matter pathways or intervening gray matter "relay stations." Even in the case of callosal section, arguably the purest disconnection syndrome, the involved interhemispheric axons support synaptic connections that represent knowledge—connections that are lost with the surgery. In the domain of language, conduction aphasia has long been viewed as a disconnection syndrome caused by damage to the arcuate

---

[1] Local representations—that is, information defined at a single discrete locus—are not found in the central nervous system. They are present only peripherally, such as when a photon of light stimulates a single retinal rod or cone or when the firing of a single muscle fiber is elicited by the firing of the terminal of its afferent axon.

fasciculus (and, perhaps, other anteroposterior white matter pathways). It certainly is true that a discontinuity exists between language zones in the posterior perisylvian region and Broca's area, and to this extent, the result of a lesion of the connecting white matter can be viewed as a disconnection syndrome. Abundant evidence, however, exists that conduction aphasia also reflects damage to the neural networks supporting phonologic sequence knowledge.

A fully neuroscientific approach to behavioral therapy for language impairment must ask what types of knowledge need to be replaced, how are they represented in the brain, and how can the brain best be coaxed into reacquiring this knowledge? The answers to these questions are not known with certainty in any cognitive domain, but we probably know more about language than about any other cognitive function. In fact, we have sufficient knowledge about the neural basis of language processes to propose some reasonable hypotheses regarding therapeutic strategies. We currently have no ability to treat components of aphasia related to disconnection (loss of access to knowledge) other than through training of networks that are still connected and have some capability for acquiring the requisite linguistic knowledge. For example, in the subject with conduction aphasia, it may be possible to enhance phonologic sequence knowledge in networks in the nondominant hemisphere, effectively bypassing the disconnection in the dominant hemisphere (see *Phonologic, Semantic, and Lexical-Semantic Processing* under *A Parallel Distributed Processing Model of Language* below).

Although a number of approaches have been taken to explain language processing (e.g., linguistic and cognitive neuropsychological), this chapter will focus heavily (but not exclusively) on parallel distributed processing models, also known as connectionist models, both because they enable us to link neural network architecture directly to complex behavior and because they incorporate many of the properties of neural systems discussed above. A specific PDP model of language will be discussed to introduce the basic concepts and to frame some later hypotheses about the domains of knowledge represented. A brief review of the unique properties and particular strengths of PDP models will follow. Subsequently, we will have cause to refer back frequently to PDP models, but we will also rely on other sources of information about the neural basis of language as it relates to speech-language therapy.

A PARALLEL DISTRIBUTED PROCESSING MODEL OF LANGUAGE

Phonological, Semantic, and Lexical-Semantic Processing

The Wernicke-Lichtheim information processing model of language function has played a dominant role in understanding aphasic syndromes (Lichtheim, 1885) and has stood the test of time in defining the topographical relationship between the modular domains (acoustic representations, articulatory-motor representations, and concept representations) underlying spoken language function. Unfortunately, the Wernicke-Lichtheim information processing model does not specify the characteristics of the representations within these domains and how they might be stored in the brain. It also does not address the means by which these domains might interact. We have proposed a parallel distributed processing (PDP) model that uses the same general topography as the Wernicke-Lichtheim model (Nadeau, 2001; Roth, Nadeau, Hollingsworth, Cimino-Knight, & Heilman, 2006), but this PDP model also specifies how representations are generated in the modular domains and how knowledge is represented in the links between these domains (Fig. 26–1). Although not tested through simulations, this model is neurally plausible and provides a cogent explanation for a broad range of psycholinguistic phenomena. More generally, connectionist concepts now are deeply embedded in—and receive enormous support from—mainstream neuroscientific research (see, e.g., Rolls & Deco, 2002; Rolls & Treves, 1998).

The PDP modification of the Wernicke-Lichtheim model posits that the acoustic domain (akin to Wernicke's area) contains large numbers of units located in auditory association cortices that represent acoustic features of

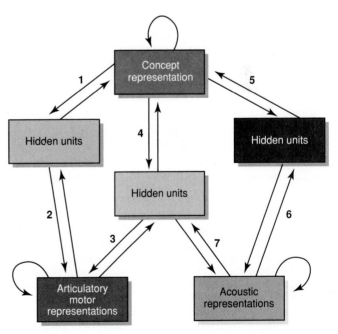

Figure 26–1. Proposed parallel distributed processing model of language. (From Roth, H. L., Nadeau, S. E., Hollingsworth, A. L., Cimino-Knight, A. M., Heilman, K. M. (2006). Naming concepts: Evidence of two routes. *Neurocase, 12*, 61–70; with permission.)

phonemes.[2] The articulatory domain (analogous to Broca's area) contains units located predominantly in the dominant frontal operculum that represent discrete articulatory features of speech, as opposed to continuously variable motor programs (e.g., phonemic distinctive features). The semantic or conceptual domain contains an array of units distributed throughout unimodal, polymodal, and supramodal association cortices that represent semantic features of concepts. For example, the representation of the concept of "house" might correspond to activation of units representing features of houses, such as visual attributes, construction materials, contents (physical and human), and so on. Each unit within a given domain is connected to many, if not most, of the other units in that same domain (symbolized by the small looping arrow appended to each domain in Fig. 26–1). Knowledge within each domain is represented as connection strengths between the units. Thus, semantic knowledge is represented as the pattern of connection strengths throughout the association cortices supporting this knowledge. Within any domain, a representation corresponds to a specific pattern of activity of all the units, hence the term "distributed representation." Each unit within each of these domains is connected via interposed hidden units to many, if not most, of the units in the other domains. During learning of a language, the strengths of the connections between the units are gradually adjusted so that a pattern of activity involving the units in one domain elicits the correct pattern of activity in the units of another domain. The entire set of connections between any two domains forms a pattern associator network. The hidden unit regions, in conjunction with nonlinear unit properties, enable the systematic association of representations in two connected domains that are arbitrarily related to one another (e.g., word sound and word meaning). The model employs left-right position in acoustic and articulatory motor representations as a surrogate for temporal order in precisely the same way as the reading model of Plaut, McClelland, Seidenberg, and Patterson (1996). Thus, acoustic-articulatory motor representations would feature positions for each output phoneme or distinctive feature, ordered as they are in the phonologic word

form. The use of left-to-right sequential order in lieu of temporal order is a device of convenience, but evidence exists for this temporal-geographic transform in the brain (Cheung, Bedenbaugh, Nagarajan, & Schreiner, 2001). During any type of language processing, initiated by input to any domain of the network, almost instantaneous engagement of all domains of the network will occur. Thus, linguistic behavior is best viewed as the emergent product of the *entire* network.

We will now focus on particular components of the network to provide a more detailed understanding of how they work and the nature of the knowledge they support.

Concepts Representations

As we have noted, the Wernicke-Lichtheim information processing model provides no insight regarding the nature of the representations in the various domains. The nature of concept representations (depicted in Fig. 26–1) can be best illustrated using a particular model developed by David Rumelhart and his colleagues (Rumelhart, Smolensky, McClelland, & Hinton, 1986). This "rooms in a house" model is comprised of 40 "feature" units, each corresponding to an article typically found in particular rooms or an aspect of particular rooms. Each unit is connected with all the other units in the network—an attribute that defines the model as an *auto-associator network*. Auto-associator networks have the capacity for "settling" into a particular state that defines a representation. Connection strengths are defined by the likelihood that any two features might appear in conjunction in a typical house. When one or more units are clamped into the "on" state (as if the network has been shown these particular features or articles), activation spreads throughout the model, and the model eventually settles into a steady state that implicitly defines a particular room in a house. Thus, clamping "oven" ultimately results in activation of all the items one would expect to find in a kitchen and thereby *implicitly* defines, via a *distributed representation*, the concept of a kitchen (Fig. 26–2). No kitchen unit *per se* is turned on. Rather, "kitchen" is defined by the pattern of feature units that are activated. The network contains the knowledge, in the totality of its connections, that enables this representation to be generated. The 40-unit model actually has the capability of generating distributed representations of a number of different rooms in a house (e.g., bathroom, bedroom, living room, or study), subcomponents of rooms (e.g., easy chair and floor lamp, desk and desk-chair, or window and drapes), and blends of rooms not anticipated in the programming of the model (e.g., clamping both bed and sofa leads to a distributed representation of a large, fancy bedroom replete with a fireplace, television, and sofa).

This auto-associator model, simple though it is, has the essential attributes of a network that might be capable of generating the distributed representations of meaning underlying semantics. The brain's semantic auto-associator obviously is comprised of vastly more that 40 features, and it

---

[2] A "unit" is the smallest functional entity within a connectionist model. It has a level of activation that is defined as a nonlinear mathematical function of its combined inputs at any one time (in many models, a sigmoidal curve that asymptotically approaches a minimum value of zero or a maximum value of one). It has an output that is a nonlinear mathematical function of its level of activation, often incorporating a threshold such that for activation levels below the threshold, no output occurs. Each unit is connected to a very large number of other units. The patterns of connectivity within a network define its functional capacity. The precise neural counterpart of a unit is uncertain and may vary from region to region. Thus, it is not implausible that single neurons function as units in the superior colliculus, whereas in the cortex, it is possible that a cortical column comes closer to meeting our definition of a unit. The neurobiology of cortical neural network function is currently understood only at the most rudimentary level.

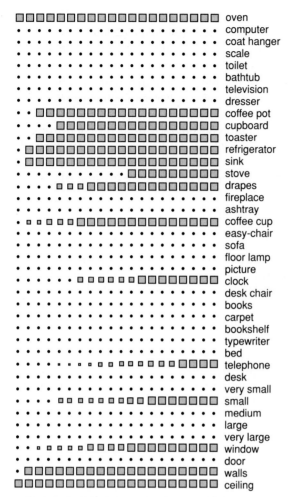

Figure 26–2. Evolution of the pattern of activation in the "rooms-in-a-house" model when the units "ceiling" and "oven" are clamped in the "on" position. Time elapses from left to right. The size of each square indicates the degree of activation of that particular feature unit. (From Rumelhart, D. E., Smolensky, P., McClelland, J. L., & Hinton, G. E. (1986). Schemata and sequential thought processes in PDP models. In J. L. McClelland, D. E. Rumelhart, & the PDP Research Group (Eds.), *Parallel distributed processing* (Vol. 2, pp. 7–57). Cambridge, Massachusetts: MIT Press; with permission.)

enables an enormous repertoire of distributed representations corresponding to the vast number of concepts we are capable of representing. This particular model network is not compartmentalized, but nothing inherent in PDP models precludes a semantic representation comprised of two or more subnetworks (see, e.g., Farah and McCelland, 1991). Good evidence suggests that in the brain, the meaning of a given word is distributed over a host of networks, depending in part on the semantic features that are most essential to that meaning. For example, visual information makes a particularly large contribution to the meaning of living things; consequently, subjects with damage to visual association cortex as a result of herpes simplex encephalitis

exhibit category-specific naming and recognition deficits for living things (Forde & Humphreys, 1999; Warrington & Shallice, 1984).

The concept of a fractionated, multi-network distributed representation of meaning is illustrated in Figure 26–3. The distributed representation of the concept "dog" has a major component in visual association cortices corresponding to knowledge of the visual appearance of dogs in general, as well as to that of particular dogs; a major component in auditory association cortices corresponding to the sounds that dogs characteristically make; a major component in the limbic system corresponding to one's feelings about dogs in general and about specific dogs; a component in somatosensory cortex corresponding to the feel of dog fur or wet tongue or cold nose; a predicative component, presumably involving the frontal cortex, corresponding to our knowledge of what dogs are likely to do; a component in the olfactory cortex corresponding to the odors of dogs; and components in the perisylvian language cortex that enable us to translate the semantic representation of "dog" into an articulatory motor representation (so we can say /dog/) or an acoustic representation (so we can understand another person saying /dog/). Not all of these subnetworks will be activated every time or in exactly the same way by everyone. Thus, we can speak in terms of *working memory*—in this case, a pattern of activity in particular subnetworks corresponding to "dog"—and we can speak in terms of *working associations*, meaning the elicitation of distributed concept representations in other connected subnetworks, either automatically or volitionally. Thus, nearly everyone would, when hearing /dog/, develop visual and limbic distributed representations, each constituting a working memory, with the two together comprising an automatic working association. The average person, however, might need to volitionally develop the working association that brings in the olfactory component of the meaning of "dog."

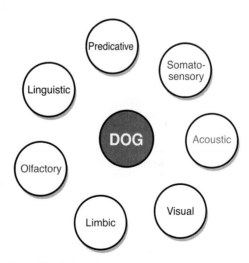

Figure 26–3. The full, multi-component, distributed representation of the concept "dog." (See text for explanation.)

The Acoustic-Articulatory Motor Pattern Associator Network

The knowledge that allows a person to translate heard sound sequences into articulatory-motor sequences and, thereby, mediates repetition of both real words and nonwords is contained in the network that connects the acoustic domain to the articulatory motor domain (the acoustic-articulatory motor pattern associator; see Fig. 26–1, pathway 7-3). Because this network has acquired, through experience, knowledge of the systematic relationships between acoustic sequences and articulatory sequences, it has learned the sound sequence regularities of the language: the phonemic sequences of joint phonemes, rhymes, syllables, affixes, morphemes, and words characteristic of the language (Nadeau, 2001). Consideration of the reading model developed by Plaut and colleagues (1996) will help to make this more transparent (see also Seidenberg & McClelland, 1989).

This reading model fundamentally recapitulates the acoustic-articulatory motor pathway of Figure 26–1, the major difference (inconsequential to this discussion) being that in place of acoustic representations, it incorporated orthographic (printed letter) representations. The model (Fig. 26–4) was composed of three layers:

1. An input layer of 105 grapheme units grouped into clusters, the first cluster including all possibilities for the one or more consonants of the onset, the second cluster including all the possible vowels in the nucleus, and the third cluster including all possibilities for the one or more consonants in the coda.
2. A hidden unit layer of 100 units.
3. An output layer of 61 phoneme units grouped into clusters, including all the possibilities for onset, nucleus, and coda, respectively (as for the graphemes).

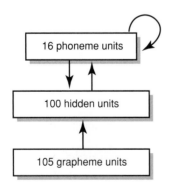

Figure 26–4. One version of the parallel distributed processing (PDP) reading model developed by Plaut and colleagues. (From Plaut, D. C., McClelland, J. L., Seidenberg, M. S., & Patterson, K. (1996). Understanding normal and impaired word reading: Computational principles in quasi-regular domains. *Psychological Review, 103,* 56–115; with permission.)

Local representations were used for the graphemes and phonemes. One-way connections from each of the grapheme input units exist to each of the hidden units, and two-way connections exist between each of the hidden units and each of the phoneme output units. Every output unit was connected to every other output unit, providing the network with the auto-associator capability for "settling into" the best solution (as opposed to its own approximate solution). The model was trained using a mathematical algorithm that incrementally alters the strengths of connections that make the biggest contribution to error, which was computed as the difference between the actual product of the network and the desired product of the network.[3] The orthographic representation of 3,000 English, single-syllable words and the corresponding phonologic forms was presented, one pair at a time, cycling repeatedly through the entire corpus. In this way, the model ultimately learned to produce the correct pronunciation of all the words it had read. One of the most striking things about the trained model is that it also was able to produce correct pronunciations of plausible English nonwords (i.e., orthographic sequences it had never encountered). How was this possible?

One might have inferred that the model was simply learning the pronunciation of all the words by rote. If this had been the case, however, the model would have been incapable of applying what it had learned to novel words. In fact, what the model learned was the relationships between *sequences* of graphemes and *sequences* of phonemes that are characteristic of the English language. To the extent that a limited repertoire of sequence types exists, the model was able to learn it and then apply that knowledge to novel forms that incorporated some of the sequential relationships in this repertoire. The information the model acquired through its long experience with English orthographic-phonologic sequential relationships, however, went considerably beyond this. Certain sequences (i.e., those most commonly found in English, single-syllable words) were more thoroughly etched in network connectivity. Thus, it was very fast with high-frequency words. It also was very fast with words having an absolutely consistent orthographic-phonologic sequence relationship (e.g., words ending in "-ust," which are always pronounced /ʌst/ [e.g., must, bust, trust, lust, or crust]). The model encountered difficulty (reflected in prolonged reading latency) only with low-frequency words, and only to the extent that it had learned different, competing pronunciations of the same orthographic sequence. Thus, it was slow to read "pint," because in every case but "pint," the sequence

---

[3] This is a highly effective but entirely heuristic means of training PDP networks. Real neural networks learn by completely different mechanisms, some of which will be discussed later in this chapter. Understanding the details of mechanisms underlying knowledge acquisition by the cerebral cortex currently poses one of our greatest neuroscientific challenges.

"int" is pronounced /Int/ (e.g., mint, tint, flint, or lint). It also was slow (but not quite so slow) to read words like "shown," because two equally frequent alternatives exist to the pronunciation of "own" (e.g., gown, down, and town vs. shown, blown, and flown). It was very slow with words that are unique in their orthographic-phonologic sequence relationship (e.g., aisle, guide, and fugue). These behaviors precisely recapitulate the behavior of normal human subjects given reading tasks.

To be more precise, the knowledge the model acquires reflects competing effects of type frequency and token frequency. If a single word is sufficiently common (high token frequency), the model acquires enough experience with it that competing orthographic-phonologic sequential relationships have a negligible impact on naming latency. If a word is relatively uncommon (e.g., pint), however, its naming latency will be significantly affected by the knowledge of other words that, although equally uncommon, together belong to a competing type (e.g., mint, flint, tint, or sprint).

The capacity of the model to read nonwords reflects its ability to capture patterns in the sequential relationships between orthographic and articulatory word forms and to apply this knowledge to novel word forms. Plaut and colleagues (1996), as well as Seidenberg and McClelland (1989) in their earlier work on this reading model, focused on differences in rhyme components of single-syllable words (the nucleus plus the coda [e.g., b<u>at</u>]), because these are the major determinants of whether a word is orthographically regular (e.g., mint) or irregular (e.g., pint). As Seidenberg and McClelland point out, however, the network architecture in these models is capable of capturing any kind of regularity in the orthographic and phonologic sequences to which it is exposed, limited only by the extent of exposure. Such regularities would include joint phonemes other than rhymes (e.g., "str-" of stream, street, stray, and strum) and, in a multi-syllabic version, syllables and morphemes (affixes and the root forms of nouns and verbs as well as functors [e.g., articles, auxiliary verbs, conjunctions, and certain prepositions]).

The acoustic-articulatory motor pathway in the model of Figure 26–1 would capture analogous patterns in the sequential relationships between acoustic and articulatory word forms (actually somewhat more redundant, because in English, acoustic-articulatory correspondences are substantially more consistent than are orthographic-articulatory correspondences). These sequential relationship patterns potentially involve sequences of varying length, from phoneme pairs (joint phonemes) and syllables up to and including whole words and, possibly, multi-word compounds. These patterns represent the repository of knowledge about subword (sublexical) entities in general as well as our knowledge of phonotactic constraints (the rules that determine whether a given phonologic sequence is permissible in a particular language). This repository of sequence knowledge also provides the basis for "neighborhood" effects (Vitevitch, 1997), which reflect the influence of variously competing pieces of sequence knowledge on the ultimate phonologic sequence selection and are demonstrated in the tendency to produce near-miss phonologic sequence errors that correspond to one of the close neighbors.

Lexicons

Understanding the meaning of a word that is heard is achieved through the connections between the domain that contains the sound features of language and the domain that contains concept features (the acoustic-concepts representations pattern associator; see Fig. 26–1, pathway 6-5). This pattern associator network corresponds to the cognitive neuropsychological concept of a phonologic input lexicon (Ellis & Young, 1988). It contains neither knowledge of acoustics nor knowledge of semantics—it serves only to translate a representation in the acoustic domain into a representation in the concepts/semantics domain, where meaning is instantiated. This conceptualization of a lexicon as a vast number of connections between two network domains, although well accepted in the connectionist literature, is not intuitive and, in fact, is strongly at odds with traditional conceptualizations of lexicons as repositories of abstract local representations of single words. It begins to make sense, however, when one recalls that all representations in the central nervous system are distributed (e.g., the "kitchen" representation), not local, and that the knowledge underlying the capacity to generate a representation lies in connection strengths and is not a piece of data at a memory location (as in a digital computer).

The knowledge that enables a person to translate a concept into a spoken word (the phonologic output lexicon) (Ellis & Young, 1988) is contained in two different pattern associator networks that connect the concept representations domain to the articulatory motor domain (Fig. 26–1, pathways 1-2 and 4-3). These two pattern associator networks support different forms of knowledge. The indirect concept representations–articulatory motor pathway (Fig. 26–1, pathway 4-3) provides a robust basis for knowledge of sequences and sublexical entities because of the sequence knowledge stored in the acoustic-articulatory motor pattern associator. The direct concept representations–articulatory motor pattern associator (Fig. 26–1, pathway 1-2) does not, however, contain much knowledge of sequences and sublexical entities, because it translates spatially distributed patterns of activity corresponding to concepts into temporally distributed sequences of activity corresponding to articulated words. This spatial-temporal translation precludes significant acquisition of sequence knowledge and makes this fundamentally a whole-word pathway. The existence of this direct, whole-word naming route finds support in studies of subjects with repetition conduction aphasia[4]; some appear to have lost most phonologic sequence knowledge (Fig. 26–1, pathways 3, 4, and 7), resulting in a severe deficit in auditory verbal short-term memory, but can speak quite well, producing few, if any, phonologic paraphasic errors; can repeat real words (with evidence of influence by semantic attributes but little influence of word length); and are severely impaired in repeating nonwords and functors (Caramazza, Basili, Koller, & Berndt, 1981; Friedrich, Glenn, & Marin, 1984; Saffran & Marin, 1975; Warrington & Shallice, 1969). It also finds some support in reports of subjects with conduction aphasia who are able to repeat words better than nonwords (Caramazza, Miceli, & Villa, 1986; Friedrich et al., 1984; McCarthy & Warrington, 1984; Saffran & Marin, 1975) and who are able to repeat words better when they are given in a sentence context than when given as a single word, thereby increasing the likelihood of engaging concept representations (McCarthy & Warrington, 1984). A model in which the only link from the concept representations domain to the articulatory motor domain is the direct one (Fig. 26–1, pathway 1-2) cannot account for observations that normal subjects exhibit phonologic slips of the tongue, and subjects with aphasia produce phonemic paraphasias in naming and internally generated spoken language quite comparable to those produced during repetition. To explain these observations, one must posit access from concept representations to phonologic sequence knowledge, as indicated in pathway 4-3 of the model (Fig. 26–1). Thus, this PDP model predicts that two pathways should be enabling the naming of concepts.

Further evidence of two pathways supporting naming of concepts has been provided by a subject who, depending on the type of verbal cue provided, could be induced to use either the whole-word (direct) naming route or the phonologic (indirect) naming route (Roth et al., 2006). This left-handed subject had a Broca's aphasia stemming from a massive infarct involving the entire left middle cerebral artery territory. His language was largely limited to single words, which he produced quite readily and with good articulation. He tended to pursue a semantic conduite d'approche, which, however, was successful only approximately 10% of the time. He made very rare phonologic paraphasic errors. When asked to name an object, such as a faucet, and given either no cue or a semantic cue, a typical response would be "dishes . . . chairs . . . dishwasher . . . shut . . . water . . . ready to go . . . water . . . shut . . . hot . . . old . . . sink . . . water . . . heavy . . . water . . . heavy . . . washer . . . tub." When given the phonemic cue "faus," however, he replied "fauwash . . . fau . . . fau . . . fauswah . . . thafaush . . . fallshine . . . fallsha . . .

fallshvine . . . fallswash . . . fallsh." These patterns of response to bedside testing suggested that he normally used a whole-word route to confrontation naming (as well as in internally generated language; see Fig. 26–1, pathway 1-2) but that by providing him with a phonemic cue, we could induce him to employ a phonologic route—a route that engaged sublexical representations implicit in his stores of phonologic sequence knowledge (Fig. 26–1, pathway 4-3). He actually was able to successfully name objects 30% of the time using this pathway, but at the cost of producing large numbers of relatively undesirable nonword errors. The dual-route naming hypothesis was further tested and validated with systematic cued naming studies.

Lexical-Semantic and Phonologic Impairment in Aphasias

At this point, we have fleshed out the essential components of the model. One might reasonably ask, how can this model account for the lexical-semantic and phonologic features of subjects with various types of aphasia and, in turn, how can the model be reconciled with what is known about correlations between lesion locus and aphasia type?

Phonologic Paraphasic Errors

Phonologic paraphasic errors generally are thought to reflect damage to dominant hemisphere networks supporting phonologic processing. In our model, this would correspond to the dominant hemisphere acoustic-articulatory motor pattern associator network (Fig. 26–1, pathway 7-3)—the repository of phonologic sequence knowledge. Nonpropositional spoken language, which often is supported by the nondominant hemisphere (Speedie, Wertman, Ta'ir, & Heilman, 1993), does reflect sequence knowledge, but discrete phrasal, lexical, or sublexical elements of this knowledge cannot be selected at will, however, as they can in propositional language processing. The subject described in the foregoing (Roth et al., 2006), who could be cued to use one or the other of the two concept-naming routes (Fig. 26–1, pathways 1-2 or 4-3), provides new insight regarding the neural basis of phonologic paraphasic errors. His left hemisphere was nearly completely destroyed. Thus, he must have been speaking with his right hemisphere, which was undamaged, and his performance when naming after phonemic cueing suggests that he was using discretely accessible phonologic sequence knowledge represented in his right hemisphere. This suggests, in turn, that deficient development of networks instantiating this knowledge (as contrasted to damage to fully developed networks) can provide an alternative basis for phonologic paraphasic errors.

Factors Influencing the Pattern of Errors in Internally Generated Language

In the two-route naming model we have introduced, three factors may influence the pattern of errors observed in internally generated spoken language in perisylvian aphasias (and

---

[4] A conduction aphasia, originally described by Warrington and Shallice (1969), in which subjects have very limited ability to repeat, have severe impairment in auditory verbal short-term memory, and make few, if any, phonologic paraphasic errors. It can be contrasted with reproduction conduction aphasia, in which subjects often make profuse phonologic paraphasic errors in repetition and, usually, in production and have variable but sometime negligible deficits in auditory verbal short-term memory.

whether this pattern is marked exclusively by impaired word retrieval or, additionally, by phonemic paraphasic errors). First, given the likely anatomical representation of the network shown in Figure 26–1, most dominant perisylvian lesions probably damage both the whole word and the phonologic output routes (Fig. 26–5), and the pattern of spoken output may reflect the relative degree to which these two-pattern associator networks are affected. This would explain why subjects with Wernicke's or conduction aphasia apparently do not have the option of relying entirely on the whole-word route. Second, these two output pattern associator networks likely are differentially represented in the two hemispheres, with the phonologic pathway being more frequently better developed in the dominant hemisphere and the whole-word pathway more equally developed in the two hemispheres. Subjects with dominant hemisphere lesions almost invariably demonstrate impaired—if not completely absent—phonologic sequence knowledge but often exhibit partial sparing of lexical-semantic knowledge. Studies of subjects with callosal disconnection demonstrate that the disconnected right hemisphere has a phonologic input lexicon and conceptual semantic knowledge but impoverished phonologic processing (Zaidel, Iacoboni, Zaidel, & Bogen, 2003). Third, there may be individual variability in the degree to which connectivity is developed in these two output routes, and this individual variability may vary as a function of hemisphere. Thus, to understand fully language production following a left hemisphere lesion, a bihemispheric language model that incorporates both developmental attributes and the impact of the lesion must be considered (Fig. 26–6).

As the case of Roth et al. (2006) suggests, in the presence of an extensive left hemisphere perisylvian lesion, deficient development of connectivity in nondominant hemisphere concept representations may lead to the generation of anomia and semantic paraphasic errors, and deficient development of connectivity in the nondominant hemisphere phonologic route may lead to the generation of phonemic paraphasic errors. The deficient development of both systems, particularly the phonologic one, may be a general characteristic of the right hemisphere, but deficient development of the phonologic

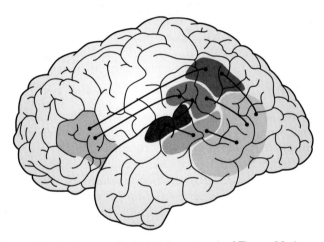

Figure 26–5. Cartoon depicting the network of Figure 26–1 mapped onto the brain. Color coding is the same as in Figure 26–1. Concept representations are assumed to be widely distributed across association cortices throughout the brain. In this cartoon, only the region of presumed interface between concept representations and the remainder of the model is depicted. Given the paucity of information about the anatomical organization of the human perisylvian region, the mapping depicted here is, at best, approximate; our goal is primarily to demonstrate the feasibility of mapping a connectionist architecture of phonologic processing to cortical anatomy. Recent magnetic resonance imaging–diffusion tensor imaging tractographic studies of deep white matter pathways, however, are shedding some light on the anatomical details. Catani, Jones, & Fytche (2005) have delineated two dominant perisylvian pathways linking Wernicke's and Broca's areas: a direct one, corresponding to the arcuate fasciculus (possibly corresponding to pathway 3 in our model), and an indirect one, projecting from Wernicke's area to the inferior parietal cortex (Brodmann's areas 39 and 40), with apparent relay to Broca's area via what likely is component III of the superior longitudinal fasciculus (Makris et al., 2005) (possibly corresponding to pathway 1-2 in our model). They concluded that the broad extent of origin and termination of these pathways and their large cross-sections favored a connectionist account. (From Roth, H. L., Nadeau, S. E., Hollingsworth, A. L., Cimino-Knight, A. M., Heilman, K. M. (2006). Naming concepts: Evidence of two routes. *Neurocase, 12,* 61–70; with permission.)

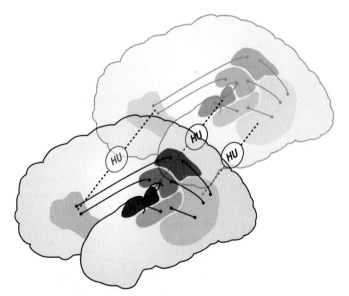

Figure 26–6. Cartoon depicting mapping of a bi-hemispheric model to the brain. This provides the basis for a fuller explanation of the results of left hemisphere lesions on language output in terms of bi-hemispheric contributions, the effect of the lesion, and the degree to which various networks are developed in each hemisphere. Color coding is the same as in Figures 26–1 and 26–5. HU = hidden units. (From Roth, H. L., Nadeau, S. E., Hollingsworth, A. L., Cimino-Knight, A. M., Heilman, K. M. (2006). Naming concepts: Evidence of two routes. *Neurocase, 12,* 61–70; with permission.)

route also may occur, to one degree or another, in the left hemisphere as a result of normal variability in phonologic network ontogenesis (Goodglass, 1993; Plaut et al., 1996).

In summary, with any given left hemisphere lesion, the actual pattern of internally generated spoken language may reflect three factors:

1. The effects of the lesion on the two output routes (phonologic and whole word).
2. The degree to which one or both of these routes is represented in the right hemisphere.
3. The degree of development of connectivity in each of the two routes in the two hemispheres.

If both naming routes are involved and the combined effect of the three factors differentially impacts the phonologic routes, the net result will be output marked predominantly by word retrieval deficits (with or without semantic paraphasic errors) as whole-word routes become the predominant means of language production (as in repetition conduction aphasia). If whole-word routes are differentially impacted, the net result will be output marked by word retrieval deficits and a substantial incidence of phonemic paraphasic errors as damaged or inadequately developed phonologic routes become the predominant means of language production.

Subjects with reproduction conduction or Wernicke's aphasia predominantly use damaged or inadequately developed phonologic pathways. Wernicke's aphasia may reflect more severe impairment and, hence, greater difficulty with word retrieval and more profuse phonemic paraphasic errors than with conduction aphasia. Subjects with Wernicke's aphasia also may have damage to acoustic representations or the acoustic representations–concept representations pathways that enable verbal comprehension. Naming difficulty may arise through mechanisms discussed in the preceding paragraph or in two additional ways. First, damage to Brodmann's areas 37 and 39 in the dominant hemisphere may be associated with word retrieval deficits (Chertkow, Bub, Deaudon, & Whitehead, 1997; Hart & Gordon, 1990; Raymer et al., 1997; Whatmough, Chaertkow, Murtha, & Hanratty, 2002). These areas may constitute the interface between association cortices throughout the brain supporting concept representations and the core language apparatus (proximal to the point at which the phonologic route provides differential access to sequence knowledge). Second, dysfunction of conceptual (semantic) networks because of left hemisphere damage and deficient development of right hemisphere networks, as in our subject, would be expected to yield naming difficulty with production of semantic paraphasic errors.

Processes Occurring During Recovery

The dual-route naming model, as elaborated in the foregoing, also can account for the patterns of evolution of internally generated spoken language observed during recovery.

First, recovery of connectivity in the dominant hemisphere phonologic route (or enhancement of deficient connectivity in phonologic routes in either hemisphere) would lead to increased naming success and a reduction in phonemic paraphasic errors. Second, because articulatory motor representations normally depend on input from both the whole-word and phonologic routes for activation, damage to either route could lead to anomia as representations fail to reach threshold for activation (a diaschisis effect).[5] Changes may occur in the connectivity within articulatory representations or in surviving connectivity within the two naming routes such that this diaschisis effect diminishes with time. Third, in normal brain development, neural network connectivity in the two hemispheres presumably evolves such that transcallosal pathways facilitate coordinated bihemispheric activity and do not impede independent unihemispheric activity. A lesion may disrupt this precise inter-hemispheric coordination (another form of diaschisis), potentially rendering transcallosal input dysfunctional until appropriate readjustment of connectivity within and between hemispheres occurs in the course of recovery. With such readjustment, word retrieval may improve as the nondominant whole-word route achieves a progressively greater transcallosal impact on dominant hemisphere spoken language output. Finally, because phonemic paraphasias have such an invidious effect on communication, subjects like the one described by Roth et al. (2006), to make themselves more readily understood, may be able to learn a strategy of using only the whole-word route and of semantically "boxing in" the concept they are trying to convey.

Why PDP Models?

Below, we will extend the model to account for grammatical function. Before doing so, however, we will briefly review particularly important features of PDP models in general and the model of phonologic, semantic, and lexical-semantic function that we have developed, because these have strong implications for the function of the model and provide major support for the application of PDP models to the under-

---

[5] Diaschisis, a concept first elaborated by von Monakow (1914), constitutes transient dysfunction of undamaged brain regions that are connected to the focus of brain damage. For example, subjects with acute middle cerebral artery (MCA) distribution strokes affecting a large extent of the dorsolateral frontal lobe often will exhibit an overwhelming tendency to direct their eyes (gaze) toward the side of the lesion and cannot be induced to look toward the opposite side. This reflects dysfunction of the frontal eye field because of diaschisis. The frontal eye field rarely is damaged by MCA distribution infarcts; however, it receives enormous, mainly excitatory input from brain regions supplied by the MCA. With the acute stroke, it no longer receives this excitatory input. Consequently, no input from other brain regions can bring the neurons in the frontal eye field up to the firing threshold. With time and neuroplasticity, these neurons adjust, and gaze substantially normalizes, typically within days.

standing of language and aphasia. Having fleshed out a concrete example of a PDP model of language, it is reasonable to take a moment to ask, why this particular approach?

Limitations of Existing Theories

Linguistic theories have not yet provided a satisfactory account for the language errors made by normal subjects or the language disorders observed in subjects with aphasia. Three major reasons can be identified:

1. Linguistic theories have been founded on the concept of serial processing, whereas abundant data suggest that language production incorporates parallel processing (Stemberger, 1985).

2. These serial processing–based theories of linguistic function have difficulty capturing effects that are easily explained by bottom-up and top-down processing interactions (Table 26–1) that are an intrinsic attribute of many PDP models (including ours), such as the occurrence of paraphasias (speech errors) that have both semantic and phonologic similarity to the target (Dell & Reich, 1981; Dell, Schwartz, Martin, Saffran, & Gagnon, 1997; Harley, 1984).

3. Linguistic theories have failed to account for how linguistic behavior might emerge from neural structure.

Cognitive neuropsychological theories incorporate, to one extent or another, information processing models—the "box and arrow" models that date back to Wernicke and

---

TABLE 26–1

Properties of Parallel Distributed Processing (PDP) Networks

The knowledge is in the connections.
  In simulated PDP models, knowledge is represented as the strength of the connections between units. In the brain, knowledge is represented as the strength of synaptic connections between neurons.

A network supports processing, working, and long-term memory.
  Like neural networks in the brain, PDP networks support the processes underlying all cognition and behavior. In both PDP and neural networks, working memory corresponds to a transient network pattern of unit/neural activity or partial neural depolarization (a mechanism not yet tested in PDP research). Long-term memory (i.e., knowledge) is represented as the sum total of unit or neural connection strengths in the network.

Hidden units plus non-linearity support associations between orthogonal representations.
  Both PDP and neural networks can translate representations in one domain into arbitrarily related representations in another, connected domain. For example, concept representations, corresponding to knowledge of word meaning, can be translated into spoken word representations.

Distributed representations bring with them several powerful emergent features.
  Content-addressable memory
    With distributed representations, engagement of a feature of a particular memory can generate the distributed representation of the entire memory. In contrast, in digital computer models, the address of a memory must be known to retrieve that memory.
  Graceful degradation
    Both PDP and neural networks can perform at close to normal levels with substantially degraded input, in part because of their ability to settle into attractor states and in part because of bottom-up/top-down processing effects (see below). Both PDP and neural networks demonstrate the same general patterns of performance even when damaged, because knowledge is represented throughout the network and because partial damage only reduces the redundancy of the knowledge and increases the probability of error or non-response.
  Inference, generalization, and confabulation
    Both PDP and neural networks naturally encode the commonalities and patterns that are implicit in the information to which they are exposed during training, thereby instantiating implicit rules. These rules can then be usefully applied to situations that have never been encountered before but that bear a resemblance to what has been experienced. The knowledge gained during training thereby generalizes. Performance based on the acquisition of implicit rules reflects the inference that the rules apply in a new, yet-to-be-experienced situation. If the rules do not apply, then the response can be characterized as confabulation.

Bottom-up and top-down processing.
  Through repeated upward and downward flow of unit/neural activity between input networks and higher-order networks (e.g., from networks supporting visual representations of orthographic input to networks supporting semantic representations), neural network systems settle into states that represent the optimal amalgamation of incoming information and existing knowledge. This enables simultaneous (but likely compromised) satisfaction of constraints provided by a multitude of different neural networks (e.g., phonologic, lexical-semantic, semantic, and syntactic—a process called parallel constraint satisfaction). It enables valid perception despite very noisy input. It also, however, carries the risk of misperception of a near-miss input as the correct input (leading, e.g., to our tendency to overlook editorial errors when proofreading).

Lichtheim. As we have seen, PDP models may be entirely consistent with information processing models with respect to the topography of processes involved—in this case, language. What PDP models provide as an added value is specificity regarding the nature of the representations in the boxes and the nature of the processes symbolized by the arrows, about which information processing models are agnostic.

PDP Models Emulate Brain

PDP models are "neural-like" in that they incorporate large arrays of simple units that are heavily interconnected with each other to form networks, like neurons in the brain (McClelland, Rumelhart, & PDP Research Group, 1986; Nadeau, 2000). Their processing sophistication stems from the simultaneous interaction of the large numbers of units (hundreds or even thousands) in these arrays. In PDP models, memories are represented as connection strengths in the same networks that support processing, just as in the brain. Thus, in PDP models of language, memories of language units (e.g., stored knowledge of phonemes, joint phonemes, syllables, words, and sentence constituents) are represented in the same neural networks that support linguistic processing. In PDP models, working memory also is represented in the same networks that support processing, as transient patterns of neural bias or firing (again, just as in the brain). The incorporation of working- and long-term memory in the same neural networks that are responsible for processing, in conjunction with processes underlying the engagement of working memory (Goldman-Rakic, 1990), eliminates the need to posit separate buffers, which are a digital computer concept. PDP models are particularly appealing in the context of language processing, because they involve simultaneous processing at a number of levels and locations, apparently mimicking what is going on in the brain (something that will become more apparent when we consider grammatical function). Finally, pure PDP models (models without incorporated digital devices), endowed with learning algorithms, can implicitly learn the rules governing the data they process in the course of their experience with that data (see, e.g., Plaut et al., 1996). In fact, they are nonpareil in extracting commonalities and patterns in the data, which form the basis for implicit rules. Thus, for example, a pure PDP model of phonology has no need to build in specific structures to account for specific phonologic phenomena. The structure of the model is defined entirely in terms of the domains of information accessible to it and the necessary topographical relationship of these domains to each other. The model learns the rest. The absence of specific, ad hoc devices motivated by models (e.g., linguistic) designed to account for particular phonologic phenomena in an orderly fashion also is crucial to the maintenance of neurologic plausibility (architectural faithfulness to neural structure). In humans, as in neurally plausible PDP models, the linguistic

phenomena we observe reflect entirely the emergent behavior of the networks.

PDP models can easily be endowed specifically with properties that emulate brain structure and function. For example, the model shown in Figure 26–1 incorporates two-way connections (the general pattern in the cerebrum), and this two-way connectivity is what enables top-down/bottom up interaction effects. These effects are enormously beneficial in enabling us to extract meaning from extraordinarily degraded input (e.g., much of the spoken language that we hear), because the input only has to be sufficiently informative to partially activate the correct target distributed representation. This target then provides top-down activation of lower-level units contributing to its activation, which, in turn, amplifies the bottom-up activation of the target. Of course, this feature can have invidious effects as well. Our great difficulty in eliminating all typographical errors from manuscripts stems from the fact that bottom-up/top-down interaction effects are quite literally leading us to see what we intended rather than what is actually there. Bottom-up/down-down interaction effects provide a powerful explanatory mechanism for many linguistic phenomenon (Dell, 1986; Dell et al., 1997; McClelland & Rumelhart, 1981; Rumelhart & McClelland, 1982).

Another useful property that can be built into PDP models is recurrent connections (as in the model shown in Fig. 26–1, symbolized by the loops at concept, articulatory motor, and acoustic representations). This feature, which also is neurologically plausible, enables the network to deal with the situation that arises when a pattern of input does not precisely correspond to one of the patterns on which the model was trained, either because the input pattern is novel or because the input is noisy. In such circumstances, a model without recurrent connections might generate a pattern of activity in the output representational field that does not correspond to any recognizable entity. Clearly, the brain has the capability for creating meaning for novel distributed representations. Equally clearly, however, we derive great advantage from the ability to translate very noisy and degraded input into something we recognize, as discussed in the context of bottom-up/top-down processing effects. This ability corresponds to a network capacity for adjusting near-miss distributed representations until they correspond to the nearest meaningful representation.[6] This capacity is achieved by creating connections between every unit within the representational field and every other unit in that field. The field is thereby transformed into what is referred to as an "auto-associator network," which is a network that tends to settle into stable states corresponding to meaningful dis-

---

[6] "Nearest" corresponds literally to the distance in n-dimensional space between the near-miss and the closest meaningful distributed representation, where n is the number of units in the representational field and "meaningfulness" is defined by the knowledge structure, latent in the network, that was acquired during the training period.

tributed representations as defined during the training period (Rumelhart et al., 1986). This feature gives the entire network what are called "attractor" properties, referring to the tendency of the network to settle into or be "attracted to" particular stable states. Attractor properties convey another very useful property in computer simulations of network behavior—that is, the time that it takes a network to "settle" into an attractor state corresponds to the response latency of that network. In this way, the attractor feature endows the network with a performance measure—namely, response latency—that precisely coincides with one of the most common dependent variables used in behavioral studies of human subjects.

PDP models provide us with the means to understand how complex behavior might emerge from neural networks, which now are accepted as the fundamental unit of cortical function (Buonomano & Merzenich, 1998). Before this approach to understanding the brain was developed, behavioral neurologists, cognitive neuropsychologists, and linguists had to accept as a matter of faith that someday, somehow, the discoveries they were making could be linked directly to neural structure. For many of us, it is stunning that this dream has been realized in our lifetime. No model represents a final answer to how the brain handles a domain of cognitive function. Rather, a particular model represents a specific hypothesis about the topographic organization of neural processes underlying a given function and the mathematical properties of the units and connections comprising the neural networks involved. It presumes the now well-established faithfulness of the PDP concept to the essential features of neural network processing, and to the extent that it successfully replicates behavior of human subjects in health and disease, it accommodates empirical data on brain function. The dialectic in the PDP literature between principles of neural network topography and mathematical function on the one hand and empirical data on language behavior on the other has proven to be a particularly fruitful one in advancing the science of language and the brain.

The Heuristic Value of PDP Modeling

The appeal of PDP modeling also derives from the fact that simulations of particular models can be run on computers, leading to the generation of vast amounts of data that can then be compared with data derived from experimental studies in animals and human subjects. It is even possible to systematically vary one or more parameters in a particular model and, thereby, generate a population of PDP "individuals" who can be simulated, thus providing a foundation for group statistics. PDP simulations have been extraordinarily successful in replicating the behavior of normal human subjects, as in the PDP reading model of Plaut and colleagues (1996; see also Seidenberg & McClelland, 1989). Simulations involving "lesioned" PDP models also have been extraordinarily successful in emulating the behavior of human subjects with

brain injury (Cohen, Johnston, & Plunkett, 2000) and even in simulating the effects of rehabilitation (Plaut, 1996).

A Paradigm Shift

PDP models invoke a scientific and philosophical paradigm shift in that they reflect chaotic order rather than deterministic order. Chaotic order (Gleick, 1987) is system order deriving from the orderly behavior of the individual units of the system, whereas deterministic order reflects the impact of an overall guiding force or principle.[7] Neural network brains, whether in *Drosophila* (100,000 neurons) or in human beings (100 billion neurons), also operate by chaotic principles. Because in PDP order emerges naturally from network properties and topography rather than being defined primarily by the structure of the model, neurologic plausibility replaces the goal of choosing the simplest of competing theories (i.e., Occam's razor) as the guiding force in the design of these models (see O'Reilly, 1998). Although the precise details of the organization of neural networks in the brain still largely elude us, it now is quite clear and well accepted that the brain incorporates PDP principles, and the related scientific field, computational neuroscience, is burgeoning (Rolls & Deco, 2002; Rolls & Treves, 1998).[8]

---

[7] Examples of chaotic order include the ornate structure of a flower and the marvelous computational machine that is the human brain; they reflect the order that emerges from the precise behavior of individual cells interacting with each other. Deterministic order is exemplified by the movement of planets in the solar system (and the satellites that we send to them), which can be explained entirely by equations that characterize the force of gravity and its effect on mass.

[8] The only major departure of neural network theory from PDP theory is that the former seeks to apply exclusively local learning processes, whereas PDP simulations employ predominantly heuristic devices that are, for the most part, not local. The prototypic example of a local learning process is Hebbian learning, named after Donald Hebb, who first elucidated the concept (Hebb, 1949). Hebb postulated that to the extent that two connected neurons are simultaneously active, the strength of the synaptic connection between them will increase. This concept has since been validated in extensive research on long-term potentiation (Buonomano & Merzenich, 1998). This work has also revealed evidence of a reciprocal process, long-term depression, which occurs to the extent that the activity of connected neurons is discrepant. Hebbian learning is intrinsically local and therefore eminently plausible neuroscientifically. It requires only a peculiar neurotransmitter receptor such as the NMDA-glutamate receptor, which functions as a detector of the coincidence of high activity of the post-synaptic neurons (reflected in a depression in membrane voltage) and high activity of the presynaptic neuron (reflected in large amounts of glutamate released from the presynaptic axon terminal). In contrast, the most common learning algorithm employed in PDP simulations is back propagation, which requires a change in the strength of inter-unit connections based upon events occurring at the output end of the network, which could be many synapses away. This intrinsically non-local learning algorithm is biologically implausible but it remains possible that some non-local learning processes are instantiated in the brain (O'Reilly, 1996). Nevertheless, there do not appear to be any fundamental scientific impediments to the realization of the language model we develop incorporating a local learning process.

Grammar

We now resume our discussion of PDP and language, extending the model to incorporate a basis for grammatical function. For purposes of discussion, we will break grammatical function down into syntax and grammatical morphology. Syntax is knowledge of acceptable word order and sentence structure. Grammatical morphology refers both to the modifications of words that are made in their use in sentences (bound grammatical morphology [e.g., affixes conveying case, number, or tense]) and to the use of individual words that, at least superficially, appear to primarily serve sentence composition rather than meaning (free grammatical morphemes [e.g., articles, auxiliary verbs, conjunctions, and certain prepositions]). We will break syntax down into (1) *sentence organization*, which encompasses such things as the necessary relationships between verbs and nouns or noun phrases in a sentence (verb argument relationships; see below), embedded clauses, and passive voice constructions and (2) *phrase structure rules*, which constrain word order at the local level (e.g., the rule that constrains articles to precede nouns). In Chomskian thinking, both of these components of syntax are thought to arise from the operational principles of a grammar generator. In contrast, we will argue that principles of sentence organization follow directly from the way in which the brain manipulates concept representations and that phrase structure rules and rules of grammatical morphology are an emergent property of the pattern associator networks responsible for articulatory and inscriptional (written) output.[9]

Syntax: Sentence Organization

It is easy to conceive of spoken, concrete nouns as being the product of distributed representations of concepts that are linked, through pattern associator networks (Fig. 26–1, pathways 1-2 and 4-3), to articulatory motor representations and, ultimately, to networks that support the sequences of oropharyngeal movements that actually produce the speech sounds of the noun, as discussed in the section on phonology. The same cannot be said about other types of words, most particularly adjectives, verbs, and abstract nouns.

Adjectives represent the simplest case and, therefore, are a reasonable place to start. In principle, the distributed representations corresponding to noun concepts are infinitely malleable. We can easily modify the general distributed representation of "dog" to capture any species of dog or any particular dog we have personally known. We can easily

contemplate the most complicated and arbitrary of distributed representations, such as "the obese, pockmarked, oily-haired, slovenly, unctuous, check-shirted, plaid-jacketed man with the striped pants, food-stained paisley tie, goatee, wire-rimmed glasses, bundle of pens in his pocket, and clip board in his hand"—a sort of Uriah Heep cum used-car salesman. The process of pairing one or more adjectives or adjectival phrases with a noun corresponds to a particular modification of the distributed representation of the noun.

Verbs are viewed as the work masters in traditional linguistic formulations, because they specify the major participants in the action that is described by the verb, thereby defining sentence structure. These participants are called the arguments of the verb. Arguments usually are noun phrases but also may be prepositional phrases, adjectival phrases, and sentential clauses. They fill argument positions (e.g., subject, object, and indirect object positions). Each argument is assigned a purpose in the sentence by the verb, referred to as its "thematic role." For example, the agent is the perpetrator of the action ("The *man* gave flowers to Mary"), the theme is the object of the verb's action ("flowers" in the preceding sentence), and the goal is the recipient of the action (Mary). Verbs differ with respect to the arguments they specify—some require only an agent; some an agent and a theme; others an agent, theme, and goal—and many verbs allow some freedom in choosing whether to include a certain argument. They also differ with respect to the nature of the arguments they can specify (e.g., "knew" easily accommodates a sentential clause in the predicate, e.g., "He knew Mary would arrive soon," whereas "hit" does not).

Does the argument specification property of verbs provide direct insight regarding the cerebral processing of verbs? To date, no one has succeeded in answering this question using a traditional linguistic formulation. How might a verb be represented in PDP terms? First, consider what might be the distributed representation of a verb, such as the verb "to shoot." What features underlie this distributed representation? A problem is immediately apparent. Our conceptualization of "shooting" actually consists of the juxtaposition of two distributed concept representations: a person who is the shooter, and a person who has been shot or is about to be shot. The sentence "the old man shot the burglar" generates two distributed concept representations: one of an old man appropriately altered to incorporate the act of shooting, and the second of a burglar appropriately altered to incorporate the fact of having been shot. Thus, "shot" achieves its meaning not through the generation of its own distributed representation but, rather, through the elicitation of two reciprocally modified distributed representations ("old man shooter" and "shot burglar") that, in addition, are meaningfully linked, in effect constituting a composite, "super-distributed" representation that incorporates the entire shooting scene. The two components of this composite representation are implicitly linked by their complementarity (shooter and

---

[9] Although the ideas proposed here are fundamentally at odds with traditional linguistic formulations, any consideration of language and the brain, including PDP, must rely heavily on the extraordinarily rich and detailed information that linguistic studies have provided about regularities in the phenomenology of languages.

shot) and their simultaneity. They become explicitly linked when this particular reciprocal pair of distributed representations generates a pattern of activation in articulatory motor cortex that will produce the sound sequence corresponding to the sentence. They also may become explicitly linked when a pattern of activity in acoustic cortex, generated by the sound of the sentence being produced by a speaker, leads to production of the reciprocal pair of distributed concept representations underlying "old man shooter" and "shot burglar."

Intransitive verbs function in a fashion essentially identical to adjectives (e.g., "the soldier salutes"). A transitive verb functions as a sort of super-adjective, reciprocally modifying the distributed representations of the concepts underlying the two or three noun phrases in the sentence and at the same time, linking them to form a new, super-distributed representation. Thus, in our new conceptualization, verbs are defined exclusively by the effect that they have on the distributed representations of the nouns they constrain, which constitutes both their grammatical and their semantic roles, and on the pattern of activity in the phonologic processing network, which constitutes their lexical-semantic role.

Any volitional alteration in distributed concept representations constitutes *concept manipulation*. Thus, even use of adjectives or intransitive verbs, which serve to modify a single distributed concept representation, can be usefully viewed as concept manipulation and, as will be discussed below, will tend to be impaired in subjects with aphasias (e.g., Broca's aphasia) that are associated with deficits in transitive verb use and argument structure. Production of the sentence "the old man shot the burglar" requires fairly symmetric manipulations of two distributed concept representations. Sentences employing adjunctive phrases, however, such as "Jones slept in the park," may demand highly asymmetric manipulation of the two distributed concept representations. In this sentence, the "Jones" concept is the object of most of the modification, and the "park" concept is only very subtly modified. This asymmetry could be dramatically altered, however, by additional information neurally defined as additional distributed concept representations—for example, "Jones was apprehended as the murderer of nighttime joggers. He slept in the park during the day."—in which case the distributed concept representation of park is substantially modified by its association with Jones the murderer.

The auto-associator network representation of a concept can be translated by the concept–articulatory motor pattern associator networks into any one of a number of different word sequences. The actual word sequence chosen will depend on several factors, including (1) the modifiability of the core distributed representation of the concept, (2) whether the modification occurs nearly simultaneously with the generation of the core distributed representation or at some later time, and (3) the availability of words to be elicited by the auto-associator network representation of the concept. To provide a sense of the concept manipulation

demands that are met by the normal brain, we will consider each of these possibilities in some detail.

Modifiability of the Core Representation

Consider the core representation of "burglar" in our previous example. "Old man shot burglar" is not likely to be a modification of the distributed representation of burglar that is readily available to us. Thus, we are forced to use a super-distributed representation to capture this concept—namely, a representation that therefore engages a verb (e.g., "The burglar that had been shot by the old man"). On the other hand, consider the concept of streets wet with rain. Here, the concept of "rain-wet streets" falls well within the various modifications of street that are readily available to us. Thus, we have a choice in expressing this idea. We can employ a single distributed representation, modified by an adjective, yielding "rain-wet streets," or we can employ a super-distributed representation, thus engaging a verb (e.g., "The streets made wet by the rain").

Simultaneous Versus Sequential Modification

Whether a modification of the distributed representation underlying a concept occurs as the concept is formed or sometime later is likely to influence the word sequence corresponding to that concept. Thus, someone viewing a romantic Parisian street in her mind's eye might incorporate "rain-wet" from the beginning, favoring the verbal product "rain-wet streets." On the other hand, the wetness modification might be conceptualized only after the street concept has been realized and verbalization has been initiated, hence "the car skidded on the street that was still wet from the rain," "the car skidded on the street because the street was still wet from the rain," or "The car skidded on the street. The street was still wet from the rain." The way the sequence of conceptual development happens to emerge probably is not the only factor at play here. We may have the luxury of shaping the conceptual stream according to our intent to place emphasis or imply causality. On the other hand, working memory capacity may limit the number and complexity of modifications we can make in a distributed representation at one time, forcing us to use a narrative stream employing multiple clauses or sentences, each further modifying the original distributed concept representation.

The Availability of Words

Word representations corresponding to certain distributed concept representations may be completely unavailable, available but inappropriate to the context, or temporarily unavailable. Each of these circumstances would necessitate a clause construction in lieu of an adjectival construction. Thus, "rain-wet" might simply not be in a person's vocabulary. Alternatively, it might be available but carry with it a sense of inappropriateness to the context (possibly a limbic component to the distributed representation generated by the word in this context). Thus, "rain-wet" is satisfactory in a novel but would sound contrived in ordinary conversation and inappropriate in formal discourse. Finally, the word may be transiently unavailable because of the "tip-of-the-tongue" phenomenon, necessitating a circumlocutory clause or sentence to convey the concept.

In this way, the aspect of syntax that we have defined as sentence organization depends not on the machinations of a sophisticated language processor but, rather, constitutes an emergent property of the distributed representations of concepts, the modification of concepts, the linking of concepts into super-distributed representations, and the interaction of network systems defining concepts with the pattern associator networks defining language output. Concept representations and their manipulations invoke association cortices throughout the brain as well as subcortical structures, such as the amygdala. Therefore, the ways in which concepts are handled provide a window on the fundamental properties of higher brain function. The grammatical properties that are common to the vast number of languages spoken on our planet (the "universal grammar") reflect the fact that, as a first approximation, the basic structure and function of the entire brain is the same in all human beings. On the other hand, because language production is a direct reflection of patterns of distributed concept manipulation, grammatical differences in language production may provide a window on cultural, genetic, and even individual differences in the way people think.

Disorders of Syntax

Two aspects of a common aphasia, Broca's aphasia, are explainable on the basis of a breakdown in the processes we have just outlined. Broca's aphasia commonly is characterized by two grammatical attributes: simplification of syntax, and a characteristic abnormality of grammatical morphology known as agrammatism—that is, the propensity for leaving out words of primarily grammatical importance, such as articles, auxiliary verbs, conjunctions, and to some extent, prepositions. These two aspects of Broca's aphasia may be dissociated: A number of cases of morphologic agrammatism without simplification of syntax have been reported, and several cases of simplification of syntax without morphologic agrammatism have been reported (Nadeau, 1988; Nadeau & Gonzalez-Rothi, 1993). As we have noted, sentence production reflects the flexible modification and manipulation of the distributed representations underlying concepts. The simplification of syntax seen with Broca's aphasia, including a paucity of embedded clauses and inability to use strings of adjectives (e.g., "big barn" or "red barn," but not "big, red barn"), can be accounted for in terms of a defect in the ability to alter the distributed representations of single or

multiple concepts at will. This may be caused by a general inability to maintain selective engagement of the specific neural networks incorporating the featural basis for the concepts and their intended nuances. Consistent with this interpretation is the fact that subjects with Broca's aphasia exhibit limited lexical priming (Prather, Zurif, Stern, & Rosen, 1992). By *selective engagement*, we mean the bringing online of selected representations in selected neural networks, either by eliciting sustained neural activity in those networks or altering the state of polarization of the neurons such that they are more susceptible to firing by other afferent input (see Chapter 19). Selective engagement is a general term that embraces the many processes by which the brain allocates resources, and it includes processes commonly referred to as working memory—the specific type of selective engagement we refer to here—as well as attention (Nadeau & Crosson, 1997). In normal subjects engaged in a lexical decision task, preceding a lexical target with a semantically related word reduces the time that is needed to determine whether the target is a word or a nonword. Seeing the semantically related word has led to the selective engagement of a number of semantically related distributed concept representations and their associated articulatory motor representations, one of which is the target. In subjects with Broca's aphasia, the range and number of the distributed concept representations selectively engaged appears to be limited, with the result that speeding of lexical decision by semantic priming is less likely to occur.

Generating verbs also normally invokes a particular form of selective engagement to modify two or more distributed representations in reciprocal fashion and link them to form a super-distributed representation. It thus makes special demands on selective engagement mechanisms. Subjects with Broca's aphasia exhibit relatively greater difficulty accessing verbs than nouns, and their production of verbs with complex argument structures is more impaired than their production of simple verbs (e.g., intransitive verbs) (Thompson, Lange, Schneider, & Shapiro, 1997)—further evidence of impairment in ability to simultaneously manipulate multiple distributed representations. Notably, the ability of subjects with Broca's aphasia to produce verbs in tasks of picture naming, whether naturally or as a result of treatment (in our nomenclature, to use verbs as adjectives), does not translate into the ability to use verbs in sentences (i.e., to link and reciprocally modify distributed concept representations), a far more demanding skill (Mitchum & Berndt, 2001).

One of the most widely accepted theories regarding the fundamental deficit in Broca's aphasia is referred to as the Mapping Deficit Hypothesis (Saffran & Schwartz, 1988; Saffran, Schwartz, & Marin, 1980; Schwartz, Linebarger, Saffran, & Pate, 1987). This hypothesis characterizes the deficit as an inability to produce ordered sentence components (e.g., noun phrase–verb–noun phrase) that reflect the underling thematic roles (e.g., agent, theme, or goal) to link sentence structure to meaning. Two components are identified: lexical, referring to argument information specified by verbs; and procedural, referring to operations governing thematic role assignment for sentences that require interpretation of structural cues (e.g., word order or verb morphology) to relate noun phrases as they literally appear in the sentence to underlying sentence meaning. For example, to understand who did what to whom in the passive-voice sentence "Joe was hit by John," one must cue not just on word order but also on the auxiliary verb "was" and the preposition "by" (we will have more to say about such words below). These mapping capacities correspond quite directly to the capacities for distributed concept manipulation and association discussed in the foregoing. The advantage of the sentence organization hypothesis we have introduced is that it relates these functions directly to neural network processes.

Syntax: Phrase Structure Rules

One of the most remarkable attributes of words in spoken language is their consistent respect for phrase structure rules (e.g., articles always precede and never follow nouns). Only in the occasional patient with jargon aphasia does this rule seem to be broken, and even then, it is far from clear whether inappropriate sequences emerge in continuous discourse or result just by happenstance, from the juxtaposition of phrase fragments. Clearly, these immutable phrase structure rules reflect some very fundamental and redundantly represented attributes of cerebral language networks that govern word sequence. To gain some insight regarding such network properties, we return to the pattern associator model of single-syllable word reading developed by Plaut and colleagues (1996; see also Seidenberg & McClelland, 1989). Had the model been designed to accommodate multi-syllable words rather than only single-syllable words, we would have seen it acquire, simply from its experience with English vocabulary, sequence knowledge about syllables, polysyllables, root forms, and affixes as they combine to form words. This sequence knowledge incorporates the sequential relationship of these various sublexical phoneme clumps to each other—the lexical equivalent of phrase structure rules.

The inferential leap we make at this point is that sequential relationships *between words* also are represented in various neural pattern associator networks in the same way that sequential relationships between phonemes *within* words are represented. Most specifically, we need to posit that, for phrase structure rules to be represented in oral language output, there needs to be a pattern associator network encoding word sequence knowledge that parallels the acoustic-articulatory motor pattern associator supporting sublexical sequence knowledge, or that a single pattern associator network incorporates sequential knowledge of both sublexical entities and short phrases. This additional pattern associator

provides the basis for a link between distributed representations of concepts underlying words, characterized by the properties of their network representation (e.g., nouns, adjectives, or verbs, as we have discussed), with distributed representations of the articulatory forms of these words in proper sequence. In effect, it is a property-sequence transducer in which the systematic relationships between concept representation properties and articulatory sequences emerge as implicit knowledge through extended experience with heard and spoken language. At first, one is inclined to protest that, because the number of possible word sequences is virtually infinite, no system, even one comprised of tens of billions of units and involving combinatorial mathematics, could possibly represent all the possibilities. The actual amount of information relevant to word sequence that is implicit in all the allowable word sequences, however, is actually much less than it seems and quite plausibly is incorporated within neural connectivity. This is because word sequence information implicitly incorporates rules governing the order of *classes* of words, precisely as a multi-syllabic phonemic processor would implicitly incorporate rules about the placement of suffixes and prefixes. Thus, in English, words that have the attribute of modifying the distributed representation of a concept (adjectives) uniformly precede nouns and knowledge about the proper order of adjective-noun sequences simply emerges from the network's experience with heard and written English. PDP networks can learn specific exceptional representations as well as patterns that are common to many representations. Thus, the reading model of Plaut and colleagues (1996) was able to learn to read such extremely exceptional words as "aisle," "guide," and "fugue." By the same token, a word sequence network should be able to learn certain sequences with very few exemplars, such as those involving the placement of articles. In fact, because articles are among the most commonly encountered words in the language, the network would be expected to instantiate the sequential relationship between articles and nouns with particular redundancy.

How long are the word sequences that are likely to be entrained by the pattern associator network contemplated here? The answer is not known. Some evidence suggests that the length of commonly used sequences grows with practice through the life span. Elderly people are relatively more likely than younger people to develop Wernicke's aphasia and relatively less likely than younger people to develop Broca's aphasia, whether the lesion is caused by stroke, neoplasm, or trauma (Basso, Bracchi, Capitani, Laiacona, & Zanobio, 1987; Brown & Grober, 1983; Kertesz & Sheppard, 1981; Miceli et al., 1981). One possible explanation for this is that elderly people are able to maintain reasonable fluency given a frontal lobe lesion because of the repertoire of word sequence knowledge that they retain in the predominantly posteriorly located pattern associator network we have described. Only when the lesion directly affects this pattern associator and/or its related phonologic pattern associator does aphasia result, and then it is a Wernicke's aphasia or a conduction aphasia, directly reflecting the impairment in sequence knowledge. This explanation does not presume superior syntactic capability by elderly subjects (in fact, the evidence is to the contrary), only greater reliance on a particular repository of knowledge than in the young.

Grammatical Morphology

Grammatical morphology refers to the use of words (free grammatical morphemes [e.g., articles, auxiliary verbs, conjunctions, and some prepositions]) and suffixes (bound grammatical morphemes [e.g., affixes specifying case, number, or tense]), the role of which appears to be primarily grammatical. The distinctiveness of these free grammatical morphemes and the apparently fundamental differences between them and major lexical items (nouns and main verbs) is further conveyed in the other terms by which they are known: functors, and closed-class words.

This way of classifying these words has a certain appeal if one posits the existence of a grammatical processor, such as that proposed by Chomsky and others. As we have noted, however, there has not been a successful effort to account for a grammatical processor in terms of known principles of neural network function. Therefore, in this section, we will continue the approach taken earlier, assuming that all aspects of language can be understood in terms of (1) the properties of distributed representations, (2) the mechanisms that manipulate distributed representations, and (3) the interface of the auto-associator network supporting semantic distributed representations with pattern associator networks that translate these semantic distributed representations into alternate forms (e.g. acoustic, orthographic, articulatory, and inscriptional) that are represented in networks supporting sequence knowledge. The essential currency of semantic distributed representations is meaning. Constraints on sequence in spoken language are provided primarily by implicit sequence rules latent in the connectivity of the acoustic-articulatory pattern associator network. We will attempt to approach the problem of grammatical morphology from the perspective of meaning constrained by sequence.

Articles

We have already noted (in the section on phrase structure rules) that representations of articles such as "the" probably are engaged, to some degree, by virtue of their incorporation in multi-word sequence knowledge. In addition, although articles have minimal meaning, they cannot be characterized as having no meaning whatsoever—they do indicate definite or indefinite. As modifiers in noun phrases, however, they differ from adjectives in that their meaning is contextual, whereas the meaning of adjectives is absolute. That is,

whether the article "a" or "the" is used depends on the preceding discourse; in contrast, the use of an adjective, such as "big," depends only on the attributes of the noun distributed representation to which it is linked. Thus, the use of articles depends, in part, on the maintenance of some working memory of what has already been said (i.e., sustained selective engagement of immediately preceding distributed concept representations and their relationship to each other). To the extent that working memory (selective engagement) mechanisms are defective, we might expect the impetus to article use from this source to be reduced. In English-speaking subjects with Broca's aphasia, as we have noted, some evidence of such a defect exists. As predicted by our hypothesis of defective selective engagement, these subjects tend to omit articles (agrammatism). In other languages (e.g., German), articles are marked for case, gender, and number—additional meaningful information that derives from the semantic representation of the nouns with which they are associated. Apparently because of these additional contributors to engagement of article representations, German subjects with Broca's aphasia are much more likely to produce incorrect articles (para-grammatisms) than to omit articles (Bates, Friederici, & Wulfeck, 1987); these substitutions can be viewed as the equivalent of syllabic sequence errors.

The essential lesion for producing agrammatism in spontaneous language appears to involve dominant postcentral perisylvian cortex (Nadeau, 1988). If our hypothesis regarding the contextual and, hence, working memory dependence of article use is correct, however, we should see some evidence of article omission in English speakers with dominant frontal lobe convexity cortex lesions. The fact that subjects with frontal lesions with sparing of postcentral perisylvian cortex are not conspicuously agrammatical may reflect two things: (1) that frontal systems engaged in working memory processes underlying article use are highly distributed, and (2) that frontal lesions spare the neural network representation of multi-word sequence knowledge (e.g., phrase structure rules). Thus, a modest lesion in postcentral perisylvian cortex may produce agrammatism (Kolk & Friederici, 1985), both because it is at the point where frontal projections converge on the pattern associator networks producing language output and because it is the locus of relevant sequence knowledge.

Auxiliary Verbs

Four attributes of auxiliary verbs (e.g., "The boy <u>was</u> fishing") might make them particularly prone to omission by subjects with Broca's aphasia given the model we have been considering. First, they are linked to the main verb. We have reasoned that main verbs function by simultaneously reciprocally modifying and linking as many as three distributed representations corresponding to the verb arguments in the sentence, a process particularly demanding of selective engagement mechanisms. Although auxiliary verbs have been consigned to the class of functors, in their use they typically act like main verbs in an adjectival way to modify distributed concept representations. For example, consider the two sentences "Mary hides the candy" and "Mary had hidden the candy." In the first, Mary is in motion, busily secreting the candy in an obscure place. In the second, Mary is static, but she has the attribute of responsibility for the current state of the candy. In the first, the candy is being carried about; in the second, the candy is still. We have already identified this process of volitional modification of distributed concept representations as one requiring frontal systems, which are consistently impaired in subjects with Broca's aphasia.

Second, the purpose of an auxiliary verb often is to convey tense. Frontal systems may provide the chief substrate for the neural instantiation of the time concept by virtue of their primary role in planning. Time-tagging of memories is impaired in subjects with frontal lobe lesions. Third, auxiliary verbs often are used only to reconcile the tense of the sentence with the tense of the preceding narrative, such as "She has a headache now. She has been having headaches for six months." That is, the inclusion and choice of auxiliary verbs are based, like those of articles, on narrative context and, hence, on working memory. Finally, auxiliary verbs may be linked to main verbs within the domain of sequence knowledge. The fact that the neural mechanisms underlying all four of these are impaired in subjects with Broca's aphasia may account for the tendency of these subjects to omit these words.

Articles and Auxiliary Verbs as Syntactic Elements

Some circumstances exist in which articles and auxiliary verbs appear to play a truly syntactic role, in which case the knowledge that supports them could be characterized as lexical-syntactic. Consider first the two dative sentences: (1) "The teacher showed the parents the student's desk," and (2) "The teacher showed the parent's student the desk." Here, the placement of the article "the" and the possessive "-'s" is critical to the meaning of the sentence. In passive-voice sentences, the presence of the "was . . . by" combination is equally essential to the meaning of the sentence.

Prepositions

Although many types of prepositions exist, we will focus only on locative prepositions (e.g., "The book is *on* the table"). These words strongly resemble main verbs in that they are the product of reciprocal alterations in the distributed representations of the concepts underlying the nouns on which they operate, coupled with linkage of these noun concepts. On this basis alone, we might expect them to be differentially affected by brain lesions that impair the selective engagement processes necessary for this to happen, as in the case of verbs.

Pronouns

Because they derive their meaning only through reference to antecedent nouns, pronouns depend on sustained engagement (working memory) of the noun representations that have been used recently. Again, to the extent that such sustained selective engagement mechanisms are impaired, one would expect defective use of pronouns. Indeed, this is the case in subjects with Broca's aphasia. By contrast, people with aphasia resulting from more posterior lesions, which leave frontally mediated selective engagement mechanisms intact, use pronouns to excess as a device to deal with their problems with lexical-semantic access.

Grammar: A Synthesis

Lexical-semantic function is based primarily on three domains of knowledge: semantic, sequence, and the pattern associators linking semantic and sequence knowledge, which provide the basis for the phonologic lexicons. In addition, it may require frontal systems involved in selective engagement (working memory) and frontal systems involved in manipulation of distributed concept representations to volitionally modify distributed concept representations corresponding to nouns.

Grammatical expression demands:

1. An elaboration of sequence knowledge to the extent that word stems may attach free-standing and bound grammatical morphemes and multi-word sequences are governed by phrase structure rules.
2. Engagement and reciprocal modification of two or more distributed concept representations employing procedures that correspond to rules of verb argument structure, further modified in a way that will support engagement of modifying auxiliary verbs.
3. Engagement by the super-distributed concept representations that instantiate verb argument structure of phonologic sequences in the acoustic-articulatory motor pattern associator that will instantiate the lexical form of the verb, with or without auxiliaries.
4. Engagement by certain super-distributed concept representations of articles and auxiliary verbs that are essential to syntax and can usefully be viewed as lexical-syntactic in nature.
5. The operation of volitional selective engagement mechanisms that will support the working memory of the modified distributed concept representations currently in play as well as recent modified representations, the recall of which is essential to correct production of articles, pronouns, and some auxiliary verbs.

Because all of the systems supporting these various aspects of grammatical function impose constraints, the process of sentence production involves parallel constraint satisfaction, a particular strength of PDP systems (Nadeau, 2000).

In this conceptualization, anomia for nouns reflects a breakdown in semantic or lexical-semantic knowledge. Curiously, difficulty modifying nouns (e.g., with adjectives) could be caused, in part, by a breakdown in syntactic function, because it also involves volitional modification of distributed concept representations. Anomia for verbs may reflect, in part, a form of breakdown in lexical-semantic knowledge in which super-distributed representations fail to elicit a pattern of activity in articulatory motor representations corresponding to the spoken form of the verb. Impaired ability to generate the super-distributed concept representations that are essential to verb production, however, also may cause difficulty with verb production as well as violation of rules of verb argument structure. Even when syntactically impaired subjects produce a relatively normal number of verbs, their verb use tends to ignore argument structure (Thompson, Shapiro, Kiran, & Sobecks, 1997). The production of articles and auxiliary verbs usually depends, in part, on the integrity of sequence knowledge but also on capacity for further, often subtle refinement of distributed or super-distributed concept representations and the engagement of working memory of recent sentences spoken or heard.

These general principles will apply to all languages. Languages differ, however, in the degree to which they rely on particular domains of knowledge, the specific content of these domains of knowledge, and the particular acquired skills in distributed concept manipulation.

MEMORY

Any behavioral therapy—language therapy included—involves the addition of new knowledge to the brain to replace that lost as a result of brain injury or disease. Because the properties of the neural systems that incorporate new knowledge have major implications for the therapeutic strategies employed in presenting that information, we will address this topic in some detail.

Language processes explicitly involve two well-known types of memory, procedural and declarative (Squire & Knowlton, 2000), and may involve other as-yet-unrecognized types of memory.

Procedural Memory

Procedural memories, often referred to as skill memories, are acquired incrementally by the neural systems representing the skills as they are practiced. For example, skill in playing tennis is enhanced gradually through extended practice as connectivity in the premotor and motor cortices, basal ganglia, cerebellum, brain stem, and spinal motor systems is incrementally modified. In language, the neural network knowledge that enables translation of continuous incoming sound into the acoustic representation of phonemes, which are discrete (i.e., not continuous), probably represents a

form of procedural knowledge. By the same token, the neural network knowledge that enables the translation of the articulatory representation of phonemes, which also are discrete, into continuous programs of movement involving pharyngeal and respiratory musculature also probably represents a form of procedural knowledge. It also seems likely that knowledge of the phonemic sequence repertoire of a given language is procedural, at least insofar as this knowledge is actually used in speech. For example, subjects with amnesia resulting from mesial temporal lobe lesions are not impaired in learning artificial "grammars" characterized by rule-bound letter strings (Squire & Knowlton, 2000). The development of phonologic awareness—that is, awareness of the discrete phoneme structure of words—may correspond to the addition of a declarative form of this knowledge.

Declarative Memory

Declarative memories, or memories for discrete facts, are acquired all at once in approximately 1 second in a process that is thought to involve fast Hebbian learning (see footnote 18) within Ammon's horn (the "cornu Ammonis") of the hippocampus (Alvarez & Squire, 1994; McClelland, McNaughton, & O'Reilly, 1995; Rolls & Treves, 1998; Squire & Zola-Morgan, 1991). Subsequently, some fairly rapid decay occurs, even in normal individuals.

This nearly instantaneous establishment of new connections between active neurons within the hippocampus serves to close long loops linking neural networks in the cerebral cortex. Cerebral association cortices project to the parahippocampal gyrus and perirhinal cortex, which, in turn, project to the entorhinal cortex and then to the dentate gyrus of the hippocampus. Dentate neurons project to the pyramidal neurons in the cornu Ammonis (CA3 and CA1 fields) of the hippocampus. The pyramidal neurons then project via the subiculum to the entorhinal cortex, which then projects back to cerebral association cortices. These circuitous new connections instantiate new knowledge. Initially, this new knowledge constitutes episodic memory in that it is memory of a particular aspect of a particular event at a particular place and time. Eventually, to one extent or another, this new knowledge may be incorporated into neural network connectivity in the cerebral cortex in a process referred to as consolidation. The process of declarative memory consolidation is not completely understood and currently is somewhat controversial. It appears that memories most likely are incorporated into cortical network connectivity to the extent they share features with knowledge already represented in the cortex. In this process of consolidation, the hippocampus appears to serve as a teacher to the cortex, repeatedly subjecting the cortex to patterns of activation congruent with the new information the hippocampus has incorporated. Growing evidence suggests that this process occurs during sleep (Power, 2004). If this theory of consolidation is correct, then it follows that memories that cannot be readily incorporated into the cortex, because they share few features with existent cortical knowledge, will remain permanently dependent on connections within the hippocampus and its immediately adjacent neural structures. This appears to be the case: Autobiographical memories generally share few features with knowledge represented in the cortex (they represent knowledge of particular places and times that are of only personal significance), and autobiographical memories are highly susceptible to disruption by lesions of the hippocampus and its associated structures.

It currently is thought that the hippocampal system is required, because in neural network simulations, the sustained presentation of new information to networks results in replacement of old knowledge already represented in the network by the new knowledge; in other words, catastrophic degradation of the old information occurs (McClelland et al., 1995; McCloskey & Cohen, 1989). If presentation of new information is interleaved with rehearsal of the old information, however, then a network is capable of instantiating both old and new knowledge simultaneously. It is thought that the hippocampal system provides the brain with a means to circumvent this impasse: It serves both as a repository of newly acquired declarative knowledge and as a teacher to the cortex that, during sleep, serves to interleave the new knowledge with rehearsal of old, related knowledge. The new knowledge is added gradually to the old knowledge, and because the changes in neural connections are made incrementally and the new is interleaved with the old, catastrophic degradation of old knowledge does not occur.

Lexical-Semantic Memory

In our discussion so far, we have suggested that knowledge underlying translation of sound sequences into phonemic acoustic representations, knowledge underlying translation of phonemic articulatory representations into motor sequences, and phonologic sequence knowledge all may constitute varieties of procedural memory. In contrast, knowledge of concepts, by virtue of being discrete and consciously accessible, is prototypic declarative knowledge. What about knowledge linking distributed concept representations to phonemic sequences or to articulatory or acoustic representations? This, the basis for lexical-semantic knowledge, spans the declarative-procedural divide. Is this knowledge declarative or procedural?

A famous paper by Vargha-Khadem and colleagues (1997) provides some hints. They reported three subjects who, early in life, had experienced severe bilateral damage to the hippocampus as a result of anoxic insults. During subsequent intensive neuropsychological testing, these subjects demonstrated expectable severe deficits in episodic memory acquisition. All three, however, had acquired language function that appeared to be nearly normal. There had been similar reports

of this phenomenon in previous case studies, but none nearly as compelling as the paper by Vargha-Khadem and colleagues. The nearly normal language function and the remarkably good general knowledge acquisition of these subjects, in conjunction with the results of studies in nonhuman primates, suggested to the authors that two separate declarative memory acquisition systems exist: one resident in the hippocampus that is essential to acquisition of episodic memories, and one in entorhinal/perirhinal cortex (relatively spared in the three subjects reported) that suffices for declarative semantic memory acquisition. This hypothesis remains to be fully tested. Furthermore, the evidence that the hippocampus and adjacent cortices are anatomically and functionally organized as a cascade system, not a binary system (McClelland et al., 1995; Rolls & Treves, 1998), as discussed in an earlier section, weighs strongly against this interpretation.

The importance of this issue for speech-language therapy is that lexical-semantic dysfunction constitutes one of the most common and disabling aspects of aphasia. Direct approaches to this problem—that is, "naming" therapies—tend to be extraordinarily inefficient. The observations of Vargha-Khadem and colleagues raise the possibility of a completely different declarative memory–like brain mechanism underlying the acquisition of lexical-semantic knowledge. If only we better understood this principle, we might be able to substantially improve the efficiency of naming therapies. The observations of Vargha-Khadem and colleagues also suggest that naming therapies might be successful even in subjects with substantial hippocampal dysfunction (e.g., because of traumatic brain injury).

Properties of Procedural and Declarative Memory Systems Relevant to Therapy for Aphasia

Both procedural and declarative memory systems have characteristic strengths and weaknesses relevant to their recruitment in therapy for aphasia. One major advantage of procedural knowledge underlying language is that it generalizes widely. For example, the acquisition of skills in decoding of sound sequences into phonemic acoustic representations (rarely a source of difficulty), of skills in translating phonemic articulatory representations into motor programs, and of a critical mass of phonemic sequence knowledge will provide the procedural knowledge basis for decoding and producing all words in the native vocabulary. Acquisition of certain skills in manipulating distributed concept representations should generalize to all distributed concept representations susceptible to those manipulations. A second major advantage is that achieving an adequate foundation of procedural language skills potentially gives the subject the tools to continue growth of language capacity on his or her own in the course of routine conversation—in direct analogy to the normal process of language acquisition in early childhood. We will discuss some specific examples of such therapies later in this chapter.

The major disadvantage of procedural knowledge acquisition is that it is incremental; therefore, the ultimate development of a useful level of skill will require extensive practice. Specific domains of procedural memory underlying language also pose their own particular problems. Successful procedural linguistic memory acquisition in the domain of phonologic knowledge would only build the phonemic/articulatory foundation for acquisition of lexical-semantic knowledge. The actual links between distributed concept representations (semantic knowledge) and phonemic/articulatory sequences that would enable naming would still have to be developed, either through further therapy or by the subject in the course of daily use of language. Fortunately, even in the context of extensive brain damage, the language brain likely is not a tabula rasa: There exist extensive remnants of previous knowledge (Plaut, 1996), and the therapist's task is to develop these remnants until they reach the critical mass needed for daily spoken communication. Acquisition of grammatical skills in distributed concept manipulation may require such extensive practice that only a very limited repertoire of such skills can be trained.

The advantage of declarative knowledge underlying language is that it can potentially be acquired all at once, but two major disadvantages also exist. First, acquisition of declarative memory is considerably less than 100% efficient in normal subjects (else all attentive students would score 100% on tests of knowledge), and its efficiency drops substantially in the face of extensive damage to cortices supporting declarative memories. Second, the potential for generalization is limited. This limitation is most serious for lexical-semantic knowledge, because little relationship exists between the meaning of a word and its sound: When you have learned one word, you have learned one word. Thus, for any therapeutic strategy that depends on acquisition of lexical-semantic knowledge to achieve practical value, the learning process must be extended to incorporate a full, useful working vocabulary for the subject—something that, remarkably, has been achieved, but only in a very unusual individual (Basso, 2003). The number of words that would be necessary for this, the demographic and cultural modifications in this vocabulary that would be needed, and the practical means for training subjects in this extended vocabulary are largely unknown. The potential for generalization of semantic knowledge may be considerably greater, because many concepts share features and, to the extent that they share features, training of one concept may benefit the ability to generate a distributed representation of another concept. We have not remotely plumbed all the possibilities for engaging shared semantic features to best advantage in therapy for aphasia.

GENERALIZATION

Generalization is the process by which the effects of therapy extend to material or circumstances not explicitly taught during speech-language therapy sessions. Generalization is essential if speech-language therapy is to have an important impact on the daily communicative lives of subjects. To date, however, evidence from clinical trials has only provided glimpses of generalization effects, and the mechanisms remain poorly understood. In the preceding section on memory, we introduced the concept of generalization in several specific contexts. In this section, we briefly consider the full spectrum of mechanisms that might underlie generalization. Seven (listed in Table 26–2) are posited:

1. **Intrinsic** Application of knowledge acquired in therapy (e.g., semantic features, phonologic sequences, phonetic sounds, or syntactic techniques) to other knowledge that shares these features or sequences or to situations that allow application of the acquired techniques (Kiran & Thompson, 2003; Thompson et al., 2003; Wambaugh, Kalinyak-Fliszar, West, & Doyle, 1998; Weinrich, Whelton, Cox, & McCall, 1997). We touched on this principle in the section on memory. Because knowledge gained about phonetics, phonologic sequences, and syntactic techniques can, in principle, be applied regardless of the subject of communication, therapies that develop this knowledge have the potential for extensive generalization. On the other hand, generalization from semantic therapy will be limited to concepts that share semantic features with the concepts actually trained. These various types of generalization stem directly from the knowledge gained in therapy.

2. **Cross-function** Development of knowledge during therapy that can be applied to multiple tasks. For example, semantic therapy could benefit oral word production, written word production, oral word comprehension, and written word comprehension, because all four capacities involve pattern associator networks linked to association cortices supporting concept representations (in traditional terms, all four capacities depend on the integrity of the semantic field).

3. **Extrinsic** Development during therapy of a knowledge acquisition/skill learning technique that subjects with motivation—and who are capable of engaging motivation to employ the technique—can use during and outside of therapy to rebuild language function (e.g., semantic therapy, phonologic sequence therapy, or syntactic therapy). Here, it is not the substantive material learned in therapy that is crucial to ongoing progress outside of therapy (although a critical mass of substantive knowledge may be necessary)—it is the acquisition of a therapeutic technique that the subject, perhaps with help from family, can continue to apply in the months and years outside of therapy. (This will be further elucidated in some of the specific examples that are discussed in the section on specific rehabilitative strategies.) For

TABLE 26–2

Mechanisms of Generalization

Mechanism	Description
Intrinsic	Application of knowledge acquired in therapy (e.g., semantic features, phonologic sequences, phonetic sounds, and syntactic techniques) to other knowledge that shares these features or sequences or to situations that allow application of the acquired techniques.
Cross-function	Development of knowledge during therapy (e.g., semantic) that can be applied to multiple functions (e.g., comprehension and production) involving verbal and orthographic modalities, because all these functions depend on the integrity of the core domain (in this case, semantics).
Extrinsic	Development during therapy of a knowledge acquisition/skill learning technique that subjects with motivation, and who are capable of engaging motivation to employ the technique, can use during and outside of therapy to rebuild language function.
Mechanistic	Development of a nonlinguistic brain resource (e.g., working memory), ability to endogenously generate distributed concept representations, or intentional bias to use language that is essential to language function.
Substrate mediated	Development of the critical mass of language skill needed to enable conversation at home and elsewhere and, thereby, further the therapeutic process.
Contextual	Acquisition of knowledge, predominantly contextual, during speech-language therapy that aids in retrieval of knowledge outside of therapy by establishing additional commonality between the training situation and the retrieval situation.
Socially mediated	Change in the perception of the subject and his or her family regarding his or her role in the family unit, with the adoption of a new/revised role that subsumes more expectation of speech, more pressure to speak, and greater language production.

example, a subject who has received semantic therapy could continue to use the techniques acquired during therapy for systematically identifying the semantic attributes of concepts, both those that can be named and those that cannot, provided that he or she has the motivation and the capacity for translating motivation into action, thereby continuing to develop the semantic field long after the conclusion of therapy. Even lexical-semantic therapy can make use of this generalization mechanism, as demonstrated by Basso (2003): Exceptionally capable subjects can be given the guidance and techniques to practice naming of the thousands of words needed to communicate in daily life. For extrinsic generalization to occur, subjects must be motivated to continue to use therapeutic techniques learned during therapy after completion of therapy, and they must have the brain mechanisms (which presumably depend, in part, on frontal systems) to translate this motivation into effective post-therapeutic practice. We have preliminary evidence from a study of semantic therapy that only subjects who demonstrate intact frontal function show widespread generalization that also impacts daily communicative behavior (Nadeau & Kendall, 2006).

4. **Mechanistic** Training of a key brain resource, essential to language processing but not fundamentally linguistic, that enables improvement in language function. Three subtypes can be postulated:

a. Development of working memory capacity needed for language, as discussed, is likely to be particularly important for normal grammatical function, in which multiple distributed concept representations need to be maintained simultaneously for sufficient time for appropriate modifications to be made, and some grammatical functions dependent on reference (e.g., articles, auxiliary verbs, or pronouns) require some recollection of what has recently been said, some of which may be represented as working memory.

b. Development of the ability to endogenously generate distributed concept representations, which is most impaired in adynamic aphasia[10] (Gold et al., 1997), may be the same as 4.a. The differences between adynamic aphasia (in which there is difficulty generating the representations) and Broca's aphasia (in which there appears to be particular difficulty in

---

[10] Subjects with adynamic aphasia characteristically are extremely non-fluent in internally generated language and, in extreme cases, may be incapable of more than occasional single-word production. In picture description tasks, however, they may perform almost normally. This suggests that when called on to generate their own distributed concept representations, they have great difficulty, but when distributed concept representations are "planted" in their brain by showing them a picture, they are capable of substantially normal language production.

modifying and manipulating the representations), however, suggest an important difference.

   c. Development of a new intentional bias that favors language use over either non-use or gestural communication, the cardinal example being constraint-induced language therapy (Maher et al., 2003; Meinzer, Djundja, Barthel, Elbert, & Rockstroh, 2005; Pulvermüller et al., 2001). The idea here is that because of frustration with language impairment that is particularly severe in the months immediately following stroke, patients develop an intentional habit of minimal effort to communicate or a habit that leads to alternative communicative modes, such as gesture. This intentional bias then persists despite substantial improvement in capacity for language and, thereby, actually inhibits linguistic communication in the long run. Training that alters the bias can enable the subject to take full advantage of partially recovered language function. There may be other mechanisms at play in mediating the effects of constraint-induced language therapy (e.g., see 7 below), but this particular one (i.e., modification of intentional bias) is the one that has motivated the development of this therapy and appears to be most responsible for the gains associated with the previously developed constraint-induced movement therapy.

5. **Substrate mediated** Development of the critical mass of language skill needed to enable conversation at home and elsewhere and, thereby, further the therapeutic process. It probably is necessary to enable intrinsic and extrinsic generalization mechanisms to operate. For example, below we will discuss our experience in using training in phonemic awareness, phoneme production, and phonologic sequence knowledge to ameliorate impairment of lexical access in aphasia. The therapy does not include training in the ability to link phonemic sequences to concepts—this must occur outside the treatment session. We presume that it can only occur if subjects have acquired a repertoire of phoneme sequence knowledge that covers most words encountered in their daily communication. Under these circumstances, the production of most words, with or without caregiver help, will provide an opportunity for strengthening connectivity between concept representations and corresponding phonemic sequences.

6. **Contextual** Acquisition of knowledge, predominantly contextual, during speech-language therapy that aids retrieval of knowledge outside of therapy (detailed in the next section). In essence, the principle is that when we learn, the knowledge acquired includes not only the intended material but also knowledge about the context. This knowledge may include attributes of other stimuli introduced during a treatment session. It also may include more general attributes of the situation (e.g., where the treatment was provided, characteristics of the treatment room and the therapist, who else was present, the mood of the participant, participant attitudes to the stroke experience and associated disability, and the strategies the participant brings to therapy). The greater the resemblance between context in the learning environment and context in the retrieval environment, the higher the likelihood of success in retrieval. Most of us have encountered the negative effects of absence of contextual similarity when we try to remember the name of a professional acquaintance during a chance encounter outside our professional environment.

7. **Socially mediated** Change in the perception of the subject and her or his family regarding his or her role in the family unit, with the adoption of a new/revised role that subsumes more expectation of speech, more pressure to speak, and greater language production (Blonder, 2000). As Blonder has shown, the alterations in lives produced by aphasia may be profound, and even if patients with stroke do not become socially isolated, the value of language facility may be fundamentally reduced. Thus, to varying degrees, restoration of daily communicative ability may require some restoration of the social context that will promote language use as an instrumental measure.

TEMPORAL SPACING, STRUCTURE, AND CONTEXT, STIMULUS PROPERTIES, AND FEEDBACK DURING THERAPY

The focus of clinical research on treatment of aphasia has overwhelmingly been on the substance of that treatment, and very little attention has been devoted to factors that might influence the acquisition of knowledge by the brain during therapy and the retention of that knowledge after the conclusion of therapy. Because, in the subject with chronic stroke, therapy for aphasia is likely to produce its effects by engaging normal learning mechanisms, the educational psychology literature can provide evidence that may be useful in the treatment of aphasia. The discoveries in this research can be related, in a cogent way, to brain structure and function. We will focus on three topics: (1) the distribution of aphasia treatment over time, (2) the structure and context of therapy for aphasia, and (3) feedback during treatment.

Distribution of Aphasia Treatment over Time

Condensed Versus Distributed Practice

The predominant focus in neurorehabilitation in general has been on knowledge or skill acquisition—in other words, the difference between performance at the end of treatment and performance at baseline. Most, however, would agree that the real measure of treatment efficacy is the knowledge and skills acquired during treatment that the subject retains through the months and years after the conclusion of treatment, which are likely to be considerably less than those acquired by the end of treatment. Only changes retained by the brain over the long run can have a lasting impact on daily performance, activity, participation, and quality of life. This suggests that our primary focus in treatment studies should be on long-term outcome—that is, the difference between performance long after the conclusion of treatment and performance at baseline—rather than on acquisition. It also poses the challenge of understanding the neural mechanisms underlying the relationship between retention and acquisition. The degree to which practice is more or less temporally condensed is very much germane to this issue.

"Massed practice" traditionally is defined as continuous practice conducted over a single day in which the stimuli or skills to be remembered are presented without any intervening irrelevant stimuli or activities. "Distributed practice" traditionally is defined as practice that is broken up into two or more sessions, each separated by an interlude of minutes, hours, or days, or a single session in which repetitions of target stimuli are separated by one or more nontarget stimuli. In speech-language therapy, target stimulus repetitions typically are separated by many intervening, nontarget stimuli, and the limits of human endurance dictate that sessions be conducted over multiple days. Thus, no speech-language therapy conforms to traditional definitions of massed practice, and our major focus here will be on evidence bearing on the impact of more or less temporally distributed therapy.

Studies of constraint-induced movement therapy for upper extremity paresis following stroke may have cultivated the notion that the case for large amounts of highly condensed practice, by virtue of the dramatic impact on outcome measures, has largely been proven (Taub, Uswatte, & Pidikiti, 1999; Taub et al., 2006). Studies have consistently demonstrated, however, a dramatic loss of constraint-induced movement therapy–associated gains over the weeks and months following treatment. Relatively little attention has been devoted to treatments after constraint-induced movement therapy that might help to sustain gains, and to our knowledge, no study has been conducted regarding the relative impact of more versus less distributed constraint-induced movement therapy schedules on long-term retention. Thus, treatment schedule density remains a matter of great scientific and clinical interest in all fields of rehabilitation, and no study that we are aware of provides definitive answers.

Studies contrasting the relative impact of massed practice and distributed practice on learning rate and knowledge retention date back to 1885 (Dempster, 1996; Donovan & Radosevich, 1999; Ebbinghaus, 1885). Literally hundreds of investigations have been conducted involving a wide range of knowledge and skill types. With very few exceptions, distributed practice has been found to be superior to massed

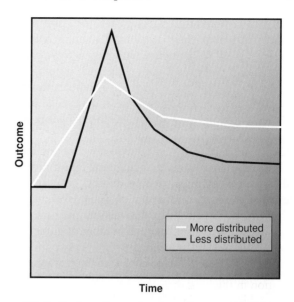

Figure 26–7. Cartoon illustrating the trajectory of skill/knowledge as a function of time with more and less condensed learning regimens. More condensed (less distributed) regimens commonly achieve greater acquisition of knowledge and skill by the end of training, but this is then followed by a higher rate of loss, with the net result that long-term retention typically is greater with less condensed (more distributed) regimens.

practice in its effects on knowledge retention, whether the training involves factual knowledge, simple motor skills, or more complex tasks involving acquisition of factual knowledge, advanced motor skills, and the development of strategies. This superiority has come to be known as the "spacing effect." Often, recall is greater at the end of the acquisition phase of more condensed training than it is after more distributed training. This superior acquisition efficacy is offset by relatively greater forgetting, however, such that long-term retention usually ends up being greater with more distributed training (Fig. 26–7).

Although these studies provide strong evidence for the superiority of modest temporal distribution of short-duration task practice on retention of knowledge and skill, they do not provide data regarding training, such as rehabilitation therapy, that must be sustained over days, weeks, or months. Unfortunately, very few studies have directly compared the impact of different degrees of distribution of practice over these more extended periods of time. Pyle (1913) compared the impact of an addition drill given to third-grade students twice a day for 5 days with the same drill given once a day for 10 days. The more distributed drill was more effective. Murphy (1916) found that training schoolgirls in a left-handed javelin throw produced a higher rate of learning if done one or three times weekly than if done daily. Shea, Lai, Black, & Park (2000) studied training on two tasks, a dynamic balance task and a calibrated sequential key-press timing task; for both tasks, training over 2 or 3 days proved to be more efficacious than distributed training over 1 day. Shebilske, Goettl, Corrington, and Day (1999) compared training distributed over 2 days with equal training distributed over 10 days on Space Fortress, a complex task involving acquisition of factual knowledge, motor skills, and strategy. Subjects trained over 10 days performed better on both acquisition and retention measures. Childers and Tomasello (2002) trained 2-year-old children on novel nouns and verbs (i.e., lexical-semantic training bridging a declarative-procedural divide). They found that production performance was better when training was distributed over 4 days compared to 1, 2, or 3 days. Two-day gaps between training sessions did not impair performance, but gaps between training sessions of 5 or 10 days were associated with poorer performance. Bahrick and Phelps (1987) found that among subjects trained on 50 English-Spanish word pairs tested 8 years later, recall was 15% among those trained with a 30-day intersession training schedule, 8% among those on a 1-day intersession interval, and 6% among those with no spacing between sessions. Baddeley and Longman (1978) trained British postal workers to type. Learning was more effective (as defined by retention up to 9 months later) when training was given 1 hour per day over 60 days than when given in two 2-hour sessions per day over 15 days. The task involves training of typographical-semantic knowledge, which is directly analogous to lexical-semantic knowledge in that it involves linking declarative knowledge to procedural knowledge. These various studies suggest that when training must be sustained over extended periods of time, very substantial degrees of temporal distribution of practice may yield superior long-term retention of knowledge and skill.

No studies provide definitive data regarding the impact of degree of distribution on training programs like speech-language therapy that involve intensive, cumulative treatment conducted up to hours at a time over many days, nor to our knowledge have any studies examined the effect of differing degrees of distribution of speech-language therapy. A recent review concluded that more concentrated therapy probably was superior, but degree of distribution was confounded with dose (shorter studies typically involved more hours of therapy) (Bhogal, Teasell, & Speechley, 2003). Thus, both studies of the impact of variable distribution of speech-language therapy over days as a function of domain of knowledge being trained as well as studies of the distribution of therapy within day are needed.

Potential Mechanisms Underling the Spacing Effect

Many theories have been offered to account for the relative superiority of distributed practice (Greene, 1989; Hintzman, 1974; Shebilske et al., 1999). Although no theory has been shown to account for all experimental results, including both declarative and procedural knowledge, and to fully accommo-

date our current understanding of the neurobiologic bases of memory, the component-levels theory of Glenberg (Glenberg, 1979; Glenberg & Lehmann, 1980) comes closest. Glenberg considered only declarative memory experiments, his own and other's, largely involving free recall of words from word lists and cued recall from word pair learning tasks. This work finds it origins in encoding variability theory (Bower, 1972; Estes, 1955; Melton, 1970). Three principles are essential to his theory. First, in a conceptualization that fully anticipates current concepts of episodic memory, Glenberg posited that when an item to be remembered is learned, three attributes of that item are encoded: (1) its *semantic attributes*; (2) attributes of the neighboring task stimuli (e.g., the neighboring words in the word list), within which it is embedded, as they are perceived and organized by the subject (*structural context*); and (3) the *general context* of the experiment (e.g., the testing environment, the cognitive and affective state and degree of fatigue of the subject, and in complex tasks, the inter-trial reminiscence of salient stimuli and strategy formation). General and structural context exert their impact by modifying the semantic representation. Thus, spacing effects in the declarative domain are attenuated with stimuli being processed only at more superficial levels (e.g., perceptual) (Craik & Lockhart, 1972). Second, a repetition is potentially effective to the degree that the second presentation allows the storage of information distinct from that stored at the first presentation. In massed practice, general and structural context are very nearly identical for every presentation of the item to be remembered. Distributed presentations generally produce differences in general and structural context. Third, the realization of the potential effect of repetition is controlled by the conditions at the time of the memory test—that is, the retrieval environment (i.e., *the spacing effect reflects a storage-retrieval context interaction effect*). Repetition will contribute to recall to the extent that structural and general context attributes associated with *each* presentation of the item to be remembered add together to increase the likelihood that some of these same attributes will be present in the recall environment, thereby increasing the probability of recall. If structural and general context are nearly identical, as in massed practice, repetition confers minimal advantage. If structural and general context differ but recall is requested shortly after the item is repeated, no spacing effect will occur, both because the general context at the time of repetition and at the time of recall are similar and because both are different from the general context at the time of the first presentation of the item (thereby largely eliminating its contribution to recall). Glenberg and Lehmann (1980) have shown that these principles apply not just to learning studies/retention probes that occur within a single day but also to learning epochs that take place a week apart with tests for retention a week later. Studies by Glenberg and others support a proportionality rule: When the retention interval is short relative to spacing intervals, performance is inversely related to spacing, and when the retention interval is long relative to spacing intervals, performance is directly related to spacing—hence the value of highly distributed training on long-term retention.

It seems likely that treatment of aphasia after stroke engages normal learning mechanisms, both declarative and procedural, even as the relative contributions of each of these two learning mechanisms to training effects in various types of therapy for various types of impairment remain uncertain. Therefore, it is worth asking whether the principles proposed by Glenberg to account for the spacing effect in declarative learning might apply to procedural learning as well. Very little data regarding this are available. The most salient difference between declarative and procedural memory that we need to contend with is that general context attributes are unlikely to be encoded as part of the procedural memory trace (because the hippocampus is not involved). Thus, there likely will be no benefit from the long spacing intervals that enhance the likelihood of change in general context attributes, a major contributor to spacing effects on declarative memory recall. Only structural context attributes are important to the spacing effect on procedural memory retention. Thus, if a particular skill to be learned can be repeated within each one of a full spectrum of *skill contexts* within a short period of time, there should be no advantage to distributing training over a longer period. Evidence suggests that procedural memory acquisition involves a consolidation phase that takes place over several hours (Brashers-Krug, Shadmehr, & Bizzi, 1996). A flurry of recent studies, however, has demonstrated a complex of further consolidative and re-consolidative processes that take place during sleep (Stickgold & Walker, 2005; Walker & Stickgold, 2004). Thus, distribution of procedural training could provide a relative advantage in retention, both because it provides a greater opportunity to train individual skills in a variety of action contexts and because it allows more occasions for sleep-associated consolidative processes to occur. The advantage of distributed over massed practice also can be seen in the superiority of "random" over blocked practice in skill learning (Schmidt & Bjork, 1992).

In the domain of procedural memory is an alternative, connectionist account for the superior retention of knowledge acquired through distributed practice (Sejinowski & Rosenberg, 1988). This account is compatible with the component-levels theory of Glenberg. A pattern associator network employing distributed representations in which extensive knowledge is already stored in its connections can readily, through massed practice, learn to achieve high performance on a particular new skill (e.g., converting a novel acoustic sequence into a novel articulatory motor sequence). When tested immediately after training, performance of the new skill will be excellent. When the network subsequently receives "refresher training" in its old knowledge repertoire, however, performance of the new skill will rapidly decline (catastrophic degradation) (McClelland et al., 1995). On the

other hand, with distributed practice, during which training in the new skill is interleaved with retraining of old skills, the new skill is retained. The explanation is this: With massed practice, connection strengths are altered in a relatively limited part of the network and in a way that supports the new skill at the expense of the old skills. With distributed practice, connection strengths are altered throughout the network in a way that optimizes encoding of attributes that both new and old skills have in common. Thus, distributed practice optimizes compatibility between new and old by distributing connection strength changes more widely through the network. This connectionist conceptualization can be viewed as the neural network embodiment of the structural context knowledge discussed above. The more widely disseminated instantiation of network knowledge of the new skill achieved with distributed practice enables better recall of the new skill under a variety of situations that do not exactly match the training situation. In a sense, with distributed practice, the network implicitly learns the rules underlying the new skill, whereas with massed practice, it learns the new skill by rote. Thus, this connectionist account also suggests that some distribution of procedural training may be superior to massed practice as traditionally defined.

Glenberg's theory also can be logically reconciled with current knowledge of the neurobiology of declarative (fact) memory acquisition. Declarative memory is acquired as episodic memory all at once, albeit with variable efficiency, through fast Hebbian learning in the hippocampus. Over time, to the extent that this knowledge has features in common with knowledge already represented in the cerebral cortex, it apparently is introduced gradually into cortical connectivity and, eventually, becomes hippocampally independent, a process referred to as "memory consolidation" (Alvarez & Squire, 1994; McClelland et al., 1995; Rolls & Treves, 1998; Squire & Zola-Morgan, 1991). Evidence is accumulating that the process of consolidation also occurs substantially during sleep (Stickgold & Walker, 2005; Walker & Stickgold, 2004). Thus, we can posit two mechanisms by which highly distributed training in declarative memory domains may enhance the likelihood of successful retrieval during retention testing: (1) It enhances the likelihood that structural and general context conditions at the time of test will share attributes with conditions at the time of learning, and (2) it increases the opportunity for memory consolidation (i.e., the conversion of episodic memory into semantic memory that is substantially independent of context effects). Because declarative memory acquisition is far less than 100% efficient, particularly in face of damaged cortical repositories for long-term memory, more paired exposure-consolidation events and more than one night of consolidation per exposure may achieve superior efficacy.

The spacing effect, reflected in the superiority of distributed over fully massed practice in inducing long-term memory, also has been observed in a number of relatively primitive organisms, such as the sea snail *Aplysia*, goldfish, *Drosophila*, crabs, a nudibranch, and honeybees (Sutton, Ide, Masters, & Carew, 2002). In many of these experimental models, the spacing effect appears to reflect the differential impact of spacing on molecular mechanisms of synaptic change, including induction of cAMP-response element–binding protein, MAP kinase, and subsequent RNA and protein synthesis. Presently, it seems unlikely that such mechanisms underlie the differential effects of more versus less distributed training over days in humans, but this possibility cannot be ruled out entirely.

The Spacing Effect: Summary

A large body of evidence regarding the psychology and neurobiology of learning, as well as connectionist work, strongly supports the superiority of more over less distributed practice in promoting long-term retention. This spacing effect appears to apply to both declarative and procedural memory retention, but for somewhat different reasons and in incompletely understood ways. Distribution of training that engages declarative (but not procedural) memory mechanisms provides the opportunity to benefit from variation in general context attributes during the course of training, and it takes full advantage of hippocampal consolidation processes that are known to continue for years. The emerging importance of brain processes occurring during sleep for memory consolidation, however, both declarative and procedural, could indicate that distribution effects will turn out to be just as important for procedural memory retention.

Very few studies have examined the spacing effect in subjects with brain damage, however, and their results have been inconclusive. A number of other factors need to be considered in this population as well. Hillary and colleagues (2003) found a significant spacing effect on a word list–learning task in subjects with traumatic brain injury. Hochhalter, Overmier, Gasper, Bakke, and Holub (2005) found no such effect on either a pill name or a nonverbal sequence–learning task in subjects with dementia. Subjects with brain injury typically have a heterogeneous mixes of deficits, variability in motivation and fatigability, and uneven support systems. The effect size of greater distribution of training thus may be too small to be of importance in the clinical population, and greater distribution may lead to greater long-term attenuation of gain than expected with less distributed practice. The potential advantages of more distributed practice may be outweighed by the effects of reduced concentration on therapy, loss of continuity, reduced practice between sessions, reduced involvement by caregivers, and reduced motivation. These factors may lead to a greater-than-expected disparity between outcomes at the end of the acquisition phase that mitigates the potential long-term advantage of more distributed practice. Only empirical studies can address these questions.

Structure and Context of Aphasia Therapy

In our preceding discussion of the spacing effect, we noted two major factors that might contribute to the relative advantage of more distributed training: (1) time for the evolution of neurobiologic processes, and (2) time for broadening of structural and general context. We have no good ideas for how to manipulate the neurobiologic processes. The broadening of structural and general context need not be left to time and accident, however; we could deliberately alter therapeutic programs in a way that will enhance structural and general context.

Structural context pertains to the content of individual therapy sessions. The spacing effect literature suggests that the richer and more variable the language contexts in a therapy session, the greater the variety of contexts in which any one fact or skill will be acquired and, therefore, the greater the likelihood of similarities between the language environment in one or more training sessions and the language environment at the time of recall, with an attendant increase in the probability of recall. We can therefore ask whether the typical current speech-language therapy session is as rich and varied as it could be, and whether we could achieve some benefits of the spacing effect by enhancing intra-session linguistic richness and variability without increasing the temporal distribution of therapy sessions.

General context pertains to the conditions of individual therapy sessions. The spacing effect literature suggests that the more variability in the general conditions in which individual therapy sessions are held, the greater will be the variety of conditions in which any one fact or skill is acquired and, therefore, the greater will be the likelihood of similarities between the therapy environment in one or more training sessions and the general environment at the time of recall, with an attendant increase in the probability of recall. We can therefore ask how much resemblance exists between the routine speech-language therapy environment and the environments in which the subject ultimately will be struggling day to day to use language to communicate. The physical environs, the people present, the mood of the subject, and strategizing by subject and caregivers between sessions all are factors to be considered. If greater similarity between general context conditions during therapy and during recall can be achieved, the need to distribute therapy over time possibly will be reduced at the same time that retention is enhanced. It also is worth noting that every successful recall by the subject that is overtly recognized by the subject and caregivers constitutes a continuation of the training process outside of therapy.

Stimulus Properties

More than 30 years ago, in a landmark paper, Craik and Lockhart (1972) argued from extensive experimental data that memory retention was strongly influenced by depth of processing of the material presented. For example, a subject who is asked to count vowels in each of a series of presented words is likely to exhibit far poorer recall of these words than if he or she is asked to make a judgment about the meaning of each word. The concepts elaborated in this chapter enable us to define depth of processing in neural network terms. Counting vowels would require a distributed representation of the orthographic form of the word in a relatively restricted part of visual association cortices. Making a judgment about the meaning of a word is more likely to engage the full, multi-component distributed representation of the word (Fig. 26–3). This would set the stage for closure of long-loop cortical–hippocampal–cortical loops involving association cortices throughout the brain, not just those involving a limited portion of visual association cortices. The much larger number of connections that are susceptible to alteration with deep processing may provide the entire basis for the superior retention of "deeply encoded" items. It also is possible, however, that certain connections, such as those to cortices supporting limbic and predicative representations, are particularly important to long-term retention.

These observations suggest that measures taken to assure multi-component distributed representations of stimuli presented during language therapy may enhance retention. Raymer and colleagues (2006) provided evidence in support of this thesis in a study of noun and verb naming treatment in nine subjects with aphasia. In nearly all the subjects, learning was markedly enhanced when picture presentation was accompanied by a pantomime of the use of the object or the motion of the verb and the subject imitated the gesture as he or she repeated the name.

Feedback during Treatment

In the preceding sections, we have presented evidence that *all* the stimuli to which a subject is exposed during a therapeutic session have the potential for altering neural network connectivity and, hence, for being remembered in some form. The therapeutic goal, however, is to assure that the stimuli targeted by the therapist are particularly well established in neural connectivity in a way that will maximize the potential for retrieval at a later time. Among the many stimuli to which a subject is exposed during therapy are those that we might classify as feedback. We define "feedback" as substantive information regarding performance provided by the therapist to the subject.

Feedback can be divided into two categories: knowledge of results, and knowledge of performance. Feedback about results consists of information provided to subjects regarding the correctness of a response at the operational level (e.g., the phoneme, word, sentence, or intonation actually produced). Such feedback might consist of responses such as "Your answer was correct" or "Your answer was incorrect; here is the correct answer." Feedback about performance

consists of information provided to subjects regarding attributes of their response that might help them to understand what was wrong with the response and what measures might be taken to improve it (Proctor & Dutta, 1995; Schmidt & Wrisberg, 2004). For example, in a lexical-semantic or semantic treatment program, the therapist might respond to an error with observations such as "The word you produced isn't exactly correct but it is related in meaning to (or it is in the same category as) the correct word" or "I think you responded too quickly and ended up just repeating your answer to the last question." In a phonologic treatment program, the therapist might seek to help subjects understand what components of the pharyngeal movement complex led to the error produced through the use of diagrams, mirrors, and palpation by subjects of their own lips and larynx. In a prosody treatment program, the therapist might show subjects the acoustic profile of their response (e.g., using Visipitch [Kay Elemetrics, Inc.]) to help the subject understand what attributes of his or her response were incorrect. Clearly, different therapies have different potential for the provision of feedback about results and performance, and motor therapies most readily lend themselves to feedback about performance (e.g., therapies for apraxia of speech or aprosodia). Any therapy in which there might be useful information in pattern of performance, however, such as semantic or syntactic therapy, might theoretically benefit from feedback about performance.

Knowledge of results generally has little potential for providing subjects with the insight regarding the causes of their errors that might engage them in the development of strategies to systematically correct them. Feedback about results provided to subjects one or more times later in a therapy session, however, or at subsequent sessions can serve to vary the structural and general context associated with that particular response and, thereby, contribute to retention, just as tests and detailed feedback about test performance can enhance retention of knowledge acquired in the classroom (via the spacing effect). Furthermore, if it is possible to provide subjects with graphic knowledge about the pattern of their responses over time, then with certain therapies this might help subjects to see a pattern in their errors and, thereby, develop a strategy for improving performance. This strategy will have the potential for directly enhancing future performance and, if encouraged, might become a useful general context attribute that may carry over to recall situations.

Knowledge of performance can benefit retention via all the mechanisms underlying the benefits of knowledge of results. In addition, it can help to focus subjects on the particular attributes of the performance that are contributing to error and to develop their own strategies, perhaps with the aid of counseling by the therapist (Proctor & Dutta, 1995; Schmidt & Wrisberg, 2004). Feedback about performance can be complicated, and considerable research will be needed to define optimal programs for individual subjects. If feedback is too complex or is presented inadequately, it may overwhelm the subject. If feedback is too focused, it may inhibit the subject from developing an understanding of the pattern of response that is leading to error (Goodman & Wood, 2004). Feedback that guides the subject to responses within a target range may be more conducive to strategy formation and constructive responses (Schmidt & Wrisberg, 2004). If feedback is too immediate or frequent, it may inhibit self-evaluation, self-judgment, and strategy formation by the subject. Fading the amount of feedback about performance over time, delaying feedback, and presenting patterns in attributes of performance may put needed pressure on the subject to make the necessary changes, develop strategies, and see whether those strategies have been effective (Knock, Ballard, Robin, & Schmidt, 2000; Swinnen, Nicholson, Schmidt, & Shapiro, 1990; Weeks & Kordus, 1998; Winstein, Merians, & Sullivan, 1999; Winstein & Schmidt, 1990).

SPECIFIC REHABILITATIVE STRATEGIES

At this point, we have developed a conceptual PDP model of language processes that subsumes phonology, semantics, lexical-semantics, and grammar. We have carefully considered the types of knowledge implicit in the various components of this model, because these have strong implications for the types of therapy we might pursue in subjects with aphasia and for the success we might expect. We have drawn particular attention to the principle of generalization and the mechanisms that might mediate it, because generalization will be absolutely essential if we are to succeed in the ultimate goal of therapy for aphasia—namely, improving the daily communicative lives of subjects. Finally, we have introduced evidence that the temporal spacing of therapy, structure and context of therapy sessions, stimulus properties, and type of feedback could profoundly influence long-term retention of therapeutic gain. We hope that our arguments have been cogent, but we concede that much of this is new theoretic territory and that vast work remains ahead to test these theories. As we will show below, aphasia treatment studies will be major contributors to this testing. Learning processes are implicit in the model (a by-product of the PDP principle that memory and processing involve the same neural network); therefore, tests of learning will be important to testing the hypotheses implicit in the model.

In this section, we will discuss some specific therapies for aphasia that receive theoretic justification from the model and, in some cases, have already provided support for the model. We hope that this discussion will help to consolidate some of the ideas we have already introduced and aid understanding by providing some concrete clinical examples. It will provide opportunities to introduce some new ideas about therapeutic approaches. Our discussion will be limited to therapies within the scope of the model. We will not, for example, discuss apraxia of speech, which we view as a disorder stemming from damage to neural networks lying between articulatory motor representations (Fig. 26–1) and projection targets of motor cortex.

Phonologic and Lexical-Semantic Impairment

Our core model (Fig. 26–1) defines three domains of knowledge: (1) sequence (latent in the acoustic-articulatory motor pathway), (2) semantic (latent in concept representations), and (3) lexical-semantic (latent in the pattern associator networks linking concept representations to the acoustic-articulatory motor pathway). Impairment of lexical access (manifested as anomia and word finding difficulty), whether in internally generated language or in naming to confrontation, is by far the most common and debilitating component of aphasia. Treatment of impairment in lexical-semantic access must directly or indirectly retrain lexical-semantic knowledge—that is, the knowledge latent in the pathways between concept representations and articulatory motor representations (Fig. 26–1, pathways 1-2 and 4-3). Traditional approaches have confronted the problem of anomia head-on, through naming therapy (re-teaching of the names of things).[11] Our core model (Fig. 26–1), however, suggests that two additional approaches may be of value in selected subjects. If naming is failing because of damage to unimodal, polymodal, and supramodal association cortices supporting distributed concept representations, then it might be improved by redeveloping the knowledge underlying these concept representations (i.e., semantic therapy; see below). If naming is failing because of impaired lexical-semantic function, the presence of two pathways linking distributed concept representations with phonologic representations suggests two potential treatment strategies. The traditional naming therapy approach might logically be directed to subjects in whom the target is the direct concept representations–articulatory motor representations pathway (Fig. 26–1, pathway 1-2). This target would be most logical in subjects with essentially no evidence of phonologic function (poor repetition, reduced auditory verbal short-term memory, no phonemic paraphasias in spontaneous language or repetition, and no improvement in naming with phonemic cues),

---

[11] We use the term "naming therapy" to designate therapeutic approaches in which re-teaching the names of objects features prominently (see Fillingham, Hodgson, Sage, & Lambon Ralph, 2003, for a relatively recent inventory). Lexical-semantic knowledge (Fig. 26–1, pathways 1-2 and 4-3) has not heretofore been commonly recognized as a separate domain of knowledge. In fact, cognitive neuropsychological models of language function, such as that of Patterson and Shewell (1987; see Raymer and Gonzalez Rothi, Chapter 23), specifically encourage one to view naming impairments as stemming exclusively from deficits in semantics or deficits in phonologic word form rather than the "arrow" that connects them. Thus, "naming therapies" also typically involve a component of semantic or phonologic treatment (Howard, Patterson, Ranklin. Orchard-Lisle, & Morton, 1985).

such as repetition conduction aphasia and some cases of deep dysphasia. On the other hand, if subjects have some evidence of phonologic function, albeit impaired, the presence of an indirect concept representations–acoustic/articulatory motor pathway suggests that phonologic therapy might improve naming. The presence of phonemic paraphasias in naming or repetition (especially nonword repetition) or evidence of improved naming with phonemic cueing would constitute evidence of some residual phonologic sequence knowledge and partial integrity of the acoustic-articulatory motor pathway.

Naming Therapy

Naming therapy, in our conceptualization, would be the only lexical-semantic therapy available to us in subjects with no phonologic function, and it might provide a useful complement to other techniques for treating lexical-semantic impairment, such as phonologic therapy (see below). The critical limitation is lack of potential for intrinsic generalization, because there is little resemblance between word meaning and word sound (except for onomatopoeic words and derivational forms). Consequently, practical and relatively inexpensive techniques will have to be developed to extend training to encompass useful working vocabularies and to carry out that training with sufficient intensity and over sufficient time to overcome the inefficiencies of naming therapies—in essence, building an extrinsic generalization process. Just how many words comprise a useful working vocabulary would need to be determined. Age-, gender-, and culture-specific vocabularies would need to be developed. An individualized, ongoing dynamic vocabulary list development project involving both subject and caregivers may be the best way to define such personal vocabularies. Once a target vocabulary starts to emerge, a training algorithm that does not require a therapist would then need to be developed, almost certainly involving caregivers and possibly using computers. This algorithm would then need to be executed over many months (and, perhaps, indefinitely) to enable maintenance and expansion of the vocabulary over time. The report of Basso (2003) is paradigmatic (but see also Hillis, 1998).

A word of caution is in order, however. In this discussion, access to articulatory motor representations during internally generated language and during naming to confrontation have been treated as if they were supported by identical neural structures. This assumption provided the basis for the implicit conclusion that if subjects are adequately trained in naming to confrontation, this capacity will generalize to internally generated language. This is not necessarily so, however. In fact, there appear to be two pathways by which we name to confrontation. In the best known (the "semantic route"), the object is seen, a concept representation is formed, and then an articulatory motor representation is elicited in one of the ways described in the foregoing.

The second pathway (the "direct route") provides the basis for directly associating an object representation in visual association cortex with an articulatory motor representation—that is, without recourse to an intervening concept or any associated meaning. For example, if you are told that the symbol is a framezoid, then if you are later shown this symbol א, you will be able to provide the correct name despite the complete absence of any meaning beyond the visual configuration. Two clinical syndromes, reflecting a double dissociation, provide support for this two-pathway confrontation naming hypothesis. Severe damage to the direct route and partial damage to the indirect route presumably provide the basis for optic aphasia; subjects with this disorder exhibit some knowledge of the object they are looking at but cannot name it. Typically, they can name the object given a definition and have relatively preserved lexical access during internally generated language (Bauer & Demery, 2003). Severe damage to the semantic route with relative preservation of the direct route presumably provides the basis for nonoptic aphasia (Shuren & Heilman, 1993). Subjects with this disorder may have difficulty describing attributes or functions of objects they see but can name them with relative facility. They typically exhibit impaired lexical access during internally generated language, presumably because of associated damage to the neural basis for concept representations. Thus, we see the risk latent in naming therapy: It might train the direct route without impacting the semantic route, the route invoking concept representations, which a subject must employ in internally generated language. The extent to which this might occur is unknown; it might depend, in part, on the degree of semantic impairment that is present. To the extent that it does occur, it might be necessary to complement confrontation naming therapy with naming to definition therapy; to train names in the context of sentences, thereby increasing the probability that concept representations will be engaged; or to provide sufficient semantic therapy to assure that the subject adopts a semantic set (see below).

Phonologic Sequence Therapy

The use of phonologic sequence therapy in the treatment of lexical-semantic deficits (specifically, impaired lexical access in internally generated language) is predicated on the existence of the indirect pathway from concepts to articulatory motor representations (Fig. 16–1, pathway 4-3), a pathway that takes advantage of the phonologic sequence knowledge embedded in the acoustic-articulatory motor pattern associator. So long as some remnants of this pathway are left after a stroke (either in the damaged hemisphere or in the normal hemisphere)—that is, so long as there remain some existing phonologic sequence knowledge and some connections between neural networks supporting concept representations and the acoustic-articulatory motor pattern associators supporting phonologic sequence knowledge—then it may be possible to improve word retrieval by enhancing phonologic sequence knowledge.

Support for this hypothesis comes from studies of language acquisition in young children. They first learn many of the various phonologic sequence regularities of their language (Gathercole, 1995; Gathercole & Martin, 1996). Subsequently, they learn to assemble these various sequences into combinations and to associate these combinations with concepts (meaning), enabling both word comprehension and word production. If this principle of language development also applies to language redevelopment after brain injury, it suggests two possibilities: (1) that effective retraining in phonologic sequence knowledge may generalize to all words containing the trained sequences, and (2) that once given an adequate repertoire of phonologic sequence knowledge during treatment, subjects with aphasia should be able to continue *after* therapy to enhance existing but inadequate connections between the substrate for concept representations and the substrate for phonologic sequence knowledge and to steadily rebuild their working vocabularies. It also is possible that training some phonologic sequences will generalize to other phonologic sequences (e.g., through shared distinctive feature and motor programming sequences).

We have recently completed a phase I study of phonologic sequence therapy for impaired lexical access (Kendall et al., in press). The operational goal of the treatment was to develop phoneme sequence knowledge, but one cannot hope to develop knowledge of sequences without neural instantiation of individual phonemes. The first phase of treatment therefore consisted of developing linked distributed representations of individual phonemes. If treatment were completely successful, insertion of any form of a phoneme into any given domain of the network would instantly generate distributed representations of all corresponding forms in all domains (conceptual, articulatory, acoustic, and orthographic).[12] For example, at the end of

completely successful training, insertion of the acoustic form of /b/ into the acoustic domain (by saying /b/ to the subject) would instantly lead to the generation of distributed representations of the articulatory form of /b/, a concept of /b/, and an orthographic representation corresponding to the letter "b" (Fig. 26–8 illustrates a mechanism by which orthographic representations might contribute to the process). Eventually, all the individual domain-specific distributed phoneme representations would be linked through the network into a multi-domain distributed representation of individual phonemes. The second phase of treatment consisted of training in the regularities of English phonologic sequences, first by inserting single syllables into the network and later by inserting two- or three-syllable nonwords into the network. Distributed representations were presumably generated in all domains and pathways of the network by this phonologic sequence input. One network, the acoustic-articulatory pattern associator network (Fig. 26–1, pathway 7-3), however, is uniquely equipped for accumulating knowledge of the regularities of phonologic sequences, because it is the only pattern associator in the phonologic network that is exposed to sequential input paired with sequential output. Thus, the second phase of treatment primarily involved building up phonologic sequence knowledge in the acoustic-articulatory pattern associator networks on the two sides of the brain.

The ultimate goal of the treatment was to enable naming via the indirect concepts–articulatory pathway (Fig. 26–1, pathway 4-3). Only the knowledge in pathway 7-3 of Figure 26–1 (not pathway 4), however, is enhanced by therapy. We assume two mechanisms by which training of only pathway 7-3, without explicit training of pathway 4, might enhance naming by the indirect pathway: (1) Training of pathway 7-3 enables better use of residual knowledge in pathway 4, and (2) training of pathway 7-3 provides adults with aphasia with a repertoire of phonologic sequences that they can then learn, *outside of therapy*, to combine and link to concept representations through further development of pathway 4. Further development of pathway 4 can occur because, when a subject hears a word, this simultaneously generates a concept representation corresponding to the meaning of the word and a phonologic sequence representation in pathway 7-3. The simultaneous engagement of these two representations enables Hebbian learning involving the connections in pathway 4 to occur. This Hebbian learning would provide the basis for continued growth in the ability to engage phonologic sequence knowledge by distributed concept representations to produce spoken words, just as appears to occur during normal language development in children.

Ten right-handed subjects (mean age, 52 years; mean time poststroke, 60 months) with anomic aphasia (Kertesz, 1982) received a total of 96 hours of therapy (2 hours/day,

---

[12] The validity of this statement requires considerable broadening of the traditional notion of concept representations (semantic knowledge). Two considerations support this broadening. First, meaning can be instantiated by very abbreviated knowledge of an object. For example, if told that a novel abstract symbol ℵ is a framezoid, we will readily be able to name this symbol if we see it again. Our knowledge of this symbol will consist entirely of the memory of the visual image of the symbol that is stored in hippocampal and visual association cortex connectivity. This type of abbreviated semantic representation could be viewed as an extreme manifestation of the heterogeneity of semantic knowledge distribution that underlies the phenomenon of category-specific recognition impairments (Forde & Humphreys, 1999). Second, if we have phonological awareness, we clearly have knowledge of any given phoneme and can respond to queries about what letters it corresponds to, whether a heard sound corresponds to that phoneme, and so on. If our knowledge of phonemes were confined to their acoustic and articulatory representations, we would not be able to speak about them or make decisions involving them.

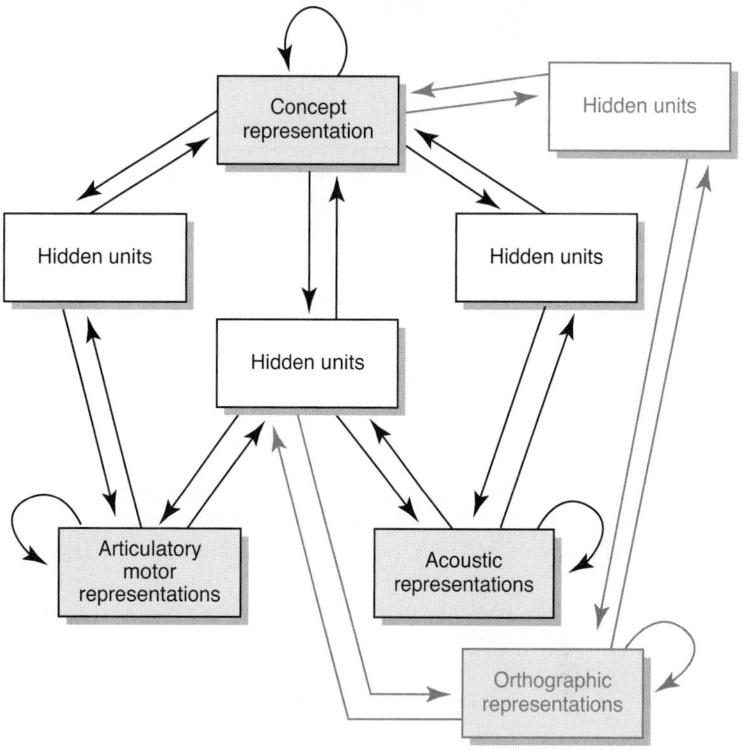

Figure 26–8. Connectionist model of phonologic processing. The core model (from Figure 26–1) is depicted in black. An elaboration of the model that includes networks supporting reading, depicted in gray, suggests a means by which letter and orthographic sequence knowledge introduced during the phonologic rehabilitation process might contribute to the development of phonologic awareness (conceptualization of discrete phonemes) and to phonologic sequence knowledge, and vice versa. (From Kendall, D. L., Rosenbek, J. C., Heilman, K. M., Conway, T. W., Klenberg, K., Gonzalez Rothi, L. J., et al. (in press). Phoneme-based rehabilitation of anomia in aphasia; Brain and Language with permission.)

4 days/week, for 12 weeks) using a modified version of the Lindamood Phoneme Sequencing Program (Lindamood & Lindamood, 1998). The group results are summarized in Tables 26–3 and 26–4. One week after completion of therapy, they demonstrated significant gains on the outcome measures most directly related to the treatment (CTOPP-PA, CTOPP-APA, and LAC); the gain on the LAC remained significant 3 months later. Subjects also demonstrated significant gains on the primary outcome measure, the Object-Action Naming Test, 1 week after completion of therapy and significant gains on the Boston Naming Test and the Controlled Oral Word Association Test 3 months after completion of therapy. Because the treatment involved no training of words, these results suggest generalization. Furthermore, the increase in Boston Naming Test and Controlled Oral Word Association Test scores between completion of therapy and 3 months later suggests that continued acquisition of lexical-semantic knowledge (Fig. 26–1, pathway 4-3) occurred after conclusion of therapy (i.e., evidence of extrinsic generalization).

This was a phase I investigation. The results suggest that a phonologic sequence therapy can be used to treat lexical-semantic deficits and provide support for the model that motivated the study, but they are not remotely definitive. If this therapy is to be viable, it must be refined and made considerably more efficient, predictors of response and predictors of extrinsic generalization need to be better

understood, and better measures of daily communication need to be employed.

Semantic Impairment

In a PDP conceptualization, anomia, to the extent that it results from semantic impairment, reflects insufficient engagement of representations of the critical features that distinguish concepts from each other (see Raymer & Rothi, 2000, for detection and quantitation of semantic impairment). The goal of therapy is to alter network connectivity such that these distinguishing features are more reliably engaged at the same time that features shared with other items are relatively disengaged. The left hemisphere perisylvian lesions that commonly are responsible for aphasia and its associated anomia frequently do not involve much of the association cortices that provide the basis for semantic representations. They may, however, damage Brodmann's area 37 and surrounding regions in the posterior temporal cortex (Fig. 26–5), which appear to provide the interface between cortices supporting semantic representations and the dominant perisylvian language cortex (producing anomia as a disconnection syndrome). One might naturally conclude that a lexical-semantic therapy is the best strategy to retrain the knowledge lost in the disconnection. To the extent that the subject has the potential for engaging right hemisphere mechanisms, semantic therapy might aid anomia in all

TABLE 26–3

Acquisition and Retention Data from Before and After Phonologic Sequence Therapy

Immediately Post-Treatment Termination – Pre-Treatment (Acquisition)				
	n	*Mean Difference*	*SD*	*p**
WAB	10	5.70	3.80	0.001
BNT	10	3.60	4.27	0.026
COWA	10	0.90	3.18	0.394
CTOPP-PA	8	7.88	8.77	0.039
CTOPP-APA	8	9.38	7.25	0.008
LAC	10	16	18.2	0.021
O-ANT	10	7.70	8.35	0.017
Post 3-Months – Pre-Treatment (Retention)				
	n	*Mean Diff*	*SD*	*p*
WAB	8	2.62	11.7	0.633
BNT	8	9.50	8.60	0.017
COWA	8	5.12	4.22	0.011
CTOPP-PA	7	5.43	10.8	0.233
CTOPP-APA	7	8.71	7.85	0.26
LAC	8	10.6	7.74	0.006
O-ANT	7	5.71	8.83	0.138

Mean Diff = mean difference; SD = standard deviation; WAB = Western Aphasia Battery; BNT = Boston Naming Test; COWA = Controlled Word Association Test; CTOPP = Comprehensive Test of Phonologic Processes; PA = phonologic awareness/real words; APA = alternate phonologic awareness/nonwords; LAC = Lindamood Auditory Conceptualization; O-ANT = Object-Action Naming Test.
*Uncorrected for multiple comparisons.
(From Kendall, D. L., Rosenbek, J. C., Heilman, K. M., Conway, T. W., Klenberg, K., Gonzalez Rothi, L. J., et al. (in press). Phoneme-based rehabilitation of anomia in aphasia; Brain and Language with permission.)

TABLE 26–4

Repeated Probe Results: Primary and Secondary Outcome Measures*

	Primary Outcome: Confrontation Naming		Secondary Outcome: Discourse Production: Word Count		Secondary Outcome: Discourse Production: Content Information Units		Secondary Outcome: Phonologic Production		Secondary Outcome: Nonword Repetition	
	Effect Size	*Visual Inspection*	*Effect Size*	*Visual Inspection*	*Effect Size*	*Visual Inspection*	*Effect Size*	*Visual Inspection*	*Effect Size*	*Visual Inspection*
After 1 week	1.63	9/10	1.49	5/8	1.71	4/8	6.88	10/10	0.95	5/6
After 3 months	1.53	7/8	1.40	1/6	1.41	4/6	5.73	5/8	1.12	5/6

*Average effect size and number of subjects with efficacy as judged by visual inspection of graphs.
(From Kendall, D. L., Rosenbek, J. C., Heilman, K. M., Conway, T. W., Klenberg, K., Gonzalez Rothi, L. J., et al. (in press). Phoneme-based rehabilitation of anomia in aphasia; Brain and Language with permission.)

affected subjects by training up inadequately trained right brain cortices supporting semantic representations. In this way, semantic therapy might have very broad applicability to the treatment of aphasia associated with significant anomia.

A variety of approaches to semantic therapy have been employed with some success (Raymer & Rothi, 2000). These have included:

1. Word-picture matching tasks using semantically related foils.
2. Answering yes/no questions about semantic features of pictured objects.
3. Semantic sorting of objects.
4. Variously cued matching of semantic associates as the number and relatedness of semantic foils is increased.
5. Correction of naming errors by provision of additional semantic information that distinguishes the erroneous response from the correct response.
6. Systematic training in the semantic features of objects.

Unlike naming therapy directed at lexical-semantic deficits, therapy directed to more purely semantic deficits might be expected to intrinsically generalize substantially, because refining featural relationships of trained items (the regularities in the knowledge implicit in the network) will benefit naming of untrained items to the extent that they share some of these featural relationships (Plaut, 1996). Counterintuitively, training on a spectrum of unusual exemplars of a category can be more effective than training on typical exemplars in inducing generalization (Plaut, 1996). This is because unusual exemplars convey information about both the core regularities defining the category, which help to distinguish it from other categories, and the greater range of regularities that are crucial in distinguishing all the different within-category exemplars from each other. Recent clinical work has confirmed this concept (Kiran & Thompson, 2003).

Even a damaged network still contains a great deal of information, so the task of therapy is to refine network knowledge rather than to reestablish it (Plaut, 1996). The distributed nature of semantics may provide some rationale for the targeting of semantic therapy at particular representational domains (e.g., representations with a substantial visual component in subjects with selective deficits in naming living things). Individualization of vocabulary development, as in therapy for lexical-semantic impairment (see above), also would be needed.

The potential for generalization using current semantic therapeutic techniques appears to be very modest unless the scope of intrinsic generalization can be expanded (and, thereby, impact a significant portion of the semantic domain used in daily life) or mechanisms for promoting extrinsic generalization can be developed. Broad intrinsic generalization is difficult to achieve for most semantic therapies, because their principle aim is to enlarge knowledge of the semantic attributes of single items, one item at a time. The extent to which this leads to incorporation of semantic features shared with other entities is largely a matter of chance. Knowledge of particular semantic domains (e.g., animals) might usefully be fleshed out in this way, especially through presentation of atypical exemplars (see above) (Kiran & Thompson, 2003; Plaut, 1996), but semantic knowledge that spans the breadth of daily life is difficult to achieve with this approach. Recently, Edmonds, Nadeau and Kiran (in preparation) have developed an innovative and fundamentally broader approach, in which therapy focuses on verb arguments. It takes advantage of the fact that many verbs admit a very broad range of possibilities for both agent and patient, thereby providing an opportunity for highly diverse modifications of the distributed concept representations of agent and patient as well as engagement of atypical exemplars of agent and patient. In this way, the therapy vastly expands the spectrum of semantic features that are incorporated in the training. The therapy also provides subjects with the opportunity to draw exemplars from daily life so long as they are acceptable agents or patients for the verb being presented. Some details about the therapy will help to illustrate.

In the first phase of therapy, subjects were presented with 10 individual verbs (e.g., "write"), one at a time, and tasked with producing three agents for each verb (e.g., author, journalist, and mother) or three patients for each verb (e.g., story, articles, and to-do list) while being cued with who or what questions. They then had to create suitable agent/patient pairs (e.g., author/story). If necessary, subjects were semantically cued through provision of appropriate targets mixed in with foils. Subjects also were asked to produce one personal response (e.g., husband/songs). In the second phase of therapy, subjects were tasked with answering when, where, and why questions about particular agent/patient pairs (an approach that might particularly invite responses related to the subject's own life, thereby facilitating generalization to daily life). In the third phase of treatment, subjects were read 12 sentences containing the target verb (three semantically correct, three containing an inappropriate agent, three containing an inappropriate patient, and three semantically correct but with agent and patient reversed). A fourth phase replicated phase 1 but without cueing. Four subjects received 2 hours of therapy per week for 4 to 6 weeks in a single-subject, multiple-baseline design. Results of therapy on measures reflecting intrinsic generalization are presented in Table 26–5. Although clearly this therapy needs to be tested in larger populations, predictors of response identified, and impact on measures of language function in daily life established, these results are very promising. They suggest that a therapy engineered to develop semantic representations in a particularly broad way, and in a way that allows subjects to explicitly connect the content of therapy to their daily lives, may achieve impressive results. The design of the therapy suggests that these results were achieved through intrinsic generalization, but of course, one cannot rule out contributions

TABLE 26–5

Results of a Broad Semantic Therapy

Subject	Aphasia Type	WAB		BNT (%)		Connected Speech*	
		Pre-Treatment	Post-Treatment	Pre-Treatment	Post-Treatment	Pre-Treatment	Post-Treatment
1	TM	76.4	82.5	71.7	81.7	52.0	82.1
2	TM	78.5	86.4	86.7	91.7	50.9	67.8
3	Conduction	73.8	81.2	40.7	58.3	62.5	90.8
4	Conduction	70.6	82.3	44.0	68.0	50.4	52.8

WAB = Western Aphasia Battery (Kertesz, 1982); BNT = Boston Naming Test (Kaplan, Goodglass, Weintraub, & Segal, 1983); TM = Transcortical motor.
*Percentage of sentences that contained subject and verb, with or without object, and were relevant to the topic. Connected speech from picture description test of the Western Aphasia Battery, the Boston Diagnostic Aphasia Examination (Goodglass & Kaplan, 2000), and the Cinderella story.
(From Edmonds, L. A., Nadeau, S. E., & Kiran, S. (in preparation). Effect of verb network strengthening treatment (vnest) on sentence production in persons with aphasia; with permission.)

from extrinsic, contextual, and mechanistic generalization mechanisms.

In our previous discussion of extrinsic generalization, we alluded to results of a trial of semantic therapy we performed that suggested that subjects with evidence of intact frontal systems function, despite the relatively modest potential for intrinsic generalization in the therapy we used, were the only ones who exhibited extensive generalization as well as gain in daily communication, as reflected in the American Speech-Language-Hearing Association Functional Aphasia Quotient (Nadeau & Kendall, 2006). These results, though very preliminary, suggest that more attention should perhaps be devoted to explicitly developing extrinsic generalization techniques on which subjects can be trained and monitored after completion of therapy.

Grammatical Impairment

For subjects who have good lexical-semantic function, impairment in grammatical function may represent only a modest handicap and, therefore, provides relatively less motivation for language therapy compared with lexical-semantic deficits. Assuming that therapy for grammatical impairment is desired, we have identified a number of facilities underlying grammatical function that may be logical targets of therapy:

• Capacity for arbitrary modification of single-noun concept representations.
• Capacity for simultaneous endogenous generation of multiple-noun concept representations.
• Capacity for maintenance of memory of the immediately preceding discourse.
• Capacity for manipulation of multiple related, modified noun concept representations to fit the particular situation.
• Multi-word sequence knowledge (underlying grammatical morphology and phrase structure rules).

The essential neural processes underlying these capacities have not yet been well defined. We suggest at least three:

1. Working memory (engagement of one or more concept representations and recall of immediately preceding linguistic history).
2. Concept manipulation (modification of individual concepts and adaptation of temporal order and content relationships of multiple concept representations to meet the situation at hand).
3. Sequence knowledge.

These essential neural processes are discussed in some detail in the following sections.

Working Memory

Working memory is an intrinsic brain function that appears to be particularly dependent on frontal lobe systems, and it likely is no accident that grammatical impairment is seen predominantly in subjects with major dominant frontal lesions. It is possible that treatment of working memory impairment relevant to language will have to be specific to particular language constructs. It may be, however, that generic improvement in working memory capacity will enable improvement in grammatical function. We suggest two possible strategies, one pharmacologic and one behavioral. The pharmacologic therapy, involving either methylphenidate or D-amphetamine, is motivated by experience with subjects with attention-deficit hyperactivity disorder (ADHD) (Heilman, Voeller, & Nadeau, 1991). These subjects appear to have a disorder involving the selection of plans for action. Plans for action may be formulated (often on the basis of memory or reflex) in more or less automatic response to environmental stimuli, a process that might be termed "reactive intention," which is driven primarily by temporoparietal and brain-stem systems. Alternatively, plans for action may be formulated deliberately as part of an ongoing problem-solving strategy, a process that might be termed "intentional intention," which is driven primarily by frontal systems. In this view, subjects with ADHD have a relative imbalance between reactive and intentional plan formulation such that their behavior is dominated by reactive planning. Treating these subjects with methylphenidate appears to redress this imbalance, enabling these subjects to achieve more balanced plan formulation and, most particularly, to sustain the intentional intention that is necessary to successfully complete tasks. We propose methylphenidate treatment of subjects with grammatical dysfunction, most particularly those with simplification of syntax and difficulty articulating complex concepts that might be related in part to working memory deficits. Because these subjects likely have multi-component deficits, methylphenidate treatment might have to be accompanied by behavioral treatment of associated deficits (see below) to demonstrate efficacy.

Our proposal for behavioral treatment of working memory deficits contributing to syntactic dysfunction also is predicated on the concept of something approaching a generic working memory capacity for language and that training of this capacity in one domain will generalize to other domains. Two tests commonly used to probe working memory, the Brown-Peterson paradigm (Peterson & Peterson, 1959) and the Paced Auditory Serial Addition Test (Gronwall, 1977), or PASAT, lend themselves to adaptation as training devices to enhance working memory capacity (the main problem being to reduce task difficulty such that subjects with aphasia can make some correct responses). Both tasks require the maintenance of two working memory compartments, one to support recall of a previous stimulus and one to support a computation (in direct analogy to the working memory demands of language). As we cautioned in the testing of methylphenidate effects, it may be necessary to couple working memory training with other behavioral training in subjects who have syntactic dysfunction before the benefit of working memory training becomes evident. The study of Stablum, Umiltà, Mogentale, Carlan, and Guerrini (2000) suggests that facility with operating two working memory compartments can be trained but provides no insight regarding how this might impact language. Those authors trained subjects with closed-head injury and subjects who have had anterior communicating artery aneurysm rupture on a dual-task paradigm in which the stimuli consisted of two letters, one above the other, placed to the right or left of the center of a display screen. Subjects had to indicate, first, the side of the stimulus (manual reaction time paradigm) and, second, whether the letters were the same or different (verbal report). The chief dependent measure was the reaction time cost of introducing the second task. With the training on this task, subjects showed significant improvement that was sustained over time (to the extent that they became indistinguishable from controls) together with comparable improvement in PASAT performance, which was highly correlated with dual-task cost. The effect on PASAT performance suggests generalization of the trained dual-task skill to other content domains.

Concept Manipulation

Concept manipulation may have declarative components that render it domain specific, but we suspect that it predominantly represents a set of skills (i.e., nondeclarative memories akin to procedural memory) (see also Ullman, 2004). This means that effective training will require extensive practice and that there should be good generalization of skills across exemplars of particular manipulations. One would not necessarily expect generalization from one type of concept manipulation to another, however, any more than one would expect much generalization from training on serves in tennis to backhand skills. Thus, the extensive practice may need to involve a variety of constructions, no less than phonologic therapy must involve a substantial portion of the repertoire of native phonemic sequences to be successful. Thompson (2001) has shown explicitly that subjects can be trained on specific distributed concept manipulation skills and show generalization to different applications of these skills but not a generic improvement in concept manipulation capacity. Subjects with syntactic impairment trained to produce who questions showed generalization to production of what questions (both involve a verb that requires an agent and a theme) but not to production of when or where questions (in which the verb does not take a theme but may take an adjunctive phrase, e.g., "He is sleeping in the bedroom" and "Where is he sleeping?"). Subjects trained to produce when questions showed generalization to where questions, which also involve verbs that take adjunctive phrases, but not to who or what questions. None of these subjects showed generalization to passive-voice sentence production. Notably, subjects trained on more complex variants of a particular distributed concept manipulation (e.g., cleft object constructions) showed generalization to simpler variants of the same manipulation (e.g., who questions) but not vice versa (Thompson et al., 2003). This suggests that training on more complex variants may constitute a more efficient therapeutic approach. What constitutes a useful repertoire of syntactic skills has not been defined, much less the extended line of therapies that would be needed to train enough of these skills to make a clinically significant difference.

Word Sequence Knowledge

To the extent that multi-word sequence knowledge is like phonologic sequence knowledge, it is procedural in nature and will require extensive practice. At first glance, it might seem that this training process would require repeated exposure to an almost infinite number of word sequences. As discussed above, however, this may not be so, because the essential memories that are being acquired are between word classes (e.g., noun, verb, and adjective) rather than between word exemplars. To the extent that word class knowledge is incorporated in distributed concept representations and their modifications, which are relatively less susceptible to the effects of discrete lesions, the size of the training task will be reduced.

Constraint-Induced Language Therapy

Up to this point, we have discussed language rehabilitation strategies that are precisely targeted at specific deficits. They are predicated on careful evaluation of the various components of the subject's aphasia, identification of the salient neural system deficits, and design of a specific treatment that takes into account the underlying mechanisms. The achievement of success with such therapies not only is clinically important but also yields scientific information about the neural basis of language processes (see, e.g., Thompson, 2001). Much work remains to refine these therapies, improve efficacy, identify predictors of response, develop variations applicable to different profiles of impairment, and fully explore their potential for elucidating the neural basis of language processes. Much further work also is in order to translate them into approaches that substantially improve the communicative lives of subjects. This will require further study of mechanisms underlying generalization (Table 26–2). Up to this point in our discussion of specific types of therapy, we have focused primarily on intrinsic and extrinsic generalization mechanisms. Any of the therapies discussed also could benefit from socially mediated generalization. In addition, any of the therapies discussed could, to one degree or another, engage a particular type of mechanistic generalization—namely, the development of an intentional bias to use language in lieu of other communicative techniques developed to compensate for aphasia. Constraint-induced language therapy (Maher et al., 2003; Meinzer et al., 2005; Pulvermüller et al., 2001) represents an approach in which the primary aim is to develop intentional bias to use language.

Constraint-induced language therapy seeks to engage subjects in intensive language production by absolutely limiting their opportunities for communication to spoken language (the constraint) and placing them in situations (e.g., partially scripted scenarios, games, or problem-solving tasks) that absolutely require verbally mediated collaboration with others, thus placing considerable pressure on subjects to speak at length. It is inspired by constraint-induced movement therapy, in which the goal is to overcome intentional bias in subjects with stroke to use the normal hand by engaging them in intensive functional task practice with the impaired hand, typically while the normal hand is constrained in a mitt. Constraint-induced language therapy does not seek to develop a corpus of language knowledge that might subserve intrinsic generalization. Its goal is narrowly construed as developing an intentional bias to use language. The efficacy reported in published trials has been sufficient to encourage further research. The most immediate challenge is how to design the process and content of therapeutic sessions to maximize efficacy and efficiency. The recruitment of caregivers into the process might provide a means of engaging extrinsic generalization, contextual generalization, and socially mediated generalization. There is nothing about constraint-induced language therapy per se that precludes incorporation of a program that would engage mechanisms of intrinsic generalization. Thus, for example, a semantic therapy could be pursued in a constraint-induced language therapy format.

Errorless Learning

Therapy employing an errorless learning feature has recently achieved some popularity as an approach to speech-language therapy (for review, see Fillingham et al., 2003). Essentially the same therapy goes under the guise of repetition priming (Best, Herbert, Hickin, Osborne, & Howard, 2002; Patterson, Purell, & Morton, 1983; Raymer, Thompson, Jacobs, & Le Grand, 1993) and its variant, contextual repetition priming (Martin, Fink, & Laine, 2004), although the principles that motivate repetition priming treatment are quite different. Here, we consider the neural rationale for treatments seeking errorless learning.

The efficacy of errorless learning was first demonstrated in studies of pigeons; later studies of human subjects with severe learning disabilities provided some further support for the concept (Jones & Eayrs, 1992). In 1994, Boddey and Wilson applied it for the first time to subjects with acquired brain damage (i.e., subjects with severe anterograde amnesia). The experimental paradigm was somewhat contrived: Subjects were presented with the first two letters of a five-letter word. In the errorful condition, they had to make three guesses regarding the word before being told the correct answer, which they were instructed to write down. In the errorless condition, they were immediately told the correct answer. Subjects trained in the errorless condition showed better retention of word knowledge given the two-letter cues. Baddeley and Wilson interpreted this as supporting their hypothesis that these patients, with their severe impairment in explicit memory function, were relying substantially on implicit memory function for performance of the task. Their results have since been replicated many times, but the implicit memory hypothesis has been successfully challenged (Hunkin, Squires, Parkin, & Tidy, 1998). Errorless learning techniques have since been tried in amnesic populations for a variety of tasks, including associating names with photos of unfamiliar people (with or without cueing with the first letter of the names), learning routes around a room defined in relationship to objects in the room, learning a route through an array of patterned stepping stones, and programming an electronic organizer (Evans et al., 2000). Errorless learning techniques facilitated cued learning of names of unfamiliar people, but it provided either no clinically important advantage or worse performance on these other tasks. A review of naming therapies for aphasia found no advantage for treatments employing error reduction techniques; too few studies have employed errorless techniques to draw any conclusions (Fillingham et al., 2003).

The errorless learning literature does not provide an adequate basis for drawing conclusions about the mechanisms by which errorless learning might or might not provide benefit, nor about the deficit domains in which it might be effective. Most important, it does not provide information regarding the potential benefit of errorless learning for patients with intact memory function who already have partial knowledge of the correct answer (simply not enough knowledge to produce the correct response reliably). This is the situation in patients with aphasia. Nevertheless, errorless learning techniques have recently gained some popularity in treatment of aphasia, at least in part on the presumption that errorless learning obeys Hebbian principles (i.e., that to the extent two connected neurons are coactive, the strength of the synaptic connection between them will increase). For example, in naming therapy, it is posited that if subjects are asked to name an object and are left to their own devices and arrive at the wrong answer, an opportunity exists for strengthening of connections between that particular concept representation and the articulatory motor representation of that wrong answer. Two immediate problems can be seen with this conceptualization. First, Hebbian learning (and the related synaptic process, long-term potentiation) is a complex and incompletely understood process that requires, among other things, a burst of acetylcholine delivered to the cortex by the nucleus basalis or to the hippocampus by the medial septal nuclei that signals the neurons in question that the activity in which they are engaged is important (Kilgard & Merzenich, 1998). This will occur only if the behavior is rewarded, which a wrong answer would not be.[13] Second, in naming therapy, the Hebbian learning rationale will apply only to the extent that auditory input delivered by the therapist elicits the correct articulatory motor representation. If the subject has no phonologic function (e.g., has repetition conduction aphasia), then simultaneous auditory presentation of the object name will not be of value, because auditory input will not elicit an articulatory motor representation except via the concept representation. If repetition commonly is associated with

production of phonemic paraphasias, then simultaneous auditory presentation might actually be dysfunctional, because it might lead to production of incorrect patterns of activity in the cortex supporting articulatory motor representations.

Under what circumstances might an errorless learning paradigm be beneficial or harmful? Because of the limitations of the literature, we can only offer some tentative hypotheses. Errorless learning might be beneficial in naming therapy (with the caveats noted in the foregoing) not so much because of its impact on Hebbian learning but, rather, because it can markedly speed therapy and cut through long, frustrating word searches and perseverative responses, thereby vastly increasing the number of stimuli presented and reducing patient frustration. In naming therapy directed at lexical-semantic deficits, only one answer is correct, and no evident reason exists why permitting the patient to struggle might be beneficial. The same may be true for phonologic therapy directed at disorders of phonemic sequencing. For other therapies, however, such as those for speech apraxia and semantic deficits, the therapeutic goal is for the patient to re-differentiate functions that have become de-differentiated because of injury. In apraxia of speech, a reduced number of crude motor responses must be differentiated into a larger number of more refined and specific responses. With semantic deficits, the various exemplars of semantic categories must be re-differentiated from the central tendency of those categories (e.g., from the general concept of "dogness" must be differentiated specific breeds of dogs and particular individual dogs, as well as wolves, coyotes, foxes, hyenas and dingoes). In the realm of syntax, there typically exist many different syntactic approaches (multiple concept manipulations) to any particular communicative problem. In patients with syntactic impairment, as in patents with semantic impairment or apraxia of speech, there may be value in allowing the patient to produce responses with successive corrections by the therapist. Feedback of some type is essential. Thus, we may tentatively posit that errorless learning may be of value when only one response is correct, as in treatment of lexical-semantic deficits, but also that it may be less effective or deleterious when re-differentiation of procedural or semantic representations is needed. These (yet unproven) hypotheses are broadly congruent with the conclusions drawn by Jones and Eayrs (1992) in their critique of errorless learning.

In considering errorful learning techniques as an approach to treatment of apraxia of speech or semantic or syntactic deficits, an important distinction needs to be made. Truly errorless learning is defined as learning in an environment in which the goal is to completely prevent erroneous responses. Errorful learning, however, need not be completely unconstrained. Guidelines, cues, vanishing cues, and prompts (error reduction techniques) can be used to constrain the domain of error, improving subject focus in a way

---

[13] The implicit memory hypothesis is important here, because it is possible —even likely—that implicit memories can be established in the absence of reward. Thus, the evidence against the implicit memory hypothesis provided by Hunkin and colleagues (1998) is directly relevant to the key hypothesis that motivates errorless learning therapies.

that will permit the subject to learn from the pattern of errors and prevent the subject from becoming overwhelmed or frustrated. In short, a profitable middle ground likely exists between errorless learning and wild guessing. Defining this middle ground and adapting it to individual subjects may be a useful topic for speech-language therapy research.

Finally, studies of neural network reorganization in the somatosensory cortex (Buonomano & Merzenich, 1998) suggest that for change to occur in response to somatosensory stimuli, those stimuli must be attended. If this is true throughout the brain, including the association cortices supporting language function, it suggests that in errorless learning paradigms, the target of the subject's attention must be adequately constrained. This should pose no major difficulty at the single-word level (barring subject fatigue and given a task paradigm that sustains subject interest, attention, and effort), but it may be a problem at the sentence level. If whole sentences are provided by the therapist in pursuit of errorless syntactic therapy, it is quite possible that the subject will attend to the phonologic sequence (i.e., performing repetition) rather than to the syntactic structure.

CONCLUSION

In this review, we have introduced a general neural network conceptualization of spoken language processes, attempting to be as specific as possible about the nature of the knowledge represented in the various domains and the neural principles underlying modification of that knowledge. A substantial body of evidence supports certain aspects of this conceptualization (particularly phonology); other aspects are somewhat more speculative (e.g., grammar). Nevertheless, all aspects of our model represent hypotheses only. The particular value of these hypotheses is that experiments testing them will challenge not just a conceptualization of language function but also a conceptualization of the neural network organization of the brain, because we have avidly sought to make these hypotheses neurally plausible (O'Reilly, 1998). As tentative as these hypotheses are, they make many specific predictions regarding approaches to be taken in language therapy, as we have discussed throughout this chapter. The success or failure of implementation of these therapeutic strategies will serve to further test these underlying hypotheses and will add specificity to their predictions (see, e.g., Thompson, 2001). In all of this, we have strived to show how conceptualizing aphasic language and language therapy in relation to neural processes, as opposed to strictly empirically defined processes, contributes to the scientific richness of linguistic inquiry.

We have given major emphasis to mechanisms of generalization, both because of their intrinsic scientific interest and because extensive generalization must occur if language therapy is to impact the daily communicative lives of subjects.

We also have devoted substantial space to the educational psychology literature, because language therapy engages normal learning mechanisms and it behooves us to determine ways of conducting language therapy that will maximize retention of knowledge in forms that are most readily retrievable by subjects in daily life.

FUTURE TRENDS

Much of what we have discussed finds support in research extending over decades (120 years in the case of the psychology of learning). Many of the ideas are new, however, and will require much study for validation. Several specific paths of research inquiry can be defined:

- Further study of neural network models of language function.
- Further study of specific language therapies with high potential for intrinsic generalization (e.g., phonologic, semantic, and syntactic).
- Further study of therapies predicated on mechanistic generalization (e.g., redevelopment of working memory capacity and constraint-induced language therapy).
- Further study of mechanisms of generalization per se.
- Further study of the impact of temporal distribution of training; structure and context of treatment sessions; properties of stimuli; and nature of feedback on long-term retention.
- Further study of error reduction and errorless learning techniques.

KEY POINTS

1. Neural networks are the essential unit of brain function.
2. Neural networks simultaneously support knowledge (long-term memory; as connection strengths), working memory (as patterns of neural activity), and processing (as transformation of input patterns into output patterns).
3. Deficits resulting from brain lesions stem predominantly from loss of knowledge represented in the synapses (neural connections) that were destroyed, although disconnection from sources of knowledge (loss of access) may play an important role in certain syndromes, often referred to as "disconnection syndromes" (e.g., alexia without agraphia because of lesions of the left occipital cortex and the splenium of the corpus callosum).
4. PDP models are particularly appealing, because their structure emulates that of the brain. They can

learn naturally from experience, as does the brain, and implicit rules emerge that represent regularities in the knowledge acquired. PDP models enable us to logically account for complex behavior in terms of brain microstructure, have a natural ability to capture bottom-up/top-down processing effects, and have been remarkably successful at emulating the behaviors of normal subjects and those with brain damage.

5. Processes underlying phonologic and lexical-semantic function can be defined in a PDP model supporting phonologic sequence, lexical-semantic, and semantic knowledge in a way that accounts for nearly all the findings of psycholinguistic studies on slips of the tongue in normal subjects and phonologic, lexical-semantic and semantic errors in subjects with aphasia.

6. Grammar can be conceptualized in PDP terms. The picture that emerges is one of multiple distributed concept representations in association cortices throughout the brain that are modified in various ways, often reciprocally, by verbs, adjectives, and prepositions. Grammatical function is based on the brain capacity for simultaneously supporting multiple distributed concept representations (as working memory), the ready capacity of PDP systems to accommodate an almost arbitrarily large number of modifications of distributed concept representations, acquired knowledge of word sequence regularities, and acquired skill in manipulating concept representations.

7. Semantic knowledge and, possibly, lexical-semantic knowledge represent fact memories that depend on hippocampal function for their acquisition. Phonetics, phonologic sequence and (to a substantial extent) word sequence knowledge, and grammatical skill likely represent procedural knowledge acquired incrementally via hippocampally independent mechanisms.

8. Generalization is the process by which the effects of speech-language therapy extend to material or circumstances not explicitly trained during therapy sessions. A number of generalization mechanisms can be defined, including intrinsic, cross-function, extrinsic, mechanistic, substrate mediated, contextual, and socially mediated.

9. Extensive studies conducted over the past 100 years indicate that a given amount of knowledge taught over a greater period of time is more likely to be retained (i.e., the "spacing effect"). This effect can be accounted for either by an interaction between conditions at the time of acquisition and conditions at the time of retrieval or by the effects of sleep processes on the consolidation of declarative and procedural memory.

10. Retention of knowledge acquired during speech-language therapy can potentially be increased not only by greater spacing of sessions but also by increasing the commonalities between the conditions of therapy and the normal living conditions of the subjects being treated.

11. Measures taken during therapy to achieve maximal extent of representation of stimuli in cerebral cortical networks (e.g., by engaging visual, auditory, tactile, predicative, and gestural representations of the object) may benefit learning by maximizing the number of neural connections that are engaged and, therefore, susceptible to modification (the depth of processing effect of Craik and Lockhart, 1972).

12. The manner and form in which feedback is provided during therapy may have a major impact on learning and retention.

13. Phonologic sequence therapy may provide a logical approach to many subjects with aphasia who have impaired lexical access, and it has the potential advantage of achieving effects that generalize widely, unlike "naming therapies."

14. Verbs might be usefully employed in semantic therapy as an effective device to achieve maximally diverse modifications of distributed concept representations and highly atypical exemplars of agent and patient, thereby maximizing the potential for generalization.

15. Training of working memory capacity per se might benefit a number of components of grammatical function.

16. Research on retraining of such grammatical capacities as the ability to generate who, what, when, and where questions from declarative sentences provides support for the PDP conceptualization of syntax as a set of skills in manipulating distributed concept representations. Individual syntactic skills are not word specific but, rather, are specific to type of sentence structure.

17. Constraint-induced language therapy might usefully be employed to induce subjects with aphasia to redevelop a natural intention to use language in the various circumstances of daily life.

18. Although the idea that completely errorless learning techniques are beneficial in aphasia therapy has neither a theoretic nor an empirical basis, varying degrees of constraint on allowable errors may be of value, and the optimal degree of constraint likely will depend on the particular aphasic deficit being rehabilitated.

ACTIVITIES FOR REFLECTION AND DISCUSSION

1. Discuss the evidence for and against the concept that aphasia reflects loss of access to knowledge rather than loss of the knowledge itself. How can this concept be reconciled with the extensive loss of neural connections that occurs with stroke? How do PDP models provide an alternative account for the evidence of partial preservation of language knowledge after stroke that has motivated the loss of access concept?

2. Discuss the various mechanisms of generalization of treatment effects and what could be done to promote these mechanisms.

3. Explain how a PDP model eliminates the need to posit the buffers and error correction devices frequently incorporated into information processing models of language.

4. Do language errors produced by subjects with aphasia support the concept of graceful degradation?

5. Discuss the ways in which a representation can be distributed. What unique properties does a network capable of supporting distributed representations confer? What are the implications of distributed semantic representations for the spectrum of category-specific naming errors?

6. Discuss the potential roles of sequence knowledge in language function.

7. Why is the traditional conceptualization of a lexicon not neurally plausible? Describe how PDP models can provide an alternate, neurally plausible account.

8. Why is it likely that we use two pathways, a predominantly whole-word pathway and a predominantly phonologic pathway, to name concepts?

9. By what mechanisms might phonemic paraphasic errors be produced?

10. Describe serial and parallel processing theories of language production, and consider how each accounts for the spectrum of observed language behavior.

11. Consider the pros and cons of Chomskian approaches to verbs and the PDP conceptualization of multi-argument verbs as "super-adjectives" that simultaneously achieve a lexical representation and act to produce reciprocal modification and binding of multiple distributed concept representations.

12. Discuss the various features of Broca's aphasia in terms of the PDP conceptualization introduced in this chapter. Are there alternate, neurally plausible accounts for any of these features?

13. Why are phrase structure rules so infrequently violated in aphasia?

14. Discuss the various factors that constrain article use in different languages and how these might influence the relative frequency of omission errors (agrammatism) and paraphasic substitutions (paragrammatism).

15. Discuss the problems with the theory that lexical semantic knowledge represents declarative knowledge whose acquisition requires the hippocampus.

16. Discuss the relative advantages and disadvantages of procedural and declarative knowledge acquisition mechanisms for aphasia treatment.

17. Discuss potential advantages and disadvantages of more versus less temporally distributed treatment of aphasia. Are their alternative approaches that could be pursued that would achieve some of the potential benefits of more temporally distributed treatment sessions while retaining a relatively condensed schedule? What is likely to be an unavoidable consequence of more condensed scheduling?

18. Discuss the depth of learning concept of Craik and Lockart and how it might be relevant to aphasia therapy?

19. Discuss ways in which feedback might be given during aphasia therapy and their potential advantages and disadvantages.

20. The ability to translate concepts into spoken word form is essential to effective verbal communication. Discuss the various reasons that training a subject to name objects may have little impact on that subject's ability to name concepts (both those corresponding to objects trained and those corresponding to objects that have not been trained).

21. Why might phonological sequence therapy, semantic therapy, and syntactic therapy generalize in ways that naming therapy cannot?

22. In what ways might improvement in working memory benefit grammatic function?

23. Consider ways that generalization of benefits from constraint induced language therapy might be increased.

24. Discuss the circumstances in which minimal and maximal constraint of error might be desirable in treatment of aphasia.

References

Alvarez, P., & Squire, L. R. (1994). Memory consolidation and the medial temporal lobe: A simple network model. *PNAS, 91,* 7041–7045.

Baddeley, A. D., & Longman, D. J. A. (1978). The influence of length and frequency of training session on the rate of learning to type. *Ergonomics, 21,* 627–635.

Bahrick, H. P., & Phelps, E. (1987). Retention of Spanish vocabulary over 8 years. *Journal of Experimental Psychology: Learning, Memory, and Cognition, 13,* 344–349.

Basso, A. (2003). *Aphasia and its therapy.* New York: Oxford University Press.

Basso, A., Bracchi, M., Capitani, E., Laiacona, M., & Zanobio, M. E. (1987). Age and evolution of language area functions. A study of adult stroke patients. *Cortex, 23,* 475–483.

Bates, E., Friederici, A., & Wulfeck, B. (1987). Grammatical morphology in aphasia: Evidence from three languages. *Cortex, 23,* 545–574.

Bauer, R. M., & Demery, J. A. (2003). Agnosia. In K. M. Heilman & E. Valenstein (Eds.), *Clinical neuropsychology* (4th ed., pp. 236–295). New York: Oxford University Press.

Best, W., Herbert, R., Hickin, J., Osborne, F., & Howard, D. (2002). Phonological and orthographic facilitation off word retrieval in aphasia: Immediate and delayed effects. *Aphasiology, 16,* 151–168.

Bhogal, S. K., Teasell, R., & Speechley, M. (2003). Intensity of aphasia therapy, impact on recovery. *Stroke, 34,* 987–993.

Blonder, L. X. (2000). Language use. In S. E. Nadeau, L. J. Gonzalez Rothi & B. Crosson (Eds.), *Aphasia and language. Theory to practice* (pp. 284–295). New York: Guilford Press.

Bower, G. H. (1972). Stimulus-sampling theory of encoding variability. In A. W. Melton & E. Martin (Eds.), *Coding processes in human memory*. Washington, D.C.: Winston.

Brashers-Krug, T., Shadmehr, R., & Bizzi, E. (1996). Consolidation in human motor memory. *Nature, 382,* 252–255.

Brown, J. W., & Grober, E. (1983). Age, sex, and aphasia type. Evidence for a regional cerebral growth process underlying lateralization. *Journal of Nervous and Mental Disease, 171,* 431–434.

Buonomano, D. V., & Merzenich, M. M. (1998). Cortical plasticity: From synapses to maps. *Annual Review of Neuroscience, 21,* 149–186.

Caramazza, A., Basili, A. G., Koller, J. J., & Berndt, R. S. (1981). An investigation of repetition and language processing in a case of conduction aphasia. *Brain and Language, 14,* 235–271.

Caramazza, A., Miceli, G., & Villa, G. (1986). The role of the (output) phonological buffer in reading, writing, and repetition. *Cognitive Neuropsychology, 3,* 37–76.

Catani, M., Jones, D. K., & Fytche, D. H. (2005). Perisylvian language networks of the human brain. *Annals of Neurology, 57,* 8–16.

Chertkow, H., Bub, D., Deaudon, C., & Whitehead, V. (1997). On the status of object concepts in aphasia. *Brain & Language, 58,* 203–232.

Cheung, S. W., Bedenbaugh, P. H., Nagarajan, S. S., & Schreiner, C. E. (2001). Functional organization of squirrel monkey primary auditory cortex: Responses to pure tones. *Journal of Neurophysiology, 85,* 1732–1749.

Childers, J. B., & Tomasello, M. (2002). Two-year-olds learn novel nouns, verbs, and conventional actions from massed or distributed exposures. *Developmental Psychology, 38,* 967–978.

Cohen, G., Johnston, R. A., & Plunkett, K. (Eds.). (2000). *Exploring cognition: Damaged brains and neural networks*. Philadelphia: Taylor and Francis Group.

Craik, F. I. M., & Lockhart, R. S. (1972). Levels of processing: A framework for memory research. *Journal of Verbal Learning and Verbal Behavior, 11,* 671–684.

Dell, G. S. (1986). A spreading-activation theory of retrieval in sentence production. *Psychological Review, 93,* 283–321.

Dell, G. S., & Reich, P. A. (1981). Stages in sentence production: An analysis of speech error data. *Journal of Verbal Learning and Verbal Behavior, 20,* 611–629.

Dell, G. S., Schwartz, M. F., Martin, N., Saffran, E. M., & Gagnon, D. A. (1997). Lexical access in normal and aphasic speakers. *Psychological Review, 104,* 801–838.

Dempster, F. N. (1996). Distributing and managing the conditions of encoding and practice. In E. L. Bjork & R. A. Bjork (Eds.), *Memory* (pp. 317–344). San Diego: Academic Press.

Donovan, J. J., & Radosevich, D. J. (1999). A meta-analytic review of the distribution of practice effect: Now you see it, now you don't. *Journal of Applied Psychology, 84,* 795–805.

Ebbinghaus, H. (1885). *Memory: A contribution to experimental psychology*. Berlin: Private Docent in Philosophy at the University of Berlin. Reprinted by Dover: NY, 1964.

Edmonds, L. A., Nadeau, S. E., & Kiran, S. (in preparation). Effect of verb network strengthening treatment (vnest) on sentence production in persons with aphasia.

Ellis, A. W., & Young, A. W. (1988). *Human cognitive neuropsychology*. Hillsdale, New Jersey: Lawrence Erlbaum.

Estes, W. K. (1955). Statistical theory of spontaneous recovery and regression. *Psychological Review, 62,* 145–154.

Evans, J. J., Wilson, B. A., Schuri, U., Andrade, J., Baddeley, A. D., Bruna, O., et al. (2000). A comparison of "errorless" and "trial-and-error" learning methods for teaching individuals with acquired memory deficits. *Neuropsychological Rehabilitation, 10,* 67–101.

Farah, M. J., & McClelland, J. L. (1991). A computational model of semantic memory impairment: Modality-specificity and emergent category-specificity. *Journal of Experimental Psychology: General, 120*(4), 339–357.

Fillingham, J. K., Hodgson, C., Sage, K., & Lambon Ralph, M. A. (2003). The application of errorless learning to aphasic disorders: A review of theory and practice. *Neuropsychological Rehabilitation, 13,* 337–363.

Forde, E. M. E., & Humphreys, G. W. (1999). Category specific recognition impairments: A review of important case studies and influential theories. *Aphasiology, 13,* 169–193.

Friedrich, F. J., Glenn, C. G., & Marin, O. S. M. (1984). Interruption of phonological coding in conduction aphasia. *Brain and Language, 22,* 266–291.

Geschwind, N. (1965). Disconnexion syndromes in animals and man. *Brain, 88,* 237–294.

Gleick, J. (1987). *Chaos: Making a new science*. New York: Viking.

Glenberg, A. M. (1979). Component-levels theory of the effects of spacing of repetitions on recall and recognition. *Memory & Cognition, 7,* 95–112.

Glenberg, A. M., & Lehmann, T. S. (1980). Spacing repetitions over 1 week. *Memory & Cognition, 8,* 528–538.

Gold, M., Nadeau, S. E., Jacobs, D. H., Adair, J. C., Gonzalez-Rothi, L. J., & Heilman, K. M. (1997). Adynamic aphasia: A transcortical motor aphasia with defective semantic strategy formation. *Brain and Language, 57,* 374–393.

Goldman-Rakic, P. S. (1990). Cellular and circuit basis of working memory in prefrontal cortex of nonhuman primates. *Progress in Brain Research, 85,* 325–336.

Goodglass, H. (1993). *Understanding aphasia*. San Diego: Academic Press.

Goodglass, H., & Kaplan, E. (2000). *Boston Diagnostic Aphasia Examination* (3rd ed.). East Moline, IL: LinguiSystems.

Goodman, J. S., & Wood, R. E. (2004). Feedback specificity, learning opportunities, and learning. *Journal of Applied Psychology, 89,* 809–821.

Greene, R. L. (1989). Spacing effects in memory: Evidence for a two-process account. *Journal of Experimental Psychology: Learn Mem Cogn, 15,* 371–377.

Gronwall, D. M. A. (1977). Paced auditory serial addition test: A measure of recovery from concussion. *Percept Motor Skills, 44,* 367–373.

Harley, T. A. (1984). A critique of top-down independent levels models of speech production: Evidence from non-plan-internal speech errors. *Cognitive Science, 8*, 191–219.

Hart, J., & Gordon, B. (1990). Delineation of single-word semantic comprehension deficits in aphasia, with anatomical correlation. *Annals of Neurology, 27*, 226–231.

Hebb, D. O. (1949). *The organization of behavior*. New York: Wiley.

Heilman, K. M., Voeller, K. S., & Nadeau, S. E. (1991). A possible pathophysiological substrate of attention-deficit-hyperactivity disorder. *Journal of Child Neurology, 6*(Suppl), S76–S78.

Hillary, F. G., Schultheis, M. T., Challis, B. H., Carnevale, G. J., Galshi, T., & DeLuca, J. (2003). Spacing of repetitions improves learning and memory after moderate and severe TBI. *Journal of Clinical and Experimental Neuropsychology, 25*, 49–58.

Hillis, A. E. (1998). Treatment of naming disorders: New issues regarding old therapies. *JINS, 4*, 648–660.

Hintzman, D. L. (1974). Theoretical implications of the spacing effect. In R. L. Solso (Ed.), *Theories in cognitive psychology: The Loyola symposium* (pp. 77–99). Potomac, MD: Lawrence Erlbaum.

Hochhalter, A. K., Overmier, J. B., Gasper, S. M., Bakke, B. L., & Holub, R. J. (2005). A comparison of spaced retrieval to other schedules of practice for people with dementia. *Experimental Aging Research, 31*, 101–118.

Howard, D., Patterson, K., Franklin, S., Orchard-Lisle, V., & Morton, J. (1985). Treatment of word retrieval deficits in aphasia. A comparison of two therapy methods. *Brain, 108*, 817–829.

Hunkin, N. M., Squires, E. J., Parkin, A. J., & Tidy, J. A. (1998). Are the benefits of errorless learning dependent on implicit memory? *Neuropsychologia, 36*, 25–36.

Jones, R. S., & Eayrs, C. B. (1992). The use of errorless learning procedures in teaching people with a learning disability: A critical review. *Mental Handicap Research, 5*, 204–212.

Kaplan, E., Goodglass, H., Weintraub, S., & Segal, O. (1983). *Boston Naming Test*. Philadelphia: Lea and Febiger.

Kendall, D. L., Rosenbek, J. C., Heilman, K. M., Conway, T. W., Klenberg, K., Gonzalez Rothi, L. J., et al. Brain & Language (in press). Phoneme-based rehabilitation of anomia in aphasia.

Kertesz, A. (1982). *Western Aphasia Battery*. New York: Grune and Stratton.

Kertesz, A., & Sheppard, A. (1981). The epidemiology of aphasic and cognitive impairment in stroke. Age, sex, aphasia type, and laterality differences. *Brain, 104*, 117–128.

Kilgard, M. P., & Merzenich, M. M. (1998). Cortical map reorganization enabled by nucleus basalis activity. *Science, 279*, 1714–1718.

Kiran, S., & Thompson, C. K. (2003). The role of semantic complexity in treatment of naming deficits: Training semantic categories in fluent aphasia by controlling exemplar typicality. *Journal of Speech, Language, and Hearing Research, 46*, 608–622.

Knock, T. R., Ballard, K. J., Robin, D. A., & Schmidt, R. A. (2000). Influence of order of stimulus presentation on speech motor learning: A principled approach to treatment for apraxia of speech. *Aphasiology, 14*, 653–668.

Kolb, B. (2004). Mechanisms of cortical plasticity after neuronal injury. In J. Ponsford (Ed.), *Cognitive and behavioral rehabilitation* (pp. 30–58). New York: Guilford Press.

Kolb, B., & Cioe, J. (2004). Neuronal organization and change after neuronal injury. In J. Ponsford (Ed.), *Cognitive and behavioral rehabilitation* (pp. 7–29). New York: Guilford Press.

Kolk, H. H. J., & Friederici, A. D. (1985). Strategy and impairment in sentence understanding by Broca's and Wernicke's aphasics. *Cortex, 21*, 47–67.

Lichtheim, L. (1885). On aphasia. *Brain, 7*, 433–484.

Lindamood, P. C., & Lindamood, P. D. (1998). *The Lindamood phoneme sequencing program for reading, spelling and speech*. Austin, TX: Pro-Ed.

Maher, L. M., Kendall, D., Swearengin, J. A., Pingel, K., Holland, A., & Roth, L. J. G. (2003). Constraint induced language therapy for chronic aphasia: Preliminary findings. *JINS, 9*, 192.

Makris, N., Kennedy, D. N., McInerney, S., Sorensen, A. G., Wang, R., Caviness, V. S., et al. (2005). Segmentation of subcomponents within the superior longitudinal fascicle in humans: A quantitative, in vivo, DT-MRI study. *Cerebral Cortex, 15*, 854–869.

Martin, N., Fink, R., & Laine, M. (2004). Treatment of word retrieval deficits with contextual priming. *Aphasiology, 18*, 457–471.

McCarthy, R., & Warrington, E. K. (1984). A two-route model of speech production. Evidence from aphasia. *Brain, 107*, 463–485.

McClelland, J. L., McNaughton, B. L., & O'Reilly, R. C. (1995). Why there are complementary learning systems in the hippocampus and neocortex: Insights from the successes and failures of connectionist models of learning and memory. *Psychological Review, 102*, 419–457.

McClelland, J. L., & Rumelhart, D. E. (1981). An interactive activation model of context effects in letter perception: Part 1. An account of basic findings. *Psychological Review, 88*, 375–407.

McClelland, J. L., Rumelhart, D. E., & PDP Research Group. (1986). *Parallel distributed processing*. Cambridge, Massachusetts: MIT Press.

McCloskey, M., & Cohen, N. J. (1989). Catastrophic interference in connectionist networks: The sequential learning problem. In G. H. Bower (Ed.), *The psychology of learning and motivation: Advances in research and theory* (pp. 109–165). San Diego: Academic Press.

Meinzer, M., Djundja, D., Barthel, G., Elbert, T. R., & Rockstroh, B. (2005). Long-term stability of improved language functions in chronic aphasia after constraint-induced aphasia therapy. *Stroke, 36*, 1462–1466.

Melton, A. W. (1970). The situation with respect to the spacing of repetitions and memory. *Journal of Verbal Learning and Verbal Behavior, 9*, 596–606.

Miceli, G., Caltagirone, C., Gainotti, G., Masullo, C., Silveri, M. C., & Villa, G. (1981). Influence of age, sex, literacy and pathologic lesion on incidence, severity and type of aphasia. *Acta Neurologica Scandinavica, 64*, 370–382.

Mitchum, C. C., & Berndt, R. S. (2001). Cognitive neuropsychological approaches to diagnosing and treating language disorders. In R. Chapey (Ed.), *Language intervention strategies in aphasia and related neurogenic communication disorders* (pp. 551–571). Philadelphia: Lippincott Williams and Wilkins.

Murphy, H. H. (1916). Distribution of practice periods in learning. *Journal of Educational Psychology, 7*, 150–162.

Nadeau, S. E. (1988). Impaired grammar with normal fluency and phonology. Implications for Broca's aphasia. *Brain, 111*, 1111–1137.

Nadeau, S. E. (2000). Connectionist models and language. In S. E. Nadeau, L. J. Gonzalez Rothi, & B. Crosson (Eds.), *Aphasia and language. Theory to practice* (pp. 299–347). New York: Guilford Press.

Nadeau, S. E. (2001). Phonology: A review and proposals from a connectionist perspective. *Brain and Language, 79,* 511–579.

Nadeau, S. E., & Crosson, B. (1997). Subcortical aphasia. *Brain and Language, 58,* 355–402.

Nadeau, S. E., Ferguson, T. S., Valenstein, E., Vierck, C. J., Petruska, J. C., Streit, W. J., et al. (2004). *Medical neuroscience.* Philadelphia: Saunders/Elsevier.

Nadeau, S. E., & Gonzalez-Rothi, L. J. (1993). Morphologic agrammatism following a right hemisphere stroke in a dextral patient. *Brain and Language, 43,* 642–667.

Nadeau, S. E., & Kendall, D. L. (2006). Significance and possible mechanisms underlying generalization in aphasia therapy: Semantic treatment of anomia. *Brain and Language, 99,* 10–11.

O'Reilly, R. C. (1996). Biologically plausible error-driven learning using local activation differences: The generalized recirculation algorithm. *Neural Computation, 8,* 895–938.

O'Reilly, R. C. (1998). Six principles for biologically based computational models of cortical cognition. *Trends in Cognitive Sciences, 2,* 455–462.

Patterson, K., Purell, C., & Morton, J. (1983). Facilitation of word retrieval in aphasia. In C. Code & D. J. Muller (Eds.), *Aphasia therapy.* London: Arnold.

Patterson, K., & Shewell, C. (1987). Speak and spell: Dissociations and word-class effects. In M. Coltheart, G. Sartori, & R. Job (Eds.), *The cognitive neuropsychology of language* (pp. 273–294). London: Lawrence Erlbaum.

Peterson, L. R., & Peterson, M. J. (1959). Short-term retention of individual verbal items. *Journal of Experimental Psychology, 58,* 193–198.

Plaut, D. C. (1996). Relearning after damage in connectionist networks: Toward a theory of rehabilitation. *Brain and Language, 52,* 25–82.

Plaut, D. C., McClelland, J. L., Seidenberg, M. S., & Patterson, K. (1996). Understanding normal and impaired word reading: Computational principles in quasi-regular domains. *Psychological Review, 103,* 56–115.

Power, A. E. (2004). Slow-wave sleep, acetylcholine, and memory consolidation. *PNAS, 101,* 1795–1796.

Prather, P., Zurif, E., Stern, C., & Rosen, T. J. (1992). Slowed lexical access in nonfluent aphasia. A case study. *Brain and Language, 43,* 336–348.

Proctor, P. W., & Dutta, A. (1995). *Skill acquisition and human performance.* Thousand Oaks, CA: Sage.

Pulvermüller, F., Neininger, B., Elbert, T., Mohr, B., Rockstroh, B., Koebbel, P., et al. (2001). Constraint-induced therapy of chronic aphasia after stroke. *Stroke, 32,* 1621–1626.

Pyle, W. H. (1913). Economical learning. *Journal of Educational Psychology, 4,* 148–158.

Raymer, A. M., Foundas, A. L., Maher, L. M., Greenwald, M. L., Morris, M., Rothi, L. J., et al. (1997). Cognitive neuropsychological analysis and neuroanatomic correlates in a case of acute anomia. *Brain and Language, 58,* 137–156.

Raymer, A. M., & Rothi, L. J. G. (2000). The semantic system. In S. E. Nadeau, L. J. G. Rothi, & B. Crosson (Eds.), *Aphasia and language: Theory to practice* (pp. 108–132). New York: Guilford.

Raymer, A. M., Singletary, F., Rodriguez, A., Ciampitti, M., Heilman, K. M., & Rothi, L. J. G. (2006). Effects of

gesture+verbal treatment for noun and verb retrieval in aphasia. *JINS, 12,* 867–882.

Raymer, A. M., Thompson, C. K., Jacobs, B., & Le Grand, H. R. (1993). Phonological treatment of naming deficits in aphasia: Model-based generalization analysis. *Aphasiology, 7,* 27–54.

Rolls, E. T., & Deco, G. (2002). *Computational neuroscience of vision.* Oxford: Oxford University Press.

Rolls, E. T., & Treves, A. (1998). *Neural networks and brain function.* New York: Oxford University Press.

Roth, H. L., Nadeau, S. E., Hollingsworth, A. L., Cimino-Knight, A. M., Heilman, K. M. (2006). Naming concepts: Evidence of two routes. *Neurocase, 12,* 61–70.

Rumelhart, D. E., & McClelland, J. L. (1982). An interactive activation model of context effects in letter perception: Part 2. The contextual enhancement effect and some tests and extensions of the model. *Psychological Review, 89,* 60–94.

Rumelhart, D. E., Smolensky, P., McClelland, J. L., & Hinton, G. E. (1986). Schemata and sequential thought processes in PDP models. In J. L. McClelland, D. E. Rumelhart, & the PDP Research Group (Eds.), *Parallel distributed processing* (Vol. 2, pp. 7–57). Cambridge, Massachusetts: MIT Press.

Saffran, E. M., & Marin, O. S. M. (1975). Immediate memory for word lists in a patient with deficient auditory short-term memory. *Brain and Language, 2,* 420–433.

Saffran, E. M., & Schwartz, M. F. (1988). 'Agrammatic' comprehension it's not: Alternatives and implications. *Aphasiology, 2,* 389–394.

Saffran, E. M., Schwartz, M. F., & Marin, O. (1980). The word order problem in agrammatism: Production. *Brain and Language, 10,* 263–280.

Schmidt, R. A., & Bjork, R. A. (1992). Common principles in three paradigms suggest new concepts for training. *Psychological Science, 3,* 207–271.

Schmidt, R. A., & Wrisberg, C. A. (2004). *Motor learning and performance* (3rd ed.). Champaign, IL: Human Kinetics.

Schwartz, M. F., Linebarger, M. C., Saffran, E. M., & Pate, D. S. (1987). Syntactic transparency and sentence interpretation in aphasia. *Language and Cognitive Processes, 2,* 85–113.

Seidenberg, M. S., & McClelland, J. L. (1989). A distributed, developmental model of word recognition and naming. *Psychological Review, 96,* 523–568.

Sejinowski, T. J., & Rosenberg, C. R. (1988). Learning and representation in connectionist models. In M. S. Gazzinaga (Ed.), *Perspectives in memory research.* Cambridge, MA: MIT Press.

Shea, C. H., Lai, Q., Black, C., & Park, J.- H. (2000). Spacing practice sessions across days benefits the learning of motor skills. *Human Movement Science, 19,* 737–760.

Shebilske, W. L., Goettl, B. P., Corrington, K., & Day, E. A. (1999). Interlession spacing and task-related processing during complex skill acquisition. *Journal of Experimental Psychology: Appl, 5,* 413–437.

Shuren, J., & Heilman, K. M. (1993). Non-optic aphasia. *Neurology, 43,* 1900–1907.

Speedie, L. J., Wertman, E., Ta'ir, J., & Heilman, K. M. (1993). Disruption of automatic speech following a right basal ganglia lesion. *Neurology, 43,* 1768–1774.

Squire, L. R., & Knowlton, B. J. (2000). The medial temporal lobe, the hippocampus and the memory systems of the brain. In M. S. Gazzaniga (Ed.), *The new cognitive neurosciences* (pp. 765–779). Cambridge: MIT Press.

Squire, L. R., & Zola-Morgan, S. (1991). The medial temporal lobe memory system. *Science, 253,* 1380–1386.

Stablum, F., Umiltà, C., Mogentale, C., Carlan, M., & Guerrini, C. (2000). Rehabilitation of executive deficits in closed head injury and anterior communicating artery aneurysm patients. *Psychological Research, 63,* 265–278.

Stemberger, J. P. (1985). An interactive activation model of language production. In A. W. Ellis (Ed.), *Progress in the psychology of language* (Vol. 1, pp. 143–186). Hillsdale, NJ: Lawrence Erlbaum.

Stickgold, R., & Walker, M. P. (2005). Memory consolidation and reconsolidation: What is the role of sleep? *TINS, 28,* 408–415.

Sutton, M. A., Ide, J., Masters, S. E., & Carew, T. J. (2002). Interaction between amount and pattern of training in the induction of intermediate- and long-term memory for sensitization in aplysia. *Learning & Memory, 9,* 29–40.

Swinnen, S. P., Nicholson, D. E., Schmidt, R. A., & Shapiro, D. C. (1990). Information feedback for skill acquisition—Instantaneous knowledge of results degrades learning. *Journal of Experimental Psychology Learning and Memory Cognition, 16,* 706–716.

Taub, E., Uswatte, G., King, D. K., Morris, D., Crago, J. E., & Chatterjee, A. (2006). A placebo-controlled trial of constraint-induced movement therapy for upper extremity after stroke. *Stroke, 37,* 1045–1049.

Taub, E., Uswatte, G., & Pidikiti, R. (1999). Constraint-induced movement therapy: A new family of techniques with broad application to physical rehabilitation—A clinical review. *Journal of Rehabilitation Research and Development, 36,* 237–251.

Thompson, C. K. (2001). Treatment of underlying forms: A linguistic specific approach to sentence production deficits in agrammatic aphasia. In R. Chapey (Ed.), *Language intervention strategies in aphasia and related neurogenic communication disorders* (4th ed., pp. 605–625). Philadelphia: Lippincott Williams and Wilkins.

Thompson, C. K., Lange, K. L., Schneider, S. L., & Shapiro, L. P. (1997). Agrammatic and non-brain damaged subjects' verb and verb argument structure production. *Aphasiology, 11,* 473–490.

Thompson, C. K., Shapiro, L. P., Kiran, S., & Sobecks, J. (2003). The role of syntactic complexity in treatment of sentence deficits in agrammatic aphasia: The complexity account of treatment efficacy (CATE). *Journal of Speech, Language, and Hearing Research, 46,* 591–607.

Ullman, M. T. (2004). Contributions of memory circuits to language: The declarative/procedural model. *Cognition, 92,* 231–270.

Vargha-Khadem, F., Gadian, D. G., Watkins, K. E., Connelly, A., Van Paesschen, W., & Mishkin, M. (1997). Differential effects of early hippocampal pathology on episodic and semantic memory. *Science, 277,* 376–380.

Vitevitch, M. S. (1997). The neighborhood characteristics of malapropisms. *Language & Speech, 40,* 211–228.

von Monakow, C. (1914). *Die lokalisation im grosshirn.* Wiesbaden: Bergmann.

Walker, M. P., & Stickgold, R. (2004). Sleep-dependent learning and memory consolidation. *Neuron, 44,* 121–133.

Wambaugh, J. L., Kalinyak-Fliszar, M. M., West, J. E., & Doyle, P. J. (1998). Effects of treatment for sound errors in apraxia of speech and aphasia. *Journal of Speech, Language, and Hearing Research, 41,* 725–743.

Warrington, E. K., & Shallice, T. (1969). The selective impairment of auditory verbal short-term memory. *Brain, 92,* 885–896.

Warrington, E. K., & Shallice, T. (1984). Category specific semantic impairments. *Brain, 107,* 829–854.

Weeks, D. L., & Kordus, R. N. (1998). Relative frequency of knowledge of performance and motor skill learning. *Research Quarterly for Exercise and Sport, 69,* 224–230.

Weinrich, M., Shelton, J. R., Cox, D. M., & McCall, D. (1997). Remediating production of tense morphology improves verb retrieval in chronic aphasia. *Brain and Language, 58,* 23–45.

Whatmough, C., Chertkow, H., Murtha, S., & Hanratty, K. (2002). Dissociable brain regions process object meaning and object structure during picture naming. *Neuropsychologia, 40,* 174–186.

Winstein, C. J., Merians, A. S., & Sullivan, K. J. (1999). Motor learning after unilateral brain damage. *Neuropsychologia, 37,* 975–987.

Winstein, C. J., & Schmidt, R. A. (1990). Reduced frequency of knowledge of results enhances motor skill learning. *Journal of Experimental Psychology Learning and Memory Cognition, 16,* 677–691.

Zaidel, E., Iacoboni, M., Zaidel, D. W., & Bogen, J. (2003). The callosal syndromes. In K. M. Heilman & E. Valenstein (Eds.), *Clinical neuropsychology* (4th ed., pp. 347–403). New York: Oxford University Press.

Chapter 27

Treatment of Syntactic and Morphologic Deficits in Agrammatic Aphasia: Treatment of Underlying Forms

Cynthia K. Thompson

OBJECTIVES

The objectives of this chapter are to present the background, methods, and efficacy data for two treatments for agrammatism. The generalization effects of these treatments to untrained structures and narrative discourse are emphasized. Neuroimaging data also are presented that show the effects of treatment on brain activity.

This chapter discusses two recently developed and researched treatments for sentence production (and comprehension) deficits in non-fluent, agrammatic aphasia. One treatment is designed for improving syntactic deficits and the other for improving grammatical morphology. Derived from mutually supportive linguistic and language processing theories, both treatments promote generalization using a "metalinguistic" training procedure, controlling the linguistic nature and complexity of structures trained based on the underlying representation of target structures. Two principles of generalization underlie these treatments: (1) generalization occurs to structures that are linguistically related to those trained but not to linguistically unrelated material, and (2) generalization is enhanced by beginning treatment with more complex rather than simple structures.

WHAT IS AGRAMMATISM?

Agrammatism is a symptom complex seen in the context of nonfluent (Broca's) aphasia. Classically, the site of lesion is associated with the frontal opercular region, occupying Brodmann's areas 44 and 45 adjacent cortical and subcortical regions (Damasio, 1991). Today, however, it is well known that agrammatic speech patterns can result from lesions

(both large and small) occupying these and other areas.[1] The disorder refers to a pattern of erroneous sentence production in which grammatical structure is diminished (or absent). Individuals with agrammatism often use strings of (primarily) content words and have greater difficulty producing verbs as compared to nouns (Kohn, Lorch, & Pearson, 1989; Kim & Thompson, 2000, 2004; Thompson et al., 1997; Zingeser & Berndt, 1990).

Even when individuals with agrammatic aphasia produce verbs, the structures in which they appear generally are simple, subject-verb-object (SVO) constructions (Caplan & Hanna, 1998; Goodglass, Christiansen, & Gallagher, 1993; Saffran, Berndt, & Schwartz, 1989). The *arguments* of the verb—that is, the participant roles required by the verb— also may be missing or mis-ordered around the verb. For example, verb-object (e.g., *fit her*) and subject-verb (e.g., *Shoe uh fit*) sequences are common. In the former, the *agent* is missing from subject position, and in the latter, the *theme* is missing from the object position. Notably, individuals with agrammatic aphasia have marked difficulty producing complex sentences in which noun phrases (NPs) have been moved out of their canonical order (i.e., SVO in English), such as "wh-" questions (e.g., *Cinderella where?* should be *Where is Cinderella?*) (Saffran et al., 1989; Thompson et al., 1995).

Another key problem in agrammatism is production of grammatical/functional morphology, including finite verb inflections (tense, agreement), complementizers (if, whether, that), and other free-standing morphemes (Benedet, Christiansen, & Goodglass, 1998; Bird, Franklin, & Howard,

---

[1] The lesion site associated with agrammatism can vary greatly. Vanier and Caplan (1990) reported lesions quantified by computed tomographic scans from 20 cross-linguistic cases of agrammatism, ranging from small lesions located in the frontal lobe or outside the frontal lobe, sparing the entirety of the perisylvian lateral cortex, to middle-sized lesions affecting both cortical and subcortical structures to large lesions affecting the entire perisylvian area and other structures in the distribution of the middle cerebral artery.

2002; Caramazza & Hillis, 1989; Druks & Carroll, 2005; Faroqi-Shah & Thompson, 2004; Goodglass, 1976; Menn & Obler, 1990). Either omission or substitution of these elements renders sentences ungrammatical (e.g., *Slipper fell* should be *The slipper is falling* or *The slipper fell*). Consider the following selected utterances produced by a 41-year-old gentleman with nonfluent Broca's aphasia illustrating many of the characteristics of agrammatic speech. He is telling the story of Cinderella:

Cinderella uh . . . scrubbing and uh . . . hard worker.
Step fa . . . mother uh go . . . but no.
Scrubbing uh uh whatchacallit uh uh working.
Stepmother really ugly.
Dress break . . . stepmother and now what dress?
Mother Teresa . . . not exactly . . . uh uh magic godmother!
Dress . . . beautiful and carriage where?
I can uh . . . pumpkin and uh . . . servants and horse and beautiful carriage and so magic. But, better midnight . . . pumpkin carriage gone.
Cinderella dance.
Midnight uh clock uh Cinderella clock!
Slipper fall.
Prince can't uh uh stepmother fitting slipper?
Cinderella where?
Well locked.
Sure enough fits because Cinderella uh . . . magic uh . . . girl.
And probably uh prince and Cinderella marrying and happy.
That's it.

Agrammatic aphasia also is associated with deficits in comprehension, although general descriptions of the disorder suggest that comprehension remains relatively spared (Goodglass, 1976; for historical review, see also de Blesser, 1987). These patients show particular difficulty comprehending noncanonical sentences, such as passive sentences and object relative clauses (e.g., *The artist was chased by the thief* or *The man saw the artist who the thief chased*), but less difficulty is noted in comprehending active sentences or those with subject relative clauses (e.g., *The thief chased the artist* or *The man saw the thief who chased the thief*) (Berndt, Mitchum, & Haendiges, 1996; Caplan & Hildebrandt, 1988; Grodzinsky, 1986). This pattern of comprehension impairment is referred to as "asyntactic comprehension." It is important to note that agrammatic patients often show particular difficulty with semantically reversible sentences (i.e., those in which two nouns are equally probable candidates for the thematic role of agent of the action).

THEORETIC UNDERPINNINGS

Several theories of agrammatism exist, both representational and processing. No one theory, however, accommodates deficits in both production and comprehension, and no one theory completely accommodates all available data regarding agrammatic speech. In this section, linguistic constructs and theories that are most relevant to the treatment approaches described below are discussed.

Treatment of underlying forms (TUF), whether focused on syntactic or morphologic deficits, is based on representational (linguistic) theory (within the framework of generative syntax; see Chomsky 1986, 1993, 1995)[2] and processing accounts of language, which suggest that agrammatic impairments are caused by faulty processing or access to relevant linguistic representations. We begin with a representational description of the syntactic tree, which provides a hierarchy of nodes describing the relation among elements, both lexical and functional, that form clauses and sentences in the English language. Tree structures are abstract descriptions, but they provide a template for well-formed sentences against which observed patterns of sentence disruption in agrammatism can be compared.

The tree diagram shown in Figure 27–1, going from the top-down, includes the complementizer phrase (CP), which is comprised of two positions from which linguistic elements project: the specifier position (Spec, CP), which accommodates "wh-" words in sentences such as *Who did the hiker follow?*, and the head position (COMP), the site for complementizers such as *if*, *that*, and *whether* in sentences with embedded clauses such as *I wonder whether the team will play next week.*[3] Thus, CP is crucial for complex sentences that often are impaired in agrammatism, like "wh-" questions and sentences with embeddings (e.g., complement clauses).

The next level is the inflection phrase (IP), which also has two major branches: the SPEC position (Spec, IP), and the INFL (the local head of IP). Spec, IP is the subject position as in *The lady chased the bartender at the party.*[4] The subject in passive sentences such as *The bartender was chased by the lady at the party* also occupies Spec, IP. The INFL position contains finite verb inflections—that is, tense and agreement information. Some linguists suggest that all inflectional morphology is projected from IP (Bobaljik & Thráinsson, 1988), while others contend that IP is subdivided into pro-

---

[2] The theoretical constructs that we exploit are integral to Government-Binding Theory, the Principles and Parameters (P & P) frameworks, and the Minimalist Program (Chomsky, 1986, 1993, 1995; Marantz, 1995), but they also have their counterparts in other linguistic theories. For example, X-bar theory, subcategorization, and argument structure are part of Generalized Phrase Structure Grammar (GPSG) (Gazdar, Klein, Pullum, & Sag, 1985) and Lexical Functional Grammar (LFG) (Bresnan, 1992). Noncontinuous dependencies of the sort that are targeted in syntactic treatment also are considered in GPSG (e.g., the category SLASH, which effectively connects one part of the tree to another) and LFG (i.e., functional control).

[3] COMP also is the landing site for auxiliary verb movement—for example, in yes/no questions such as *Are you going to the opera tonight?*

[4] According to current theory, the subject is generated within the verb phrase (Koopman & Sportiche, 1991), and moves to Spec, CP.

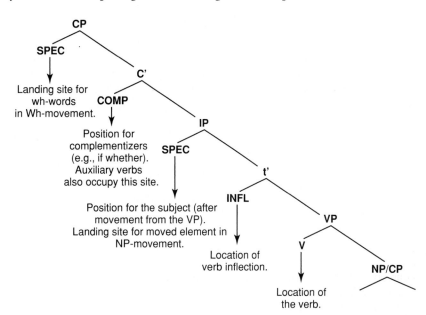

Figure 27–1. General linguistic tree structure, illustrating positions for various structures in the English language. Shown are local trees headed by CP (complementizer phrase), IP (inflection phrase), and VP (verb phrase). Going from the top down, the *specifier* position of CP (Spec, CP) is the landing site for "wh-" words. The head of CP (C', COMP) is the position for complementizers, such as *if*, *that*, *whether*. The auxiliary verb in subject-auxiliary inversion (i.e., verb movement) also takes this position. The next level down is IP. Its *specifier* position (Spec, IP) is the subject position. The local head INFL contains verb tense and agreement information. Finally, verbs and other lexical material are generated in VP.

jections for a tense phrase (TP), negative phrase, and agreement phrase (AgrP) (Pollock, 1989).[5] Because many agrammatic speakers have selective deficits producing verb inflections, the configuration of IP is relevant to treatment.

The next level in the tree is the verb phrase (VP). The VP is associated with basic lexical categories (e.g., nouns, verbs, adjectives, or adverbs). The main verb projects from the head of VP, and in its sister position are verb complements—that is, internal arguments of the verb—which can be either NPs (theme arguments) or CPs (sentential complements). Thus, the VP accommodates sentence elements that are impaired in agrammatism as discussed below.

Canonical Sentence Computation: The Role of the Verb

The *canonical* (usual) form of sentences in the English language is SVO, with the verb serving as the core of the sentence. Agrammatic speakers have difficulty producing verbs as well as the arguments that go with them, rendering their sentences ungrammatical. That is, the verb provides the scaffolding of grammatical sentences; without a verb, a word string does not qualify as a sentence. In addition, the verb selects and assigns associated syntactic and semantic features, including argument structure and thematic roles. These features also must be present in grammatical sentences. For example *the fairy Godmother fixes.* and *The stepsisters put Cinderella.* are ungrammatical, because all of the arguments of the verb are not represented.

Importantly, several types of verbs are defined by their syntactic and semantic features. Consider the following sentences:

1. Everyday, <u>the parrot</u> AGENT *laughs*
2. Everyday, <u>the dancer</u> AGENT *fixes* <u>her shoes</u> THEME
3. Everyday, <u>the artist</u> AGENT *puts* <u>fresh flowers</u> THEME <u>in the studio</u> GOAL

The verb *laugh* (sentence 1) is a one-argument (pure intransitive) verb. This means that only one participant role is required: agent. *Fix* is a two-argument verb as in sentence 2; it assigns two thematic roles: agent and theme. The verb *put* assigns three-arguments (agent, theme, and goal). Other verbs, such as *wonder*, *care*, *see*, or *believe*, are complement verbs that assign sentential complements as in sentence 4 below:

4. Everyday, <u>the editor</u> AGENT *wonders* <u>whether the writer finished the article</u> SENTENTIAL COMPLEMENT/INTERROGATIVE

Research in agrammatism shows that the number and type of arguments required by the verb influence production. As argument structure becomes more complex, production ability decreases: Three-argument verbs are more difficult to produce than two- or one-argument verbs, and when these verbs are produced in sentence contexts, obligatory arguments often are omitted. This pattern has been noted in English as well as in Dutch, German, Italian, and Hungarian agrammatic speakers (de Bleser & Kauschke, 2000; Jonkers & Bastiaanse, 1998; Kemmerer & Tranel, 2000; Kim & Thompson, 2000, 2004; Kiss 2000; Luzzatti et al., 2002; Thompson et al., 1997). Further, complement verbs such as *wonder* are difficult for patients with Broca's

---

[5] The status of IP (i.e., split or unsplit) likely is language specific.

aphasia (Thompson et al., 1997), and intransitive unaccusative verbs such as *melt* and *amuse*-type psychological verbs, which involve complex syntactic and/or semantic computations, are more difficult to produce than agentive intransitive such as *sleep* and *admire*-type psychological verbs, which do not (Bastiaanse & van Zonneveld, 2005; Lee & Thompson, 2004; Thompson, 2003).

Some theories of agrammatic production attribute sentence deficits to verbs and verb argument structure. Bastiaanse and van Zonneveld (2005) found that speakers with Broca's aphasic are better at producing unaccusative verbs like *melt* in transitive sentence frames (e.g., *The sun melted the snowman*) than in intransitive frames (e.g., *The snowman melted*), because the latter word order involves movement of the theme argument (*snowman*) to the subject position of the sentence. Similarly, the Argument Structure Complexity Hypothesis suggests that verbs with more complex argument structure (considering both the number and type of arguments in the lexical entry of the verb) are more difficult than those with less complex argument structure, because the former entail greater phrase structure building demands (Thompson, 2003). Other theories point to representational deficits, such as the Tree Pruning Hypothesis (TPH; discussed in detail below) (Friedmann 2002; Friedmann & Grodzinsky 1997), whereas resource-based accounts suggest that agrammatism results from reduced short-term working memory or limited processing capacity (Goodglass 1976; Kolk 1987; Kolk & Heeschen, 1990).

Phrase Structure Building

Theoretic accounts of phrase structure building suggest that the verb guides this process. In the Minimalist Program, a syntactic operation, Merge, serves to amalgamate two categories to yield a higher-order category, and a series of Merge operations builds the syntactic structure of sentences (Chomsky, 1995, 1993; Marantz, 1995; see also Adger, 2003). Simply put, a lexical item (e.g., a verb) is selected from the lexicon and combines with other selected items to form a higher-order category. So, for example, considering the two-argument verb *chase* and its thematic grid (agent, theme), agent is assigned to the subject position, and theme is assigned to the direct object position. Figure 27–2 demonstrates how this occurs in a sentence such as *The dog chased the cat*. The verb (*chase*) merges with a determiner phrase (DP; *the cat*) to yield V' and assigns the thematic role theme. The V' then merges with another DP (*the dog*), assigning the role of agent and forming a VP. The VP then merges with higher nodes in the syntactic tree. The number of arguments selected by the verb affects phrase structure operations: The greater the number of arguments, the more steps required to build phrase structural frames. (For further discussion of phrase structure building operations, see Lee & Thompson, 2004.)

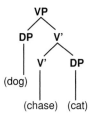

Figure 27–2. Schematic representation of merge within the verb phrase (VP). DP = determiner phrase; V = verb.

Psycholinguistic and neurolinguistic research findings indicate that verb argument structure also influences sentence processing. Both normal and agrammatic speakers appear to access not only the verb but also its thematic representations when listening to sentences (see, e.g., Shapiro, Gordon, Hack, & Killacky, 1993; Shapiro & Levine, 1990; Shapiro, McNamara, Zurif, Lanzoni, & Cermak, 1991). Using a cross-modal lexical decision task, Shapiro and colleagues found that reaction times for complex verbs (i.e., those with more dense argument structure entries) are longer than for simple verbs. These findings suggest that when the verb is accessed during the temporal unfolding of a sentence, so, too, are its thematic properties. The fact that individuals with Broca's aphasia retain this ability after brain damage is important in the treatment of agrammatism.

Noncanonical Sentence Computation

As noted above, the *canonical* form of sentences in the English language is SVO, such as *Zack climbed Mt. Katadin*. Of course, many sentences do not follow this simple pattern (see sentences 5–8 below). Theoretically, however, all sentences are derived from their underlying SVO representation, a pure representation of lexical information, and despite appearing in different positions, *Zack* is the agent (the person doing the climbing) and *Mt Katadin* (or what) is the theme (the thing that was climbed) in all sentences:

5. What mountain did Zack climb? (object "wh-" question)
6. It was Mt. Katadin that Zack climbed. (object cleft)
7. Mt. Katadin was climbed by Zack. (passive)
8. Zack seems to have climbed Mt. Katadin. (subject raising structure)

By displacement—*movement*—of sentence constituents from their underlying position to a different location in the sentence, a new surface form is derived. Two types of movement are relevant to agrammatism: *Wh-movement*, and *NP-movement*. Wh-movement is involved in wh-questions (sentence 5) and object clefts (sentence 6); NP-movement is involved in passives (sentence 7) and subject raising sentences (sentence 8).

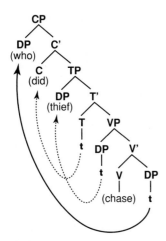

Figure 27–3. Tree diagram illustrating Wh-movement in "wh-" questions, such as *Who did the thief chase?* Movement is from the direct object position to the Spec, CP. Subject-auxiliary verb inversion also is depicted.

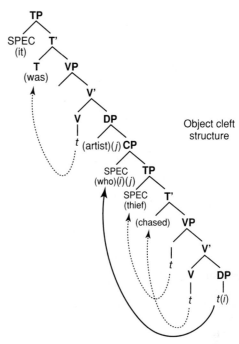

Figure 27–4. Tree diagram illustrating Wh-movement in object cleft structures, such as *It was the artist who the thief chased.* Movement is from the direct object position to Spec, CP, as in "wh-" questions. Importantly, movement occurs in an embedded clause. Note that there is a co-referential relation between the moved element (e.g., *who*) and the head noun of the main clause (*the artist*), marked by subscripted j.

Wh-Movement

Consider the Wh-movement structures in sentences 5 and 6 above. Indeed, on the face of it, these two sentences appear to be quite different. They are fundamentally similar, however, in that both involve Wh-movement. Consider sentences 9a and 9b below; sentence 9a is an approximation of the underlying representation of sentence 9b:

9a. Zack $_{\text{AGENT}}$ climbed what $_{\text{THEME}}$
9b. What$_{i\ \text{THEME}}$ did Zack $_{\text{AGENT}}$ climb [t$_i$]

In sentence 9a, *what* is in the direct object position and is assigned the thematic role of theme by the verb *climb*. To derive the noncanonical surface form, *what* is moved to the sentence initial position, leaving behind a *copy or trace* (*t*) in the direct object argument position, as illustrated in sentence 9b. Because the object or theme argument moves from the object position to the subject position, the derived structure is called an object "wh-" question.[6] Figure 27–3 illustrates this movement from the direct object position to Spec, CP, a non-argument position.[7]

Object cleft structures as in sentence 6 above also are formed by movement of the direct object (theme) to Spec, CP. Consider the underlying form (sentence 10a) and surface form (sentence 10b) of an object cleft construction:

10a. Zack $_{\text{AGENT}}$ climbed Mt. Katadin $_{\text{THEME}}$
10b. It was Mt. Katadin$_{i\ \text{THEME}}$ that Zack $_{\text{AGENT}}$ climbed [t$_i$]

The crucial difference between object "wh-" questions and object clefts is that in the latter, movement occurs within an embedded clause, as shown in Figure 27–4. This property of object clefts renders them more complex than object "wh-" questions. The issue of structural complexity is addressed further below.

NP-Movement

NP-movement forms, as in sentences 7 and 8 above, are quite different from Wh-movment forms. Unlike Wh-movement, which involves movement from an argument (i.e., theme) position to a non-argument position (Spec, CP), NP-movement involves displacement of an argument (i.e., theme) to another argument position (Spec, IP; the subject position of the sentence). To illustrate the NP-movement involved in passive sentences, consider again the underlying form of sentence 7 approximated in sentence 11a below:

11a. ɸ was climbed Mt. Katadin $_{\text{THEME}}$ by the Zack $_{\text{AGENT}}$
11b. Mt. Katadin$_{i\ \text{THEME}}$ was climbed [t$_i$] by Zack $_{\text{AGENT}}$

---

[6] Subject "wh-" questions do not involve Wh-movement (e.g., *Who climbed Mt. Katadin?*).

[7] The example above (sentence 9b) illustrates movement of an argument, the direct object NP. Wh-movement also can apply to adjuncts, as in *Matt fixed the car [in the garage] -> Where did Matt fix the car?* In this example, the moved element, *where*, corresponds to a locative adjunct prepositional phrase, *in the garage*.

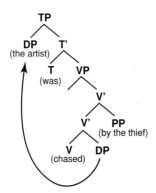

Figure 27–5. Tree diagram illustrating NP-movement in passives, as in *The artist was chased by the thief*. Note that the landing site for movement is the subject position.

To derive the passive, the direct object NP, theme, (i.e., *Mt. Katadin*) in sentence 11a is moved, and a trace of this movement is left behind. The landing site of the moved NP is the empty subject position (φ, Spec, TP)*, as in sentence 11b. This movement is illustrated in Figure 27–5.

NP-movement also is involved in subject-raising constructions (see sentence 8 above). In this type of sentence, movement is from the subject position of a sentential complement (subordinate clause) to the empty subject position of the matrix sentence, as in sentences 12a and 12b (Fig. 27–6):

12a. φ seems Zack to have climbed Mt. Katadin
12b. Zack$_i$ seems [t$_i$] to have climbed Mt. Katadin

The linear order of constituents in a sentence affects both sentence production and comprehension. When producing

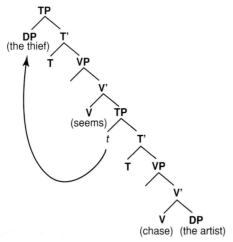

Figure 27–6. Tree diagram illustrating NP-movement in subject raising structures, as in *The thief seems to have chased the artist*. Note that the moved element lands in the subject position (Spec, TP), as in passive constructions.

---

*IP is replaced by TP when the inflection phrase is split.

or listening to sentences in which constituents are not in their canonical form, greater processing resources are required as compared to when the ordering of constituents is canonical. When individuals without brain damage process noncanonical sentences with movement, it appears that they "reaccess" the moved element in the vicinity of the trace—well after it has occurred in the sentence. That is, they "hold on to" the moved constituent such that it can be assigned its proper thematic role once the verb in the sentence is heard. Some debate exists regarding whether agrammatic speakers retain the ability to do this. Some researchers have shown that they do not (Swinney & Zurif, 1995; Zurif, Swinney, Prather, Solomon, & Bushell, 1993), but others have found that these speakers show normal online processing of complex, noncanonical sentences despite their inability to comprehend or produce them (Blumstein et al., 1998; Dickey, Choy, & Thompson, 2007).

Some theories of agrammatism suggest that the source of asyntactic comprehension relates to an inability to form traces (or copies) of movement and/or failure to establish co-referential relations between moved constituents and the trace/copy—for example, the Trace Deletion Hypothesis and its variants (e.g., The Trace Based Account) (Grodzinsky, 1986, 1995, 1990) and the Double Dependency Hypothesis (Mauner, Fromkin, & Cornell, 1993). Others suggest that, rather than a representational deficit, the problem is related to processing deficiencies. The Slow-Syntax Hypothesis claims, for example, that comprehension of complex sentences results from delayed processing (Burkhardt, Piñango, & Wong, 2003; Piñango, 2000; Prather, Zurif, Love, & Brownell, 1997; Swinney, Prather, & Love, 2000). On this account, traces are present in the syntactic representation, and their antecedents are "reactivated" at the trace site. The problem is that this reactivation is delayed. Another theory, the Mapping Deficit Hypothesis, suggests that the problem lies in mapping semantic representations onto the syntax, based on the observation that some agrammatic speakers have little difficulty determining the grammaticality of sentences but still show comprehension problems (Linebarger, Schwartz, & Saffran, 1983). This latter theory is similar to the Argument Linking Hypothesis (Piñago, 2000), which suggests that the deficit relates to difficulty coordinating semantic and syntactic linking.

Grammatical Morphology

One representational theory of agrammatism, The Tree Pruning Hypothesis (TPH), suggests that functional categories projecting from higher nodes in the syntactic tree are more at risk than those projecting from lower nodes (Friedmann & Grodzinsky, 1997; Hagiwara 1995). Impairment may occur at any level of the tree, but it will necessarily result in deficits at all higher levels. Accordingly, an IP impairment would also impair CP structures.

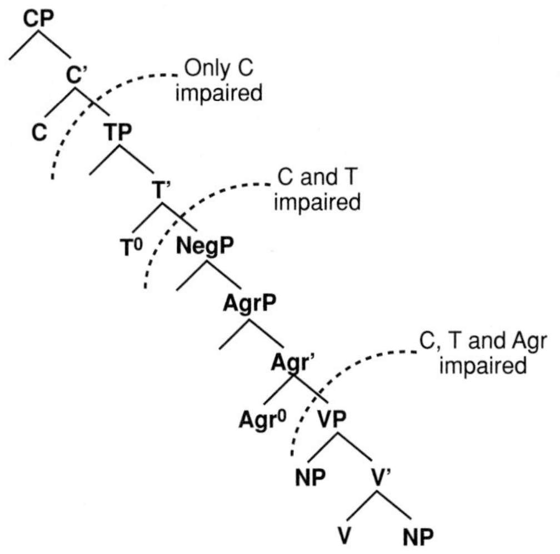

Figure 27–7. Illustration of ways that the syntactic tree can be "pruned" according to the Tree Pruning Hypothesis, which assumes a "split-IP." Functional category members—C (complementizers), T (tense), or Agr (agreement)—may be impaired or underspecified. When a node is impaired, all nodes above the pruned one will be impaired as well.

As discussed previously, Pollock (1989) suggested that IP is "split" into separate tense and agreement nodes. Thus, the TPH also predicts that morphology associated with tense should be more impaired than agreement, because the TP is higher in the tree than the agreement phrase (AgrP). Supporting data have come from Hebrew and Palestinian Arabic (Friedmann, 2002; Friedmann and Grodzinsky, 1997) and Spanish agrammatic speakers (Benedet et al., 1988). For example, Friedmann & Grodzinsky (1997) describe a Hebrew patient with agrammatic aphasia who showed intact representation of lower nodes within IP (AgrP) but selective impairment in higher ones (TP). In addition, their subject showed difficulty with complementizers and embeddings, indicating impaired CP as well (Fig. 27–7).

The validity of the THP, however, has been challenged by research showing patterns of impairment in agrammatism that do not follow the proposed hierarchies in Korean (Lee 2003), German (Burchert, Swobody-Moll, & de Bleser, 2005), and English (Lee & Thompson, 2005). Lee and Thompson (2005), for example, studied four English-speaking patients with agrammatism with spared CP but impaired IP. None of these patients showed more difficulty with tense as compared to agreement inflection. Finally, the participants showed variability in their production ability, indicating retention of partial knowledge rather than a complete loss of ability, which would be expected if a syntactic node or nodes were simply absent of "pruned." These data suggest that the impairment is more likely the result of faulty processing or access to relevant representation (for a discussion of processing accounts, see Arabatzi & Edwards, 2002).

Considering recovery of grammatical morphology, the TPH suggests that training higher nodes will improve structures projected from lower ones. That is, training CP structures should improve IP structures, and within IP, training tense should improve agreement. Training IP structures should have no effect on CP structures, however, and training agreement should not influence tense. In our functional category (grammatical morphology) treatment, we use the syntactic tree to select treatment targets and to generate hypotheses about generalization within and across functional category members. We also, however, consider the processing mechanisms engaged in accessing and producing them.

TREATMENT OF AGRAMMATISM

Treating agrammatic aphasia is a challenge. Few treatments have been developed for improving grammatical deficits in aphasia, and of these, most are focused on improving syntactic deficits, with fewer being concerned with improving grammatical morphology. In addition, the extent to which these treatments improve language or result in generalization to untrained language structures and/or language use in untrained contexts is not always clear. Indeed, generalization has become the gold standard for efficacious treatment; without it, treatment may be deemed ineffective. In addition, few published tests are available for detailing syntactic and morphological impairments seen in agrammatism. In this section, a short overview of assessment tools is presented, followed by discussion of the treatment for syntactic and morphological impairments in agrammatism, respectively.

Assessment of Agrammatic Deficits

Agrammatism exists within the context of nonfluent (Broca's) aphasia, which can be diagnosed by administration of a standardized aphasia test battery, such as the Western Aphasia Battery (Kertesz, 2006) or the Boston Diagnostic Aphasia Examination, 3rd Edition (BDAE-3; Goodglass, Kaplan, & Barresi, 2000). Additional measures are required, however, to detail verb and verb argument structure deficits, comprehension and production of canonical and noncanonical sentences, and deficits in grammatical morphology.

In recent years, several measures have been published for testing verb comprehension and production, including one subtest of the BDAE-3 (Goodglass et al., 2000), the Action Naming Test (Druks & Masterson, 2002), and the Verbs and Sentences Test (Bastiaanse, Edwards, & Rispens, 2002). The latter, developed for Dutch speakers and translated into English, also evaluates comprehension and production of sentence types that are compromised in agrammatism. One drawback of these tests is that they are not completely controlled for argument structure.

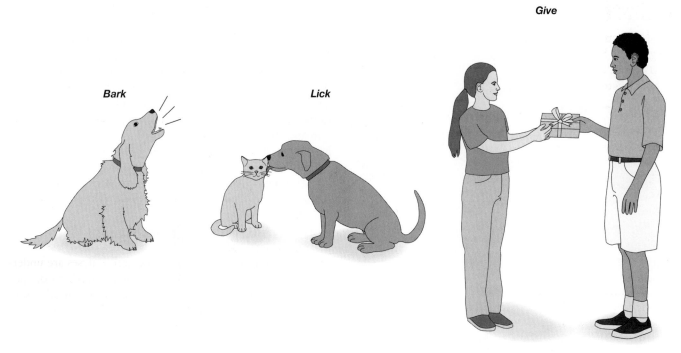

Figure 27–8. Sample picture stimuli for testing production of one-, two-, and three-argument verbs using the Northwestern Assessment of Verbs and Sentences (NAVS). *Bark* is a one-argument verb, *lick* a two- argument verb, and *give* a three-argument verb.

The Northwestern Assessment of Verbs and Sentences (Thompson), in preparation is a battery of tests developed particularly for evaluating agrammatic aphasia. The measure consists of five tests: (1) the Test of Verb Comprehension, (2) the Test of Verb Production, (3) the Verb Argument Structure Production Test, (4) the Sentence Comprehension Test, and (5) the Sentence Production Priming Test. The verb tests examine one-argument (i.e., intransitive), obligatory two-argument verbs (i.e., transitive), and three-argument verbs (ditransitive both obligatory and optional)[8] using action pictures (Table 27–1). To test comprehension, subjects are asked to point to the verb named (out of four pictures), and to assess verb naming, they are asked to name the action depicted. Verb argument structure production is tested by adding arrows to denote objects or people in the picture that represent arguments of the verb. Sample stimuli used to elicit production of verbs and verb arguments are shown in Figures 27–8 and 27–9.

The Sentence Comprehension and Sentence Production Priming Tests examine actives, passives, yes/no questions, object "wh-" questions, subject "wh-" questions, object relatives, and subject relative constructions (see Table 27–2 for

sample sentences of each type). In both tests, action picture pairs depicting semantically reversible scenes with transitive (two-argument) verbs are used. Comprehension is tested using a sentence-picture matching task: A picture pair is presented, and the one corresponding to a spoken sentence is selected. The Sentence Production Priming Test elicits sentences by the examiner modeling the target sentence type using one of the pictures in the pair and asking the patient to

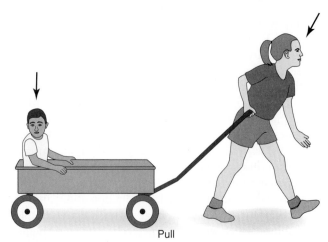

Figure 27–9. Stimulus used in the Argument Structure Production Test for production of sentences with two-argument verbs on the Northwestern Assessment of Verbs and Sentences (NAVS). Arrows refer to arguments of the verb.

[8] Obligatory three-argument verbs are those that require all arguments be overtly represented in sentences (e.g., *put*). Optional three-arguments verbs allow omission of an argument, even though it is part of the verb's lexical entry (e.g., *send*).

TABLE 27–1

Verbs Tested for Comprehension, Production, and Argument Structure Production (in Simple Sentences) in Tests 1, 2, and 3, Respectively, on the Northwestern Assessment of Verbs and Sentences

One-Argument Verbs	Two-Argument Verbs, Obligatory (Ob)	Three-Argument Verbs, Obligatory (Ob) and Optional (Op)
bark	cut	build (Op)
crawl	kiss	deliver (Op)
dive	lick	give (Ob)
howl	pinch	put (Ob)
laugh	pull	read (Op)
sit	shove	send (Op)
sleep	stir	throw (Op)
swim	tickle	write (Op)

produce a sentence of the same type with the other, target picture. A sample picture pair and instructions used to test comprehension and production are shown in Figure 27–10. On these tests, agrammatic speakers show relatively intact comprehension of canonical sentences (i.e., actives, subject "wh-" questions, and subject relatives) and poorer comprehension of noncanonical sentences (i.e., passives, object "wh-" questions, and object relatives). A similar pattern often is seen in production, in which canonical forms are less impaired than noncanonical structures, although as noted above, some canonical forms also present difficulty for some patients.

Virtually no published tests are available for evaluating functional category deficits in aphasia. We, therefore, are in

the processing of developing the Northwestern Assessment of Verb Inflection (Thompson, in preparation), which examines production of finite (inflected) and nonfinite verb forms (Table 27–3). Finite forms include present singular, present plural, and past tense. Nonfinite forms include: present progressive (aspectual ing) and the infinitive. To elicit these forms, a sentence completion task and action pictures are used. The task requires production of the missing verb with the correct verb form.

Analysis of spontaneous discourse also is crucial for uncovering grammatical deficits in agrammatism. Saffran and colleagues (1989) recommend using a story-retelling task to collect language sample. The samples are then coded for utterance type, word class, verb inflections, and so on (Rochon, Saffran, Berndt, & Schwartz, 2000). Sentence constituents (e.g., NPs or VPs) also are coded, and from these data, both lexical and sentence structural analyses are undertaken to derive information such as noun-to-verb ratio, open class–to–closed class ratio, number of words produced in sentences, and proportion of utterances with complete sentences.

Thompson and colleagues (1995) developed a similar method. Patients are asked to tell the story of Cinderella or Red Riding Hood. We also have asked individuals to watch a silent Charlie Chaplin film and then tell about it and describe pictures depicting a sequence of events. Notably, regardless of elicitation condition, individuals with agrammatic aphasia show very similar patterns of language production. Once the sample is collected, it is transcribed and segmented into utterances based on syntactic, prosodic, and semantic criteria. Each utterance then is coded at five levels:

1. The Utterance Level, where codes for a sentence or non-sentence are entered (utterances without verbs are not sentences).
2. The Sentences Level, where sentences are coded by type and as simple or complex.

TABLE 27–2

Sentences Tested for Comprehension (Test 4) and Production (Test 5) in the Northwestern Assessment of Verbs and Sentences

Sentence Type	Sample Stimulus	Semantically Reversed
Active	The girl tickled the boy.	The boy tickled the girl.
Passive	The boy was tickled by the girl.	The girl was tickled by the boy.
Object "wh-" question	Who did the girl tickle?	Who did the boy tickle?
Subject "wh-" question	Who tickled the boy?	Who tickled the girl?
Yes/no question	Did the girl tickle the boy?	Did the boy tickle the girl?
Object relative	I see the boy who the girl tickled.	I see the girl who the boy tickled.
Subject relative	I see the girl who tickled the boy.	I see the boy who tickled the girl.

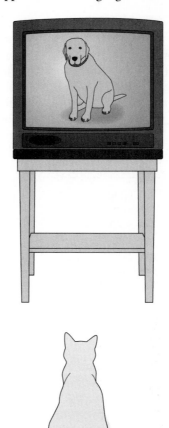
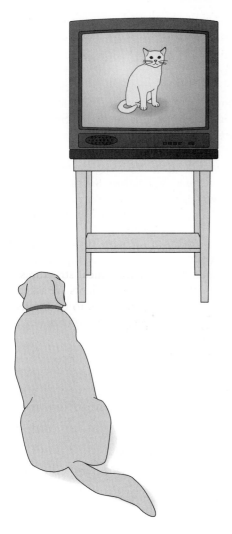

Figure 27–10. Picture pair used to test sentence comprehension and production on the Northwestern Assessment of Verbs and Sentences (NAVS). For comprehension, the examiner says, "Point to, the dog was watched by the cat." For production elicitation, the examiner says, "For this picture [pointing to the picture on the left], you could say, *The cat was watched by the dog*; for this picture [pointing to the picture on the right], you could say . . ." (Expected response: *The dog was watched by the cat.*)

3. The Lexical Level, where all lexical items are coded by word class.
4. The Bound Morpheme Level, where codes for inflectional morphemes are entered.
5. The Verb Level, which details verbs by type and argument structure.

TABLE 27–3

Northwestern Assessment of Verb Inflection Sores for an Agrammatic Speaker

Verb Inflection Condition	Percent Correct
Present singular: The cat watches the dog.	0
Present plural: The cats watch the dog.	20
Regular past tense: The cat watched the dog.	0
Present progressive: The cat is watching the dog.	80
Infinitive: The cat will watch the dog.	80

The analysis yields data such as mean length of utterance, the proportion of grammatical sentences, open class–to–closed class ratio, noun-to-verb ratio, the proportion of verbs produced with correct arguments, and the proportion of verbs and nouns produced with correct inflection. Although this coding system is quite complex, it is worthwhile for clinicians to become familiar with analyses of this type not only to diagnose the patient but also because changes in these language variables often are seen with treatment. Table 27–4 presents a typical spontaneous language profile for an agrammatic aphasic speaker (compared to unimpaired speakers).

Treatment of Syntactic Deficits

Few treatments for improving sentence structural (syntactic) deficits in aphasia are available, and of those, several focus on instruction and practice in producing the surface form of certain types of sentences. The Helm-Estabrooks Language Program for Syntax Stimulation (Helm-Estabrooks, 1981;

TABLE 27–4

Sample Spontaneous Language Profile for an Agrammatic Speaker (AS)

	AS	Normal*
Mean length of utterance	4.75	14.5 (2.2)
Open to closed class ratio	1.73	0.91 (0.08)
Noun to verb ratio	2.12	1.21 (0.25)
Proportion of grammatical sentences	0.19	0.89 (0.08)
Proportion of verbs with correct arguments	0.50	>0.95
Proportion of correctly inflected verbs	0.57	NA

Key: NA = data unavailable.

*Values are for normal speakers and are presented as the mean (standard deviation). Data from Kim and Thompson (2000).

Helm-Estabrooks & Ramsberger, 1986), for example, is focused on training a set of sentences shown by Goodglass, Gleason, Bernholtz, & Hyde (1972) to be difficult for individuals with agrammatic aphasia to produce (Table 27–5). One sentence type is trained at a time, beginning with that considered to be the easiest (e.g., imperative intransitives [e.g., *Sit down*]). Research concerned with establishing the efficacy of this approach has indicated that patients improve in their ability to produce trained sentences; however, less impressive findings have been reported with regard to generalization across sentence types (Doyle, Goldstein, & Bourgeois, 1987; Fink et al., 1995).

Rather than focusing on the surface form of sentences, other approaches exploit processes thought to be operating in normal sentence processing and production. For example,

TABLE 27–5

Helm-Elicited Language Program for Syntax Stimulation Sentence Types

Sentence Type	Sample Sentence
Imperative intransitive	Sit down.
Imperative transitive	Drink your milk.
"Wh-" interrogative	Where are my shoes?
Declarative transitive	He teaches school.
Declarative intransitive	He swims.
Comparative	He's taller.
Passive	The car was towed.
Yes/no questions	Did you watch the news?
Direct and indirect object	He brings his mother flowers.
Embedded sentences	She wanted him to be rich.
Future	He will sleep.

Loverso, Prescott, & Selinger (1986) developed a method known as "Verb as Core" treatment, based on the premises that, first, access to verbs often is disrupted in agrammatic aphasia and, second, verbs are required for grammatical sentences. Patients are trained to produce verbs together with specific sentence constituents (usually NPs) that are assigned various thematic roles by the verb (e.g., agent and theme) in simple, active sentences. Little research examining this approach is available.

Another treatment designed to improve both comprehension and production of sentences is Mapping Therapy (Byng, 1988; Rochon, Laird, Bose, & Scofield, 2005; Schwartz, Saffran, Fink, Myers, & Martin, 1994). Like Verb as Core training, this approach is theoretically motivated, based on the Mapping Deficit Hypothesis discussed above. Treatment focuses on verbs and the thematic role of sentence NPs in both canonical and noncanonical structures. Presented with sentences in written form, patients are asked to underline the agent and theme in response to questions concerning the logical subject and the logical object (e.g., "Which one is doing the chasing?" and "What/who is she/he chasing?"). Results of research using this method have shown improved comprehension of both canonical and noncanonical sentence forms. Like Syntax Stimulation, however, improvement is constrained largely to the types of sentences entered into treatment. In a recent study directly comparing Mapping Therapy to TUF, we (Thompson, Shapiro, Kiran, & Mass, in preparation) found that both approaches improve comprehension and production of sentence types trained. But the generalization patterns differed for the two treatments; a greater number of participants showed generalization across sentences resulting from TUF as compared to MT.

Treatment of Underlying Forms for Syntax (TUF$_{SYNTAX}$) exploits the fact that individuals with agrammatic aphasia have normal access to verbs and thematic information; however, they do not always assign thematic roles normally, nor do they use them fully in sentence production. Further, these patients have difficulty comprehending sentences with movement, TUF$_{SYNTAX}$ uses the active form of target sentences as a starting point for treatment, and tasks are directed toward establishing and improving knowledge of and access to the thematic role information entailed in target verbs. Then, instructions as to how various sentence constituents move to derive the surface form of target sentences, while retaining their thematic roles, are provided (see Appendix 27-1 for detailed treatment protocols).

In a series of studies, it has been shown that this approach improves sentence production and comprehension. Crucially, treatment results in successful generalization to structures that are related linguistically to the structures trained. Ballard & Thompson, 1999; Jacobs & Thompson, 2000; Thompson et al., 1993, 1996; Thompson, Shapiro et al, 1997.

As noted above, a distinction exists among certain sentence types, depending on whether they involve the syntactic operations of Wh- or NP-movement. Object "wh-" questions and object clefts are Wh-movement structures, whereas passive sentences and subject raising forms are NP-movement structures. What do these linguistic descriptions have to do with treatment and recovery of language in aphasia? In sentence production and comprehension work, we have found that sentences that are linguistically related recover together (see Thompson, Shapiro et al., 1997). For example, training object cleft sentences improves both object who and what questions. Similarly, training subject raising structures improves not only untrained subject raising structures but also passive sentences.[9]

For example, in a study examining the relation between Wh- and NP-movement (Thompson, Shapiro et al., 1997), the Wh-movement structures selected for treatment included "wh-" questions, as in sentence 13 below, and object cleft sentences, as in sentence 14 below. In addition, NP-movement structures were selected for treatment and generalization testing. These included passives and subject-raising sentences as in sentences 15 and 16, respectively, below. Individuals with agrammatic Broca's aphasia were trained to produce one of these sentence types at a time using active sentences, as in sentence 17 below, and TUF$_{SYNTAX}$ protocols:

13. Who did the boy pinch? (object "wh-" question)
14. It was the teacher who the boy pinched. (object cleft)
15. The teacher was pinched by the boy. (passive)
16. The boy seems to have pinched the teacher. (subject raising)
17. The boy pinched the teacher. (active)

Results showed that training Wh-movement structures improved both trained and untrained Wh-movement structures—that is, generalization from object clefts to "wh-" questions was found. The Wh-movement treatment, however, had little influence on production of NP-movement structures. Similarly, when NP-movement structures were trained, generalization occurred to other NP-movement structures (e.g., generalization occurred from subject raising to passives), but no change in production of object clefts or object "wh-" questions was seen.

Ballard and Thompson (1999) as well as Jacobs and Thompson (2000) found a similar dissociation between Wh- and NP-movement sentences. Ballard and Thompson (1999) trained five patients to produce object clefts and/or "wh-" questions and tested passives. All subjects improved in production of Wh-movement structures, but no change in passive forms was seen. Jacobs and Thompson (2000)

trained both object clefts and passive sentences in four patients. Again, all improved on the structures trained, but none showed generalization from object clefts to passives or from passives to object clefts.

Another finding is that generalization is enhanced if the direction of treatment is from more complex to less complex structures. Close examination of data reported in earlier studies (Thompson & Shapiro, 1994; Thompson, Shapiro et al., 1997) showed that for subjects who received Wh-movement training, better generalization was noted from object clefts to object "wh-" questions than from object "wh-" questions to object clefts. In consideration of the complexity of these structures, object clefts are the most complex. The two structures are similar in that they both require Wh-movement; however, as pointed out above, the movement in object clefts is within an embedded clause. The movement in object "wh-" questions occurs in the matrix clause; no embedding is required.

Results of studies directly examining the effects of complexity showed that, indeed, generalization occurs more readily from object clefts to "wh-" questions than vice versa (Thompson, Ballard, & Shapiro, 1998). Further, training even more complex sentences with Wh-movement, object relative clause structures, as in sentence 18 below, results in generalization to both object clefts, as in sentence 19 below, and "wh-" questions, as in sentence 20 below. Generalization from simpler "wh-" question structures (sentence 20), however, does not improve object clefts (sentence 19) or object relative clause constructions (sentence 18) (Thompson, Shapiro, Kiran, & Sobecks, 2003). Figure 27–11 illustrates the collective results of training more than 30 subjects with agrammatic aphasia. Most participants trained to produce and comprehend complex structures show generalization to simpler structures (86%), whereas fewer show generalization in the opposite direction (from simple to complex structures; 17%):

18. The chef saw the busboy who the waitress kissed.
19. It was the busboy who the waitress kissed.
20. Who did the waitress kiss?

Training complex structures before training simpler ones may seem counterintuitive, but these studies, as well as those in other language domains, indicate that optimal generalization results from this approach (Thompson 2007). For discussion of complexity in treatment of phonological, semantic, and syntactic deficits, see Gierut (2007), Kiran (2007), and Thompson and Shapiro (2007), respectively.

Summary of Syntax Training Effects

Work concerned with examining Wh- and NP-movement shows that they are functionally independent. That is, generalization is not seen from sentences relying on one type of movement to sentences relying on the other. Importantly, however, sentences that rely on the same type of movement form a functional class; generalization across from one form

[9] Also see Thompson, Shapiro, and Roberts (1993); Thompson & Shapiro (1994); and Thompson, Shapiro, Tait, Jacobs, and Schneider (1996) for studies training object (argument) "wh-" questions (e.g., who and what) and adjunct "wh-" questions (e.g., where and when).

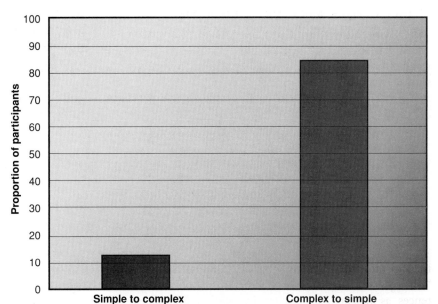

Figure 27–11. Proportion of participants showing successful generalization from less complex to more complex structures, and vice versa.

to others within the same movement class, even when sentences are very different in their surface form. Further, generalization is enhanced when complex, rather than simple, structures are used as the starting point for treatment as long as the simpler structures are related to the more complex ones. These data show that the linguistic underpinnings of sentences are important to consider in treatment of syntactic deficits in aphasia.

Treatment of Grammatical Morphology (Functional Categories)

Treatment research concerned with establishing methods for improving access to grammatical morphemes—either bound or free-standing—is limited to a handful of studies (see, e.g.,, Cannito & Vogel, 1987; Kearns & Salmon, 1984). These treatments can be considered surface form approaches, because the underlying representation and processing demands of the grammatical morphemes trained were not completely considered.

Treatment of Underlying Forms for grammatical morphology or functional categories (TUF_{FUNCAT}) considers both functional category projections from the syntactic tree as well as computational processes involved in producing grammatical morphemes in sentences. Consider the following sentences:

21. The people wonder *if/whether* the boy is ticking the girl.
22. The boy tickl*ed* the girl.
23. The boy tickl*es* the girl.

The complementizer *if/whether* in sentence 21 as well as morphemes marking verb tense and agreement in sentences 22 and 23, respectively, are functional category members. From a linguistic representational point of view, sentence 21 is more difficult than either sentence 22 or sentence 23. As

noted above, the TPH suggests this because complementizers occupy a higher node (i.e., CP) in the syntactic tree compared with tense or agreement (i.e., IP). Further, the TPH holds that tense (sentence 22) is more vulnerable than agreement (sentence 23), again because tense is higher in the tree than agreement (Fig. 27–11). The position of tense and agreement in the syntactic tree is debatable: Some suggest that:

1. Both are subsumed under IP (Bobaljik & Thráinsson, 1998).
2. Tense is above agreement (Pollock, 1989).
3. Agreement is above tense (Chomsky, 1993).

In addition, the computational routines and processing demands required for sentences with complementizers differ from those involved in marking tense/agreement features. Complementizers (*whether, if, that*) are free-standing morphemes that introduce a complement or subordinate clause. They are strongly syntactically constrained, because they are directly selected for by complement verbs, such as *know, wonder, see,* and *care*. Conversely, tense and agreement are bound grammatical morphemes that rely on processes such as grammatical encoding and well-formedness constraints (Arabatzi & Edwards, 2002; Faroqi-Shah & Thompson, 2007; Halle & Marantz, 1993). Past tense, for example, requires encoding a past-tense meaning (provided by the temporal adverb *yesterday* or by other contextual information). Verb tense, however, is only indirectly constrained by the adverb: The adverb introduces information about the temporal context, but it does not *select* the verb's tense in the same way that complement verbs select complement clauses.

Why are these distinctions important for treatment of agrammatism? Simply put, both representation and processing accounts suggest that complementizers are more difficult (or complex) than tense or agreement. Because the underlying representation as well as the processing routines involved in the two structures are different, however, they are linguistically distinct, even though both are functional category members. Given this, training complementizers should have no effect on production of verb tense or agreement, and training verb tense and agreement should have no effect on complementizers.

Predicting generalization from tense to agreement or from agreement to tense is more difficult, however. Both forms involve attachment of inflections to base-form verbs, which likely entail similar computations. They may or may not occupy different nodes in the syntactic tree, however, and one may occupy a higher node than the other. Thus, a functional relationship between tense and agreement is predicted, but no specific prediction regarding the direction of generalization can clearly be made.

We recently trained 12 participants to produce complementizers, tense, and agreement and examined generalization across structures (Thompson et al., 2006). The three structures were trained, one at a time, using TUF$_{FUNCAT}$, with the order of structure trained counterbalanced across participants. As in TUF$_{SYNTAX}$, TUF$_{FUNCAT}$ considers the underlying form of target structures. For complementizers, this is approximated in sentence 24a below, with two separate clauses; sentence 24b below shows the surface from, which results from combining the two clauses with the complementizer + **that**. For tense and agreement, the underlying and surface forms are approximated in sentences 25 and 26, respectively:

24a. [$_{IP}$ the people [$_{VP}$ see [$_{DP/CP}$ something]]] [$_{IP}$ the bride [$_{VP}$ is carrying [$_{DP}$ the groom]]]
24b. [$_{IP}$ the people [$_{VP}$ see [$_{CP}$ **that** [$_{IP}$ the bride [$_{VP}$ is carrying [$_{DP}$ the groom]]]]]]
25a. [$_{IP}$ the bride [$_{VP}$ is carrying [$_{DP}$ the groom]]]
25b. Yesterday [$_{IP}$ the bride [$_{VP}$ carry +**ed** [$_{DP}$ the groom]]]
26a. [$_{IP}$ the bride [$_{VP}$ is carrying [$_{DP}$ the groom]]]
26b. Nowadays [$_{IP}$ the bride [$_{VP}$ carry +**s** [$_{DP}$ the groom]]]

Treatment involved the use of written-sentence constituent cards corresponding with the active sentence(s) for each target as well as cards for [if], [that], [whether], [ed], or [s], depending on the grammatical morpheme in training. Each training trial consisted of:

1. Thematic role training of constituents in the matrix clause and for complementizers in the embedded clause as well.
2. Introduction of the grammatical morpheme, its function, and its placement in the sentence.
3. Reassembly of scrambled written sentence constituent cards.

Participants read or repeated the target sentence at each step.

Results showed that all participants improved on trained forms following low and stable baseline performance. Three of four participants trained on complementizers showed no generalization to tense or agreement, and zero of eight par-

ticipants trained on tense or agreement showed improvement on complementizers. These data suggest that even though complementizers and verb inflections are functional category members, they are not functionally related to one another, thus, training one did not influence the other. This finding is similar to that derived from our Wh- and NP-movement studies; even though sentences with both types of movement are noncanonical and difficult for patients with agrammatic aphasia, they involve different types of movement. Thus, a functional relationship does not exist between them. Generalization from tense to agreement or from agreement to tense was seen, however, for 7 of 11 participants. These findings suggest that the two inflected forms are functionally related to one another; however, one is not necessarily more complex than the other.

Effects of Treatment on Discourse Patterns

Changes in discourse characteristics have resulted from both syntactic and morphologic treatment in many participants, with increases in mean length of utterance, the proportion of grammatical sentences produced, and the proportion of verbs (as compared to nouns). Syntactic treatment also improves the proportion of verbs produced with correct argument structure, and treatment focused on grammatical morphology increases the proportion of correctly inflected verbs. Notably, Ballard and Thompson (1999) found improvements in informativeness and efficiency of production following syntactic treatment using the analysis system of Nicholas and Brookhire (1993). This latter finding indicates that treatment focused on structural deficits impacts functional language use.

Neural Mechanisms of Recovery

The language improvement resulting from both TUF$_{SYNTAX}$ and TUF$_{FUNCAT}$ affects the neural mechanisms of language. Using functional magnetic resonance imaging, we find two patterns of recovery: Some participants show increases in areas of the brain that are active during language processing, and others show decreases following treatment. In one study of TUF$_{SYNTAX}$, participants received treatment focused on Wh-movement structures, including object–relative clause constructions, object clefts, and object-extracted "wh-" questions, with all showing improved production and comprehension of all forms. Before and following treatment, the patients were scanned while performing a sentence-picture matching task in which object cleft sentences, such as "It was the judge who the lawyer tripped," and simpler subject cleft sentences, such as "It was the judge who tripped the lawyer," were tested. Two (of three) participants showed decreased neural activity following treatment; whereas the third participant showed more widespread activation following treatment. Regardless of the amount of active tissue, however, the final

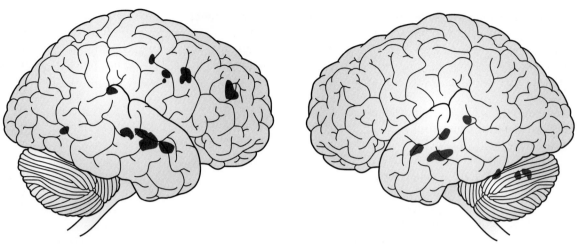

Figure 27–12. Areas of significant activation found in post-treatment scans that were not active in pre-treatment scans. Note that treatment resulted in increased activation in the left and right perisylvian regions.

scans for all participants showed recruitment of perisylvian tissue, which was not active during pre-scanning. Figure 27–12 shows post-treatment activation for one participant which was not seen on his pre-treatment scan. Before treatment, activation was limited to small clusters of active tissue in the right superior parietal and the middle temporal gyri. No activation was seen in the left hemisphere.

A similar pattern was found for participants receiving TUF$_{FUNCAT}$. Of 12 patients studied, five underwent pre- and post-treatment scanning. Four of these five participants showed improved production of grammatical morphology with treatment, whereas one did not. The scan task involved production of verbs in their base form (e.g., *save*) or inflected for tense (e.g., *saved*) or agreement (e.g. *saves*). Results showed that the four patients who improved with treatment showed a decrease in activation following treatment. Figure 27–13 shows this pattern for one patient. Interestingly, the gentleman who did not improve with treatment showed an increase in

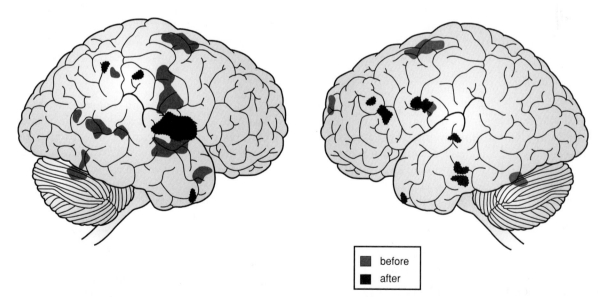

| before |
| after |

Figure 27–13. Areas of significant activation before (grey) and after (black) treatment of grammatical morphology for one agrammatic participant. The activation shown reflects the following contrast: production of ((tense + agreement) − bare stem). This participant showed a decrease in activation following treatment. Before treatment, widespread, primarily right hemisphere activation was noted, whereas following treatment, a shift to more focal right perisylvian and left perilesional activation was found. Note that this participant had a large left hemisphere lesion that encompassed the inferior frontal area and extended to superior and anterior temporal regions.

cortical tissue engaged while performing the task, with all activity in the right hemisphere both before and following treatment.

CONCLUSION

Findings from our work in developing and testing the effects of treatment for agrammatism indicate that treatment for sentence production deficits in patients with agrammatic aphasia is efficacious when the linguistic underpinnings of the language deficit exhibited by the individual with aphasia, the sentences selected for treatment, and the treatment strategy used are considered. When lexical and syntactic properties of sentences are not considered, generalization effects are considerably diminished—or even absent. That is, little or no discernible improvement in sentence production beyond constructions trained is found. We also find that the complexity of structures trained is a factor that needs to be considered in facilitating generalization.

The results of our work have important clinical implications. Because of restrictions in health care presently imposed for individuals with aphasia, it is essential that clinicians provide treatment that will result in optimal generalization. Our data suggest that optimal generalization results from treatment when structures that are linguistically similar are selected as treatment targets and when treatment is applied to the most complex of these structures first. While additional data are needed to further substantiate the latter, we conclude that linguistically based treatment can be used successfully for training sentence production in individuals with aphasia who present with deficits like those seen in our subjects.

In conclusion, treatment of both syntactic and morphological aspects of sentence production requires careful analysis of *how* and in *what ways* the sentence processing/production system has been affected with brain damage. Application of treatment explicitly designed to address these deficits is recommended. Indeed, the more we learn about the linguistic and psycholinguistic underpinnings of sentence production and comprehension and in what ways these are disrupted in aphasia, the more detailed we can be about the design of treatment.

▶ *Acknowledgment*—The work reported here was funded by the National Institutes on Deafness and other Communication Disorders (NIDCD) grant RO1-DC01948, for which the author is very grateful. Special thanks are extended to the aphasic participants and their family members, postdoctoral fellows (Drs. Steve Fix, Miseon Lee, and Lisa Milman), and research assistants involved in this work, and colleagues and collaborators, particularly Drs. Michael Walsh-Dickey and Lew Shapiro, for their invaluable contributions.

KEY POINTS

1. The literature indicates that individuals with agrammatic aphasia show particular deficit patterns that must be carefully tested before application of treatment.
2. Consideration of the lexical and morphosyntactic properties of sentences selected for treatment and for generalization analysis is important for obtaining optimal generalization.
3. Generalization from one structure to another occurs when sentences are linguistically related to one another. When sentences are not linguistically related, generalization is limited.
4. Generalization may be enhanced by training more complex structures first. Generalization from more complex to simple structures occurs when simple structures involve common linguistic representations and psycholinguistic processes.
5. Treatment improves the grammar, content, and efficiency of spontaneous discourse.
6. Neural correlates of treatment-induced behavioral changes can be mapped onto the brain.

ACTIVITIES FOR DISCUSSION AND REFLECTION

1. Two types of generalization occur: generalization to untrained language structures (response generalization), and generalization to untrained contexts (stimulus generalization). Provide examples of both. Discuss why generalization is important for successful treatment and what can be done if generalization does not occur.
2. Beginning treatment with complex structures is counterintuitive, but it has been shown to be successful for treatment of both naming and sentence comprehension/production in aphasia. Consider one of your current or previous clients with aphasia, and create a treatment plan for this client using this concept.
3. Code the language sample presented in section 2 of this chapter. Use the methods described under *Assessment of Agrammatic Deficits* (see p. 741) for coding the Utterance Level and Lexical Level. Calculate the following: mean length of utterance, the proportion of grammatical sentences, open class–to–closed class ratio, and noun-to-verb ratio. Do your results match those of other students in the class? For advanced students, try coding the Sentence Level, Bound Morpheme Level, and Verb Levels.
4. Based on the results of coding (in activity 3 above), develop a treatment plan for this client. Discuss how you will evaluate the effects of treatment.

5. Converging data suggest that the neural networks for language are influenced by aphasia treatment. Discuss the following questions: Do you think that different treatments might result in different patterns of neural recruitment? If so, why? Do you think that some treatments might impede recovery of the neural networks for language? If so, what treatments might have this effect? Is the neurobiology of recovery important? Why, or why not?

6. Administration of treatments that are theoretically based (as are TUF$_{\text{SYNTAX}}$ and TUF$_{\text{FUNCAT}}$) is difficult for some clinicians because of limits in their knowledge about theories and data pertaining to normal language representation and processing? Do you think it is important for clinicians to have this knowledge? Is so, how can it be obtained? If not, why not?

References

Adger, D. (2003). *Core syntax: A minimalist approach*. New York: Oxford University Press.

Arabatzi, M., & Edwards, S. (2002). Tense and syntactic processes in agrammatic speech. *Brain and Language, 80*, 314–327.

Ballard, K. J., & Thompson, C. K. (1999). Treatment and generalization of complex sentence production in agrammatism. *Journal of Speech, Language, and Hearing Research, 42*, 690–707.

Bastiaanse, R., Edwards, S., & Rispens, J. (2002). *Verb and Sentence Test* (VAST). Harcourt Assessment.

Bastiaanse, R., & van Zonneveld, R. (2005) Sentence production with verbs of alternating transitivity in agrammatic Broca's aphasia. *Journal of Neurolinguistics, 18*, 57–66.

Benedet, M. J., Christiansen, J. A., & Goodglass, H. (1998). A cross-linguistic study of grammatical morphology in Spanish- and English-speaking agrammatical patients. *Cortex, 34*, 309–336.

Berndt, R. S., Mitchum, C. C., & Haendiges, A. N. (1996). Comprehension of reversible sentences in "agrammatism": A meta-analysis. *Cognition, 58*, 289–308.

Bird, H., Franklin, S., & Howard, D. (2002). 'Little words'–not really: Function and content words in normal and aphasic speech. *Journal of Neurolinguistics, 15*, 209–237.

Blumstein, S. E., Byma, G., Kurowski, K., Hourihan, J., Brown, T., & Hutchinson, A. (1998). On-line processing of filler-gap construction in aphasia. *Brain and Language, 61*, 149–68.

Bobaljik, D. B., & Thráinsson, H. (1998). Two heads aren't always better than one. *Syntax, 1*, 37–71.

Bresnan, J. (Ed.). (1992). *The mental representation of grammatical relations*. Cambridge, MA: MIT Press.

Burchert, F., Swoboda-Moll, M., & de Bleser, R. (2005). Tense and agreement dissociations in German agrammatic speakers: Underspecification vs. hierarchy. *Brain and Language, 94*, 188–199.

Burkhardt, P., Piñango, M. M., & Wong, K. (2003). The role of the anterior left hemisphere in real-time sentence comprehension: Evidence from split intransitivity. *Brain and Language, 86*, 9–22.

Byng, S. (1988). Sentence processing deficits: Theory and therapy. *Cognitive neuropsychology, 5*, 629–676.

Cannito, M. P., & Vogel, D. (1987). Treatment can facilitate reacquisition of a morphological rule. In R. H. Brookshire (Ed.), *Clinical aphasiology: Conference proceedings* (pp. 23–28). Minneapolis: BRK.

Caplan, D., & Hanna (1998). Sentence production by aphasic patients in a constrained task. *Brain and Language, 63*, 184–218.

Caplan, D., & Hildebrandt, N. (1988). Specific deficits in syntactic comprehension. *Aphasiology, 2*, 255–258.

Caramazza, A., & Hillis, A.E. (1989). The disruption of sentence production: Some dissociations. *Brain and Language, 36*, 625–650.

Chomsky, N. (1986). *Knowledge of language: Its nature, origin, and use*. New York: Praeger. (Ed.), *Principles and parameters in comparative grammar*. Cambridge, MA: MIT Press.

Chomsky, N. (1993). A minimalist program for linguistic theory. In K. Hale & S. J. Keyser (Eds.), *The view from building 20*. Cambridge, MA: MIT Press.

Chomsky, N. (1995). Bare phrase structure. In G. Webelhuth (Ed.), *Government and binding theory and the minimalist program*. London: Basil Blackwell.

Damasio, H. (1991). Neuroanatomical correlates of the aphasias. In M. T. Sarno (Ed.), *Acquired aphasia* (2nd ed.). New York: Academic Press.

De Bleser, R., & Kauschke, C. (2003). Acquisition and loss of nouns and verbs: Parallel or divergent patterns? *Journal of Neurolinguistics, 16*, 213–229.

Dickey, M. W., Choy, J., & Thompson, C. K. (2007). Real-time comprehension of wh-movement in aphasia: Evidence from eyetracking while listening. *Brain and Language, 100*, 1–22.

Doyle, P. J., Goldstein, H., & Bourgeois, M. (1987). Experimental analysis of syntax training in Broca's aphasia: A generalization and social validation study. *Journal of Speech and Hearing Disorders, 52*, 143–155.

Druks, J., & Carroll, E. (2005). The crucial role of tense for verb production. *Brain and Language, 94*, 1–18.

Druks, J., & Masterson, J. (2002). *An object and action naming battery*. Routledge: Taylor and Francis.

Faroqi-Shah, Y., & Thompson, C. K. (2004). Semantic, lexical, and phonological influences on the production of verb inflections in agrammatic aphasia. *Brain and Language, 89*, 484–498.

Faroqi-Shah, Y., & Thompson, C. K. (2007). Verb inflections in agrammatic aphasia: Encoding of tense features. *Journal of Memory and Language, 56*, 129–151.

Fink, R. B., Schwartz, M. F., Rochon, E., Myers, J. L., Socolof, G. S., & Bluestone, R. (1995). Syntax stimulation revisited: An analysis of generalization of treatment effect. *American Journal of Speech Language Pathology, 4*, 99–104.

Friedmann, N. (2002). Question production in agrammatism: The tree pruning hypothesis. *Brain and Language, 56*, 397–425.

Friedmann, N., & Grodzinsky, Y. (1997). Tense and agreement in agrammatic production: Pruning the syntactic tree. *Brain and Language, 56*, 397–425.

Gazdar, G., Kein, E., Pullum, J., & Sag, I. (1985). *Generalized phrase structure grammar*. Cambridge, MA: Harvard University Press.

Gierut, J. (2007). Phonological complexity and language learnability. *American Journal of Speech and Language Pathology, 16*, 6–17.

Goodglass, H. (1976). Agrammatism. In H. Whitaker & H. A. Whitaker (Eds.), *Studies in neurolinguistics* (Vol. 1, pp. 237–260). New York: Academic Press.

Goodglass, H., Christiansen, J. A., & Gallagher, R. (1993). Comparison of morphology and syntax in free narrative and structured tests: Fluent vs. nonfluent aphasics. *Cortex, 29,* 377–407.

Goodglass, H., Gleason, J. B., Bernholtz, N. D., & Hyde, M. K. (1972). Some linguistic structures in the speech of a Broca's aphasic. *Cortex, 8,* 191–212.

Goodglass, H., Kaplan, E., & Barresi, B. (2000). *Boston Diagnostic Aphasia Examination-3rd ed.* (BDAE-3). Philadelphia: Lea & Febiger.

Grodzinsky, Y. (1986). Language deficits and syntactic theory. *Brain and Language, 27,* 135–159.

Grodzinsky, Y. (1990). *Theoretical perspectives on language deficits.* Cambridge, MA: MIT Press.

Grodzinsky, Y. (1995). A restrictive theory of agrammatic comprehension. *Brain and Language, 50,* 27–51.

Hagiwara, H. (1995). The breakdown of functional categories and the economy of derivation. *Brain and Language, 50,* 92–116.

Halle, M., & Marantz, A. 1993. Distributed morphology and the pieces of inflection. In K. Hale & S. J. Keyser, *The view from building 20: Essays in honor of Sylvian Bromberger* (pp. 111–176). Cambridge, MA: MIT Press.

Helm-Estabrooks, N. (1981). *Helm Elicited Language Program for Syntax Stimulation.* Austin, TX: Exceptional Resources.

Helm-Estabrooks, N., & Ramsberger, G. (1986). Treatment of agrammatism in long-term Broca's aphasia. *British Journal of Disorders of Communication, 21,* 39–45.

Jacobs, B. J., & Thompson, C. K. (2000). Cross-modal generalization effects of training noncanonical sentence comprehension and production in agrammatic aphasia. *Journal of Speech, Language, and Hearing Research, 43,* 5–20.

Jonkers, R., & Bastiaanse, R. (1998). How selective are selective word class deficits? Two case studies of action and object naming. *Aphasiology, 12,* 245–256.

Kearns, K. P., & Salmon, S. (1984). An experimental analysis of auxiliary and copula verb generalization in aphasia. *Journal of Speech and Hearing Disorders, 49,* 152–163.

Kemmerer, D., & Tranel, D. (2000). Verb retrieval in brain-damaged subjects: I. Analysis of stimulus, lexical, and conceptual factors. *Brain and Language, 73,* 347–392.

Kertesz, A. (2006). *The Western Aphasia Battery.* New York: Grune & Stratton.

Kim, M., & Thompson, C. K. (2000). Patterns of comprehension and production of nouns and verbs in agrammatism: Implications for lexical organization. *Brain and Lanaguage, 74,* 1–25.

Kim, M., & Thompson, C. K. (2004). Verb deficits in Alzheimer's disease and agrammatism: Implications for lexical organization. *Brain and Language, 88,* 1–20.

Kiran, S. (2007). Complexity in treatment of naming deficits. *American Journal of Speech and Language Pathology, 46,* 773–787.

Kiss, K. (2000). Effects of verb complexity on agrammatic aphasics' sentence production. In R. Bastiaanse & Y. Grodzinsky (Eds.), *Grammatical disorders in aphasia* (pp. 123–151). London: Whurr.

Kohn, S. E., Lorch, M. P., & Pearson, D. M. (1989). Verb finding in aphasia. *Cortex, 25,* 57–69.

Kolk, H. H. J. (1987). A theory of grammatical impairment in aphasia. In G. Kempen (Ed.), *Natural language generation: New results in artificial intelligence, psychology and linguistics.* Dordrecht: Martinus Nijhoff.

Kolk, H. H. J., & Heeschen, C. (1990). Adaptation symptoms and impairment symptoms in Broca's aphasia. *Aphasiology, 4,* 221–231.

Koopman, H., & Sportiche, D. (1991). The position of subjects. *Lingua, 85,* 211–258.

Lee, J., & Thompson, C. K. (2005). Functional categories in agrammatic speech. *LSO Working papers in linguistics 5: Proceedings of WIGL,* 107–123.

Lee, M. (2003). Dissociations among functional categories in Korean agrammatism. *Brain and Language, 84,* 170–188.

Lee, M., & Thompson, C. K. (2004). Agrammatic aphasic production and comprehension of unaccusative verbs in sentence contexts. *Journal of Neurolinguistics, 17,* 315–330.

Linebarger, M. C., Schwartz, M. F., & Saffran, E. M. (1983). Sensitivity to grammatical structure in so-called agrammatic aphasics. *Cognition, 13,* 361–394.

Loverso, F. L., Prescott, T. E., & Selinger, M. (1986). Cueing verbs: A treatment strategy for aphasic adults. *Journal of Rehabilitation Research, 25,* 47–60.

Luzzatti, C., Raggi, R., Zonca, G., Pistarini, C., Contardi, A., & Pinna, G. D. (2002). Verb-noun double dissociation in aphasic lexical impairments: The role of word frequency and imageability. *Brain and Language, 81,* 432–444.

Marantz, A. (1995). The minimalist program. In G. Webelhuth (Ed.), *Government and binding theory and the minimalist program.* London: Basil Blackwell.

Mauner, G., Fromkin, V., & Cornell, T. (1993). Comprehension and acceptability judgments in agrammatism: Disruption in the syntax of referential dependency. *Brain and Language, 45,* 340–370.

Menn, L., & Obler, L. (Eds.). (1990). *Agrammatic aphasia: A cross-language narrative sourcebook.* Amsterdam: Benjamins.

Nicholas, L. E., & Brookshire, R. H. (1993). A system for quantifying the informativeness and efficiency of the connected speech of adults with aphasia. *Journal of Speech and Hearing Research, 36,* 338–350.

Piñango, M. M. (2000). On the proper generalization for Broca's aphasia comprehension pattern: Why argument movement may not be at the source of the Broca's deficit. *Behavioral and Brain Sciences, 23,* 48–49.

Pollock, J.- Y. (1989). Verb movement, universal grammar, and the structure of IP. *Linguistic Inquiry, 20,* 365–424.

Prather, P., Zurif, E., Love, T., & Brownell, H. (1997). Speed of lexical activation in non-fluent Broca's aphasia and fluent Wernicke's aphasia. *Brain and Language, 59,* 391–411.

Rochon, E., Laird, L., Bose, A., & Scofield, J. (2005). Mapping Therapy for sentence production impairments in nonfluent aphasia. *Neuropsychological Rehabilitation, 15,* 1–36.

Rochon, E., Saffran, E. M., Berndt, R. S., & Schwartz, M. F. (2000). Quantitative analysis on aphasic sentence production: further development and new data. *Brain and Language, 72,* 193–218.

Saffran, E. M., Berndt, R. S., & Schwartz, M. F. (1989). The quantitative analysis of agrammatic production: Procedure and data. *Brain and Language, 37,* 440–479.

Schwartz, M. F., Saffran, E. M., Fink, R. B., Myers, J. L., & Martin, N. (1994). Mapping Therapy: A treatment programme for agrammatism. *Aphasiology, 8,* 19–54.

Shapiro, L., Gordon, B., Hack, N., & Killackey, J. (1993). Verb-argument structure processing in complex sentences in Broca's and Wernicke's aphasia. *Brain and Language, 45,* 423–447.

Shapiro, L. P., & Levine, B. A. (1990). Verb processing during sentence comprehension in aphasia. *Brain and Language, 38,* 21–47.

Shapiro, L. P., McNamara, P., Zurif, E., Lanzoni, S., & Cermak, L. (1991). Processing complexity and sentence memory: Evidence from amnesia. *Brain and Language, 42,* 431–453.

Swinney, D., Prather, P., & Love, T. (2000) The time course of lexical access and the role of context: Converging evidence from normal and aphasic processing. In Y. Grodzinsky, L. P. Shapiro, & D. Swinney (Eds.), *Language and the brain: Representation and processing.* Academic Press, New York.

Swinney, D., & Zurif, E. (1995). Syntactic processing in aphasia. *Brain and Language, 50,* 225–239.

Thompson, C. K. (2003). Unaccusative verb production in agrammatic aphasia: The argument structure complexity hypothesis. *Journal of Neurolinguistics, 16,* 151–167.

Thompson, C. K. (2007). Complexity in language learning and treatment. *American Journal of Speech and Language Pathology, 16,* 3–5.

Thompson, C. K. (in preparation for publication). *The Northwestern Assessment of Verbs and Sentences.*

Thompson, C. K. (in preparation for publication). *The Northwestern Assessment of Verb Inflection.*

Thompson, C. K., Ballard, K. J., & Shapiro, L. P. (1998). The role of syntactic complexity in training wh- movement structures in agrammatic aphasia: Optimal order for promoting generalization. *Journal of the International Neuropsychological Society, 4*(6), 661–674.

Thompson, C. K., Lange, K. L., Schneider, S. L., & Shapiro, L. P. (1997). Agrammatic and non-brain damaged subjects' verb and verb argument structure production. *Aphasiology, 11,* 473–490.

Thompson, C. K., Milman, L. H., Dickey, M. W., O'Connor, J. E., Bonakdarpour, B., Fix, S. C., et al. (2006). Functional category production in agrammatism: Treatment and generalization effects. *Brain and Language, 99,* 79–81.

Thompson, C. K., & Shapiro, L. P. (1994). A linguistic-specific approach to treatment of sentence production deficits in aphasia. In P. Lemme (Ed.), *Clinical aphasiology* (Vol. 21). Austin, TX: Pro-Ed.

Thompson, C. K., & Shapiro, L. P. (2007). Complexity in treatment of syntactic deficits. *American Journal of Speech and Language Pathology, 16,* 30–42.

Thompson, C. K., Shapiro, L. P., Ballard, K. J., Jacobs, B. J., Schneider, S. L., & Tait, M. E. (1997). Training and generalized production of wh- and NP- movement structures in agrammatic aphasia. *Journal of Speech and Hearing Research, 40,* 228–244.

Thompson, C. K., Shaprio, L, Kiran, S., & Maas, E. (manuscript in preparation). *Mapping Therapy and treatment of underlying forms: A comparison of treatment effect.*

Thompson, C. K, Shapiro, L., Kiran, S., & Sobecks, J. (2003). The role of syntactic complexity in treatment of sentence deficits in agrammatic aphasia: The complexity account of treatment efficacy (CATE). *Journal of Speech, Language, and Hearing Research, 42,* 690–707.

Thompson, C. K., Shapiro, L. P., & Roberts, M. M. (1993). Treatment of sentence production deficits in aphasia: A linguistic-specific approach to wh- interrogative training and generalization. *Aphasiology, 7,* 111–133.

Thompson, C. K., Shapiro, L. P., Tait, M. E., Jacobs, B., Schneider, S. L., & Ballard, K. J. (1995). A system for the linguistic analysis of agrammatic language production. *Brain and Language, 51,* 124–129.

Thompson, C. K., Shapiro, L. P., Tait, M. E., Jacobs, B., & Schneider, S. S. (1996). Training wh- question production in agrammatic aphasia: Analysis of argument and adjunct movement. *Brain and Language, 52,* 175–228.

Vanier, M., & Caplan, D. (1990). CT-scan correlates of agrammatism. In L. Menn & L. Obler (Eds.), *Agrammatic aphasia: A cross-language narrative sourcebook* (pp. 37–114). Amsterdam/Philadelphia: John Benjamins.

Zingeser, L., & Berndt, R. S. (1990). Retrieval of nouns and verbs in agrammatism and anomia. *Brain and Language, 39,* 14–32.

Zurif, E., Swinney, D., Prather, P., Solomon, J., & Bushell, C. (1993). On-line analysis of syntactic processing in Broca's and Wernicke's aphasia. *Brain and Language, 45,* 448–464.

APPENDIX 27.1
Treatment Protocols[1]

Protocol for Training Object Clefts

Pre-Trial Probe Task

A randomly selected, semantically reversible picture pair is presented, such as, (a) girl kissing a boy and (b) boy kissing a girl. Object cleft production and comprehension are tested using sentence-picture matching and sentence production priming (see *Assessment of Agrammatic Deficits* on p. 741).

TREATMENT STEP 1: THEMATIC ROLE TRAINING

The clinician says, "Let's work on that sentence." Sentence constituents comprising the active form of the target sentence are presented on individual cards under the target picture. For example, [THE BOY] [IS] [KISSING] [THE GIRL] is placed below the boy-kissing-girl picture. The client reads aloud or repeats the active sentence. Additional cards for [WHO] and [IT WAS] are placed next to the picture. The verb and verb arguments (thematic roles) are identified by the examiner in the following manner: Pointing to the verb, the examiner explains, "This is *kissing*; it is the action of the sentence"; pointing to the Agent (subject NP), the examiner explains, "This is *the boy*; he is the person kissing"; pointing to the Theme (object NP), the examiner explains, "This is *the girl*; she is the person being kissed." The client is then asked to point to and name the Agent/Action/Theme. The client reads aloud or repeats the active sentence again.

TREATMENT STEP 2: SENTENCE BUILDING

The examiner first explains, "We are going to make a new sentence to go with this picture using these cards." The [WHO] card is placed next to the Theme card [THE GIRL]. The clinician explains that to make a new sentence, [WHO] is added next to [THE GIRL], because the girl is the person who is kissed. The client is instructed to read aloud/repeat the sentence in the order of the cards: [THE BOY] [KISSED] [THE GIRL] [WHO].

The Theme [THE GIRL] and the [WHO] cards are moved to the sentence initial position, creating the following word string: [THE GIRL] [WHO] [THE BOY] [KISSED]. The examiner explains, "To make the new sentence, these words are moved to the beginning of the sentence. They move together because the girl is the person who is kissed."

The examiner explains that to make a correct sentence, the [IT WAS] card needs to be added "because it was the man who the

woman kissed." The [IT WAS] card is placed at the beginning of the sentence. The client reads aloud/repeats the target sentence: [IT WAS] [THE MAN] [WHO] [THE WOMAN] [KISSED].

TREATMENT STEP 3: THEMATIC ROLE TRAINING

The examiner explains that the agent/action/theme are the same in the new sentence as in the old one. The client is asked to point to and name the Agent/Action/Theme. The client reads aloud or repeats the target sentence again.

TREATMENT STEP 4: PRACTICE

Sentence constituents are rearranged in active sentence form, together with [WHO] and [IT WAS] cards (as in Treatment Step 1). The client moves the cards to form the target object cleft sentence. Assistance is provided as needed.

Post-Trial Probe Task

The same procedures as in the *Pre-Trial Probe Task* are used.

Object "Wh-" Questions

Pre-Trial Probe Task

A randomly selected, semantically reversible picture pair is presented, such as (a) girl kissing a boy and (b) boy kissing a girl. "Wh-" question production and comprehension are tested using sentence-picture matching and sentence production priming (see *Assessment of Agrammatiic Deficits* on p. 741).

TREATMENT STEP 1: THEMATIC ROLE TRAINING

The clinician says, "Let's work on that sentence." Sentence constituents comprising the active training sentence are presented on individual cards under the target picture. For example, [THE BOY] [IS] [KISSING] [THE GIRL] is placed under the boy-kissing-girl picture. The client reads aloud or repeats the active sentence. Additional cards, [WHO] and [?], are put next to the picture. The verb and verb arguments (thematic roles) are identified by the examiner in the following manner: Pointing to the verb, the examiner explains, "This is *kissing*; it is the action of the sentence"; pointing to the Agent (subject NP), the examiner explains, "This is *the boy*; he is the person doing the kissing"; pointing to the Theme (object NP), the examiner explains, "This is *the girl*; she is the person being kissed," The client is then asked to point to and name the Agent/Action/Theme. The client reads aloud or repeats the active sentence again.

---

[1] Computerized protocols (**Sentactic®**) for training three Wh-movement sentences, object relative clause structures, object clefts, and object "wh-" questions have been developed and are currently being studied. For description of the program and updates, go to http://cslr.colorado. edu/beginweb/sentactics/sentactics.html.

TREATMENT STEP 2: SENTENCE BUILDING

The examiner first explains, "We are going to make a new sentence, a question, to go with this picture using these cards." The Theme [THE GIRL] card is replaced by [WHO], and the examiner explains that this is done because *the girl* is WHO is kissed. The question mark card then is placed at the end of the card string, forming an echo question: [THE BOY] [IS] [KISSING] [WHO][2] [?]. The clinician explains that the [?] card is needed to make a question sentence. The client reads aloud or repeats the echo questions.

Subject/auxiliary verb inversion is demonstrated, resulting in the following string: [IS] [THE BOY] [KISSING] [WHO] [?]. The clinician says, "To make the question sentence, we need to switch [THE BOY] and [IS]."

---

[2] We recognize that proper English requires *whom* rather than *who* in the object position. We use *who* for simplification; we also note that who in the object position is now accepted.

Movement of [WHO] to the sentence initial position is demonstrated, as the examiner explains that the question starts with [WHO]: [WHO] [IS] [THE BOY] [KISSING] [?]. The client reads/repeats the question.

TREATMENT STEP 3: THEMATIC ROLE TRAINING

The examiner explains that the Agent/Action/Theme are the same in the new sentence as in the old one. The client is asked to point to and name the Agent/Action/Theme. The client reads aloud or repeats the target sentence again.

TREATMENT STEP 4: PRACTICE

Sentence constituents are rearranged in active sentence form, together with the [WHO] and [?] cards (as in Treatment Step 1). The client moves the cards to form the target "wh-" question, then reads or repeats it. Assistance is provided as needed.

Post-Trial Probe Task

The same procedures as in the *Pre-Trial Probe Task* are used.

Chapter 28

Language-Oriented Treatment: A Psycholinguistic Approach to Aphasia

Donna L. Bandur and
Cynthia M. Shewan

OBJECTIVES

The objectives of this chapter are:

- To define Language-Oriented Treatment (LOT)
- To outline the implementation of LOT
- To describe the benefits of an LOT approach
- To highlight the functional aspects of LOT
- To demonstrate the efficacy of LOT

Language-Oriented Treatment (LOT) is a psycholinguistic approach to the treatment of aphasia. As such, it strives to enable a person with aphasia to use a language processing system at its maximum functional level. This language-oriented approach is based on the application of psycholinguistic research evidence to treatment, reflecting how language normally is processed and how it is altered in the presence of aphasia. Because of the neurolinguistic underpinnings of LOT with respect to theory, application, and evolution, Helm-Estabrooks (1988) categorized LOT as a neurolinguistic approach to treatment. Shewan (1977) developed LOT during the 1970s, over a 2-year period, with the aim of creating an approach consisting of a structured methodology coupled with content based on research data from normal and disordered language. To acquaint the reader with the climate in which LOT was conceived, a brief history of aphasia treatment will be reviewed.

HISTORY OF APHASIA TREATMENT

Little in the way of what we now know as orthodox treatment for aphasia appeared before the beginning of the 20th century. In the early 1900s, the literature reported a few studies describing treatment (Franz, 1906, 1924; Frazier & Ingham, 1920; Mills, 1904; Weisenburg & McBride, 1935), and even as far back as this, questions were raised, although not answered, relative to the efficacy of treatment.

After World War II, interest regarding aphasia treatment surged because of the number of war veterans with aphasia as a result of trauma. The focus of these rehabilitation efforts was on reeducation, the approach developed for treatment. Because of the effects of trauma on the personality of these individuals, many psychotherapy groups became a part of rehabilitation efforts (Backus, 1952; Blackman, 1950). Reportedly, these groups provided support and positively influenced both communication and personality adjustment (Aronson, Shatin, & Cook, 1956; Blackman & Tureen, 1948). With the exceptions of Eisenson (1949) and Wepman (1951), however, data were primarily anecdotal and not statistically supported. In addition, the data focused on trauma rather than on stroke.

In the 1950s, aphasia treatment shifted, focusing on individuals who developed aphasia as a result of stroke. Schuell's work, both in this era and in the 1960s, predominated (Schuell, Jenkins, & Jimenez-Pabon, 1964). The data published about treatment were controversial, and whether aphasia treatment was efficacious remained an issue. On the one hand, Vignolo's study (1964) reported the significantly positive effects of treatment, but the study by Sarno, Silverman, and Sands (1970) failed to show the positive effects of language treatment.

The 1970s and early 1980s witnessed the publication of several studies, some with and some without control groups, that supported the efficacy of language treatment in patients with aphasia (Basso, Capitani, & Vignolo, 1979; Basso, Faglioni, & Vignolo, 1975; Broida, 1977; Dabul & Hanson, 1975; Deal & Deal, 1978; Hagen, 1973; Prins, Snow, & Wegenaar, 1978; Sefer, 1973; Shewan & Kertesz, 1984; Smith, Champoux, Leri, London, & Muraski, 1972; Wertz et al., 1978, 1981). The ideal study, using a randomized no-treatment control group, had not been completed, and some believed that only this study would put to rest their doubts about the efficacy of aphasia treatment. Despite some studies that disputed the efficaciousness of language treatment (David, Enderby, & Bainton, 1982; Meikle et al., 1979), enough evidence had been gathered by 1982 for Darley (1982) to conclude that the foregoing collage of studies "collectively provides a series of answers and together lays our doubt about efficacy to rest" (p. 175).

Darley's proclamation did not, however, convince everyone, and efficacy studies continued throughout the 1980s and into the next decade, with the majority favoring the significant and positive effects of treatment (Brindley, Copeland, Demain, & Martyn, 1989; Holland & Wertz, 1988; Poeck, Huber, & Willmes, 1989; Schonle, 1988; Springer, Glindemann, Huber, & Willmes, 1991; Wertz et al., 1986; Whitney & Goldstein, 1989). In summarizing the results of most large group studies, Holland, Fromm, De Ruyter, and Stein (1996) described them as demonstrating the value of aphasia treatment, particularly when therapy is frequent and conducted over a lengthy interval. The authors also highlighted the contributions made in recent years by small-group, single-subject experimental studies and individual case studies. These investigations have provided more detailed descriptions about the efficacy of specific approaches when applied to particular language problems. Because the individuals studied in these reports generally have been in the chronic stages of their recovery, the language gains realized are not likely to be attributed to spontaneous recovery.

More recently, Bhogal, Teasell, and Speechley (2003) reviewed the aphasia literature for language treatment studies reported from January 1975 through May 2002 to determine the possible relationship between intensity of therapy and language outcomes as assessed using the Porch Index of Communicative Abilities, or PICA, and the Functional Communication Profile, or FCP. The authors found that studies with positive treatment results were associated with greater than 2 hours of therapy per week. Our work would support the idea that further studies employing carefully tailored, intensive treatment approaches directed at addressing the underlying nature and complexity of the behavioral symptoms will best delineate what specific approaches work best for whom.

EVOLUTION OF LANGUAGE-ORIENTED TREATMENT

From the foregoing summary, one can see how both the study and our understanding of aphasia have evolved. With pressures not only to demonstrate that therapy results not only in improved linguistic performance but also in meaningful functional outcomes, we are compelled to examine and describe what processes we are addressing that result in these positive changes. When LOT was first conceptualized, the aphasia literature contained few descriptions of treatment that were sufficiently detailed to assure clinicians they were, indeed, actually replicating that treatment. The predominant type of treatment was stimulation therapy, but there remained many patients for whom this approach did

not bring about significant change. The need for alternative methods, which incorporated the accumulating research data regarding how individuals with and without aphasia process language and which could be clearly defined for replication, became apparent. Because clinicians were being pressured to reexamine their treatment approaches and accompanying rationales, it became imperative that theoretical information be incorporated into designing therapy and be described in such a way as to be systemically applied across patients. Subsequently, LOT was designed, outlining a structured methodology in which an individual progressed through steps of increasing difficulty, with the content of therapy based on psycholinguistic research data. Next, LOT was pilot tested (Shewan, 1977) with a small group of patients. The resulting data were promising and led to a full-scale clinical trial (described later in this chapter). A decade passed from ideational conception to the publication of a book fully describing LOT, complete with treatment guidelines, treatment materials, and efficacy data (Shewan & Bandur, 1986). Ongoing research has necessitated modifications, particularly to the content of LOT.

The 21st century has witnessed a surge in the use of technology, with advances in neuroimaging techniques. Positron-emission tomography and functional magnetic resonance imaging have enabled the growth in our understanding of how those with and without aphasia process and produce language (Gernsbacher & Kaschak, 2003; Martin, 2003). Information derived from these avenues of research can complement the work of those addressing psycholinguistic measures of language to assist clinicians in better understanding the neural basis of language and cognition and how those functions may be altered in the presence of lesions in various areas of the human brain. With this understanding, greater customization of assessment tools, treatment goals, and strategies is possible, which in turn can positively impact our clinical efficiency and outcomes. Studies demonstrating the brain's plasticity and ability to adjust to injury have been emerging and lend further support for the importance of our language interventions (Belin et al., 1996; Calvert et al., 2000; Cao, Vikinstad, George, Johnson, & Welch, 1999; Cappa, 2000; Leger et al., 2002; Thiel et al., 2001; Thomas, Altenmuller, Marckmann, Kahrs, & Dichgans, 1997; Warburton, Price, Swinburn, & Wise, 1999).

As our understanding of normal language processing has advanced, along with greater specification of language impairments and their functional impact on those with aphasia, LOT has been refined. As additional research findings emerge, LOT will continue to evolve.

Philosophy and Rationale

Aphasia treatments typically are based on a theoretic construct of aphasia, and LOT is no exception. As defined here, aphasia represents impairment in the language system and in access to the language system. Processes for understanding and producing language thereby are affected. This theoretic view of aphasia is derived from the work of Zurif and his colleagues (Zurif and Caramazza, 1976; Zurif, Caramazza, & Myerson, 1972; Zurif, Green, Caramazza, & Goodenough, 1976). It is proposed that the linguistic or conceptual knowledge base is not lost in aphasia but, rather, no longer can be accessed automatically, at an unconscious level. Language, or at least certain aspects of language, must be mediated by more conscious and explicit mechanisms (Byng & Black, 1995).

In the LOT method, the content of language treatment is extremely important, with the ultimate goal being to provide the patient with a language-processing system that operates at its maximum functional level by applying neurolinguistic findings to treatment. This approach is in contrast to that of providing indiscriminant stimulation of the language system, with expectations that exposure to a variety of tasks will facilitate change in performance. For example, workbook activities selected to match symptoms can lead to frustration and discouragement when responding appears to be inconsistent, when difficulty levels may be inappropriate, and when changes in communicative performance ultimately are not realized.

Language-Oriented Treatment is designed to provide a highly individualized and tailored approach to treatment based on the language profile, the interests, and the goals of the patient. Guidelines are detailed to assist with organizing and implementing therapy but are not intended to be prescriptive in nature. An effort has been made to maintain a high degree of flexibility with the approach while providing enough structure to allow effective replication.

Content

Implementation of LOT requires careful analysis and understanding of the pattern of deficits presented by a particular individual. A hypothesis regarding the underlying nature of the problems is based on available information from normal language processing and that found in those with aphasia. A psycholinguistic approach emphasizes the need for clinicians to ensure that their interpretation of symptoms is guided by theoretic hypotheses rather than relying on intuition and that treatment is individualized with respect to the symptoms displayed by the specific person being treated (Albert, 1998; Byng, 1992). To provide a system whereby the content of language can be described comprehensively and to facilitate data collection, LOT divides the communication system into five modalities, which are non-overlapping and mutually exclusive (Fig. 28–1). The five modalities are (1) auditory processing, (2) visual processing,

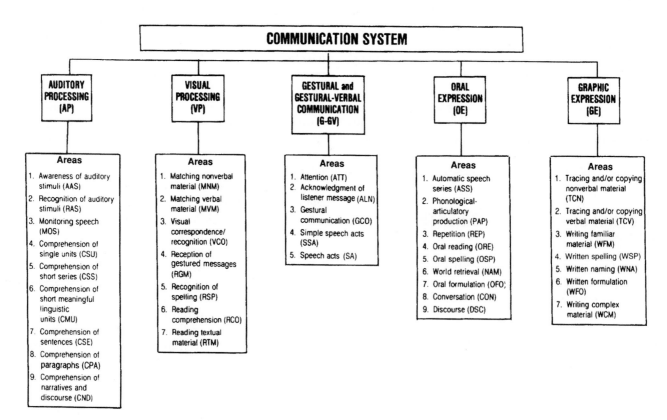

Figure 28–1. Schematic model of the language modalities and areas within these modalities that make up the communication system.

(3) gestural and combined gestural-verbal communication, (4) oral expression, and (5) graphic expression.

Each modality is further subdivided into mutually exclusive areas that, collectively, encompass the entire modality. With each modality segmented into component parts, a clinician can clearly specify the content of treatment being provided. Rather than advocating a particular breakdown of the communication system, the division is intended to facilitate specification of the content of treatment and to permit its replication.

Within each area of a modality (e.g., comprehension of sentences within the Auditory Processing modality) treatment materials are organized according to the level of difficulty based on available data from research literature. The goal of language treatment is to improve a patient's language deficits by presenting material that increases in difficulty level at a pace that the individual can accommodate.

Although the modalities have been delineated to assist in outlining LOT content and areas for potential treatment, treatment within one modality or area may be targeted to facilitate performance in another. For example, within the Oral Expression modality, oral reading rarely would be chosen as a goal in and of itself. Instead, an oral reading task may be selected to achieve a variety of objectives, such as self-monitoring, auditory processing, reading comprehension, and so forth. When selecting an activity within an area, it is essential that it correspond to the established goal, and how responses within an activity, area, or modality might reflect or challenge other language processes must be considered.

The content areas within each modality are considered to be the base in treatment or guidelines for consideration, but they are not necessarily arranged in a hierarchical order or intended for use with every patient. As our understanding of aphasia evolves, along with our knowledge about the effectiveness of specific treatment techniques, these advancements can be incorporated into the content of LOT.

Because LOT was designed to be flexible and promote the use of procedures that facilitate optimal responding by the patient, more than one modality typically are treated simultaneously, either within the same session or even within the same activity. To this end, the clinician must be cognizant of the many variables that impact performance, design tasks that can meet the goals selected, and organize them in ways that allow changes to be measured and documented.

Methodology

The methodology of LOT has adopted a paradigm in which the major components are stimulus, response, and reinforcement. In contrast to operant conditioning, however, the goal is not to learn specific stimulus–response connections, such as certain words in a word retrieval task or specific sentences in a sentence formulation task. Rather, the paradigm of presenting stimuli followed by responses with accompanying descriptive feedback enables patients to process or use language at levels appropriate, yet challenging, given their current capabilities. To enhance correct responding, modifications may be made to the stimuli or task requirements because difficulties are encountered. Facilitated Problem Solving has been used to describe treatment that is characterized by the relationship between a narrow focus in the materials used, what the patient is required to do with them, and the interaction with the clinician (Byng & Black, 1995). This process of adjusting the task in response to the patient at a given point in time has been proposed to be one of the critical elements of therapy.

Approaching treatment from a stimulus–response–reinforcement construct enables the clinician to collect data about performance and provides objective feedback to both the clinician and the patient about progress over time on particular tasks and/or areas. Because improvements in treatment may not be immediately reflected in changes on standardized test measures, demonstration of steady gains across a hierarchy of activities can be an invaluable source of reinforcement for the patient, significant others, and those who may be challenging the value of financial support for ongoing treatment. Alternatively, this method provides objective information, in a timely manner, regarding when a task or procedure should be modified or, perhaps, even abandoned.

Difficulty Levels

In LOT, activities are presented in order of increasing difficulty to optimize opportunities for success and minimize feelings of frustration and failure on the part of the patient. Several variables can affect the difficulty level of a task, such as type of materials incorporated, mode of presentation, complexity of response required, and amount of clinician support provided. Difficulty levels may be based on an analysis of results from standardized testing and systematic probing in concert with information from research literature regarding normal and/or disordered language functioning.

The stimuli and their responses in treatment are presented in blocks of 10 items each. To advance the level of a task, a patient must achieve 70% or more correct responses on two consecutive blocks of items at the same level of difficulty. When this criterion is met, the difficulty of the task is increased to the next level in the hierarchy. If the 70% correct criterion is not achieved, the block of 10 stimulus items is repeated. The difficulty level of the task is decreased if the patient is unable to meet the 70% criterion, followed by discontinuation of the task should the alteration in task difficulty not produce the desired outcome. A criterion of 70% correct was chosen to allow flexibility in response performance and to accommodate some error without unduly delaying progress in treatment. If a particular patient demonstrates the need for a higher criterion, it can be altered, although the efficacy data reported later in this chapter reflects the use of the 70% criterion.

Cueing

If a patient cannot generate an independent response, the clinician may incorporate the presentation of cues within an activity, with a hierarchy of difficulty levels established, based on the amount of support provided by the clinician. The goal in implementing a cueing system is to determine which cues are facilitative, to develop the individual's awareness of those that are effective, to transfer the responsibility for initiating and providing cues from the clinician to the patient, and to increase the production of independent responses, with self-cueing as needed.

Criterion Response and Branching

Defining the elements of a correct response is required to advance the level of difficulty. As described earlier, the clinician decides what constitutes a correct response. Because flexibility in establishing this decision is available, the definition of a correct response may differ for each task. In most tasks, many different levels of response are possible, and what is accepted as correct may change with time and as improvement occurs. For example, early during treatment, a clinician may decide that, in a naming task, a recognizable production meets criterion. Later, however, a phonetically correct response may be required to score it as meeting criterion.

When the difference between two adjacent levels of difficulty proves to be too great for a patient to master, the clinician can create levels of intermediate difficulty (branching). Branching constructs a link between the initial task and assists the patient in advancing to the next level. Another situation requiring branching may arise when a clinician determines that dividing a large group of equally difficult material into two subgroups might be advantageous in providing additional language processing opportunities with each subgroup rather than omitting some of the material.

Feedback

Feedback is a key aspect to the implementation of LOT. Information regarding the correctness and quality of a response promotes a better understanding of the language impairment and the factors influencing performance. By engaging in mutual problem-solving exchanges and encouraging self-evaluation, the patient becomes a more active participant in treatment. The patient can serve as an invaluable source of information and insight for the clinician, with a personal and, many times, richer perspective, through indicating or describing how a particular response has occurred and/or was facilitated.

Recording Data

Because the patient's performance dictates when tasks should be increased or decreased in difficulty, recording data is an important component in LOT. Two forms can be helpful in this respect. A LOT Goals Form (Appendix 28-1) may be used for each area in each modality. The difficulty level, stimuli, presentation method, type of cueing, criterion for a correct response, and response method are recorded, with space for additional observations. A LOT Data Record Form (Appendix 28-2) specifies the amount of time spent in each session for each area and modality, difficulty level of the task, number of items presented, data collected, and any other pertinent observations that a clinician may wish to record. Both forms are useful in charting the course of treatment and highlighting for the clinician when difficulty levels or tasks might be altered.

Patient–Clinician Relationship

Although LOT is structured in content and methodology, it is carried out within a caring and positive interpersonal environment. Albert (1998) describes the loss of ability to communicate as being tantamount to the loss of personhood, and evidence suggests that the self-esteem of individuals who have suffered strokes can contribute to their functional abilities, at least during the early phases of recovery (Chang & MacKenzie, 1998). Le Dorze and Brassard (1995) have reported on the impact of aphasia on both patients and their significant others. Negative communication consequences include increased effort, irritation, frustration, and fatigue in communication, with language disabilities having a marked impact on interpersonal relationships.

Sarno (1997) has described how intensive, long term rehabilitation that addresses language, communication strategies, functional communication, and psychosocial issues for the first year positively impacts the quality of life of persons with aphasia. In this context, the importance of the patient–clinician relationship cannot be overstated. Understanding and respecting premorbid personality and lifestyle characteristics of patients are the first steps in developing collaborative, supportive relationships both with them and with their significant others. Creating a climate for an open and honest exchange of ideas and feelings is needed to facilitate mutual goal setting and a sense of partnership. Skilful clinicians are mindful of how central the therapeutic relationship is to the treatment of aphasia. Helping patients and their support systems understand the loss accompanying aphasia is a necessary component of treatment. In turn, this creates the foundation for working through the many challenges and, sometimes, disappointments that are encountered throughout the rehabilitation process.

Language-Oriented Treatment employs a structured methodology of stimulus–response–reinforcement, in concert with clearly defined hierarchies and scoring systems, but this approach does not preclude the establishment of a patient-centered milieu in treatment. The patient and significant others play integral roles in determining goals and activities based on their needs, interests, and abilities. To facilitate the transfer of skills to more functional aspects of the patient's life, the clinician must develop an understanding about the impact of aphasia on the whole person and the world in which he or she participates. Chapey and colleagues (2000) described the importance of a life participation approach to aphasia, or LPAA. Those authors suggested that, at every step of the rehabilitation process, the clinician needs to understand and address the impact of aphasia on the attainment of the patient's personal goals and direct treatment to identify the supports needed to enable participation in his or her environment as a competent individual.

IMPLEMENTATION OF LANGUAGE-ORIENTED TREATMENT

Guiding Principles

In the following sections, a description of each modality will be provided. It is not possible to address all the areas within the confines of this chapter, so only some of them will be highlighted, particularly as they reflect current practice or changes since the inception of LOT. The reader is referred to *Treatment of Aphasia: A Language-Oriented Approach* (Shewan & Bandur, 1986). A complete listing of the areas incorporated in each of the modalities also is found in Figure 28–1. It is worth noting that this chart reflects the content of LOT at the time of its original development. Since then, approaches to treatment have been refined in some areas, and these new or expanded treatment applications will be discussed in the descriptions of the modalities that follow.

Consideration of lesion site and an understanding of that area's role in cognitive and linguistic processes are essential in guiding a comprehensive assessment. The decision regarding which modalities and areas to introduce initially during treatment can be made once a hypothesis as to the nature of the underlying deficits is established. Only with integration of knowledge about neural substrates and psycholinguistic principles can we inform our treatment decisions and educate our patients regarding prognostic implications.

At the conclusion of the treatment section, some case illustrations will be provided to demonstrate the practical applications of LOT with patients exhibiting a range of aphasic deficits. These descriptions provide evidence that systematically addressing the underlying problems results in functional improvements.

The Role of Computers

Generally, therapy for aphasia takes place in a face-to-face setting between the clinician and the patient, with the clinician presenting activities and related feedback while modifying tasks according to the response characteristics of the patient. Advances in computer technology and its increased accessibility have lead investigators to explore computer applications in aphasia management. The role of the computer in delivering therapeutic tasks and in serving both as an alternative-augmentative communication system and as a tool for work and recreational activities has been examined.

The literature reflects varying degrees of improvement in language functioning related to implementation of computerized programs. When evaluating the results of an unsupervised home-based computer program, Petheram (1996) failed to find a relationship between progression through a hierarchy of tasks and improvements on formalized language measures. Amount of time spent on the computer varied widely and appeared to be associated with less frequent opportunities for hobbies or other forms of social interaction.

Weinrich, McCall, Boser, and Virata (2002) examined the impact of Computerized Visual Communication (Steele, Weinrich, Wertz, Kleczewsda, & Carlson, 1989), or C-VIC, training on sentence production and discourse in five patients with nonfluent aphasia. They found an improvement in sentence formulation skills on a picture description task both in oral and C-VIC formulation for trained items and, to a lesser extent, for untrained vocabulary. Procedural and narrative discourse performance proved to be similar. Spoken was described as less accurate than C-VIC productions, which the investigators attributed to the increased cognitive load required in the former task.

Greater success with computerized treatment has been reported in the realm of word retrieval. Doesborgh and colleagues (2004) described positive changes in naming performance by a group of patients with chronic aphasia, following implementation of a computer-based treatment program. With Multicue (Van Mourik & Van de Sandt-Koenderman, 1992), opportunities for the user to independently determine and select cues to facilitate naming of both high- and low-frequency pictured words were provided. Improvements in word retrieval were found on standardized testing at the end of a 2-month period. Positive gains in naming skills in a group of patients with chronic aphasia also were reported by Aftonomos, Steele, and Wertz (1997) through coupling home- and clinic-based computer instruction. Icons associated with natural lexical items, representing various categories, were manipulated in a range of activities. The amount of daily home practice (mean, 2.04 hours) was judged to be a significant contributor to the treatment outcome.

Mortley, Wade, and Enderby (2004) used their computer-based treatment program to target word retrieval skills in a group of patients, again, with chronic aphasia, implementing a home-practice paradigm that was monitored through the Internet and telephone interviews. Significant improvements in naming scores were found after a 27-week period of home practice, with the participants spending, on average, 2 hours and 45 minutes per week engaged in the computer activities. Other stated benefits were family and patient reports of the improved confidence and independence in everyday communication exchanges exhibited by the patients.

Others have studied the treatment of syntactic comprehension deficits through application of computerized tasks. Beveridge and Crerar (2002) reported on the use of Multimedia Microworld, a program based on a mapping therapy protocol (Schwartz, Saffran, Fink, Myers, & Martin, 1994). Active, passive, and object cleft sentences were produced by the computer in written form, accompanied by auditory presentation, with the subjects required to arrange pictorial elements to represent the sentences. Eight 1-hour treatment sessions were provided, with minimal clinician input. At the conclusion of therapy, all three patients demonstrated significant improvement in written sentence comprehension for trained sentence forms, along with variable improvement in auditory processing.

Positive treatment outcomes in reading comprehension also were reported by Katz and Wertz (1997), employing a hierarchy of activities from simple letter matching to sentence comprehension tasks. Following therapy, consisting of 3 hours of practice per week over the course of 26 weeks, those who had received reading comprehension training demonstrated significantly more improved scores on overall language measures than those who were provided with only computer stimulation tasks.

Wertz and Katz (2004) reviewed the literature for reports on treatment outcomes in patients with aphasia through the use of computers. Studies were evaluated with respect to the model of Robey, Schultz, Crawford, & Sinner (1998), defining outcome, efficacy, effectiveness, and efficiency, along with a five-phase outcome research model. The American Academy of Neurology's 1994 level of evidence scale also was incorporated into evaluating the findings. Only the Katz and Wertz (1997) study met the criterion of Class 1 evidence (i.e., evidence from one or more well-designed, randomized, controlled clinical trials), with the remainder providing Class 3 evidence (i.e., expert opinion, nonrandomized historical controls, or one or more case reports obtained in Phase 1 and 2 investigations).

With many individuals now having computers in their homes, development of carefully structured treatment activities using a hierarchy of difficulty levels may well be incorporated into the LOT approach, providing additional avenues for practice. The previous studies suggest that reading comprehension and naming activities might well be areas of consideration for supplementation with computer assignments. Construction and processing of electronic mail

(e-mail) could be effectively incorporated into a treatment hierarchy and bridge the gap between structured therapeutic tasks to those of a more functional nature.

The use of both low and high-tech Alternative and Augmentative Communication (AAC) strategies to support communication in those with aphasia was reviewed by Van de Sandt-Koendermann (2004). Overall, Van de Sandt-Koendermann suggested the lack of advancement within the field of AAC to be attributed to the few published case reports with respect to design and efficacy, which then places the burden on clinicians to establish time-consuming alternatives, with limited resources for a heterogeneous population. Challenges with implementation of low-tech devices include factors such as the severity of the language disorder and, perhaps, cognitive impairments faced by the individuals most in need of them, in addition to the issues of acceptance by the user and/or communication partner.

The C-VIC was designed both for treatment and as a method of communication for those with agrammatism. Although it has proven to be effective in improving oral sentence formulation skills, success in establishing online communication exchanges or transfer of skills outside the clinical environment has not been demonstrated. More recently, a Personal Communication Assistant for Dysphasic People, or PCAD, has become available. Van de Sandt-Koendermann described it as a small, portable device that is individually configured according to the modules that might be appropriate for the user. A hierarchy of options is available, including words, drawings, photographs, and pictograms, along with a voice output option. In a later study of 28 patients with aphasia, with time post-onset ranging from 3 months to 13 years, Van de Sandt-Koendermann, Wiegers, and Philippa (2005) determined that PCAD could be used as a functional communication system in the environment. In their investigation, which excluded those with cognitive impairment and poor auditory comprehension, 77% of the participants reported use of the device outside of the therapy sessions. Those who were most successful were older. The authors suggested that acceptance of a communication device might occur only when patients are in the more chronic phase of their disability and have accepted their limitations with oral speech. Because of the increasing popularity and familiarity of handheld devices in the general population, this option may hold further promise for at least some individuals with aphasia.

Wade, Petheram, and Cain (2001) considered whether voice recognition software could be a tool to assist those with aphasia in functions such as dictation and use of environmental controls and, potentially, as an input modality for treatment. They studied six individuals with a range in severity of aphasic deficits along with a control group and examined their success, over a period of five sessions, in training the software to recognize 50 words and 24 phrases. A great amount of variability was found in both groups during single-word training, with the phrase training demonstrating even greater variation in the group with aphasia. Not unexpectedly, the lowest accuracy levels were associated with greater levels of severity in speech production.

The introduction of voice recognition software also was explored for a patient with problems involving word finding and expression of complex information following a left parietal stroke (Bruce, Edmundson, & Coleman, 2003). Although reading skills were relatively well preserved, written spelling was significantly impacted. At the conclusion of 8 months of training and practice with the system, written skills had improved, and the patient reported using the system for constructing e-mail, letters, and lists. The investigators postulated that the system's success depends on an individual's ability to manage the large number of errors during the recognition training of the system. Some partially preserved spelling skills also were judged to be important in error correction. From these studies, one might conclude that as the technology undergoes further refinement, a future role exists for voice recognition software in assisting those with milder forms of aphasia.

A more recent focus in computer use by those with aphasia has been placed on facilitating Internet access, with the goal of broadening opportunities for communication exchanges. Sohleberg, Ehlhardt, Fickas, and Sutcliffe (2003) conducted a study to examine e-mail training with a small group of subjects having varying neurologic etiologies, including right and left hemisphere strokes. They concluded that the major barriers were lack of computer familiarity and difficulty with learning to operate the mouse/cursor functions. Problems with generating ideas for message construction, lack of error detection, and subsequent limitations in editing also were apparent. Overall, however, the participants proved to be highly enthusiastic and motivated to develop their abilities to formulate and send e-mails.

Egan, Worrall, and Oxenham (2004) examined whether patients could be taught to access the Internet through development of a written guide and a series of six training sessions provided by a volunteer. A range of tasks was included, such as turning on and off the computer, searching the World Wide Web, constructing e-mail, and so on. Before training, the subjects were found to have a low level of independence with computer tasks, with 8 of 20 patients ultimately achieving a high level of independence on the specified tasks. E-mail use proved to be the most popular function for all subjects.

Given that many people with aphasia are able to access—or have the potential for learning to access—information from the Internet, aphasia Web sites have more recently drawn attention. The accessibility and quality of Web sites for those with aphasia were examined by Ghidella, Murray, Smart, McKenna, and Worrall (2005) through ratings given by samples of patients with aphasia and speech-language pathologists. The speech-language pathologists judged

www.aphasiahelp.org as being the one containing the highest quality of information and accessibility. Those with aphasia ranked www.speakability.org.uk as being the most accessible site, although www.aphasiahelp.org also proved to be highly rated. Other aphasia Web sites included www.aphasiocenter.org, www.aphasiahope.org., and www.aphasia.org.

Cognition and Language

The relationship between cognition and language has been of long-standing debate in the aphasia literature. The roles of attention and memory in aphasia are intertwined with the impaired language system, making it challenging to separate their potential effects. Burgio and Basso (1997) have described long-term problems with verbal memory associated with even mild aphasia. Although memory problems were found across all of their subjects in the acute phase, some individuals showed improved performance over time with story retelling as compared to word list (paired associate) learning. These findings indicate that tasks dependent on verbal memory may not all be equal and may reflect that differing processes are at work.

Evidence suggests that some individuals with aphasia may experience problems even with tasks that involve orienting, sustaining, focusing, or dividing their attention and that these difficulties may occur with both visual and auditory input (Murray, 1999). Especially with patients who have more severe impairments and are unresponsive to auditory and/or visual input, directly addressing attentional skills may be the first avenue of treatment. A specific cognitive approach to treatment was reported by Helm-Estabrooks (1998) to meet with success. Attention and concentration activities included cancellation tasks, repeating and alternating graphomotor patterns, and trail making. Other cognitive tasks were incorporated that addressed visual memory, visuoperception, judgment, and semantic knowledge. Post-treatment testing revealed significant gains with auditory comprehension.

Advancing her claims that aphasia therapy outcomes are dependent on cognitive processes, Helm-Estabrooks (2002) cited five domains of cognition—attention, memory, executive functions, language, and visuospatial skills—as important areas to consider in developing therapeutic approaches. She designed the Cognitive Linguistic Quick Test, or CQLT, to screen for problems in cognition that potentially impact linguistic performance (Helm-Estabrooks, 2001), with findings indicating that impairments of executive functions were the cognitive skills most often associated with aphasia.

Murray (2004) posited that, because of common lesion sites, attention and working memory may be disturbed in those with aphasia and may, in fact, intensify the actual language symptoms. Successful remediation approaches have heretofore not been well documented. Although developed for the population with acquired brain injury, Attention Processing Training-11 (Sohlberg, Johnson, Paule, Raskin, & Mateer, 2001), or APT, was used by Murray, Keeton, and Karcher (2006) with a patient demonstrating long-standing conduction aphasia. The APT hierarchy did not correspond to the patient's hierarchy of task difficulty. After 50 hours of treatment, modest improvements in attention and memory scores were reported, with no changes in auditory comprehension other than improved latencies in listening to paragraphs. The patient and caregiver reported no positive changes from a functional perspective.

Baldo and colleagues (2005) explored the relationship between language and problem solving in those with normal language skills and in those with aphasia. Using the Wisconsin Card Sorting Test (Heaton, Chelune, Talley, Kay, & Curtis, 1993), or WCST, they found a consistent correlation between this measure and comprehension and naming scores in the patients with aphasia. These findings were most evident in those with Wernicke's aphasia. When the subjects with normal language skills were required to vocalize during administration of the WCST, their performance became significantly impaired. The authors hypothesized that as tasks become particularly complex, one relies on covert vocalization to aid performance. When access to "inner" speech is disrupted, a reduced working memory capacity may therefore occur. The investigators further suggested that verbal working memory is a "specialized form of covert verbalization that allows one to rehearse/maintain information online, whereas covert verbalization is a more general capacity for subvocalizing ongoing thought processes" (p. 248). Another possible explanation may be the existence of a general working memory or attentional allocation system that underlies both language and problem solving.

Auditory Processing

General Considerations

Various types of auditory processing problems occur in aphasia, including auditory imperception, pure-word deafness, and auditory agnosia. The most prominent difficulties, however, generally are associated with auditory comprehension and, consequently, have received the most attention in designing treatment strategies. In LOT, auditory processing has been divided into two major categories: Auditory Perceptual Processing Deficits, and Auditory Comprehension Deficits. Generally, auditory perceptual activities are introduced only if success cannot be attained with auditory comprehension tasks. By developing auditory perceptual skills, the patient may learn to tune into the auditory modality and prepare this mechanism for comprehension activities.

Auditory Perception

Auditory perceptual deficits are addressed in three areas:

1. Awareness of Nonspeech and Speech Stimuli
2. Recognition of Nonspeech and Speech Stimuli
3. Monitoring Speech

In establishing awareness of nonspeech and speech stimuli, the patient is required only to respond differentially, but not necessarily to demonstrate recognition of the stimuli. Environmental sounds, music, familiar and unfamiliar speakers, and foreign languages may be used. In the second area, Recognition of Nonspeech and Speech Stimuli, however, the patient must attach meaning to the stimuli presented, such as matching a telephone ring to its corresponding referent.

In the final area, Monitoring Speech, activities are incorporated to develop the patient's ability to monitor the accuracy and/or meaningfulness of speech stimuli, whether these stimuli are his or her own productions or those of others. It has been suggested that auditory comprehension may not be tied directly to monitoring skills or, at least, may not totally account for the monitoring problems encountered by patients (Marshall, Robson, Pring, & Chiat, 1998). In this account, ability to detect neologisms was purported to be affected by impaired access to the phonologic output lexicon from semantics. Following a course of treatment designed to improve semantic associations between written words and related pictures, significantly improved judgments regarding the accuracy of verbal responses were noted. This approach might be used with those patients who are able to identify clinician errors as well as errors in their own productions off-line but who persist with erroneous online judgments.

Auditory Comprehension

Treatment for auditory comprehension has been divided into five areas:

1. Comprehension of Single Units
2. Comprehension of Short Series
3. Comprehension of Short Meaningful Linguistic Units
4. Comprehension of Paragraphs
5. Comprehension of Narratives and Discourse

Comprehension of Single Units involves stimuli at the single-word level. In designing activities, some important factors related to vocabulary selection are frequency of occurrence, grammatical class, and semantic category. Depending on the type of aphasia, various hierarchies may be established through systematic alteration of both stimuli and response variables. A hierarchy for semantic word categories for three types of aphasia is illustrated in Figure 28–2 (Goodglass, Klein, Carey, & Jones, 1966; Goodglass & Wingfield, 1993). It has been proposed that auditory comprehension of visually presented stimuli may be negatively

	Broca's	Wernicke's	Anomic
Easy	Body parts	Body parts	Body parts
↓	Actions	Actions	Objects
	Objects	Objects	Actions
	Numbers	Numbers	Numbers
	Colors	Letters	Colors
	Letters	Colors	Letters
Difficult	Geometric forms	Forms	Forms

Figure 28–2. Hierarchies in difficulty levels, showing differences according to semantic categories.

impacted if the items depicted represent functionally conceived, man-made objects (e.g., furniture) rather than those that are visually conceived or based on physical properties (e.g., animals) (Goodglass, 1993). Finally, evidence from lexical decision tasks indicates that both normal controls and subjects with aphasia experience greater priming for concrete versus abstract word pairs, suggesting that abstract words may be less rich in semantic representations, thereby making them more difficult to access (Tyler, Moss, & Jennings, 1995). In addition to carefully selecting and ordering stimuli, manipulating response variables such as picture relatedness and number of response choices can increase task difficulty (Pierce, Jarecki, & Cannito, 1990).

Comprehension of Short Series might be introduced when memory variables need to be stressed, because the word series themselves do not form a syntactic unit. For example, when presenting a group of numbers, the patient must attend to each item in order to identify the series correctly. Syntactic units are incorporated in the area of Comprehension of Short Meaningful Linguistic Units, where variables such as word frequency and topic familiarity are important to consider.

Individuals with aphasia have demonstrated superior performance on language tasks, including comprehension of yes/no questions (Wallace & Canter, 1985) when personally relevant material is used. Other issues to be considered include situational context, speech rate, emotional content, and topic familiarity.

Particularly with sentences, stress as a suprasegmental cue has been found to influence performance (Goodglass, 1975, 1976; Kellar, 1978; Pashek & Brookshire, 1980). Patients with severe comprehension problems may obtain information from intonational contour to differentiate among questions, statements, and commands (Boller & Green, 1972; Green & Boller, 1974). Word frequency has been shown to affect comprehension in sentences, with common, frequently occurring vocabulary items facilitating processing.

Sentences that are longer and reflect more complex syntax tend to be more difficult (Shewan, 1979). Altering the canonicity of thematic roles (i.e., agent, theme, and goal) or

incorporating a second verb or proposition in a sentence has been shown to negatively impact comprehension in aphasia (Caplan, Waters, & Hildebrandt, 1997). Patients also may benefit from the use of context in sentence comprehension activities (Pierce, 1988). Cannito, Hough, Vogel, and Pierce (1996) found that patients in the post-acute phase (5 weeks to 6 months) of their recovery experienced a facilitative effect in processing reversible passive sentences when they followed a paragraph of a predictive nature. Patients in the chronic stages of recovery (>6 months) benefited equally from both predictive and non-predictive paragraphs preceding sentence presentation. Repetition of key lexical items in the paragraph was believed to reduce the semantic processing load for the target sentences so that more resources could be assigned to understanding the relationships between the nouns. Decreased verbal memory span also was associated with those who were able to make the best use of context. With these findings in mind, sentence comprehension activities might incorporate a hierarchy of sentence types in concert with a presentation of predictive and non-predictive paragraphs, teaching the patient to recognize salient or redundant cues in the narratives and then use them to assist with sentence processing.

Although sentence comprehension is influenced by word frequency and syntactic complexity, these variables have less impact on discourse processing (Nicholas & Brookshire, 1995b). In addition, a weak link between comprehension of individual sentences and comprehension of discourse has been offered. In analyzing discourse, comprehension has been shown to be superior for main ideas as compared to details, and directly stated information is recalled with greater accuracy than implied information, by both normal subjects and those with aphasia.

Pierce and Grogan (1992) describe a number of factors that normally are involved in narrative comprehension. Briefly, they identify the microstructure (words and their relationship to the text) and macrostructure (gist) as the two major text components. Bringing one's own formulation of goals, expectations, and previous experience to the interpretation of the narrative forms a schema. Schemas will vary among individuals, and the macrostructure that is formed is influenced by situational variables (e.g., listening to a news broadcast versus a classroom lecture). Finally, the authors point out that while a text base (meaning of the narrative) is being developed, the listener brings his or her own knowledge and opinions to the topic, which assists with inferencing. In aphasia, it is suggested that with greater coherence or a strong relationship between propositions, comprehension and retention are facilitated. Knowledge about the topic increases inferencing, coherence, and ultimately, comprehension. Less cohesive narratives may be better understood by providing a topic theme. Alternatively, using narratives with several topic changes can facilitate recall of details.

Some patients may experience difficulty in comprehending referents from contextual information (Chapman & Ulatowska, 1989) and may benefit from specific instruction for processing them. More errors in recalling details of high-ratio dialogues (i.e., ones in which the amount of speaking between the participants is significantly disproportionate) also have been noted. Finally, mode of presentation may affect performance such that audiotape, videotape, and live presentations can have varying impacts, depending on the individual.

When addressing Comprehension of Paragraphs and Comprehension of Narratives and Discourse, many of the above variables can be manipulated to form individualized hierarchies depending on the nature and degree of the impairment. Identification of the gist, main ideas, and details in narratives of increasing length and decreasing personal relevance could be considered. Other tasks might include those directed at improving inferencing skills by capitalizing on the patient's knowledge of scripts and developing awareness and use of contextual cues. Altering the amount of cohesion and/or redundancy within narratives and discourse could be additional factors to control while varying the response requirements.

Case Example

SK is a 24-year-old, male university student. Following excision of a left temporo-occipital arteriovenous malformation, he demonstrated fluent aphasia characterized by moderate anomia, auditory and visual processing problems, and mild agraphia. Formalized testing included administration of the Boston Diagnostic Aphasia Evaluation, the Auditory Comprehension Test for Sentences, the Revised Token Test, and the Boston Naming Test.

Auditory comprehension problems were initially found in SK's comprehension of material at the paragraph level and in his processing of linguistically complex, lengthy instructions. The first treatment area selected was comprehension of paragraphs. Further probing revealed that SK experienced increased difficulty when required to make inferences and when the number of facts included within a paragraph was substantially increased.

For the first level of difficulty, the clinician aurally provided short paragraphs consisting of a high degree of redundancy, with SK required to answer inferential questions. When a 70% success rate was achieved at this level, more facts were included in the paragraphs to increase difficulty. As treatment progressed, difficulty levels were further adjusted by altering topic familiarity. More complex responses on the part of the patient were gradually required so that, before questioning by the clinician, SK was asked to recall as many details as possible from the paragraph. Further information was then extracted through use of either factual or inferential questions.

Comprehension of Narratives and Discourse was next developed. Short radio broadcasts were presented, followed by videotaped news segments and lengthier documentaries. Task difficulty was again altered by increasing the complexity of the response and varying the degree of topic familiarity.

SK was an active participant in developing treatment goals and hierarchies. He provided detailed feedback regarding the variables that he found affected his performance and reported on written spelling. SK returned to university to complete his Master's degree.

Sample Activities

Level 1
Stimuli: Paragraphs 60 to 80 syllables in length, high degree of redundancy, and high degree of topic familiarity.
Procedure: The paragraph is read aloud by the clinician, followed by inferential questions requiring a yes/no response.

Level 2
Stimuli: Paragraphs 60 to 80 syllables in length, low degree of redundancy, and high degree of topic familiarity.
Procedure: The paragraph is read aloud by the clinician, followed by inferential questions requiring a yes/no response.

Level 3
Stimuli: Paragraphs 60 to 80 syllables in length, low degree of redundancy, and low degree of topic familiarity.
Procedure: The paragraph is read aloud by the clinician, followed by inferential questions requiring a yes/no response.

Visual Processing

General Considerations

Visual processing refers to the processing of information presented in pictorial, gestural, and/or written forms. As with the auditory modality, this area can be subdivided into visual perception and reading comprehension. Patients with aphasia demonstrate reading impairments of varying degrees. Those with the most severe language impairments can experience limitations with visual recognition such that even matching objects, drawings, forms, colors, letters, and words may be compromised. Visual acuity and field deficits also can affect performance, resulting in problems with visual attention, scanning, and tracking.

Inability to comprehend written material because of brain damage is referred to as alexia. When applied to those with aphasia, this term is used only when particular patterns are observed. Alexia without agraphia, or pure alexia, consists of reading problems with preserved writing. Patients may have difficulty recognizing words, although identification of high-frequency vocabulary and letters may be superior. Reading usually is accomplished using a letter-by-letter approach, making longer words more difficult to decode because of memory load (Goodglass, 1993). Comprehension of oral spelling typically is intact, and words traced in the palm of the hand or palpated often can be recognized. Although no accompanying agraphia is present, the patient is unable to read his or her own writing. Both color naming and color name recognition can be impaired.

Alexia with agraphia is characterized by a severe reading impairment, often along with problems in reading musical notes and numbers, and a calculation deficit. Those affected are unable to recognize orally spelled words and to spell words aloud. Tracing or palpating letters is not facilitative (Lecours, 1999). Marked writing problems usually are found in conjunction with a right homonymous hemianopsia.

Although the area of Oral Reading was initially included under the Oral Expression modality, it will be addressed here for ease of description and application. Three disorders of oral reading have been described because of their unique pattern of errors (Goodglass, 1993; Webb & Love, 1994). The most salient feature of deep dyslexia is substitution of semantically related words bearing no structural or phonologic similarity to the targets, with functor words typically being substituted or omitted. From easiest to most difficult to read are nouns, verbs, and adjectives. Failure to read pseudo-words also is encountered. Some consider deep dyslexia to be a variant of phonologic alexia (Friedman, 1995), which is characterized by disruption in applying grapheme-to-phoneme correspondence rules to enable the reading of pseudo-words. Errors involving visually similar words may be encountered.

Various patterns of symptoms have been associated with surface dyslexia. Commonalities reflect impairments in effectively accessing semantics and whole-word phonology along with an overuse and faulty application of phoneme-to-grapheme conversion rules.

Another reported syndrome, although rare, is visual agnosia. Patients experience difficulty recognizing material presented visually (Benson & Geschwind, 1969; Eisenson, 1984), but presentation of stimuli through another modality (e.g., touch and hearing) can meet with success. Breakdown occurs for both verbal and nonverbal material.

More current approaches in studying reading impairments in aphasia tend to focus on construction of a model for reading that details the effects of breakdowns at the various levels or stages of processing. Hillis, Kane, Barker, Beauchamp, and Wityk (2001) identified the processes that most researchers agree are involved in reading. Briefly summarized, the orthographic input lexicon (OIL) is accessed when irregularly spelled vocabulary is introduced. The meaning of a word is derived from the lexical-semantic level, which is activated by the OIL. Once the lexical-semantic level is sufficiently activated, it in turn provides input to the phonological output lexicon if reading aloud of irregularly spelled vocabulary is required. Orthography-to-phonology conversion (OPC) is responsible for one's ability to read aloud pseudo-words or regularly spelled vocabulary, which do not need to rely on meaning or activation of OIL. The final stage, which is activated for all spoken tasks, involves motor planning and articulation.

In attempting to determine the neural correlates of reading, Hillis and colleagues (2001) assessed hypoperfusion of cortical areas in patients during the hyperacute stages of stroke. They determined that some regions were responsible for more than one component of the reading system, whereas some individual components were associated with more than one cortical area. Disruption of OPC and OIL mechanisms were associated with hypoperfusion of the angular gyrus, although access to the OIL also was negatively impacted by hypoperfusion of the posterior middle temporal gyrus. Lexical-semantic impairments were noted in four areas: the left angular and supramarginal gyri and middle temporal gyrus, with the most important role being played by Wernicke's area.

Hillis and colleagues (2005) later studied the contribution of the visual word form area, or the left midfusiform gyrus (BA 37), to reading because of its known consistent activation during reading tasks. Hypoperfusion of BA 37 was associated with impairments in oral and written naming, whereas difficulty with word comprehension was related to hypoperfusion in the left posterior, superotemporal, and angular gyri. The investigators hypothesized that both the right and left midfusiform gyri play roles, although only one is essential, in the prelexical activity of forming a representation of a sequence of graphemes, called the "graphemic description" (p. 554). The left angular gyrus relies on stored knowledge for OPC, with the modality-independent lexical representations required for output being subsumed by BA 37. A cortical network, involving frontal, temporal, parietal, and occipital cortices, was considered to be essential for various aspects of reading, depending on factors such as spelling regularity, word familiarity, rate of presentation, and level of an individual's reading skills.

Berndt, Haendiges, and Mitchum (2005) summarized the reading impairments of left dominant hemisphere individuals to be caused by impairment of a possible lack of availability of grapheme-to-sound conversion, reducing sublexical activation, which in turn impacts formulation of the abstract sequential code for graphemes required for accessing the graphemic lexicon. These investigators found that more than half of the errors in oral reading consisted of word substitutions, and the majority of these items were visually similar to their targets. Although some individual variation was noted, letter errors increased from the beginnings to the ends of words. Because subjects without neurologic impairment demonstrate faster reaction times in naming words that have several orthographic neighbors, the authors contend that a tendency exists for those with left hemisphere dysfunction to substitute their targets with words that have letter overlap in the early part of the word. This hypothesis was supported by earlier work (Whitney & Berndt, 1999) demonstrating that, in reading, activation levels are highest at the beginning of a word, followed by a gradual decline because of the activation of subsequent letters and then an increase at the final letter position because no additional letters follow.

Under normal conditions, processing of single words, sentences, and narratives reflects changes in neural circuitry (Xu, Kemeny, Park, Fratali, & Braun, 2005). In narrative processing, the left hemisphere activations have been found to be stronger, with involvement of the temporal, parietal, and opercular areas at the beginning of a story. These regions are deemed to be implicated in the processing of the factual aspects of a narrative, such as setting, characters, and time. The right hemisphere activations are heightened toward the ends of the narratives, when information is being synthesized and conclusions are being drawn. Others have examined "theory of mind," or the ability to understand the behavior of others based on interpretation of, for example, feelings, intent, and motivation (Fletcher et al., 1995). Activation has been found bilaterally in the temporal poles, in the left superior temporal gyrus and the posterior cingulate cortex, during narrative processing tasks. The theory of mind tasks, however, implicated the left medial frontal gyrus, with further analysis revealing that more complex social interactions were found in those stories.

Many factors, such as the individual's educational level, occupation, and avocational interests, are considered in determining the extent to which the visual modality is addressed during treatment. In addition, with patients demonstrating severe impairments, this modality may be better preserved than others (Helm & Barresi, 1980; Helm-Estabrooks, 1983) and can serve as an appropriate entry point in treatment.

Visual Perception

Treatment of visual processing is divided into six areas. Three of these areas fall under the category of visual perception, with the first specifically addressing visual perceptual deficits.

Area 1, Matching Nonverbal Material, requires the patient to match objects, pictures, and geometric forms. In developing a hierarchy of difficulty, picture complexity and degree of stylization can be adjusted (in addition to altering the stimulus category). The task may then be made more difficult by requiring category recognition.

Area 2 incorporates Matching of Verbal Material, such as numbers, letters, and words. Individual hierarchies are established considering variables of length, visual similarity, and size of the stimuli. To tax attention and memory, a series of these items may be introduced.

Area 3, Visual Correspondence/Recognition, demands that the patient recognize different visual forms of the same stimulus. For example, the task may require matching a printed word to a corresponding object, or matching trademarks to referents. Other activities in this area might attempt to strengthen semantic activation through having the patient make decisions about subordinate–superordinate relationships. Individuals with aphasia may experience even more difficulty in performing categorization tasks that involve functional relationships (e.g., things that write) as opposed to those consisting of superordinate relations (McCleary & Hirst, 1986).

Visual Comprehension

Two areas for treatment of visual processing fall under the category of visual comprehension. Area 4 focuses on Reception of Gestured Messages. Although gesture recognition may be a less impaired modality (Porch, 1967), patients with aphasia, as a group, tend to perform more poorly in interpreting pantomimes than do those with normal language abilities. A strong relationship has been found between gesture recognition and the ability of the person with aphasia to imitate non-meaningful movements (Wang & Goodglass, 1992). Pantomime recognition and production are correlated with each other and with auditory comprehension, but not with a global measure of aphasia.

One hierarchy that has been suggested for developing comprehension of gestures, in increasing order of difficulty, is associating object, action picture, object picture, and line drawing to corresponding gestures (Daniloff, Noll, Fristoe, & Lloyd, 1982; Netsu & Marguardt, 1984). Typically, this area would be developed in the context of preparing a patient for a gestural production system. Additional detail will therefore follow in discussion of the Gestural and Gestural-Verbal Communication modality.

Recognition of Spelling is addressed in Area 5. Tasks may involve proofreading activities that include presentation of the patient's written production or those of others for correction. This activity might be considered a form of monitoring for those who rely heavily on written communication. Also, individuals with surface dyslexia may benefit from sentence judgment tasks requiring homophone recognition (e.g., *We took our/hour car*) (Scott & Byng, 1989).

Reading Comprehension

In the final area for treatment of visual processing, or Area 6, Reading Comprehension activities are initiated in which stimuli may consist of single words, phrases, sentences, or paragraphs. Treatment of single-word reading deficits has received the most attention in the literature and will be addressed in greater detail. Many treatment methods have been designed for those who demonstrate features of pure alexia or letter-by-letter reading. Investigators tend to agree that the deficits found in pure alexia are associated with prelexical problems and, typically, intact lexical-orthographic and phonologic knowledge (Arguin & Bub, 1994; Coslett, Saffran, Greenbaum, & Schwartz, 1993). It has been hypothesized that the encoding of printed words is forced to be accomplished by the right hemisphere, which is unable to encode individual letters and has limited ability to process low-imageability words, morphemes, and functors (Burbaum & Coslett, 1996). This, in turn, forces the patient to analyze individual letters rather than using a more holistic approach in reading words. Additionally, more difficulty in reading lowercase as compared to uppercase letters may be encountered. One therapeutic approach (Arguin & Bub, 1994) addressed what those authors posited as being the underlying problem of pure alexia, the failure of the patient to encode abstract letter types. Uppercase and lowercase letters of varying fonts were used in matching tasks, followed by speeded reading of pronounceable four-letter strings consisting of uppercase letters and a font resembling script. Improvements were reported for matching tasks, in addition to increased speed and accuracy of reading letter strings.

Another method in treating pure alexia has been to capitalize on the tactile-kinesthetic feedback that the patient may be able to use (Lott, Friedman, & Linebaugh, 1994). A treatment hierarchy was established, starting with copying sets of individual letters in a uniform way, first, in the palm of the hand, followed by naming of the target and then presentation of cards with printed words for copying and oral production. Reading of both trained and untrained word lists improved with this therapy.

Beeson and colleagues (2003) examined the natural recovery and treatment response of a letter-by-letter reader through implementation of a program involving multiple oral reading trails (Moyer, 1979) to improve the reading rate of text. Treatment was not initiated until 22 weeks poststroke, although performance was monitored before this time to assess changes as a result of spontaneous recovery. Spontaneous recovery of letter naming and single-word reading accuracy did occur, with a slow reading rate of text persisting until the initiation of therapy. The improvement in reading rate after treatment was threefold greater than the gains made during the period (1–3 months) associated with the most significant improvements resulting from spontaneous recovery (Robey et al., 1998). By week 54, the length effect in reading single words was no longer present. Although reading rate continued to be slow, the patient reported being able to once again read for pleasure.

An errorless learning approach has been applied to treating letter-by-letter reading (Sage, Hesketh, & Ralph, 2005).

Errors in reading words of increased length and reduced familiarity were described in a patient with some preserved ability to make semantic judgments of concrete words. The first treatment method was designed to facilitate whole-word reading by having the patient listen to production of a word along with simultaneous visual presentation of its printed form. Repetition of the word was then required until the word was read spontaneously with 80% accuracy. Tactile and visual cues were introduced later to assist in meeting the criterion. At the end of 7 weeks, significant improvement in reading of the trained set occurred, with no generalization to the control items. The second treatment method was implemented in an attempt to improve the accuracy and speed of the patient's letter-by-letter reading. The instructor identified the individual letters of printed words while tracing them in the subject's hand. Gradually, support was withdrawn, with independent oral reading then being required. At the end of 7 weeks, improvements in both the trained and untrained word sets were realized. Although an overall decrease occurred in the number of errors after the implementation of both methods, the investigators noted that the patient's reading pattern evolved to resemble that of deep dyslexia, with an increase in semantic and visual errors. Specific treatment techniques also have been applied to the problems associated with surface dyslexia (Nickels, 1995). In surface dyslexia, in which the impairment is believed to occur at the lexical level, pairing words with mnemonic aids such as pictures improved oral reading of irregularly spelled words, using a whole-word approach, with generalization to untrained items. Another patient was provided with sentence completion tasks involving homophone selection to establish the route from the visual input lexicon to the semantic system. Improvements were particularly evident with treated homophones and, to a lesser extent, with those that were untreated.

Individuals with deep dyslexia are impaired in using grapheme-to-phoneme correspondence rules and in using the whole-word reading route (orthographic input to phonologic output lexicons) and must access the semantic route for reading. Closed class words and pseudo-words are read more poorly than open class words, but semantic value does not appear to be the sole contributing factor (Siverberg, Vigliocco, Insaluco, & Garrett, 1998). Greater accuracy in oral reading was found when comparing list to text forms of presentation, particularly for closed class words. Bound class morphemes were read more accurately than free class morphemes, especially in the list format, although again, both benefited from text presentation. Those authors suggested that treatment emphasizing reading in context might be more advantageous than single-word reading or the training of phoneme-to-grapheme correspondence rules. Teaching grapheme-to-phoneme correspondence rules, however, has been used successfully in some patients with deep dyslexia. Patients were taught to link letters of the alphabet with specific words that they had selected and then to sound out letters of simple words and nonwords using these established associations (Nickels, 1995).

Stadie and Rilling (2006) compared two forms of treatment for deep dyslexia in a single case study. The first treatment applied was lexically based, with the underlying premise being that greater activation of the target word could be achieved by priming, with presentation of semantically and/or phonologically related words. Prime words were presented on a computer screen, followed by their targets. Feedback and additional cues were provided as needed. After 10 sessions, reading accuracy for trained items had significantly improved, although generalization to untrained vocabulary did not occur. The investigators did note that a part of speech effect no longer was apparent following therapy. The second phase of treatment was non-lexical, teaching grapheme-phoneme correspondence rules by initially pairing graphemes with specific words selected by the patient. Following 19 sessions, reading significantly improved from pre-treatment measures for both trained and untrained vocabulary. Particular gains were found in the reading of content words. Because lexical and sublexical reading processes overlapped in time course, the authors speculated that a combined lexical and non-lexical approach might prove to be the most beneficial.

From the foregoing descriptions of treatment approaches for some of the more clearly defined and studied forms of alexia, efforts have been made to associate the symptomatology with a breakdown in one or more aspects of a model for processing written words. Treatment hierarchies can then be established by altering vocabulary and contextual variables that are known to play specific roles in each of these disorders based on site of lesion. When phrases and sentences are introduced, other factors such as syntax and number of content words relevant to length may be considered. Similar to performance in listening, patients benefit from the presentation of predictive and non-predictive preceding paragraphs to facilitate comprehension of at least certain complex sentence forms (Germani & Pierce, 1992). Altering the degree of redundancy and amount of context can be used in developing a hierarchy for treating various sentence types.

At the paragraph level, overall length can be systematically adjusted while varying individual sentence length, complexity, vocabulary difficulty, and thematic content. In developing or selecting paragraphs, one strives for high passage dependency, which reflects the degree to which accurate responses to questions about the paragraph are dependent on having read the paragraph and not on previous knowledge (Thomas & Jackson, 1997). Other issues affecting passage dependency are the relatedness of the test questions to each other and the plausibility of the answers given a multiple-choice sentence format. Questions involving little known facts and those requiring more detailed answers would be

harder to answer without having read the paragraph on which they are based. It is suggested that if the patient is able to answer less than half the questions without having read the paragraph, higher passage dependency is indicated.

Area 7 completes this modality with Reading Textual Material. As empirical data are limited, individual hierarchies must be developed considering variables such as overall length, vocabulary, redundancy, grammatical complexity, amount of cohesion, use of anaphoric reference, and familiarity (Shewan & Bandur, 1986).

As well, many of the factors outlined in auditory comprehension of narratives and discourse could be applied to and incorporated in this section.

Case Example

NH is a 69-year-old homemaker who suffered from multiple strokes resulting in left frontal and right parietal occipital lobe infarcts. Administration of the Western Aphasia Battery, or WAB, and of the Auditory Comprehension Test for Sentences and the Boston Naming Test revealed a mild auditory processing problem, a mild verbal dyspraxia, anomia, and moderate visual processing and graphic expression difficulties. Because the patient reported being an avid reader up until the time of her most recent stroke, visual processing activities were introduced simultaneously with activities from other modalities.

Language testing suggested good single-word reading comprehension and ability to read short, simple paragraphs. Additional probing demonstrated reading comprehension to be compromised above a Grade 3 readability level. Degree of abstractness also significantly affected performance. The first difficulty level involved presentation of short paragraphs with a readability level of Grade 3 to Grade 4. The patient was required to read the paragraphs and to reformulate them orally using printed who, what, when, where, and why/how prompts. Once NH was successful in recounting the significant points from the paragraphs at this level, the same length of paragraph was used, but the grade level was increased to Grade 5. Over time, paragraph length, abstractness, and grade level were systematically increased. Newspaper articles and short stories were gradually introduced, with the patient eventually reporting success in reading romance novels for enjoyment.

Sample Activities

Level 1

Stimuli: Paragraphs 75 to 100 syllables in length, Grade 3 to Grade 4 readability, and printed who, what, when, where, and why/how cards.

Procedure: The patient reads the paragraph and orally responds to who, what, when, where, and why/how prompts.

Level 2

Stimuli: Paragraphs 75 to 100 syllables in length, Grade 5 readability, and printed who, what, when, where, and why/how prompts.

Procedure: The patient reads the paragraph and orally responds to who, what, when, where, and why/how prompts.

Level 3

Stimuli: Paragraphs 75 to 100 syllables in length, Grade 5 readability, and no printed cues.

Procedure: The patient reads the paragraph and orally provides the relevant information.

Gestural and Gestural-Verbal Communication

General Considerations

Gestural production may prove to be an alternative mode of communication for some patients with severe aphasic impairments or may be used to augment verbal expression attempts. For others, this modality may serve as a starting point in treatment, with gradual transition to oral expression activities.

As noted in the previous section, the gestural modality tends to be less affected than others in aphasia (Porch, 1967), although individuals with more severe impairments have been shown to use fewer complex gestural forms spontaneously in their communication attempts, with gestures becoming nonspecific and unclear (Glosser, Wiener, & Kaplan, 1986). As a group, patients with severe aphasia communicate more often and for longer periods of time through nonverbal means than their communication partners (Herrmann, Reichle, Lucius-Hoene, Wallesch, & Johannsen-Horbach, 1988). Pantomime production is reportedly infrequent, but at least in untrained users, a greater use of codified gestures has been observed, suggesting, perhaps, that they require less creativity and praxis skills. Wang and Goodglass (1992) found a strong correlation between auditory comprehension skills and measures of pantomime recognition and expression. Pantomime performance also was strongly linked to the ability to produce meaningless gestures on imitation. Duffy, Watt, and Duffy (1994) have proposed that both language and neurophysiologic motor and visual processing disorders are tied to pantomime deficits.

Individuals with significant language limitations may be able to acquire some single signs, and patients with less involvement may, perhaps, be capable of acquiring and generalizing simple grammars (Coelho, 1990). Ability to generalize signs has been inversely related to severity of aphasia (Coelho & Duffy, 1987). Aphasia severity may, in fact, be the most significant determinant of successful sign use (Coelho & Duffy, 1986). Some positive effects on the reception and production of gestures through pantomime training have been described (Schlanger & Freemann, 1979). The American-Indian (Amer-Ind) Sign System (Skelly, 1979) has been used with varying reports of success. Rao (1994) has suggested that possible prognostic indicators for success with Amer-Ind code include good pantomime recognition and that limb apraxia is not severe and predominantly ideomotor rather than ideational in nature. Rose and Douglas (2003) studied the relationship between limb apraxia and gestural use in seven patients with nonfluent aphasia, all of whom had demonstrated a limb apraxia on formalized testing. Conversational samples were elicited and analyzed for the presence of gestures. Despite the presence of an identified limb apraxia on test measures, the patients demonstrated several instances of gestural use to supplement or replace their oral speech attempts. These investigators concluded that the highly conscious nature of the testing, requiring abstract thought, in addition to the removal of meaningful context negatively impacted the patients' performance on those measures. They suggested that gestural training and/or enhancement might best be targeted in naturalistic settings, capitalizing on opportunities to provide reinforcement, modeling, and shaping of behaviors.

Finally, use of gestures can facilitate oral speech production for some patients by serving as a cue for word retrieval or by adding greater descriptive value to verbal output. Individuals may not automatically use this strategy, so specific instruction and coaching may be required for it to be successfully incorporated into communication exchanges.

Social Signals

Area 1 of gestural and gestural-verbal communication, Attention, is an elementary step in gestural communication. The patient learns to obtain the attention of a communication partner through eye contact, touch, vocalization, gesture, or a combination of these.

With Area 2, Acknowledgment of the Message Received, some form of gesture, such as a head nod, is developed to indicate that a message has been received, although not necessarily understood.

Gestures

Single gestures and combinations of gestures are used in Area 3, Gestural Communication. Some investigators have found propositional gestures to be more difficult to acquire than nonpropositional ones (Buck & Duffy, 1980). A possible hierarchy might consist of appropriate facial expressions, conventional gestures, and propositional gestures.

Successful outcomes have been described with Visual Action Therapy, or VAT, in improving both apraxia and gestural communication abilities (Helm-Estabrooks, Fitzpatrick, & Barresi, 1982). In this nonvocal, visual/gestural program, a hierarchy of activities, ranging from tasks such as requiring the patient to match objects and pictures to gesturing the use of items hidden from view, is used. Modifications to VAT were based on the finding that patients experience less difficulty using gestures representing objects involving proximal movements compared with those involving distal movements (Helm-Estabrooks, Ramsberger, Brownell, & Albert, 1989). With patients demonstrating severe language problems, VAT may serve as the initial phase in treatment, advancing to implementation of Amer-Ind code training.

Communicative importance or personal relevance is one factor that may affect the ease of sign acquisition (Coelho & Duffy, 1986). Patients also have a tendency to experience less difficulty in learning signs that have a high degree of iconicity—that is, those for which the meaning is evident based on their physical or structural characteristics (Coelho & Duffy, 1986). Other important variables to consider are the stimuli selected to teach the gestures. Objects and action pictures have been found to evoke superior gestural performance to line drawings (Netsu & Marguardt, 1984).

A treatment hierarchy has been described by Rao (1994) for training patients with aphasia in the use of Amer-Ind code. It consists of a continuum of tasks: demonstration, recognition, imitation, replication, consolidation, retrieval, and initiation. Additional strategies to ensure generalization include involving significant others in the program and encouraging some risk taking on the part of the patient.

Speech Acts

Area 4, Simple Speech Acts, incorporates both message content (proposition) and intent of the speaker (elocutionary force). Elocutionary force is communicated with gestures and/or vocalization to signal a command, statement, or question. Simple pointing gestures may be used to communicate content, such as indicating the action, agent, or object. Area 5, Speech Acts, includes a combination of verbal and nonverbal communication. Gestures continue, however, to carry the burden of communication, although some verbalization may be produced.

Case Example

AG is a 62-year-old, retired political consultant who suffered a stroke, with a large left middle cerebral artery infarct, resulting in global aphasia and a right hemiplegia. Initially, the Boston Assessment of Severe Aphasia was administered. Relative strengths were found in the areas of oral-gestural expression, gesture recognition, and visuospatial tasks. Various treatment strategies were used to develop oral expression skills, including VAT and Melodic Intonation Therapy as well as LOT naming and sentence formulation activities. Functional oral communication skills, however, remained severely limited.

The Amer-Ind Sign System (Skelly, 1979) was next introduced. Because this treatment approach focuses on new learning as opposed to stimulation of previously learned material, a strict LOT paradigm could not apply. Ten common agents and actions were chosen for training. Initially, the clinician provided a gesture along with an array of four action pictures from which the patient was to select the one associated with the gesture. Once recognition was established, AG was required to produce the gesture in response to an action picture. In the next phase of treatment, situations were simulated in which AG provided the gesture in the absence of the action picture.

The subsequent difficulty level involved encouraging the use of trained gestures in conversational attempts. AG consistently progressed through his treatment program, successfully producing gestures that had not even been trained. Continuous encouragement and counseling were needed, however, because AG was reluctant to use gestural communication as a substitute for oral speech, even several months poststroke.

Sample Activities

Level 1
Stimuli: Ten pictured actions, along with 20 foils.
Procedure: The clinician presents an array of four pictures to the patient and produces a gesture corresponding to one of the actions depicted. The patient points to the appropriate picture.

Level 2
Stimuli: The 10 action pictures used in Level 1 for identification.
Procedure: The pictures are presented one at a time, and the patient is required to produce the associated gesture.

Level 3
Stimuli: The 10 action pictures used in Levels 1 and 2.
Procedure: A sentence or brief story is aurally presented, and the patient is required to complete the sentence with the appropriate gesture (e.g., *When you are hungry, you*).

Oral Expression

General Considerations

Oral expression problems vary with respect to both nature and severity in aphasia. Although oral expression patterns differ among types of aphasia, many patients share common impairments. Problems may be encountered with highly overlearned or automatic speech, phonologic articulatory skills, repetition, oral reading, naming, sentence formulation, and discourse planning/production. Because these areas are not mutually exclusive, limitations involving one area may directly affect another. Treatment therefore may simultaneously incorporate two or more areas. In developing a therapeutic plan, the areas of deficit, along with their nature and severity, are carefully examined.

Automatic Speech

Area 1 of Oral Expression addresses development of Automatic Speech Series. Activities are designed to facilitate oral speech in those patients with very limited verbal output. Stimuli such as greetings, number sequences, poems, days of the week, months of the year, and letters of the alphabet may be incorporated.

Voluntary Control of Involuntary Utterances, or VCIU, is a treatment approach designed for patients with nonfluent aphasia that attempts to use their stereotypic expressions as a step to develop meaningful propositional speech (Helm & Barresi, 1980). It incorporates a progression through oral reading, confrontation naming, and conversation involving production of the stereotypic words and phrases.

Phonological-Articulatory Production

Misarticulations that occur with aphasia may be the result of phonological problems, articulatory problems, or a combination of both. Phonologic-articulatory impairment resulting from an anterior left hemisphere lesion, in and surrounding Broca's area, most often is termed verbal dyspraxia. Posterior left hemisphere lesions also may result in sound production errors, generally in the form of literal or phonemic paraphasias.

Language-Oriented Treatment activities in Area 2, Phonologic-Articulatory Production, are based on Shewan's (1980) Content Network for treating verbal dyspraxia. Separate hierarchies for presentation method, stimulus characteristics, type of response, and facilitation of response variables have been constructed according to difficulty levels. These hierarchies are based on data provided by a variety of researchers. A step-by-step progression toward the goal of achieving spontaneous production of propositional speech is used, as the patient can accommodate. Support provided by the clinician is gradually reduced to ensure that the patient develops more independence in oral speech.

In selecting treatment stimuli, several variables may be critical. At the phoneme level, vowels are easier to produce than consonants, and highly frequent consonants are less difficult than those of low frequency. Distinctive feature characteristics also play a role in ease of production, with nasality and voicing features being less problematic than manner and place. In phoneme selection, the clinician therefore can establish a hierarchy incorporating all of these parameters.

When introducing single words, performance is influenced positively by concrete, functional words. Additional variables that may be important to control are word fre-quency and length. Howard and Smith (2002) examined a group of 12 individuals with aphasia who demonstrated phonologic errors in repetition. They found that two-syllable words with word final stress were most likely to be impaired in both repetition and naming tasks. When they did occur, errors were significantly more frequent on production of the second syllable. In repetition, the majority of errors of stress assignment were produced on words with weak-strong stress patterns. In both picture naming and repetition, three-syllable words with primary stress on the second syllable were the most affected. In conclusion, those authors found that weak-stress and weak-strong-weak patterns were less likely to be produced correctly. They hypothesized that stress-related errors are related to problems with phonologic assembly when stress does not automatically occur on the first syllable.

Beyond single words, phrase/sentence length, stress pattern, and linguistic complexity may be systematically varied to increase the difficulty levels in treatment. Differing presentation methods also can be incorporated into a hierarchy. Combined auditory-visual presentation may facilitate correct speech production more easily than either auditory or visual presentation in isolation.

The clinician may alter the type of response required, such as production following a model, unison production, or production requiring a number of consecutive responses. Facilitating response variables can be manipulated to elicit more accurate productions. For example, associated movements, such as finger tapping, may accompany speech. Inserting a schwa (/ə/) between consonants in a cluster may enhance performance. Facilitating responses may be used temporarily by some and be required as long-term strategies by others.

As the patient advances within the treatment hierarchy, additional response complexity can be required while maintaining the presentation method, stimuli, and facilitating response variables constant. More spontaneous productions are incorporated, with the clinician gradually withdrawing assistance.

Repetition

Although the ability to repeat is not an end goal in treatment, this skill is described in Area 3, to facilitate performance of other related speech-language behaviors. For example, repetition tasks may be used in treating verbal dyspraxia and play an important component of Melodic Intonation Therapy, which consists of a hierarchy of three levels in which multisyllabic words and short, high-probability phrases are musically intoned, followed by longer, phonologically complex sentences (Sparks, Helm, & Albert, cited in Helm-Estabrooks & Albert, 1991).

When preparing stimuli for repetition activities, many factors can influence performance. Single-word repetition is affected by phonologic complexity, frequency of occurrence, semantic class, and if the stimulus is a foreign or pseudo-word (Ramsberger, 1996). When abstractness and frequency are controlled, repetition of emotional words is superior to that of nonemotional vocabulary. High probability (Goodglass & Kaplan, 1972, 1983) and personally relevant material (Wallace & Canter, 1985) are easier to repeat, as are shorter items (Gardner & Winner, 1978). When sentence-level material is introduced, a hierarchy that varies sentence forms (Goodglass 1968, 1976) can be used, because patients demonstrate repetition difficulty with increasing syntactic complexity.

Response variables can affect accuracy and/or ease of production. For some individuals, use of a delay before initiation of a response can facilitate performance, although for others, this strategy may have a negative impact (Gardner & Winner, 1978). It therefore is important for the clinician to determine the direction of this effect before its implementation in treatment.

Oral Reading and Spelling

Area 4, Oral Reading, most often is used as a vehicle for treating other aspects of speech-language skills, as Area 3 is. Improvements in language functioning, such as reading comprehension, oral expression, auditory comprehension, and written expression, have been described (Cherney, Merbitz, & Grip, 1986; Tuomainen & Laine, 1991). Oral reading of sentences and paragraphs, whether in unison and independently, has resulted in improved language skills in those with fluent and those with nonfluent aphasia. Presentation of scrambled written sentences for oral reading can be used with patients who may demonstrate impulsive responding and poor self-monitoring skills. They can be required to point to each word in the sentence while reading aloud, with sentences being systematically adjusted for length and syntactic complexity.

Some forms of dyslexia have been characterized by differences in oral reading performance. These were described in detail in the discussion of the Visual Processing modality, within the area of Reading Comprehension. Area 5, Oral Spelling, may be used as an activity to enhance written spelling skills and be practiced as a strategy for word retrieval with some patients.

Word Retrieval

Word-finding problems are associated with all types of aphasia and also may occur in patients with non-aphasic disorders. Anomic aphasia has been associated with lesions outside the perisylvian region in the anterior or inferior temporal regions. For example, Damasio, Tranel, Grabowski, Adolphs, and Damasio (2004) examined the naming of specific categories in individuals with brain damage. In their investigations, errors in naming unique persons were associated with lesions primarily in the left temporal pole; errors in naming of animals with lesions in the left anteroinferior temporal lobe, anterior insula, and dorsal temporo-occipital junction; and errors in naming of tools in the posterolateral temporo-occipito-parietal junction. These investigators proposed that although the perisylvian structures are involved in the transient reconstruction and explicit phonemic representation of word forms, additional neural sites mediate between those that support conceptual knowledge and the perisylvian structures, triggering and conducting the process of reconstruction. They claimed that no single mediational site exists for words but, rather, that separable regions exist within a large network, which would preferentially assist in the processing of words denoting varied kinds of entities (e.g., unique persons).

Having an appreciation for a model of lexical processing and formulating hypotheses regarding the cause of word retrieval symptoms in a given patient can lead to the design of individualized treatment procedures. Responses can be analyzed more effectively; not only enabling the clinician to successively respond online but also, with explanation, enabling the patient to develop a greater understanding of how and when errors may be generated.

The generally agreed-on cognitive processes involved in single-word production are semantic or meaning-based, involving word selection to convey a concept, and phonologic, which is used to access phonemes (Goldrick & Rapp, 2002). Researchers disagree concerning the degree to which these two processes interact (Dell, Schwartz, Martin, Saffran, & Gagnon, 1997; Levelt, Roelofs, & Myers, 1999). The model of Goldrick and Rapp (2002) is termed a restricted interaction account of spoken word production. In the first stage, a concept activates numerous semantic features, with the activation spreading to the next level (L-Level or lexical representations), with the target word and its neighbors that share semantic and/or syntactic information being activated. Activation also spreads to the phoneme level, again activating the target word and its related neighbors. In turn, the phoneme level provides feedback to the L-Level, activating the target and competitors that are phonologically similar. The most active unit, as compared to its neighbors, at the L-Level is chosen and feeds information down to the phoneme level, along with weaker activation of its competitors. Continued feedback from the phoneme level to the L-Level eventually results in the most appropriate word being selected from those with competing semantic and syntactic information.

Martin and Saffran (2002) examined the outcomes of investigations concerning the relationship between input and output phonologic processing and tested their hypothesis that such a relationship exists. On measures of phoneme discrimination and on rhyming judgment tasks, those with poor performance also made more nonword but phonologically related errors on picture naming. During comprehension, acoustic information is mapped to phonologic and then to lexical, followed by semantic and then conceptual, representations. The top-down lexical-semantic processing could help to compensate for an impaired phonologic network. The authors proposed that, in production, impairment of a single phonologic network would create a greater challenge, because the benefit from lexical-semantic feedback is less than that provided during the input process.

These models can be used to account for the various error types found in aphasia (Goldrick & Rapp, 2002). Damage to the semantic or L-Levels results in production of semantic errors, with impairment at the phoneme level causing multiple error types. The effect is postulated to be comparable to introducing noise into the processing system. If noise affects the L-Level, various errors can occur because of decreased activation of the target, allowing an opportunity for increased activation of semantically related and unrelated neighbors. Disrupted feedback to the phoneme level can result in nonword errors being produced from the lack of signal strength of the appropriate phonemes.

Nickels (2002) reviewed the aphasia literature addressing word retrieval treatment methods described through single-case studies. Findings indicated the positive effects of treatment but left unanswered specifically what form of treatment might work best for a given individual and how these improvements can be generalized to functional language use. It might be argued that greater specificity regarding selection and control of vocabulary as well as cueing strategies might be better delineated according to the specific word retrieval problem of the individual patient. Methods of strengthening activation patterns at the levels of disruption during the naming process need to be explored so that the underlying nature of the deficit can be treated with greater precision.

In creating activities in Area 6, the goal is to facilitate the actual word retrieval process rather than to teach specific vocabulary items. The clinician first attempts to determine the nature of the word retrieval problem or where in the process the breakdown appears to occur, establishes the vocabulary level and type with which the patient experiences errors, and determines whether patterns of performance vary across picture description, confrontation naming, and conversational activities.

Selecting vocabulary and developing a hierarchy includes consideration of the lesion site and its known impact on naming, including word characteristics. Differences in the ability to recall living (e.g., animals, food, flowers, or body parts) as opposed to non-living object labels have been described (De Renzi & Lucchelli, 1994). One explanation is that members of living categories are discriminated among each other based on visual features, rendering them more difficult to name, whereas identification of tools is based on functional characteristics. Others argue that when con-

founding effects are controlled, animacy and operativity do not play significant roles in word retrieval (Howard, Best, Bruce, & Gatehouse, 1995). A trend does, however, appear to exist for objects experienced through multiple senses to be better named. Many patients also demonstrate greater success in naming objects that are not embedded in a physical context (e.g., doorknob) or are separate from their environment.

In other activation studies involving normal subjects, Damasio and colleagues (2004) found a small area of activation in the temporal lobe for naming unique persons, animals, and tools. Increases also were found in rCBF in the left temporal pole for persons; animals and tools activated the left posteroinferior temporal region, with tool naming activation noted in the posterior middle and inferior temporal gyri. Bandur, Parrent, and Steven (2006) studied intraoperative naming errors in patients undergoing dominant anterior temporal lobectomies for epilepsy. During electrical stimulation, naming errors were incurred at sites located more anterior to those identified during implementation of traditional language mapping tasks. Of those sites, the majority included naming errors involving unique persons, which is consistent with results from lesion studies and activation findings in normal subjects.

It has been purported that word retrieval of common nouns in conduction and Broca's aphasia can occur late in lexical retrieval once semantic activation has occurred and some indication of word form has been established or, in some instances, may reflect unsuccessful lemma retrieval (Beeson, Holland, & Murray, 1997). Reporting on the frequently observed tip-of-the-tongue phenomenon, the authors found that these two groups were more successful than chance in identifying the initial letters of target words (names of famous faces). Alternatively, more limited evidence exists to suggest that word form knowledge is intact for patients with Wernicke's and anomic aphasia.

The influence of grammatical class on naming has been examined in neurologically intact subjects using positron-emission tomography. Tranel, Martin, Damasio, Grabowski, and Hichwa (2005) reported that areas associated with action naming were the left frontal operculum and the left posterior middle temporal region. The middle temporal area was more activated in naming actions than in naming tools. The naming of homonymous verbs (e.g., comb) resulted in less activation of the frontal operculum and middle temporal area. The homonymous nouns activated the frontal operculum and the left inferior temporal area, but the non-homonymous nouns only produced activation in the left inferior temporal lobe. The authors concluded that grammatical class does play a role in word retrieval.

Berndt, Burton, Haendiges, and Mitchum (2002) studied the effect of word class on word retrieval of nouns and verbs in aphasia and a matched normal control group through use of various elicitation contexts. When matched for frequency, both patients with aphasia and controls demonstrated more difficulty in naming pictured actions using latency measures. The authors judged that imageability was not a contributing factor. The poorer naming performance of verbs by patients correlated with poor sentence production skills. This group also tended to substitute nouns for verbs across all the tasks as compared to those with anomia.

Some investigators have reported that semantic and grammatical categories may be differentially affected depending on the type of aphasia (Berndt, Mitchum, Haendiges, & Sandson, 1997; Goodglass et al., 1966). Noun impairments have been specifically associated with severe anomia, although verb retrieval deficits can occur with both Broca's and Wernicke's aphasia. Lu and colleagues (2002) studied the controversy regarding whether category-specific naming deficits are attributed to grammatical or semantic category specifications. They found that patients who had undergone left anterior temporal lobectomies performed more poorly than those who had undergone right temporal lobectomies and that both groups were less successful at naming actions than at naming objects. It also was noted that patients in the left anterior temporal lobectomy group demonstrated better naming of objects defined by visual attributes compared with those associated more with human action.

Within the grammatical category of verbs, other factors also may affect performance. Light verbs (e.g., have, do, and come), although frequently used, may generate a number of meanings when activated, which, in turn, render them more difficult to retrieve compared with heavy or more complex verbs (e.g., run, hit, and stop) (Breedin, Saffron, & Schwartz, 1998). Lambon-Ralph, Braber, McClelland, and Patterson (2005) studied a group of patients with nonfluent aphasia to compare production of regular and irregular verb forms. They found that those patients demonstrating the most consistent problem in producing regular past tense verbs were those who were most impacted by phonologic complexity (consonant clusters) and atypicality (syllabic stress falling on the second syllable).

Finally, some additional stimulus variables to consider are word length, frequency, and concreteness. An item may be easier to name if its label is of low uncertainty. Uncertainty indicates the consistency with which an item is called a particular name. Some individuals may be sensitive to prototypicality, or the degree to which an item is characteristic of its class.

Once stimuli have been selected, effective cueing strategies are determined for each patient. Best, Herbert, Hickin, Osborne, and Howard (2002) studied a group of 11 individuals with aphasia to examine the effects of training with cues including repetition, rhyme, and phonemic and orthographic cues. All cue conditions were effective, and they remained so for a period of 10 minutes. The authors did not find a relationship between degree of impairment and the ultimate size of the facilitation effect. The largest cue effects were found in those whose impairments did not lay at either the semantic or phonologic levels but appeared to be associated with mapping between the two levels.

Patients with anomia also seem to demonstrate a preference for semantic cues (Li & Williams, 1990) when verbs are presented. Wambaugh (2003) compared the use of phonologic and semantic cues in the treatment of one patient with chronic anomia. Although both types of cues proved to be beneficial, a greater and sustained effect after 6 weeks was found with the lists trained using semantic cues.

Some findings (Stimley & Noll, 1991) indicate that presentation of semantic cues increases the number of semantic paraphasias, with a decrease in unrelated word errors. Phonemic cue presentation, on the other hand, may increase the number of phonemic paraphasias. Another factor to consider in cue presentation is the use of simultaneous cues (e.g., initial syllable combined with sentence completion format). Particularly with those who demonstrate more severe impairments, combined presentation may be most effective (Huntley, Pindzola, & Werdner, 1986). Marshall, Karow, Freed, and Babcock (2002) examined the facilitation effects of personalized cues on naming in a group of unimpaired speakers and in a group with patients with aphasia. Each group was required to learn a list of names from a subordinate category (dogs) by developing their own cues that would potentially aid recall. Training sessions occurred three times per week over a 4-week period. For the group without brain damage, no effect for cue type on learning was found. The group with aphasia, however, demonstrated a positive effect for semantic as compared to only phonologic information.

Hickin, Best, Herber, Howard, and Osborne (2002) studied the long-term effectiveness of phonologic and orthographic cueing in facilitating word retrieval with 8 patients who demonstrated difficulty mapping semantics to phonology. In this study, patients were given the choice of cues that they wished to be presented. Seven of the eight patients demonstrated a significant improvement on a 200-word naming task at the end of 8 weeks of treatment conducted once weekly. No one cue was found to be more effective, which could reflect the fact that both cues were trained within the same sessions. The authors suggested that the success of their study might be related to the patients choosing the cues, perhaps signaling more active reflection during the tasks. The three individuals who benefited most from therapy were those with good repetition and oral reading skills.

The hierarchy shown in Figure 28–3 is an attempt to integrate the findings of various researchers. A number of activities and contexts may be employed to assist the patient in developing an understanding of the effectiveness and use of cues. Less difficulty may be encountered in naming pictured stimuli than in providing responses to definition or sentence

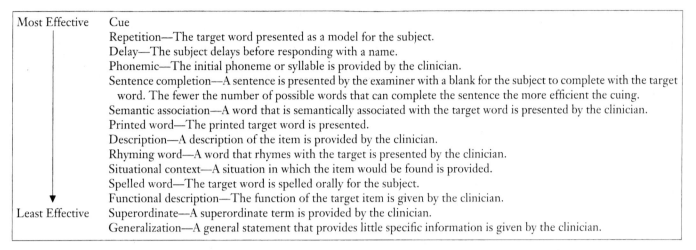

Most Effective	Cue
	Repetition—The target word presented as a model for the subject.
	Delay—The subject delays before responding with a name.
	Phonemic—The initial phoneme or syllable is provided by the clinician.
	Sentence completion—A sentence is presented by the examiner with a blank for the subject to complete with the target word. The fewer the number of possible words that can complete the sentence the more efficient the cuing.
	Semantic association—A word that is semantically associated with the target word is presented by the clinician.
	Printed word—The printed target word is presented.
	Description—A description of the item is provided by the clinician.
	Rhyming word—A word that rhymes with the target is presented by the clinician.
	Situational context—A situation in which the item would be found is provided.
	Spelled word—The target word is spelled orally for the subject.
	Functional description—The function of the target item is given by the clinician.
Least Effective	Superordinate—A superordinate term is provided by the clinician.
	Generalization—A general statement that provides little specific information is given by the clinician.

Figure 28–3. Hierarchy of cues according to effectiveness level.

completion tasks (Berndt et al., 1997), particularly in the presence of auditory comprehension problems. Patients with anomia, on the other hand, may benefit from the presentation of a sentence frame containing a word semantically related to the target (McCall, Cox, Shelton, & Weinrich, 1997). Both the syntactic context and/or syntactic constraints imposed, supplemented by semantic information, appear to be facilitative.

Differing findings regarding the use of real objects, colored photos, or line drawings have been cited, so the clinician may need to alter this presentation variable on an individual basis (Benton, Smith, & Lang, 1972; Bisiach, 1966).

As patients advance along a hierarchy—that is, using increasingly difficult levels of vocabulary and cue presentation—responsibility for cueing is shifted from the clinician to the patient. Ultimately, tasks should be implemented that allow practice to occur in meaningful, naturalistic situations. For example, application of Promoting Aphasics' Communicative Effectiveness (Davis & Wilcox, 1981), or PACE, which encourages patients to use multiple channels to communicate, has met with some success in developing effective cueing strategies (Li, Kitselman, Dusatko, & Spinelli, 1988).

Sentence Formulation

Area 7, Sentence Formulation, focuses on the generation of meaningful units at the phrase and sentence levels. A hierarchy of sentence types may be established, such as that found in the Helm Elicited Language Program for Syntax Stimulation (Helm-Estabrooks, 1981), or HELPSS. This approach was developed for patients with nonfluent aphasia to improve their use of syntax by training 11 sentence types with a story completion format. Sentence types range from the imperative intransitive to use of the future verb tense.

A hierarchy of sentence types for training also might be created based on order of reappearance in language samples

(Ludlow, 1973) elicited from those with aphasia. Difficulty levels can be developed by varying the uses of morphological markers (Goodglass & Berko, 1960) and by varying phrase/sentence length. The stress pattern of a sentence may influence performance of some individuals. Patients with Broca's aphasia, for example, tend to initiate utterances with stressed words. Use of stress in these cases would be an important variable to include in the treatment hierarchy.

Another highly researched approach in treating agrammatism has been mapping therapy (Byng, Nickels, and Black, 1994; Marshall, 1995; Schwartz et al., 1994; Thompson & Shapiro, 1995). The mapping deficit hypothesis suggests that some patients are unable to relate sentence form to meaning (Marshall, 1995). The problem can arise from a lexical deficit in which the verb fails to provide information about its thematic structure (goal or agent) or a procedural deficit in which the rules assigning thematic roles to moved argument structures are lost. These limitations occur in both comprehension and production, although patients generally are able to carry out grammaticality judgments, perhaps related to residual syntactic skills. No one particular application of mapping therapy has proven to result in qualitatively or quantitatively similar outcomes for all patients, requiring highly individualized implementation. Typically, treatment involves both comprehension and production tasks to encourage explicit analysis of verb-noun relational structures in canonical (e.g., subject-verb-object) and noncanonical sentence types (Schwartz et al., 1994). Colored lines may be drawn on cards to represent syntactic class (noun phrase and verb), with the patient required to select the appropriate color-coded written phrases to match the cards and corresponding pictured representation (Byng et al., 1994). Eventually, the patient is required to produce the sentence, with prompts from the clinician to enable the development and use of self-monitoring and problem-solving skills. Byng and colleagues (1994) described increased verb retrieval with their patients using this method. Other improvements were noted but varied with individuals, perhaps reflecting differing patterns of deficits and/or a need for more customized approaches. Although no specific training in production was provided to their group with chronic, nonfluent aphasia, Schwartz and colleagues (1994) found that the majority of patients improved on one or more of their production measures following a course of mapping therapy.

Mapping therapy for sentence production has been investigated by Rochon, Laird, Bose, and Scofield (2005). Improvements on all trained sentence structures were found with varied degrees of generalization. The authors commented that performance might have been reflective of the heterogeneous skills with thematic role mapping demonstrated by the participants, even before the beginning of treatment. Thompson and Shapiro (1994) concerned that treatment approaches for sentence formulation were targeting only the surface forms of sentences and not their linguistic and psycholinguistic underpinnings developed a Linguistic-Specific Approach (LST). They proposed that by addressing the underlying representations and processes of sentence formulation, generalization to untrained items could be enabled. The LST was applied to training of sentences in which noun phrases (NPs) had been moved out of their canonical positions. The investigators initiated treatment with more complex forms: NP-Verb-NP-PP (e.g., *The mother is taking flowers from her son*) vs. NP-Verb (copula)-NP (e.g., *Flowers are plants*). They found generalization to the less complex sentences of the same type and, in three of the eight patients, generalization to untrained sentence types. The authors claimed that improvement on untrained sentence types resulted because they involved similar underlying forms and processes. Individual differences were noted across patients, indicating that other variables may need to be considered, such as lesion site and/or psychological factors. In a study conducted to validate the generalization findings from complex to less complex structures (Thompson, Shapiro, Kiran, & Sobecks, 2003), the authors again revealed this phenomenon with significantly less generalization occurring when simpler forms were trained first. They also found an improvement in comprehension skills, although a similar generalization pattern was not apparent. Other noteworthy findings were an increase in utterance length and in the proportion of grammatical sentences documented in narrative analysis.

Generalization of LST treatment gains to discourse was further studied by Thompson and Shapiro (1995). At the completion of treatment, they found that more complex sentences in discourse were evident, along with an increase in the number of verbs produced. Ballard and Thompson (1999) determined this approach to be successful in a group of five patients with Broca's aphasia; those with the least severe impairments benefited most, with narrative produc-

tions becoming more informative and efficient. Jacobs (2001) further detailed discourse changes following LST and found that communicative efficiency improved, with only a positive trend in informativeness for four of the five patients studied. Significant improvements in grammar were not shown, although listener comfort was rated as being higher post-treatment. In summary, the application of a systematic psycholinguistic approach, such as LST, to address the underlying nature of agrammatism has shown promising results. This approach challenges our thinking in the development of sentence hierarchies, and it leads us to reexamine the complexity factor within that context.

The use of C-VIC has been widely investigated, particularly with respect to its use with patients exhibiting nonfluent aphasia. In this system (Weinrich, McCall, Weber, Thomas, & Thornburg, 1995), patients were introduced to a lexicon consisting of animate nouns, common nouns, verbs, prepositions, and modifiers. Icons with printed words were available to be inserted into slots provided for the patient and clinician/interactant to form simple syntactic constructions. Employing comprehension and formulation tasks, while encouraging subsequent verbalization, subject-verb-object constructions improved both when using C-VIC and in spontaneous speech. Improvements also were noted in the use of locative prepositional phrases (e.g., in, on, and by). Some patients have demonstrated a positive response through C-VIC training that targets tense inflection (Weinrich, Shelton, Cox, & McCall, 1997). Gains in retrieving verbs also were a by-product of this approach. To date, successful attempts to facilitate the generalization of single sentence production in C-VIC to narrative production have not been reported (Weinrich, Shelton, McCall, & Cox, 1997).

The C-VIC training might be employed as a branch step in LOT to facilitate oral sentence forms with those who are unable to make gains in these abilities using the methods described previously. For some with severe aphasic limitations, C-VIC might serve as a more permanent avenue of communication. Naeser and colleagues (1998) studied a group of patients with severe aphasia to isolate factors that might play a role in determining successful candidacy for C-VIC. These authors concluded that the best outcome (ability to initiate communication with C-VIC) was associated with a lesion sparing large portions of either the posterior or anterior systems involved in language recovery. Inability to use C-VIC was associated with bilateral lesions. Overall test scores on the Boston Assessment of Severe Aphasia (Helm-Estabrooks, Ramsberger, Morgan, & Nicholas, 1989b) also were good indicators of response to C-VIC when considered along with lesion data.

Finally, in selecting treatment tasks and or materials, the impact of contextual variables, such as use of pictured stimuli or conversation, needs to be considered in terms of how they may be impact responses. Some patients produce a greater number of major utterances (subject-predicate) in response to pictures compared with the number in conversation (Easterbrook, Brown, & Perera, 1982); others may produce more words, depending on the gender bias of the picture (Correia, Brookshire, & Nicholas, 1990).

Conversation and Discourse

Current practice delineates four categories of discourse: conversational, expository, procedural and narrative. Although conversation is formally addressed in Area 8, many of the parameters affecting performance also apply to other forms of discourse (Area 9) and will be outlined in that section. Unique to conversation, however, are the roles of turn taking and repair (Ferguson, 1998). Turn taking was found to be unimpaired in a sample of speakers with fluent aphasia when conversing with both familiar and unfamiliar communication partners. Perkins (1995) suggested that conversational partners respond based on the amount of shared knowledge, degree of linguistic impairment, and individual discourse styles. For example, the presence of significant difficulties in oral expression in the context of shared knowledge regarding a particular topic may result in glossing over of problematic aspects in conversation rather than in working to modify them through collaborative repair. Variability of tolerance for pauses also can be found among communication partners, which can impact turn taking and repair.

Successful use of the involvement of significant others in treating conversation has been reported by authors incorporating different approaches. Conversational coaching (Holland, 1991) uses prepared scripts, requiring the patient, with initial support from the clinician, to communicate the story to a significant other. The clinician assists the communication partner in identifying opportunities for and practicing implementation of effective strategies to facilitate the exchange. Hopper, Holland, and Rewega (2002) studied the efficacy of conversational couching with two couples. Ten treatment sessions were provided in which communication strategies were described, modeled, and then practiced by the pairs. Following treatment, the patients demonstrated an increase in the number of main ideas conveyed in telling stories to their partners. The investigators suggested that developing an understanding of the couples' communication patterns and styles before treatment were important factors in facilitating conversational success.

Using a modified approach in a case report, Boles (1998) selected three aspects of a spouse's conversational style for intervention. With the spouse reducing her rate of speech, percentage of talking turns, and topic shifts, the patient participated more effectively and to a greater extent in conversation.

Kagan, Black, Duchan, Simmons-Mackie, and Square (2001) reported on the effectiveness of teaching conversa-

tional strategies to communication partners of those with aphasia called Supported Conversation for Adults with Aphasia, or SCA. The program was designed to assist those with aphasia to express, verbally and/or nonverbally, their knowledge, thoughts, and feelings by directly training others to enhance communication opportunities, both as a listener and as an enabler for more successful communication attempts. The volunteer training program consisted of a 1-day workshop focusing on behaviors that assist in both acknowledging and revealing the competence of those with aphasia, followed by conversational opportunities, in which the volunteers' skills were rated and compared to those of an untrained, matched control group. This approach was proven to be effective in improving the skills of the volunteers and the effectiveness of conversations in those with aphasia.

Simmons-Mackie, Kingston, and Schultz (2004) studied the conversational interactions of a patient when the communication partner was successful in using a variety of behaviors, such as eye gaze, posture, and introduction of contextual referents to enable the person to successfully convey his or her message. The authors maintained that, although some individuals might intuitively adopt these behaviors, others benefit from more direct training.

Another form of communication, collaborative referencing, has been examined in the context of aphasia (Hengst, 2003). This process was examined in a group of patients with aphasia and familiar communication partners when they were jointly performing a complex task. The couples demonstrated a number of different verbal and nonverbal means to communicate information, perspectives, and goals. It was observed that the pairs relied on their shared personal histories to frame their communication, and over the course of the trials, communication became less effortful and overt, a pattern similar to that found in those without aphasia. These patients were in the chronic stage of aphasia, so it was difficult to determine the role that treatment may have played in enabling them to use various strategies with their routine communication partners. The study does, however, demonstrate that even those with moderate to severe aphasia can learn and modify behavior through collaborative referencing tasks, and this area may be an important one to address in establishing more functional communication exchanges and/or in attempting to generalize targeted areas in treatment.

Reported speech is a common form of conversation and one that may be enhanced in those with aphasia to promote more functional communication. Hengst, Frame, Neuman-Strizel, and Gannaway (2005) described reported speech to be an act of discourse for quoting or paraphrasing an individual's words from another point in time. The rephrasing and/or restating may consist of the production of one's own words or of someone else's. In examining the conversational patterns of seven individuals with aphasia who had either completed or were in the course of the therapy, the investigators found that reported speech was used by those with aphasia and actually provided contextual information to their partner for them to successfully communicate despite syntactic and linguistic errors. The authors suggested that measures of reported speech could be used for documenting functional changes in communication over time and could be included as a goal in therapy. Five forms of reported speech were described and coded: direct (direct quotation), indirect (paraphrased), projected (suggesting what someone should have said or to speak for animals/objects), indexed (not stated directly or indirectly but "pointed to," e.g., *That's what I heard*), and undecided (unable to categorize). The first two forms of reported speech are the ones used most often and may be appropriate tasks for treatment. The value of a shared history was an important factor in reported speech, so involving significant others in this aspect of treatment would be especially important.

Drawing on the work of the previously mentioned authors, one might develop a hierarchy of activities in enhancing conversational exchanges between patients and significant others. Communication partners might benefit from specific instruction in dealing appropriately with pauses in conversation, altering their rate of speech, effectively introducing new topics, and modifying their turn taking. Various forms of conversation also could be introduced, in which the amount of shared knowledge or new information is controlled. Although pragmatic deficits in conversation have been documented less frequently in those with aphasia, some may require instruction and practice in turn taking, topic maintenance, seeking clarification, and initiating repairs. Treatment in the area of conversation also may focus on the generalization of specific linguistic skills, such as word retrieval, gestural production, or writing, to everyday communication situations.

A model for evaluating discourse can be useful for both assessment and planning intervention in Area 9. Chapman and Ulatowska (1992) described discourse as involving an interaction between cognition and language and detailed the components of discourse production. Superstructure refers to elements such as setting (e.g., characters, time, and place), complicating action (sequence of events), and resolution. The global meaning or semantic content is termed macrostructure, which is closely tied to cognition and, to a lesser degree, linguistic performance. Tasks that address this aspect of discourse may include summarizing the story, selecting the main idea/gist, identifying the main hero, formulating a title, and deriving a lesson/moral. As the complexity and degree of abstraction are increased with these activities, opportunities for incorporating more linguistically complex sentence forms become available.

The ability of the speaker to maintain coherence or a unified theme depends not only on the macrostructure but also on the microstructure components of discourse (Hough & Pierce, 1994). Microstructure coherence deals with the conceptual links that are established between sentences or propositions. Appropriate use of pronouns (with corresponding referents), articles, and ellipsis (the sentence construction is incomplete, but the intent is understood) signal that the speaker is aware of when information is novel or has, in some way, already been communicated to the listener. Coherence also is aided by inclusion of cohesive ties between sentences such as coreference and anaphora.

When developing a hierarchy for discourse production, many variables can be altered, depending on the particular profile of the patient. One might initiate treatment with tasks that require identification of the components of the superstructure in relation to a particular topic. Practice in identifying the main concepts can be followed by development of accuracy and completeness of information. Nicholas and Brookshire (1995a) determined that the presence, completeness, and accuracy of main concepts in connected speech were related to the severity of aphasia. Patients with less severe aphasia generally were found to have fewer absent main concepts and more accurate/complete main concepts than those with more severe aphasia when a variety of speech samples were studied. When analyzing speech samples for number of words spoken per minute and percentage of words that are correct information units, Brookshire and Nicholas (1994) concluded that it is important to elicit samples from different forms of discourse and that a total sample of 300 to 400 words leads to more reliable interpretation.

The difficulty level can further be increased by requiring the sequencing of information and the establishment of coherence at the macro- and microstructure levels. Specific instruction in the use of pronouns and other devices for maintaining cohesion may be needed. When constructing tasks to improve grammatical form or word retrieval skills in discourse, the context might be altered to promote greater opportunities for practice. Patients may demonstrate varying degrees of grammatical complexity in relation to the type of discourse involved. Expository discourse (related to a particular topic, as in picture description), procedural discourse (consisting of steps, either conceptually or chronologically associated), and narrative discourse (information about an event, or story retelling) have been compared (Li, Volpe, Ritterman, & Williams, 1996). The most complex grammar was elicited through picture description, followed by the procedural discourse task and then the story retelling condition. In contrast, however, a significantly higher percentage of content words was found with story retelling as compared to expository and procedural discourse, suggesting that the patients were conveying the informational load through lexical rather than grammatical avenues.

In some instances, topic familiarity may play a role with grammatical complexity in discourse production. When provided with less familiar topics, grammatical complexity can increase for procedural discourse but appears to have no similar effect for story retelling (Williams, Li, Volpe, & Ritterman, 1994). In that study, the number of content words increased with both procedural discourse and story retelling conditions involving familiar topics. Listener familiarity evidenced no impact on discourse production.

Picture description and procedural discourse tasks involving less familiar topics might be chosen when the emphasis on discourse production is to improve grammatical form. Alternatively, story retelling and procedural discourse tasks incorporating familiar topics could be presented when one is attempting to elicit a greater number of content words.

Because the interplay between cognition and language is particularly evident in discourse, some of the mental operations (Chapey, 2001) associated with language processing and production are considered in this section. Convergent thinking or the development of logical conclusions based on information provided is involved in tasks such as explaining similarities and differences between concepts, retelling stories, describing procedures, making inferences, and organizing ideas in a logical order for expression. Divergent thinking demands the production of alternatives from given information, with an emphasis on quantity, elaboration, and originality. In discourse, this skill might be reflected by producing alternate perspectives, presenting a variety of ideas, predicting different outcomes or solutions, and changing the direction of one's responses. A hierarchy of tasks could be constructed addressing all these parameters, in addition to varying the degree of abstractness and the familiarity of the stimuli.

Chapey also highlighted the role of evaluative thinking or judgment. Some aspects included in discourse are selecting the best word to fit the situation; determining an appropriate metaphor, idiom, or proverb; and judging what can and cannot be said in various contexts with different communication partners.

The processing and production of figurative language are integral to discourse. In addressing these aspects of communication, however, several factors must be considered. The ability to provide correct idiom interpretation has been correlated with years of formal education and auditory comprehension skills (Tompkins, Boada, & McGarry, 1992). Accurate explanation of proverbs also tends to be related to educational level and age (Nippold, Uhden, & Schwarz, 1997), with highly educated subjects without brain damage performing better than their peers in all age groups. Performance has been shown to peek at 20 years and declines significantly after 70 years of age. Those with higher verbal ability demonstrate less of a decline with age compared to those with lower verbal ability. In examining proverb interpretation and explanation abilities in patients with fluent aphasia and relatively high auditory comprehension skills, comprehension of proverbs proved to be relatively intact (Chapman et al., 1997). This performance is in contrast to the significantly impaired performance of subjects in providing explanations for both familiar and unfamiliar proverbs. Interpretation and explanation of idioms and proverbs can be used as higher-level, cognitive-linguistic tasks with patients experiencing problems in conveying information of a more abstract nature. In selecting stimuli, however, the patient's age, educational background, and familiarity with the stimuli must be considered.

Finally, strategies may be introduced to facilitate self-evaluation, such as monitoring for inclusion of and appropriate sequencing of relevant details and checking for redundancy and tangential or off-topic remarks. The use of written stimuli can be particularly beneficial in this area, either by having the patient write his or her narrative when possible or by having the clinician transcribe it for review and editing.

Case Example

LP is a 44-year-old engineer who underwent a craniotomy with resection of a left frontal glioma. The WAB, the Auditory Comprehension Test for Sentences, and the Boston Naming Test were administered. A nonfluent aphasia was exhibited, with oral speech limited to sentence fragments and frequent word retrieval problems. Auditory and reading comprehension were both mildly impaired. Written output paralleled spoken speech.

Along with activities targeting other areas, word retrieval was chosen for treatment. Probing revealed that LP was 80% successful in naming pictured objects characterized by monosyllabic word forms using Grade 1 and Grade 2 vocabulary levels. Polysyllabic nouns were named spontaneously, with 50% accuracy at these grade levels. No successful responses were elicited when pictured actions were presented.

Subsequent testing determined that the most effective cues for LP were presentation of the initial phoneme, description of physical and/or functional properties, and provision of the situational context (i.e., the situation in which the item may be found). Because the clinician believed that phonemic cueing would be a difficult process to transfer from the clinician to the patient, use of description and situational contexts was emphasized.

In the first stage of the treatment hierarchy, specific training in the area of providing physical and functional descriptions and identifying situational contexts for pictured polysyllabic objects at a Grade 1 to a Grade 3 level was provided. Written prompts were used on individual cards to remind the patient of the various physical and functional attributes. For example, the phrases *What color?*, *What size?*, *What shape?*, and *What material?* were printed on one card, and on another, the question *What is it used for?* was printed. Once LP achieved a 70% success rate in providing the required information, another series of stimuli at the same level of difficulty was presented. In this activity, the patient, by providing descriptions and situational contexts, was required to help the clinician identify pictured objects hidden from her view.

When the provision of the cues became more automatic for LP, confrontation naming tasks were used, in which he provided needed cues only when naming was not spontaneous. To limit the patient's reliance on the clinician, the pictured items were again seen only by LP. Difficulty levels also were systematically increased by introducing advanced vocabulary grade levels and other grammatical form classes (e.g., verbs and adjectives). In addition, practice with implementing self-cueing strategies was provided in various conversational activities. When treatment was discontinued, LP was a highly functional communicator, encountering word-finding problems primarily beyond a Grade 6 vocabulary level. His self-cueing strategies usually proved to be successful in assisting him to retrieve the intended word.

Sample Activities

Level 1
Stimuli: Grade 1 to Grade 3 polysyllabic pictured objects and printed cue cards (*What color?, What size?, What shape?, What material?,* and *What is it used for?*).

Procedure: The patient is required to provide oral responses to information requested on the cue cards.

Level 2
Stimuli: Grade 1 to Grade 3 polysyllabic pictured objects and printed cue cards (*What color?, What size?, What shape?, What material?,* and *What is it used for?*).

Procedure: The pictures are hidden from the clinician's view. The patient provides information prompted by the cue cards to enable the clinician to guess the identity of the pictures.

Level 3
Stimuli: Grade 1 to Grade 3 polysyllabic pictured objects and printed cue cards (*What color?, What size?, What shape?, What material?,* and *What is it used for?*).

Procedure: The pictures are hidden from the clinician's view. The patient first attempts to name the object spontaneously. If unsuccessful, he or she provides the information prompted by the cue cards to facilitate self-retrieval or identification by the clinician.

Graphic Expression

General Considerations

Graphic Expression refers to the written output of communication through the use of graphemes (letters) or drawing.

Writing frequently is the most severely affected modality in aphasia. Historically, varying patterns of writing problems or agraphia have been described in the literature, along with a number of classification systems (Benson, 1979; Ellis, 1982; Goodglass, 1993; Margolin, 1984). They include pure agraphia, in which writing defects occur in relative isolation of other language impairments, and agraphia with alexia, in which patients are unable to retrieve the graphic form of letter strings and, sometimes, even individual letters. Differing symptoms and localization have been noted in pure agraphia. Signs may include the inability to write words, as compared to individual letters, although oral spelling is intact.

More recent research trends have focused on developing computational models to describe the various processes involved in writing, with attempts being made to relate disruption at or between given levels to specific cortical regions. It generally is agreed that the writing of a familiar word first involves activation of the semantic system or the word meaning, and then its spelling, through access of its orthographic representation in the orthographic output lexicon (OOL), Maintenance and sequencing of these graphemes are the responsibility of the graphemic buffer until written production is completed through allographic conversion and a motor response. In the writing of less familiar vocabulary and pseudo-words, phonology-to-orthography conversion rules are implicated (Hillis, Change, Breese, & Heider, 2004; Hillis et al., 2002).

In studying patients during the hyperacute phases of their strokes, Hillis and colleagues (2002) were able to associate patterns of written performance with areas of cortical dysfunction. Impairments with semantic-lexical processes were reflected in the production of semantic errors in writing, resulting from hypoperfusion/infarct in the following areas: Wernicke's (BA 22), posterior middle and inferior temporal gyrus (BA 37), angular gyrus (BA 39), supramarginal gyrus (BA 40), and visual association cortex (BA 19). Patients experiencing difficulty accessing their semantic systems demonstrate imageability effects (Schmalzl & Nickels, 2006). Specific damage to the lexical route of spelling has been termed lexical or surface dysgraphia (Beeson et al., 2003; Schmalzl & Nickels, 2006). Errors, although sparing phoneme-to-grapheme conversion (PGC) rules, involve irregularly spelled vocabulary and demonstrate a word frequency effect. Hillis and colleagues (2002) noted regularization errors and/or omissions in spelling familiar words, with involvement of Broca's area (BA 44 and 45), although accurate spelling of pseudo-words was possible. More recently, a relationship was identified between hypoperfusion/infarcts in BA 44, 45, and 6 and three cases of pure agraphia, with disrupted access to lexical orthographic representations (Hillis et al., 2004). Verbs proved to be particularly error-prone, as were the skills required for conversion of graphemes to letters during writing. Weekes,

Davies, and Parris (2003) found that in their subjects with surface agraphia, words that were learned earlier in life were better spared. Rapcsak and Beeson (2004) discovered an association between lexical agraphia and damage to the left fusiform gyrus and inferior temporal gyrus (BA 37 and 20). Co-occurring impairments consisted of alexia and naming problems, leading the investigators to conclude that BA 37 and 20 may be involved in a variety of language tasks that require integration of semantic, phonologic-lexical, and orthographic information, impacting multiple modalities.

Phonologic dysgraphia, with damage to the angular gyrus, is characterized by disrupted phoneme-to grapheme conversion. Although real words may be accessed through the lexical output system, spelling of pseudo-words and unfamiliar words is negatively impacted. Impairments to both the OOL and to the phonology-orthography levels, with production of semantic substitutions, has been termed deep agraphia.

Graphemic buffer deficits as a result of injury to BA 39 include word length effects, letter substitutions, omissions, and sequencing errors, and yet accurate copying. Ellis (1988) detailed a number of stages that intervene between selection of graphemes and handwriting. The allographic system is responsible for selecting letter case and style. For example, Del Grosso Destreri and colleagues (2000) described a patient with severe alexia and agraphia subsequent to a left temporoparieto-occipital hemorrhage. Better preserved spelling of lowercase versus uppercase letters and impaired letter substitutions resembling the physical forms of their targets were noted.

With activation of graphomotor patterns, letter stroke sequences can be specified in detail. Partial activation of neighbors with similar strokes also occurs so that disruption at this level can result in substitution of visually similar letters. Production of poorly formed or illegible letters are claimed to be related to impairment of additional components of the graphomotor pattern that affect size, orientation, and order of strokes and has been termed apractic agraphia. Allographic conversion, dependent on the use of skilled hand movements, has been associated with hypoperfusion/infarct in the area anterior and posterior to Broca's area (Exner's area; BA 6) (Hillis et al., 2004).

The premorbid skills and interests of the patient will dictate the degree to which the Graphic Expression modality will be incorporated into or, perhaps, even be the sole focus of treatment. In some instances, writing can be facilitative for oral naming or can be targeted simultaneously when sentence or discourse formulation skills are being developed.

The final portion of this section will briefly address the use of drawing in aphasia. This channel for expression might be considered as a compensatory form of communication, with varying degrees of success being reported in its implementation.

Graphomotor Access

Areas 1 and 2 focus on establishing graphic and graphemic motor patterns, with Area 3 stressing the recall of highly overlearned grapheme motor patterns. In Area 1, Tracing and/or Copying Nonverbal Material, two- and three-dimensional representations of nonverbal material are used. Task difficulty may be increased by altering the complexity of the designs in producing geometric forms and objects. Letters, numbers, and words are introduced in Area 2, Tracing and/or Copying Verbal Material. Activities are designed to address such problems as incorrect letter elements, inappropriate spatial positioning, rotation of letters/elements, and repetition of elements/letters. Some patients have demonstrated better ability to print in uppercase letters than to write in cursive script (Goodglass, 1993; Hanley & Peters, 1996), so this variable also might be included in designing tasks or considering response variables. Single items may be practiced, followed by those in a series (e.g., letters and numbers). In Area 3, Writing Familiar Material, highly overlearned stimuli, such as the patient's name, address, and telephone number, are incorporated.

Word Orthography

Areas 4 and 5, Written Spelling and Naming, may include activities such as writing to dictation, oral spelling, and written naming. A hierarchy can be established by selection of vocabulary across several dimensions. Word frequency, imageability, concreteness, emotionality, and grammatical class may influence the accuracy of the patient's performance. When a part-of-speech effect is observed, spelling of nouns is more readily available than verbs, followed by adjectives and grammatical functors (Goodglass, 1993).

Length is an important variable to alter, because shorter words occasion fewer errors than longer ones do (Friederici, Schonle, & Goodglass, 1981). Stimuli containing the most regular expression of phoneme-to-grapheme correspondence rules are easier than those in which letter combinations are a less frequent realization of sounds (e.g., /f/ in telephone) (Friederici et al., 1981). Although order of difficulty varies among patients and types of aphasia, double vowels, double consonants, and regular versus irregular spelling may be incorporated into a treatment hierarchy. Words containing suffixes may prove to be more difficult for patients (Langmore & Canter, 1983), as may production of homonyms and homophones.

In the last number of years, treatment approaches directed at addressing breakdowns within the various levels of the orthographic output model have been detailed (Hillis, 1992). With a patient demonstrating deficits within the semantic system, therapy was designed to teach semantic distinctions. Generalization of improved written naming to untrained items was found within the same semantic category. Another successful approach, with a different patient, involved implementation of a cueing hierarchy for written naming incorporating anagrams and initial letter cues. Schmalzl and Nickels (2006) applied two types of therapy to address a semantic spelling deficit, with impaired access to output orthography and suspected degradation within the OOL in a patient with a left temporal lobe infarction. Two-hundred irregularly spelled words were chosen for remediation, with attempts made to strengthen or improve access to their orthographic representations. The first phase of the treatment program consisted of the patient studying a word presented on a card, copying it, and then rewriting it once the card was removed after a 5-second delay. The second phase incorporated the use of mnemonics. Only the set of words trained with mnemonics improved, with no evidence of generalization to untreated items found. Another noteworthy finding was the reduction of phonologically related errors at the conclusion of treatment. Persisting errors resembled the orthographic representations of their targets, suggesting increased attempts to access the lexical route of spelling.

Problems arising from the OOL, in the context of intact PGC skills, may result in errors that are phonologically plausible (Hillis, 1992). In this instance, treatment targeting production of homophones could be beneficial. If disruption to the PGC mechanism is invoked with an intact OOL, spelling of nonwords is problematic. Hillis reported successful outcomes with tasks designed to develop the PGC system using cueing hierarchies. In one example, self-cueing was established for a patient with verbal apraxia, and in another, written monitoring of semantic errors was facilitated. Although the goals of addressing the impaired PGC system were different in these patients, systematic approaches to treating the disorder produced positive functional changes in other areas.

Raymer, Cudworth, and Haley (2003) examined the effectiveness of a treatment program for a patient who demonstrated impairments in the grapheme buffer characterized by spelling errors, increasing with word length, and omission of letters in the latter halves of words, along with letter substitutions, transpositions, and insertions. The OOL also demonstrated disruption, with regular and irregular words being error-prone, along with a frequency effect. The treatment method consisted of copying and recall of printed word lists. Initially, the patient was required to copy a presented written word, with the clinician then covering the first two letters and requiring the patient to recall and reproduce the letters. The clinician continued to conceal additional letters until the entire word was hidden and reproduction required. The word sets crossed a number of grammatical classes and were controlled for frequency and length. At the conclusion of treatment, which had been supplemented by home practice, a significant improvement in spelling to dictation was found, along with greater accuracy in writing narratives. The investigators cited evidence that the treatment had impacted both the graphemic buffer and the OOL deficits. Generalization to at least some sets of untreated words suggested increased capacity of the graphemic buffer, whereas transfer of spelling knowledge from the trained words to at least some untrained items with similar spellings indicated improvements in the OOL.

Rapp and Kane (2002) treated two patients who had selective deficits in the OOL and the graphemic buffer using the same approach to better understand the underlying cognitive deficits and how they respond to treatment. The first patient, with lesions involving the left posterior parietal and temporal areas, exhibited an agraphia impacting the OOL. The second patient, whose lesion involved the left anterior parietal region, experienced a consequent graphemic buffer impairment. The overall severity of the agraphia was similar in both patients. Three sets of words were developed that were matched according to frequency and length. Most items were nouns, with the remainder consisting of verbs and adjectives. The therapy paradigm consisted of auditory presentation of the stimulus, followed by repetition and attempted written spelling by the patient. If unsuccessful, the clinician provided the written word, identified each of the letters, removed the card, and asked the patient to write the word. Therapy concluded when the subjects had achieved a 95% success rate in writing the treated words. The patient with OOL deficits demonstrated a significant improvement on treated items at the conclusion of therapy, with no signs of generalization. Generalization to untreated items, however, was noted in the patient with the graphemic buffer deficit.

Treatment of writing also has been investigated to promote more functional communication. Robson, Marshall, Chiat, and Pring (2001) examined the potential for developing written communication in a group of patients with jargon aphasia. A personalized vocabulary consisting of 20 common and 20 proper nouns was used as stimuli. Initially, twice-weekly, 45- to 60-minute treatment sessions were conducted that incorporated a number of tasks, such as word-picture matching, completion of anagrams, delayed copying, and written naming. Four patients made significant improvements, although all patients demonstrated some treatment gains after approximately 12 sessions, with more correct responses and closer approximations to the targets. Generalization to the control sets or to use in conversation was not found. A second stage of therapy was introduced to three of the participants. Each received six 45-minute sessions of "message therapy" incorporating treated vocabulary. The patients and their partners were instructed on the utility of writing words to convey information in conversation and were provided with strategies to facilitate more meaningful exchanges. Follow up assessment of conversations and partner interviews revealed that patients were using writing in these contexts, with untreated words being incorporated in this functional activity.

Clausen and Beeson (2003) targeted writing to develop conversational exchanges in a small group of subjects with chronic aphasia. In their study, they trained four patients with global aphasia to write a list of personally relevant words pertaining to family, work, personal history, and interests, with the goal of establishing conversation in a group setting. The vocabulary was not controlled for frequency, grammatical class, or spelling regularity. Copy and recall training was provided, with the subjects required to write a word in response to a picture representation accompanied by auditory presentation. If unsuccessful, a model was provided for copying until success was achieved spontaneously in response to the picture stimulus. Thirteen weeks of individual treatment were provided, followed by weekly group sessions with the four patients. A facilitator attempted to provide a natural communication setting for the subjects to practice their trained vocabulary in the absence of any pictured stimuli. Each of the participants was encouraged to provide written responses or questions to the other members of the group. The writing of four out of five words in a set by an individual in the group session was the measure of success required before proceeding to training of the next set of words. Once criterion was reached in the group setting, a conversational interaction was arranged with a novel communication partner. The authors reported that the patients demonstrated improved pragmatic use of the written words in the group setting and demonstrated support for one another. Although written words were used frequently in that more routinized context, production with an unfamiliar communication partner was more limited, with earlier trained words being better maintained than those more recently targeted.

Text

Grammatical structures are first introduced in Area 6, Written Formulation, in which material at the phrase, sentence, and paragraph levels may be used. Sentence complexity and length may be altered, along with topic familiarity. Many of the same variables found to influence oral expression can be incorporated into this area and developed simultaneously. At the paragraph level, a hierarchy can be established focusing on the structure of the text (Labov, cited in Freedman-Stern, Ulatowska, Baker, & Delacoste, 1984) such that task requirements might include mention of time, place, participants, complicating action, and result/resolution. Once the patient is successful in including these obligatory elements, optional ones, such as coda/moral of the story, may be required. Instruction in the use of cohesive devices, such as anaphoric reference, relative clauses, and temporal ordering, can be systematically approached, perhaps initially through identifying their application in read-ing comprehension activities and then by their incorporation in written output.

In addition to the variables stated above, in Area 7, Writing Complex Material, a response hierarchy that addresses the purpose and complexity of the text can be established. A possible progression from easy to difficult is narrative, letter, and expository (Freedman-Stern et al., 1984). This aspect of treatment requires a highly individualistic application given the diversity of functions that writing may serve in a patient's day-to-day activities.

Case Example

BC is a 64-year-old, self-employed business consultant. A left hemisphere stroke resulted in an infarct involving the white matter in the region of the superior temporal lobe and angular gyrus, with extension into the white matter in the left corona radiata. The WAB, the Auditory Comprehension Test for Sentences, and the Boston Naming Test were administered. A fluent aphasia, characterized by moderately impaired auditory comprehension, with paraphasic speech production, anomia, mildly impaired reading comprehension, and agraphia were revealed.

At the time of initial testing, BC successfully wrote his name but not his address. Only a portion of the alphabet and numbers to 20 were correctly written. Writing single words to dictation resulted in no correct responses. Letter substitutions and additions made words, for the most part, unidentifiable. Over the course of the next 2 weeks, however, spontaneous improvement was noted such that short sentence formulation was possible, with word-finding problems identical to those in oral speech.

Spelling errors were found mainly at the ends of words, where letter substitutions were noted. Irregularly spelled words occasioned the most errors. Further probing revealed that written naming was 50% successful using Grade 7 and Grade 8 polysyllabic, irregularly spelled words. Oral naming, followed by oral spelling, proved to be effective cues for BC to write the word correctly.

BC identified graphic expression as an important focus in treatment. His daily work activities relied heavily on written skills, particularly related to correspondence.

Because oral naming activities were being used in treatment, Area 5, Written Naming, was simultaneously developed. Once BC was able to write stimuli at the Grade 7 and Grade 8 levels successfully, including polysyllabic, regularly spelled nouns, and the difficulty level was increased by using nouns with irregular spelling, followed by other word classes, such as adjectives and verbs. Eventually, the vocabulary level was altered, along with grammatical form class, word length, and degree of imageability. Written naming activities were later incorporated into Area 7, Writing Complex Material, in preparation for the patient's eventual return to work.

Sample Activities

Level 1
Stimuli: Grade 7 and Grade 8 polysyllabic, regularly spelled nouns.

Procedure: A written sentence is presented with the stimulus word omitted. The patient orally provides the word, spells it aloud, and finally writes it.

Level 2
Stimuli: Grade 7 and Grade 8 polysyllabic, irregularly spelled nouns.

Procedure: A written sentence is presented with the stimulus word omitted. The patient orally provides the word, spells it aloud, and finally writes it.

Level 3
Stimuli: Grade 7 and Grade 8 polysyllabic, regularly spelled verbs.

Procedure: A written sentence is presented with the stimulus word omitted. The patient orally provides the word, spells it aloud, and finally writes it.

Compensatory Communication

Back to the Drawing Board is an approach that was designed as a tool for communication by patients with severe limitations in their oral expression abilities (Morgan & Helm-Estabrooks, cited in Helm-Estabrooks & Albert, 1991). Uncaptioned cartoons are presented for copying from memory until the patient is able to produce triple-panel sequences. The clinician provides coaching to elicit drawings that are recognizable, with productions including main ideas and essential details. During the later phase of treatment, practice in conveying information to significant others is incorporated.

Lyon (1995) considered drawing as an augmentative form of communication, not as a replacement for language, for those who have retained inner thought. Hypothetical situations are posed, with the patient encouraged to respond through drawing. The clinician aids in correcting or expanding portions that may be unidentifiable through questions and/or adding features to the drawings. As skills are developed, more complex topics are introduced, along with strategies to reflect different time periods. Involving significant others in communication exchanges through drawing and teaching them to interpret and probe for more information are viewed as key components in this treatment approach.

The development of drawing in LOT may provide an avenue of communication for those who are unable to access communication through more conventional means. Some patients may encounter success in combining drawing with their limited written output to facilitate meaningful oral output. Because the drawings of patients with

aphasia initially may be simplistic (Lyon, 1995), implementation of a treatment hierarchy to improve the complexity of both the drawings and their communicative intents could be advantageous.

EFFICACY STUDY

The LOT subjects for whom the efficacy data are reported here were part of a larger project designed to study the efficacy of three different types of aphasia treatment. The LOT subjects were drawn from a population in London, Ontario, and the surrounding southwestern Ontario region in Canada. Table 28–1 shows the entry criteria that were met by all subjects. Only adult subjects were included (i.e., individuals between the ages of 18 and 85 years). The upper cutoff of 85 years was used to eliminate subjects at high risk of not being available for the 1-year treatment duration provided in the study. Only literate subjects and those with a single, unilateral stroke and whose symptoms had lasted for at least 5 days were included in the sample.

Subjects who had a medical condition that interfered with testing or survival were eliminated, as were subjects with a hearing impairment or blindness. Subjects were included if they were referred and tested within 2 to 4 weeks poststroke. Native speakers of English and competent bilinguals for whom treatment in English was appropriate were included. Subjects who achieved an initial WAB Aphasia Quotient score of less than 93.8, the cutoff score defining normal performance, were included in the study.

Random assignment to treatment type resulted in 28 subjects being assigned to LOT. To avoid an imbalance in terms of severity or type of aphasia, assignment was stratified for these variables. Because patients with hemorrhagic strokes appeared to behave differently from those with ischemic stroke, the subject with a hemorrhagic stroke was excluded from data analysis.

Demographic Data of LOT Subjects

Ages of the subjects with aphasia ranged from 28 to 82 years, with a mean age of 62.3 years (Table 28–2). Education ranged from 4 to 21 years of formal education, with a mean of 9.85 years. (In Ontario, 9 years represents completion of the first year of high school.) Socioeconomic status was measured using the Blishen Scale (Blishen & McRoberts, 1976), which rates 500 occupations based on income and education. The mean rating of 38.92 was similar to the mean for a group of 60 older, normal subjects gathered in the area (Shewan & Henderson, 1988). This suggested that the socioeconomic status of the LOT group was similar to that of the general older population. The LOT group was composed of 17 male subjects and 10 female subjects. This ratio of 1.7:1.0 was similar to ratios in other literature reports

TABLE 28–1

Entry and Exit Criteria for Aphasic Subjects

Criterion Variable	Entry Criteria
Age	18–85 years
Education	Literacy by history
Etiology	Infarcts
	Stable intracerebral hemorrhages
	Excluded hemorrhages because of:
	Arteriovenous malformation
	Subarachnoid hemorrhage
	Aneurysm
	Single unilateral strokes
	Transient ischemic attacks (≤5 days) excluded
Medical status	Excluded unstable medical illnesses interfering with testing or survival
Sensory status	Passed hearing screening for age appropriateness
	Blind patients (defined clinically) excluded
	Tactile dysfunction not excluded
Time post-onset	2–4 weeks poststroke
Language severity	Native speakers of English or competent bilinguals for whom treatment in English was appropriate
	Severe language barrier or accent excluded

Criterion Variable	Exit Criteria
Language recovery	Western Aphasia Battery Language Quotient of 94.0 or above
Death	Subject died
Second stroke	Neurologic deficit persisting longer than 5 days
Prolonged illness	Absence or illness longer than 3 weeks duration
Geographic relocation	Subject moved
Voluntary withdrawal	Subject did not wish further treatment and/or tests
Termination of project	Data collection terminated at end of funding period

Treatment of aphasia. A language-oriented approach (p. 246). Austin, TX: Pro-Ed.

(Abu-Zeid, Choi, & Nelson, 1975; Kurtzke, 1976). Most subjects were right-handed, with one left-handed and one ambidextrous person in the group. All subjects received treatment in English. For 22 subjects, English was their only language; five subjects spoke two or more languages, one of which was English.

TABLE 28–2

Demographic Data for 27 LOT Subjects[a]

Variable	Value
Age (years)	
Mean	62.33
Median	63.0
Range	28–82
Education (years)	
Mean	9.85
Median	9.0
Range	4–21
Socioeconomic status	
Mean	38.92
Sex	
Male	17
Female	10
Handedness	
Right	25
Left	1
Ambidextrous	1
Language	
English	22
Polyglot	5
Etiology	
Infarction	27

Treatment of aphasia. A language-oriented approach (p. 249). Austin, TX: Pro-Ed.

Methods and Procedures

All LOT subjects met the entry criteria (Table 28–1) and were tested at periodic intervals by trained, reliable test administrators who were independent of the clinicians providing treatment in the study. Tests occurred 2 to 4 weeks poststroke (Entry Test) and at 3, 6, and 12 months after the first test. A follow-up test at 6 months after termination of treatment also was completed for as many subjects as possible.

The test battery included the WAB (Kertesz & Poole, 1974); the Auditory Comprehension Test for Sentences (Shewan, 1979), or ACTS; Raven's Colored Progressive Matrices (Raven, 1956), or RCPM; and a neurologic examination, with the site and side of lesion confirmed by computed tomography or isotope brain scan. Twenty-six subjects had left-sided lesions, and one had a right-sided lesion. Seventeen subjects showed some hemiplegia, eight were hemianoptic, and 11 demonstrated some hemisensory loss.

Speech and language treatment was initiated as soon after administration of the Entry Test as possible, and always within 7 weeks postonset of aphasia. Treatment was controlled for both duration and intensity. Subjects received treatment for 1 year unless they exited from the study before that time (for exit criteria, see Table 28–1). Intensity of treatment was controlled by providing three 1-hour sessions weekly. The LOT subjects received a mean of 55.3 sessions, with a range of 1 to 118 sessions. Only subjects who received at least 3 months of treatment were included in the efficacy evaluation. Six subjects were lost to follow-up: One died, two relocated geographically, and three withdrew voluntarily.

Treatment was provided by trained speech-language pathologists. Each clinician was trained by C. M. Shewan, the developer of LOT. Before providing LOT in the study, each clinician demonstrated the competence to plan LOT. Competence was assessed by having each clinician design a 1-month LOT patient treatment plan, which passed evaluation by CMS and an independent, external evaluator. At 6-month intervals, each clinician was evaluated by a second independent, external evaluator to ensure that LOT was the treatment type being provided.

Efficacy Data

The efficacy of LOT was demonstrated by comparing the LOT subjects with a no-treatment control (NTC) group. The NTC group contained 22 subjects with aphasia who did not wish to or could not attend treatment. The NTC group was comparable with the LOT group for age, education, socioeconomic status, handedness, language, and etiology. Unlike the LOT group, however, the NTC group contained an equal number of men ($n = 11$) and women ($n = 11$).

Whether LOT resulted in significantly greater language gains compared with no treatment was examined using analysis of covariance, controlling for the initial severity of language impairment. The dependent variable in the comparison was the final test Language Quotient (LQ) score (LQLAST) on the WAB for each subject. The LQ score is a composite of the WAB oral and written language tests (Shewan, 1986). Initial severity was controlled through covarying for initial WAB LQ score (LQENTRY), because the LQ score was designed to be a measure of severity of language impairment, which, in turn, is known to affect language outcome. The LOT had significant positive effects compared with no treatment (Table 28–3) when the Entry Test and the Last Test were compared. The estimate of the difference between LOT and NTC group means, after adjusting for entry score and educational level, was 11.50, with a standard error of 4.71. When age and sex (variables that could possibly influence outcome results) were added as concomitant variables in the analysis of covariance, the results remained essentially the same.

To control for the effects of spontaneous recovery, additional analyses of covariance were performed comparing LQTEST 2 (3 months after the Entry Test) with LQLAST. Again, controlling for initial severity, the analysis of covariance indicated the gains for the LOT group were significantly greater than those for the NTC group (Table 28–3).

TABLE 28–3

Summary of Analyses of Covariance for Language Quotient (LQ) Outcome Measure for Language-Oriented Therapy (LOT) and No-Treatment Control (NTC) Groups[a]

ρ	Estimate of Adjusted Mean Difference	Standard Error
	Entry—Last Test	
≤0.02	11.50	4.75
	Entry—Test 2	
≤0.43	3.93	4.90
	Test 2—Last Test	
≤0.02	5.86	2.19

Treatment of aphasia. A language-oriented approach (p. 254). Austin, TX: Pro-Ed.

The number of subjects within each aphasia type was too small to permit statistical comparisons among groups. Tracking the LQ scores over the course of treatment and through follow-up, however, showed some interesting recovery curves. Because the number of subjects who contributed to the mean LQ score at each test could be different as a result of subjects exiting from the group, the subjects were grouped according to the number of tests that they received and were followed accordingly in streams (Fig. 28–4). When the entire LOT group was considered, gains in the streams were greatest within the first 3 months of treatment. Substantial gains were noted at each test thereafter, and the gains were maintained for the most part for 6 months following treatment. The LQ mean at Test 5 (follow-up) was only 1.4 points lower than that at Test 4 (treatment termination).

Type of Aphasia

For subjects with global aphasia, gains were greatest during the first 3 months, although gains were substantial during the second 3 months as well. After this time, LQ scores plateaued. For the three subjects with follow-up tests, the gains from treatment were maintained. As seen in Figure 28–4, although those with global aphasia did make notable gains, these subjects both started and ended with lower LQ scores compared with those of subjects who had the other types of aphasia.

The subjects with Broca's aphasia made gains throughout the treatment period. As with other groups, the largest gains were during the first 3 months. At follow-up, scores were slightly lower than those at the end of treatment (2.4 points).

The group of subjects with Wernicke's aphasia contained only four subjects, who made substantial gains in the first 3 months of treatment. Because scores for only one subject were available beyond that point, no generalizations can be

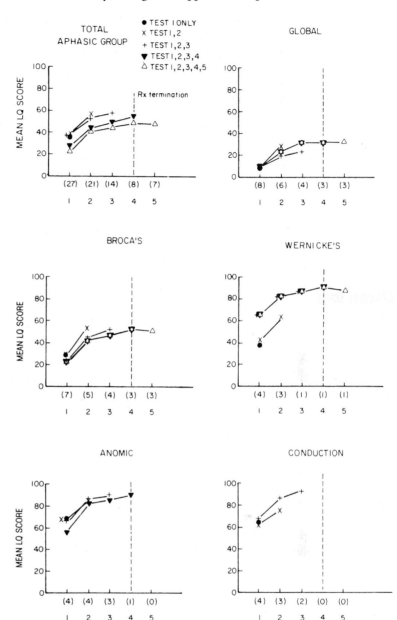

Figure 28–4. Mean Language Quotient (LQ) scores at Tests 1, 2, 3, 4, and 5 for the total Language-Oriented Treatment (LOT) group and the five types of aphasia: global, Broca's, Wernicke's, anomic, and conduction. Patients have been grouped into streams according to the number of tests received. The numbers in parentheses refer to the number of patients included at each test. Termination of treatment (Rx termination) is represented with a dashed line. Test 5 is a follow-up test conducted 6 months after the termination of treatment.

made. This subject did make gains in all treatment periods and showed a slight decline during the 6-month follow-up period.

Subjects with anomic aphasia, as with the other groups, made their greatest gains during the first 3 months, although gains also were substantial during the next 3-month treatment period. The single subject remaining beyond that time made additional gains during the 6- to 12-month period, although no scores at follow-up were available. Overall, gains for the subjects with anomia were nearly 20 LQ points; in general, these subjects were less severely impaired than the subjects with Broca's, Wernicke's or global aphasia.

Individuals with conduction aphasia were among the less severely impaired subjects, as might be expected. In concert with other groups, they made the greatest gains during the first 3 months of treatment. The two subjects remaining at Test 3 (6-month test) were approaching complete recovery (LQ > 94). No scores were available beyond this point.

Severity of Aphasia

The subjects with aphasia were separated into mild, moderate, and severe groups on the basis of the initial test battery, and subjects in these groups were followed in streams,

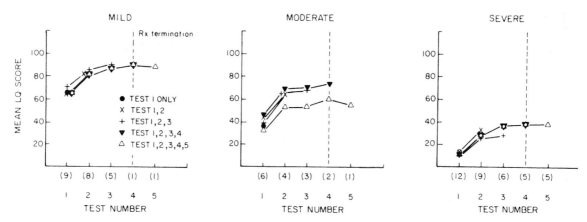

Figure 28–5. Mean Language Quotient (LQ) scores at Tests 1, 2, 3, 4, and 5 for the mild, moderate, and severe groups. Patients have been grouped into streams according to the number of tests received. The numbers in parentheses refer to the number of patients included at each test. Termination of treatment (Rx termination) is represented with a dashed line. Test 5 is a follow-up test conducted 6 months after the termination of treatment.

similar to the analysis for type of aphasia (Fig. 28–5). The group with mild aphasia made visible gains throughout the treatment period, averaging 24.8 LQ points. The greatest gains occurred during the first 3 months of treatment. The single subject with aphasia remaining for the follow-up test showed only a slight decline from the termination of treatment.

Subjects with moderate aphasia showed the greatest LQ gains during the first 3-month period (at least 20 LQ points on average). Scores stabilized for the next 3 months and increased again for the 6-to 12-month treatment period. The mean overall gain for the group was 33.8 LQ points. The one subject available at follow-up showed a moderate decline in the LQ score from the termination of treatment.

The group with severe aphasia, despite obtaining the lowest scores overall, did improve an average of 24.8 points on the LQ. Although greatest in the first 3 months, gains also were seen during the second 3-month treatment period, after which scores leveled off. These gains were maintained at the follow-up test.

FUTURE TRENDS

Language Oriented Treatment was conceived at a time when detailed descriptions of language therapy and its efficacy were sparse. It evolved primarily out of a need to demonstrate that speech-language interventions served as more than just a vehicle for providing emotional and social support to those suffering from aphasia and that our treatment was, in fact, based on scientific principles. Over the last two decades, numerous advances have been made in our understanding of the complexities of the language system,

its interplay with cognition, and how it becomes altered in the face of neurologic insult.

Some of the most exciting discoveries in our field have occurred through the development of technology as it relates to neuroimaging. We are now provided with rich opportunities to better visualize brain lesions and determine how cortical and subcortical areas contribute to language. It remains critical that speech-language pathologists demonstrate a comprehensive understanding of the neural substrates and their relationship to speech and language processes, both in those with intact communication functioning and in those who have been affected by aphasia. As we implement various treatment methods with patients, we have come to observe more directly their impact on the brain's plasticity and the positive outcomes of our therapy.

The fundamental principles of LOT have not changed over time, although the content has become enriched by the proliferation of studies examining language in highly specified ways. An analytical framework continues to be imperative in breaking down the components that underlie the behavioral symptoms of aphasia so that we provide treatment that is customized to the needs of our patients. Most importantly, communication is a highly dynamic and intimate reflection of our personhood, which can and does remain at the forefront of our efforts, even within the context of this highly structured and systematic approach to treatment. Bridging the gap between therapeutic tasks and functional communication can be accomplished through flexibility, ingenuity, and successful engagement of our patients and their significant others in achieving mutually determined and achievable goals.

1. Aphasia represents impairment in the processes for understanding and producing language.
2. Language-Oriented Treatment is a psycholinguistic approach to intervention, applying research information about normal language processing and the impairments associated with aphasia.
3. Identification and understanding of the substrates affected by neurologic damage and their contribution to language are fundamental in developing a treatment plan that is customized for the patient.
4. The patient and significant others play central roles in determining treatment goals, activities and expectations.
5. Language-Oriented Treatment is organized according to content, reflecting potential areas of focus within five language modalities.
6. Activities incorporate a hierarchy of difficulty levels, both within and across areas, based on the analysis of strengths and deficits.
7. Treatment approaches that have proven to be beneficial in large and small group investigations as well as in single-case studies are incorporated when applicable to a particular patient.
8. Language-Oriented Treatment was proven to be efficacious in a full-scale clinical trial incorporating a NTC group.
9. Through systematic treatment of the underlying deficits, functional improvements in language can result from a LOT approach.

References

Abu-Zeid, H. A. H., Choi, N. W., & Nelson, N. A. (1975). Epidemiologic features of cerebrovascular disease in Manitoba: Incidence by age, sex and residence, with etiologic implications. *Canadian Medical Association Journal, 113,* 379–384.

Aftonomos, L. B., Steele, R. D., & Wertz, R. T. (1997). Promoting recovery in chronic aphasia with an interactive technology. *Archives of Physical Medicine and Rehabilitation, 78,* 841–846.

Albert, M. (1998). Treatment of aphasia. *Archives of Neurology, 55,* 1417–1419.

Arguin, M., & Bub, D. (1994). Pure alexia: Attempted rehabilitation and its implications for interpretation of the deficit. *Brain and Language, 47,* 233–268.

Aronson, M., Shatin, L., & Cook, J. (1956). Sociopsychotherapeutic approach to the treatment of aphasia. *Journal of Speech and Hearing Disorders, 21,* 325–364.

Backus, O. (1952). The use of a group structure in speech therapy. *Journal of Speech and Hearing Disorders, 17,* 116–122.

Baldo, J. V., Dronkers, N. F., Wilkins, D., Ludy, C., Raskins, P., & Kim, J. (2005). Is problem solving dependent on language? *Brain and Language, 92,* 240–250.

Ballard, K. J. & Thompson, C. K. (1999). Treatment and generalization of complex sentence production in agrammatism. *Journal of Speech, Language and Hearing Research. 42*(3),690–707.

Bandur, D. L., Parrent, A. G., & Steven, D. A. (2006). A tailored approach to language mapping in epilepsy surgery: Some preliminary findings. *Journal of Medical Speech-Language Pathology, in press.*

Basso, A., Capitani, E., & Vignolo, L. A. (1979). Influence of rehabilitation on language skills in aphasia patients: A controlled study. *Archives of Neurology, 36,* 190–196.

Basso, A., Faglioni, P., & Vignolo, L. A. (1975). Etudee controlee de la reeducation du language dans l'aphasie: Comparaison entre aphasiques traites et nontraites. *Revue Neurologique, 131,* 607–614.

Beeson, P. M., Rapcsak, S. Z., Plante, E., Chargualaf, J., Chung, A., Johnson, S. C., et al. (2003). The neural substrates of writing: A functional magnetic resonance imaging study. *Aphasiology, 17*(6/7), 647–665.

Beeson, P. M., Holland, A. L., & Murray, L. L. (1997). Naming famous people: An examination of tip-of-the-tongue phenomena in aphasia and Alzheimer's disease. *Aphasiology, 11,* 323–336.

Belin, P., Van Eekhout, P., Zilbovicius, M., Remy, P., Francois, C., Guillaume, S., et al. (1996). Recovery from nonfluent aphasia after melodic intonation therapy: A PET study. *Neurology, 47*(6), 1504–1511.

Benson, D. F. (1979). *Aphasia, alexia, and agraphia.* New York: Churchill Livingstone.

Benson, D. F., & Geschwind, N. (1969). The alexias. In P. J. Vinken & G. Bruyn (Eds.), *Handbook of clinical neurology* (Vol. 4). Amsterdam: North Holland.

Benton, A. L., Smith, K. C., & Lang, M. (1972). Stimulus characteristics and object naming in aphasic patients. *Journal of Communication Disorders, 5,* 19–24.

Berndt, R. S., Haendiges, A. N., & Mitchum, C. C. (2005). Orthographic effects in the word substitutions of aphasic patients: An epidemic of right neglect dyslexia? *Brain and Language, 93,* 55–63.

Berndt, R. S., Burton, M. W., Haendiges, A. N., & Mitchum, C. (2002). Production of nouns and verbs in aphasia: Effects of elicitation context. *Aphasiology, 16*(1/2), 83–106.

Berndt, R. S., Mitchum, C. C., Haendiges, A., & Sandson, J. (1997). Verb retrieval in aphasia. *Brain and Language, 56,* 68–106.

Best, W., Herbert, R., Hickin, J., Osborne, F., & Howard, D. (2002) Phonological and orthographic facilitation of word-retrieval in aphasia: Immediate and delayed effects. *Aphasiology, 16*(1/2), 151–168.

Beveridge, M. A., & Crerar, M. A. (2002). Remediation of asyntactic sentence comprehension using a multimedia microworld. *Brain and Language, 82,* 243–295.

Bhogal, S. K., Teasell, R., & Speechley, M. (2003). Intensity of aphasia therapy, impact on recovery. *Stroke, 34,* 987–992.

Bisiach, E. (1966). Perceptual factors in the pathogenesis of anomia. *Cortex, 2,* 90–95.

Blackman, N. (1950). Group psychotherapy with aphasics. *Journal of Nervous and Mental Disorders, 111,* 154–163.

Blackman, N., & Tureen, L. L. (1948). Aphasia-psychosomatic approach in rehabilitation. *Transactions of the American Neurology Association, 73,* 193–196.

Blishen, B. R., & McRoberts, H. A. (1976). A revised socioeconomic index for occupations in Canada. *Canadian Review of Sociology and Anthropology 13*, 71–73.

Boles, L. (1998). Conducting conversation: A case study using the spouse in aphasia treatment. *Neurophysiology and Neurogenic Speech and Language Disorders (Newsletter)*, September, 24–30.

Boller, F., & Green, E. (1972). Comprehension in severe aphasia. *Cortex, 8*, 382–394.

Breedin, S., Saffron, E., & Schwartz, M. (1998). Semantic factors in verb retrieval: An effect of complexity. *Brain and Language, 63*, 1–31.

Brindley, P., Copeland, M., Demain, C., & Martyn, P. (1989). A comparison of the speech of ten chronic Broca's aphasics following intensive and non-intensive periods of therapy. *Aphasiology, 3*, 695–707.

Brookshire, R. H., & Nicholas, L. E. (1994). Speech sample size and test-retest stability of connected speech measures for adults with aphasia. *Journal of Speech, Language, and Hearing Research, 37*, 399–407.

Broida, H. (1977). Language therapy effects in long term aphasia. *Archives of Physical Medicine and Rehabilitation, 58*, 248–253.

Bruce, C., Edmundson, A., & Coleman, M. (2003). Writing with voice: An investigation of the use of a voice recognition system as a writing aid for a man with aphasia. *International Journal of Language and Communication Disorders, 38*(2), 131–148.

Burbaum, L. J. & Coslett, H. B. (1996). Deep dyslexic phenomena in a letter-by-letter reader. *Brain and Language, 54*, 136–167.

Buck, R., & Duffy, R. J. (1980). Nonverbal communication of affect in brain-damaged patients. *Cortex, 16*, 351–362.

Burgio, F., & Basso, A. (1997). Memory and aphasia. *Neuropsychologia, 35*, 759–766.

Byng, S. (1992). Testing the tried: Replicating sentence-processing therapy for agrammatic Broca's aphasia. *Clinical Communication Disorders, 2*, 34–42.

Byng, S., & Black, M. (1995). What makes a therapy? Some parameters of therapeutic intervention in aphasia. *European Journal of Disorders of Communication, 30*, 303–316.

Byng, S., Nickels, L., & Black, M. (1994). Replicating therapy for mapping deficits in agrammatism: Remapping the deficit? *Aphasiology, 8*, 315–341.

Calvert, G. A., Brammer, M. J., Morris, R. G., Williams, S. C. R., King, N., & Mattews, P. M. (2000). Using fMRI to study recovery from acquired dysphasia. *Brain and Language, 71*, 391–399.

Cannito, M. P., Hough, M., Vogel, S., & Pierce, R. S. (1996). Contextual influences on auditory comprehension of reversible passive sentences in aphasia. *Aphasiology, 10*, 235–251.

Cao, Y., Vikingstad, E. M., George, P., Johnson, A., & Welch, K. M. A. (1999). Cortical language activation in stroke patients recovering from aphasia with functional MRI. *Stroke, 30*, 2331–2340.

Cappa, S. F. (2000). Recovery from aphasia: Why and how? *Brain and Language, 71*, 39–41.

Caplan, D., Waters, G., & Hildebrandt, N. (1997). Determinants of sentence comprehension in aphasic patients in sentence picture matching tasks. *Journal of Speech, Language, and Hearing Research, 40*, 542–555.

Chang, A., & MacKenzie, A. (1998). State self-esteem following stroke. *Stroke, 29*, 2325–2328.

Chapey, R. (2001). Cognitive stimulation: Stimulation of recognition/comprehension, memory, and convergent, divergent, and evaluative thinking. In R. Chapey (Ed.), *Language intervention strategies in aphasia and related neurogenic communication disorders*. (pp. 397–434). Baltimore, MD: Lippincott Williams & Wilkins.

Chapey, R., Duchan, J. F., Elman, R. J., Garcia, L. J., Kagan, A., Lyon, J., et al. (2000). Life participation approach to aphasia: A statement of values for the future. *The ASHA Leader, 5*(3), 4–6.

Chapman, S. B., & Ulatowska, H. K. (1989). Discourse in aphasia: Integration deficits in processing reference. *Brain and Language, 36*, 651–669.

Chapman, S. B. & Ulatowska, H. K. (1992). Methodology for discourse management in the treatment of aphasia. *Clinical Communication Disorders, 2*, 64–81.

Chapman, S. B., Ulatowska, H. K., Franklin, L. R., Shobe, A. E., Thompson, J. L., & McIntire, D. D. (1997). Proverb interpretation in fluent aphasia and Alzheimer's disease: Implications beyond abstract thinking. *Aphasiology, 11*, 337–350.

Cherney, L. R., Merbitz, C. T., & Grip, J. C. (1986). Efficacy of oral reading in aphasia treatment outcome. *Rehabilitation Literature, 47*(5–6), 112–118.

Clausen, N. S. & Beeson, P. M. (2003). Conversational use of writing in severe aphasia: A group treatment approach. *Aphasiology, 17*(6/7), 625–644.

Coelho, C. A. (1990). Acquisition and generalization of simple manual sign grammars by aphasic subjects. *Journal of Communication Disorders, 23*, 383–400.

Coelho, C. A., & Duffy, R. J. (1986). Effects on iconicity, motoric complexity, and linguistic function on sign acquisition in severe aphasia. *Perceptual and Motor Skills, 63*, 519–530.

Coelho, C. A., & Duffy, R. J. (1987). The relationship of the acquisition of manual signs to severity of aphasias: A training study. *Brain and Language, 31*, 328–345.

Correia, L., Brookshire, R. H., & Nicholas, L. E. (1990). Aphasic and non-brain-damaged adults' descriptions of aphasic test pictures and gender biased pictures. *Journal of Speech and Hearing Disorders, 55*, 713–720.

Coslett, H. B., Saffran, E. M., Greenbaum, S., & Schwartz, H. (1993). Reading in pure alexia. *Brain, 116*, 21–37.

Dabul, B., & Hanson, W. R. (1975, October). *The amount of language improvement in adult aphasics related to early and late treatment*. Paper presented at the annual convention of the American Speech Language and Hearing Association, Washington, DC.

Damasio, H. Tranel, D., Grabowski, T., Adolphs, R., & Damasio, A. (2004). Neural systems behind word and concept retrieval. *Cognition, 92*, 179–229.

Daniloff, J. K., Noll, J. D., Fristoe, M., & Lloyd, L. L. (1982). Gestural recognition in patients with aphasia. *Journal of Speech and Hearing Disorders, 47*, 43–49.

Darley, F. L. (1982). *Aphasia*. Philadelphia: W. B. Saunders.

David, R., Enderby, P., & Bainton, D. (1982). Treatment of acquired aphasia: Speech therapists and volunteers compared. *Journal of Neurology, Neurosurgery, and Psychiatry, 45*, 957–961.

Davis, G. A., & Wilcox, M. J. (1981). Incorporating parameters of natural conversation in aphasia treatment. In R. Chapey (Ed.), *Language intervention strategies in adult aphasia*. Baltimore, MD: Lippincott Williams & Wilkins.

De Renzi, E., & Lucchelli, F. (1994). Are semantic systems separately represented in the brain? The case of living category impairment. *Cortex, 30,* 3–25.

Deal, J. L., & Deal, L. A. (1978). Efficacy of aphasia rehabilitation: Preliminary results. In R. H. Brookshire (Ed.), *Clinical aphasiology: Conference proceedings* (pp. 66–77). Minneapolis: BRK.

Del Grosso Destreri, N., Farina, E., Alberoni, M., Pomati, S., Nichelli, P., & Mariani, C. (2000). Selective uppercase dysgraphia with loss of visual imagery of letter forms: A window on the organization of graphomotor patterns. *Brain and Language, 71,* 353–372.

Dell, G. S., Schwartz, M. F., Martin, N., Saffran, E. M., & Gagnon, D. A. (1997) Lexical access in aphasic and nonaphasic speakers. *Psychological Review, 104,* 801–838.

Doesborgh, S. J. C., Van de Sandt-Koenderman, W. M., Dippel, D. W. J., van Harshamp, F., Koudstaal, P. J., & Visch-Brink, E. G. (2004). Cues on request: The efficacy of multicue, a computer program for wordfinding therapy. *Aphasiology, 18*(3), 213–222.

Duffy, R., Watt, J., & Duffy, J. R. (1994). Testing causal theories of pantomimic deficits in aphasia using path analysis. *Aphasiology, 8,* 361–379.

Easterbrook, A., Brown, B. B., & Perera, K. (1982). A comparison of the speech of adult aphasic subjects in spontaneous and structured interactions. *British Journal of Disorders of Communication, 17,* 93–107.

Egan, J., Worrall, L., & Oxenham, D. (2004). Accessible internet training package helps people with aphasia cross the digital divide. *Aphasiology 18*(3), 265–280.

Eisenson, J. (1949). Prognostic factors related to language rehabilitation in aphasic patients. *Journal of Speech Disorders, 14,* 262–264.

Eisenson, J. (1984). *Adult aphasia* (2nd ed.). Englewood Cliffs, NJ: Prentice-Hall.

Ellis, A. W. (1982). Spelling and writing (and reading and speaking). In A. W. Ellis (Ed.), *Normality and pathology in cognitive functions.* London: Academic Press.

Ellis, A. W. (1988). Normal writing processes and peripheral acquired dysgraphias. *Language and Cognitive Processes, 3*(2), 99–127.

Ferguson, A. (1998). Conversational turn-taking and repair in fluent aphasia. *Aphasiology, 12,* 1007–1031.

Fletcher, P. C., Happe, F., Frith, U., Baker, S. C., Dolan, R. J., Frackowiak, R. S. J., et al. (1995). Other minds in the brain: A functional imaging study of "theory of mind" in story comprehension. *Cognition, 57,* 109–128.

Franz. S. I. (1906). The reeducation of an aphasic. *Journal of Philosophy, Psychology and Scientific Methods, 2,* 589–597.

Franz, S. I. (1924). Studies in re-education: The aphasics. *Journal of Comparative Psychology, 4,* 349–429.

Frazier, C. H., & Ingham, D. (1920). A review of the effects of gunshot wounds of the head. *Archives of Neurology and Psychiatry, 3,* 17–40.

Freedman-Stern R., Ulatowska, H. K., Baker, T., & Delacoste, C. (1984). Description of written language in aphasia: A case study. *Brain and Language, 22,* 181–205.

Friederici, A. D., Schonle, P. W., & Goodglass, H. (1981). Mechanisms underlying writing and speech in aphasia. *Brain and Language, 13,* 212–222.

Friedman, R. (1995). Two types of phonological alexia. *Cortex, 31,* 397–403.

Gardner, H., & Winner, E. (1978). A study of repetition in aphasic patients. *Brain and Language, 6,* 168–178.

Germani, M. J., & Pierce, R. S. (1992). Contextual influences in reading comprehension in aphasia. *Brain and Language, 42,* 308–319.

Gernsbacher, M. A., & Kaschak, M. P. (2003). Neuroimaging studies of language production and comprehension. *Annual Review of Psychology, 54,* 91–114.

Ghidella, C. L., Murray, S. J., Smart, M. J., McKenna, K. T., & Worrall, L. E. (2005). Aphasia websites: An examination of their quality and communicative accessibility. *Aphasiology, 19*(12), 1134–1146.

Glosser, G., Wiener, M.. & Kaplan, E. (1986). Communicative gestures in aphasia. *Brain and Language, 27,* 345–359.

Goldrick, M., & Rapp, B. (2002). A restricted interaction account (RIA) of spoken word production: The best of both worlds. *Aphasiology, 16*(1–2), 20–55.

Goodglass, H. (1968). Studies on the grammar of aphasics. In S. Rosenberg & J. Koplin (Eds.), *Developments in applied psycholinguistic research* (pp. 77–208). New York: Macmillan.

Goodglass, H. (1975). Phonological factors in aphasia. In R. H. Brookshire (Ed.), *Clinical aphasiology: Conference proceedings* (pp. 132–144). Minneapolis: BRK.

Goodglass, H. (1976). Agrammatism. In H. Whitaker & H. A. Whitaker (Eds.), *Studies in neurolinguistics* (Vol. 1, pp. 237–260). New York: Academic Press.

Goodglass, H. (1993). *Understanding aphasia.* San Diego: Academic Press.

Goodglass, H., & Berko, J. (1960). Aphasia and inflectional morphology in English. *Journal of Speech and Hearing Research, 10,* 257–262.

Goodglass, H., & Kaplan, E. (1972). *The assessment of aphasia and related disorders.* Philadelphia: Lea & Febiger.

Goodglass, H., & Kaplan, E. (1983). *The assessment of aphasia and related disorders* (2nd ed.). Philadelphia: Lea & Febiger.

Goodglass, H., Klein, B., Carey, P. W., & Jones, K. J. (1966). Specific semantic word categories in aphasia. *Cortex, 2,* 74–89.

Goodglass, H., & Wingfield, A. (1993). Selective preservation of a lexical category in aphasia: Dissociations in comprehension of body parts and geographical place names following focal brain lesion. *Memory, I*(4), 313–328.

Green, E., & Boller, F. (1974). Features of auditory comprehension in severely impaired aphasics. *Cortex, 10,* 133–145.

Hagen, C. (1973). Communication abilities in hemiplegia: Effect of speech therapy. *Archives of Physical Medicine and Rehabilitation, 54,* 454–463.

Hanley, J. R. & Peters, S. (1996). A dissociation between the ability to print and write cursively in lower-case letters. *Cortex, 32,* 737–745.

Heaton, R., Chelune, G. J., Talley, J. L., Kay, G. G., & Curtis, G. (1993). *Wisconsin Card Sorting Test (WCST) manual: Revised and expanded.* Odessa, FL: Psychological Assessment Resources.

Helm, N. A., & Barresi, B. (1980). Voluntary control of involuntary utterances: A treatment approach for severe aphasia. In R. Brookshire (Ed.), *Clinical aphasiology: Conference proceedings.* Minneapolis: BRK.

Helm-Estabrooks, N. (1981). *Helm elicited language program for syntax simulation.* Austin, TX: Exceptional Resources.

Helm-Estabrooks, N. (1983). Approaches to treating subcortical aphasias. In W. Perkins (Ed.), *Current therapy of communication disorders* (pp. 97–103). New York: Thieme-Stratton.

Helm-Estabrooks, N. (1988). The application of neurobehavioral research to aphasia rehabilitation. *Aphasiology, 2,* 303–308.

Helm-Estabrooks, N. (1998). A cognitive approach to treatment of an aphasic patient. In N. Helm-Estabrooks & A. L.Holland (Eds.). *Approaches to the treatment of aphasia.* San Diego: Singular.

Helm-Estabrooks, N. (2001) *Cognitive Linguistic Quick Test.* San Antonio, TX: The Psychological Corporation.

Helm-Estabrooks, N. (2002). Cognition and aphasia: A discussion and a study. *Journal of Communication Disorders, 35,* 171–186.

Helm-Estabrooks, N., & Albert, M. (1991). *Manual of aphasia therapy.* Austin, TX: Pro-Ed.

Helm-Estabrooks, N., Fitzpatrick, P., & Barresi, B. (1982). Visual action therapy for global aphasia. *Journal of Speech and Hearing Disorders, 44,* 385–389.

HeIm-Estabrooks, N., Ramsberger, G., Brownell, H., & Albert, M. (1989). Distal versus proximal movement in limb apraxia (Abstract). *Journal of Clinical and Experimental Neuropsychology, 7,* 608.

Helm-Estabrooks, N., Ramsberger, G., Morgan, A., & Nicholas, M. (1989). *Boston Assessment of Severe Aphasia.* Austin, TX: Pro-Ed.

Hengst, J. (2003). Collaborative referencing between individuals with aphasia and routine communication partners. *Journal of Speech, Language and Hearing Research.* 46, 831–848.

Hengst, J. A. Frame, S. R., Neuman-Strizel, T., & Gannaway, R. (2005). Using others' words: Conversational use of reported speech by individuals with aphasia and their communication partners. (2005). *Journal of Speech, Language and Hearing Research.* 48(1), 137–156.

Herrmann, M., Reichle, T., Lucius-Hoene, G., Wallesch, C.- W., & Johannsen-Horbach, H. (1988). Nonverbal communication as a compensatory strategy for severely nonfluent aphasics? A quantitative approach. *Brain and Language, 33,* 41–54.

Hickin, J., Best, W., Herber, R., Howard, D., & Osborne, F. (2002). Phonological therapy for word-finding difficulties: A re-evaluation. *Aphasiology 16(10/11),* 981–900.

Hillis, A. (1992). Facilitating written production. *Clinical Communication Disorders, 2,* 19–33.

Hillis, A. E., Kane, A., Barker, P., Beauchamp, B. G., & Wityk, R. (2001). Neural substrates of the cognitive processes underlying reading: Evidence from magnetic resonance perfusion imaging in hyperacute stroke. *Aphasiology, 15(10/11),* 919–931.

Hillis, A. E., Kane, A., Turfiash, E., Beauchamp, B. G., Barker, P., Jacobs, M. A., & Wityk, R. J. (2002). Neural substrates of the cognitive processes underlying spelling: Evidence from MR diffusion and perfusion imaging. *Aphasiology, 16(4/5/6),* 425–438.

Hillis, A. E., Chang, S., Breese, E., & Heider, J. (2004). The crucial role of posterior frontal regions in modality specific components of the spelling process. *Neurocase, 10(2),* 175–187.

Hillis, A. E., Newhart, M., Heidler, J., Barker, P., Herskovits, E., & Degaonkar, M. (2005). The role of the "visual word form area" in reading. *Neuroimage, 24,* 548–559.

Holland, A. (1991). Pragmatic aspects of intervention in aphasia. *Journal of Neurolinguistics, 6,* 197–211.

Holland, A. L., Fromm, D. S., De Ruyter, F., & Stein, M. (1996). Treatment efficacy: Aphasia. *Journal of Speech, Language, and Hearing Research, 39,* S27–S36.

Holland, A. L., & Wertz, R. T. (1988). Measuring aphasia treatment effects: Large-group, small-group, and single-subject designs. In F. Plum (Ed.), *Language, communication, and the brain.* New York: Raven Press.

Hopper, T., Holland, A., & Rewega, M. (2002). Conversational coaching: Treatment outcomes and future directions. *Aphasiology, 16(7),* 745–761.

Hough, M. S. & Pierce, R. S. (1994). Pragmatics and treatment. In R. Chapey (Ed.), *Language intervention strategies in adult aphasia* (pp. 246–268). Baltimore, MD: Lippincott Williams &Wilkins.

Howard, D., Best, W., Bruce, C., & Gatehouse, C. (1995). Operativity and animacy effects in aphasic naming. *European Journal of Disorders of Communication, 30,* 286–302.

Howard, D., & Smith, K. (2002). The effects of lexical stress in aphasic word production. *Aphasiology, 16(1/2),* 198–237.

Huntley, R. A., Pindzola, R., & Werdner, W. (1986). The effectiveness of simultaneous cues on naming disturbance in aphasia. *Journal of Communication Disorders, 19,* 261–270.

Jacobs, B. (2001). Social validity of changes in informativeness and efficiency of aphasic discourse following Linguistic Specific Treatment (LST). *Brain and Language 78,* 115–127.

Kagan, A., Black, S. E., Duchan, J. F., Simmons-Mackie, N., & Square, P. (2001). Training volunteers as conversation partner using "Supported Conversation for Adults with aphasia" (SCA): A controlled trial. *Journal of Speech, Language and Hearing Research, 44,* 624–638.

Katz, R., & Wertz, R. T. (1997). The efficacy of computer-provided reading treatment for chronic aphasic adults. *Journal of Speech, Language, and Hearing Research, 40,* 493–507.

Kellar, L. A. (1978). *Stress and syntax in aphasia.* Paper presented at the Academy of Aphasia, Chicago, IL.

Kertesz, A., & Poole, E. (1974). The aphasia quotient: The taxonomic approach to measurement of aphasic disability. *Canadian Journal of Neurological Sciences, 1,* 7–16.

Kurtzke, J. F. (1976). An introduction to the epidemiology of cerebrovascular disease. In P. Scheinberg (Ed.), *Cerebrovascular diseases: Tenth Princeton Conference.* New York: Raven Press.

Lambon Ralph, M., Braber, N., McClelland, J. L., & Patterson, K. (2005). What underlies the neuropsychological pattern of irregular:regular past-tense verb production? *Brain and Language, 93,* 106–119.

Langmore, S. E., & Canter, G. J. (1983). Written spelling deficit of Broca's aphasics. *Brain and Language, 18,* 293–314.

Le Dorze, G., & Brassard, C. (1995). A description of the consequences of aphasia on aphasic persons and their relatives and friends, based on the WHO model of chronic diseases. *Aphasiology, 9,* 239–255.

Lecours, A. R. (1999). Frank Benson's teachings of acquired disorders of written language (with addenda). *Aphasiology, 13,* 21–40.

Leger, A., Demonet, J.- F., Ruff, B., Aithamon, B., Touyeras, B., Puel, M., et al. (2002). Neural substrates of spoken language rehabilitation in an aphasic patient: An fMRI study. *NeuroImage. 17,* 174–183.

Levelt, W. J. M., Roelofs. A., & Myers, A. S. (1999). A theory of lexical access in speed production. *Behavioral and Brain Sciences, 22,* 1–75.

Li, E. C., Kitselman, K., Dusatko, D., & Spinelli, C. (1988). The efficacy of PACE in remediation of naming deficits. *Journal of Communication Disorders, 21*, 491–503.

Li, E. C., Volpe, A. D., Ritterman, S., & Williams, S. E. (1996). Variations in grammatic complexity across three types of discourse. *Journal of Speech-Language Pathology and Audiology, 30*, 180–186.

Li, E. C., & Williams S. E. (1990). The effects of grammatic class and cue type on cueing responsiveness in aphasia. *Brain and Language, 38*, 48–60.

Lott, S. L., Friedman, R. B., & Linebaugh, C. W. (1994). Rationale and efficacy of a tactile-kinesthetic treatment for alexia. *Aphasiology, 8*, 181–195.

Lu, L. H., Crosson, B., Nadeau, S. E., Heilman, K. M., Gonzalez-Rothi, L. J., Raymenr, A., et al. (2002) Category-specific naming deficits for objects and actions: semantic attribute and grammatical role hypotheses. *Neuropsychologia, 40*, 1608–1621.

Ludlow, C. L. (1973). *The recovery of syntax in aphasia: An analysis of syntactic structures used in connected speech during the initial recovery period.* Unpublished doctoral dissertation. New York University.

Lyon, J. G. (1995). Drawing: Its value as a communication aid for adults with aphasia. *Aphasiology, 9*, 33–50.

Margolin, D. I. (1984). The neuropsychology of writing and spelling: Semantic, phonological, motor and perceptual processes. *Quarterly Journal of Experimental Psychology, 36A*, 459–489.

Marshall, J. (1995). The mapping hypothesis and aphasia therapy. *Aphasiology, 9*, 517–539.

Marshall, R. C., Karow, C. M., Freed, D. B., Babcock, P. (2002). Effects of personalized cue form on the learning of subordinate category names by aphasic and non-brain-damaged subjects. *Aphasiology, 16(7)*, 763–771.

Marshall, J., Robson, J., Pring, T., & Chiat, S. (1998). Why does monitoring fail in jargon aphasia? Comprehension, judgment and therapy evidence. *Brain and Language, 63*, 79–107.

Martin, N., & Saffran, E., (2002). The relationship of input and output phonological processing: An evaluation of models and evidence to support them. *Aphasiology, 16 (1/2)*, 107–150.

Martin, R. C. (2003). Language processing: Functional organization and neuroanatomical basis. *Annual Review of Psychology, 54*, 55–89.

McCall, D., Cox, D. M., Shelton, J. R., & Weinrich, M. (1997). The influence of syntactic and semantic information on picture-naming performance in aphasic persons. *Aphasiology, 11*, 581–600.

McCleary, C., & Hirst, W. (1986). Semantic classification in aphasia: A study of basic superordinate and functional relations. *Brain and Language, 27*, 199–209.

Meikle, M., Wechsler, E., Tupper, A., Benenson, M., Butler, J., Mulhally, D., & Stern, G. (1979). Comparative trial of volunteer and professional treatments of dysphasia after stroke. *British Medical Journal, 2*, 87–89.

Mills, C. K. (1904). Treatment of aphasia by training. *Journal of American Medical Association, 43*, 1940–1949.

Mitchum, C. C., & Berndt, R. S. (1995). The cognitive neuropsychological approach to treatment of language disorders. *Neuropsychological Rehabilitation, 5*, 1–16.

Mortley, J., Wade, J., & Enderby, P. (2004). Superhighway to promoting a client-therapist partnership? Using the internet to deliver word-retrieval computer therapy, monitored remotely with minimal speech and language therapy input. *Aphasiology 18(3)*, 193–211.

Moyer, S. B. (1979). Rehabilitation of alexia: A case study. *Cortex, 15(1)*, 139–144.

Murray, L. (1999). Attention and aphasia: Theory, research, and clinical implications. (Review). *Aphasiology, 13*, 91–111.

Murray, L. L. (2004). Cognitive treatments for aphasia: Should we and can we help attention and working memory problems? *Journal of Medical Speech-Language Pathology, 12(3)*, xxv–xi.

Murray, L. L., Keeton, R. J., & Karcher, L. (2006). Treating attention in mild aphasia: Evaluation of attention process training-11. *Journal of Communication Disorders, 39*, 37–61.

Naeser, M. A., Baker, E. H., Palumbo, C., Nicholas, M., Alexander, M. P., Samaraweera, R., et al. (1998). Lesion site patterns in severe, nonverbal aphasia to predict outcome with a computer-assisted treatment program. *Archives of Neurology, 55*, 1438–1448.

Netsu, R., & Marguardt, T. P. (1984). Pantomime in aphasia: Effects of stimulus characteristics. *Journal of Communication Disorders, 17*, 37–46.

Nickels, L. (1995). Reading too little into reading?: Strategies in the rehabilitation of acquired dyslexia. *European Journal of Disorders of Communication, 30*, 37–50.

Nickels, L. (2002) Therapy for naming disorders: Revisiting, revising, and reviewing. *Aphasiology, 16(10/11)*, 935–979.

Nicholas, L. E., & Brookshire, R. H. (1995a). Presence, completeness, and accuracy of main concepts in the connected speech of non-brain-damaged adults and adults with aphasia. *Journal of Speech, Language, and Hearing Research, 38*, 145–156.

Nicholas, L. E., & Brookshire, R. H. (1995b). Comprehension of spoken narrative discourse by adults with aphasia, right-hemisphere brain damage or traumatic brain damage. *American Journal of Speech-Language Pathology, 4*, 69–81.

Nippold, M. A., Uhden, L. D., & Schwarz, I. E. (1997). Proverb explanation through the lifespan: A developmental study of adolescents and adults. *Journal of Speech, Language, and Hearing Research, 40*, 245–253.

Pashek, G. V., & Brookshire, R. H. (1980). Effects of rate of speech and linguistic stress on auditory paragraph comprehension of aphasic individuals. In R. H. Brookshire (Ed.), *Clinical aphasiology: Conference proceedings* (pp. 64–65, Abstract). Minneapolis: BRK.

Perkins, L. (1995). Applying conversation analysis to aphasia: Clinical implications and analytic issues. *European Journal of Disorders of Communication, 30*, 372–383.

Petheram, B. (1996). Exploring the home-based use of microcomputers in aphasia therapy. *Aphasiology, 10*, 267–282.

Pierce, R. S. (1988). Influence of prior and subsequent context on comprehension in aphasia. *Aphasiology, 2(6)*, 577–582.

Pierce, R., & Grogan, S. (1992). Improving listening comprehension of narratives. *Clinical Communication Disorders, 2*, 54–63.

Pierce, R. S., Jarecki, J., & Cannito, M. (1990). Single word comprehension in aphasia: Influence of array size, picture relatedness and situational context. *Aphasiology, 4(2)*, 155–156.

Poeck, K, Huber, W., & Willmes, K. (1989). Outcome of intensive language treatment in aphasia. *Journal of Speech and Hearing Disorders, 54*, 471–478.

Porch, B. E. (1967). *Porch index of communicative ability.* Palo Alto, CA: Consulting Psychologists Press.

Prins, R. S., Snow, C. E., & Wagenaar, E. (1978). Recovery from aphasia: Spontaneous speech versus language comprehension. *Brain and Language, 6,* 192–211.

Ramsberger, G. (1996). Repetition of emotional and nonemotional words in aphasia. *Journal of Medical Speech-Language Pathology, 4,* 1–12.

Rao, P. L. (1994). Use of amer-ind code by persons with aphasia. In R. Chapey (Ed.), *Language intervention strategies in adult aphasia* (pp. 359–367). Baltimore, MD: Lippincott Williams & Wilkins.

Rapcsak, S. Z., & Beeson, P. M. (2004). The role of left posterior inferior temporal cortex in spelling. *Neurology, 62,* 2221–2229.

Rapp, B., & Kane, A. (2002). Remediation of deficits affecting different components of the spelling process. *Aphasiology, 16*(4/5/6), 439–454.

Raven, J. (1956). *Coloured Progressive Matrices: Sets A, A, B (revised order).* London: Lewis and Company Limited.

Raymer, A. M., Cudworth, C., & Haley, M. A. (2003). Spelling treatment for an individual with dysgraphia: Analysis of generalization to untrained words. *Aphasiology, 17*(6/7), 607–624.

Robey, R. R., Schultz, M. C., Crawford, A. B., & Sinner, C. A. (1998). Single-subject clinical-outcome research: Designs, data, effect sizes, and analyses. *Aphasiology, 13,* 445–473.

Robson, J., Marshall, J., Chiat, S., & Pring, T. (2001). Enhancing communication in jargon aphasia: A small group study of writing therapy. *International Journal of Language and Communication Disorders, 36*(4), 471–488.

Rochon, E., Laird, L., Bose, A., & Scofield, J. (2005). Mapping therapy for sentence production impairments in nonfluent aphasia. *Neuropsychological Rehabilitation, 15*(1), 1–36.

Rose, M., & Douglas, J. (2003). Limb apraxia, panatomine, and lexical gesture in aphasic speakers: Preliminary findings, *Aphasiology, 17*(5), 453–464.

Sage, K., Hesketh, A., & Ralph, M. A. L. (2005). Using errorless learning to treat letter-by-letter reading: Contrasting word versus letter-based therapy. *Neuropsychological Rehabilitation, 15*(5), 616–642.

Sarno, M. T. (1997). Quality of life in aphasia in the first post-stroke year. *Aphasiology, 11,* 665–679.

Sarno, M. T., Silverman, M., & Sands, E. S. (1970). Speech therapy and language recovery in severe aphasia. *Journal of Speech and Hearing Research, 13,* 607–623.

Schlanger, P. H., & Freemann, R. (1979). Pantomime therapy with aphasics. *Aphasia-Apraxia-Agnosia, 1,* 34–39.

Schmalzl, L., & Nickels, L. (2006). Treatment of irregular word spelling in acquired dysgraphia: Selective benefit from visual mnemonics. *Neuropsychological Rehabilitation, 16*(1), 1–37.

Schonle, P. W. (1988). Compound noun stimulation: An intensive treatment approach to severe aphasia. *Aphasiology, 2*(3–4), 401–404.

Schuell, H., Jenkins, J. J., & Jimenez-Pabon, E. (1964). *Aphasia in adults: Diagnosis, prognosis, and treatment.* New York: Harper & Row.

Schwartz, M. F., Saffran, E. M., Fink, R. B., Myers, J. L., & Martin, N. (1994). Mapping therapy: A treatment programme for agrammatism. *Aphasiology, 8,* 19–54.

Scott, C., & Byng, S. (1989). Computer assisted remediation of homophone comprehension disorder in surface dyslexia. *Aphasiology, 3*(3), 301–320.

Sefer, J. W. (1973). A case study demonstrating the value of aphasia therapy. *British Journal of Disorders of Communication, 8,* 99–104.

Shewan, C. M. (1977). *Procedures manual for speech and language training: Language-Oriented Therapy (LOT).* Unpublished manuscript. The University of Western Ontario, London, Ontario.

Shewan, C. M. (1979). *Auditory Comprehension Test For Sentences (ACTS).* Menomonee, WI: Biolinguistics Clinical Institutes.

Shewan, C. M. (1980). Verbal dyspraxia and its treatment. *Human Communication, 5,* 3–12.

Shewan, C. M. (1986). The Language Quotient (LQ): A new measure for the Western Aphasia Battery. *Journal of Communication Disorders, 19,* 427–439.

Shewan, C. M., & Bandur, D. L. (1986). *Treatment of aphasia: A language-oriented approach.* Austin, TX: Pro-Ed.

Shewan, C. M., & Henderson, V. L. (1988). Analysis of spontaneous language in the older normal population. *Journal of Communication Disorders, 21,* 139–154.

Shewan, C. M., & Kertesz, A. (1984). Effects of speech and language treatment on recovery from aphasia. *Brain and Language, 23,* 272–299.

Silverberg, N., Vigliocco, G., Insaluco, D., & Garrett, M. (1998). When reading a sentence is easier than reading a little word: The role of production processes in deep dyslexics reading aloud. *Aphasiology, 12,* 335–356.

Simmons-Mackie, N., Kingston, D., & Schultz, M. (2004). "Speaking for another": The management of participant frames in aphasia. *American Journal of Speech-Language Pathology, 13,* 114–127.

Skelly, M. (1979). *Amer-Ind gestural code.* New York: Elsevier.

Smith, A., Champoux, R., Leri, J., London, R., & Muraski, A. (1972). *Diagnosis, intelligence and rehabilitation of chronic aphasics.* University of Michigan, Department of Physical Medicine and Rehabilitation. Social and Rehabilitation Service (Grant No. 14-P-55198/5-01).

Sohlberg, M. M., Ehlhardt, L. A., Fickas, S., & Sutcliffe, A. (2003). A pilot study exploring electronic (or e-mail) mail in users with acquired cognitive-linguistic impairments. *Brain Injury, 17*(7), 609–629.

Sohlbergh, M. M., Johnson, L., Paule, L., Raskin, S. A. & Mateer, C. A. (2001). *Attention process training-11: A program to address attentional deficits for persons with mild cognitive dysfunction* (2nd ed). Wake Forest, NC: Lash & Associates.

Springer, L., Glindemann, R., Huber, W., & Willmes, K. (1991). How efficacious is PACE-therapy when Language Systematic Training is incorporated? *Aphasiology, 5,* 391–399.

Stadie, N., & Rilling, E. (2006). Evaluation of lexically and nonlexically based reading treatment in a deep dyslexic. *Cognitive Neuropsychology, 23*(4), 643–672.

Steele, R. D., Weinrich, M., Wertz, R. T., Kleczewsda, M. K., & Carlson, G. S. (1989). Computer-based visual communication in aphasia. *Neuropsychologia, 27,* 409–426.

Stimley, M. A., & Noll, J. D. (1991). The effects of semantic and phonemic prestimulation cues in picture naming in aphasia. *Brain and Language, 41,* 496–509.

Thiel, A., Herholz, K., Koyuncu, A., Ghaemi, M., Kracht, L.W., Habedank, B., et al. (2001). Plasticity of language networks in patients with brain tumors: A positron emission tomography activation study. *Annals of Neurology, 50,* 620–629.

Thomas, C., Altenmuller, E., Marckmann, G., Kahrs, J., & Dichgans, J. (1997). Language processing in aphasia: Changes in lateralization patterns during recovery reflect cerebral plasticity in adults. *Electroencephalography and clinical neurophysiology, 102,* 86–97.

Thomas, C. A., & Jackson, S. T. (1997). The validity of reading comprehension therapy materials. *Journal of Communication Disorders, 30,* 231–243.

Thompson, C. K., & Shapiro, L. P. (1994). A linguistic-specific approach to treatment of sentence production deficits in aphasia. *Clinical Aphasiology, 22,* 307–323.

Thompson, C. K., & Shapiro, L. P. (1995). Training sentence production in agrammatism: Implications for normal and disordered language. *Brain and Language, 50,* 201–224.

Thompson, C. K., Shapiro, L. P., Kiran, S., & Sobecks, J. (2003). The role of syntactic complexity in treatment of sentence deficits in agrammatic aphasia: The complexity account of treatment efficacy (CATE). *Journal of Speech, Language and Hearing Research, 46,* 591–607.

Tompkins, C. A., Boada, R., & McGarry, K. (1992). The access and processing of familiar idioms by brain-damaged and normally aging adults. *Journal of Speech, Language, and Hearing Research, 35,* 626–637.

Tranel, D., Martin, C., Damasio, H., Grabowski, T. J., & Hichwa, R. (2005). Effects of noun-verb homonymy on the neural correlates of naming concrete entities and actions. *Brain and Language, 92,* 288–299.

Tuomainen, J., & Laine, M. (1991). Multiple oral reading technique in rehabilitation of pure alexia. *Aphasiology, 5*(4–5), 401–409.

Tyler, L. K., Moss, H. E., & Jennings, F. (1995). Abstract word deficits in aphasia: Evidence from semantic priming. *Neuropsychology, 9,* 354–363.

Van de Sandt-Koenderman, W. M. (2004). High, tech AAC and aphasia. Widening the horizons? *Aphasiology, 18*(3), 245–263.

Van de Sandt-Koenderman, W. M., & Visch-Brink, E. G. (1993). Experiences with multi-cue. In F. J. Stachowiak, R. De Bleser, G. Deloche, R. Kaschel, H. Kremin, P. North, et al. (Eds.), *Developments in the assessment and rehabilitation of brain-damaged patients* (pp. 347–351). Tubingen: Gunter Narr Verlag.

Van de Sandt-Koenderman, W. M., Wiegers, J., & Philippa, H. (2005). A computerized communication aid for people with aphasia. *Disability and Rehabilitation, 27*(9), 529–533.

Van Mourik, M., & Van de Sandt-Koenderman, W. M. (1992). Multicue. *Aphasiology, 6,* 179–183.

Vignolo, L. A. (1964). Evolution of aphasia and language rehabilitation: A retrospective exploratory study. *Cortex, 1,* 344–367.

Wade, J., Petheram, B., & Cain, R. (2001). Voice recognition and aphasia: Can computers understand aphasic speech? *Disability and rehabilitation, 23*(14), 604–613.

Wallace, G. L., & Canter, G. J. (1985). Effects of personally relevant language materials on the performance of severely apha-sic individuals. *Journal of Speech and Hearing Disorders, 50,* 385–390.

Wambaugh, J. L. (2003). A comparison of the relative effects of phonologic and semantic cueing treatments. *Aphasiology, 17*(5), 433–444.

Wang, L., & Goodglass, H., (1992). Pantomime, praxis, and aphasia. *Brain and Language, 42,* 402–418.

Warburton, E., Price, C. J., Swinburn, K., & Wise, R. J. S. (1999). Mechanisms of recovery from aphasia: Evidence from positron emission tomography studies. *Journal of Neurology, Neurosurgery, and Psychiatry, 66,* 155–161.

Weekes, B., Davies, R., & Parris, B. (2003). Age of acquisition effects on spelling in surface dysgraphia. *Aphasiology, 17*(6/7), 563–584.

Webb, W., & Love, R. (1994). Treatment of acquired reading disorders. In R. Chapey (Ed.), *Language intervention strategies in adult aphasia* (pp. 446–457). Baltimore, MD: Lippincott Williams and Wilkins.

Weinrich, M., McCall, D., Boser, K. K., & Virata, T. (2002). Narrative and procedural discourse production by severely aphasic patients. *Neurorehabilitation and Neural Repair 16*(3), 249–274.

Weinrich, M., McCall, D., Weber, C., Thomas, K., & Thornburg, L. (1995). Training on an iconic communication system for severe aphasia can improve natural language production. *Aphasiology, 9,* 343–364.

Weinrich, M., Shelton, J. R., Cox, D. M., & McCall, D. (1997). Remediating production of tense morphology improves verb retrieval in chronic aphasia. *Brain and Language, 58,* 23–45.

Weinrich, M., Shelton, J. R., McCall, D., & Cox, D. M. (1997). Generalization from single sentence to multisentence production in severely aphasic patients. *Brain and Language, 58,* 327–352.

Weisenburg, T., & McBride, K. E. (1935). *Aphasia.* New York: Hafner.

Wepman, J. M. (1951). *Recovery from aphasia.* New York: Ronald Press.

Wertz, R. T., Collins, M., Weiss, D., Brookshire, R. H., Friden, T., Kurtzke, J. F., & Pierce, J. (1978). *Preliminary report on a comparison of individual and group treatment.* Paper presented at the annual meeting of the American Association for the Advancement of Science, Washington, DC.

Wertz, R. T., Collins, M., Weiss, D., Kurtzke, J. F., Frident, T., Brookshire, R. H., et al. (1981). Veterans Administration cooperative study on aphasia: A comparison of individual and group treatment. *Journal of Speech and Hearing Research, 24,* 580–594.

Wertz, R. T., & Katz, R. C. (2004). Outcomes of computer-provided treatment for aphasia. *Aphasiology, 18*(3), 229–244.

Wertz, R. T., Weiss, D. G., Aten, J. L., Brookshire, R. H., Garcia-Bunuel, L., Holland, A. H., et al. (1986). Comparison of clinic, home, and deferred language treatment for aphasia. *Archives of Neurology, 43,* 653–658.

Whitney, C., & Berndt, R. S. (1999). A new model of letter string encoding: Simulating right neglect dyslexia. In J. A. Reggia, E. Ruppin, & D. Glansman (Eds.), *Progress in brain research* (Vol. 121, pp. 143–163). Amsterdam: Elsevier.

Whitney, J. L., & Goldstein, H. (1989). Using self-monitoring to reduce disfluencies in speakers with mild aphasia. *Journal of Speech and Hearing Disorders, 54,* 576–586.

Williams, S. E., Li, E. C., Volpe, A. D., & Ritterman, S. (1994). The influence of topic and listener familiarity on aphasic discourse. *Journal of Communication Disorders, 27,* 207–222.

Xu, J., Kemeny, S., Park, G., Fratali, C., & Braun, A. (2005). Language in context: Emergent features of word, sentence, and narrative comprehension. *NeuroImage, 25,* 1002–1015.

Zurif, E. B., & Caramazza, A. (1976). Psycholinguistic structures in aphasia. In H. Whitaker & H. A. Whitaker (Eds.), *Studies in Neurolinguistics* (Vol. 1). New York: Academic Press.

Zurif, E. B., Caramazza, A., & Myerson, R. (1972). Grammatical judgments of agrammatic aphasics. *Neuropsychologia, 10,* 405–417.

Zurif, E. B., Green, E., Caramazza, A., & Goodenough, C. (1976). Grammatical intuitions of aphasic patients: Sensitivity to functors. *Cortex, 12,* 182–186.

APPENDIX 28.1
Language-Oriented Treatment Goals Form

MODALITY: _____   CLIENT: _____

AREA: _____   CLINICIAN: _____

GOAL: _____   **LOT GOALS**

Level	Stimulus	Presentation Method	Cuing Provided	Criterion Correct Response	Response Method	Additional Responses

APPENDIX 28.2
Language-Oriented Treatment Data Record Form

MODALITY: _____   CLIENT: _____

AREA: _____   **LOT DATA RECORD**   CLINICIAN: _____

Session No.	Date	Time (minutes)	Difficulty Level	No. of items	Data and Comments

Chapter 29

Treatment of Aphasia Subsequent to the Porch Index of Communicative Ability (PICA)

Bruce E. Porch

OBJECTIVES

The major objective of this chapter is to demonstrate that the nature of response behavior is indicative of the status of the brain's circuits and systems. The following main arguments are presented to help the clinician appreciate the importance of this concept to the understanding of brain function and to the development of viable plans for treatment of aphasia.

1. The brain survives best when its circuits and systems function quickly and easily and when it stores information that is accurate. When these circuits and systems are damaged, information is processed more slowly and inefficiently, more circuits are required to do simpler tasks, and information is treated as tentative and not stored.
2. The patient's response behavior reflects these changes in the brain circuitry's reduced efficiency. Because response changes, such as delayed responses, self-corrections, and requests for repetition of the stimulus, signal significant changes within the brain systems, the use of plus-minus scoring in testing or treatment is not appropriate, and multidimensional scoring or some other method of observing small behavioral changes is necessary clinically.
3. Treatment planning based on this model therefore is directed at assisting the patient in achieving easy, immediate responses on progressively more difficult tasks.
4. Decisions about the patient's potential for change as a result of treatment should be made on the basis of a psychometric sampling of the patient processing.

Before initiating treatment, and at various critical points during the therapeutic process, the clinician must answer a series of critical questions about the conduct of that treatment. The issues of major concern are how the brain lesion has affected the communicative ability of the patient; whether those deficits are treatable; what modalities, tasks, and stimuli should be used in treatment; what behavior should be reinforced; and when should treatment be terminated. Traditionally, answers to these problems are evolved empirically during treatment through trial-and-error methods or are arbitrarily determined because of the clinician's bias for certain techniques and methods. In recent years, the tendency among clinicians who use the Porch Index of Communicative Ability (Porch, 2001), or PICA, to rely on the test results to help with the therapeutic decision making has been growing.

The discussion that follows will consider some of these treatment issues and will illustrate how PICA test results and PICA theory can assist the clinician in planning therapy. Much of this material is drawn from basic and advanced training courses that are designed to prepare the clinician for use of the test. Therefore, although it is hoped that the concepts presented here are useful to a general audience, the full application of some of these methods will necessarily be limited to PICA-trained clinicians who have demonstrated accuracy in the use of this multidimensional scoring system.

A SYSTEMS ANALYSIS APPROACH TO APHASIA TREATMENT

The principle of the brain as survival mechanism is fundamental to understanding the brain, why it does what it does in both normal and damaged states, and how to treat it. The ways in which the brain processes information, reacts to stimuli, and responds to damage are all biased by the ultimate effect of that moment on its capacity to survive. This principle pervades every aspect of treatment and must be used by the clinician to anticipate what must be done, and what must be avoided, while treating the patient.

A second principle essential to the development of an appropriate sequence of treatment is that all the systems of the brain and their components are intimately interrelated and that no part of a system can be affected positively or negatively without affecting all systems. A brief look at a hypothetical brain circuit might illustrate the practical implications of these two principles and serve as an introduction to PICA theory as applied to treatment.

At the simplest level, a brain circuit may be viewed as being made of a series of modules, each of which processes data from the previous module and then sends the processed information on to the next module in the circuit. Each module has the capacity to enhance the information, reject it as inaccurate, or mark it as a survival message. For example, the auditory processing circuit shows three levels of modules between the input of each bit of raw data to the circuit and the output of the circuit to other circuits or integrators. When the input pathway sends basic data from the input transducers, such as the ears, or from other circuits to the feature detection modules, the data are stored temporarily in processing storage. The module then scans its data banks, or operational storage, to determine if the raw data have been processed before and if some information exists about the data that can further define that data, especially in terms of its significance to survival. This information is moved to the comparator to verify that the retrieved data explain or define the raw data stored in processing storage. If the comparator finds a good match between the input data and the retrieved data, it allows the combined product to be sent on to the next module in the circuit, which in this simple circuit is "pattern recognition." After storing the output of the features module in its processing storage, this next module scans its operational storage to see if the features coming in have a pattern that was processed previously as valid information. It then compares the retrieved information from its storage, compares it with the input data in processing storage, and if it matches, sends it to the signal processing module to determine if the recognized patterns have a specific significance, especially to survival. If the significance of the patterns is established, the processed information may now be sent on to other circuits, or to integrators that combine information from multiple circuits.

The storage units in this model are conceived of as an access core that defines the nature of the information stored around it, and each core has a "surround" made of data, subcores, and subsurrounds, all of which share a common relationship to the access core. The more important that information is to survival, and the more frequently that it is used, the closer it is to the core or subcore and, therefore, the more retrievable it is, because it requires less switching to reach it. Another interesting characteristic of these storage units (operational and permanent cores and surrounds) is that they tend not to store tentative or nonverified information. Processing storage and a general persistence in the circuit will maintain data temporarily. Only when a bit of data is processed immediately and accurately is it considered to be appropriate for operational, long-term storage. Usually, operational storage is achieved through processing a data bit enough times to verify it is both accurate and useable or when the data bit has high impact, in terms of survival, so

that it must be remembered after one exposure to it and trial-and-error learning is not conducive to survival. If a caveman with friends was walking down a path lined with bushes and a saber-toothed tiger jumped out and devoured one of the group, for example, it would be important to remember that path and those bushes after one exposure rather than repeating the walk and watching friends disappear over the next few days!

Feedback loops may be used when a module finds that it does not have sufficient information to complete the processing of a data bit sent to it and, therefore, needs the previous module to send more data. These feedback loops also can inform the previous modules that the information being processed is the first in a series that is well known, so no need exists to process the rest of the series. This frees the previous modules for processing new and less familiar data and reduces the circuitry necessary to process familiar data to a minimum. Thus, circuitry reduction results in more efficient, faster processing of familiar data and allows the circuit to use its energy on more complex, unique, or "danger" kinds of data. The immature brain uses many circuits to carry out relatively simple tasks. The mature brain reduces the number of circuits necessary to carry out a task to a minimum. The damaged brain is less efficient, must once again use its circuits to cope with less complex tasks, and is challenged by previously easy tasks. The goal of treatment is to restore circuitry efficiency.

A final important observation has to do with the interconnectedness of the brain's circuits and systems and why damage has such widespread implications in the brain. If, in our theoretic circuit, the processing storage in the pattern recognition module fails to function, the raw data enter the module, scanning in memory occurs, and the comparator attempts to match the retrieved information with the original input data. Nothing is stored in processing storage, however, and comparison is impossible. The comparator must then request that the input data be sent again from the previous module, or it must rescan memory in an attempt to verify the information. The comparator's other options are to simply stop functioning or to assume that the retrieved information is accurate and send it on to the next module. While all this is going on in the pattern recognition module, the features recognition module is waiting to send the next bit of data forward, and the signal processing module is waiting for the patterns module to send it some data. The entire circuit is locked up, because one small part of one module is broken. Furthermore, previous circuits are waiting for this circuit to accept information, and succeeding circuits are waiting for the output of this circuit. The entire system is affected, and this system is interlocked with all other systems.

In summary, this systems analysis model that we will be applying to treatment of aphasia suggests that the brain is made of complex, interlocked, interrelated modules and circuits that are survival biased. Survival is facilitated by

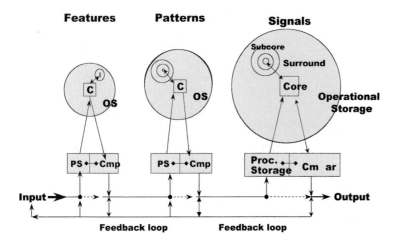

Figure 29–1. Multidimensional binary-choice scoring system.

maximizing the efficiency of these circuits by permanently storing only verified information that is not tentative. The efficiency of a circuit is further increased by circuitry reduction that allows fewer modules or fewer circuits to be necessary to quickly process accurate and familiar data entering the system. The clinical caution here is that both operational storage and circuitry reduction do not occur if any aspect of processing is not easy and immediate. What constitutes "easy and immediate" brings us to a consideration of the patients' response behavior and why the use of plus-minus scoring during treatment of aphasia is both impractical and unproductive.

Multidimensional Scoring

The circuitry within the brain defies direct observation; therefore, the clinician must infer what is going on in a system by carefully observing the patient's response behavior during a treatment task. A wide range of behavior is possible in a response to a given stimulus and task, depending on how the involved circuits are able to process the data. Several examples of response behavior to follow will illustrate this and will show how PICA multidimensional scoring is used to quantify behavior.

Returning to the theoretic circuit described earlier, when data move through each of the modules of a circuit both easily and immediately and produce an accurate, well-produced output from the circuit, those data are permanently stored in operational storage, and circuitry reduction may occur for those data. Use of the multidimensional, binary-choice PICA scoring system shown in Figure 29–1 would score such responses as accurate, responsive, complete, prompt, and efficient (score of 15). During treatment, it is these 15-type responses that are the target behavior the clinician strives for on every response.

In contrast to an "easy" response, a patient might retrieve inaccurate or incomplete information when scanning operational storage. When the retrieved information is sent to the comparator, the discrepancy between this retrieved information and what is stored in processing storage is noted. This necessitates looping back to operational storage to retrieve a better match. When the comparator finds that the second information is accurate, it sends it on to the next module for processing. Such double looping appears, behaviorally, as a brief hesitancy or processing delay (score of 13) but is significant clinically, because that bit of information is still considered to be tentative by the circuit and, therefore, is not stored in operational storage (Aaronson, 1974). It still requires total, not reduced, circuitry for its processing. This is why any response other than an easy, accurate, immediate response (score of 15) means further treatment is necessary on that item.

Let us examine this double-looping example for other types of behavior that could have resulted. After double looping, a damaged comparator might accept incorrect information from storage and send it on to the next module. If this incorrect information produces an error response but the response reenters the circuit, is recognized as being inaccurate, and is then changed to be accurate, the clinician observes this use of an external comparator as a self-correction (score of 10). If the comparator recognized that the stored information in that module was inadequate, it might feed back to earlier modules or to sensory transducers a request for additional information about the data bit (score of 8) or for the same data to be sent through again (score of 9). If such information is not available earlier in the circuit, the comparator might just send on the erroneous information to produce an incorrect response (score of 6), or the comparator might stop all processing and accept that it cannot produce a response, with the patient rejecting the item by saying, "I don't know" (score of 5).

Although this scoring system was developed for sensitively and reliably quantifying subtle changes in a patient's test behavior, it has proven to be equally vital in documenting the response characteristics during treatment. A final benefit of multidimensional scoring is that it forces the clinician to be sensitive to small, but important, changes in behavior.

Internal Consistency of Tasks

The PICA is designed so that all the subtests revolve around 10 common objects. This has the psychometric advantage of holding content constant across subtests and, therefore, making it possible to compare the patient's skill across modalities and tasks. It also produces subtests that have very high internal consistency, with all the items on a subtest being relatively equal in difficulty for the patient. Under these conditions, it is possible to detect patterns of response that normally are obscured by conventional aphasia tests beginning with easy items and getting progressively more difficult.

Table 29–1 shows how having stimuli that are relatively equal in difficulty will reveal various types of processing problems during testing or treatment. In this simple example, we see the scores for three different patients on a task involving 10 items of relatively equal difficulty. Patient A rejects the first item but is able to respond to the next few items after the stimulus is repeated or cued or after a significant delay. Eventually, he begins to respond at normal levels and receives scores of 15. With Patient A, it is apparent that he had trouble tuning into the task and adjusting his system to perform adequately during the first part of the task, but eventually, he reached fully operational levels. Patient B starts out with no difficulty but gradually has decreasing scores and tunes out on the task, suggesting that he lacks the ability to keep his system locked into the task or to handle cumulative noise that might build up during the task. Patient C has a performance that is very homogeneous and shows no variation from item to item.

TABLE 29–1

Examples of Patterns of Response

Stimulus	Patient		
	A	B	C
Cat	5	15	11
Dog	8	15	11
Boy	9	15	11
Apple	10	15	11
Cup	13	15	11
Shoe	15	13	11
Car	15	10	11
Soup	15	9	11
Ball	15	8	11
Pie	15	5	11
Mean score	11.0	11.0	11.0

We see in the bottom row of Table 29–1 that all three patients got a mean score of 11.0, indicating that they were all functioning at about the same communicative level on this task. Clearly, however, the type of processing difficulties that each manifests is quite different. In addition, patients A and B demonstrate several fully operational responses, suggesting that their circuits have the capacity to carry out the task once the processing problems are resolved. Although Patient C got all 10 items correct on a plus-minus basis, he showed no ability to do the task at operational levels. His system is indicating that, at least at this point in time, it is performing the task as well as it can.

Because the PICA has high internal consistency, it is able to give some indication about these types of processing problems, and it indicates potential levels of ability that a patient may have on a given task (Disimoni, Keith, & Darley, 1983). These same principles can be employed in treatment if the clinician will take the time to ensure that the stimulus items used on the task are relatively equal in difficulty.

DESIGNING A PLAN OF TREATMENT

Once the clinician has gained a thorough familiarity with the patient and his or her history, has completed comprehensive testing, and has found that the patient's condition is no longer changing dramatically from day to day, treatment planning can be initiated. The usual sequence of considerations at this point is to determine if the patient is a suitable candidate for treatment, to choose the tasks and stimuli to be used during treatment, to decide on which types of behavior will be reinforced on each task, and finally, to determine when treatment should be terminated.

Selecting Patients for Treatment

Determining whether a patient is treatable is a relatively new concern, arising in recent years as treatment has become more expensive and available funding for treatment scarce. During the 1960s, Schuell, Jenkins, and Jiminez-Pabon (1964) did some work on prognosis that assigned postrecovery, stabilized patients to one of five major or two minor prognostic groups. More recently, in an effort to develop earlier predictions, Porch, Wertz, and Collins (1974) as well as Porch, Collins, Wertz, and Friden (1980) have described other prognostic studies that attempted to develop more accurate predictions of eventual recovery levels; however, these studies employing multiple discriminate analysis have not yet been validated for clinical use.

Perhaps the most widely used clinical method currently is the high-overall-prediction (HOAP) method (Porch, 1970) that was developed during the late 1960s as an interim approach to prediction but proved to be reasonably accurate and simple to use and, therefore, has persisted for three decades. In this method, it was theorized that the capacity of the patient's total communicative system was indicated by the highest scores or peak abilities. Therefore, the clinician could estimate the maximum potential for communication by using the average of the nine highest subtest scores achieved on the PICA or by using the highest modality score, whichever was the greatest. Appropriate tables or graphs enable the clinician to convert these scores into an estimate of the eventual outcome level and, thereby, make appropriate plans regarding treatment of the patient. Because this HOAP method may be applied as early as 1 month post-onset in most cases, and because it takes into consideration the normal recovery stages, the clinician is in a better position to select the patients who are most treatable and to counsel families and physicians regarding the eventual recovery levels (Porch & Callaghan, 1981).

For clinicians who use the PICA to test their patients early in the recovery process, another prognostic indicator is the acceleration rate of recovery. This is determined by subtracting the 1-month post-onset PICA Overall percentile from the 2-month post-onset PICA Overall percentile. Patients who improve more than 12 percentile points during this period tend to exceed the HOAP target percentile by the time they reach 6 months post-onset. Those with slower early recovery tend to not reach the early PICA predictions.

Estimating treatment potential is equally important later in the course of recovery. Eventually, the patient's condition seems to stabilize, and the clinician must decide whether to continue treatment. Once again, PICA scores are helpful in several ways for making this decision. First, discrepancies between the patient's overall score and the high modality score indicate the amount of potential change that remains. Second, after the patient is past the acute stage, it is expected that when he or she is at maximum recovery, his or her subtest percentiles will be approximately equal; therefore, differences between the nine highest subtest percentiles and the nine lowest subtest percentiles also will suggest a range of possible change or the lack of it.

These same principles hold true within subtests. The PICA scoring system provides 16 possible scores for any given response; therefore, it is not unusual for a patient to obtain a wide range of item scores. As a patient undergoes treatment for aphasia, the intrasubtest variability of scores gradually reduces until all the item scores within the subtests are quite homogeneous, indicating no peaks or depressions of ability on the task. This homogeneity suggests that the patient, at least at that point in time, is functioning at near-maximum ability on that particular task. The circuits necessary to carry that task are consistently performing at their highest current potential levels of efficiency: There are no low responses that might be brought up to the patient's average level, and there are no higher scores that might serve as a target level toward which to strive. When the patient demonstrates homogeneity in all modalities on the PICA, his or her brain is indicating that it is performing communicatively and cybernetically near its maximum potential level of functioning and that further treatment of the processing problems may not be fruitful. At that point, the clinician may evolve new treatment goals to maximize the patient's use of his or her functional systems, to modify the patient's environment to facilitate his or her communication, and to educate the people in his or her environment about the status of the patient's abilities and deficits and how to assist that patient.

In summary, an ideal treatment candidate is a cooperative patient whose medical condition is stable, who has a predicted overall percentile significantly above his or her present overall score, and who exhibits variation on item scores within subtests in some modalities.

Selecting Treatment Tasks

Before the discussion on treatment can continue, it is necessary to introduce some concepts and terminology related to PICA theory. As we see in Figure 29–2, we may visualize a continuum of communicative tasks, ranging from the most simple vegetative communicative processes to the most complex learned processes. The ordinate represents the response continuum, ranging at the top from the most complex levels of responses to the bottom of the continuum, where the patient fails to attend or give any type of response.

The PICA samples a test field somewhere in the middle of the task continuum. The tasks that were sampled range from relatively simple tasks in which only the most involved patients have difficulty to moderately challenging tasks in which even mild patients demonstrate some processing problems. The standard PICA test battery samples 18 points in the test field and establishes the subject's capacity to carry out tasks of varying difficulty.

The PICA tests have demonstrated that the interaction between the task and the response continua is best depicted by a sigmoidal function curve. If one were to test a normal subject longitudinally from infancy to adult levels of communication, this sigmoidal function curve would move from right to left on the task continuum and, finally, stabilize at some fairly high level of communicative ability. When a normal brain is damaged, its circuits are less efficient, it must use more circuits to carry out simpler tasks (the reverse of circuitry reduction), and it treats more entering data as tentative and, therefore, does not store it easily in operational storage. Because of these changes, the sigmoidal function curve shifts negatively to the right. The PICA locates the position of that response curve on the task continuum and, as indicated above, predicts how far positively that curve can be shifted with treatment.

Returning to our premise that aphasia represents a reduction in the processing efficiency of the brain, we can see that the sigmoidal function curve depicts the individual's processing abilities on a series of tasks that are ranked according

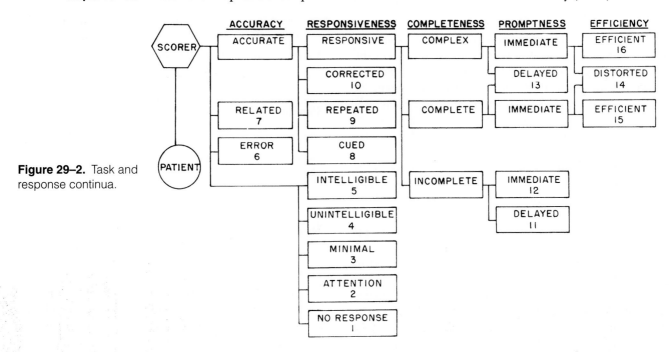

Figure 29–2. Task and response continua.

to their level of difficulty. The tasks to the right of the curve are all within the capacity of the individual's circuits and are carried out accurately, responsively, completely, promptly, and efficiently; therefore, they do not require treatment. As the tasks become a little more complex and require more communicative ability, the test responses are performed accurately but with some delays, self-corrections, or distortions, so the response curve begins to descend. As we will see, this area is referred to as the fulcrum of the curve, and it is the primary focus of treatment.

Referring again to Figure 29–2, note that as the tasks become increasingly complex, the curve begins to drop more precipitously as the person being tested begins to make errors and requires more information or more assistance to respond. To put it in terms of circuit theory, the circuits necessary for doing these tasks require the participation of more basic circuitry, such as those that are active at the fulcrum of the curve. These circuits are not yet operational, however, and cannot participate in more complex processing. Finally, as the tasks become even more complex, the sigmoidal curve bottoms out at the lower end of the response continuum, indicating that all tasks on the task continuum beyond this point are beyond the capacity of that person at that time.

Using this schema, the problem of task and modality selection is greatly simplified for the clinician, because the patient's system indicates precisely those tasks that need immediate attention. Once the PICA has been administered and the results plotted to indicate the patient's response curve, it is quite apparent which tasks are already operational and do not require treatment, which are on the fulcrum of

the curve and should be treated, and which are beyond the capacity of the patient's system at this time and should be excluded from the treatment format.

The reader should not confuse the concept of the fulcrum of the curve with the earlier suggestion that tasks on which the patient has the greatest item variability have the most potential for change and, therefore, assume that these tasks should be chosen for treatment. Tasks on which the patient has a large variety of scores, including high target scores and low scores that may be improved, have good potential for eventual change, but such tasks are too far down the curve. Attempts at treatment produce some errors, suggesting either that the circuits involved are getting insufficient information to perform the task or that more efficiency in the circuit needs to be developed by using tasks more within the capacity of the circuits (i.e., farther up the curve). In general, errors during treatment usually suggest either that the task selected is too difficult at this point in time or that the stimuli have been poorly chosen. The patient does not have enough information to monitor the developing processing before responding by using internal comparators or to evaluate the output after responding using external comparators.

Selecting Treatment Stimuli

After the tasks in various modalities have been selected from the fulcrum of the curve, it is necessary to select appropriate treatment stimuli to serve as vehicles for resolving the patient's processing problems on those tasks. Although it is common practice for clinicians to select stimuli on some a priori basis and then proceed with treatment, expecting the patient to do as well with whatever stimuli are selected is dangerous, because it does not take into consideration the specific type of processing problem the patient has. Stimuli that are too difficult and overdrive the patient's system, or those that are too "noisy" and interfere with processing, not only may reduce the amount of positive results from treatment but actually may produce problems rather than resolve them.

The danger of using inappropriate stimuli can be obviated by testing their appropriateness on selected tasks. The PICA score sheet may have already indicated to the clinician that the patient has more difficulty on certain types of stimuli, such as polysyllabic words, words with consonant blends, or words that are too short to provide adequate clues for decoding. This type of information might be used in assisting in the selection of the repertoire of stimuli that the clinician plans to use for the treatment tasks. It remains important, however, to verify the selected stimuli under the actual treatment conditions.

Stimulus verification is done through the use of PICA scoring, because the classic plus-minus scoring is relatively insensitive to processing disorders. Having selected 20 or 30 stimuli that seem to be appropriate for the task, the clinician explains to the patient what the task is and what he or she is expected to do. It also is useful to explain to the patient that the clinician will be scoring the responses so as to determine which stimuli will be the best to use in subsequent treatment sessions. Each stimulus, which has been listed on a treatment score sheet, is presented in order, and the patient's responses are scored for later analysis. After all the stimuli have been presented once, it usually is informative to present them again after a brief rest period to see how consistent the patient's processing is on each stimulus.

Table 29–2 shows how a few stimuli might be scored during a stimulus verification session. The clinician has selected some common nouns for treatment stimuli and has presented the list twice. In addition to the specific item scores the patient received, some other, more general observations may be made about these two trials. First, the patient tends to improve slightly on the second trial, demonstrating a good potential for improving after repeated trials. Second, it appears that the patient does somewhat better on polysyllabic words, thus suggesting that the auditory system may not be able to decode short stimuli rapidly enough and that the longer duration and increased information in longer words makes it easier to process them. Finally, it does not appear that, as one scans down the column of scores for both trials, that any orderly changes occurred. It is not unusual to find some patients whose scores gradually increase during a trial, suggesting that it takes several items for them to make the necessary adjustments to carry out the task. Other patients may start out a given trial with high scores and then, suddenly, have decreasing scores as the trial proceeds, indi-

TABLE 29–2

Verification of Treatment Stimuli

Stimulus	Trial	
	First	Second
Apple	8	9
Hammer	13	15
Shoe	10	13
Cup	6	6
Baseball	15	15
Hat	9	9
Bicycle	15	15
Car	7	10
Window	13	13
Bus	9	10

cating that they are unable to lock their system into the task, and they gradually tune out on the succeeding stimuli. In the example in Table 29–2, these types of trends are not seen; therefore, the variation in scores probably is attributable to the stimuli themselves.

Having made these general observations, the clinician is now ready to decide on which stimuli he or she will use in subsequent treatment sessions. The first rule here is to drop any stimuli on which the patient received errors (i.e., scores of seven or below). The fact that the patient got error scores on one of the trials on those stimuli indicates that they are either too noisy or too difficult to be used in treatment and can only interfere with processing and progress. Too often, the inexperienced clinician will attempt to "teach" these words to the patient but, instead, ends up putting more noise into his or her system along with practicing errors. A second consequence of using error-type responses is that not only do you prohibit the facilitation of good switching on these stimuli, the effect spreads to other stimuli on the list, and it creates a spread of poor processing to other stimuli in the treatment trial (Brookshire, 1976). When a clinician is treating the processing problems of the patient, no given stimulus can be considered as sacred, and whenever one presents a problem, it should be dropped out of the program.

This concept of dropping error items or stimuli also should be incorporated into the stimulus verification process, because items that are too difficult may have an interaction effect on other items. It generally is a good policy when running such trials to eliminate any error items from second and third trials to rule out possible interactions. In addition, the items that produce errors should be analyzed carefully for characteristics that are in contrast with items that invariably elicit 15-level responses Such an analysis will give the clinician important information about what variables affect the circuits involved and what type of stimuli should be avoided in treatment.

It should be apparent that plus-minus scoring is too gross to yield meaningful information about the patient's system, and that PICA scoring should be used if possible. Clinicians who are not trained in PICA methods, however, may achieve similar results by sorting stimuli into three categories: "easy"—items that the patient has responded to accurately, without effort or delay and in a manner that might be referred to as "normal"; "medium"—items that are responded to accurately, but only after processing delays, self-corrections, or repeats of the stimuli or after cues or additional information are given; and "hard"—items that yield error responses. When using this system, it is customary to designate the type of response as E, M, or H (or as 3, 2, and 1), or the stimuli may be sorted into three separate piles if card-type stimuli are used.

At this point, after all the sorting and analyzing of stimuli is complete, it would seem that the selection of tasks and stimuli is complete and the actual treatment might begin, but one more preliminary step is quite informative. Having selected a treatment task on which the patient gets 9- to 15-type scores (easy and medium responses), the clinician, instead of simply presenting the task multiple times to eventually achieve all "easy" responses, should manipulate some single variable of the task in a way that will immediately produce higher scores. If a particular manipulation does, in fact, improve responses, the clinician has discovered an important factor about the patient's system and what helps it to function successfully. By the same token, if the manipulation produces lower scores, evidence is obtained as to what variables have negative effects on the system. No change in responses as a result of the manipulation signifies that variable is not a relevant factor in the patient's performance of the task.

A simple auditory task might illustrate how one carries out this probe technique. The clinician has selected a task that involves placing six pictures of common things in front of the patient and having him point to the one that is named. The clinician on the initial presentation obtained three easy responses (scores of 15), a correct response after a repeat of the stimulus (score of 9), a self-correction (score of 10), and a delayed response (score of 13). The question now is how may the task be modified to produce all easy-type responses immediately? Several possibilities exist—reduce the number of items from six to four to simplify the task and reduce visual loading, use a carrier phrase before the noun (e.g., "Point to the . . .") to negate rise-time problems, add the printed word for the noun (e.g., "car") to the picture to add visual information to assist the auditory system, give an arousal signal (e.g., "Ready? . . . Car") for system activation or attention problems, and so on.

Gradually, as various modifications of the task succeed, the patient is able to come to all easy responses until he or she finally achieves all scores of 15. During the process, the clinician learns what factors make the patient's processing more or less efficient, which is information that will assist in this and future therapeutic tasks. In addition, possible tasks for subsequent treatment have been documented. As the original probe task that started out down the curve was manipulated, it gradually moved up the curve until it reached the all-15 level. With each change, the clinician documented the location of the various modifications of the task on the curve during this upward movement. Therefore, the clinician may, by working in reverse order down the curve, move from one task to the next in that sequence documented during the probe. As each task is raised to the all-easy level, the circuits under treatment become available for assisting the processing of other tasks down the curve, and the entire response curve moves toward the more complex end of the task continuum.

Treatment Format

Once the tasks and the stimuli have been selected for treatment, the clinician is now ready to organize them into a treatment format that is designed to present a consistent presentation of tasks that will facilitate the patient responding at the all-15 level. In other words, the goal of the clinician and the patient, working as a team, is to have the patient eventually respond to every stimulus on the task without requiring cues, repeats, self-corrections, or significant delays. Not only is this type of treatment designed to be error free, but as much as possible, it tries to facilitate the patient's responses so that they are produced easily and without any processing difficulty.

All these principles discussed thus far are roughly what is meant by "treating on the fulcrum of the curve." Processes in which the patient demonstrates delays and self-corrections are tentative processes that break down when used in more complex tasks employed farther down the curve. If these minor processing problems are cleared up and the patient reaches the all-15 level in carrying out the processes, then these become available farther down the curve, and all the more complex processes can take advantage of the now normal, simpler processes. This phenomenon may explain, in part, why so many times we see tasks improving in the clinic that have not been treated directly during the therapeutic process. This schema also makes clear why it is so inappropriate to treat tasks too far down the response curve—because we are expecting the patient to carry out complex processes that require other basic processes that are not yet available to him or her.

Finally, in connection with this issue of the dangers of overdriving the patient's systems, we should note how different the fulcrum of the multidimensional curve is from the plus-minus curve. If you refer again to Figure 29–2, you will note that the response curve for the average patient with aphasia is in the middle of the test field. This response curve, however, is a multidimensional response curvethat drops off on the tasks on which the patient first begins to have some delays, self-corrections, or repeats. In plus-minus scoring, these behaviors are ignored; therefore, the plus-minus response curve would not begin to drop until the patient gets some responses wrong. The plus-minus fulcrum of the curve would be equivalent to a point far down the multidimensional curve, a point at which tasks tend to be beyond the capacity of the patient's circuits.

When setting up the sequence of presentation for treatment activities, realize that the goal of treatment is to assist the patient in mastering noisy, inadequate circuits and switching. Because sudden changes in tasks, target behavior, or methods of reinforcement invariably produce distraction and noise in the patient's communicative system, it is advisable to establish an orderly and fairly fixed treatment format. If patients can anticipate the treatment events and have time to make leisurely transitions from task to task, they will maintain a more efficient, quieter system.

A useful format for ensuring adequate stimulation of the patient's system without producing noise or overload might be summarized as follows:

1. Adjustment period (clearing out)
2. General activation (warmer upper)
3. Consolidation (old stuff)
4. Modification (new stuff)
5. Consolidation (old stuff)
6. Modification (new stuff)
7. Conclusion (winder upper)

Adjustment Period: Checking and Clearing Out Circuits

The adjustment period that initiates the treatment session is a brief, but important, time. After the patient enters the room and sits down at the treatment table, the clinician greets him or her and simply asks a broad, nondirective question, such as "How's everything?" or "What's new?" This is designed to give the patient the opportunity to clear out his or her system and to tell the clinician about any special occurrences, problems, or questions that may have arisen since the last session. It also gives the patient an opportunity to try out, in a free-speech situation, some of the processes that he or she has been working on previously. The clinician, on the other hand, is trying to observe several things about the patient.

First, any significant difference between how the patient currently appears compared with how he or she appeared in previous sessions should be noted. If he or she is markedly improved, it may be necessary to redesign the treatment session or to retest the patient to determine his or her new level of functioning. If the patient is functioning poorly compared with previous sessions, it may be necessary to probe into the

cause of the problem or to discuss the matter with the family to see if there has been an exacerbation of the patient's medical problem. Sometimes, the patient has less serious problems, such as headache, shoulder pain, or some psychological or social issue that produces a depression in his or her ability and may make it necessary to be somewhat less adventurous in the treatment session on that day. Finally, while the patient is gradually adjusting his or her system to the room and to the clinician and is getting prepared for more difficult treatment tasks, the clinician is carefully noting the quality of the patient's communication and observing how much carryover has occurred from those processes that are being attacked during treatment to a spontaneous speech situation.

General Activation: Turning On and Warming Up Systems

Once it is certain that the patient is functioning adequately and has cleared his or her storage systems in preparation for treatment, the clinician can begin to focus the patient's attention on treatment-type tasks. For this purpose, a task is selected from the highest, or consolidated, part of the patient's response curve. This fairly easy, all-15-type task is for activating the patient's communicative systems and warming them up and for furnishing the patient with a gradual transition into the more difficult tasks. This activation period also will provide the clinician with a second check on the patient's general level of functioning on that day, and it gets the patient off to a successful start in the treatment session.

When initiating treatment with a new patient, information about what might be suitable warm-up tasks might be obtained from the PICA score sheet if one looks at the all-15 items on the easiest subtests. In the case of a patient who has been treated for a period of time, the clinician may elect tasks that, at one time, were on the fulcrum of the curve but that, eventually, become fully operational. Selecting these old tasks serves to verify that the patient is maintaining skills that were worked on formerly.

If, after a short period of general activation, the patient seems to be responding easily to simpler processing tasks, the clinician is ready to move on to the next step in treatment.

Just as in testing, where making a definite and clear transition in between tasks is important, the change between one step in treatment to the next should be made obvious to the patient so that he or she can clear out his or her system and make the necessary switching adjustments for the new task. This is done by giving the patient a general positive reinforcement for his or her efforts on the previous task and then suggesting that the patient just relax for a moment while the clinician makes notes about what has occurred in the session until that point. Then, the clinician announces to the patient that they are going to be doing something different. The clinician should explain what the task will be and what the patient is expected to do, and then the first item of that task should be demonstrated for the patient. When it is apparent that the patient understands the task, that task should then be started with the demonstration item so that the patient's system is gently eased into the task. Generally, following this type of transition will minimize the amount of noise in the patient's system and greatly reduce his or her anxiety and fatigue.

Consolidation: Pushing for All "Easy" Responses on Old Stuff

Having moved through the adjustment and activation steps, the patient and clinician now are ready to begin the first of several treatment modules. A treatment module is a series of tasks directed at a given modality or process. Depending on how many steps are in each module and how much time the total program takes, there may be two or three modules in a 1-hour treatment session. For instance, the first module might be devoted to consolidating and modifying auditory processing, and the clinician may then move on to the second module for consolidating and modifying verbal processing and, finally, turn to work on reading or writing as a third module. A module usually is begun with a task that the clinician is trying to consolidate and make fully operational. This task is quite high on the fulcrum of the curve, which on the first presentation has occasional delays in it but by the second or third presentation is all scores of 15. If, in a given session, it is found that this task is done at the all-15 level on the first presentation, the clinician might consider using that task as a warm-up in the future. If, on the other hand, the patient has continuing difficulty and cannot get to the all-15 level even after several presentations, it generally means that he or she is not ready to proceed to new tasks in that module. If, after a few presentations, the patient is able to get all 15s, the clinician should do the task several times to consolidate those 15s and then prepare to move on to the next step in the module.

Modification: Moving Down the Curve to New Tasks

As the patient approaches the point at which he or she is fully operational on a given task, it becomes appropriate to think about modifying that task slightly so that it involves some new aspect of switching or storage. For instance, if, on an auditory task that requires the patient to point to one of four pictures after the clinician says the noun, the task might be modified by using six pictures, by having the patient point to two pictures instead of one, or by not allowing the patient to see the pictures while the clinician is saying the noun. Any of these changes probably would produce an increase in the number of delays or self-corrections that the patient might have on the task. The goal then would be to increase the patient's performance until he or she achieves all 15s on the new task. If the clinician makes what is considered to be a

small modification in the task and the patient begins to make errors or requires multiple repeats and cues before he or she gets a correct response, the modification is larger than expected, and the task should move more in the direction of the consolidation task.

If the patient does fairly well with the new material and seems to understand it after several trials, he or she should be given a brief rest period in preparation for the next module. Usually, shifting to a new modality means shifting to new stimuli and treatment materials, but once again, the transition should be verbalized to help the patient readjust his or her system for the new task. This same general procedure is then followed, beginning with old material in the modality that needs to be consolidated and then, if appropriate, moving on to some new modifications of the task to increase the patient's processing capabilities.

Conclusion: A Positive Wind Up to the Treatment Session

The final step in the treatment format should involve a fairly easy task at the all-15 level. The patient and the clinician have moved through a variety of fairly arduous tasks during the previous hour and have just completed a relatively new modification task that has been somewhat difficult, and concluding the treatment session on that note would be psychologically undesirable. Therefore, the clinician should select a task from the easy, consolidated part of the curve, which will assure winding up the session on a successful note. The clinician also may use this final step as a verification that the patient is maintaining his or her skills on one of the earlier treated processes. In addition, it is a nice technique to use wind-up tasks from one day's session for a warm-up task on the next day's session. This helps the patient to get back to the same point at which he or she was at during the previous session, and it reduces intersession regression.

To summarize this section on the treatment format, the tasks are selected and sequenced in such a way as to maximize the efficiency of the patient's communicative systems and to minimize noise. Treatment of a given process or modality is begun with tasks selected from the consolidated, all-15 part of the curve to prepare those circuits for the more difficult tasks. Next, slightly more difficult tasks are selected from the fulcrum of the curve, and these are worked on until the patient eventually reaches the all-15 level. At that point, these newly consolidated processes are available for use on other tasks; therefore, the patient's response curve moves positively toward the predicted target level.

TREATMENT PRINCIPLES

Patient–Clinician Team

Implicit in the treatment method being described here is the involvement of the patient in the conduct of the treatment process. The patient should understand that the clinician is not trying to teach the patient words but, rather, is attempting to return him or her to "easy" processing—that is, free of self-corrections, repeats, and delays. The patient must be taught what this behavior feels like. It sometimes is helpful in teaching what is meant by "easy" processing to present the task using all "medium" items first and then to repeat the task with all "easy" items so that the patient can get the feel of the contrast between the two levels of performance. Once this distinction is clear to the patient, he or she also must be taught to advise the clinician when a response is tentative or slightly off-target so that it can be consolidated. In this sense, the two people become a team in which the patient relies on the clinician to assist with selecting the tasks and stimuli and in which the patient keeps the clinician informed as to the impact of those items on his or her system.

Setting Treatment Priorities

The establishment of the specific modalities and processes to be treated is facilitated by careful examination of the PICA score sheet. All-15 tasks are selected for warm-up and wind-up tasks, 13- to 15-level tasks should be treated, and 9- to 13-level tasks, when slightly simplified, may soon be appropriate as modification tasks in the format.

In general, it is best to first treat processing problems that are not stimulus related. This includes difficulty in shifting tasks, tuning in, cumulative noise, and tuning out. These problems are diagnosed when a series of homogeneous items are presented on a task and the patient always has trouble (e.g., repeats, self-corrections, or delays) with the first few items or tunes out the last few, regardless of the order of stimulus presentation. When these temporal problems occur, a specific program may be designed to overcome them. For instance, the goal of eliminating tuning out might be achieved by discussing the problem with the patient and then presenting stimuli that generally elicit 15-type responses. At first, only a few stimuli are used, and these are worked on until the patient achieves all 15s. The number then is gradually increased until the patient can keep his or her system locked in to the task for a full complement of stimuli.

If the patient has problems that are more random or are stimulus related, those problems are overcome by getting the circuits necessary for the task to the 15 level and then processing multiple times at that level. The circuits for the task are facilitated and will store processing information once the 15 level is achieved. Therefore, as treatment proceeds, those items on which the patient scored below 15 should be repeated until a score of 15 is achieved and then repeated some more so that the circuit can sense what 15-level processing entails and can store that information.

Very often, clinicians move through a series of stimuli and score responses without repeating items enough for success to occur. This is essentially testing rather than treating, because the patient's circuits never have the opportunity to experience the target behavior and achieve fully operational circuits. It probably is more beneficial to move lower scores to 15 and then practice the 15s if stable improvement is desired.

Criteria for Shifting Tasks

By this point in the discussion, it should be apparent that plus-minus scoring is completely inadequate for carrying out this type of treatment and that a more detailed type of scoring, such as a PICA scoring system, must be used. Second, the clinician must mentally score every response of every task to decide whether he or she should repeat the item or move on to the next one. Some clinicians like to write down every score for every response during the session so that they have a running account of exactly what happened in the patient's system. In that way, they can make the correct adjustments in the program, and they can document the patient's change very precisely over time. Another approach is to record the scores on the first presentation of the task to establish a baseline, then to work on the task for a period of time, and then rescore to measure change. Still other clinicians, who plan their treatment for a longer period of time and change the format less frequently, prefer to score the responses at the beginning of the treatment week and then rescore them at the end of the week to see what changes have taken place. Specific application of PICA scoring has been described by Bollinger and Stout (1974) in their discussion on response-contingent, small-step treatment; by LaPointe (1974), who gives examples of PICA scoring as used in Base 10 Program Stimulation; and by Brookshire (1973) in his general consideration regarding treatment of aphasia.

Some of the major differences between these types of programs and the PICA program described here are the criteria for selecting tasks and stimuli and the criteria for shifting to new tasks or terminating tasks. Many programs suggest a criterion of 80% or 90% correct as an indication that the patient is ready to proceed to more difficult tasks. This is undoubtedly too low, because this would allow the patient to have repeats, self-corrections, or delays on every item and still meet the criterion. Even a standard of 95% 13s (delays) or better allows the patient to have significant problems with 5% of the items. When this amount of interference in processing occurs, the information being processed probably is considered by the system as being tentative and, therefore, is not stored for long-term use. In turn, this means that the process being treated is not fully consolidated and is not available for use on tasks farther down the curve.

The PICA theory, therefore, suggests that the target for changing or terminating tasks is all-15 responses. This may seem to be overly idealistic but, in fact, is realistic and essential. Such a goal is attainable, because the tasks and the stimuli used have been carefully chosen and verified through the patient's system.

The second reason that all-15 responses are an appropriate treatment goal is that this type of processing seems to transfer better and is more resistant to regression. Unless a task is fully consolidated, it will tend to deteriorate in a normal life situation or in a more difficult treatment task. Cued (8) to self-corrected (10) responses often become errors, and delayed responses (13) shift to lower, more tentative scores. For this reason, transfer of these skills rarely occurs, because they are not operational. Conversely, if the patient develops a good awareness of what "easy" responses are and achieves them on all the items on the task, transfer can be maximized and regression prevented.

REINFORCEMENT OF RESPONSES

One of the advantages in using an error-free program is that the focus of the patient and the clinician is on achieving an "easy" 15-type response as opposed to delays, self-corrections, and so on. As the clinician presents stimuli, all responses are correct but may or may not be easy. Whenever either the patient or the clinician feels that the response was not easy, it should be repeated until the response is easy, and it should be reintroduced into that module later to verify that the response is still easy. Unlike doing plus-minus treatment, in which the use of tangible reinforcements, verbal praise, and so on are necessary because the stimuli are too complex for the patient to evaluate, such rewards are not required, useful, or even desirable, because they tend to interrupt processing and to distract the patient, who must concentrate on improving processing. When the clinician simply presents the next stimulus, this indicates to the patient that the last response appeared to be easy. If the stimulus is repeated, the patient knows that the response was not easy and needs more effective processing.

FUTURE TRENDS

The treatment methods based on PICA test results and multidimensional scoring described in this chapter offer several advantages over less structured approaches. In starting treatment, the clinician and the patient are offered a specific target level of overall communicative ability to work toward, and this can be computed quite early during the course of recovery. The treatment, once initiated, focuses on modalities and processes that the patient's own communicative systems have indicated are appropriate to modify at that point in time, and the exact difficulty levels of the tasks, the stimuli, and the target behavior are prescribed and verified by the level of multidimensional scores the patient achieves. All this evolves naturally out of a treatment format that maximizes the patient's processing efficiency yet minimizes the possibility that the clinician is misdesigning the treatment. Finally, the predictive formulas and the measures of intrasubtest variability indicate when the patient is at last functioning at his or her highest possible levels so that plans for terminating treatment may be made.

In contrast to these advantages, the PICA approach to treatment has disadvantages. It requires training to see the response behavior in detail and to convert the behavior into scores: It requires careful preparation and planning based on the patient's responses at every stage of treatment; necessitates accurately recording and analyzing of the response scores; and because of the emphasis on systems analysis rather that on language per se, requires that the clinician always be sensitive to the many variables that affect the patient's processing.

To clinicians who have not been trained in using the PICA, these approaches to treatment of aphasia can seem both demanding and complicated. In fact, it recently was suggested by Odekar and Hallowell (2005) that using such multidimensional methods is cumbersome, time-consuming, and may not be efficient and cost-effective within many current service-delivery contexts. Those authors recommend plus-minus scoring as a faster, less expensive method. Perhaps, someday, someone will demonstrate that it is not clinically important to recognize and quantify all the types of behavior that the patient with aphasia can show during a treatment task. Goldstein (1945) may have been wrong when he said, "If the results are viewed as so many pluses and minuses, as often is the case, no real insight is gained as to what the patient can still do and what he can no longer do." It may be that Schuell and colleagues (1964) erred when they considered the necessity to have a stimulus repeated, a response behavior that generally was ignored at the time, as being so significant that they scored it as an error. It could be that the treatment using multidimensional scoring described in this chapter will be superceded by other methods that use less complicated scoring. It appears, however, that the current trend is not toward simplified scoring. If one peruses the literature, not only in aphasiology but in many other fields, one will discover that an increasing number of multidimensional scoring systems or category scoring methods are replacing simpler scoring systems that have been found to be imprecise. In the future, the PICA scoring system probably will be just one of many multidimensional scoring systems the clinician will find in the clinical armamentarium.

KEY POINTS

1. An efficient brain processes information both quickly and accurately and only stores information that it can trust for survival.
2. The inefficient brain must use its circuits for simpler tasks, and it does the tasks less quickly and efficiently.
3. This reduced processing efficiency is evident in the response behavior of the individual.
4. The clinician must be able to discern and document all the behaviors that distinguish an easy, immediate response, which is the goal of treatment, from less efficient responses.
5. Multidimensional scoring, or some other method that distinguishes easy responses from less efficient responses, is necessary in treatment of aphasia, because both the patient and the clinician must make these distinctions. Plus-minus scoring fails to make these distinctions and is not useful in treatment.
6. Treatment should focus on those tasks and stimuli on which the patient produces accurate but not easy responses. Error responses suggest that that item, task, or stimulus is beyond the capacity of the patient's circuits at that time and is not appropriate now.
7. Once tasks and stimuli that are appropriate for the patient's circuits and systems have been selected, a treatment format should be organized to maximize the probability that the patient will achieve easy responses on items that previously were tentative.
8. Decisions about the reasonableness of treating or continuing to treat a patient should be made on a psychometric basis, which samples the patient's processing potential.

ACTIVITIES FOR **REFLECTION AND DISCUSSION**

1. Discuss how a cybernetic, systems analysis view of aphasia contrasts with the one using the classic subtypes of aphasia (e.g. Wernicke's or Broca's).
2. Why would it be impossible for a clinician to do the kind of treatment described in this chapter using plus-minus scoring?
3. What is the danger in having a clinician select tasks and stimuli a priori without verifying that they are appropriate for the patient?
4. Several psychometric reasons exist for an aphasia test having high internal consistency. Can you describe some clinical reasons why using homogeneous items in testing or treatment might be preferable to using items of undetermined difficult or items going from easy to difficult?

5. Considering this discussion on PICA treatment, how should you react to these clinicians' statements:
   - "I like to make my therapy sessions interesting by doing a variety of different things and by always trying new activities to surprise my patients."
   - "I don't go on to a new task in treatment until he gets them all right."
   - "He's doing pretty well on that task. I think I'll go on to something else."
   - "When he has to point to one of six pictures I name, I use poker chips as reinforcement so he knows if he's right or wrong."
   - "I don't have time to test my patients. I can find out how the patient is doing while I'm doing treatment."
6. Improving your clinical skills: Have a group of students and/or clinicians watch a videotape of a patient with aphasia doing some test or treatment tasks. For a short period of time, score each response using plus-minus scoring. Next, replay the same responses, but use the multidimensional scoring system shown in Figure 29–2 to score each response. Saying the scores out loud as they occur will give everyone some immediate feedback as to what response behavior is occurring and how well each person is seeing delays, self-corrections, rule breaking, repeated stimuli, related errors, distorted responses, and so on.

References

Aaronson, D. (1974). Stimulus factors and listening strategies in auditory memory: A theoretical analysis. *Cognitive Psychology, 6,* 108–132.

Bollinger, R., & Stout, C. E. (1974). Response contingent small step treatment. In B. E. Porch (Ed.), *Clinical aphasiology: Conference proceedings.* Albuquerque, NM: VA Hospital.

Brookshire, R. H. (1973). *An introduction to aphasia.* Minneapolis, MN: BRK.

Brookshire, R. H. (1976). Effects of task difficulty on sentence comprehension performance of aphasic subjects. *Journal of Communication Disorders, 9,* 167–173.

Disimoni, F. G., Keith, R. L., & Darley, F. L. (1983). "Tuning in" and "tuning out": Performance of aphasic patients on ordering PICA subtests. *Journal of Communication Disorders, 16,* 31–40.

Goldstein, K. (1948). *Language and language disturbances.* New York: Grune and Stratton.

LaPointe, L. L. (1974). Base 10 "programmed-stimulation": Task specification, scoring, and plotting performance in aphasia therapy. In B. E. Porch (Ed.), *Clinical aphasiology: Conference proceedings.* Albuquerque, NM: VA Hospital.

McNeil, M. R. (1979). The Porch index of communicative ability. In F. L. Darley (Ed.), *Evaluation of appraisal techniques in speech and language pathology.* Cambridge, MA: Addison-Wesley.

Odekar, A., & Hallowell, B. (2005) Comparison of alternatives to multidimensional scoring in the assessment of language comprehension in aphasia. *American Journal of Speech-Language Pathology, 14,* 337–345.

Porch, B. E. (1970). *PICA interpretation: Recovery and treatment (video training tape).* Albuquerque, NM: VA Hospital.

Porch, B. E. (1971). Multidimensional scoring in aphasia testing. *Journal of Speech and Hearing Research, 14,* 777–792.

Porch, B. E. (1981). *The Porch index of communicative ability.* Palo Alto, CA: Consulting Psychologists Press.

Porch, B. E. (2001). *The Porch index of communicative ability.* Albuquerque: Pica Programs.

Porch, B. E., & Callaghan, S. (1981). Making predictions about recovery: Is there HOAP? In R. H. Brookshire (Ed.), *Clinical aphasiology: Conference proceedings.* Minneapolis, MN: BRK.

Porch, B. E., Collins, M., Wertz, R. T., & Friden, T. P. (1980). Statistical prediction of change in aphasia. *Journal of Speech and Hearing Research, 23,* 312–321.

Porch, B. E., Wertz, R. T., & Collins, M. (1974). Statistical and clinical procedures for predicting recovery from aphasia. In B. E. Porch (Ed.), *Clinical aphasiology: Conference proceedings.* Albuquerque, NM: VA Hospital.

Schuell, H., Jenkins, J., & Jiminez-Pabon, E. (1964). *Aphasia in adults.* New York, Harper & Row.

D. Specialized Interventions for Patients with Aphasia

Chapter 30

Communication-Based Interventions: Augmentative and Alternative Communication for People with Aphasia

Karen Hux, Kristy Weissling, and Sarah Wallace

OBJECTIVES

This chapter introduces readers to the variety of augmentative and alternative communication (AAC) options available to support the communicative interactions of people with aphasia. Readers will learn about barriers and assets regarding the incorporation of AAC into communication-based interventions for people with aphasia; partner-dependent, transitional, and partner-independent communicators within the population of adults with aphasia; various types of assessment procedures that allow practitioners to match cognitive and linguistic strengths and challenges with AAC methods; and various AAC techniques and strategies for use with people with aphasia.

"In all but the most transient of aphasia, and perhaps its mildest forms, there is little reason to believe that aphasia therapy 'removes' the aphasia" (Holland & Beeson, 1993, p. 582). This statement highlights a major problem with which aphasiologists have long struggled: Existing interventions do not always restore the abilities of people with aphasia to their premorbid levels and, hence, leave some people with unmet communication and social needs (LaPointe,

2005). This does not mean that therapy for aphasia is ineffective in facilitating linguistic improvements in many people with aphasia (Holland, Fromm, DeRuyter, & Stein, 1996; Robey, 1998). Months or even years of speech and language intervention services, however, do not spare some people with aphasia from facing futures in which communication challenges repeatedly prevent or impede full participation in the social roles, activities, and relationships that they enjoyed previously.

The Holland and Beeson (1993) statement also reinforces another well-known phenomenon concerning aphasia recovery: People with mild aphasia typically have better outcomes and are more likely to regain functional communication skills compared to people with severe aphasia. Those with initial aphasia severity levels that are moderate or worse may make gains in recovering some aspects of language functioning, but they frequently experience a degree of chronic aphasia. The persistent struggles these people face demand a flexible clinical approach that takes into account the complexities of augmenting impaired symbolic processing systems.

Despite these phenomena, a strong inclination to restore impaired language underlies the efforts of many speech-language pathologists working with people who have aphasia. Traditional therapy for aphasia has, at its core, the notion that providing systematic and extensive language stimulation to people with aphasia, especially during the acute stage of recovery, will help to re-establish language processing, either through recovery of language-specific brain regions or through recruitment of alternate brain regions to assume language functions. Indeed, the rapid changes observed in many people during the first several weeks or months following the onset of aphasia support the notion that language restoration is a viable goal. Total restoration may not be realized, especially by those who are faced with moderate or severe aphasia. For them, additional compensation-oriented interventions, such as those associated with augmentative and alternative communication (AAC) devices, strategies, and techniques, are needed.

We believe that practitioners can improve the long-term outcomes of people with aphasia by providing early supplementation of restorative intervention approaches with ones that are compensatory in nature. Early introduction of compensatory AAC strategies and techniques supports the residual verbal comprehension and expression of people with aphasia. The alternative strategy—namely, providing only restorative intervention initially and, when insufficient gains signal that natural speech will not reach functional levels, belatedly introducing AAC interventions, or even dismissing clients from therapy altogether—is unlikely to support functional communication. Given the limited reimbursement that insurance companies currently provide for speech and language services, the early introduction of AAC interventions is important to allow adequate time for people with aphasia to adjust to, practice, refine, master, and begin to generalize compensatory strategies to a variety of communication situations.

To compensate for the persistent communication challenges they face, people with aphasia need instruction about multi-modal communication strategies that include the use of residual speech and language as well as compensatory strategies and techniques that support communicative interactions across diverse settings and with multiple partners. Speech-language pathologists have the challenging job of designing and implementing intervention programs to assist people with aphasia in mastering these compensatory behaviors. The purpose of this chapter is to provide speech-language pathologists with the information they need to make informed decisions about the types of AAC devices, strategies, techniques, and applications most likely to benefit people who display various communicative capabilities and needs associated with differing types and severities of aphasia.

Information in this chapter is organized into five sections. First, we provide an overview of the relation between AAC and aphasia, highlighting the complexity of implementing AAC interventions with individuals who have weakened symbol processing abilities. Second, we address AAC assessment issues by providing guidelines for determining the clinical profiles of people with aphasia regarding their communicative capabilities and needs. This includes distinguishing partner-dependent, transitional, and partner-independent communicators and aligning them with traditional types of aphasia classification. Third, we present intervention procedures associated with communication-based AAC strategies and techniques that support the residual speech and language capabilities of people with aphasia. Fourth, we discuss the generalization and application of AAC systems, techniques, and strategies to the variety of communication situations and interactions encountered by people with aphasia. Finally, we address future trends concerning the integration of AAC interventions into standard clinical practice for people with aphasia. Throughout this chapter, we provide case examples to illustrate the application of specific aspects of AAC systems to people with varying types and severities of aphasia.

RELATION BETWEEN AAC AND APHASIA

Rehabilitation professionals have long recognized the potential for exploring AAC interventions for people with aphasia (Beukelman, Yorkston, & Dowden, 1985; Jacobs, Drew, Ogletree, & Pierce, 2004; Kraat, 1990; van de Sandt-Koenderman, 2004). Discussion about adapting existing AAC interventions or creating new strategies and techniques to meet the needs of people with aphasia has appeared periodically in professional journals. A consistent theme across these discussions is that AAC holds considerable promise for supporting individuals with aphasia. Improved communication outcomes for people with chronic aphasia are likely as speech-language pathologists increasingly (a) introduce compensatory techniques as early supplements to restorative approaches, (b) develop and refine AAC interventions to address the specific needs and capabilities of people with aphasia, and (c) promote greater AAC acceptance by other practitioners both within and outside the profession, the lay public, and people with aphasia.

The successful development and implementation of AAC interventions for people with aphasia requires that speech-language pathologists have accurate information regarding two issues: the nature of AAC interventions for people with aphasia as multifaceted systems geared toward maximizing functional and effective communication, and the symbolic processing weaknesses that underlie aphasia and that influence the design and application of AAC interventions. These issues are discussed separately in the following sections.

Multifaceted AAC Interventions

As stated in the American Speech-Language-Hearing Association Technical Report, "AAC is best thought of as a system, as opposed to a single entity" (2004, p. 4). The development and maintenance of successful AAC systems for people with aphasia almost invariably require multi-modal approaches that combine several strategies, need frequent updating to meet changing needs, and provide a means of facilitating ongoing partner support of communicative interactions. For people with aphasia, AAC is most effective when it is multifaceted, dynamic, and adaptable.

By viewing AAC as a combination of strategies and techniques geared toward minimizing barriers to successful communicative interactions, speech-language pathologists can create systems that address the multiple challenges faced by people with aphasia when they attempt to participate in activities. For example, to communicate during a social gathering of friends, a person with severe, chronic aphasia may need compensatory strategies to assist with understanding verbal statements made by others as well as with relating details about recent personal experiences. This may mean using a combination of spoken and written language, gestures, self-generated drawings, and references to pre-stored information or remnants. Because multiple challenges associated with aphasia (e.g., auditory comprehension limitations, word retrieval problems, production of jargon, verbal perseveration, and agrammatism) could potentially contribute to communication breakdowns, reliance on only one communication modality or a single type of compensatory strategy or device is unlikely to foster sufficient success for a person with aphasia to engage in this type of social event. Hence, it is crucial that speech-language pathologists teach people with aphasia and their communication partners multiple strategies that they can employ systematically to minimize communication breakdowns interfering with either transactional (i.e., transmitting specific information from one person to another) or interactional (i.e., developing and maintaining interpersonal relationships) communication goals (Simmons-Mackie & Damico, 1997).

Viewing Aphasia as a Symbolic Processing Weakness

One of the biggest challenges to designing and implementing AAC interventions for people with aphasia relates to the nature of aphasia as a symbolic processing weakness. Aphasia is not simply a language disorder; rather, it is a problem that limits an individual's ability to process all types of symbolic information. McNeil (1988) provided a definition of aphasia highlighting the symbolic nature of the underlying deficit that is experienced: "Aphasia is a multimodality physiological inefficiency with verbal symbolic manipulations (e.g., association, storage, retrieval, and rule implementation). . . . It is affected by and affects other physiological information processing and cognitive processes to the degree that they support, interact with, or are supported by the symbolic deficits" (p. 739).

Certain features of this definition have particular importance regarding AAC applications. First is the stipulation that people with aphasia are inefficient, rather than deficient, in manipulating verbal symbols (McNeil & Pratt, 2001). People who are inefficient in verbal symbol manipulation are not totally devoid of this ability. Hence, they are likely to benefit from compensatory strategies that provide

redundancy through the presentation of information in multiple modalities. The devices, strategies, and techniques of AAC can provide this type of informational redundancy.

A second important feature of McNeil's (1988) definition concerns the notion that people with aphasia have information processing challenges that not only include language but also extend beyond language to the processing of all types of symbols (McNeil & Pratt, 2001). The fact that people with aphasia have difficulty processing all symbol types means that simply substituting one symbol for another (e.g., substituting the written word *drink* or a line drawing of a person lifting a cup to his mouth for the spoken word, *drink*) will not provide sufficient support or compensation. The problem stems from the fact that many existing AAC systems designed for people with disabilities other than aphasia resemble "language in a box"—that is, the systems have isolated and decontextualized representations of language concepts (i.e., individual verbal symbols) arranged in separate compartments of a grid for use to construct linguistic structures (Light et al., 2004). This occurs because, when designing a system, AAC specialists rely on their own fully developed, unimpaired language systems as the basis for organization and structure. Hence, many current AAC technologies reflect how people without language impairments use language. This strategy does not work well for most people with aphasia precisely because they are inefficient in accessing and using symbolic elements, and their challenges extend across all symbol systems. For AAC to benefit people with aphasia, professionals need novel approaches to system design, organization, and structure that extend beyond the mere substitution of one symbol system for another and that do not use normal language processing as the underlying framework.

In summary, the need for improved outcomes in overall communication—including goals relating to interactional as well as transactional functions—has been a driving force behind the development of AAC strategies for individuals with aphasia. Within the realm of designing and teaching compensatory strategies, two types of approaches exist for using AAC to support the residual speech and language capabilities of people with aphasia. First, professionals can design systems that supplement a person's inefficient language processing by providing informational redundancy. This means that, through the use of multiple modalities and contextual supports, people with aphasia and their communication partners promote redundancy by presenting a single message through simultaneous or sequential use of speech, gestures, written language, drawing, or reference to environmental cues, low-tech communication books, or high-tech communication devices. Such informational redundancy increases the likelihood of accurate comprehension and expression of intended meanings. Second, professionals can design systems that minimize reliance on linguistic or symbolic processing. This approach will be discussed in the portion of this chapter that explains the incorporation of visual scenes into low-tech and high-tech communication systems. The basic premise with this approach is that people with aphasia communicate most effectively when relying on cognitive processes that are non-symbolic in nature, such as visual perception, memory for important life events, and holistic processing of contextual information.

To date, AAC professionals and aphasiologists have succeeded primarily in developing treatment approaches corresponding with the first of these strategies—that is, by uncovering innovative ways of supporting the weakened language systems of people with aphasia through provision of informational redundancy. Recent advances, however, also have revealed new possibilities for bypassing sole dependence on linguistic elements and symbolic processing by, instead, increasing reliance on other, relatively preserved cognitive processes. By combining existing knowledge about systems supporting language processing with development of systems minimizing reliance on symbolic processing, AAC and aphasia specialists have an array of communication-based treatments from which to choose when supplementing the restorative intervention approaches commonly used to assist people with aphasia. The remainder of this chapter provides information to assist speech-language pathologists in deciding which AAC techniques and strategies are most likely to be effective with people displaying different aphasia characteristics and severities as well as information about how to design and implement a variety of communication-based AAC intervention strategies.

ASSESSING PEOPLE WITH APHASIA FOR SELECTION OF AAC INTERVENTIONS

Attempting to determine which of the many possible AAC intervention techniques will help a particular person with aphasia is a complex undertaking. The primary goal during AAC assessment for people with aphasia is the development of a clinical profile of capabilities and needs. This profile, once developed, can be matched against clinical trials with various AAC strategies and devices to determine those that hold the most promise for generalization into real communication contexts.

Capability Profile

Historically, constructing a capability profile of a person with communication needs is a starting point for developing an AAC treatment plan. Often, scores reflecting previous administration of a standard aphasia battery are available to begin formulation of the capability profile; if not, clinicians may wish to administer such a battery. In addition, if desired, clinicians can supplement these scores with administration of additional measures looking at specific cognitive functions

and/or specific AAC assessment measures to provide a more complete profile of a client's capabilities.

Aphasia Batteries

Speech-language pathologists can choose from several standardized assessment tools to help determine current linguistic and symbolic processing abilities of a person with aphasia. Some of the more commonly used options include the Boston Assessment of Severe Aphasia (Helm-Estabrooks, Ramsberger, Morgan, & Nicholas, 1989), or BASA; the Boston Diagnostic Aphasia Examination–3rd Edition (Goodglass, Kaplan, & Barresi, 2001), or BDAE-3; the Western Aphasia Battery (Kertesz, 1982), or WAB; and the Porch Index of Communicative Ability (Porch, 1967), or PICA. Clinicians may find the BASA particularly useful for people displaying very limited communication behaviors, because this tool provides a means of acknowledging non-spoken responses, assessing both linguistic and paralinguistic skills, and observing and identifying some AAC strategies spontaneously used by the person with aphasia (Nicholas, Helm-Estabrooks, Ward-Lonergan, & Morgan, 1993). For individuals who retain greater linguistic processing abilities, clinicians may prefer assessment measures that provide a means of observing behaviors across the modalities of listening, speaking, reading, writing, and gesturing. Most standardized aphasia batteries allow clinicians to identify areas of preserved strength relative to overall linguistic functioning.

Many comprehensive aphasia tests allow the classification of aphasia by type. Classification of aphasia types has a long history and broad appeal among speech-language pathologists and other rehabilitation medicine professionals. In particular, the clinical applicability of the Boston Classification System has made it popular among clinicians (Kertesz & Poole, 2004). In part, this appeal is because this provides a consistent vocabulary for discussing the clinical features of subgroups of people. Terms such as Broca's aphasia, Wernicke's aphasia, and anomic aphasia convey information about the status of a person's retrieval of words, fluency in speaking, comprehension of auditory messages, and repetition of utterances produced by others. These labels, however, may provide little practical information to guide practitioners in selecting and applying appropriate AAC interventions.

Beukelman and Garrett (1998) and, more recently, Garrett, Lasker, and Fox (2007; see also Garrett & Lasker, 2005a; Lasker & Garrett, 2004) suggested an alternate classification system placing greater emphasis on the partner-independent/dependent status with which a person who has aphasia communicates and less emphasis on the modality-specific language characteristics that he or she displays. For AAC purposes, this type of classification system can be a beneficial supplement to help speech-language

TABLE 30–1

Characteristics of Partner-Independent and Partner-Dependent Communicators

Partner-Independent Communicator	Partner-Dependent Communicator
• Initiates communicative interactions with others frequently and independently • Uses both natural modalities (e.g., speaking and gesturing) and AAC strategies to communicate • Experiences frequent communication breakdowns leading to inconsistent success communicating messages • Recognizes when communication breakdowns occur • Combines some symbols (e.g., spoken words, pictures, written words) to create simple and some complex messages • Displays relatively good pragmatic behaviors during conversational interactions • Has relatively good comprehension skills	• Needs assistance from a partner to initiate and maintain communicative interactions • Does not use AAC strategies without support and may not search, or searches ineffectively, for ways to communicate • Relies on a partner to interpret most, if not all, intents to others • Does not consistently recognize errors in communication • May have difficulty using symbols of any kind • May not engage in appropriate turn-taking during conversation • May require support for comprehension and/or expression of messages

Key: AAC = augmentative and alternative communication.

pathologists make decisions about communication-based treatment approaches. As implied by the label, partner-independent communicators are ones who communicate independently in many situations, without the need for assistance from others. Some partner-independent communicators use pre-stored messages, whereas others generate their own novel messages. In contrast, partner-dependent communicators require assistance from others to convey and comprehend messages and to reveal their communicative competence. Table 30–1 summarizes some of the common characteristics distinguishing partner-independent and partner-dependent communicators (Garrett & Lasker, 2005a).

Clinicians familiar with the Boston Classification System may find it helpful to consider how the corresponding aphasia types relate to partner-independent and partner-dependent communicators. Over the years, many aphasiologists have come to view the Boston Classification System as a severity continuum (Kertesz & Poole, 2004). This, in fact, is the underlying premise of the Aphasia Quotient score derived from administration of the WAB (Kertesz, 1982). Similarly, aphasia severity has a large impact on a person's classification as a partner-independent versus a partner-dependent communicator; however, severity by itself is an insufficient indicator (Garrett & Lasker, 2005a). Other factors, such as awareness of production errors and motivation to communicate, also contribute to determination of a person's partner-dependency status. Specifically, people exhibiting those types of aphasia identified through the Boston Classification System as being severe (e.g., such as global or mixed transcortical aphasia) or people having those aphasia types that correspond to severe comprehension problems and limited awareness of production errors (e.g.,

Wernicke's, transcortical sensory, or subcortical sensory aphasia) tend to be partner-dependent communicators. People with less severe types of aphasia and good awareness of their challenges, such as those with Broca's, conduction, or anomic aphasia, tend to be partner-independent communicators.

Of note, many individuals with aphasia fall somewhere in the middle of the partner-independent/dependent continuum. These individuals may be independent communicators in some instances but, at other times, may rely heavily on partner support to convey intents, comprehend others, and engage in meaningful communicative interactions. The label transitional communicator serves to describe the communicative competence displayed by these individuals. Indeed, many partner-dependent communicators evolve into transitional communicators as they gain skill and confidence applying AAC strategies and techniques to a variety of situations and with multiple communication partners.

Supplemental Cognitive Assessments

In addition to determining aphasia characteristics, clinicians may wish to assess cognitive skills if they feel this information will add meaningfully to a client's profile. Tools such as the Cognitive Linguistic Quick Test (Helm-Estabrooks, 2001), Raven's Progressive Matrices (Raven, Raven, & Court, 1998), and Wisconsin Card Sorting Test (Heaton, 1981) may be useful for assessing such skills. These measures give clinicians information about nonverbal processing and executive functions.

Helm-Estabrooks (2002) attempted to determine the correspondence between aphasia battery scores and scores

---

Box 30–1

Case Study 1

Tom sustained a left hemisphere cerebrovascular accident (CVA) 9 years ago, at the age of 52 years. Before his stroke, he lived by himself and worked as a photographer. As an adult, he had traveled throughout much of the world, both for his own enjoyment and as part of his vocation.

Following his stroke, Tom had frequent word finding difficulties, used several stereotypic phrases repeatedly during conversational interactions, and perseverated on certain ideas and verbal responses. His language production was nonfluent in nature, with poor verbal repetition skills. Tom's auditory comprehension skills surpassed his verbal expression abilities. A typical utterance follows, illustrating the nature of Tom's stereotypies and word retrieval challenges: "Well / let's see / I see a / I see a / you know I have a problem / I really do / I am bad / it's really bad / I see a / no that's not it / well it floats / and kids and things / you know I really have a problem / I really do."

Tom's language characteristics are consistent with moderate to severe Broca's aphasia, a diagnosis confirmed by his achieved scores on subtests of the Western Aphasia Battery (Kertesz, 1982) (i.e., Fluency = 4; Comprehension = 7; Repetition = 0.9; Naming = 2.3), yielding an Aphasia Quotient of 38.4. Tom's performance on Raven's Colored Progressive Matrices (Raven, Raven, & Court, 1998) placed him at the 25th percentile, and his performance on the Test of Nonverbal Intelligence (Brown, Sherbenou, & Johnsen, 1997) placed him in the 39th percentile. According to Garrett and Lasker's (2005a) classification system, Tom is a partner-independent, generative communicator.

Tom uses multiple AAC materials to support his communicative interactions. These include (a) two low-tech communication books differing in size and complexity; (b) a business card organizer for discussion of health care, financial concerns, and other matters involving interactions with professionals; (c) remnants about current events/activities in the form of news articles, advertisements, restaurant napkins, and so on that he stores in a shoulder pouch; and (d) paper and pencil for writing first letters or partial words and for drawing simple pictures. His ongoing intervention goals include (a) further development and expansion of use of low-tech communication books; (b) refinement of an organizational strategy for business cards and remnants; (c) expansion of his use of writing, including introduction of a spelling board for cueing production of more content words; and (d) mastery of conversational repair strategies related to misunderstandings by communication partners.

on assessments of non-linguistic functions. She found no consistent pattern of performance regarding the relation between linguistic and non-linguistic skills. Instead, individuals with aphasia appear to have unique profiles of cognitive strengths and weaknesses that are not predictable based on language test results. Helm-Estabrooks postulated that differences in the long-term outcomes of individuals with similar aphasia severities may stem from discrepancies in their cognitive abilities—specifically, within the realm of executive functions that allow flexibility and performance of goal-directed behaviors. Therefore, administration of assessments to measure the status of these functions may provide additional important information for consideration when developing a profile of a person with aphasia.

Aphasia-Based AAC Assessments

The specific assessment of the AAC strategy as used by people with aphasia is a relatively new undertaking. In recent years, some tools for examining these skills have emerged. For example, Garrett and Beukelman (1998) originally developed—and Garrett and Lasker (2005b) later updated—a communication assessment measure relating specifically to use of AAC by people with aphasia. This assessment, the Multi-Modal Communication Screening Task for Persons with Aphasia (available at http://aac.unl.edu/screen/screen.html) assesses a person's ability to communicate with an external system, search pictures, categorize, combine symbols, combine communication modalities, and use symbols for story telling or to convey a message (Garrett & Lasker, 2005b; Lasker & Garrett, 2004). Information gathered through administration of this tool assists clinicians in making decisions about the viability of using aided communication systems with specific individuals who have aphasia. The tool includes eight activities:

1. Selecting a symbol to request a basic need or provide a response to a biographical question.
2. Selecting two or more symbols to convey a specific message.
3. Choosing symbols that are exemplars of a given category.
4. Using symbols to complete a transaction and to converse with another person.
5. Pointing to sequential pictures to tell a story.
6. Listening to a clinician tell a story, and then retelling it using pictures or other available materials.
7. Using a map to provide information about places.
8. Spelling to supplement communication attempts.

When administering the tool, a clinician marks the type and frequency of cueing that a person needs to perform specific tasks. A summary score sheet allows clinicians to interpret test results with regard to an individual's communication partner-dependency.

Another way of collecting this partner-dependency information is to engage the person with aphasia in spontaneous communication using activities such as responding to open-ended questions (e.g., *What is your typical day like?*) or describing contextually rich pictures. While eliciting such a sample, the clinician provides alternative means with which the person who has aphasia can communicate by making tools, such as pencil and paper and a spelling board, readily available. Then, by watching and listening as the person with aphasia engages in the communication process, the clinician can make a judgment about partner-dependency, paying particularly attention to spontaneous uses of speech, gestures, drawing, writing, and spelling as well as to the person's overall comprehension level. This information, combined with results from other assessment procedures, may provide a sufficient basis for determining partner-dependency during communication attempts.

Needs Profile

A needs profile involves identifying all the contexts and interactions in which a person desires to communicate; the term should not be limited to requests for objects or actions. A needs profile include both transactional (i.e., transmitting specific information from one person to another) and interactional (i.e., developing and maintaining interpersonal relationships) activities. Beyond meeting basic needs, people communicate for a variety of purposes, including sharing information, establishing social closeness, and maintaining social etiquette (Light, 1988). Communication checklists and informal interviews are common ways of obtaining this type of information.

Checklists completed by caregivers provide a means of obtaining information about the needs and abilities of people with aphasia regarding use of AAC. Although experienced clinicians may prefer to gather such information through informal interviews, checklists provide a systematic way of collecting information about a person's functional and routine behaviors and needs. In particular, checklists provide clinicians with a means for amassing information about the communication roles, functions, and modes routinely used. For example, the Aphasia Needs Assessment (Garrett & Beukelman, 1997) (available at http://aac.unl. edu/screen/screen.html) includes items relating to a variety of communication needs that an individual with aphasia may experience. Administering the Partner Skill Screening Form and Partner Attitudinal Survey (Garrett & Beukelman, 1992) to family or caregivers may assist in delineating strengths of the communication partners regarding the facilitation of comprehension and expression by people with aphasia. Additionally, having a family member complete the Inventory of Topics (Garrett & Beukelman, 1992) may assist clinicians in identifying potential communication topics.

Strategy and Device Trials

The final aspect of assessing people with aphasia for AAC interventions involves the implementation of communication strategy and device trials. To perform such trials, a clinician first must identify a cluster of potentially useful strategies for exploration by matching a person's clinical profile to available strategies. This can be guided by identification of the person's independent-, transitional-, or dependent-communicator status. If initial trials are unsuccessful, alternate strategies should be explored. (Approaches that are appropriate for independent and dependent communicators are summarized in Communication-Based Interventions for People with Aphasia.)

Once a clinician has generated a list of potential strategies, he or she introduces them to a person with aphasia to determine which are used with ease, which are viable options for further training, and which the person with aphasia is not yet ready to attempt. People with aphasia and the professionals working with them sometimes require only a single session to decide whether a particular strategy or device has potential value; more frequently, however, experimentation and implementation over multiple sessions is necessary. Clinicians should judge the usefulness of particular strategies based on the person's responsiveness in terms of ability, engagement, willingness, and comfort.

Additional Considerations

Most people with aphasia have sustained strokes or acquired brain damage from other types of acute incidents. A subgroup of individuals, however, has a progressive form of aphasia—primary progressive aphasia (PPA)—associated with a decline in communicative function over time. These people have unique needs regarding AAC assessment, because over time, they will show the opposite shift regarding their partner-dependency status compared to people with acutely acquired aphasia. Specifically, during early stages of the disease process, people with PPA function as independent communicators. As the disease progresses, however, people with PPA become transitional communicators and then, eventually, partner-dependent communicators. This deterioration in communication independence has implications regarding the introduction and application of AAC strategies and devices that differ from those relevant to people with aphasia resulting from acute events. An overriding strategy regarding people with PPA is to provide instruction early during the disease process, when the individual still has adequate language and cognitive skills to understand and master compensatory strategies. The same philosophy extends to instruction regarding AAC strategies, techniques, and device usage (King, Alarcon, & Rogers, in press). Specifically, to maintain maximum communicative performance for as long as possible, practitioners should teach AAC strategies that are appropriate for transitional and partner-dependent communicators while the individual with PPA is still functioning as an independent communicator.

COMMUNICATION-BASED INTERVENTIONS FOR PEOPLE WITH APHASIA

This section presents information about multiple AAC interventions designed to promote successful interactions among people with aphasia and their communication partners.

Augmented Input/Augmented Comprehension

Augmented input, also called augmented comprehension, refers to a set of compensatory strategies that speech-language pathologists can teach to family, friends, and caretakers of partner-dependent and transitional communicators. The purpose of augmented input is to increase the ease and accuracy with which a person who has aphasia understands the verbalizations of others (Beukelman & Garrett, 1998; Garrett & Beukelman, 1992). Thus, the focus of augmented input is on improving receptive, rather than expressive, aspects of language processing, although it is easily paired with other AAC techniques, such as the written choice communication strategy, targeting the expression of communicative intents. Augmented input is appropriate for use with any individual who has reduced auditory-verbal comprehension.

Augmented input is multi-modal by nature. Communication partners of people with aphasia use drawing, writing key words, gesturing, referencing readily available contextual information in the environment, and providing prosodic emphasis to supplement spoken words as a means of communicating. These multiple-input modalities typically occur in combination with spoken messages.

The following example shows augmented input in an interactional exchange. Note that the communication partner uses augmented input to verify the person's response as well as to convey the initial question. As is typical of augmented input, the communication partner verbalizes the question in its entirety but only augments key elements:

Communication partner Did you go to your sister's [writes, *sister?*] on Sunday [points to *Sunday* on calendar]?
Person with aphasia [nods head]
Communication partner So, yes [nods head], you did go to your sister's [points to word, *sister*] on Sunday [points to *Sunday* on calendar].
Person with aphasia [nods head vigorously]

Communication Books

Communication books are used with many populations of people who have communication disorders. Regarding people with aphasia, communication books can be helpful to individuals across the spectrum of partner-dependency, although the type, complexity of information, and format will vary substantially based on capabilities, needs, aphasia severity, and partner-dependency status. Dependent communicators are most likely to benefit from communication books that include instructions to others about ways to foster communicative interactions along with relatively simple, contextually organized pages providing information about frequently discussed topics as well as topics of high interest. Independent communicators benefit from access to multiple types of conversational supports, such as maps of buildings or local areas, places for collecting and storing important remnants from recent events (e.g., newspaper clippings, ticket stubs, and business cards), and pages for drawing or writing to supplement verbalizations. Regardless of content or organization, communication books are relatively inexpensive ways of allowing people with aphasia to communicate about subjects that a clinician, caretaker, or family member anticipates will be frequent or desirable topics, and they are ways of providing tools for generative communication. They are among the most commonly used of all AAC strategies for people with aphasia, although the success that individuals experience when using them varies widely, depending on the content, organization, and instruction provided.

Communication Book Content

Inexperienced clinicians may believe that the intent of communication books is to provide people who have aphasia with a method of requesting attention to basic wants and needs. Although some people with aphasia require an AAC strategy to express basic needs, staff and family members often anticipate these needs, thus eliminating the necessity for communicating directly about them. For example, a person residing in a long-term care facility may have meals delivered at routine times and water available at all times on a bedside table, thus eliminating the need to request food or liquids; a person living at home may not need assistance dressing, toileting, or grooming, thus eliminating the need to communicate with another person about these activities. Because of this, not all people with aphasia use communication books to express basic needs, and communication books that solely provide a means of expressing such information generally are unsatisfactory.

Communication books have many potential uses other than the expression of basic wants and needs and, depending on their content, can be used to assist with communicative interactions in a wide variety of contexts. For example, a communication book may include content specifically targeting communication with grandchildren while babysitting, requesting directions to sale items in a store when shopping, or relaying personal information about an individual, his or her family, and interests when meeting new acquaintances. Determination of content and the context for use of communication books stems from careful consideration of an individual's needs and communication desires. Interviewing key people and reviewing information in the case history are good ways to make initial decisions about content and context.

Among the major goals of communication books are the provision of means to establish social closeness through small talk and storytelling, share information through generation of unique messages, make communication repairs, and use a variety of communication registers to indicate different social relationships with others (Stuart, Lasker, & Beukelman, 2000). The failure of clinicians to include ways of engaging in communication acts beyond requesting assistance to provide for basic wants and needs is one of the prime reasons that people with aphasia sometimes reject their communication books. Communication is about forming social relationships with other people, and communication books need to allow people with aphasia to do that through the development of conversations, the exchange of information, the opportunity to tell stories, and the chance to relate personal experiences and opinions.

Another important aspect of communication book content is to provide instructions about methods of facilitating communicative interactions to people who are not familiar with aphasia. Inclusion of simple messages explaining why an individual struggles with speaking or ways of helping to determine communicative intents can minimize the embarrassment that people with aphasia may experience when their communication attempts are less than perfect or the discomfort that others may feel when they do not know any strategies for facilitating communication. A sample message might be "I have aphasia, and I use this book to help me communicate. I can understand what you say if you speak slowly. Please be patient." Specific directions to write down words or repeat utterances also may be helpful in setting the context for a communication exchange.

As more pages and additional types of information are added to a communication book, the clinician may need to divide it into sections to foster easy location of material. Organizational strategies need careful consideration and adjustment, however, to ensure that they are logical to the person with aphasia and do not require symbolic or linguistic processing beyond the person's capabilities. (Ideas about how to organize books are provided in *Communication Book Organization*.)

Finally, communication books need to be dynamic in nature—that is, they should change in content and complexity to meet the changing needs of a person with aphasia. Once use of a communication book has been established, a family member, staff member, or other person should assume responsibility for updating the book as needed after

Box 30–2

Case Study 2

John had severe Broca's aphasia resulting from a stroke. He could say only a few words, although he often understood comments made by others when the topics were familiar and predictable. He used a communication book along with a collection of remnants to support many of his communicative interactions.

John lived with his wife in a small, rural community. One of his favorite activities was accompanying his wife to town to purchase groceries or run errands. John used these trips as an opportunity to catch up with friends and acquaintances by sitting in the car while his wife shopped. Because John had spent most of his adult life living and working in the town, he knew most of the people who passed by, and he enjoyed hearing the latest news about their families or projects at work.

Unfortunately, John's chats with friends frequently were followed by difficult conversations with his wife. Having visited with several friends and acquaintances, John was eager to share the latest news with his wife. Although he could often use his communication book and remnant collection to indicate the topics of his conversations, he struggled to tell his wife with whom he had talked—a problem exacerbated by the fact that John knew many people who his wife knew by name only. To solve this dilemma, John's clinician added a sign-in sheet and written instructions to the front of John's communication book. After talking with someone, John simply presented his communication partner with the sign-in sheet so that the person could write his or her name and the topic discussed.

the termination of formal speech and language intervention. For this to be successful, a speech-language pathologist must teach the designated individual how to make such additions and changes to the existing book.

Communication Book Organization

Categorical organization, based on either semantic or syntactic features, is common in AAC devices for people with communication disorders other than aphasia. Comprehension of traditional categorical organization may be difficult for people with aphasia, however, because organization by category requires symbolic abilities that often are impaired following strokes to the language-dominant hemisphere. For this reason, communication books in which pages are organized according to topic (e.g., eating, playing, or getting ready for work) or location (e.g., office at work or bedroom at home)—as is common for some children needing AAC materials—or according to syntactic categories (e.g., nouns, verbs, or adjectives)—as may be appropriate for literate adults—are not beneficial to some people with aphasia. These strategies require rather complex linguistic processes involving the recall of specific lexical items and the association of those items with either semantic or syntactic categories. Because these types of semantic and syntactic associations are difficult for people with symbolic deficits, communication books using semantic or syntactic categorical organization, regardless of the pictorial or lexical nature of individual items, may not provide as much benefit as communication books using other organizational schemes to people with aphasia.

Because of the nature of aphasia, an alternate organizational strategy not reliant on symbolic or linguistic processing may help when structuring communication books and other AAC devices for people with aphasia. The use of contextualized photographs and visual scene displays are ways of accomplishing this. A contextualized photograph shows an activity or experienced event in which familiar and personally relevant people, animals, and objects appear in a setting that is congruent with the depicted activity or event (McKelvey, Dietz, Hux, Weissling, & Beukelmen, 2007). Contextualized photographs contrast with portraits or isolated pictures of objects in that they include contextual or environmental content, show an ongoing activity or important life experience that is conducive to relating a story, and suggest the type or nature of relationships among people. For comparison purposes, consider the photographs displayed in Figure 30–1. Figure 30–1a shows a typical portrait in which a person not engaged in an activity appears against a neutral background. Although the image is clear and the pose is typical of static portraits, the photograph is of little use communicatively other than to identify the individual. Similarly, Figure 30–1b shows a family picture with little meaningful contextual information and no action or implied story. Again, the communicative potential relating to the image is limited. These pictures contrast with the contextualized photograph shown in Figure 30–1c. Here, a considerable amount of informational content is available to foster communication about the depicted individuals, the relationship among them, and the activity in which they are engaged.

Figure 30–1. Examples of non-contextual and contextual photographs.

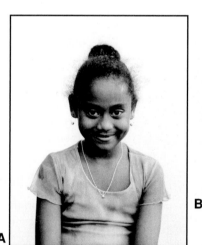

Non-contextualized individual portrait

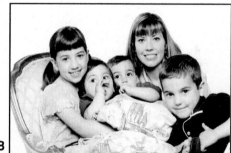

Non-contextualized family portrait

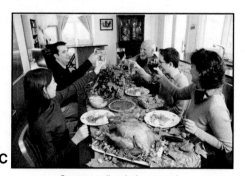

Contextualized photograph

Using contextualized photographs to organize communication books can be an effective strategy for people with aphasia. Incorporating one or more contextualized photographs into the display of a visual scene that incorporates digital reproductions of personally relevant photographs from an individual's private collection, written words, phrases, or sentences relating to the content depicted, as well as supplemental organizational strategies such as color coding or highlighting, can result in highly personalized support to the conversational interactions of a person with aphasia. An example of a visual scene display for incorporation into a low-tech communication book of a person with aphasia appears in Figure 30–2. Templates providing potential layouts for making visual scene displays to include in low-tech communication books are available at http://aac.unl.edu.

Recognizing pictures of familiar people and events is a relatively preserved cognitive skill for most people with aphasia (Fox & Fried-Oken, 1996). Using highly contextualized photographs in visual scene displays capitalizes on the intact visual processing and memory skills of people with aphasia as well as on the holistic nature of contextually rich pictures to organize content information and support conversation (McKelvey et al., 2007). As noted by Wilkinson and Jagaroo (2004), consideration of visual processing abilities is important when determining what type of AAC layout will best support

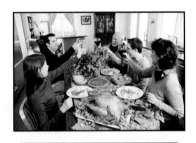

We went to my son Jack and daughter-in-law Becky's home for Thanksgiving.

Becky's decoration of the table is a tradition.

The family really looks forward to seeing what she does with the table each year.

To get started, ask me about:
• What I did for Thanksgiving
or
• My daughter-in-law

Figure 30–2. Sample visual scene display from a low-tech device.

an individual's attempts at communication. A potential advantage exists in using visual scene displays, rather than the traditional grid layouts common to many AAC systems, when dealing with people with aphasia, because grid processing requires individuals to evaluate all items in a grid both individually and equally, without the benefit of contextual support. In contrast, processing information contained in a visual scene display allows recognition of natural relations among objects displayed in a cohesive, holistic, and familiar context. People process visual scenes in a "gist" format that does not require full comprehension of all depicted elements to interpret meaning; hence, people with aphasia may benefit more from AAC systems that use visual scene displays compared with those that use traditional grid formats.

Instruction in Using Communication Books

Introducing the concept of using a communication book early in the treatment process may improve overall communication as well as allow a person with aphasia and his or her family to become accustomed to the idea of using AAC strategies to support natural speech. Delays in implementing communication books may contribute to their eventual rejection, both because the person with aphasia has not had sufficient time to master use of the book and because the clinician has not had sufficient time to make the necessary adjustments to maximize communication. Success most often occurs when practitioners introduce and teach the use of communication books in therapeutic activities that mirror real contexts. This allows the clinician to gauge an individual's feelings about using the communication book as well as to monitor his or her success. It allows the person with aphasia to practice using the book in a supportive setting and to participate in decision making about changes or additions to its structure and content.

High-Tech Devices

In the past, the use of high-tech AAC devices by people with aphasia has met with only limited success. A few anecdotal reports and case studies exist suggesting that some individuals—often those with motor speech challenges masking relatively intact residual language abilities—are successful in using high-tech devices to support communication attempts in real-life situations extending beyond the therapeutic environment (Garrett & Lasker, 2005a; Lasker & Garrett, 2003, 2004). The most common scenario, however, is that such a device is used only for a limited number of situational contexts (e.g., ordering at a restaurant or getting tickets at a box office). The goal of using high-tech AAC to support spontaneous generative communication remains elusive to most people with aphasia. The problem that people with aphasia face when attempting to use high-tech communication devices is circumventing their symbolic processing challenges.

Simply substituting an alternate symbol system for spoken language does not change the underlying symbolic processing problems. Hence, although people with aphasia may benefit from the multiple modalities that are presented on displays with written words, pictures of items, or alphabet letters, using such symbols to construct linguistically based generative messages remains difficult. Furthermore, the expense associated with purchasing and maintaining high-tech devices persuades most clinicians, family members, and people with aphasia to select low-tech options providing comparable features.

Despite the challenges experienced in the past, new advances incorporating visual scene displays hold considerable promise for facilitating the use of high-tech AAC devices by people with aphasia. As with low-tech communication books, high-tech devices displaying personally relevant, highly contextualized photographs along with related words or phrases and color-coding to assist recognition and navigation emphasize reliance on the intact visual processing and memory skills of people with aphasia while simulta-

neously minimizing the need for symbolic processing. In addition, high-tech applications of visual scene display offer advantages over their low-tech counterparts in that they allow digitized or synthetic speech output and increased amounts and complexity of included information. Use of miniaturized pictures (i.e., signature pictures) revealing the content/topics of hidden levels and touch-screen technology simplify organization, navigation, and access within the device. Researchers working on the development and implementation of high-tech AAC devices using visual scene displays have reported success by people with chronic aphasia in navigating their systems, using them to communicate stories to unfamiliar communication partners, and improving the overall quality of their communicative interactions as reported by family members (Dietz, McKelvey, & Beukelman, 2006; Dietz, McKelvey, Beukelman, Weissling, & Hux, 2005; McKelvey, Dietz, Hux, Weissling, & Beukelman, 2005, 2007). An example of a screen from a high-tech device showing a visual scene display appears in Figure 30–3. The large pictures in the center region of the

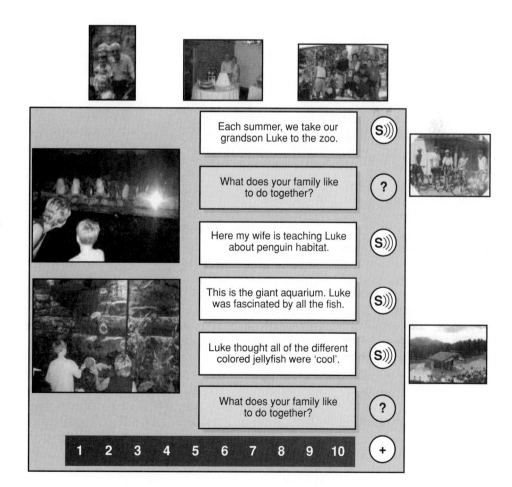

Figure 30–3. Sample visual scene display from a high-tech device. Printed with permission. Copyright Beukelman, 2007.

screen correspond with the selected topic, written text, and available digitized speech. The icons, when touched, allow navigation to higher or lower levels within the selected topic as well as triggering production of digitized messages, and the signature pictures around the perimeter of the screen, when touched provide access to screens relating to other conversational topics or other supplements to convey communicative intents or resolve communication breakdowns (e.g., maps, calendars, rating scales, or instructions to communication partners).

Basic guidelines for introducing high-tech AAC devices to people with aphasia are available (Garrett & Lasker, 2005a; Lasker & Garrett, 2004). First, the optimal size and number of symbols per page needs specification. Second, a practitioner needs to explore the impact of using devices with synthetic versus digitized speech. Third, the clinician should develop a scenario to assess the person's use of the device to relate stories and communicate novel messages, such as placing a phone call to order clothing from a mail-order catalogue or asking a stranger for directions to locate a store. Because people with aphasia have difficulty using symbols to encode and represent content, they may have difficulty with complex encoding strategies. When assessing the usefulness of a high-tech AAC device, it has been suggested (Garrett & Lasker, 2005a; Lasker & Garrett, 2004) to record information about the number of times that a person (a) uses the device successfully to communicate part or all of a message, (b) initiates communicative interactions, (c) integrates aided and unaided communication strategies, (d) navigates from one section or level of the device to another, (e) uses organizational strategies to search for items, and (f) resolves communication breakdowns. Clinicians also need to observe the competence with which the person handles control features for turning the device on and off, adjusting the volume, and troubleshooting unanticipated problems.

Virtually all people with aphasia who use high-tech AAC devices also employ multiple other strategies to support their communication attempts. These include both spontaneous, natural communication strategies, (e.g., gesturing and using facial expressions) as well as more formal, augmentative communication strategies, (e.g., referring to remnants, low-tech communication books, and lists). When used in combination, the multi-modal nature of these strategies is paramount in making them beneficial to people with aphasia. Limiting AAC strategies to a single device or modality does not maximize a person's use of residual cognitive recognition and problem-solving skills.

Drawing

Given appropriate instruction, people with aphasia can learn to use drawings to express simple thoughts and ideas, make requests, and gain social closeness; drawings also are beneficial when used by communication partners as a type of augmented input. The value of communicative drawing stems from two features: first, its provision of a permanent or semi-permanent record, providing additional time for people with aphasia to co-construct messages or revise communication attempts, and second, its lack of reliance on the processing of linguistic symbols (Lyon, 1995a, 1995b). Although drawings are symbolic in nature, people with aphasia may interpret the non-linguistic symbols used in drawings more easily than the linguistic symbols used in spoken and written messages.

Effective communicative drawing by people with aphasia requires good visual attention, relatively intact visual memory, and the ability to copy one-dimensional shapes (Helm-Estabrooks & Alberts, 2004). Despite frequent preservation of these skills, however, many people with aphasia do not spontaneously use drawing to convey ideas (Lyon, 1995a, 1995b). This is not surprising, because most people without communication challenges do not routinely incorporate drawing in their communication attempts. Hence, people do not automatically recognize the potential for communicative drawing, and direct instruction often is necessary to encourage its use. In particular, clinicians need to allay the concerns of both people with aphasia and their communication partners relating to limited artistic ability or coordination challenges resulting from use of the nondominant hand. Because of the simplistic nature of drawings required for communicative purposes, neither concern should limit exploration of the potential benefits of using drawing to supplement other modes of communication.

In addition to the creation of simple illustrations, communicative drawing can include graphic elements. Graphic elements are non-text symbols that do not convey meaning in isolation but that, when added to illustrations, can extend or clarify an intended meaning (Boling, Eccarius, Smith, & Frick, 2004). For example, a drawing of a car might connote a stopped car or one that is moving at either a fast or a slow rate of speed. The addition of three lines (i.e., movement lines) behind the vehicle provides the impression that the car is moving quickly. Movement lines, as well as other examples of graphic elements that people with aphasia and their communication partners can use to supplement drawings, are presented in Figure 30–4.

People with aphasia may initially benefit from a drawing program specifically geared toward improving communicative drawing (see, e.g.,Helm-Estabrooks & Albert, 2004; Lyon, 1995, 1995b). Because communicative drawing typically uses simple line drawings and stick figures, drawing intervention programs for people with aphasia are not expected to increase artistic talent. Instead, the prime objectives of drawing programs are, first, to correct or expand drawings so they better convey their intended meaning and, second, to augment unrecognizable portions of drawings through clinician feedback and implementation of additional drawing strategies, such as enlargement of main ideas and inclusion of graphic elements.

Box 30–3

Case Study 3

Mary acquired severe Broca's aphasia as a result of a cerebrovascular accident when she was 58 years old. Following the stroke, Mary's verbalizations were limited primarily to automatic speech and stereotypic and perseverative responses; she sometimes was successful in writing simple words or the first few letters of the words she wished to say.

Because of the severity of her expressive language challenges, Mary and her speech-language pathologist devoted a portion of their individual therapy time to improving Mary's generation of drawings as a means of supplementing her limited verbal and written output. First, Mary practiced identifying key shapes (e.g., square, circle, or triangle) in simple line drawings. Then, she traced these shapes, and after demonstrating adequate tracing skills, she copied shapes of increasing complexity. Eventually, the copied shapes became sufficiently complex so that they resemble objects. The next treatment step involved Mary's completion of drawings made by her clinician but lacking key elements. Only after repeated success with this activity did Mary's clinician engage her in communication-based tasks during which Mary had to use drawing to convey information displayed on cards visible to her but not to her communication partner.

Eventually, Mary independently initiated drawing as a supplement to verbalizations and/or written words or parts of words to convey communicative intents to others. She generated the drawing shown below to express her frustra-

tion with not being included in a women's discussion group following a recent church service.

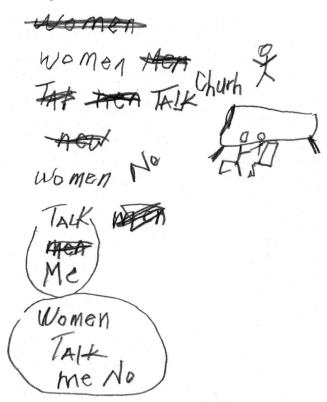

Communicative drawing serves to augment communication, not replace it. People with aphasia may shift between drawing and using other forms of communication, such as speaking, gesturing, and writing. As with many aphasia treatments and supports, use of communicative drawing during therapeutic contexts does not guarantee its use during natural communication settings. Only when others are supportive of the inclusion of drawing in communication attempts and encourage and embrace its use are people with aphasia likely to generalize it to natural settings.

Particularly for dependent communicators, communicative drawing is highly dependent on the ability of a communication partner to interpret a drawing. Some communication partners and people with aphasia find that using a drawing as a basis for a dynamic communicative interaction is beneficial. This means that each person intermittently contributes features or details to a shared drawing during the course of an interaction. In this manner, communication partners draw, interpret, correct, and probe while jointly creating an image along with a person who has aphasia. Especially when a person with aphasia does not draw to initiate communication of an intended message, the partner may need to start the process by making a guess about an intended message. By describing details while they draw, communication partners foster comprehension through provision of information in multiple modalities. Then, the person with aphasia may add to a partial drawing or answer simple yes/no questions to confirm the drawing's accuracy or appropriateness concerning the intended message. This approach also provides a way for the communication partner to model the use of drawing as a supplement to other modes of communication.

Written Choice Communication

Garrett and Beukelman (1992) developed the written choice communication strategy as a means for partner-dependent individuals with severe aphasia to express personal ideas, preferences, and opinions. The strategy capitalizes on the observation that people with aphasia benefit from informational redundancy and comprehend better when information is presented through multiple modalities rather than a

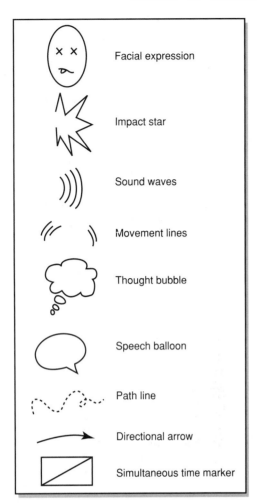

Figure 30–4. Examples of graphic elements. Printed with permission. Eccarius, M (2004). Using graphic elements in cartoon sequences to improve written narratives of hard of hearing students. Unpublished doctoral dissertation, University of Nebraska-Lincoln.

single modality. Residual skills and competencies of partner-dependent communicators become evident when communication partners present spoken questions simultaneously with written key words and followed by possible responses, again presented both in spoken and written modalities. To initiate an interaction, a communication partner and person with aphasia determine a topic of mutual interest. This is achieved by the communication partner asking a question such as *What topic would you like to talk about?*, printing and underlining the word *Topic* at the top of a piece of paper visible to the person with aphasia, and suggesting several possible topics. As the partner suggests each topic, he or she prints a key word or phrase relating to that topic and preceded by a bullet on the piece of paper. For example, as shown in Figure 30–5, the partner might suggest talking about events that occurred the previous weekend during a family visit, the performance of a favorite team in a recent

sporting event, or plans the individual has for returning home after completing his or her stay at a rehabilitation hospital. Usually, a communication partner presents three to five options from which the person with aphasia can choose, with one option being *Something else* or *Other*, in case the person with aphasia has a topic in mind other than those initially suggested. The person with aphasia responds to the question by pointing to one of the printed options. The communication partner then confirms the selection by circling it on the piece of paper and verbalizing it (e.g., *You want to talk about your family's visit last weekend*). The communication partner presents subsequent questions and potential answers relating to the selected topic in the same manner, with the interaction continuing until the topic is exhausted.

Many variations in applying the written choice communication strategy make it adaptable to the needs of a particular person with aphasia. For example, the number of possible responses that a communication partner proposes for questions can vary according to a person's ability to manage multiple potential answers (Garrett, 1993; Garrett & Beukelman, 1995). Also, some people with aphasia do not need the support of written key words and can use the strategy by having the communication partner simply write numbers or signal, with his or her fingers, a number to correspond with each verbalized option (Lasker, Hux, Garrett, Moncrief, & Eischeid, 1997). In addition, the strategy works well to elicit opinions or ratings corresponding to a continuum of responses presented on Likert-type response scales (e.g., a scale ranging from 1 to 5, with 1 corresponding to a very negative response and 5 corresponding to a very positive response). Other variations involve altering the pace of an interaction through inclusion of additional repetitions by a communication partner of questions or response choices. Finally, a communication partner or person with aphasia can supplement the written choice communication strategy, with drawings or gestures serving as forms of augmented input or alternative forms of expression.

As shown in the example illustrated in Figure 30–5, a key advantage of the written choice communication strategy is that it allows a person with severe aphasia to express personal desires and opinions—a communication skill that often eludes such patients. The quality of interactions using the written choice strategy, however, largely is dependent on the skill of the communication partner. Speech-language pathologists must ensure that family members, friends, and caretakers of a person with aphasia receive instruction and structured practice using the technique.

Gestures

Gestures are a standard supplement to most people's natural speech production. Although some people with aphasia retain some spontaneous use of gestures as supplements to speaking, most struggle with using gestures, comparable to their challenges with other forms of linguistic and symbolic

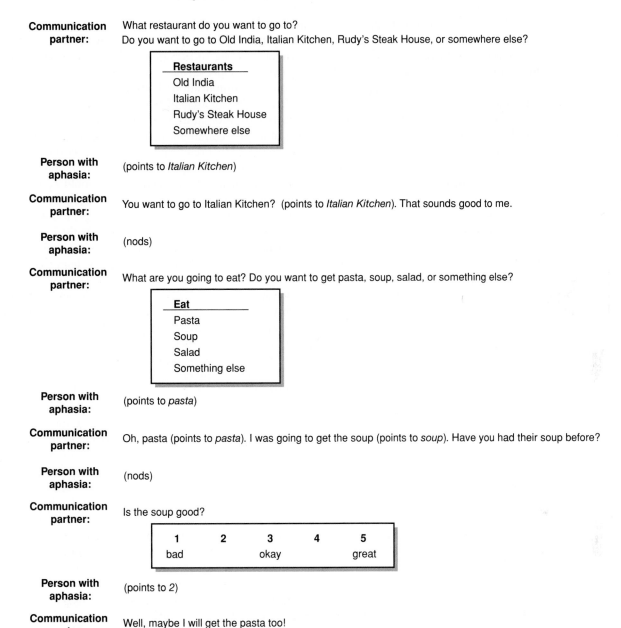

Communication partner: What restaurant do you want to go to?
Do you want to go to Old India, Italian Kitchen, Rudy's Steak House, or somewhere else?

> **Restaurants**
> Old India
> Italian Kitchen
> Rudy's Steak House
> Somewhere else

Person with aphasia: (points to *Italian Kitchen*)

Communication partner: You want to go to Italian Kitchen? (points to *Italian Kitchen*). That sounds good to me.

Person with aphasia: (nods)

Communication partner: What are you going to eat? Do you want to get pasta, soup, salad, or something else?

> **Eat**
> Pasta
> Soup
> Salad
> Something else

Person with aphasia: (points to *pasta*)

Communication partner: Oh, pasta (points to *pasta*). I was going to get the soup (points to *soup*). Have you had their soup before?

Person with aphasia: (nods)

Communication partner: Is the soup good?

> | 1 | 2 | 3 | 4 | 5 |
> |---|---|---|---|---|
> | bad | | okay | | great |

Person with aphasia: (points to 2)

Communication partner: Well, maybe I will get the pasta too!

Figure 30–5. Sample interaction using the written choice communication strategy.

systems. In general, practitioners need to provide direct instruction to encourage use of gestures as an AAC strategy for people with aphasia (Collins, 1986).

Gestures can serve many purposes during interactions. Common examples include:

1. Waving a hand, touching another person's arm, or establishing joint eye contact to gain a person's attention.
2. Pointing to a desired object to replace a verbal request for the item.

3. Using iconic or charade-like movements to express needs or transfer information (e.g., raising a hand to the mouth in imitation of holding a glass and drinking from it).
4. Affirming or refuting statements made by others through head nods and shakes.
5. Indicating feelings, opinions, or reactions through facial expressions and standardized gestures (e.g., raising the eyebrows to indicate surprise, shrugging the shoulders to indicate indecision or doubt, or pointing the thumb up or down to indicate approval or disapproval, respectively).

Clinician- and researcher-developed treatment programs exist that specifically target the use of gestures by people with aphasia. One such training program is Visual Action Therapy developed by Helm-Estabrooks, Fitzpatrick, and Barresi (1982). The intent of Visual Action Therapy is to decrease the effects of apraxia of speech, improve verbal expression, and improve the use of gestures for communicative purposes by people with severe aphasia (Helm-Estabrooks & Albert, 2004). The program includes three phases, focusing on development of proximal limb, distal limb, and oral gestures. Various stimuli (e.g., real objects, line drawings, and pictures) are presented to elicit responses following a hierarchy that begins with matching objects to pictures and concludes with independent use of gestures to represent objects unknown to a communication partner.

Coelho and Duffy (1986) developed another gesture training program that included levels of imitation, recognition, and production. During the imitation level, a practitioner shows a person with aphasia a picture and a corresponding gesture or sign for imitation. During the recognition level, the clinician signs a referent, and the person with aphasia matches the gesture to the appropriate picture given a group of four choices. During the production level of training, the person with aphasia practices making appropriate signs or gestures when presented with a pictures of referents.

Concerns exist about the generalization of gesture use to communicative interactions outside of structured treatment sessions both for Visual Action Therapy (Helm-Estrabrooks et al., 1982) and Coelho and Duffy's (1986) gesture-training program (Coelho, 1990; Coelho & Duffy, 1987). To address this concern, Cubelli, Trentini, and Montagna (1991) used Promoting Aphasic's Communicative Effectiveness (Davis & Wilcox, 1985), or PACE, procedures in which, given a picture of an object or action, a person with aphasia pantomimes an intended message to his or her communication partner or clinician. Questions and cues from the listener prompt the person with aphasia to provide increasingly specific gestures. After successful conveyance of the intended meaning, a review of distinctive features, function, or form provides a platform for refinement and practice generating appropriate gestures, although the emphasis remains on message communication rather than on perfection in performance of gestures.

Although the various gesture training programs differ somewhat in their instructional methods, they face similar challenges regarding effectiveness. The success of gesture use by people with aphasia depends on factors such as the amount of contextual support available; the presence of limb apraxia, facial apraxia, or other motor impairments; and the iconicity of selected gestures. Context affects how people interpret gestures. For example, two fingers held in a "V" shape can mean *peace* or *two*, depending on the context. Gestures used without a pre-established topic may be ambiguous to communication partners because of multiple possible interpretations. Also, attempts at gestural communication relating to previous or future activities or objects not physically present are considerably more difficult than gestural communication about current events (Glennen & DeCoste, 1997). In addition, motor impairments in the form of paresis or apraxia complicate the acquisition and use of gestures for communicative purposes. Clinicians typically find that gestures requiring only simple motor movements are the easiest for people with aphasia to master (Coelho & Duffy, 1986). In addition, clinicians should consider location, hand shape, movements associated with the sign, spatial orientation, and handedness of the person with aphasia when selecting gestures for training. Finally, iconicity is an important factor for consideration when selecting gestures to include in an intervention program. Iconicity refers to how apparent the meaning of a gesture is based on its resemblance to a physical entity. For example, pantomimes are highly iconic movements designed to be direct, concrete portrayals of an intended message; socially or culturally recognizable gestures, such as waving or saluting, also have a high degree of iconicity for members within a society or social group (Glennen & DeCoste, 1997). Highly iconic gestures typically are easier for people with aphasia to master as compared to those with low iconicity (Coelho & Duffy, 1986). Again, however, motor impairments may impede acquisition and use of even highly iconic gestures.

As a rule, dependent and transitional communicators use gestures less frequently and less effectively compared with independent communicators. For most individuals with aphasia, spontaneous gesture use is roughly comparable to residual verbal output (Glosser, Wiener, & Kaplan, 1986); hence, dependent communicators with limited effective verbal output also may have a limited repertoire of interpretable gestural communication. Because of this, direct instruction in use of gestures is particularly important for dependent and transitional communicators. Independent communicators who routinely rely on gestures as a communication supplement may find it helpful to carry a dictionary of gestures with them to help partners interpret specific, idiosyncratic gestures.

Aphasia-Friendly Environments

In addition to the specific AAC strategies and techniques described in the previous sections, the notion of aphasia-friendly environments warrants attention. The development of aphasia-friendly environments is an overarching principle governing the incorporation of AAC strategies, techniques, and devices into communication-based interactions involving people with aphasia who function as partner-dependent, transitional, or partner-independent communicators. Aphasia-friendly environments refer to settings that are conducive to maximizing the effectiveness of people with aphasia by increasing situational supports and decreasing barriers interfering with the success of communication attempts (Howe, Worrall, & Hickson, 2004). Howe and colleagues (2004) relate the components of aphasia-friendly environments to the five domains identified in the International Classification of Functioning, Disability, and Health Environmental Factors Model (World Health Organization, 2001):

1. Support and relationships
2. Attitudes
3. Products and technology
4. Natural environments and human-made changes to the environment
5. Services, systems, and polices

Regarding the first two domains, aphasia-friendly environments are ones in which partners acknowledge the competence of people with aphasia by including them in decision-making activities and by using simple, adult language with extended processing time for language comprehension and formulation. Members of society demonstrate accepting attitudes by facilitating the participation of people with aphasia in novel as well as established activities and by encouraging people with aphasia to interact with familiar as well as unfamiliar partners. The third domain—products and technology—affects the establishment of aphasia-friendly environments through the development of programs and products that are easily accessed by people with aphasia, minimize challenges associated with aphasia, and serve to educate others about aphasia. This includes a wide diversity of items, ranging from specially adapted computer applications to public-information materials describing the strengths and challenges experienced by people with aphasia. Regarding the domain of the natural environment and human-made changes to the environment, aphasia-friendly settings are conducive to optimizing communicative interactions through strategies such as eliminating competing background noises and distractions. The final domain—services, systems, and policies—is evident in aphasia-friendly environments through the availability of support groups, transportation services, and communication services to aid people with aphasia as they participate in daily activities, such as running errands, attending meetings/appointments, placing telephone calls, and responding to written correspondence.

For dependent communicators, two domains are of particular importance: support and relationships, and the natural environment and human-made changes to the environment. These domains are especially important because dependent communicators rely heavily on family members and friends to modify various aspects of the environment for facilitation of effective communication. Hence, professionals must ensure that communication partners of people with aphasia are adept in supporting conversation. A skilled communication partner must know how to use strategies such as

writing key words (i.e., providing augmented input), providing written choices, and referencing contextually rich pictures to present information through multiple modalities and to enhance comprehension and expression. Elaboration about implementing each of these strategies is provided in the following sections.

Independent communicators may rely on some of the same types of supports that are used by dependent communicators; in addition, however, they benefit from attention to the domains of attitudes, products and technology, and services, systems, and policies. Changes in these domains reflect modifications affecting the whole of society rather than individual people. For example, as society becomes more accepting of and educated about people with communication challenges, more support groups and services in the community will become accessible and, hence, more widely used. Given proper support, independent communicators may even be the individuals responsible for organizing support groups or rallying for services not otherwise provided. In addition, technologic advances may provide the basis for environmental supports, allowing independent communicators to maintain their independence. Independent communicators are the subset of people with aphasia most likely to benefit from traditional high-tech communication systems. Other AAC strategies that are particularly helpful for independent communicators (and reviewed in the following sections) focus on the incorporation of multiple communication modalities through drawing, gesturing, writing, and accessing low-tech and high-tech communication books incorporating visual scenes.

Computer-Based Treatment Approaches

A final issue warranting attention concerns the development and use of computer-based treatment approaches. Compensatory, communication-based, AAC interventions differ from computer-based treatment approaches in important ways. Computer-based treatment approaches allow the provision of intervention services in a manner that contrasts with or supplements traditional aphasia intervention services in which a professional interacts during individualized or group therapy sessions with one or more people who have aphasia. A professional's goal when applying a computer-based treatment approach is to facilitate language restoration by providing opportunities for massed practice, nonjudgmental feedback, the possibility of practicing outside formal speech-language therapy sessions, real-time task modification to meet individual needs, and reduced time pressure (Wallesch & Johannsen-Horbach, 2004). In contrast, a professional's goal when applying AAC interventions is to teach people with aphasia and their communication partners the strategies that will support communication in diverse settings and with a wide variety of people. By teaching AAC techniques, strategies, or device usage, a professional strives to help a person with aphasia compensate for persistent communication challenges. Both computer-based treatment approaches and AAC have important contributions to make in the field of aphasiology and warrant the attention of speech-language pathologists and other rehabilitation specialists; however, recognition of the differences between the two approaches is important.

As covered more extensively in this book's chapter about computer-based treatment approaches, professionals have designed several types of technology-based programs to support treatment of aphasia. Computer-based interventions vary in their status as sole methods of treatment or as parts of comprehensive programs, in the extent to which they are client- or therapist-directed, and in the type and number of treatment goals that are targeted. For example, some programs are designed to function as replacements for spoken language (Steele, Kleczewska, Carlson, & Weinrich, 1992), although people with aphasia often do not have sufficient linguistic competence to use such systems in multidimensional ways that extend beyond treatment settings. Other computer-based treatments support only one aspect of language performance, such as word retrieval (Adrian, Gonzalez, & Buiza, 2003; Fink, Brecher, Sobel, & Schwartz, 2005) or sentence-level auditory comprehension (Crerar, Ellis, & Dean, 1996). Differences regarding client/therapist direction and support during practice sessions range from programs allowing people with aphasia to engage in independent practice using specific linguistic structures (Mortley, Wade, & Enderby, 2004; Petheram, 1996) to programs requiring professional input to guide intervention and monitor progress (Aftonomos, Steele, & Wertz, 1997; Crerar et al., 1996).

A major concern expressed by some aphasia specialists is that computer-based treatments provide little opportunity for generalizing learned skills to communicative interactions and limited, if any, improvement in functional communication. Instead, observed improvements following application of computer-based treatment approaches almost invariably take the form of higher scores on formal aphasia assessments (Aftonomos et al., 1997). Although such a change may indicate overall improvement in language processing, it does not ensure generalization to conversational interactions with other people. The opposite, however, is true of AAC interventions: By definition, AAC interventions aim to support a person's real-life communicative interactions in diverse settings and with multiple partners.

Recognizing potential limitations associated with computer-based treatments is important. Computer-based systems can be expensive and time-consuming, with mastery only occurring after many hours of work with a speech-language pathologist over a period of weeks or even months (Wallesch & Johnnsen-Horbach, 2004). In additional, computer-based approaches that emphasize massed practice may have the unintended negative effect of increasing isolation and reducing time spent engaging in other activities or interacting with others (Wade, Mortley, & Enderby, 2003; Wallash & Johannsen-Horbach, 2004). Given the large investment in time and/or money needed to pursue computer-based approaches and the lack of evidence documenting generalization to real-life conversational interactions, careful and individualized weighing of the risk–benefit ratio is necessary before embarking on extensive programs using computers solely for treatment purposes. As long as professionals recognize that computer-based treatment approaches have limitations as well as advantages, however, and that they are distinct from AAC interventions, people with aphasia and those who interact with them are likely to benefit from advances regarding both types of treatment.

GENERALIZATION OF AAC STRATEGIES AND TECHNIQUES

The generalization of AAC systems into everyday, meaningful communication activities is the desired outcome of such intervention. Generalization is unlikely, however, unless a therapist strategically plans for it from the inception of treatment. Conceptually, generalization is a four-step process involving (1) planning, (2) providing intervention services to a person with aphasia and instruction to family members or caretakers, (3) designing a home program, and (4) performing monitoring activities to make adjustments as appropriate.

Generalization planning involves identifying immediate, short-term, and long-term goals that a person with aphasia can achieve through application of specific AAC techniques and strategies. By engaging in a planning process, clinicians construct ideas about generalization at the outset of treatment. For example, regarding instruction about using written choice as a communication strategy, a clinician first might plan activities that require a small number of exchanges and for which family members may have preexisting knowledge about probable preferences. To achieve this short-term goal, the clinician might teach family members to use written choice as a communication strategy when providing choices to a person with aphasia about the day's meals. Initial activities such as this are ones in which people with aphasia and their caretakers are likely to experience success, thus encouraging continued use of the AAC strategy to attempt more substantive interactions. The clinician's plan for long-term generalization of the written choice strategy might involve progress toward using it for more generalized and conversational purposes, such as talking about an upcoming grandchild's dance recital or discussing events of the past week. The long-term goal is to facilitate expression of intents to a variety of familiar and unfamiliar communication partners across multiple settings to enhance an individual's formation and maintenance of relationships with others. The key to the planning stage is that the clinician considers generalization issues at the start of strategy instruction rather than waiting for mastery first.

After the planning stage, intervention targets both family and client development of the skills needed to meet treatment goals. The combination of skilled intervention for a person with aphasia and instruction to family members about AAC strategies is important for successful generalization. Although such dual instruction is well-established when treatment involves children with AAC needs (Bruno & Dribbon, 1998), the concept of providing instruction to family members often is overlooked when dealing with adults with aphasia.

Once both family members and a person with aphasia can successfully implement AAC strategies and techniques to perform tasks presented within structured therapeutic settings, home assignments encourage generalization of the learned skills. Not waiting too long to transfer skills to settings outside of therapy is important. Otherwise, people may view the techniques as only applying to therapy and may not attempt their use in real-world situations. In addition, to facilitate generalization, therapists need to model AAC strategy use whenever possible before, during, and after treatment sessions and not restrict it to treatment time devoted specifically to practicing AAC techniques. Regarding home assignments, specific instructions about when and where to implement certain techniques is initially beneficial. For example, a clinician might instruct a person with aphasia to use drawing to facilitate his or her communication during dinner with a granddaughter the following evening or when having coffee with a neighbor the next morning. Later, the clinician can provide more generalized instructions, such as telling the person with aphasia to find two people with which to use the drawing strategy within the next week.

Arranging outings and accompanying people to specific locations are other ways of providing highly structured homework tasks. Examples include planning a trip to a local store to allow interaction with a clerk, using an AAC device to place a phone call, or interacting with a receptionist or other employee of a health care facility with which the person with aphasia is familiar. As people with aphasia experience success, they often think of additional ideas on their own and report back about their independent success.

The last step in establishing a generalization program is to arrange a method for monitoring progress and refining AAC skills as needed. Adjustments to the home program and overall plan may be necessary if a person with aphasia experiences multiple communication breakdowns or encounters resistance from others in certain settings. Again, clinicians must keep in mind the goal of providing ways for people with aphasia to convey communicative intents, allowing the formation and maintenance of relationships with others.

FUTURE TRENDS

Advances in AAC and in aphasiology largely have occurred independently from each other. Few AAC specialists consider themselves to be experts in aphasia, and few aphasiologists feel comfortable implementing a wide variety of AAC strategies and techniques. Likewise, few empirical research articles appearing in aphasia journals have addressed the application of AAC interventions, and equally few articles appearing in AAC journals have reported the effectiveness of implementing such interventions for people with aphasia. The melding of assessment and intervention strategies that support both restoring speech and language functions to the greatest extent possible and compensating for persistent challenges holds considerable promise regarding the development of innovative and effective communication-based approaches for people with aphasia. For this to occur, however, practitioners need to maintain their focus on designing and implementing strategies and techniques that apply to interactions extending beyond the confines of treatment sessions and that address the day-to-day interactional and transactional needs of adults with aphasia. In particular, interventions must be directed toward decreasing the social isolation that people with aphasia commonly experience. A goal of all aphasia-based interventions—whether they involve AAC strategies, devices, and techniques or rely on other language restoration strategies—must be greater social reintegration of people with aphasia through increased opportunities and participation in social activities.

New interventions are likely to include the development of new AAC devices and strategies specifically taking into consideration the preserved and impaired aspects of cognitive functioning displayed by people with aphasia. These applications will exploit relatively preserved cognitive skills, such as memory and visual perception, while minimizing reliance on linguistic and symbolic processing. In addition, these applications will foster the provision of communicative information through multiple modalities to maximize the likelihood of comprehension and expression by people with aphasia.

Clinical professionals have a responsibility to be familiar and comfortable with the notion of AAC for people with aphasia, with existing communication-based AAC strategies and devices, and with new AAC applications as they become available. With this knowledge, early introduction of compensatory and communication-based AAC interventions will be more likely, in turn promoting greater skill acquisition and acceptance of compensatory strategy use by people with aphasia, their family members, other rehabilitation professionals, and society in general. This type of treatment advance, coupled with increased attention regarding the training of communication partners for people with aphasia and the establishment of aphasia-friendly environments, could substantially impact the overall effectiveness of aphasia intervention.

1. Many people with aphasia—particularly those with more severe forms of the disorder—experience chronic communication challenges that negatively impact their participation in social roles, activities, and relationships.

2. In addition to restorative treatment approaches, people with aphasia can benefit from exposure to AAC interventions during all stages of recovery—including the acute stages—to ensure sufficient time and opportunity to practice and refine strategies that will help them to compensate for persistent communication challenges.

3. For people with aphasia, AAC is most effective when it is conceptualized as a combination of procedures and processes that are multi-modal, compensatory, adaptable, and geared toward minimizing communication breakdowns.

4. Aphasia is a weakness of symbolic processing and, as such, requires innovative and non-symbolic approaches to the design, organization, and application of AAC interventions.

5. Two types of approaches exist for using AAC to support the communication efforts of people with aphasia:
   a. AAC systems can supplement a person's inefficient language comprehension and production by providing informational redundancy through the use of multiple modalities and contextual supports.
   b. AAC systems can minimize reliance on linguistic or symbolic processing by incorporating contextual scenes or visual scene displays into low-tech or high-tech devices.

6. Practitioners can obtain important information about a person's communicative capabilities and needs as well as their potential to use various AAC strategies and techniques effectively by administering and interpreting results from aphasia batteries, supplemental cognitive assessments, communication checklists, and aphasia-based AAC assessments and by implementing strategy and device trials.

7. For AAC purposes, practitioners need to consider the partner-dependent, transitional, or partner-independent status of the communication attempts of individuals with aphasia.

8. Specific AAC strategies and techniques for people with aphasia include the use of augmented input, high- and low-tech communication books and devices, drawing, written choice communication, and gestures.

9. Computer-based treatment approaches differ from AAC interventions, and although they provide for massed, non-judgmental, and untimed practice, they may not necessarily generalize to communication used for interactive purposes.

10. Aphasia-friendly environments are crucial to the successful incorporation of AAC strategies, techniques, and devices into communication-based treatments for people with aphasia.

11. AAC approaches hold considerable promise for supporting individuals with aphasia, but professionals need to continue working on generalizing use of AAC to natural contexts and everyday settings.

1. Why are AAC systems that provide symbols (in any form) as substitutions for spoken words only partially beneficial to people with aphasia?

2. How does partner-dependency status impact a practitioner's selection of AAC strategies and techniques to try with a person who has aphasia?

3. What are the key characteristics of an aphasia-friendly environment?

4. How can augmented input facilitate comprehension by a person with aphasia?

5. What distinguishes a portrait from a contextual scene?

6. Why should family members and caretakers of people with aphasia learn AAC strategies and techniques?

7. What are the characteristics of a person with aphasia who might benefit from written choice communication?

8. What AAC strategies and techniques provide informational redundancy to support either the receptive or expressive communication attempts of people with aphasia?

9. What are the relatively intact cognitive processes retained by many people with aphasia that allow them to benefit from communication book or device organization using contextually rich photographs or visual scene displays?

References

Adrian, J. A., Gonzalez, M., & Buiza, J. J. (2003). The use of computer-assisted therapy in anomia rehabilitation: A single-case report. *Aphasiology, 17,* 981–1002.

Aftonomos, L. B., Steele, R. D., & Wertz, R. T. (1997). Promoting recovery in chronic aphasia with an interactive technology. *Archives of Physical Medicine and Rehabilitation, 78,* 841–846.

American Speech-Language-Hearing Association [ASHA] (2004). Roles and responsibilities of speech-language pathologists with respect to augmentative and alternative communication: Technical report. *ASHA Supplement, 24,* 1–17.

Beukelman, D. R., & Garrett, K. L. (1998). Adults with severe aphasia. In D. R. Beukelman & P. Mirenda (Eds.), *Augmentative and alternative communication management of severe communication* disorders in children and adults (pp. 467–504). Baltimore, MD: Paul H. Brookes.

Beukelman, D. R., Yorkston, K., & Dowden, P. (1985). *Communication augmentation: A casebook of clinical management.* San Diego: College Hill Press.

Boling, E., Eccarius, M., Smith, K., & Frick, T. (2004). Instructional illustrations: Intended meanings and learner interpretations. *Journal of Visual Literacy, 24,* 185–204.

Brown, L., Sherbenou, R., & Johnsen, S. (1997). *Test of Nonverbal Intelligence* (3rd ed.). Austin, TX : Pro-Ed.

Bruno, J., & Dribbon, M. (1998). Outcomes in AAC: Evaluating the effectiveness of a parent training program. *Augmentative and Alternative Communication, 14,* 59–70.

Coelho, C. A., & Duffy, R. J. (1986). Effects of iconicity, motoric complexity, and linguistic function on sign acquisition in severe aphasia. *Perceptual and Motor Skills, 63,* 519–530.

Coelho, C. A., & Duffy, R. J. (1987). The relationship of the acquisition of manual signs to severity of aphasia: A training study. *Brain and Language, 31,* 328–345.

Coelho, K. M. (1990). Acquisition of generalization of simple manual sign grammars by aphasia subjects. *Brain and Language, 31,* 328–345.

Collins, M. (1986). *Diagnosis and treatment of global aphasia.* San Diego: College Hill Press.

Crerar, M. A., Ellis, A. W., & Dean, E. C. (1996). The mediation of sentence processing deficits in aphasia using a computer-based microworld. *Brain and Language, 52,* 229–275.

Cubelli, R., Trentini, P., & Montagna, C. G. (1991). Re-education of gestural communication in a case of chronic global aphasia and limb apraxia. *Cognitive Neuropsychology, 8,* 369–380.

Davis, G., & Wilcox, M. (1985). *Adult aphasia rehabilitation: Applied pragmatics.* San Diego, CA: College-Hill Press.

Dietz, A., McKelvey, M., & Beukelman, D. R. (2006). Visual Scene Display (VSD): New AAC interface for persons with aphasia. *Perspectives in Augmentative and Alternative Communication, 15,* 13–17.

Dietz, A., McKelvey, M., Beukelman, D. R., Weissling, K., & Hux, K. (2005). *Visual scenes: An AAC prototype for people with aphasia.* Paper presented at the meeting of the American Speech-Language-Hearing Association, San Diego, CA.

Fink, R. B., Brecher, A., Sobel, P., & Schwartz, M. F. (2005). Computer-assisted treatment of word retrieval deficits in aphasia. *Aphasiology, 19,* 943–954.

Fox, L. E., & Fried-Oken, M. (1996). AAC Aphasiology: Partnership for future research. *Augmentative and Alternative Communication, 12,* 257–271.

Garrett, K. (1993). *Changes in conversation participation of individuals with severe aphasia given three types of partner support.* Unpublished doctoral dissertation, University of Nebraska-Lincoln.

Garrett, K., & Beukelman, D. (1992). Augmentative communication approaches for persons with severe aphasia. In K. Yorkston (Ed.), *Augmentative communication in the medical setting* (pp. 245–338). Tucson, AZ: Communication Skill Builders.

Garrett, K., & Beukelman, D. (1995). Changes in the interaction patterns of individuals with severe aphasia given three types of partner support. *Clinical Aphasiology, 23,* 237–251.

Garrett, K., & Beukelman, D. R. (1997). *Aphasia needs assessment.* Retrieved June 9, 2005 from http://aac.unl.edu/screen/screen.html.

Garrett, K., & Beukelman, D. R. (1998). Adults with severe aphasia. In D. R. Beukelman & P. Mirenda (Eds.), *Augmentative and alternative communication: Management of severe communication disorders in children and adults* (2nd ed., pp. 465–499). Baltimore, MD: Paul H. Brookes.

Garrett, K., & Lasker, J. (2005a). AAC for adults with severe aphasia. In D. R. Beukelman & P. Mirenda (Eds.), *Augmentative & alternative communication: Supporting children & adults with complex communication needs* (3rd ed., pp. 467–504). Baltimore, MD: Paul H. Brookes.

Garrett, K., & Lasker, J. (2005b). *The multimodal screening task for persons with aphasia.* Retrieved June 9, 2005 from http://aac.unl.edu/screen/screen.html.

Garrett, K., Lasker, J., & Fox, L. (2007). Severe aphasia. In D. R. Beukelman, K. Garrett, & K. Yorkston (Eds.), *Augmentative communication in the medical setting.* Tucson, AZ: Communication Skill Builders.

Glennen, S., & DeCoste, D. (1997). *The handbook of augmentative and alternative communication.* San Diego, CA: Singular.

Glosser, G., Wiener, M., & Kaplan, E. (1986). Communicative gestures in aphasia. *Brain and Language, 27,* 345–359.

Goodglass, H., Kaplan, E., & Barresi, B. (2001). *The assessment of aphasia and related disorders* (3rd ed.). Philadelphia: Lippincott, Williams & Wilkins.

Heaton, R. K. (1981). *Wisconsin Card Sorting Test.* Odessa, FL: Psychological Assessment Resources.

Helm-Estabrooks, N. (2001). *Cognitive Linguistic Quick Test.* San Antonio, TX: Psychological Corporation.

Helm-Estabrooks, N. (2002). Cognition and aphasia: A discussion and a study. *Journal of Communication Disorders, 35,* 171–186.

Helm-Estabrooks, N., & Albert, M. (2004). *Manual of aphasia therapy* (2nd ed.). Austin, TX: Pro-Ed.

Helm-Estabrooks, N., Fitzpatrick, P. M., & Barresi, B. (1982). Visual action therapy for global aphasia. *Journal of Speech and Hearing Disorders, 47,* 385–389.

Helm-Estabrooks, N., Ramsberger, G., Moragan, A. R., & Nicholas, M. (1989). *Boston Assessment of Severe Aphasia.* Chicago: Riverside.

Holland, A., & Beeson, P. (1993). Finding a new sense of self: What the clinician can do to help. A reply to Brumfitt's Losing one's sense of self following stroke. *Aphasiology, 7,* 569–591.

Holland, A. L., Fromm, D. S., DeRuyter, F., & Stein, M. (1996). Treatment efficacy: Aphasia. *Journal of Speech & Hearing Research, 39,* S27–S36.

Howe, T. J., Worrall, L. E., & Hickson, L. M. H. (2004). What is an aphasia-friendly environment? *Aphasiology, 18,* 1015–1037.

Jacobs, B., Drew, R., Ogletree, B. T., & Pierce, K. (2004). Augmentative and alternative communication (AAC) for adults with severe aphasia: Where we stand and how we can go further. *Disability and Rehabilitation, 26,* 1231–1240.

Kertesz, A. (1982). *The Western Aphasia Battery.* New York: Grune & Stratton.

Kertesz, A., & Poole, E. (2004). The aphasia quotient: The taxonomic approach to measurement of aphasic disability. *Canadian Journal of Neurological Sciences, 31,* 175–184.

King, J., Alarcon, N., & Rogers, M. (2007) in Beukelman, D., Garrett, K., & Yorkston, K. (Eds.), *Augmentative communication strategies for adults with acute or chronic medical conditions.* Baltimore: Paul H. Brookes Publishing Co.

Kraat, A. W. (1990). Augmentative and alternative communication: Does it have a future in aphasia rehabilitation? *Aphasiology, 4,* 321–338.

LaPointe, L. (2005). Foundations: Adaptation, accommodation, aristos. In L. LaPointe (Ed.), *Aphasia and related neurogenic language disorders* (2nd ed., pp. 1–18). New York: Thieme.

Lasker, J., & Garrett, K., (2003). *Cognitive-linguistic profiles of aphasic communicators who use AAC.* Paper presented at the American Speech-Language-Hearing Association annual convention, Chicago, IL.

Lasker, J., & Garrett, K. (2004). *Alternative communication options for aphasia: Cognitive behavioral assessment protocol.* Paper presented at the American Speech-Language-Hearing Association, Philadelphia annual convention, PA.

Lasker, J., Garrett, K., & Fox, L. (2007) in Beukelman, D., Garrett, K., & Yorkston, K. (Eds.), *Augmentative communication strategies for adults with acute or chronic medical conditions.* Baltimore: Paul H. Brookes Publishing Co.

Lasker, J., Hux, K., Garrett, K., Moncrief, E., & Eischeid, T. (1997). Variations on the written choice communication strategy for individuals with severe aphasia. *Augmentative and Alternative Communication, 13,* 108–116.

Light, J. (1988). Interaction involving individuals using augmentative and alternative communication systems: State of the art and future directions. *Augmentative and Alternative Communication, 4,* 66–82.

Light, J., Drager, K., McCarthy, J., Mellott, S., Millar, D., Parrish, C., et al. (2004). Performance of typically developing four- and five-year-old children with AAC systems using different language organization techniques. *Augmentative and Alternative Communication, 20,* 63–88.

Lyon, J. G. (1995a). Communicative drawing: An augmentative mode of interaction. *Aphasiology, 9,* 84–94.

Lyon, J. G. (1995b). Drawing: Its value as a communication aid for adults with aphasia. *Aphasiology, 9,* 33–50.

McKelvey, M. L., Deitz, A. R., Hux, K., Weissling, K., & Beukelman, D. R. (in press). *Performance of a person with chronic aphasia using a visual scene display prototype. Journal of Medical Speech-Language Pathology, 15*(3), 305–313.

McKelvey, M. L., Dietz, A. R., Hux, K., Weissling, K., & Beukelman, D. R. (2005). *Performance in people with chronic aphasia using a visual scenes display.* Paper presented at the American Speech-Language-Hearing Association annual convention, San Diego, CA.

McNeil, M. R. (1988). Aphasia in the adult. In N. J. Lass, L. V. McReynolds, J. L. Northern, & D. E. Yoder (Eds.), *Handbook of speech-language pathology and audiology* (pp. 738–786). Philadelphia, PA: W. B. Saunders.

McNeil, M. R., & Pratt, S. R. (2001). Defining aphasia: Some theoretical and clinical implications of operating from a formal definition. *Aphasiology, 15,* 901–911.

Mortley, J., Wade, J., & Enderby, P. (2004). Superhighway to promoting a client-therapist partnership? Using the Internet to deliver word-retrieval computer therapy, monitored remotely with minimal speech and language therapy input. *Aphasiology, 18,* 193–211.

Nicholas, M. L., Helm-Estabrooks, N., War-Lonergan, J., & Morgan, A. R. (1993). Evolution of severe aphasia in the first two years post onset. *Archives of Physical Medicine and Rehabilitation, 74,* 830–836.

Petheram, D. (1996). The behaviour of stroke patients in unsupervised computer-administered aphasia therapy. *Disability and Rehabilitation, 18,* 21–26.

Porch, B. E. (1967). *The Porch index of communicative ability.* Palo Alto, CA: Consulting Psychologists.

Raven, J., Raven, J. C., & Court, J. H. (1998). *Coloured progressive matrices.* Oxford: Oxford Psychologists Press.

Robey, R. R. (1998). A meta-analysis of clinical outcomes in the treatment of aphasia. *Journal of Speech and Hearing Research, 41,* 172–187.

Simmons-Mackie, N. N., & Damico, J. S. (1997). Reformulating the definition of compensatory strategies in aphasia. *Aphasiology, 11,* 761–781.

Steele, R. D., Kleczewska, M. K., Carlson, G. S., & Weinrich, M. (1992). Computers in the rehabilitation of chronic, severe aphasia: C-VIC 2.0 cross-modal studies. *Aphasiology, 6,* 185–194.

Stuart, S., Lasker, J., & Beukelman, D. R. (2000). AAC message management. In D. R. Beukelman, K. M. Yorkston, & J. Reichle (Eds.), *Augmentative and alternative communication for adults with acquired neurologic disorders* (pp. 25–54). Baltimore, MD: Paul H. Brookes.

van de Sandt-Koenderman, M. W. M. E. (2004). High-tech AAC and aphasia: Widening horizons? *Aphasiology, 18,* 245–263.

Wade, J., Mortley, J., & Enderby, P. (2003). Talk about IT: Views of people with aphasia and their partners on receiving remotely monitored computer-based word finding therapy. *Aphasiology, 17,* 1031–1056.

Wallesch, C. W., & Johannsen-Horbach, H. (2004). Computers in aphasia therapy: Effects and side-effects. *Aphasiology, 18,* 223–228.

Wilkinson, K. M., & Jagaroo, V. (2004). Contributions of principles of visual cognitive science to AAC system display design. *Augmentative and Alternative Communication, 20,* 123–136.

World Health Organization. (2001). *International classification of functioning, disability, and health.* Geneva: Author.

Chapter 31

Melodic Intonation Therapy

Robert W. Sparks

OBJECTIVES

The objectives of this chapter are to instruct the clinician in the technique of melodic intonation, describe the verbal behavior of both good candidates and poor candidates for melodic intonation therapy (MIT), discuss the administration of the MIT hierarchy, offer suggestions for involving the families of those with aphasia who are selected for exposure to this language intervention strategy, and suggest future trends in further development of MIT.

Numerous studies have indicated that an unimpaired right cerebral hemisphere is dominant for music in right-handed persons. This explains why persons with aphasia can sing the melody of a familiar song. Their accurate emission of the words of the song is of greater interest, however, because of its contrast with their inability to communicate the most basic needs. This preserved skill also includes recitation of prayers, some social gesture phrases, and premorbid use of profanity. Jackson (1931) classified such utterances as nonpropositional language, because they do not involve encoding of a message that contains specific information. He theorized that such utterances are processed in an undamaged, so-called nondominant hemisphere of a person with aphasia. Today, we can produce no better word to describe such language, although we no longer label the right hemisphere as being a nondominant one. Indeed, research indicates that the right hemisphere is involved in processing the prosody of propositional language.

Sparks, Helm, and Albert (1974) reviewed some of the literature on right hemisphere processing of the prosodic elements of speech. Their analysis suggests that, in normal right-handed persons and many left-handed persons, the right hemisphere functions in a tandem relationship with the left hemisphere both for encoding and for emission of propositional language. The final integrative process, however, takes place in the temporal lobe of the left hemisphere.

Reorganization of this interhemispheric process with increased participation of the right hemisphere probably occurs only when recovery is slow and incomplete. Of equal importance in this reorganization are preserved interhemispheral pathways for language. Indeed, Gordon (1972) states that a long period may be involved in increasing the function of the right hemisphere. The reader is referred to Code's discussion of the role of the right hemisphere in the treatment of aphasia. The probability that this is increased by melodic intonation therapy (MIT) is even more likely when we consider the right hemisphere's dominance for music. Studies of adult aphasia that have described language performance from a phonologic model have included Blumstein (1973), Martin and Rigrodsky (1979), and Whitaker (1970).

Melodic intonation therapy involves singing, and the specific techniques that we call intonation are described in some detail later in the chapter. This type of singing is an ancient form, dating back at least to the Judeo-Christian period. It is distinct from other forms of singing in that each intoned utterance is based on the melody pattern, the rhythm, and the points of stress in the spoken model. Use of an intoned utterance that resembles a familiar song may produce disastrous results, therapeutically speaking. The familiar melody will stimulate recall of the nonpropositional words of that song.

PRINCIPLES OF LANGUAGE THERAPY AFFECTING MIT

Objectives of MIT

The original intention for developing MIT for those with severe nonfluent aphasia was to achieve at least a basic recovery of the ability to use some language accurately. Good candidates demonstrate extreme paucity of speech and show concern about such an incapacity. Reasonable priorities of therapeutic purpose for such patients would relegate the quality of articulation and syntax to secondary consideration. Emphasis on the linguistic or semantic aspects of verbal utterances for these persons with aphasia is the primary goal of MIT. Some clinicians, however, are using the technique as a more phonologic intervention for verbal apraxia. A review of our physiological model implies that the right hemisphere controls prosody. This, then, justifies the use of MIT for the phonologic defects of such patients.

Speech Pathology Principles Applied to MIT

The Examination

A preference as to standardized aphasia examinations that are used to evaluate a potential candidate for MIT is not an issue. Sparks (1978) has presented guidelines for supplementary para-standardized examination of persons with aphasia that make it possible to investigate more specific language skills in addition to those sampled by standardized examination batteries. In any event, MIT depends on evidence from the examination that the aphasic candidate has a distinct potential for some recovery of language.

Eight Principles of Language Therapy Involved in MIT

1. The first principle is concerned with gradual progression of the length and difficulty of the tasks in the therapeutic hierarchy. Such progression involves the type of linguistic material used, a gradual withdrawal of participation by the clinician in that are purely repetition, and reduction of reliance on melodic intonation in the last level of the MIT hierarchy.

2. The second principle—one endorsed by Schuell, Jenkins, & Jimenez-Pabon (1964)—maintains that direct attempts to correct the verbal errors of the person with aphasia fail because he or she cannot recall the specific nature of his errors. Attempts to correct errors accomplish little, and even may do some harm, if they detract from the smooth progression of the hierarchy. The person severely handicapped by aphasia who is considered to be a candidate seldom can effectively correct his or her verbal errors by retrial. Such retrials often result in a perseverated repetition of the error, which thus reinforces it. During MIT, attempts are made to achieve correct responses by means of a second trial that involves the technique of "backup." Specifically, when the person with aphasia fails a step, he or she is immediately guided through a repetition of the previous step and then a second attempt of the step that he or she failed. The person with aphasia may or may not be aware of the purpose of this procedure, but it is not drawn to his or her attention. A second backup retrial is never attempted if failure occurs again.

3. The third principle maintains that repetition is a highly effective therapeutic device. Repetition serves as the core of MIT. Actually, repetition involves a rather complex process. The fact that normal persons can repeat familiar or simple sentences more efficiently than they can more difficult sentences suggests that a process of decoding the stimulus and then re-encoding it for emission is involved. Accurate repetition deteriorates in longer units. The paraphrased repetition of the longer sentence, however, does not alter the meaning. The stimulus has been accurately received and decoded, but some word substitutions have been used for the restatement. Perhaps the most difficult repetition task involves unknown words of another language or nonsense syllables. In this task, the usual decode–encode process is less efficient. As stated previously, the use of repetition in MIT gradually decreases as the level of difficulty of tasks increases.

4. The fourth principle is concerned with latencies of response. One such control is use of latency between completion of stimulus presentation by the clinician and permission for response by the person with aphasia so that the complete stimulus is received and decoded. Another use of latency is between the completion of one sentence-item progression in the hierarchy and the beginning of the next.

5. The fifth principle is avoidance of practice effect by using the same material or carrier phrases repeatedly. This often is tedious and not therapeutically effective. A well-constructed program of intervention will include many useful high-probability utterances that trigger recall of premorbid language skills. Language that is alien to the person with aphasia should not be used. Therefore, enough variety of meaningful material is encouraged for MIT so that no utterance is used more often than every ninth or tenth session of therapy.

6. The sixth principle maintains that the clinician should pay scrupulous attention to the purpose and semantic value of each of his or her verbal utterances. For example, exuberant reinforcements within a sequence of steps are disruptive. A smile of encouragement will serve just as well or better. This is not an indictment of a warm, holistic approach to therapeutic intervention in general; however, clinicians should practice restraint during MIT.

7. The seventh principle maintains that written or pictorial materials should not be used as added stimuli. We believe the presumption that such material is supportive to the auditory stimulus is very suspect. Our premise is that these materials actually distract rather than support the MIT therapeutic process. This is particularly true of good candidates for MIT who have auditory comprehension that permits them to understand and retain spoken stimuli in a variety of contexts. Persons with aphasia and severe auditory deficits may respond better to auditory stimuli when they are accompanied by pictures; however, such patients are not candidates for MIT.

8. The eighth principle pertains to the frequency of therapy sessions. Twice-daily treatment sessions are essential for the person with aphasia and severe impairment

of language. When restrictions of time, resources, or transportation are involved, the training of family members to function as assistants in the MIT program may be very effective.

CANDIDACY FOR MIT

Assessment regarding the efficacy of MIT has proved that no single language intervention strategy for aphasia is a panacea. Indeed, MIT is effective for only a portion of the aphasic population. This, then, implies a need for careful evaluation of each person with aphasia who is being considered for exposure to this method. Chapter 3 of this text described computed tomographic findings of cortical and subcortical lesions as predictions of candidacy for MIT. Such studies contribute much. Language profiles of both good and poor candidates are presented here as guides for selection. Emphasis is placed on auditory comprehension, several aspects of verbal expression, and nonlanguage behavior.

The Good Candidate

Auditory Comprehension

Examination of auditory comprehension indicates that the good candidate's understanding and retention of spoken language are essentially normal in a variety of contexts. It is simplistic to presume that the process of monitoring one's own verbal utterances is solely through auditory feedback. Actually, kinesthetic feedback probably alerts us to phonologic or semantic errors immediately before the auditory feedback has commenced. In any event, evidence of preserved self-criticism in the good candidate is important.

Verbal Language

The clinical impression of the good candidate is that of a person with aphasia and a marked paucity of any kind of verbal output. In other words, he or she is a nonfluent aphasic. This is accompanied by demonstration of frustration and despondency concerning his or her language impairment. A curious and enigmatic perseveration of a neologistic utterance has been observed in some persons with aphasia who have subsequently responded well to MIT. It is enigmatic because it is similar to the stereotypical jargon utterances of some patients with global aphasia, but two points of difference are notable. First, good candidates will modify the prosody of the utterance so that it reflects their intention to make a declarative, interrogative, or forceful imperative statement. Second, they < will be annoyed by the meaningless morphology of the utterance. With the exception of such stereotyped jargon utterances, little speech is initiated except for an occasional, single substantive word that is always an appropriate communication.

Phonologic performance by the good candidate who has no language impairment other than speech production includes effortful but indistinct speech that is interrupted by pauses for attempted initiation of each utterance and attempts to correct himself or herself. Speech is phonologically distorted. When the articulation is analyzed, a systematic reorganization of sound patterns may seem to occur.

A summary of the results from examination of verbal expression produces a profile of the good candidate as follows:

1. Almost no responses occur in confrontation naming, responsive naming, word and phrase repetition, or sentence completion. An occasional response, however, will be poorly articulated but accurate enough to indicate correct encoding of the target word.
2. Effort at self-correction often is vigorous. This is to be expected in persons with aphasia who are acutely aware of making errors in their verbal output. Unfortunately, the product usually is not improved by this effort.

Nonverbal Behavior

Good candidates often are reasonably depressed, but they almost always are emotionally stable, with a mature response to counseling by the clinician. They manifest a strong desire to enter into intensive efforts to rehabilitate their speech, and they accept MIT.

Concurrent Abnormalities

The good candidate usually demonstrates a significant buccofacial apraxia and has a hemiplegia that is more severe in the arm than in the leg.

Language Profile after MIT

A diagnosis of "classical" this or "classical" that usually is careless, but it is tempting to describe the verbal output of the person with aphasia after MIT as having evolved into that of a person with classical Broca's aphasia. Some of the person's utterances continue to be poorly articulated and agrammatical but telegraphically appropriate. An example is "Home—weekend—Saturday and Sunday. Hospital—you;—Monday." Considering the graduate's almost total inability to communicate before the therapy, this telegram is a triumph.

Further Improvement after MIT

The question as to whether achieved language improvement will be retained by the person with aphasia following successful MIT produces some concern for clinicians. Fortunately, follow-up examinations of MIT graduates have shown that not only do they maintain their new competency, they also continue to improve in their own home environment.

Syntactic substance begins to appear in their verbal output. Graduates of MIT and their families should be advised that a review of the final steps of the hierarchy will be beneficial in the continuing improvement. The clinician should discuss the extent of the family's participation and be available as a continuing consultant.

The Poor Candidate

Three aphasic syndromes are not responsive to the present form of MIT—namely, Wernicke's, transcortical, and global aphasia. The labels are not as important as brief reviews of the verbal behavior involved in each of the three types. All are clearly distinct from the profile of the good candidate that has been presented.

Wernicke's Aphasia

Achieving therapeutic success in those with Wernicke's aphasia is a very difficult and challenging task. Concerted effort by some speech pathologists to produce more effective language therapy for persons with this type of aphasia is essential. The following characteristics of those with Wernicke's aphasia are in marked contrast to those of the good candidate:

1. Auditory comprehension is poor and variable. Those with Wernicke's aphasia show no evidence of being aware that they fail to be understood. In fact, they usually reject language therapy, and their reaction to MIT is either explosive or one of amused condescension.
2. Verbal utterances are overly fluent, syntactically normal, and clearly articulated. They include abundant paraphasic errors for the substantive words, however, and the end result is bizarre and meaningless.
3. Those with Wernicke's aphasia are often emotionally unstable, often hostile, but sometimes extremely cordial. The application of MIT techniques to patients with Wernicke's aphasia has produced poor results. These patients accurately duplicate intonation patterns, including the melody, rhythm, and points of stress. This is in contrast to their replacement of the words in the stimulus model with their own paraphasic jargon.

Transcortical Aphasia

The person with aphasia demonstrating this profile may be similar in some ways to the good candidate and in other ways to the person with Wernicke's aphasia. The important feature of this form of aphasia is an isolated skill at accurately repeating long phrases and sentences, seemingly without the normal decoding process mentioned earlier. The person with aphasia performs perfectly in MIT, but no carryover to improved functional language occurs. Investigation of repetition skill as a candidacy factor would suggest that the ability to repeat even single words may be a negative prognostic factor for MIT candidacy.

Global Aphasia

The history of language therapy for persons with global aphasia indicates that such therapy has been unsuccessful in improving their functional verbal language. This was pointed out by Albert and Helm-Estabrook (1988); by Sarno, Silverman, and Sands (1970); and by Schuell and colleagues (1964). In fact, MIT is no more effective than other language therapy in reestablishing any useful verbal communication.

MELODIC INTONATION

Sparks and Holland (1976) briefly describe the difference between songs and melodic intonation. Specifically, songs have distinct melodies. In contrast, melodic intonation is based solely on the spoken prosody of verbal utterances. The latter uses a vocal range that is limited to three or four whole notes; this is all that is necessary to achieve an adequate variety of melodic patterns. The range is about the same as that of the melodic line of speech.

This limited range of sung notes is comfortable for the untrained voice of adults. It is important to point out the necessity of avoiding melodic intonation patterns that are similar to those of long-lasting popular songs.

The Form of Melodic Intonation

Melodic intonation is based on three elements of spoken prosody:

1. The melodic line or variation of pitch in the spoken phrase or sentence.
2. The tempo and rhythm of the utterance.
3. The points of stress for emphasis.

Certainty regarding the appropriateness of the intonation pattern is essential in MIT. The need for this appropriateness becomes essential in the final level of the hierarchy, when intoned utterances gradually are transposed back to spoken prosody.

Some exaggeration of the three elements of a spoken prosody model occurs when that utterance is intoned. First, the tempo is lengthened to a more lyrical utterance. Second, the varying pitch of speech is reduced and stylized into a melodic pattern involving the constant pitch of intoned notes. Third, the rhythm and stress are exaggerated for emphasis; this usually involves increased loudness and elevation of intoned notes. These three modifications of spoken prosody serve as a means for emphasizing the prosodic structure of the utterance.

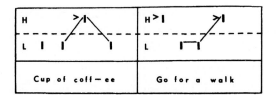

Figure 31–1. Prosodic patterns of speech. H indicates higher pitch; L indicates lower pitch. A single-syllable word is indicated by a single vertical bar. Vertical bars that are connected represent multi-syllabic words or clusters of words. An arrow preceding a vertical bar indicates stress on that word or syllable.

Acceptable Variety of Melodic Patterns and Regional Differences

Several alternative prosody patterns exist for any verbal utterance. The clinician must exercise his or her judgment as to which one will be used for a phrase or sentence in any one session of language therapy. Using a different intonation pattern in a subsequent session is a means for achieving variety of stimulation. Two such variations are illustrated in Figure 31–1.

Regional differences of speech prosody sometimes are quite pronounced. This is not a matter of concern if the clinician and the person with aphasia come from, and are in, the same region. The emigration of a clinician from one prosodically distinct area to another, however, implies that he or she must make an adjustment when MIT is involved. Samples of regional differences are presented in Figure 31–2.

Plotting Spoken Prosody Patterns

Two illustrations of the method of graphically plotting verbal utterances along with an explanation of the plotting technique are presented in Figure 31–1. This method, an adaptation of the one developed at the Kodaly Musical Training Institute and presented by Knighton (1973), will be used in all subsequent illustrations.

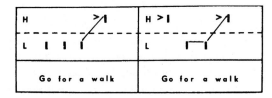

Figure 31–2. Two equally acceptable spoken prosody patterns. H indicates higher pitch; L indicates lower pitch. A single-syllable word is indicated by a single vertical bar. Vertical bars that are connected represent multi-syllabic words or clusters of words. An arrow preceding a vertical bar indicates stress on that word or syllable.

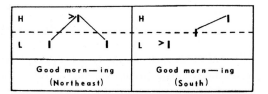

Figure 31–3. Regional differences in patterns of spoken prosody for one sentence.

In the first phrase shown in Figure 31–1, "cup of coffee," the utterance starts on a lower pitch for "cup," but the substantive importance of the word places it alone. This is followed by the cluster of words, "of coffee." Emphasis stress is on the first syllable of "coffee," along with the higher pitch that such stress produces. The last syllable of this declarative phrase has the customary drop in pitch. In the second illustration, "Go for a walk," the stress is on "go," with an accompanying higher pitch, then a drop in pitch for the two functor words in the cluster, then a return to the higher pitch along with stress for the substantive word, "walk."

Figure 31–2 plots the difference of two variations for the phrase "Go for a walk." The first is as illustrated in Figure 31–1. The second illustrates a model in which the word "for" is detached from the rest of the cluster that follows. This may be desirable as the person with aphasia improves and the clinician thinks that therapy should begin to attack the absence of functor or relational words in the patient's speech.

In Figure 31–3, a comparison of prosody for the social gesture utterance "good morning" shows a rise–fall melody pattern of the northeastern parts of the United States and a gradually rising inflectional pattern of at least some parts of the South.

Transposing Speech to Intonation

Illustrations of the transposition of plotted speech prosody models into melodic intonation are presented in Figure 31–4

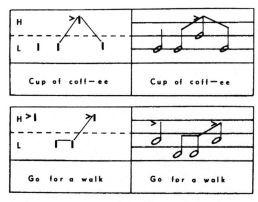

Figure 31–4. Transposition of spoken prosody models to melodic intonation. Key of C in treble cleff is used for illustration. No attempt is made to present accurate musical tempo.

using the phrases illustrated in Figure 31–1. The placing of the notes on a musical staff in these illustrations does not imply that ability to read music is a prerequisite to administering MIT, although such skill is an advantage. The primary purpose here is to duplicate graphically the pattern of spoken prosody that has served as the model. Considerable musical license has been taken—and musicians are requested not to take issue. For those who are interested, however, the key of C is used in the illustrations so that variations of sung note combinations may be demonstrated.

Sprechgesang

The fading of melodic intonation and a return to spoken prosody occurs in the fourth level of the MIT hierarchy. It is a technique that lies halfway between speech and singing. It is used in choral reading but more lyrically by Schoenberg in his *Ode to Napoleon* and *Pierrot Luraire*. Schoenberg defined the technique as sprechgesang, or "spoken song."

The exaggerated tempo, rhythm, and points of stress in sprechgesang are the same as in the intoned model. The more variable pitch of speech, however, replaces the more constant pitch of intoned notes. The utterance is lyrical but spoken rather than sung.

The senior author lays claim to the use of this art form as a bridging technique in the MIT hierarchy after having heard a performance of *Ode to Napoleon* by the Boston Symphony Orchestra in 1973. He will furnish a cassette sample of sprechgesang on request, provided that the request is accompanied by phrases to be illustrated and a cassette.

LINGUISTIC CONTENT

The importance of a linguistically sophisticated control of the grammatical structure of phrases and sentences used in MIT depends largely on the severity of the individual person with aphasia's inability to communicate and the usefulness of the verbal material. The selection of phrases and short sentences should be high-priority communication. This involves investigation of basic aspects of the patient's premorbid milieu that may be used and then some creativity on the part of the clinician to produce stimulating material. In other words, all material should be egocentric for the individual person with aphasia. This should be the case in all therapy for the traumatized person with aphasia, but it is particularly important as a counterbalance during MIT, in which the technique is so atypical of normal verbal behavior. Information about such things as basic family routines, family relationships and customs, personal needs, and personal likes and dislikes will suggest an abundance of material with both universal and individual appeal. Clusters of sentences that have a spherical relationship add an even greater significance. This is illustrated in Figure 31–5, which

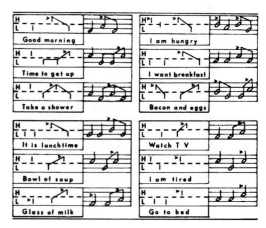

Figure 31–5. Four thematic, three-item illustrations of melodic intonation material using the same figure legend presented in Figure 31–1.

presents four three-item themes as an illustration of thematic relationship of therapeutic material along with further illustration of melodic intonation plotting. Additional illustration of the thematic arrangement of material presented by Sparks and Holland (1976) is included here with the permission of the senior author of that article:

---

3. Look at the Sports Page 6. Time to Go to Bed

Sample Material for Level II

1. twelve o'clock	6. apple pie
2. time for lunch	7. glass of milk
3. bowl of soup	8. I am sleepy
4. salt and pepper	9. take a nap
5. ham sandwich	

Sample Material for Levels III and IV

1. Sit down in a chair.	6. I am very tired.
2. Read the newspaper.	7. It is getting late.
3. Look at the sports page.	8. Time to go to bed.
4. Turn on the TV.	9. It is ten o'clock.
5. Go for a walk.	

Meaningful stimulus items for the aphemic candidate who has no impairment other than phonologic errors should, in addition to being meaningful for the individual patient, focus on facilitating more intelligible speech. The creative clinician will meet with the candidate and family and explain the importance of gaining information about specific linguistic preferences that the patient used in his or her premorbid speech. Therapeutic concern for consistent phonologic errors makes it more difficult to select meaningful material. Table 31–1 illustrates the use of phonologic patterns in selecting stimulus materials.

TABLE 31-1

Sample Phonologic Patterns for Melodic Intonation Therapy Stimuli

Facilitation of Velar Production		
cup of coffee	corn on the cob	piece of cake
calico cat	good cookie	call a cab
make music	big lake	can of coke

Facilitation of Cluster Production		
ask the man	pass the salt	small price
stamp please	go back home	last street
deep snow fall	spare room	sports coat

Facilitation of Syllable Sequencing		
build a snowman	light the Christmas trees	more ice cubes
it's a democracy	open the refrigerator	fix the machine
read it in the paper	time for breakfast	play the music box

MELODIC INTONATION HIERARCHY

The hierarchy of MIT is highly structured for gradual progression of difficulty. Therefore, it is presented in explicit detail, because attention to every specification has contributed to its success. We are sympathetic with those clinicians who prefer less structured language intervention strategies, and we assure them that their reservations about using hierarchies is understood. Sparks and Holland (1976) referred to the dilemma of presenting a hierarchy in a way that is too detailed and seemingly dogmatic for some clinicians and, perhaps, not explicit enough for others. The presentation here will include a description of the technique of intoning, a detailed and illustrated discussion of the four levels of the hierarchy, and a suggested method of scoring each MIT session.

Specific Aspects of the Technique

Discussion of the hierarchy will be made more explicit by first describing the several techniques that are involved.

Use of Verbal Cueing

Phonemic cues, along with their important visual components, are used in the second level of the program and, to a lesser extent, in the subsequent levels. The use of such cues is limited to assisting those with aphasia in the initiation of their responses when it is apparent that they are having difficulty. It is never used as a means of repeating the task for purposes of correcting errors in the responses of the person with aphasia.

Backups and Patient's Failures

A means of attempting indirect correction of errors, called "backups," is used in the third and fourth levels of the program. If the response of the person with aphasia in any step is not considered to be adequate, the clinician has the person repeat the preceding step and then attempt the failed step again. This second trial often is effective in producing the correct response without distracting the patient or making him or her directly aware of the error. As illustrated, if the third step of a level is failed, the second is repeated and the third is then attempted again. If the fourth step is failed, the third is repeated as a backup, and so forth. If the person with aphasia again repeats the error or produces a different one after a backup sequence, the clinician terminates any further effort with that sentence-item and proceeds to the first step of the level with a new sentence. This is consistent with the concept that overt attempts to correct errors are not useful with the type of aphasia that indicates a patient is a candidate for MIT.

Hand Tapping and Control by Hand Signals

It is recommended that the clinician seat himself or herself across the table from the patient with aphasia so that his or her participation is visible to the patient and the patient's performance is clearly visible to him or her. The clinician grasps the patient's left hand so that he or she can engage it in tapping out the rhythm of the stimulus as it is presented and then the rhythm of the responses. Many subjects begin to exercise some control of the hand tapping. This should be encouraged provided that it is accurate. The clinician's participation may then be faded to that of monitoring accuracy while continuing to hold the patient's hand. Hand tapping has proved to be an important and effective supportive stimulus. It has a cueing value that often seems to be as effective as the verbal component it accompanies.

The clinician's use of his or her left hand as a means of controlling onset of the patient's responses is recommended as a nonverbal and nondistracting means of exercising such control. Held up, the left hand advises the patient to remain silent and listen. Dropped with a finger pointed at the patient, it signals him or her to respond. This method is useful in enforcing latency if it is used consistently. The clinician may feel like a traffic officer and may wish that he or she could develop a means of also using his or her feet.

Unison Repetition and Fading Participation by the Clinician

An early step in all levels of the hierarchy involves clinician—patient unison repetition of the stimulus that the clinician has just presented. The clinician fades his or her participation, first the audible and then the visible component, so that the patient is repeating the sentence "solo." It often is necessary for the clinician to rejoin the patient when it is evident that the patient is not quite ready to proceed in the repetition on his or her own.

Adapting to the Patient's Modification of Melody Patterns

The clinician should be prepared to change the key of the melody to that of the person with aphasia's inadvertent modification. Attempts to correct such modifications is an unnecessary distraction. Rather, accurate repetition of the verbal material is the primary goal. Modification of the rhythm or number of intoned syllables, however, cannot be permitted because of their effect on the substance of the sentence.

MIT Session Scoring

The best way to judge the effectiveness of any highly structured form of language therapy for aphasia is to use or develop an objective system of scoring each therapy session. This principle is recommended for MIT as a means of measuring the efficiency of the method for producing steady improvement by any one patient. The method suggested here involves a two-point score for an accurate response that has not required a phonemic cue to initiate a response or a backup, a one-point score for an accurate response achieved with cueing or after a backup, and a reduction of the maximum possible score for any sentence-item if steps have not been completed.

The Hierarchy of MIT

The discussion of each of the four levels of the MIT hierarchy will include a fully detailed description, and Table 31–5 will provide a quick reference. A second table for each level presents a sample therapy session that includes management of errors and scoring, and a review of the types of errors most frequently encountered.

Level I

The first level is a one-step, preliminary means of establishing a set for holding hands and, as far as the person with aphasia may see it, singing odd little nothings. The melodies are those that are used for intoning phrases and sentences. They should increase in length and complexity of melody and stress points as the person with aphasia adapts to the technique. A good candidate usually can be introduced to the idea by a simple description of the process and its purpose. The clinician hums a melody twice while hand tapping the rhythm-tempo-stress pattern with the patient. Humming is suggested rather than a vowel of "la-la" because of its less distinct phonemic quality. Melody patterns similar to those illustrated in Figure 31–5 should be used. Second, the clinician signals the patient to join him or her in unison humming of the melody along with the hand tapping. The patient may use a more phonemic verbal utterance when he or she joins in with the clinician. This is acceptable in this first nonverbal level. When the clinician thinks the patient is ready for a solo effort, the clinical fades his or her vocal participation but continues hand tapping with the patient. When the patient has completed his unaccompanied repetition, the clinician reinforces the performance by saying "good" and proceeding to the next melody pattern. No scoring takes place in Level I. The time required to complete this first level varies from 15 minutes for some patients to two full therapy sessions for others. In any event, moving to the second level occurs as soon as the patient is comfortable in the set of intoning, hand tapping, and complying with the hand-signal controls of the clinician.

Level II

In Level II, linguistic material is added to the type of intonation patterns introduced in the first level. Each of the four steps in the level is presented in detail below. The model presented by Sparks and Holland (1976) had five steps. The present model has combined the first two steps of that model. The use of phonemic cueing is indicated when applicable. Scoring involves two points for a response from the patient that does not require a cue to initiate it and one point if the response is acceptable when initiated by a cue from the clinician. Hand tapping by the clinician and the patient occurs in all stimuli and responses.

Step 1

The clinician hums the melody-tempo-stress intonation pattern that is to be used with the sentence while hand tapping it with the patient, then repeats it with the sentence added. The clinician pauses briefly and then repeats it again. Next, the clinician signals the patient to join him or her in unison repetition of the intoned sentence. If the patient's performance is acceptable, the clinician proceeds to Step 2. If the patient's performance is not acceptable, the clinician pauses for several seconds to produce decay of the strength of the stimulus and then proceeds to the next sentence. The maximum score for an acceptable performance by the patient is one point.

Step 2

After a brief pause, the clinician and the patient begin a unison intoning of the same sentence along with hand tapping. The clinician then fades his or her verbal participation in the manner described earlier but continues to hand tap the rhythm stress pattern with the patient. An acceptable performance implies progression to the third step, and the maximum score is again one point. An unacceptable performance terminates further progression; the clinician pauses for several seconds and then proceeds to the next sentence to be attempted.

Step 3

The patient is signaled to listen. Then, the clinician presents the same intoned sentence. This is accompanied by the hand tapping. Next, the patient is signaled to repeat it, unaccompanied by the clinician except for the clinician's participation in the hand tapping. If the patient has difficulty initiating the repetition, the clinician gives a phonemic cue for the first phoneme of the sentence. Again, this is accompanied by the hand tapping, and hopefully, the patient will respond to the cue accurately. If this third step is completed without cueing, the score is two points; if it is unacceptable only after cueing for initiation, the score is one point. Failure to initiate the utterance after one cueing effort or to produce it accurately enough to be acceptable terminates progression to the fourth step. After a suitable pause, the clinician proceeds to the next sentence.

Step 4

In the final step of the second level, the clinician, without hand tapping, intones the question "What did you say?" immediately after successful completion of the third step. The clinician then signals the patient to repeat the intoned sentence. Cueing along with the hand tapping is offered once if the patient is having difficulty initiating the repetition. Occasionally, the patient may modify the sentence slightly by omitting a functor word or by a slight paraphrase of the sentence. This may be acceptable to the clinician. We maintain that any appropriate near-target response is evidence of progress. Scoring is the same as that of the third step. Two points are given for an acceptable uncued response; only one point is given when a cue was necessary for initiation. The patient is reinforced if he or she successfully completes the four steps for the sentence.

Level II Accomplishment

The patient who succeeds in Level II has acquired the skill of repeating intoned sentences immediately after hearing the model and then in response to a question. The latter is more difficult, however, because the question not only acts as a masking intrusion but also initiates the process of reencoding the stimulus for responsive speech. Attention to this becomes progressively more active in the subsequent levels.

The Most Common Errors Occurring in Level II

First, the patient may be so surprised by his or her solo repetition when the clinician fades his or her participation that the patient will falter. The clinician should be generous in reentering the unison repetition as much as he or she considers it to be useful in producing improvement of the patient's performance. Second, increasing repetition skill may disclose significant evidence of poor articulation, and this will continue throughout the MIT program for that patient. As stated previously, we give greater priority to increasing linguistic skill.

Sample MIT Session and Scoring for Level II

A brief, five-item therapy session and its scoring is presented in Table 31–2 to illustrate management of errors in the patient's performance.

Level III

The third level actually is a liaison between the recovery by the patient with aphasia of his or her ability to repeat during participation in Level II and the return to speech prosody and responsive speech in the fourth level. Latency of permitted responses and less specific questions in the last step

---

TABLE 31–2

Sample Melodic Intonation Therapy Level II Session With Step and Summation Scores

Patient Performance	Scores			
	Step 1	*Step 2*	*Step 3*	*Step 4*
First sentence: Patient succeeds in all steps. Maximum scores attained.	1	1	2	2
Second sentence: Patient succeeds in all steps but requires a cue to initiate response in Steps 3 and 4.	1	1	1	1
Third sentence: Patient succeeds in Steps 1 and 2, requires a cue to initiate response in Step 3, and fails Step 4 because of an unacceptable response after backup.	1	1	1	0
Fourth sentence: Patient succeeds in Steps 1 and 2, requires a cue to initiate response in Step 3, and requires a backup to initiate Step 4.	1	1	1	1
Fifth sentence: Patient succeeds in Step 1 but fails in Step 2. Progression is stopped, and no scores are given for Steps 3 and 4.	1	0	—	—
Scores	5/5	4/5	5/8	4/6
Total	18/24 (75%)			

begin to put more stress on the encoding of responsive speech. In this level, phonemic cueing by the clinician is replaced by the backup system already discussed. In addition to their use as an aid for initiation of responses, backups also are used as an indirect means of correcting an error in a response. As in cueing, only one backup and retrial of a failed step is permitted if the hierarchy is followed without modification. Again, the Sparks and Holland (1976) hierarchy has been modified by combining their first and second steps into one. The detailed description of this third level follows.

Step 1

The clinician presents the intoned sentence with the usual hand tapping once, then signals the patient to join in unison intoning and hand tapping the sentence. As the patient shows evidence that he or she can continue, the clinician fades his or her verbal participation, returning briefly if necessary and then fading again until the patient can continue alone. The maximum score is one point for acceptable performance, and the clinician proceeds to Step 2. It would be unusual for the patient to fail this step, but if he or she does, the progression for that sentence is discontinued.

Step 2

The clinician intones the same sentence once with the usual patient–clinician hand tapping. The patient's response will be intoned repetition, but delay in his or her response of 1 or 2 seconds is imposed by a hand signal from the clinician. Then, the clinician signals the patient to repeat the intoned sentence. Failure involves an immediate backup to Step 1 (i.e., unison intoning with clinician fading) and then retrial of the second step. If the step is completed without a backup, the score is two points. One point is given for an adequate response following a backup if it is necessary. Failure after one retrial terminates progression to the third step for that sentence.

Step 3

No hand tapping is performed in this step. The clinician intones a question asking for a substantive response concerning some element of information in the sentence that has been presented. For instance, if the sentence used in the preceding steps was "I want some pie," the question for Step 3 could be "What kind of pie?" Perhaps the encouraging early indications of language recovery during MIT are the occasional appropriate, but nondirected, responses to the question. Such responses seem to be ahead of any other evidence of recovery in the patient's functional language. Such responses please and surprise the patient and reward the clinician. These responses usually are uttered in normal speech prosody, and they certainly should be accepted. Failure to respond appropriately to the question implies an immediate backup to Step 2 (i.e., delayed repetition) and then a retrial of

Step 3. The clinician should not solicit some response of his or her own choosing. Scores are the same as for Step 2: two points without a backup, and one point after a backup.

Level III Accomplishment

Satisfactory completion of this third level of MIT has begun the modification of the patient's responses from simpler repetition that is well supported by the clinician's participation to more difficult responses involving some retrieval and a beginning of attempts at encoded responses to specific questions.

The Most Common "Errors" Occurring in Level III

The patient's burgeoning confidence and enthusiasm may prompt him/her to respond before the clinician has signaled him/her to do so, particularly when delayed response is required. This is not, strictly speaking, a verbal error, but because of the increasing difficulty of the tasks, the clinician must insist on compliance with his or her controls. The patient also may omit an occasional functor word. Perhaps this is an error of omission, but we believe that any improvement should be free of criticism and should not be inhibited by too much attention to syntax at this point in the progression of the hierarchy. Finally, the variety of appropriate but unanticipated responses to the question in Step 3 should be praised even though they may not be what was expected. They are not errors, particularly if the questions are open-ended enough to make it possible for a variety of responses to occur.

Sample MIT Session and Scoring of Level III

As in Level II, a brief, five-item therapy session and its scoring are presented in Table 31–3 to illustrate management of errors.

Level IV

In this last level, the return to normal speech prosody by way of the sprechgesang technique described earlier occurs for each sentence used, longer delays are imposed by the clinician before he or she permits the person with aphasia to respond, and more spontaneous and appropriate verbal intrusions by the person with aphasia may be expected.

Step 1

The clinician signals the patient to listen, then intones the sentence. The clinician then pauses briefly and presents the sentence twice in sprechgesang accompanied by hand tapping with the patient. He or she then invites the patient to join him or her in unison sprechgesang repetition of the sentence with continued hand tapping. Failure of the patient to respond appropriately calls for a backup to the clinician's solo presentation accompanied by hand tapping, then a second trial of the unison repetition. A second failure terminates

TABLE 31–3

Sample Melodic Intonation Therapy Level III Session with Step and Summation Scores

Patient Performance	Scores		
	Step 1	Step 2	Step 3
First sentence: Patient succeeds in all steps. Maximum scores attained.	1	2	2
Second sentence: Patient succeeds in all steps but requires backups for Steps 2 and 3.	1	1	1
Third sentence: Patient succeeds in Step 1, requires a backup to initiate Step 2, and succeeds in Step 3.	1	1	2
Fourth sentence: Patient succeeds in Step 1, requires a backup for Step 2 because of inaccurate response, and fails to initiate response in Step 3 after a backup.	1	1	0
Fifth sentence: Patient succeeds in Step 1, fails to repeat accurately in Step 2, and fails after a backup. Progression is stopped, and no score may be given for Step 3.	1	0	—
Scores	5/5	5/10	5/8
Total	15/23 (65%)		

further effort with that sentence. If the step is completed without a backup, the score is two points; the score is one point if a backup is necessary.

Step 2

The clinician again signals the patient to listen. Then, the clinician presents the same sentence in sprechgesang with hand tapping, delays permission for the patient to respond for 2 or 3 seconds, and then signals the patient to repeat it in sprechgesang with hand tapping. Failure involves an immediate backup to the first step (i.e., unison repetition in sprechgesang with hand tapping and fading participation by the clinician) and then a retrial of Step 2. If the step is completed without a backup, the score is two points; if a backup is necessary to get an acceptable response, the score is one point. Failure to respond appropriately after one backup terminates progression to the third step for that sentence.

Step 3

Hand tapping is now discontinued for the remainder of Level IV for each sentence. The clinician signals the patient to listen, then presents the same sentence twice but now in normal speech prosody. After delaying permission to respond for 1 or 2 seconds, the clinician signals the patient to repeat the sentence as presented in normal speech prosody. The length of the delay may be lengthened as the patient develops proficiency. Failure involves a backup to the second step (i.e., delayed repetition in sprechgesang, with hand tapping) and then a retrial of Step 3. Scoring is the same: Two points without a backup, and one point after a backup that produces an acceptable response. Failure after a backup terminates progression to the fourth step for that sentence.

Step 4

As in the last step of the third level, the clinician asks questions concerning substantive information contained in the same sentence immediately after successful completion of Step 3, but the number of such questions may be increased. Then, the clinician asks questions that are more associative in nature. As illustration, the following example is given:

Sentence

I want to watch TV.

(a) What do you want to watch? (b) Who wants to? (c) When do you like to do that? (d) What programs do you enjoy most?

The guidelines for decisions regarding what may be considered to be acceptable responses and when a backup should be used are less specific as this last step in the hierarchy becomes less rigidly structured. One suggested solution is to demand accurate responses to the specific questions based on material in the sentence and reward the patient with extra credit for appropriate responses to the less specific questions. Backups should be used only for failures to initiate responses to the specific questions or when such responses are inferior to the patient's current ability. Principles of suggested scoring are modified to conform to the above guidelines for acceptability of responses. If a backup is used, it will be Step 3 (i.e., delayed repetition of the sentence in normal speech prosody) and then a retrial of this fourth step. Backups should be restricted to use with the first specific questions, because responses to the less specific questions are bonus items. Response to the specific questions yields two points for each one, but only one point if a backup was necessary. Response to one or more of the less specific questions would yield a single score of three points, an added bonus that is a nice reinforcement the patient will enjoy.

This last level of the MIT hierarchy is more permissive than the first three and demands significantly more from the patient because he or she has recovered enough speech to reach it. The somewhat less stringent form lends itself to transition to any other language therapies that the clinician may want to employ after completion of MIT.

Level IV Accomplishments and Post-MIT Therapy

The patient who has completed the MIT program has maintained the skills that he or she acquired earlier in the program and has carried them over to normal speech prosody, along with an ongoing recovery of ability to encode and emit at least basic verbal communication. Perhaps this recovery now exceeds, or will exceed, the limits of what MIT currently is designed to offer. Some clinicians may think that the goals should be expanded to help the patient with aphasia and less severe impairment, whose language profile is essentially that of the good candidate but with less acute impairment. This would place the method alongside other techniques that are concerned with improving syntax, articulation, and efficiency of retrieval. The MIT might be used concurrently with these techniques in post-MIT language therapy. Many of us have modified the hierarchy for limited use after completion of the four levels. The issue could be raised as to how long language therapy should continue when the improving patient reaches a point at which he or she can experience some continuing recovery in his or her own milieu. That discussion, however, does not belong here.

A fifth, less structured postgraduate step has been used to retire melodic intonation. Its design includes only sprechgesang and normal speech prosody repetition, along with an increased emphasis on answering questions, such as those used in Step 4 of the last level. It is useful to encourage the patient to use sprechgesang as an auto-therapy when he or she is experiencing difficulty with word finding and the phonemic structure of words. Most MIT graduates find it difficult to use the technique unless some prompting takes place before final discharge from the realm of MIT.

Sample MIT Session and Scoring for Level IV

A five-item therapy session with scoring for the fourth level is presented in Table 31–4.

Quick Reference Guide for the Hierarchy

The four levels of the MIT hierarchy are presented in Table 31–5 for the convenience of the clinician during administration of the therapy.

Concurrent Language Therapies

Because MIT involves a marked departure from normal speech, and because of its carefully planned program of progression, we recommend that no other therapy that is directed specifically to improved verbal output be used concurrently. The patient may easily be confused if one form demands intoning all verbal output, and another uses a procedure involving normal speech prosody. The gradual transition in MIT to therapy that involves normal prosody makes it

---

TABLE 31–4

Sample Melodic Intonation Therapy Level IV Session with Step and Summation Scores

Patient Performance	Scores			
	Step 1	*Step 2*	*Step 3*	*Step 4*
First sentence: Patient succeeds in Steps 1 and 2 requires a backup to initiate normal prosody in Step 3. Patient succeeds in Step 4, but no bonus because of failure on last associative question.	2	2	1	2
Second sentence: Patient succeeds in Step 1 but requires backups for Steps 2 and 3. Patient succeeds with bonus in Step 4.	2	1	1	3
Third sentence: Patient requires a backup to succeed in Step 1 and then succeeds in subsequent steps.	1	2	2	3
Fourth sentence: Patient succeeds in Steps 1, 2, and 3 but requires a backup for Step 4 and fails to answer any associative question.	2	2	2	1
Fifth sentence: Patient succeeds in Steps 1, 2, and 3 and requires a backup for one specific question in Step 4 but answers all associative questions.	2	2	2	2
Scores	9/10	9/10	8/10	11/15
Total	37/45 (82%)			

TABLE 31–5

Quick Reference Hierarchy Guide Melodic Intonation Therapy Levels I to IV

LEVEL I
Single Step
  C (HT) hums melody twice.
  C and **A** (U) hum melody twice. **C** fades.
  Score and progression: No score. Proceed to next melody.

LEVEL II
Step 1
  C (HT) hums melody → intones sentence.
  C signals **A**.
  C and **A** (HT) (U) intone sentence.
  Score and progression:
    Acceptable—1 point. Proceed to Step 2, same sentence.
    Unacceptable—Discontinue progress for sentence.
Step 2
  C (HT) hums melody → intones same sentence.
  C signals **A**.
  C and **A** (HT) (U) intone sentence. **C** fades.
  Score and progression:
    Acceptable—1 point. Proceed to Step 3, same sentence.
    Unacceptable—Discontinue progression for sentence.
Step 3
  C (HT) intones same sentence → **C** signals **A**.
  C and **A** as **A** intones sentence. **C** intones sentence. **C** intones cue if necessary.
  Score and progression:
    Acceptable without cue—2 points. Proceed to Step 4, same sentence.
    Acceptable with cue—1 point. Proceed to Step 4, same sentence.
    Unacceptable—Discontinue progression for sentence.
Step 4
  C intones "What did you say?" → **C** signals **A**.
  A repeats intoned sentence. **C** intones cue if necessary.
  Score and progression:
    Acceptable without cue—2 points.
    Acceptable with cue—1 point.
    Proceed to Step 1 for next sentence.

LEVEL III
Step 1
  C (HT) intones sentence → **C** signals **A**.
  C and **A** (HT) (U) intone sentence. **C** fades.
  Score and progression:
    Acceptable—1 point. Proceed to Step 2, same sentence.
    Unacceptable—Discontinue progression for sentence.
Step 2
  C intones same sentence → **C** signals **A** to wait.
  C signals **A** after 1 or 2 seconds.
  A (HT) repeats intoned sentence.
  (B) to Step 1 if **A** fails → retrial of Step 2.
  Score and progression:
    Acceptable without (B)—2 points. Proceed to Step 3, same sentence.
    Acceptable after (B)—1 point. Proceed to Step 3, same sentence.
    Unacceptable after (B)—Discontinue progression for sentence.

TABLE 31–5

Quick Reference Hierarchy Guide Melodic Intonation Therapy Levels I to IV (continued)

Step 3
   C intones a question → **C** signals **A.**
   A gives an appropriate answer, intoned or spoken.
   (B) to Step 2 if **A** fails → retrial of Step 3.
   Score and progression:
      Acceptable after (B)—2 points.
      Acceptable after (B)—1 point.
      Proceed to Step 1 for next sentence.

LEVEL IV
Step 1
   C (HT) intones sentence → **C** signals **A** to wait.
   C (HT) presents sentence twice in sprechgesang.
   C signals **A.**
   C and **A** (HT) (U) sprechgesang of sentence.
   (B) to **C** (HT) presentation in sprechgesang if aphasic fails.
   Retrial of **C** and **A** (HT) (U) sprechgesang.
   Score and progression:
      Acceptable sprechgesang—2 points. Proceed to Step 2, same sentence.
      Acceptable after (B)—1 point. Proceed to Step 2, same sentence.
      Unacceptable—Discontinue progression for sentence.
Step 2
   C (HT) presents same sentence in sprechgesang → **C** signals
      A to wait.
   C signals **A** after 2 or 3 seconds.
   A (HT) repeats sentence in sprechgesang.
   (B) to Step 1 if **A** fails → retrial of Step 2.
   Score and progression:
      Acceptable without (B)—2 points. Proceed to Step 3, same sentence.
      Unacceptable—Discontinue progression for sentence.
Step 3
   No hand tapping.
   C presents same sentence twice in normal speech prosody.
   C signals **A** to wait 2 or 3 seconds → then signals to repeat.
   A repeats sentence in normal speech prosody.
   (B) to **C** presentation in normal speech prosody if **A** fails.
   Retrial of **A** repetition.
   Score and progression:
      Acceptable without (B)—2 points. Proceed to Step 4, same sentence.
      Acceptable after (B)—1 point. Proceed to Step 4, same sentence.
      Unacceptable—Discontinue progression for sentence.
Step 4
   C Question about substantive content, same sentence.
   A Any appropriate response.
   (B) to Step 3 if response is unacceptable → retrial of Step 4.
   C Questions about associative information.
   A Any appropriate responses.
   Score and progression:
      2 points without (B), substantive content, 1 point after (B).
      3 bonus points, one or more responses to associative questions.
   Proceed to next sentence.

Key: **A** = patient with aphasia; **C** = clinician; (HT) = hand tapping by clinician with patient; (B) = backup; (U) = unison.

possible to transfer to other language intervention strategies easily after completion of the hierarchy, as discussed earlier.

Progression from One Level to the Next One

Progression from Level II to Level III, from Level III to Level IV, or from Level IV to post-MIT therapy should occur after sufficient evidence shows that the patient has developed a stable proficiency. Our hypothesis that increased participation of the right hemisphere occurs in MIT implies that a somewhat prolonged process is involved. Whether the clinician who uses MIT agrees with our hypothesis is less essential than whether he or she progresses slowly, to ensure that improvement from this method is maintained. Actually, the rate of progress made by the good candidate will be slow.

Suggested Means of Controlling Rate of Progression

We recommend that moving from one level to the next higher one should occur only after a mean score of 90% or better for 10 consecutive therapy sessions has been achieved. When we consider the usual fluctuation of performance in those with aphasia from day to day, this often may involve some approach-retreat before the 90% mean is achieved.

Participation of the Family During and After Clinical MIT

Much emphasis is placed on members of the person with aphasia's family participating in the process of attempted rehabilitation of his or her language. Participation of the family during the early period, however, when the focus is entirely on intonation and accuracy of intonation patterns, is viewed with reservations unless supervision is provided by the clinician. The family should be encouraged to assist in selection of useful phrases used frequently by themselves and the patient premorbidly. It is important that these lists be extensive to provide great variety of word orders. Experience with this selective process makes it possible for the patient and his or her family to offer information and vocabulary based on observations and experience in their daily activities.

The role of the family to encourage sprechgesang as a means of word-retrieval efficiency for the patient in the home and among selected friends is strongly recommended for words and phrases that have a high frequency of use in the household.

SUMMARY

In summary, six major elements of MIT are covered in this chapter:

1. A discussion of certain principles of language therapy for aphasia and associated phonologic disorders that have influenced the design of the MIT strategy.

2. A discussion of the candidacy that contrasts the language profiles of good and poor candidates for this type of language intervention.
3. A description of the technique of intoning and plotting intonation patterns.
4. A detailed instruction of administration of the MIT hierarchy.
5. A discussion of post-MIT strategies.
6. A discussion of participation by family members during clinical intervention and after its completion.

FUTURE TRENDS

The family of the person with aphasia who is receiving, or has received, MIT should be systematically involved as a support team. Future development of MIT should include the development of published guidelines that the family may use. Their support is particularly essential when the patient is receiving less than one therapy session each day with the clinician.

Further collection of data regarding candidacy is essential as a means of providing further evidence of the efficacy of MIT. The contributions of careful language examination and scientific studies are of equal importance.

References

Albert, M. L., & Helm-Estabrook, N. (1988). Diagnosis and treatment of aphasia, Part II. *Journal of the American Medical Association, 259*, 1208–1209.

Blumstein, S. E. (1973). *A phonological investigation of aphasic speech.* The Hague: Mouton.

Gordon, H. W. (1972). *Verbal and non-verbal cerebral processing in man for audition.* Doctoral thesis, California Institute of Technology.

Jackson, H. (1931). *Selected writings of John Hughlings Jackson.* London: Hodder & Stoughton.

Knighton, K. (1973). *Beginning teaching techniques: Teaching music at beginning levels.* Wellesley, MA: Kodaly Musical Training Institute.

Martin, A. D., & Rigrodsky, S. (1979). An investigation of phonological impairment in aphasia, Part I. *Cortex, 10,* 318–328.

Sarno, M., Silverman, M., & Sands, E. (1970). Speech therapy and language recovery in severe aphasia. *Journal of Speech and Hearing Research, 13,* 607–623.

Schuell, H., Jenkins, H., & Jimenez-Pabon, E. (1964). *Aphasia in adults.* New York: Harper & Row.

Sparks, R. (1978). Parastandardized examination guidelines for adult aphasia. *British Journal of Disorders of Communication, 41,* 135–146.

Sparks, R., Helm, N., & Albert, M. (1974). Aphasia rehabilitation resulting from melodic intonation therapy. *Cortex, 10,* 303–316.

Sparks, R. & Holland, A. (1976). Method: Melodic intonation therapy. *Journal of Speech and Hearing Disorders, 41,* 287–297.

Whitaker, H. A. (1970). A model for neurolinguistics. Occasional Papers.

Chapter 32

Computer Applications in Aphasia Treatment

Richard C. Katz

OBJECTIVES

The objects of this chapter are:

1. To familiarize reader with the various applications of computers and related technology in the rehabilitation of adults with aphasia.
2. To discuss the strengths and limitations of computerized aphasia treatment.
3. To describe classic and recent research literature demonstrating the efficacy of computerized aphasia treatment.
4. To evaluate the effectiveness and appropriateness of treatment software for patients with aphasia.
5. To incorporate computers and related technology when appropriate into the diagnostic and treatment process for people with aphasia.

DEFINITIONS

"Computerized aphasia treatment" refers to the systematic use of computers and software to improve communication skills in people with aphasia. The roles that computers play in aphasia treatment can be described as three discontinuous categories.

The first, computer-only treatment (COT) software, is designed to allow a patient, as part of a clinician-provided treatment program, to practice alone at the computer, without the simultaneous ("online") supervision or direct assistance of the clinician or others (e.g., spouse or speech-pathology assistant). The clinician later reviews patient performance ("off-line") by examining task performance scores saved on disk by the program for later review, by directly observing performance using the software during a subsequent treatment session, or by measuring generalization to related, non-computer activities or tests. Operation of the program should be familiar and intuitive for patients, particularly those who cannot read extensive instructions or other text. In addition, clinicians and programmers cannot anticipate every possible cue or strategy that may be helpful to every patient, resulting in simplistic or nonexistent intervention components. Consequentally, COT software usually consists of convergent tasks with simple, obvious goals (e.g., drills) and supplementary tasks designed to reinforce or help generalize recently learned skills.

The second, computer-assisted treatment (CAT) software, is presented on a computer by a clinician working at the same time ("side-by-side") with the patient. The role of the computer is limited to elements of basic task structure, such as presenting stimuli, storing responses, and summarizing performance, whereas the clinician provides special instruction, intervention, additional cueing, and other information to modify the activity to accommodate the patient's needs in the same way as during tradition, clinician-provided treatment. This symbiotic relation between clinician and computer permits considerable flexibility, thus compensating for the limitations inherent in the COT approach. In addition to treatment programs written specifically for use with clinicians, other software, such as COT, word processing, or video game programs, can be used in this manner as long as the clinician provides the patient with the additional information needed to perform the task. Fink, Brecher, Schwartz, and Robey (2002) compared the benefits of the same computerized treatment for naming disorders under two conditions, partial independence (similar to COT) and full clinician guidance (similar to CAT), and found that training-specific learning for adults with chronic aphasia was demonstrated under both conditions.

The third, alternative and augmentative communication (AAC), usually, in aphasia treatment, refers to small computers functioning as sophisticated "electronic pointing boards." Unlike the devices used by patients with severe dysarthria or other speech problems, patients with aphasia cannot simply type the words they want to say. The AAC devices designed for speakers with aphasia may incorporate digitized speech, text, pictures, and animation. Some allow both communication partners to use the device to exchange messages during conversations.

The organization and semantic content of the AAC devices frequently can be modified for each patient's particular needs and abilities. In addition to providing an alternative mode of communication, some researchers attribute improved performance on standardized tests and in "natural language" (e.g., speaking and listeing) to treatment involving AAC devices (Aftonomos, Steele, & Wertz, 1997).

A BRIEF HISTORY OF COMPUTERS

A mechanical computer was first built by an English mathematician almost 200 years ago (Babbage, 1822), but the technology for building electronic devices recognizable to us as computers did not exist until the 20th century. Another English mathematician, Alan Turing (1936), described a device similar to a typewriter that used a "contingency table" (criteria and algorithms) to perform complex calculations that, until then, had been completed only by specially trained personnel. The concept of a machine capable of complex decision making without human intervention was revolutionary (Turing, 1950). In the 1950s, computers were large, electronic calculating machines that filled rooms with switches, vacuum tubes, and mechanical relays and that read rolls of punch tape and, later, reels of electronic tape. Only banks, large corporations, and civilian and military governmental agencies could afford to purchase and operate these machines. Over the years, however, computers grew smaller, more reliable, and less expensive. "Microcomputers" were first sold in the mid to late 1970s to hobbyists and other technology enthusiasts who programmed the machines to perform specialized tasks, such as controlling all the lights in a house or measuring rainfall. As computers began to show up in offices and homes, software developers saw a market for functional and entertaining programs for the general public: games, word processing, spreadsheet, data base, graphics, communications (modem), financial planning, will writing, and so on. Today's multimedia desktop, laptop, and palm-size personal computers that access information from the World Wide Web are only the latest stage in this evolution. Looking back on the recent rapid growth—or, some might say, intrusion—of technology, it is understandable why many expect an imminent breakthrough that will abruptly change our lives for the better, a promise that the computer industry's sales force has made since the mid-1950s. People with aphasia and their families may be particularly vulnerable to the unsubstantiated promises made by an avid computer industry intent on increasing sales. While the world rushes forward to embrace technology, those of us engaged in rehabilitation should step cautiously and apply accepted standards to determine the value of computer applications for each patient with aphasia.

LIMITATIONS OF COMPUTERIZED TREATMENT SOFTWARE

A speech-language pathologist, educated in communication theory and sufficiently experienced in both the clinic and real-life, can generate an infinite number of novel and relevant treatment stimuli and recognize, evaluate, and modify treatment activities in response to previously unacknowledged associations and unanticipated responses. In contrast, computer-provided treatment is based on a finite set of rules that are stated explicitly to specify actions likely to occur at particular points during a future treatment session. Limitations in modalities (e.g., computers cannot understand speech or writing very well) ensure that computerized treatment will be a subset of clinician-provided treatment and supplemental to treatment provided by properly trained clinicians.

Computers cannot be all things to everyone. Bolter (1984) described four general properties of computers and computer programming that can be used to illustrate the limitations inherent in the application of computers to aphasia treatment: (1) discrete, (2) conventional, (3) finite, and (4) isolated.

Discrete

Because computers acknowledge and manipulate discrete (i.e., digital) units, qualitative description and decisions are difficult to make. Events must first be separated into distinct, unconnected elements before they can be acted on by a computer. Face-to-face communication is a complex act described as our "oldest and highest bandwidth technology" (Rheingold, 1991, p. 216). Many elements of language and communication are not well deliniated or even universally recognized. In summarizing research concerning perception of the meaning of words versus the message's affect (i.e., the emotional content) for listeners during face-to-face communication, Mehrabian (1968) estimated that 55% of a message's affect is communicated via facial cues, 38% vocally, but only 7% by the actual words. Although individual language tasks can be programmed, applying computer technology appropriately to aphasia rehabilitation requires an appreciation of the intricacies and interdependence of elements within verbal (i.e., language) and nonverbal (e.g., kinesics and proxemics) channels of communication (Egolf & Chester, 1973; Katz, LaPointe & Markel, 1978, 2005; Katz, LaPointe, Markel, & Silkes, 2005).

Conventional

Computers apply predetermined rules to symbols that have no effect on the rules. Regardless of the value of the symbols or the outcome of the program, the rules never change. Although a consensus exists for some fundamental guidelines of aphasia treatment, all the rules are not known, however, and those that are accepted may not be right under all conditions (Rosenbek, 1979). Computer-only treatment does not follow the clinical cycle of (a) administer treatment, (b) measure performance, (c) modify treatment, and (d) re-administer treatment and, therefore, is not adequately responsive to the dynamics of patient performance.

Finite

The rules and symbols that control computer-provided treatment are limited to those that are defined within the program. Except for the most sophisticated (i.e., "artificial intelligence") programs (see, e.g., Guyard, Masson, & Quiniou, 1990), unforeseen problems and associations do not result in the creation of new rules and symbols. Therapy presents the opposite case. Not all therapeutically relevant behaviors are identified, and those that have often vary in importance between patients and situations. Computer-provided learning commonly defers decisions to software designers and programmers who are not physically present during the session but who must plan in advance how to handle the intervention and code these steps into a computer program (c.f., Odor, 1988).

Isolated

Problems and their solutions presented by computers exist within the computer's own parameters, apart from the real world. Problems are stated in a way such that symbols can be manipulated to solve the problem by following an algorithm—that is, a finite series of steps described with adequate detail to guide the program to respond to input, answer questions, or solve problems. This lack of "world knowledge" is, perhaps, the most significant impedance to comprehensive computer-provided treatment. Language tasks as presented by computers essentially differ from the meaningful, pragmatic setting in which communication occurs among people. Computers, therefore, only consider problems in which all the variables and rules are known ahead of time and can be solved in a step-by-step procedure with a finite number of steps, much like a game of chess. Learning to solve linguistic riddles on a computer program may lead to better scores on conventional aphasia tests; however, improving communication is quite another matter.

Treatment is recognized as a multi-level, interactive behavioral exchange. Not all therapeutically relevant behaviors have been identified; many that have (e.g., functionality) are influenced by internal (e.g., idiopathic) and external (e.g., environmental) factors and cannot be controlled effectively by a computer. In addition, whereas many basic parameters of therapy and fundamental skills of clinicians have been identified (Goldberg, 1997), all the rules are not known, and those on which we agree may not be correct (Rosenbek, 1979). For example, use of linguistic models to construct software to diagnose and treat aphasia is appealing (see, e.g., Guyard et al., 1990) and, ultimately, can teach us much about language (see, e.g., Fenstad, 1988) and aphasia (see, e.g., Wallich, 1991). Some researchers (see, e.g., Katz, 1986, 1990; Kotten, 1989), however, believe that the pathologic language behavior of people with aphasia also is influenced by a variety of other factors, including cognition (e.g., attention, vigilance, memory, and resource allocation), cybernetics (e.g., slow rise time, noise buildup, and intermittent imperception), behavioral factors (e.g., discriminatory stimuli, chaining, and extinction), pragmatics (e.g., functionality and social status), and emotion (e.g., interest, relevance, novelty, and enjoyment). No single therapeutic approach currently encompasses all known intervening variables.

If a program were written that could completely represent clinician-provided treatment, the software would be massive and exceed the capacity of modern personal computers. By reducing the scope of the problem to a size that is manageable for the computer, treatment software has been squeezed and shaped to imitate cognitive and language therapy in small, trivial, and predominantly symbolic activities. Rather than emphasize state-of-the-art aphasia treatment, the resultant computerized activity highlights the technical limitations of the computer medium. Odor (1988) referred to this problem when he wrote that computer intervention defers decisions to programmers who are not physically present during the session, but must gather and send information only through the computer medium, plan in advance how to handle the learning interaction, and then encode these steps into a computer program. Consequently, the scope of treatment software is limited, because computer programs are not powerful enough to represent every potentially relevant nuance of interaction during therapy. Odor concluded that computer-assisted instruction often is based on convergent rather than divergent theories of learning. Most computer treatment studies reported in the aphasia research literature describe convergent activities, particularly drills, in which specific responses are learned. Dean (1987) stated that the inability to incorporate divergent strategies in computer programs severely limits their value and application to treatment of patients with aphasia, particularly those with chronic aphasia, for whom such treatment appears promising (Chapey, Rigrodsky, & Morrison, 1976). Divergent treatment software is becoming commercially available, such as Language Activities of Daily Living (Learning Systems), but as of this writing, no data exist to support efficacy. The adaptation of divergent therapy to computer-provided treatment continues to remain a challenge for contemporary software developers.

TREATMENT

The earliest applications of computers to aphasia rehabilitation owe much to behavior modification and the development of instrumental learning devices or "teaching machines" (Skinner, 1958). Some of these devices were prototypes and experimental (see, e.g., Keith & Darley, 1967), whereas others were commercially available and widely used, such as the Language Master (Keenan, 1967) and the Programmed Assistance to Learning filmstrip projector (Pfau, 1974). Following the introduction of small mainframe computers ("minicomputers"), reports began to appear in professional journals describing attempts by researchers and clinicians to use computers to meet the needs of patients with aphasia. For example, Vaughn (1980) incorporated small, microprocessor-driven auditory, visual, and writing devices and minicomputers (e.g., the PDP-11) to provide treatment to outpatients over the telephone (telecommunicology). By the time that personal computers (then called "microcomputers") were introduced in the mid to late 1970s, sufficient interest had grown among clinicians and researcher to develop treatment protocols for specific patients and types of problems (see, e.g., Schwartz, 1984).

Speed, accuracy, reliability, and ease of use are valued characteristics wherever personal computers are used, but the power of computers in rehabilitation is not simply the result of faster microprocessors or larger storage devices. Schuell, Jenkins, and Jiménez-Pabón (1964) stated that principles of aphasia treatment should be used throughout our increasing repertoire of clinical techniques. The role of computers will evolve as the technology improves. In many areas, computers have the potential to become significant tools for treating aphasia.

Supplementary Treatment

Supplementary treatment in the form of workbooks and other structured activities has always been a useful option for clinicians (Brubaker, 1996; Dressler, 1991; Eisenson, 1973). Patients can work longer and more often on a variety of activities designed to stabilize, maintain, or generalize newly acquired skills. Contemporary commercial treatment and educational software extend controlled, treatment-related language and cognitive activities beyond the confines of the treatment session if they are presented in a structured setting that incorporates important therapeutic principles and factors, such as control of stimulus characteristics and response requirements and recording of session performance for later review. Programs can vary along a continuum according to structure and content, ranging from simple, repetitive drills to interactive tasks that not only evaluate individual responses but also measure overall performance and adjust the type and degree of intervention provided (see, e.g., Katz & Wertz, 1997).

Treatment Efficacy and Prognosis

Measuring the effects of intervention on aphasia is an essential part of any treatment regimen. Speech-language pathologists assess the influences of various linguistic, psychological, and physical variables on communication and task performance to evaluate the effectiveness of a treatment approach or activity (Darley, 1972). Computers present treatment activities in a standard manner and routinely store performance data for later descriptive and statistical analysis. Additionally, computers can help clinicians to develop local and national prognostic data bases to predict with confidence that, for example, a 55-year-old adult with Broca's aphasia who 1-year post-onset is at the 50th percentile on the Porch Index of Communicative Ability (Porch, 1981), or PICA, will require between 125 and 150 trials to learn to write or print 10 functionally relevant words at the third-grade level (LaPointe, 1977). This benchmark of prognostic resolution would serve as an invaluable clinical yardstick against which the success of treatment could be measured (see, e.g., Matthews & LaPointe, 1981, 1983).

The widely used health care assessment tool, the SF-36 Health Survey, is available for downloading from the Internet (http://www.sf-36.com). Like the print version of the SF-36, this version can be used for assessing effects from clinical trials, monitoring outcomes in clinical practice, and screening medical patients for mental health referral. It provides measures of physical functioning, bodily pain, general health, vitality, social functioning, emotional role functioning, mental health, and reported health transition. Translations of the SF-36 are being tested in more than 40 countries as part of the International Quality of Life Assessment Project. The face validity of this tool is impressive for clinicians and researchers interested in investigating quality of health care across health disciplines, especially as it relates to the construct of quality of life. The SF-36 software that provides administration, scoring, and data export for research support is available for Windows.

Generalization

"Prepare for rather than pray for generalization" (Rosenbek, LaPointe & Wertz, 1989, p. 138). Ultimately, the value of aphasia treatment is measured by the degree to which skills acquired in treatment are observed in real-life situations. It is imperative that the clinician actively train generalization. Computer-provided treatment is an environment very different from real-life communication. Generalization can be aided by the computer, which can administer some aspects of treatment without the familiar presence and constant conscious (and unconscious) control of the clinician. On fulfilling criteria for a computer task, a similar task should be presented without the computer—for example, writing instead of typing, or performing the actual functional activity rather than a computer simulation. Rosenbek and colleagues (1989) recommended a series of clinical activities to increase the likelihood of generalization. Several of the recommendations appear well suited for the computer:

1. Expose each patient to numerous repetitions.
2. Train a large number of items in a given category.
3. Extend treatment outside of the clinic.
4. Organize treatment to maximize independence so that patients learn to use treated responses when they want to rather than when told to by the clinician.

Programs like MultiCue (Van de Sandt-Koenderman, 1994) and Visual Confrontation Naming (Parrot Software) help to teach the patient a strategy to stimulate or compensate for word-finding problems by selecting among possible cues. MultiCue offers several different strategies simultaneously, whereas Visual Confrontation Naming provides cues that are audible (i.e., first sound) and visual (e.g., first letter, description, and multiple-choice list containing the word). The CD-ROM version has more than 500 target words with pictures that aid in generalization of self-cueing strategies. Ideally, patients should develop and practice their own self-cueing strategies that have been shown to be effective in treatment.

Independence and Emotional Factors

To foster independence, minimize dependency and depression, and help patients to develop insight regarding their communication problems, patients should be able to use treatment software with minimal assistance from others. The required computer skills include turning on the computer system; selecting the treatment program from a removable disk, hard drive, or the Internet; and following the protocol for each particular program. Patients themselves can then determine when and how often they participate in supplementary language activities. This is consistent with Wertz's (1981) statement that we should allow patients to maintain as much independence as possible and that a long-term goal of aphasia treatment is to have patients become their own best therapists. The insight that patients have regarding *their* problems and *their* strengths can be used instead of ignored, and in this way, patients can take a more active role in their recovery.

Factors such as motivation, dependency, and quality of life are concerns that may become increasingly important to people with aphasia and their families as recovery slows and the degree of disability and its subsequent effect on life become more apparent. Under conditions of perceived helplessness and hopelessness, people frequently become depressed (Seligman, 1975) and have greater difficulty coping with and adapting to changes and problems (Coelho, Hamburg & Adams, 1974). Bengston (1973), Langer and Rodin (1976), Schulz (1976), and others have shown that giving some options and responsibilities to persons in otherwise

dependent situations (e.g., the institutionalized elderly) can have a strong, positive effect on their satisfaction and physical well-being. Decision making and expression of personal preferences by each patient should be a basic part of any treatment program. Computerized activities can address this aspect of treatment by providing patients with aphasia a degree of control over the content and frequency of treatment.

Administrative Functions

Currently, computers are assisting clinicians in the performance of administrative and clinical duties, and in all likelihood, they will soon to do even more (Hallowell & Katz, 1999). Morrison (1998a) describes an active role for computers and related technology in the evaluation of many factors essential to the delivery of services and quality of care. Large-scale systems are expensive to set up and maintain, so it is essential to plan carefully and consult with information technology specialists who are experienced in health care before attempting to integrate technology and clinical and support staff (Morrison, 1998b). On a smaller scale, many clinicians use computers to gather, organize, and report case history information (Silverman, 1997). As is the case for many other professions, general purpose programs have useful applications for clinicians working with patients—for example, report and letter writing (word processing programs); organizing, recording, and recalling information (database programs); and organizing, calculating, and projecting values (spreadsheet programs). Innovations include the use of voice recognition in report writing to increase the speed of generating reports (Tonkovich, Horowitz, Kawahigashi, Krainen, & Kronick, 1991) and the use of authoring systems to customize data base entry and retrieval. One of the most comprehensive systems is Computerized Patient Records System (Kolodner, 1997), which enables clinicians using PCs in every medical center in the Department of Veterans Affairs (the "VA") to access patient records not only within their own medical centers but also from others. This ability saves time and greatly simplifies the process of retrieving and updating patient records, especially for patients who are treated at different facilities across the country. The VA officials have developed a system that many believe could be the low-cost foundation of a nationwide electronic health record system.

Commercially available software provide another path to incorporating technology into administrative activities. Chart Links (Chart Links) is a commercially available system that is based on electronic patient medical records. It creates a record for each patient and tracks reports of each patient encounter, lab report, team report, medical diagnosis, recommended treatment, and treatment schedule. Workflow applications allow charting, sorting, organizing, filing, report writing, and automated review of patient information. Chart Links is based on Lotus Notes, which allows advantageous communication and security features. Therapist Helper (Therapist Helper) is another clinical practice management software developed to facilitate patient and insurance billing transactions and accounting as well as report writing.

Recreational Activities

Commercial recreational programs (e.g., arcade and adventure games) have long found a limited but useful role in treatment (Lynch, 1983). Enderby (1987) discussed the possibility of computers in this role providing a path toward social and intellectual stimulation for patients with aphasia. Many educational and treatment programs use familiar game formats to minimize learning time and heighten enjoyment (e.g., Laureate Learning Systems). Recreation therapy, a valuable service for many patients, is outside of our scope of practice, but speech-language clinicians can incorporate computer game activities, educational software programs, and even the Internet to help promote intellectual stimulation and social interaction in a novel and entertaining manner for patients with aphasia.

MODALITY CONSIDERATIONS

Conversation (i.e., talking and listening), whether face-to-face or via cell phones, is our primary mode of communication. Management of auditory and verbal skills therefore is central to the concept of aphasia rehabilitation (see, e.g., Schuell et al., 1964). Listening and talking are the communicative behaviors used to classify most types of aphasia (Goodglass & Kaplan, 1983; Kertesz, 1982) and are the focus of most therapy for aphasia. Listening and talking, more than other language modalities, affect the likelihood of a person with aphasia's successful reintegration into the community—the final demonstration of the success of therapy. For most patients, and for their families, friends, and physicians, the *perception* of recovery and treatment success is driven by improvement in listening and talking.

Contemporary treatment software offers little assistance to clinicians treating the speaking and listening problems that occur during conversation for patients with aphasia. Speech recognition is limited and unreliable for multiple speakers (as would be the situation found in the treatment rooms of any clinic) and for speakers who produce variable errors, such as apraxia of speech and phonemic paraphasia. High-quality digital speech is common on today's multimedia computer systems, but programs that merely repeat object names or offer nonlinguistic visual cues are of limited value to patients with auditory comprehension deficits. Listening drills are promising, but the potential to developing automated, complex listening task that address specific patterns of auditory problems has not yet been realized.

The major contribution of computers to aphasia treatment currently appears to be in the areas of reading and writing. Computers are basically visuomotor, graphic-oriented machines. Information from the user normally is entered by typing on a keyboard; the output of the computer is displayed on the monitor screen and read by the user. This makes the computer well suited for presenting reading tasks and, through typing, writing tasks. Reading and writing skills appear to be an appropriate focus of computerized aphasia treatment for several reasons. Most patients with apashia have problems reading (Rosenbek et al., 1989) and writing (Geschwind, 1973). Reading requires minimal response from the patient. Programs for treating reading can run on standard personal computers, without expensive modification or specialized peripheral devices. Typing on the keyboard can be used to address many aspects central to writing (Selinger, Prescott, & Katz, 1987), with the obvious exception of the mechanics of handwriting. Also, reading and writing as communicative acts usually are done alone; having greater interpersonal distance, they are in many ways less direct and responsive than speaking and listening. As such, reading and writing are appropriate communication (as opposed to therapeutic) activities for people with aphasia to practice on computers. Computerized reading and writing treatment tasks can free up valuable treatment time so that face-to-face, individual therapy can emphasize complex elements of auditory comprehension and verbal output skills that computers do not address. The computer can provide valuable reading and writing activities (see, e.g., Scott and Byng, 1989), but clinicians also should provide additional non-computerized reading and writing treatment that is individualized to each patient's particular need beyond the capacity of computer software.

STRUCTURE OF TREATMENT ACTIVITIES

Many elements are common to the structure of all treatment activities regardless of the underlying principles or mode of delivery, and although some are obvious, none are trivial. An understanding of these task components is useful for describing, developing, and evaluating treatment activities for the computer.

All tasks have a goal, which usually is an intermediate step toward a major or long-term treatment goal. To understand the goal of the task, the patient should recognize both the objective of the task (what is being required) and the underlying purpose of the task (why the task is being required). Equally important, the patient should be aware from the beginning of the steps within the task that advance toward the goal. The clinician should provide the patient with instructions so that the patient knows from the beginning what is expected. The stimuli used and the desired responses should be consistent with the purpose of the task. In many instances, responses should be described and quantified using a multi-dimensional scoring system (LaPointe, 1977; Porch, 1981) to identify and measure the occurrence of salient behaviors within the task (accuracy being only one). Care should be taken that the patient is not burdened with additional, unnecessary response requirements that could confound performance, such as requiring a typing response (i.e., word retrieval, spelling ability, and motor skills) instead of a simple two key (yes/no) response on a comprehension task. Responses should be as simple as possible to reflect accurately the performance of the target behavior. General feedback (Stoicheff, 1960) to encourage the patient and specific feedback to describe the most recent response should be readily provided. The clinician should provide an intervention (strategy or cue) to improve performance as needed. Teaching specific responses may be the goal of some tasks (e.g., associate printed names of family members to their pictures); a more valuable goal commonly is to develop a task to help the patient learn a strategy (i.e., self-cue or compensatory) to improve communication during actual, functional situations (e.g., point to name on card when referring to particular family member). Criteria for termination of the task should be specified to provide a target against which the patient can measure progress. Responses and performance scores should be stored for later review and analysis. The patient's performance and the intervention can be evaluated using various techniques (LaPointe, 1977; Matthews & LaPointe, 1981, 1983; McReynolds & Kearns, 1983, Prescott & McNeil, 1973). Finally, the intervention may be modified or the activity discontinued, as indicated.

MODELS FOR COMPUTER REHABILITATION

In contrast to the considerable attention afforded the arrival of new treatment programs, software developers rarely provide thorough descriptions of the treatment models influencing software evolution. As described by Wolfe (1987), early reports of computerized aphasia treatment (see, e.g., Katz & Nagy, 1982, 1983, 1984, 1985; Mills, 1982) provided no explicit models of rehabilitation from which the software could be evaluated. Recent studies have reversed the trend (see, e.g., Katz & Wertz, 1997; Loverso, Prescott, Selinger, Wheeler, & Smith, 1985; Scott & Byng, 1989). Bracy (1986) was among the first to explicitly incorporate the work of Luria (1973, 1980) in the development of rehabilitation software. Having an explicit model facilitates the systematic development of software and provides a basis for clinicians selecting software for their patients. Three general models of rehabilitation provide clinicians with the structure to develop and evaluate software. Although they are not mutually exclusive, the models offer a basis from which the role of computers in aphasia rehabilitation can be directed and examined.

Brain-Behavior Relationships

Bracy (1986) described four theories accounting for the recovery of cognitive functions, but the theory that function recovers through the retraining process is the most closely allied to the modern concept of rehabilitation. Luria (1963, 1973) believed the return of skills involved a reorganization of brain functions so that new methods existed of performing behaviors previously executed through the damaged structures ("intersystemic reorganization"). One function of computerized treatment therefore is to provide the patient with the direction and opportunity to retrain skills through the reorganization.

Behavior Modification

Behavior modification (operant conditioning and instrumental learning) describes the process of either teaching a new behavior or eliminating an established one through the systematic application of consequences (Goldberg, 1997). The principles of behavior modification are thoroughly woven into the fabric of human behavior—simply put, people tend to do things that result in rewards and avoid behaviors that result in punishment (Skinner, 1948). [According to Skinner (1957), these principles even guide the way in which we communicate and use language.] The frequency of occurrence, duration (e.g., exposure time), and other parameters (e.g., size, color, and loudness) of elements central to behavior modification (e.g., stimulus characteristics and reinforcement schedules) can be monitored and controlled with a computer. Many computer programs control some aspect of stimulus characteristics and provide reinforcement to patients in the form of corrective and general feedback.

Educational Models

Lepper (1985) contrasted three approaches to learning with direct application to treatment software: (1) individualized drill and practice, (2) educational games, and (3) simulations. Drill and practice capitalize on the computer's advantages in providing immediate feedback, sustained attention, data analysis, and highly individualized instruction. Educational games stimulate a person's interest through game-like activities. Educational simulations, also called microworlds, involve the patient in a series of problems in an imaginary environment. The contingencies between actions and outcome should lead the patient to an understanding of basic principles relevant to real-world environments. These programs assume that active, inductive, "discovery-based" learning is better for learning general skills compared with direct, didactic approaches, which seem to be more effective when learning highly specified information. The three programs that make up the Language Activities of Daily Living (Laureate

Learning Systems) are examples of computer software that represent microworlds in which the patient is free to explore the total simulated environment rather than respond to specific stimuli.

TYPES OF COMPUTERIZED TREATMENT TASKS

Four major types of treatment activities are appropriate for presentation on the computer: (1) stimulation, (2) drill and practice, (3) simulations, and (4) tutorials. This list is not exhaustive, and types are not mutually exclusive. One treatment activity may have several purposes and demonstrate characteristics of more than one type—for example, stimulation and drill and practice (see, e.g., Seron, Deloche, Moulard, & Rouselle, 1980).

Stimulation

As described by Schuell and colleagues (1964), stimulation activities offer the patient numerous opportunities to respond quickly and, usually, correctly over a relatively long period of time for the purpose of maintaining and stabilizing the underlying processes or skills rather than simply learning a new set of responses. The process therefore is the focus of the task. Stimuli are not selected primarily for informational content (e.g., interest and relevance) but, rather, for salient stimulus characteristics (e.g., length, number of critical elements, complexity, and presentation rate). Computer programs can easily be designed that contain a large database of stimuli and control these variables as a function of the patient's response accuracy. Overall accuracy and other salient response characteristics (e.g., latency) usually are displayed at the end of the task. An early example of a computer stimulation task is the auditory comprehension task described by Mills (1982).

Drill and Practice

The goal of drill and practice exercises is to teach specific information so that the patient is able to—or appears able to—function more independently. Stimuli are selected for a particular patient and goal, so an authoring or editing mode is needed to modify stimuli and target responses. A limited number of stimuli are presented and are replaced when criterion is reached. Because response accuracy is the focus of the task, the program should present an intervention or cues to help shape the patient's response toward the target response. Drill and practice exercises therefore are convergent tasks, because the accurate response must match the target response exactly. Results are displayed or stored on disk and show the effectiveness of the intervention. Examples of drill and practice programs are described by Katz and Nagy

(1984); Katz, Wertz, Davidoff, Schubitowski, and Devitt (1989); Katz and Wertz (1997); and Seron and colleagues (1980).

Simulations

Simulations (i.e., microworlds) are programs that present the patient with a structured environment in which a problem or problems are presented and possible solutions are offered. Simulations may be simple, such as presenting a series of paragraphs describing stages of a problem and listing possible solutions. Complex programs more closely simulate a real-life situation by using pictures and sound. The term "virtual reality" (Rheingold, 1991) describes a totally simulated environment created through the interaction of a computer and a human along both verbal and nonverbal channels. Simulations have been used in fields such as chemistry, geology, meteorology, and astrophysics to test conditions that are impossible to experience or to train people in situations that otherwise would be too dangerous to experience firsthand. Simulations provide the opportunity to design divergent treatment tasks that could address real-life problem-solving strategies more fully than those addressed by more traditional, convergent computer tasks—for example, by including several alternative but equally correct solutions to a problem, such as during Promoting Aphasics Communicative Effectiveness, or PACE, therapy (Davis & Wilcox, 1985). The question of whether computer simulations can improve generalization of newly acquired behavior to real-life settings as well as or better than traditional methods remains to be tested.

Tutorials

Some authors (see, e.g., Eisenson, 1973) have suggested that patients with aphasia are best served by modification of their communication environment. In that respect, tutorials offer valuable information regarding communication and quality of life to the family, friends, and others who influence the patient's world. At the most fundamental level, the computer tutorial could present information commonly found in patient information pamphlets in an interactive format, with additional modules provided when needed or requested. This type of self-paced, informational program can be appropriately realized in a hypertext format, such as found on the World Wide Web, where a family member can navigate through text, pictures, animation, and sound describing relevant aspects of aphasia and communication. The tutorial program could incorporate features of an expert system, in which detailed information is provided in response to a patient/family profile, and function as a source of information for family members in the future when new problems and questions arise.

CANDIDACY FOR THERAPY

Most patients with aphasia can benefit from the thoughtful application of appropriate treatment software used in a supplementary role. Prognostic indicators common to patients with aphasia in general will apply, such as etiology and site of lesion, age, time post-onset, educational level, and so on (Eisenson, 1973). Cognitive factors, like those described for patients suffering right hemisphere damage (Myers, 1999) or bilateral brain damage (Goldstein, 1942, 1948), also should be considered. Many factors influence which patients benefit most from computerized aphasia treatment, but the most critical factors are severity, modality, sensory and physical impairments, independence, and self-monitoring. Severely impaired patients may be limited to simple treatment drills, providing little real value or generalization, whereas the meta-communication needs of mildly impaired patients may not be served by complex, problem-oriented software. These patients may benefit from more direct, clinician-provided treatment. Patients with problems involving reading, writing, and to some extent, listening can practice and maintain skills and compensatory strategies learned from the clinician by using various computer programs. Hemianopsia, visual neglect, or simply changes in visual acuity can interfere with the patient's ability to view material on the computer display, whereas right hemiparesis can prevent a patient from easily using the computer mouse, typing on the keyboard, or even sitting comfortably in front of a computer for an extended period of time (Petheram, 1988). Many patients look forward to working with their clinicians, who they see as supportive and sympathetic—feelings that patients do not get from working with a computer. Others may not have sufficient initiative or discipline to maintain a treatment program without the continual watchful eye of the clinician. Perhaps most critically, patients who are unable to monitor their own performance (e.g., detect errors after feedback or modify subsequent responses) will gain little or no value from working independently on a computer.

EFFICACY OF APHASIA TREATMENT SOFTWARE

Treatment efficacy considers whether outcomes are improved as a result of a specific intervention (McGlynn, 1996). According to Rosenbek (1995), efficacy is improvement resulting from treatment applied in a rigidly controlled design when treatment and no-treatment conditions are compared. Wolfe (1987) found that early reports of computerized aphasia treatment did not provide explicit models of rehabilitation from which the software could be evaluated. In an extensive review of the literature, Robinson (1990) reported that the efficacy of computerized treatment for aphasia as well as other cognitive disorders had not been demonstrated. The research studies reviewed suffered from inappropriate experimental designs, insufficient statistical analyses, and other deficiencies. Since Robinson's critique, a number of publications have described the effect of particular computerized interventions (see, e.g., Crerar, Ellis, & Dean, 1996; Katz & Wertz, 1992, 1997; Loverso, Prescott, & Selinger, 1992), whereas others have surveyed trends reported in the research literature (Cicerone et al., 2000; Wertz & Katz, 2004).

According to Loverso (1987), most computer advocates focus on "appealing" features of computers, such as cost-effectiveness and operational efficiency, but the real issue that demands attention from clinicians is treatment effectiveness. In other words, treatment activities must be effective before they can be efficient. Ineffective treatment programs would be damaging to the overall quality of treatment provided to patients with aphasia. If computerized treatment is to continue to develop and improve, it should undergo the same scientific scrutiny and systematic modification as all other aspects of treatment do.

Software, however, cannot reproduce every process, variable, and nuance that occur during treatment, so computerized treatment in this sense will never be as efficacious as clinician-provided treatment. One way clinicians can increase the likelihood that software is efficacious is to develop and test their own treatment programs. Mills (1988) accurately suggested that clinicians with only limited programming skills tend to produce programs with only limited therapeutic value. It is equally important that programmers have more than a superficial understanding of treatment principles if treatment software is not to be limited in its effectiveness.

A range of support for the clinical application of computers exists in aphasiology. Dean (1987) wrote that existing computer treatment programs "are not firmly grounded in a theoretical rationale for remediation" (p. 267), thus limiting their potential. To Katz (1984, 1986) as well as Loverso, Prescott, Selinger, and Riley (1988), most contemporary treatment software consisted of drills with no explicitly stated intervention goals; their use should be conservative and practical. Other authors (see, e.g., Bracy, 1983; Lucas, 1977; Skilbeck, 1984) advocated the computer rather than the clinician as the primary treatment medium, and a few (see, e.g., Rushakoff, 1984) described the development of clinician-independent, autonomous computerized aphasia treatment programs. Early literature reviews resulted in conflicting opinions of the efficacy of computers (see, e.g., Katz, 1987; Robinson, 1990). Robinson (1990), issued a strong statement, arguing that research evidence was simply not available to support the use of computers for most language and cognitive problems. Robinson claimed that many researchers obscured the basic issue of whether computerized treatment is effective by asking what works with whom under what conditions, as Darley (1972) suggested. He concluded that computers are prematurely promoted in clinical work and that their routine clinical use may be causing patients more harm than good. A decade and half later, Wertz and Katz (2004) evaluate examples of reports concerning the computerized treatment for aphasia outcomes in the research literature by applying precise definitions of the treatment outcome research terminology, placing the examples within the context of the five-phase treatment outcomes research model (Robey, 1998; Robey & Shultz, 1998), applying a level-of-evidence scale to rate the evidence provided by the selected examples (American Academy of Neurology Therapeutics and Technology Assessment Subcommittee, 1994), and speculating where we are and where we may need to go to demonstrate the influence of computer-provided treatment on improvement in aphasia.

No substitute exists for carefully controlled, randomized studies, the documentation of which has become the scientific foundation of aphasiology. Research reported over the last 15 years has incorporated increasingly sophisticated designs and greater numbers of subjects to assess the efficacy of computerized aphasia treatment (Wertz & Katz, 2004), ranging from simple Phase I and II studies, A-B-A designs, and comparisons of pre- and post-treatment testing (Katz & Nagy, 1982, 1983, 1984, 1985; Mills, 1982) to large, randomly assigned single-subject studies (Loverso et al., 1992) and Phase III clinical trials incorporating randomly assigned treatment and no-treatment groups (Katz & Wertz, 1992, 1997). Efficacy of computerized aphasia treatment is being addressed one study at a time.

Auditory Comprehension

Few studies have investigated the effects of computerized treatment drills on auditory comprehension problems. Until recently, high-quality digitized speech was costly and difficult to include in the computer systems found in most clinics. Also, agreement on treatment approaches was limited by the varied, complex, and transient nature of auditory comprehension problems. Mills (1982) first used computer-controlled digitized speech to provide one-, two-, and three-part auditory "pointing" commands in a simple drill to a patient with chronic aphasia. Intervention was limited to repetitions of the auditory stimulus. Improvement was noted on pre- and post-treatment testing and on PICA (Porch, 1981) and Token Test (De Renzi & Vignolo, 1962) scores. The influence of other factors (e.g., placebo effect) should not be discounted, because no withdrawal or multiple-baseline, single-subject research strategies were used. Even so, the study is a good first step toward adapting auditory comprehension activities to the computer.

Verbal Output

Researchers apply technology to dysnomia in different ways. Colby and colleagues made extensive use of computers and speech synthesizers in attempts to increase verbalization and communication in autistic and other "non-speaking" children (see, e.g., Colby & Kraemer, 1975; Colby & Smith, 1973). Later, Colby, Christinaz, Parkison, Graham, and Karpf (1981) built and programmed a small, portable microcomputer carried by a subject with dysnomia on a sling and shoulder-strap combination, thus allowing use of the device in actual communicative situations. When the subject experienced word-finding problems (Brown & Cullinan, 1981), she pushed keys in response to prompts from the computer. On a small liquid crystal display (LCD) screen, the computer printed a series of questions designed to help the individual with dysnomia identify the forgotten word—for example, "Do you remember the first letter of the word?", "...the last letter?", "...any other letters?", and "...any other words that go with the forgotten word?" The subject's answers were applied according to an algorithm outlined in the program, and a list of possible words was produced and displayed across the computer screen, beginning with the most "probable" words. When the patient recognized the forgotten word, she pressed a button, and the word was produced via synthesized speech. [Most patients with dysnomia usually can recognize the correct word and say it after a visual or auditory model (see, e.g., Benson, 1975).] The authors reported that the subject was cued successfully by the portable computer in real-life situations that were functional and communicatively stressful. Although their computer may be viewed as strictly an AAC device, Christinaz (personal communication) reported that the cueing algorithm subsequently generalized to non-computer settings. Patients reported after several weeks of using the computer that they no longer required it, instead asking themselves the same series of questions previously displayed by the computer. Christinaz reasoned that the subjects had "internalized the algorithm" and now cued themselves without the need of external prompts. The frequency and success of this observation was not reported, but the implication of Christinaz's statement is certainly relevant and potentially significant. As more powerful portable computers are used as compensatory devices, acquisition and generalization of functional communication behaviors may occur if these or similar devices modeled self-cueing strategies for patients during actual communicative situations.

Van de Sandt-Koenderman (1994) described a computer program, Multicue, that is designed to help patients with dysnomia identify and select self-cueing and compensatory strategies for word-finding problems. A picture is presented in the left upper quarter of the computer screen, and the patient's goal is to type the appropriate name. If the patient does not know the name (or cannot type it), various cues can be selected (e.g., word meaning, word form, and sentence completion) to help the patient retrieve the word. The goal of the program is to allow the patient to evaluate and practice several word-finding strategies, ultimately changing the process of word-finding for the patient. The effectiveness of Multicue in a controlled study has not been reported.

Naming continues to be the most frequent aspect of verbal output studied by researchers developing aphasia treatment software. Fink and colleagues (2002) compared outcomes of the same computerized treatment ("hierarchical phonologic cueing") for naming disorders under two conditions, "partial independence" (similar to COT) and "full clinician guidance" (similar to CAT), and found that training-specific learning was demonstrated under both conditions. Laganaro, Di Pietro, & Schnider (2003) reported that "computerized treatment of anomia" resulted in item-specific improvement for four subjects with chronic aphasia but only three of seven subjects with acute aphasia. Adrian, Gonzalez, & Buiza (2003) described the Computer-Assisted Anomia Rehabilitation Program that used semantic, phonologic, written, and semantic/phonologic cueing to facilitate naming in a speaker with aphasia. They reported that 30 days after administration of the 12-day treatment program, performance of the practiced words improved 17% (from 53% to 70%), and the performance of untrained words doubled (from 32.5% to 65.8%), suggesting the patient's internalization of the strategies provided during treatment. All researchers recognize the necessity of further testing their software using additional subjects and more sophisticated experimental designs.

Reading Comprehension

Early work by Katz and Nagy (1982, 1983, 1984, 1985) demonstrated various functions that computers could provide when treating reading problems in patients with aphasia, although interpretation of the results must be tempered because of small sample sizes and limited research designs. Katz and Nagy (1982) described a program designed to test reading and provide reading stimulation for patients with aphasia. Five subjects with aphasia ran the computer programs two to four times per week for 8 to 12 weeks. Although several subjects demonstrated improved accuracy, decreased response latency, and increased number of attempted items on some computer tasks, changes in pre- and post-treatment test performance were minimal. The following year, Katz and Nagy (1983) reported a drill and practice computer program for improving word recognition in patients with chronic aphasia. The program was designed to accomplish a task that is difficult to undertake for a clinician and used the advantages of a computer. The program presented 65 words that occur frequently in text and varied the rate of exposure as a function of accuracy of response. The goal of the program was to help increase and stabilize the subject's sight vocabulary, but no changes were observed on pre- and post-treatment measures for the five subjects with chronic aphasia. Later, Katz and Nagy (1985) described a self-modifying drill and practice computerized reading

program for severely impaired adults with aphasia. The objective of the study was to improve functional reading, and a program was developed to teach subjects to read single words without intensive clinician involvement. The program also generated, through a printer, homework (writing activities) that corresponded to the subject's performance. Four of the five subjects demonstrated pre- to post-treatment changes on the treatment items that ranged from 16% to 54%.

Scott and Byng (1989) tested the effectiveness of a computer program designed to improve comprehension of homophones (similar-sounding words) for a 24-year-old subject who suffered traumatic head injury and underwent subsequent left temporal lobe surgery. Eight months after the accident, the subject continued to demonstrate aphasic symptoms as well as surface dyslexia and surface dysgraphia. Reading was slow and labored; she was able to understand printed words by sounding them out, presenting particular problems with homophones. The computer program, based on an information processing model, was designed to focus on this particular aspect of the subject's reading problem. The subject demonstrated steady improvement on the 136-item treatment program, which was run 29 times over a 10-week period. The subject improved in recognition and comprehension of treated ($p < 0.001$) and untreated ($p < 0.002$) homophones used in sentences. Improvement also was demonstrated on recognition of isolated homophones that were treated ($p < 0.05$) and on defining isolated treated ($p < 0.03$) and untreated homophones ($p < 0.02$). Recognition of isolated untreated homophones and spelling of irregular words showed no improvement.

Katz and Wertz (1997) conducted a longitudinal group study to investigate the effects of computerized language activities and computer stimulation on language test scores for adults with chronic aphasia. Fifty-five subjects with chronic aphasia who were no longer receiving speech-language therapy were randomly assigned to one of three conditions: (a) 78 hours of Computer Reading Treatment, (b) 78 hours of Computer Stimulation ("non-language" activities), or (c) No Treatment. The Computer Reading Treatment software consisted of 29 activities, each containing eight levels of difficulty, totaling 232 different tasks. Treatment tasks required visual-matching and reading comprehension skills, displayed only text (no pictures), and used a standard, match-to-sample format with two to five multiple choices. Treatment software automatically adjusted task difficulty in response to subject performance by incorporating traditional treatment procedures, such as hierarchically arranged tasks and measurement of performance on baseline and generalization stimulus sets, in conjunction with complex branching algorithms. Software used in the Computer Stimulation condition was a combination of cognitive rehabilitation software and computer games that used movement, shape, and/or color to focus on reaction time, attention span, memory, and other skills that did not overtly require language or other communication abilities. Subjects in the two computer conditions worked on the computer for 3 hours per week for 26 weeks. Clinician interaction during the two computer conditions was minimal. Subjects from all three conditions were tested using the PICA and Western Aphasia Battery, or WAB, at baseline, 3 months, and 6 months. Significant improvement over the 26 weeks occurred on five language measures for the Computer Reading Treatment group, on one language measure for the Computer Stimulation group, and on none of the language measures for the No Treatment group. The computer reading treatment group displayed significantly more improvement on the PICA Overall and Verbal modality percentiles and on the WAB Aphasia Quotient and Repetition subtest compared with the other two groups. The results suggest that (1) computerized reading treatment can be administered with minimal assistance from a clinician, (2) improvement on the computerized reading treatment tasks generalized to non-computer language performance, (3) improvement resulted from the language content of the software and not stimulation provided by a computer, and (4) the computerized reading treatment we provided to patients with chronic aphasia was efficacious.

Writing: Typing and Spelling Words

Many reading comprehension activities are easily transferred to the computer. Writing activities, however, are less easily adapted. The most obvious problem is the inability of the common computer to evaluate handwriting and printing. The computerized writing treatment programs described in the literature substitute typing for writing during the intervention. In a comparison of writing and typing abilities of subjects with aphasia, Selinger, Prescott, & Katz (1987) examined seven subjects with left hemisphere damage to assess differences between PICA graphic scores on subtests A through E using standardized PICA graphics responses and PICA responses typed on a computer. No differences were found between scores on the PICA subtests as generated with a pencil and paper and PICA responses typed on a computer. These results suggest that the graphic language abilities of brain-damaged adults are equally represented by the two output systems.

Several investigators have incorporated complex branching algorithms in computerized writing programs to provide multilevel intervention. Seron and colleagues (1980) described a minicomputer/clinician combination that helped patients with aphasia learn to type words to dictation. The clinician said the target word and the subject typed a response on the computer keyboard. (The clinician had to know in advance the order of the stimuli programmed in the computer.) Intervention consisted of three levels of feedback: (1) the number of letters in the target word, (2) whether the letter typed was in

the word, and (3) when the correct letter was typed, regardless of whether that letter was in the correct position. The five subjects completed the program in 7 to 30 sessions. Pre- and post-treatment tests required the subjects to write a generalization set of single words to dictation. A decrease ($p < 0.05$) in the number of misspelled words and in the total number of errors made on the post-treatment test suggested that the computer program had improved spelling of words written by hand. Four of the five subjects maintained improved performance on a second post-treatment test administered 6 weeks later.

Katz and Nagy (1984) used complex branching steps to evaluate responses and provide patients with specific feedback in a computerized typing/handwriting confrontation/spelling task. A stimulus was randomly selected by the program, and a drawing representing the stimulus was displayed on the computer screen. The subject responded by typing on the keyboard. Feedback consisted of auditory sounds and text printed on the screen. Single and multiple cues from a hierarchy of six cues were selected by the program in response to the number of errors made for each of 10 stimuli. A seven-point multi-dimensional scoring system was used to describe performance and track the effectiveness of the various cues. Additional feedback included repetition of the successful and most recently failed cues. At the end of the computer session, pencil and paper copying assignments automatically generated via the computer printer were completed by the subject. Pre- and post-writing tests revealed improved spelling of the target words for seven of the eight subjects with aphasia ($p < 0.01$).

Glisky, Schlacter, and Tuving (1986) reported the ability of four memory-impaired subjects without aphasia to type words in response to definitions displayed on the computer screen. Cues included displaying the number of letters in the word and displaying the first and subsequent letters in the word, one or all at a time, as needed. Cues continued until either the patient typed the word correctly or the program displayed the entire word. All patients improved in the ability to type the target words without cues. Patients maintained their gains after a 6-week period of no treatment and demonstrated generalization to another typing task, although generalization to writing was not measured.

Katz and colleagues (1989) developed and tested a computer program designed to improve written confrontation naming of animals for nine subjects with minimal assistance from a clinician. The treatment program required subjects to type the names of 10 animals in response to pictures displayed on the computer monitor. If the name was typed correctly, feedback was provided, and another picture was displayed. If an error was made, hierarchically arranged cues were presented, and response requirements were modified. Five of the nine subjects achieved criterion for success within six treatment sessions, and the performance of all nine subjects improved an average of 40% on the computer task ($p < 0.0001$). In addition, improvement was measured on non-computerized written naming tasks, such as written confrontation naming of the treatment stimuli and written word fluency for animal names ($p < 0.001$). The PICA Writing modality score improved by +4.1 percentile points ($p < 0.05$). Improvement did not extend to PICA Overall and Reading scores. Because the goal of the program was to teach subjects the 10 names, improvement did not—and was not expected to—generalize to written word fluency for an unrelated category. The lack of change in these latter language activities for these 10 subjects with chronic aphasia contrasts with their improved performance on treated words.

Deloche, Dordain, and Kremin (1993) developed software to treat oral and written modality differences in confrontation naming for two subjects with aphasia, a surface dysgraphic and a conduction aphasic. The intervention focused on written naming from the keyboard. Both subjects maintained improvements 1 year following therapy. Mortley, Enderby, and Petheram (2001) used the computer as "a tool to facilate repetitive practice" and to "encourage the independent use" of the treatment strategy for an adult who, despite his chronic dysgraphia, was able to spell target words orally. Computer practice was part of a more comprehensive regime, including a specially designed word processing program to help with carryover and use of a dictionary to support the spelling strategy. The patient was able to move from non-functional tasks to more functional activities as a result of the treatment.

Augmentative Communication Device

Published reports from Gardner and Gardner (1969), Premack (1970), and others involved in animal communication described success teaching non-human primates (e.g., chimps and apes) the use of nonverbal, language-like symbolic communication systems. These reports stimulated efforts to teach visually based, alternative communication systems to people with severe aphasia (see, e.g., Gardner, Zurif, Berry, & Baker, 1976). Developing the concept further, Steele, Weinrich, Kleczewska, Wertz, and Carlson (1987); Weinrich and colleagues (1989); and Steele, Weinrich, Wertz, Kleczewska, and Carlson (1989) developed and tested a graphically oriented, computer-based alternate communication system called the Computer-Aided Visual Communication, or C-VIC, system for adults with chronic global aphasia. The C-VIC is an interactive pointing board that runs on a Macintosh computer and uses a picture-card design, or metaphor. Subjects use the mouse to select one of several pictures, called icons, each of which represents a general category. The selected icon then "opens up" to reveal pictures of the items within the selected category. After selecting the desired item, the picture is added to a sequence of other selected pictures; this "string" of pictures

represents the message. The message can be read via the sequence of icons, words printed below the sequence, or in some cases, heard through digitized speech. Much attention is given to the selection of icons. Weinrich and colleagues (1989) reported that concrete icons were learned and generalized faster than abstract icons, but that neither type of icon generalized well to new situations. The empirical evidence to support the efficacy of C-VIC was collected in a series of single-case studies (Steele et al., 1987; Weinrich et al., 1989, 1993). Steele and colleagues (1987) noted that, although globally impaired subjects with aphasia using C-VIC improve on expressive and receptive tasks, communication through more traditional modes of communication remains unchanged. Weinrich, McCall, Weber, Thomas, and Thornburg (1995), however, trained two subjects with Broca's aphasia in the production of locative prepositional phrases and Subject-Verb-Object (S-V-O) sentences on C-VIC and reported that their verbal ability improved considerably. In subsequent reports (see, e.g., McCall, Shelton, Weinrich, & Cox, 2000), Weinrich and colleagues continued to develop and test C-VIC as a potential therapeutic approach to improve the communication and natural language of adults with aphasia.

A commercial version of C-VIC, called Lingraphica, incorporates animation and digitized speech on a Macintosh Powerbook computer. Lingraphica is an integrated, computerized communication system that combines spoken words, printed words, pictures (icons), and text processing. Patients use a mouse device to select one of several icons, each of which represents a general category. The selected icon then "opens up" to reveal pictures of the items within the selected category. After selecting the desired item, the picture is added to a sequence of other selected pictures; this "string" of pictures represents the message, which can be read via the sequence of icons and words printed below the sequence or can be heard through digitized speech. Aftonomos and colleagues (1997) used Lingraphica with 20 subjects and reported improvement in multiple modalities, including verbal, for most subjects. Clearly, further single-subject and group research using standardized measurements is needed to test the effectiveness of new computer technology adapted to the communicative needs of patients with aphasia. The treatment approach refered to in Aftonomos and colleagues (1997) formed the basis of multimodal treatment for aphasia administered by speech-language pathologists using Lingraphica at Lingraphi Care clinics.

Other researchers have taken different approaches to the application of AAC to aphasia. Van de Sandt-Koenderman (2004) reviewed the state of the art in AAC applications for aphasia and suggested that lack of motivation, inadequate vocabulary, insufficient training, and limitations in cognition and language abilities are major obstacles to the functional use of assistive technology in the aphasic population. She points to the relatively frequent appearance of small, portable devices with ready-made messages tailored to specific communicative situations and calls for more research to refine these devices and improve their adaptability to the needs of individual patients. Linebarger, Schwartz, and Kohn (2001) described a computerized intervention that incorporated speech recognition software with software that allowed patients to construct spoken sentences "piecemeal" for later use. They reported that their five patients with agrammatism patients, using one or both programs, showed gains in language after independent home use of the software, and they concluded that this improvement may have resulted from training during therapy followed by practice under "normal" communication settings.

Artificial Intelligence

Reports by Guyard and colleagues (1990) represent the beginnings of new stage in the development of treatment software by integrating artificial intelligence (AI) programming and computer-assisted instruction (CAI) for the rehabilitation of patients with aphasia. Researchers (see, e.g., Barr & Geigenbaum, 1982) described this union between AI and CAI as "Intelligent CAI" (ICAI). In their view, ICAI can expand the scope, responsiveness, and flexibility of software for aphasia therapy so that a computer program would determine the type, sequence, and rate of stimuli presented based on evaluation of the patient's responses. While valued in education, ICAI has met with limited success in aphasia rehabilitation, primarily because of two factors: the heterogeneity of the aphasic population, and the complexity of aphasia therapy (Katz, 1990).

Simulations

Roth (1992) as well as Gadler and Zechner (1992) have described computer-simulated worlds (NeueWEGE and AUSWEGE, respectively) in which patients, guided by their clinicians, explore a microworld, making decisions, "traveling," and taking chances without any real physical or interpersonal risks. Topics of tasks are familiar and function to patients (e.g., planning a vacation). To my knowledge, however, no controlled study measuring efficacy has been reported. Crerar and Ellis (1995) described the "Microworld Project," a computer system based on sound neuropsychological and psycholinguistic theory and designed to treat impairments in sentence processing. Concepts such as agent, action, object, and spatial relations were manipulated to improve sentence comprehension. A series of experiments (Crerar & Ellis, 1995; Crerar, Ellis, & Dean, 1996) demonstrated improvement in subjects with chronic aphasia after a relatively short duration of treatment.

Telemedicine

American Speech-Language-Hearing Association teleseminars and videoconferences as well as the Telerounds series sponsored by the National Center for Communication Disorders are good signs that telecommunications technology is coming of age in our own discipline (Duffy, 1998). This technology permits improved access to health services, especially for remote and underserved populations. The use of telecommunications technology to provide clinical services has numerous potential advantages, but many factors must be carefully evaluated, such as image quality, appropriateness of the fields of view, training requirements, user preferences, cost, and reliability and validity of the diagnostic findings using such technology (Peters & Peters, 1998).

Technology has been used in the past to provide assessment and treatment for patients with communication impairments who live in remote locations. Tele-Communicology (Vaughn, 1980; Vaughn et al., 1987) incorporated small, microprocessor-driven auditory, visual, and writing devices placed in the homes of patients and remote computers to provide assessment and treatment over the telephone. Wertz, Dronkers, Knight, Shenaut, and Deal (1987) compared the effectiveness of closed-circuit television, computer-controlled video laserdisc, and traditional face-to-face interaction for providing appraisal and treatment of patients with aphasia in remote settings. Subjects in all three treatment conditions demonstrated clinically significant improvement as indexed by scores on the PICA (Porch, 1981). No significant differences among the three conditions were observed. The results suggest that television and video laserdisc transmitted over telephone lines could be employed to provide services for patients who live where services do not exist. Brodin and Magnusson (1994) reported numerous studies conducted in Sweden demonstrating the feasibility of treatment provided over telephone lines for patients with aphasia in rural settings.

Duffy, Werven, and Aronson (1997) summarized results of telemedicine evaluations of speech and language disorders in patients of a small, rural hospital and large, multidisciplinary medical practices. They concluded that telemedicine evaluations can be reliable, beneficial, and acceptable to patients with a variety of acquired speech and language disorders, both in rural settings and within large, multi-disciplinary medical settings. To date, no explicit technical or clinical national standards or guidelines exist for the use of telecommunications to deliver services in the field of speech-language pathology. Although Medicare does provide coverage for some telehealth services (c.f., Goldberg, 1997), no explicit provision involves coverage for speech-language pathology services at this time.

Comparison of Traditional and Computer Mediums

Comparing the effect of similar treatment activities provided by two different mediums should improve understanding about the influence of the medium and the relative effectiveness of the treatment. Many researchers are attempting to simulate accepted testing and treatment protocols on the computer. Some researchers think that, because of their speed, reliability, and relative autonomy, computers are ideally suited to administer tests to patients with aphasia, who can then work at their own pace and without embarrassment or fear of humiliation (e.g., Enderby, 1987). Odell, Collins, Dirkx, and Kelso (1985) developed two computerized versions of the Raven Colored Progressive Matrices (Raven, 1975). The program used high-resolution graphics and a touch screen input device to administer and analyze test performance quickly and accurately, with minimal supervision from a clinician. The authors compared the two computerized versions of the Raven matrices with a traditional, clinician-controlled, paper booklet administration of the test. The performances of 16 subjects with aphasia were essentially equivalent under all three conditions, leading the authors to conclude that the computer testing conditions did not present greater visual or cognitive demands on the subjects.

Wolfe, Davidoff, and Katz (1987) compared the real-object and computer simulation performances of adults without brain damage and adults with aphasia on another nonverbal problem-solving task, "The Towers of Hanoi" puzzle, originally administered to subjects with aphasia by Prescott, Loverso, and Selinger (1984). The performances of 19 subjects with aphasia and 19 subjects without brain damage were compared using two different methods of presentation: two-dimensional color computer simulation of the puzzle versus the manipulation of the actual wooden model. Subjects without brain damage performed equally well under both conditions. As in the study by Odell and colleagues (1985), subjects with aphasia demonstrated similar performance on the task under both conditions. These same subjects, however, required more time to complete the puzzle in the computer condition than when manipulating the actual wooden model. The results suggest that, although the computer medium did not affect the accuracy of performance for the subjects with aphasia, task completion took longer and was less efficient under the computer condition.

The effectiveness of closed-circuit television, computer-controlled video laserdisc, and traditional face-to-face interaction for providing appraisal and treatment to patients with aphasia in remote settings as measured by Wertz and colleagues (1987) was described earlier. Results suggested no significant differences among the three conditions in the diagnoses assigned to subjects; additionally, subjects in all three treatment conditions demonstrated clinically significant change (between 12 and 17 percentile points on the PICA). No significant differences in improvement among the three treatment groups were observed, indicating that patients with aphasia could benefit from treatment provided in any of the three conditions.

An excellent example of the process of demonstrating efficacy in a computerized treatment program involves 14 years of published research by Loverso and colleagues, who have documented a series of data-based reports describing the development and testing of a model-driven, clinician-provided treatment approach—the "verb as core"—from its origins as a "clinician-delivered therapy" (Loverso, Selinger, & Prescott., 1979; Loverso, Prescott, & Selinger, 1988) to its encoding and refinement as a computer/clinician-assisted program (Loverso et al., 1985, 1988, 1992).

Loverso and colleagues (1979, 1988) and Selinger, Prescott, Loverso, and Fuller (1987) initially developed and tested a treatment protocol for patients with aphasia in which verbs were presented as starting points and paired with different "wh-" question words to provide cues to elicit sentences in an actor-action-object framework. Thirty verbs were used at each of six modules. The hierarchy was divided into two major levels, each consisting of an initial module and two submodules that provided additional cueing for subjects unable to achieve 60% or better accuracy on the initial module. Level I presented stimulus verbs and the question words "who" or "what" to elicit an actor-action sentence. Level II elicited actor-action-object sentences by presenting stimulus verbs and the question words "who" or "what" for the actor and the question words "how," "when," "where," and "why" for the object. Subjects responded verbally and graphically and were scheduled for treatment three to five times per week. During each session, 30 stimulus verbs were presented for generation of sentences. Statistically significant improvement ($p < 0.05$) was demonstrated on the PICA following 3.5 months of treatment for each of the two subjects with aphasia.

Later, Loverso and colleagues (1985) compared the effects of the same treatment approach when treatment was provided by a clinician versus when it was provided by a computer and speech synthesizer assisted by a clinician. The subject with aphasia responded in the clinician-only condition by speaking and writing and in the clinician–computer condition by speaking and typing. Stimulus presentation and feedback in the clinician–computer condition normally was provided only by the computer. The clinician intervened only if the patient's typed response was correct but the spoken response was in error. The subject improved on the task under both conditions but took longer to reach criteria under the computer–clinician condition. Based on the subject's improvement, both on the treatment task and on "clinically meaningful" changes during successive administrations of the PICA ($p < 0.01$), the authors concluded that their listening, reading, and typing activities under the clinician–computer condition had a positive influence on the patient's language performance. They suggested that, although still in the early stages of development, aphasia treatment administered by computers is practical and has the capacity for success. Loverso and colleagues (1988) replicated the study by Loverso and colleagues (1985) with five subjects having fluent and five subjects having confluent aphasia for the purpose of examining whether treatment provided under the computer–clinician condition was as effective as a clinician alone when treating various types and severities of aphasia using their cueing-verb-treatment technique. The 10 subjects required 28% more sessions ($p < 0.05$) to reach criteria under the computer–clinician condition than under the clinician-only condition. Subjects with fluent aphasia required 24% more sessions, and subjects with nonfluent aphasia required 33% more sessions, under the computer–clinician conditions than under the clinician-only condition. Of the 10 subjects, eight showed significant improvement ($p < 0.05$) on the PICA Overall percentile measure, on the Verbal modality measure, and on the Graphic modality measure. All subjects maintained gains after a maintenance phase of 1 month post-treatment or longer. Similar results were reported following a replication of the study using 20 subjects (Loverso et al., 1992).

EXAMPLES OF COMMERCIALLY AVAILABLE SOFTWARE

Auditory Comprehension

Although developed for primarily for children, three programs under the title Language Activities of Daily Living (Laureate Learning Systems)—My House, My Town, and to a lesser extent, My School—are good examples of software that can be used to provide stimulation treatment for adults with aphasia. For example, in My House, rooms within a house can be viewed, along with many items typically found in the rooms. For example, the bedroom contains a bed, end table, lamp, bureau, closet, clothes, and so on. A natural-sounding, digitized voice identifies the target item by name or function (pre-elected by the clinician). After the patient uses the mouse (or touch screen, if available) to designate an item, the program indicates accuracy visually and/or auditorally. Text (name or function) also can be displayed, as selected by the clinician. The program provides repetitions when requested by the patient and options for repetitions and nonlinguistic (visual) cues following incorrect responses to help the patient complete the item successfully. Items are drawn with color and charm.

Verbal Output

Technology has been more readily adapted to motor speech problems than to the complex and less completely understood language formulation problems of adults with aphasia; however, some recent programs show promise. Visual Confrontation Naming (Parrot) helps to teach the patient a strategy to stimulate or compensate for word-finding problems by selecting among possible cues. Cues may be audible (i.e., first sound) or visual (e.g., first letter, description, or multiple-choice list containing the word). Ideally, patients should develop self-cueing strategies using the most successful cue. The CD-ROM version has more than 500 target words with pictures. Verbal Picture Naming Plus (Parrot) recognizes spoken words by using sophisticated speech recognition technology. The patient is prompted to name a picture displayed by the computer. The computer then evaluates the verbal response and, if that response is incorrect, prompts the patient to repeat the word after it is verbally presented. The task requirements for patients are not unusual, but clinicians may wish to determine for themselves whether the voice recognition software is sufficiently accurate for the needs of each patient. Also, be aware that speech recognition software designed for some versions of Windows (e.g., Windows 95/98) may not work for others (e.g., Windows NT, Window Vista).

Aphasia Tutor 0: Sights 'n Sounds (Bungalow) is a word repetition task that displays a word or picture while presenting the word using digitized speech. The patient's repetition is recorded, and both the computer model and the patient's response are played back for comparison. The software provides more than 400 words, and clinicians can add their own words (in the "Professional version").

Reading Comprehension

Treatment of reading problems using computers appears to be particularly appropriate when considering the nature of patients, activities, interventions, and computers. Most people with aphasia—even mild, residual aphasia—report problems understanding long or complex text. Because reading is a task that we typically engage in alone, it is socially appropriate to practice alone. Reading requires minimal responses by the patient, thus simplifying software development. These programs can run on minimally configured, less expensive systems.

Reading Comprehension Adults (Parrot) presents single-page short stories written to be of interest to adults. AphasiaTutor (Bungalow) is a series of programs that provide reading exercises to improve reading comprehension, allowing progression from letters to words to sentences to paragraphs. It also includes a module allowing "practical reading" of items, such as newspapers, product labels, and bills. For patients who drive or hope to drive again, Traffic Sign Tutor (Bungalow) may complement functional reading as well as symbolic comprehension goals. This program allows interactive practice with traffic sign recognition and response to written hypothetical driving scenarios.

Writing: Typing and Spelling

Computers also are an appropriate medium for treating writing disorders, a common and persistent problem in patients with aphasia. Like reading, writing tasks usually are done alone. It is unexpected for computers to improve the mechanics of writing, but they can provide tasks that are designed to improve other components of written language, such as spelling and grammar. Word processing software, such as Word (Microsoft), offers many features that could assist mildly impaired patients, such as spelling check, grammar check, thesauraus, templates, and the "Assistant," which automatically provides guidance when writing letters or performing other common functions.

Brubaker on Disk: Database of Customized Language and Cognitive Exercises (Parrot) contains more than 1,500 exercises that can be arranged and printed to create personalized activities or workbooks for patients to complete either during treatment sessions or as homework. The clinician uses a mouse to select among different language and cognitive tasks, difficulty levels, response types, print size, and type face. The program uses these choices to select exercises from a large data base. The clinician then reviews on screen the selected exercises and prints what he or she wants to include in a personalized workbook.

Cognitive Problems

Treatment efficacy for computerized cognitive retraining is less clearly documented than that for speech and language treatment (Robinson, 1990), but researchers are striving to better assess efficacy. Two multi-level computerized cognitive treatment programs that are shared among professionals in neuropsychology and speech-language pathology are Captain's Log (BrainTrain) and PSSCogReHab (Psychological). Captain's Log includes 33 separate computer programs that focus on visuomotor, conceptual, and numeric skills as well as on attention. It allows tracking of performance across several sessions and includes reaction time measures and analyses of error responses. PSSCogReHab (Psychological) includes a set of eight software packages with treatment activities focused on attention, executive skills, visuospatial and memory skills, and problem solving. Many other programs are designed to help treat specific problems. For example, Conditional Statements (Parrot) presents, either visually or auditorally, a hierarchy of conditional statements. Responses are indicated by pointing and dragging icons on-screen with the mouse. Clinicians also may build

their software libraries by subscribing to the *Journal of Cognitive Rehabilitation* (Psychological). Each monthly issue includes a 3.5-inch disk that contains Soft Tools, a treatment program (frequently, a "game") designed for the PC to focus on a different cognitive problem, such as memory or visual spatial skills.

Additionally, many devices are designed to help patients with cognitive impairments cope with complex daily activities. Electronic scheduling and reminding devices as well as computerized calendars (c.f., Herrmann, Yoder, Wells, & Raybeck, 1996) are increasingly affordable for integration into cognitive rehabilitation programs. PocketCoach (Ablelink Technologies) is a portable voice recorder designed to help patients with cognitive problems complete complex, real-life tasks. Using his or her own voice, the clinician records a series of instructions or steps into the device. The patient then plays back the steps, one at a time, until the task is completed.

Alternative and Augmentative Communication Devices

Lingraphica as a compensatory device was described earlier. Steele and colleagues recently have redirected their efforts; as LingraphiCARE America, they have begun to establish a network of specialized "Language Care Centers" for treatment of adults with aphasia by combining the use of Lingraphica technology with standardized clinical treatment strategies and a growing patient data base containing demographics and outcome measures. Although preliminary outcome data have been reported (Aftonomos et al., 1997), further single-subject and group research using standardized measurements is needed.

Another example of an AAC device is the DynaVox 2c, a lightweight (approximately 6 pounds) system designed for children and adults. The device uses a color display and text-to-speech conversion. It has built-in infrared environment control capabilities that permit the user to easily transmit files between the DynaVox and a desktop PC. Infrared capability also permits control of televisions, VCRs, and other appliances, thus providing more independence for the user. DynaVox software uses symbol and word prediction capability and a searchable "concept tagged" vocabulary list, enabling faster programming and automatically generated "pages" or screens of associated pictures and words.

FUTURE TRENDS

The computer can become a very powerful clinical tool by incorporating what we know about aphasia, treatment, and technology. Multimedia PCs are now common, providing better platforms for treatment software focusing on problems of auditory comprehension and verbal output. Improved speech recognition, a goal for the entire computer industry, can result in an entirely new generation of treatment programs and AAC devices. Replacing traditional, static, still images with dynamic digital video segments in treatment software increases interest and relevance for many patients. Affordable digital still and video cameras increase the ease with which software can be individualized for each patient's needs and interests. Palm-size PCs will influence the development of AAC devices and computers in rehabilitation in the same manner that laptop computers did just a few years ago. Eisenson (1973) suggested that clinicians consider changes the environment of patients with aphasia to maximize their communicative potential. Technology is helping us do that.

The most influential element, however, is not technological but, instead, clinical. In all computerized aphasia treatment studies cited in this chapter, clinicians selected and tested the patients, designed the treatment plans, designed and modified the treatment tasks, trained the patients to use the computers, and measured treatment efficacy. Computers, programmers, publishers, or researchers are not responsible for treatment effectiveness; clinicians are. Because treatment cannot be effectively "prescribed" like medicine, software should be viewed as supplementary treatment, with the clinician providing critical intervention as indicated by performance and other considerations. The role of computers and treatment software, like that of all tools, should extend the abilities of the clinician, allowing clinicians to intervene when skills, experience, and flexibility are required. Rather than emphasize what computers can or cannot do better than clinicians, our focus should be on an intelligent division of labor between computers and clinicians—a combination that can do more than either one alone. The real danger comes from a failure to appreciate the scope and depth of clinical work. An autonomous, robotic therapist, representing the knowledge and experience of a competent aphasia clinician, is a fantasy dreamed up by people who focus too much on the *costs* of care and not enough on the *efficacy* of care. Until we can describe to others precisely how to treat specific problems in individual patients, it is unreasonable, unethical, and a misrepresentation of the complexity of therapy for aphasia to assume that, at this time, a machine can perform the functions of a clinician.

The true value of computers in the rehabilitation of patients with aphasia continues to be studied. Just like the question of efficacy itself in aphasia rehabilitation (Darley, 1972; Fitz-Gibbon, 1986; Howard, 1986) the effectiveness of computer use in aphasia treatment cannot be answered with a simple "yes" or "no." More work is needed. Treatment software may always be an imperfect reflection of clinician-provided therapy, but by improving the software, clinicians and programmers will learn more about how and why treatment works. In the best tradition of scientific and rehabilitative efforts, aphasiologists can work together to shape this tool of technology for the development of their professions and the benefit of all patients.

KEY POINTS

1. What is believed about aphasia and treatment should be reflected in treatment software and not diminished by the limitations of computers.

2. Four properties of computers and computer programming that illustrate the limitations inherent in the application of computers to aphasia treatment are discrete (quantity rather than quality), conventional (pre-applied, unchanging rules), finite (cannot anticipate every possibility), and isolated (artificial rather than real world).

3. Major areas in which computers have the potential to become significant tools for treating patients with aphasia include providing supplemental treatment, measuring efficacy, making prognoses, helping generalization, fostering independence and a more active role in treatment, providing recreational activities, and performing administrative functions.

4. Contemporary multi-media computers are ideal for providing auditory stimulation, reading treatment, and to a lesser extend, writing treatment (through typing).

5. Speech recognition software has improved in recent years but is still inadequate for most clinical applications in aphasia because of poor ability to understand multiple, different speakers as well as speakers with variable phonologic errors (as in aphasic paraphasias and apraxia of speech).

6. Clinicians should assess the following components of any treatment software considered for use by patients with aphasia: goal, instructions, stimulus characteristics, response requirements, scoring system, general feedback, specific ("corrective") feedback, type and degree of intervention, criteria for termination, and scores stored for later analysis.

7. Treatment software, like all treatment activities, should be based on a treatment model or models. Three basic models are brain–behavior relationships, behavior modification, and educational models

8. Four basic types of treatment software are stimulation, drill and practice, simulation, and tutorial.

9. Treatment efficacy refers to whether outcomes are improved as a result of a specific intervention.

10. A large body of research published in peer-reviewed journals demonstrates the effectiveness of aphasia treatment—and of computerized aphasia treatment—for various populations of people with aphasia.

11. The value of aphasia treatment is measured by the degree to which skills acquired during treatment are observed in real-life situations. Generalization can be aided by the computer, which can administer some aspects of treatment without the familiar presence

and constant conscious (and unconscious) control of the clinician.

12. Success of treatment for adults with chronic aphasia depends more on their acceptance of their residual disabilities and their social re-integration than on periodic but minimal gains in language tasks. Technology can assist patients with aphasia in these goals by helping them gain new language skills, by modifying and helping them grain control of their environment, and by providing them with options to improve their communication and quality of life.

ACTIVITIES FOR REFLECTION AND DISCUSSION

1. Review treatment software in your clinic. Evaluate the programs as though they were clinician-provided treatment activities. How do they measure up to the treatment you provide your patients?

2. Critically review treatment software described in commercial catalogs. Are expectations stated or implied that seem a little too good to be true? Do the tasks seem to be worthwhile as treatment activities or supplementary activities?

3. Under what circumstances could a person with aphasia improve talking, listening, reading, and/or writing by using an AAC device?

4. What are some of the major limitations of computer-provided treatment? How can you, as a clinician, overcome these limitations with your patients?

5. What would you like to see computers do in aphasia treatment? Describe a program that helps a clinician to improve a patient's reading comprehension.

6. Design a computer program based on a favorite or familiar treatment activity. Incorporate options that allow the clinician to modify task requirements for patients with different types or severities of aphasia.

References

Adrian, J. A., Gonzalez, M., & Buiza, J. J. (2003). The use of computer-assisted therapy in anomia rehabilitation: A single-case report. *Aphasiology, 17*, 981–1002.

Aftonomos, L. B., Steele, R. D., & Wertz, R. T. (1997, August). Promoting recovery in chronic aphasia with an interactive technology. *Archives of Physical Medicine, 78*, 841–846.

American Academy of Neurology Therapeutics and Technology Assessment Subcommittee (1994). Assessment: Melodic intonation therapy. *Neurology, 44*, 566–568.

Babbage, C. (1822). A note respecting the application of machinery to the calculations of mathematical tables. *Memoirs of the Astronomical Society, 1*, 309.

Barr, A., & Geigenbaum, E. A. (Eds.). (1982). *The handbook of artificial intelligence*. Stanford, CA: HeurisTech Press.

Bengston, V. L. (1973). Self-determination: A social psychologic perspective on helping the aged. *Geriatrics, 28*(12), 1118–1130.

Benson, D. F. (1975). Disorders of verbal expression. In D. F. Benson & D. Blumer (Eds.), *Psychiatric aspects of neurologic disease* (pp. 121–137). New York: Grune & Stratton.

Bolter, J. D. (1984). *Turing's man: Western culture in the computer age.* Chapel Hill: University of North Carolina Press.

Bracy, O. L. (1983). Computer based cognitive rehabilitation. *Cognitive Rehabilitation, 1*(1), 7–8, 18–19.

Bracy, O. L. (1986). Cognitive rehabilitation: A process approach. *Cognitive Rehabilitation, 4*, 10–17.

Brodin, J., & Magnusson, M. (1994). Videotelephony and disability: A bibliography. *Technology, Communication and Disability (Report No. 5)*. Stockholm: Department of Education, Stockholm University.

Brown, C. S., & Cullinan, W. L. (1981). Word-retrieval difficulty and dysfluent speech in adult anomic speakers. *Journal of Speech and Hearing Research. 24*, 358–365.

Brubaker, S. H. (1996). *Basic level workbook for aphasia.* Detroit: Wayne State University Press.

Chapey, R., Rigrodsky, S., & Morrison, E. (1976). Divergent semantic behavior in aphasia. *Journal of Speech and Hearing Research, 19*, 664–677.

Cicerone, K. D., Dahlberg, C., Kalmar, K., Langenbahm, D. M., Malec, J. F., Bergquist, T. F., et al. (2000). Evidence-based cognitive rehabilitation: Recommendations for clinical practice. *Archives of Physcial Medicine and Rehabilitation, 81*, 1596–1615.

Coelho, G. V., Hamburg, D. A., & Adams, J. E. (1974). *Coping and adaptation.* New York: Basic Books.

Colby, K. M., Christinaz, D., Parkison, R. C., Graham, S., & Karpf, C. (1981). A word-finding computer program with a dynamic lexical-semantic memory for patients with anomia using an intelligent speech prosthesis. *Brain and Language, 14*, 272–281.

Colby, K. M., & Kraemer, H. C. (1975). An objective measurement of nonspeaking children's performance with a computer-controlled program for the stimulation of language behavior. *Journal of Autism and Childhood Schizophrenia, 5*(2), 139–146.

Colby, K. M., & Smith, D. C. (1973). Computers in the treatment of nonspeaking autistic children. In J. H. Masserman (Ed.), *Current psychiatric therapies* (Vol. 11, pp. 1–17). New York: Grune & Stratton.

Crerar, M. A., & Ellis, A. W. (1995). Computer-based therapy for aphasia: Towards second generation clinical tools. In C. Code & D. Müller (Eds.), *Treatment of aphasia: From theory to practice* (pp. 223–250). London: Whurr.

Crerar, M. A., Ellis, A. W., & Dean, E. C. (1996). Remediation of sentence processing deficits in aphasia using a computer-based microworld. *Brain and Language, 52*, 229–275.

Darley, F. L. (1972). The efficacy of language rehabilitation in aphasia. *Journal of Speech and Hearing Research, 37*, 3–21.

Davis, G. A., & Wilcox, M. J. (1985). *Adult aphasia rehabilitation: Applied pragmatics.* Austin, TX: Pro-Ed.

Dean, E. C. (1987). Microcomputers and aphasia. *Aphasiology, 1*(3), 267–270.

Delouche, G., Dordain, M., & Kremin, H. (1993). Rehabilitation of confrontational naming in aphasia: Relations between oral and written modalities. *Aphasiology*, 7, 201–216.

De Renzi, E., & Vignolo, L. A. (1962, December). The Token Test: A sensitive test to detect receptive disturbances in aphasics. *Brain*, 85, 665–678.

Dressler, R. A. (1991). *Beyond workbooks: The computer as a treatment supplement.* Poster session presented at the American Speech-Language Hearing Association Annual Convention, Atlanta, GA, November 24, 1991.

Duffy, J. R. (1998, June). *Telehealth practice applications.* ASHA Leadership Inservice Delivery Conference. Tucson, AZ.

Duffy, J. R., Werven, G. W., & Aronson, A. E. (1997). Telemedicine and the diagnosis of speech and language disorders. *Mayo Clinic Proceedings*, 72, 1116–1122.

Egolf, D. B., & Chester, S. L. (1973). Nonverbal communication and the disorders of speech and language. *Asha*, 15, 511–518.

Eisenson, J. (1973). *Adult aphasia.* New York: Appleton-Century-Crofts.

Enderby, P. (1987). Microcomputers in assessment, rehabilitation and recreation. *Aphasiology*, 1(2), 151–166.

Fenstad, J. E. (1988). Language and computations. In R. Herken (Ed.), *The universal Turing machine: A half-century survey* (pp. 327–348). New York: Oxford University Press.

Fink, R. B., Brecher, A., Schwartz, M. F., & Robey, R. R. (2002). A computer-implemented protocol for treatment of naming disorders: Evaluation of clinician-guided and partially self-guided instruction. *Aphasiology*, 16, 1061–1086.

Fitz-Gibbon, C. T. (1986). In defense of randomized controlled trials, with suggestions about the possible use of meta-analysis. *British Journal of disorders of Communication*, 21, 117–124.

Gadler, H. P., & Zechner, K. (1992). AUSWEGE—WEGE in Osterreich [AUSWEGE—WEGE in Austria]. In V. M. Roth (Ed.), *Computer in der sprachtherapie* [Computers in speech-language therapy] (pp. 147–160). Tubingen: Gunter Narr Verlag.

Gardner, H., Zurif, E., Berry, T., & Baker, E. (1976). Visual communication in aphasia. *Neuropsychologia*, 14, 275–292.

Gardner, R., & Gardner, B. (1969). Teaching sign language to a chimpanzee. *Science*, 165, 664–672.

Geschwind, N. (1973). *Writing and its disorders.* Paper presented at the Second Pan-American Congress of Audition and Language, Lima, Peru.

Glisky, E. L., Schlacter, D. L., & Tuving, E. (1986). Learning and retention of computer-related vocabulary in memory-impaired patients: Method of vanishing cues. *Journal of Clinical and Experimental Neuropsychology*, 8(3), 292–312.

Goldberg, S. A. (1997). *Clinical skills for speech-language pathologists.* San Diego: Singular.

Goldstein, K. (1942). *After-affects of brain injury in war.* New York: Grune & Stratton.

Goldstein, K. (1948). *Language and language disturbances.* New York: Grune & Stratton.

Goodglass, H., & Kaplan, E. (1983). *Boston Diagnostic Aphasia Examination.* Philadelphia: Lea & Febiger.

Guyard, H., Masson, V., & Quiniou, R. (1990). Computer-based aphasia treatment meets artificial intelligence. *Aphasiology*, 4(6), 599–613.

Hallowell, B., & Katz, R. C. (1999). Technological applications in the assessment of acquired neurogenic communication and swallowing disorders in adults. *Seminars in Speech, Language and Hearing*, 20(2), 149–167.

Herrmann, D., Yoder, C. Y., Wells, J., & Raybeck, D. (1996). Portable electronic scheduling/reminding devices. *Cognitive Technology*, 1, 19–24.

Howard. D. (1986). Beyond randomized controlled trials: The case for effective case studies of the effects of treatment in aphasia. *British Journal of Disorders of Communication*, 21, 89–102.

Katz, R. C. (1984). Using microcomputers in the diagnosis and treatment of chronic aphasic adults. *Seminars in Speech, Language and Hearing*, 5(l), 11–22.

Katz, R. C. (1986). *Aphasia treatment and microcomputers.* New York: Taylor & Francis.

Katz, R. C. (1987). Efficacy of aphasia treatment using microcomputers. *Aphasiology*, 1(2), 141–150.

Katz, R. C. (1990). Intelligent computerized treatment or artificial aphasia therapy. *Aphasiology*, 4(6), 621–624.

Katz, R. C., LaPointe, L. L., & Markel, N. N. (1978). Coverbal behavior and aphasic speakers. In R. H. Brookshire. (Ed.), *Clinical aphasiology: Conference proceedings* (pp. 164–173). Minneapolis: BRK.

Katz, R. C., LaPointe, L. L., & Markel, N. N. (2005). Coverbal behavior and aphasic speakers. *Aphasiology*, 18(12), 1213–1220.

Katz, R. C., LaPointe, L. L., Markel, N. N., & Silkes, J. (2005). Coverbal behavior and aphasic speakers: Revised. *Aphasiology*, 18(12), 1221–1225.

Katz, R. C., & Nagy, V. T. (1982). A computerized treatment system for chronic aphasic adults. In R. H. Brookshire (Ed.), *Clinical aphasiology: Conference proceedings* (pp. 153–160). Minneapolis, MN: BRK.

Katz, R. C., & Nagy, V. T. (1983). A computerized approach for improving word recognition in chronic aphasic patients. In R. H. Brookshire (Ed.), *Clinical aphasiology: Conference proceedings* (pp. 65–72). Minneapolis, MN: BRK.

Katz, R. C., & Nagy, V. T. (1984). An intelligent computer-based task for chronic aphasic patients. In R. H. Brookshire (Ed.), *Clinical aphasiology: Conference proceedings* (pp. 159–165). Minneapolis, MN: BRK.

Katz, R. C., & Nagy, V. T. (1985). A self-modifying computerized reading program for severely-impaired aphasic adults. In R. H. Brookshire (Ed.), *Clinical aphasiology: Conference proceedings* (pp. 184–188). Minneapolis, MN: BRK.

Katz, R. C., & Wertz, R. T. (1992). Computerized hierarchical reading treatment in aphasia. *Aphasiology*, 6, 165–177.

Katz, R. C., & Wertz, R. T. (1997). The efficacy of computer-provided reading treatment for chronic aphasic adults. *Journal of Speech, Language and Hearing Research*, 40(3), 493–507.

Katz, R. C., Wertz, R. T., Davidoff, M., Schubitowski, Y. D., &. Devitt, E. W. (1989). A computer program to improve written confrontation naming In aphasia. In T. E. Prescott (Ed.), *Clinical aphasiology: Conference proceedings* (pp. 321–338). Austin, TX: Pro-Ed.

Keenan, J. S. (1967). *A language rehabilitation program—Aphasia.* Chicago: Bell and Howell.

Keith, R. L., & Darley, F. L. (1967). The use of a special electric board in rehabilitation of the aphasic patient. *Journal of Speech and Hearing Disorders*, 32(2), 148–153.

Kertesz, A. (1982). *Western Aphasia Battery.* New York: Grune & Stratton.

Kolonder, R. M. (Ed.) (1997). *Computering Large Integrated Health Networks.* New York: Springer-Verlag.

Kotten, A. (1989). Aphasia treatment: A multidimensional process. In E. Perecman (Ed.), *Integrating theory and practice in neuropsychology* (pp. 293–315). Hillsdale, NJ: Lawrence Erlbaum.

Laganaro, M., Di Pietro, M., & Schnider, A. (2003). Computerized treatment of anomia in chronic and acute aphasia: An exploratory study. *Aphasiology, 17,* 709–721.

Langer, E. J., & Rodin, J. (1976). The effect of choice and enhanced personal responsibility for the aged: A field experiment in an institutional setting. *Journal of Personality and Social Psychology, 34,* 191–198.

LaPointe, L. L. (1977). Base-10 "programmed stimulation": Task specification, scoring and plotting performance in aphasia therapy. *Journal of Speech and Hearing Disorders, 42,* 90–105.

Lepper, M. R. (1985). Microcomputers in education: Motivational and social issues. *American Psychologist, 40,* 1–18.

Linebarger, M. C., Schwartz, M. F., & Kohn, S. E. (2001). Computer-based training of language production: An exploratory study. *Aphasiology, 11,* 57–96.

Loverso, F. L. (1987). Unfounded expectations: Computers in rehabilitation. *Aphasiology, 1*(2), 157–160.

Loverso, F. L., Prescott, T. E., & Selinger, M. (1988). Cueing verbs: A treatment strategy for aphasic adults. *Journal of Rehabilitation Research and Development, 25,* 47–60.

Loverso, F. L., Prescott, T. E., & Selinger, M. (1992). Microcomputer treatment applications in aphasiology. *Aphasiology, 6*(2), 155–163.

Loverso, F. L., Prescott, T. E., Selinger, M., & Riley, L. (1988). Comparison of two modes of aphasia treatment: Clinician and computer-clinician assisted. In T. E. Prescott (Ed.), *Clinical aphasiology* (Vol. 18, pp. 297–319). Austin, TX: Pro-Ed.

Loverso, F. L., Prescott, T. E., Selinger, M., Wheeler, K. M., & Smith, R. D. (1985). The application of microcomputers for the treatment of aphasic adults. In R. H. Brookshire (Ed.), *Clinical aphasiology: Conference proceedings* (pp. 189–195). Minneapolis, MN: BRK.

Loverso, F. L., Selinger, M., & Prescott, T. E. (1979). Application of verbing strategies to aphasia treatment. In R. H. Brookshire (Ed.), *Clinical aphasiology: Conference proceedings* (pp. 229–238). Minneapolis, MN: BRK.

Lucas, R. W. (1977). A study of patients' attitudes to computer interrogation. *International Journal of Man-Machine Studies, 9,* 69–86.

Luria, A. R. (1963). *Restoration of function after brain injury.* New York: Macmillan.

Luria, A. R. (1973). *The working brain.* New York: Basic Books.

Luria, A. R. (1980). *Higher cortical functions in man* (2nd ed.). New York: Basic Books.

Lynch, W. J. (1983). Cognitive retraining using microcomputer games and commercially-available software. *Cognitive Rehabilitation, 1,* 19–22.

Matthews, B. A. J., & LaPointe, L. L. (1981). Determining rate of change and predicting performance levels in aphasia therapy. In R. H. Brookshire (Ed.), *Clinical aphasiology: Conference proceedings* (pp. 17–25). Minneapolis, MN: BRK.

Matthews, B. A. J., & LaPointe, L. L. (1983). Slope and variability of performance on selected aphasia treatment tasks. In R. H. Brookshire (Ed.), *Clinical aphasiology: Conference proceedings* (pp. 113–120). Minneapolis, MN: BRK.

McCall, D., Shelton, J. R., Weinrich, M., & Cox, D. (2000). The utility of computerized visual communication for improving natural language in chronic global aphasia: Implications for approaches to treatment in global aphasia. *Aphasiology, 14,* 795–826.

McGlynn, E. A. (1996). Domains of study and methodological challenges. In L. I. Sederer & B. Dickey (Eds.), *Outcomes assessment in clinical practice* (pp. 19–24). Baltimore: Williams & Wilkins.

McReynolds, L. V., & Kearns, K. P. (1983). *Single-subject experimental designs in communicative disorders.* Baltimore, MD: University Park Press.

Mehrabian, A. (1968). Communication without words. *Psychology Today, 2,* 52–55.

Mills, R. H. (1982). Microcomputerized auditory comprehension training. In R. H. Brookshire (Ed.), *Clinical aphasiology: Conference proceedings* (pp. 147–152). Minneapolis, MN: BRK.

Mills, R. H. (1988). Book review (*Aphasia treatment and microcomputers*). *Journal of Computer Users in Speech and Hearing, 41*(1), 40–41.

Morrison, M. H. (1998a). Information technology for medical rehabilitation, Part 1: An overview. In E. A. Dobrzykowski (Ed.), *Essential readings in rehabilitation outcomes measurements: Application, methodology, and technology* (pp. 255–257). Gaithersburg, MD: Aspen.

Morrison, M. H. (1998b). Information technology for medical rehabilitation, Part 2: Requirements. In E. A. Dobrzykowski (Ed.), *Essential readings in rehabilitation outcomes measurements: Application, methodology, and technology* (pp. 258–261). Gaithersburg, MD: Aspen.

Mortley, J., Enderby, P., & Petheram, B. (2001). Using a computer to improve functional writing in a patient with severe dysgraphia. *Aphasiology, 15,* 443–461.

Myers, P. S. (1999). *Right hemisphere damage.* San Diego: Singular.

Odell, K., Collins, M., Dirkx, T., & Kelso, D. (1985). A computerized version of the Coloured Progressive Matrices. In R. H. Brookshire (Ed.), *Clinical aphasiology: Conference proceedings* (pp. 47–56). Minneapolis, MN: BRK.

Odor, J. P. (1988). Student models in machine-mediated learning. *Journal of Mental Deficiency Research, 32,* 247–256.

Peters, L. J., & Peters, D. P. (1998). Telehealth. Part II. A total system approach. *Asha, 40*(2), 31–33.

Petheram, B. (1988). Enabling stroke victims to interact with a minicomputer—Comparison of input devices. *International Disabilities Studies, 10*(2), 73–80.

Pfau, G. S. (1974). *Instruction manual for the General Electric / Project LIFE program: Programmed Assistance to Learning (PAL).* Ballston Lake, NY: Instructional Industries.

Porch, B. E. (1981). *The Porch index of communicative ability: Administration, scoring and interpretation* (Vol. 1, 3rd ed.). Palo Alto, CA,: Consulting Psychologists Press.

Premack, D. (1970). The education of Sarah: A chimp learns the language. *Psychology Today, 4,* 55–58.

Prescott, T. E., Loverso, F. L., & Selinger, M. (1984). Differences between normals and left brain damaged (aphasic) subjects on a nonverbal problem solving task. In R. H. Brookshire (Ed.), *Clinical aphasiology: Conference proceedings* (pp. 235–240). Minneapolis, MN: BRK.

Prescott, T. E., & McNeil, M. R. (1973). *Measuring the effects of treatment of aphasia.* Paper presented at the Third Conference on Clinical Aphasiology, Albuquerque, MM.

Raven, J. C. (1975). *Coloured progressive matrices.* Los Angeles, CA: Western Psychologic Services.

Rheingold, H. (1991). *Virtual reality*. New York: Summit Books.

Robey, R. R. (1998). A meta-analysis of clinical outcomes in the treatment of aphasia. *Journal of Speech, Language, and Hearing Research, 41,* 172–187.

Robey, R. R., & Schultz, M. C. (1998). A model for conducting clinical-outcome research: Adaptation of the standard protocol for use in aphasiology. *Aphasiology, 12,* 787–810.

Robertson, I. (1990). Does computerized cognitive rehabilitation work? A review. *Aphasiology, 4*(4), 381–405.

Rosenbek, J. C. (1979). Wrinkled feet. In R. H. Brookshire (Ed.), *Clinical aphasiology: Conference proceedings* (pp. 163–176). Minneapolis, MN: BRK.

Rosenbek, J. C. (1995). Efficacy in dysphagia. *Dysphagia, 10,* 263–267.

Rosenbek, J. C., LaPointe, L. L., & Wertz, R. T. (1989). *Aphasia: A clinical approach*. Austin, TX: Pro-Ed.

Roth, V. M. (1992). SICH-ÄUSSERNDES Verstehen NeueWEGE [Understanding SICH-ÄUSSERNDES: NeueWEGE]. In V. M. Roth (Ed.), *Computer in der sprachtherapie* [Computers in speech-language therapy] (pp. 187–214). Tubingen: Gunter Narr Verlag.

Rushakoff, G. E. (1984). Clinical applications in communication disorders. In A. H. Schwartz (Ed.), *Handbook of microcomputer applications in communication disorders* (pp. 148–171). San Diego, CA: College Hill Press.

Schuell, H., Jenkins, J. J., & Jiménez-Pabón, E. (1964). *Aphasia in adults*. New York: Harper & Row.

Schulz, R. (1976). Effects of control and predictability, on the physical well being of the institutionalized aged. *Journal of Personality and Social Psychology, 33,* 563–573.

Schwartz, A. H. (1984). *Handbook of microcomputer applications in communication disorders*. San Diego: College-Hill Press.

Scott, C., & Byng, S. (1989). Computer-assisted remediation of a homophone comprehension disorder in surface dyslexia. *Aphasiology, 3*(3), 301–320.

Seligman. M. (1975). *Helplessness: On depression, development and death*. San Francisco, CA: Freeman.

Selinger, M., Prescott, T. E., & Katz, R. C. (1987). Handwritten versus typed responses on PICA graphic subtests. In R. H. Brookshire (Ed.), *Clinical aphasiology: Conference proceedings* (pp. 136–142). Minneapolis, MN: BRK.

Selinger, M., Prescott, T. E., Loverso, F. L., & Fuller, K. (1987). Below the 50th percentile: Application of the verb as core model. In R. H. Brookshire (Ed.), *Clinical aphasiology: Conference proceedings* (pp. 55–63). Minneapolis, MN: BRK.

Seron, X., Deloche, G., Moulard, G., & Rouselle, M. (1980). A computer-based therapy for the treatment of aphasic subjects with writing disorders. *Journal of Speech and Hearing Disorders, 45,* 45–58.

Silverman, F. H. (1997). *Computer applications for augmenting the management of speech, language, and hearing disorders*. Boston: Allyn and Bacon.

Skilbeck, C. (1984). Computer assistance in the management of memory and cognitive impairment. In B. A. Wilson & N. Moffat (Ed.), *Clinical management of memory problems*. Rockville, MD: Aspen.

Skinner, B. F. (1948). *Walden two*. New York: Macmillan.

Skinner, B. F. (1957). *Verbal behavior*. New York: Appleton-Century-Crofts.

Skinner, B. F. (1958). Teaching machines. *Science, 128,* 969–977.

Steele, R. D., Weinrich, M., Kleczewska, M. K., Wertz, R. T., & Carlson, G. S. (1987). Evaluating performance of severely aphasic patients on a computer-aided visual communication system. In R. H. Brookshire (Ed.), *Clinical aphasiology: Conference proceedings* (pp. 46–54). Minneapolis, MN: BRK.

Steele, R. D., Weinrich, M., Wertz, R. T., Kleczewska, M. K., & Carlson, G. S. (1989). Computer-based visual communication in aphasia. *Neuropsychologia, 27,* 409–427.

Stoicheff, M. L. (1960). Motivating instructions and language performance of dysphasic subjects. *Journal of Speech and Hearing Research, 3,* 75–85.

Tonkovich, J. D., Horowitz, D. M., Kawahigashi, J. N., Krainen, G. H., & Kronick, D. (1991). *An application of voice recognition technology for clinical documentation*. Computer poster session presented at the 1991 American Speech-Language-Hearing Association Annual Convention, Atlanta, GA.

Turing, A. M. (1936). On computable numbers, with an application to the Entscheidungs problem. *Proceedings of the London Mathematical Society, 42*(2), 230–265.

Turing, A. M. (1950). Computing machinery and intelligence. *Mind, 59*(236), 433–460.

Van de Sandt-Koenderman, M. (1994). Multicue, a computer program for word finding in aphasia, 1. *International Congress Language-Therapy-Computers*, Graz, Austria: University of Graz.

Van de Sandt-Koenderman, M. (2004). High-tech AAC and aphasia: Widening horizons? *Aphasiology, 18,* 245–263.

Vaughn, G. R. (1980, August). *REMATE (Remote Machine Assisted Treatment and Evaluation): Communication outreach innovative health care delivery system for persons with communicative disorders workshop*. Birmingham: Veterans Administration Medical Center.

Vaughn, G. R., Amster, W. W., Bess, J. C., Gilbert, D. J., Kearrns, K. P., Rudd, A. K., et al. (1987). Efficacy of remote treatment of aphasia by TEL-Communicology. *Journal of Rehabilitative Research and Development, 25*(1), 446–447.

Wallich, P. (1991, October). Digital dyslexia: Neural network mimics the effects of stroke. *Scientific American, 265*(4), 36.

Weinrich, M., McCall, D., Shoosmith, L., Thomas, K., Katzenberger, K., & Weber, C. (1993). Locative prepositional phrases in severe aphasia. *Brain and Language, 45,* 21–45.

Weinrich, M., McCall, D., Weber, C., Thomas, K., & Thornburg, L. (1995). Training on an iconic communication system for severe aphasia can improve natural language production. *Aphasiology, 9,* 343–364.

Weinrich, M., Steele, R. D., Kleczewska, M., Carlson, G. S., Baker, E., & Wertz, R. T. (1989). Representation of "verbs" in a computerized visual communication system. *Aphasiology, 3*(6), 501–512.

Wertz, R. T. (1981). Aphasia management: The speech pathologist's role. *Seminars in Speech, Language and Hearing, 2,* 315–331.

Wertz, R. T., Dronkers, N. F., Knight, R. T., Shenaut, G. K., & Deal, J. L. (1987). Rehabilitation of neurogenic communication disorders in remote settings. *Journal of Rehabilitative Research and Development, 25*(l), 432–433.

Wertz, R. T., & Katz, R. C. (2004). Outcomes for computer-provided treatment for aphasia. *Aphasiology, 18,* 229–244.

Wolfe, G. R. (1987). Microcomputers and treatment of aphasia. *Aphasiology, 1*(2), 165–170.

Wolfe, G. R., Davidoff, M., & Katz, R. C. (1987). Nonverbal problem-solving in aphasic and non-aphasic subjects with computer presented and actual stimuli. In R. H. Brookshire (Ed.), *Clinical aphasiology: Conference proceedings* (pp. 243–248). Minneapolis, MN: BRK.

APPENDIX 32.1
Clinical Examples

Example 1: Auditory Comprehension

MODALITY:	Listening
DESIGN:	Stimulation
GOALS:	To maintain accuracy, self-monitoring, and attention as response time decreases
TASK:	Using digitized speech, the computer states the name (or function) of an item in a complex scene containing several functionally related items displayed on the monitor. The patient selects the correct item with the mouse.
SOFTWARE:	Language Activities of Daily Living: My House (Laureate Learning Systems)
PROCEDURE:	The clinician selects a response time (e.g., 10 seconds) that permits the patient to respond to all items with 100% accuracy. Response time is reduced for subsequent trials until the patient begins to make errors.
INTERVENTION:	Keep response time at the level when errors first occurred. Reduce the number of items to two, and identify those two items for the patient before beginning (e.g., "The computer is going to ask you to point to only this one or that one."). When 100% accurate for three consecutive trials, increase number of items to three, four, and so on until all items are presented.
SCORING:	1 point per correctly selected item

Example 2: Writing/Printing Personal ID Information

MODALITY:	Writing (typing)
DESIGN:	Drill and practice
GOAL:	To improve the ability to write or print personal information for a chronic, severely impaired, predominantly nonverbal patient with aphasia using a typing drill
TASK:	Type name, address, and telephone number in response to a diminishing set of cues
SOFTWARE:	Word processor
PROCEDURE:	The clinician creates a series of word processing documents with diminishing cues (e.g., Document 1 has the intact model for simple copying, Document 2 has every third letter or number missing, Document 3 has every other word missing, and so on.) The diminishing cues can take any form thought useful by the clinician. From either the word processing program or from within a Windows (or Macintosh) folder, the patient selects the document containing the level of cueing needed to successfully type the personal information. The patient can save the file, or the "autosave" option can be invoked, for later review of performance by the clinician. To aid in generalization, the documents are printed, and the patient practices writing (printing) at home directly on the same pages.
INTERVENTION:	The clinician dictates error items to the patient. If errors persist, the clinician provides models or other cues as needed.
SCORING:	Number of correctly spelled words, legible words, etc.

APPENDIX 32.2
Sources for Software and Other Relevant Technology

AbleLink Technologies
528 North Tejon Street, Suite 100
Colorado Springs, CO 80903
(719) 592-0347
www.ablelinktech.com

Avaaz Innovations
258 Beckley Lane
P.O. Box 1055
Dublin, OH 43017-6055
614-932-0757
www.avaaz.com

BrainTrain
727 Twin Ridge Lane
Richmond, VA 23235
800-822-0538
www.braintrain.com

Bungalow Software
5390 NE Stanchion Court
Hillsboro, OR 97124
800-891-9937
www.BungalowSoftware.com

Chart Links
74 Forbes Avenue
New Haven, CT 06512
203-469-0707
www.chartlinks.com

Communication Skill Builders/
The Psychological Corporation
555 Academic Court
San Antonio, TX 78204-2498
800-211-8378
800-232-1223

Don Johnston
1000 North Rand Road, Bldg. 115
P.O. Box 639
Wauconda, IL 60084-0639
800-999-4660
www.donjohnston.com

Gus Communications
1006 Lonetree Court
Bellingham, WA 98226
360-715-8580
www.gusinc.com

IBM
New Orchard Road

Armonk, NY 10504
800-426-4968
www.ibm.com

Interactive Learning Materials
150 Croton Lake Road
P.O. Box S
Katonah, NY 10536
(914) 232-4682

Laureate Learning Systems, Inc.
110 East Spring Street
Winooski, VT 05404-1898
800-562-6801
www.llsys.com

The Learning Company
One Athenaeum Street
Cambridge, MA 02142
617-494-5700
www.learningco.com

LingraphiCARE
20 Nassau Street, Suite 235
Princeton, NJ 08542
888-274-2742
www.aphasia.com

Madentec Limited
4664 99th Street
Edmonton, Alberta
T6E 5H5, Canada
877-623-3682
www.madentec.com

Mayer-Johnson Co.
P.O. Box 1579
Solana Beach, CA 92075-1579
800-588-4548
www.mayer-johnson.com

Medical Software Products
6415 Oak Hill Drive
Granite Bay, CA 95746-8909
916-797-2363
www.medsoftware.com

Microsoft
One Microsoft Way
Redmond, WA 98052-6399
425-882-8080
www.microsoft.com/ms.htm

Parrot Software
P.O. Box 250755
West Bloomfield, MI 48325
800-PARROT-1
www.parrotsoftware.com/index.html

Prentke Romich Company
1022 Heyl Road
Wooster, OH 44691
800-262-1984
www.prentrom.com

Pro-Ed
8700 Shoal Creek
Austin, TX 78758-6897
800-897-3202
www.proedinc.com

Psychological Software Services
6555 Carrollton Avenue
Indianapolis, IN 46220

317-257-9672
www.neuroscience.cnter.com

Sunburst Communications
1550 Executive Drive
Elgin, IL 60123-9979
800-321-7511
www.store.sunburst.com

SPSS
233 South Wacker Drive
Chicago, IL 60606
312-651-3000
www.spss.com

Therapist Helper Brand Software
600 West Cummings Park
Suite 3450
Woburn, MA 01801
800-343-5737
www.helper.com

APPENDIX 32.3
Web Sites of Interest

Academy of Aphasia
http://www.academyofaphasia.org

Academy of Neurologic Communication Disorders and Sciences
(ANCDS)
www.ancds.org

American Stroke Association (American Heart Association)
http://www.strokeassociation.org

American Medical Association (AMA) Insight: Atlas of the
Human Body
http://www.ama-assn.org/insight/gen_hlth/atlas/atlas.htm

American Speech-Language-Hearing Association (ASHA)
www.asha.org

Brain Injury Associations, Inc.
www.biausa.org

CenterNet Homepage (National Center for Neurogenic
Communication Disorders at the University of Arizona)
http://cnet.shs.arizona.edu/cnet

Communication Disorders and Sciences Home Page (resource
center by Judith Kuster)
http://www.mnsu.edu/comdis/kuster2/welcome.html

Clinical Aphasiology Conference
www.clinicalaphasiology.org

Mayo Clinic: Cardiology and Vascular Medicine
http://www.mayoclinic.org/cardiovascular-rst

Mayo Clinic: Rehabilitation After Stroke
http://www.mayoclinic.org/stroke/rehabilitation.html

National Aphasia Association (NAA)
www.aphasia.org

National Institutes of Health (NIH)
www.nih.gov

National Institute of Neurologic Diseases and Stroke (NINDS)
http://www.ninds.nih.gov

National Resource Center for Traumatic Brain Injury
www.neuro.pmr.vcu.edu

National Stroke Association
www.stroke.org

Neurology Web Forums at Massachusetts General Hospital
http://neuro-www.mgh.harvard.edu/forum/

Section V

Therapy for Associated Neuropathologies of Speech- and Language-Related Functions

Chapter 33

Communication Disorders Associated with Traumatic Brain Injury

Mark Ylvisaker, Shirley F. Szekeres, and
Timothy Feeney

OBJECTIVES

The reader will be able to:

1. Describe epidemiologic trends related to traumatic brain injury (TBI).
2. Describe central themes in the pathophysiology of TBI, including both primary injuries (e.g., diffuse axonal injury and focal damage related to irregular surfaces on the floor of the skull) and secondary injuries (e.g., associated with elevated pressure, swelling, bleeding, neurotransmitter surges, and others).
3. Describe risk factors for TBI and the relation between preinjury factors and long-term outcome.
4. Describe central tendencies in long-term outcome from the perspectives of communication, cognition, executive functions, and behavior.
5. Describe central themes in rehabilitation and ongoing support for individuals with chronic cognitive, communication, and behavioral impairment after TBI.
6. Offer several rationales for a context-sensitive, everyday, routine-based approach to intervention.
7. Describe procedures associated with ongoing, context-sensitive, collaborative hypothesis testing assessment, and give a rationale for this approach to assessment for planning intervention.
8. Create functional, individualized rehabilitation plans in the domains of executive functions/self-regulation, cognition, social communication, and behavior.
9. Describe executive function routines, and give illustrations for individuals at varied stages of recovery.
10. Give reasons for avoiding process-specific cognitive exercises.
11. Create functional cognitive rehabilitation and support plans.
12. Implement self-coaching procedures for individuals with social communication problems.
13. Distinguish between antecedent-focused and consequence-focused behavior management, and offer a rationale for antecedent-focused approaches for individuals with TBI.
14. Create functional intervention plans designed to teach positive communication alternatives to negative behavior.
15. Offer several rationales for collaborating with everyday people, and describe effective ways to create such collaborative relationships.

In this chapter, we offer a functional and highly context-sensitive perspective on assessment and intervention for individuals with chronic cognitive and behavioral impairments, which underlie the most common and most debilitating communication-related disabilities after traumatic brain injury (TBI; i.e., damage to the brain caused by external forces acting on the skull). The perspective is based on (1) our combined 85 years of clinical experience in the field, (2) current theory and research in cognitive neuroscience, (3) a considerable body of efficacy research in related disability fields, and (4) a growing body of efficacy literature in TBI rehabilitation. The importance of the approach to cognitive rehabilitation described in this chapter is underscored by pessimistic reviews concerning the effectiveness of restorative, decontextualized cognitive and executive function exercises, possibly combined with neuropharmacologic management.

The length of this chapter is dictated by our attempt to address many critical themes associated with an increasingly important disability group for specialists in cognitive, behavioral, and communication disorders. Because readers tend to use this textbook as an ongoing resource, we have included a large number of tables, figures, and appendices designed to organize and summarize large quantities of information for easy access. The chapter is divided into eight sections:

1. Epidemiology
2. Pathophysiology
3. Disability associated with TBI, including frequently used measures of disability, considerations associated with prediction of outcome, stages of improvement, and commonly occurring communication consequences of TBI
4. Framework for everyday, routine-based intervention, including theoretical, neuropsychological, and economic rationales
5. Functional assessment for planning intervention
6. Intervention for self-regulatory impairments: cognitive and executive function disorders associated with TBI
7. Intervention for self-regulatory impairments: social-communication and behavioral disorders associated with TBI
8. Collaboration among professional clinicians, the person with disability, and the everyday people in that person's life.

Throughout the chapter, we highlight the role of the self-regulatory/executive system because of its vulnerability after frontal lobe injury and its significance in relation to successful outcome in the domains of rehabilitation discussed in this chapter. In other publications, we have developed these themes in greater detail than is possible here (see, e.g., Feeney & Ylvisaker, 1995, 1997; Szekeres, Ylvisaker, & Cohen, 1987; Ylvisaker, 2003, 2006; Ylvisaker & Feeney, 1996, 1998a, 1998b, 2000a, 2000b; Ylvisaker, Feeney, & Feeney, 1999; Ylvisaker, Feeney, & Szekeres, 1998; Ylvisaker, Szekeres, & Feeney, 1998; Ylvisaker, Szekeres, & Haarbauer-Krupa, 1998).

EPIDEMIOLOGY OF TBI

Incidence and Prevalence

According to the Centers for Disease Control and Prevention (CDC; 2001), at least 1.5 million TBIs occur in the United States annually, resulting in approximately 50,000 deaths and 235,000 hospitalizations. Of the 1.5 million injured people, 80,000 are expected to experience persisting disability, yielding a prevalence estimate of 5.3 million Americans living with TBI-related disability. These estimates are lower than previously reported (Kraus, 1993), possibly representing a positive trend in highway safety and increasingly restrictive criteria for hospital admission. Because of the relative youth of most individuals with TBI, prevalence-to-incidence ratios are much higher than those for neurogenic disorders associated with aging. Approximately 80% of those hospitalized with TBI have mild injuries, with an expectation of excellent recovery in most, but not all, cases (80%–90% excellent recovery) (Kraus & Nourjah, 1988; Ruff, 2005). Many more cases of mild injury are uncounted, either because those affected do not seek medical attention or because the brain injury is masked by more pressing medical concerns (e.g., high spinal cord injury). Direct medical costs (acute hospitalization and rehabilitation) have been estimated at $48.3 billion per year, not including the enormous financial and psychological costs associated with ongoing support and reduced employability (AHCPR, 1999).

Risk Factors

The incidence of TBI is highest among young people, with 15- to 24-year-old males being most vulnerable. Secondary peaks have been identified in people older than 65 years and in children 5 years or younger (CDC, 1997; Kraus, Rock, & Hemyari, 1990). With the introduction of TBI as an educational disability category in the revised Individuals with Disability Education Act (IDEA: Federal Register, 1991), children have received increasing attention in the clinical and education literatures. In contrast, elderly individuals, who also are at risk both for TBI and for relatively severe consequences of the injury, continue to be under-represented in the literature (Goldstein & Levin, 1995; Payne, 1999).

Several risk factors in addition to age have been identified. Historically, males have been said to have twice the rate of TBI as females, with this ratio being even higher (3:1 or 4:1) for the highest risk group of older adolescents and young adults (Kraus, 1993). More recent CDC estimates place the male-to-female ratio at closer to 1.5:1. Clinicians often characterize the highest risk group as including adolescent and young adult males from lower socioeconomic groups, whose preinjury lives may have been characterized by some degree of risk-taking behavior, poor academic and vocational achievement, and greater-than-average use of alcohol and recreational drugs. Supporting this stereotype, incidence studies have suggested that TBI appears to be especially common in lower socioeconomic groups, among people with less than a high school education, and among those with a history of poor academic performance (Fife, Faich, Hollinshead, & Boynton, 1986: Haas, Cope, & Hall, 1987; Sosin, Sniezek, & Thurman, 1996). Alcohol often is a contributing factor in the occurrence of TBI, strongly associated with both motor vehicle–related injuries and with falls in both young adults and the elderly (Hartshorne, Harruff, & Alvord, 1997; Kraus, 1993; Santora, Schinco, & Trooskin, 1994; U.S. Department of Transportation, 1995). Previous TBI increases the risk of subsequent TBI by threefold (Annegers, Grabow, Kurland, & Laws, 1980; Gerberich, Priest, Boen, Staub, & Maxwell, 1983). Previous TBI also may increase the negative consequences of subsequent TBI (Collins et al., 1999; Gronwall & Wrightson, 1975).

Not all epidemiologic reports, however, are consistent with the stereotype. For example, in two Australian studies, Tate (1998) failed to find a high rate of pretrauma social maladjustment in her cohort and, more surprisingly, did find that such maladjustment, when present, appeared not to have a pronounced effect on outcome. In contrast to Tate, our experience with several hundred young adults referred for neurobehavioral support as a result of behavior-related community reintegration problems suggests that preinjury factors play a significant role in outcome, with preinjury developmental and adjustment problems often exacerbated by the injury (Ylvisaker & Feeney, 2000a).

With respect to the cause of injury, transportation-related events account for approximately 50% of TBI cases (CDC, 1997), followed by falls (slightly more than 20% of the total, but much higher in young children and the elderly), assaults (approximately 20%), and finally, sports-related injuries and other causes. Tragically, abuse is a major factor in infants and the elderly. Consideration of the causes of TBI reveals that this is a largely preventable epidemic. With concerted efforts to improve automobile safety, reduce alcohol-impaired driving, enhance safety measures in sports, and eliminate child and elder abuse, the epidemiology of TBI could be dramatically changed.

PATHOPHYSIOLOGY OF TBI

The term "traumatic brain injury" refers to damage to the brain caused by external forces. Traumatic brain injuries can be open, involving penetration of the dural covering of the brain, or closed. Penetrating missile injuries, in which focal damage is related to the site of penetration and trajectory of the missile, are more strongly associated with aphasia than is closed head injury (CHI) (Newcomb, 1969). Generally, CHI refers to brain injuries in which the primary mechanism of damage is a blunt blow to the head or rapid changes of skull motion, both of which are associated with acceleration/deceleration forces acting on the brain (Levin, Benton, & Grossman, 1982). In special education discussions of students with brain injury, acquired brain injury often is used to identify an even broader pathophysiologic category, including stroke, tumor, anoxia, toxic encephalopathy, meningitis, encephalitis, and other causes of noncongenital brain impairment. Federal education law, PL 101-476 (Individuals with Disabilities Education Act, 1990; amended 1997), defined TBI in relation to external causes, but some state departments of education use TBI as a synonym for acquired brain injury.

Primary Impact Damage

Primary and secondary injuries associated with TBI are summarized in Figures 33–1 and 33–2 (information taken from Alexander, 1987; Katz, 1992; Pang, 1985; Povlishock & Katz., 2005; Young, 1999). Contact of a moving skull with a stationary surface may cause skull distortion and fracture and, traditionally, is thought to be responsible for coup (site of contact) and contrecoup (opposite side) brain contusion and cavitation injury (Fig. 33–3). Neurobehavioral deficits associated with lesions that vary with the site of impact cannot explain central tendencies within the population as a whole. Rather, damage associated with differential tissue movements within the skull, both brain—skull and brain—brain movements created by inertial forces (especially rotational inertia), often plays the greatest role in determining outcome and best explains population commonalities. This type of injury is possible even in the absence of a blow to the head if the skull is accelerated and/or decelerated rapidly (e.g., shaken baby syndrome) (Gennarelli et al., 1982).

In severe CHI, brain–skull differential movement in the area of bony prominences within the skull can cause surface contusion and laceration as well as deeper shearing of axons (diffuse axonal injury) and blood vessels (subdural and intracerebral hematoma) (Povlishock & Katz, 2005). Regardless of site of impact in high-speed CHI, focal contusion as well as axon shearing often are concentrated within anterior and inferior frontal and temporal lobe structures bilaterally because of their adjacency to sharp, irregular surfaces inside the skull (Alexander, 1987; Courville, 1937; Katz, 1992) (Figs. 33–4 and 33–5). Damage to these areas explains many of the commonly observed behavioral symptoms that negatively affect communication after CHI, including (a) depressed executive control over cognitive and communicative functions (prefrontal damage), (b) impaired social perception and social reactivity (prefrontal and frontolimbic damage, particularly right hemisphere), and (c) generally reduced behavioral self-regulation (prefrontal, frontolimbic, and anterior temporal lobe damage). Diffuse neuronal shearing also often is concentrated in subcortical white matter, brain stem, and corpus callosum, contributing to initial coma and subsequent arousal/attentional deficits as well as slowed mental processing (Adams, Graham, Murray, & Scott, 1982). Over the weeks and months after severe TBI, diffuse axonal injury can continue to contribute to degeneration at nerve terminals. Characteristic stages of recovery are related to diffuse rather than focal injuries (Povlishock & Katz, 2005). The relative infrequency of specific aphasic syndromes in CHI is, in part, a consequence of the smooth interior surface of the skull adjacent to the traditional perisylvian language centers in the brain.

Secondary Damage

Secondary damage in TBI is associated with slowly developing hemorrhages and localized or widespread swelling and edema, both of which contribute to increased intracranial pressure, which can be acutely life-threatening and contribute to morbidity in those who survive. In addition,

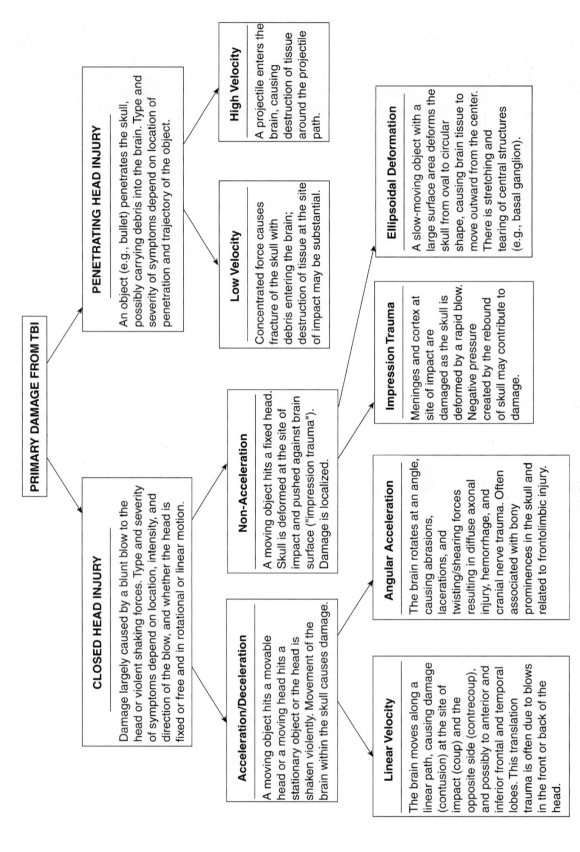

Figure 33–1. Mechanisms of immediate injury in closed and open traumatic brain injuries.

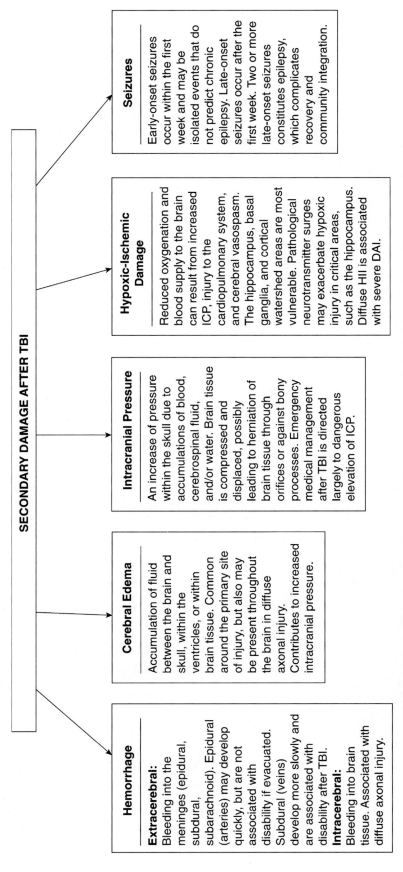

Figure 33–2. Pathologic events that often follow severe traumatic brain injury and contribute to impairment.

SECONDARY DAMAGE AFTER TBI

Hemorrhage

Extracerebral: Bleeding into the meninges (epidural, subdural, subarachnoid). Epidural (arteries) may develop quickly, but are not associated with disability if evacuated. Subdural (veins) develop more slowly and are associated with disability after TBI. **Intracerebral:** Bleeding into brain tissue. Associated with diffuse axonal injury.

Cerebral Edema

Accumulation of fluid between the brain and skull, within the ventricles, or within brain tissue. Common around the primary site of injury, but also may be present throughout the brain in diffuse axonal injury. Contributes to increased intracranial pressure.

Intracranial Pressure

An increase of pressure within the skull due to accumulations of blood, cerebrospinal fluid, and/or water. Brain tissue is compressed and displaced, possibly leading to herniation of brain tissue through orifices or against bony processes. Emergency medical management after TBI is directed largely to dangerous elevation of ICP.

Hypoxic-Ischemic Damage

Reduced oxygenation and blood supply to the brain can result from increased ICP, injury to the cardiopulmonary system, and cerebral vasospasm. The hippocampus, basal ganglia, and cortical watershed areas are most vulnerable. Pathological neurotransmitter surges may exacerbate hypoxic injury in critical areas, such as the hippocampus. Diffuse HII is associated with severe DAI.

Seizures

Early-onset seizures occur within the first week and may be isolated events that do not predict chronic epilepsy. Late-onset seizures occur after the first week. Two or more late-onset seizures constitutes epilepsy, which complicates recovery and community integration.

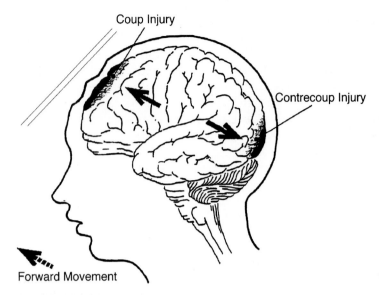

Figure 33–3. Representation of coup injury (i.e., contusion and cavitation at the site of impact) and contrecoup injury (i.e., contusion and cavitation at the opposite side of the brain). (Adapted with permission from Walker & the North Carolina State Board of Education, 1997; with permission.)

hypoxic-ischemic injury and pathologic neurotransmitter surges (specifically glutamate), both of which are common secondary consequences of severe TBI, often pick out specific vulnerable structures, notably the hippocampus bilaterally, thereby contributing to memory and new learning problems after the injury (Katz, 1992). This is an especially ominous consequence for young people who face substantial new learning challenges in school and on the job. Tragically, the vast majority of individuals with TBI are children, adolescents, and young adults. Post-traumatic seizures, including both early onset (within the first week) and late onset (appearing after the first week), also can complicate recovery and become a major concern if epilepsy persists.

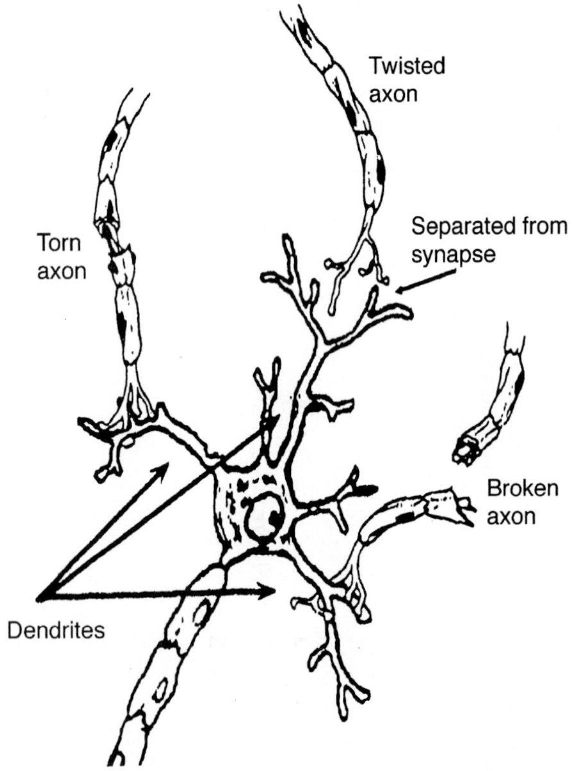

DISABILITY FOLLOWING TBI

Predictable inconsistencies are found in the published descriptions of disability following TBI. Because of the extended period of neurologic improvement, the time postinjury at which consequences of the injury are assessed influences the description of central tendencies in the population.

Figure 33–4. Diffuse axonal injury: twisting, tearing, and breaking of axons associated with primary impact damage in traumatic brain injury.

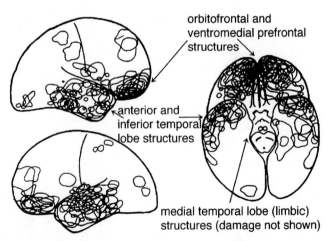

Figure 33–5. Contusions after traumatic brain injury, based on 40 consecutive cases, clearly depict the tendency for maximum pathology in the orbitofrontal and temporal regions. (Reprinted from Courville, 1937; with permission.)

Variation in the severity mix from study to study also adds to variation in this outcome picture. Furthermore, as increasingly valid language and cognitive assessments have become available (e.g., sensitive analysis of extended discourse versus aphasia batteries developed for a different clinical population) (Coehlo, Ylvisaker, & Turkstra, 2005), increasing numbers of individuals with TBI have been shown to have language and more general cognitive processing and self-regulatory difficulties. Finally, because of the variable associations among impairment, activity/participation, and context, different outcome profiles inevitably emerge depending on which domain is assessed.

The World Health Organization International Classification of Functioning

Throughout the chapter, we use the World Health Organization (WHO) framework of body structure and function (previously impairment), activity/participation (previously disability and handicap), and environmental context (WHO, 2001). Disorders of body structure and function include the underlying physiological or psychological ("in the head") impairments traditionally measured by office-bound test batteries (e.g., slowed processing, memory impairment, loss of organizing schemata, disruption of phonologic or grammatical systems, and hemiplegia). Disorders at the level of activity and participation, which may or may not be directly associated with the underlying impairment, refer to reduced ability to successfully perform activities that are important in the individual's life (e.g., difficulty maintaining a conversation, problems comprehending school textbooks, difficulty remaining focused and organized at work, and impulsive or aggressive interaction under stress). This level also includes the individual's potential educational, vocational, and social losses as a result of the disability, including loss of work, educational opportunity, friends, living situation, avocational pursuits, social status, community mobility, and the like. Context or environmental factors include potential barriers or facilitators in the physical and social environments. For example, ramps are a positive environmental factor for people with physical disability. Well-oriented and trained communication partners, on-the-job supports, and understanding work supervisors are examples of positive context factors for individuals with cognitive and communication disability.

Many of the changes in rehabilitation over the past two decades have been associated with an increasing emphasis on functional activities and participation (Level 2 of the WHO classification system) and context/environmental supports for social, educational, vocational, and avocational participation (Level 3), in contrast to the primary focus on the underlying impairment, as with traditional rehabilitation. Clearly, the relationships among the three levels are complex and relative to individuals and their contexts in life. For example,

the same underlying impairment can result in dramatically different types and degrees of activity and participation limitations in different individuals with varying activity and environmental demands, compensatory strategies, emotional adjustment, and social/educational/vocational supports. Furthermore, as we argue later in this chapter, intervention that begins with a focus on context supports, and then emerging into an activity/participation-oriented focus on compensatory strategies, can ultimately result in reduced impairment as the individual practices supported compensatory procedures until they become habitual and automatic aspects of information processing.

Measures of Injury and Disability Severity

Several rating scales have enjoyed increasing popularity as measures of initial severity of injury, ongoing improvement, and chronic disability. These scales are not intended for use in planning interventions with specific individuals; sensitive, individualized assessments are needed for that purpose. Furthermore, rating scales rarely are sufficient to measure the effectiveness of intervention in individual cases. For that purpose, no substitute exists for objective documentation of progress toward or achievement of individualized functional objectives directly related to important personal life goals.

General rating scales, however, have become part of the lingua franca of medical rehabilitation, are useful in capturing severity of injury and disability in general terms, and often are used in epidemiologic and program evaluation studies. Table 33–1 includes descriptions of commonly used scales. Many other functional scales have been developed, attesting to the shortcomings of impairment-oriented tests for measuring functional disability after TBI. These include the Patient Competency Rating Scale (Prigatano & Altman, 1990), Mayo-Portland Adaptability Inventory (Malec & Thompson, 1994), Neurobehavioral Functioning Inventory (Kreutzer, Marwitz, Seel, & Serio, 1996), Supervision Rating Scale (Boake, 1996), and BIRCO-39 Scales (Powell, Beckers, & Greenwood, 1998).

Prediction of Outcome

Many studies suggest a general "dose–response" relation between injury severity and long-term outcome (Katz & Alexander, 1994). Most studies correlating injury severity and outcome after TBI, however, use broad severity categories (e.g., four or five grades of severity, based on Glasgow Coma Scale score, duration of coma, or duration of post-traumatic amnesia, possibly combined with focal neurologic signs) and broad outcome categories (e.g., the five grades of outcome defined by the Glasgow Outcome Scale). Although useful for epidemiologic purposes, these studies must be interpreted cautiously by rehabilitation clinicians. First, correlation studies will always contain individuals who deviate

TABLE 33–1

Assessments Commonly Used to Measure Injury Severity and Associated Disability

Assessment Procedure	Description
Glasgow Coma Scale (GCS) (Teasdale & Jennett, 1974)	A three-category (eye opening, motor response, and verbal response), 15-point scale commonly used to measure the initial severity of TBI. Scores of 8 or lower within the first several hours after injury typically are classified as severe injuries, scores of 11 or 12 as moderate, and scores of 13–15 as mild.
Duration of Coma	Generally based on time from injury to eye opening and resumption of normal sleep–wake cycles. Measured in minutes or hours for mild to moderate injuries and in days, weeks, or months for severe injuries. Sometimes used more informally to refer to the period of significantly altered consciousness.
Duration of Post-Traumatic Amnesia	Based on time from injury to resumption of orientation and integration of day-to-day memories. Very hard to establish with precision in severe cases.
Galveston Orientation and Amnesia Test (GOAT) (Levin, O'Donnell, & Grossman, 1979)	A 10-question test of orientation to person, place, and time and of memory for recent, postinjury events as well as for most recent preinjury events.
Glasgow Outcome Scale (Jennett & Bond, 1975)	A five-category global outcome scale: death, persistent vegetative state, severe disability (conscious but disabled and dependent), moderate disability (disabled but independent), and good recovery (relatively normal life but possibly with ongoing minor impairment).
Rancho Los Amigos Levels of Cognitive Functioning (Hagen, 1981)	An eight-level scale of cognitive recovery based on observation of responsiveness, purposeful activity, orientation, memory, self-regulation, spontaneity, and independence. Levels: no response, generalized response, localized response, confused-agitated, confused-nonagitated, confused-appropriate, automatic-appropriate, and purposeful-appropriate.
Disability Rating Scale (Rappaport, Hall, Hopkins, Belleza, & Cope, 1982)	A rating scale developed to track improvement of people with TBI from coma to community. Includes subscales for impairment (similar to GCS), disability (cognitive ability for feeding, toileting, and grooming), and handicap (level of community functioning, and employability).
Functional Assessment Measure (FIM+FAM) (Hall, 1992)	A rating scale that adds 12 domains for disability rating to the 12 domains of the older Functional Independence Measure (FIM). The additional items, added specifically for individuals with brain injury, include swallowing, reading, writing, orientation, attention, safety judgment, emotional status, and adjustment to limitations.
Community Integration Questionnaire (Willer, Ottenbacher, & Coad, 1994)	A 15-item questionnaire designed to assess home and social integration and productivity in the following domains: household activities, shopping, errands, and leisure activities.
American Speech-Language-Hearing Association FACS	A rating scale designed to assess functional communication with greater precision than is possible with most general disability rating tools.
Communication Effectiveness Survey (Beukelman, 1998)	A survey designed to assess functional communication in natural contexts.
LaTrobe Communication Questionnaire (Douglas, O'Flaherty, & Snow, 2000)	A 30-item questionnaire divided into six communication domains: conversational tone, effectiveness, flow, engagement, partner sensitivity, and attention/focus. Self and "close other" forms are available.

Key: TBI = traumatic brain injury.

sharply from the general population relationships (Ponsford, Olver, Current, & Ng, 1995), and these exceptional individuals and their families often are those with whom clinicians interact in their everyday clinical practice. Second, within broad severity of injury and outcome categories is substantial individual variation, rendering specific predictions hazardous and leaving room for optimism regarding the potential effectiveness of intervention efforts. For example, two individuals in the good outcome category can be extremely different with respect to (a) their level of success measured in relation to preinjury success, (b) the effort required to maintain that level of functioning, (c) the level of supports they require and the associated caregiver burden, and (d) their subjective level of satisfaction and adjustment to life after the injury. Because of these sources of variability, intervention that fails to change a person's outcome category may, nevertheless, be very effective for the individual and caregivers alike.

Patterns and Stages of "Recovery"

In the heading, the word *recovery* is in quotation marks because it is a frequent source of miscommunication. In ordinary language, "to recover" is to return to normal. In contrast, rehabilitation professionals typically use the word to refer to gradual improvement, without intending to suggest that improvement will continue until a full recovery is achieved. Indeed, full recovery is rare following TBI with coma of a few days or more. Therefore, *improvement* may be a better choice of words to communicate what professionals often intend with *recovery* (Kay & Lezak, 1990).

Most individuals with severe TBI experience a large number of distinct stages or levels of cognitive and self-regulatory functioning over the course of their spontaneous neurologic improvement and rehabilitation. In many cases, improvement is characterized by a stairstep pattern rather than a smooth recovery curve, as commonly is observed following ischemic stroke (Brookshire, 1997). Furthermore, spontaneous neurologic improvement may continue for many months and, in some cases, even years (at decreasing rates of improvement) after severe TBI.

The popular Rancho Los Amigos Hospital Levels of Cognitive Functioning (see Table 33–1) organizes cognitive and behavioral recovery into eight relatively distinct levels. An understanding of typical levels of improvement helps treatment staff, family members, and individuals with TBI to place in perspective behaviors that would otherwise be distressing (e.g., agitation associated with Level IV) and to organize their rehabilitative efforts effectively. For purposes of discussing broadly different focuses of assessment and intervention—and, importantly, different levels and types of support provided to the patient by rehabilitation staff and families—we have collapsed the eight Rancho Los Amigos levels into three broadly distinct stages of recovery (Szekeres, Ylvisaker, & Holland, 1985) that also can be understood in

terms of the amount and types of support needed by the individual to function. Any discussion of stages, however, must be sensitive to the varied patterns and rates of improvement experienced by specific individuals and to the many small changes in functioning, required supports, and appropriate expectations that are more properly represented as a continuum rather than a series of qualitatively different stages.

Early Stage: Intensive Cognitive Supports

This stage begins with the first generalized responses to environmental stimuli and ends with stimulus-specific responses (e.g., visual tracking or localizing to sound), recognition of some common objects through appropriate use of the object (if motorically capable), and comprehension of some simple commands in context. From a cognitive perspective, this stage often is called the sensory or coma stimulation stage of rehabilitation, a controversial and hotly debated field of intervention. Zasler, Kreutzer, and Taylor (1991) presented a useful review of these themes and a conservative approach to coma management. From the perspective of performance of everyday activities (e.g., self-care), individuals at this stage require intensive levels of support.

Middle Stage: Moderate Cognitive Supports

This stage begins with heightened alertness and increased activity combined with some degree of confusion and disorientation, which may include agitated behavior unrelated to environmental provocation. This stage ends with a reduction in confusion, which is manifested by adequate orientation and behavior that generally is goal directed in a familiar environment. Most individuals experience gradual improvement in focused attention and episodic (autobiographical) memory, but memory impairment may remain a residual deficit. Behavior, including social communication, may continue to be impulsive; lack of initiation is an alternative possibility. Most individuals have difficulty with organizing complex tasks, including discourse tasks, and with planning how to achieve their goals.

During this stage, individuals require moderate, but systematically decreasing, levels of support to succeed at everyday tasks. The rehabilitation (or home) environment as well as group and individual therapy sessions are simplified, structured, focused, and rich in external compensatory supports so as to reduce confusion, facilitate improved and increasingly independent performance of functional activities (including relevant social, educational, and vocational activities), and promote adaptive behavior and a progressively increasing ability to process information and communicate effectively.

Late Stage: Minimal and Variable Cognitive Supports

This stage begins with an adequate, though perhaps superficial and fragile, orientation to important aspects of life, and it ends with the individual's ultimate level of neurologic improvement, which may or may not include cognitive and communicative impairments that are functionally disabling. Environmental supports are gradually withdrawn to help individuals become maximally independent and learn how to compensate for and adjust to their residual deficits. This stage also is the stage of refinement of skills, with a focus on effective information processing and social communication in real-world settings and with real-life demands (e.g., school, work, and social life). No specific upper limit exists to learning, compensation, and adjustment that can be facilitated by creative clinicians and, thereby, substantially improve real-world success.

Sequence of Service Settings

Severe TBI typically is associated with many service settings and sets of service providers. Emergency medical services routinely are administered at the site of the injury and during transport to a trauma center. Emergency room care largely is devoted to managing life-threatening increases in intracranial pressure as well as treating other injuries (e.g., orthopaedic injuries and internal organ injuries) that frequently accompany TBI. Following initial stabilization, patients are transferred to the intensive care unit for ongoing management of critical intracranial dynamics. Stabilization of intracranial pressure often is followed by transfer to the hospital's neurologic care floor and the beginning of early rehabilitation. Speech-language pathologists may be members of the early rehabilitation team, often focusing their efforts on resumption of oral feeding, development of simple communication systems, and family education and support.

In the event of slow recovery, patients may be transferred to a rehabilitation unit or free-standing rehabilitation hospital for intensive acute rehabilitation. When cognitive, behavioral, physical, and general medical needs reach a level at which the person can be cared for in a less restrictive setting, the individual is discharged to home—and, often, ongoing outpatient or community support services—or to a community reintegration post-acute rehabilitation facility. Individuals with ongoing intense medical needs (e.g., respirator-dependent patients) or severe and unchanging cognitive impairment (e.g., persistent unresponsiveness) may be discharged to a long-term care nursing facility, with the possibility of resuming aggressive rehabilitation if signs of neurologic improvement are noted.

Individuals with concussion (i.e., traumatically induced alteration in mental status not necessarily resulting in loss of consciousness) or mild TBI (i.e., brief loss of consciousness or initial Glasgow Coma Scale score of 13–15) may be examined in a physician's office, observed in a hospital emergency room, admitted briefly, or not come to the attention of medical professionals at all. In most cases (approximately 80%–90%), mild TBI is associated with excellent recovery within a few days to a few weeks (Ruff, 2005). Persistent, serious disability is possible, however, requiring professional support and possible work or school accommodations. Individuals with a history of previous concussion or other neurologic vulnerability (e.g., learning disabilities or neurologic impairment associated with aging) are at increased risk for persistent symptoms (Collins et al., 1999; Gronwall & Wrightson, 1975; Rimel, Giordani, Barth, Boll, & Jane, 1981).

Long-Term Communication-Related Outcome

Earlier, we stated that the relation between injury severity and outcome is, at best, very general. Many factors interact to determine a person's ultimate level of impairment; ability to perform activities of daily living; ability to maintain desired levels of participation in social, educational, vocational, and avocational pursuits; level of personal satisfaction with life after the injury; and level of support required from everyday people in the environment. In addition to the injury itself, these factors include preinjury and postinjury variables summarized in Figures 33–6 and 33–7.

Given preinjury variability (Fig. 33–6) and the variety of pathophysiologic mechanisms in TBI (Figs. 33–1 and 33–2), some of which are related to site of impact, it is understandable that no consistent outcome profiles exist with respect to communication. Constellations of communication-related strengths and weaknesses potentially associated with TBI are extremely varied, depending on the nature, location, and severity of the injury as well as on the characteristics of the individual who is injured and post-trauma supports. Indeed, many professionals consider TBI to be, at best, misleading as a disability category, because it actually is an etiologic category, identifying a potential cause of varied disabilities and not the disability itself. In this respect, TBI is comparable to stroke or perinatal asphyxia, neurologic events that may or may not produce varied disabilities. Therefore, clinicians should expect not only great diversity within this group but also possible overlap between TBI and other categories of adult neurogenic communication disorder, such as aphasia, dementia, and the so-called right hemisphere syndrome.

As indicated in Figures 33–6 and 33–7, heterogeneity within the population is increased by diversity in pretraumatic intelligence, educational and vocational levels, age, personality, and coping styles as well as by variation in post-traumatic environments, support systems, and emotional and behavioral reactions of the individual. Despite many commonalities among survivors of severe TBI (described below), these considerations underscore the importance of customizing assessment procedures as well as intervention goals and methods for this diverse clinical population.

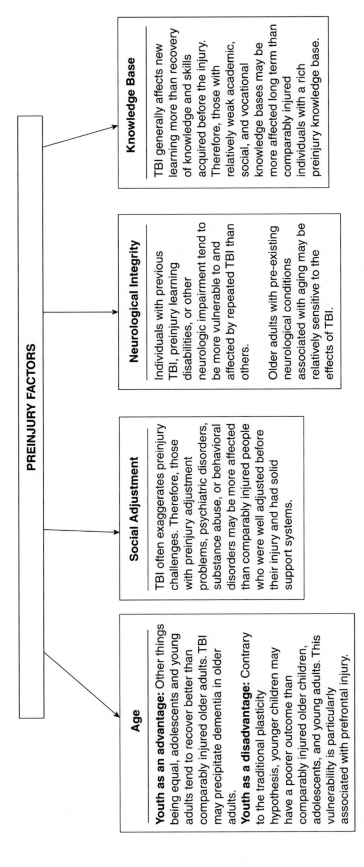

PREINJURY FACTORS

Age

Youth as an advantage: Other things being equal, adolescents and young adults tend to recover better than comparably injured older adults. TBI may precipitate dementia in older adults.

Youth as a disadvantage: Contrary to the traditional plasticity hypothesis, younger children may have a poorer outcome than comparably injured older children, adolescents, and young adults. This vulnerability is particularly associated with prefrontal injury.

Social Adjustment

TBI often exaggerates preinjury challenges. Therefore, those with preinjury adjustment problems, psychiatric disorders, substance abuse, or behavioral disorders may be more affected than comparably injured people who were well adjusted before their injury and had solid support systems.

Neurological Integrity

Individuals with previous TBI, preinjury learning disabilities, or other neurologic impairment tend to be more vulnerable to and affected by repeated TBI than others.

Older adults with pre-existing neurological conditions associated with aging may be relatively sensitive to the effects of TBI.

Knowledge Base

TBI generally affects new learning more than recovery of knowledge and skills acquired before the injury. Therefore, those with relatively weak academic, social, and vocational knowledge bases may be more affected long term than comparably injured individuals with a rich preinjury knowledge base.

Figure 33–6. Factors that often are present before traumatic brain injury and that may contribute to outcome.

889

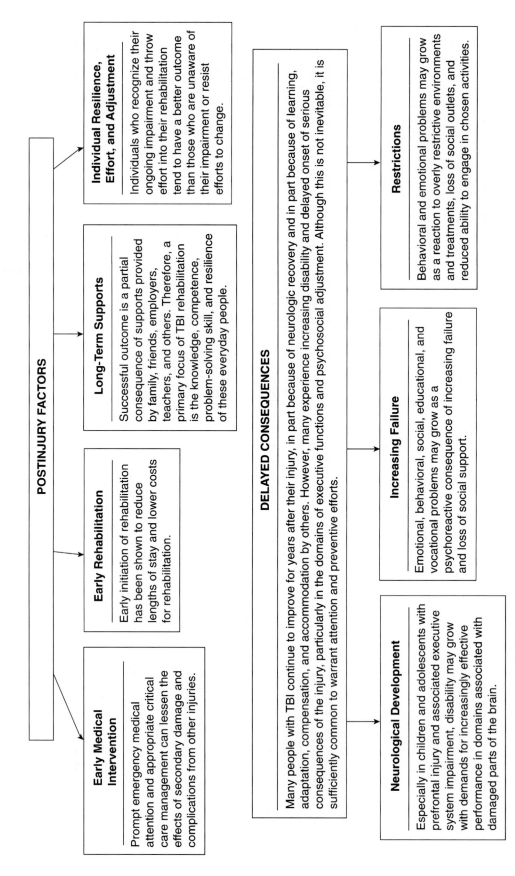

POSTINJURY FACTORS

Early Medical Intervention

Prompt emergency medical attention and appropriate critical care management can lessen the effects of secondary damage and complications from other injuries.

Early Rehabilitation

Early initiation of rehabilitation has been shown to reduce lengths of stay and lower costs for rehabilitation.

Long-Term Supports

Successful outcome is a partial consequence of supports provided by family, friends, employers, teachers, and others. Therefore, a primary focus of TBI rehabilitation is the knowledge, competence, problem-solving skill, and resilience of these everyday people.

Individual Resilience, Effort, and Adjustment

Individuals who recognize their ongoing impairment and throw effort into their rehabilitation tend to have a better outcome than those who are unaware of their impairment or resist efforts to change.

DELAYED CONSEQUENCES

Many people with TBI continue to improve for years after their injury, in part because of neurologic recovery and in part because of learning, adaptation, compensation, and accommodation by others. However, many experience increasing disability and delayed onset of serious consequences of the injury, particularly in the domains of executive functions and psychosocial adjustment. Although this is not inevitable, it is sufficiently common to warrant attention and preventive efforts.

Neurological Development

Especially in children and adolescents with prefrontal injury and associated executive system impairment, disability may grow with demands for increasingly effective performance in domains associated with damaged parts of the brain.

Increasing Failure

Emotional, behavioral, social, educational, and vocational problems may grow as a psychoreactive consequence of increasing failure and loss of social support.

Restrictions

Behavioral and emotional problems may grow as a reaction to overly restrictive environments and treatments, loss of social outlets, and reduced ability to engage in chosen activities.

Figure 33–7. Factors that occur after traumatic brain injury and that contribute to outcome.

Infrequency of Aphasia

Although symptoms of aphasia often are present early in recovery and, in some cases, specific language impairment does persist, aphasia, as defined in terms of the classical syndromes, is relatively uncommon after TBI in adults (Heilman, Safran, & Geschwind, 1971; Sarno, 1980, 1984; Sarno, Buonaguro, & Levita, 1986) and children (Chapman, 1997; Ylvisaker, 1993). Anomia, which can be associated with a wide variety of brain lesions, often is reported to be the primary residual aphasic symptom in the absence of general cognitive disruption (Heilman et al., 1971; Levin, Grossman, Sarwar, & Meyers, 1981; Sarno, 1980, 1984; Thomsen, 1975). Generalized and persistent expressive and receptive language impairment usually is associated with widespread diffuse injury that also produces global cognitive deficits (Levin et al., 1981). If aphasia is present, clinicians should apply the assessment and intervention frameworks presented elsewhere in this text.

Non-Aphasic Communication Disorders: Executive Functions, Cognition, Behavior, and Communication

Communication challenges following TBI most often are "non-aphasic" in nature; that is, they co-exist with intelligible speech, reasonably fluent and grammatical expressive language, and comprehension adequate to support everyday interaction. Depending on the severity of injury, stage of recovery, and particular focus of research, the characteristic communication profiles following TBI have been variously referred to as "the language of confusion" (early in recovery) (Halpern, Darley, & Brown, 1973), "non-aphasic language disturbances" (Prigatano, 1986; Prigatano, Roueche, & Fordyce, 1985), "cognitive-language disturbances" (Hagen, 1981), and "subclinical aphasia" (Sarno, 1980, 1984). Sarno (1984) found that, although a distinct minority of a consecutive series of 69 severely injured individuals admitted to an inpatient rehabilitation facility could be diagnosed with aphasia, all of the patients were found to have some combination of language deficits that were not apparent in everyday interaction. These included impaired confrontation naming, word fluency, and comprehension of complex oral commands. Sarno did not evaluate their interactive competence with increasing cognitive and social demands, social competence, or behavioral self-regulation—factors that clinicians, teachers, family members, and recent investigators often identify as major contributors to communication breakdowns after TBI.

The overlapping collections of communication deficits highlighted by these investigators have been grouped by the American Speech-Language-Hearing Association (ASHA) under the heading "cognitive-communication impairment" (ASHA, 1988) and are all associated with frontolimbic damage, the most common damage in CHI. These impairments are included in Table 33–2, which also includes lists of impairments under three additional headings: executive system, cognitive, and psychosocial/behavioral impairments. In important respects, these four lists are descriptions of the consequences of the same underlying impairments, using four distinct professional frameworks. The extent of overlap in deficit domains underscores the importance of professionals from different clinical fields collaborating in their approach to assessment and intervention.

Communication Disorders Associated with Executive Function/Self-Regulatory Impairment

The same executive function/self-regulatory (EF/SR) skills underlie emotional/social/behavioral self-regulation (e.g., controlling affective states, inhibiting impulses, deferring gratification, communicating respectfully, and benefitting from feedback) (Vohs & Ciarocco, 2004) and cognitive-vocational-academic self-regulation (e.g., planning a work task, reading strategically, studying efficiently, and taking responsibility for vocational and academic success) (Meichenbaum & Biemiller, 1998) and, thus, should be viewed within one consistent intervention framework (Ylvisaker, Jacobs, & Feeney, 2003). Consistent with our previous work on the subject, we have chosen a functional definition of the construct, based on an analysis of prerequisites for successful performance of any difficult task (Ylvisaker & Feeney, 1998a; Ylvisaker, Szekeres, & Haarbauer-Krupa, 1998). These include: (1) some degree of awareness of ones strengths and weaknesses (thereby enabling a judgment of task difficulty) and (2) an ability to set reasonable goals, (3) organize plans to achieve the goals, (3) initiate goal-directed behavior, (4) inhibit impulses that interfere with goal achievement, (5) monitor behavior and (6) evaluate it in relation to the goals, (7) benefit from feedback, (8) flexibly select and modify strategies in response to performance feedback, and (9) flexibly perceive situations from a variety of possible perspectives. Each of these components falls on a continuum of performance and develops gradually during childhood, in dynamic interaction both with each other and with related domains of cognitive and social development (Flavell, Miller, & Miller, 2002). Because the term "self-regulation" is better understood by those who are unfamiliar with neuropsychological discussions of the topic, and because that term brings to the table a large literature in related fields of psychology, we have chosen to combine the terms to form the general construct, EF/SR.

The growing literature on self-regulation has close theoretic ties with psychological theory construction regarding the self and clinical ties with fields such as substance abuse, eating disorders, health problems, crime, motivation, procrastination, and the like (Baumeister & Vohs, 2004). Self-regulation and self-determination also have come to be used as the central terms within theory construction and research related to intrinsic motivation (Ryan & Deci, 2002). The literature on executive functions has close theoretic ties with neuropsychological investigations and clinical ties with

TABLE 33–2

Vulnerable Frontolimbic Structures and Frequently Associated Impairments

Frontolimbic Injury and Executive System Impairment
- Reduced awareness of personal strengths and weaknesses
- Difficulty setting realistic goals
- Difficulty planning and organizing behavior to achieve the goals
- Impaired ability to initiate action needed to achieve the goals
- Difficulty inhibiting behavior incompatible with achieving the goals
- Difficulty self-monitoring and self-evaluating
- Difficulty thinking and acting strategically and solving real-world problems in a flexible and efficient manner
- General inflexibility and concreteness in thinking, talking, and acting

Frontolimbic Injury and Cognitive-Communication Impairment
- Disorganized, poorly controlled discourse or paucity of discourse (spoken and written)
- Inefficient comprehension of language related to increasing amounts of information to be processed (spoken or written) and to rate of speech imprecise language and word retrieval problems
- Difficulty understanding and expressing abstract and indirect language
- Difficulty reading social cues, interpreting speaker intent, and flexibly adjusting interactive styles to meet situational demands in varied social contexts
- Awkward or inappropriate communication in stressful social contexts
- Impaired verbal learning

Frontolimbic Injury and Cognitive Impairment
- Reduced internal control over all cognitive functions (e.g., attentional, perceptual, memory, organizational, and reasoning processes)
- Impaired working memory
- Impaired declarative and explicit memory (encoding and retrieval)
- Disorganized behavior related to impaired organizing schemes (managerial knowledge frames, such as scripts, themes, schemas, and mental models)
- Impaired reasoning
- Concrete thinking
- Difficulty generalizing

Frontolimbic Injury and Psychosocial/Behavioral Impairment
- Disinhibited, socially inappropriate, and possibly aggressive behavior
- Impaired initiation or paucity of behavior
- Inefficient learning from consequences
- Perseverative behavior
- Impaired social perception and interpretation

Adapted from Ylvisaker, Feeney, & Feeney, 1999; with permission.

rehabilitation for individuals who have frank neurologic impairment (Burgess & Robertson, 2002; Cicerone, 2005; Shallice & Burgess, 1991; Ylvisaker, Szekeres, & Feeney, 1998). In educational psychology and special education, the term "meta-cognition" has, historically, been used to refer to "executive self-regulatory" control over cognitive processes in the context of learning and academic performance (Flavell, Miller, & Miller, 2002); today, however, "self-determined learning" is increasingly used to describe these approaches (Martin et al., 2003; Meichenbaum & Beimiller, 1998). Finally, the term "self-determination" commonly is used to

cover much the same ground in discussions of developmental disabilities (Wehmeyer, Agran, & Hughes, 1998). We have attempted to mine all these fields in formulating a theoretically informed but practice-based approach to serving children and adolescents with EF/SR impairment.

Pathophysiological Bases: Frontolimbic Injury

It has long been known that prefrontal or frontolimbic structures are most vulnerable in CHI (Adams, Graham, Scott, Parker, & Doyle, 1980; Levin, Goldstein, Williams, &

Eisenberg, 1991; Mendelsohn et al., 1992; Mesulam, 2002; Povlishock & Katz, 2005; Varney & Menefee, 1993). Although it certainly is possible to escape frontolimbic injury in TBI, its frequency and profound impact on communicative effectiveness combine to give it—and its general neurobehavioral correlate, EF/SR dysfunction—an important heuristic role in organizing intervention planning (Ylvisaker, 1992). In recent years, investigators have increasingly differentiated varied frontal and limbic functions and have loosened, to some degree, the connection between frontal lobe functions and executive functions (Stuss, 1999a, 1999b). The most common communication-related themes after TBI, however, continue to be associated with frontolimbic injury.

Indeed, all the symptoms listed in Table 33–2 are associated with damage to the frontal lobes, limbic structures, and/or the critical axonal connections between prefrontal and limbic structures (Alexander, Benson, & Stuss, 1989; Povlishock & Katz, 2005; Stuss & Benson, 1986). For example, both right and left hemisphere prefrontal structures are associated with self-regulation (e.g., initiation, inhibition, and direction) of behavior, including communication behavior; with organization of language into coherent discourse; and with control over attentional and memory processes to make them useful in daily life. Both left and right hemisphere orbital frontal damage have been associated with personality changes, including disinhibition, volatility, and verbal "dysdecorum" (Alexander et al., 1989). Right frontal lobe damage has been associated with more specific pragmatic deficits, such as (1) decreased ability to produce appropriate para-linguistic accompaniments to speech, including gesture and facial expression as well as prosody in speech; (2) decreased ability to comprehend prosodic features in the speech of others and to interpret indirect pragmatic intents, including humor, sarcasm, metaphor, and other indirect meanings (McDonald, 2005); and (3) inattention to context, including social context, resulting in socially inappropriate behavior (Alexander et al., 1989; Shammi & Stuss, 1999; Stuss & Alexander, 1999).

Damage to the hippocampus and surrounding limbic tissue is associated with impaired declarative and explicit memory—roughly, memory for facts rather than procedures, combined with a subjective sense that one possesses the memory (Schacter, 1996; Squire, 1992). Because of the extreme vulnerability of the hippocampus to postinjury anoxia, new learning problems are very common after TBI, despite potentially good recovery of pretraumatically acquired and effectively stored knowledge and skills. Damage to other limbic structures and frontolimbic connections contribute to the transient or persistent difficulty with emotional and behavioral self-regulation commonly seen after TBI (Izard, 1992; Ledoux, 1991, 1996).

Discourse Impairment

Discourse impairment (i.e., difficulty organizing language over more than one utterance for production or comprehen-sion) probably has received more attention than other communication-related deficits in the recent TBI research literature (Coehlo et al., 2005). Both adults and children with TBI have been found to be impaired relative to controls on many measures of interactive (conversational) and noninteractive (monologic) discourse (Biddle, McCabe, & Bliss, 1996; Chapman, 1997; Chapman, Levin, Matejka, Harward, & Kufera, 1995; Chapmen et al., 1992, 1997; Coelho, Liles, & Duffy, 1991; Dennis, 1991, 1992; Dennis & Barnes, 1990; Dennis, Barnes, Donnelly, Wilkinson, & Humphreys, 1996; Dennis & Lovett, 1990; Ehrlich, 1988; Groher, 1990; Hagen, 1981; Hartley, 1995; Hartley & Jenson, 1991; Liles, Coelho, Duffy, & Zalagens, 1989; McDonald, 1992a, 1992b; 1993; McDonald & Pearce, 1998; Mentis & Prutting, 1991; Pearce, McDonald, & Coltheart, 1998; Sarno et al., 1986; Togher, Hand, & Code, 1997; Turkstra & Holland, 1998; Ylvisaker, 1992, 1993).

Discourse impairment in the presence of adequate vocabulary, grammar, and motor speech ability often can be understood as a language consequence of more general cognitive disruption—that is, the loss or inaccessibility of the knowledge structures needed to organize thought units across multiple utterances (sometimes referred to as ideational apraxia). Alternatively, discourse impairment may be a consequence of failure to select and implement the appropriate organizing schemas when they are needed (sometimes referred to as frontal apraxia), or to maintain directed attention to the organizing scheme in a conversation or monolog, and monitor success of the communication. The latter phenomenon sometimes is referred to as impairment of the supervisory attentional system, which is the component of the executive system responsible for controlling behavior-regulating schemas in nonroutine contexts (Shallice, 1982). In most cases, discourse impairment after TBI represents a failure of executive control over cognitive and linguistic organizing processes rather than a linguistic impairment per se (Schwartz, 1995; Schwartz, Mayer, FitzpatrickDeSalme, & Montgomery, 1993). Alexander (2002) refers to the disorder as impaired action planning in the verbal domain.

In the intervention section of this chapter, we focus on organizational functioning in part because of its important relation to these common discourse impairments. According to many cognitive theories, the same cognitive macrostructures or managerial knowledge units (e.g., scripts, themes, schemas, plans, and mental models) that guide organized thinking, remembering, reasoning, and acting also guide organized talking, writing, and comprehension of lengthy discourse. According to one leading neuropsychological theory, such managerial knowledge units are stored in prefrontal parts of the cortex, explaining the frequency of organizational impairment in TBI (Grafman, 1995; Grafman, Sirigu, Sepctor, & Hendler, 1993), particularly with left hemisphere dorsolateral prefrontal involvement. Thus, discourse is one of the critical points of intersection between language and cognition, mandating an informed cognitive focus during intervention and collaboration among professionals who address the cognitive dimensions of behavior.

Communication Disability Related to Memory/Retrieval Impairment

Memory deficits are among the most commonly reported problems after TBI. Encoding of new information into memory often is impaired, either as a result of damage to the vulnerable hippocampal system responsible for consolidating new declarative memories (Giap, Jong, Ricker, Cullen, & Zafonte, 2000) or of damage to the frontal lobes (especially left hemisphere), resulting in poorly focused attention and/or shallow, nonstrategic organization and elaboration of information during its initial processing (Anderson, Damasio, Tranel, & Damasio, 1988; Brazzeli, Colombo, DellaSala, & Spinnler, 1994; Cabeza & Nyberg, 1997; Gluck & Myers, 1995; Schacter, 1996; Squire, Knowlton, & Musen, 1993). Encoding new memories for facts and events (declarative memory) often is more severely impaired than encoding for procedures (procedural memory); similarly, memories stored with some awareness of the memory (explicit memory) often are more vulnerable than those stored without such awareness (implicit memory) (Ewert, Levin, Watson, & Kalisky, 1989; Schacter, 1996). Procedural and implicit memory often are run together in the TBI literature but, in fact, are neuropsychologically distinct (Salmon & Butters, 1995). Storage over time is less commonly impaired in TBI; once information is adequately processed and encoded, it is unlikely to decay rapidly, as is the case in degenerative diseases, such as Alzheimer's.

Retrieval may be impaired in TBI as a result of posterior damage that reduces the number of retrieval routes in the networks of neural connections that compose the storage system (Buschke & Fuld, 1974). More commonly, however, word and information retrieval is impaired as a result of frontal lobe injury, which can result in nonstrategic searches of memory (Petrides, 1995; Schacter, 1996; Shimamura, 2002) and degraded managerial knowledge units being used to direct those searches (Grafman, 1995, 2002). For example, when looking for car keys, people characteristically focus their search around organized routines of everyday life. Similar organizational schemas are used to guide internal searches of memory, which therefore are rendered ineffective in the presence of degraded schemas. Recent positron-emission tomographic investigations of explicit retrieval of information have isolated important contributions of left lateral prefrontal cortex, right anterior frontopolar cortex, and anterior cingulate gyrus (Buckner et al., 1995; Shimamura, 2002). Retrieval of episodic memories is differentially impaired by right frontal lobe damage, even if encoding of that same information may have made greater use of left frontal lobe systems (Schacter, 1996; Tulving,

Kapur, Craik, Moscovitch, & Houle, 1994). Meta-cognitive skills, particularly the ability to monitor memory searches, are required for effective retrieval and are an aspect of executive functioning that often is impaired in TBI (Hanton, Bartha, & Levin, 2000; Kennedy & Yorkston, 2000).

These memory problems affect communication in a variety of ways. Inefficient information and word retrieval slows interaction and can be socially distracting. Failure to recall information can result in tedious repetition during conversation and embarrassing social breakdowns. Impaired verbal learning has an obvious negative impact on return to school or to a job that requires new learning, possibly resulting in failure that may lead to social withdrawal. Impaired prospective memory without effective compensation creates substantial everyday difficulties as the individual misses appointments or other scheduled activities, forgets medication, and the like.

Communication Disability Associated with Psychosocial and Behavioral Impairment

Any combination of the deficits listed in Table 33–2 can substantially affect life after TBI. Often, however, it is the communication-related personality and psychosocial changes that most profoundly influence the individual's social, vocational, familial, and academic reintegration. For example, families routinely report that it is easier to adjust to physical disability in a loved one than to personality changes manifested in stressful and unsatisfying communication; employers often highlight communication-related obstacles to maintenance of employment; and teachers frequently identify social and behavioral changes as most problematic in school reentry (Bond, 1990; Brooks, Campsie, Symington, Beattie, Bryden, & McKinley, 1987; Brooks & McKinlay, 1983; Brooks, McKinlay, Symington, Beattie, & Campsie, 1987; Brown, Chadwick, Shaffer, Rutter, & Traub, 1981; Filley, Cranberg, Alexander, & Hart, 1987; Fletcher, Levin, & Butler, 1995; Hall et al., 1994; Jacobs, 1993; Klonoff, Costa, & Snow, 1986; Lezak, 1986; 1987; Livingston & Brooks, 1988; McKinlay, Brooks, Bond, Martinage, & Marshall, 1981; Morton & Wehman, 1995; Perlesz, Kinsella, & Crowe, 2000; Prigatano, 1986; Taylor et al., 2002; Thomsen, 1974, 1984, 1987; Weddell, Oddy, & Jenkins, 1980; Ylvisaker et al., 2001). Social communication and general psychosocial problems were found to be critical predictors of vocational failure and poor quality of adult life in two groups of young adults who were injured as children and followed into adulthood (Cattelani, Lombardi, Brianti, & Mazzuchi, 1998; Nybo & Koskiniemi, 1999).

These social communication problems are common in both children and adults with TBI, and they often are associated with personality changes, including increases in negative behavior and awkward or impulsive social communication (see the review by Ylvisaker, Jacobs, & Feeney, 2003). Among children and adolescents with severe TBI, estimates of new persisting behavior and psychosocial problems (i.e., those not predating the injury) range from approximately 35% (Max et al., 1997) to a high of 70% (Costeff, Grosswasser, Landmen, & Brenner, 1985). Behavior and social-communication problems also are common among adults with TBI and remain at high levels at long-term follow-up (Baguley, Cooper, & Felmingham, 2006). Preexisting behavior and social interaction problems, which are common among both children (Cattelani et al., 1998) and adults (MacMillan, Hart, Martelli, & Zasler, 2002), add to this already alarming total. The intensity of behavior and psychosocial disorders has been associated in some studies with the severity of injury (Schwartz et al., 2003) and with preinjury problems (MacMillan et al., 2002).

Personality changes frequently highlighted in the TBI literature include irritability, impatience, frequent loss of temper, emotional volatility, egocentrism, impulsiveness, anxiety, depression, loss of social contact, lack of interests, and reduced initiation. Blumer and Benson (1975) summarized the inhibition-related and initiation-related personality changes associated with frontal lobe injury with the labels pseudo-psychopathic and pseudo-depressed personalities, respectively. Mesalum (2002) used the terms "frontal disinhibition syndrome" and "frontal abulic syndrome" to cover much the same territory. For communication specialists, these psychosocial and behavioral themes typically are grouped under the heading "pragmatics of language."

Aggressive, poorly controlled, or otherwise awkward social behavior has been linked to disruption in a variety of frontal lobe or frontolimbic circuits, which often are injured in TBI (Scheibel & Levin, 1997), but most often to orbitofrontal damage and/or connections between these areas and limbic structures (e.g., the amygdala). Furthermore, damage to prefrontal areas, in association with the amygdala, insula, anterior cingulate gyrus, and basal ganglia (right hemisphere more than left), results in difficulty interpreting the emotional states of others and in "reading" the non-literal aspects of their communication (McDonald, 2005). Difficulty with interpreting sarcasm (and, possibly, other non-literal meanings) and with recognizing vocal expressions of emotions is common in TBI and has a negative impact on social communication (Channon, Pellijeff, & Rule, 2005; Milders, Fuchs, & Crawford, 2003). Brothers (1997) used the term "damaged social editor" to characterize the functional consequences of damage to a circuit that includes the orbitofrontal cortex, amygdala, anterior cingulate gyrus, and temporal poles; the individual has difficulty "editing" social behavior because of impairment in the ability to read social situations and interpret the emotional states of others (i.e., impaired "theory of mind"). Commonly occurring cognitive and executive function impairments (in the domains of attention, memory, organization, planning,

flexible problem solving, self-awareness, and the like) can further reduce social effectiveness directly and also indirectly by contributing to failure and frustration.

Variability in Performance

Teachers, family members, work supervisors, and others often emphasize a frustrating inconsistency in performance when describing people with TBI. An uncharitable but common interpretation of this variability is that the person is unmotivated (i.e., lazy) or excessively moody, perhaps even depressed. Although these characteristics may be present, neuropsychological investigations have found relatively extreme variability in performance to be associated with frontal lobe injury, particularly injury to the right frontal lobes (Stuss, 1999b; Stuss, Pogue, Buckle, & Bondar, 1994). Variability is increased with increasing task demands and with aging. This inconsistency in performance is one of several reasons for caution when interpreting the results of standardized tests with this population (see below).

FRAMEWORK FOR COGNITIVE AND PSYCHOSOCIAL REHABILITATION

Our goal in this section is to explain and offer a rationale for an approach to intervention that deviates in important ways from traditional approaches to medical rehabilitation for individuals with severe TBI. In addition, we offer operational definitions of cognition and executive functions, two of the primary targets of intervention for individuals with TBI. Later in this chapter, we offer procedural detail in four overlapping domains: (1) executive functions/self-regulation, (2) specific aspects of cognition, (3) social communication, and (4) behavioral self-regulation.

Appendix 33-2 contrasts central tendencies in two generally different approaches to communication, behavioral, and cognitive rehabilitation for people with TBI. We have labeled these approaches conventional and functional, with the caveat that any approach to rehabilitation that is successful as measured by real-world indices is functional. Therefore, the appropriateness of these labels depends, in part, on relatively disappointing results of TBI efficacy research conducted within the traditional or conventional paradigm (Carney et al., 1999; Cicerone et al., 2005; Park & Ingles, 2001; Ylvisaker, 2003) and on the accumulation of supporting research conducted within the functional paradigm (Feeney et al., 2001; Park & Ingles, 2001). What we refer to as the conventional approach has a long history in medical speech-language pathology (and other fields), featuring restorative services offered in clinical settings and dominated by massed practice of hierarchically organized, decontextualized training exercises. In this section, we explain the general approach referred to as "functional" in Appendix 33-2.

Positive, Everyday Routine-Based Intervention

Central to the functional approach outlined in Appendix 33–2 is the concept of positive, supported, everyday routines of action and interaction. From a behavioral perspective, a "routine" is a behavior chain in which each link—that is, each discrete behavior—is a discriminative stimulus for the next link and a conditioned reinforcer for the previous link (Halle & Spradlin, 1993). The goal of intervention, from this perspective, is to help people acquire flexible and situationally successful behavior chains (defined by stimulus and response classes) that include observable as well as internal (cognitive and emotional) behaviors as links in the chains—that is, successful routines of everyday life.

From a cognitive perspective, a routine is a concrete structured event complex (Grafman et al., 1993), which, at a more general level, becomes a script, which is an organized internal (mental) representation of a type of event complex that includes the people, places, associated objects, associated language, and their organization. Everyday routines and scripts are those that occur during the course of everyday social, familial, vocational, recreational, and educational life and involve everyday communication partners (ECPs), including family members, friends, work supervisors, and teachers. The organized knowledge that enables one to be oriented and behave successfully in a variety of restaurants, from McDonald's to fine restaurants, is an example of a fairly general script. From a cognitive perspective, a primary goal of rehabilitation is to help people with TBI acquire and apply appropriate scripts and other general knowledge structures (or Managerial Knowledge Units) (Grafman et al., 1993) to guide successful thinking, remembering, problem solving, decision making, talking, and acting in social context.

We highlight the word "routine" for several reasons. First, routine suggests habit—that is, behavior that does not require effortful deliberation or planning. With frontal lobe injury and associated executive function impairment, habitual behavior often is relatively unaffected, whereas behavior that requires a novel plan for unfamiliar circumstances may be severely impaired (Mesulam, 2002; Stuss & Benson, 1986). Later in this chapter, we suggest that executive functions themselves, including planning, organizing, and problem solving, can become routine with extensive coached practice of executive function routines within everyday action contexts. Second, routine suggests normal activities of life, motivating clinicians to move beyond commercial therapeutic materials, generic therapeutic activities, and exclusively clinical intervention settings and, instead, capitalizing on the activities that are routine for the individual and using ECPs as collaborators in intervention. Countless studies of generalization and maintenance of learned behaviors with many disability groups support the conclusion that adequate performance of targeted skills in a treatment setting—even after mastery of the skill using personally meaningful activities—is no guarantee for ongoing use of the skill in the routines of everyday life (Detterman & Sternberg, 1993).

Supports (Scaffolding)

Within an everyday, routine-based approach to intervention, the technical term "support" designates a pivotal concept, connected with a Vygotskyan approach to cognitive and behavioral intervention (discussed later). To say that routines of action or interaction are positive and supported is to say that people with disability are provided with the supports or "scaffolding" (Wood, Bruner, & Ross, 1976) that they need to be successful. Table 33–3 lists examples of supports commonly used to facilitate success with cognitively demanding tasks ("supported cognition") (Ylvisaker & Feeney, 1996) and with behaviorally stressful tasks ("supported behavioral self-regulation") (Ylvisaker, Jacobs & Feeney, 2003). In both cases, supports can be understood using the more familiar model of supported employment, wherein workers with disability are enabled to perform otherwise difficult work tasks because they have the help of a job coach or designated peer, use customized equipment and strategies to compensate for their disability, and/or rely on other environmental supports. Supported employment has enjoyed considerable success among adults with TBI (Curl, Fraser, Cook, & Clemmens, 1996; Wehman, West, Kregel, Sherron, & Kreutzer, 1995; Wehmen et al., 1993) and is one of the few areas of TBI rehabilitation found by a government-sponsored, systematic evidence review to have a solid research base (National Institutes of Health, 1999).

Progression of Intervention

Table 33–4 outlines a progression of intervention that is consistent with a context-sensitive, everyday, routine-based approach to cognitive, psychosocial, and communication rehabilitation. First, staff and everyday people (ideally including the person with disability) collaborate to identify what is and is not working in the everyday routines of life.

Second, the same group of collaborators identifies what changes in everyday routines (including context supports) could quickly produce increases in domains of activity and participation and, in the longer run, in reduction of disability (i.e., improved performance of functional activities) and, ultimately, in reduction of the underlying impairment. Systematic hypothesis testing (described in the next section) often is required to identify the source of the manifest problem and, therefore, to identify the most useful and positive changes in everyday routines.

Third, the same stakeholders collaborate to identify the supports needed for positive changes in everyday routines and ways to motivate these changes for the person with disability and for others in the environment. Often, this stage

TABLE 33–3

Antecedent Procedures for Supporting Individuals with Cognitive and Behavioral Impairment

Supported Cognition
1. Ensure do-ability of tasks; eliminate unreasonable demands.
2. Create facilitative work/study environment.
3. Ensure orientation to setting and tasks; use clear, facilitative instructions.
4. Induce positive internal setting events (see section on behavioral intervention) before cognitively demanding tasks:
    • Positive behavioral momentum (see section on behavioral intervention).
    • Choice and control.
    • Rest, relaxation, absence of pain.
5. Establish well-rehearsed routines and scripts.
6. Use advance organizers (e.g., organizationally clear graphic organizers) for complex tasks.
7. Use appropriate cognitive prosthetics as needed (e.g., memory aids, electronic pager/reminder systems, organization aids, and attention aids).
8. Use collaboration to complete difficult tasks (e.g., cooperative work/learning groups; buddy system).
9. Ensure that communication partners use elaborative and collaborative conversational competencies (see later in this chapter).
10. Ensure that communication partners use supportive cognitive scripts (see later in this chapter).
11. Desensitize the individual to events and tasks that cause anxiety.
12. Help the individual to manage cognitive antecedents.

Supported Behavioral Self-Regulation
1. Eliminate unreasonable provocation, including unreasonable demands.
2. Ensure orientation to setting and task.
3. Ensure do-ability of tasks.
4. Induce positive internal setting events before stressful tasks:
    • Positive behavioral momentum.
    • Choice and control.
    • Rest, relaxation, absence of pain.
5. Teach positive communication alternatives to negative behavior.
6. Establish alternative scripts to negative behavior (e.g., give the individual a positive role that requires responsible behavior).
7. Ensure that the individual has positive, meaningful roles to play and goals to achieve.
8. Desensitize the individual to events that cause anxiety.
9. Help the individual to manage behavioral antecedents (e.g., avoid overly stressful tasks, create scripts for potentially negative interactions, and alert friends and supervisors to how they might help during a stressful experience).

Adapted from Ylvisaker and Feeney, 1998a; with permission.

requires considerable creativity and flexibility. No rehabilitation textbook can prescribe the unique combinations of supports that often are needed in people's real-world contexts or can show how these changes in everyday routine can be motivating for everyone involved.

Fourth, systems of support are implemented so that everyday routines of action and interaction are successful and that important skills, possibly including compensatory skills, can be practiced extensively in real-world contexts.

Finally, levels of support are systematically reduced as the individual becomes more successful at everyday tasks and/or habituates the use of compensatory procedures; at the same time, contexts of successful action and interaction are systematically increased. Later in this section, we illustrate how the process of modification and reduction of supports applies across the continuum of recovery after severe TBI.

This context-sensitive, everyday, routine-based approach to rehabilitation reverses the traditional "first impairment, then disability (functional activities), then handicap (participation), finally context" hierarchy in rehabilitation. Table 33–5 outlines this reversal. Within traditional rehabilitation, the initial goal generally has been to eliminate or reduce the

TABLE 33–4

Progression of Intervention Within a Functional Everyday Approach to Rehabilitation

Step 1	Identify successful and unsuccessful routines of everyday life: What is working, and what is not working?
Step 2	Identify what changes (including changes in the environment, in the behavior of others, and in the individual's own behavior) hold the potential to transform negative, unsuccessful routines into positive, successful routines and to build repertoires of positive behavior.
Step 3	Identify how those changes in everyday routines can be become motivating for the individual and for critical everyday people in that environment.
Step 4	Implement whatever supports are necessary for intensive practice of positive routines in real-world contexts.
Step 5	Systematically withdraw supports and expand contexts as it becomes possible to do so.

From Ylvisaker and colleagues (1999); with permission.

underlying impairment with decontextualized exercises or medical interventions. If these efforts are insufficiently successful, the intervention has tended to shift to attempts to equip the individual with compensatory behaviors to perform functional activities and overcome the ongoing disability. Finally, in the event of insufficiently successful disability-oriented interventions, the focus again shifts, this time to attempts to increase the individual's participation possibilities by focusing on the environmental context: simplifying tasks, modifying the environment, and increasing the support behaviors of others in the environment. This traditional approach often is most efficient in the case of physical restoration—and in other domains as well, if reason exists to believe that decontextualized, restorative, impairment-oriented interventions are effective. Research and clinical experience, however, give little reason for such optimism in the case of individuals with significant chronic cognitive and psychosocial impairment after TBI.

Reversing the traditional hierarchy does not imply abandoning the goal of reducing the individual's underlying impairment. Rather, impairment is potentially reduced as a result of internalizing habits of action and interaction that may have originated as deliberate compensations for chronic impairment. For example, a person who uses a graphic organizer to succeed in complex vocational planning tasks or discourse tasks may internalize the organizer so that it becomes an automatically applied knowledge structure, thereby reducing the original underlying impairment. Several case illustrations have been presented in which impairment reduction was a long-term outcome of intervention that

TABLE 33–5

Two Perspectives on Relations Between Impairment-Oriented, Disability-Oriented, and Handicap-Oriented Interventions for People with Chronic Cognitive, Communication, and Behavioral Impairment after Brain Injury

I. **THE TRADITION IN REHABILITATION**
   First: Attempt to eliminate the individual's underlying impairment with impairment-oriented treatments.
   - Medical treatments (e.g., neuropharmacology, surgery)
   - Impairment-oriented exercises
   Second: Attempt to improve performance of daily activities and increase participation if impairment-oriented treatment is insufficiently successful.
   - Practice with compensatory procedures
   - Extensive practice of specific functional activities
   Third: Attempt to modify the social, vocational, or educational contexts if impairment- and disability-oriented interventions are insufficiently successful.
   - Modification of tasks, routines, and the environments in which they take place
   - Modification of the support behaviors of other people in the environment
   - Modification of the attitudes of important people in the environment

II. **AN ALTERNATIVE PERSPECTIVE**
   First: Increase participation by modifying everyday routines, including the support provided by everyday people in the environment.
   Second: Potentially, improve performance of daily activities by including functional compensatory procedures in the individual's everyday routines and ensuring intensive context-sensitive practice in the use of those compensatory procedures.
   Third: Potentially reduce the underlying impairment by ensuring that the individual practices compensatory procedures—in increasingly varied contexts—to the point at which they are internalized and become components of his or her automatic cognitive or self-regulatory mechanism.

From Ylvisaker and colleagues (1999); with permission.

began with participation-oriented and context supports for successful performance of everyday activities (Ylvisaker & Feeney, 1998a, 2000a; Ylvisaker et al., 1999).

Rationale for a Context-Sensitive, Everyday, Routine-Based Approach to Executive System, Cognitive, Social, and Behavioral Rehabilitation

Theoretical Support: Developmental Cognitive Psychology

For many years, our work in cognitive, social, and behavioral intervention for children and adults with TBI has been guided, in part, by the theoretic formulations of the great Russian psychologist Lev Vygotsky. Over the past 30 years, his work has enjoyed a striking renaissance in many applied fields, including educational psychology (see, e.g., Brown, Campione, Weber, & McGilly, 1992; Campione & Brown, 1990), developmental cognitive psychology (see, e.g., Berk, 2001; Flavell et al., 2002), reading instruction (see, e.g., Palinscar & Brown, 1989), early childhood education (see, e.g., Berk & Winsler, 1995; Bodrova & Leong, 1996), special education (see, e.g., Ashman & Conway, 1989; Evans, 1993), child language disorders (see, e.g., Schneider & Watkins, 1996; Westby, 1994), and other professions. In light of Vygotsky's lifelong influence on the work of his colleague, Alexander Luria (Luria, 1979), it is rather surprising that relatively little attention has been paid to Vygotsky's work in adult neurologic rehabilitation (Ylvisaker & Feeney, 1998a).

According to Vygotsky, internal cognitive and self-regulatory functions, beyond those that are instinctive or purely sensorimotor, are derived in childhood (and later) from internalization/appropriation of interaction with others who are more competent within the context of social-communication routines. "Higher mental functions evolve through social interactions with adults; they are gradually internalized as the child becomes more and more proficient and needs less and less cueing and other support from the adult" (Vygotsky, 1981, p. 261). Thus, cognitive processes like remembering, organizing, and problem solving, as well as self-regulatory processes like self-instructing, first exist as supported interpsychological processes—that is, as interaction between a child or other "apprentice-in-thinking" and a more mature thinker. Gradually, the processes are internalized and become internal, or intrapsychological, processes. Within cognitive and psychosocial rehabilitation, clinicians and other ECPs play a role comparable to expert-parents in relation to apprentice-children, with the goal of equipping the client with the cognitive, communication, and self-regulatory skills needed for success in his or her chosen contexts of life.

The apprenticeship metaphor, which often is used to capture the spirit of Vygotsky's theories (Rogoff, 1990), helps in translating a developmental theory into operational terms during adult rehabilitation. Table 33–6 contrasts two different approaches to teaching: the traditional behavioral training model, and a Vygotskyan apprenticeship model. The latter underpins interventions described later in this chapter.

Theoretical Support: Cognitive Neuroscience and Neuropsychology

Commonly observed neuropsychological profiles following TBI—and most leading neuroscience theories designed to explained these profiles—can be understood as lending support to an everyday, routine-based approach to rehabilita-

tion. For example, Damasio's frontal lobe injury dilemma can be resolved with supported everyday routines of action and interaction as the basis for learning and successful behavior. Context dependence, highlighted by Mesulam and others as being central to the diverse manifestations of frontal lobe injury, yields an alternative neuropsychological rationale for a context-sensitive, everyday, routine orientation to rehabilitation. Grafman's theory of executive processes as complex representations stored in the prefrontal cortex lends further support for a systematic, routine-based approach to rehabilitation. The limitations of information processing capacity associated with diffuse injury as well as with frontal lobe injury can similarly be addressed with automatized routines of action and interaction in everyday contexts. Finally, increasing evidence supports errorless learning practices with individuals who have severe memory impairments associated with TBI-related damage to the hippocampus. Real-world apprenticeship teaching offers the possibility of rehabilitation interventions that are, at the same time, ecologically valid as well as designed to minimize errors.

A Rehabilitation Dilemma and Its Resolution

Ylvisaker and Feeney (1998a) borrowed from the work of Antonio Damasio in building neuropsychological support for an everyday, routine-based approach to rehabilitation after TBI. In his classic book *Descartes Error*, Damasio (1994) sketched an apparently destructive dilemma associated with frontolimbic injury. To be successful in everyday activities, it appears that one must either (1) make good decisions, based on careful consideration of the information available and memory for past successes and failures (the "high reason" approach), or (2) act on the basis of learned behaviors derived from one's personal history of reinforcement (the operant or "somatic marker" approach). Unfortunately, frontolimbic injury jeopardizes both routes to successful action.

Success via high reason presupposes reasonable planning skill, adequate space in working memory for consideration of many relevant factors, adequate explicit memory for past actions and their consequences, reasonable ability to inhibit impulsive action, and an ability to flexibly transfer learning from one context to another. People with significant frontolimbic injury tend to be impaired in all of these cognitive functions, jeopardizing the high reason approach to successful decision making and action.

Success via learning from consequences presupposes reasonable intactness of the neural circuits that are responsible for connecting two types of memory: memory for the factual aspects of past behavior, and memory for the "somatic markers" or feeling states associated with the consequences of those behaviors. Without such connections in memory (however unconscious they may be), past rewards and

TABLE 33–6

Features of Teaching Tasks: Traditional Training Model Versus Vygotskyan Apprenticeship Model

Traditional Training Model

Context
- Training takes place outside of a natural setting.
- Performance of the learner is demanded by the trainer.
- Performance is solo, not social.
- Tasks and components of tasks are hierarchically organized.

Task structure
- The trainer requests performance of a specific task.
- The trainer may model performance.
- The learner performs.
- If the performance is adequate, the learner is reinforced.
- If the performance is inadequate, the trainer either:
  - Requests a hierarchically easier task.
  - Reduces the difficulty of the task.
  - Provides needed cues, prompts, shaping procedures.
- When performance is adequate, repeated practice is required to habituate the learned behavior.
- Systematic transfer procedures are then applied.

Vygotskyan Apprenticeship Model

Context
- Learning (ideally) takes place in a natural setting for the behavior or skill that is to be learned.
- Learning takes place within the context of projects designed to achieve a meaningful goal.
- Performance is not demanded from the learner; rather, the task is completed collaboratively.
- Completion of the task is social, not solo.
- The learner is not expected to fail; the collaborator is available to contribute whatever the learner cannot contribute to successful completion of the task.
- Tasks are not necessarily organized hierarchically; the learner can learn aspects of difficult tasks by participating with a collaborator.

Task structure
- The teacher (facilitator, collaborator) introduces a task and engages the learner in guided observation (not necessarily task specific).
- The teacher engages the learner in collaborative, functional, goal-oriented, project-oriented work.
- The learner contributes what he or she can contribute.
- The teacher coaches (including suggestions, modeling, brainstorming, cues, feedback, and encouragement) and continues to collaborate as the learner accomplishes more components of the task.
- As the learner improves, supports are systematically withdrawn, the task is made more difficult, or both.
- The teacher continues to provide ongoing incidental coaching.
- Transfer is guaranteed because it is part of the context-sensitive teaching process from the outset of the teaching process.

From Ylvisaker and Feeney (1998a); with permission.

punishments lack the power to drive future decision making and behavior. Extensive investigations of adults with frontal lobe injury have convinced Damasio and colleagues that ventromedial prefrontal lesions, which are very common in CHI, weaken the ability to connect these two types of memory, resulting in the common clinical profile of people who respond immediately to rewards and punishments but whose behavior in the long run is inefficiently shaped by the organized arrangement of such consequences (Damasio, 1998; Damasio, Tranel & Damasio, 1990, 1991; Tranel, 2002).

Some clinicians respond to this dilemma by suggesting (a) that consequences must be much more extreme than is commonly necessary or (b) that individuals with significant frontolimbic injury may require a substantial degree of external control indefinitely. In our view, escaping through the horns of this dilemma requires the development of contextually relevant cognitive, communication, and behavioral habits, acquired with the help of antecedent-focused apprenticeship procedures (see Tables 33–3 and 33–6 for operational definitions) rather than relying on consequences to shape behavior, as in traditional training models of intervention and traditional behavior management. In the section on behavioral and psychosocial rehabilitation (below), we return to this theme of relative inefficiency in learning from consequences.

Related to the somatic marker theory is Roll's view, based on extensive research with primates and humans, that the key function of ventral prefrontal cortex, in particular the orbitofrontal cortex, is to distinguish rewarding consequences and to modify behavior in relation to changing contingencies (Rolls, 2002). This explains the observed phenomenon of individuals with frontal lobe injury failing to learn from the consequences of their behavior. Rolls also attempts to bring more general frontal lobe phenomena under this reinforcement-learning umbrella, including difficulty sorting, shifting, and changing direction; perseverating; euphoria; irresponsibility; lack of affect; lack of concern/egocentrism; socially inappropriate and disinhibited behavior; and impaired perception/identification of facial and voice emotion—with associated alteration of emotional processing and increased disinhibition and behavioral problems. The theory of Rolls, like that of Damasio and colleagues, provides a comfortable theoretical home for intervention based on the creation of positive, everyday, context-sensitive routines of action and interaction.

Context Dependence and Frontal Lobe Injury

Mesulam's (2002) review of frontal lobe function and dysfunction highlights, as its central theme, that the frontal lobes enable humans to transcend "the default mode" of inflexible stimulus–response linkages tied to the immediate stimulus environment. From this central theme evolve the commonly observed deficits associated with frontal lobe injury:

1. Poor working memory (i.e., difficulty expanding consciousness beyond the here and now)
2. Distractibility, perseveration, and disinhibition
3. Difficulty with decision making in novel situations
4. Impaired integration of reason, experience, and emotion
5. Inflexibility, insensitivity to contextual subtleties, failure to appreciate ambiguity, and difficulty with abstract thinking
6. Cognitive egocentrism or difficulty switching perspectives (otherwise known as impaired "theory of mind")

Each of these themes is addressed within an intervention perspective that is context sensitive and attempts to build repertoires of successful behavior, thinking, and self-regulation triggered by environmental stimuli specifically relevant to the individual being served. Mesulam also uses his default mode theory to explain the well-documented ecological invalidity of office-bound assessments. (We will return to this theme in the section on assessment.)

Executive Dysfunction as Impairment of Structured Event Complexes

Grafman's theory of prefrontal function proposes that executive processes really are complex mental representations ("structured event complexes") at greater or lesser levels of generality (Grafman, 2002). Thus, "executive direction" of complex activities, understood neurologically, is activation of a complex knowledge structure that represents that activity. These representations or knowledge structures are strengthened by multiple experiences with activities in the world. Like the previous theories, Grafman's view supports an approach to rehabilitation that attempts to strengthen these complex knowledge structures by creating routines of action and interaction triggered by contextually appropriate environmental stimuli.

Limited Processing Capacity

Individuals with frontal lobe or diffuse neuronal pathology, both of which are common in TBI, often have limited processing resources (Schmitter-Edgecombe, 1996). These limited resources are easily exhausted, particularly in the context of novel, complex, or inadequately rehearsed activities. When additional demands are placed on those resources, activity failures and contextually inappropriate behaviors are likely to occur. Thus, we argue later that everyday activities as well as scripts of self-regulation should be practiced to habituation. Furthermore, this practice should take place within the context of everyday activities so that the environmental triggers are those that the individual will encounter in everyday life. The clinical need to automatize self-regulation scripts is based on studies (see review by Schmeichel & Baumeister, 2004) showing that self-regulatory resources are depleted with effortful self-regulation.

Procedural Memory, Implicit Memory, and Errorless Learning

The superiority of implicit memory and learning over explicit memory and learning in many individuals with TBI provides additional support for an everyday, routine-based approach to rehabilitation and errorless teaching procedures. As we describe apprenticeship teaching, the teaching/learning process can be conducted either in a trial-and-error manner or in an errorless manner. Individuals with significant memory disorders associated with damage to the hippocampus benefit from errorless teaching procedures (described below). Thus, everyday habits and procedures of action and interaction can be learned without error and triggered by environmental stimuli, assuming that the teaching was adequately sensitive to context.

Empirical Support: Transfer (Generalization) and Maintenance

Decades of experimental studies of generalization and maintenance offer yet another support for a richly context-sensitive, everyday, routine-based approach to intervention. Many investigators in behavioral, cognitive, and educational psychology have amassed large quantities of evidence that yields the following heuristic principle: *Behaviors or skills acquired in a laboratory or training context are unlikely to transfer to functional application contexts and be maintained over time without heroic efforts to facilitate that transfer and maintenance* (Detterman & Sternberg, 1993; Horner, Dunlap, & Koegel, 1988; Martin & Pear, 1996; Morris, 1992; Singley & Anderson, 1989). Recognition of the impact of this principle has led to the development and validation of increasingly context-sensitive interventions in many clinical fields, including vocational rehabilitation (see, e.g., Wehman et al., 1993, 1995), special education (see, e.g., Giangreco, Cloninger, & Iverson, 1993), strategy intervention for students with and without specific disability (see, e.g., Baker, Gersten, & Scanlon, 2002; Pressley, 1995; Sweet & Snow, 2002), behavioral intervention (see, e.g., Carr et al., 1994; Carr, Reeve, & Magito-McLaughlin, 1997; Kennedy, 1994; Koegel, Koegel, & Dunlap, 1997; Reichle & Wacker, 1993), and language and social skills intervention (see, e.g., Fey, 1986; Gresham, Sugai, & Horner, 2001; Koegel & Koegel, 1995; MacDonald, 1989; Walker, Schwarz, Nippold, Irvin, & Noell, 1994; Wiener & Harris, 1998).

In our judgment, the use of decontextualized cognitive retraining exercises (popular during the 1980s for TBI rehabilitation and still used today by some practitioners) is insensitive to this important principle. Isolating components of cognition (e.g., selective attention, working memory, sequential or categorical organization, and deductive rea-

soning) and engaging people in massed learning trials with tasks largely unrelated to functional application tasks falls squarely in the tradition of decontextualized cognitive training that has been found to be relatively ineffective with many disability groups, including mental retardation (Mann, 1979), learning disabilities (Kavale & Mattson, 1983), and TBI (Carney et al., 1999; Cicerone et al., 2005; Park & Ingles, 2001), as well as in people without disability (Singley & Anderson, 1989). More than 100 years ago, William James made the same observation in connection with memory training: "the retention of particular things" but not "general physiological retentiveness," can be improved with practice (James, 1890, p. 665). The systematically increasing use of everyday contexts for cognitive and behavioral interventions bears testimony to these concerns about transfer (Ylvisaker, 2003; Ylvisaker et al., 2003).

Economic Support: Managed Care and the Demand for Efficient Rehabilitation

A fourth category of support for an everyday, routine-based approach to rehabilitation is provided by the fierce economic realities that have come to play a prominent role in rehabilitation planning. Managed care and cutbacks in federal supports for rehabilitation have dramatically shortened the lengths of inpatient rehabilitation stay and reduced access to outpatient services (AHCPR, 1999; Johnson, 1999). Some funders routinely deny reimbursement for interventions, such as cognitive rehabilitation, that are said to have an inadequate research base. At the same time, funders increasingly demand improved functional outcomes in return for their limited support of rehabilitation (Henri & Hallowell, 1999; Schmidt, 1997).

Meanwhile, the prevalence of TBI-related disability continues to increase because of the population's relative youth at the time of injury. For example, over the past 10 years, the New York State Department of Health Neurobehavioral Resource Project has served more than 1,000 young adults who have a history of TBI and ongoing difficulty with community reintegration, often many years after their injury. This Medicaid waiver community support program was designed specifically for individuals with serious, chronic cognitive and behavioral impairment after TBI. Feeney and colleagues (2001) found that the program not only yielded positive outcomes for the participants but also proved to be cost-effective, yielding substantial savings for the New York State Department of Health. Under these stressful economic circumstances, it is critical for rehabilitation specialists to creatively design ways to accomplish more with less, to achieve positive outcomes with fewer resources. Inviting specialists to intensify their collaboration with everyday people (e.g., family members, direct care staff, job coaches, and others) so that long-term rehabilitation can be provided in large part in the context of the everyday routines of life

TABLE 33–7

Rationale for an Everyday, Routine-Based Approach to Intervention for Individuals with TBI

From the Perspective of Executive Functions
A. *Threat to Social Success*: Difficulty making good decisions based on thoughtful consideration of consequences and other relevant factors.
   Possible Solution: Provide needed supports in everyday routines, stopping short of a degree of support that creates learned helplessness or oppositional behavior.
B. *Threat to Social Success*: Reduced inhibition.
   Possible Solutions: (1) Create everyday routines that include ample antecedent supports, such as positive setting events and avoidance of identified triggers; (2) help the individual self-manage antecedents.
C. *Threat to Social Success*: Reduced initiation.
   Possible Solution: Create everyday routines that include initiation supports, such as initiation scripts, initiation cues (e.g., alarm watch), and peer support for initiation.

From the Perspective of Cognition
A. *Threat to Social Success*: Impaired working memory.
   Possible Solutions: (1) Practice positive everyday routines so that they come to be elicited by everyday environmental cues, obviating the need for complex thought processes; (2) create prosthetic reminder systems (e.g., pager systems); (3) Create positive metaphors that package several pieces of information into one thought unit.
B. *Threat to Social Success*: Impaired explicit and strategic memory; difficulty remembering past successes and failures.
   Possible Solution: Proceduralize positive context-sensitive routines using implicit versus explicit memory processes, procedural versus declarative memory systems, and involuntary versus strategic or effortful learning tasks.
C. *Threat to Social Success*: Reduced organizational skills.
   Possible Solution: Create positive, everyday routines that include external organizers, possibly including graphic advance organizers.
D. *Threat to Social Success*: Difficulty transferring newly acquired skills from training to application contexts.
   Possible Solution: Facilitate acquisition of social competencies in the context of everyday social interaction.

From the Perspective of Behavior Management
A. *Threat to Social Success*: Inefficiency in learning from consequences.
   Possible Solution: Build repertoires of positive behaviors using antecedent supports versus relying on consequences to shape positive behaviors.
B. *Threat to Social Success*: Oppositional behavior.
   Possible Solutions: (1) As much as possible, work within the individual's world of meaning and personal goals; (2) tie interventions to positive personal metaphors or life narratives.

From Ylvisaker and Feeney (2000a); with permission.

represents a positive response to the crisis of funding for rehabilitation.

Summary

Table 33–7 summarizes ways in which an everyday, routine-based approach to rehabilitation addresses chronic obstacles to social success after TBI. Obstacles are grouped under the headings of executive functions, cognition, and behavior. Some of the solutions are elaborated later in this chapter.

ASSESSMENT FOR PLANNING FUNCTIONAL, CONTEXT-SENSITIVE INTERVENTION

Cognitive and communication assessments may be conducted for several distinct purposes, including (a) diagnosing a disorder, (b) formulating a prognosis, (c) generating epidemiologic information, (d) preparing for legal testimony, (e) acquiring services or funding, (f) developing an intervention plan, and (g) monitoring the results of intervention. Specific assessment procedures may be valid for some, but not all, purposes of assessment. For example, a standardized aphasia battery may be useful in diagnosing a specific language impairment but offers little help in identifying the associated activity reductions (i.e., degree of difficulty following directions at work), participation limitations, and context facilitators and barriers. Furthermore, the tests may offer little guidance in creating the most fruitful approach to reducing the individual's impairment and increasing activity and participation domains.

Over the past 15 years, several standardized tests have been developed for use with adults who have TBI, including the Scales of Cognitive Ability for Traumatic Brain Injury

(Adamovich & Henderson, 1992); Ross Information Processing Assessment (Ross-Swain, 1996), or RIPA-2; Brief Test of Head Injury (Helm-Estabrooks & Hotz, 1991), or BTHI; Behavior Rating Inventory of Executive Function –Adult Version (Roth, Isquith, & Gioia, 2005); Behavioral Assessment of the Dysexecutive Syndrome (Wilson, Alderman, Burgess, Elmslie, & Evans, 1996); Measure of Cognitive-Linguistic Abilities (Ellmo, Graser, Krchnavek, Hauck, & Calabrese, 1995); Functional Assessment of Verbal Reasoning and Executive Strategies (MacDonald, 2005); Rivermead Behavioral Memory Test (Wilson, Cockburn, Baddeley, 1985); and others. Turkstra, Coehlo, and Ylvisaker (2005) discussed the strengths and limitations of standardized testing for individuals with TBI.

Standardized assessments can serve a variety of useful purposes. In this chapter, however, we restrict our discussion to assessment for purposes of planning, monitoring, and modifying individualized intervention. Functional intervention often is directed at reducing disability by improving compensatory behavior in specific functional contexts of activity or at increasing participation either by modifying the environment or by improving the support behaviors of others. In these cases, standardized, office-bound assessments are not particularly helpful.

In Table 33–8, we present categories of assessments, grouped under the headings of impairment, activity/participation, and context. This scheme for classifying assessment procedures may help clinicians to avoid the common pitfall of attempting to achieve an assessment goal by administering a type of assessment designed for other purposes. Furthermore, static versus dynamic assessments are contrasted. Whereas static assessment often is used for diagnosis, classification, and outcome monitoring, dynamic hypothesis-testing assessment is designed to identify the intervention and support procedures that hold the greatest promise for rehabilitation of the individual.

Functional, Collaborative, Context-Sensitive, Hypothesis-Testing Assessment for Planning Intervention

Elsewhere, we have described and illustrated an experimental approach to assessment that is consistent with the functional, everyday approach to intervention described in this chapter (Ylvisaker & Feeney, 1998a; Ylvisaker & Gioia, 1998). In the case of individuals with complex impairment and disability in the domains addressed in this chapter, assessment for purposes of planning intervention is ongoing, context-sensitive, collaborative, and based on careful tests of hypotheses. This approach to assessment has its historical roots in Vygotsky's dynamic assessment (Vygotsky, 1978), as elaborated by Feuerstein (1979) and, more recently, by many practitioners in educational psychology (see, e.g., Palinscar, Brown, & Campione, 1994), special education, speech-language

---

TABLE 33–8

Approaches to Communication Assessment for People with Traumatic Brain Injury

Impairment-Oriented Assessment

Purpose:	For diagnosis: to identify underlying neuropsychological, including linguistic and motor, strengths and weaknesses
Static:	Standardized neuropsychological tests and test batteries
	Standardized aphasia tests and test batteries
	Standardized motor speech tests
Dynamic:	Process assessment: to identify what intact neuropsychological process explains successful performance and what affected processes explain unsuccessful performance, using systematic hypothesis-testing modification of test items (Kaplan, 1988)

Activity/Particiaption-Oriented Assessment

Purposes:	For diagnosis: to identify possible effects of neuropsychological impairments on real-world performance of functional activities and associated limitations of social, vocational, and educational participation
	For treatment planning: to identify everyday activities that require intervention and to identify strategies that may improve performance
Static:	Customized: Observation of performance of functional tasks of everyday life
	Standardized: Functional scales (e.g., American Speech-Language-Hearing Association FACS, FIM, and DRS)
Dynamic:	Experimentation with strategies and supports that hold the potential to improve performance of daily activities (OCCHTA)

Context-Oriented Assessment

Purposes:	For treatment planning: to identify facilitators and barriers in the environment; to identify environmental modification strategies that may enhance participation; to identify strengths and needs of everyday communication partners (e.g., family members, friends, job supervisors, and teachers) relative to their ability to serve as supports for the individual with ongoing disability; and to identify changes in the behavior of communication partners that may enhance successful participation
Static:	Standardized: Quality-of-life inventories
	Customized: Observation of and interviews regarding level of participation and level of success in social, familial, academic, and vocational pursuits and roles
Dynamic:	Context-sensitive experimentation with environmental supports and with potentially helpful changes in the support behaviors of others (OCCHTA)

pathology, and other fields. Behavioral psychologists have a long history of assessment by means of experimental analysis of variables that potentially influence behavior (Iwata, Vollmer, & Zarcone, 1990; Kern, Childs, Dunlap, Clarke, & Falk, 1994). Our goal in this section is restricted to presenting a brief rationale for this type of assessment and an outline of the steps of functional, hypothesis-testing assessment (Ylvisaker et al., 1999).

Rationale

Why Ongoing?

Following severe TBI, individuals can continue spontaneous neurologic recovery for months and, in some cases, years. This by itself mandates ongoing assessment. In addition, changes in environmental and task demands, in the individual's ability levels and psychoreactive responses, and in the skill levels of everyday people in the environment all contribute to ongoing unpredictability in evolving outcome, inviting ongoing assessment to ensure that services and supports are maximally effective.

Why Context Sensitive?

The ecological validity of office-bound, standardized tests of cognitive and communication functioning for individuals with TBI (or, more specifically, frontal lobe injury) has been challenged by the results of many neuropsychological studies (Anderson, Damasio, Tranel, & Damasio, 2000; Benton, 1991; Burgess, Alderman, Evans, Emslie, & Wilson, 1998; Crépeau, Scherzer, Belleville, & Desmarais, 1997; Dennis, 1991; Dywan & Segalowitz, 1996; Eslinger & Damasio, 1985; LeBlanc, Hayden, & Paulman, 2000; Rath, Simon, Langenbahn, Sherr, & Diller, 2000; Stuss & Benson, 1986; Stuss & Buckle, 1992; Tranel, 2002; Turkstra et al., 2005; Varney & Menefee, 1993). Some individuals with impairment of executive function perform better on standardized tests than one would expect based on real-world performance, because the tests are externally structured and impose few demands in the areas of goal setting, task identification, initiation, self-monitoring, or real-world strategic thinking. Others perform surprisingly poorly on standardized tests, because the tasks are novel and the familiar stimulus cues of everyday life are not present to support performance. In either case, tests must be supplemented by effective use of real-world contexts in functional assessment.

Why Collaborative?

Collaboration increases the number of observations that can be made, the number of real-world contexts that can be explored, and the number of functional experiments that can be performed. In addition, when many people collaborate in assessment, the likelihood that these same people will collaborate in implementing the intervention plan resulting

from the assessment is increased. Participation in collaborative assessment also is an ideal way for everyday people to learn about the realities associated with the disability. Finally, asking professional colleagues, aides, family members, and others to become collaborators in assessment is a profound statement of respect and, therefore, contributes to team building.

Why Tests of Hypotheses?

Many capacities, processes, and skills are involved in most human behavior. Therefore, if a person has trouble with a task, there typically are scores of potential explanations for that difficulty. Similarly, when a person succeeds, that success may be a product of varied strategies (Kaplan, 1988). If specialists in rehabilitation do not know why people succeed when they succeed or what underlying impairment explains failure when they fail, these specialists are not in a position to create a meaningful, appropriately targeted intervention program. Therefore, alternative hypotheses must be tested.

Assessment Process

Ylvisaker and Feeney (1998a) illustrated the processes of collaborative, context-sensitive hypothesis-testing assessment. In each case, the process included collaborative identification of the problem, collaborative formulation, selection and testing of hypotheses, and collaborative interpretation of the findings in relation to planning interventions and supports.

Collaboratively Identify the Problem

In some cases, little difficulty exists in identifying the functional problem that calls for intervention. In other cases, however, it is not so easy. For example, the same behavioral issue may be identified by one person as defiance, by another as withdrawal, and by still others as lack of initiation or laziness. In these cases, it is critical to agree to a neutral description of the problem behavior before proceeding.

Collaboratively Formulate Hypotheses

Hypotheses may be derived from neurodiagnostic information, neuropsychological or other testing, clinical experience with similar individuals, or real-world interaction with the person whose intervention plan is being developed. Typically, teams of professionals and others have little difficulty in generating possible explanations for the person's behavior or proposing intervention plans. It may not be as easy to label one's favored explanation as a hypothesis and then subject it to testing along with other hypotheses. This is precisely the process, however, that enables teams to move beyond conflict over treatment plans and to identify interventions that have a demonstrable effect.

Collaboratively Select Hypotheses to Test

Some hypotheses may be easier to test than others, and some may have greater face validity than others, more interesting implications for intervention than others, and be embraced by more members of the team than others. Selecting hypotheses to test—and the order in which to test them—requires balancing these considerations. In general, it is important to start with hypotheses that are readily testable, with results that will be recognized and accepted by all members of the team.

Collaboratively Test Hypotheses

In some cases, several hypotheses can be tested within a short period of time and, possibly, within a controlled assessment setting; in other cases, the process extends for weeks and mandates exploration in several real-world settings. In some cases, hypothesis testing is designed to explore the impact of hypothesized variables one at a time; in other cases in which the issue to be explored is serious (e.g., aggressive behavior) and requires immediate attention, it may be desirable to combine hypotheses—that is, to experiment with a multifaceted intervention. If the complex hypothesis is confirmed (i.e., if the intervention is successful), it may not be possible to know which individual hypotheses were confirmed and in what combination, but at least the clinical problem is solved. Feeney and Ylvisaker (1995) presented three single-subject experimental designs that fit this description.

Collaboratively Interpret the Results and
Formulate an Intervention Plan

In many cases, the test is, in effect, a trial intervention. If the trial intervention works well, then the treatment plan may follow in a relatively automatic manner. In other cases, the treatment plan may be an elaboration of the initial experiments. When people have chronic disability in the executive system, cognitive, communication, and behavioral domains, intervention often takes the form of supportive modifications of everyday routines—modifications that were identified as positive by means of hypothesis testing (Ylvisaker & Feeney, 1998a).

Context-Sensitive, Experimental Assessment in the Early and Middle Stages of Recovery

Early in neurologic recovery, context-sensitive experimental assessment from the perspective of cognition, communication, and behavior is designed, in part, to identify the conditions under which the individual is maximally alert, externally focused, and responsive to environmental stimuli. Variables that need to be explored include time of day; the sensory environment (e.g., lighting, auditory stimuli, and

tactile responsiveness); responses to positioning, movement (e.g., rocking) and temperature (e.g., warm bath); levels of medication; and differential responses to people and their communication styles. The goal of this systematic exploration is to maximize the amount of time the individual spends at the highest levels of responsiveness, to minimize stimulation associated with pathologic responses or withdrawal, and to encourage basic levels of communication (e.g., reaching for desired objects or pushing undesired objects away). In addition, staff explore ways in which the individual can be supported in participating in activities of everyday life (e.g., self-care, turning on and off lights, and controlling sources of stimulation like tape-recorded music). Once appropriate supports are identified, family members and nursing staff are encouraged to engage the individual frequently in meaningful activities of everyday life, even if the individual appears to give little response at the time.

During the middle stage of recovery, context-sensitive experimental assessment from the perspective of cognition, communication, and behavior largely is designed to identify the environmental and task supports that are needed to perform adaptively on activities of daily living as well as on personally meaningful communication, educational, vocational, recreational, and social tasks. The supports and scaffolding highlighted later in this chapter (Table 33–9) often are the variables manipulated experimentally to identify the nature of the disability and the supports that are useful in increasing participation and improving everyday functional activities (Table 33–9).

Illustration of Context-Sensitive, Collaborative Hypothesis Testing

Sue incurred severe TBI at age 35 in a motor-vehicle crash. In addition to diffuse injury, neurodiagnostic imaging revealed significant left hemisphere frontotemporal damage. Before her injury, Sue was employed as a laborer in a large factory. She had a history of marital conflict, and her two children had been removed from her home as a result of neglect and suspected abuse.

At the time of our involvement, Sue was 47 years old and had been a resident of a nursing home for 12 years. She had been diagnosed with serious cognitive-language impairment (including anomia, circumlocution, and wandering, tangential discourse), disorganized behavior in all domains of life, episodic and semantic memory impairment, reduced anger control, and physically aggressive behavior. With newly available community support funding through a Medicaid waiver program, she was placed in a supported apartment and given a job in a developmental disabilities sheltered workshop. In the social environment of that work setting, Sue's aggression escalated.

Local staff proposed that she be returned to the nursing home until she demonstrated the communication and anger

TABLE 33–9

Illustration of Functional, Content- and Context-Sensitive Executive Function/Cognitive Rehabilitation Through the Continuum of Recovery: Organization, Memory, Language, and Executive Functions

Client: Tom is a 30-year-old, married father of two with a pretrauma avocational and vocational interest in baseball cards. He collected cards and traded them at shows and on the Internet. Residual impairment in the areas of executive functions (e.g., self-awareness, planning, organizing, and self-monitoring), memory, and organization of language were associated with frontolimbic injury.

Long-Term Goal: The client will regulate his behavior adequately to manage his baseball card collection and resume trading with minimal assistance.

Facilitators: Therapists, family members, direct care staff, friends.

Early Stages (Maximal Support)	Middle Stages (Moderate Support)	Late Stages (Relative Independence; Support as Needed)
EF-Cognitive-Language Goals: • Increase alertness and arousal. • Improve external focus. • Increase recognition of objects and people. • Increase engagement in overlearned activities. • Improve basic communication: comprehension of simple, everyday language; expression of basic wants, needs, and reactions.	**EF-Cognitive-Language Goals:** • Increase duration of attention; ability to shift attention from object to object and activity to activity; ability filter out distractions. • Improve perceptual scanning abilities. • Use organizing schemes, including external organizers, to complete functional tasks. • Use a prosthetic log/memory system to aid orientation, organization, memory, and self-management. • Improve organization of spoken and written discourse, with external supports. • Improve awareness of needs and strategies to compensate for deficits.	**EF-Cognitive-Language Goals:** • Improve awareness of self as a thinker, learner, communicator, and self-manager. • Increase independent use of strategies to compensate for ongoing cognitive deficits. • Improve organization of discourse with decreasing use of external organizers. • Improve comprehension of vocabulary and extended texts related to vocational and avocational interests. • Improve independent goal setting, planning, initiating, and self-evaluating. • Increase independent creation, implementation, review, and revision of compensatory strategies.
Meaningful Activities/ Everyday Routines: • Turn pages of a baseball card album or collector book. • Move cards in and out of album sleeves. • Stack cards as others look at them. • Find particular cards on the page. • Help find all the cards from a team. • On request, hand the cards to visitors to see. • Place cards into rows for viewing. **Transfer Activities:** • With support, participate in self-care activities and other activities of daily living. • With prompts, activate switches to control electronic devices (e.g., TV or tape recorder).	**Meaningful Activities/Everyday Routines:** • Organize cards by team or value. • Write names of players on each team. • Show and describe cards to others, including children. • Read/write short narratives or biographical sketches about players; describe players to others (e.g., in group therapy). • Determine value of cards and list prices. • Role play selling cards at a show; determine costs for purchase of various combinations of cards. • Explain features of card trading to peers in group therapy; prepare script in advance with the help of a graphic organizer. **Transfer Activities:** • Use graphic organizers and written reminders for other tasks (e.g., activities of daily living on the nursing unit, writing letters to family members). • Plan menus, prepare own lunch. • Organize narratives and descriptions of experiences to offer visitors.	**Meaningful Activities/Everyday Routines:** • Use sales books and the Internet to determine availability and cost of cards. • Purchase and organize new cards in the collection. • Keep financial records. • Read and write articles about baseball card collecting. • Create organized displays for card shows. • Set up a display at a card show. • Interact with visitors at a card show. • Help his children with their collections. **Transfer Activities:** • Assist other individuals with traumatic brain injury at an earlier stage of recovery or with greater disability. • Work with his children in the use of organizing systems for their homework. • Develop strategies and organizers for other demanding activities (e.g., banking or shopping).

(continued)

TABLE 33–9

Illustration of Functional, Content- and Context-Sensitive Executive Function/Cognitive Rehabilitation Through the Continuum of Recovery: Organization, Memory, Language, and Executive Functions (continued)

- Review family picture albums.
- Look at greeting cards.

- Play simple card games with children.
- Write letters, thank you cards.
- Use goal-plan-do-review format in all therapies, including physical therapies.

- Continue to use goal-plan-do-review format for major life activities.

Facilitator Expectations and Mediation:

- Facilitator is responsible for modifying the environment and stimulus presentation to fit Tom's response potential.
- Facilitator treats Tom's actions, even if accidental, as meaningful and makes them seem appropriate to the situation (e.g., touching a card is interpreted as a request).
- Facilitator associated simple language with actions (e.g., "Let's see if we can find a Yankee; no, that's a Dodger.").

Scaffolding:

- Facilitator may be required to perform all components of the task, but collaboratively engaging Tom in any way possible (e.g., hand-over-hand joint performance of the task).

Facilitator Expectations and Mediation:

- Facilitator ensures that the environment is appropriate for efficient information processing.
- Facilitator gradually turns over more components of tasks to Tom.
- Facilitator changes prompts from physical (e.g., hand-over-hand) to verbal (simple instructions) to graphic (e.g., graphic organizers such as price sheets, inventory sheets, discourse guides for narrative and biographical sketches, feature analysis guide for organizing full descriptions and practicing organized word retrieval).
- Facilitator begins all activities with identification of the goal and formulation of a plan (e.g., use of an organizer), monitors progress ("Let's make sure we're getting the job done right."), ends all sessions with review of achievement ("Did you finish? How'd you do?") and usefulness of supports (e.g., "Did this organizer help?"), and helps Tom record important information in a memory book for future reference.
- Facilitator highlights improvements and the value of the supports that are used, helping Tom gain greater insight into his strengths and needs.

Scaffolding:

- In addition to cues and organizers, the facilitator uses verbal mediation to highlight the important aspects of each component of the task, routinely reviews the goal, plan, and progress, models organized thinking, makes connections to related activities.

Facilitator Expectations and Mediation:

- Tom increasingly assumes responsibility for creating organizing systems to accomplish home and work tasks; facilitator (e.g., therapist, Tom's wife) may simply play a monitoring role.
- Tom assumes responsibility for independent use of memory aids; facilitator engages Tom in brainstorming if systems fail.
- Tom assumes responsibility for independent use of organizing systems (e.g., graphic organizers; prepared scripts) to communicate (speak and write) in an organized manner; facilitator provides feedback.
- Tom assumes primary responsibility for self-management (e.g., sets goals, makes plans, initiates work, evaluates self and products, and chooses strategic compensations); facilitator encourages daily use of executive function routines and brainstorms with Tom about strategies.

Scaffolding:

- Facilitator plays an ongoing role as coach (if necessary), consultant, and source of emotional support. As a consultant, the facilitator helps Tom identify barriers to success (e.g., inattention to scheduled responsibilities, reading comprehension problems, disorganized record keeping, gaps in his knowledge base) and develop customized strategies to overcome them.

Log/Journal/Memory Book:
Facilitators keep a log of Tom's significant experiences and progress. The system is used, in part, to help facilitators identify factors that promote improved cognitive and adaptive functioning and to communicate with one another. Facilitators review the log with Tom with the ultimate goal of improving recall of daily events and establishing a routine of review.

Log/Journal/Memory Book:
Tom gradually assumes greater responsibility for management of the log/memory book system. He begins to write his own entries, with guidance. The book plays a meaningful role in helping Tom stay oriented, know his schedule, plan activities, remember important events, and keep track of goals and assignments. Photographs of staff, well-organized schedules, and graphic organizers for important tasks are included in the book.

Log/Journal/Memory Book:
Tom has primary responsibility for upkeep and use of the book, which may become more like a traditional day planner to organize daily events and facilitate memory. An outline of needs and strategies may continue to be included. An electronic pager system and/or computer memory system may be used.

management skills as well as the positive attitude needed to live and work in the community. Sue's opposing view, which she offered in emotionally strong language, was that she would do fine if she had a meaningful life, including work in a "real" work setting. The staff insisted that she must first demonstrate work and interpersonal skills in a sheltered setting. With considerable encouragement, staff were convinced to treat Sue's proposal as a testable hypothesis. With the approval of her preinjury boss, Sue was placed in her old job with detailed, negotiated plans for asking for help when needed and for anticipating and dealing with frustration. Relevant employees in the factory were oriented to Sue's cognitive and communication deficits and given scripts to negotiate routine, work-related interaction. A job coach was used for less than a month. Four years later, Sue continues to be successful in her nonsupported job and community living—an achievement made possible, in part, by framing alternative recommendations (those of the staff versus that of Sue) as hypotheses to be tested collaboratively and using real-world routines as the context for those tests.

TBI REHABILITATION: EXECUTIVE FUNCTIONS/SELF-REGULATION AS THE UNIFYING THEME

In our discussion of disability associated with TBI, we offered a definition of executive functions, tied it to the more general concept of self-regulation (using the hybrid term "executive functions/self-regulation" [EF/SR]), and stated that we would organize the intervention sections of the chapter around this unifying concept. Most cognitive problems of people with TBI (e.g., poorly controlled attention, weak encoding and retrieval of new information, and impaired planning and organizing), communication problems (e.g., disorganized discourse and impulsive or otherwise unsuccessful social communication), and behavioral problems (e.g., aggression and sexually inappropriate behavior) can be traced to weak executive control over their cognition, communication, and behavior as opposed to problems specific to the domain. This is not universally true, however, and in our discussion below, we do address memory problems that are not a consequence of frontal lobe injury and, therefore, could be seen as independent of the EF/SR system. Yet even in these cases, the most common approach to intervention is compensation for the problem as opposed to restoration of function. Therefore, the EF/SR system again becomes the key to successful rehabilitation.

Following general comments about executive functions/self-regulation, our discussion of intervention is divided into four main sections:

1. EF/SR interventions, including the processes of facilitating compensatory strategies in general and discourse strategies specifically.

2. Cognitive rehabilitation, including a critique of traditional processes-specific cognitive retraining and discussions of memory aids, errorless learning for individuals with severe memory impairment, and the use of virtual reality (VR) in rehabilitation.
3. Social communication intervention, including a critique of traditional social skills and pragmatics training.
4. Behavioral intervention, including a critique of traditional contingency management, a discussion of positive behavior supports, and a special focus on teaching positive communication alternatives to negative behavior.

Executive Functions/Self-Regulation: An Intervention-Relevant Operational Definition

In Appendix 33.1, the executive system is included as a component of cognition. In this limited and "cold" sense of the term (Denckla, 1996), executive functions direct and regulate cognitive processes. Thus, people with frontal lobe injury may perform well on tests of intelligence and may appear to attend, perceive, organize, learn, and reason adequately under highly structured and externally directed conditions but, because of executive system impairment, fail to use their cognitive processes effectively under real-world conditions.

In discussions of TBI and frontal lobe injury, executive functions often are highlighted for separate consideration in their role as planner, initiator, and regulator of all aspects of behavior, not just cognitive processes. Understood most generally, the executive self-regulatory system includes those mental functions involved in formulating goals, planning how to achieve them, carrying out the plans, and revising those plans in response to feedback (Lezak, 1982; Luria, 1966). In this broad sense, the same set of control functions directs all deliberate, nonroutine behavior, including cognitive (e.g., paying attention in the presence of distractions), emotional (e.g., controlling anger), communication (e.g., planning an effective way to express a complex or sensitive thought), social (e.g., inhibiting aggressive behavior when provoked), educational (e.g., using effective reading and writing strategies), and vocational (e.g., planning a day at work to complete a large number of assigned tasks). Earlier in this chapter, we explicitly tied our discussion of EF/SR to important literatures in related fields. Table 33–10 offers a functional operational definition of the executive system, based in part on analysis of the characteristics (beyond intellectual, linguistic, and motor skills) that enable successful people to be successful—that is, to make efficient real-world use the abilities and knowledge that they possess.

In discussions of neuropsychological rehabilitation, executive functions often are characterized as being high on a hierarchy of cognitive functions and, therefore, an inappropriate target for intervention until late in recovery after most aspects of cognition have undergone substantial recovery.

TABLE 33–10

A Functional Operational Definition of the Executive System

1. Awareness of strengths and limitations, and associated understanding of the difficulty level of tasks.
2. Based on this awareness, an ability to:
   - Set reasonable goals.
   - Plan and organize behavior designed to achieve the goals.
   - Initiate behavior toward achieving goals.
   - Inhibit behavior incompatible with achieving those goals.
   - Monitor and evaluate performance in relation to the goals.
   - Benefit from feedback.
   - Flexibly revise plans and strategically solve problems in the event of difficulty or failure.
3. Ability to assume a non-egocentric perspective and "read" others' mental states.
4. Ability to think abstractly and transfer skills from training to application contexts.

Unfortunately, this hierarchical view is insensitive to developmental studies of both immature primates (Goldman, 1971) and humans (Bjorklund, 1990; Bronson, 2000; Welsh & Pennington, 1988). Recent work in developmental cognitive psychology strongly suggests a developmental course for executive functions characterized by early onset of development (in infancy); slow maturation of functions (continuing through the adolescent years); dynamic interaction with other aspects of cognitive, linguistic, and social development; and modifiability of development with experience and training (Bjorklund, 1990; Bronson, 2000; Tranel, Anderson, & Benton, 1995; Welsh & Pennington, 1988). Indeed, one of the most popular and successful curricula for preschoolers with and without disability, the High Scope Curriculum, organizes preschool activities around a simple, executive function, goal-plan-do-review routine (Schweinhart & Weikart, 1993). Recognizing the profound importance of executive functions for success in life and with these developmental themes as background, we introduce executive functions as a rehabilitation target relatively early in recovery, along with all other aspects of cognition (see Table, 33–9 and 33–11).

Executive Function Intervention Themes

Executive Function/Self-Regulatory Scripts and Development of Autonomy

Ylvisaker, Szekeres, and Feeney (1998) described a variety of interventions that address specific components of executive functioning. Our goal in this section is to highlight the core of EF/SR intervention by describing routines or scripts of interaction organized in such a way that the individual gradually internalizes the script as automatic, self-regulatory self-talk. Thus, the theme is facilitation of automatic self-regulation or EF/SR habits via internalized, self-regulatory self-talk (Ylvisaker & Feeney, in press). The section ends with a discussion of empirical evidence.

The general notion that thinking, including self-regulatory self-talk, is internalized speech has a varied and venerable lineage, including classical philosophy (see, e.g., Plato in the *Phaedrus*), classical behavioral psychology (see, e.g., Skinner, 1953), and classical developmental cognitive psychology (see, e.g., Vygotsky, 1934). Often, the operation of these self-regulatory executive functions is assumed to be conscious and deliberate. Indeed, many theorists draw a sharp contrast between self-regulated behavior on the one hand and automatic or habitual behavior on the other. Fitzsimons and Bargh (2004) disputed this dichotomy by summarizing evidence showing that self regulation—that is, "the capacity of individuals to guide themselves . . . toward important goal states" (p. 151)—can be active, dynamic, complex, *and automatic*. Automatic EF/SR behavior in adults is illustrated by the habit or automatically triggered routine of fastening the seat belt when entering an automobile. The clinical need to automatize EF/SR scripts is based on studies (for review, see Schmeichel & Baumeister, 2004) showing that self-regulatory resources are depleted with effortful self-regulation. Individuals with frontal lobe or diffuse neuronal pathology often have limited processing resources even without placing additional demands on those resources with deliberate self-regulation (Schmitter-Edgecombe, 1996).

Consistent with the Vygotskyan theme of thinking as self-talk internalized from interaction with more competent members of the culture, Landry and colleagues recently documented a significant association between parents' interactive style and growth in the preschool child's executive self-regulatory functions, specifically problem-solving skills (Landry, Miller-Loncar, Smith, & Swank, 2002; Landry, Smith, Swank, Assel, & Vellet, 2001; Landry, Smith, & Swank, 2003). Effective parental scaffolding (including hints, prompts, and other verbal supports) at age 3 predicted high scores on executive function measures at age 6. In educational psychology, teacher "scaffolding" for problem solving (i.e., hints that facilitate success without taking over the problem-solving activity) have been shown to facilitate self-determined learners (Reeve, 2002; Reeve, Bolt, & Cai, 1999). Because many professionals take over the executive, self-regulatory aspects of functioning for individuals with disability, they should be alerted to the importance of engaging their clients in scripted EF/SR routines, providing whatever support may be necessary but stopping short of threatening the development of learned helplessness. Larsen and Prizmic (2004) reviewed the available developmental evidence regarding affect-regulation strategies, including self-talk strategies, that might be encouraged within these everyday routines of interaction.

Table 33–11 includes examples of specific EF/SR scripts as well as the most general goal-obstacle-plan-do-review

TABLE 33-11

Examples of Executive Function/Self-Regulation (EF/SR) Scripts of Interaction Designed to be Used at Appropriate Times in Real-World Contexts with the Goal of Having the Individual Internalize EF/SR Self-Talk

The words can be customized for specific individuals, and delivery should be conversational, non-punitive, and motivating. Questions can be used rather than statements if you are confident that the individual can answer the question.

General EF/SR Script: Goal-Obstacle-Plan-Do-Review
1. This is the goal (what do you want to accomplish, make happen; what will it look like when you're done?).
2. This might be hard because . . . So you need a plan; how about . . .?
3. Do it.
4. Review it: How did it work out? What worked for you? What didn't work? What adjustments need to be made?

Hard/Easy Script
1. This seems to be kind of hard (or easy) for you (or Hard or easy for you?).
2. I think it's hard (easy) because . . . (or Why do you think it's hard/easy?).
3. Because it's hard, you should probably . . . (or What do you think you can do?).
4. There's always something that works.

Ready/Not Ready Script
1. I think you are ready now (or You ready?).
2. You look ready because . . . (or What makes you think you're ready?).
3. Because you're ready, you can . . . (or What do you think you should do?).
4. There's always something that works.

Problem-Solving Script
1. This seems to be a problem.
2. It's a problem because . . . (or Why is this a problem?).
3. Let's see if this works . . . (or What do you want to try to solve the problem?).
4. There's always something that works.

Big Deal/Little Deal Script
1. I think this is a big deal (or not a big deal) (or Is this a big deal?).
2. It's a big (or little) deal because . . . (or Why is it a big deal?).
3. Because it's a big (little) deal, you . . . (or What do you think you should do?).
4. There's always something that works.

Scary/Not Scary (Dangerous/Not Dangerous) Script
1. This is kind of dangerous (or not dangerous) (or Do you think this might be dangerous?).
2. It's dangerous (or not) because . . . (or Why dangerous?).
3. Because it's dangerous, you . . . (or What do you think you should do?).
4. There's always something that works.

What About You Script
1. It's important to know what John thinks/John feels (or What's John's perspective?).
2. It's important because . . . (or Why should you try to get into John's head?).
3. Here's a way to find out (or How can you find out what John's perspective is?).
4. There's always something that works.

Experimental Script
1. You and I have different ideas about how to get this done.
2. We disagree because . . . (or Why do you suppose we disagree?).
3. Let's try it both ways and see what works best.
4. There's always something that works.

script, listed first because it is a simple operational definition of executive self-regulatory functioning that should pervade the facilitation process from preschool through adulthood. As a rule, successful people facing important decisions (a) make choices about what they wish to accomplish, (b) set reasonable goals for themselves (based on their understanding of their strengths and limitations), (c) identify obstacles to achieving the goals, (d) create intelligent plans for achieving the goals (possibly predicting their level of success), (e) act on the plans, and (f) review their performance, profiting from the feedback they receive (what worked and what did not work) (Meichenbaum & Biemiller, 1998). Often, these processes operate in a relatively automatic manner (Bargh & Chartrand, 1999). These same self-regulatory processes can—and should—become routine for people with disability, from preschoolers through adults. Clearly, people with significant impairment of executive function require considerable support from others to engage in these intellectual processes and, ultimately, make them habitual. Precisely such habits, however, are the goal of executive function intervention.

Figure 33–8 presents a guide for addressing the executive components of any task. With relevant modifications (e.g., simplifying the routine for people with substantial impairment), this general schema can be used to incrementally improve everyday routines of self-regulation. To remind individuals with disability and their caregivers to use the routine, we frequently post brightly colored reminders with the words GOAL-OBSTACLE-PLAN-DO-REVIEW and help family members, staff, and the person with TBI to become comfortable with simple, conversational use of the routine.

Scripts similar to those listed in Table 33–11 can be devised for strategy exploration routines, social self-control, and the like. The goal is to associate the scripts with the everyday occurrences for which that self-regulatory thought process would be helpful. With repetition and gradual reduction of supports, these scripts can then be internalized as relatively automatic, self-regulatory thought processes triggered by relevant environmental events. For some individuals, the scripts can be framed as questions (e.g., "Is this a big deal or a little deal?"); for others, questions should be avoided, particularly for those individuals whose anxiety is aroused by questions or who would have difficulty answering the question accurately. In some cases, it is important for clinicians to formulate the script for the individual carefully. In each case, the scripts should be delivered in a supportive, conversational manner using language that the person understands and reacts to positively. Ideally, these scripts are used frequently (while avoiding boredom and nagging) and within everyday action contexts when the person ideally should have use of the script as self-regulatory self-talk. To avoid negative associations with the scripts, the positive versions (e.g., easy, little deal, not a problem, and not scary) should predominate early in the facilitation process.

For many adolescents and young adults, particularly those with experience in sports (strongly valued in many cultures), we have framed this self-regulatory self-talk as self-coaching (Ylvisaker, 2006). Individualized self-regulatory (self-coaching) "plays" can be negotiated with the person and then videotaped during role-playing activities in which the words of the "self-coach" are used by the client, and perhaps, negotiated cueing words can be used by staff or other ECPs. The video also should include a meaningful rationale for the "play," possibly including relevant information about brains as well as about situations in which the play is important. In other words, the goal is not only to improve self-regulation of behavior and emotions but also to increase understanding of the personal and social worlds—all within the compelling context of personally meaningful sports metaphors. The video can then be repeatedly viewed, much as an athlete views game films, to improve performance by internalizing the self-coaching script.

Commonly used adolescent and young adult "self-coaching plays," in addition to those core plays listed in Table 33–11, include the following:

1. "Am I sure?" For example, am I sure that John is angry at me; did I interpret his behavior correctly? (Sports: Has the quarterback called the right play for this defense, or should he change the play at the line of scrimmage?)
2. "What exactly am I trying to accomplish?" For example, do I have a major test to study for or an important project at work? (Sports: Who's the opponent this week?)
3. "What's the game plan? What do I need to do to win?" For example, what do I need to do to prepare for this test? (Sports: What's the game plan?)
4. "How'd I do?" For example, did I get a low grade because I didn't study enough? What will I do the next time? (Sports: Review the game films.)
5. "Call time out! Spike the ball! Get organized!" For example, I feel overwhelmed, but maybe if I just stop and organize my tasks, I'll get back on track. (Sports: Call time out.)
6. "Let's think about that." For example, I feel like smacking him, but maybe I'd better get the facts. (Sports: Should the coach throw the replay flag or not?)

For sports-minded adolescents and young adults, sports metaphors should be used liberally to create positive associations with effortful self-regulation. For those who are not sports minded, a variety of other positive metaphors are available, such as "self-direction" (drama, film), "self-guiding" (hiking), "self-choreographing" (dance), "self-supervising" (business), and "self-conducting" (music).

Evidence for Self-Regulatory/Self-Talk Interventions

Self-talk interventions have been studied with a variety of disability populations, mainly children and adolescents.

Goal
What do I want to accomplish?

Obstacle
What might stand in the way of achieving my goal?

Plan
How am I going to accomplish my goal?

Materials/equipment	**Steps/assignments**
1.	1.
2.	2.
3.	3.
4.	4.

Predict
How well will I do? How much will I get done?

Choose
Do

Problems arise?	**Formulate solutions!**
1.	1.
2.	2.
3.	3.

Review

How did I do?

Self rating:

1   2   3   4   5   6   7   8   9   10

Other rating (teacher, therapist, peer, family member)

1   2   3   4   5   6   7   8   9   10

What worked?	**What didn't work?**
1.	1.
2.	2.
3.	3.

What will I try differently next time?

Figure 33–8. A guide for explicitly teaching or highlighting the executive components of any task. This form can be simplified to goal-obstacle-plan-do-review for ease of remembering. (Reproduced from Ylvisaker, Szekeres, and Feeney, 1998; with permission.)

Although this book is devoted to interventions for adults, evidence from the adolescent literature is relevant in this chapter, because many of the patients and clients in adult TBI programs are adolescents or young adults. The most thoroughly studied self-talk/self-regulation intervention is cognitive behavior modification (CBM) (Meichenbaum, 1977). Barkley (2004) reviewed the reviews and meta-analyses of CBM applied to adolescents with attention-deficit/hyperactivity disorder (ADHD; understood as an EF disorder) and concluded that, despite documentation of statistically significant improvements, the literature has failed to demonstrate clinically meaningful outcomes. Missing from Barkley's review, however, was a meta-analysis in which the investigators restricted their review to studies in which the intervention was delivered in the setting in which the problems were occurring. Robinson, Smith, Miller, and Brownell (1999) wisely restricted the scope of their meta-analysis to studies implemented in everyday school settings for adolescent students with aggressive behavior associated with ADHD. Twelve studies (with 36 effect size measures) yielded a large mean effect size of 0.64, or a 24-percentile rank increase for the CBM subjects compared to controls.

It is reasonable to interpret this positive meta-analysis—particularly in contrast to earlier pessimistic reviews—as underscoring the importance of a culture in which the interventions are embedded within the routines of everyday life, especially for children and adolescents with EF/SR impairment. Consistent with this interpretation, Berk (2001) pointed out that clinic-based CBM is not consistent with its purported Vygotskyan roots. Rather, modeling and coaching for self-regulatory self-talk should be provided within the individual's authentic tasks and settings. The approach described in this chapter is fully consistent with Berk's authoritative advice.

Reid, Trout, & Schartz (2005) completed a meta-analysis of peer-reviewed studies that examined the effectiveness of more specific self-regulation interventions for children with ADHD. The four interventions examined were self-monitoring training, self-monitoring plus reinforcement, self-reinforcement, and self-management (combining self-monitoring, self-rating, and self-evaluating). Each of these interventions can be readily incorporated within the scripts listed in Table 33–11. The 16 studies, which included 51 participants, were mainly single-subject experiments with elementary school students, implemented in their educational setting. Large effect sizes (greater than 0.8) were found for most of the interventions in relation to most of the outcome variables: on-task behavior, socially appropriate behavior, and academic accuracy and productivity. Furthermore, the self-regulation interventions showed a strong additive effect in those cases in which the children were simultaneously treated pharmacologically. Averaging across all interventions and outcomes, the effect sizes were greater than 1.0.

The meta-analysis of Reid and colleagues (2005) regarding executive function interventions for children with ADHD contrasts sharply with the results of a randomized, controlled clinical trial reported a year earlier by Abikoff and colleagues (Abikoff et al., 2004; Hechtman et al., 2004). These investigators found that none of the behavioral or psychosocial interventions for students with ADHD added to the effect size produced by medication alone. These contradictory findings can, perhaps, be explained by some combination of the following two differences: (1) The behavioral and social interventions in the study by Abikoff and colleagues were decontextualized and, therefore, poorly conceived in relation to what is known about the underlying impairment; and (2) the positive meta-analysis of Reid and colleagues mainly considered single-subject experiments. Single-subject studies tend to use highly individualized and context-sensitive interventions (in contrast to group intervention protocols like those used in the Abikoff et al. study), to select subjects likely to benefit from the intervention, and to terminate the study in the event of likely failure of the intervention.

Graham and Harris (2003) presented results of meta-analysis of 18 experimental studies that yielded large to very large effect sizes across a variety of outcome measures using their executive function academic curriculum, self-regulated strategy development. This program embeds several self-regulation scripts within its teaching routines. At least two additional studies have evaluated the effectiveness of teaching-learning routines in which the adolescent student is trained to use something like the goal-obstacle-plan-do-review EF/SR routine described in Table 33–11. Martin and colleagues (2003) found that a plan-work-evaluate-adjust routine, delivered in the context of everyday academic lessons, improved the self-regulated learning of intellectually normal students in a residential school for students with severe emotional and behavioral problems.

Wehmeyer, Palmer, Agran, Mithaug, & Martin (2000) evaluated the effectiveness of the Self-Determined Learning Model as applied to 40 adolescents with mild mental retardation, learning disabilities, or emotional/behavioral disturbance. Teaching-learning routines included 12 self-addressed questions that the students used to guide their learning behavior. Again, the goal-obstacle-plan-do-review EF/SR routine described in Figure 33–8 was represented in these questions:

- **Goal** "What do I want to learn?"
- **Obstacle** "What could keep me from taking action?"
- **Plan** "What can I do to make this happen?"
- **Do** "When will I take action?"
- **Review** "Do I now know what I want to know?"

Teacher facilitation of these self-talk questions resulted in goal attainment beyond teacher expectations and improvements on standardized measures of self-determination. No significant differences were found among the three disability groups, suggesting equal effectiveness across disabilities.

The lesson to be derived for clinicians from the variety of overlapping studies is that an underlying intervention theme can be operationalized in a variety of ways in a variety of settings with a variety of individuals. Therefore, rigid adherence to a specific model is clinically dangerous.

Functional Approaches to Executive Function and Cognitive Processes and Systems through the Continuum of Recovery

In Table 33–9, we present a plan for improving cognitive functioning for a specific individual who improved slowly after TBI and retained residual cognitive impairment. The focus of intervention in this case included organization, memory, language, and general executive functions, although any aspect of cognition could be targeted within this everyday, routine-based framework. The table includes appropriate goals, activities, and daily routines within which the intervention plan was implemented (including transfer activities) as well as a description of the types of mediation and support used at each phase. Project-oriented rehabilitation was used with Tom (Table 33-9) during both the middle and late stages of his cognitive recovery. Ylvisaker, Feeney, and Capo (2007) explore project-oriented interventions and supports in post-acute rehabilitation. We use the term "facilitator" to refer to people who have regular interaction with the person with disability (e.g., family members, direct care staff, therapists, teachers, job coaches, friends, co-workers, and others) and who therefore are in a position to use everyday activities and routines of life to facilitate improved cognitive functioning. Table 33–9 also suggests evolving uses for a log or memory book system over the continuum of recovery.

Clearly, specific activities and routines as well as specific intervention emphases within the broad domain of cognition vary from individual to individual. Our goal in offering the detailed intervention plan in Table 33–9 is to encourage clinicians to similarly apply, in an individualized manner, the intervention framework described earlier to specific individuals, integrating their goals, interests, needs, support systems, and routines of life.

Compensatory Strategies and Strategic Behavior

In the general five-step template for functional, everyday, routine-based intervention (Table 33–4) and also in the description of Tom's cognitive and executive function intervention (Table 33–9), we highlighted the use of compensatory procedures. Compensatory strategies are procedures—sometimes unconventional—that an individual deliberately uses to achieve goals that cannot be achieved without such special effort. Although the ultimate goal of intervention is habituation ("routinization") of the procedures so that their use need not consume limited attentional resources, we emphasize the word "deliberate" to distinguish this sense of "strategy" from the general notion of organized behavior, which often is referred to as a strategy, even if not

deliberate, and from instructional or treatment strategies, which are procedures used by therapists and teachers.

Strategies designed to compensate for cognitive deficits may involve the use of external aids (e.g., memory book, printed reminders, maps, task guide, alarm watch, electronic organizer, or pager system). External memory aids are discussed in the section on cognitive rehabilitation. Alternatively, a person might compensate using overt behavior (e.g., requesting clarification or repetition) or covert behavior (e.g., self-reminders, mental rehearsal or elaboration, or structured thinking procedures). Appendix 33–3 includes a large number (by no means exhaustive) of strategic procedures that appropriately selected individuals can use to compensate for selected cognitive and communicative deficits.

Compensatory strategies may be used temporarily in the case of transient impairment. Alternatively, they may be used indefinitely to reduce the functional disability of people with chronic impairment. Compensatory procedures may require effort initially but, with sufficient practice, become a routine component of the individual's automatic processing system, thereby possibly reducing the underlying impairment. Unfortunately, as discussed in earlier sections, the parts of the brain associated with strategic thinking and behavior (i.e., the frontal lobes) are particularly vulnerable in TBI. Therefore, intervention designed to equip individuals with strategic procedures for overcoming obstacles is, at the same time, extremely important and extremely tricky.

It is tempting to conceive of strategy intervention as being no different from other teaching—that is, the clinician identifies the client's needs, selects an appropriate strategy, selects appropriate teaching procedures, teaches the strategy, and then monitors and evaluates the outcome. The client's role is, therefore, to follow the clinician's lead and acquire the strategic procedure. If strategies are what strategic people do, however, then this model of teaching must be thought of as *antistrategic* **strategy intervention,** because all the truly strategic, problem-solving behavior is assumed by the clinician. In denying the client the right to participate in the strategic aspects of strategy learning, the clinician might inadvertently contribute to the client's learned helplessness—that is, passive reliance on others to solve critical problems posed by cognitive and communicative weakness. Furthermore, not only does this model of teaching fail to promote truly strategic behavior, it also has been found to fail the litmus tests of generalization and maintenance when applied to a variety of populations of impaired learners (Flavell, Miller, & Miller, 2002; Meichenbaum & Beimuller, 1998; Pressley, 1995; Pressley & Associates, 1990).

Following Pressley's advice to structure strategy intervention around a model of a good strategy user (Pressley, Borkowski, & Schneider, 1989), therefore, has clinical wisdom. Such a model serves not only to identify a variety of diverse goals that may be components of this intervention but also helps to separate reasonable from risky candidates for strategy intervention. Truly strategic people have the following characteristics:

- They have goals to which strategies are relevant.
- They know that their performance needs to be enhanced, that strategies enhance performance, and that they are capable of using strategies.
- They know when, where, and why to use specific strategic procedures.
- They monitor and evaluate the effectiveness of their performance so that being strategic is its own reward.
- They know a number of strategic procedures, can select the procedure most relevant to a particular challenge, and can flexibly modify it as needed or create new procedures.
- They use strategic procedures frequently so that they become relatively automatic and require little effort or planning.
- They have adequate "space" in working memory so that they can think about the task at hand and the strategic procedures at the same time (assuming that the strategies have not become automatic).
- They are not so impulsive that they habitually act before considering a strategic maneuver. (Context-sensitive automatization may overcome this obstacle.)
- They are not so anxious that they neglect strategic behavior because of their focus on fear of failure.
- They have the support of teachers, employers, and family members to use strategies.
- They know enough about the subject at hand that they can meaningfully use strategies to learn more.

Ideal candidates for strategy intervention are individuals who have specific goals; are aware of their needs; have sufficient meta-cognitive maturity to think about thinking, communicating, and other cognitive issues; are disposed to strategic behavior (e.g., like to play games of strategy); have adequate attentional resources; are motivated; have reasonable self-control; and live in supportive environments. College students returning to school after a mild to moderate injury often fall into this category. At the other extreme, individuals who are extremely weak in many of these dimensions may require considerable support to use all but the most simple external aid strategies (e.g., printed schedules or maps). For most people with TBI, strategy intervention includes attempts to improve functioning in a variety of domains (outlined above) that are related to strategic behavior.

Selection of the areas for compensation and of specific strategic procedures must involve active engagement of the client, which frequently includes a tension between his or her natural strategic inclinations and the judgment of the clinician. Brainstorming and experimentation with alternative strategies (Table 33–12) help to resolve this tension. The ultimate test of the appropriateness of the strategy is spontaneous, automatic use and improved performance in natural

settings. Intervention will inevitably fail if clients do not see the usefulness of the strategy relative to their goals or if the strategy does not fit the individual's overall style of learning, interacting, and coping. For example, it is quixotic at best to expect shy and generally noninteractive individuals to enthusiastically adopt an input control strategy that requires them to request that speakers slow down or clarify and simplify their language. Variables to be reviewed in negotiating the selection of strategies include:

- Whether the procedure is used spontaneously
- Whether its degree of complexity and abstractness fits the client's cognitive level
- How difficult the procedure is to use relative to its payoff
- Whether it fits the client's profile of neuropsychological strengths
- Whether it fits the client's personality
- Whether it specifically addresses obstacles to the individual's concrete goals

In Table 33–12, we outline intervention procedures that we have found to be useful in working with individuals who have TBI. The three components are very roughly sequential but should not be considered as mutually exclusive or hierarchical. For example, attempts to promote improved awareness of strengths and weaknesses (part of Component I) often continue throughout a client's entire rehabilitation program. In addition, work on generalization (Component IV) should begin early, before a procedure is habituated in a clinical setting.

In summary, our experience in helping individuals with TBI to become increasingly strategic underscores the importance of the following principles of strategy intervention:

1. Intervention should be embedded in natural, meaningful activities and settings, with strategic procedures specifically related to the client's goals.
2. The individual should be maximally engaged in experimenting with strategies, using the general goal-obstacle-plan-do-review format, selecting the strategies to use, and monitoring their effectiveness.
3. Intervention should be intensive and long term.
4. Goals should be modest.
5. Other things being equal, simple, low-tech options often are preferable to complicated, high-tech options, and external supports (e.g., graphic organizers for complex tasks or memory books) often are preferable to internal elaboration and organization strategies (Evans, Needham, Wilson, & Brentnall, 2003).
6. The environment as a whole should be supportive of and promote strategic thinking and strategic behavior.

In the absence of sensitivity to these principles, strategic compensations for cognitive or others impairments are unlikely to be maintained over time (Wilson & Watson,

TABLE 33–12

Teaching Compensatory Strategies

Note: These components of intervention are not necessarily hierarchical or mutually exclusive.

Component I: General Strategic thinking

A. Meta-cognitive Awareness
Goals: Clients will discriminate effective from ineffective performance; become increasingly aware of their strengths and needs; recognize implications of their deficits.
Rationale: Given the frequency of frontolimbic and right hemisphere damage in TBI, self-awareness is frequently compromised. Individuals are unlikely to acquire and use procedures designed to compensate for problems that they do not recognize as problems.
Procedures:
1. **Objective:** Improve the client's perception of successful versus unsuccessful task performance.
   Procedures: Illustrate successful and unsuccessful performance of a functional task through role play or on videotape. With the client, analyze the performances in sufficient detail that the client can identify the features that account for successful versus unsuccessful performance.
2. **Objective:** Improve the client's ability to perceive functional impairments.
   Procedures: Individually, request that the client make note of specific deficits of other clients in the program or of individuals observed on tape. Discuss these observations. Planned peer teaching is useful. Discuss the effects of TBI on cognitive and social functioning. If appropriate, read and discuss literature on the effects of TBI.
3. **Objective:** Improve the client's awareness of his or her own strengths and weaknesses.
   Procedures: Videotape the client in activities designed to reveal strong and weak areas of functioning. (Alternatively, use role play.) Review the tapes (beginning with strong performance), first without commentary, subsequently inviting comments about what was done well and what needs improvement. Gradually turn over to the client the responsibility for stopping the tape when problems are noted. **Note:** Considerable desensitizing may be needed before video self-viewing is possible.
4. **Objective:** Improve the client's understanding of the relation between deficits and long-term goals.
   Procedures: Discuss in concrete detail the individual's long-term goals and expectations. Jointly create a list of specific skills and resources needed to achieve these goals. Jointly identify the skills that are present and those that are weak relative to this goal.
Note: These meta-cognitive discoveries are facilitated if the activities are personally meaningful and intimately connected to the client's goals.
B. Value of Being Strategic
Goal: Clients will recognize the importance of being strategic and will identify the characteristics of strategic people.
Rationale: Since the ultimate goal of this intervention is to promote strategic thinking and strategic behavior in general—not simply to teach specific strategic behaviors as routines—it is important that the client understand what it is to be strategic and that these are valuable attributes.
Procedures:
1. **Objective:** Improve the client's understanding of strategy.
   Procedures: Using games, sports, or other relevant model, clarify the concept of strategy as something that one does to achieve goals when there are obstacles.
2. **Objective:** Heighten the client's appreciation of strategic behavior.
   Procedures: Together with the client, identify several individuals who are known to be very strategic (e.g., sports heroes or military heroes). Discuss why they are considered to be heroic. Clinicians also should clearly model their own strategic behavior and discuss the value of their own strategies.
3. **Objective:** Improve the client's understanding of the behaviors that are part of being strategic.
   Procedures: Using models relevant to the client (e.g., military, sports, or business analogies), brainstorm about the characteristics of people who are known to be very strategic. Include high level of motivation and initiative; ability to identify and clarify obstacles to goals; ability to plan procedures to overcome obstacles; ability to monitor and evaluate performance; willingness to engage in ongoing problem solving.

Component II: Selecting Specific Strategic Procedures
Goal: Clients will identify specific procedures useful in overcoming important personal obstacles.
Rationale: It is important that clients participate in the selection of strategic procedures that they will use and that the procedures be truly useful in achieving their goals.

(continued)

TABLE 33–12

Teaching Compensatory Strategies (continued)

Procedures:
1. Use group brainstorming procedures to identify possible strategies.
2. Use "product monitoring" tasks to test the value of strategies: Have the client perform a task with and without the strategy or with a variety of different strategies. Objectively compare the results. (Video analysis may be useful here.)
3. Have advanced clients demonstrate the value of certain procedures or offer testimonials.
4. Discuss the widespread use of compensatory procedures (e.g., lists, memos, tape recorders, and so forth) by people who do not have brain injury.

Component III: Teaching Specific Strategies
Note: If the discovery procedures in Component II (e.g., brainstorming and product monitoring) are effective, there may be little need for specific teaching procedures.
Procedures:
A. **Modeling:** The steps in the strategy can be modeled by the therapist, by a peer, or by means of videotape or other media. Modeling is initially accompanied by overt verbalization of the strategy by the model. The client then rehearses the strategy with gradually decreasing cues and self-talk.
B. **Direct Instruction:** The carefully programmed behavioral teaching procedures of direct instruction can be used to teach strategies. If this is the only approach used, however, the best result likely will be the acquisition of a learned sequence of behaviors (which may be a desirable outcome) without positive movement in the direction of becoming a strategic person.
C. **Functional Practice:** However the strategy is acquired, it must be frequently rehearsed in natural settings using functional activities.

Component IV: Generalization and Maintenance
Generalization of strategic behavior beyond the context of training is a combined consequence of the perceived utility of the strategy for the individual, the inherent generalizability and utility of the strategy, widespread environmental support for strategic behavior and thinking, intensive practice in a variety of real-world contexts, and specific teaching procedures designed to enhance generalization.
Note 1: Generalization includes generalized use of specific strategies as well as strategic behavior in general.
Note 2: Generalization may not be a separate phase if the acquisition stage takes place in the context of functional activities and natural settings. This is particularly important for very concrete people.
Note 3: Generalization may be a relatively unimportant phase of intervention if the individual has acquired a strategic attitude and actively seeks occasions for transfer.
Note 4: Some individuals may need environmental reminders indefinitely to use their strategic procedures.
1. **Objective:** Improve the client's discrimination of situations that require or do not require a given strategy.
   Procedures: Use videotaped scenes or role playing to illustrate the correct use of a strategy in an appropriate situation, inappropriate use of the strategy, and failure to use the strategy when appropriate. Discuss the conditions that require the strategy. Use short videotaped scenes to train the client in efficient and accurate judgments as to whether a strategy is appropriate in a context.
2. **Objective:** Increase the client's spontaneous use of strategies in varied situations.
   Procedures: Include family members, work supervisors, and teachers in strategy intervention to (1) provide varied opportunities for the use of specific strategies and of strategic behavior in general, (2) reinforce the client's use of strategies, and (3) model strategic behavior themselves. Ask clients to keep a log in which they record their successes and failures in strategy use. Make generalization an explicit goal.
3. **Objective:** Increase the client's acceptance of strategic behavior.
   Procedures: Ensure that the client is successful using strategies. Promote emotional acceptance of strategic behavior by using whatever motivating procedures work (e.g., personal images or metaphors, testimonials, and the like).

Key: TBI = traumatic brain injury.
Modified from Haarbauer-Krupa, Henry, Szekeres, and Ylvisaker (1985); with permission.

1996). The TBI literature contains an increasing number of reports regarding the effectiveness of compensatory strategy intervention (Carney et al., 1999; Cicerone et al., 2005; Kennedy et al., 2007, accepted), but a much larger evidence base exists in educational psychology (Baker et al., 2002; Gersten, Fuchs, Williams, & Baker, 2001; Martin et al., 2003; Pressley & Associates, 1990; Resnick, 1987; Sweet & Snow, 2002), which Pressley (1993) has attempted to apply to the field of cognitive intervention after TBI. Meichenbaum (1993) discussed the application of a related set of intervention procedures, CBM, to TBI rehabilitation.

Strategies and Discourse Impairment

For language specialists, discourse represents the intersection of language skill, cognitive/organizational schemas, facility with perspective taking (to be sensitive to the needs of communication partners), and strategic direction of organizing schemas to specific contexts and material. Effective discourse requires action planning in the verbal domain (Alexander, 2002). Organizational difficulties, as a component of executive function impairment, often result in difficulty organizing thoughts and behavior for effective learning and performance of activities of daily living, complex work activities, efficient word retrieval, expressive discourse tasks (speaking and writing), extended text comprehension, and other complex social, educational, or vocational tasks that require organization.

Grafman's neuropsychological theory of specific event complexes and managerial knowledge units (Grafman, 2002, 1995; Grafman et al., 1993) maintains that the foundation for focused attention, organized thinking and talking, efficient remembering, effective planning, and success with any organizationally demanding task lies in the effective use of organized knowledge structures (schemas) of greater or lesser generality with respect to domains of content. "Managerial knowledge unit" is a particularly felicitous phrase in its identification of the need for neurologic management of complex behavior. Discourse, understood as the organization of language over many sentences, requires management for successful communication of complex ideas. Effective application of these knowledge schemas relies on the development of domain-specific knowledge and intactness of frontal lobe structures, explaining much of the disorganized discourse of individuals with impairment of executive function associated with prefrontal brain pathology.

Some discourse schemas or managerial knowledge units are tightly structured, such as the organizational structure of scientific reports, basic narratives, and menus. Others are less structured, such as describing a vacation or persuading a friend to give up smoking. Left hemisphere dorsolateral prefrontal damage tends to result in discourse that is impoverished in both words and themes. Individuals with right hemisphere damage may be verbose, tangential, and socially awkward in their discourse. Impaired theory of mind, associated with prefrontal damage (more right than left), causes inattention to the needs and tolerance of listeners and, therefore, socially ineffective discourse (Alexander, 2002).

Ylvisaker, Szekeres, and Haarbauer-Krupa (1998) discussed organizational impairment within a neuropsychological framework and presented a variety of intervention and support approaches. Advance organizational supports for complex tasks, including graphic organizers of a variety of types, have become an evidence-based standard of practice in many settings in which disorganized individuals are supported. Bulgren and Schumaker (2006) reviewed 19 successful studies of advance organizers, all with adolescent participants with or without disability. Graphic organizers also are commonplace supports for nondisabled adults, including maps, blueprints, and sequences of pictures to guide individuals through the assembly of products that are sold unassembled.

Perhaps the most studied discourse structure in both children and adults is narrative structure or story grammar. Elementary students benefit from a clear flow diagram that includes the components of a narrative as they attempt to comprehend and produce stories more effectively. We have used a similar graphic organizer for adults with TBI in a literacy group. The organizer has three side-by-side boxes at the top for characters, place, and time. The remaining boxes progress downward in a linear manner and include the initiating event (that starts the narrative action), the main characters' reactions to that event, the plan that is developed, the ensuing action, and the resolution. Because this also is the organization of the mental representation of everyday events in life, this organizer is particularly important. As the components of narrative structure are internalized, the diagram can be gradually faded. Ylvisaker, Szekeres, and Haarbauer-Krupa (1998) presented a variety of graphic advance organizers and procedures for their implementation. A critical feature of organizers is that they accurately capture the organization of that which is to be organized. Many graphic organizers available in special education materials are visually attractive but fail to meet this obvious standard (e.g., representing a narrative as circular rather than linear).

Specific Cognitive Interventions

Cognitive rehabilitation, in a meaningful and broad sense of the term, includes all the interventions described in the previous sections under the heading of executive functions. For purposes of exposition in this chapter, we have separated out specific cognitive themes for discussion in the current section. After offering a functional operational definition of cognition, we present a critique of traditional, process-specific cognitive retraining exercises. We then discuss themes in cognitive rehabilitation that have received special attention over the past decade, memory aids, errorless learning, and the use of virtual reality in rehabilitation.

Cognition: An Intervention-Relevant Operational Definition

Because of the complexity of cognition and the relationships among its components, as well as the variety of theoretical descriptions of cognition and its development in childhood (see, e.g., Ashcraft, 1994; Barsalou, 1992; Dodd & White, 1980; Flavell, Miller, & Miller, 2002; Siegler & Alibali, 2004), the construction of a coherent and manageable framework for cognitive-communication intervention becomes a major challenge. Just such a framework is critical, however, because it helps clinicians to avoid a haphazard and inefficient "workbook" approach to treatment, facilitates communication among professionals and between clinicians and clients, promotes systematic observation and program evaluation, and serves as a source of intervention principles and procedures.

Appendix 33.1 presents a scheme for organizing descriptions of behavior from a cognitive perspective. The scheme is based generally on information processing theories of cognition, wherein cognition is viewed broadly as the processing of information for particular purposes within specific mental structures and environmental constraints and directed by the executive control system (Dodd & White, 1980). In our clinical work, we have found it productive to describe cognitive functioning and recovery in terms of three general aspects of cognition: (1) processes, (2) systems, and (3) functional-integrative performance. Each of the processes and systems relates, in identifiable ways, to language and communication.

Profiles of cognitive impairment after TBI can be varied and complex, requiring thorough exploration with formal neuropsychological assessments and, more importantly for treatment purposes, context-sensitive hypothesis-testing, as described earlier. Treatment decisions are further driven by decisions about relationships among cognitive processes and systems. For example, a person with TBI may process information slowly, appear to be inattentive, forget easily, show evidence of disorganized thinking and behavior, misperceive social cues, respond impulsively, and appear to have lost social and vocational knowledge. These may be separate impairments, but more likely, at least some are related. For example, problems with memory, organization, and social perception all may be secondary to attentional impairment. Alternatively, difficulty attending and slowed processing may be caused, in part, by loss of organizing schemes and preinjury knowledge, which also may reduce memory efficiency. Hypothesis testing with alternative support strategies helps to answer these questions, which often are left unanswered by comprehensive neuropsychological assessment.

An understanding of cognition from a developmental perspective (Flavell, Miller, & Miller, 2002; Siegler & Alibali, 2004) is useful in avoiding common pitfalls in cognitive rehabilitation for adults. Clinicians who believe that cognitive processes are serially ordered in development are naturally inclined to embrace a hierarchical progression in rehabilitation, first addressing components of attention and then, perhaps, perception, organization and memory, and finally, executive control over cognitive processes. This model is inconsistent with the essential interrelations among components of cognition that dominate cognitive development in children and yields an inefficient and misguided approach to intervention.

Decontextualized Cognitive Retraining

In the early period of program development for survivors of severe TBI, cognitive rehabilitation was understood by many practitioners as being an enterprise that involved (a) hierarchical organization of cognitive processes and subprocesses (e.g., attention is more basic than organization, and maintaining attention is more basic than shifting attention), (b) creation of cognitive exercises that targeted specific aspects of cognition in a hierarchical manner, and (c) efficient delivery of exercises using massed learning trials outside the context of functional application of the cognitive processes being trained (Ben-Yishay & Diller, 1983; Ben-Yishay, Piasetsky, & Rattok, 1987; Sohlberg & Mateer, 1987). In the 1970s, customized retraining devices were designed for the delivery of cognitive exercises. In the 1980s, these devices largely were replaced by cognitive retraining software.

These early developments in TBI rehabilitation were remarkably similar in theory and practice to unsuccessful attempts in the early 20th century to cure mental retardation with hierarchically organized cognitive exercises and to largely unsuccessful efforts in the 1950s, 1960s, and 1970s to cure learning disabilities with decontextualized cognitive exercises (Kavale & Mattson, 1983; Mann, 1979). In both of these older fields of intervention (based on the 19th-century concept of separate "faculties of the mind" that can be strengthened with exercises), decontextualized cognitive training tasks have largely given way to context-sensitive efforts to improve cognitive processing and self-regulated learning within the context of meaningful academic, social, vocational, and other daily activities.

This sea change in cognitive rehabilitation has been motivated, in part, by a growing experimental literature documenting the failure of transfer from improvements on decontexualized training tasks to everyday performance in everyday settings. Park and Ingles (2001) subjected studies concerning the effectiveness of decontextualized attention process training in TBI rehabilitation to a meta-analysis and concluded that well-controlled studies showed a minimal effect size, whereas efforts to improve attention within the context of specific everyday activities demonstrated a substantial effect size. Thus, general attention process training has given way to a focus on attention within the context of specific tasks that require attentional skill, such as driving (Park & Ingles, 2001), or attention training with a metacognitive or compensatory strategy focus (Cicerone, 2002; Cicerone et al., 2005).

Similarly, efforts to improve memory functioning with decontextualized memory exercises have been found to be ineffective at any stage of recovery after TBI (Baddeley, 1999; Cicerone et al., 2005; Schacter, 1996; Thoene, 1996; Wilson, 1995). In recent years, memory rehabilitation therefore has focused on the use of external memory aids, internal memory strategies, and errorless teaching/learning procedures specifically designed for individuals with severe memory impairment (discussed below). As often is the case, practice in the field of cognitive rehabilitation has not kept up with research. Thus, many practitioners continue to use exercise-oriented, cognitive retraining computer programs as well as workbooks with page after page of exercises in cognitive skills, such as sequencing, categorizing, associating, and the like, despite the well-documented failure of improvements with these exercises to transfer to everyday tasks (Carney et al., 1999; Ylvisaker, 2003).

Memory Aids

External memory aids are widely considered to be the most commonly used—and the most effective—intervention for chronic memory impairments (Evans, 2003; Wilson, 1992). External aids include environmental modifications (e.g., labeling rooms, cupboards, etc.; color coding; positioning to-be-remembered items; and training communication partners to be effective memory prosthetics), memory prosthetics actively used by the individual (e.g., memory books, appointment books/calendars, and electronic memory aids), and memory prosthetics requiring no activation by the person (e.g., pager systems).

Sohlberg and colleagues (2007) reviewed 19 studies concerning the effectiveness of memory aids involving 267 participants, all with significant memory impairments. Although most of the studies were single-subject designs or case studies, sufficient evidence was found for the authors to conclude that provision of memory aids to individuals with memory impairment after TBI should be considered a practice guideline. The most commonly used was the memory notebook, which also was the most commonly studied (nine studies). Training methods often were unspecified, and considerable variation existed among those studies that did describe the training.

Evans and colleagues (2003) studied the use of memory aids in 94 individuals with memory impairment, mainly associated with TBI. The most commonly used aids were a calendar or wall chart (68/94), memory notebook (60/94), lists (59/94), appointment diary (41/94), and asking others for reminders (46/94). Uncommonly used aids or procedures included electronic organizer (7/94), tape recorder (2/94), visual imagery (9/94), first-letter mnemonics (5/94), rhymes (2/94), and "chunking" (1/94). These numbers are worth attending to, because rehabilitation professionals often are drawn to sophisticated electronic devices (rarely used) and superficial internal mnemonics (rarely used). The infrequent use of internal mnemonics, however, may be an artifact of the participants (e.g., relatively few students who need to study for exams) and of the mnemonics sampled. Studies in educational psychology indicate that elaborative encoding strategies that go beyond superficial rhyming and first-letter mnemonics are useful in deepening comprehension and, thereby, in facilitating retrieval.

Forty-seven percent of the 94 participants were considered to be independent in the sense that they worked for pay, were full-time students, lived alone, and/or played a major role in running a household and caring for children. Evans and colleagues (2003) identified a statistically significant association between independence and regular use of three or more memory aids. Thus, it may be that clinicians need to equip individuals who have memory impairment with a variety of memory aids or strategies to be used for specific material or on specific occasions. Those participants who maintained regular use of six or more types of memory aids tended to be younger, more recently injured, higher in intellectual ability, better at attending, and more aware of and distressed about their memory impairment. Higher executive function scores predicted more effective use of aids (versus simply more use).

Many people with memory impairment predictably forget to use their memory prostheses (Kapur, 1995). Therefore, reminder systems have been developed that do not rely on the individual's initiation or ability to remember to use the system. "Passive" systems of this sort are comparable to passive restraints in automobiles, such as air bags, that (unlike seat belts) do not rely on the individual to do anything to be protected. For example, NeuroPage is an integration of computer and paging technologies that enables people with memory, planning, organization, attention, or initiation problems to receive pre-dictated reminders at specified times through an alphanumeric pager (Hersh & Treadgold, 1994). The reminders can be typed into the system by the individual or a caregiver. This system has been sufficiently effective that it is covered by the British health system (Wilson, Emslie, Quirk, & Evans, 2001).

For people who cannot read effectively or who have other impairments that interfere with attending to a pager screen, voice reminder systems are available. Van den Broek, Downes, Johnson, Dayus, and Hilton (2000) found that the Voice Organizer, a hand-held, dictaphone-type voice output reminder device, benefitted five of five patients with prospective memory impairment. Yasuda and colleagues (2002) found that the recently developed Sony IC Recorder, a voice output memory aid capable of producing approximately 300 spoken messages (48 minutes) at programmed times, served as a successful prompt for five of eight patients with prospective memory impairment, creating a dramatic improvement in their everyday lives.

Intelligently prescribed passive reminder systems are capable of reducing caregiver burden, increasing the likelihood that people with memory impairment will stay healthy by eating and taking prescribed medications at appropriate times and improving quality of life by reducing painful reliance on others. However, a minimal level of initiation, motivation, and self-awareness likely is necessary for such systems to succeed (Yasuda et al., 2002).

Implicit Memory and Errorless Learning

The practice of teaching habits (routines) of thought, communication, and social conduct using antecedent supports is additionally bolstered by recent findings in the areas of implicit and procedural memory and errorless learning. Significant damage to the hippocampus and para-hippocampal structures (common in TBI) typically impairs declarative memory (i.e., remembering that such and such is the case) and explicit memory (i.e., having a subjective sense that one possesses the memory) but may leave procedural memory (i.e., remembering how to do something, including motor sequences, skilled operations, or other habits) and implicit memory (i.e., possessing a memory trace that influences future behavior but lacking a subjective sense that one remembers) relatively intact (Bachman, 1992; Izard, 1992; Pascual-Leone, Grafman, & Hallett, 1995; Schacter, 1996; Squire, 1992).

In their now-classic studies, Glisky and Schacter (1988, 1989) have found that people with apparently dense amnesia after brain injury are still capable of implicit memory and procedural learning. Similarly, Shum, Sweeper, and Murray (1996) found that subjects with TBI performed relatively poorly on explicit memory tasks but comparable to controls on implicit memory tasks. In their "good guy/bad guy" experiments, Tranel and Damasio (1993) found that individuals with severe amnesia associated with damage to para-hippocampal structures nevertheless create implicitly stored affective memories about people with whom they have had positive or negative experiences despite no explicit memories for those people.

In the presence of such neuropsychological profiles, which are common in varying degrees after TBI, Barbara Wilson, Jonathan Evans, and others have found errorless learning procedures to be a critical component of rehabilitation (Evans et al., 2000; Kessels & De Haan, 2003; Kessels et al., 2005; Riley & Heaton, 2000; Tailby & Haslam, 2005; Wilson & Evans, 1996; Wilson, Baddeley, Evans, & Shiel, 1994). Therapy tasks for individuals with significant memory problems should be organized in such a way that potential errors are anticipated and prevented with advance cues. Apprenticeship ("scaffolded") teaching procedures can achieve this goal as the teacher/collaborator ensures successful and error-free performance during learning tasks. Similarly, the need for error-free learning is one of the supports for VR technology in rehabilitation. Cues can be given before a response and then systematically withdrawn (Brooks et al., 1999; Rizzo, Schulteis, Kerns, & Mateer, 2004). In the case of less severe memory impairment, trial-and-error learning may be preferable to errorless learning, because it encourages deeper processing and improved explicit memory (Squires, Hunkin, & Parkin, 1997).

When people with severe explicit and declarative memory impairment make errors and experience a rush of embarrassment or anger when those errors are corrected, they are likely to store the erroneous response, but not associated with an awareness of the response as an error. Thus, the erroneous memory influences future behavior in an insidious manner. That is, people who seem to have severe memory impairment may encode and store some memories effectively, particularly when associated with strong emotional reactions—and errors often elicit strong emotional reactions. Under these circumstances, clinicians must ensure that the information being processed and the behaviors being rehearsed are the correct information and the desired behaviors. These neuropsychological considerations have revived a decades-old tradition of errorless learning in animal training (Terrace, 1963) and in developmental disabilities (Sidman & Stoddard, 1967), and they serve as an additional buttress for a supported, everyday, routine-based approach to rehabilitation for people with significant cognitive impairment after TBI.

Virtual Reality and Cognitive Rehabilitation

Rizzo and colleagues (2004) summarized the potential benefits of VR technology in neuropsychological rehabilitation. The central theme of VR as applied to cognitive rehabilitation is ecological validity and context-sensitivity of the training tasks and task environments, thereby addressing the failure of much traditional rehabilitation at the level of transfer of treatment gains to real-world settings and activities. Current applications of VR technology (in research centers) enable the creation of real-world virtual environments, including virtual cities, supermarkets, homes, kitchens, school environments, workspaces, and more. Within these realistic environments, a variety of ecologically valid assessment and training tasks can be constructed.

Compared with both traditional artificial tasks and real-world tasks, advantages of VR intervention include the following (as summarized by Rizzo et al., 2004):

1. Precise presentation and control of dynamic multi-sensory, three-dimensional stimulus environments. For example, it is possible to gradually build up complexity of tasks within a realistic VR environment for development of compensatory strategies or just practice under increasingly complex circumstances (e.g., driving, meal preparation).
2. Advanced methods for recording behavioral responses and delivering immediate performance feedback.
3. Provision of pre-planned systematic cueing to support error-free learning.
4. Potential for "after-action reviews" from a variety of virtual perspectives.

5. Safe testing and training environments.

6. Improved access to assessment and training for persons with sensorimotor impairments via adapted interface devices and tailored sensory modality presentations.

7. Increasingly realistic virtual human representations (avatars). This technologic development may create the possibility of VR training in social interaction, naturalistic communication, and awareness of social cues. Related procedures are now used in treating anxiety disorders and public speaking phobias.

Evaluation of the effectiveness of VR interventions is in its infancy; however, preliminary studies are promising, with documented success, including transfer of training, on tasks such as meal preparation (Fidopiastis et al., 2006), route finding (Brooks et al., 1999), and driving (Schulteis & Mourant, 2001). Until such procedures are well validated and the technology reasonably priced, VR may remain only a promise in TBI rehabilitation.

Behavioral and Psychosocial Rehabilitation

Importance of Behavioral and Psychosocial Issues

In the earlier section on outcome, we highlighted the frequency of personality changes, behavioral problems, and associated social interactive weakness after TBI. Difficulties in this domain may be a result of the injury but often are complicated by preinjury challenges and postinjury social, academic, and vocational failure and consequent adjustment problems. Our work with several hundred adolescents and young adults with chronic school and work problems and general community reintegration difficulty suggests that behavioral and psychosocial themes often are at the core of these problems, although in most cases, complex patterns of interaction exist between cognitive and behavioral consequences of the injury.

Furthermore, costs associated with failure of rehabilitation and community support efforts are staggering. In recent years, we have served more than 1,000 young adults through a New York State community support project for individuals with TBI, some degree of chronic behavioral impairment, and demonstrated lack of success in community reintegration using standard services and supports. Conservative Department of Health estimates regarding the cost of serving these individuals without a targeted community support program, based on expenses for the year before their introduction to the program, exceed $40,000,000 annually. Because most of the people served by the program were more than 5 years postinjury at the time of referral and had failed in previous rehabilitation attempts, the state had projected enormous lifetime costs for this population (Feeney et al., 2001).

Speech-language pathologists have a natural role in this domain of service delivery under the headings of pragmatics of language and teaching positive communication alternatives to challenging behavior. Pragmatics has a long history within the profession—and in other professions—under the label of social skills. The role of speech-language pathologists in behavior management may be somewhat more controversial but is included in the ASHA's scope of practice and has become commonplace in many settings where individuals with developmental disabilities are served (Carr et al., 1994; Reichle & Johnston, 1993; Reichle & Wacker, 1993; Ylvisaker & Feeney, 1994). In this section, we outline and offer a rationale for a context-sensitive, self-coaching approach to social skills weakness; a positive, antecedent-focused approach to challenging behavior; and a collaborative, context-sensitive approach to teaching positive communication alternatives to negative behavior.

Building Repertoires of Positive Social Communication Routines

Traditional Social Skills (and Pragmatics) Training

Social skills include general competencies (e.g., self-control), personal attributes (e.g., concern for others), and situationally relative social behaviors (e.g., communication scripts appropriate for the workplace, classroom interaction, church groups, bar room conversations, and others) that enable a person to be socially successful in selected settings. Historically, social skills intervention, a component of which is pragmatics training, has been understood as an effort to equip individuals with knowledge of social rules, roles, and routines along with the communication competencies that are components of those routines. Thus, the primary goal of the service is to impart social knowledge, both declarative (knowing that certain behaviors are desirable in specific contexts) and procedural (knowing how to perform the behaviors).

Traditional social skills training (SST) often takes place in social skills or pragmatics groups—outside of the context of real social interaction—guided by a curriculum that specifies the social competencies needed by the group members and the types of modeling and role playing that are used to teach and rehearse the skills. Many structured SST programs have been developed for individuals representing varied populations (see, e.g., Goldstein, Sprafkin, Gershaw, & Klein, 1980; Sheinker & Sheinker, 1988; Waksman, Messmer, & Waksman, 1989; Walker et al., 1988; Walker, Todis, Holmes, & Horton, 1988). Designed for children, adolescents, or adults from culturally diverse backgrounds or with developmental disabilities, learning problems, or psychiatric disorders, the programs are organized around training groups within which the participants practice social behaviors considered to be relevant to their social success. Such training programs differ with respect to the degree to which they emphasize discrete trial training or social problem solving. The common thread, however, is repeated practice in a socially decontextualized training setting.

In part because of the logistical ease with which such group SST can be implemented in rehabilitation hospitals and outpatient clinics, SST or pragmatics groups enjoy considerable popularity in TBI rehabilitation. Limited evidence suggests that SST of this sort can be somewhat effective with some adolescents and young adults with TBI, particularly with an emphasis on self-monitoring (Braunling-McMorrow, Lloyd, & Fralish, 1986; Brotherton, Thomas, Wisotzek, & Milan, 1988; Gajar, Schloss, Schloss, & Thompson, 1984; Johnson & Newton, 1987). Concerns about the usefulness of decontextualized role play–based SST, however, arise at several levels.

First, traditional SST (defined above) has received little support in the many experimental studies of its use with a variety of clinical populations. Gresham and colleagues (2001) reviewed several narrative reviews and meta-analyses of this extensive research literature and concluded that "SST has not produced large, socially important, long-term, or generalized changes in the social competence of students with high-incidence disabilities" (p. 331). Specifically, they described two meta-analyses. The first included 99 studies of SST applied to students with emotional and behavioral disturbance, with a small mean effect size of 0.20. The second included 53 studies of SST applied to students with learning disabilities, with a similarly small mean effect size of 0.21. Likewise, the randomized, controlled clinical trial by Abikoff and colleagues of interventions for students with ADHD (a population similar in pathophysiology and symptomatology to those with TBI) found that decontextualized SST added nothing to the effect size produced by medication alone (Abikoff et al., 2004; Hechtman et al., 2004).

Second, even at the level of theoretical rationale, a clear disconnect exists between traditional SST and the types of social interaction problems that are common after TBI. The success of traditional SST groups (including pragmatics groups typically led by speech-language pathologists) assumes that the participants (1) lack knowledge of relevant social rules, roles, and routines; (2) are motivated to change their social behavior; (3) possess the capacity to transfer skills acquired in a training setting to varied real-world application settings; (4) modify their behavior in response to planned contingencies; and (5) are reasonably self-regulated. Unfortunately, the profile of many individuals with TBI is the opposite of that suggested by these assumptions. With relatively damaged anterior brain structures and relatively preserved posterior structures, individuals with a common profile after TBI typically possess relevant declarative social knowledge but are poorly regulated, have difficulty transferring social knowledge to daily living, respond inefficiently to behavioral contingencies, and may lack the motivation to change, particularly if the injury has reduced their awareness

of their interactive social competence and the effects of their behavior on others. Thus, no reason exists to believe that traditional SST (or pragmatics training) holds promise for those individuals with TBI with the most common neuropsychological profiles. Rather, the combination of inhibition, initiation, planning, working memory, and resource allocation impairments common in TBI lends itself to intervention designed to create positive habits of interaction in the social contexts in which the skills in question are needed. Creation of positive habits of interaction requires individualized selection of teaching targets and extensive coached practice in context.

Self-Coaching and Scripts of Social Interaction

Since the early 1980s, Ylvisaker and colleagues have used self-coaching as a metaphor and set of procedures in TBI rehabilitation (see, e.g., Ylvisaker & Holland, 1985). Because TBI disproportionately affects active young people who typically have personal experiences and positive associations with sports as participants or fans, the self-coaching metaphor yields insight regarding self-regulatory/executive system concerns and potential social strategies. Individuals who have self-regulatory impairment but desire higher levels of success in their social, educational, and vocational lives often agree to organize themselves around self-coaching procedures ("plays") despite possible opposition to other intervention approaches. The term "play" refers to an organized strategy, plan, or script, such as that performed during a football game or other athletic contest.

The general goal of self-coaching is to improve planful goal-oriented and, ultimately, successful behavior while decreasing impulsive and reactive behavior. Applied to social interaction, self-coaching plays include specific scripts that enable a person to successfully negotiate personally relevant social environments. Self-coaching has its historical roots in the view that self-regulation is, at its core, self-regulatory self-talk, even if that self-talk is automatic and minimally conscious.

As a psychological therapy, self-coaching most closely resembles cognitive-behavior therapy and, more specifically, cognitive-behavior modification (Meichenbaum, 1977), but with the important caveat that self-coaching is, ideally, an everyday, context-sensitive (versus clinic-bound) intervention, with "plays" that also specify roles for ECPs. According to Berk (2001), this "everyday routine" approach to self-regulatory self-talk is consistent with the views of Vygotsky, which were distorted when self-talk therapies became clinical interventions delivered in a manner insensitive to everyday contextual realities.

Self-coaching plays (including self-regulatory self-talk scripts) can be designed to address a variety of obstacles common after TBI: poorly controlled emotions, impulsive or otherwise ineffective social interaction, difficulty interpreting others' social behavior and reading others' emotional states, difficulty managing everyday routines, problems at work or school, personal goals (e.g., sobriety, money management, hygiene, and weight loss), and others. The key procedural concepts are:

- Negotiate personally appealing and effective plays/scripts of self-regulation or interaction designed to solve specific problems or overcome specific obstacles.
- Associate those plays/scripts with compelling images, goals, heroes, and the like to make their meaning clear and personally appealing.
- Rehearse the plays/scripts repeatedly, possibly using video learning trials ("game films"), with the goal of automatic elicitation of the self-coaching play by natural everyday stimuli.
- Negotiate acceptable reminder plays or partner scripts that can be used by ECPs.
- Try the plays in real "games" (i.e., real-world interaction), and evaluate their effectiveness and comfort level.
- Modify the plays, or design new plays, in the event of failure, frustration, or discomfort.
- Ensure celebration of everyday successes that result from using the self-regulatory self-coaching plays/scripts successfully.

Table 33–13 lists the principles underlying this self-coaching approach. All self-coaching interventions are organized within the general goal-obstacle-plan-do-review framework discussed earlier. That is, participants are encouraged to (1) describe what they want to accomplish or get better at (goal), (2) identify what is blocking successful achievement of that goal (obstacle), (3) create a play (plan, script), (4) try it under highly supported and then real-world conditions (do), and (5) review what is working and what is not working, making modifications as needed (review).

Particularly for individuals with limited space in working memory and weak online decision making, habituating or automatizing the self-coaching plays and scripts is critical. Furthermore, the plays need to be automatized within the settings and routines in which the difficulties arise. Thus, the intervention must take into account the routines of everyday life and ensure considerable practice with the self-coaching scripts within those routines. This is one of the reasons for the involvement of ECPs. Ideally, relevant ECPs understand the plays and their rationale, know and are comfortable with their roles (e.g., prompting the play), and can execute their roles without irritating or boring the person with brain injury. The need for automatization also is one of the reasons for using self-coaching videos to ensure large numbers of learning trials for habituation. These short videos typically include content outlined in Table 33–14 but can be customized to meet individual needs.

If well constructed, the self-coaching videos serve three purposes beyond habituation of the plays. First, following

TABLE 33–13

Principles of Self Coaching as a Social Competence Intervention

1. **Automatic Self-Regulation:** The ultimate goal of self-coaching is to create situations in which relevant environmental cues automatically trigger effective self-regulatory/self-coaching thoughts and behaviors rather than triggering poorly controlled, impulsive, negative, unsuccessful, or self-destructive behavior.
2. **Participant Involvement:** Self-coaching requires creative and respectful collaboration with the participants in identifying difficult situations and negative behaviors, personally meaningful goals, useful self-talk plays/scripts, and acceptable supports from others.
3. **Specificity of Real-World Needs:** Self-coaching targets specific issues that have a direct and measurable effect on the quality of the individual's life.
4. **Negotiation of Scripts and Metaphors:** Plays/scripts and metaphors are individually negotiated to be as personally meaningful as possible.
5. **Motivating Associations:** The self-regulatory plays/scripts should be creatively associated with motivating images, people, or other symbols of strength and success.
6. **Self-Coaching Plays/Scripts and Communication Partner Scripts:** Ideally, "coaching" scripts are negotiated and developed for the individual (self-coaching scripts) and also for everyday communication partners (e.g., how to cue self-coaching without eliciting oppositional responses).
7. **Practice:** Automaticity of self-coaching "plays" cannot be achieved without a great deal of practice. One of the reasons for video self-modeling is that many of these learning trials can be logged as the individual watches the video ("the game film").
8. **Monitoring, Revisions, and Celebration:** The effectiveness of self-coaching plays must be carefully monitored, with revisions as necessary and ample celebration of success.

From Ylvisaker (2006); with permission.

TBI, many people have relatively weak self-monitoring and self-awareness, both of which might be improved with video self-observation. These self-coaching videos allow the participants to observe themselves being successful using the self-coaching plays and scripts. In some cases, they allow the participants to observe themselves being unsuccessful without the self-coaching play/script. Because self-observation can be emotionally challenging, authorization for self-observation should be granted by a relevant clinician (e.g., clinical psychologist, psychiatrist, or social worker).

Second, the video can include the negotiation and agreements that led to the play. This short circuits later objections based on faulty recollection of the rationale for the play.

Third, the videos can contain simple educational content about the person's injury and its effects. When we create

TABLE 33–14

Possible Content for Self-Coaching Videos

1. Introduction to the concept and importance of self-coaching. This may be a videotaped live discussion within the group and then used as the introduction to many or all of the individual self-coaching videos. Brain injury–related information may be included in this segment, ideally using a model of the brain to make the information as concrete as possible.

2. Explanation of the individual's specific difficulty that requires self-coaching. Often, this statement is made collaboratively by the person and the therapist. Person-specific brain injury information may be included in this segment—again using a model of the brain. If an appropriate level of comfort and mutual respect has been established in the group, then statements about the person's difficulty can and should be clear and direct—for example, "Bob, you see this part of the brain? It helps us to control our impulses. Your brain is injured here; that's why you're an impulsive guy. You have a hard time stopping yourself from doing or saying the first thing that pops into your head, right? But that doesn't mean you can't be successful. Think about Ben Rothlisburger, quarterback of the Pittsburgh Steelers. Last week he had a banged up knee and broken thumb, but he still played and played very well. But he had to wear special equipment, use special strategies, and accept special help—and it wasn't easy. But he did it. It's not easy for you to control your impulses; that's why we're working out these special plays; and that's why you're going to get the video and watch it many times to make the plays automatic!"

3. Brief vignette demonstrating what the difficult social situation looks like without self-coaching (e.g., participant loses his temper, or the participant misinterprets another person's behavior).

4. Brief vignette demonstrating what the difficult social situation looks like with the self-coaching script—that is, successful negotiation of the difficult situation. This segment could include an admired peer using the self-coaching script so that it has positive associations as it is viewed on the video.

5. Possibly an everyday communication partner demonstrating an acceptable cue for the participant to use self-coaching script.

6. Possibly a description of what changes in behavior will demonstrate success of the self-coaching script.

7. Possibly some "cheerleading" from group members for motivational purposes.

8. For some individuals, it may be desirable to include in the video the entire discussion and negotiation that leads to the scripts. This may be particularly valuable for those with significant memory impairment.

From Ylvisaker (2006); with permission.

self-coaching videos, we routinely begin with a few minutes of educational content about brain injury and the individual's specific injury. During these few minutes of presentation, we typically sit next to the participant and, while holding a model of a brain, point out relevant areas and their importance. Participants who are many years post-injury often report that this information is new and important for them and their ECPs.

Behavior Management and Communication

Concerns About Traditional Consequence-Based Behavior Management

Traditional operant applications of applied behavior analysis, dating back to Skinner's early work (Skinner, 1938), have explained behavior as a consequence of both antecedents and consequences but have placed the major burden on manipulation of consequences in teaching new behaviors or modifying undesirable behavior. Within this tradition, intervention strategies largely are reactive, specifying positive consequences for desirable behavior and negative or no consequences for undesirable behavior. Furthermore, to the extent that antecedents are targeted in behavior management, it largely has been the immediate and observable antecedents (e.g., the trainer's commands, cues, and prompts as well as environmental stressors at the time of the behavior). An enormous literature and impressive technology of behavioral change have evolved within this tradition. Furthermore, reports have documented some success with traditional consequence management applied to both adults (see, e.g., Alderman, 2003; Alderman & Ward, 1991; Pace & Ivancic, 1994; Wood, 1987, 1990) and children (see, e.g., Slifer, Cataldo, & Kurtz, 1995; Slifer et al., 1996) with TBI.

Unfortunately, clinicians who work with individuals who have frontal lobe impairment, whether congenital (e.g., ADHD) or acquired (e.g., TBI), often report a frustrating lack of success or, at best, inefficiency in their implementation of primarily consequence-oriented behavior modification programs (Barkley, 1987; Hallowell & Ratey, 1994). This inefficiency has been documented in the frontal lobe research literature, which offers at least four potential explanations, which are summarized in Table 33–15. Damasio and colleagues (Bechera, Damasio, Damasio, & Anderson, 1994; Bechera, Tranel, Damasio, & Damasio, 1996; Damasio, 1994; Damasio et al., 1991; Tranel, 2002) have suggested that favorable or unfavorable consequences of behavior can influence future behavior only if somatic markers, or feeling states, are associated with the stored representation of the original behavior. Their neuropsychological investigations indicate that ventromedial prefrontal cortex is critical to laying down somatic markers and connecting them to memories of past

TABLE 33–15

Possible Explanations for Inefficiency of Consequence-Oriented Behavior Management in Rehabilitation of Traumatic Brain Injury

Hypothesis	Discussion
Disinhibition Hypothesis (Rolls et al., 1994)	Because of the high frequency of orbitofrontal injury in TBI, impulsiveness is a common impairment. People who are impulsive, like young children, are capable of learning from consequences, but immediate impulses easily overwhelm learned behaviors on the occasion of action.
Working Memory Hypothesis (Alderman, 1996)	Because of the relative frequency of dorsolateral prefrontal injury in TBI, reduced working memory is a common impairment. Alderman found a correlation between impaired working memory and difficulty learning from consequences, perhaps suggesting that reasonably adequate working memory is needed for correct selection of learned responses.
Somatic Marker Hypothesis (Damasio, 1994)	Because of the high frequency of ventromedial prefrontal injury in TBI, attachment of somatic markers (feeling states associated with rewards and punishments) to stored representations of past experiences is inefficient. According to this theory, somatic marker storage is critical to learning from consequences and is weak in individuals with ventromedial prefrontal damage.
Initiation Hypothesis (Stuss & Benson, 1986)	Because of the relative frequency of dorsal (especially dorsomesial) prefrontal injury in TBI, some individuals lack organically based initiation/activation capacity to act in situations in which they have learned the correct behavior and are adequately motivated to act.
Infantilization and Oppositionality Hypothesis (Ylvisaker & Feeney, 1998a)	Because many people with TBI, especially adolescents and young adults, react negatively to attempts by others to manage their behavior with consequences, traditional behavior management systems may be counterproductive. The common complaint is that reward and punishment systems are child-like or that external manipulation beyond their control and approval is in general offensive to them.

Key: TBI = traumatic brain injury.

behavior, thereby explaining the inefficiency of consequence-oriented behavior management in many people with CHI, given its high frequency of ventral prefrontal damage.

Rolls (2002) as well as Rolls, Hornak, Wade, & McGrath (1994) highlighted inflexibility in response to changing contingencies and impulsiveness, associated with orbitofrontal lesions, as a hypothesis capable of explaining the maintenance of behaviors that have resulted in a history of seriously punishing consequences. Alderman (1996) concluded that weakness in the central executive component of working memory may explain the failure of many individuals with frontal lobe injury to respond to traditional operant training techniques, including reinforcement, extinction, and time-out interventions. In some cases, reduced initiation/activation, associated with dorsal (especially dorsomesial) prefrontal injury, may explain failure to act despite possession of the appropriate learned response (Stuss & Benson, 1986). In individual cases, a satisfactory explanation for the inefficiency of traditional behavior management may include a combination of these four phenomena, possibly exacerbated by oppositionality, which may grow in response to ineffective consequence-oriented management (Ylvisaker & Feeney, 2000a). For our purposes, the research literature at least directs clinicians to focus their attention on both immediate and remote antecedents of behavior.

Positive, Antecedent-Focused Behavior Management

In Table 33–16, we outline alternative approaches to the role of antecedent manipulation in behavior management (based on Carr, Carlson, Langdon, Magito-McLaughlin, & Yarbrough, 1998). Historically, the narrow "molecular" approach co-existed with a primary focus on consequences. Until recently, relatively little attention has been paid to remote events (e.g., an unpleasant interaction earlier in the day) or internal states of the individual (e.g., anger resulting from loss of friends, anxiety over lost skills, or frustration associated with an unsatisfying job or no meaningful role in life) as potentially modifiable antecedents that increase or decrease the likelihood of certain behaviors.

Over the past 20 years, momentum has grown within the field of applied behavior analysis favoring an approach to teaching and supporting individuals with challenging behavior that places greatest emphasis on the manipulation of antecedents, including immediate and remote as well as observable and unobservable antecedents (the "molar" approach in Table 33–16). Although most of the research and clinical discussions within this new tradition address behavioral issues associated with developmental disabilities (Carr, et al., 1999), application of antecedent technologies has entered the experimental and clinical literatures in TBI rehabilitation (Feeney & Ylvisaker, 1995, 1997; Jacobs, 1993; Ylvisaker et al., 2003; Ylvisaker & Feeney, 1996, 1998a, 2000a; Ylvisaker, Turkstra et al. (2007), Zencius, Wesolowski, Burke, & McQuade, 1989). Furthermore, the molar approach to antecedent-focused behavior management is completely consistent with the theoretical and procedural discussion of positive, everyday, routine-based intervention presented earlier.

Building Positive, Everyday Behavioral and Communication Routines

Earlier, we offered a rationale for a positive, everyday, routine-based approach to rehabilitation equally applicable to intervention for individuals with chronic cognitive, behavioral, and communication impairment. Behavior management within this approach can be divided into two overlapping efforts: preventing negative behaviors, and building repertoires of positive behaviors, including communication routines.

Preventing Negative Behavior with Antecedent Manipulations

Part 2 of Table 33–3 in *Framework for Cognitive and Psychosocial Rehabilitation* lists several categories of antecedent procedures designed, in part, to avoid negative behavioral routines and increase the likelihood that positive behaviors will become habitual. Critical to antecedent management is the concept of "setting events" (Michael, 1982, 1993), which are potentially remote occurrences or conditions that increase or decrease the likelihood of a behavior and deter-

---

TABLE 33–16

Behavior Management Via Control of Antecedents: Alternative Approaches

Molecular Approach to Antecedent Control: The Tradition in Applied Behavior Analysis

Antecedents: Discrete measurable stimuli that precede a behavior and increase or decrease its likelihood of occurrence (e.g., a specific instruction, cue, warning, or promise).

Assessment: To identify these antecedents for purposes of control (a-b-c analysis, including active experimentation with antecedents), often in controlled settings (i.e., analog assessment).

Intervention: To increase or decrease specific behaviors by manipulating the specific immediate antecedents related to the behavior (e.g., eliminate triggers, modify antecedents, and fade antecedents in or out).

Molar Approach To Antecedent Control

Antecedents: Broad, potentially continuous, often hard to measure variables that may increase or decrease the likelihood of occurrence of positive or negative behavior:
- Internal states (e.g., illness).
- Living arrangements.
- Social relationships.
- Education (e.g., placement, demands, and level of success).
- Work (e.g., placement, demands, level of success, and perceived meaningfulness).
- Leisure (frequency and quality of enjoyable activities).
- The relation between the person's needs, competencies, and environmental demands.
- Self-perception, including implicit metaphors that guide thinking and behavior.

Assessment:
- To identify the background antecedents or non-immediate "setting events" that may be related to positive or negative behaviors, generally in natural settings.
- To assess the "goodness of fit" between the person's needs, competencies, and social, educational, and vocational demands.

Intervention:

Primary Purpose: To influence major background setting events and conditions with the goal of helping the individual to create a satisfying lifestyle:
- May be most efficiently met by educating and training everyday communication partners and, in other ways, creating a "best fit" between the individual and his or her living, work, social, and/or educational environments and activities.

Secondary Purpose: To indirectly increase desirable and decrease undesirable behaviors.

Based on Carr and colleagues (1998). From Ylvisaker & Feeney (2000a); with permission.

TABLE 33–17

Categories and Examples of Setting Events that Potentially Influence Behavior

Internal States of the Individual

- **Neurologic States**
  Positive setting events: normal neurology.
  Negative setting events: overactivity of the limbic regions; seizures; neurotransmitter disruption; decreased cerebral blood flow.
- **Other Physiologic States**
  Positive setting events: rest, relaxation, satiation, and appropriate levels of medication.
  Negative setting events: pain, illness, hunger, over medication, under medication, motor deficits, and sensory deficits.
- **Cognitive States**
  Positive setting events: orientation to task, familiarity with routine, adequate recall of relevant events, and adequate recognition of things and people.
  Negative setting events: confusion, disorientation, frustration, and inadequate recall and recognition.
- **Emotional States**
  Positive setting events: sense of accomplishment, success, achievement, acceptance by others, respect from others, meaningful role, sense of self consistent with life circumstances, and feeling in control.
  Negative setting events: anxiety, anger, depression, and sense of loss and failure.
- **Perception of Task Meaningfulness and Difficulty**
  Positive setting events: belief that assigned tasks are meaningful and can be accomplished.
  Negative setting events: belief that assigned tasks are meaningless, infantilizing, or impossible.

External Events and Conditions

- **Living Arrangement**
  Positive setting events: living in a self-selected environment without excessive restrictions.
  Negative setting events: living in an excessively restrictive setting; living at home with parents after having lived independently.
- **Presence or Absence of Specific People**
  Positive setting events: presence of preferred people and reciprocal friendships.
  Negative setting events: absence of preferred people, loss of friends, and presence of nonpreferred people.
- **Recent History of Interaction**
  Positive setting events: recent positive and pleasurable interactions.
  Negative setting events: recent conflict or disrespectful interaction.
- **Other Environmental Stressors**
  Positive setting events: appropriate and desirable environmental stimulation.
  Negative setting events: irritating environmental stimulation (e.g., ambient noise, improper lighting, and other distractors).
- **Time of Day**
  Positive setting events: alertness; best time of day relative to the individual's natural cycles.
  Negative setting events: bad time of day relative to the individual's natural cycles.

From Ylvisaker and Feeney (1998a); with permission.

mine whether a specific behavioral intervention will be effective (Baer, Wolf, & Risley, 1987). Because the concept of setting events is unfamiliar to some rehabilitation specialists and bears meaning that is not transparent (e.g., "event" is not restricted to temporally discrete occurrences but, rather, can include internal states and conditions), we include in Table 33–17 a list of positive and negative setting events that can be used as a checklist in working with individuals with difficult behavior after TBI.

Attention to setting events is particularly critical in working with people who have acquired brain injury because of the cumulative negative effect on behavior of chronic discomfort, restrictions on activities and choices, limited control over major life events, frequent changes in living situation and

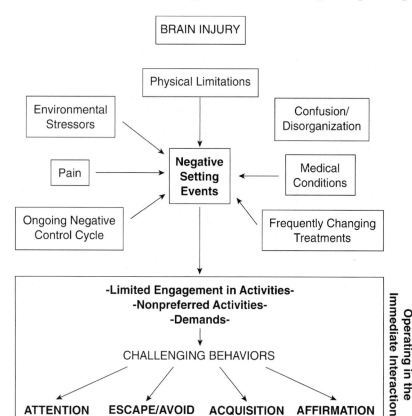

Figure 33–9. Relationship between negative setting events and challenging behavior. (Modified from Feeney & Ylvisaker, 1997; with permission.)

routines, and perhaps most critically, failure to achieve goals consistent with preinjury expectations and aspirations. A background of negative setting events lowers behavioral thresholds that, as a result of the injury, already may be low (Fig. 33–9). Conversely, a background of positive setting events elevates those thresholds and increases the likelihood that the individual will become productively engaged in difficult tasks (Fig. 33–10). The developmental disabilities behavioral litera-

ture is rich in reports of experiments demonstrating the positive effects on behavior of inducing positive setting events, including creating positive behavioral momentum before introducing difficult tasks (Carr et al., 1997; Fowler, 1996; Kennedy, Itkonen, & Lindquist, 1995; Mace et al., 1988, 1990; Mace, Mauro, Boyajian, & Eckert, 1997) and offering choice and control (Bannerman, Sheldon, Sherman, & Harchik, 1990; Brown, Belz, Corsi, & Wenig, 1993; Dunlap

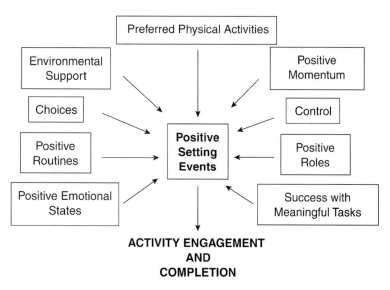

Figure 33–10. Relationship between positive setting events and positive behavior. (Modified from Feeney & Ylvisaker, 1997; with permission.)

et al., 1994; Harchik, Sherman, & Bannerman, 1993). Harchik and colleagues (1993) reviewed more than 100 experimental reports in the developmental disabilities literature and concluded that increasing an individual's opportunities for choice and control decreases challenging behavior, increases participation, and increases subjective reports of satisfaction derived from that participation.

The Role of Consequences

In emphasizing antecedents in behavior management for people with TBI, we do not wish to recommend inattention to consequences. First, many people with TBI escape frontolimbic injury entirely and, therefore, can be expected to be as efficient as their uninjured peers at learning from consequences. Furthermore, the frontolimbic threats to efficiency of consequence-oriented behavior management come in degrees and, in individual cases, may not be serious. Third, the positive, everyday routines that antecedent supports are designed to facilitate are positive, in part, because they result in extrinsic or intrinsic rewards for the person. Fourth, the possibility of serious punishment (e.g., jail) may serve as motivation for participation in the development of antecedent-supported routines. Finally, even those who are inefficient at learning from consequences benefit from a positive culture in which there is ample noncontingent reinforcement, successful performance is greeted with encouragement and praise, and failure and negative behavior elicit efforts to help the person succeed rather than punishment that may breed anger and additional failure.

In using consequences, some basic rules apply. First, individuals who are impulsive and concrete in their thinking need consequences that are immediate (versus delayed) and salient. As cognition improves, consequences can become progressively more delayed and less salient.

Second, with the goal of helping people to succeed in the real world, rewards and punishments should be as natural and logically related to the individual's behavior as possible. For example, a good grade is a natural and logical consequence of effective preparation for a test; a raise or promotion is a natural and logical consequence of hard work on the job; and an enjoyable social interaction is a natural and logical consequence of socially appropriate initiation. On the punishment side, cleaning one's room is a natural and logical consequence of "trashing" the room during a tantrum, and receiving a poor grade is a natural and logical consequence of failing to prepare for an examination. In contrast, the following contingent responses are not related in a natural and logical way to the behavior and, therefore, are not likely to help shape enduring, positive behaviors:

- "Nice talking, John."
- "I liked the way you responded to Jeremy; I'll give you a point for that."

- "That's not an appropriate way to request cigarettes; you will not be allowed to go on the outing tonight."

Token economies, which are popular components of consequence-oriented behavioral programs, often fail to promote understanding of natural and logical relationships in the real world. For example, if an appropriate conversational bid from a person known for acting out sexually is rewarded with a token that can be exchanged later for a cigarette, the natural connection between appropriate conversational openers and subsequent satisfying conversations is violated. Furthermore, liberal use of extrinsic rewards can create dependence on such rewards and interfere with internally driven motivation, a finding that has been replicated many times in many contexts over the past 30 years (Deci, 1995; Deci & Ryan, 2002). Finally, our experience suggests that many oppositional young people become increasingly oppositional in an environment that they perceive as being dominated by arbitrary authority figures who arbitrarily dispense rewards and punishments that are not personally meaningful.

Teaching Positive Communication Alternatives to Challenging Behavior

Behavior management and SST come together in the process of helping people with challenging behavior to substitute a socially acceptable mode of communication for behavior that is unsuccessful or considered to be inappropriate in their social contexts. As an organized approach to behavior management, positive communication training has its roots in work with individuals who have mental retardation, autism, or other developmental disabilities (Bird, Dores, Moniz, & Robinson, 1989; Carr & Durand, 1985; Carr et al., 1994; Donnellan, Mirenda, Mesaros, & Fassbender, 1984; Doss & Reichle, 1989; Reichle & Wacker, 1993). Functional analysis of problem behavior in those groups typically indicates that the behavior serves a communication function, often expressing an intention to gain access to a desired activity, person, thing, or place or to escape an activity, person, demand, or place. Organized procedures for assessing the communication value of challenging behavior (see, e.g., Durand & Crimmins, 1992) and for teaching positive alternatives are available in the developmental disabilities literature, along with evidence of the effectiveness of these efforts.

In Table 33–18, we present a summary of the communication approach to behavior management, including the premises underlying the approach, considerations in assessment, preteaching activities, categories of teaching procedure, and finally, obstacles to success, along with suggestions for overcoming the obstacles. Elsewhere, we have discussed, illustrated, and demonstrated the effectiveness of this approach to behavior management for individuals with TBI in greater detail (Feeney & Ylvisaker, 1995, 1997, 2003;

TABLE 33–18

Behavior as Communication: Teaching Positive Communication Alternatives to Challenging Behavior

Premises

1. All behaviors (potentially) communicate something to someone. One cannot not communicate, although not all communication is intentional.
2. Few behaviors are truly maladaptive; most apparently maladaptive behaviors (e.g., aggression, self-injury, and withdrawal) achieve a social, communication goal.
3. The messages communicated with challenging behavior often can be understood as communicating the individual's need to escape (e.g., escape a task, person, place, or activity), to access/acquire (e.g., access a task, person, place, activity, thing, form of stimulation, or attention from others), or to protest (e.g., protest restrictions on behavior or disrespectful interaction).
4. The behavior of communication partners is a critical part of the context of behavior (antecedent conditions and consequences that potentially elicit and maintain types of behavior) and must figure prominently in intervention efforts.
5. Clearly defined communication routines of everyday life, supported by well-trained everyday communication partners, are the ideal context within which communication and behavior goals are optimally achieved.
6. Communication specialists and behavior specialists play essentially the same role in helping individuals with communication-related behavioral problems.

Assessment

1. Collaboratively identify and describe the unacceptable behavior and the contexts in which it occurs.
2. Collaboratively interpret the meaning of the challenging behavior:
   a. Systematic, passive observation: What are the stimuli and responses that trigger and maintain the undesirable behavior in varied everyday contexts?
   b. Systematic, active experimentation with hypotheses regarding the meaning/purpose of the challenging behavior (e.g., if communication partners routinely reward verbal requests for a desirable activity, does the challenging behavior disappear? If so, the meaning/purpose of the challenging probably was "I want that activity!").
   (See also Durand & Crimmins, 1992, and the discussion of collaborative, context-sensitive, hypothesis-testing assessment earlier in this chapter.)
3. Collaboratively explore potential positive alternatives to the challenging behavior.

Preteaching

1. Collaboratively decide under what circumstances the individual will be allowed to control tasks and settings with positive communication (e.g., escape undesirable tasks, people, settings; gain access to desirable tasks, people, settings).
2. Collaboratively select a positive communication alternative to the negative behavior. Ideally, the communication alternative should have the following characteristics:
   • Easy to produce: If the alternative is harder for the individual to produce than the behavior it is intended to replace, it is unlikely to be adopted.
   • Satisfying: The positive communication alternative should fit the person's personality and communication milieu.
   • Effective: The alternative must be at least as effective for the individual as the negative behavior it is replacing.
   • Promptable: There is an advantage to physically promptable communication alternatives (e.g., signing, gesturing, or pointing to a picture on a board) versus those that are not promptable (e.g., talking) during the initial stages of teaching, but this often is not possible.
   • Interpretable: The communication must be interpretable by all relevant communication partners.

Teaching the Positive Communication Alternative

1. Collaboratively ensure many successful positive communication routines daily (i.e., successful, rewarded use of the positive communication alternative) throughout the day and in a variety of contexts:
   a. Naturally occurring opportunities.
   b. Contrived opportunities.
2. Initially attempt to achieve a high ratio of positive communication alternatives to challenging behavior (e.g., 10:1), with prompts and other supports as necessary.
3. Gradually reduce prompts and other supports.
4. Gradually re-introduce normal demands:
   a. This may require explicit teaching of the difference between choice and no-choice situations.
   b. This may require considerable focus on antecedent supports (e.g., positive behavioral momentum or other positive setting events) to ensure that the individual does not revert to challenging behavior during stressful tasks.
5. Monitor and modify as necessary.

(continued)

TABLE 33–18

Behavior as Communication: Teaching Positive Communication Alternatives to Challenging Behavior (continued)

Obstacles to Teaching Communication Alternatives

1. **Staff Insularity:** The success of this teaching depends on all or most everyday communication partners being generally consistent in their communication with the person with challenging behavior.
   Possible Solutions:
   a. Try to include everybody in the initial functional assessment of behavior.
   b. Negotiate the behavior plan so that all relevant people agree that the plan is reasonable and do-able.
2. **Concern about Contributing to the Behavior Problem:** Many staff and family members are concerned that rewarding positive escape or access-motivated behavior will give the individual too much control.
   Possible Solutions:
   a. Point out research and experience that shows that this natural fear is unfounded if the teaching is implemented correctly.
   b. Emphasize that normal demands will be reintroduced once the challenging behavior is substantially eliminated.
3. **Concern that Some Activities Are Mandatory, Others Forbidden.**
   Possible Solutions:
   a. Try to achieve agreement about those activities that are mandatory and, therefore, cannot be escaped (e.g., taking medication) and those that are forbidden and, therefore, cannot be chosen (e.g., harming others, interacting with dangerous materials, and placing oneself at risk).
   b. Try to help all everyday communication partners agree that improving behavior and communication is a high priority at this time, necessitating considerable control by the individual using positive communication alternatives.
4. **No Choice Times Heavily Outweigh Choice Times:** It is unlikely that the individual will change old communication habits in the absence of a large number of meaningful, successful, rewarded learning trials with the positive alternative.
   Possible Solutions:
   a. Create—artificially if necessary—a large number of choice occasions so that the individual has many opportunities to practice and be rewarded for the positive communication alternative.
5. **Behavior Management Is Somebody Else's Job:** Some people believe that behavioral problems should be dealt with by behavior specialists and not by others.
   Possible Solutions:
   a. Ensure that all relevant communication partners are involved in identifying the need for behavioral change, in implementing the functional analysis of behavior, and in modifying everyday routines of communication so that the individual has many opportunities to practice positive communication alternatives.
6. **Difficulty with Timing.**
   Possible Solutions:
   a. Ensure that communication partners know that they must respond to the positive communication alternative promptly—knowing that if they wait, the individual is likely to revert to the challenging behavior—and will likely be unintentionally rewarded for the challenging behavior.
7. **Concern about Power/Authority Roles:** Some adults, particularly those who are personally insecure, resist creating the impression that a client or student or employee is in a position of power or authority over them.
   Possible Solutions:
   1. Work with resistive staff to help them understand that this teaching strategy ultimately gives them more, not less, authority.
   2. Help everybody to understand the importance of substituting positive for negative communication and that this may require giving the individual a sense of power with positive communication.
   3. Help everybody to understand that normal expectations will be re-instituted once the challenging behavior is under adequate control.

2006; Ylvisaker & Feeney, 1994, 1998a; Ylvisaker et al., 1999; Ylvisaker, Feeney, & Szekeres, 1998).

We have used the approach outlined in Table 33–18 with a large number of children and adults who show challenging behavior after TBI. In some cases, particularly people with significant cognitive, behavioral, and possibly also motor impairment, the messages communicated in problematic ways were relatively simple to decipher (e.g., a desire to escape demands), and the intervention process was not unlike that described in the developmental disabilities literature. In other cases, particularly people with relatively good cognitive and motor recovery but complex behavioral and emotional profiles both before and after their injuries, the messages delivered in challenging ways were more complex, and the process of intervention involved a higher level of collaboration with the individual. In these cases, motivation and negotiation (discussed in the next section) are central to the intervention.

Behavioral Interventions: Evidence

In a systematic review of the evidence regarding behavioral interventions for individuals with behavioral problems after TBI, Ylvisaker, Turkstra, and colleagues (2007 located 65 studies with a total of 172 participants). Two of the studies were randomized, controlled trials (Class I), 2 were group studies with inadequate controls (Class II), 36 were well-controlled, single-subject experiments (Class III), and 25 were case studies or poorly designed, single-subject experiments (Class IV). All the studies showed positive effects of the intervention, supporting the conclusion that behavioral intervention in general (i.e., not a specific intervention protocol) for behavioral problems after TBI in both children and adults should be considered as a practice guideline at both acute and post-acute stages of recovery. The authors concluded that individuals with challenging behavior after TBI should be provided with systematically organized behavioral interventions and supports consistent with the available evidence and based on individualized functional behavior assessments. Furthermore, specific behavioral interventions grouped under the headings of traditional contingency management and positive behavior interventions and supports can be considered as evidence-based treatment options. Because most of the evidence is Class III or Class IV, and because intervention protocols vary from study to study, stronger recommendations (i.e., practice standards or intervention guidelines) for specific behavioral intervention protocols cannot be supported by the available evidence. Interestingly, the review documented a sharp movement in the direction of positive behavior interventions and supports over the past 30 years.

The Role of Individual and Group Therapy within an Everyday Rehabilitation Framework

In highlighting the importance of context and the role of supported routines of everyday life as the core of rehabilitation for individuals with chronic cognitive, psychosocial, and communication impairment after TBI, we do not wish to suggest that both individual and group therapy have no role. First, many of the traditional roles played by speech-language pathologists in relation to swallowing, motor speech, and aphasic deficits are appropriate and necessary for some individuals with TBI.

Second, the meaning of "context" is not restricted to setting. Clinicians can contextualize therapy sessions with personally meaningful activities and materials (e.g., academic texts and tasks for a college student) and also people (e.g., including family members in communication therapy sessions).

Third, individual and group therapy sessions can be used to brainstorm about and explore the usefulness of alternative

strategies, supports, or self-coaching "plays" (Step 2 of everyday intervention in Table 33–4). Having identified what works—and what does not work—under controlled conditions, plans can be implemented for context-sensitive practice in the routines of everyday life, possibly supported by everyday people and even self-managed.

Fourth, the intimacy of individual therapy sessions often is necessary to address the sensitive issue of self-awareness of ongoing impairment.

Finally, individual or group sessions are a useful venue for the motivational and supportive interaction needed by individuals who struggle to maintain the level of effort needed to be successful after their injury (Step 3 of everyday intervention in Table 33–4).

Having highlighted the potential value of therapy sessions, however, we wish to stress the goal of transforming every hour of reimbursed therapy into several hours of well-conceived rehabilitation by virtue of effective alliances with everyday people and creative use of the routines of everyday life.

Motivation, Metaphor, and Collaboration with the Person with Disability

In the case of adolescents and young adults who are struggling unsuccessfully to reestablish preinjury activities and levels of success, challenging behaviors such as aggression, withdrawal, sexual acting out, and others often communicate messages like the following:

- "You just treated me disrespectfully and I won't take it!"
- "I know I can't do this and it's driving me crazy, but it's just too hard to ask for help!"
- "I find you very attractive, and I would like to spend time with you."

Because loss of friends, difficulty maintaining work, and increasingly stressful family interaction may be the result of negative communication behavior, intervention designed to substitute positive alternatives can be critical to social, vocational, and familial success. Proud and oppositional adolescents and young adults, however, particularly those from cultural backgrounds in which communication often is somewhat unrefined, are most unlikely to accept alternatives such as the following:

- "Excuse me, but I think we need to spend some quality time working on our relationship because I find your attitude unacceptable."
- "Since my accident I have a hard time doing even simple things. I need a lot of help. Please help me."
- "Is there any chance we could spend some time talking? I would like to get to know you better."

In our experience, the most critical component of intervention is the negotiation that leads to communication scripts or a general communication style enabling the person to be successful in chosen educational, vocational, and social contexts and that is, at the same time, consistent with his or her sense of self (Step 3 of the intervention sequence outlined in Table 33–4). Often, this negotiation is facilitated by collaborative identification of a positive role model or metaphor that can help the individual to overcome emotional barriers to positive communication alternatives to negative behavior.

Compelling metaphors have the added advantage that they combine into one thought unit a set of social behaviors or scripts that otherwise could be difficult to remember when considered separately, particularly under stress. Thus, for one young adult with a post-injury history of aggressive behavior and multiple psychiatric hospitalizations and incarcerations, calling up the image of Clint Eastwood when stressed yielded a compelling image of self-control as well as a script that included a few words designed to extricate himself from potentially volatile situations. At the same time, the Clint Eastwood metaphor motivated positive, self-regulated behavior and compensated for reduced space in working memory. Functioning in this manner, effective metaphors are components of the "implicational code" or organized set of "emotional beliefs," as those concepts have recently emerged in new interpretations of cognitive psychotherapy (Teasdale, 1997).

Ylvisaker and Feeney (2000a) explored the facilitating role played by positive metaphors for individuals with cognitive impairment and oppositional behavior following TBI. They illustrated this role by describing their intervention for a fiercely oppositional adolescent who had been in serious trouble with the law and threatened several staff members in his residential program. His initial resistance to any intervention was overcome by hiring him as a consultant to develop a training video about oppositionality. In his capacity as a paid consultant, he revealed that his overriding goal in interacting with authority figures and many peers was to avoid being a "suck up" (his term). The only "non-suck-up" role with which he was familiar was that of a fiercely oppositional and defiant bulldog, which he played effectively—and which routinely got him into serious trouble. He agreed to refer to this role with a vulgar metaphor (to cast it in a negative light) and worked with the clinicians to identify a third way of acting, that of "winners"—successful people who are not suck ups but, rather, who do what needs to be done to achieve their goals. He then agreed to practice negotiating many everyday social interactions in three ways: (1) as a suck up, (2) as his traditional defiant self, and (3) as a winner. These interactions were videotaped (as part of developing the training program), and he reviewed the tapes as part of his responsibilities as a consultant to the project and as part of his communication therapy.

During his context-sensitive practice, a social skills coach (speech-language pathology intern) mediated his experience with discussion of which of these three interactive styles were comfortable for him (predictably, the suck-up style was never comfortable) and which were successful (the defiant style was never successful). Success and adequate comfort came to be associated with a wide range of positive ("winner") interactive behaviors. Social cues could then be reduced to one positive reminder—"You can be a winner"—as opposed to the top-down admonitions that he had routinely interpreted as nagging and to which he had routinely reacted with oppositional behavior. Perhaps more important, success came to be associated with a conviction that "winner behavior" was his route to freedom, a good job, and other personally significant goals. This metaphorical transformation at least brought him onto the playing field of successful social interaction, which he continued to practice with considerable success.

Other metaphors described by Ylvisaker and Feeney (2000a) and used successfully in TBI rehabilitation include:

1. **Social skills as basketball plays.** A former basketball player whose impulsiveness had led to substance abuse and serious trouble with the authorities came to agree that he needed "to be like Mike [Michael Jordan] and use set plays rather than running around the court like a crazy kid." Social skills training then became a process of defining successful plays, putting them in his play book, and videotaping him while engaged in these plays so that he could review the game films as part of routinizing the plays. Social cues for this extremely disinhibited person were then reduced to the nonthreatening "What's the play?" and "Is this play in the play book?" as opposed to the cues (i.e., nagging) that staff had previously used and that had routinely elicited oppositional behavior.

2. **Requests for clarification as journalistic behavior.** A well-educated young woman with a commitment to feminism before her injury overcame her reluctance to asking communication partners for clarification of their message (and increasing social withdrawal) once she associated these requests for clarification with the journalistic practices of her heroine, the well-known feminist and journalist Gloria Steinem.

3. **Cognitive prostheses as common workplace practices.** A young man who before his injury had been a truck driver at a gravel pit overcame his resistance to compensatory procedures, such as a small memory notebook, when he connected these strategies with the common practice at his former job site of having unused trucks and drivers available for emergency purposes if the others broke down.

4. **Risk-taking behavior as red-card violations in soccer.** A former soccer player, who had been arrested twice on drug charges after his injury, began to work hard on his recovery after formulating the following

metaphorical insight: "I want to play the game, but I have two yellow cards. The next time, it's a red card, and I'm off the field. But my teammates will still be playing—and playing at a disadvantage because I got myself thrown out of the game. I can play and enjoy playing and win, but I've got to pay attention to the rules."

5. **Ignoring provocation as cool behavior.** A young adult who before his injury was a drug user and drug dealer in New York City was placed in a developmental disabilities workshop as part of his community reintegration plan. John routinely reacted with physical and verbal aggression when co-workers irritated him at work. His resistance to ignoring these provocations was overcome after discussion of his hero, the rap musician LL Cool J, who not only delivers fiery lyrics in his performances but also is a successful and self-controlled businessman and family man. Ignoring provocation at work came to be seen not as weakness but, rather, as an aspect of the strength of LL Cool J.

In a self-advocacy videotape that we helped John (see illustration 5 above) produce and that he asked his work supervisor to watch, he explained that it was difficult to overcome instincts and communication styles fashioned during his years on the streets. He described his efforts to resist impulsive aggressive responses and to use the behavior that he had chosen as a substitute (a somewhat sarcastic, dismissive comment, followed by turning away). He ended his video with a plea to the supervisor, "Please, let me be me." Subsequently, this supervisor used a subtle written cue ("Cool J") at the first sign of John's loss of control, resulting in his successful effort to regain control because of its association with his positive self-metaphor.

People will be who they are. With this in mind, one responsibility of rehabilitation professionals is to assist people in becoming who they are. It is not the job of communication specialists to force individuals to communicate in ways that are foreign to their understanding of who they are but, rather, to help them communicate in ways that contribute to the achievement of meaningful goals in their lives, consistent with the needs of others. That this aspect of communication intervention enters the domain of self-discovery and self-acceptance counseling should not frighten away communication specialists inadequately trained as counselors but, rather, cause them to redouble their collaboration with other rehabilitation professionals. Through such collaborative efforts, including collaboration with colleagues, the person with disability, and everyday people in the environment, functional intervention is allowed to take root in the real world, facilitated by positive alliances among all relevant stakeholders. These intervention themes are further elaborated by Ylvisaker and Feeney (2000b).

COLLABORATION WITH EVERYDAY PEOPLE THROUGHOUT RECOVERY

In this chapter, we have placed major emphasis on the role played by everyday people (e.g., family members, direct care staff, teachers, work supervisors, coworkers, friends, and others) in the long-term rehabilitation of individuals with chronic cognitive, communication, and behavioral impairment after TBI. This emphasis is motivated, in part, by the economic realities governing neurologic rehabilitation at the turn of the century but also, in part, by the enduring principles of sound, appropriately context-sensitive intervention. Rehabilitation within this framework mandates effective collaborative alliances with everyday people. In Appendix 33.4, we list reasons for such alliances, along with obstacles to establishing collaborative alliances, strategies for overcoming the obstacles, characteristics of effective everyday coaches/facilitators, and training and support options.

In medical rehabilitation, many obstacles to the creation of such collaborative alliances exist. Appendix 33.4 lists some of these obstacles and offers a menu of strategies to overcome them. In our experience, managers in rehabilitation facilities play a critical role in supporting a culture of rehabilitation that values alliances with everyday people. In such facilities, therapists' schedules are creatively designed so that they have natural opportunities to interact collaboratively with one another, nursing staff (in an inpatient facility), assistant-level staff, and family members. In addition, training opportunities and materials (e.g., peer coaching and customized training videos) are available for orientation of staff who did not learn collaborative principles and procedures in their professional training programs.

Appendix 33.4 includes a list of characteristics of people who are effective in their role as everyday coach and facilitator for people with chronic impairment after TBI. Some family members, therapists, direct care staff, work supervisors, and others have these characteristics in abundance. Others need considerable help to play their role effectively. Appendix 33.4 concludes with a list of procedures that can be used to put everyday people in a position to play this role. Traditional training procedures (e.g., brief in-services for direct care staff and family conferences) are notoriously insufficient. Situational coaching and support typically are necessary to change behavior (just as clinical practicum experiences are critical for clinicians in training). Strong support systems are critical for people whose resilience and optimism become severely strained. Specific scripts may be needed by those people who are not, by nature, flexible or enthusiastic problem solvers but, rather, who need to create everyday routines of flexibility and effective problem solving. Because of their expertise in communication, speech-language pathologists often play a central role in developing interaction scripts and in general staff and family training.

Ylvisaker and Feeney (1998a, 1998b) explored these themes in greater detail.

Communication Partner Conversational Support Competencies

Speech-language pathologists often are called on to train direct care staff and others in the interactive competencies needed to communicate effectively with patients in neurologic rehabilitation settings (Ylvisaker, Feeney, & Urbanczyk, 1993a). It is less common, however, for communication partner training to be considered as a critical component of cognitive rehabilitation. Recent research in developmental cognitive psychology has emphasized the role of parent–child conversations about the past in facilitating children's development of thought organization and autobiographical memory (Fivush, 1991; Fivush & Fromhoff, 1988; Fivush & Haden, 2003; Fivush & Reese, 1992; Haden, Haine, & Fivush, 1997; Hudson, 1990; Lucariello, Hudson, Fivush, & Bauer, 2004; McCabe & Peterson, 1991; Nelson, 1992; Reese & Fivush, 1993; Reese, Haden & Fivush, 1993). The evolving view is that parents who interact frequently with their preschool children in a collaborative, elaborative, and socially enjoyable way have children who develop internal cognitive organization and autobiographical memory more effectively than comparable children whose parents interact with them less frequently or in a way that is not similarly supportive. Although these interactions can focus on a variety of topics, developmental investigations in this area largely have targeted parent–child interaction while jointly talking about events that they have experienced together— that is, socially co-constructed narratives about the past.

In Appendix 33.5, we attempt to capture the competencies associated with a cognitively facilitative style under two general headings: collaboration and elaboration. In other words, conversation partners who are effective in facilitating cognitive growth in children or people with cognitive impairment tend to participate with them in conversation rather than demand performance from them. In addition, facilitators use conversational procedures to help their conversation partner understand how things, people, and events in the world are organized—that is, they gradually clarify the many ways in which things in the world go together. In effect, within this Vygotskyan framework, facilitative conversationalists, whether parents, teachers, therapists, aides, or others, are able to teach their partner how to think and how to organize their thoughts while, at the same time, enjoying pleasant conversations about topics of mutual interest.

We have used the competencies listed in Appendix 33.5 in the training of family members and staff serving children and adults with cognitive impairment after TBI. In addition to enhancing the cognitive value of everyday interaction, these competencies often have the effect of reducing tension between people with TBI and staff members. In our experi-ence, many well-meaning people interact with adults who have cognitive impairment in an inquisitorial and nonelabo-rative manner, a style of interaction that tends to elicit negative behavioral responses and that is the opposite of facilitative from a cognitive perspective. An additional component of staff communication training, associated with an every-day, routine-based approach to intervention, is the development of scripts that promote problem solving and flexibility in individuals who otherwise are rigid and disorganized in their approach to everyday problems. Appendix 33.5 concludes with examples of such scripts.

Self-Advocacy Videotapes

As part of a general focus on collaboration and executive functions in rehabilitation, it is useful to engage individuals with TBI, working collaboratively with staff and family members, in the production of a videotape that has as its primary purpose to orient and train future (or current) staff in how to teach, help, coach, and otherwise work with the person. This can be a project for the last 2 or 3 weeks of the inpatient rehabilitation program or at any time when such a training vehicle may be useful. The person with disability is engaged in a meaningful and important project that has a concrete and very legitimate goal—namely, to help others understand their strengths and needs and become oriented to the teaching or support procedures that are most helpful.

This project also has several secondary purposes, including consolidation of collaborative alliances through product-oriented efforts. Furthermore, this process helps the person with disability, family members, and other relevant everyday people to gain insight regarding postinjury issues. Their learning often is enhanced when important information and procedures are processed to teach someone else. A general protocol (that can and should be modified to meet the needs of specific individuals and situations) and its rationale are presented in Table 33–19. In at least two New York State TBI community support programs, protocols are in place that enable all participants to create and use self-advocacy videotapes.

CLINICAL DECISION MAKING IN THE FACE OF INCOMPLETE EVIDENCE

Throughout this chapter, we have cited key pieces of experimental literature and general reviews of the efficacy literature in TBI rehabilitation and, importantly, in closely related fields of intervention. In our view, serious consideration of these literatures, combined with clinical experience in many practice settings, supports the general approach to intervention described in this chapter. At this time, however, evidence from well-designed clinical trials with large numbers of subjects is insufficient to draw strong conclusions. Therefore, clinicians must make responsible clinical judgments in the absence of accepted standards of practice.

TABLE 33–19

Transitional/Self-Advocacy Video: Rationale and Procedures

Goals

Primary Goal: To produce a videotape that can be used to orient and train people (e.g., school staff, employers, family members, home health aides, and others) who may need to be trained in how to teach, interact with, or otherwise support the person with disability.

Important Associated Goals:

The individual with disability will:

• Gain a sense of empowerment.
• Gain progressively more insight regarding their strengths and needs.
• Progressively become more strategic in their thinking about themselves and their rehabilitation and school careers.

Family members will:

• Gain a sense of empowerment.
• Gain progressively more insight regarding the child's strengths and needs and share their insights with staff.
• Gain an appreciation of the importance of executive functions and the student's participation in goal setting, planning, and strategic thinking.

Staff will:

• Strengthen their collaborative relationships with other team members (including parents) as they work together to produce the video.
• Gain greater appreciation for the perspective of students and parents.

Procedures (Subject to Considerable Variation in Individual Cases)

1. Several weeks before a substantial transition (e.g., discharge from inpatient rehabilitation, return to work or school) staff, individual with disability, and family members hold a **planning meeting**. The purposes of this meeting are:
   a. To decide what **content** would be most important to demonstrate on video. This could include:
      • **Physical** strengths, weaknesses and intervention/support issues (e.g., seating, positioning, mobility, dressing, and eating).
      • **Cognitive** strengths, weaknesses. and intervention/support issues (e.g., types of advance organizers needed; types of environmental or materials modifications needed because of attentional, perceptual, or other processing problems; types of cues and prompts needed).
      • **Communication** strengths, weaknesses, and intervention/support issues (e.g., use of an augmentative communication system; demonstration of partner communication styles that facilitate comprehension).
      • **Behavioral/social** strengths, weaknesses, and intervention/support issues (e.g., procedures for preventing behavioral problems, ways to diffuse behavioral outbursts, and ways to facilitate peer interaction).
      It is critical that both **strengths** and the **goals of the individual with disability and family members** be highlighted.
   b. To decide what **format and scripts** would be most effective in demonstrating critical points:
      1. It often is effective to show the individual (1) succeeding at a task that he or she is good at; (2) failing at an important but difficult task when appropriate procedures, modifications, or equipment are **not** in place; and then (3) succeeding when they are in place.
      2. It often is effective to communicate content by means of a **conversation** between individual with disability and staff or between staff and family members, as opposed to simply videoing a "talking head."
      3. It is ideal to videotape the individual's own orientation to and commentary about the video segments and then edit these into the tape as orientation for the viewer. This videoing can be made after the person has watched the other segments.
   c. To decide **who should play what role** in the video. If possible, the person with disability should play a leading role (possibly with considerable support). If the person is extremely impaired, family members can play a leading role.
   d. To work out **logistics** of videoing and editing.
   The individual and family members may be more or less involved in this planning, depending on many factors.
2. During the following weeks, the planning of video demonstrations can be included in therapy sessions. For example, development of scripts can be part of speech-language therapy sessions; development of presentation of strengths and needs can be part of counseling sessions; and development of physical demonstrations can be part of PT, OT, ST, and other therapies.
3. The actual videotaping may be no more than a camera in a therapy session capturing an important demonstration. If other individuals are present, they must have signed releases. The videotape may or may not be edited, depending on the skills of staff and time available.

(continued)

TABLE 33-19

Transitional/Self-Advocacy Video: Rationale and Procedures (continued)

Advantages of this Transitional/Self-Advocacy Routine
Beyond the obvious goal of orienting future staff and caregivers, the transitional, self-advocacy videos serve a number of purposes:
1. **Incidental Learning: Individual with Disability**—People acquire important information about themselves and about their rehabilitation program by being engaged in a fun, product-oriented activity.
2. **Incidental Learning: Staff**—Staff members acquire important information about the person with disability, the family, and their own program by being engaged in a fun, product-oriented activity.
3. **Incidental Learning: Family Members**—Family members acquire important information about the individual and the intervention program by being engaged in a fun, product-oriented activity.
4. **Efficient Cross-Training:** Staff currently working with the person may learn important things from other staff or from family members without the stigma associated with being singled out for remedial instruction.
5. **Development of a Shared Conceptual Framework:** The intervention team refines its own shared conceptual framework by being engaged in a fun, product-oriented activity.
6. **Fun:** Producing this video can be fun.
7. **Permanent Record:** If this practice becomes routine, the person with disability and family will have an invaluable permanent record of the recovery process.
8. **Costumer Satisfaction:** In general, people with disability and family members are pleased when staff accord them the respect that is implicit in this activity. Indeed, this can be a vehicle for overcoming an adversarial relationship if that exists.

Modified from Ylvisaker, Szekeres, Feeney (1998); with permission.

In domains of impairment in which the need for clinical services is undeniable but published experimental guidance is, at best, incomplete, responsible clinicians make decisions about intervention for specific individuals with disability based on informed consideration of the following factors (Ylvisaker et al., 2002):

- Is the proposed intervention supported by any intervention outcome studies with subjects who have TBI and who possess the same impairments and needs as the client?
- Is the proposed intervention supported by intervention outcome studies with related populations (e.g., those with learning disabilities, developmental disabilities, ADHD, or behavioral disorders)?
- Is the proposed intervention supported by trial intervention with the client?
- Is the proposed intervention supported by extensive clinical experience with clients who have TBI?
- Is the proposed intervention supported by theory, including neuropsychological, cognitive, behavioral, pedagogical, and other theories?
- Is the proposed intervention supported by negotiation with the client and relevant stakeholders in the client's life?
- Is the proposed intervention consistent with known constraints, including expertise of service providers, availability of support personnel, time to complete the intervention, and adequate resources?
- Can the proposed intervention be judged as preferable to known alternatives—in relation to predicted functional outcome for the client—based on the previous considerations?

- Is the proposed intervention humane, morally justifiable, and consistent with the scope of practice and relevant licensing laws governing the provider of services?

In our experience with several hundred children, adolescents, and adults who have chronic disability after TBI—disability in the territory in which communication, cognition, executive functions, and behavior overlap and interact—the approach outlined and illustrated in this chapter requires creative effort, but can be effective and functional, based on all these considerations. Furthermore, data from our work with the New York State Department of Health TBI Medicaid Waiver Program demonstrates the cost effectiveness of this approach (Feeney et al., 2001).

FUTURE TRENDS

At the beginning of the 21st century, managed care and associated reductions in funding for rehabilitation have become thoroughly established as dominant themes in adult neurogenic rehabilitation. Inpatient lengths of stay have decreased dramatically over the past 20 years, and funding for traditional outpatient therapies also has been substantially reduced (AHCPR, 1999). The staggering cost of catastrophic neurologic rehabilitation, which was estimated in 1993 to be approximately $4 billion a year, increasing at a rate of 15% a year (Cope & O'Lear, 1993), has motivated draconian cost-cutting measures. Even as they cut funding, however, funders of services increasingly demand meaningful evidence of improved functional outcomes. Clinicians, attempting to meet the challenge of having a greater effect with fewer resources, have attempted to create efficiencies in the form of increased use of group therapy and indirect therapy using adequately trained support staff, volunteers, family members, and others. Reason exists to believe that these trends will continue.

We urge professionals in brain injury rehabilitation to increasingly look to other disability groups for insights regarding the provision of effective, community-based services and supports. Community-based models of service delivery have a longer (although not uniformly successful) history in developmental disabilities, mental health, and spinal cord injury compared with brain injury rehabilitation. More generally, professionals serving other populations of people with chronic cognitive, communication, and behavioral impairment may offer wisdom regarding the process of contextualizing and "de-medicalizing" long-term services and supports.

Although driven by economic forces, some of the new directions in service delivery may simply be good practice finally come of age. Following severe TBI, even the best combination of medical and other clinically based interventions generally leave survivors with some degree of impairment and associated disability. Because a majority of these people are relatively young, the ongoing impairments affect social life, work, family life, and community living in dynamic and evolving ways. Therefore, we believe that demands will continue to increase for community-based services and supports, including appropriate supported housing and work, recreational possibilities, behavioral services, and family supports. Cognitive, behavioral, and communication competence plays a critical role in real-world success in these domains. Therefore, specialists trained in community-based cognitive, behavioral, and communication intervention likely will be in increasing demand.

In our experience, delivery of services and supports becomes increasingly challenging years after the injury, particularly if the person with TBI has experienced considerable failure in attempting community reintegration and, possibly, has made unfortunate choices, such as abuse of alcohol and drugs, to escape the pain of ongoing failure. We expect that more states will recognize the combined rehabilitative, humanistic, and budgetary advantages of long-term community support services, like those provided through the New York State TBI Medicaid Waiver Program, for individuals with TBI who are particularly difficult to serve (Feeney et al., 2001; Ylvisaker, 1999; Ylvisaker, Feeney, & Capo, 2007). Potentially lifelong supports through community support agencies, including the services of professionals with expertise in cognition, communication, and behavior, will be found cheaper and more effective than periodic crisis services (e.g., psychiatric hospitalization or jail). Communication specialists will need to be comfortable delivering services

within teams that necessarily include the person with disability and in nonstandard venues, such as the workplace, private residences, and other community settings. Furthermore, specialists in rehabilitation will increasingly deliver their services indirectly, through everyday people in the life of the person with disability.

Developing technologies continue to hold promise for individuals with disability. In particular, the world of electronic communication and access to the Internet have been opened to individuals with varying cognitive disabilities. Sohlberg, Fickas, Ehlhardt, and Todis (2005) evaluated the effectiveness of adapted e-mail access for four adults with severe cognitive impairments after TBI and associated social isolation. The investigators found that all four participants became independent users of the system and continued to e-mail at a 9-month follow-up. The participants endorsed the benefits of e-mailing and reported feeling more connected with family and friends. Earlier, we described the promise that VR technology holds in potentially providing ecologically valid training within a clinical setting.

Reports from animal laboratories regarding the potential usefulness of neuropharmacologic agents in the treatment of individuals with TBI continue to be promising. Despite the trumpeting of this promise for at least two decades, however, "there are currently no drugs available that are of demonstrated benefit in promoting cognitive and motor recovery from TBI" (National Institutes of Health, 1999, p. 269). Clinicians are well advised to remain alert to developments in this field and to ensure that significantly impaired individuals receive needed evaluations from a physician with expertise in TBI pharmacology. Hopefulness, however, must be muted by the realistic expectation that, into the foreseeable future, the greatest effects for individuals with chronic impairment will be derived from a combination of behavioral interventions and environmental supports.

KEY POINTS

1. Because most individuals with severe TBI are relatively young and, therefore, live for several decades with ongoing impairment, the prevalence of TBI is high, and the costs to society are extraordinary.

2. Although virtually any combination of preserved and impaired functions is technically possible after TBI, there are central tendencies within the population, associated, in large part, with damage to the vulnerable frontal lobes, limbic structures, and neural connections among these regions.

3. TBI does not randomly select its victims. Disproportionately large numbers of people with TBI are adolescents or young adults and, in many cases, had preinjury predisposing factors, including

weak academic and vocational histories, risk-taking behavior, and possibly, substance abuse.

4. Among the common consequences of TBI is weak executive control over behavior, including cognition, communication, and social behavior generally.

5. Historically, the dominant intervention approach in medical rehabilitation has been characterized by a focus on reducing the underlying impairment with decontextualized exercises administered by specialists in specialized treatment settings. An alternative approach that has gained increasing acceptance focuses flexibly on impairment, activity/participation, and context—often starting with context modifications (or threats to participation)—involves context-sensitive practice of successful everyday routines and is supported, in large part, by everyday people.

6. Context-sensitive, everyday, routine-based intervention has its rationale in the special needs of people with frontal lobe injury, in recent developments in learning theory, and in the economic realities of neurologic rehabilitation.

7. Context-sensitive, everyday, routine-based intervention is associated with an approach to assessment that is ongoing, sensitive to real-world contexts, and collaborative and that involves the testing of intervention hypotheses.

8. At the center of executive system intervention is the concept of an executive function routine, wherein the individual with disability contributes as much as possible to identifying goals and potential obstacles to achieving the goals, creating plans for achieving the goals, reviewing the usefulness of the plans, and reflecting on what does and does not work for that person in attempting to achieve his or her goals.

9. Functional, individualized rehabilitation plans are centered around goals and activities that are important to the individual, with varied impairments and disabilities targeted within the context of these activities in an attempt to routinize improved cognitive functioning.

10. For reasons that are in part neuropsychological and in part psychological, behavior plans for individuals with TBI should be largely antecedent-focused, understanding antecedents broadly to include both immediate and remote setting events.

11. Communication/behavior plans for individuals with TBI often focus on teaching positive communication alternatives to negative behavior. Positive communication scripts must be integrated into the individual's sense of personal identity that may have to be revised after the injury.

12. Helping individuals with TBI to increase their participation in chosen life activities, improve performance of activities of everyday life, and ultimately, reduce their impairments (i.e., improve neurologically mediated processing) frequently requires massive amounts of supported practice in the routines of everyday life. In turn, ensuring adequate amounts of practice requires that specialists collaborate with everyday people who become the primary facilitators of improved performance.

ACTIVITIES FOR REFLECTION AND DISCUSSION

1. Explain the difference between incidence and prevalence.
2. Explain why TBI is associated with extraordinary societal costs.
3. Why are the frontal lobes especially vulnerable in TBI? List and explain common communication-related impairments associated with frontal lobe injury.
4. What are the most important reasons for contextualizing assessment for individuals with TBI?
5. List and explain several possible hypotheses that could explain why a specific individual with TBI speaks very little and only when spoken to. How would you test the hypotheses?
6. List and explain several possible hypotheses that could explain why a young adult with TBI becomes verbally aggressive when reminded to perform a routine task. How would you test the hypotheses?
7. List and explain several possible hypotheses that could explain why a specific individual with TBI speaks in a way that is disorganized, tangential, and verbose? How would you test the hypotheses?
8. What are the most important reasons for contextualizing intervention for individuals with TBI?
9. Describe differences in executive function routines for people in the middle and late stages of recovery from TBI.
10. What is meant by "supported cognition," and why is it important?
11. What are the most important reasons for focusing on antecedents in TBI behavior management?
12. Why is it important for speech-language pathologists to be included on behavior management teams?
13. Describe strategies for maximizing the effects that can be obtained from shrinking resources available for long-term rehabilitation.

References

Abikoff, H., Hechtman, L., Klien, R. G., Gallagher, R., Fleiss, K., Etcovitch, J., et al. (2004). Social functioning in children with ADHD treated with long-term methylphenidate and multimodal psychosocial treatment. *Journal of the American Academy of Childhood and Adolescent Psychiatry, 43*(7), 820–829.

Adamonovich, B., & Henderson, J. (1992). *Scales of cognitive ability for traumatic brain injury.* Chicago, IL: Riverside.

Adams, J. H., Graham, D. I., Murray, L. S., & Scott, G. (1982). Diffuse axonal injury due to non-missile head injury in humans: An analysis of 45 cases. *Annals of Neurology, 12,* 557–563.

Adams, J. H., Graham, D. I., Scott, G., Parker, L. S., & Doyle, D. (1980). Brain damage in fatal non-missel head injury. *Journal of Clinical Pathology, 33,* 1132–1145.

AHCPR (1999). *Rehabilitation for traumatic brain injury: Evidence report/technology assessment Number 2* (Agency for Health Care Policy and Research Publication No. 99-E006). Author.

Alderman, N. (1996). Central executive deficit and response to operant conditioning methods. *Neuropsychological Rehabilitation, 6,* 161–186.

Alderman, N. (2003). Contemporary approaches to the management of irritability and aggression following traumatic brain injury. *Neuropsychological Rehabilitation, 13*(1–2), 211–240.

Alderman, N., & Ward, A. (1991). Behavioral treatment of the dysexecutive syndrome: Reduction of repetitive speech using response cost and cognitive overlearning. *Neuropsychological Rehabilitation, 1,* 65–80.

Alexander, M. (1987). Syndromes in the rehabilitation and outcome of closed head injury. In H. S. Levin, J. Grafman, & H. M. Eisenberg (Eds.), *Neurobehavioral recovery from head injury* (pp. 192–205). New York: Oxford.

Alexander, M. P. (2002). Disorders of language after frontal lobe injury: Evidence for the neural mechanisms of assembling language. In D. T. Stuss & R. T. Knight (Eds.), *Principles of frontal lobe function* (pp. 159–167). New York: Oxford University Press.

Alexander, M. P., Benson, D. F., & Stuss, D. T. (1989). Frontal lobes and language. *Brain and Language, 37,* 656–691.

American Speech-Language-Hearing Association (ASHA) (1988, March). The role of speech-language pathologists in the identification, diagnosis, and treatment of individuals with cognitive-communicative impairments. *ASHA, 30,* 79.

Anderson, S.W., Damasio, H., Tranel, D., & Damasio, A. R. (1988). Neuropsychological correlates of bilateral frontal lobe lesions in humans. *Society for Neuroscience, 14,* 1288.

Anderson, S. W., Damasio, H., Tranel, D., & Damasio, A. R. (2000). Long-term sequelae of prefrontal cortex damage acquired in early childhood. *Developmental Neuropsychology, 18*(3), 281–296.

Annegers, J. F., Grabow, J. D., Kurland, L. T., & Laws, E. R. (1980). The incidence, causes, and secular trends of head trauma in Olmsted County, Minnesota, 1935-1974. *Neurology, 30,* 912–919.

Ashcraft, M. (1994). *Human memory and cognition.* Reading, MA: Addison-Wesley, Longman.

Ashman, A. F., & Conway, R. N. F. (1989). *Cognitive strategies for special education.* London: Routledge.

Bachman, D. L. (1992). The diagnosis and management of common neurologic sequelae of closed head injury. *Journal of Head Trauma Rehabilitation, 7,* 50–59.

Baddeley, A. D. (1999). *Essentials of human memory.* East Sussex, UK: Psychology Press.

Baer, D. M., Wolf, M. M., & Risley, T. R. (1987). Some still current dimensions of applied behavior analysis. *Journal of Applied Behavior Analysis, 20,* 313–327.

Baguley, I. J., Cooper, J., & Felmingham, K. (2006). Aggressive behavior following traumatic brain injury: How common is common? *Journal of Head Trauma Rehabilitation, 21*(1), 45–56.

Baker, S., Gersten, R., & Scanlon, D. (2002). Procedural facilitators and cognitive strategies: Tools for unraveling the mysteries of comprehension and the writing process, and for providing meaningful access to the general curriculum. *Learning Disabilities Research & Practice, 17*(1), 65–77.

Bannerman, D. J., Sheldon, J. B., Sherman, J. A., & Harchik, A. E. (1990). Balancing the right to habilitation with the right to personal liberties: The rights of people with developmental disabilities to eat too many doughnuts and take a nap. *Journal of Applied Behavior Analysis, 23,* 79–89.

Bargh, J. A., & Chartrand, T. L. (1999). The unbearable automaticity of being. *American Psychologist, 54,* 462–479.

Barkley, R. A. (1987). *Defiant children: A clinician's manual for parent training.* NY: The Guilford Press.

Barkley, R. A. (2004). Adolescents with attention-deficit/hyperactivity disorder: An overview of empirically based treatments. *Journal of Psychiatric Practice, 10*(1), 39–56.

Barsalou, L. W. (1992). *Cognitive psychology: An overview for cognitive scientists.* Hillsdale, NJ: Lawrence Erlbaum.

Baumeister, R. F., & Vohs, K. D. (2004). *Handbook of self-regulation: Research, theory, and applications.* New York: Guilford Press.

Bechara, A., Damasio, A. R., Damasio, H., & Anderson, S. W. (1994). Insensitivity to future consequences following damage to the human prefrontal cortex. *Cognition, 50,* 7–12.

Bechara, A., Tranel, D., Damasio, H., & Damasio, A. (1996). Failure to respond autonomically to anticipated future outcomes following damage to prefrontal cortex. *Cerebral Cortex, 6,* 215–225.

Benton, A. (1991). Prefrontal injury and behavior in children. *Developmental Neuropsychology, 7*(3), 275–281.

Ben-Yishay, Y., & Diller, L. (1983). Cognitive remediation. In M. Rosenthal, E. Griffith, M. Bond, & J. D. Miller (Eds.), *Rehabilitation of the head injured adult* (pp. 367–380). Philadelphia: F. A. Davis.

Ben-Yishay, Y., Piasetsky, E. B., & Rattok, J. (1987). A systematic method for ameliorating disorders in basic attention. In M. J. Meier, A. L. Benton, & L. Diller (Eds.), *Neuropsychological Rehabilitation* (pp. 165–181). New York: Churchill Livingstone.

Berk, L. E. (2001). *Awakening children's minds: How parents and teachers can make a difference.* New York: Oxford University Press.

Berk, L. E., & Winsler, A. (1995). Scaffolding children's learning: Vygotsky and early childhood education. *NAEYC Research and Practice Series, 7.* Washington, D.C.: National Association for the Education of Young Children.

Beukelman, D. R. (1998). Communication Effectiveness Survey. In D. R. Beukelman, P. Mathy, & K. Yorkston (1998). Outcomes measurement in motor speech disorders. In C. M. Frattali (Ed.), *Measuring outcomes in speech-language pathology* (pp. 334–353). New York: Thieme Medical.

Biddle, K. R., McCabe, A., & Bliss, L. S. (1996). Narrative skills following traumatic brain injury in children and adults. *Journal of Communication Disorders, 29*(6), 447–470.

Bird, F., Dores, P. A., Moniz, D., & Robinson, J. (1989). Reducing severe aggressive and self-injurious behaviors with functional communication training: Direct, collateral, and generalized results. *American Journal of Mental Retardation, 94,* 37–48.

Bjorklund, D. F. (1990). *Children's strategies: Contemporary views of cognitive development.* Hillsdale, NJ: Lawrence Erlbaum.

Blumer, D., & Benson, F. (1975). Personality changes with frontal and temporal lobe lesions. In D. F. Benson & D. Blumer (Eds.), *Psychiatric aspects of neurologic disease* (pp. 151–170). New York: Grune & Stratton.

Boake, C. (1996). Supervision Rating Scale: A measure of functional outcome from brain injury. *Archives of Physical Medicine and Rehabilitation, 77,* 765–772.

Bodrova, E., & Leong, D. J. (1996). *Tools of the mind: The Vygotskyan approach to early childhood education.* Englewood Cliffs, NJ: Prentice-Hall.

Bond, M. (1990). Standardized methods of assessing and predicting outcome. In M. Rosenthal, E. R. Griffith, M. R. Bond, & J. D. Miller (Eds.), *Rehabilitation of the adult and child with traumatic brain injury.* Philadelphia: F. A. Davis.

Braunling-McMorrow, D., Lloyd, K., & Fralish, K. (1986). Teaching social skills to head injured adults. *Journal of Rehabilitation, 52,* 39–44.

Brazzeli, M., Colombo, N. DellaSala, S., & Spinnler, H. (1994). Spared and impaired cognitive abilities after bilateral frontal lobe damage. *Cortex, 30,* 27–51.

Bronson, M. B. (2000). *Self-regulation in early childhood.* New York: Guilford Press.

Brooks, B. M., McNeil, J. E., Rose, F. D., Greenwood, R. J., Attree, E. A., & Leadbetter, A. G. (1999). Route learning in a case of amnesia: A preliminary investigation into the efficacy of training in a virtual environment. *Neuropsychological Rehabilitation, 9,* 63–76.

Brooks, D. N., Campsie, L., Symington, C., Beattie, A., Bryden, J., & McKinley, W. (1987). The effects of severe head injury upon patient and relative within seven years of injury. *Journal of Head Trauma Rehabilitation, 2,* 1–13.

Brooks, D. N., & McKinlay, W. (1983). Personality and behavioral change after severe blunt head injury—A relative's view. *Journal of Neurology, Neurosurgery, and Psychiatry, 46,* 336–344.

Brothers, L. (1997). *Friday's footprint: How society shapes the human mind.* New York: Oxford University Press.

Brotherton, F. A., Thomas, L. L., Wisotzek, I. E., & Milan, M. A. (1988). Social skills training in the rehabilitation of patients with traumatic closed head injury. *Archives of Physical Medicine and Rehabilitation, 69,* 827–832.

Brown, A. L., Campione, J. C., Weber, L. S., & McGilly; K. (1992). *Interactive learning environments: A new look at assessment and instruction.* Berkeley: University of California, Commission on Testing and Public Policy.

Brown, F., Belz, P., Corsi, L., & Wenig, B. (1993). Choice diversity for people with severe disabilities. *Education and Training in Mental Retardation, 28,* 318–326.

Brown, G., Chadwick, O., Shaffer, D., Rutter, M., & Traub, M. (1981). A prospective study of children with head injuries. III. Psychiatric sequelae. *Psychological Medicine, 11,* 63–78.

Brookshire, R. H. (1997). *Introduction to neurogenic communication disorders* (5th ed.). St. Louis, MO: Mosby.

Buckner, R. L., Peterson, S., Ojemann, J., Miezin, F., Squire, L., & Raichle, M. (1995). Functional anatomical studies of explicit and implicit memory. *Journal of Neuroscience, 15,* 12–29.

Bulgren, J. A., & Schumaker, J. B. (2006). Teaching practices that optimize curriculum access. In Deshler, D. D., & Schumaker, J. B. (Eds.), Teaching adolescents with disabilities: Accessing the general curriculum (pp. 79–120). Thousand Oaks, CA: Corwin Press.

Burgess, P., Alderman, N., Evans, J., Emslie, H., & Wilson, B. (1998). The ecological validity of tests of executive function. *Journal of the International Neuropsychological Society, 4,* 547–558.

Burgess, P. W., & Robertson, I. H. (2002a). Principles of the rehabilitation of frontal lobe function. In D. T. Stuss & R. T. Knight (Eds.), *Principles of frontal lobe function* (pp. 557–572). New York: Oxford University Press.

Burgess, P. W., & Robertson, I. H. (2002b). Principles of the rehabilitation of frontal lobe function. In D. T. Stuss & R. T. Knight (Eds.), *Principles of frontal lobe function* (pp. 557–572). New York: Oxford University Press.

Buschke, H., & Fuld, P. A. (1974). Evaluating storage, retention, and retrieval in disordered memory and learning. *Neurology,* 1019–1025.

Cabeza, R., & Nyberg, L. (1997). Imaging cognition: An empirical review of PET studies with normal subjects. *Journal of Cognitive Neuroscience, 9,* 1–26.

Campione, J. C., & Brown, A. L. (1990). Guided learning and transfer. In N. Fredrickson, R. Glaser, A. Lesgold, & M. Shafto (Eds.), *Diagnostic monitoring of skill and knowledge acquisition* (pp. 114–172). Hillsdale, NJ: Lawrence Erlbaum.

Carney, N., Chesnut, R. M., Maynard, H., Mann, N. C., Patterson, P., & Helfand, M. (1999). Effect of cognitive rehabilitation on outcomes for persons with traumatic brain injury: A systematic review. *Journal of Head Trauma Rehabilitation, 14,* 277–307.

Carr, E. G., Carlson, J. I., Langdon, N. A., Magito-McLaughlin, D., & Yarbrough, S. C. (1998). Two perspectives on antecedent control. In J. K. Luiselli & M. J. Cameron (Eds.), *Antecedent control: Innovative approaches to behavioral support* (pp. 3–28). Baltimore: Paul H. Brookes.

Carr, E. G., & Durand, V. M., (1985). Reducing behavior problems through functional communication training. *Journal of Applied Behavior Analysis, 18,* 111–126.

Carr, E. G., Horner, R. H., Turnbull, A. P., et al. (1999). *Positive behavior support for people with developmental disabilities: A research synthesis.* Washington, D.C.: American Association of Mental Retardation.

Carr, E. G., Levin, L., McConnachie, G., Carlson, J. I, Kemp, D. C., & Smith, C. E. (1994). *Communication-based intervention for problem behavior: A user's guide for producing positive change.* Baltimore, MD: Paul Brookes.

Carr, E. G., Reeve, C. E., Magito-McLaughlin, D. (1997). Contextual influences on problem behavior in people with developmental disabilities. In L. K. Koegel, R. L. Koegel, & G. Dunlap (Eds.), *Positive behavioral support: Including people with difficult behavior in the community* (pp. 403–423). Baltimore: Paul H. Brookes.

Cattelani, R., Lombardi, F., Brianti, R., & Mazucchi, A. (1998). Traumatic brain injury in childhood: Intellectual, behavioral and social outcome into adulthood. *Brain Injury, 12* (4), 283–296.

Centers for Disease Control and Prevention. (1997). Traumatic brain injury—Colorado, Missouri, Oklahoma, and Utah, 1990-1993. *MMWR, 46,* 8-11.

Centers for Disease Control and Prevention. (Jan. 16, 2001). Traumatic brain injury in the United States: A report to congress. *www.cdc.gov.*

Channon, S., Pellijeff, A., & Rule, A. (2005). Social cognition after head injury: Sarcasm and theory of mind. *Brain and Language, 93*, 123–134.

Chapman, S., Culhane, K., Levin, H., Harward, H., Mendelsohn, D., Ewing-Cobbs, L., et al. (1992). Narrative discourse after closed head injury in children and adolescents. *Brain and Language, 43*, 42–65.

Chapman, S. B. (1997). Cognitive-communication abilities in children with closed head injury. *American Journal of Speech-Language Pathology, 6*, 50–58.

Chapman, S. B., Levin, H. S., Matejka, J., Harward, H. N., & Kufera, J. (1995). Discourse ability in head injured children: Consideration of linguistic, psychosocial, & cognitive factors. *Journal of Head Trauma Rehabilitation, 10*, 36–54.

Chapman, S. B., Watkins, R., Gustafson, C., Moore, S., Levin, H. S., & Kufera, J. A. (1997). Narrative discourse in children with closed head injury, children with language impairment, and typically developing children. *American Journal of Speech-Language Pathology, 6*, 66–76.

Cicerone, K. D. (2002). Remediation of 'working attention' in mild traumatic brain injury. *Brain Injury, 16*, 185–195.

Cicerone, K. (2005). Rehabilitation of executive function deficits. In W. M. High, A. M. Sander, M. A. Struchen, & K. A. Hart (Eds.), *Rehabilitation interventions following traumatic brain injury: State of the science* (pp. 71–87). New York: Oxford University Press.

Cicerone, K. D., Dahlberg, C., Malec, J. F., Langenbbahn, D. M., Felicetti, T., Kneipp, S., et al. (2005). Evidence-based cognitive rehabilitation: Updated review of the literature from 1998 through 2002. *Archives of Physical Medicine & Rehabilitation, 86*(8), 1681–1692.

Coelho, C., Ylvisaker, M., & Turkstra, L. (2005). Non-standardized assessment approaches for individuals with traumatic brain injuries. *Seminars in Speech and Language, 26*(4), 223–241.

Coelho, C. A., Liles, B. Z., & Duffy, R. J. (1991). Analysis of conversational discourse in head-injured clients. *Journal of Head Trauma Rehabilitation, 6*, 92–99.

Collins, M. W., Grindel, S. H., Lovell, M. R., Dede, D. E., Moser, D. J., Phalin, B. R., et al. (1999). Relationship between concussion and neuropsychological performance in college football players. *Journal of the American Medical Association, 282*(10), 964–970.

Cope, D. N., & O'Lear, J. (1993). A clinical and economic perspective on head injury rehabilitation. *Journal of Head Trauma Rehabilitation, 8*, 1–14.

Costeff, H., Grosswasser, Z., Landman, Y., & Brenner, T. (1985). Survivors of severe traumatic brain injury in childhood: I. Late residual disability. *Scandinavian Journal of Rehabilitation Medicine, 12*(suppl), 10–15.

Courville, J. (1937). *Pathology of the central nervous system.* Mountain View, CA: Pacific.

Crépeau, F., Scherzer, B. P., Belleville, S., & Desmarais, G. (1997). A qualitative analysis of central executive disorders in a real-life work situation. *Neuropsychological Rehabilitation, 7*(2), 147–165.

Curl, R. M., Fraser, R. T., Cook, R. G., & Clemmons, D. (1996). Traumatic brain injury vocational rehabilitation: Preliminary findings for the coworker as trainer project. *Journal of Head Trauma Rehabilitation, 11*, 75–85.

Damasio, A. R. (1994). *Descartes error.* New York: Harper-Collins.

Damasio, A. R. (1998). The somatic marker hypothesis and the possible functions of the prefrontal cortex. In A. C. Roberts, T. W. Robbins, & L. Weiskrantz (Eds.), *The prefrontal cortex: Executive and cognitive functions* (pp. 36–50). Oxford: Oxford University Press.

Damasio, A. R., Tranel, D., & Damasio, H. (1990). Individuals with sociopathic behavior caused by frontal lobe damage fail to respond automatically to socially charged stimuli. *Behavioral Brain Research, 14*, 81–94.

Damasio, A. R., Tranel, D., & Damasio, H. (1991). Somatic markers and the guidance of behavior: Theory and preliminary testing. In H. S. Levin, H. M. Eisenberg, & A. L. Benton (Eds.), *Frontal lobe function and dysfunction* (pp. 217–229). New York: Oxford University Press.

Deci, E. L. (1995). *Why we do what we do: Understanding self-motivation.* New York: Penguin Books.

Deci, E. L., & Ryan, R. M. (Eds.) (2002). *Handbook of self-determination research.* Rochester, NY: University of Rochester Press.

Denckla, M. B. (1996). Research on executive function in a neurodevelopmental context: Application of clinical measures. *Developmental Neuropsychology, 12*, 5–15.

Dennis, M. (1991). Frontal lobe function in childhood and adolescence: A heuristic for assessing attention regulation, executive control, and the intentional states important for social discourse. *Developmental Neuropsychology, 7*(3), 327–358.

Dennis, M. (1992). Word-finding in children and adolescents with a history of brain injury. *Topics in Language Disorders, 13*, 66–82.

Dennis, M., & Barnes, M. (1990). Knowing the meaning, getting the point, bridging the gap, and carrying the message: Aspects of discourse following closed head injury in childhood and adolescence. *Brain and Language, 39*, 428–446.

Dennis, M., Barnes, M. A., Donnelly, R. E., Wilkinson, M., & Humphreys, R. P. (1996). Appraising and managing knowledge: Metacognitive skills after childhood head injury. *Developmental Neuropsychology, 12*, 77–103.

Dennis, M., & Lovett, M. (1990). Discourse ability in children after brain damage. In Y. Joanette & H. H. Brownell (Eds.), *Discourse ability and brain damage: Theoretical and empirical perspectives* (pp. 199–223). New York: Springer Verlag.

Detterman, D. K., & Sternberg, R. J. (Eds.). (1993). *Transfer on trial: Intelligence, cognition, and instruction.* Norwood, NJ: Ablex.

Dodd, D., & White, R. M. (1980). *Cognition: Mental structures and processes.* Boston, MA: Allyn & Bacon.

Donnellan, A. M., Mirenda, P. L., Mesaros, R. A., & Fassbender, L. L. (1984). Analyzing the communicative functions of aberrant behavior. *Journal of the Association for Persons with Severe Handicaps, 9*, 201–212.

Doss, S., & Reichle, J. (1989). Establishing communicative alternatives to the emission of socially motivated excess behavior: A review. *Journal of the Association for Persons with Severe Handicaps, 14*, 101–112.

Douglas, J. M., O'Flaherty, C. A., & Snow, P. C. (2000). Measuring perception of communicative ability: The development and evaluation of the La Trobe communication questionnaire. *Aphasiology, 14*(3), 251–268.

Dunlap, G., dePerczel, M., Clarke, S., Wilson, D., Wright, S., White, R., et al. (1994). Choice-making to promote adaptive behavior for students with emotional and behavioral challenges. *Journal of Applied Behavior Analysis, 27*, 505–518.

Durand, V. M., & Crimmins, D. B. (1992). *The Motivation Assessment Scale.* Topeka, Kansas: Monaco.

Dywan, J., & Segalowitz, S. J. (1996). Self- and family-ratings of adaptive behavior after traumatic brain injury: Psychometric scores and frontally generated RRPs. *Journal of Head Trauma Rehabilitation, 11*(2), 79–75.

Ehrlich, J. S. (1988). Selective characteristics of narrative discourse in head-injured and normal adults. *Journal of communication Disorders, 21*, 1–9.

Ellmo, W. J., Graser, J. M., Krchnavek, B., Hauck, K., & Calabrese, D. B. (1995). *Measure of Cognitive-Linguistic Abilities.* Florida: The Speech Bin.

Eslinger, P. J., & Damasio, A. R. (1985). Severe disturbance of higher cognition following bilateral frontal lobe oblation: Patient EVR. *Neurology, 35*, 1731–1741.

Evans, J. J., Needham, P., Wilson, B. A., & Brentnall, S. (2003). Which memory impaired people make good use of memory aids? Results of a survey of people with acquired brain injury. *Journal of the International Neuropsychological Society, 9*, 925–935.

Evans, J. J., Wilson, B. A., Schuri, U., Andrade, J., Baddeley, A., Bruna, O., et al. (2000). A comparison of "errorless" and "trial-and-error" learning methods for teaching individuals with acquired memory deficits. *Neuropsychological Rehabilitation, 10*(1), 67–101.

Evans, P. (1993). Some implications of Vygotsky's work for special education. In H. Daniels (Ed.), *Charting the agenda: Education activity after Vygotsky.* London: Routledge.

Ewert, J., Levin, H. S., Watson, M. G., & Kalisky, Z. (1989). Procedural memory during posttraumatic amnesia in survivors of severe closed head injury: Implications for rehabilitation. *Archives of Neurology, 46*, 911–916.

Feeney, T., Ylvisaker, M., Rosen, B., & Greene, P. (2001a). Community supports for individuals with challenging behavior after brain injury: An analysis of the New York State Behavioral Resource Project. *Journal of Head Trauma Rehabilitation, 16*(1), 61–75.

Feeney, T. J., & Ylvisaker, M. (1995). Choice and routine: Antecedent behavior interventions for adolescents with severe traumatic brain injury. *Journal of Head Trauma Rehabilitation, 10*, 67–86.

Feeney, T. J., & Ylvisaker, M. (1997). Communication-based approaches to challenging behaviors after brain injury. In G. H. S. Singer, A. Glang, & B. Todis (Eds.), *Traumatic brain injury: The school's response* (pp. 229–254). Baltimore: Brookes.

Feeney, T., & Ylvisaker, M. (2003). Context-sensitive behavioral supports for young children with TBI: Short-term effects and long-term outcome. *Journal of Head Trauma Rehabilitation, 18*(1), 33–51.

Feeney, T., & Ylvisaker, M. (2006). Context-sensitive behavioral supports for young children with TBI: A replication study. *Brain Injury, 20*(6), 629–645.

Feeney, T., Ylvisaker, M., Rosen, B., & Greene, P. Cost effectiveness of community supports for individuals with challenging behavior after TBI: Public policy implications. *Journal of Head Trauma Rehabilitation, 16*(1), 61–75.

Feuerstein, R. (1979). *The dynamic assessment of retarded performers: The Learning Potential Assessment Device, theory, instruments, and techniques.* Baltimore, MD: University Park Press.

Fey, M. (1986). *Language intervention with young children.* San Diego: College-Hill Press.

Fidopiastis, C. M., Stapleton, C. B., Whiteside, J. D., Hughes, C. E., Fiore, S. M., Martin, G. M., et al. (2006). Human experience modeler: Context-driven cognitive retraining to facilitate transfer of learning. *CyberPsychology & Behavior, 9*(2), 183–187.

Fife, D., Faich, G., Hollinshead, W., & Boynton, W. (1986). Incidence and outcome of hospital-treated head injury in Rhode Island. *American Journal of Public Health, 77*, 810–812.

Filley, C. M., Cranberg, M. D., Alexander, M. P., & Hart, E. J. (1987). Neurobehavioral outcome after closed head injury in childhood and adolescence. *Archives of Neurology, 44*, 194–198.

Fitzsimons, G. M., & Bargh, J. A. (2004). Automatic self-regulation. In R. F. Baumeister & K. D. Vohs (Eds.), *Handbook of self-regulation: Research, theory and applications* (pp. 151–170). New York: Guilford Press.

Fivush, R. (1991). The social construction of personal narratives. *Merrill-Palmer Quarterly, 37*(1), 59–81.

Fivush, R., & Fromhoff, F. A. (1988). Style and structure in mother-child conversations about the past. *Discourse Processes, 11*, 337–355.

Fivush, R., & Haden, C. A. (2003). *Autobiographical memory and the construction of a narrative self: Developmental and cultural perspectives.* Mahaw, NJ: Lawrence Erlbaum.

Fivush, R., & Reese, E. (1992). The social construction of autobiographical memory. In M. A. Conway, D. C. Rubin, H. Spinnler, & W. A. Wagenaar (Eds.), *Theoretical perspectives on autobiographical memory* (pp. 115–132). The Netherlands: Kluwer Academic.

Flavell, J., Miller, P., & Miller, S. (2001). *Cognitive development* (4th ed.). Englewood Cliffs, NJ: Prentice Hall.

Fletcher, J. M., Levin, H. S., & Butler, I. J. (1995). Neurobehavioral effects of brain injury on children: Hydrocephalus, traumatic brain injury, and cerebral palsy. In M. C. Roberts (Ed.), *Handbook of pediatric psychology* (2nd ed., pp. 362–383). New York: Guilford Press.

Fowler, R. (1996). Supporting students with challenging behaviors in general education settings: A review of behavioral momentum techniques and guidelines for use. *The Oregon Conference Monograph, 8*, 137–155.

Gajar, A., Schloss, P. J., Schloss, C. N., & Thompson, C. K. (1984). Effects of feedback and self-monitoring on head trauma youths' conversation skills. *Journal of Applied Behavior Analysis, 17*, 353–358.

Gennarelli, T. A., Thibault, L. E., Adams, J. H., Graham, D. I., Thompson, C. J., & Marcincin, R. P. (1982). Diffuse axonal injury and traumatic coma in the primate. *Annals of Neurology, 12*, 564–574.

Gerberich, S. G., Priest, J. D., Boen, J. R., Staub, C. P., & Maxwell, R. E. (1983). Concussion incidences and severity in secondary school varsity football players. *American Journal of Public Health, 73*, 1370–1375.

Gersten, R., Fuchs, L. S., Williams, J. P., & Baker, S. (2001). Teaching reading comprehension strategies to students with learning disabilities: A review of research. *Review of Educational Research, 71*(2), 279–320.

Giangreco, M. F., Cloninger, C. J., & Iverson, V. S. (1993). *Choosing Options and Accommodations for Children (COACH): A guide to planning inclusive education.* Baltimore: Paul H. Brookes.

Giap, B. T., Jong, C. N., Ricker, J. H., Cullen, N. K., & Zafonte, R. D. (2000). The hippocampus: Anatomy, pathophysiology, and regenerative capacity. *Journal of Head Trauma Rehabilitation, 15*(3), 875–894.

Glisky, E. L., & Schacter, D. L. (1988). Acquisition of domain-specific knowledge in patients with organic memory disorders. *Journal of Learning Disabilities, 21,* 333–339, 351.

Glisky, E. L., & Schacter, D. L. (1989). Models and methods of memory rehabilitation. In F. Boller & J. Grafman (Eds.), *Handbook of neuropsychology: Memory and its disorders* (Vol. 3, Sec. 5., pp. 233–246). Amsterdam: Elsevier Science.

Gluck, M. A., & Myers, C. E. (1995). Representation and association in memory: A neurocomputational view of hippocampal function. *Current Directions in Psychological Science, 4,* 23–29.

Goldman, P. S. (1971). Functional development of the prefrontal cortex early in life and the problem of neural plasticity. *Experimental Neurology, 32,* 366–387.

Goldstein, A. P., Sprafkin, R. P., Gershaw, N. J., & Klein, P. (1980). *Skillstreaming the adolescent: A structured learning approach to teaching prosocial skills.* Champaign, IL: Research Press.

Goldstein, F. C., & Levin, H. S. (1995). Neurobehavioral outcome of traumatic brain injury in older adults: Initial findings. *Journal of Head Trauma Rehabilitation, 10,* 57–73.

Grafman, J. (1995). Similarities and distinctions among current models of prefrontal cortical functions. In J. Grafman, K. J. Holyoak, & F. Boller (Eds.), *Structure and function of the human prefrontal cortex* (pp. 337–368). New York: The New York Academy of Sciences.

Grafman, J. (2002). The structured event complex and the human prefrontal cortex. In D. T. Stuss & R. T. Knight (Eds.), *Principles of frontal lobe function* (pp. 292–311). New York: Oxford University Press.

Grafman, J., Sirigu, A., Spector, L., & Hendler, J. (1993). Damage to the prefrontal cortex leads to decomposition of structured event complexes. *Journal of Head Trauma Rehabilitation, 8,* 73–87.

Graham, S. & Harris, K. R. (2003). Students with learning disabilities and the process of writing: a meta-analysis of SRSD studies. In H. L. Swanson, K. R. Harris, & S. Graham (Eds.), *Handbook of Learning Disabilities* (pp. 323–344.) New York: Guilford Press.

Gresham, F. M., Sugai, G., & Horner, R. H. (2001). Interpreting outcomes of social skills training for students with high-incidence disabilities. *Exceptional Children, 67*(3), 331–344.

Groher, M. (1990). Communication disorders in adults. In M. Rosenthal, E. Griffith, M. Bond, & J. D. Miller (Eds.), *Rehabilitation of the adult and child with traumatic brain injury* (pp. 148–162). Philadelphia: F. A. Davis.

Gronwall, D., & Wrightson, P. (1975). Cumulative effect of concussion. *Lancet, 2,* 995–997.

Haarbauer-Krupa, J., Henry, K., Szekeres, S., & Ylvisaker, M. (1985). Cognitive rehabilitation therapy: Late stages of recovery. In M. Ylvisaker (Ed.), *Head injury rehabilitation:*

Children and adolescent. Boston: College-Hill Press/Little, Brown & Co.

Haas, J., Cope, D. N., & Hall, K. (1987). Premorbid prevalence of poor academic performance in severe head injury. *Journal of Neurology, Neurosurgery, and Psychiatry, 50,* 52–56.

Haden, C. A., Haine, R. A., & Fivush, R. (1997). Developing narrative structure in parent-child reminiscing across the preschool years. *Developmental Psychology, 33,* 295–307.

Hagen, C. (1981). Language disorders secondary to closed head injury. *Topics in Language Disorders, 1,* 73–87.

Hall, K. M. (1992). Overview of functional assessment scales in brain injury rehabilitation. *NeuroRehabilitation, 2,* 98–113.

Hall, K. M., Karzmark, P., Stevens, M., Englander, J., O'Hare, P., & Wright, J. (1994). Family stressors in traumatic brain injury: A two-year follow-up. *Archives of Physical Medicine and Rehabilitation, 75,* 876–884.

Halle, J. W., & Spradlin, J. E. (1993). Identifying stimulus control of challenging behavior: Extending the analysis. In J. Reichle & D. P. Wacker (Eds.), *Communicative alternative to challenging behavior: Integrating functional assessment and intervention strategies* (pp. 83–109). Baltimore: Paul H. Brookes.

Hallowell, E. M., & Ratey, J. J. (1994). *Driven to distraction.* New York: Touchstone.

Halpern, H. Darley, F. L., & Brown, J. R. (1973). Differential language and neurologic characteristics in cerebral involvement. *Journal of Speech and Hearing Disorders, 38,* 162–173.

Hanton, G., Bartha, M., & Levin, H. (2000). Metacognition following pediatric brain injury: A preliminary study. *Developmental Neuropsychology, 18,* 383–398.

Harchik, A. E., Sherman, J. A., & Bannerman, D. J. (1993). Choice and control: New opportunities for people with developmental disabilities. *Annals of Clinical Psychiatry, 5,* 151–162.

Hartley, L. L. (1995). *Cognitive-communicative abilities following brain injury: A functional approach.* San Diego: Singular.

Hartley, L. L., & Jensen, P. J. (1991). Narrative and procedural discourse after closed head injury. *Brain Injury, 5,* 267–285.

Hartshorne, N. J., Harruff, R. C., & Alvord, E. C. (1997). Fatal head injuries in ground-level falls. *American Journal of Medical Pathology, 18,* 258–264.

Hechtman, L., Abikoff, H., Klien, R. G., Weiss, G., Respitz, C., Kouri, J., et al. (2004). Academic achievement and emotional status of children with ADHD treated with long-term methylphenidate and multimodal psychosocial treatment. *Journal of the American Academy of Childhood and Adolescent Psychiatry, 43*(7), 812–819.

Heilman, K. M., Safran, A., & Geschwind, N. (1971). Close head trauma and aphasia. *Journal of Neurology, Neurosurgery, and Psychiatry, 34,* 265–269.

Helm-Estabrooks, N., & Hotz, G. (1991). *Brief Test of Head injury (BTHI).* Chicago, IL: Riverside.

Henri, B. P., & Hallowell, B. (1999). Mastering managed care: Problems and possibilities. In B. Cornett (Ed.), *Clinical practice management in speech-language pathology: Principles and practicalities* (pp. 3–28). Gaithersburg, MD: Aspen.

Hersh, N. A., & Treadgold, L. G. (1994). NeuroPage: The rehabilitation of memory dysfunction by prosthetic memory and cueing. *NeuroRehabilitation, 4,* 187–197.

Horner, R. H., Dunlap, G., & Koegel, R. L. (Eds.). (1988). *Generalization and maintenance: Lifestyle changes in applied settings.* Baltimore: Paul H. Brookes.

Hudson, J. A. (1990). The emergence of autobiographical memory in mother-child conversations. In R. Fivush & J. A. Hudson (Eds.), *Knowing and remembering in young children* (pp. 166–196). New York: Cambridge University Press.

IDEA: Federal Register (1991, August). *Public Law 101-476: Individuals with disabilities education act.* Department of Education.

Iwata, B. A., Vollmer, T. R., & Zarcone, J. R. (1990). The experimental (functional) analysis of behavior disorders: Methodology, applications, and limitations. In A. C. Repp & N. N. Singh (Eds.), *Perspectives on the use of nonaversive and aversive interventions for persons with developmental disabilities* (pp. 301–330). Sycamore, IL: Sycamore.

Izard, C. E. (1992) Four systems for emotion activation: Cognitive and noncognitive. *Psychological Review, 100,* 68–90.

Jacobs, H. E. (1993). *Behavior analysis guidelines and brain injury rehabilitation: People, principles, and programs.* Gaithersburg, MD: Aspen.

James, W. (1890). *Principles of psychology* (Vol. 1). New York: Dover.

Jennett, B., & Bond, M. (1975). Assessment of outcome after severe brain damage: A practical scale. *Lancet, 1,* 480–484.

Johnson, A. (1999). Speech-language pathology in health settings: A view of the future. In B. Cornett (Ed.), *Clinical practice management in speech-language pathology: Principles and practicalities* (pp. 219–242). Gaithersburg, MD: Aspen.

Johnson, D. A., & Newton, A. (1987). Social adjustment and interaction after severe head injury: II. Rationale and bases for intervention. *British Journal of Clinical Psychology, 26,* 289–298.

Kaplan, E. (1988). A process approach to neuropsychological assessment. In T. Boll & B. K. Bryant (Eds.), *Clinical neuropsychology and brain function: Research, measurement, and practice* (pp. 129–167). Washington, D.C.: American Psychological Association.

Kapur, N (1995). Memory aids in the rehabilitation of memory disordered patients. In A. D. Baddeley, B. A. Wilson, & F. N. Watts (Eds.), *Handbook of memory disorders* (pp. 533–556.) New York: Wiley.

Katz, D. I. (1992). Neuropathology and neurobehavioral recovery from closed head injury. *Journal of Head Trauma Rehabilitation, 7,* 1–15.

Katz, D. I., & Alexander, M. P. (1994). Traumatic brain injury. In D. C. Good & J. R. Couch (Eds.), *Handbook of neurorehabilitation* (pp. 493–549). New York: Decker.

Kavale, K., & Mattson, P. (1983). "One jumped off the balance beam": Meta-analysis of perceptual-motor training. *Journal of Learning Disabilities, 16,* 165–173.

Kay, T., & Lezak, M. (1990). The nature of head injury. In D. W. Corthell (Ed.), *Traumatic brain injury and vocational rehabilitation* (pp. 21–65). Menomonie, WI: University of Wisconsin, Stout.

Kennedy, C. H. (1994). Manipulating antecedent conditions to alter the stimulus control of problem behavior. *Journal of Applied Behavior Analysis, 27,* 161–170.

Kennedy, C. H., Itkonen, T., & Lindquist, K. (1995). Comparing interspersed requests and social comments for increasing student compliance. *Journal of Applied Behavior Analysis, 28,* 97–98.

Kennedy, M. R. T., Coelho, C., Ylvisaker, M., Sohlberg, M. M., Turkstra, L., Avery, J., & Yorkston, K. (2007, accepted). A systematic review of treatments for disorders of executive function and metacognition after traumatic brain injury: Technical report and clinical recommendations. *Neuropsychological Rehabilitation.*

Kennedy, M., & Yorkston, K. (2000). Accuracy of metamemory after traumatic brain injury: Predictions during verbal learning. *Journal of Speech, Language, and Hearing Research, 43,* 1072–1086.

Kern, L., Childs, K. E., Dunlap, G., Clarke, S., & Falk, G. D. (1994). Using assessment based curricular intervention to improve the classroom behavior of a student with emotional and behavioral challenges. *Journal of Applied Behavior Analysis, 27,* 7–19.

Kessels R. P. C., Boekhorst, S. & Postma, A. et al. (2005) The contribution of implicit and explicit memory to the effects of errorless learning: A comparison between young and older adults. *Journal of the International Neuropsychological Society 11,* 144–151

Klonoff, P. S., Costa, L. D., & Snow, W. G. (1986). Predictors and indicators of quality of life in patients with closed-head injury. *Journal of Clinical and Experimental Neuropsychology, 8,* 469–485.

Koegel, L. K., Koegel, R. L., & Dunlap, G. (1997). *Positive behavioral support: Including people with difficult behavior in the community.* Baltimore, MD: Paul Brooks.

Koegel, R., & Koegel, L. K. (1995). *Teaching children with autism: Strategies for initiating positive interactions and improving learning opportunities.* Baltimore: Paul H. Brookes.

Kraus, J. F. (1993). Epidemiology of head injury. In P. R. Cooper (Ed.), *Head injury* (3rd ed.). Baltimore: Williams & Wilkins.

Kraus, J. F., & Nourjah, P. (1988). The epidemiology of mild, uncomplicated brain injury. *Journal of Trauma, 28,* 1637–1643.

Kraus, J. F., Rock, A., & Hemyari, P. (1990). Brain injuries among infants, children, adolescents, and young adults. *American Journal of Diseases of Childhood, 144,* 684–691.

Kreutzer, J. S., Marwitz, J. H., Seel, R., & Serio, C. (1996). Validation of a neurobehavioral inventory for adults with traumatic brain injury. *Archives of Physical Medicine and Rehabilitation, 77,* 116–124.

Landry, S. H., Miller-Loncar, C. L., Smith, K. E., & Swank, P. R. (2002). The role of early parenting in children's development of executive processes. *Developmental Neuropsychology, 21*(1), 15–41.

Landry, S. H., Smith, K. E., & Swank, P.R. (2003). The importance of parenting during early childhood for school-age development. *Developmental Neuropsychology, 24*(2/3), 559–591.

Landry, S. H., Smith, K. E., Swank, P. R., Assel, M. A., & Vellet, S. (2001). Does early responsive parenting have a special importance for children's development or is consistency across early childhood necessary? *Developmental Psychology, 37,* 387–403.

Larsen, R. J., & Prizmic, Z. (2004). Affect regulation. In R. F. Baumeister & K. D. Vohs (Eds.), *Handbook of self-regulation: Research, theory and applications* (pp. 40–61). New York: Guilford Press.

LeBlanc, J. E., Hayden, M. E., & Paulman, R. G. (2000). A comparison of neuropsychological and situational assessment for predicting employability after closed head injury. *Journal of Head Trauma Rehabilitation, 15*(4), 1022–1040.

LeDoux, J. E. (1991). Emotion and the limbic system concept. *Concepts in Neuroscience, 2,* 169–199.

LeDoux, J. E. (1996). *The emotional brain.* New York: Touchstone.

Levin, H. S., Benton, A. L., & Grossman, R. G. (1982). *Neurobehavioral consequences of closed head injury.* New York: Oxford University Press.

Levin, H. S., Goldstein, F. C., Williams, D. H., & Eisenberg, H. M. (1991). The contribution of frontal lobe lesions to the neurobehavioral outcome of closed head injury. In H. S. Levin, H. M. Eisenberg, & A. L. Benton (Eds.), *Frontal lobe function and dysfunction* (pp. 318–338). New York: Oxford University Press

Levin, H. S., Grossman, R. G., Sarwar, M., & Meyers, C. A. (1981). Linguistic recovery after closed head injury. *Brain and Language, 12,* 360–374.

Levin, H. S., O'Donnell, V. M., & Grossman, R. G. (1979). The Galveston Orientation and Amnesia Test: A practical scale to assess cognition after head injury. *Journal of Nervous and Mental Diseases, 167,* 675–684.

Lezak, M. (1982). The problem of assessing executive functions. *International Journal of Psychology, 17,* 281–297.

Lezak, M. (1986). Psychological implications of traumatic brain damage for the patient's family. *Rehabilitation Psychology, 31,* 241–250.

Lezak, M. (1987). Relationships between personality disorders, social disturbances, and physical disability following traumatic brain injury. *Journal of Head Trauma Rehabilitation, 2,* 57–69.

Liles, B. J., Coelho, C. A., Duffy, R. J., & Zalagens, M. R. (1989). Effects of elicitation procedures on the narratives of normal and closed head-injured adults. *Journal of Speech and Hearing Disorders, 54,* 356–366.

Livingston, M. G., & Brooks, D. N. (1988). The burden on families of the brain injured: A review. *Journal of Head Trauma Rehabilitation, 3,* 6–15.

Lucariello, J. M., Hudson, J. A., Fivush, R., & Bauer, P. J. (Eds.). (2004). *The development of the mediated mind: Sociocultural context and cognitive development.* Mahwah, NJ: Lawrence Erlbaum.

Luria, A. R. (1966). *Higher cortical functions in man.* NY: Basic Books.

Luria, A. R. (1979). *The making of mind: A personal account of soviet psychology.* Cambridge, MA: Harvard University Press.

Mace, F. C., Hock, M. L., Lalli, J. S., West, B. J., Belfore, P., Pinter, E., et al. (1988). Behavioral momentum in the treatment of noncompliance. *Journal of Applied Behavior Analysis, 21,* 123–132.

Mace, F. C., Lalli, J. S., Shea, M. C., Lalli, E. P., West, B. J., Roberts, M., et al. (1990). The momentum of human behavior in a natural setting. *Journal of the Experimental Analysis of Behavior, 54,* 163–172.

Mace, F. C., Mauro, B. C., Boyajian, A. E., & Eckert, T. L. (1997). Effects of reinforcer quality on behavioral momentum: Coordinated applied and basic research. *Journal of Applied Behavior Analysis, 30,* 1–20.

MacDonald, J. (1989). *Becoming partners with children: From play to conversation.* Chicago: Riverside.

MacDonald, S. (2005). *Functional Assessment of Verbal Reasoning and Executive Strategies.* Guelph, Ontario: CCD.

MacMillan, P. J., Hart, R. P., Martelli, M. F., & Zasler, N. D. (2002). Pre-injury status and adaptation following traumatic brain injury. *Brain Injury, 16*(1), 41–49.

Malec, J. F., & Thompson, J. M. (1994). Relationship of the Mayo-Portland Adaptability Inventory to functional outcome and cognitive performance measures. *Journal of Head Trauma Rehabilitation, 9,* 1–11.

Mann, L. (1979). *On the trail of process: A historical perspective on cognitive processes and their training.* New York: Grune and Stratton.

Martin, G., & Pear, J. (1996). *Behavior modification: What it is and how to do it* (5th ed.). Upper Saddle River, NJ: Prentice Hall.

Martin, J. E., Mithaug, D. E., Cox, P., Peterson, L. Y., Van Dyke, J. L., & Cash, M. E. (2003). Increasing self-determination: Teaching students to plan, work, evaluate, and adjust. *Exceptional Children, 69*(4), 431–447.

Max, J. E., Robin, D. A., Lingren, S. D., Smith, W. L., Sato, Y., Mattheis, P. J., et al. (1997). Traumatic brain injury in children and adolescents: Psychiatric problems at two years. *Journal of the American Academy of Child and Adolescent Psychiatry, 36,* 1278–1285.

McCabe, A., & Peterson, C. (1991). Getting the story: A longitudinal study of parental styles in eliciting narratives and developing narrative skills. In A. McCabe & C. Peterson (Eds.), *New directions in developing narrative structure.* (pp. 217–253). Hillsdale, NJ: Erlbaum.

McDonald, S. (1992a). Communication disorders following closed head injury: New approaches to assessment and rehabilitation. *Brain Injury, 6,* 283–292.

McDonald, S. (1992b). Differential pragmatic language loss following severe closed head injury: Inability to comprehend conversational implicature. *Applied Psycholinguistics, 13,* 295–312.

McDonald, S. (1993). Pragmatic language loss following closed head injury: Inability to meet the informational needs of the listener. *Brain and Language, 44,* 28–46.

McDonald, S. (2005). Are you crying or laughing? Emotion recognition deficits after severe traumatic brain injury. *Brain Impairment, 6*(1), 56–67.

McDonald, S., & Pearce, S. (1998). Requests that overcome listener reluctance: Impairment associated with executive dysfunction in brain injury. *Brain and Language, 61,* 88–104.

McKinlay, W. W., Brooks, D. N., Bond, M. R., Martinage, D. P., & Marshall, M. M. (1981). The short-term outcome of severe blunt head injury as reported by relatives of the injured persons. *Journal of Neurology, Neurosurgery, and Psychiatry, 44,* 529.

Meichenbaum, D. (1977). *Cognitive behavior modification: An integrative approach.* New York: Plenum Press.

Meichenbaum, D. (1993). The "potential" contributions of cognitive behavior modification to the rehabilitation of individuals with traumatic brain injury. *Seminars in Speech and Language, 14,* 18–30.

Meichenbaum, D., & Biemiller, A. (1998). *Nurturing independent learners: Helping students take charge of their learning.* Cambridge, MA: Brookline Books.

Mendelsohn, D., Levin, H. S., Bruce, D., Lilly, M. A., Harward, H., Culhane, K., et al. (1992). Late MRI after head injury in children: Relationship to clinical features and outcome. *Child's Nervous System, 8*, 445–452.

Mentis, M., & Prutting, C. A. (1991). Analysis of topic as illustrated in a head-injured and a normal adult. *Journal of Speech and Hearing Research, 34*, 583–595.

Mesulam, M. (2002). The human frontal lobes: Transcending the default mode through contingent encoding. In D. T. Stuss & R. T. Knight (Eds.), *Principles of frontal lobe function* (pp. 8–30). New York: Oxford University Press.

Michael, J. (1982). Distinguishing between discriminative and motivational functions of stimulus. *Journal of the Experimental Analysis of Behavior, 37*, 33–44

Michael, J. (1993). Establishing operations. *Behavior Analyst, 16*, 191–206.

Milders, M., Fuchs, S., & Crawford, J. R. (2003). Neuropsychological impairments and changes in emotional and social behavior following severe traumatic brain injury, *Journal of Clinical and Experimental Neuropsychology, 25*(2), 157–172.

Milton, S. B., & Wertz, R. T. (1986). Management of persisting communication deficits in patients with traumatic brain injury. In B. P. Uzzell & Y. Gross (Eds.), *Clinical Neuropsychology of Intervention*. Boston: Martinus Nijhoff.

Morris, E. K. (1992). The aim, progress, and evolution of behavior analysis. *The Behavior Analyst, 15*, 3–29.

Morton, V. M., & Wehman, P. (1995). Psychosocial and emotional sequelae of individuals with traumatic brain injury: A literature review and recommendations. *Brain Injury, 9*, 81–92.

Nelson, K. (1992). Emergence of autobiographical memory at age 4. *Human Development, 35*(3), 172–177.

Newcomb, F. (1969). *Missel wounds of the brain*. London: Oxford University Press.

National Institutes of Health. (1999). *Report of the Consensus Development Conference on the rehabilitation of persons with traumatic brain injury*. National Institutes of Health: Author.

Nybo T., & Kosklniemi, M. (1999) Cognitive indicators of vocational outcomes after severe traumatic brain injury in childhood. *Brain Injury, 13*(10), 759–766.

Pace, G. M., & Ivancic, M. T. (1994). Stimulus fading as treatment for obscenity in a brain-damaged client. *Journal of Applied Behavior Analysis, 27*, 302–305.

Palinscar, A. S., & Brown, A. L. (1989). Classroom dialogues to promote self-regulated comprehension. In J. Brophy (Ed.), *Teaching for understanding and self-regulated learning* (Vol. 1). Greenwich, CT: JAI Press.

Palinscar, A. S., Brown, A. L., & Campione, J. C. (1994). Models and practices of dynamic assessment. In G. P. Wallach & K. G. Butler (Eds.), *Language learning disabilities in school-age children and adolescents* (pp. 132–134). New York: Macmillan.

Pang, D. (1985). Pathophysiologic correlates of neurobehavioral syndromes following closed head injury. In M. Ylvisaker (Ed.), *Head injury rehabilitation: Children and adolescents* (pp. 3–70). Newton, MA: Butterworth-Heinemann.

Park, N. W., & Ingles, J. L. (2001). Effectiveness of attention rehabilitation after an acquired brain injury: A meta-analysis. *Neuropsychology, 15*(2), 199–210.

Pascual-Leone, A., Grafman, J., & Hallett, M. (1995). Procedural learning and prefrontal cortex. In J. Grafman, K. J. Holyoak, & F. Boller (Eds.), *Structure and function of the human prefrontal cortex* (pp. 61–70). New York: The New York Academy of Sciences.

Payne, J. C. (1999). *Adult neurogenic language disorders: Assessment and treatment*. San Diego: Singular.

Perlesz, A., Kinsella, G., & Crowe, S. (2000). Psychological distress and family satisfaction following traumatic brain injury: Injured individuals and their primary, secondary, and tertiary carers. *Journal of Head Trauma Rehabilitation, 15*(3), 909–929.

Pearce, S., McDonald, S., & Coltheart, M. (1998). Ability to process ambiguous advertisements after frontal lobe damage. *Brain and Cognition, 38*, 150–164.

Petrides, M. (1995). Functional organization of the human frontal cortex for mnemonic processing. In J. Grafman, K. J. Holyoak, & F. Boller (Eds.), *Structure and function of the human prefrontal cortex* (pp. 85–96). New York: The New York Academy of Sciences.

Ponsford, J. L., Olver, J. H., Curren, C., & Ng, K. (1995). Prediction of employment status two years after traumatic brain injury. *Brain Injury, 9*, 11–20.

Powell, J. H., Beckers, K., & Greenwood, R. J. (1998). The measurement of progress and outcome in community rehabilitation after brain injury: A new assessment measure, the BICRO-39 Scales. *Archives of Physical Medicine and Rehabilitation*, 1213–1225.

Povlishock, J. T., & Katz, D. I., (2005). Update on neuropathology and neurological recovery after traumatic brain injury. *Journal of Head Trauma Rehabilitation, 20*(1), 76–94.

Pressley, M. (1993). Teaching cognitive strategies to brain-injured clients: The good information processing perspective. *Seminars in Speech and Language, 14*, 1–16.

Pressley, M. (1995). More about the development of self-regulation: Complex, long-term, and thoroughly social. *Educational Psychology, 30*, 207–212.

Pressley, M., and Colleagues (1990). *Cognitive strategy instruction that really improves children's academic performance*. Cambridge, MA: Brookline Books.

Pressley, M., Borkowski, J. G., & Schneider, W. (1989). Good information processing: What is it and what education can do to promote it. *International Journal of Educational Research, 13*, 857–867.

Prigatano, G. P. (1986). *Neuropsychological rehabilitation after brain injury*. Baltimore: Johns Hopkins University Press.

Prigatano, G. P., & Altman, I. M. (1990). Impaired awareness of behavioral limitations after traumatic brain injury. *Archives of Physical Medicine and Rehabilitation, 71*, 1058-1064.

Prigatano, G. P., Roueche, J. R., & Fordyce, D. J. (1985). Nonaphasic language disturbances after closed head injury. *Language Sciences, 1*, 217–229.

Rappaport, M., Hall, K. M., Hopkins, H. K., Belleza, T., & Cope, D. N. (1982). Disability Rating Scale for severe head trauma: Coma to community. *Archives of Physical Medicine and Rehabilitation, 63*, 118–123.

Rath, J. F., Simon, D., Langenbahn, D. M., Sherr, R. L., & Diller, L. (2000). Measurement of problem-solving deficits in adults with acquired brain damage. *Journal of Head Trauma Rehabilitation, 15*(1), 724–733.

Reese, E., & Fivush, G. (1993). Parental styles of talking about the past. *Developmental Psychology, 29,* 596–606.

Reese, E., Haden, C. A., & Fivush, R. (1993). Mother-child conversations about the past: Relationships of style and memory over time. *Cognitive Development, 8,* 403–430.

Reeve, J. (2002). Self-determination theory applied to educational settings. In E. L. Deci & R. M. Ryan (Eds.), Handbook of self-determination research (pp. 183–203). Rochester, NY: University of Rochester Press.

Reeve, J., Bolt, E., & Cai, Y. (1999). Autonomy-supportive teachers: How they teach and motivate students. *Journal of Educational Psychology, 91,* 537–548

Reichle, J., & Johnston, S. S. (1993). Replacing challenging behavior: The role of communication intervention. *Topics in Language Disorders, 13,* 61–76.

Reichle, J., & Wacker, D. P. (Eds.). (1993). *Communicative alternatives to challenging behavior.* Baltimore: Brookes.

Reid, R., Trout, A. L., & Schartz, M. (2005). Self-regulation interventions for children with attention deficit/hyperactivity disorder. *Exceptional Children, 71*(4), 361–377.

Resnick, L. B. (1987). *Education and learning to think.* Washington, DC: National Academy Press.

Riley, G. A., & Heaton, S. (2000). Guidelines for the selection of a method of fading cues. *Neuropsychological Rehabilitation, 10*(2), 133–149.

Rimel, R. W., Giordani, B., Barth, J. T., Boll, T. J., & Jane, J. A. (1981). Disability caused by minor head injury. *Neurosurgery, 9,* 221–228.

Rizzo, A. A., Schulteis, M., Kerns, K. A., & Mateer, C. (2004). Analysis of assets for virtual reality applications in neuropsychology. *Neuropsychological Rehabilitation, 14*(1/2), 207–239.

Robinson, T. R., Smith, S. W., Miller, M. D., & Brownell, M. T. (1999). Cognitive behavior modification of hyperactivity/impulsivity and aggression. A meta-analysis of school-based studies. *Journal of Educational Psychology, 91,* 195–203.

Rogoff, B. (1990). *Apprenticeship in thinking: Cognitive development in social context.* New York: Oxford University Press.

Rolls, E. T. (2002). The functions of the orbitofrontal cortex. In D. T. Stuss & R. T. Knight (Eds.), *Principles of frontal lobe function* (pp. 354–375). New York: Oxford University Press.

Rolls, E. T., Hornak, J., Wade, D., & McGrath, J. (1994). Emotion-related learning in patients with social and emotional changes associated with frontal lobe damage. *Journal of Neurology, Neurosurgery, and Psychiatry, 57,* 1518–1524.

Ross-Swain, D. (1996). *Ross Information Processing Assessment* (RIPA-2). Austin, TX: Pro-Ed.

Roth, R. M., Isquith, P. K., & Gioia, G. A. (2005). *Behavior Rating Inventory of Executive Function-Adult Version.* Lutz, FL: Psychological Assessment Resources.

Ruff, R., (2005). Two decades of advances in understanding mild traumatic brain injury. *Journal of Head Trauma Rehabilitation, 20*(1), 5–18.

Ryan, R. M., & Deci, E. L. (2002). Overview of self-determination theory: An organismic dialectical perspective. In E. L. Deci & R. M. Ryan (Eds.), *Handbook of self-determination research* (pp. 3–33). Rochester, NY: University of Rochester Press.

Salmon, D. P., & Butters, N. (1995). Neurobiology of skill and habit learning. *Current Opinion in Neurobiology, 5,* 184–190.

Santora, T. A., Schinco, K. A., & Trooskin, S. Z. (1994). Management of trauma in the elderly patient. *Surgical Clinics of North America, 74,* 164–186.

Sarno, M. T. (1980). The nature of verbal impairment after closed head injury. *Journal of Nervous and Mental Disease, 168,* 685–692.

Sarno, M. T. (1984). Verbal impairment after closed head injury: Report of a replication study. *Journal of Nervous and Mental Disease, 172,* 475–479.

Sarno, M. T., Buonaguro, A., & Levita, E. (1986). Characteristics of verbal impairment in closed head injured patients. *Archives of Physical Medicine and Rehabilitation, 67,* 400–405.

Schacter, D. L. (1996). *Searching for memory: The brain, the mind and the past.* New York: Basic Books.

Scheibel, R. S., & Levin, H. S. (1997). Frontal lobe dysfunction following closed head injury in children and adults. In N. A. Krasnegor, G. R. Lyon, & P. S. Goldman-Rakic (Eds.), *Development of the prefrontal cortex: Evolution, neurobiology, and behavior* (pp. 241–263). Baltimore, MD: Paul Brookes.

Schmeichel, B. J., & Baumeister, R. F. (2004). Self-regulatory strength. In R. F. Baumeister & K.D. Vohs (Eds.), *Handbook of self-regulation: Research, theory and applications* (pp. 84–98). New York: Guilford Press.

Schmidt, N. D. (1997). Outcome-oriented rehabilitation: A response to managed care. *Journal of Head Trauma Rehabilitation, 12,* 44–50.

Schmitter-Edgecombe, M. (1996). Effects of traumatic brain injury on cognitive performance: An attentional resource hypothesis in search of data. *Journal of Head Trauma Rehabilitation, 11*(2), 17–30.

Schneider, P., & Watkins, R. (1996). Applying Vygotskyan developmental theory to language intervention. *Language Speech, and Hearing Services in the Schools, 27,* 157–170.

Schulteis, M. T., & Mourant, R. R. (2001). Virtual reality and driving: The road to better assessment of cognitively impaired populations. *Presence: Teleoperators and Virtual Environments, 10,* 436–444.

Schwartz, L., Taylor, H. G., Drotar, D., Yeates, K. O., Wade, S. L., & Stancin, T. (2003). Long-term behavior problems following pediatric traumatic brain injury: Prevalence, predictors, and correlates. *Journal of Pediatric Psychology, 28,* 251–263.

Schwartz, M. F. (1995). Re-examining the role of executive functions in routine action production. In J. Grafman, K. J. Holyoak, & F. Boller (Eds.), *Structure and function of the human prefrontal cortex* (pp. 321–335). New York: The New York Academy of Sciences.

Schwartz, M. F., Mayer, N. H., FitzpatrickDeSalme, E. J., & Montgomery, M. W. (1993). Cognitive theory and the study of everyday action disorders after brain damage. *Journal of Head Trauma Rehabilitation, 8*(1), 59–72.

Schweinhart, L. J., & Weikart, D. P. (1993). Success by empowerment: The High/Scope Perry preschool study through age 27. *Young Children, 49,* 54–58.

Shallice, T. (1982). Specific impairments of planning. *Philosophical Transactions of the Royal Society of London, 298,* 199–209.

Shallice, T., & Burgess, P. W. (1991). Deficits in strategy application following frontal lobe damage in man. *Brain, 114,* 727–741.

Shammi, P., & Stuss, D. T. (1999). Humour appreciation: A role of the right frontal lobe. *Brain, 122,* 657–666.

Sheinker, J., & Sheinker, A. (1988). *Metacognitive approach to social skills training.* Rockville, MD: Aspen.

Shimamura, A. P. (2002). Memory retrieval and executive control processes. In D. T. Stuss & R. T. Knight (Eds.), *Principles of frontal lobe function* (pp. 210–220). New York: Oxford University Press.

Shum, D., Sweeper, S., & Murray, R. (1996). Performance on verbal implicit and explicit memory tasks following traumatic brain injury. *Journal of Head Trauma Rehabilitation, 11,* 43–53.

Sidman, M., & Stoddard, L. T. (1967). The effectiveness of fading in programming simultaneous form discrimination for retarded children. *Journal of Experimental Analysis of Behavior, 10,* 3–15.

Siegler, R. S., & Alibali, M. W. (2004). *Children's thinking* (4th ed.). Upper Saddle River, NJ: Prentice Hall.

Singley, M. K., & Anderson, J. R. (1989). *Transfer of cognitive skill.* Cambridge, MA: Harvard University Press.

Skinner, B. F. (1938). *The behavior of organisms: An experimental analysis.* New York: Appleton.

Skinner, B. F. (1953). *Science and human behavior.* New York: Free Press.

Slifer, K. J., Cataldo, M. D., Kurtz, P. F. (1995). Behavioral training during acute brain trauma rehabilitation: An empirical case study. *Brain Injury, 9,* 585–593.

Slifer, K. J., Tucker, C. L., Gerson, A. C., Cataldo, M. D., Sevier, R. C., Suter, A. H., et al. (1996). Operant conditioning for behavior during posttraumatic amnesia in children and adolescents with brain injury. *Journal of Head Trauma Rehabilitation, 11,* 39–50.

Sohlberg, M., Kennedy, M., Avery, J., Coehlo, C., Turkstra, L., Ylvisaker, M., et al. (2007). Evidence-based practice for the use of memory aids as a rehabilitation technique. *Journal of Medical Speech-Language Pathology,*

Sohlberg, M., & Mateer, C. (1987). *Introduction to cognitive rehabilitation: Theory and practice.* New York: Guilford Press.

Sohlberg, M. M., Fickas, S., Ehlhardt, L., & Todis, B. (2005a). The longitudinal effects of accessible email for individuals with severe cognitive impairments. *Aphasiology, 19*(7), 651–681.

Sohlberg, M. M., Fickas, S., Ehlhardt, L., & Todis, B. (2005b). The longitudinal effects of accessible email for individuals with severe cognitive impairments. *Aphasiology, 19*(7), 651–681.

Sosin, D. M., Sniezek, J. E., & Thurman, D. J. (1996). Incidence of mild and moderate brain injury in the United States, 1991. *Brain Injury, 10,* 47–54.

Squire, L. R. (1992). Memory and the hippocampus: A synthesis from findings with rats, monkeys, and humans. *Psychological Review, 99,* 195–231.

Squire, L. R., Knowlton, B., & Musen, G.(1993). The structure and organization of memory. *Annual Review in Psychology, 44,* 453–495.

Squires, E. J., Hunkin, N. M., & Parkin, A. J. (1997). Errorless learning of novel associations in amnesia. *Neuropsychologia, 35,* 1103–1111.

Stuss, D. T. (1999a, October). *New data on frontal functioning— Localization and assessment.* Workshop presented at the 20th Annual Neurorehabilitation Conference on Traumatic Brain Injury and Stroke, Boston, MA.

Stuss, D. T. (1999b, October). *Variability in performance and outcome after brain injury.* Plenary lecture presented at the 20th Annual Neurorehabilitation Conference on Traumatic Brain Injury and Stroke, Boston, MA.

Stuss, D. T., & Alexander, M. P. (1999). Affectively burnt in: A proposed role of the right frontal lobe. In E. Tulving (Ed.), *Memory, consciousness and the brain: The Tallinn Conference* (pp. 215–227). Philadelphia: Psychology Press.

Stuss, D. T., & Benson, D. F. (1986). *The frontal lobes.* New York: Raven Press.

Stuss, D. T., & Buckle, L. (1992). Traumatic brain injury: Neuropsychological deficits and evaluation at different stages of recovery and in different pathologic subtypes. *Journal of Head Trauma Rehabilitation, 7,* 40–49.

Stuss, D. T., Pogue, J., Buckle, L., & Bondar, J. (1994). Characterization of stability of performance in patients with traumatic brain injury: Variability and consistency on reaction time tests. *Neuropsychology, 8,* 316–324.

Sweet, A. P., & Snow, C. (2002). Reconceptualizing reading comprehension. In C. C. Block, L. B. Gambrell, & M. Pressley (Eds.), *Improving comprehension instruction: Rethinking research, theory, and classroom practice* (pp. 17–53). San Francisco, CA: John Wiley & Sons (Jossey-Bass).

Szekeres, S., Ylvisaker, M., & Holland, A. (1985). Cognitive rehabilitation therapy: A framework for intervention. In M. Ylvisaker (Ed.), *Head injury rehabilitation: Children and adolescents.* Boston: College-Hill Press/Little, Brown & Co.

Szekeres, S., Ylvisaker, M., & Cohen, S. (1987). A framework for cognitive rehabilitation therapy. In M. Ylvisaker & E. Gobble (Eds.), *Community re-entry for head injured adults.* Boston: College-Hill Press/ Little, Brown & Co.

Tailby, R, & Haslam, C. (2005). An investigation of errorless learning in memory-impaired patients: Improving the technique and clarifying theory. *Neuropsychologia, 41,* 1230–1240.

Tate, R. L. (1998). "It is not only the kind of injury that matters, but the kind of head": The contribution of premorbid psychosocial factors to rehabilitation outcomes after severe traumatic brain injury. *Neuropsychological Rehabilitation, 8,* 1–18.

Taylor, H. G., Yeates, K. O., Wade, S. L., Drotar, D., Stancin, T., & Minich, N. (2002). A prospective study of short- and long-term outcomes after traumatic brain injury in children: Behavior and achievement. *Neuropsychology, 16*(1), 15–27.

Teasdale, G., & Jennett, B. (1974). Assessment of coma and impaired consciousness. *Lancet, ii,* 81–84.

Teasdale, J. D. (1997). The transformation of meaning: The interacting cognitive subsystems approach. In M. Power & C. R. Brewin (Eds.), *The transformation of meaning in psychological therapies* (pp. 141–156). New York: John Wiley & Sons.

Terrace, H. S. (1963). Discrimination learning with and without "errors." *Journal of Experimental Analysis of Behavior, 6,* 1–27.

Thoene, A. (1996). Memory rehabilitation—Recent developments and future directions. *Restorative Neurology and Neuroscience, 9,* 125–140.

Thomsen, I. V. (1974). The patient with severe head injury and his family. *Scandinavian Journal of Rehabilitation and Medicine, 6,* 180–183.

Thomsen, I. V. (1975). Evaluation and outcome of aphasia in patients with severe head trauma. *Journal of Neurology, Neurosurgery, and Psychiatry, 38,* 713–718.

Thomsen, I. V. (1984). Late outcome of very severe blunt head trauma: A 10-15 year second follow-up. *Journal of Neurology, Neurosurgery, and Psychiatry, 47*, 260–268.

Thomsen, I. V. (1987). Late psychosocial outcome in severe blunt head trauma. *Brain Injury, 1*, 131–143.

Thomsen, I. V. (1989). Do young patients have worse outcome after severe blunt head trauma? *Brain Injury, 3*, 157– 162.

Togher, L., Hand, L., & Code, C. (1997). Analysing discourse in the traumatic brain injury population: Telephone interactions with different communication partners. *Brain Injury, 11*, 169–189.

Tranel, D. (2002). Emotion, decision making, and the ventromedial prefrontal cortex. In D. T. Stuss & R. T. Knight (Eds.), *Principles of frontal lobe function* (pp. 338–353). New York: Oxford University Press.

Tranel, D., Anderson, S. W., & Benton, A. I. (1995). Development of the concept of executive function and its relationship to the frontal lobes. In F. Boller & J. Grafman (Eds.), *Handbook of neuropsychology* (pp. 125–148). Amsterdam: Elsevier.

Tranel, D., & Damasio, A. (1993). The covert learning of affective valence does not require structures in hippocampal system or amygdala. *Journal of Cognitive Neuroscience, 5*, 79–88.

Tulving, E., Kapur, S., Craik, F. I. M., Moscovitch, M., & Houle, S. (1994). Hemispheric encoding/retrieval asymmetry in episodic memory: Positron emission tomography findings. *Proceedings of the National Academy of Sciences, USA, 91*, 2016–2020.

Turkstra, L. S., Coehlo, C., & Ylvisaker, M. (2005). The use of standardized tests for individuals with cognitive-communication disorders. *Seminars in Speech and Language, 26*(4), 215–222.

Turkstra, L. S., & Holland, A. L. (1998). Assessment of syntax after adolescent brain injury: Effects of memory on test performance. *Journal of Speech, Language, and Hearing Research, 41*, 137–149.

U.S. Department of Transportation (1995). *Traffic safety facts 1994: Older population*. Washington, D.C.: National Highway Traffic Safety Administration.

Van den Broek, M. D., Downes, J., Johnson, Z., Dayus, B., & Hilton, N. (2000). Evaluation of an electronic memory aid in the neuropsychological rehabilitation of prospective memory deficits. *Brain Injury, 14*, 455–462.

Varney, N. R., & Menefee, L. (1993). Psychosocial and executive deficits following closed head injury: Implications for orbital frontal cortex. *Journal of Head Trauma Rehabilitation, 8*, 32–44.

Vohs, K. D., & Ciarocco, N. J. (2004). Interpersonal functioning requires self-regulation. In R. F. Baumeister & K. D. Vohs (Eds.), *Handbook of self-regulation: Research, theory and applications* (pp. 392–407). New York: Guilford Press.

Vygotsky, L. S. (1962). *Thought and language*. A. Kozulin (Trans.). Cambridge, MA: M.I.T. Press. Original work published 1934.

Vygotsky, L.S. (1981). The genesis of higher mental functions. In J. V. Wertsch (Ed.), *The concept of activity in Soviet psychology* (pp. 144–189). Armonk, NY: M. E. Sharps.

Vygotsky, L. S. (1978). *Mind in society: The development of higher psychological processes*. M. Cole, V. John-Steiner, S. Scribner, & E. Souberman (Eds. & Trans.). Cambridge, MA: Harvard University Press.

Waksman, S., Messmer, C. L., & Waksman, D. D. (1989). *The Waksman Social Skills Curriculum: An assertive behavior program for adolescents*. Austin, TX: Pro-Ed.

Walker, H. M., McConnell, S. M., Holmes, D., Todis, B., Walker, J., & Golden, N. (1988). *The Walker Social Skills Curriculum: The ACCEPTS program*. Austin, TX: Pro-Ed.

Walker, H. M., Todis, B., Holmes, D., & Horton, G. (1988). *The Walker Social Skills Program: The ACCESS program: Adolescent curriculum for communication and effective social skills*. Austin, TX: Pro-Ed.

Walker, H. M., Schwarz, I. E., Nippold, M. A., Irvin, L. K., & Noell, J. W. (1994). Social skills in school-age children and youth: Issues and best practices in assessment and intervention. *Topics in Language Disorders, 14*, 70–82.

Walker, W., and the North Carolina State Board of Education. (1997). *Best Practices in Assessment and Programming for Students with Traumatic Brain Injury*. Raleigh, NC: State Board of Education.

Weddell, R., Oddy, M., & Jenkins, D. (1980). Social adjustment after rehabilitation: A two year follow-up of patients with severe head injury. *Psychological Medicine, 10*, 257–263.

Wehman, P., Kregel, J., Sherron, P., Nguyen, S., Kreutzer, J., Fry, R., et al. (1993). Critical factors associated with the successful supported employment of patients with severe traumatic brain injury. *Journal of Head Trauma Rehabilitation, 7*, 31–44.

Wehman, P., West, M. D., Kregel, J., Sherron, P., & Kreutzer, J. S. (1995). Return to work for persons with severe traumatic brain injury: A data-based approach to program development. *Journal of Head Trauma Rehabilitation, 10*, 27–39.

Wehmeyer, M., & Schwartz, M. (1997). Self determination and positive adult outcomes: A follow-up study of youth with mental retardation or learning disabilities, *Exceptional Children, 4*, 245–255.

Wehmeyer, M. L., Agran, M., & Hughes, C. (1998). *Teaching self-determination to students with disabilities: Basic skills for successful transition*. Baltimore: Paul H. Brookes.

Wehmeyer, M. L., Palmer, S. B., Agran, M., Mithaug, D. E., & Martin, J. E. (2000). Promoting causal agency: The self-determined learning model of instruction. *Exceptional Children, 66*(4), 439–453.

Welsh, M. C., & Pennington, B. F. (1988). Assessing frontal lobe functioning in children: Views from developmental psychology. *Developmental Neuropsychology, 4*, 199–230.

Westby, C. E. (1994). The effects of culture on genre, structure, and style of oral and written texts. In G. P. Wallach & K. G. Butler (Eds.), *Language learning disabilities in school-age children and adolescents* (pp. 180–218). New York: Merrill.

Wiener, J., & Harris, P. J. (1998). Evaluation of an individualized, context-based social skills training program for children with learning disabilities. *Learning Disabilities Research and Practice, 12*, 40–53.

Willer, B., Ottenbacher, K. J., & Coad, M. L. (1994). The Community Integration Questionnaire. *American Journal of Physical and Medical Rehabilitation, 73*, 103–107.

Wilson, B. (1992) Memory therapy in practice. In B. Wilson & N. Moffat (Eds.), *Clinical management of memory problems* (2nd ed., pp. 120–153). San Diego: Singular.

Wilson, B., & Watson, P. (1996). A practical framework for understanding compensatory behaviour in people with organic memory impairment. *Memory, 4*(5), 465–486.

Wilson, B. A. (1995). Management and remediation of memory problems in brain-injured adults. In A. D. Baddeley, B. A. Wilson, & F. N. Watts (Eds.), *Handbook of memory disorders* (pp. 452–479). New York: John Wiley & Sons.

Wilson, B. A., Alderman, N., Burgess, P. W., Elmslie, H., & Evans, J. J. (1996). *Behavioural Assessment of the Dysexecutive Syndrome*. Bury St. Edmunds, England: Thames Valley Test Company.

Wilson, B. A., Baddeley, A. D., Evans, J. J., & Shiel, A. (1994). Errorless learning in the rehabilitation of memory-impaired people. *Neuropsychological Rehabilitation, 4*, 307–326.

Wilson, B., Cockburn, J., & Baddeley, A. (1985), *The Rivermead Behavioural Memory Test*. Bury St. Edmonds: Thames Valley Test Company.

Wilson, B. A., Emslie, H. C., Quirk, K., & Evans, J. J. (2001). Reducing everyday memory and planning problems by means of a paging system: A randomised control crossover study. *Journal of Neurology, Neurosurgery and Psychiatry, 70*, 477–482.

Wilson, B. A., & Evans, J. J. (1996). Error-free learning in the rehabilitation of people with memory impairments. *Journal of Head Trauma Rehabilitation, 11*, 54–64.

Wood, D., Bruner, J., & Ross, G. (1976). The role of tutoring in problem solving. *Journal of Child Psychology and Psychiatry, 17*, 89–100.

Wood, R. L. (1987). *Brain injury rehabilitation: A neurobehavioral approach*. London: Croom-Helm.

Wood, R. L. (Ed.). (1990). *Neurobehavioral consequences of traumatic brain injury*. London: Taylor and Francis.

World Health Organization (2001). *International classification of functioning, disability and health:* Final Draft. [http://www.who.int/icidh].

Yasuda, K., Misu, T., Beckman, B., Watanabe, O., Ozawa, Y., & Nakamura, T. (2002). Use of an IC recorder as a voice output memory aid for patients with prospective memory impairment. *Neuropsychological Rehabilitation, 12*(2), 155–166.

Ylvisaker, M. (1992). Communication outcome following traumatic brain injury. *Seminars in Speech and Language, 13*, 239–251.

Ylvisaker, M. (1993). Communication outcome in children and adolescents with traumatic brain injury. *Neuropsychological Rehabilitation, 3*, 367–387.

Ylvisaker, M. (1999). A contextualized and routine-based approach to cognitive and behavioral rehabilitation: A historical perspective. In *Report of the NIH Consensus Development Conference on the rehabilitation of persons with traumatic brain injury*. Bethesda, MD: National Institutes of Health.

Ylvisaker, M. (2003). Context-sensitive cognitive rehabilitation: Theory and practice. *Brain Impairment, 4*(1), 1–16.

Ylvisaker, M. (2006). Self-coaching: A context-sensitive approach to social communication after traumatic brain injury. *Brain Impairment, 7*, 246–258.

Ylvisaker, M., Coelho, C., Kennedy, M., Sohlberg, M. M., Turkstra, L., Avery, J., et al. (2002). Reflections on evidence-based practice and rational clinical decision making. *Journal of Medical Speech-Language Pathology, 10*(3), xxv–xxxiii.

Ylvisaker, M., Feeney, J., & Feeney, T. (1999). An everyday approach to long-term rehabilitation after traumatic brain injury. In B. Cornett (Ed.), *Clinical practice management in speech-language pathology: Principles and practicalities* (pp. 117–162). Gaithersburg, MD: Aspen.

Ylvisaker, M., & Feeney, T. (1996). Executive functions after traumatic brain injury: Supported cognition and self-advocacy. *Seminars in Speech and Language, 17*, 217–232.

Ylvisaker, M., & Feeney, T. (1998a). *Collaborative brain injury intervention: Positive everyday routines*. San Diego: Singular.

Ylvisaker, M., & Feeney, T. (1998b). Everyday people as supports: Developing competencies through collaboration. In M. Ylvisaker (Ed.), *Traumatic brain injury rehabilitation: Children and adolescents* (Revised ed., pp. 429–464). Boston: Butterworth Heinemann.

Ylvisaker, M., & Feeney, T. (2000a). Reflections on Dobermanns, poodles, and social rehabilitation for difficult-to-serve individuals with traumatic brain injury. *Aphasiology, 14*, 407–431.

Ylvisaker, M., & Feeney, T. (2000b). Construction of identity after traumatic brain injury. *Brain Impairment, 1*, 12–28.

Ylvisaker, M., & Feeney, T. (In press). Helping children without making them helpless: Facilitating development of executive self-regulation in children and adolescents. In V. Anderson, R. Jacobs, & P. Anderson (Eds.), *Executive functions and the frontal lobes: A lifespan perspective.*

Ylvisaker, M., Feeney, T. (2006). Helping children without making them helpless: Facilitating development of executive self-regulation in children and adolescents. In V. Anderson, R. Jacobs, & P. Anderson (Eds.), *Executive functions and the frontal lobes: A lifespan perspective.*

Ylvisaker, M., Feeney, T. & Capo, M. (2007). Long-term community supports for individuals with co-occurring disabilities: Cost effective and project based intervention *Brain Impairment, 8*, (2),1–17.

Ylvisaker, M., Feeney, T., & Szekeres, S. (1998). A social-environmental approach to communication and behavior. In M. Ylvisaker (Ed.), *Traumatic brain injury rehabilitation: Children and adolescents* (Revised ed., pp. 271–302). Boston: Butterworth-Heinemann.

Ylvisaker, M., Feeney, T., & Urbanczyk, B. (1993a). Developing a positive rehabilitation culture for communication. In C. Durgin, N. Schmidt, & J. Freyer (Eds.), *Brain injury rehabilitation: Clinical intervention and staff development techniques*. Baltimore: Aspen.

Ylvisaker, M., & Feeney, T. J. (1994). Communication and behavior: Collaboration between speech-language pathologists and behavioral psychologists. *Topics in Language Disorders, 15*, 37–54.

Ylvisaker, M., & Gioia, G. (1998). Comprehensive cognitive assessment. In M. Ylvisaker (Ed.), *Traumatic brain injury rehabilitation: Children and adolescents* (Revised ed., pp. 159-179). Boston: Butterworth-Heinemann.

Ylvisaker, M., & Holland, A. (1985). Coaching, self-coaching, and the rehabilitation of head injury. In D. Johns (Ed.), *Clinical management of neurogenic communicative disorders* (pp. 243–257). Boston: Little-Brown.

Ylvisaker, M., Jacobs, H., & Feeney, T. (2003). Positive supports for people who experience disability following brain injury: A review. *Journal of Head Trauma Rehabilitation, 18*(1), 7–32.

Ylvisaker, M., Sellars, C., & Edelman, L. (1998). Rehabilitation after traumatic brain injury in preschoolers. In M. Ylvisaker

(Ed.), *Traumatic brain injury rehabilitation: Children and adolescents* (Revised ed., pp. 303–329). Boston: Butterworth-Heinemann.

Ylvisaker, M., Szekeres, S. F., & Feeney, T. (1998). Cognitive rehabilitation: Executive functions. In M. Ylvisaker (Ed.), *Traumatic brain injury rehabilitation: Children and adolescents* (Revised ed., pp. 221–269). Boston: Butterworth-Heinemann.

Ylvisaker, M., Szekeres, S. F., & Haarbauer-Krupa. J. (1998). Cognitive rehabilitation: Organization, memory and language. In M. Ylvisaker (Ed.), *Traumatic brain injury rehabilitation: Children and adolescents* (Revised ed., pp. 181–220). Boston: Butterworth-Heinemann.

Ylvisaker, M., Todis, B., Glang, A., Urbanczyk, B., Franklin, C., DePompei, R., et al. (2001). Educating students with TBI: Themes and recommendations. *Journal of Head Trauma Rehabilitation*, *16*(1), 76–93.

Ylvisaker, M., Turkstra, L., Coehlo, C., Yorkston, K., Kennedy, M., Sohlberg, M., & Avery, J. (2007). Behavioral interventions for individuals with behavior disorders after TBI: A systematic review of the evidence. *Brain Injury*, *21*(8), 769–805.

Young, P. H. (1999, October). *Anatomy and pathophysiology of traumatic brain injury and stroke*. Presented at the 20th Annual Neurorehabilitation Conference on Traumatic Brain Injury and Stroke. Boston, MA.

Zasler, N. D., Kreutzer, J. S., & Taylor, D. (1991). Coma stimulation and coma recovery: A critical review. *NeuroRehabilitation*, *1*, 33–40.

Zencius, A. H., Wesolowski, M. D., Burke, W. H., & McQuade, D. (1989). Antecedent control in the treatment of brain injured clients. *Brain Injury*, *3*, 199–205.

APPENDIX 33.1
Aspects of Cognition

COMPONENT SYSTEMS

WORKING MEMORY (system for holding and acting on information in consciousness)

- Structural capacity (7 ± 2 units of information) versus functional capacity (information organized for efficient processing)
- Phonologic, visuospatial, and other holding spaces versus supervisory control system

KNOWLEDGE BASE (system for long-term storage of information, rules, schemas, word meanings, and other memories)

- Episodic (autobiographical) versus semantic memory
- Declarative (remembering that . . .) versus procedural (remembering how to . . .) memory
- Explicit (including awareness of the memory) versus implicit (no awareness) memory
- Remote memory (memory for preinjury events, associated with retrograde amnesia) versus recent memory (memory for postinjury events, associated with anterograde amnesia)

EXECUTIVE SYSTEM (system for initiating, directing, and regulating all cognitive processes)
RESPONSE SYSTEM (system for expressing knowledge, including speech, writing, and other modalities)

COMPONENT PROCESSES

ATTENTION

- Arousal and alertness
- Preparing attention
- Maintaining/sustaining attention
- Selecting a focus of attention (concentrating attention)
- Suppressing/filtering distractions
- Shifting/switching attention
- Dividing/sharing attention

PERCEPTION

MEMORY AND LEARNING

- Encoding (placing items in memory), storage (holding memories over time), and retrieval (retrieving items from memory)

- Involuntary (memory as a by-product of functional activity) versus deliberate (effortful or strategic) memory
- Retrospective (memory for the past) versus prospective (memory for appointments and other future events) memory
- Verbal versus nonverbal memory
- Sensory modality–specific (e.g., auditory versus verbal) memory

ORGANIZATION

- Feature identification
- Organization by categories
- Organization by temporal sequences
- Organization by analysis into parts
- Organization by integration into wholes, main ideas, themes, and scripts

REASONING

- Deductive (formal inference) versus inductive (inference from experience) reasoning
- Analogical reasoning (drawing indirect inferences from experience, perceiving relationships)
- Evaluative reasoning (value judgments)
- Convergent (identifying main ideas and themes) versus divergent (exploring possibilities) thinking

FUNCTIONAL INTEGRATIVE PERFORMANCE

EFFICIENCY of information processing

- Rate of performance
- Amount accomplished

SCOPE of processing, including settings and knowledge domains in which processing is efficient
MANNER of processing, including impulsive/reflective, dependent/independent, rigid/flexible, active/passive processing
LEVEL: Developmental, academic, linguistic, or vocational level at which information can be processed

APPENDIX 33.2
Conventional Versus Functional Approaches to Intervention after Brain Injury: Communication, Behavior, and Cognition*

Scope of Intervention

Conventional Approach

1. **Speech-Language Pathology.** The focus is on speech and specific aspects of linguistic competence (semantics, syntax, morphology).
2. **Behavioral Psychology.** The focus is on management of specific problem behaviors in a narrow sense.
3. **Cognitive Rehabilitation.** The focus is on neuropsychological assessment and intervention that sequentially targets separate components of cognition, arranged in a hierarchy for treatment purposes.

Functional Approach

1. The focus of each profession is on helping individuals with brain injury achieve their real-world goals in real-world contexts, including academic, vocational, and social success.
2. Correctly understood, applied behavior analysis in psychology, pragmatics in speech-language pathology, and social-cognitive intervention in cognitive rehabilitation are essentially the same service, necessitating close collaboration among service providers.
3. Each profession recognizes the overarching importance of executive or self-control functions for academic, vocational, and social success.

Integration of Intervention: Collaboration

Conventional Approach

1. Cognition, communication, and behavior are targeted for assessment and intervention by separate professionals working in relative isolation.
2. Evaluation reports, including proposed goals, objectives, and plans to achieve the objectives, are produced separately by three professionals.

Functional Approach

1. Although behavioral psychologists, cognitive rehabilitation specialists (including special educators), and speech-language pathologists are recognized as possessing special and unique expertise, the important overlap in their services is explicitly acknowledged.
2. Assessments are conducted, and plans for intervention are developed in an integrated manner. Ideally, reports are written as integrated, cross-disciplinary documents.

*Modified from Ylvisaker and Feeney (1998a); with permission.

3. Individuals with disability and significant everyday people in their lives are included as contributing members of the collaborative assessment and intervention teams.

Orientation of Intervention: Deficits and Strengths

Conventional Approach: Deficit Orientation

1. The cognitive rehabilitation specialist attempts to remediate cognitive deficits and restore specific preexisting cognitive skills in areas of impairment.
2. The speech-language pathologist attempts to remediate communication deficits and restore specific preexisting speech and language skills in areas of impairment.
3. The behavioral psychologist attempts to eliminate undesirable behaviors (e.g., noncompliance, agitation, and combativeness) and increase specific desirable behaviors (e.g., participation and "socially appropriate" behaviors).

Functional Approach: Strength Orientation

1. Each professional begins with existing strengths and builds on them with:
   a. Attempts to ensure success in functional activities at the individual's current level of capacity.
   b. Apprenticeship procedures (including chaining and shaping).
   c. Compensatory strategies, using strengths to compensate for weaknesses.
2. Success is a goal throughout intervention, using whatever antecedent supports may be necessary to succeed at functional tasks at the individual's current level of ability.
3. Undesirable and challenging behaviors, including explicitly communicative behaviors, are never simply extinguished without an attempt to substitute a positive alternative that achieves the same goal.
4. Preservation and enhancement of the individual's self-esteem is a background goal for all professionals.

Service Delivery: Settings and Activities

Conventional Approach

1. The speech-language pathologist uses repetitive drill and practice in isolated settings that bear little resemblance to real-world communication settings (e.g., pull-out therapy). Activities in therapeutic settings are not necessarily related to real-world communication activities.
2. The cognitive rehabilitation specialist uses repetitive drill and practice in isolated settings that bear little resemblance to real-world settings (e.g., pull-out therapy using workbook or computer exercises that are insensitive to context and to personally meaningful content). Activities in therapeutic settings

are not necessarily related to real-world activities that require the targeted cognitive skill.

3. The behavioral psychologist delivers targeted behavioral services on a behavior unit, in a neurobehavioral rehabilitation facility, or in a behavior classroom, with little opportunity to facilitate transfer of training to real-world settings and tasks.

Functional Approach

1. Each profession focuses on real-world needs in real-world contexts. This focus includes supports for achieving real-world goals in real-world contexts and practice of functional communication, social, and cognitive skills in real-world contexts. Specific aspects of the individual's environments and demands in those environments are considered in choosing objectives.

2. As much as possible, communication and behavioral services are delivered in meaningful social groups, in settings that resemble settings in which the skills will need to be used, and in the context of meaningful activities.

3. Pursuit of cognitive, executive function, communication, and behavioral goals largely is in the context of everyday routines, involving modification of those routines with supports that gradually are withdrawn as the individual's skills improve.

Providers of Service: Involvement of Everyday Communication Partners

Conventional Approach

1. Professionals are considered to be the primary agents of change in the individual with disability.

2. Each profession focuses primarily on remediation of deficits in the individual; that is, the intervention is impairment oriented.

Functional Approach

1. Each profession focuses on improvement of function within everyday routines. Therefore, everyday communication partners (e.g., family members, paraprofessional aides, supervisors, teachers, coworkers, and friends) are critical deliverers of rehabilitation services and supports.

2. A primary role of rehabilitation specialists is to train and provide ongoing supports for everyday communication partners. Within a rehabilitation facility, evening and weekend staff are recognized as being particularly critical to the development of a positive and therapeutically efficient rehabilitation environment.

Source of Control

Conventional Approach

1. There is near total reliance on external control of behavior. Little emphasis is placed on helping the individual to set goals and make good choices, plan how to achieve selected goals, monitor and evaluate behavior in relation to those goals, and make strategic decisions in the face of failure. Professionals assume responsibility for most executive dimensions of behavior.

2. The individual with disability is not included as a member of the team of people who perform assessments, select goals and objectives, plan intervention, monitor and evaluate performance, and create strategic solutions to problems as they arise over the course of intervention.

Functional Approach

1. The ultimate goal is to ensure that the individual controls his or her behavior as much as possible by means of effective decision making, strategic thinking, self-regulation of behavior, and self-regulated control over environmental contingencies.

2. The individual with disability is included as a member of the team of people who perform assessments, select goals and objectives, plan intervention, monitor and evaluate performance, and create strategic solutions to problems as they arise over the course of intervention.

Intervention Procedures

Conventional Approach

1. Prescriptive behavioral objectives specify isolated targets; for example, specific language behaviors are selected for training.

2. Modification of behavior largely is a result of manipulating the consequences of behavior. Within training tasks, correct performance of the target behavior is consequated with presumably desirable objects or events; failure to use the target behavior is followed by a withholding of rewards, a cost of some kind, removal from the situation, or some other neutral or undesirable consequence.

Functional Approach

1. The goal is an acceptable range of behaviors (versus a specific behavior) that may vary in their effectiveness in achieving the communicative objective.

2. Modification of behavior (including cognitive and social behavior) is considered to be a result of manipulating the consequences as well as antecedents of the behavior, but the focus is on antecedents. Antecedent-control procedures include creating environmental supports, avoiding triggers for negative behavior, inducing positive setting events, generating positive momentum, creating opportunities for choice and control, establishing familiar, positive routines and effective procedures for deviating from routines, providing advance organizers for difficult tasks, teaching scripts for negotiating difficult social situations, and ensuring that the individual has maximal self-management skills.

3. Contingency management (i.e., manipulation of consequences of behavior) focuses on positive consequences for desirable behavior (versus punishing consequences and "time out" for negative behavior) and on natural contingencies (versus artificial rewards).

   a. As much as possible, rewards are internally related to the action performed (e.g., when people request something appropriately, they get it; when people initiate social interaction, they are rewarded with a pleasant interaction; and when people use strategies, they succeed in their endeavors).

   b. As much as possible, feedback (positive or negative) is given by natural communication partners (e.g., peers or family members).

4. As much as possible, teaching and learning take place within an apprenticeship relationship. The teacher and the learner are jointly engaged in projects designed to achieve meaningful goals. Initially, the teacher assumes much of the responsibility for achieving the goal, but he or she turns over responsibility to the learner/apprentice as soon as possible.

APPENDIX 33.3
Examples of Compensatory Strategies for Individuals with Cognitive Impairments*

Attention and Concentration

External Aids

- Use a timer or alarm watch to focus attention for a specified period.
- Organize the work environment to reduce distractions.
- Use a written or graphic task planner, with built-in rest periods and reinforcement; move a marker along to show progress.
- Place a symbol or picture card in an obvious place in the work area as a reminder to maintain attention.
- Alternate low-interest tasks with high-interest tasks.

Internal Procedures

- Set increasingly demanding goals for self, including work time.
- Self-instruct (e.g., "Am I wandering? What am I supposed to do? What should I be doing now?"). Written cue cards may be needed.

Orientation (To Time, Place, Person, and Events)

External Procedures

- **Time.** Use a watch that included day and date.
- **Schedule.** Use a daytimer or other user-friendly schedule form; use an alarm watch or pager system to stay oriented to schedule.
- **Person.** Use photos of persons not readily identified (e.g., in log book).
- **Place.** Refer to customized maps or diagrams for spatial orientation; label places or routes.
- **Event.** Use a log book or journal or tape recorder to record significant information and events of the day.

Internal Procedures

- Select anchor points or events during the week, and then attempt to reconstruct previous or subsequent points in time (e.g., "My birthday was yesterday—Wednesday—so today must be Thursday and I have to go to work.").
- Request time, date, and other information from others.
- Scan environment for landmarks.

Input Control/Comprehension

External Procedures

- Give feedback to speakers (e.g., "Slow down; speed up; break that down for me").
- Request repetition in another form (e.g., "Could you write that down please?").
- Request longer viewing time or repeated readings.
- Create charts or graphs to assist in comprehending complex material.
- Use a finger or index card to assist in scanning and reading.
- Use symbols to mark right and left margins of written material.
- Use large-print books.
- Use books on tape; request a verbal description if reading is weak.
- Place items to be viewed in the best visual field and eliminate visual distractions.
- Turn head to compensate for visual field cut.

Internal Procedures

- Use self-questioning (e.g., "Do I understand? Do I need to ask a question? How is this meaningful to me? How does this fit with what I know?").
- Prepare self for new information by presetting with questions and building frames of relevant background information.
- Attempt to summarize and explain information to oneself; check with speaker or source.
- Use a study guide for complex material (e.g., SQ3R: survey, question, read, recite, and review).
- Impose organization using diagrams or other advance organizers (see below).

Memory

External Procedures

- **Retrospective memory.:** Use a log book, journal, tape recorder, or computerized information storage system to record significant information and events of the day.
- **Prospective memory.**
  Nonelectronic. Use memos, pictures, post-it notes, calendars, graphic time lines, and the like as self-reminders.
  Electronic. E-mail self reminders. Use pager system, telememo watch, beeping watch, or handheld personal information storage system.
- **Encoding.** See attention, comprehension, and organization strategies.
- Keep items in a designated place (e.g., keys). Label the places.

*Please see text for suggestions and cautions about the teaching and facilitating process.
Modified from Ylvisaker, Szekeres, Henry, Sullivan, and Wheeler (1987); with permission.

Internal Procedures

- See attention, comprehension, and organization strategies.
- Rehearse to-be-remembered information (covert or overt; pantomime).
- Instruct self about when and why the information will be needed.
- Relate information to personal life experiences and current knowledge.
- Use knowledge of common scripts to reconstruct to-be-remembered events.
- Use mnemonics (e.g., meaningful/novel imagery, method of loci, and rhymes).
- Visualize verbal information; verbalize visuospatial information.
- At the time of retrieval, reconstruct the environment at the time of encoding.

Word Retrieval

External Procedures

- Circumlocute, describing the items in an organized way (e.g., "What kind of thing is it? What does it do? What is it used for? What are its parts? What are its attributes? Where is it found? What do I associated with it?").
- Use gestures of signs.
- Start a sentence with a carrier phrase (e.g., "I eat with a . . .").
- Attempt to write the word.

Internal Procedures

- Search lexical memory using an organized feature analysis system (e.g., "What kind of thing is it? What does it do? What is it used for? What are its parts? What are its attributes? Where is it found? What do I associated with it?").
- Attempt to cue self with phoneme cues, proceeding through the alphabet (slow, and appropriate only for items in a limited category, such as proper names).
- Create an image of the item in a scene, then attempt to describe the scene.
- Attempt to retrieve the overlearned opposite.
- Engage in free association, having an image in mind.
- Associate person's names with physical characteristics or a known person of the same name.

Thought Organization, Task Organization, and Organized Expression

External Procedures

- Use a graphic organizer or flow chart appropriate for the task or content.
  - **Task organizer.** Goal, materials needed, people and their responsibilities, sequence of steps, timeline, and evaluation of results.

- **Narrative discourse organizer.** People, places, time; initiating event, main character's response, plan, action, and resolution.
- Prepare work space; assign space as task demands.
- Construct a timeline to maintain appropriate sequence of events.
- Alert others before shifting topic in conversation.
- Watch others for feedback in conversation; ask, "Am I being clear?"
- Use outlining software

Internal Procedures

- Use a mental representation of a graphic organizer or flow chart appropriate for the task or content.
- Use knowledge scripts (e.g., discourse scripts like narrative form; event scripts like going out to eat, applying for a job, visiting a doctor scripts).
- Note topics in conversation; self-question about the main point.
- Rehearse important comments; listen to self.
- Set limits of time or allowable sentences in any turn of conversation.

Reasoning, Problem Solving, and Judgment

External Procedures

- Ask others for advice or problem-solving guidance.
- Use others for reality checks.
- Post important social rules to follow

Internal Procedures

- Use an organized problem-solving guide (e.g., "What exactly is the problem? What do I need to know in order to solve it? What are some possible solutions? What are the pro's and con's of each? Which is best? [Following action] How'd I do").
- Use self-questioning for alternative courses of action or consequences.
- Examine possible courses of action from at least two perspectives.
- Scan environment for cues to appropriateness of action.

Self-Monitoring and Self-Evaluating

- Post reminder: goal-plan-do-review.
- Post reminders or use alarms that mean "Pause and review: How am I doing?"
- Place monitoring reminder cards in books, at work station, and wherever needed (e.g., "How am I doing?" or "Summarize what you have read or done.").
- Set aside a review time at the end of the day or at the end of the workday.

APPENDIX 33.4
Rationale for Collaborative Relationships with Everyday People

Purposes Served by Collaboration with Everyday People

1. To communicate respect.
2. To integrate useful insights and skills of everyday people.
3. To increase the intensity, consistency, and duration of services by ensuring concordance among all relevant people.
4. To enhance generalization and maintenance of treatment gains.
5. To infuse reality, common sense, and functional goals into professional practice.
6. To ensure appropriate services and supports over the long term as unpredictable problems are encountered (often associated with major life transitions).
7. To enhance community inclusion by creating networks of community support. (Individuals rely more on community supports than on rehabilitation professionals over the long term.)
8. To stretch limited professional resources in an era of managed care.
9. To increase the amount of available data on the basis of which intervention decisions are made.

Obstacles to Collaborative Alliances with Family Members and Other Everyday People

1. Distrust; adversarial relationships based on:
   * Judgmental attitudes (staff or everyday people).
   * Failure to respect the other's perspective.
2. Professional self-perception that as experts, they do not collaborate with everyday people.
3. Insufficient access to everyday people, possibly because services are provided entirely outside of natural contexts.
4. Potential barriers to learning:
   * Quantity and complexity of information and skills.
   * Family: accepting need to learn is a threat to hope.
   * Family: severely competing priorities: exhaustion and stress.
   * Time.
5. Conflict of priorities between rehabilitation professionals and everyday people.
6. Language barriers: vocabulary, cross-cultural barriers.

Strategies to Overcome Obstacles to Alliances with Everyday People

1. Be available to interact with everyday people in contexts that facilitate collaborative activity.
2. Listen actively and nonjudgmentally.
3. Be respectful: "I am a guest in your home."
   * Respect diversity.
   * Seek capacity.
   * Respect expertise.
   * Be sensitive to differences in behavior in different circumstances.
   * Acknowledge mistakes.
   * Understand grieving.
   * Identify effective communicator.
   * Ensure that everyday people are supported.
4. Clarify roles and expectations.
5. Collaborate in assessment (see section on collaborative assessment).
6. Use in vivo coaching—demonstrate competence in context.
7. Provide training videos.
   * Generic videos.
   * Customized videos.
   * Collaboratively produced transitional/self-advocacy videos.

Characteristics of Effective Everyday Coach/Facilitator

1. Knowledge
2. Interactive competence
3. Competence in facilitation procedures
4. Optimism
5. Flexibility
6. Creativity
7. Problem-solving ability and enthusiasm
8. Maturity, nondefensiveness
9. Sense of humor
10. Empathy based on rich experience with the realities of the individual's life

Collaborating with Everyday People: Training and Support Options

1. Informational in-services
2. Family conferences
3. Creation of support networks
4. Competency-based training sessions
5. Apprenticeship teaching
   * Teaching in vivo
   * Self-observation on video
   * Collaborative formulation of scripts, including problem-solving, flexibility, and optimism scripts
   * Community meetings
   * Peer teaching and support
     * Staff and family training chains
     * Child peers
6. Training videos
   * Generic videos
   * Customized videos
   * Collaboratively produced transitional/self-advocacy videos

APPENDIX 33.5
Communication-Partner Competencies for Supporting and Improving Cognition in Individuals with Cognitive Impairment*

These conversational support procedures are designed to ensure participation (overcome handicap) and, with repetition, improve cognitive function (reduce impairment). Illustrations of associated interactive scripts also are provided.

Collaboration Procedures

Implicit message: "We are doing this together as a cooperative project"

Supportive Collaborative Style	Noncollaborative Style
Collaborative Intent • Shares information • Uses collaborative talk (e.g., "Let's think about this.") • Communicates understanding of partner's contribution • Invites partner to evaluate own contribution • Confirms partner's contributions • Shows enthusiasm for partner's contributions • Makes effort to establish equal leadership roles	*Noncollaborative (e.g., Teaching, Testing) Intent* • Demands information • Talks as teacher or trainer • Fails to communicate understanding of partner's contribution • Fails to invite partner to evaluate own contribution • Fails to confirm partner's contribution • Expresses lack of enthusiasm • Takes leadership role, despite other's attempt to contribute
Cognitive Support • Gives information when needed (within statements or questions) • Makes available memory and organization supports (e.g., calendar, photos, memory book, gestures) • Gives cues in a conversational manner • Responds to errors by giving correct information in a non-threatening, nonpunitive manner	*Lack of Cognitive Support* • Does not give information when needed; continues to quiz • Fails to use cognitive supports at appropriate times • Fails to give necessary cues • Corrects errors in a punishing manner
Emotional Support • Communicates respects for other's concerns, perspectives, and abilities • Explicitly acknowledges difficulty of the task (e.g. "It's hard to put all these things in order, isn't it?")	*Lack of Emotional Support* • Fails to communicate respect for other's concerns, perspectives, and abilities • Fails to acknowledge difficulty of the task
Questions: Positive Style • Questions in a nondemanding manner • Questions in a supportive manner (e.g., questions include needed cues, such as "Do you need a wake-up call in the morning?")	*Questions: Negative Style* • Questions in a demanding manner (i.e., performance-oriented quizzing) • Questions in a nonsupportive manner (e.g., questions lack needed cues, such as "How are you going to get that done?")
Collaborative Turn Taking • Takes appropriate conversational turns • Helps partner express thoughts when struggle occurs (e.g. word finding difficulties)	*Noncollaborative Turn Taking* • Interrupts in a way that disrupts partner's thought process and statements • Fails to help partner when struggle occurs

Elaboration Procedures

Implicit message: "I am going to help you organize and extend your thinking"

Positive Elaborative Style	Nonelaborative Style
Elaboration of Topics • Introduces/initiates topics of interest with potential for elaboration • Maintains topic for many turns • Contributes many pieces of information to topic • Invites elaboration (e.g., "I wonder what happened . . .")	***Nonelaboration of Topics*** • Introduces topics of marginal interest, with little potential for elaboration • Changes topic frequently • Fails to add adequate information to topic • Fails to invite other to add information
Elaborative Organization • Conversationally organizes information as clearly as possible: 　• Sequential order of events (e.g., "First we . . ., then we . . .") 　• Physical causality (e.g., "The radio's not working because it got wet.") 　• Psychological causality (e.g., "Maybe you're avoiding it because you're scared.") 　• Similarity and difference (e.g., "Yes, they're similar because . . .") 　• Analogy and association (e.g., "That reminds me of . . . because . . .") • Reviews organization of information • Makes connections when topics change • Makes connections among day to day conversational themes	***Nonelaborative Organization*** • Fails to organize information • Fails to review organization of information • Fails to make connections explicit when topics change • Fails to make connections among day to day conversational themes; meaning is vague
Elaborative Explanation • Conversationally adds explanation for events (e.g., "Maybe the fact that you were drunk at the time had something to do with it.") • Invites explanations for events • Invites discussion of problems and solutions (e.g., "I wonder whether we can think of a better way to handle this if it comes up again."); invites partner to address problems and solutions • Reflects on other's physical and psychological status (e.g., "You must have felt miserable about that."), and invites other to reflect on his or her physical and psychological states	***Nonelaborative Explanation*** • Offers few explanations • Fails to invite explanations • Does little problem solving or all of the problem solving; fails to invite partner to address problems and solutions • Fails to reflect on or invite the other to reflect on other's physical or psychological status

Problem-Solving Conversation Script

Problem arises:

Staff or Person with TBI Identifies the problematic issue.

Staff Invites reflection about what might work (e.g., "Let's see; there's gotta be something that can be done about this.").

Person with TBI Expresses frustration.

Staff Outlines a few possible solutions.

Person with TBI Rejects one or more.

Staff Continues review of possibilities until person with TBI chooses one to try.

Staff Facilitates an experimental attitude, reflection about what does and does not work.

Flexibility Conversation Script

Person with TBI resists an activity:

Staff "Alright, maybe my idea wasn't such a good one. There's got to be another way to do this. Let's try your idea. (*OR* Let's think about it . . .) What are we trying to make happen here? You're trying to be successful at . . . ? Am I right?"

Alternatively, person with TBI perseverates on an action or thought:

Staff: "This isn't working real well. You have another thought? (*OR* Here's another way (or thought) . . .and another.)"

*Modified from Ylvisaker, Sellars, and Edelman (1998); with permission.

Chapter 34

Communication Disorders Associated with Right-Hemisphere Damage

Penelope S. Myers and
Margaret Lehman Blake

OBJECTIVES

Upon completion of this chapter, readers will be able to (1) describe the major communication deficits associated with acquired right-hemisphere damage (RHD) and apply that knowledge to clinical work; (2) recognize the impact of deficits in arousal, orienting, vigilance, and selective attention on the communicative performance of adults with RHD; (3) explain the potential impact of neglect on discourse as well as on reading and writing in adults with RHD; (4) describe the extralinguistic deficits associated with RHD and their impact on communication; (5) distinguish cognitive from true affective deficits caused by RHD; (6) describe deficits in specific prosodic parameters and recognize that prosodic production and comprehension can be impaired independently of one another; (7) distinguish process-oriented from task-oriented treatment strategies and apply that knowledge to management of RHD deficits; and (8) generate appropriate stimuli, and apply various treatment suggestions and scoring systems to their clinical work with adults with RHD.

Patients with damage confined to the right hemisphere (RH) may have a variety of processing deficits, including impairments in attention, visual perception, cognition, and communication. Not all patients with right-hemisphere damage (RHD) have communication impairments, but it is generally accepted that those who do are not aphasic. Their command over basic linguistic structures is usually adequate, and they may do well in superficial or straightforward conversation. Their communication problems typically become apparent in more complex communicative events in which verbal and nonverbal contextual cues must be used to assess and convey communicative intent. Before discussing these problems in detail, it might be useful to draw a very general portrait of a typical patient with RHD, Mr. Smith.

An initial and fairly casual encounter with Mr. Smith may leave the visitor with an overly optimistic picture of his cognitive and communicative capacity. Questions about the weather, treatment by the hospital staff, the quality of the food, and so on will elicit responses that seem not only linguistically accurate, but appropriate as well. He may seem a bit less responsive, and may speak in a monotone, but these characteristics might easily be attributed to fatigue and to the general effects of his recent trauma. The visitor may even be cheered by Mr. Smith's occasional jocularity and blithe assurances about resuming all aspects of his former life.

During subsequent visits, however, the very factors that led to a firm belief in his full recovery seem suspect. He may deny a need for rehabilitative services, refusing to take his physical limitations seriously. His assessment of his capabilities may be at odds with his progress in simple self-care. He may be unable to groom himself properly or to figure out how to put on his shirt. He may talk about returning to work next week, yet be unable to transfer himself from bed to wheelchair. Once in his wheelchair, he may demonstrate difficulty finding his way to the nearby nurses station, or back to his room.

Mr. Smith may have trouble recognizing friends and may deny that they have visited him before. In extended conversation he may seem excessively bound up in himself. He may not respect conversational rules. He may interrupt, fail to assess, and appear not to care about his listener's reaction. He may not maintain eye contact, and he may seem unresponsive to the emotional tone of verbal and nonverbal messages. His tendency to personalize abstract topics, his seeming difficulty in grasping the point of a conversation, and his tendency to digress furthers the impression that he is either confused or that he operates in isolation during conversation.

His jocularity will now strike a discordant note, and he may trivialize topics and focus on tangential and unnecessary detail. Although quick to provide a response, he may take an excessive amount of time to actually answer substantive questions. He may seem verbose and disorganized. His responses, then, may seem inefficient and lacking an organizational base. His ready answers may seem impulsive, produced without internal reflection.

In short, despite an apparently adequate linguistic system, many patients with RHD neither respond to nor participate in communicative events as they once did. The near-universal refrain of friends and families associated with communicatively impaired adults with RHD is, "He (she) can talk, but it isn't the same."

As this portrait suggests, individuals with RHD not only have communication impairments, but may also suffer from a variety of other cognitive impairments. Regardless of whether these deficits affect communication directly or indirectly, the clinician must recognize their potential impact on the patient.

NONLINGISTIC DEFICITS

Nonlinguistic deficits associated with RHD include left-sided neglect, attentional deficits, and visuoperceptual problems. Neglect and attention can affect communication and are discussed below.

Neglect

Unilateral or hemispatial neglect is a complex disorder in which patients fail to report, respond, or orient to stimuli on the side opposite their brain lesion (the contralesional side), despite the motor and sensory capacity to do so (Heilman, Watson, Valenstein, & Damasio, 1983). Although it may occur with left-hemisphere damage (LHD), neglect is usually longer-lasting, more severe, and more common in individuals with RHD lesions (Bowen, McKenna, & Tallis, 1999; Mesulam, 1985). Neglect most often occurs with lesions of the *frontal, temporal,* or *parietal* cortex (Buxbaum et al., 2004; Mesulam, 1981, 1985; Vallar, 1993; Vallar & Perani, 1986), but can occur as well with subcortical lesions, specifically in the *thalamus* (Hillis, Newhart, Heidler, Barker, Herskovits, & Degaonkar, 2005; Rafal & Posner, 1987; Vallar & Perani, 1986) and the *basal ganglia* (Buxbaum et al., 2004; Damasio, Damasio, & Chui, 1980). Hillis and colleagues (2005) have suggested that neglect due to subcortical lesions may be related to decreased perfusion to distant cortical areas. Neglect may occur in the visual, tactile, auditory, or olfactory senses, or in combinations thereof, but it is most commonly observed in the visual modality.

Patients with RHD with neglect fail to attend to left-sided input; that is, to input from contralesional space. They may not eat food on the left side of their trays, nor notice people on the left side of their beds, nor localize sounds to their left (and thus may look to the right when a phone rings on the left). Neglect can differentially affect body space

(e.g., lack of grooming or dressing the left side of the body), peri-personal space (within arms' reach), or far space (Appelros, Nydevik, Karlsson, Throwalls, & Seiger, 2004; Buxbaum, 2004). More severe manifestations of neglect may co-occur with somatoparaphrenia, which is the failure to recognize paralyzed or weakened limbs as one's own ("I'd be all right if I had my own arm."). This type of delusion can be part of a more generalized disorder called "anosognosia," which is a lack of awareness of illness. Denial of neglect and other deficits is characteristic of patients with neglect.

Patients with neglect have difficulty processing stimuli to the left of their midline, a difficulty that can extend to the left side of any item, regardless of where it appears in the environment (Duncan, Bundesen, Olson, Humphreys, Chabada, & Shibuya, 1999; Gainotti, D'Erme, Monteleone, & Silveri, 1986). The imaginary line dividing their world into neglected and non-neglected space can also shift based on how many things are in the environment and on instructions or cues given. It can be worse in the lower quadrants of space than in the upper quadrants.

Neglect can have a motor as well as a sensory component. According to Mesulam (1981), neglect may disrupt the motor sequences (including eye movements) necessary for exploring and manipulating stimuli in contralesional space. Thus, patients with neglect may fail to perform tasks that require visual exploration or movements on both sides of the body. They may not include left-sided detail in their drawings (sometimes called "constructional apraxia"). They may not be able to dress or groom themselves properly because they fail to reach over to the contralesional side of their bodies.

Reduced attention to the left may be combined with a "magnetic attraction" to stimuli on the right (Bartolomeo & Chokron, 1999), making it difficult to disengage attention when it is captured by right-sided stimuli (Posner, 1980; Posner, Walker, Friedrich, & Raphal, 1984). For example, subjects with RHD canceled more lines in a cancellation task when asked to erase (rather than cancel) the lines, thus removing the attention-attracting right-sided stimuli as they progressed through the task (Mark, Kooistra, & Heilman, 1988). This phenomenon can occur in the auditory as well as the visual modality (Farah, Wong, Monheit, & Morrow, 1989; Robin & Rizzo, 1989). Magnetic attraction may be related to the phenomenon of "extinction," in which the presence of bilateral competing stimuli can increase the severity of neglect (DiPellegrino & DeRenzi, 1995; Duncan et al., 1999). Clinicians should take the level of right-sided stimulation into account in tasks designed to measure or alleviate left-sided neglect.

Most theories of neglect hold that it is a deficit in attention, and many types of attention are implicated, including (1) arousal (Coslett, Bowers, & Heilman, 1987; Heilman, Schwartz, & Watson, 1978, Heilman, Valenstein, & Watson, 1984); (2) sustained attention (Bub, Audet, & Lecours, 1990;

Duncan et al., 1999); (3) the capacity to disengage attention from ipsilesional space (Heilman, Bowers, Coslett, Whelan, & Watson, 1985; Posner et al., 1984); and (4) selective and directed attention (Bartolomeo, Sieroff, Chokron, & Decaix, 2001; Mesulam, 1981; Rapcsak, Verfaellie, Fleet, & Heilman, 1989).

Neglect may be one manifestation of a larger, more generalized attentional impairment (Cherney, 2002; Duncan et al., 1999; Husain & Rorden, 2003; Mesulam, 1985; Myers 1999a). Attention has an obvious impact on cognition. Some studies have reported that neglect has significant negative ramifications for the recovery of independence (Buxbaum et al., 2004, Jehkonen et al., 2001; but see Odell, Wollack, & Flynn, 2005). It may also interfere in some of the cognitive operations involved in communication (Myers & Brookshire, 1996; Rivers & Love, 1980), and even if recovered, individuals initially diagnosed with neglect often demonstrate greater cognitive-communicative deficits than those who never had neglect (Myers & Brookshire, 1996; Tompkins, Bloise, Timko, & Baumgaertner, 1994).

Evaluation of Neglect

Professionals participating in the evaluation of neglect include physicians, occupational therapists, neuropsychologists, and speech-language pathologists. The presence of neglect can be established by published tests or by the informal tasks described below.

Typical paper-and-pencil tests of neglect include *cancellation, line bisection, scanning,* and *drawing* tasks. Cancellation tasks require patients to look at an array of stimuli (e.g., lines, letters, numbers, or shapes) that are distributed in equal numbers on the left and right across a sheet of paper (Albert, 1973). The patient is asked to make a mark through ("cancel") all occurrences of the stimuli. Neglect is measured by comparing the number of left-sided to the number of right-sided stimuli missed by the patient. Generalized attention can be measured by the total number missed, regardless of their spatial location. Because the target stimuli do not differ from each other, this type of cancellation task is considered *simple*.

Complex cancellation tasks involve selective attention. The stimuli may differ in shape, size, or color. The patient is asked to cancel instances of a particular target in a field of foils (e.g., red triangles in an array of red and blue triangles and squares). Selective attention deficits may exacerbate neglect in complex visual search and cancellation tasks. Thus, a patient may not only omit left-sided stimuli, but may miss targets on the right and may miss more targets on the left in a complex compared to a simple cancellation task. By using both simple and complex cancellation tasks, one can assess the influence of selective attention on a patient's neglect. Task difficulty can be increased by increasing the field density, by placing targets and foils in random arrays

(versus rows), and/or by having targets and foils differ in more than one feature, such as shape and color (Myers, 1999a).

Line bisection requires patients to bisect a horizontal line by making a vertical mark through its center. Performance on line bisection helps determine the degree to which the patient's sense of space is skewed to the right by measuring how far to the right of center the patient's vertical line is placed. Several studies have found that there is wide variability in the normal population in accuracy of line bisection and that deviations of approximately 1/4 inch on a 10.5-inch line can be considered within normal limits. In general, the shorter the line, the more accurate people are in judging its center (Halligan, Manning, & Marshall, 1990; Halligan & Marshall, 1988; Marshall & Halligan, 1989; Tegner, Levander, & Caneman, 1990).

Scanning tasks, used to assess the influence of neglect on reading, require patients to scan an array of letters, numbers, or shapes in which instances of a target stimulus are embedded in a row of foils (e.g., finding all the instances of the letter "A" in a line of letters). Neglect is measured by the number of target stimuli missed to the left of the midline.

Patients can also be asked to read compound words, sentences, or paragraphs presented at their visual midline. The longer the material, the more likely neglect will surface in the form of left-sided omissions (e.g., "able" for "table") or inaccuracies (e.g., "tree" for "three"). A particularly sensitive test requires the patient to read a paragraph in which the left margin is randomly indented from 2 to 25 spaces (Caplan, 1987). The unpredictability of the left margin makes this test well-suited to detecting mild neglect. The score consists of the number of words read aloud by the patient.

The effect of neglect on writing can be assessed by asking patients to write or copy sentences or a short paragraph. Patients may omit the left half of sentences and words (e.g., "house" for "greenhouse"), and their writing samples may contain excessive left-sided margins, iterations and/or omissions of letters and words, and words trailing down the right side of the page.

Finally, patients may be asked to draw from memory or copy symmetrical objects such as a flower, a man, or a geometric form. Neglect is measured by comparing the number of left-sided details to those included on the right in the patient's rendition (see Myers, 1999a, for a scoring method for scene-copying). Drawings can also be inspected for overall structure and integration of object parts. Typically, drawings from patients with LHD are somewhat primitive. Those from patients with RHD may not only be primitive, but also disorganized and disconnected.

Several researchers (Beis et al., 2004; Horner, Massey, Woodruff, Chase, & Dawson, 1989; Ogden, 1985) have reported that because no one task is substantially better than another at detecting neglect, combinations of tasks should be administered. Severity can be estimated by combining scores across tasks. Establishing the presence of neglect helps clarify whether or not reading and writing deficits are linguistically based. It helps establish the patient's capacity to attend to stimuli in other diagnostic and therapeutic material. Finally, as a reflection of a general attention deficit, neglect may signal a decrease in the patient's general level of arousal and his or her readiness to respond and to produce and sustain effortful, directed attention during complex communicative events.

Treatment of Neglect

There have been many studies of treatment for neglect, and several reviews of the efficacy of treatment of neglect (Calvanio, Levine, & Petrone, 1993; Cicerone et al., 2000, 2005; Manly, 2002). Scanning treatments generally are effective, although generalization of gains to functional tasks such as reading and writing does not always occur.

Management of neglect revolves around the issue of treating the symptoms versus the cause. Symptomatic treatment attempts to compensate for neglect by external aids that are meant to encourage leftward scanning. However, verbally cuing the patient to look to the left, highlighting stimuli on the left (e.g., drawing a red line down the left margin of a printed page), and other external reminders to increase visual scanning are rarely effective because while they may improve performance in therapy, they rarely translate into internal self-cues or generalize to more functional tasks (Calvanio et al., 1993; Halper & Cherney, 1998; Manly, 2002; Tompkins & Lehman, 1998).

Examples of tasks that are thought to encourage internal self-cuing include (a) internally motivated leftward search tasks and (b) tasks designed to stimulate unconscious perception (see Myers, 1999a and 1999b for specific tasks). For example, one can present a very simple leftward search task in which patients are required to find only one or two target objects (e.g., colored cubes) within specified borders. Because the number of targets is low, patients typically continue the search voluntarily until the total number is found. Cubes can be placed on a flat board that has been divided into quadrants. One may begin such a search-and-find task with as few as two cubes of a single color. Task difficulty can be increased by changing cube placement (e.g., placing cubes to the left as well as the right of midline, then in the lower-left quadrant as well as the upper-left quadrant), by increasing the number of cubes, and by having target cubes differ in color from foils. This type of task has been described in detail by Myers (1999a) and Myers and Mackisack (1990). The underlying theory is that by enlisting voluntary attention without external cuing, the potential for generalization of leftward search increases. A second advantage, noted clinically, is that it appears to increase patients' general level of attention and thus may be a good start-up task for cognitive and communication therapy.

Tapping into unconscious perception of left-sided details is another potential way to stimulate leftward movement of attention without external monitoring. The literature contains numerous examples of the phenomenon of unconscious perception, the most common of which is letter substitution (versus omission) in single-word reading (e.g., reading "table" and not "able" for "sable"), which demonstrates that patients have processed left letters at some early level of processing. For example, stimuli that are contiguous, such as a person on the right side of a page holding hands with someone on the left side, can encourage movement of attention leftward such that the patient reports two people in the drawing, unconsciously perceiving them as a single object. Other tasks of this type are described by Myers (1999a) and Brooks, Wong, & Robertson (2005). Leftward search and unconscious processing tasks are theoretically motivated, but their efficacy has yet to be evaluated.

Finally, if one accepts that various types of attention are a significant factor in neglect and in RHD deficits in general, it makes sense to work on attention directly in tasks designed to increase the level of arousal, vigilance, and selective attention capacity. One such treatment with demonstrated generalization requires the clinician to knock loudly on the table and say "ATTEND!" at random times during a scanning task. This cue is then shared with the patient (he or she says "attend" when the clinician knocks), and eventually internalized by the patient (he or she subvocally says "attend" during tasks) (Robertson, Tegner, Tham, Lo, & Nimmo-Smith, 1995).

Clinicians should counsel patients about their neglect and its effects on activities of daily living, including communication, and if necessary, demonstrate the problems in a way that enables patients to overcome possible denial. Families should be included in understanding neglect as an attention disorder and its effects on communication.

Attention Deficits

Patients with RHD with and without demonstrable neglect may have attention deficits. Each type of RHD attention disorder is discussed briefly in the sections that follow.

Arousal and Orienting

Individuals with RHD are sometimes called "hypoaroused," and studies comparing them to those with LHD suggest they are generally less attentive and less alert (Coslett et al., 1987; Davidson, Fedio, Smith, Aureille, & Martin, 1992). Behavioral, anatomical, neurochemical, and autonomic evidence suggests that the right hemisphere (RH) plays a special role in arousal and in orienting to the external environment (Corbetta, Kincade, & Shulman, 2002; Sturm, Longoni, Weiss, Specht, Herzog, & Vohn, 2004; also see Myers, 1999a, for a review). Unlike the left hemisphere (LH), the

RH appears to be able to orient attention to both right and left hemispace. Evidence suggests that neurotransmitter pathways supporting arousal are to some extent lateralized to the right (Oke, Keller, Medford, & Adams, 1978; Oke, Lewis, & Adams, 1980; Posner & Petersen, 1990; Robinson, 1985; Tucker & Williamson, 1984). Physiologic correlates of arousal, such as electrodermal activity or galvanic skin response, indicate that subjects with RHD have significantly lower physiologic responses to pain and to emotional material than those with LHD or those without brain damage (Davidson et al., 1992; Heilman et al., 1978; Zahn, Grafman, & Tranel, 1999). Individuals with RHD also have slower reaction times in response to simple visual and auditory stimuli, such as a point of light or a simple tone (Ladavas, Del Pesce, & Provinciali, 1989; Yokoyama, Jennings, Ackles, Hood, & Boller, 1987), suggesting a reduction in arousal or general attention. Finally, neglect may inhibit the scanning necessary to generate the broad-based view that is fundamental to environmental scanning and for which the arousal and orienting systems are critical.

In functional terms, patients with RHD may need more intense stimulation or more time to get ready to attend than other populations of brain-damaged patients with focal lesions. They may not be as attuned to the environment, nor able to expand attention beyond a narrow focus. A narrowed focus of attention and poor orienting, characteristic of neglect, can reduce sensitivity to environmental cues that carry important pragmatic information.

Vigilance and Sustained Attention

Vigilance is a state of alertness in anticipation of an event. Reaction-time tasks have been conceptualized as measures of general attention and/or of vigilance. Participants must be ready to respond to stimuli that occur at unpredictable or random intervals. To measure attention adequately, reaction-time tasks elicit many responses that require sustained attention over long periods of time. Studies have found that the performance of participants with RHD is poorer than that of individuals with LHD (Sturm & Willmes, 1991), and deteriorates over time (Bub et al., 1990; Koski & Petrides, 2001) and with longer interstimulus intervals (Wilkins, Shallice, & McCarthy, 1987).

Studies of healthy adults indicate a RH dominance for sustained attention (Arruda, Walker, Weiler, & Valentino, 1999; Coull, Frith, Frackowiak, & Grasby, 1996; but see Audet, Mercier, Collard, Rochette, & Herbert, 2000, for conflicting results) and vigilance (Cherry & Hellige, 1999), and increased metabolic activity in the RH during vigilance tasks (Cohen, Semple, Gross, Holcomb, Dowling, & Nordahl, 1988; Deutsch, Papanicolaou, Bourbon, & Eisenberg, 1987; Pardo, Fox, & Raichle, 1991). Results from a recent study using functional magnetic resonance imaging (fMRI) suggest that RH attentional networks are activated

first in focused attention tasks, with recruitment of specific LH areas only with increased task difficulty (Nebel, Wiese, Stude, deGreiff, Deiner, & Keidel, 2005).

These results support the clinical impression that some patients with RHD have difficulty sustaining attention and remaining vigilant, factors that may affect their progress in therapy. Their level of attention during any demanding communicative situation can fluctuate such that they may not process crucial information even when prepared to do so.

Selective Attention

Selective attention enables one to screen out distracting stimuli and to recognize stimulus significance. It can be automatic or voluntary, and is dependent on the arousal, orienting, and vigilance systems. Studies suggest that the RH is particularly important for selective attention. For example, positron emission tomography (PET) studies have found prominent activation of the right anterior cingulate gyrus (Bench et al., 1993; Pardo, Pardo, Janer, & Raichle, 1990), and in the right as opposed to the left frontal cortex of non–brain-damaged (NBD) participants (Deutsch et al., 1987). In reaction-time tasks calling for selective attention patients with right frontal lesions performed slower and less accurately than those with lesions in other cortical areas (Ruff, Nieman, Allen, Farrow, & Wylie, 1992; Stuss, Toth, Franchi, Alexander, Tipper, & Craik, 1999).

In addition, neglect increases as the selective attention demands of tasks increase (Kaplan, Verfaillie, Meadows, Caplan, Peasin, & de Witt, 1991; Rapcsak et al., 1989; Riddoch & Humphreys, 1987). These findings support the notion that neglect is a symptom of a larger attentional deficit.

Effect of Attention Deficits on Communication

Attentional impairments have cognitive consequences that may affect all levels of experience, including communication. Attention deficits may impair the appreciation of the verbal and visual cues that specify the context within which communication takes place. Patients may be less able to shift attention, actively or covertly, during conversations. They may be less able to sustain attention to stimuli anywhere in the environment and to filter out distracters. Thus, they may not be able to attend selectively to important information during communicative events. Finally, attention deficits may place demands on patients' internal resources such that as interactions become more complex and demanding, cognitive resources are strained and patients become overwhelmed. These effects will be addressed more thoroughly in the section on extralinguistic disorders.

Evaluation and Treatment

It should be emphasized that most individuals with RHD will have some type of impaired attention, regardless of the presence of neglect. Thus, all patients with RHD should be tested for attentional deficits, and the results should be included in family counseling and taken into account in evaluating and treating RHD communication impairments. Tests of attention and treatment techniques can be found in some of the RHD batteries, as well as in published materials designed for patients with traumatic brain injury and in the literature on cognitive rehabilitation (e.g., Turkstra et al., 2005).

Evidence of treatment efficacy is available primarily in the literature on traumatic brain injury (Cappa, Benke, Clarke, Rossi, Stemmer, & van Heugten, 2005; Sohlberg et al., 2003). Direct attention training is effective, although generalization to more functional tasks is limited. Tasks that require attention over time to the occurrence of simple but unpredictable stimuli may increase the capacity for vigilance (e.g., listening for a target word in a word list or monitoring a computer screen for the appearance of a target). Sturm and colleagues (Sturm, Longoni, Fimm et al., 2004) reported improvements in internal alertness in a computerized task with concomitant changes in the function of RH attentional networks, as observed on PET and fMRI scans. Selective attention may be addressed by modifying the complex cancellation tasks designed for evaluating neglect (Myers, 1999a). Additional tasks for treating attentional deficits subsequent to brain injury can be found in commercial materials, including computer software designed for attention training. Research is needed on the efficacy and generalization of attention treatments specifically for adults with RHD.

LINGUISTIC DEFICITS

Pure linguistic deficits are not considered a source of RHD communication impairments. It is true that some individuals with RHD may make errors on straightforward expressive and receptive language tasks such as naming, word discrimination, following simple commands, word definitions, verbal fluency, and reading and writing. However, the available data suggest that the problems are relatively mild, are not characteristic of aphasia, and rarely affect communication significantly (Archibald & Wepman, 1968; Deal, Deal, Wertz, Kitselman, & Dwyer, 1979; Eisenson, 1962). In addition, visuospatial deficits, neglect, and attentional impairments have been cited as possible contaminating factors in some studies investigating linguistic disorders in adults with RHD (Adamovich & Brooks, 1981; Archibald & Wepman, 1968; Swisher & Sarno, 1969).

In general, patients with RHD are able to structure sentences and paragraphs according to the rules of their language. They do not have particular problems in retrieving words, and they rarely make paraphasic errors. However, their control over linguistic structure may belie a more general problem with language use at the narrative and discourse level of communication, as discussed in the section on extralinguistic deficits.

Evaluation and Treatment

If a true linguistic problem is suspected, subtests from aphasia batteries, designed to test language in constructions that are essentially context-free, are useful in assessing linguistic comprehension (e.g., following verbal commands rather than interpreting paragraphs) and expression (e.g., object naming rather than scene description). Errors should be examined in light of visuoperceptual and attentional deficits. If the clinician feels certain that the patient has a language problem rather than, or in addition to, signs of RHD, treatment should follow the traditional approaches used in the management of aphasia. It is important to remember that language is not always lateralized to the LH, particularly in left-handed people. Thus, although extremely rare, a patient with RHD could have aphasia.

EXTRALINGUISTIC DEFICITS

Although individuals with RHD typically do not have aphasia, many of them do have communication disorders. Extralinguistic deficits represent the heart of RHD communication problems. The term "extralinguistic" refers to factors that affect communication but are not strictly linguistic in nature. The extralinguistic and pragmatic aspects of communication specify the context within which communication takes place and allow one to understand and convey intentions, emotional tone, and implied meaning. These aspects of communication extend communicated meaning beyond the literal or surface structure of words and sentences. Context is conveyed through an array of sensory cues such as gesture, body language, facial expression, and prosodic contour, as well as through the choice and grouping of words themselves. Extralinguistic cues allow us to interpret intended meaning (what is meant from what is said) and to understand the relative formality and emotional tone of discourse, the roles played by participants in a conversation (e.g., peer versus subordinate), and whether someone is being funny or sarcastic or serious. These same cues help us express our own intended meanings.

Some patients with RHD appear to have difficulty using these cues to understand the implied meaning of complex discourse and narratives. Thus, they may miss the theme or point of a story. They may not recognize relationships among characters, their emotional state, and/or the motives behind their actions. In conversation they may not understand humor or the subtleties of irony. They may miss the main points a speaker is making because they focus on unimportant details and have difficulty integrating information into an overall theme. They may not attend to a speaker's facial expression, the prosodic cues that convey emotion and emphasis, or to the physical setting in which the communicative act takes place.

Patients with RHD may also have difficulty expressing their own intended meaning. Their speech may be inefficient and uninformative, and lack specificity. They may have problems getting to the point they are trying to make. Finally, they may have difficulty using the extralinguistic cues that convey emotion and intention through gesture and prosody.

It is of note that we still use the term "right-hemisphere communication disorders" to describe these symptoms, a label that refers to a location in the brain rather than the nature of the problem. However, it has only been in the past 25 years that the notion of communication disorders associated with "minor" hemisphere damage gained credence. Early studies focused on describing the deficits and the conditions under which deficits may be observed. With descriptions more firmly established, studies have now begun to address underlying cause in a systematic way. By addressing the mechanisms of the impairments, we may eventually arrive at a more appropriate term to capture the nature of the extralinguistic deficits associated with RHD (see Myers, 2001, for further discussion of this topic). Hypotheses about underlying mechanisms will move management toward treating the cause, rather than the symptoms. Certainly, impaired attentional mechanisms contribute to all levels of cognitive processing, including communication. In addition, there may be specific *semantic* deficits that have an impact on the RHD communicative impairments.

Discourse Deficits

Macrostructure Deficits

A macrostructure is the overall theme, central message, or main point of narratives, pictured scenes, situations, or discourse. Individuals with RHD may have difficulty generating macrostructures in comprehension and expression of complex communication. They may miss the point of conversation and be unable to stick to the point or convey the gist of their own messages. They may produce fewer core concepts, have problems giving titles to or choosing a summary statement for story contents, and have difficulty extracting story morals and themes in linguistic and pictured stories (Benowitz, Moya, & Levine, 1990; Gardner, Brownell, Wapner, & Michelow, 1983; Hough, 1990; Joanette, Goulet, Ska, & Nespoulous, 1986; Lojek-Osiejuk, 1996; Mackisack, Myers, & Duffy, 1987; Moya, Benowitz, Levine, & Finklestein, 1986; Myers & Brookshire, 1996; Rehak, Kaplan, Weylman, Kelly, & Brownell, 1992; Wapner, Hamby, & Gardner, 1981).

Generating a macrostructure depends on the capacity to draw inferences or interpret information. According to Myers (1992), "an inference is a hypothesis about sensory data such that input is not only sensed, but interpreted" (p. 9). Inferences about individual features must be integrated within the entire context to produce the overall theme we call a macrostructure. Initial inferences are beliefs or hypotheses about sensations. Later-stage inferences are hypotheses based on those initial beliefs. Thus, a viewer might interpret a picture of a man in a purple robe, wearing a crown, and holding a scepter as a king. The conclusion that he is a king is a hypothesis about the intended meaning of the visual image.

There are many levels of inference. In the above example, organizing the visual image into the form of a human is an inference, and determining that the image is that of a man is another inference. In general, the type of communication impairments experienced by adults with RHD suggests that inference breaks down at a later stage of processing, rather than at the level of translating light rays into shapes or sound waves into phonemes, or even linking pronouns to their antecedents (Leonard, Waters, & Caplan, 1997a, 1997b). The process of inferencing does not end once an inference is generated. The inference may have to be maintained in working memory until required for selection from one of several possible interpretations when more than one inference is generated (Blake & Lesniewicz, 2005).

Generation of inferences depends on at least four operations: (1) attention to individual cues; (2) selection of relevant cues; (3) integration of relevant cues with one another; and (4) association of cues with prior experience. In the above example, the color of the man's hair would be considered an irrelevant cue. Relevant cues include the crown, the robe, and the scepter, and perhaps the color purple. These combined cues create the context from which the inference of royalty is made. That is, the elements must not only be recognized, but must be sorted for relevance, and those considered relevant must be combined or integrated to create a context or pattern or meaning beyond the superficial recognition of color, form, light, and shadow. The cues also must be associated with prior experience. These operations are not necessarily ordered sequentially, but more likely occur in parallel.

In similar fashion, recognizing the intended meaning of verbal communication requires that one go beyond the superficial, literal, or referential meaning of individual words to their implied or inferred meaning. In general, adults with RHD do not have difficulty with simple or automatic inferences (Brownell, Potter, Bihrle, & Gardner, 1986; Lehman & Tompkins, 2000; McDonald & Wales, 1986). They may have more difficulty with "elaborative inferences," which expand or embellish information and place demands on processing resources (McKoon & Ratcliff, 1989). Making predictions and determining the emotions or motives of story characters or conversational partners are elaborative inferences. Despite the fact that these inferences can be cognitively demanding, they can be generated by adults with RHD when they are strongly suggested or supported by a context (Blake & Lesniewicz, 2005; Lehman-Blake & Tompkins, 2001). More likely, inferencing problems tend to arise when correct interpretations rely on integrating multiple cues or selecting one of several possible interpretations. These deficits are discussed below.

Selection and Integration Deficits

Problems generating an organizing principle or macrostructure for narrative discourse may be related to deficits in integrating contextual information (Hough, 1990; Wapner et al., 1981). As explained by Hough (1990) and Brownell (1988), understanding the theme or overall gist of narratives involves the extraction of meaning from individual sentences and the integration of their meaning into the context supplied by the other sentences. One must often infer the semantic links between sentences because not all the links are explicitly stated (Brownell, 1988; Joanette et al., 1986). Narrative discourse, then, requires the extraction and integration of individual units of meaning (explicit and implicit) into a larger whole. Similarly, interpreting pictured scenes or real situations involves the extraction of key individual objects and their integration with one another.

Impaired ability to extract and integrate selected bits of information can be demonstrated by patient descriptions of the familiar "cookie theft" picture (Fig. 34–1) from the Boston Diagnostic Aphasia Examination (Goodglass, Kaplan, & Barresi, 2001). Adequate interpretation of the scene (i.e., the overall implication of disaster) requires selecting and integrating relevant cues to build elaborative

inferences about individual elements upon which the overall theme or macrostructure rests. For example, calling the woman a mother (versus a woman) is an inference based on recognizing and integrating the appliances that suggest a kitchen, her apron, and the children behind her. Determining that the children are not just reaching for cookies, but stealing them, requires the integration of the action of the boy reaching in the cookie jar with the action of the girl who has her finger to her mouth in the gesture of "shhh." Adults with RHD may say the boy has his hand in the jar, and the girl has her finger to her mouth without combining the two actions into the inference of "stealing."

Clinical experience suggests that individuals with RHD often begin their descriptions of this picture by discussing irrelevant details such as the garden outside the window or the cups on the counter. This problem in selecting relevant information alters the overall interpretation. Myers (1979, 2005), and Myers and Linebaugh (1980) found that subjects with RHD produced significantly fewer inferential concepts in describing the "cookie theft" picture compared to NBD controls, and noted that they tended to list items without explicitly connecting them to each other or to the central action. Much of what they did list was irrelevant, an observation also documented in a study using Norman Rockwell illustrations in which subjects with RHD labeled more than twice as many items as did NBD controls (Mackisack et al., 1987).

Selection and integration deficits have also been reported in verbal-comprehension studies. Hough (1990) asked subjects to interpret the theme of short narratives and found that those with RHD tended to list information and "retained isolated pieces of paragraph data rather than

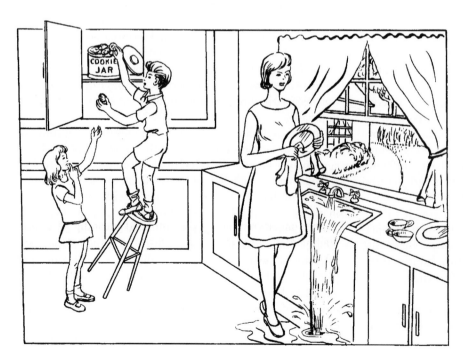

Figure 34–1. Cookie Theft Picture from the Boston Diagnostic Aphasia Examination (Goodglass, Kaplan, & Barresi, 2001)

integrating this information to deduce the meaning of the narratives" (p. 271). Brownell and colleagues (Brownell, Pincus, Blum, Rehak, & Winner, 1997; Brownell & Stringfellow, 1999; Kaplan, Brownell, Jacobs, & Gardner, 1990; Winner, Brownell, Happe, Blum, & Pincus, 1998) have demonstrated that adults with RHD have difficulty using cues such as familiarity between characters, relationships (friends vs. enemies), status (e.g., employer vs. co-worker), and understanding of another's knowledge (sometimes referred to as "theory of mind") to determine speakers' intents and generate appropriate responses. They also may not use contextual cues effectively to constrain the generation of elaborative inferences. For example, they have been found to generate multiple possible predictions about a story's outcome regardless of how specific the context is about the most plausible outcome (Blake & Lesniewicz, 2005).

Integration deficits also surface when adults with RHD are asked to organize printed sentences into paragraphs (Delis, Wapner, Gardner, & Moses, 1983) and to name object categories (Myers & Brookshire, 1995). Deficits in all of these tasks support the notion that although the command over basic narrative structure (i.e., script knowledge) is intact (Lojek-Osiejuk, 1996; Ostrove, Simpson, & Gardner, 1990; Rehak, Kaplan, & Weylman et al., 1992), RHD can interfere in integrating isolated pieces of information.

Macrostructure deficits can be influenced by other problems associated with RHD. For example, integration deficits also occur at the perceptual level. Piecemeal processing in the visuospatial realm is thought to be a factor in "constructional apraxia." That is, a patient may draw a chimney extending straight out from the side of a house or the petals of a flower trailing away from the stem, suggesting that the patient grasps the components, but cannot put them together into a coherent structure. Benowitz and colleagues (1990) found a relationship between difficulty organizing spatial relations and problems integrating verbal information in subjects with RHD. Selective attention deficits may inhibit the ability to filter irrelevant information and recognize important contextual cues. As a result, individuals with RHD may have difficulty not only comprehending *external* information, but also in filtering, integrating, and organizing *internal* information in such a way as to generate efficient narrative expression.

Producing Informative Content

The conversational expression of some patients with RHD has been described as hyperfluent and digressive; that of others as truncated and abrupt (Myers, 1999a; Roman, Brownell, Potter, Seibold, & Gardner, 1987; Sherratt & Penn, 1990; Trupe & Hillis, 1985). These opposing patterns of output occur with approximately the same frequency (Blake, Duffy, Myers, & Tompkins, 2002). Patients with unelaborated output (paucity of speech) often seem perfunc-

tory, giving the most immediate response without reflection about or interest in its accuracy or adequacy. Excessive output (verbosity) is characterized as digressive and tangential.

Individuals with RHD may produce as many or more words than NBD adults, but what they say may convey less information. Studies investigating informative content have found that subjects with RHD produce narratives that contain fewer concepts, less relevant concepts, and less specific information than those of NBD participants (Bartels-Tobin & Hinckley, 2005; Bloom, Borod, Obler, & Gerstman, 1992; Cimino, Verfaellie, Bowers, & Heilman, 1991; Diggs & Basili, 1987; Joanette et al., 1986; Myers & Brookshire, 1996; Urayse, Duffy, & Liles, 1991). For example, Tompkins and Flowers (1985) noted that low concept scores were overwhelmingly associated with excessive verbal output, reflecting "repetitiveness," and "irrelevant comments" (p. 529). As one of the first author's patients said, "I know the point I want to reach, but as I get there my mind, like a vacuum cleaner, sucks up every thought along the way and spews it out."

Tangential comments may not be off the topic altogether, but their presence signals difficulty in getting to the point. For example, asked what had happened to her and why she was in the hospital, one patient responded:

"My husband saw I wasn't in bed, and he found me in the clothes that I came to the hospital in, same robe and gown and everything. And we have a very thick rug, what they call a sculptured pattern with swirls and all that. It goes down to the base—fiber base, about two, more than two inches down deep . . ."

Her comments about the carpet continued. They are tangential, but related—related to the fact that although she had fallen on the floor, the cause of her hospitalization was a stroke, not the blow to her head, because the carpet softened the fall. She was unable to make her point explicitly, and thus her listener was burdened with having to fill in the missing information.

Digressive and inefficient output may be related to impaired appreciation of listener needs. Rehak, Kaplan, and Gardner (1992) found that individuals with RHD were impaired in judging the effects of tangentiality on conversational partners. Their lack of sensitivity to the interference of other people's tangential remarks seems to mirror insensitivity to their own tendencies in this direction.

Occasionally, tangential or irrelevant output appears to reflect uncertainty about the intended meaning of events. Failing to infer the examiner's intended meaning when asked to describe a pictured scene, or perhaps confused by its contents, one patient with RHD discussed the size and weight of the paper, its plastic coating, and the type of ink used to create the drawing, without ever describing the action depicted in the picture. Sometimes, individuals with RHD confabulate when faced with uncertainty or nonsensical information. For example, when re-telling stories with surprise or nonsensical endings, subjects with RHD made up details to make the events more plausible (Wapner et al., 1981). This same tendency can be seen in everyday situations when, for example, patients confabulate reasons for impaired performance.

It is possible that narratives based on visual stimuli contain less informative content because adults with RHD have problems perceiving what is in the pictures. However, several studies of scene description have demonstrated that individuals with RHD do not have problems recognizing objects and people in scenes as visually complex as Norman Rockwell illustrations and that the level of inference required to interpret a scene significantly affected performance, while levels of visual complexity did not (Mackisack et al., 1987; Myers & Brookshire, 1996). Reduced informative content has also been found in response to verbally presented narrative passages (Cimino et al., 1991; Wapner et al., 1981), suggesting that problems with content extend beyond visual material.

Generating Alternative Meanings

It often happens that we must generate different, less familiar, or alternative meanings during discourse. Sometimes this occurs because we need to accommodate new information that alters our original interpretation. Sometimes we need to call on a less familiar meaning for a word or set of words. For example, if we walk in on a conversation as someone says, "He was really flying," we might assume that he was talking about someone going at great speed. If we listen further and find it is a discussion about the Wright brothers and their first aircraft, we would have to revise our initial assumption and reinterpret the phrase to mean the person really *was* flying—in an airplane. Individuals with RHD have been found to have difficulty producing alternate meanings under effortful processing conditions.

Connotative and Metaphoric Meanings

Individual words may evoke a denotative or connotative meaning. Denotative meanings are like dictionary definitions and are appropriate for words taken out of context where further interpretation is not called for. Connotative meanings refer to alternative, nonliteral, or interpretive meanings. Thus, for example, the denotative meaning of the word "lion" is "large animal that lives in Africa." Its connotative meanings may include "regal," "king of the jungle," "ferocious," or even "MGM." Figurative language and idiomatic phrases have two meanings—the literal face value of the words, and the metaphoric meaning. Either meaning may be called upon, depending on the context.

Studies have demonstrated RHD impairments in generating connotative meanings for single words that are not embedded in context (Brownell, Potter, Michelow, & Gardner, 1984; Brownell, Simpson, Bihrle, Potter, & Gardner, 1990; Gardner & Denes, 1973), and in appreciating both metaphoric and nonmetaphoric alternative meanings for sentences and phrases (Brownell et al., 1990; Myers & Linebaugh, 1981; Van Lancker & Kempler, 1987; Winner & Gardner, 1977) and indirect requests (Foldi, 1987; Hirst, LeDoux, & Stein, 1984; Weylman, Brownell, Roman, & Gardner, 1989). As Brownell and colleagues (1990) suggest, these impairments "may not be restricted to metaphor; rather they may be but one reflection of a more pervasive impairment affecting appreciation of different types of alternative meanings" (p. 376).

Revising Initial Interpretations

Sometimes, one must change one's original interpretation of sentences or events to accommodate new information. Impaired ability to revise expectations may be a factor in problems with following everyday conversation. For example, Kaplan and colleagues (1990) found subjects with RHD impaired in interpreting whether or not conversational remarks between two speakers were to be taken literally. Nonliteral remarks occurred when one speaker was making fun, being sarcastic, or telling a white lie. Understanding the intended meaning of these nonliteral remarks required reinterpreting them in light of previous information.

Similarly, Brownell and Tompkins and their colleagues (Brownell et al., 1986; Tompkins, Baumgaertner, & Lehman, 2000; Tompkins, Lehman-Blake, Baumgaertner, & Fassbinder, 2001) found subjects with RHD impaired in interpreting the meaning of sentence pairs when misleading information was presented in the first as opposed to the second sentence, as in the example, "Barbara became too bored to finish the history book. She had already spent five years writing it." Taken in isolation, the first sentence implies that Barbara is reading a book, rather than writing one. When misleading information was presented first, RHD subjects had more difficulty than the NBD group in revising their original interpretations to accommodate the information contained in the second sentence. Impairments in revision have even been found in a lexical task that required revising the lexical function of a single word (Schneiderman & Saddy, 1988).

We are continually confronted with new information that alters our original interpretations as we negotiate the twists and turns in everyday events and conversations. For the person with RHD such seemingly automatic revisions may overtax resources, so that new information is processed inadequately and entire meanings are missed.

Explanatory Theories: Activation and Suppression Deficit

It has been postulated that the intact RH is more adept at processing multiple, alternate, less familiar, more loosely connected meanings than the LH, and that the LH is more adept at automatic processing of dominant single meanings or several meanings that are tightly overlapped (Beeman, 1993; Brownell et al., 1984, 1990; Burgess & Simpson, 1988; Chiarello, Burgess, Richards, & Pollock, 1990). Two opposing theories have been proposed to accommodate impaired ability to manage alternative meanings and to revise initial interpretations (see Myers, 1999a, for a review).

The *activation theory* holds that brain damage impairs the normal RH functions noted above, such that patients have difficulty in activating multiple, distant, or subordinate meanings (Beeman, 1993). It may take more effort than normal to generate alternate meanings during discourse, interfering with efficient and accurate processing.

The *suppression theory* holds that individuals with RHD are able to activate multiple meanings, but have difficulty suppressing (versus activating) the less likely meanings for a concept. Continued activation of meanings that are not appropriate to the context interferes in the selection of the particular alternate meaning that is *most* appropriate (Tompkins et al., 2000, 2001).

More studies are needed to sort out which hypothesis best explains the problems adults with RHD have with alternate meanings. For now, it appears that RHD can interfere in the semantic processing of alternate meanings. This problem can disrupt the ability to manage complex discourse that contains ambiguities and/or requires revising initial impressions.

Summary

Problems in generating elaborative inferences, integrating information, and generating or selecting the most plausible meaning(s) can contribute to impaired discourse processing in adults with RHD. They may have problems inferring the links among sentences, integrating verbal information into an overall structure and theme, filtering unnecessary information, and revising original interpretations as new information unfolds. As a result they may fixate on irrelevant details and be vague, nonspecific, and uninformative. They may have problems selecting, integrating, and organizing information and be digressive and verbose. In some circumstances, they may not appreciate figurative and other nonliteral forms of language. Finally, they may have difficulty accommodating new, ambiguous, or seemingly conflicting information.

Evaluation of Discourse Deficits

Not every person with RHD has communication impairments (estimates range from 50% to 90%; Blake et al., 2002; Joanette & Goulet, 1994), so the primary goal in evaluation is establishing the presence or absence of deficits. Commercially available assessment tools can be used in conjunction with the informal approaches described below. Most, if not all, of these tools have weaknesses in reliability or validity, and so must be carefully evaluated and selected. Additionally, many published tests are not sensitive enough to measure mild deficits associated with RHD.

Discourse and pragmatics are often assessed using informal tasks. It is important to obtain information from the patient's family as part of this assessment. There is a wide range of "normal" conversational and pragmatic behavior, and it is essential to determine which aspects are idiosyncratic to a patient's pre-stroke personality and which ones may be a result of brain damage. For example, Baron, Goldsmith, and Beatty (1999) reported that speech-language pathologists often rated pragmatic behaviors as inappropriate, while family members reported that these same behaviors were typical of the patient prior to the stroke.

Patient Interview

The purpose of the interview is to establish rapport and to obtain a sample of the patients' conversational speech, which can be assessed for content and structure. Establishing rapport is crucial for several reasons. First, patients with RHD may not recognize or may deny their problems. They may wonder why they are seeing a speech-language clinician when their speech sounds fine to them. Second, families often support the patient's denial unwittingly by exhibiting their relief that the patient "can talk." If patients have communication problems, families may not be immediately aware of them. One way of addressing denial is to explain in the initial interview that all stroke patients are tested for communication deficits, to agree with patients that they may not have any problems, and to explain that communication consists of more than speech and language.

Another reason patients may be resistant is that they are aware of some of their deficits (perhaps they have trouble following television shows and complex conversations, or have noticed problems in reading). They may be afraid to admit to these problems in the face of family relief that they can talk (and hence, "do not have communication problems"). They may fear they are mentally unbalanced or generally confused. Their fears can be allayed by clinician assurances that there may be very specific reasons why they are having difficulty that have nothing to do with their mental stability. The clinician can help patients overcome denial by demonstrating some specific problems they may have and by explaining that help is available. Explaining and demonstrating problems to the patient can decrease fear, make problems seem more manageable, and increase insight and cooperation.

The second goal of the interview is to obtain a sample of conversational speech on audio- or videotape that can be reviewed for structure and content. Questions should address patients' orientation, their assessment of their problems, their daily activities, something about their work history or personal lives, and their plans for the future. The interview thus addresses memory, orientation, and insight. Responses can be assessed for the degree to which they observe pragmatic rules of conversation (e.g., turn-taking, listener burden, etc.), and the degree to which content is informative, accurate, organized, and efficient.

Picture Description

A pictured scene that tells a story or depicts a situation can be used to elicit narrative discourse for the evaluation of macrostructure and integration deficits. Commercially available pictures that require elaborative inferences, such as the "cookie theft" picture from the Boston Diagnostic Aphasia Examination (Goodglass et al., 2001) can be used. A picture-description task enables the clinician to quickly assess the patient's abilities to attend to and interpret contextual or extralinguistic information. The advantages over asking patients to retell stories are that it elicits a more spontaneous production, it does not involve memory, and missed or inaccurate concepts can be pointed out by directing the patient's attention to the visually present contextual cues.

The patient's response can be scored in several ways. For example, the number of inferential concepts generated can be compared to the number of noninferential concepts. Such a scoring system for the "cookie theft" picture has been developed (Myers, 1999a). It can be adapted as clinicians see fit and used during treatment as a probe task to measure progress in therapy.

Transcribed picture descriptions can also be evaluated by techniques of discourse analysis (see Sherratt & Penn, 1990; Urayse et al., 1991) or other types of concept analysis (see Cherney & Canter, 1993; and Nicholas & Brookshire, 1993, 1995; also see Myers, 1999a, for a review of the advantages and disadvantages of these scoring systems). Pragmatic rating scales can assess problems in recognizing the limits of shared knowledge, turn-taking, topic maintenance, eye contact, and other pragmatic deficits.

Treatment of Extralinguistic Deficits

Management of extralinguistic deficits usually consists of a combination of functional or task-oriented and process-oriented methods (see Myers, 1999a and 1999b, for reviews of these two methods for deficits associated with RHD). Task-oriented treatments typically attempt to retrain performance on a specific task—usually through compensation—and address symptoms, rather than the underlying cause of deficits. Process-oriented treatments, on the other hand, address underlying processes and attempt to stimulate recovery of function. For that reason they may have greater potential for generalization across tasks. No studies have been conducted on treatment outcomes for extralinguistic deficits associated with RHD. As a result, therapy for these

problems relies on clinical experience and our current understanding of the deficits and their underlying cause.

One way of stimulating recovery of function for many of the extralinguistic deficits associated with RHD is to work directly on attention and neglect. One should also work on increasing informative content, on generating elaborative inferences, and on generating or selecting alternate meanings and inference revisions.

Clinicians must be creative in designing tasks and evaluating their impact on communication. Treatment tasks that are grounded in theory can be found in Myers (1999a, 1999b), Tompkins (1995), and Tompkins and Baumgaertner (1998). It is assumed that clinicians will use the techniques mentioned elsewhere in this book to establish cuing hierarchies and to probe patient progress. The next sections provide some general directions for designing therapy techniques for RHD discourse deficits.

Inference and Macrostructure Generation

Macrostructure tasks include asking patients to report the overall themes of pictured scenes, stories, or conversational interactions. This can be done by asking them to produce titles for pictures, headlines for news stories, or to state the main theme of the stimulus item. Task difficulty depends on the complexity of the inference to be generated. The less explicit or concrete the theme, the more difficult the inference. By manipulating the level of inferential complexity, one can stimulate the process of inference generation through repeated trials at a level at which the patient reaches a pre-set accuracy criterion.

One can also guide inference generation by working on scenes or stories for which the patient was not able to arrive at an inference. In this process, the clinician attempts to facilitate the patient's conscious control over what was once a more automatic task. Patients can be asked to (1) label items in a scene; (2) specify the relevant or significant items in a scene; (3) point to items that are related; and (4) explain the relationships among items or some variant thereof. Obviously, to understand the significant items, one must have a sense of the overall theme in a "chicken-egg" conundrum. However, often the process of asking the patient to overtly specify significant items usually helps him or her come closer to the overall theme. For example, in the "cookie theft" picture, the insignificance of the bushes beyond the window and the dishes on the counter to which patients with RHD are often so attracted becomes clear when one asks, "What are the most important items in the picture?" Typically, patients will point to the mother and children and to the water overflowing from the sink and from there arrive at an integrated concept of the picture's meaning.

Integration tasks include asking patients to organize printed sentences into a story or pictures into a logical sequence. Stimuli can vary in number of details and in how explicit or implicit the content is. Tasks that require patients to recognize commonalities may also improve integration skills. Patients can be asked to group pictured objects, scenes, or printed words into categories. Categories can range from concrete (e.g., foods, tools, vehicles) to more abstract themes for pictured scenes (e.g., celebrations, disasters, suspicion). Prior to sorting, the clinician can identify the categories, or require the patient to generate them.

At the perceptual level, integration can be addressed in tasks that require patients to arrange puzzle pieces or identify fragmented objects from their individual parts. To make such materials, one can simply photocopy large line drawings of common objects, cut them into several pieces, and rearrange and re-photocopy them.

In addition, patients can be asked to provide an opinion for open-ended questions on current topics of interest. One-minute answers can be tape recorded, transcribed, and rated according to how integrated, complete, efficient, relevant, and coherent the answer is. Impairments in each of these areas can then be worked on separately. Audio or video recording of conversational interactions is a useful way to review various pragmatic deficits (e.g., topic maintenance, turn-taking).

Managing Alternative Meanings

Improving the ability to manage alternative meanings can be addressed in several ways. If one subscribes to the *activation deficit* hypothesis, one can ask the patient to provide two meanings for homographs (e.g., bank, bat, choke, knot, dough) or to group sets of words according to their denotative or connotative meanings.

If one subscribes to the *suppression deficit* theory, one can help the patient enlist conscious control over the suppression of alternate meanings by putting an ambiguous word or sentence into context. The different meanings of the ambiguity can be discussed; the clinician can then help the patient identify contextual cues that lead to the most appropriate interpretation, followed by a discussion of why the original interpretation was no longer accurate.

Tasks designed to improve the ability to formulate revisions may include presenting patients with two-sentence stories, the first of which leads one to a faulty conclusion unless it is reevaluated in light of the second sentence. For example, the sentence, "Ella grabbed her bag and rushed to the gate" might lead one to picture an airport scene until the second sentence, "Once there, she pulled out her key and unlocked it" leads to a different conclusion (Myers, 1999a, p. 106) (see Bloise & Tompkins, 1993; Brownell et al., 1986; Kaplan et al., 1990; and Tompkins & Baumgaertner, 1998, for other examples). Another type of stimulus is a brief story that ends in a statement by the main character. The final statement may be either congruent or incongruent with the preceding information (Brownell et al., 1997; Brownell & Stringfellow, 1999). Stories can be followed by inferential questions that probe patients' abilities to revise their initial impressions of story content, and their ability to use cues within the text (e.g., familiarity between speakers, and character attitudes or emotions [Kaplan et al., 1990]).

Processing Emotional Content

Individuals with RHD may have difficulty interpreting and expressing emotional content. This can be seen in use and comprehension of (1) facial expression, (2) emotional prosody (aprosodia), and (3) emotionally laden words. In a recent study, reduced affective response was diagnosed in 30% of patients with RHD on a rehabilitation unit, and aprosodia specifically was diagnosed in 20% of the same population (Blake et al., 2002). Although it may seem logical that the two deficits might have similar underlying emotional processes, Blake and colleagues found that they did not frequently co-occur.

Several investigators have suggested that the RH plays a special role in processing emotional content (Bear, 1983; Borod, 1992; Silberman & Weingartner, 1986; Tucker, 1981). It is not clear whether these impairments are the result of an altered internal experience of emotion, reduced levels of arousal, cognitive interference, or some combination thereof. Evidence of an association between altered internal emotional states and site of lesion following stroke is inconclusive (Folstein, Maiberger, & McHugh, 1977; Robinson, Kubos, Starr, Rao, & Price, 1984; Robinson, Starr, Lipsey, Rao, & Price, 1984; Sinyor, Jacques, Kalpoupek, Becker, Goldenberg, & Coopersmith, 1986), although a recent study suggests that emotional deficits most commonly occur when lesions affect both basal ganglia and cortical structures (Karow, Marquardt, & Marshall, 2001). In adults with RHD, what is known as "indifference" and "flattened affect" may be associated with reduced arousal (Heilman et al., 1978). That is, these individuals may be less aware of and less responsive to external stimuli, including the cues that signal emotions. Cognitive-processing deficits may also interfere in emotional processing. Comprehension of emotion requires generation of elaborative inferences using contextual and other extralinguistic cues that enable us to recognize emotional states of story characters and conversational partners.

It is important to remember that "flat affect," reduced responsivity, and flattened prosodic production also can be signs of depression. Other signs of depression include feelings of hopelessness, sleep disturbance, reduced concentration, loss of energy, psychomotor slowing or agitation, and significant changes in weight. Depression occurs in 30% to 60% of stroke survivors in the acute phase (Andersen, Vestergaard, Riis, & Lauritzen, 1994; Cummings, 1994; Iacoboni, Padovani, DiPiero, & Lenzi, 1995; Ng, Chan, &

Straughan, 1995; Ramasubbu & Kennedy, 1994). Obviously, if other signs of depression are present or if depression is suspected in addition to the clinical signs of RHD, a referral for psychiatric evaluation should be made.

Facial Expression Deficits

Comprehension of Facial Expression

Decreased arousal and attention may affect patients' responses to the nonverbal cues that signify emotional expression. Numerous studies have reported that adults with RHD have difficulty interpreting facial expressions depicting emotions (Adolfs, Damasio, & Tranel, 2002; Benowitz, Bear, Rosenthal, Mesulam, Zaidel, & Sperry, 1983; Blonder, Bowers, & Heilman, 1991; Borod, Koff, Lorch, & Nicholas, 1986; Bowers, Bauer, Coslett, & Heilman, 1985; Cancelliere & Kertesz, 1990; Cicone, Wapner, & Gardner, 1980; DeKosky, Heilman, Bowers, & Valenstein, 1980; Karow et al., 2001). Areas of the brain thought to be important in recognizing facial expression include the amygdala, orbitofrontal regions, basal ganglia, and RH neocortex and somatosensory-related areas (Adolphs et al., 2002). The basal ganglia appears to play an important role in interpretation of emotional material (Karow et al., 2001), and some researchers speculate that emotional processing relies on a hierarchy ranging from low-level perception to cognitive selection and interpretation (Blonder et al., 1991; Karow et al., 2001).

Most studies investigating the interpretation of facial expression present faces in isolation without other contextual cues to specify the emotion. The expression must thus be determined by inspection and analysis of the spatial characteristics of facial features such as how close the eyebrows are, how wide open the eyes are, the degree to which the corners of the mouth are upturned, and so on. This type of perceptual-feature analysis depends on spatial or "metric" judgments that may be in the province of the intact RH (Kosslyn, 1987, 1988). Furthermore, individual features must be combined with one another to arrive at an accurate judgment. Thus, feature integration may also play a role.

Production of Facial Expression

Even in patients without "flat affect," facial expressivity may be reduced. Studies of spontaneous facial expression have found that subjects with RHD had reduced facial expression in response to slides depicting emotional situations in comparison to NBD subjects (Mammucari et al., 1988) and subjects with LHD (Borod et al., 1986; Buck & Duffy, 1981). Blonder and colleagues (2005) also reported reduced facial expression in subjects with RHD during casual conversation. While the earlier studies did not control for the effects of facial paresis, in the latter study subjects with LHD were more likely to have facial paresis but also to produce more facial expression.

Comprehension of Verbal Emotional Content

Comprehension of emotion has been assessed by asking patients to identify emotions depicted in pictures or described in sentences or stories, or to match emotional words (Blonder et al., 1991; Bloom et al., 1992; Borod, 1992; Cancelliere & Kertesz, 1990; Cicero et al., 1999; Cicone et al., 1980). Subjects with RHD are impaired relative to NBD controls primarily when tasks are more complex (Borod, 1992; Cicero et al., 1999), or when responses require conscious thought, such as answering questions or making explicit judgments (Rehak, Kaplan, Weylman et al., 1992).

Determining the emotional valance of situations, expressions, and narratives requires generation of elaborative inferences. For example, "He went into the house" is inferentially less complex than "He stole into the house." Most studies documenting problems in inferring emotions from stimuli have not included comparable tasks designed to test subjects' capacity to infer nonemotional or neutral content. Studies that have done so have produced mixed results. Thus, it is difficult to know whether the findings relate to emotional content independent of inferential complexity.

Verbal Expression of Emotional Content

Most studies of the verbal expression of emotional content involve a comprehension task, so it is difficult to know whether impairments are based on failure to comprehend emotions, failure to express emotions, or both. Some studies without a comprehension component still reported deficits in adults with RHD. For example, Cimino and colleagues (1991) asked subjects to recall episodes from their own lives in response to a cue word that was either emotional or neutral. Not surprisingly, the responses of subjects with RHD were rated as less specific than those from the NBD group regardless of the type of cue word. Although the emotional cue words produced higher emotionality ratings than neutral cues for both groups, the responses from the RHD group were significantly less emotional than those of the NBD group. Similarly, Bloom, Borod, Obler, and Koff (1990) and Borod, Koff, Lorch, and Nicholas (1985) found that adults with RHD used fewer and less intense emotional words when they described pictures.

Summary

Individuals with RHD may have problems both in interpreting and in expressing emotional content. However, it is not clear that they have an affective disorder per se. Studies investigating emotional status following stroke have produced conflicting results. Emotional "indifference" may be a component of a more general attention deficit that reduces responsiveness to the external environment, or it may be related to a patient's denial or lack of awareness of his or her deficits. Reduced responsivity may impair the appreciation of the extralinguistic cues from which one can infer the emotional valance of situations and narratives. In addition, perceptual impairments in spatial judgment and feature integration may contribute to impaired ability to identify emotional facial expression.

Prosodic Processing

The prosodic features of speech convey both emotional and linguistic information. Alterations in pitch, volume, and the duration of utterances and pause time between words create intonational patterns that add extralinguistic information to linguistic content. Linguistic prosody disambiguates word and sentence types, distinguishing noun phrases from compound nouns (e.g., "green house" from "greenhouse") and interrogative from declarative sentences, and clarifies meaning through the use of stress ("Joe loves *Ella*," versus "*Joe* loves Ella."). Emotional prosody captures not only emotional states, but intents such as sarcasm and irony.

Adults with RHD may be impaired in their appreciation and expression of these prosodic features of speech, a disorder termed "aprosodia" (Ross, 1981). One theory suggests that linguistic prosody is processed primarily by the LH, while emotional prosody is processed primarily by the RH, or by bilateral frontal regions (Van Lancker, 1980). One limitation of many studies designed to describe or explain the nature of prosodic deficits associated with RHD is that they generally test a group of individuals with damage to the RH, regardless of whether or not they have been screened for prosodic deficits. The group results may not be reflective of individuals, a minority of whom may actually have aprosodia. The results provide general information about incidence, but not necessarily about the characteristics of prosodic impairments in those who have them.

Prosodic Comprehension

A variety of tasks have been used to examine comprehension of both linguistic and emotional prosody. Recent studies suggest that adults with RHD are able to use prosody to identify word meaning (e.g., OBject versus obJECT), aid in syntactic parsing ("listen to the choir, boy" versus "listen to the choirboy"), and to differentiate questions from statements (Heilman, Bowers, Speedie, & Coslett, 1984; Walker, Daigle, & Buzzard, 2002; Weintraub, Mesulam, & Kramer, 1981).

Adults with RHD generally demonstrate more difficulty with emotional than with linguistic prosody. Compared to both healthy adults and individuals with LHD, they are less accurate in making same/different judgments, identifying emotion (e.g., sad versus happy), and in detecting or rating the amount of emotion conveyed prosodically. They also have been found to have impairments in discriminating emotions when speech was filtered so that prosodic features

remained while words did not (Denes, Caldognetto, Semenza, Vagges, & Zettin, 1984; Heilman, Bowers et al., 1984; Tompkins & Flowers, 1985) and in identifying emotional prosody in nonsense sentences (Pell, 2006).

The cause of impaired prosodic comprehension is uncertain. Wunderlich, Ziegler, and Geigenberger (2003) suggest three components influence interpretation of prosody: (1) input—the type of perceptual processing required, either tonal/rhythmic or fast/spectral; (2) the processing components or complexity of the task, including linguistic and cognitive demands; and (3) the processing mode, be it explicit (and effortful), or implicit. These will be discussed in turn.

Prosodic-comprehension deficits may be related to a perceptual deficit in detecting changes in tonal patterns. The RH is thought to be more adept at processing nontemporal properties of spectral information, pitch, and harmonic structure, whereas the LH is specialized for processing temporal order, sequence, sound duration, and intervals between sound (Chobor & Brown, 1987; Robin et al., 1990; Sidtis & van Lancker-Sidtis, 2003). Pitch perception has been found to be selectively impaired subsequent to RHD (Chobor & Brown, 1987; Robin, Tranel, & Damasio, 1990; Sidtis & Van Lancker-Sidtis, 2003; Tompkins, 1991a; Tompkins & Flowers, 1985). Another hypothesis suggests that the LH is dominant for processing prosody at the word level, while the RH is involved with larger regions, such as phrases and sentences (Baum & Pell, 1999; Behrens, 1988).

Another processing component that may affect task performance is sustained attention. In many studies participants must listen to sentences but dissociate meaning from tone, forcing them to divide their attention in a rather unnatural task. Considering that neglect is associated with attention deficits, it is surprising to note that neglect is not often tested or reported in studies of prosody (even those that use picture stimuli). Some studies that have evaluated neglect report that subjects with RHD and neglect have difficulty with prosodic tasks (Heilman, Scholes, & Watson, 1975; Tompkins & Flowers, 1985; Tucker, Watson, & Heilman, 1977), while those without neglect may not (Schlanger, Schlanger, & Gerstman, 1976).

Another aspect of processing complexity involves determining communicative intent when the prosodic and linguistic meanings differ. Adults with RHD demonstrate a greater prosodic comprehension deficit when prosody is in conflict with linguistic meaning (e.g., hearing "I lost my purse" spoken in a happy voice). Other evidence comes from Tompkins (1991b), who found that increased semantic redundancy in the form of a word suggesting a given emotion improved accuracy of LHD, RHD, and NBD participants in judging the mood conveyed in a short paragraph. The redundancy also improved the RHD groups' prosodic judgments of neutral sentences that followed the paragraphs.

The last component, processing mode, refers to whether the task is explicit, and requires off-line, metalinguistic responses, or whether it measures more on-line, automatic responses from which comprehension of prosodic meaning can be inferred. Wunderlich and colleagues (2003) suggest that the task demands may increase the influence of the non-prosodic (linguistic and cognitive) factors. Most studies have used explicit tasks (e.g., point to the picture that matches the emotion), so it is difficult to determine the effect of task demands. However, given that such demands influence performance on a variety of other tasks (e.g., Tompkins & Baumgaertner, 1998), they likely play a role in prosody too.

The extent to which patients suffer from difficulty in prosodic comprehension in everyday conversation is not clear. Laboratory investigations of prosodic deficits attempt to control the variables that operate in natural conversation. Subjects with RHD are impaired in tasks that force them to select and detect relevant features, to attend to two things at once, and to ignore one thing while attending to another. Thus, it is uncertain whether or not prosodic impairments in the laboratory reflect true deficits in processing prosodic aspects of conversations in which multiple cues signal meaning and emotional content. It is likely that some individuals with RHD may not be able to mount the resources to attend to these important extralinguistic cues, and that they may have specific problems with pitch perception. The severity of the deficit may vary with the level of redundancy of contextual information specifying the speaker's intended meaning.

Prosodic Production

Emotional and linguistic prosodic production has been tested by asking subjects to repeat or read neutral sentences with a specified emotional tone, imitate the prosodic production of a speaker, and/or spontaneously produce emphatic stress. Prosodic productions have been analyzed perceptually and acoustically. The findings, particularly in studies using acoustic analysis, have been mixed. Adults with RHD who have prosodic production deficits (aprosodia) tend to rely less on pitch variation and more on shifts in intensity or volume to signal emotions, and tend to use consistent duration and pause time, giving a robotic quality to their speech. Patients with mild prosodic production impairments may sound fatigued. In more severe cases, they may sound mechanical and stilted.

Individuals with RHD generally do not have problems producing linguistic prosodic contours to distinguish noun phrases from compound nouns, to signal syntactic boundaries, or to differentiate statements from questions (Shah, Baum, & Dwivedi, 2006; Walker, Pelletier, & Reif, 2004). Acoustic examinations of speech waves suggest that individuals with RHD may have a fast rate, reduced acoustic contrast, and reduced energy in frequencies above 500 Hz (Kent & Rosenbek, 1982). Other studies report no significant differences between individuals with and without RHD in

terms of duration, amplitude, fundamental frequency, and pause duration on tasks requiring manipulation of linguistic prosody (Shah et al., 2006; Walker et al., 2004).

In general, it appears that damage to the RH can result in reduced use of pitch variation and increased use of intensity to convey emphatic emotional stress (Colsher, Cooper, & Graff-Radford, 1987; Ross, Edmondson, Seibert, & Homan, 1988; Ryalls, 1986). Of note, pitch variation is one of the most critical prosodic features used to distinguish emotional tone in NBD speakers (Shapiro & Danly, 1985; Van Lancker & Sidtis, 1992). Thus, attenuated pitch variation has the potential to have a negative impact on the production of emotional prosody.

Patients with RHD with prosodic-production impairments may complain of difficulty getting emotional tone into their speech (Ross & Mesulam, 1979; Ryalls, Joanette, & Feldman, 1987). A patient seen by the first author stated that she tried to get more inflection into her speech, but that it required "a lot of concentration" and was often ineffective. Patients in the Ryalls (1987) study reported a sense of reduced volume and pitch range and that their voices sometimes felt "hoarse" and "strangled." These findings, combined with problems in voluntary control over prosody, suggest that impaired prosodic production subsequent to RHD may be in part a motor execution disorder (i.e., a form of dysarthria).

Summary

Prosodic comprehension and production deficits may occur subsequent to RHD. Comprehension impairments may include both emotional and linguistic prosodic deficits, and may be related to impaired pitch perception and/or to attentional deficits in response to tasks designed to isolate prosodic from linguistic information. Whether or not prosodic-comprehension deficits found in the laboratory translate into similar deficits in natural conversation is not clear.

Prosodic-production impairments may also exist in some individuals with RHD. Clinical impressions of impaired prosody have been difficult to quantify. Patients tend to be aware of, but unable to correct, these deficits. It is possible that dysarthria plays a role in prosodic-production impairments in some adults with RHD, although this possibility has not been formally addressed.

Evaluation

Emotional prosodic comprehension can be assessed by asking patients to identify the emotion (happy, sad, angry) conveyed in prerecorded sentences with neutral content (e.g., "The boy came home"). For linguistic prosody, patients can be asked to match a spoken word to one of a set of two that vary in stress placement (e.g., "hot dog" versus "hotdog").

Prosodic production can be difficult to assess. Patients can be asked to produce or imitate prosodic contour that distinguishes words or phrases from one another either in mood or in emphatic stress. Productions should be tape recorded and played for judges (e.g., other staff) who try to identify the emotion the patient was attempting to express. This method can be cumbersome, and it provides information only about how well a person can volitionally control and produce emotional prosody, which may be different from the spontaneous expression of emotion through prosody. Acoustic measures are more objective, but may not be available to clinicians, and there is uncertainty about whether acoustic measures translate into clinical relevance.

Treatment

Treatment for prosodic deficits may not be a priority in patient management if the patient has other extralinguistic deficits. However, prosodic impairment can occur in patients with few other RHD problems, and it may interfere in the resumption of their daily lives and work. Recent studies of treatment for aprosodia have been developed to treat the disorder as if it were a cognitive deficit (Leon et al., 2005; Rosenbek et al., 2004) or a purely motoric disorder (e.g., similar to a dysarthria) (Leon et al., 2005; Rosenbek et al., 2004; Stringer, 1996). The cognitive treatment is based on the theory that aprosodia is caused by reduced access to emotional words and prosody. Patients are asked to explain the prosodic characteristics used to convey specific emotions, and to match prosody to facial expressions. The motoric treatment involves imitation of productions of different emotions. Preliminary data suggest that both treatments are effective in increasing expressive prosody.

When using a motoric approach, clinicians should remember that such training is not like accent reduction therapy. Although aware of their deficit, patients may not have voluntary control over their production or the ability to improve, particularly if the effort required diverts resources from other types of extralinguistic processing. If the patient is free of other impairments, such training may be worth the attempt. In addition, patients and family members should be counseled about the problem, and the patient can be trained to state more explicitly the emotion they are trying to convey in everyday conversations.

FUTURE DIRECTIONS

We hope that the description of deficits and the framework in which they have been laid out in this chapter will help clinicians recognize and understand RHD communication disorders and design innovative therapy techniques for them. Improved treatment rests on clinical insights and on continued research aimed at:

(1) mechanisms that underlie identified communication and cognitive deficits;

(2) potential connections between nonlinguistic and extralinguistic deficits;

(3) prognosis and recovery patterns subsequent to RHD;

(4) incidence and prevalence of identified deficits;

(5) theory-driven assessment tools based on new research findings; and

(6) treatment efficacy.

Defining Core Deficits

Research and practice would both benefit from consensus about the core deficits that define communication disorders associated with RHD and an operational definition and label that adequately captures them. To understand how essential this is, one need only imagine the term "LHD communication impairment" to describe aphasia. There are many things that aphasia is and many that it is not (a motor speech disorder, for example), but as often as it may occur with LHD, its diagnosis does not rest on lesion localization. It is a condition that includes some features and excludes others—a disorder with some predictable consequences and defined subtypes. "RHD communication impairment," on the other hand, identifies a location in the brain, but there is no common, agreed-upon understanding of the behavioral deficits it includes and excludes. Joanette and Ansaldo (1999) suggested the term "pragmatic aphasia." Myers (2001) argued against the term "aphasia" and suggested instead "apragmatism," because "pragmatics" relates to communicative intent, an apparently central feature of the extralinguistic deficits associated with RHD. Both terms avoid "RHD" in the label in recognition that not all those with RHD have communication disorders. Perhaps a term such as "cognitive-communication disorder of the RHD type" better captures the broad range of communication deficits that may be present with RHD.

In clinical work, lack of an adequate label that reflects an agreed-upon set of defining features makes it difficult to communicate about the disorders with colleagues, including other speech-language pathologists, rehabilitation professionals, neurologists, and other physicians. It makes it difficult to raise public awareness and to gain recognition from third-party payors. It makes it difficult to explain the deficits to families and patients, who often equate the ability to speak with adequate communication.

Research Needs

Arriving at the core deficits that define a label is the more difficult and vexing problem—one which requires continued research. In a chicken-egg conundrum, researchers would benefit from having a list of operationally defined core deficits for purposes of subject selection, and it is research that will lead us toward that list.

In the past, subjects were often selected only on the basis of a lesion site confined to the RH. While appropriate for studies of incidence or prevalence, it is reasonable to ask if we now know enough about the disorders to move beyond lesion lateralization for subject selection when the research goal is to delineate the nature of a single disorder or group of RHD communication deficits. To understand the importance of subject selection for studies of this type, one need only consider how potentially misleading a study on the nature of anomia would be if subjects were selected on the basis of unilateral LHD, regardless of whether they had anomia or even aphasia.

How can we best achieve subject selection without reliable and valid measures of RHD communication disorders or an agreed-upon definition of them? We can start by using tasks from the literature that have demonstrated sensitivity to RHD communication deficits and/or to the specific deficit under study. Tests of cognitive function, neglect, and/or attention that have good psychometric properties can also be used. Subjects can be grouped according to the presence or absence or severity of the specific deficit under study or related deficits either á priori or during the study. Including subjects who do and do not have the deficits under study, but do have some related cognitive or communicative disorders, allows for examination of relationships among deficits. However, individuals with RHD who are free of any signs of communication impairment should be included only as a control group when the research goal is to further our understanding of RHD *communication* disorders.

Summary

We have made great strides over the past 30 years in recognizing that the RH, this once "silent" hemisphere, plays a role in communication and that damage to it can affect communicative function. We look to a future in which continued clinical insight and informed research bring us to a comprehensive definition of the core deficits, better understanding of their natural history and cause, and, most importantly, improved patient care.

KEY POINTS

1. This chapter is focused on the nature and characteristics of communication impairments that can occur subsequent to RHD. It is important to remember that not every person with RHD has communication impairment and that while we have come a long way in our understanding of these disorders, a core set of deficits that define "RHD communication impairment" has yet to be determined.

2. Neglect can occur across modalities, in ipsilesional as well as in contralesional space. As an attentional deficit, neglect may affect cognitive processing, and hence communicative ability as well as recovery of independence.

3. Attentional deficits associated with RHD include hypoarousal and deficits in orienting, vigilance, maintenance, and selective attention. These deficits may have a significant negative impact on the cognitive processes that contribute to the pragmatic and extralinguistic aspects of communication.

4. Basic linguistic performance (e.g., word retrieval, sentence structure) is rarely affected by unilateral RHD.

5. RHD discourse impairments tend to be cognitively based and include deficits in generating a macrostructure, integrating information, disambiguating information, and drawing complex inferences based on contextual cues. These deficits may result in reduced levels of informative content in discourse production and reduced sensitivity to shades of meaning in discourse comprehension.

6. RHD may include pragmatic deficits in recognizing speaker intentions, understanding the internal motivations of others, and following conversational conventions.

7. RHD may affect the capacity to process alternative meanings in discourse, a capacity for which the intact RH is thought to be dominant.

8. RHD may reduce sensitivity to emotional content and can affect the ability to express emotion in facial expression, body language, gesture, and written and spoken discourse.

9. Prosodic impairments may include emotional and nonemotional prosodic comprehension and expression. They may occur independently of the nonlinguistic and extralinguistic deficits described in this chapter. They should be managed according to patient need relative to other potentially more pressing communicative impairments and the patient's ability to exert volitional cognitive or motor control over prosodic features.

10. Assessment for extralinguistic deficits should consist of an initial screening that includes an interview, tests of neglect, and a discourse sample, followed by further testing using informal and/or formal measures.

11. Patient management should include task-oriented (i.e., functional) and process-oriented treatment approaches as well as patient and family counseling.

12. Treatment for discourse deficits should include tasks to reduce neglect and attentional deficits, as well as tasks to stimulate integration abilities, increase the ability to process alternate meanings and generate inferences, and improve the use of contextual cues.

ACTIVITIES FOR REFLECTION AND DISCUSSION

1. Compare and contrast the communication deficits associated with RHD with those commonly associated with other neurologic disorders, such as aphasia, dementia, or traumatic brain injury.
2. List how deficits in various types of attention (e.g., arousal, vigilance, sustained attention) might affect a person's ability to communicate effectively in various situations, such as during a language evaluation, a conversation with a spouse, or a team conference at a rehabilitation center.
3. Imagine you are talking to a patient's family and have to describe visuospatial neglect. How would you explain the difference between visual neglect and homonymous hemianopsia? Think about the neurophysiologic bases for the disorders and the behavioral consequences of them.
4. Define "extralinguistic," explain why such factors are vital for effective communication, and describe three ways in they may be compromised in patients with RHD.
5. List the different ways that affect is portrayed in everyday communication situations. Discuss how you might conduct treatment to address deficits in each area of affective communication.
6. Select one attentional and one language goal for a hypothetical patient. Describe how you would design treatment to achieve each goal through (a) process-oriented treatment, (b) task-oriented treatment, and (c) a combination of the two methods.
7. Given the paucity of evidence-based practice data for deficits associated with RHD, discuss ways to evaluate and select appropriate treatments for patients with RHD.

References

Adamovich, B. L., & Brooks, R. L. (1981). A diagnostic protocol to assess the communication deficits of patients with right hemisphere damage. In R. H. Brookshire (Ed.), *Clinical aphasiology: Conference proceedings* (pp. 244–253). Minneapolis: BRK.

Adolphs, R., Damasio, H., & Tranel, D. (2002). Neural systems for recognition of emotional prosody: A 3-D lesion study. *Emotion, 2*, 23–51.

Albert, M. L. (1973). A simple test of visual neglect. *Neurology, 23*, 658–664.

Andersen, G., Vestergaard, K., Riis, J. O., & Lauritzen, L. (1994). Incidence of post-stroke depression during the first year in a large unselected stroke population determined using a valid standardized rating scale. *Acta Psychiatrcia Scandinavica, 90*, 190–195.

Appelros, P., Nydevik, I., Karlsson, G. M., Throwalls, A., & Seiger, A. (2004). Recovery from unilateral neglect after right-hemisphere stroke *Disability & Rehabilitation, 26*, 471–477.

Archibald, T. M., & Wepman, J. M. (1968). Language disturbances and nonverbal cognitive performance in eight patients following injury to the right hemisphere. *Brain, 91*, 117–130.

Arruda, J. E., Walker, K. A., Weiler, M. D., & Valentino, D. A. (1999). Validation of a right hemisphere vigilance system as measured by principal component and factor analyzed quantitative electroencephalogram. *International Journal of Psychophysiology, 32*, 119–128.

Audet, T., Mercier, L., Collard, S., Rochette, A., & Hebert, R. (2000). Attention deficits: Is there a right hemisphere specialization for simple reaction time, sustained attention, and phasic alertness? *Brain and Cognition, 43*, 17–21.

Baron, C., Goldsmith, T., & Beatty, P. W. (1999). Family and clinician perceptions of pragmatic communication skills following right hemisphere stroke. *Topics in Stroke Rehabilitation, 5*, 55–63.

Bartels-Tobin, L. R., & Hinckley, J. J. (2005). Cognition and discourse production in right hemisphere disorder. *Journal of Neurolinguistics, 18*, 461–477.

Bartolomeo, P., & Chokron, S. (1999). Left unilateral neglect or right hyperattention? *Neurology, 53*, 2023–2027.

Bartolomeo, P., Sieroff, E., Chokron, S., & Decaix, C. (2001). Variability of response times as a marker of diverted attention. *Neuropsychologia, 39*, 358–363.

Baum, S. R., & Pell, M. D. (1999). The neural bases of prosody: Insights from lesion studies and neuroimaging. *Aphasiology, 13*, 581–608.

Bear, D. M. (1983). Hemispheric specialization and the neurology of emotion. *Archives of Neurology, 40*, 195–202.

Beeman, M. (1993). Semantic processing in the right hemisphere may contribute to drawing inferences from discourse. *Brain and Language, 44*, 80–120.

Behrens, S. J. (1988). The role of the right hemisphere in the production of linguistic stress. *Brain and Language, 33*, 104–127.

Beis, J. M., Keller, C., Morin, N., Bartolomeo, P., Bernati, T., Chokron, S., et al. (2004). Right spatial neglect after left hemisphere stroke: Qualitative and quantitative study. *Neurology, 63*, 1600–1605.

Bench, C. J., Frith, C. D., Grasby, P. M., Friston, K. J., Paulesu, E., Frackowiak, R. S. J., & et al. (1993). Investigations of the functional anatomy of attention using the Stroop Test. *Neuropsychologia, 31*, 907–922.

Benowitz, L. I., Bear, D. M., Rosenthal, R., Mesulam, M. M., Zaidel, E., & Sperry, R. W. (1983). Hemispheric specialization in nonverbal communication. *Cortex, 19*, 5–11.

Benowitz, L. I., Moya, K. L., & Levine, D. N. (1990). Impaired verbal reasoning and constructional apraxia in subjects with right hemisphere damage. *Neuropsychologia, 28*, 231.

Blake, M. L., Duffy, J. R., Myers, P. S., & Tompkins, C. A. (2002). Prevalence and patterns of right hemisphere cognitive/communicative deficits: Retrospective data from an inpatient rehabilitation unit. *Aphasiology, 16*, 537–548.

Blake, M. L., & Lesniewicz, K. (2005). Contextual bias and predictive inferencing in adults with and without right hemisphere brain damage. *Aphasiology, 19*, 423–434.

Bloise, C. G. R., & Tompkins, C. A. (1993). Right brain damage and inference revision revisited. *Clinical Aphasiology, 21*, 145–155.

Blonder, L. X., Bowers, D., & Heilman, K. M. (1991). The role of the right hemisphere in emotional communication. *Brain, 114*, 1115–1127.

Blonder, L. X., Heilman, K. M., Ketterson, T., Rosenbek, J., Raymer, A., Crosson, B., et al. (2005). Affective facial and lexical expression in aprosodic versus aphasic stroke patients. *Journal of the International Neuropsychological Society, 11,* 677–685.

Bloom, R. L., Borod, J. C., Obler, L. K., & Gerstman, L. J. (1992). Impact of emotional content on discourse production in patients with unilateral brain damage. *Brain and Language, 42,* 153–164.

Bloom, R. L., Borod, J. C., Obler, L. K., & Koff, E. (1990). A preliminary characterization of lexical emotional expression in right and left brain-damaged patients. *International Journal of Neuroscience, 55,* 71–80.

Borod, J. (1992). Interhemispheric and intrahemispheric control of emotion: A focus on unilateral brain damage. *Journal of Consulting and Clinical Psychology, 60,* 339–348.

Borod, J. C., Koff, E., Lorch, M. P., & Nicholas, M. (1985). Channels of emotional expression in patients with unilateral brain damage. *Archives of Neurology, 42,* 245–348.

Borod, J. C., Koff, E., Lorch, M. P., & Nicholas, M. (1986). The expression and perception of facial emotion in brain-damaged patients. *Neuropsychologia, 24,* 169–180.

Bowen, A., McKenna, K., & Tallis, R. C. (1999). Reasons for variability in the reported rate of occurrence of unilateral spatial neglect after stroke. *Stroke, 30,* 1196–1202.

Bowers, D., Bauer, R. M., Coslett, H. B., & Heilman, K. M. (1985). Processing of faces by patients with unilateral hemisphere lesions. *Brain and Cognition, 4,* 258–272.

Brooks, J. L., Wong, Y., & Robertson, L. C. (2005). Crossing the midline: Reducing attentional deficits via interhemispheric interactions. *Neuropsychologia, 43,* 572–582.

Brownell, H. H. (1988). The neuropsychology of narrative comprehension. *Aphasiology, 2,* 247–250.

Brownell, H. H., Pincus, D., Blum, A., Rehak, A., & Winner, E. (1997). The effects of right-hemisphere brain damage on patients' use of terms of personal reference. *Brain and Language, 57,* 60–79.

Brownell, H. H., Potter, H. H., Bihrle, A. M., & Gardner, H. (1986). Inference deficits in right brain-damaged patients. *Brain and Language, 27,* 310–321.

Brownell, H. H., Potter, H. H., Michelow, D., & Gardner, H. (1984). Sensitivity to lexical denotation and connotation in brain damaged patients: A double dissociation? *Brain and Language, 22,* 253–265.

Brownell, H. H., Simpson, T. L., Bihrle, A. M., Potter, H. H., & Gardner, H. (1990). Appreciation of metaphoric alternative word meanings by left and right brain-damaged patients. *Neuropsychologia, 28,* 375–383.

Brownell, H. H., & Stringfellow, A. (1999). Making requests: Illustrations of how right-hemisphere brain damage can affect discourse production. *Brain and Language, 68,* 442–465.

Bub, D., Audet, T., & Lecours, A. R. (1990). Re-evaluating the effect of unilateral brain damage on simple reaction time to auditory stimulation. *Cortex, 26,* 227–237.

Buck, R., & Duffy, R. J. (1981). Nonverbal communication of affect in brain-damaged patients. *Cortex, 6,* 351–362.

Burgess, C., & Simpson, G. B. (1988). Cerebral hemispheric mechanisms in the retrieval of ambiguous word meanings. *Brain and Language, 33,* 86–103.

Buxbaum, L. J., Ferraro, M. K., Veramonti, T., Farne, A., Whyte, J., Ladavas, E., et al. (2004). Hemispatial neglect: Subtypes, neuroanatomy, and disability. *Neurology, 62,* 749–756.

Calvanio, R., Levine, D., & Petrone, P. (1993). Elements of cognitive rehabilitation after right hemisphere stroke. *Behavioral Neurology, 11,* 25–57.

Cancelliere, A. E. B., & Kertesz, A. (1990). Lesion localization in acquired deficits of emotional expression and comprehension. *Brain and Cognition, 13,* 133–147.

Caplan, B. (1987). Assessment of unilateral neglect: A new reading test. *Journal of Clinical and Experimental Neuropsychology, 9,* 359–364.

Cappa, S. F., Benke, T., Clarke, S., Rossi, B., Stemmer, B., & van Heugten, C. M. (2005). EFNS guidelines on cognitive rehabilitation: Report of an EFNS task force. *European Journal of Neurology, 12,* 665–680.

Cherney, L. R. (2002). Unilateral neglect: A disorder of attention. *Seminars in Speech and Language, 23,* 117–128.

Cherney, L. R., & Canter, G. J. (1993). Informational content in the discourse of patients with probable Alzheimer's disease and patients with right brain damage. *Clinical Aphasiology, 21,* 123–133.

Cherry, B. J., & Hellige, J. B. (1999). Hemispheric asymmetries in vigilance and cerebral arousal mechanisms in younger and older adults. *Neuropsychology, 13,* 111–120.

Chiarello, C., Burgess, C., Richards, L., & Pollock, A. (1990). Semantic and associative priming in the cerebral hemispheres: Some words do, some words don't . . . sometimes, in some places. *Brain and Language, 38,* 75–104.

Chobor, K. L., & Brown, J. W. (1987). Phoneme and timbre monitoring in left and right cerebrovascular accident patients. *Brain and Language, 30,* 278–284.

Cicero, B. A., Borod, J. C., Santschi, C., Erhan, H. M., Obler, L. K., Agosti, R. M., et al. (1999). Emotional versus nonemotional lexical perception in patients with right and left brain damage. *Neuropsychiatry, Neuropsychology, and Behavioral Neurology, 12,* 255–264.

Cicerone, K. D., Dahlberg, C., Kalmar, K., Langenbahn, D. M., Malec, J. F., Bergquist, T. F., et al. (2000). Evidence-based cognitive rehabilitation: recommendations for clinical practice. *Archives of Physical Medicine and Rehabilitation, 81,* 1596–1615.

Cicerone, K. D., Dahlberg, C., Malec, J. F., Langenbahn, D. M., Felicetti, T., & Kneipp, S., et al. (2005). Evidence based cognitive rehabilitation: Updated review of the literature from 1998 through 2002. *Archives of Physical Medicine and Rehabilitation, 86,* 1681–1692.

Cicone, M., Wapner, W., & Gardner, H. (1980). Sensitivity to emotional expressions and situations in organic patients. *Cortex, 16,* 145–158.

Cimino, C. R., Verfaellie, M., Bowers, D., & Heilman, K. M. (1991). Autobiographical memory: Influence of right hemisphere damage on emotionality and specificity. *Brain and Cognition, 15,* 106–118.

Cohen, R. M., Semple, W. E., Gross, M., Holcomb, H. J., Dowling, S. M., & Nordahl, S. (1988). Functional localization of sustained attention. *Neuropsychiatry, Neuropsychology, and Behavioral Neurology, 1,* 3–20.

Colsher, P. L., Cooper, W. E., & Graff-Radford, N. (1987). Intonational variability in the speech of right-hemisphere damaged patients. *Brain and Language, 32,* 379–383.

Corbetta, M. J., Kincade, M., & Shulman, G. (2002). Neural systems for visual orienting and their relationships to spatial working memory. *Journal of Cognitive Neuroscience, 14,* 508–523.

Coslett, H. B., Bowers, D., & Heilman, K. M. (1987). Reduction in cerebral activation after right hemisphere stroke. *Neurology, 37,* 957–962.

Coull, J. T., Frith, C. D., Frackowiak, R. S. J., & Grasby, P. M. (1996). A fronto-parietal network for rapid visual information processing: A PET study of sustained attention and working memory. *Neuropsychologia, 34,* 1085–1095.

Cummings, J. L. (1994). Depression in neurological disease. *Psychiatric Annals, 24,* 525–531.

Damasio, A. R., Damasio, H., & Chui, H. C. (1980). Neglect following damage to frontal lobe or basal ganglia. *Neuropsychologia, 18,* 128–132.

Davidson, R. A., Fedio, P., Smith, B. D., Aureille, E., & Martin, A. (1992). Lateralized mediation of arousal and habituation: Differential bilateral electrodermal activity in unilateral temporal lobectomy patients. *Neuropsychologia, 30,* 1053–1063.

Deal, J., Deal, L., Wertz, R. W., Kitselman, K., & Dwyer, C. (1979). Right hemisphere PICA percentiles: Some speculations about aphasia. In R. H. Brookshire (Ed.), *Clinical aphasiology: Conference proceedings* (pp. 30–37). Minneapolis: BRK.

Denes, G., Caldognetto, E. M., Semenza, C., Vagges, K., & Zettin, M. (1984). Discrimination and identification of emotions in human voice by brain-damaged subjects. *Acta Neurologica Scandinavica, 69,* 154–162.

DeKosky, S. T., Heilman, K. M., Bowers, D., & Valenstein, E. (1980). Recognition and discrimination of emotional faces and pictures. *Brain and Language, 9,* 206–214.

Delis, D., Wapner, W., Gardner, H., & Moses, J. (1983). The contribution of the right hemisphere to the organization of paragraphs. *Cortex, 19,* 43–50.

Deutsch, G., Papanicolaou, A. C., Bourbon, T., & Eisenberg, H. M. (1987). Cerebral blood flow evidence of right cerebral activation in attention demanding tasks. *International Journal of Neuroscience, 36,* 23–28.

Diggs, C., & Basili, A. G. (1987). Verbal expression of right cerebrovascular accident patients: Convergent and divergent language. *Brain and Language, 30,* 130–146.

DiPellegrino, G., & DeRenzi, E. (1995). An experimental investigation on the nature of extinction. *Neuropsychologia, 33,* 153–170.

Duncan, J., Bundesen, C., Olson, A., Humphreys, G., Chavada, S., & Shibuya, H. (1999). Systematic analysis of deficits in visual attention. *Journal of Experimental Psychology: General, 128,* 450–478.

Eisenson, J. (1962). Language and intellectual modifications associated with right cerebral damage. *Language and Speech, 5,* 49–53.

Farah, M. J., Wong, A. B., Monheit, M. A., & Morrow, L. A. (1989). Parietal lobe mechanisms of spatial attention: Modality-specific or supramodal? *Neuropsychologia, 27,* 461–470.

Foldi, N. S. (1987). Appreciation of pragmatic interpretation of indirect commands: Comparison of right and left hemisphere brain-damaged patients. *Brain and Language, 31,* 88–108.

Folstein, M. R., Maiberger, R., & McHugh, P. R. (1977). Mood disorder as a specific complication of stroke. *Journal of Neurology, Neurosurgery, and Psychiatry, 40,* 1018–1020.

Gainotti, G., D'Erme, P., Monteleone, D., & Silveri, M. C. (1986). Mechanisms of unilateral spatial neglect in relation to laterality of cerebral lesions. *Brain, 109,* 599–612.

Gardner, H., Brownell, H. H., Wapner, W., & Michelow, D. (1983). Missing the point: The role of the right hemisphere in the processing of complex linguistic materials. In E. Perecman (Ed.), *Cognitive processing in the right hemisphere* (pp. 169–191). New York: Academic.

Gardner, H., & Denes, G. (1973). Connotative judgments by aphasic patients on a pictorial adaptation of the semantic differential. *Cortex, 9,* 183–196.

Goodglass, H., Kaplan, E., & Barresi (2001). *The Boston Diagnostic Aphasia Examination* (3rd ed.). Baltimore: Lippinott Williams & Wilkins.

Halligan, P. W., Manning, L., & Marshall, J. C. (1990). Individual variation in line bisection: A study of four patients with right hemisphere damage and normal controls. *Neuropsychologia, 28,* 1043–1051.

Halligan, P. W., & Marshall, J. C. (1988). How long is a piece of string? A study of line bisection in a case of visual neglect. *Cortex, 24,* 321–328.

Halper, A. S., & Cherney, L. R. (1998). Cognitive-communication problems after right hemisphere stroke: A review of intervention studies. *Topics in Stroke Rehabilitation, 5,* 1–10.

Heilman, K. M., Bowers, D., Coslett, H. B., Whelan, H., & Watson, R. T. (1985). Directional hypokinesia: Prolonged reaction times for leftward movements in patients with right hemisphere lesions and neglect. *Neurology, 35,* 855–859.

Heilman, K. M., Bowers, D., Speedie, L., & Coslett, H. B. (1984). Comprehension of affective and nonaffective prosody. *Neurology, 34,* 917–921.

Heilman, K. M., Scholes, R., & Watson, R. T. (1975). Auditory affective agnosia. *Journal of Neurology, Neurosurgery, and Psychiatry, 38,* 69–72.

Heilman, K. M., Schwartz, H. D., & Watson, R. T. (1978). Hypoarousal in patients with the neglect syndrome and emotional indifference. *Neurology, 28,* 229–232.

Heilman, K. M., Valenstein, E., & Watson, R. T. (1984). Neglect and related disorders. *Seminars in Neurology, 4,* 209–219.

Heilman, K. M., Watson, R. T., Valenstein, E., & Damasio, A. (1983). Localization of lesions in neglect. In A. Kertesz (Ed.), *Localization in neuropsychology* (pp. 471–492). New York: Academic.

Hillis, A. E., Newhart, M., Heidler, J., Barker, P. B., Herskovits, E. H., & Degaonkar, M. (2005). Anatomy of spatial attention: Insights from perfusion imaging and hemispatial neglect in acute stroke. *The Journal of Neuroscience, 25,* 3161–3167.

Hirst, W., LeDoux, J., & Stein, S. (1984). Constraints on the processing of indirect speech acts: Evidence from aphasiology. *Brain and Language, 23,* 26–33.

Hough, M. (1990). Narrative comprehension in adults with right and left hemisphere brain-damage: Theme organization. *Brain and Language, 38,* 253–277.

Horner, J., Massey, E. W., Woodruff, W. W., Chase, K. N., & Dawson, D. V. (1989). Task-dependent neglect: Computed tomography size and locus correlations. *Journal of Neurological Rehabilitation, 3,* 7–13.

Husain, M., & Rorden, C. (2003). Non-spatially lateralized mechanisms in hemispatial neglect. *Nature, 4,* 26–36.

Iacoboni, M., Padovani, A., DiPiero, V., & Lenzi, G. L. (1995). Post-stroke depression: Relationships with morphological damage and cognition over time. *International Journal of Neurological Science, 16,* 209–216.

Jehkonen, M., Ahonen, J. P., Dastidar, P., Koivisto, A. M., Laippala, P., Vilkki, J., et al. (2001). Predictors of discharge to home during the first year after right hemisphere stroke. *Acta Neurologica Scandinavica, 104,* 136–141.

Joanette, Y., & Ansaldo, A. (1999). Acquired pragmatic impairments and aphasia. *Brain and Language, 68,* 529–534.

Joanette, Y., & Goulet, P. (1994). Right hemisphere and verbal communication: Conceptual, methodological, and clinical issues. *Clinical Aphasiology, 22,* 1–23.

Joanette, Y., Goulet, P., Ska, B., & Nespoulous, J.- L. (1986). Informative content of narrative discourse in right-brain-damaged right-handers. *Brain and Language, 29,* 81–105.

Kaplan, J., Brownell, H. H., Jacobs, J. R., & Gardner, H. (1990). The effects of right hemisphere damage on the pragmatic interpretation of conversational remarks. *Brain and Language, 38,* 315–333.

Kaplan, R. F., Verfaillie, M., Meadows, M. E., Caplan, L. R., Peasin, M. S., & de Witt, D. (1991). Changing attentional demands in left hemispatial neglect. *Archives of Neurology, 48,* 1263–1266.

Karow, C. M., Marquardt, T. P., & Marshall, R. C. (2001). Affective processing in left and right hemisphere brain-damaged subjects with and without subcortical involvement. *Aphasiology, 15,* 715–729.

Kent, R. D., & Rosenbek, J. C. (1982). Prosodic disturbance and neurologic lesion. *Brain and Language, 15,* 259–291.

Koski, L., & Petrides, M. (2001). Time-related changes in task performance after lesions restricted to the frontal cortex. *Neuropsychologia, 39,* 268–281.

Kosslyn, S. M. (1987). Seeing and imagining in the cerebral hemispheres: A computational approach. *Psychological Review, 94,* 148–175.

Kosslyn, S. M. (1988). Aspects of a cognitive neuroscience of mental imagery. *Science, 240,* 1621–1626.

Ladavas, E., Del Pesce, M., & Provinciali, L. (1989). Unilateral attention deficits and hemispheric asymmetries in the control of visual attention. *Neuropsychologia, 27,* 353–366.

Lehman, M. T., & Tompkins, C. A. (2000). Inferencing in adults with right hemisphere brain damage: An analysis of conflicting results. *Aphasiology, 14,* 485–499.

Lehman-Blake, M. T., & Tompkins, C. A. (2001). Predictive inferencing in adults with right hemisphere brain damage. *Journal of Speech, Language and Hearing Research, 44,* 639–654.

Leon, S. A., Rosenbek, J. C., Crucian, G. P., Hieber, B., Holiway, B., Rodriguez, A. D., et al. (2005). Active treatments for aprosodia secondary to right hemisphere stroke. *Journal of Rehabilitation Research and Development, 42,* 93–102.

Leonard, C. L., Waters, G. S., & Caplan, D. (1997a). The use of contextual information by right-brain damaged individuals in the resolution of ambiguous pronouns. *Brain and Language, 57,* 309–342.

Leonard, C. L., Waters, G. S., & Caplan, D. (1997b). The use of contextual information related to general world knowledge by right-brain damaged individuals in pronoun resolution. *Brain and Language, 57,* 343–359.

Lojek-Osiejuk, E. (1996). Knowledge of scripts reflected in discourse of aphasics and right-brain-damaged patients. *Brain and Language, 53,* 58–80.

Mackisack, E. L., Myers, P. S., & Duffy, J. R. (1987). Verbosity and labeling behavior: The performance of right hemisphere and non-brain-damaged adults on an inferential picture description task. In R. H. Brookshire (Ed.), *Clinical aphasiology* (Vol. 17, pp. 143–151). Minneapolis: BRK.

Mammucari, A., Caltagrione, C., Ekman, P., Friesen, W., Gianotti, G., Pizzamiglio, L., et al. (1988). Spontaneous facial expression of emotions in brain-damaged patients. *Cortex, 24,* 521–533.

Manly, T. (2002). Cognitive rehabilitation for unilateral neglect: Review. *Neuropsychological Rehabilitation, 12,* 289–310.

Mark, V. W., Kooistra, C. A., & Heilman, K. M. (1988). Hemispatial neglect affected by non-neglected stimuli. *Neurology, 38,* 1207–1211.

Marshall, J. C., & Halligan, P. W. (1989). When right goes left: An investigation of line bisection in a case of visual neglect. *Cortex, 25,* 503–515.

McDonald, S., & Wales, R. (1986). An investigation of the ability to process inferences in language following right hemisphere brain damage. *Brain and Language, 29,* 68–80.

McKoon, G., & Ratcliff, R. (1989). Semantic associations and elaborative inference. *Journal of Experimental Psychology: Learning, Memory, and Cognition, 15,* 326–338.

Mesulam, M.- M. (1981). A cortical network for directed attention and unilateral neglect. *Annals of Neurology, 10,* 307–325.

Mesulam, M.- M. (1985). Attention, confusional states, and neglect. In M. Mesulam (Ed.), *Principles of behavioral neurology* (pp. 125–168). Philadelphia: F. A. Davis.

Moya, K. L., Benowitz, L. I., Levine, D. N., & Finklestein, S. P. (1986). Covariant deficits in visuospatial abilities and recall of verbal narrative after right hemisphere stroke. *Cortex, 22,* 381–397.

Myers, P. S. (1979). Profiles of communication deficits in patients with right cerebral hemisphere damage. In R. H. Brookshire (Ed.), *Clinical aphasiology: Conference proceedings* (pp. 38–46). Minneapolis: BRK.

Myers, P. S. (1992). *The effect of visual and inferential complexity on the verbal expression of non-brain-damaged and right-hemisphere-damaged adults.* Unpublished doctoral dissertation, University of Minnesota, Minneapolis.

Myers, P. S. (1999a). *Right hemisphere damage: Disorders of communication and cognition.* San Diego: Singular.

Myers, P. S. (1999b). Process-oriented treatment of right hemisphere communication disorders. *Seminars in Speech and Language, 20,* 319–334.

Myers, P. S. (2001). Toward a definition of RHD Syndrome. *Aphasiology, 15,* 913–918.

Myers, P. S. (2005). Profiles of communication deficits in patients with right cerebral hemisphere damage: Implications for diagnosis and treatment. CAC CLASSICS. *Aphasiology, 19,* 1147–1160.

Myers, P. S., & Brookshire, R. H. (1995). Effects of noun type on naming performance of right-hemisphere-damaged and non-brain-damaged adults. *Clinical Aphasiology, 23,* 195–206.

Myers, P. S., & Brookshire, R. H. (1996). Effect of visual and inferential variables on scene descriptions by right-hemisphere-damaged and non-brain-damaged adults. *Journal of Speech and Hearing Research, 39,* 870–880.

Myers, P. S., & Linebaugh, C. W. (1980, November). *The perception of contextually conveyed relationships by right brain-damaged patients.* Paper presented at the American Speech-Language-Hearing Association Convention, Detroit, MI.

Myers, P. S., & Linebaugh, C. W. (1981). Comprehension of idiomatic expressions by right-hemisphere-damaged adults. In

R. H. Brookshire (Ed.), *Clinical aphasiology: Conference proceedings* (pp. 254–261). Minneapolis: BRK.

Myers, P. S., & Mackisack, E. L. (1990). Right hemisphere syndrome. In L. L. LaPointe (Ed.). *Aphasia and related neurogenic language disorders* (pp. 177–195). New York: Thieme.

Nebel, K., Wiese, H., Stude, P., deGreiff, A., Deiner, H.- C., & Keidel, M. (2005). On the neural basis of focused and divided attention. *Cognitive Brain Research, 25,* 760–776.

Ng, K. C., Chan, K. L., & Straughan, P. T. (1995). A study of post-stroke depression in a rehabilitative center. *Acta Psychiatrica Scandanavica, 92,* 75–79.

Nicholas, L. E., & Brookshire, R. H. (1993). A system for quantifying the informativeness and efficiency of the connected speech of adults with aphasia. *Journal of Speech and Hearing Research, 36,* 338–350.

Nicholas, L. E., & Brookshire, R. H. (1995). Presence, completeness, and accuracy of main concepts in the connected speech of non-brain-damaged adults and adults with aphasia. *Journal of Speech and Hearing Research, 38,* 145–157.

Odell, K. H., Wollack, J. A., & Flynn, M. (2005). Functional outcomes in patients with right hemisphere brain damage. *Aphasiology, 19,* 807–830.

Ogden, J. A. (1985). Anterior-posterior interhemispheric differences in the loci of lesions producing visual hemineglect. *Brain and Cognition, 4,* 59–75.

Oke, A., Keller, R., Medford, I., & Adams, R. (1978). Lateralization of norepinephrine in human thalamus. *Science, 200,* 1411–1413.

Oke, A., Lewis, R., & Adams, R. N. (1980). Hemispheric asymmetry of norepinephrine distribution in rat thalamus. *Brain Research, 188,* 269–272.

Ostrove, J. M., Simpson, T., & Gardner, H. (1990). Beyond scripts: A note on the capacity of right hemisphere-damaged patients to process social and emotional content. *Brain and Cognition, 12,* 144–154.

Pardo, J. V., Fox, P. T., & Raichle, M. E. (1991). Localization of a human system for sustained attention by positron emission tomography. *Nature, 349,* 61–64.

Pardo, J. V., Pardo, P. J., Janer, K. W., & Raichle, M. E. (1990). The anterior cingulate cortex mediates processing selection in the Stroop attentional conflict paradigm. *Proceedings of the National Academy of Science, USA, 87,* 256–259.

Pell, M. D. (2006). Cerebral mechanisms for understanding emotional prosody in speech. *Brain and Language, 96,* 221–234.

Posner, M. I. (1980). Orienting of attention. *Quarterly Journal of Experimental Psychology, 32,* 3–25.

Posner, M. I., & Petersen, S. E. (1990). The attention system of the human brain. *Annual Review of Neuroscience, 13,* 25–42.

Posner, M. I., Walker, J. A., Friedrich, F. J., & Raphal, R. D. (1984). Effects of parietal lobe injury on convert orienting of visual attention. *Journal of Neuroscience, 4,* 1863–1864.

Rafal, R. D., & Posner, M. E. (1987). Deficits in human visual spatial attention following thalamic lesions. *Proceedings of the National Academy of Science, USA, 84,* 7349–7353.

Ramasubbu, R., & Kennedy, S. H. (1994). Factors complicating the diagnosis of depression in cerebrovascular disease. Part I: Phenomenological and nosological issues. *Canadian Journal of Psychiatry, 39,* 596–607.

Rapcsak, S. Z., Verfaellie, M., Fleet, W. S., & Heilman, K. M. (1989). Selective attention in hemispatial neglect. *Archives of Neurology, 46,* 178–182.

Rehak, A., Kaplan, J. A., & Gardner, H. (1992). Sensitivity to conversational deviance in right-hemisphere-damaged patients. *Brain and Language, 42,* 203–217.

Rehak, A., Kaplan, J. A., Weylman, S. T., Kelly, B., Brownell, H. H. (1992). Story processing in right-hemisphere-brain damaged patients. *Brain and Language, 42,* 320–336.

Riddoch, M. J., & Humphreys, G. W. (1987). Perceptual action systems in unilateral neglect. In M. Jeannerod (Ed.), *Neurophysiological and neuropsychological aspects of spatial neglect* (pp. 151–181). Amsterdam: Elsevier.

Rivers, D. L., & Love, R. J. (1980). Language performance on visual processing tasks in right hemisphere lesion cases. *Brain and Language, 10,* 348–366.

Robertson, I. H., Tegner, R., Tham, K., Lo, A., & Nimmo-Smith, I. (1995). Sustained attention training for unilateral neglect: Theoretical and rehabilitation implications. *Journal of Clinical and Experimental Neuropsychology, 17,* 416–430.

Robin, D. A., & Rizzo, M. (1989). The effect of focal cerebral lesions on intramodal and cross modal orienting of attention. In T. Prescott (Ed.), *Clinical aphasiology* (Vol. 18, pp. 61–74). Austin, TX: Pro-Ed.

Robin, D. A., Tranel, D., & Damasio, H. (1990). Auditory perception of temporal and spectral events in patients with focal left and right cerebral lesions. *Brain and Language, 39,* 539–555.

Robinson, R. G. (1985). Lateralized behavioral and neurochemical consequences of unilateral brain injury in rats. In S. G. Glick (Ed.), *Cerebral lateralization in nonhuman species* (pp. 135–156). Orlando, FL: Academic Press.

Robinson, R. G., Kubos, K. L., Starr, L. B., Rao, K., & Price, T. R. (1984). Mood disorders in stroke patients: Importance of location of lesion. *Brain, 107,* 81–93.

Robinson, R. G., Starr, L. B., Lipsey, J. R., Rao, K., & Price, T. R. (1984). A two-year longitudinal study of post-stroke mood disorders: Dynamic changes in associated variables over the first six months of follow-up. *Stroke, 15,* 510–517.

Roman, M., Brownell, H. H., Potter, H. H., Seibold, M. S., & Gardner, H. (1987). Script knowledge in right hemisphere-damaged and normal elderly adults. *Brain and Language, 31,* 151–170.

Rosenbek, J. C., Crucian, G. P., & Leon, S. A., Hieber, B., Rodriguez, A. D., Holiway, B., et al. (2004). Novel treatments for expressive aprosodia: A phase I investigation of cognitive linguistic and imitative interventions. *Journal of the International Neuropsychological Society* (Vol 10, pp. 786–793).

Ross, E. D. (1981). The aprosodias. *Archives of Neurology, 38,* 561–569.

Ross, E. D., Edmondson, J. A., Seibert, G. B., & Homan, R. W. (1988). Acoustic analysis of affective measures of prosody during right-sided Wada test: A within-subjects verification of the right hemisphere's role in language. *Brain and Language, 33,* 128–145.

Ross, E. D., & Mesulam, M.-M. (1979). Dominant language functions of the right hemisphere? Prosody and emotional gesturing. *Archives of Neurology, 36,* 561–569.

Ruff, R. M., Nieman, H., Allen, C. C., Farrow, C. E., & Wylie, T. (1992). The Ruff 2 and 7 Selective Attention Test: A neuropsychological application. *Perceptual and Motor Skills, 75,* 1311–1319.

Ryalls, R. (1986). What constitutes a primary disturbance of speech prosody? A reply to Shapiro and Danly. *Brain and Language, 29,* 183–187.

Ryalls, R., Joanette, Y., & Feldman, L. (1987). An acoustic comparison of normal and right-hemisphere-damaged speech prosody. *Cortex, 23,* 685–694.

Schlanger, B. B., Schlanger, P., & Gerstman, L. J. (1976). The perception of emotionally toned sentences by right hemisphere-damaged and aphasic subjects. *Brain and Language, 3,* 396–403.

Schneiderman, E. I., & Saddy, J. D. (1988). A linguistic deficit resulting from right-hemisphere damage. *Brain and Language, 34,* 38–53.

Shah, A. P., Baum, S. R., & Dwivedi, V. D. (2006). Neural substrates of linguistic prosody: Evidence from syntactic disambiguation in the productions of brain-damaged patients. *Brain and Language, 96,* 78–89.

Shapiro, B. E., & Danly, M. (1985). The role of the right hemisphere in the control of speech prosody in propositional and affective contexts. *Brain and Language, 25,* 19–36.

Sherratt, S. M., & Penn, C. (1990). Discourse in a right-hemisphere brain-damaged subject. *Aphasiology, 4,* 539–560.

Sidtis, J. J., & Van Lanker-Sidtis, D. (2003). A neurobehavioral approach to dysprosody. *Seminars in Speech and Language, 24,* 93–105.

Silberman, E. K., & Weingartner, H. (1986). Hemispheric lateralization of functions related to emotion. *Brain and Cognition, 5,* 322–353.

Sinyor, D., Jacques, P., Kaloupek, D. G., Becker, R., Goldenberg, M., & Coopersmith, H. (1986). Poststroke depression and lesion location: An attempted replication. *Brain, l09,* 537–546.

Sohlberg, M. M., Avery, J., Kennedy, M., Ylvisaker, M., Coelho, C., Turkstra, L., et al. (2003). Practice guidelines for direct attention training. *Journal of Medical Speech-Language Pathology, 11,* xix–xxxix.

Stringer, A. Y. (1996). Treatment of motor aprosodia with pitch biofeedback and expression modeling. *Brain Injury, 10,* 583–590.

Sturm, W., Longoni, F., Fimm, B., Dietrich, T., Weis, S., Kemna, S., et al., (2004). Network for auditory intrinsic alertness: A PET study. *Neuropsychologia, 42,* 563–568.

Sturm, W., Longoni, F., Weis, S., Specht, K., Herzog, H., & Vohn, R. (2004). Functional reorganisation in patients with right hemisphere stroke after training of alertness: A longitudinal PET and fMRI study in eight cases. *Neuropsychologia, 42,* 434–450.

Sturm, W., & Willmes, K. (1991). Efficacy of a reaction training on various attentional and cognitive functions in stroke patients. *Neuropsychological Rehabilitation, 1,* 259–280.

Stuss, D. T., Toth, J. P., Franchi, D., Alexander, M. P., Tipper, S., Craik, F. I. M. (1999). Dissociation of attentional processes in patients with focal frontal and posterior lesions. *Neuropsychologia, 37,* 1005–1027.

Swisher, L. P., & Sarno, M. T. (1969). Token test scores of three matched patient groups: Left brain-damaged, right brain-damaged without aphasia, and non-brain-damaged. *Cortex, 5,* 264–273.

Tegner, R., Levander, M., & Caneman, G. (1990). Apparent right neglect in patients with left visual neglect. *Cortex, 26,* 455–458.

Tompkins, C. A. (1991a). Automatic and effortful processing of emotional intonation after right or left hemisphere brain damage. *Journal of Speech and Hearing Research, 34,* 820–830.

Tompkins, C. A. (1991b). Redundancy enhances emotional inferencing by right- and left-hemisphere-damaged adults. *Journal of Speech and Hearing Research, 34,* 1142–1149.

Tompkins, C. A. (1995). *Right hemisphere communication disorders: Theory and management.* San Diego, CA: Singular.

Tompkins, C. A., Baumgaertner, A., & Lehman, M. T. (2000). Mechanisms of discourse comprehension impairment after right hemisphere brain damage: Suppression in lexical ambiguity resolution. *Journal of Speech, Language, and Hearing Research, 43,* 62–78.

Tompkins, C. A., & Baumgaertner, A. (1998). Clinical value of online measures for adults with right hemisphere brain damage. *American Journal of Speech-Language Pathology, 7,* 68–74.

Tompkins, C. A., Bloise, C. G. R., Timko, M. L., & Baumgaertner, A. (1994). Working memory and inference revision in brain-damaged and normally aging adults. *Journal of Speech and Hearing Research, 37,* 896–912.

Tompkins, C. A., & Flowers, C. R. (1985). Perception of emotional intonation by brain-damaged adults: The influence of task processing levels. *Journal of Speech and Hearing Research, 28,* 527–538.

Tompkins, C. A., & Lehman, M. T. (1998). Interpreting intended meanings after right hemisphere brain damage: An analysis of evidence, potential accounts, and clinical implications. *Topics in Stroke Rehabilitation, 5,* 29–47.

Tompkins, C. A., Lehman-Blake, M. T., Baumgaertner, A., & Fassbinder, W. (2001) Mechanisms of discourse comprehension impairment after right hemisphere brain damage: Suppression in inferential ambiguity resolution. *Journal of Speech, Language and Hearing Research, 44,* 400–415.

Trupe, E. H., & Hillis, A. (1985). Paucity vs. verbosity: Another analysis of right hemisphere communication deficits. In R. H. Brookshire (Ed.), *Clinical aphasiology* (Vol. 15, pp. 83–96). Minneapolis, MN: BRK.

Tucker, D. M. (1981). Lateral brain function, emotion, and conceptualization. *Psychological Bulletin, 89,* 19–46.

Tucker, D. M., Watson, R. T., & Heilman, K. M. (1977). Discrimination and evocation of affectively intoned speech in patients with right parietal disease. *Neurology, 27,* 947–950.

Tucker, D. M., & Williamson, P. A. (1984). Asymmetric neuronal control systems in human self-regulation. *Psychological Review, 91,* 185–215.

Turkstra, L. S., Ylvisaker, M., Coelho, C., Kennedy, M., Sohlberg, M. M., Avery, J., et al. (2005). Practice guidelines for standardized assessment for persons with traumatic brain injury. *Journal of Medical Speech-Language Pathology, 13,* ix–xxxviii.

Urayse, D., Duffy, R. J., & Liles, B. Z. (1991). Analysis and description of narrative discourse in right-hemisphere-damaged adults: A comparison with neurologically normal and left-hemisphere-damaged aphasic adults. In T. Prescott (Ed.), *Clinical aphasiology* (Vol. 19, pp. 125–138). Austin, TX: Pro-Ed.

Vallar, G. (1993). The anatomical basis of spatial hemi-neglect in humans. In I. H. Robertson & J. C. Marshall (Eds.), *Unilateral neglect: Clinical and experimental studies.* Hillsdale, NJ: Lawrence Erlbaum.

Vallar, G., & Perani, D. (1986). The anatomy of unilateral neglect after right-hemisphere stroke lesions: A clinical/CT-scan correlation study in man. *Neuropsychologia, 24,* 609–622.

Van Lancker, D. (1980). Cerebral lateralization of pitch cues in the linguistic signal. *International Journal of Human Communication, 13,* 201–227.

Van Lancker, D. R., & Kempler, D. (1987). Comprehension of familiar phrases by left- but not by right hemisphere damaged patients. *Brain and Language, 32,* 265–277.

Van Lancker, D. R., & Sidtis, J. J. (1992). The identification of affective prosodic stimuli by left and right-hemisphere damaged subjects: All errors are not created equal. *Journal of Speech and Hearing Research, 35,* 963–970.

Walker, J. P., Daigle, T., & Buzzard, M. (2002). Hemispheric specialisation in processing prosodic structures: Revisited. *Aphasiology, 16,* 1155–1172.

Walker, J. P., Pelletier, R., & Reif, L. (2004). The production of linguistic prosodic structures in subjects with right hemisphere brain damage. *Clinical Linguistics & Phonetics, 18,* 85–106.

Wapner, W., Hamby, S., & Gardner, H. (1981). The role of the right hemisphere in the appreciation of complex linguistic materials. *Brain and Language, 14,* 15–33.

Weintraub, S., Mesulam, M. M., & Kramer, L. (1981). Disturbances in prosody: A right-hemisphere contribution to language. *Archives of Neurology, 38,* 742–744.

Weylman, S. T., Brownell, H. H., Roman, M., & Gardner, H. (1989). Appreciation of indirect requests by left- and right-brain-damaged patients: The effects of verbal context and conventionality of wording. *Brain and Language, 36,* 580–591.

Wilkins, A. M., Shallice, T., & McCarthy, R. (1987). Frontal lesions and sustained attention. *Neuropsychologia, 25,* 359–365.

Winner, E., Brownell, H., Happe, F., Blum, A., & Pincus, D. (1998). Distinguishing lies from jokes: Theory of mind deficits and discourse interpretation in right hemisphere brain-damaged patients. *Brain and Language, 62,* 89–106.

Winner, E., & Gardner, H. (1977). The comprehension of metaphor in brain damaged patients. *Brain, 100,* 719–727.

Wunderlich, A., Ziegler, W., & Geigenberger, A. (2003). Implicit processing of prosodic information in patients with left and right hemisphere stroke. *Aphasiology, 17,* 861–879.

Yokoyama, K., Jennings, R., Ackles, P., Hood, B. S., & Boller, F. (1987). Lack of heart rate changes during an attention-demanding task after right hemisphere lesions. *Neurology, 37,* 624–630.

Zahn, T. P., Grafman, J., & Tranel, D. (1999). Frontal lobe lesions and electrodermal activity: Effects of significance. *Neuropsychologia, 37,* 1227–1241.

Chapter 35

Management of Neurogenic Communication Disorders Associated with Dementia

Tammy Hopper and Kathryn A. Bayles

OBJECTIVES

After reading this chapter, the reader will be able to:

1. Define the dementia syndrome and commonly associated diseases.
2. Describe memory and the pattern of spared and impaired memory functions in dementia.
3. Explain the effects of memory impairment on cognitive-communication abilities of individuals with dementia.
4. Discuss assessment of individuals with dementia.
5. Design treatment programs based on principles of dementia management.

Older adults (65+ years) comprise the fastest growing segment of the world's population, with the oldest old (85+) increasing most rapidly (Kinsella & Velkoff, 2001). This tremendous growth in the number of older adults translates to an increased incidence and prevalence of individuals with dementia. In 2000, an estimated 4 million people in the U.S. were living with Alzheimer's disease (AD), the leading cause of dementia, and this number is predicted to increase to 13.2 million by 2050 (Hebert, Scherr, Bienias, Bennett, & Evans, 2003) unless a cure or effective prevention is found.

Understanding the pathogenesis of AD and other diseases that cause dementia, and developing pharmacologic and behavioral strategies for improving quality of life for affected individuals, are national research priorities. The cognitive-communication difficulties experienced by individuals with dementia, and the contribution of these deficits to diminished quality of life, necessitate speech-language pathology services (ASHA, 2005a, b). The purpose of this chapter is to define the dementia syndrome, explain common causes of dementia, discuss the effects of dementia on

communication, and outline principles for cognitive-communication assessment and treatment. The chapter will conclude with examples of evidence-based treatment programs that promote clinically significant changes in individuals with dementia.

THE DEMENTIA SYNDROME

Dementia is a clinical syndrome defined by deterioration of memory and at least one other cognitive function that is severe enough to interfere with daily life activities. The *Diagnostic and Statistical Manual of Mental Disorders* (4th ed., Text Revision) (DSM-IV-TR; American Psychiatric Association, 2000) specifies certain criteria that must be met for a diagnosis of dementia. Specifically, a patient must have multiple cognitive deficits that include both (1) evidence of short and long-term memory impairment, and (2) at least one of the following conditions: aphasia, apraxia, agnosia, or impaired executive functioning. These deficits must result in significant problems with employment and social functioning, not occur exclusively with delirium, and represent a significant decline from premorbid levels of functioning. Dementia is associated with many diseases, infections, trauma, and toxins, and although many cases of dementia are reversible, speech-language pathologists primarily deal with patients who have irreversible dementia caused by degenerative neurologic disease.

The cognitive-communication problems of dementia are a direct result of deterioration in higher cognitive processes, most notably memory. Therefore, understanding memory systems, and their neuroanatomy, is necessary to understanding why and how communicative functioning is affected in individuals with dementing diseases.

MEMORY

Memory can be defined as stored representations and the processes of encoding, consolidation, and retrieval through which knowledge is acquired and manipulated (Baddeley, 1999; Bayles & Tomoeda, 1997). Memory is not a unitary phenomenon, but is better characterized as comprising multiple systems. Although the systems are interrelated, some degree of modularity exists. For example, patients with neurologic disease or injury that affects specific brain regions may demonstrate relative preservation of one type of memory whereas another memory system is severely impaired. The idea of memory systems is not without controversy; however, the distinction between short- and long-term memory systems is generally accepted.

Short-term, or working, memory is the system responsible for activating and retrieving information, holding information in consciousness, and focusing attention (Baddeley, 1986), and is thought to be subserved by the dorsolateral prefrontal cortex. Working memory is described as comprising a central executive control system, and two "slave" or buffer systems: the phonologic loop and the visuospatial scratchpad (Baddeley & Hitch, 1974). In Baddeley's model, the central executive system functions to integrate sensory input, coordinate and allocate processing resources, and plan and control actions. The phonologic loop and the visuospatial scratchpad are buffers for acoustic and visual information, respectively. Working memory not only integrates sensory information from the environment, but also is involved in processing of information retrieved from long-term memory.

Long-term memory can be conceptualized as being declarative or nondeclarative (Squire, 1994). Declarative memory is memory for factual information, and comprises semantic, lexical, and episodic subsystems. Semantic memory refers to general conceptual knowledge, whereas lexical memory comprises knowledge for words. Tulving (1983) defines episodic memory as an individual's autobiographical memory, encoded in a temporal/spatial context. Declarative memory is assessed routinely using explicit memory tasks that require recall or recognition of past episodes or specific facts (Schacter & Tulving, 1994). Declarative memory is dependent upon the hippocampus and adjacent structures and connections of the medial temporal lobe (Broadbent, Clark, Zola, & Squire, 2002) as well as areas of prefrontal cortex that are active during encoding and retrieval (Schacter, 1996). Patients with damage to these neuroanatomic areas have difficulty with explicit memory. However, implicit memory expression may be preserved.

Implicit memory is the "unintentional or nonconscious use of previously acquired information" (Schacter & Tulving, 1994, p. 12). For example, patients with dementia may be unable to recall consciously a previous learning episode in which several words were practiced. However, if given the first few letters or stem of the practiced word, the practiced word may come to mind. This exemplifies how knowledge gained in the training sessions is expressed through improved performance rather than conscious recollection (Squire, 1994). This facilitated performance, following exposure to a related stimulus, is referred to as positive

"priming" and is inferred from decreased response time and/or increased response accuracy. The occurrence of priming in individuals with deficits in explicit memory suggests that priming depends on different neuroanatomic and functional systems than those that support explicit, declarative memory (Butters, Heindel, & Salmon, 1990; Schacter & Tulving, 1994).

Nondeclarative memory consists of verbal and motor procedural memory subsystems, reflexes, and habit memory (Squire, 1994). Procedural motor memory refers to knowledge for motor procedures, such as playing tennis or shoveling snow. Importantly, learning of procedures may not require conscious recollection of previous study episodes. Rather, motor learning can be implicit, and is demonstrated by behavioral change rather than explicit recall (Squire, 1994). The anatomic systems underlying procedural memory include the basal ganglia, cerebellum, and other neuromotor regions and connections (Daselaar, Rombouts, Veltman, Raaijmakers, & Jonker, 2003; Doyon & Ungerleider, 2002).

The vunerability of declarative and nondeclarative memory systems varies by disease. Those diseases that primarily affect cortical structures are more likely to produce declarative memory deficits. Diseases that primarily affect subcortical structures, such as the basal ganglia, produce nondeclarative memory impairments. The memory and language profiles of four common diseases associated with progressive dementia will be presented in the following section (Table 35–1).

ALZHEIMER'S DISEASE

The most common cause of irreversible dementia is Alzheimer's disease (Katzman & Bick, 2000). Diagnosis of AD can only be made upon postmortem examination of the brain; however, while an individual is alive, the diagnosis of probable AD can be made by exclusion. The criteria for diagnosis are specified in the DSM-IV-TR (APA, 2000) and include gradual onset of cognitive deficits that progressively worsen and are not due to other central nervous system etiologies, systemic conditions, or substance-induced conditions; neither do they result from a psychiatric disorder such as schizophrenia or depression.

Neuropathologic and neurochemical changes play a role in the development of AD (Fig. 35–1). Neuropathologic changes are characterized by neurofibrillary tangles and neuritic plaques that are distributed initially in the entorhinal cortex (adjacent to the hippocampus), spreading in stages to the hippocampus, inferior and lateral temporal lobes, and eventually other neocortical association areas (temporoparietal and frontal regions) (Braak & Braak, 1991, 1997). Changes are less apparent in primary sensorimotor (Braak & Braak, 1997) and occipital (Tomlinson, 1982) areas.

TABLE 35-1

Common Etiologies of Irreversible Dementia and Associated Cognitive Profiles

Alzheimer's disease	• Early stage: deficits in episodic and working memory • Later stage: impairments in semantic memory • Relatively spared procedural memory in early to middle stages of disease
Cerebrovascular disease	• Cognitive signs and symptoms are heterogeneous depending on lesion distribution • Cortical lesions are associated with amnesia, visuospatial deficits, and aphasia • Subcortical lesions (common in the periventricular white matter and basal ganglia) are associated with impairments of memory, executive functions, attention, and motor function
Lewy body disease	• Fluctuating presentation of cognitive symptoms • Procedural memory and learning deficits may occur with subcortical pathology • Declarative memory systems may be impaired with cortical pathology
Parkinson's disease	• Procedural memory impairment • Declarative memory deficits when cortical lesions exist

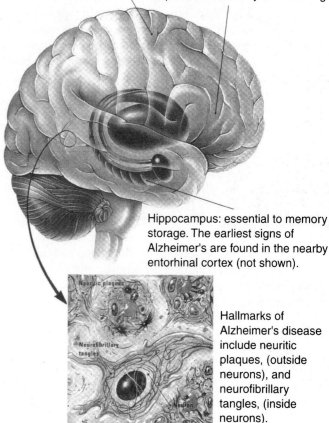

Cerebral cortex: involved in conscious thought and language.

Basal forebrain: has large numbers of neurons containing acetylcholine, a chemical important in memory and learning.

Hippocampus: essential to memory storage. The earliest signs of Alzheimer's are found in the nearby entorhinal cortex (not shown).

Hallmarks of Alzheimer's disease include neuritic plaques, (outside neurons), and neurofibrillary tangles, (inside neurons).

Figure 35–1. Neuropathological changes associated with Alzheimer's disease. Nerve cells (neurons) in several regions of the brain are affected. Illustration by Lydia Kibiuk. (Reprinted with permission from Alzheimer's disease: Unraveling the mystery. NIH Publication #96-3782. National Institutes of Health, 1995.)

Neurofibrillary tangles are intracellular deposits that occur when fibers within the neuron become twisted in a helical fashion. Scientists have provided evidence to suggest that these paired helical filaments are composed of the protein tau in an abnormally phosphorylated state (Goedert, 1993). Neuritic plaques are extracellular deposits best described as aggregations of neurons with an amyloid core surrounded by a ring of granular material. It is not clear how amyloid deposition is related to AD; it may be an inert byproduct of neuronal death, or a causative agent in neuronal degeneration (Goldman & Côté, 1991; Uylings & de Brabander, 2002).

General overall neuronal atrophy also is present in the brains of individuals with AD, and is seen in areas that have plaque and tangle pathology (Goldman & Côté, 1991). Neuronal degeneration in AD is marked by a loss of synapses and "presynaptic marker proteins" in the neocortex

and hippocampus (Goldman & Côté, 1991). Taken together, these neuropathologic changes interfere with axonal transport and cause synaptic dysfunction. It is important to note that researchers have discovered the presence of neurofibrillary tangles and neuritic plaques in sufficient numbers to warrant a definite neuropathologic diagnosis of AD in individuals who did not meet the criteria for a diagnosis of probable AD while alive (Davis, Schmitt, Wekstein & Markesbery, 1999).

Neurochemical deficiencies, specifically in the cholinergic system, also contribute to the disruption of nerve transmission at the cellular level. The cholinergic system is a neuronal network that transmits nerve impulses through acetylcholine. Enzymes necessary for the manufacture of acetylcholine, choline acetyltransferase, and acetylcholinesterase have been found to be reduced by 80% in individuals with AD (Bowen, Davison, & Sims, 1981; Davies, 1983). Of interest to scientists is the connection between cortical changes and subcortical nuclei containing cholinergic neurons, particularly the nucleus basalis of Meynert (Coyle, Price, & DeLong, 1983). This nucleus is a major component of the substantia innominata located beneath the globus pallidus. In individuals with AD, extensive reduction of cholinergic neurons has occurred within the nucleus basalis, a finding that has led researchers to theorize a relation between lack of cortical cholinergic input and the development of neuritic plaques and neurofibrillary tangles. Consistent with the cholinergic hypothesis is the observation that drugs that interfere with acetylcholine can produce memory impairment and confusion in normal individuals (Drachman & Leavitt, 1974; Goldman & Côté, 1991). In addition to the loss of acetylcholine, reductions are apparent in other neurochemicals, among them dopamine and serotonin.

Although specific causative factors of AD have not been determined, certain risk factors have been identified (Salmon & Bondi, 1997). Besides age, which is the most important risk factor, a genetic contribution to the development of late-onset AD is now recognized. Apolipoprotein E (ApoE), a protein involved in cholesterol transport, is associated with an increased risk of AD. The gene for ApoE is found on chromosome 19 and exists in three common allelic forms in humans: ApoE-2, ApoE-3, and ApoE-4 (National Institute on Aging/Alzheimer's Association Working Group, 1996). Individuals having one or two alleles for the e4 form are at a greater risk for developing AD than those who do not have the e4 allele (Honig, 1997), and the e4 form has been found to exist about three times more frequently in individuals with AD than among age-matched controls (National Institute on Aging/Alzheimer's Association Working Group, 1996). Despite the genetic risk factor of ApoE-4 presence, late-onset AD is not characterized as an "inherited" disorder. Only a small proportion of AD cases (approximately 5%) are transmitted by autosomal dominant inheritance (van der Flier & Scheltens, 2005).

Memory Deficits of Individuals with AD

The neuropathology of AD begins and is distributed most densely in areas of the brain important to episodic memory. Not surprisingly, therefore, the most commonly reported initial symptom is difficulty remembering recent events. Individuals with early AD consistently perform poorly on tests of episodic memory, such as verbal recall tasks, which are useful for early differential diagnosis. Working memory also is impaired in AD. Deficits in verbal and visuospatial span tasks have been reported (Spinnler, Della Sala, Bandera, & Baddeley, 1988), and individuals with AD have

demonstrated diminished performance on tasks of central executive function (e.g., dual task performance) compared to control subjects (Baddeley, Bressi, Della Sala, Logie, & Spinnler, 1991).

Semantic memory, on the other hand, is not always impaired in early AD. Hodges and Patterson (1995) reported that individuals with early-stage AD exhibited variability in their performance on semantic memory tasks, with some participants even demonstrating intact abilities as compared to healthy control participants. Other evidence for relative preservation of semantic memory comes from the literature on priming. As mentioned earlier, priming occurs when a response is facilitated by previous exposure to a related stimulus. Some researchers have found that individuals with AD demonstrate intact priming (Lustig & Buckner, 2004; Nebes, 1994; Nebes, Boller, & Holland, 1986; Nebes, Martin, & Horn, 1984), although others report negative effects (Salmon, Shimamura, Butters, & Smith, 1988). Nevertheless, the presence of positive priming supports the notion of gross preservation of semantic memory at least in the early stages of AD.

Of course, as dementia severity increases semantic memory is affected. Individuals with AD have particular difficulty on tasks that require the use of conceptual information, such as naming, category knowledge, attribute knowledge, and verbal fluency (Bayles & Kaszniak, 1987). However, the exact nature of the breakdown in semantic memory is debatable. Some researchers have argued that it occurs from the "bottom up," with knowledge of attributes of objects being lost before generic categorical knowledge (Martin & Fedio, 1983; Warrington, 1975). Evidence from this hypothesis comes from the misnamings of individuals with AD who often give the name of another item in the same category, such as "orange" for "lemon." The argument is that individuals with AD lose knowledge of the attributes that distinguish "orange" from "lemon," but retain the categorical knowledge that they are "fruit." Several investigators have challenged the "bottom-up" deterioration theory (Cox, Bayles, & Trosset, 1996; Nebes & Brady, 1988), showing that individuals with AD are as likely to give attributes as category information when asked to define words.

Other types of memory that may be spared in AD include nondeclarative types of memory such as motor procedural memory. On implicit memory tasks of motor learning, individuals with AD in the mild to moderate stages have been shown to improve task performance over time (Heindel, Salmon, Shults, Walicke, & Butters, 1989), or demonstrate the ability to acquire and retain a skill (Dick, Nielson, Beth, Shankle, & Cotman, 1995). These types of memory are preserved relative to declarative memory because the basal ganglia, cerebellum, and other neuromotor areas are relatively spared throughout much of the course of the disease.

CEREBROVASCULAR DISEASE

Cerebrovascular disease (CVD) is increasingly common and may be the second most common cause of dementia (Dubois & Hébért, 2001). When CVD causes dementia, it is referred to as vascular dementia (VaD). In addition to the basic criteria for dementia, the DSM-IV-TR (2000) specifies that a diagnosis of VaD be based upon presence of the following: focal neurologic signs and symptoms (e.g., weakness of an extremity), or laboratory evidence (i.e., neuroimaging results of multiple infarctions involving cortex and underlying white matter). However, the diagnosis of VaD remains controversial owing to its various causes and differing clinical manifestations.

VaD can be caused by ischemia (and less frequently by hemorrhage) in large arteries and in smaller, penetrating arteries (McPherson & Cummings, 1997). In the case of large-vessel disease, patients often have thrombosis or embolism in cerebral arteries that causes a single "strategic" infarct in cortical areas important for cognition and language or multiple, recurrent infarcts in these same areas (Román, 2005). In small-vessel disease, deep, penetrating arteries or arterioles are most affected, causing infarcts in subcortical structures and pathways (e.g., periventricular white matter, basal ganglia) (Mungas, 2005).

Cognitive signs and symptoms associated with VaD are heterogeneous and depend on the distribution and type of lesions involved. Small-vessel disease is considered the most common cause of VaD and is marked by multiple cognitive deficits in attention, executive functions, memory, language, and motor skills (see Jefferson, Brickman, Aloia, & Paul, 2005 for a review; McPherson & Cummings, 1997). The prominence of dysexecutive syndrome in individuals with subcortical VaD (Kramer, Reed, Mungas, Weiner, & Chui, 2002) has prompted researchers to call for revised diagnostic criteria that include dysexecutive syndrome as a cardinal feature of VaD (Jefferson, Brickman, Aloia, & Paul, 2005). The clinical course of subcortical VaD also resembles AD in that it is chronic and progressive; however, deterioration can occur in a stepwise fashion, with marked fluctuations in cognitive and functional abilities (Hachinski et al., 1975).

Individuals who suffer from acute strokes, as in large-vessel disease, may not always present with prominent memory problems and may have a stable or improving progression of symptoms (Román, 2005). In these cases, patients may not meet the DSM-IV-TR (2000) criteria for dementia, despite the demonstration of other cognitive deficits and evidence of cerebrovascular disease.

One of the most important developments in research on VaD is the recognition that VaD may actually moderate the expression of AD when the diseases co-occur ("mixed dementia"). Specifically, the presence of cerebrovascular lesions may actually promote clinical expression of AD

symptomatology (Snowdon, Grenier, Mortimer, Riley, & Markesbery, 1997; Román, 2003, 2005).

LEWY BODY DISEASE

Dementia with Lewy bodies (DLB) rivals VaD as the second most common type of dementia. Although DLB commonly co-occurs with AD, and is considered by some researchers to occur most often as a variant of AD (LBV of AD), others report that it is neuropathologically distinct from AD (Cercy & Bylsma, 1997) and can occur in isolation ("pure" DLB).

The neuropathology of DLB is marked by protein deposits (Lewy bodies) in neuronal-cell bodies. The pathologic distribution of Lewy bodies can be classified as brainstem predominant, limbic, and neocortical (McKeith et al., 1996; McKeith & O'Brien, 1999). According to McKeith and colleagues (2005), certain features, called "central features," are essential for a diagnosis of possible or probable DLB. These include presence of dementia with a progressive cognitive decline of sufficient magnitude to interfere with normal social or occupational function; prominent or persistent memory impairment that may not necessarily occur in the early stages but is usually evident with progression; and prominent deficits on tests of attention, executive function, and visuospatial ability. Other features (classified as core, suggestive, and supportive) can help contribute to the certainty of a possible or probable diagnosis. Core features of fluctuating cognition with pronounced variations in attention and alertness, recurrent visual hallucinations that are typically well-formed and detailed, and spontaneous features of parkinsonism are considered sufficient for a probable (in the case of two or more) or possible (if one feature is present) DLB.

Continued research with larger samples is needed to further elucidate the cognitive and linguistic characteristics of DLB. Researchers have noted, however, that patients with DLB have marked deficits in visuospatial and construction abilities that are not typically present in individuals with early AD (Calderon, Perry, Erzinclioglu, Berrios, Dening, & Hodges, 2001; Connor, Salmon, Sandy, Galasko, Hansen, & Thal, 1998; McKeith & O'Brien, 1999; Salmon et al., 1996; Tiraboschi, Salmon, Hansen, Hofstetter, Thal, & Corey-Bloom, 2006).

PARKINSON'S DISEASE

Idiopathic Parkinson's disease (PD) accounts for most cases of parkinsonism. The classic signs of rigidity, resting tremor, and bradykinesia are consequent with deterioration of dopaminergic neurons in the basal ganglia. The basal ganglia are important in the control of movement, and dopamine is a neurotransmitter involved in the initiation of movement. As a result of decreased levels of dopamine, patients with PD have difficulty initiating movement and commonly exhibit a slow, shuffling gait, flexed posture, and an inexpressive, mask-like face.

Increasingly, the term "Parkinson's disease with dementia" (PDD) is being used to describe those individuals with PD who develop dementia over the course of the disease process. The prevalence of dementia among individuals with PD has been reported to range from 10% to 20% (Tison, Dartigues, Auriacombe, Letenneur, Boller, & Alperovitch, 1995) up to 70% (Aarsland, Andersen, Larsen, Lolk, & Kragh-Sorensen, 2003).

Lewy bodies are present in all patients with PD (both with and without dementia) and are a prerequisite for postmortem diagnosis of PD (Braak, Del Tredici, Rüb, de Vos, Jansen Steur, & Braak, 2003). However, in PD without dementia the distribution of the Lewy bodies tends to be confined to subcortical areas, in particular the substantia nigra, whereas in PDD the distribution of Lewy bodies is more diffuse (Emre, 2003). Unsurprisingly, then, both groups of individuals with PD demonstrate difficulties with procedural memory and learning (Saint-Cyr, Taylor, & Lang, 1988). The neuropsychological profiles of individuals with PDD greatly resemble those of individuals with DLB (Noe, Marder, Bell, Jacobs, Manly, & Stern, 2004) and are sometimes clinically indistinguishable. These similarities between PDD and DLB have led some researchers to conclude that PDD is a subtype of DLB (Press, 2004). However, researchers have also found AD-type pathology in the brains of individuals with PDD; thus, AD cannot be ruled out as the cause of dementia among patients with PD (Braak et al., 2003; SantaCruz et al., 1999).

EFFECTS OF MEMORY DEFICITS ON COMMUNICATION ABILITY OF INDIVIDUALS WITH ALZHEIMER-TYPE DEMENTIA

Intact cognition is necessary for normal communication abilities. As a result of memory and other cognitive impairments, individuals with dementia have considerable difficulty communicating. Most of the research on communication in dementia has been conducted with individuals with AD. Early in the disease, individuals with AD become repetitious and forget what they have heard or read. Over time, the discourse of individuals with AD becomes impoverished and fragmented (Tomoeda & Bayles, 1993), and is characterized by a lack of coherence (Ripich & Terrill, 1988), tangentiality (Obler, 1983), and perseverations (Hier, Hagenlocker, & Shindler, 1985). The ability to formulate ideas and express them orally and in writing diminishes (Bayles & Kaszniak, 1987). Auditory comprehension of language also is impaired because memory for what was recently seen or heard fades rapidly. Nonetheless, phonology and syntax are relatively preserved into the advanced stages of the disease. The following discourse samples are

from a patient with AD who was followed for several years. His responses to the same stimulus picture reveal the disease effects on linguistic communication. The devastation of semantic content and verbal output is apparent. Note, however, the relative preservation of grammar.

Sample 1—Year 1

Examiner (E): Now I'd like you to look at that picture there.

Subject (S): Too many children.

E: Yes, I'd like you to tell me everything you can about that. Describe what's happening in the picture.

S: Well, here's a man reading something. It's happening, but he's not looking at the reading. See he's looking someplace else, and he's he's talking to these beautiful ladies here, and also reading his own paper beside. And here's his little boy. Isn't he cute?

E: Describe what's happening there.

S: Well the father's gotten a little tired of reading all this, see, so he's just getting rid of that, one at a time as they march past him going to their own reading or whatever else they do. (laugh) That's real good. And he has his own great big, great great big newspaper. And then he has a few down here like this. Two feet for all that. That's a cute thing right there. (laughing)

E: Okay, do you want to say anything else about that?

S: No, I don't think anything needs to be seen on it.

E: Okay, great.

S: There's a man that thinks maybe something else might be, but he's left everything alone except his newspaper. So everything is all right with him. Don't you think?

E: Yeah.

S: He's he's keeping some of the papers with his teeth. (laughs)

E: All right, thanks.

Sample 2—Year 2

E: Describe what's going on in this picture, and say what you would like to about that.

S: Well, they look like the pictures that uh don't want to be pick-picketed or or made made up into an odd creature in in the meantime.

E: Is there anything else that you want to say about that?

S: Yes, they do. They they they they they actually look so actable that it makes you want to run away for some reason or other. But um they have their their special aqualelge over. The way people take uh take uh an (actoba) that they don't even know anything about. But they just don't try to bother with these other people who have their.

E: Okay, great, thank you.

Sample 3—Year 3

E: Tell me about this picture. What can you tell me about that picture?

S: Yes. Mmhm. It must be a ah, ah, somebody that really thought themselves really gone and close way.

E: What's happening in this picture?

S: No.

E: What's happening in this picture?

S: Well, there's that's something that we'd be supplied with it, but usually goes away with a

E: Okay. good.

ASSESSMENT

Clinicians need to evaluate for the presence of dementia and its effect on communication skills. To detect dementia, the clinician will benefit from case history information about any neuropsychological changes. Interviewing the primary caregiver, usually the spouse, is advantageous. As part of a longitudinal study of the effects of AD on language, the primary caregivers of 99 individuals with AD were interviewed about early linguistic and nonlinguistic symptomatology (Bayles, 1991). Caregivers commonly reported memory deficits, word-finding problems, difficulty with finances, and trouble writing letters as antedating the medical diagnosis of the disease.

Identifying the presence of dementia demands consideration of whether current behavior is congruent with the individual's premorbid intellectual ability. For example, an individual whose clinical performance on intellectual tasks was average, but who was a Phi Beta Kappa in college, would be suspect. Such an individual would be expected to perform above average. Premorbid intelligence can be estimated using demographic information (Barona, Reynolds, & Chastain, 1984; Wilson, Rosenbaum, & Brown, 1979). Because individuals with dementia are older, hearing and visual problems may exist and can confound the dementia diagnosis. Polypharmacy also can confound the diagnosis because many drugs affect mental status.

Another condition that can cause the performance of the individual to mimic dementia is depression, often referred to as pseudodementia. Consider screening for depression using one of the many depression scales, such as the Hamilton Rating Scale (Hamilton, 1960), and the Beck Depression Inventory (Beck, Ward, Mendelson, Mock, & Erbaugh, 1961). The Hamilton Rating Scale is an interview-based rating scale composed of a 17-item inventory of symptoms, both physical and psychological, that are rated for severity by one or two clinicians. The Beck Depression Inventory is a self-report instrument comprising 21 items, and has been used extensively in research and screening applications with elderly adults (Gallagher, Breckenridge, Steinmetz, & Thompson, 1983; Miller & Seligman, 1973).

As mentioned previously, AD and VaD commonly co-occur in individuals with dementia, making it important to consider the possibility of cerebrovascular disease in patients suspected of having dementia. The Hachinski Ischemic Scale (Hachinski et al., 1975) is widely used to identify individuals with symptoms typically associated with vascular disease and stroke. The scale comprises 13 features associated with vascular disease and stroke, such as history of hypertension, focal neurologic signs, and abrupt onset. Each feature is evaluated and points are accumulated for those present. Individuals who have seven or more points are considered at risk for VaD.

Neuropsychological Tests Sensitive to Dementia

The neuropsychological test most sensitive to early dementia is the episodic memory test. However, because dementia is by definition the loss of multiple cognitive abilities, neuropsychologists typically evaluate attention, problem-solving, reasoning, and other intellectual functions in addition to memory. It is beyond the scope of this chapter to review all of the neuropsychological tests used with individuals with dementia. Instead, the focus will be on measures of cognitive-linguistic function that can be used to screen for dementia, stage dementia severity, and comprehensively evaluate the communicative abilities of individuals with dementia (Table 35–2).

Screening Tests

Tasks most sensitive to the dementia syndrome are those that are active, nonautomatic, or generative, and ones that depend on logical reasoning. Active nonautomatic tasks require the patient's mental and linguistic involvement in a creative way, such as in retelling a story or generating names of items in a category.

The Story Retelling subtest of the Arizona Battery for Communication Disorders of Dementia (ABCD; Bayles & Tomoeda, 1993) is an effective screening tool. In this test, subjects are asked to tell a short story immediately after hearing it and again after an imposed delay. The subtest takes about 5 minutes to administer, and has high sensitivity (i.e., correctly classifies adults who have dementia as having dementia) and specificity (i.e., correctly classifies adults who are not demented as being nondemented) (Bayles & Tomoeda, 1993). The scores of individuals with mild and moderate AD and the scores of individuals with PD (with

---

TABLE 35–2

Summary of Assessment Measures

Screening
  Story Retelling Subtest, Arizona Battery for
    Communication Disorders of Dementia (Bayles &
    Tomoeda, 1993)
  FAS Verbal Fluency Test (Borkowski et al., 1967)
Staging Severity
  Mini-Mental State Examination (Folstein et al., 1975)
  Global Deterioration Scale (Reisberg et al., 1982)
Comprehensive Assessment of Cognitive-Communicative
  Functioning
  The Arizona Battery for Communication Disorders of
    Dementia (Bayles & Tomoeda, 1993)
  The Functional Linguistic Communication Inventory
    (Bayles & Tomoeda, 1994)

TABLE 35-3

Mean Scores and Standard Deviations of Normal Elders (NC), Mild and Moderate Alzheimer's Disease (AD) Patients, and Parkinson's Disease Patients with and without Dementia on Story Retelling in the Immediate and Delayed Conditions

	Old NC	Mild AD	Mod AD	NPD*	DPD*
Story Retelling, Immediate	14.0 (2.3)	7.3 (4.1)	2.6 (3.0)	13.8 (2.5)	7.3 (4.1)
Story Retelling, Delayed	12.4 (4.5)	1.0 (2.6)	0.0 (0.0)	12.9 (3.9)	4.1 (6.3)

*NPD = nondemented Parkinson's disease; DPD = demented Parkinson's disease (Reprinted with permission from Bayles, K. A., & Tomoeda, C. K. (1997). *Improving function in dementia and other cognitive-linguistic disorders.* Austin, TX: Pro-Ed.

and without dementia) are shown in Table 35–3. Note that individuals with moderate AD remember nothing about the story in the delayed condition.

Generative naming or verbal fluency tests also are sensitive to the presence of dementia (Chertkow & Bub, 1990; Ober, Dronkers, Koss, Delis, & Friedland, 1986). When individuals have to conceive of and produce, either in writing or orally, a series of related ideas of examples of objects in a category, they are performing a generative task. The two most common types of fluency tasks are semantic and letter tests.

Semantic verbal fluency requires that individuals produce words in a specific category, such as animals. The Boston Diagnostic Aphasia Examination (Goodglass & Kaplan, 1983), and the Arizona Battery for Communication Disorders of Dementia (Bayles & Tomoeda, 1993) both contain semantic verbal fluency tests. Letter-fluency tasks involve the production of words that begin with a target letter. An example of a letter task is the FAS Verbal Fluency Test or the Controlled Oral Word Association Test (Borkowski, Benton, & Spreen, 1967), in which an individual must think of as many words as possible beginning with the letters F, A, and S in 1 minute. Individuals with AD have been reported to be deficient in performing both types of verbal fluency tests, likely because of frontal-lobe damage. Patients with PD and those with DLB also are reported to be deficient on generative naming tasks (Salmon et al., 1996; Bayles, Trosset, Tomoeda, Montgomery, & Wilson, 1993). Because verbal-fluency performance involves recruitment of multiple cognitive systems, it is an extremely sensitive indicator of the cognitive impairments of individuals with dementia (Azuma & Bayles, 1997).

The Mini-Mental State Examination (MMSE; Folstein, Folstein, & McHugh, 1975) is a widely used screening instrument. The MMSE comprises 11 items related to orientation, attention, calculation, language, memory, and visuospatial construction, and takes 5 to 10 minutes to administer. Although education may influence examinee performance, reliability and validity of the measure for assessing mental status have been reported to be high (Farber, Schmitt, & Logue, 1988; Foreman, 1987), and age- and education-adjusted norms have been reported (Crum, Anthony, Bassett, & Folstein, 1993).

Staging Severity

One of the most commonly used scales to stage dementia severity is the Global Deterioration Scale (GDS; Reisberg, Ferris, deLeon, & Crook, 1982). An observation scale, it is composed of seven stages that include detailed descriptions of functional deficits typical of individuals at each stage of disease severity. An extension of the GDS, the Functional Assessment Staging Scale (FAST; Reisberg, Ferris, & Franssen, 1985), was developed to better characterize the functional abilities (e.g., dressing, communication) of individuals in the more severe stages of cognitive decline.

Comprehensive Evaluation of Cognitive-Communicative Functioning

Although individual tests are appropriate for domain-specific assessment, a comprehensive evaluation of language and communication abilities is best accomplished with a battery of tests. A battery for testing the communicative functions of individuals with dementia must contain measures of the effects of cognitive deterioration, particularly memory deficits, on communication.

Pragmatic and semantic skills are more vulnerable to deficits in higher cognitive functions than phonologic and syntactic skills. This is understandable because the content of language and the purpose for which it is used require conscious thought, memory, and planning. The rules of phonology and syntax are finite, predictable, and typically do not require conscious attention. For this reason, measures of semantic and pragmatic reasoning should be included in a test battery for patients with dementia.

A relatively short test that is being increasingly used in clinical settings to assess the cognitive and language abilities of individuals with AD is the Cognitive Subscale of the Alzheimer's Disease Assessment Scale (ADAS-Cog; Rosen, Mohs, & Davis, 1984). This test includes items related to attention, memory, reasoning, praxis, language production (naming), and comprehension (following commands). Although not considered a comprehensive evaluation measure, administration of the ADAS-Cog may yield information on cognition and language useful in structuring further in-depth assessment.

Bayles and Tomoeda (1993) designed the Arizona Battery of Communication Disorders of Dementia (ABCD) for the purpose of quantifying the communication disorders associated with mild to moderate dementia. The battery contains 14 subtests that yield information about five cognitive constructs: linguistic expression, linguistic comprehension, verbal episodic memory, mental status, and visuospatial construction. Raw scores are obtained from individual subtests and are converted to summary scores to allow comparisons between subtests. Summary scores can be converted to construct scores, for interconstruct comparisons, and construct scores can be summed to obtain a total score for the complete test (Bayles & Tomoeda, 1997). The validity and reliability have been reported to be high, and the test has been standardized on individuals with AD, PD, and healthy young and elderly control subjects in the United States, Great Britain (Armstrong, Bayles, Borthwick, & Tomoeda, 1996) and Australia (Moorhouse, Douglas, Panaccio, & Steel, 1999).

For the patient with more severe dementia, a second test battery was developed, the Functional Linguistic Communication Inventory (FLCI; Bayles and Tomoeda, 1994). The FLCI has 10 components that allow quantification of linguistic communication. Subtests include tasks such as greeting and naming, writing, reminiscing, comprehending signs, and gesturing. The test battery is sensitive to differences in patients with moderate, moderately severe, severe, and very severe dementia (Bayles & Tomoeda, 1994), and has established reliability and validity. Additionally, patterns of responses to test questions can be profiled to determine intra-individual communication strengths and weaknesses. These profiles are extremely useful for completing the Minimum Data Set (MDS; Morris et al., 1990) and developing care plans, as well as for designing individualized stimulation and activity programs for individuals with moderate and severe dementia.

BEHAVIORAL TREATMENT FOR INDIVIDUALS WITH AD

The functional deficits that individuals with dementia experience in communication, activities of daily living, and quality of life result directly from the cognitive impairments that define dementia. As mentioned previously, the pattern of these impairments depends upon the distribution of the neuropathology associated with different diseases that cause dementia. In AD, certain aspects of cognitive processing remain relatively preserved, despite severe impairments in other cognitive areas. Recognition of residual capacities in addition to diminished abilities will provide the basis for successful interventions for individuals with dementia.

Principles for Successful Intervention

Bayles and Tomoeda (1997) propose several principles for improving function in individuals with AD. Clinicians should first reduce demands on episodic and working memory systems. Second, increase reliance on nondeclarative memory systems. Third, provide activities that strengthen lexical and conceptual associations, and fourth, provide sensory cues that will evoke positive fact memory, action, and emotion.

Application of these principles to treatment can help to improve or maintain cognitive-linguistic abilities of individuals with AD. In the following section, several recent studies are reviewed in which one or more of these principles has been utilized to improve functioning of individuals with AD or related dementias.

Spaced-Retrieval Training

Spaced-retrieval training (SRT) is a technique used to teach new and forgotten information and behaviors to patients with dementia. In SRT, a patient is told a piece of information and then is asked to recall that information repeatedly and systematically over time. Intervals are manipulated to facilitate production of a high number of correct responses to the stimulus question and retention of information over increasingly longer periods of time. SRT is considered to require little cognitive effort (Schacter, Rich, & Stampp, 1985), and can occur without the patient having explicit recall of the training situation. Also, because strength of association between concepts in semantic memory depends on how often they are activated, repeatedly bringing into consciousness these associations will result in their increased accessibility (Bayles & Tomoeda, 1997). Therefore, SRT involves strengthening of associations, increasing reliance on implicit memory expression (Camp, Foss, O'Hanlon, & Stevens, 1996), and reducing demands on episodic and working memory.

Clinicians may use SRT to teach individuals with dementia new information and helpful behaviors. Camp and colleagues (1996) assessed the effectiveness of SRT to teach calendar use for improving prospective memory performance. Also of interest to these investigators was whether the effects of the calendar intervention would be maintained at least 6 months after training. Treatment sessions lasted approximately 30 minutes and continued for 10 weeks. Each session started with the prompt question "How are you going to remember what to do each day?" The participant had to answer "Look at my calendar" to be correct. If the response was correct, a delay was followed by another recall trial. Intervals were increased if the participant continued with correct responses. If a response was incorrect on any trial, the experimenter provided the correct answer and then immediately repeated the prompt question. When the participant could recall the strategy after a 1-week interval, SRT was terminated.

Once calendar training was successful, up to 5 weeks of additional therapy, one session per week, was provided to teach each patient to complete two tasks on each page of the daily calendar. In this way, the investigators were able to teach the implementation of the skill and evaluate its usefulness in aiding performance of prospective memory tasks in daily life (e.g., walk the dog, write a letter).

Results indicated that the individuals with mild, moderate, and moderately severe dementia were able to recall the calendar strategy over a 1-week period, and some participants used the calendar to remember to perform daily tasks. Although participants did not consistently perform tasks on each day, they showed improvement in using the calendar to carry out the majority of the noted tasks. Six-month follow-up visits showed that calendar use continued well after completion of the study.

McKitrick, Camp, and Black (1992) also conducted a study in which prospective memory was targeted. Four individuals with mild to moderate dementia participated. Sessions were conducted once weekly, and involved teaching subjects verbal and motor responses necessary to redeem a coupon for money. SRT was used to first teach participants a verbal response to the prompt question "What are you going to do when I come back next week?" ("Give you the [pink] coupon"). The motor response consisted of having the subject select the correct coupon and hand it to the examiner. To be successful, the participant had to hand the coupon to the experimenter at the start of the following week's session. In return, the participant was given a dollar. Different colored coupons were trained to criterion successively.

The results again showed that individuals with AD could learn to perform a task following intensive training. Three of the participants required only one session of therapy, whereas one subject required five training sessions. Two of the participants, who had the lowest cognitive functioning scores, actually performed better on the task than the two with higher scores. This finding suggests that level of cognitive function may not be the only predictor of performance on the SRT task and that more severe memory dysfunction does not prevent the learning of some types of factual and procedural information.

Other functional information also has been taught to individuals with dementia using SRT. Vanhalle, Van der

Linden, Belleville, and Gilbert (1998) used SRT to teach face–name associations to a dementia patient. Although they found that the patient was affected by proactive interference (i.e., learning of previous items interfered with the learning of subsequent items), the SRT technique was successful in teaching the patient to recall new names.

SRT can be implemented in the context of other activities, such as speech-language therapy sessions. To demonstrate the utility of SRT in this context, Brush and Camp (1998) conducted a study with nine participants: seven with memory deficits resulting from dementia, and two patients with memory disorders resulting from stroke. The goal was to assess the effect of SRT with memory disordered patients of different etiologies, and to examine the application of SRT within the speech-language therapy session.

Three pieces of information were taught to each participant: the therapist's name, a personal fact that was considered important to the person (e.g., wife's birthday, room number), and a compensatory technique that was being practiced in speech-language therapy sessions (e.g., using a louder voice, describing an item when unable to name it). Successful recall of the information at the beginning of two consecutive sessions was criterion for completion of the SRT for each piece of information. The three pieces of information were taught sequentially.

Five of the participants with dementia completed the study. All learned the three pieces of information but had varying levels of recall of the information at 4 weeks posttherapy. The two patients who had suffered strokes also successfully completed the study and demonstrated consistent recall of the information at the 4-week follow-up probe.

The aforementioned studies were included in a systematic review of the literature on SRT conducted by Hopper and colleagues (2005). The researchers reviewed 15 studies that were judged to provide Class II and III research evidence (Miller et al., 1999) for SRT with people who have AD or a related dementia. In conclusion, using SRT to teach compensatory strategies that enhance communication is a promising technique for speech-language pathologists. Although patients may not remember the specific episodes of learning, they may show an increase in the number of correct responses produced and exhibit a change in the trained behavior.

Capitalizing on Spared-Memory Processes

Treatment approaches that draw on spared abilities, specifically procedural memory skills, have been shown to be effective when used with individuals with AD. Zanetti, Binetti, Magni, Rozzini, Bianchetti, and Trabucchi (1997) assessed the effects of procedural-memory stimulation on performance of activities of daily living (ADLs) of individuals with mild to moderate AD. Ten individuals with AD were trained to perform different basic and instrumental ADLs, such as washing the face and using the telephone. Twenty activities were chosen for treatment and divided into two sets. Over 3 weeks, five patients were trained on the first set of 10 activities, and the other five patients were trained on activities in the second set. Training sessions were structured such that performance would be more dependent on procedural rather than episodic memory processes (Zanetti et al., 1997). Specifically, verbal cues and prompts were provided during tasks, and patients were not asked to remember how to perform any task. The time taken for patients in both groups to perform the trained and untrained activities was recorded. Other outcome measures included performance on neuropsychological batteries, including tests of skill-learning, word-stem completion (a measure of lexical priming), and paired-associate learning (a test of episodic memory). These measures were given at the beginning and end of the treatment program.

After 3 weeks of training, patients performed the trained tasks in significantly less time than they did at baseline testing. They also showed a significant improvement in the time taken to perform untrained tasks. No significant differences between scores on neuropsychological tests administered before and after treatment were obtained, although a statistical trend for improvement by patients on the lexical priming tests was reported. Although limited by the absence of a control group, these preliminary results provide evidence that ADL training that is focused on the motor or procedural aspects of tasks may be an effective technique for improving performance of individuals with AD. The improvement on the untrained tasks may have resulted from generalization from trained activities, although practice effects may have contributed to improved performance.

Another technique that capitalizes on spared memory systems and that may be beneficial for promoting new learning by individuals with AD is errorless learning. Errorless learning involves minimization of the number of errors that are allowed to occur during learning trials. This approach differs from usual protocols for rehabilitation of memory and language deficits in that it does not involve "trial and error" techniques to promote learning. Baddeley and Wilson (1994) suggest that individuals with episodic memory impairment have difficulty eliminating errors made during learning trials because they cannot explicitly recall the learning experience. Therefore, these individuals continue to make the same errors on subsequent trials, rather than learning from the errors and making corrections.

The errorless learning technique has been used successfully with amnesic patients (Baddeley & Wilson, 1994; Wilson, Baddeley, Evans, & Shiel, 1994), and recently the technique has been applied to memory rehabilitation with individuals who have AD. Clare, Wilson, Breen, and Hodges (1999) used errorless learning principles, in conjunction with several other techniques, to teach a 72-year-old man with early AD to learn the names and faces of members of his social club. The subject learned the name–face associations, demonstrated some generalization from the pictures to real faces in the environment, and retained the information for 9 months. Although the design of the study makes it difficult to attribute the improved performance solely to reduced errors during learning trials, errorless learning principles were the core component of the instruction and clearly contributed to learning and retention of new information. Subsequent studies have been conducted and positive results of errorless learning paradigms reported by the authors (Clare, Wilson, Carter, Breen, Gosses, & Hodges, 2000; Winter & Hunkin, 1999).

The term "errorless learning" does not connote a standardized treatment program but a practice achieved through manipulation of stimulus characteristics and response contingencies. For example, spaced-retrieval training may constrain errors through practice of correct responding over several trials. Also, memory books for individuals with dementia contain printed and pictorial materials to reduce effort and errors associated with free recall of personally relevant information.

Reducing Demands on Episodic and Working Memory Systems: Using Recognition Memory

Bourgeois (1990, 1992) has improved the functioning of individuals with dementia by capitalizing on spared recognition memory and decreasing demands on impaired episodic and working memory systems. In 1990, she studied the effect on conversational ability of providing stimulus materials in the form of wallets with photographs. Three subjects and their spouses participated in the study. An individualized memory wallet was assembled for each AD subject, consisting of pictures of events and persons the patient could not remember. Caregivers were trained to use the memory wallets in conversation with the subjects, and data were collected on communicative behaviors that occurred when the wallets were used in conversation. When caregivers used the memory wallets in conversation, subjects made significantly more statements of fact and fewer ambiguous utterances.

In a second study, Bourgeois (1992) sought to replicate the treatment effects of the first study, and to investigate whether training the use of the wallets was necessary for patients to use them effectively. Initially, six patients with AD and their caregivers were trained to use the memory wallets in conversation. Positive treatment effects were obtained, with patients making more novel, on-topic statements and fewer ambiguous statements when wallets were used in conversation. Next, three additional participants with AD were given memory wallets without any specific training. The experimenter served as the communication partner during this phase of the study. Two of the participants generated more novel, on-topic utterances when the wallets were used in conversation, although the third participant's behavior was more variable. Generally, the results were positive, suggesting that the use of memory wallets improved communication even when participants were not trained in their use.

Positive results have been reported in subsequent studies by Bourgeois and other researchers (Hoerster, Hickey, & Bourgeois, 2001; Holmes, 2000). The memory wallets used by individuals with AD and communication partners acted as tangible stimuli that remained visible in a conversation, alleviating the demands that conversation typically places on working memory. Additionally, the photographs stimulated recognition of episodes and people in the patients' lives, reducing the reliance on free recall that usually occurs during conversations about remote and recent events (episodic memory). The use of pictures and sentences about familiar people and places in patients' lives capitalizes on often spared reading ability and may promote positive reminiscence and emotion.

Using Sensory Stimulation to Evoke Positive-Fact Memory, Action, and Emotion

Providing sensory stimulation to evoke positive-fact memory, action, and emotion is an important principle in the management of individuals with dementia. Frequently, people with AD in the more moderate to advanced stages are given stuffed animals as companions or decorations in their rooms. Results of several case studies and anecdotal reports support the use of such stimuli to improve communicative function of individuals with AD. Bailey, Gilbert, and Herweyer (1992) observed improved levels of alertness, increased smiling and nodding, and decreased agitation when four patients with AD were given dolls and stuffed animals. Other researchers have noted similar outcomes (Francis & Baly, 1986; Milton & MacPhail, 1985).

In a single-subject experiment, Hopper, Bayles, and Tomoeda (1998) showed that using toy stimuli improved the amount and quality of language produced by four females with moderate to moderately severe dementia. In response to questions, the subjects produced more information units when toy stimuli were present than when they were absent. The results lend support to the use of tangible stimuli, individualized according to patient preferences, when attempting to improve conversation and social interaction.

Multicomponent Treatment Programs

A program that is based on several of the aforementioned treatment principles and that capitalizes on the life experience of individuals with AD is the Montessori-based intervention developed and described by Camp and colleagues (1997). Montessori activities were originally developed for children and include materials and tasks that require active participation. The use of Montessori programming promotes learning through procedural memory processes, utilizes concrete everyday stimuli to facilitate action and memory, and reduces demands on episodic and working memory by using structured tasks and repetition.

Camp and colleagues (1997) describe intergenerational Montessori programming between individuals with dementia and children, and the positive results from a pilot study. In the study, adults and children were matched according to cognitive level, with the adult being more advanced cognitively than the child. This pairing allowed the adult to act as a mentor and teacher to the child during the Montessori activities (e.g., matching, sorting, reading aloud). The primary measure of interest was "disengagement." Disengagement was defined as time spent staring into space for at least 10 seconds or sleeping (Camp & Brush, 1998). Five-minute observation intervals were used to record data on the amount of time individuals with AD were disengaged. Results showed that when the adults were working with the children, no instances of disengagement were observed, in contrast to the times when adults were not working with the children and episodes of disengagement were common.

Camp and Brush (1998) also reported on the use of Montessori-type tasks in group activities for individuals with dementia in skilled-nursing facilities. In these group activities, engagement was a primary treatment outcome measure (see Orsulic-Jeras, Judge, & Camp, 2000). Investigators collected data on the amount of time individuals spent in active engagement (defined as verbal or motor activity focused on the environment) and passive engagement (defined as passively observing what is going on in the environment) during Montessori activities, and compared those instances to the time spent actively and passively engaged during regular adult day-care activities. Results showed that individuals participating in the Montessori group activities were more actively engaged than those who participated in the regular programming.

Mahendra, Hopper, Bayles, Azuma, Cleary, and Kim (2006) conducted a systematic review of Montessori techniques conducted individually and in groups for individuals with dementia. Five studies met criteria for inclusion in the review and were judged to provide Class II and III evidence for the use of Montessori programming for individuals with AD or a related dementia.

In another type of multicomponent treatment program, Santo Pietro and Boczko (1998) compared the effectiveness of different group therapies for individuals with AD. Outcomes of a group communication therapy called the "Breakfast Club" were compared to those of "standard" conversational group therapy. Four groups of five mid-stage individuals with AD participated in the Breakfast Club, five days per week for 12 weeks, and four matched control groups participated in conversation groups at the same frequency and duration.

Activities in the Breakfast Club were based on facilitation of procedural memory, stimulation of positive emotions, and strengthening of associations, and included a 10-step protocol to facilitate communication. Topics related to breakfast were introduced and the group members engaged in the familiar task of choosing and preparing a breakfast. Throughout, language was elicited by the clinician who "facilitated" conversation using visual cues, semantic associations, and paired-choice questions during meal preparation, eating, and clean-up.

Individuals in the control conversation group sat at a table with a clinician who facilitated conversation by introducing a topic for discussion. Language was elicited using open-ended questions, paired choices, and key-word visual prompts. Social conversation was encouraged during greeting and leave-taking.

Group differences were compared using pre- and post-treatment scores on the Arizona Battery for Communication Disorders of Dementia (Bayles & Tomoeda, 1993), and the Communication Outcomes of Communicative and Functional Independence Scale (COMFI; Santo Pietro & Boczko, 1997), a caregiver rating scale with 20 items related to cognition, psychosocial behavior, communication and conversation, and meal-time independence. Also, the number of incidents of "cross-conversation" between members within a group was compared. Cross-conversation was defined as any utterance between one group member and another, and was used as a measure of social awareness and communicative ability. Results showed that individuals in the Breakfast Club exhibited significantly improved language skills, improved functional independence, and increased use of cross-conversation as compared to members in the standard conversation groups who showed no improvement on any measure. Several other within-group improvements for Breakfast Club participants were noted, including increased interest and involvement in meal-time activities.

The multifaceted approaches underlying the Montessori group activities and the Breakfast Club were effective in promoting meaningful change in the cognitive and communicative abilities of individuals with mild to moderate AD. Most investigators have favored procedures and programs that focus on relatively preserved skills and have not attempted to directly stimulate the cognitive processes impaired in dementing diseases. However, some recent research provides encouragement for cognitive-stimulation programs.

Strengthening Associations through Cognitive Stimulation

Quayhagen, Quayhagen, Corbeil, Roth, and Rodgers (1995) produced preliminary evidence that intensive cognitive therapy may slow the general cognitive and behavioral decline associated with dementia. These researchers sought to determine the impact on individuals with AD of a home-based intervention program of active cognitive stimulation provided by family caregivers. Pairs of individuals with AD and their primary caregivers were assigned to experimental, placebo, and control groups. Families in the experimental group were trained to provide 60 minutes of "active" cognitive stimulation. The cognitive-stimulation program consisted of memory, problem-solving, and conversation activities in which the patient had to participate actively. Memory techniques were characterized by the recall and recognition of verbal and visual information. The placebo group engaged in more "passive" interventions that were designed to match experimental interventions, and yet not require active participation by the subject. For example, patients might watch "Wheel of Fortune" in the placebo group instead of playing the game "Hangman" in the experimental group. The control-group families were placed on a wait list for therapy sessions after the study was completed. Multiple behavioral and cognitive measures were used to assess intervention effects on memory, verbal fluency, problem-solving, and attention. Patients in all three groups were tested at three points in time: on entrance into the study, after 12 weeks of treatment, and 6 months after completion (Quayhagen et al., 1995).

The individuals with AD who received the active cognitive stimulation showed no decline from pre to post-testing on the measures of global cognitive functioning, whereas the control group declined on all measures. The placebo group declined on some measures and remained stable on others. Interestingly, the experimental group improved on some measures throughout treatment and for a period after treatment, and maintained their pre-treatment level of cognitive function on others, although their performance returned to baseline levels at the 9-month probe.

Bach, Bach, Bohmer, Fruhwald, and Grilc (1995) also compared the effects of two treatments on the function of 44 individuals with mild to moderate dementia. The subjects were randomly assigned to a control group or a treatment group. The control group received 24 weeks of "functional" rehabilitation, including tasks from occupational, physical, and speech therapists. The treatment group received the same functional treatment, in addition to twice-weekly small-group treatment consisting of memory training, manual/creative activities, and self-management tasks. Several measures were used to assess change as a result of treatment, including cognitive tests, measures of psychosocial function, and measures of depression. The results showed that both groups had significantly higher levels of cognitive performance and a decrease in depressive symptoms after 24 weeks of treatment. However, the patients in the treatment group had significantly better scores than the people in the functional group on measures of cognition, psychosocial functioning, subjective well-being, and depression (Bach et al., 1995).

The recognition that cognitive-stimulation programs have beneficial effects for individuals with AD has led researchers to investigate the combined effects of these programs in conjunction with commonly prescribed medications to treat AD. Chapman, Weiner, Rackley, Hynan, and Zientz (2004) recruited 54 patients with mild to moderate AD to participate in a study to assess the effects of combining cognitive-communication stimulation with donepezil, an acetylcholinesterase inhibitor prescribed for people with AD. The participants were randomly assigned to a control group (donepezil only; $n = 28$) and a treatment group (donepezil plus stimulation group; $n = 26$). The cognitive-communication stimulation program consisted of activities implemented in a group format for 12 hours over a 2-month period. The tasks included discussions about current events, information related to AD, life stories (i.e., personal narratives with pictures), and life-interest topics (e.g., hobbies or work).

The investigators followed the participants for 1 year and measured aspects of cognition, communication, emotional symptoms, and quality of life at baseline, 4 months (1 month after the end of the 2-month stimulation program), 8 months, and 12 months. Participants in the treatment group demonstrated a slower rate of decline than did participants in the control group on caregiver interview and standardized measures of discourse abilities, ADLs, and overall functioning.

Promoting Generalization

A primary goal of any cognitive-communication intervention is the generalization of treatment effects and their continuance after the intervention is discontinued. Little research has been conducted to determine the factors that promote generalization and maintenance of behaviors in individuals with dementia. Further, the progressive nature of dementia leads clinicians to think that generalization over time is unrealistic. However, the duration of dementia can be quite long, sometimes more than 10 years, and change in cognitive status occurs gradually. A treatment that improves function for several months can improve quality of life and reduce demands on caregivers, and therefore is worth investigating. To assess generalization and maintenance of treatment effects, consider evaluating behaviors that reflect stimulus generalization rather than response generalization.

Stimulus generalization is the occurrence of trained behaviors in nontraining conditions that include different people, situations, or materials than those used in treatment sessions (Olswang & Bain, 1994; Thompson, 1989). The trained response, or treatment behavior, generalizes to different stimulus conditions. For example, stimulus generalization is exhibited by the patient with dementia who is taught a strategy for requesting help in a treatment session with the clinician, who later asks for help outside of the treatment session, showing transfer of the trained response to an untrained context.

Response generalization is the occurrence of untrained responses or behaviors as a result of training other, related responses or behaviors (Thompson, 1989). For example, Lowell, Beeson, and Holland (1995) taught patients with aphasia to use a semantic-features diagram to aid in self-cueing and naming. Two of the three subjects used the schema to improve naming of trained items as well as to "generate semantic information regarding any word they wished to retrieve" (p. 110), thus demonstrating response generalization.

Stimulus generalization may be the more appropriate measure for documenting the effects of treatment of individuals with dementia, as the multiple cognitive deficits associated with dementia may prevent robust response generalization. Treatment and measurement of generalization should be focused on trained responses, such as names of family members, that can be used in different stimulus situations.

Clinicians need to program for generalization. The "train and hope" (Stokes & Baer, 1977) method, in which clinicians conduct treatment and hope for functional effects, is a commonly used, yet frequently ineffective, procedure for facilitating generalization. Stokes and Baer (1977) recommend several techniques for facilitating generalization, among them the introduction of natural contingencies and the use of common stimuli during treatment. Introducing natural maintaining contingencies involves teaching the patient behaviors that will be reinforced in the natural environment. Choosing treatment behaviors that are functional and important to patients and caregivers increases the likelihood that these behaviors will be maintained outside of the treatment situation (Bourgeois, 1991). Similarly, the use of common stimuli increases the probability that the individual with dementia will exhibit trained behaviors in other contexts.

Given the importance of generalization, it is highly desirable to include caregivers in the treatment program. They can learn to promote generalization and provide patients with opportunities to strengthen their communication skills.

Caregiver Training Programs

Nash, Koury, and Lubinski (1991) have evaluated different methods of training nursing staff to communicate effectively with individuals with dementia. These researchers investigated the effect of two training programs on nursing assistants' interactions with patients, their knowledge of geriatric communication disorders, and their problem-solving skills. Program A was traditional in-service training (i.e., 1-hour lecture format) and Program B involved in-service role-playing (i.e., 1-hour training with the focus on enacting situations and problem solving). One group of nursing assistants received no training.

Outcome scores on a test of knowledge of geriatric communication disorders and strategies for improving communication were compared before and after treatment. Results revealed that role-playing was more effective than lecture for promoting a change in employee behavior, although nursing assistants in the lecture group also showed improved test performance. These findings underscore the importance of staff training in creating a supportive communication environment and improved quality of care for institutionalized individuals with dementia.

Ripich (1994) developed a functional communication program for training caregivers of individuals with AD. The seven-step program is called "FOCUSED." Each letter in the word FOCUSED refers to a strategy for improving communication: (F) functional and face-to-face; (O) orient to topic; (C) continuity of topic and concrete topics; (U) unstick any communication blocks; (S) structure with yes/no and multiple-choice questions; (E) exchange conversation and encourage interaction; and (D) direct, short, simple sentences. The FOCUSED training program is divided into six, 2-hour modules designed for family and "formal" caregivers. To test its effectiveness, a pilot study was conducted. Seventeen nursing assistants completed the FOCUSED training program. Knowledge of communication strategies was measured before and after completion of the training. The participants demonstrated increased knowledge of communicative strategies following training, and anecdotally reported increased satisfaction during interactions with individuals with AD (Ripich, 1994). Further positive treatment effects associated with FOCUSED were noted by Ripich, Wykle, and Niles (1995) and Ripich and Ziol (1999). For a review of caregiver education and training programs and the evidence for their use with caregivers of individuals with AD and related dementias, see Zientz and colleagues (2006).

Functional Maintenance Therapy

The primary avenue of service delivery for speech-language pathologists who work with individuals with dementia in skilled-nursing facilities under Medicare reimbursement policies is through functional maintenance therapy (FMT). Glickstein and Neustadt (1995) define FMT as a program for individuals with chronic conditions who need intervention by skilled professionals. FMT typically consists of an evaluation by the rehabilitation professional, followed by the development, establishment, and short-term implementation of a treatment program. As speech-language pathologists and other rehabilitation professionals increasingly provide services to individuals with dementia in a consultant role, caregivers must be trained to carry out treatment prescribed by clinicians. Functional maintenance therapy and other short-term treatment programs necessitate early planning and inclusion of caregivers for carry-over of treatment behaviors to the natural environment. Such an approach is preferable to one in which the planning takes place only when the patient is discharged from therapy.

An example of a functional maintenance program for an individual (BW) with moderately severe dementia (Mini-Mental State Examination score of 9/30) (Folstein et al., 1975) was reported by Bayles, Hopper, Gillespie, Mahendra, Cleary, and Tomoeda (1998). BW was living at home with 24-hour care, until he fractured his hip while transferring from his chair to the bed. BW was admitted to the hospital for 3 days, and then discharged to a skilled-nursing facility for short-term rehabilitation. The speech-language pathologist evaluated BW and spoke with caregivers about techniques to improve communication during transfers. Caregivers were concerned that his dementia, coupled with a moderate hearing loss, would make it impossible for them to teach him transfer strategies. The speech-language pathologist worked with the physical therapist and the family caregivers, using the spaced-retrieval training (SRT) technique, to teach a "safe transfer" maneuver. The patient was prompted with the stimulus question, "You are standing up. You go to sit down. What do you do with your hands?" which was used consistently during training. Initially, the patient responded with statements such as "put them in my pockets" or "put them on my lap." However, after only eight sessions of SRT, and correct responding in the therapy sessions, he learned to reach back with his hands and generalized this strategy to everyday situations when cued by caregivers. This case illustrates the benefit of collaborating with caregivers to promote improved functioning after discharge from treatment.

Use of Volunteers in Treatment with Dementia

Collaborations with activities personnel and recruitment of volunteers are two other ways to extend services to individuals with AD following skilled treatment. Arkin (1995) provided a model for the use of volunteers with her Volunteers in Partnership (VIP) program. Individuals with mild to moderate dementia are paired with university students who assist them in performing weekly volunteer services and who provide memory and language stimulation. Volunteer activities are tailored to each patient's preferences, and include helping at day-care centers, working at animal shelters, and assisting other residents in nursing homes. Memory and language tasks are designed by the clinician and students are trained in their implementation. Audio-taped quiz tasks (Arkin, 1992) are used to teach factual information, and language is stimulated through activities such as association, picture description, solicitation by the student of opinions or advice about how to solve real-life problems, and reading short passages of text. In a pilot program, seven of eleven patients produced more on-topic utterances in response to questions about specific topics, such as President Kennedy's assassination. Eight patients produced more information units during picture description, and three of four patients, who used memory tapes, substantially increased their recall of biographical facts (Arkin, 1995). Doing volunteer work in partnership with university students not only stimulates individuals with dementia, it provides respite for family caregivers.

Measurement Issues

Measuring the effects of treatment for individuals with dementia is especially challenging because intellectual deterioration is progressive. However, as Camp and colleagues (1996) have noted, individuals with AD can demonstrate improvement on specific treatment tasks, despite exhibiting an overall decline in cognitive function. Assessment of change as a result of treatment should include consideration of activities and participation levels of functioning (World Health Organization, 2001). Evaluating change in one dimension of function, such as degree of memory impairment, will be insufficient. Specifically, assessing change with only pre- and post-standardized tests of memory and language will not capture the improvement that individuals with dementia may exhibit in conversational ability, affect and level of engagement, and skills or behaviors taught in treatment sessions. However, measures of quality of life, quality and quantity of communicative interactions, level of engagement and activity participation, and change in behavior may reveal the positive impact of treatment. Focusing solely on improvement in the amount or degree of deficit as a means of demonstrating improvement in therapy is inadequate with patients whose impairments are progressive. Inclusion of multiple measures allows the clinician to determine treatment effects by providing converging evidence of behavioral change.

FUTURE TRENDS IN TREATMENT RESEARCH

In 1991, Bourgeois reviewed the meager literature on behavioral treatments for individuals with dementia. Since 1991, however, interest in treating the cognitive-communication problems of individuals with dementia has increased and results of studies to date suggest that many older adults with dementia can improve function and maintain abilities longer when they participate in cognitive-communication treatment. In fact, enough literature exists to support the development of practice guidelines for speech-language pathologists working with individuals with dementia (see Bayles et al., 2005), and ASHA has published a position statement and technical report (ASHA, 2005 a, b) regarding the roles of SLPs working with individuals who have dementia and the theory and evidence for clinical work with this population. Future researchers should continue to focus on factors that influence patient performance in behavioral therapy, including stage of cognitive decline, type of dementing illness, profile of cognitive deficits, degree of caregiver support, and type of living situation.

Data are needed from large numbers of individuals with dementia to support treatment for individuals at different stages of decline. Generally, most of the treatment studies reported in this chapter involved participants with mild to moderate dementia. Future research should examine treatment of individuals with moderate and moderately severe dementia. Also, differences exist between institutionalized and non-institutionalized individuals, making it difficult to extend results from working with individuals who reside at home to patients living in long-term-care centers. Characteristics of the learning environment, particularly frequency, intensity, and type of therapy, as well as the educational background and expertise of the person providing the therapy still require systematic investigation.

Speech-language pathologists can make important contributions to the well-being of individuals with dementia. With knowledge of preserved abilities and effective intervention principles, the cognitive-communication deficits of individuals with dementia can be minimized. Positive outcomes of behavioral treatment are promising and provide the foundation for continued investigation of effective therapeutic interventions.

KEY POINTS

1. Dementia is a syndrome associated with several different causes, the most common of which is Alzheimer's disease.
2. Individuals with dementia are the profession's fastest growing clinical population.
3. Individuals with dementia develop multiple cognitive deficits and therefore problems in communicating.
4. The distribution of neuropathology of the various dementing diseases explains the patterns of spared and impaired cognitive abilities.
5. Knowledge of these patterns is necessary to provide appropriate assessment and treatment services.
6. The functioning of individuals with dementia can be improved by capitalizing on spared memory systems and reducing demands on impaired memory systems.
7. Individuals with dementia can learn new information and behaviors with appropriate therapeutic techniques.
8. To measure change as a result of therapy, clinicians must evaluate patient function in personal activities and participation in daily life, rather than focusing solely on level of cognitive impairment.

ACTIVITIES FOR REFLECTION AND DISCUSSION

1. Explain the difference between dementia and AD. What are other diseases that cause dementia?
2. What kind of memory is used when a person (a) explains the steps in changing a tire; (b) tells when and where he

or she graduated from high school; and (c) explains what he or she did last Friday night?

3. Discuss the relation between cognition and communication. What effect would a deficit in the following have on communication: episodic memory, lexical memory, procedural memory?

4. Should the communication disorder associated with AD be called aphasia? Why? Why not? Should the communication disorder associated with multiple stroke and vascular disease be called aphasia? Why? Why not?

5. Describe cognitive-communication function of individuals with mild, moderate, and severe AD.

6. What aspects of communication and cognition are important to assess in individuals with AD? What standardized tests might you use to assess these abilities?

7. Explain the principles of successful intervention for individuals with dementia. How is intervention for individuals with irreversible dementia different than intervention for individuals with nonprogressive neurologic conditions?

8. Discuss several behavioral interventions for individuals with dementia and the research evidence associated with these interventions. Think about how you would measure change in a treatment program using one or more of these interventions.

References

Aarsland, D., Andersen, K., Larsen, J. P., Lolk, A., & Kragh-Sorensen, P. (2003). Prevalence and characteristics of dementia in Parkinson's disease: An 8-year prospective study. *Archives of Neurology, 60,* 387–392.

American Psychiatric Association (2000). *Diagnostic and Statistical Manual of Mental Disorders–Text Revision* (DSM-IV-TR) (4th ed.). Washington, DC: Author.

American Speech-Language-Hearing Association. (2005a). *The roles of speech-language pathologists working with individuals with dementia: Position statement.* Rockville, MD: Author.

American Speech-Language-Hearing Association. (2005b). *The roles of speech-language pathologists working with individuals with dementia: Technical report.* Rockville, MD: Author.

Arkin, S. M. (1992). Audio-assisted memory training with early Alzheimer's patients: Two single-subject experiments. *Clinical Gerontologist, 12*(2), 77–96.

Arkin, S. M. (1995). Volunteers in partnership: A rehabilitation program for Alzheimer's patients. (J. Chitwood, Director). In C. K. Tomoeda (Producer), *Telerounds.* Tucson, AZ: The University of Arizona.

Armstrong, L., Bayles, K. A., Borthwick, S. E., & Tomoeda, C. K. (1996). Use of the Arizona Battery for Communication Disorders of Dementia in the UK. *European Journal of Disorders of Communication, 31,* 171–180.

Azuma, T., & Bayles, K. A. (1997). Memory impairments underlying language difficulties in dementia. *Topics in Language Disorders, 18*(1), 58–71.

Bach, D., Bach, M., Bohmer, F., Fruhwald, T., & Grilc, B. (1995). Reactivating occupational therapy: A method to improve cognitive performance in geriatric patients. *Age and Ageing, 24,* 222–226.

Baddeley, A. (1986). *Working memory.* Oxford, England: Oxford University Press.

Baddeley, A. (1999). *Essentials of human memory.* Hove, East Sussex: Psychology Press.

Baddeley, A. D., Bressi, S., Della Sala, S., Logie, R., & Spinnler, H. (1991). The decline of working memory in Alzheimer's disease: A longitudinal study. *Brain, 114,* 2521–2547.

Baddeley, A. D., & Hitch, G. (1974). Working memory. In G. A. Bower (Ed.), *The psychology of learning and motivation* (pp. 47–89). New York: Academic Press.

Baddeley, A. D., & Wilson, B. A. (1994). When implicit learning fails: Amnesia and the problem of error elimination. *Neuropsychologia, 32*(1), 53–68.

Bailey, J., Gilbert, E., & Herweyer, S. (1992, July). To find a soul. *Nursing,* 63–64.

Barona, A., Reynolds, C., & Chastain, R. (1984). A demographically based index of premorbid intelligence for the WAIS-R. *Journal of Clinical Consulting Psychology, 52,* 885–887.

Bayles, K. A. (1991). Alzheimer's disease symptoms: Prevalence and order of appearance. *Journal of Applied Gerontology, 10,* 419–430.

Bayles, K. A., Hopper, T., Gillispie, M., Mahendra, N., Cleary, S., & Tomoeda, C. K. (1998, November). *Improving the functioning of individuals with dementia: An emerging science.* Paper presented at the annual meeting of the American Speech-Language-Hearing Association, San Antonio, TX.

Bayles, K. A., & Kaszniak, A. W. (1987). *Communication and cognition in normal aging and dementia.* Boston, MA: College-Hill Press.

Bayles, K. A., Kim, E. S., Azuma, T., Chapman, S. B., Cleary, S., Hopper, T., Mahendra, N., et al. (2005). Developing evidenced-based practice guidelines for speech-language pathologists serving individuals with Alzheimer's dementia. *Journal of Medical Speech-Language Pathology, 13*(4), xiii–xxv.

Bayles, K. A., & Tomoeda, C. K. (1993). *The Arizona Battery for Communication Disorders of Dementia.* Austin, TX: Pro-Ed.

Bayles, K. A., & Tomoeda, C. K. (1994). *The functional linguistic communication inventory.* Austin, TX: Pro-Ed.

Bayles, K. A., & Tomoeda, C. K. (1997). *Improving function in dementia and other cognitive-linguistic disorders.* Austin, TX: Pro-Ed.

Bayles, K. A., Trosset, M. W., Tomoeda, C. K., Montgomery, E. B, & Wilson, J. (1993). Generative naming in Parkinson's disease patients. *Journal of Clinical and Experimental Neuropsychology, 15*(4), 547–562.

Beck, A. T., Ward, C. H., Mendelson, M., Mock, J., & Erbaugh, J. (1961). An inventory for measuring depression. *Archives of General Psychiatry, 4,* 53.

Borkowski, J. G., Benton, A. L., & Spreen, O. (1967). Word fluency and brain damage. *Neuropsychologia, 5,* 135–140.

Bourgeois, M. S. (1990). Enhancing conversation skills in patients with Alzheimer's disease using a prosthetic memory aid. *Journal of Applied Behavior Analysis, 23*(1), 29–42.

Bourgeois, M. S. (1991). Communication treatment for adults with dementia. *Journal of Speech and Hearing Research, 34*(4), 831–844.

Bourgeois, M. S. (1992). Evaluating memory wallets in conversations with persons with dementia. *Journal of Speech and Hearing Research, 35*(6), 1344–1357.

Bowen, D. M., Davison, A. N., & Sims, N. (1981). Biochemical and pathological correlates of cerebral aging and dementia. *Gerontology, 27,* 100–101.

Braak, H., & Braak, E. (1991). Neuropathological staging of Alzheimer-related changes. *Acta Neuropathologica, 82,* 239–259.

Braak, H., & Braak, E. (1997). Staging of Alzheimer-related cortical destruction. *International Psychogeriatrics, 9*(Suppl 1), 257–261.

Braak, H., Del Tredici, K., Rüb, U., de Vos, R. A. I., Jansen Steur, E. N. H., & Braak, E. (2003). Staging of brain pathology related to sporadic Parkinson's disease. *Neurobiology of Aging, 24,* 197–211.

Broadbent, N. J., Clark, R. E., Zola, S., & Squire, L. R. (2002). In L. R. Squire & D. L. Schacter (Eds.), *Neuropsychology of memory* (3rd ed., pp. 3–23) New York: Guilford Press.

Brush, J. A., & Camp, C. J. (1998). Using spaced-retrieval as an intervention during speech-language therapy. *Clinical Gerontologist, 19*(1), 51–64.

Butters, N., Heindel, W. C., & Salmon, D. P. (1990). Dissociation of implicit memory in dementia: Neurological implications. *Bulletin of the Psychonomic Society, 28,* 359–366.

Calderon, J., Perry, R. J., Erzinclioglu, S. W., Berrios, G. E., Dening, T. R., & Hodges, J. R. (2001). Perception, attention, and working memory are disproportionately impaired in dementia with Lewy bodies compared with Alzheimer's disease. *Journal of Neurology, Neurosurgery and Psychiatry, 70,* 157–164.

Camp, C. J., & Brush, J. A. (1998). Montessori-based interventions for persons with dementia. (J. Chitwood, Director). In C. K. Tomoeda (Producer), *Telerounds.* Tucson, AZ: The University of Arizona.

Camp, C. J., Foss, J. W., O'Hanlon, A. M., & Stevens, A. B. (1996). Memory intervention for persons with dementia. *Applied Cognitive Psychology, 10,* 193–210.

Camp, C. J., Judge, K. S., Bye, C. A., Fox, K. M., Bowden, J., Bell, M., et al. (1997). An intergenerational program for persons with dementia using Montessori methods. *The Gerontologist, 37*(5), 688–692.

Cercy, S. P., & Bylsma, F. W. (1997). Lewy bodies and progressive dementia: A critical review and meta-analysis. *Journal of the International Neuropsychological Society, 3,* 179–194.

Chapman, S. B., Weiner, M. F., Rackley, A., Hynan, L. S., & Zientz, J. (2004). Effects of cognitive-communication stimulation for Alzheimer's disease patients treated with donepezil. *Journal of Speech, Language, and Hearing Research, 47,* 1149–1163.

Chertkow, H., & Bub, D. (1990). Semantic memory loss in dementia of Alzheimer type: What do various measures measure? *Brain, 113,* 397–417.

Clare, L., Wilson, B. A., Breen, K., & Hodges, J. R. (1999). Errorless learning of face-name associations in early Alzheimer's disease. *Neurocase, 5*(1), 37–46.

Clare, L., Wilson, B. A., Carter, G., Breen, K., Gosses, A., & Hodges, J. R. (2000). Intervening with everyday memory problems in dementia of the Alzheimer type: An errorless learning approach. *Journal of Clinical and Experimental Neuropsychology, 22*(1), 132–146.

Connor, D. J., Salmon, D. P., Sandy, T. J., Galasko, D., Hansen, L. A., & Thal, L. J. (1998). Cognitive profiles of autopsy-confirmed Lewy body variant vs pure Alzheimer disease. *Archives of Neurology, 55,* 994–1000.

Cox, D. M., Bayles, K. A., & Trosset, M. W. (1996). Category and attribute knowledge deterioration in Alzheimer's disease. *Brain and Language, 52,* 536–550.

Coyle, J. T., Price, D. L., & DeLong, M. R. (1983). Alzheimer's disease: A disorder of cortical cholinergic innervation. *Science, 219,* 1194–1219.

Crum, R. M., Anthony, J. C., Bassett, S. S., & Folstein, M. F. (1993). Population-based norms for the Mini-Mental State examination by age and educational level. *Journal of the American Medical Association, 269*(18), 2386–2391.

Daselaar, S. M., Rombouts, S. A., Veltman, D. J., Raaijmakers, J. G., & Jonker, C. (2003). Similar network activated by young and old adults during the acquisition of a motor sequence. *Neurobiology of Aging, 24,* 1013–1019.

Davies, P. (1983). An update on the neurochemistry of Alzheimer disease. In R. Mayeux & W. G. Rosen (Eds.), *The dementias.* New York: Raven Press.

Davis, D. G., Schmitt, F. A., Wekstein, D. R., & Markesbery, W. R. (1999). Alzheimer neuropathologic alterations in aged cognitively intact subjects. *Journal of Neuropathology and Experimental Neurology, 58*(4), 376–388.

Dick, M. B., Nielson, K. A., Beth, R. E., Shankle, W. R., & Cotman, C. W. (1995). Acquisition and long-term retention of a fine motor skill in Alzheimer's disease. *Brain and Cognition, 29,* 294–306.

Doyon, J., & Ungerleider, L. G. (2002). Functional anatomy of motor skill learning. In L. R. Squire & D. R. Schacter (Eds.), *Neuropsychology of memory* (3rd ed., pp. 225–238). New York, NY: Guilford Press.

Drachman, D. A., & Leavitt, J. (1974). Human memory and the cholinergic system: A relationship to aging. *Archives of Neurology, 30,* 113–121.

Dubois, M. F., & Hébért R. (2001). The incidence of vascular dementia in Canada: A comparison with Europe and East Asia. *Neuroepidemiology, 20,* 179–187.

Emre, M. (2003). Dementia associated with Parkinson's disease. *Lancet Neurology, 2,* 229–237.

Farber, J. F., Schmitt, F. A., & Logue, P. E. (1988). Predicting intellectual level from the Mini-Mental State Examination. *Journal of the American Geriatrics Society, 36,* 509–510.

Folstein, M. F., Folstein, S. E., & McHugh, P. R. (1975). "Mini-Mental State": A practical method for grading the cognitive state of patients for the clinician. *Journal of Psychiatric Research, 12,* 189–198.

Foreman, M. D. (1987). Reliability and validity of mental status questionnaires in elderly hospitalized patients. *Nursing Research, 36,* 216–220.

Francis, G., & Baly, A. (1986). Plush animals—Do they make a difference? *Geriatric Nursing, 74*(9), 140–143.

Gallagher, D., Breckenridge, J., Steinmetz, J., & Thompson, L. (1983). The Beck Depression Inventory and research diagnostic criteria: Congruence in an older population. *Journal of Consulting and Clinical Psychology, 51,* 945.

Glickstein, J. K., & Neustadt, G. K. (1995). *Reimbursable geriatric service delivery: A functional maintenance therapy system.* Gaithersburg, MD: Aspen.

Goedert, M. (1993). Tau protein and the neurofibrillary pathology of Alzheimer's disease. *TINS, 16*(1), 460–465.

Goldman, J., & Côté, L. (1991). Aging of the brain: Dementia of the Alzheimer's type. In E. R. Kandel, J. H. Schwartz, & T. M. Jessell (Eds.), *Principles of neural science* (3rd ed.). New York: Elsevier Science.

Goodglass, H., & Kaplan, E. (1983). *Boston Diagnostic Aphasia Examination.* Philadelphia: Lea and Febiger.

Hachinski, V. C., Iliff, L. D., Zilhka, E., duBoulay, G. H. D., McAllister, B. L., Marxhall, J., et al. (1975). Cerebral blood flow in dementia. *Archives of Neurology, 32,* 632–637.

Hamilton, M. (1960). A rating scale for depression. *Journal of Neurological Neurosurgery and Psychiatry, 23,* 56.

Hebert, L. E., Scherr, P. A., Bienias, J. L., Bennett, D. A., & Evans, D. A. (2003). Alzheimer disease in the U. S. population: Prevalence estimates using the 2000 census. *Archives of Neurology, 60*(8), 1119–1122.

Heindel, W. C., Salmon, D. P, Shults, C. W., Walicke, P. A., & Butters, N. (1989). Neuropsychological evidence for multiple implicit memory systems: A comparison of Alzheimer's, Huntington's, and Parkinson's disease patients. *Journal of Neuroscience, 9,* 582–587.

Hier, D. B., Hagenlocker, D., & Shindler, A. G. (1985). Language disintegration in dementia: Effects of etiology and severity. *Brain and Language, 25,* 117–133.

Hodges, J. R., & Patterson, K. (1995). Is semantic memory consistently impaired early in the course of Alzheimer's disease? Neuroanatomical and diagnostic implications. *Neuropsychologia, 33*(4), 441–459.

Hoerster, L., Hickey, E. M., & Bourgeois, M. S. (2001). Effects of memory aids on conversations between nursing home residents with dementia and nursing assistants. *Neuropsychological Rehabilitation, 11*(3/4), 399–427.

Holmes, T. (2000). Use of a memory notebook to help Alzheimer's caregivers manage behavioral excesses. *Physical and Occupational Therapy in Geriatrics, 17*(3), 67–80.

Honig, L. S. (1997). Genetics of Alzheimer's disease. *Neurophysiology and Neurogenic Speech and Language Disorders, 7*(4), 6–10.

Hopper, T., Bayles, K. A., & Tomoeda, C. K. (1998). Using toys to stimulate communicative function in individuals with Alzheimer's disease. *Journal of Medical Speech-Language Pathology, 6*(2), 73–80.

Hopper, T., Mahendra, N., Kim, E., Azuma, T., Bayles, K. A., Cleary, S., et al. (2005). Evidence-based practice recommendations for individuals working with dementia: Spaced-retrieval training. *Journal of Medical Speech-Language Pathology, 13*(4), xxvii–xxxiv.

Jefferson, A. L., Brickman, A. M., Aloia, M., & Paul, R. H. (2005). The cognitive profile of vascular dementia. In R. H. Paul, B. R. Ott, & R. Cohen (Eds.), *Vascular dementia: Cerebrovascular mechanisms and clinical management* (pp. 131–144). Totowa, NJ: Humana Press.

Katzman, R., & Bick, K. (Eds.). (2000). *Alzheimer disease: The changing view.* Orlando, FL: Academic Press.

Kinsella, K., & Velkoff, V. A. (2001). U.S. Census Bureau, Series P95/01-1. *An Aging World: 2001.* U.S. Government Printing Office, Washington, DC.

Kramer, J. H., Reed, B. R., Mungas, D., Weiner, M. W., & Chui, H. C. (2002). Executive dysfunction in subcortical ischaemic vascular disease. *Journal of Neurology, Neurosurgery and Psychiatry, 72,* 217–220.

Lowell, S., Beeson, P. M., & Holland, A. L. (1995). The efficacy of a semantic cueing procedure on naming performance of adults with aphasia. *American Journal of Speech-Language Pathology, 4*(4), 109–114.

Lustig, C., & Buckner, R. L. (2004). Preserved neural correlates of priming in old age and dementia. *Neuron, 42,* 865–875.

Mahendra, N., Hopper, T., Bayles, K. A., Azuma, T., Cleary, S., & Kim, E. (2006). Evidence-based practice recommendations for working with individuals with dementia: Montessori-based interventions. *Journal of Medical Speech-Language Pathology, 14*(1), xv–xxv.

Martin, A., & Fedio, P. (1983). Word production and comprehension in Alzheimer's disease: The breakdown of semantic knowledge. *Brain and Language, 19,* 124–141.

McKeith, I. G., Dickson, D. W., Lowe, J., Emre, M., O'Brien, J. T., et al. (2005). Diagnosis and management of dementia with Lewy bodies: Third report of the DLB consortium. *Neurology, 65,* 1863–1872.

McKeith, I. G., Galasko, D., Kosaka, K., Perry, E. K., Dickson, D. W., Hansen, L. A., et al. (1996). Consensus guidelines for the clinical and pathologic diagnosis of Dementia with Lewy Bodies (DLB): Report of the consortium on DLB international workshop. *Neurology, 47,* 1113–1124.

McKeith, I. G., & O'Brien, J. T. (1999). Dementia with Lewy bodies. *Australian and New Zealand Journal of Psychiatry, 33*(6), 800–808.

McKitrick, L. A., Camp, C. J., & Black, F. W. (1992). Prospective memory intervention in Alzheimer's disease. *Journal of Gerontology: Psychological Sciences, 47*(5), 337–343.

McPherson, S. E., & Cummings, J. L. (1997). Vascular dementia: Clinical assessment, neuropsychological features and treatment. In P. D. Nussbaum (Ed.). *Handbook of neuropsychology and aging.* New York, NY: Plenum Press.

Miller, R. G., Rosenberg, J. A., Gelinas, D. F., Mitsumoto, H., Newman, D, Sufit, R, et al. (1999). Practice parameter: The care of the patient with amyotrophic lateral sclerosis (an evidence-based review). *Neurology, 52,* 1311–1325.

Miller, W. R., & Seligman, M. E. P. (1973). Depression and the perceptions of reinforcement. *Journal of Abnormal Psychology, 82,* 62.

Milton, I., & MacPhail, J. (1985). Dolls and toy animals for hospitalized elders: Infantilizing or comforting? *Geriatric Nursing,* 204–206.

Moorhouse, B., Douglas, J., Panaccio, J., & Steel G. (1999). Use of the Arizona Battery for Communication Disorders of Dementia in an Australian context. *Asia Pacific Journal of Speech Language and Hearing, 4,* 93–107.

Morris, J. N., Hawes, C., Fries, B. E., Phillips, C. D., Mor, V., Katz, S., et al. (1990). Designing the national resident assessment instrument for nursing homes. *The Gerontological Society of America, 30*(3), 293–302.

Mungas, D. (2005). Contributions of subcortical lacunar infarcts to cognitive impairment in older persons. In R. H. Paul, B. R. Ott,

& R. Cohen (Eds.), *Vascular dementia: Cerebrovascular mechanisms and clinical management.* (pp. 211–222). Totowa, NJ: Humana Press.

Nash Koury, L., & Lubinski, R. (1991). Effective in-service training for staff working with communication impaired patients. In R. Lubinski (Ed.), *Dementia and communication.* Philadelphia, PA: B. C. Decker.

National Institute on Aging/Alzheimer's Association Working Group. (1996). Apolipoprotein E genotyping in Alzheimer's disease. *The Lancet, 347*(9008), 1091–1095.

Nebes, R. D. (1994). Contextual facilitation of lexical processing in Alzheimer's disease: Intralexical priming or sentence-level priming? *Journal of Clinical and Experimental Neuropsychology, 16*(4), 489–497.

Nebes, R. D., Boller, F., & Holland, A. (1986). Use of semantic context by patients with Alzheimer's disease. *Psychology and Aging, 1*(3), 261–269.

Nebes, R. D., & Brady, C. B. (1988). Integrity of semantic fields in Alzheimer's disease. *Cortex, 24,* 291–300.

Nebes, R. D., Martin, D. C., & Horn, L. C. (1984). Sparing of semantic memory in Alzheimer's disease. *Journal of Abnormal Psychology, 93*(3), 321–330.

Noe, E., Marder, K., Bell, K. L., Jacobs, D. M., Manly, J. J., & Stern, Y. (2004). Comparison of dementia with Lewy bodies to Alzheimer's disease and Parkinson's disease with dementia. *Movement Disorders, 19*(1), 60–67.

Ober, B. A., Dronkers, N. F., Koss, E., Delis, D. C., & Friedland, R. P. (1986). Retrieval from semantic memory in Alzheimer-type dementia. *Journal of Clinical and Experimental Neuropsychology, 8,* 75–92.

Obler, L.K. (1983). Language and brain dysfunction in dementia. In S. Segalowitz (Ed.), *Language functions and brain organization* (pp. 267–282). New York: Academic Press.

Olswang, L., & Bain, B. (1994). Data collection: Monitoring children's treatment progress. *American Journal of Speech Language Pathology, 3,* 55–66.

Orsulic-Jeras, S., Judge, K., & Camp, C. (2000). Montessori-based activities for long-term care residents with dementia: Effects on engagement and affect. *The Gerontologist, 40*(1), 107–111.

Press, D. Z. (2004). Parkinson's disease dementia: A first step? *New England Journal of Medicine, 351*(24), 2547–2549.

Quayhagen, M. P., Quayhagen, M., Corbeil, R. R., Roth, P. A., & Rodgers, J. A. (1995). A dyadic remediation program for care recipients with dementia. *Nursing Research, 44*(3), 153–159.

Reisberg, B., Ferris, S. H., deLeon, M. J., & Crook, T. (1982). The Global Deterioration Scale (GDS): An instrument for the assessment of primary degenerative dementia (PDD). *American Journal of Psychiatry, 139*(1), 136–139.

Reisberg, B., Ferris, S. H., & Franssen, E. (1985). An ordinal functional assessment tool for Alzheimer's type dementia. *Hospital and Community Psychiatry, 36,* 939–944.

Ripich, D. N. (1994). Functional communication training with individuals with AD: A caregiver training program. *Alzheimer Disease and Associated Disorders, 8*(3), 95–109.

Ripich, D. N., & Terrell, B. Y. (1988). Patterns of discourse cohesion and coherence in Alzheimer's disease. *Journal of Speech and Hearing Disorders, 53,* 8–19.

Ripich, D. N, Wykle, M., & Niles, S. (1995). Alzheimer's disease caregivers: The FOCUSED program. *Geriatric Nursing, 16*(1), 15–19.

Ripich, D. N., & Ziol, E. (1999). Training Alzheimer's disease caregivers for successful communication. *Clinical Gerontologist, 21,* 37–56.

Román, G. C. (2003). Stroke, cognitive decline and vascular dementia: The silent epidemic of the 21st century. *Neuroepidemiology, 22,* 161–164.

Román, G. C. (2005). Clinical forms of vascular dementia. In R. H. Paul, B. R. Ott, & R. Cohen (Eds.), *Vascular dementia: Cerebrovascular mechanisms and clinical management* (pp. 7–22). Totowa, NJ: Humana Press.

Rosen, W. G., Mohs, R. C., & Davis, K. L. (1984). A new rating scale for Alzheimer's disease. *American Journal of Psychiatry, 141,* 1356–1364.

Saint-Cyr, J. A., Taylor, A. E., & Lang, A. E. (1988). Procedural learning and neostriatal dysfunction in man. *Brain, 111,* 941–959.

Salmon, D. P., & Bondi, M. W. (1997). The neuropsychology of Alzheimer's disease. In P. D. Nussbaum (Ed.), *Handbook of neuropsychology and aging.* New York: Plenum Press.

Salmon, D. P., Galasko, D., Hansen, L. A., Masliah, E., Butters, N., Thal, L. F., et al. (1996). Neuropsychological deficits associated with diffuse Lewy body disease. *Brain and Cognition, 31,* 118–165.

Salmon, D. P, Shimamura, A. P., Butters, N., & Smith, S. (1988). Lexical and semantic priming deficits in patients with Alzheimer's disease. *Journal of Clinical and Experimental Neuropsychology, 10,* 477–494.

SantaCruz, K., Pahwa, R., Lyons, K., Troster, A., Handler, M., Koller, W., et al. (1999). Lewy body, neurofibrillary tangle and senile plaque pathology in Parkinson's disease patients with and without dementia. *Neurology, 52,* A476–A477.

Santo Pietro, M. J., & Boczko, F. (1997). *The Communication Outcome Measure of Functional Independence: COMFI scale.* Vero Beach, FL: The Speech Bin.

Santo Pietro, M. J., & Boczko, F. (1998, May/June). The Breakfast Club: Results of a study examining the effectiveness of a multimodality group communication treatment. *American Journal of Alzheimer's Disease.*

Schacter, D. L. (1996). *Searching for memory.* New York: Basic Books, HarperCollins.

Schacter, D. L., Rich, S. A., & Stampp, M. S. (1985). Remediation of memory disorders: Experimental evaluation of the spaced-retrieval technique. *Journal of Clinical and Experimental Neuropsychology, 7,* 79–96.

Schacter, D. L., & Tulving, E. (Eds.). (1994). *Memory systems.* Cambridge, MA: MIT Press.

Snowdon, D. A., Grenier, L. H., Mortimer, J. A., Riley, K. P., & Markesbery, W. R. (1997). Brain infarction and the clinical expression of Alzheimer disease. The Nun study. *Journal of the American Medical Association, 277,* 813–817.

Spinnler, H., Della Sala, S., Bandera, R., & Baddeley, A. D. (1988). Dementia, aging, and the structure of human memory. *Cognitive Neuropsychology, 5,* 193–211.

Squire, L. R. (1994). Priming and multiple memory systems: Perceptual mechanisms of implicit memory. In D. L. Schacter & E. Tulving (Eds.), *Memory systems.* Cambridge, MA: MIT Press.

Stokes, T. F., & Baer, D. M. (1977). An implicit technology of generalization. *Journal of Applied Behavior Analysis, 10,* 349–367.

Thompson, C. K. (1989). Generalization in the treatment of aphasia. In L. V. McReynolds & J. Spradlin (Eds.), *Generalization strategies in the treatment of communication disorders.* Lewiston, NY: B.C. Decker.

Tiraboschi, P., Salmon, D. J., Hansen, L. A., Hofstetter, R. C., Thal, L. J., & Corey-Bloom, J. (2006). What best differentiates Lewy body from Alzheimer's disease in early-stage dementia? *Brain, 129,* 729–735.

Tison, F., Dartigues, J. F., Auriacombe, S., Letenneur, I., Boller, F., & Alperovitch, A. (1995). Dementia in Parkinson's disease: A population based study in ambulatory and institutionalized individuals. *Neurology, 45,* 705–708.

Tomlinson, B. E. (1982). Plaques, tangles, and Alzheimer's disease. *Psychological Medicine, 12,* 449–459.

Tomoeda, C. K., & Bayles, K. A. (1993). Longitudinal effects of Alzheimer disease on discourse production. *Alzheimer Disease and Associated Disorders, 7*(4), 223–236.

Tulving, E. (1983). *Elements of episodic memory.* Oxford: Oxford University Press.

Uylings, H. B. M., & de Brabander, J. M. (2002). Neuronal changes in normal human aging and Alzheimer's disease. *Brain and Cognition, 49,* 268–276.

Van der Flier, W. M., & Scheltens, P. (2005). Epidemiology and risk factors of dementia. *Journal of Neurology, Neurosurgery and Psychiatry, 76,* 2–7.

Vanhalle, C., Van der Linden, M., Belleville, S., & Gilbert, B. (1998). Putting names on faces: Use of a spaced-retrieval strategy in a patient with dementia of the Alzheimer type. *Neurophysiology and Neurogenic Speech and Language Disorders, 8*(4), 17–21.

Warrington, E. K. (1975). The selective impairment of semantic memory. *The Quarterly of Experimental Psychology, 27,* 635–657.

Wilson, B. A., Baddeley, A., Evans, J., & Shiel, A. (1994). Errorless learning in the rehabilitation of memory impaired people. *Neuropsychological Rehabilitation, 4*(3), 307–326.

Wilson, R. S., Rosenbaum, G., & Brown, G. (1979). The problem of premorbid intelligence in neuropsychological assessment. *Journal of Clinical Neuropsychology, 1,* 49–53.

Winter, J., & Hunkin, N. M. (1999). Re-learning in Alzheimer's disease [Letter to Editor]. *International Journal of Geriatric Psychiatry, 14,* 983–990.

World Health Organization. (2001). *International Classification of Functioning, disability and health (ICF).* Geneva, Switzerland: WHO.

Zanetti, O., Binetti, G., Magni, E., Rozzini, L., Bianchetti, A., & Trabucchi, M. (1997). Procedural memory stimulation in Alzheimer's disease: Impact of a training program. *Acta Neurologica Scandinavica, 95,* 152–157.

Zientz, J., Rackley, A., Chapman, S. B., Hopper, T., Mahendra, N., Kim, E. S., Cleary, S. (2007). Evidence-based practice recommendations for dementia: Educating caregivers on Alzheimer's disease and training communication strategies. *Journal of Medical Speech Language Pathology, 15*(1), liii–lxiv.

Chapter 36

The Nature and Management of Neuromotor Speech Disorders Accompanying Aphasia

Julie Wambaugh and Linda Shuster

OBJECTIVES

The primary objective of this chapter is to provide the clinician with the information needed to understand the neuromotor speech disorders that co-occur with aphasia and to make appropriate management decisions based upon the current available evidence. To achieve this overarching goal, the following objectives were specified:

1. To provide readers with an understanding of the role of the left cerebral cortex in the control of movement, specifically speech movement.
2. To demonstrate, based upon functional neuroanatomy, that neuromotor speech impairments are probable in many patients with acquired brain damage that produces aphasia, most probably because of the overlap of several of the neural substrates mediating linguistic and motor behaviors.
3. To provide evidence from the literature that argues for the hypothesis that motor speech deficits resulting from damage to the dominant hemisphere are likely to be heterogeneous because of the varied roles that different brain networks play in speech production.
4. To provide suggestions for assessment of apraxia of speech (AOS) for the purposes of developing treatment programs and measuring treatment effects.
5. To provide a summary of the techniques and treatments available for AOS along with a description of the rationale underlying those treatments.

Damage to the language-dominant hemisphere may result not only in aphasia but also in neuromotor speech disorders. Previous editions of this text have provided summaries of early reports of neuromotor speech disorders associated with dominant-hemisphere damage (Square & Martin, 1994; Square, Martin, & Bose, 2001), and the reader is referred to those sources for historical accounts of these disorders. Whereas it is well accepted that the dominant hemisphere is crucial for both language and motor-speech functioning (Square et al., 2001), our knowledge concerning the structural and functional neuroanatomy associated with speech and language is rapidly expanding and changing. In keeping with previous editions of this text, this chapter will provide the reader with current information concerning developments in our understanding of the underlying neurologic bases of motor-speech production. Progress has also been made relative to the management of neuromotor speech disorders in aphasia, and this chapter will serve to inform the reader about treatment advances.

MOTOR-SPEECH DISORDERS ACCOMPANYING APHASIA: STRUCTURAL AND FUNCTIONAL NEUROANATOMY

In the past few years, there has been an explosion of studies using a variety of (mainly noninvasive) technologies to investigate the structural and functional neuroanatomy underlying speech and language. These technologies include positron emission tomography (PET; e.g., Schulz, Varga, Jeffires, Ludlow, & Braun, 2005), functional magnetic resonance imaging (fMRI; e.g., Bohland & Guenther, 2006; Shuster & Lemieux, 2005), transcranial magnetic stimulation (TMS; Watkins & Paus, 2004), diffusion tensor imaging (DTI; Catani, Jones, & ffytche, 2005), and magnetoencephalography (MEG; Gunji, Hoshiyama, & Kakigi, 2001). Each of these technologies has its drawbacks; however, they are powerful tools for studying speech behavior in humans in vivo.

These new studies, as well as scores of earlier lesion, animal, and post-mortem studies on humans, have revealed a speech production network that includes the primary motor (M1) cortex, the left posterior inferior frontal gyrus, lateral premotor areas (PM), medial premotor areas, the left insula, the left parietal cortex, the left superior temporal gyrus (STG), the basal ganglia, the cerebellum, and the thalamus.

1009

Moreover, evidence continues to accumulate in support of the view, proposed by investigators such as Liberman and Mattingly (1985), that there is a tight coupling between the networks involved in speech perception and speech production (Watkins & Paus, 2004). While there is still much to be learned, we do have some idea of the role that each of these areas plays in speech production, as well as how lesions to these areas affect speech production. We describe the cortical areas of the network and their functions below.

Primary Motor Area (M1)

The primary motor area (M1) is located in the anterior bank of the precentral sulcus in area 4 of Brodmann's cytoarchitectonic map of the human cortex (Fig. 36–1). M1 receives direct inputs from somatosensory regions in the parietal lobe,

including Brodmann's area (BA) 1, 2, 3a, and 3b, as well as from BA 5 in the posterior parietal lobe (Ghez & Krakauer, 2000; Purves, Augustine, & Fitzpatrick, 2001). In primates, it also receives direct inputs from four premotor regions: the dorsal and ventral premotor areas on the lateral surface of the hemisphere and the supplementary and cingulate motor areas on the medial surface of the hemisphere. M1 receives indirect inputs from the basal ganglia and cerebellum via the ventrolateral thalamus. In a recent study using cortical stimulation in patients with epilepsy who were undergoing surgery, Greenlee and colleagues (2004) provided evidence of a connection between the orofacial region of M1 and the inferior frontal gyrus (Broca's area). M1 provides direct outputs to cranial-nerve nuclei in the brain stem via the corticobulbar tract and to spinal motor neurons in the spinal cord via the corticospinal tract. The pyramidal cells (also called Betz cells)

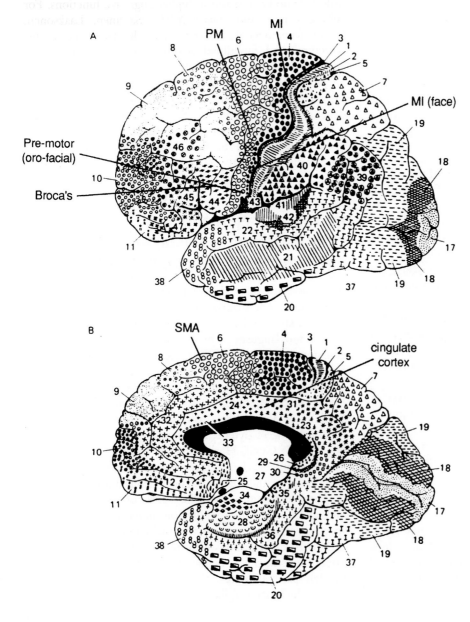

Figure 36–1. Brodmann's areas of the human cerebral cortex. A. Lateral view. B. Medial view. Cortical motor fields are also indicated. MI = primary motor cortex; SMA = supplementary motor area; PM = premotor cortex; Area 44 = Broca's area. (Adapted from Brodmann 1909, 2006, with permission.)

in cortical layer V of M1 that give rise to these tracts are referred to as upper motor neurons. Importantly, these cells also have extensive horizontal connections within M1 (Ghosh & Porter, 1988; Huntley & Jones, 1991).

Our conceptualization of M1 as an area that simply initiates voluntary movements has undergone considerable revision in recent years. Evidence suggests that it participates in motor-learning and cognitive behaviors (Sanes & Donoghue, 2000), and that it can undergo rapid plastic changes, which may underlie both motor learning and recovery of function after a lesion (Classen, Liepert, Wise, Hallett, & Cohen, 1998). Much of our knowledge regarding the functional organization of M1 comes from studies of limb (particularly upper limb) movement (Sanes & Donoghue, 2000). To a large extent, this is because animals can be studied more easily using invasive techniques, such as single-unit recording. However, so far, the general principles underlying movement in primates appear to be universal across body divisions (arm, leg, etc.; Sanes & Donoghue, 2000).

We have known, since John Hughlings Jackson's observations of patients during seizures in the late 19th century, that M1 is organized somatotopically (Jackson, 1931). That is, there are different, separable regions of M1 that represent the body's musculature from head to feet, with the head being represented more laterally and the feet being represented on the medial surface of the hemispheres (Asanuma & Rosen, 1972; Penfield & Roberts, 1959). However, there is considerable evidence to show that, although there are separable motor regions in M1 for the major body divisions (i.e., arm, leg, face, etc.), there is considerable overlap in the representation within these divisions (Barinaga, 1995; Graziano, Taylor, & Moore, 2002; Huang, Sirisko, Hiraba, Murray, & Sessle, 1988, 1989; Sanes, Donoghue, Thangaraj, Edelman, & Warach, 1995). M1 is not organized as a one-to-one mapping of cortical neurons to individual muscles. Rather, cortical neurons act on multiple muscles that behave together in a synergistic way to allow the performance of complex movements (Cheney & Fetz, 1985; Graziano et al., 2002), and to inhibit muscles that perform the opposite movements. Graziano and colleagues (2002) found that electrical microstimulation to the face area of M1 in monkeys evoked complex mouth movements, and the final position of the mouth at the end of the movement was the same for a given site, regardless of the starting position of the mouth. These data show that M1 is organized to allow us to achieve particular movement goals and that the nature of this organization permits us to achieve the same goal in a variety of different ways. Thus, humans adjust their speech movements remarkably well in response to perturbations, such as having a bite block clenched between their teeth while speaking (Warren, Allen, & King, 1984).

Another aspect of the organization of M1 is that, similar to auditory neurons, which are tuned to specific frequencies, and visual neurons, which are tuned to particular visuospatial orientations, motor neurons that are involved in reaching are tuned to particular higher level movement parameters, such as direction (Naselaris, Merchant, Amirikian, & Georgopoulos, 2006), distance (Paninski, Fellows, Hatsopoulos, & Donoghue, 2004), and target position (Paninski et al., 2004).

M1 demonstrates plasticity, and this is thought to be driven by synaptic changes in the horizontal connections within M1 (Sanes & Donoghue, 2000). This plasticity is believed to contribute to both motor learning and recovery of function after a brain lesion, and the plastic changes can occur quite rapidly. For example, Classen and colleagues (1991) used TMS to elicit thumb movements that were consistently in a particular direction. They then asked subjects to practice movements in the opposite direction for 30 minutes. After the practice, the TMS evoked the same thumb movement, but in the opposite direction from the original movement that was elicited, illustrating the rapid use–dependent plasticity of M1. Finally, M1 is thought to be involved in higher cognitive functions. For example, in a study using MEG, Saarinen, Laaksonen, Parviainen, and Salmelin (2006) found that face motor cortex participates in processes such as visuomotor mapping (e.g., learning to make a particular movement in response to a visual symbol) and movement sequencing.

At least since the time of Broca and Wernicke, we have parceled speech production and speech perception into two separate processes. Recent studies, however, suggest that these processes are not so easily separable. Watkins and Paus (2004) found that listening to but not watching speech resulted in larger motor evoked potentials recorded from the orbicularis oris muscle. In an fMRI study, Wilson, Saygin, Sereno, and Iacoboni (2004) found that listening to speech activated motor areas, including M1.

Lesions to M1 result in a variety of symptoms, including spasticity, hyporeflexia, and the loss of the ability to produce fine movements (Purves et al., 2001). Individuals with a unilateral lesion to the face region demonstrate an inability to move their lower faces voluntarily or in response to command, while maintaining the ability to move involuntarily, under conditions such as laughing or crying. In the Mayo nomenclature of dysarthria, lesions to speech areas of M1 produce spastic dysarthria (Darley, Aronson, & Brown, 1975; Duffy, 2005).

Premotor Areas

There are six premotor areas on the lateral and medial surfaces of the hemispheres that have been well defined in monkeys (Picard & Strick, 1996, 2001). In human beings, we have learned about these areas mainly through imaging studies (Schubotz & von Cramon, 2003), and our knowledge is continuing to evolve. The medial areas include the supplementary motor area (SMA, BA 6), the pre-SMA, and three areas in the cingulate sulcus (the cingulate motor area [CMA]): the rostral cingulate motor area (CMAr), the dorsal cingulate motor area (CMAd), and the ventral cingulate motor area (CMAv) (Picard & Strick, 2001). The lateral areas in humans include dorsal (PMd) and ventral (PMv) premotor areas (also BA 6), which lie immediately anterior to the precentral gyrus (Picard & Strick, 2001; Schubotz & von Cramon, 2003).

Medial Premotor Areas

The supplementary motor area (SMA) has been subdivided into two areas (possibly three, see Vorobiev, Govoni, Rizzolatti, Matelli, & Luppino, 1998) based on functional and anatomical differences. They are the SMA proper and the pre-SMA (Picard & Strick, 1996, 2001). The boundary between the SMA and the pre-SMA is the verticofrontal (VCA) line, which is an imaginary vertical line passing through the anterior commissure, perpendicular to the anterior-posterior commissure line (Picard & Strick, 1996, 2001; Talairach & Tournoux, 1988). The SMA projects directly to M1 and to the spinal cord, while the pre-SMA does not. Conversely, the pre-SMA, but not the SMA, is interconnected with the prefrontal cortex. In a recent study using DTI in humans (which permits visualization of the white-matter pathways), Lehéricy and colleagues (2004) found that the SMA and the pre-SMA also project to different areas of the striatum. The pre-SMA projects to the middle portion of the putamen, while the SMA (and M1) project to the posterior portion of the putamen. Like M1, SMA is organized somatotopically, while the pre-SMA is not (Picard & Strick, 2001). Finally, there is little interconnection between the pre-SMA and the SMA.

The role of the pre-SMA was originally thought to be in learning sequential movements; however, it has been shown that it is active during cognitive tasks, such as those involving attention and working memory. In light of these findings, Picard and Strick (2001) suggested that it might be functionally considered to be a part of the prefrontal cortex, rather than being a motor area. Alario, Chainay, Lehéricy, and Cohen (2006) suggested, based on an fMRI study of speech production, that the pre-SMA could be subdivided. They found that the anterior pre-SMA was active during effortful word selection. Activation in the posterior pre-SMA revealed an interaction between factors of word familiarity and word length, which they suggested revealed "a marker of the post-selection encoding processes that precede articulatory execution" (p. 135).

The role of the SMA is related to movement. Intracortical stimulation to the SMA produces movements of the head, forelimbs, and hindlimbs in somatopic order (Picard & Strick, 1996). Alario and colleagues (2006), in the fMRI study described above, found that the SMA was active during word articulation. Lesions to either the left or right SMA from surgical resection lead to a cluster of deficits called the "SMA syndrome" (Krainik et al., 2003, 2004). The resulting speech impairments range in severity from complete mutism to reduced spontaneous speech output. However, complete or nearly complete recovery occurs within a few weeks or months (Krainik et al., 2003, 2004). The basis for this recovery seems to be in the recruitment of the SMA in the contralesional hemisphere (Krainik et al., 2004).

Three cingulate motor areas within the cingulate sulcus have been identified in primates: the rostral cingulate motor area (CMAr), the ventral cingulate motor area (CMAv), and the dorsal cingulate motor area (CMAd). Picard and Strick (2001) proposed that humans have corresponding areas and refer to these as the rostral cingulate zone (RCZ), which is further subdivided into anterior (RCZa) and posterior (RCZp) zones, and the caudal cingulate zone (CCZ). However, there is considerable variability in the configuration of the human cingulate sulcus (Paus et al., 1996). Paus and colleagues found that, although the cingulate sulcus (CS) was continuous in the majority of subjects they studied, a "significant number" had a CS that was divided into two or three segments. Moreover, they observed two secondary sulci, the paracingulate sulcus (PCS), which was present in most subjects, and the intra-limbic sulcus, which was rare. Paus and colleagues also found left-right asymmetries. The CS was more likely to be divided and the PCS to be present in the left hemisphere than in the right hemisphere. These anatomical variations suggest that we need to be cautious in interpreting group data from functional imaging studies of the CS. With regard to function, the CCZ appears to be involved in motor execution, while the RCZa and the RCZp appear to be involved in conflict monitoring and response selection, respectively.

In an fMRI study of word generation by category, Crosson and colleagues (2001) found that the pattern of brain activation (which was analyzed individually for each subject) was dependent on whether a subject did or did not have a prominent PCS. In the majority of subjects who had a PCS, there was activation in the PCS during the word-generation task that did not extend into the CS. However, in subjects who did not have a prominent PCS, the activation did extend into the CS. Kremer, Chassagnon, Hoffman, Benabid, and Kahane (2001) used electrical stimulation to stimulate the ventral bank of the CS in a patient undergoing surgery for epilepsy. The stimulation produced an urge to grasp an object (although there was no object present). The patient was able to describe both her urge to grasp and her inability to resist the urge.

Lateral Premotor Areas

The lateral premotor area (BA 6) lies immediately anterior to the precentral gyrus. BA 44 is sometimes included as part of this area; however, we will discuss BA 44 along with BA 45 in the section on the inferior frontal cortex. The lateral premotor areas are divided, based on both anatomical and functional differences, into dorsal (PMd) and ventral (PMv) regions. However, the precise locations and boundaries of human PMd and PMv are not certain (Picard & Strick, 2001; Schubotz & Yves von Cramon, 2003). The PMd can be further subdivided, also based on anatomical and functional differences, into a rostral and a caudal division. The differences between rostral and caudal PMd are similar to those that underlie the pre-SMA/SMA distinction (Picard & Strick, 1996, 2001). Like the SMA, caudal PMd projects directly to M1 and the spinal cord, while rostral PMd does not. Like the pre-SMA, rostral PMd has connections with the prefrontal cortex, suggesting that it may be involved in cognitive rather than motor functions (Picard & Strick, 1996, 2001; Schubotz & von Cramon, 2003). Schubotz and von Cramon (2003), in their summary of functional imaging studies of the PM, described three functional trends related to the rostral-caudal anatomical gradient in the PMd: one from complex to simple execution, one from the intention to move to the execution of movement, and one from early to late sensorimotor learning stages. In a recent study using MRI, Amiez, Kostopoulos, Champod, and Petrides (2006) found considerable variability in the morphology of human PMd. In the same study, using fMRI, they found activation in the PMd when subjects performed a conditional motor-response task in which they had to push a particular computer mouse button, depending on what color they saw on the computer screen.

In monkeys, the ventral premotor area (PMv) consists of two fields, F4 and F5. It is currently not clear whether there is a human equivalent of F4. It has been proposed that BA 44 (often considered to be part of Broca's area) is the equivalent of monkey F5 (Rizzolatti & Arbib, 1998). This is discussed in further detail below. The PMv appears to be particularly involved during manipulation of objects by the hands. For example, it is active when subjects alter the force of their grip on an object (Ehrsson, Fagergren, & Forssberg, 2001).

Lesions to the PMd in monkeys and man affect the ability to perform conditional motor learning tasks, that is, to select a movement based on a (typically visual) cue (Halsband & Freund, 1990; Purves, Augustine, & Fitzpatrick, 2001). Transcranial magnetic stimulation (TMS, which produces a temporary lesion effect) of the PMd in human subjects disrupted movement selection at an early stage of performance (Schluter, Rushworth, Passingham, & Mills, 1998).

Left Posterior Inferior Frontal Gyrus (IFG)

The posterior inferior frontal gyrus consists of the pars opercularis and the pars triangularis. This region is also known as Broca's area, since Broca originally proposed that this region was the seat of "articulate language" (Broca, 1861). In Brodmann's map, opercularis and triangularis are BA 44 and 45, respectively. Studies have shown that the borders of human BA 44 and 45 vary greatly (Amunts et al., 1999, 2004; Amunts, Schleicher, Ditterich, & Zilles, 2003; Tomaiuolo et al., 1999; Uylings, Jacobsen, Zilles, & Amunts, 2006). BA 44 generally occupies the pars opercularis, but it may encroach on pars triangularis. Similarly, while BA 45 occupies pars triangularis, it may encroach on pars opercularis. There are asymmetries in the size of right and left IFG, and these differences are obvious in children as young as 1 year of age (Amunts et al., 2003). Moreover, the asymmetry in cytoarchitecture continues to change throughout life, suggesting that this region demonstrates plasticity. In a recent postmortem study of 10 brains (five male and five female), Uylings and colleagues (2006) measured the number of neurons and the volume of BA 44 and 45. They found that the volume in left BA 44 was greater than that of right BA 44 in all 10 cases. In addition, all five females and one male showed greater volume of BA 45 in the left hemisphere than in the right, although this asymmetry reached statistical significance only in the females. The total number of neurons was significantly greater in left than in right male BA 44. The number was greater in the left than in the right in female subjects, but the difference did not reach statistical significance. Although the study had a limited number of subjects, these data suggest that investigators who are using neuroimaging to study speech may want to analyze the data of male and female subjects individually, in addition to analyzing the data from the whole group.

Anwander, Tittgemeyer, von Cramon, Friederici, and Knösche (2006) used DTI to study connectivity in Broca's area. They found evidence for three separate anatomical regions, based on white-matter connections, that corresponded to the deep frontal operculum, BA 44, and BA 45. The deep frontal operculum projected through the anterior subinsular white matter and the external capsule to the temporal isthmus and continued to the anterior temporal lobe, into the inferior occipitofrontal fascicle and the inferior longitudinal fascicle. In five of the six subjects, the deep frontal operculum was also connected to the anterior temporal lobe via the uncinate fasciculus. Both BA 44 and 45 displayed the same connections through the inferior external capsule as the deep frontal operculum did. Moreover, they projected to the parietal lobe and the perisylvian region via the arcuate fasciculus in four subjects and to the dorsomedial prefrontal cortex and the ventral portion of the precentral gyrus in all six subjects. Anwander and colleagues also found that the arcuate fasciculus was more dominant in BA 44, while dorsomedial and external capsule connections were more dominant in BA 45. They suggested that their structural data support the conclusions of functional-imaging investigations that have proposed that Broca's area can be parceled into functional subdivisions (e.g., Devlin, Matthews, & Rushworth, 2003; Friederici, 2002).

Imaging studies have shown that IFG is active during a variety of different speech and language tasks, including syntactic tasks such as asking subjects to compare more or less syntactically complex sentences (Friederici, 2002); semantic tasks, such as asking subjects to determine whether a word represented a man-made object (Devlin et al., 2003); phonologic tasks, such as asking subjects to segment words into phonemes (LoCasto, Krebs-Noble, Gullapalli, & Burton, 2004); and speech articulation (Binkofski & Buccino, 2004).

In 1992, Giacomo Rizzolatti and colleagues (de Pellegrino, Fadiga, Fogassi, Gallese, & Rizzolatti, 1992) reported that neurons in F5 in the premotor cortex of monkeys fired both when the monkey performed an action and when the monkey observed a similar action performed by the experimenter. They called these neurons "mirror" neurons and proposed that these neurons "represent" the observed action. Rizzolatti and colleagues argued that the function of mirror neurons is in movement preparation. In particular, they suggested that observation of a movement elicits automatic preparation to perform the same movement, which, in turn, allows the monkey to become faster at executing the movement and to prevail on possible competitors (Rizzolatti, Fadiga, Gallese, & Fogassi, 1996). Based on a subsequent study of humans using TMS, they concluded that humans also possessed a mirror neuron system in BA 44, which they argued is the equivalent of monkey F5 (Fadiga, Fogassi, Pavesi, & Rizzolatti, 1995). Moreover, they suggested that the mirror neuron system provides evidence that modern language abilities arose from a more primitive gestural communication system mediated by F5 in primates. One piece of evidence that is often offered for this claim is human beings' ubiquitous use of gestures while speaking (Rizzolatti & Arbib, 1998).

Since the initial work by Rizzolatti and colleagues, there have been numerous imaging studies of the mirror neuron system that are designed to explore the role in human behavior, particularly speech and language (e.g., Binkofski & Buccino, 2004; see Nishitani, Schürmann, Amunts, & Hari, 2005, for a review). However, contrary to the claims of mirror neuron mechanism supporters, some investigators have argued that Broca's area is not crucial for imitation (Makuuchi, 2005). Moreover, Schütz-Bosbach, Mancini, Aglioti, and Haggard (2006) noted that an important aspect of the putative mirror neuron mechanism is its implication that humans (and other primates) represent their own actions in the same way that they represent the actions of others. However, their study suggested that this is not the case. Finally, the suggestion that the mirror neuron system is important for human speech and language discounts the fact that much of speech articulation is hidden in the mouth and invisible to the listener, and that individuals who are congenitally blind acquire speech and language with little difficulty. Binkofsky and Buccino (2004) suggested that, rather than being specific to speech and language functions, posterior BA 44 is "a high level sensorimotor interface integrating sensory stimuli and cognitive tasks with the related motor representation of hand- and face-related actions" (p. 366). If there is a mirror neuron system that is critical for speech and language, it is more likely to be an auditory mirror neuron system, something that will be discussed below.

As mentioned above, it has been suggested that the IFG plays a role in syntax, semantics, phonology, and articulation. In some studies, these functions have been localized to particular subdivisions of the IFG, while in others, investigators have reported activation simply in Broca's area of the IFG. For example, Friederici (2002) proposed a neurocognitive model of auditory sentence processing in which specific areas of the IFG play particular roles in auditory comprehension. According to the model, the superior-posterior region of BA 44 is involved in phonologic memory, and the superior-anterior and inferior BA 44 are involved in memory of syntactic structure, while BA 45/47 and BA 44/45

work to assign thematic structure based on semantic and morphosyntactic features. Burton, Small, and Blumstein (2000) observed activation in the left IFG when subjects had to separate an initial consonant from a consonant-vowel-consonant (CVC) word stimulus; however, they did not localize the activation to a specific region with the IFG.

The IFG has also been shown to play a role in speech articulation. Based on a meta-analysis of functional imaging studies of speech and language, Indefrey and Levelt (2004) argued that the posterior IFG is involved in syllabification, or the process of clustering segments into syllables. Levelt has also suggested that this area houses a repository of the motor patterns for all of the syllables that a speaker knows, or what he calls the "mental syllabary" (Levelt, 2001). Guenther and colleagues (Bohland & Guenther, 2006; Guenther, Ghosh, & Tourville, 2006) proposed the DIVA (Directions Into Velocities of Articulators) model of speech acquisition and production. In the model's most recent incarnation, each cell in its speech sound map is hypothesized to correspond to neurons in the left PMv and/or posterior Broca's area (Guenther et al., 2006). The cells in the speech map represent different speech sounds. According to Guenther and colleagues, PMv was chosen for the location of the speech sound map cells because of the cells' functional correspondence with mirror neurons. Moreover, Guenther and colleagues have proposed that the speech sound map cells form the mental syllabary of Levelt.

Lesions to the IFG can produce apraxia of speech (Duffy, 2005; Hillis, Work, Barker, Jacobs, Breese, & Maurer, 2004; Mohr et al., 1978). They can also produce aphasia; however, it is the case that lesions that produce persistent aphasia usually involve a large region of the IFG and often encompass the underlying white matter, insula, and basal ganglia (Alexander, Naeser, & Palumbo, 1990; Naeser & Hayward, 1978).

Parietal Lobe

The anterior parietal lobe contains the primary somatosensory cortex, BA 1, 2, 3a, and 3b, or S1. BA 1 lies in the crown of the central sulcus, while BA 3a and 3b lie in the fundus and the rostral bank, respectively. BA 2 lies in the caudal bank of the postcentral gyrus (Geyer, Schleicher, & Zilles, 1999). Studies that have investigated the cytoarchitecture of human S1 have shown that, while there is similarity regarding the location of these areas across brains, there is intersubject variability in their extent (Geyer, Schormann, Mohlberg, & Zilles, 2000). Like M1, S1 is organized somatotopically. The subdivisions of S1 generally respond to different stimuli. BA 1 and 3b neurons respond to cutaneous stimulation, while BA 3a neurons respond to proprioceptive stimulation, and BA 2 responds to both tactile and proprioceptive stimulation (Purves et al., 2001). S1 receives direct input from the thalamus. It projects to more posterior areas in the parietal lobe. In a recent study in monkeys, Simonyan and Jürgens (2005) found that all four subdivisions of S1 projected to the larynx representation in M1. Electrical stimulation to S1 in humans usually produces a tingling or numbness sensation in the representative body part on the contralateral side, rather than the kinds of feeling natural stimuli produce (Nolte, 1993).

There is a secondary somatosensory area (S2) in the parietal operculum, including BA 43 and a small portion of BA 40. S2 is also somatotopically organized (Eickhoff, Amunts, Mohlberg, & Zilles, 2006; Eickhoff, Schleicher, Zilles, & Amunts, 2006). This region has been shown to be responsive to light touch, pain perception, and visceral sensation.

The area of the parietal lobe posterior to the postcentral gyrus is divided into two regions: the superior parietal lobule and the inferior parietal lobule (IPL). The boundary between these areas is the intraparietal sulcus (IPS). The IPL is further subdivided into the supramarginal gyrus (BA 40) and the angular gyrus (BA 39). These areas are connected with the pulvinar and the lateral posterior nuclei of the thalamus (Nolte, 1993). Catani, Jones, and ffytche (2006) used DTI to study the white-matter connections of perisylvian language areas. They discovered a previously undescribed indirect pathway passing through the inferior parietal cortex parallel to the arcuate fasciculus. There was an anterior segment that connected IPL to "Broca's territory" and a posterior segment that connected IPL to "Wernicke's territory." In another recent study using DTI, Rushworth, Behrens, and Johansen-Berg (2006) found that BA 40 and the IPS were connected to the PMv via the arcuate fasciculus, while posterior BA 39 was connected with the parahippocampal gyrus.

Since the seminal work of Liepmann (1913), limb apraxias have been attributed to lesions of the left IPL. Liepmann proposed that space–time plans underlie the performance of skilled movement and that apraxias are a disruption of these plans (Assmus, Marshall, Ritzl, Noth, Zilles, & Fink, 2003). Neuroimaging studies in humans have supported this notion. The right parietal cortex also appears to play a role in these plans. It is involved in processing spatial aspects of movement, while the IPL is involved in processing temporal aspects, such as rhythm (Assmus et al., 2003; Schubotz & von Cramon, 2003). Rushworth, Johansen-Berg, Göbel, and Develin (2003) suggested that the role of the IPL is in motor attention, which they describe as movement preparation or redirection. Assmus and colleagues (2003) proposed that the IPL is involved not only in the computation and storage of space–time plans, but also in processing aspects of movements, so that the plans can, if necessary, be modified.

In the literature on vision, multiple, parallel neural pathways have been identified for processing visual objects. These include a "what" pathway (for identifying an object) and a "where" pathway (for identifying the location of an object in space). Similar pathways have been proposed for speech and language (Guenther et al., 2006; Hickok & Poeppel, 2004; Poeppel & Hickok, 2004; Scott & Wise, 2004). These investigators have suggested that there is an auditory "how" pathway that involves the IPL, in particular the temporoparietal junc-

tion. The role of this pathway (which projects to frontal-lobe regions) is to map "speech sounds on to motor representations of articulation" (Scott & Wise, 2004, p. 15). This pathway would be particularly important for behaviors such as imitation. In the DIVA model (Guenther et al., 2006) a component of the model, the somatosensory error map, lies within the IPL. The role of this component is to compare speech-motor and somatosensory information for the purposes of speech learning and feedback-based motor control.

Kimura and Watson (1989) suggested that the left parietal cortex is involved in selecting movements for movement sequences. In a recent study using fMRI, Shuster and Lemieux (2005) found greater activation in the left parietal cortex when subjects produced longer words (something individuals with AOS putatively have more difficulty with), as compared to when they produced shorter words. Bohland and Guenther (2006) found activation in posterior parietal regions when subjects produced more complex syllable sequences, as opposed to simpler sequences. Longer words and more complex syllable sequences would require more sequencing, so the data from these studies are compatible with Kimura and Watson's view. Like limb apraxias, speech apraxias have been attributed to parietal-lobe lesions (Buckingham, 1979; Duffy, 2005; Kimura & Watson, 1989; Square, Roy, & Martin, 1997; Square-Storer & Apeldoorn, 1991).

Insula

The insula lies hidden beneath the frontal, temporal, and parietal opercula. In Brodmanns' map, it is areas 13 to 16 (Augustine, 1996; Dupont, Bouilleret, Hasboun, Semah, & Baulac, 2003). In monkeys, the insula is divided into three cytoarchitectonic areas. The cytoarchitectonic regions are related to different functions, including olfactory, gustatory, somatosensory, auditory, and visual functions. The insula projects to the cerebral cortex (including the SMA, pre-SMA, S2, and the anterior cingulate gyrus), the basal ganglia, and limbic areas (Augustine, 1996). It receives inputs from a variety of areas, including S1, the superior temporal sulcus, the basal ganglia, and the thalamus.

The insula has been implicated in language function for many years (e.g., Freud, 1891). Functional imaging studies of speech have confirmed this. In an fMRI study of the overt and covert (silent) repetition of mono- and multisyllabic words, Shuster and Lemieux (2005) found that there was greater activation in the left insula during overt production than during covert production. In a study of bilingual individuals, Chee, Soon, Lee, and Pallier (2004) found that the left insula appeared to be involved in phonologic working memory, and that better phonologic working memory correlated with better second-language development.

Although lesions to the left insula were thought to produce AOS (Dronkers, Redfern, & Shapiro, 1993), the insula received considerably more attention in this regard after the publication of a study by Dronkers in 1996. In this study, she found that 25 patients who had been diagnosed with AOS all had lesions encompassing the left anterior insular cortex, while 19 patients who had been diagnosed with aphasia, but not AOS, did not have left insula lesions. This paper has had a significant influence on many investigators' views of AOS and of normal speech production, both because of the double dissociation that she observed, and also because some investigators believe that lesion studies, unlike neuroimaging investigations, reveal brain areas that are *necessary* for the normal performance of a behavior, rather than the areas that are involved in the performance of a behavior but might not be *critical* for that behavior (although cf. Hillis et al., 2004; Marshall & Fink, 2003).

Superior Temporal Gyrus

The superior temporal gyrus (STG) is the location of the primary auditory cortex (A1), as well as Wernicke's area (in the posterior left STG), which has long been associated with the comprehension of spoken language (Wernicke, 1874, 1885). In Brodmann's map, A1 is BA 41 and Wernicke's area is posterior BA 22. The STG is connected to the frontal lobe via the arcuate, uncinate, and inferior occipitofrontal fasciculi, the parietal lobe via the arcuate fasciculus, and the occipital lobe via the inferior occipitofrontal fasciculus (Nolte, 1993). Functional imaging data are changing our view that the STG is only involved in speech reception (Wise, Scott, Blank, Mummery, Murphy, & Warburton, 2001). Wise and colleagues performed a re-analysis of four previous PET studies. They found that the most posterior part of the STG was active during speech production, rather than speech perception. They found that the posterior left superior temporal sulcus was active when subjects listened to the speech of others and during recall of lists of words during verbal fluency tasks. These data suggest that left STG, like the left IFG, is involved in a variety of different receptive and expressive speech and language behaviors.

We have not explicitly described the role of the right cerebral hemisphere (RH) in speech and language behavior. This is not because the RH does not make an important contribution to normal communicative function (Hickok & Poeppel, 2004; Pell, 2006). Such a discussion is simply beyond the scope of this chapter.

Summary and Implications for a Model of Motor-Speech Disorders Accompanying Aphasia

In summary, our views of the role of different brain regions in speech production is changing. Broca's area is not limited to speech production, and Wernicke's area is not limited to speech perception. Moreover, nearly every one of the brain regions that we reviewed has been shown to be involved in speech, language, and cognitive-linguistic functions. This is probably why it has been so difficult to find individuals who demonstrate a pure AOS. It also may be why there has not been universal agreement on the characteristics and labels for the speech disorders that accompany aphasia. Moreover, rather than a strict separation, as some have argued, evidence suggests that the processes of speech production and speech perception are tightly coupled. Studies are finding that there is a great deal of intersubject variability in the size and location of different brain regions, and the functional consequences of these anatomical differences require further exploration.

Developing a model of motor-speech disorders presents some difficulties. As mentioned above, the brain regions involved in speech and language are multifunctional. Data from functional neuroimaging studies can be used to develop such a model, but while these data tell us which areas are involved in a behavior, they do not tell us which areas are critical for the normal performance of that behavior. One way to overcome this problem is to combine imaging technologies (e.g., fMRI and TMS), something that is occurring more and more frequently. An exciting development that will also help are new data-analysis methods, which provide information regarding the temporal characteristics of the activation patterns found with technologies such as fMRI.

The use of lesion studies to develop a model also poses problems. The assumption underlying lesion studies—that if a lesion to a particular area disrupts a function, that area must be responsible for that function—may be erroneous. As Hillis and colleagues (2004) noted, these studies typically assess the probability that a patient with a particular deficit has a lesion in a certain area, rather than assessing how many patients with a lesion to that area demonstrate that particular deficit. The consequence of this is, for example, that ". . . it is possible that all patients with apraxia of speech have insular damage, but that few patients with insular damage have apraxia of speech" (p. 1480).

Despite the difficulties described above, we can make an attempt to develop such a model. A lesion that encompasses the IFG may result in speech sound-substitution errors. These could result from problems such as the incorrect selection of syllables from the mental syllabary, or a disruption of phonologic processes. A lesion to this region might also result in difficulties with producing longer words, which would require greater syllabification. A lesion that encompasses face areas of M1 may result in speech that has a paretic quality. A lesion encompassing the left IPL may result in distortion errors, due to an impairment of motor sequencing, or to an inability to determine how well the somatosensory feedback matches the intended movement. These distortion errors could be perceived as substitution errors at times, due to what Buckingham and Yule (1987) have called "phonemic false evaluation," or an inability to detect subphonemic features (see Shuster & Wambaugh, 2000 for a further discussion of this issue). This could also result in greater difficulties in producing longer words, since they require more motor planning/programming and sequencing.

DISORDERS OF MOTOR-SPEECH PRODUCTION ACCOMPANYING APHASIA: DEFINING FEATURES

A focal lesion in the language-dominant hemisphere that results in aphasia may also result in a neuromotor speech disorder (or disorders). The neuromotor speech disorders most likely to be associated with such a lesion are apraxia of speech (AOS) and unilateral upper motor neuron dysarthria (UUMN dysarthria; Duffy, 2005).

We consider the speech production errors observed in AOS and UUMN dysarthria to be nonaphasic in nature. Square and colleagues (2001) provided a discussion of "speech errors in aphasia" and noted that a significant amount of research has been dedicated to determining whether speech errors in aphasia are motoric (phonetic) or linguistic (phonologic) in nature. As summarized by Square and others (Blumstein, 2001; Kurowski, Hazen, & Blumstein, 2003), persons with "anterior" aphasia tend to evidence phonetic-level disruptions realized as errors in various aspects of articulation. Although sound errors in "posterior" aphasia are generally considered to be phonologic in nature and phonetically intact, some subtle temporal speech differences have been reported (see Square et al., 2001, for a review).

It is not the purpose of this chapter to engage in a discussion of the nosology of speech errors associated with aphasia. Whereas some authors consider phonetic-level disruptions to be symptoms of aphasia (Blumstein, 2001; Kurowksi et al., 2003), we believe phonetic-level errors such as sound distortions and slow rate of production are necessarily motoric disturbances and, even when observed in persons with aphasia, are most likely the result of neuromotor speech disorders. Descriptions of the defining characteristics and symptoms of AOS and UUMN dysarthria are provided in the following sections.

Apraxia of Speech

The speech behaviors considered to define AOS have undergone considerable revision since Darley and colleagues' early description of the disorder (Darley et al., 1975). We agree with Croot (2002) that our current understanding of AOS is a "work in progress" (p. 268), which includes our knowledge of the symptoms that define the disorder. We ascribe to the diagnostic criteria advanced by McNeil, Robin, and Schmidt (1997) and elaborated by Wambaugh, Duffy, McNeil, Robin, and Rogers (2006a). These criteria reflect a carefully considered synthesis of classic and current perceptual, acoustic, and physiologic evidence concerning behaviors observed in individuals with AOS. As described by McNeil and colleagues (1997), the speech characteristics considered to be necessary for a diagnosis of AOS include slow speech rate (lengthened segments and intersegment durations), sound distortions, distorted sound substitutions, sound errors that are relatively

consistent in type and location on repeated productions, and prosodic abnormalities. Symptoms that are consistent with a diagnosis of AOS, but do not allow a differential diagnosis in and of themselves include articulatory groping, perseverations, speech-initiation problems, awareness of errors, repeated attempts, and increasing errors with increasing length or complexity of utterances. Behaviors that are more likely attributable to a language disruption than to AOS would include transposition and anticipatory errors. Behaviors such as normal prosody or consistently normal or fast rate of speech production would contraindicate a diagnosis of AOS.

UUMN Dysarthria

Our understanding of the clinical characteristics and pathophysiology of UUMN dysarthria is also a work in progress. The reader is referred to Duffy (2005) for a concise summary of the speech characteristics observed in UUMN which reflects findings from Duffy and Folger's (1996) retrospective study supplemented by additional confirmatory reports. As reported by Duffy (2005), the most frequently occurring speech deficit observed in UUMN dysarthria has been a disruption of articulation, primarily in the form of imprecise consonants. Disturbances in speech alternate-motion rates (AMRs) were the second most commonly occurring speech disorder seen in UUMN dysarthria, with slow rate reported most often (note: imprecise and irregular AMRs were each reported in approximately one-third of Duffy and Folger's cases). Disorders of phonation were also reported in a relatively high percentage of cases, with harshness being the most frequently reported symptom. Mildly slowed rate and mild hypernasality and/or nasal emission were noted in 18% and 14% of cases, respectively (Duffy, 2005).

MANAGEMENT OF NEUROMOTOR SPEECH DISORDERS ACCOMPANYING APHASIA

As discussed in the previous section, AOS and UUMN dysarthria are the neuromotor speech disorders most likely to accompany aphasia. Although other dysarthrias may co-exist with aphasia, in most cases additional neurologic conditions beyond that which resulted in aphasia would probably be present.

In the remainder of this chapter, we will focus on the treatment of AOS rather than the dysarthrias. Our decision to limit discussion of the management of the dysarthrias was made for several reasons. First of all, UUMN dysarthria may often be mild and relatively transient in terms of clinical presentation (Duffy, 2005). In addition, Duffy notes that "when UUMN dysarthria is the primary communication deficit, aphasia, apraxia of speech, and nonaphasic communication deficits are frequently not present" (p. 260). Furthermore, published investigations of treatment for UUMN dysarthria are not currently available.

To reiterate, other types of dysarthria may be present with aphasia, but rarely will be the result of the same neurologic event that caused the aphasia. Treatment for the dysarthrias is a complex subject; a superficial review of the topic would be of little use to the reader, and a thorough consideration of the topic is beyond the scope of this chapter. The reader is directed to recent publications concerning the management of dysarthria and is encouraged to take note of the treatment guidelines provided by the Academy of Neurologic Communication Disorders and Sciences (ANCDS; www.ancds.org) (Duffy, 2005; Duffy & Yorkston, 2003; Hanson & Yorkston, 2004; Spencer, Yorkston, & Duffy, 2003; Yorkston, Hakel, Beukelman, & Fager, 2006; Yorkston et al., 2001; Yorkston et al., 2003).

Considerations in the Treatment of AOS

The development, testing, and reporting of treatments for AOS began in 1973 with Rosenbek, Lemme, Ahern, Harris, and Wertz's influential report of the effects of their eight-step task continuum. Since that time, considerable progress has been made and a substantial body of literature now exists documenting the benefits of AOS treatments. The Academy of Neurologic Communication Disorders and Sciences (ANCDS) Writing Committee of Treatment Guidelines for AOS recently reviewed and evaluated the existing evidence base for AOS treatments and concluded that "taken as a whole, the AOS treatment literature indicates that individuals with AOS may be expected to make improvements in speech pro-duction as a result of treatment, even when AOS is chronic" (Wambaugh, Duffy, McNeil, Robin, & Rogers, 2006b, p. lxiii).

Despite advances in understanding the effects of various AOS treatments, a technology of AOS treatment, per se, does not exist. Limited data are available to guide the clinician in the selection of a specific treatment for a specific patient. Outcome prediction is extremely limited for most AOS approaches, particularly with respect to functional outcomes. We will provide a summary of the available AOS treatment approaches along with considerations for selecting appropriate treatments and documenting treatment effects. As noted by Wambaugh and colleagues (2006b), the treatment of individuals with AOS requires integration of objective evidence, knowledge gained through clinical experience, theoretical rationale, and consideration of patient requirements and wishes.

In the previous edition of this text, Square and colleagues noted that recommendations for selection of treatment interventions for AOS had historically been based upon AOS severity (see Table 36-1; Square et al., 2001). They questioned the appropriateness of such an approach and instead, proposed that the presumed underlying pathophysiologies should guide treatment selection. Specifically, Square and colleagues suggested that three types of deficits related directly to three types of interventions: (1) postural shaping; (2) production of functional units (coordinative structures); and (3) rhythm and pacing. Accordingly, as seen in Table 36-1, they specified levels of intervention at which various treatment techniques were considered to operate.

TABLE 36–1

Traditional Approaches for Patients with Apraxia of Speech of Different Degrees of Severity with Speculated Level of Intervention

Severity Level	Recommended Approaches	Level of Intervention
Severe	Segmental/syllabic level imitation with • Imitation • Phonetic placement • Phonetic derivation • Derivation plus placement	Postural shaping (spatial targeting) and/or production of functional units of speech (coordinative structures)
	• Key-word technique Imitation of contrasts Contrastive stress drills	Rate and melodic flow
Moderate	Intersystemic facilitators • Tapping foot • Tapping leg • Finger counting • Finger tapping	Rate and melodic flow
	Intrasystemic facilitators Pacing board	
Mild	Expanded contrastive stress drills	Rate and melodic flow

(From Square, P. A., .)

We would argue that the choice of a treatment approach should take into consideration both the theorized pathophysiology and the level of severity. For example, an individual with AOS may present with difficulties in transitioning between sounds/syllables only in the context of multisyllabic words containing consonant clusters. Another individual may evidence difficulty in transitioning between sounds in monosyllabic words. Although both individuals demonstrate difficulties in coordination of movements, the level of disruption in terms of severity obviously differs and so should the treatment approach. A disruption of coordinated production at the syllabic level would likely require significant direction from the clinician and necessitate techniques such as phonetic placement, modeling, and practice with integral stimulation. A disruption of coordinated production at the multisyllabic level may require minimal clinician instruction and may benefit from reducing the rate of production.

The reader may have noted a "mismatch" in suggested technique and presumed pathophysiology for the less severe patient in the preceding paragraph. That is, a rate and melodic flow technique (i.e., rate control) was suggested for a problem of coordination. This suggestion was made to illustrate the point that at present, the impact of most treatments for AOS on the underlying speech disruption is not well understood. Rate and melodic flow treatments (to be termed "rate/rhythm treatments" in subsequent discussions) have been shown to improve articulation (i.e., spatial targeting and/or production of functional units of speech) (Wambaugh & Martinez, 2000). It is not unlikely that articulation-oriented treatments will eventually be shown to have a positive influence on rate and melodic flow. For example, Croot, van Heyst, Deacon, and Law (2006) provided preliminary findings suggesting that an articulatory-kinematic treatment was associated with a reduction in multiple attempts in a speaker with AOS. Therefore, the reader should recognize that presently it is not possible to establish empirically a clear correspondence between pathophysiology and purported level of intervention for a given AOS treatment. Until treatment outcomes are demonstrated across a range of behaviors for a specific AOS treatment, the clinician should understand the theoretical mechanisms by which a treatment operates (i.e., treatment rationale) and determine whether those mechanisms are compatible with the patient's pathophysiology. The AOS Treatment Guidelines Technical Report: Evidence Table (ANCDS, 2006) is a comprehensive resource for reviewing the rationales for the AOS treatments included in the development of the guidelines.

The selection of a treatment should entail more than a determination of severity and probable pathophysiology. A thorough assessment should not only assist in making the preceding determinations, but should also lead to the identification of appropriate treatment targets, outcome measures, and viable treatment techniques. As noted by Square and colleagues (2001), neuromotor speech disorders associated with aphasia are not homogeneous. Consequently, assessment and treatment should be tailored to the individual.

Assessment for Treatment Planning

Errors in sound production are a defining feature of AOS and articulatory precision is often the focus of AOS treatments (Wambaugh et al., 2006a). As such, the clinician should have thorough knowledge of the patient's strengths and weaknesses in terms of sound production. In our experience, only rarely in cases of severe AOS or extremely mild AOS are all sounds produced with equal difficulty or ease. It is strongly suggested that an inventory of sound production be conducted, with multiple exemplars of all sounds elicited at levels that are appropriate for the patient. The level at which sound production becomes problematic for the individual should be apparent from initial contacts and assessments. For example, some patients may produce few sound errors with individual mono- and bi-syllabic words, but produce increasing numbers of errors with three- or four-syllable words or with phrases containing mono- and bi-syllabic words. To be able to structure therapy to include opportunities for success as well as for challenges, the clinician should have data available for production contexts that are easy for the patient as well as for those that are difficult. An example of items used to elicit production of most consonants in the initial and final syllables of monosyllabic words is shown in Appendix 36.1. A useful Internet resource for selecting words on the basis of factors such as phonemes, syllable structure, length, stress patterns, word type, and word frequency is the MRC Psycholinguistic Database (2006). Phoneme frequency may also be of interest in assessing and selecting sounds for treatment, and the reader is referred to Mines, Hanson, and Shoup (1978). An example of multisyllabic words that were selected to be balanced in terms of syllable shape and phoneme type and position, and that reflect a range of phoneme frequency, is provided by Mauszycki (2006) (Appendix 36.2).

The way in which items are presented to elicit productions can affect performance (Wambaugh, Nessler, Bennett, Mauszycki, 2004). Therefore, consideration should be given to the structuring of the stimuli used in elicitation of sound productions. Randomized presentations, wherein exemplars of target sounds are not presented sequentially, are likely to be more challenging than blocked presentations, in which all exemplars of a sound are presented in order.

Productions may be elicited through various modes, such as immediate repetition, delayed repetition, oral reading, sentence completion, confrontation naming, and discourse. Because most individuals with AOS will also have aphasia, elicitation modes may be constrained by language factors such as limited reading ability and significant word-retrieval deficits. Unfortunately, there are no data indicating how well different elicitation modes approximate spontaneous productions in AOS. Intuitively, it would seem that modes that are highly constrained and have maximal clinician input, such as repetition and modeling, may not be the most desirable. However, this notion may not be correct, and the patient's language disturbances may necessitate constrained elicitation conditions. Although analysis of sound production in discourse may have appeal in terms of ecologic validity, reliable methods for eliciting adequate numbers of productions of significant sounds have not yet been developed.

Examples of sentence-completion items used to elicit words containing specific sounds of interest are provided in Appendix 36.3. Sentence-completion elicitation does not entail provision of a clinician model, which may serve to make it a more valid indicator of the patient's true production abilities. Difficulties in word retrieval may be minimized if sentences are constructed for maximal cueing (i.e., if sentences are heavily semantically loaded). However, it may be difficult to construct sentences that are appropriate for less frequently occurring words, and such words may be necessary when targeting sound production at a multisyllabic level of production. Furthermore, word-retrieval problems may be severe enough to prohibit sentence completion. Utilizing sentence completion in a delayed-repetition format may allow the clinician to work around the preceding problems. That is, by providing the desired response prior to the sentence-completion request, it is more likely that the factors of low frequency of occurrence and word-retrieval deficits will not prohibit production of the desired word. To use this elicitation mode, the clinician first provides an explanation of the task, then models the desired response, and finally provides the incomplete sentence for the patient to complete. Several practice trials may be necessary to establish the correct pattern of responding.

Example 1

Clinician: "I'm going to say a sentence and I'd like you to focus on the word at the end of the sentence. I'm going to repeat the sentence leaving off the last word. I would like you to finish the sentence for me, using that word."
Clinician: "My dog is very sick, so I'm going to take him to the VET. Now you finish the sentence for me. My dog is very sick, so I'm going to take him to the _____."

Example 2

Clinician: "I'm going to say a sentence and ask you to finish it for me. But first, I'll say the whole sentence so you know what to say when it's your turn."
Clinician: "To get the news, I like to read a newspaper or a MAGAZINE. Now you finish the sentence that I'm going to start. To get the news, I like to read a newspaper or a _____."

After obtaining adequate samples of sound production at appropriate levels of complexity, performance should be summarized by sound, sound class, word position, complexity level, and patterns of errors. Any error patterns are likely to be unique to the individual; consequently, error analysis should be individualized.

Beyond sound production, AOS treatments may also target and/or impact durational aspects of speech (Wambaugh et al., 2006a). The clinician may wish to measure various durations that may be germane to treatment. For example, rate of speech in syllables per second may be of interest. Whole-word durations as well as relative durations of syllables within words may be useful measures for planning and measuring the effects of rate/rhythm control treatments. Durational measures of individual sound segments and interword intervals may reveal information pertinent to treatment. The preceding types of measures are easily conducted using relatively inexpensive speech-analysis software (e.g., Multi-Speech™, Model 3700 [Kayelemetrics, 2006]).

Other behaviors that are frequently observed with AOS, such as false starts, silent or audible groping, filled or silent pauses, starters, and motor perseverations may serve as treatment targets and/or outcomes. Difficulty with speech production may affect an individual's willingness to initiate speech. As such, quantification of speech initiations may also be considered for inclusion during assessment. Reliable measurement contexts and procedures have not been developed for the preceding behaviors associated with AOS. However, as noted by Wambaugh, "the current unavailability of such measures should not prohibit . . . (one) . . . from attempting to estimate the effects of treatment at such levels; however, caveats regarding reliability should be provided when interpreting findings" (Wambaugh, 2006, pp. 320–321).

Measures of intelligibility and comprehensibility should always be considered for inclusion in pretreatment assessment. Tests designed to assess intelligibility in dysarthria, such as the Word Intelligibility Test (Kent, Weismer, Kent, & Rosenbek, 1989) and the Assessment of Intelligibility of Dysarthric Speech (Yorkston & Beukelman, 1989) are appropriate for assessing intelligibility in AOS. Qualitative ratings, such as those described by Duffy (2005) are also appropriate, as are ratings of comprehensibility (Duffy, 2005).

Variability in speech production across different sampling occasions may or may not affect assessment for treatment planning. The extent to which productions vary from day to day is likely to be a factor that differs for each individual with AOS. To ensure that appropriate treatment goals and stimuli are selected, the clinician may wish to conduct repeated measures of sound production. Of course, upon selection of treatment targets and outcome measures, the clinician would be well advised to establish a baseline of performance that can be used to estimate the effects of treatment. This would necessitate repeated measurement of the outcomes of interest prior to the initiation of treatment.

As noted in the AOS treatment guidelines report (Wambaugh et al., 2006a), there are virtually no data to guide the clinician in the selection of one treatment approach over another. We, like other authors (Square et al., 2001; Wertz et al., 1984) advocate a period of trial therapy to assist in selecting a treatment approach.

Theraputic Approaches for the Treatment of AOS

The extant AOS treatment literature provides examples of many different treatment techniques. The AOS Treatment Guidelines Committee reported that existing AOS treatments generally fell into one of the following categories of general approaches: (1) articulatory-kinematic treatments, (2) rate/rhythm control treatments, (3) intersystemic facilitation/reorganization treatments, and (4) alternative augmentative communication (AAC) approaches (Wambaugh et al., 2006a).

The AOS guidelines report provided effectiveness determinations for each of the preceding treatment categories on the basis of the quality of the evidence available through December, 2003. The AOS committee concluded that "articulatory kinematic approaches were determined to be 'probably effective'; rate/rhythm control approaches and intersystemic approaches were considered to be 'possibly effective'; and AAC approaches could not be rated in terms of likelihood of benefit" (Wambaugh et al., 2006b; p. lxii). The report also provided recommendations concerning the clinical utilization of the different AOS approaches. The strength of the recommendation is an important component of the recommendation. Effectiveness determinations coincide with recommendation strength in that the extent and quality of the evidence supporting treatment approaches serves as the basis for the designation of both.

The AOS guidelines report used the recommendation scheme employed by the American Academy of Pediatrics (Marcuse et al., 2004) with potential recommendations being *strong recommendations, recommendations, options,* and *no recommendation*. Recommendation-strength designations are intended as translational aids for clinicians (Marcuse et al., 2004). That is, the strength of the recommendation serves as a guide for the clinician in terms of importance of adherence to the recommendation. A strong recommendation reflects the guidelines committee's belief that the evidence supporting a treatment approach is of high quality. Strong recommendations should be followed unless there are strong contraindications for a particular patient. None of the AOS treatment approaches had enough empirical support to warrant a strong recommendation.

Recommendations are assigned when the committee considers the evidence to be less strong, but still substantial, and benefits clearly exceed risks (Marcuse et al., 2004). Clinicians should typically follow recommendations, but should consider patient preferences and be alert to new evidence concerning the approach. Articulatory-kinematic approaches were recommended for use "with individuals with moderate

to severe AOS who demonstrate disrupted communication due to disturbances in the spatial and temporal aspects of speech production" (Wambaugh et al., 2006b; p. lxii).

Options are used as the designation for treatments when the evidence base is relatively weak or when benefits do not clearly outweigh risks (Marcuse et al., 2004). Clinicians should be aware of such treatments as having potential utility, but clinician judgment and patient preference should play important roles in selecting treatment. Clinicians should be watchful for new evidence relevant to the treatment option. AOS rate/rhythm control approaches, intersystemic treatments, and AAC approaches were designated as treatment options in the AOS guidelines report.

The following sections describe treatment techniques for AOS that have been reported in the literature. The general treatment approaches identified in the AOS treatment guidelines will be used as the organizing framework (Wambaugh et al., 2006a). The presumed mechanisms for treatment effects will be discussed for each general approach so that the reader may relate the information to presumed pathophysiology. Treatment targets and candidacy issues will also be discussed so that the issue of severity may be taken into account.

Articulatory-Kinematic Approaches

Approximately half of the treatment investigations that were included as the evidence base for the AOS treatment guidelines report were characterized as articulatory-kinematic in nature (Wambaugh et al., 2006a). That is, articulatory-kinematic treatments "were those in which the therapy techniques were used to facilitate improved movement and/or positioning of the articulators in an attempt to promote better speech production" (Wambaugh et al., 2006a; p. xix). The terminology utilized in Square and colleagues' (2001) previous version of this chapter to describe the foci of these types of techniques in terms of presumed pathophysiology was "enhancing postural shaping and re-establishing functional units of speech" (p. 864).

Numerous techniques have been used to promote improved spatial or temporal aspects of speech production. Many of the articulatory-kinematic techniques have been extensively written about in the speech literature since the 1930s (Van Riper, 1939). Explanations of these facilitative techniques used with AOS and aphasia are presented in detail by Wertz and colleagues (1984) and Square-Storer (1989).

An underlying theme crossing virtually all articulatory-kinematic approaches is that repeated, motoric practice of speech targets is a necessary component of treatment. Furthermore, most of the articulatory-kinematic treatment approaches included in the AOS guidelines utilized modeling/repetition to elicit desired productions. A potentially powerful variant of modeling/repetition, originally described by Rosenbek, Lemme, Ahern, Harris, and Wertz (1973), which has been incorporated into several treatment hierarchies, is integral stimulation, in which the patient is instructed to "watch me, listen to me, and say it with me" (Deal & Florance, 1978; Florance & Deal, 1977; LaPointe, 1984; Rosenbek et al., 1973; Wambaugh, Kalinyak-Fliszar, West, & Doyle, 1998a; Wambaugh, Martinez, McNeil, & Rogers,1999; Wambaugh, West, & Doyle, 1998b; Wertz et al., 1984). Integral stimulation attempts to bring to a conscious level of awareness the "look" and "sound" of the movement pattern, while combining this awareness with simultaneous practice.

Other techniques used to stimulate awareness of articulatory postures and movements are phonetic placement and phonetic derivation. Phonetic-placement techniques involve the use of descriptions of where (place) and how (manner, voice) sounds are made, with descriptions provided as verbal explanations, with or without visual modeling (Wambaugh et al., 1998a, 1998b, 1999), drawings (Raymer, Haley, & Kendall, 2002), videotaped models (Aten, 1986), and/or manipulation of the orofacial musculature by the clinician (Square et al., 2001). Phonetic derivation and shaping techniques (Wertz et al., 1984; Knock, Ballard, Robin, & Schmidt, 2000) are those that build upon an articulatory or orofacial skill already in the patient's repertoire. That is, instructions or models are provided regarding how to modify existing productions to obtain different or improved productions. For instance, if the patient can produce nonspeech lip popping, this action may serve as the basis for providing both place and manner of production for /p/ and /b/. Or, using speech, a patient may be able to produce /s/ but not /ʃ/; /ʃ/ may be derived from /s/ by having the patient slowly draw his or her tongue posteriorly along the palate.

The key-word technique is related to phonetic derivation. In this approach, a word that the patient can produce acceptably and that contains the target sound being worked upon is produced by the patient while the clinician calls to his or her attention the feel (tactile and kinesthetic) of the sound. For instance, if the goal is volitional control over the production of /s/, and the patient can produce her husband's name, 'Sam,' the name would be used to enhance the feel of /s/ so that this movement can be produced volitionally in other words.

Another method of improving speech production in AOS is to provide "enhanced sensory feedback through the pairing of dynamic tactile-kinesthetic input with auditory and visual stimulation" (Square et al., 2001; p. 866). Prompts for Restructuring Oral and Muscular Phonetic Targets (PROMPT; Chumpelik, 1984; Hayden, 1999; Square et al., 2001) is a highly developed system for providing instruction for articulatory movements and speech production in the treatment of AOS. PROMPT utilizes combinations of auditory, visual, tactile, and kinesthetic cues that are "dynamic in nature and are designed to provide sensory input regarding the place of articulatory contact, extent of mandibular opening, presence and manner of articulation, and/or coarticulation" (Bose, Square, Schlosser, & van Lieshout, 2001; p. 769). PROMPT is described more thoroughly in Square et al. (2001) and is discussed further in the subsequent section "Formalized Treatment Programs with Supporting Evidence."

Enhanced feedback and cueing in the form of visual displays of tongue-to-palate contacts are treatment techniques made available through electropalatography (EPG). With EPG, the patient (and usually the clinician as well) wears a pseudopalate embedded with electrodes that detect contact of the tongue. A pseudopalate is custom-made from an impression of the individual's hard palate (typically obtained through a dental service) and bears similarities to the palatal portion of a dental retainer. Electrodes embedded in the plastic pseudopalate feed information about tongue contact to computer-based software. Thus, a computerized, visual display is provided in real time, depicting tongue-to-palate contacts. The clinician may provide visual and acoustic models for the patient, who then receives visual feedback concerning the accuracy of his or her tongue placement in target productions. Little research exists to support the use of EPG in the treatment of AOS. Howard and Varley (1995) reported improvements in articulation in a case study with an individual with AOS. It is expected that the decreasing costs and increasing availability of EPG (e.g., EPG3 – Articulate Instruments, 2007; LogoMetrix, 2005) will lead to additional information concerning the potential benefits of EPG for AOS. Electromagnetic articulography (EMA) is another method by which visual biofeedback of tongue movement may be provided. Articulator movements are tracked through the use of magnetic fields and receiver coils that are attached to the articulators. Katz, Bharadwaj, and Carstens (1999) demonstrated the utility of EMA in improving /ʃ/ - /tʃ/ contrasts in an individual with AOS. Unfortunately, EMA is prohibitively costly for most clinical use. As with EPG, additional research is required to document the benefits of EMA for the treatment of AOS.

In a recent investigation, Rose (2006) compared three methods of providing information concerning articulation in a speaker with chronic, moderate AOS and aphasia. The three treatments all involved contrasting target and error productions, providing information about manner and place of production, imitation, and reinforcement. The treatments differed in terms of how the articulatory information was delivered, with "verbal" treatment utilizing verbal and graphic information, "gestural" treatment employing gesturally cued articulation, and "combined" treatment involving all techniques used in the other two treatments. Results revealed that all treatments resulted in significant improvements in production, with no difference in performance noted between treatments. Although the findings of this investigation require replication, they suggest that for this speaker, the nature of the information provided in treatment was more important than the modality of delivery. This study highlights the critical need for comparative investigations of treatment techniques.

All of the preceding techniques, with the exception of repeated practice, are designed to provide additional stimulation in various forms to the speaker to facilitate accuracy of articulation. This is consistent with the concept of AOS reflecting a disruption in the process of translation of correctly selected sounds to previously learned articulatory-kinematic parameters (McNeil et al., 1997). That is, there is an assumption that speakers with AOS are lacking information concerning either the general or specific aspects of sensorimotor specifications necessary for carrying out intended speech movements. Whether the lack of information stems from difficulty in accessing such information or from a loss of the information is debatable. Regardless, these types of articulatory-kinematic treatment techniques seek to provide movement information that is presumed to be lacking or incorrect. The treatments may be considered a form of meta-speech in that they require conscious processing of various cues associated with speech production.

The techniques described thus far have been applied at various levels of production, including individual movements and sounds (Holtzapple & Marshall, 1977; Square et al., 1985); syllables (Knock et al., 2000); monosyllabic words (Kahn, Stannard, & Skinner, 1998; Raymer et al., 2002; Wambaugh & Nessler, 2004); and multisyllabic words, phrases, and sentences (Bose et al., 2001; Wambaugh et al., 1998b).

Whereas techniques such as phonetic placement, phonetic derivation, PROMPT, and EPG provide relatively direct information about production of specific speech targets, indirect information concerning production is provided in the form of imitation of contrasts (Wertz, Rosenbek, & LaPointe, 1984). Wertz and colleagues (1984) suggested beginning with imitation of syllables in which the target sound is paired with different vowels (e.g., /se/-/si/-/su/). Following mastery at this elementary level, they recommended practice in contrasting the target sound with dissimilar sounds (e.g., /se/ - /pe/; /si/ - /fi/). Wertz and colleagues suggested further increasing the difficulty of the contrasts by utilizing sounds that are more similar to the target (e.g., /shu/ - /chu/) or utilizing a more difficult production environment for the target sound (e.g., "tight - tyke"). Wambaugh and colleagues have also used contrastive practice in the form of minimal pair words, with the target sound paired with the patient's typically replacing sound (Wambaugh et al., 1998a, 1999, 2004). Minimal pair words have also been used with electropalatographic feedback to practice contrasting tongue contacts (Howard & Varley, 1995). Additionally, Square and colleagues (1986, 1989) employed minimal pairs during PROMPT treatment and have reported that PROMPT should be utilized to contrast articulatory movements (Square et al., 2001). Contrastive practice may allow the speaker to experience the difference in the sensorimotor specifications related to the contrasting productions.

The use of contrastive practice relates to the motor-learning concepts of variable practice and the scheduling of variable practice (e.g., random practice versus blocked practice) (Schmidt & Lee, 1999). According to Schmidt and Lee, an important aspect of learning a task is being capable of coping with novel situations. Of course, every new speech event is presumably a novel situation. Wertz and colleagues'

notion of varying the phonetic environment of a target sound is consistent with the principle of variable practice. How the variable practice is scheduled has been shown to be important for limb learning in terms of retention and transfer of behaviors (see Schmidt & Lee, 1999 and Knock et al., 2000 for discussions and reviews). When all practice trials with one target behavior occur together (i.e., sequentially), the practice is termed "blocked." When trials of all targeted behaviors are randomly interspersed, the practice is termed "random." For instance, if two sounds have been targeted for treatment, blocked practice would require that one sound be practiced first for X number of trials, followed by practice of the remaining sound (e.g., 100 trials of /r/, followed by 100 trials of /k/). Random practice would involve practice of both sounds concurrently, with the order of the items being randomized (e.g., /r/-/k/-/r/-/r/-/k/-/r/-/k/-/k/-/r/). The literature on limb motor learning indicates that blocked practice promotes more rapid acquisition of motor behaviors, but random practice results in better retention and transfer (see Schmidt & Lee, 1999, for a review).

Although the application of principles of motor learning such as variable practice and blocked versus random practice have intuitive appeal for application to motor-speech treatment, only limited data exist concerning their utility with AOS. Knock and colleagues (2000) examined the effects of blocked and random practice on production of stops and fricatives in syllables and monosyllabic words with two participants with severe AOS. Their results were not consistent with the literature on limb motor learning in terms of acquisition of behaviors during treatment, but did suggest that for one participant, random practice resulted in superior retention.

Other issues related to articulatory-kinematic treatments, such as selection of stimuli, outcome measures, and utilization of feedback, have been discussed elsewhere (Odell, 2002; Wambaugh et al., 2006b) and will not be reiterated here. The reader is strongly encouraged to consult such resources and to take into consideration these issues when planning therapy.

As noted previously, the majority of the evidence supporting treatment for AOS has taken the form of investigations of articulatory-kinematic treatments. Wambaugh and colleagues (2006b) reported that of the 87 AOS participants studied in articulatory-kinematic investigations for whom severity ratings were available, "84% were provided a severe rating, 5% a moderate-severe rating, 9% a moderate rating, and 2% a mild-moderate rating. In comparison to the total group of 146 AOS participants studied across all investigations, the participants in the articulatory-kinematic investigations were more frequently rated as severe and none received a mild severity rating" (p. xlvii). Thus, it appears that increased severity is associated with the selection of articulatory-kinematic approaches. It may be the case that disruptions in spatial and temporal aspects of sound production occur more frequently in cases of severe AOS or are

TABLE 36–2

Rate- and Rhythm-Control Approaches for the Treatment of AOS

Treatment Type	Reference	Brief Treatment Description
Metronomic pacing	Dworkin, Abkarian, and Johns (1988)	Following tasks practiced with a metronome at slowed rates of production: nonspeech tasks with bite-block, AMRs, multisyllabic words, sentence repetition; rates were gradually increased
Metronomic pacing	Dworkin and Abkarian (1996)	Practice of vowels, vowel sequences, and vowel - /h/ sequences with metronome at slowed rate with gradual increasing of rate
Metronomic pacing plus hand tapping	Wambaugh and Martinez (2000)	Repeated production of multisyllabic words with metronome and hand tapping. Clinician modeling and unison production used initially, but faded. Rate increased and syncopation added.
Metronomic pacing plus hand tapping	Mauszycki (2006)	Repeated practice of multisyllabic words at increased rates of production in time with metronome, accompanied by hand tapping
Rhythmic control	Brendel, Ziegler, and Deger (2000)	Production of target utterances in time with computerized, rhythmic signals
Stress patterning	Tjaden (2000)	Practice of reiterant speech (e.g., DAdada) and multisyllabic words with modeling, waveform and auditory feedback, feedback of relative syllable durations, and finger tapping
Rate control	McHenry and Wilson (1994)	Rate reduction with syllable-by-syllable production. Clinician cueing used initially, then faded. Pacing board added. Feedback about rate provided. Tasks progressed from imitation of functional phrases and multisyllabic words to structured responses/conversation to unstructured conversation.
Rate control	Southwood (1987)	Prolonged speech produced in oral reading at reduced rates with rate controlled by video display.

Key: AMRs = "alternating motion rates (e.g., pataka) (e.g., puh puh puh puh)

perceived as being more disruptive of communication in severe AOS. Unfortunately, there currently are no agreed-upon, data-based methods for documenting AOS severity and determining the contribution of underlying pathophysiology to perceived severity. Or, it may be the case that behaviors in severe AOS (versus moderate or mild AOS) are more amenable to experimental control (e.g., perhaps more likely to result in stable baselines) and, thus, the existing literature may reflect conscious or unconscious experimenter bias. Regardless of the cause for the preponderance of severe cases in the articulatory-kinematic literature, it is clear that these treatments may be expected to result in improved accuracy of speech production for individuals with significant sound errors. In only one report were negative treatment findings reported (Aten, 1986), although other investigators have reported that some sounds seem to be more resistant than others for some speakers (Raymer et al., 2002; Wambaugh et al., 1998a). More data are required to document the effects of articulatory-kinematic treatments on speech production in speakers with moderate and mild AOS.

Rate- and Rhythm-Control Approaches

Another general approach to AOS treatment identified in the AOS treatment guidelines was rate and rhythm control. Rate- and rhythm-control approaches involve manipulations of rate and/or rhythm, with both often being impacted. To date, only a few investigations have reported the effects of such treatments. As seen in Table 36–2, the techniques included in this general approach include rate control through metronomic pacing, hand-tapping, prolonged speaking, clinician instruction, and utilization of a pacing board, and rhythmic manipulation through computerized control and feedback.

A basic assumption associated with rate- and rhythm-control approaches is that AOS reflects an underlying disruption in the timing of speech production. There are many theorized mechanisms by which rate- and rhythm-control treatments are thought to impact AOS, none of which have been confirmed or disproved. Use of rhythmic treatments with AOS have typically involved rate reduction (although see Mauszycki & Wambaugh, 2006). Slowing of speech production, even in speakers who already exhibit reduced rate, is thought to allow additional time for motor planning and/or programming and processing of feedback. It has also been suggested that the entrainment provided by rhythmic sources (e.g., metronome or hand-tapping) may serve to facilitate or restore internal oscillatory mechanisms that may be involved in speech production (Dworkin & Abkarian, 1996). Rate and rhythm controls may also provide a mediating function with respect to attention. For example, Dworkin and colleagues (1998) hypothesized that use of a metronome may have helped to focus the patient's attention on the need for increased precision during speech production. Brendel, Ziegler, & Deger (2000) suggested a different attentional mechanism; they proposed that their rhythmic-control treatment may have drawn attention toward the externally controlling stimulus and away from speech movements.

Of the relatively few investigations designed to examine the effects of rate- and rhythm-control treatments, half have been focused on metronomic pacing (Dworkin & Abkarian, 1996; Dworkin et al., 1988; Wambaugh & Martinez, 2000; Mauszycki & Wambaugh, 2006). With metronomic pacing, speech productions are produced to the beat of a metronome, usually at a rate of one syllable or movement per beat. Most often, the beat of the metronome has been set at a rate that is considerably slower than the habitual rate used by the speaker. Dworkin and colleagues (1988, 1996) initiated practice with the metronome set at extremely slow rates (e.g., 12, 15, or 30 beats per minute [bpm]) and gradually increased rates to 120 bpm. Wambaugh and Martinez selected a rate that reflected a 50% reduction in the participant's typical speaking rate. They also gradually increased rate and added a syncopated rhythm at the participant's request.

The behaviors that have been practiced with pacing have varied. Dworkin and Abkarian (1996) utilized stimuli designed to promote increased volitional control over phonation. Specifically, the patient practiced production of individual vowels, vowel sequences, and vowel - /h/ alternations. Dworkin, Abkarian, and Johns (1988) employed a non–speech activity (raising and lowering the tongue tip to the alveolar ridge with a bite block in place) as well as speech activities (e.g., SMRs and multisyllabic word productions). Wambaugh and Martinez (2000) trained multisyllabic word productions that were grouped according to stress pattern. Mauszycki and Wambaugh (2006) utilized multisyllabic words and phrases in their practice, which involved increasing rates of production with a speaker with mild AOS.

In the investigations by Dworkin and colleagues (1988, 1996), it appeared that little clinical instruction was involved. That is, practice was largely independent and patient controlled. In contrast, Wambaugh and Martinez (2000) and Mauszycki and Wambaugh (in press) utilized clinician modeling in early treatment phases, with clinician involvement being gradually withdrawn. The treatment protocol used by Wambaugh and Martinez is shown in Appendix 36.4. Furthermore, both investigations combined hand-tapping with the metronomic pacing. Specifically, the patients were required to tap along with the beat of the metronome while performing the speech tasks. The rationale for inclusion of the hand-tapping was that the tapping (1) could serve as a self-initiated mediating device that could be used when the metronome was not present and (2) provided additional rhythmic stimulation.

Dworkin and colleagues reported positive changes for all trained behaviors in terms of reduced presence of symptoms

of apraxia (Dworkin & Abkarian, 1988; Dworkin et al., 1996). Dworkin and colleagues (1988) reported that training effects at beginning levels of practice generalized to more complex behaviors. In contrast, Dworkin and Abkarian (1988) reported a lack of generalization of treatment effects to untrained behaviors (e.g., treatment of tongue-tip raising did not result in improved performance with AMRs). Generalization to untrained behaviors was also reported by Wambaugh and Martinez (2000) in that untrained words improved with respect to articulatory accuracy, although improvements were slightly less than those observed with trained words. It is important to note that Wambaugh and Martinez provided no training for articulation and provided no feedback relative to articulatory accuracy. Mauszycki and Wambaugh (2006) also noted increased articulatory accuracy following practice with metronomic pacing and hand-tapping.

Rate of production (Southwood, 1987) and rhythm of production (Brendel et al., 2000; Tjaden, 2000) have been controlled/trained through visual displays and/or feedback. In a facilitation study (i.e., not a true treatment investigation), Southwood (1987) encouraged use of a prolonged manner of speaking and used a video display to present words for oral reading at specified rates (30-130 words per minute). Brendel and colleagues (2000) also used a video display to have speakers match their productions to computer-generated "rhythmic cues," which were controlled for rate and metrical form. Additionally, Tjaden (2000) used a waveform display, auditory feedback, and a numerical indicator of relative syllable durations to treat stress patterning, Whereas Southwood and Brendel and colleagues reported positive outcomes, Tjaden reported negative results for a generalization measure of stress patterning.

McHenry and Wilson (1994) used a combination of techniques to reduce rate. They provided clinician cueing, which was gradually faded, along with use of a pacing board, which is a board divided horizontally into sections by raised dividers. Patients are trained to touch each consecutive section on the board for each unit of speech. Such devices have been recommended for use (Wertz et al., 1984), but little data exist concerning their utility. Although McHenry and Wilson's rate-control treatment was described only briefly, they provided descriptions of a task continuum progressing from imitation of functional phrases and multisyllabic words to structured responses in conversation to unstructured conversation.

Another technique that may act at the level of rate/rhythm modification is the application of surface prompts. Surface prompts are those that highlight tempo and stress patterns. Investigations focused on the rate and rhythmic facilitative effects of surface prompts have not yet been reported. Surface prompts are discussed further in "Formalized Treatment Programs with Supporting Evidence."

Another technique that may function at the level of rate/rhythm that has not received direct investigation is contrastive stress drills. Such drills have been advocated for treatment of AOS (e.g., Rosenbek, 1983; Wertz et al., 1984) and use emphatic stress to facilitate speech production. An additional potential benefit is that repeated productions with varied stress provide a form of variable practice. Question-and-answer dialogues that consist of short phrases centered on one or two target words are used. Questions are manipulated to require stress to be placed on a particular word in the response. The reader is directed to Wertz, et al., (1984) or Square Martin & Bose (2001) and their colleagues for further discussion.

Additional techniques that may be considered rate and rhythm techniques include finger counting (Simmons, 1978) and vibrotactile stimulation (Rubow, Rosenbek, Collins, & Longstreth, 1982). However, these approaches will be discussed in the next section, because their developers considered their therapeutic effects to derive from intersystemic reorganization.

Intersystemic Facilitation/Reorganization Approaches

Intersystemic reorganization entails the utilization of a relatively intact system/modality to promote functioning of an impaired system/modality (Rosenbek et al., 1976). The AOS Treatment Guidelines Committee added the term "facilitation" to the description of these approaches because the intent as well as the outcome of the treatments appeared to be facilitation of speech rather than necessarily reorganization of communication. The rationales for the treatments described in this section carried no assumptions about presumed pathophysiology associated with AOS. Few theories have been advanced regarding the possible mechanisms by which intersystemic facilitators/reorganizors effect changes in speech. Rubow and colleagues (1982) suggested that additional afference provided through the engagement of additional systems may play a role. Additionally, Rubow and colleagues theorized that gestural reorganization techniques may provide an organizational framework for speech production.

Utilizing gestures to enhance speech production has been the technique most often studied in terms of AOS intersystemic facilitation/reorganization (Wambaugh et al., 2006a). Both iconic (e.g., Amer-Ind gestural code; Skelly, 1979) and nonmeaningful (e.g., finger-counting; Simmons, 1978) gestures have been studied. With gestural facilitation/reorganization, gestural production is typically paired with verbal production of targets such as words or sentences (Code & Gaunt, 1986; Raymer & Thompson, 1991; Simmons, 1978; Skelly et al., 1974; Wertz et al., 1984). Dowden, Marshall, and Tompkins (1981) trained only gestural production but measured the effects of treatment on verbal production. Improvements were reported for all of the investigations in which gestures were paired with verbalizations. Improvements were noted in terms of improved articulation (Raymer & Thompson, 1991; Rubow et al., 1982; Wertz et al., 1984) as well as increases in test scores (Simmons, 1978; Skelly et al., 1974). When gestures were trained without being paired with verbalization (Dowden et al., 1981) no verbal changes were reported (i.e., PICA verbal scores). An added benefit of gestural plus verbal training may be improvements in gestural productions (Code & Gaunt, 1986; Raymer & Thompson, 1991).

Other techniques included in this general approach are the provision of vibrotactile stimulation (Rubow et al., 1982) and singing (Keith & Aronson, 1975). Rubow and colleagues applied a vibratory source to a participant's finger during production of polysyllabic words. Words beginning with fricatives received vibrotactile plus imitation treatment, while words beginning with plosives received imitation-only treatment. Although a superior treatment effect was found for the vibrotactile treatment, the potential inequality in difficulty of the word lists served as a confound. Keith & Aronson reported a case of singing as therapy which involved choral singing of a familiar song and production of object names and functional phrases in song. Facilitative effects of singing were reported, although quantitative data were not provided.

Alternative/Augmentative Communication Approaches

The remaining general approach to the treatment of AOS identified in the AOS guidelines report was AAC (Wambaugh et al., 2006b). As noted in the AOS guidelines, "the common motivation for the eight treatment investigations involving alternative/augmentative approaches was the perceived need to improve communication through the use of modalities other than speech. That is, verbal communication was judged to be less than optimally effective and consequently, methods for either circumventing or supplementing speech were devised" (Wambaugh et al., 2006b; p. lvi).

Reports of AAC training with persons with AOS and aphasia have included development of a comprehensive communication system (Yorkston & Waugh, 1989), development of a total communication approach (Fawcus & Fawcus, 1990), instruction in use of voice-output communication aids (Lasker & Bedrosian, 2001; Rabidoux, Florance, & McCauslin, 1980), and training in use of Blissymbols (Bailey, 1983; Lane & Samples, 1981).

Lasker and Bedrosian (2001) noted that AAC options may not be adopted by potential users or may be used ineffectively because of problems with acceptance. They described a case in which an individual with chronic aphasia and AOS demonstrated unwillingness to use an AAC device beyond the confines of the speech-and-language clinic. To work through this problem, they implemented a community-based treatment program utilizing role play and outings.

The literature concerning AAC and AOS consists primarily of cases in which AOS was accompanied by significant aphasia. It is impossible to determine the contribution of the co-occurring disorders to the need for AAC in these cases. However, in terms of selecting the specific AAC approach and designing treatment, the language disturbance may be the primary consideration. The reader is directed to Chapter 30 in this text for information concerning AAC and aphasia.

Two reports of AAC approaches that were designed specifically to circumvent problems resulting specifically from AOS are available (Lustig & Tompkins, 2002; Marshall, Gandour, & Windsor, 1988). Marshall and colleagues reported on a case in which apraxia was considered to have selectively affected motor programming of the larynx. In this case, the patient was provided with an electrolarynx to compensate for the deficits in phonation. Lustig and Tompkins (2002) designed a treatment for an individual with AOS and aphasia who had developed an unproductive communicative pattern of persistent verbal struggle. That is, when the participant had difficulty in verbal expression, she produced excessive verbal reattempts that were disruptive of communication. Lustig and Tompkins applied treatment that required the participant to use a written response upon the occurrence of spoken production that occurred with struggle behavior. The reader is referred to Lustig and Tompkins (2002) for a complete explanation of treatment and description of comprehensive outcome measures.

Formalized Treatment Programs with Supporting Evidence

As described in the previous sections, many techniques are available for the treatment of AOS. In the following sections, three treatment programs are described. These are treatments that are relatively more developed than others available for AOS. Of importance is the fact that their effects have been replicated in two or more investigations. A weakness of the existing AOS treatment literature is a lack of replications of positive treatment findings (Wambaugh, 2002; Wambaugh et al., 2006b). It is not the case that negative findings have been reported in subsequent investigations; rather, it is that replications have not been attempted for the majority of AOS treatment reports. For the treatments that follow, repeated study of the treatments has provided a more substantial evidence base than exists for most AOS treatments. However, even the following treatments require substantial additional research to address remaining questions regarding treatment outcomes and optimal conditions of application.

Eight-Step Continuum

Appendix 36.5 shows the treatment protocol described by Rosenbek and colleagues (1973), called the eight-step task continuum. The treatment was originally described along with a report of three cases in which it was applied with individuals with severe, chronic (i.e., longer than 1 year post-onset) AOS and moderate aphasia. The treatment entails selecting a limited set of target utterances for the client; Rosenbek and colleagues chose five, functional target utterances, varying in length from one to seven words, which were individualized for each client (e.g., "My name is _____."; "home"; "It's time to go."). Target productions are entered

into the continuum one at a time, beginning at Step 1. Criterion for moving to the next step is 80% correct in 20 consecutive treatment trials. In the Rosenbek report, clinician judgment apparently served as the primary determinant of correctness, with communicative adequacy being stressed.

Rosenbek and colleagues (1973) noted that various response facilitators were necessary and were individualized according to client needs. That is, in addition to the steps of the continuum, additional therapeutic techniques were employed. Presentation facilitators such as slowed presentation, increased stress, and exaggerated articulation were reported. In addition, production facilitators such as utilization of a mirror and phonetic placement cueing were used.

The continuum begins with steps at which the clinician exerts a relatively high degree of control. Clinician cues are faded as the steps progress and ultimately, the target utterances are elicited in simulated, naturalistic communication situations. Steps of the continuum may be skipped to accommodate different types of treatment stimuli (e.g., some single words may not be appropriate for Steps 7 and 8) and rapid response to treatment (e.g., generalization may permit skipping steps).

In the original report concerning the eight-step continuum, positive results were reported for the three participants. In a follow-up investigation, Deal and Florance (1978) reported successful application of a modified version of the continuum with four participants with severe AOS, three of whom had chronic AOS. Simmons (1980) used a withdrawal design to study the effects of a modified version of the continuum with an individual with moderate AOS and aphasia. The participant, who had been blind from birth, was trained on production of 10 sentences under two training conditions: one without Braille and one with Braille. The participant improved under both conditions, but demonstrated superior performance when Braille was utilized in the continuum. In summary, data from seven cases and one experimental study indicate that individuals with AOS and aphasia may benefit from application of the eight-step continuum in terms of acquisition of limited sets of functional words/phrases/sentences. More experimental investigations of this treatment are required to further specify its effects, especially in terms of generalization to untrained items and to different stimulus conditions.

PROMPT

PROMPT was developed by Chumpelik (Hayden) (1984) as a dynamic method for delivering tactile cues concerning articulation (i.e., place of articulation, timing, transitioning, and amount and type of contraction) to children with severely impaired speech. Application of PROMPT to adult speakers with AOS and aphasia began during the 1980's through collaborative efforts of Square, Chumpelik (Hayden), and colleagues (Square, Chumpelik, & Adams, 1985; Square, Chumpelik, Morningstar, & Adams, 1986).

Since its initial description (Chumpelik, 1984), PROMPT has been developed into a comprehensive approach to the management of speech-production disorders in children (see Hayden, 2004, for a thorough review of the history, conceptual framework, and description of PROMPT). It appears from the extant literature concerning PROMPT applied to AOS that selected techniques rather than the entire treatment approach have been utilized.

Because of the complexity of PROMPT, clinician training is recommended for its correct administration (www. promptinstitute.com). Therefore, the following brief description of its techniques is meant to provide the reader with the basic concepts associated with PROMPT, not to provide instruction in its application. PROMPT uses a combination of proprioceptive, pressure, and kinesthetic cues that are "designed to heighten sensory input regarding the place of articulatory contact, extent of mandibular opening, presence and extent of labial rounding and retraction, voicing, muscle tension, time of segments, manner of articulation, and/or coarticulation" (Bose & Square, 2001, p. 5). Treatment is individualized, and PROMPT can be applied at various levels of production ranging from movement parameters such as jaw opening to sentence productions. Different types of prompts are available for use depending upon the level of support required: parameter prompts, complex prompts, and surface prompts. For a detailed description of the different types of prompts as well as the contextual application of PROMPT see Square and colleagues (2001).

The use of PROMPT is supported by the findings of several investigations (Bose et al., 2001; Freed, Marshall, & Frazier, 1997; Square et al., 1985, 1986; Square-Storer & Hayden, 1989). Initial research concerning the application of PROMPT with speakers with AOS suggested that application of PROMPT resulted in positive changes in production of trained individual sounds, single words, minimally contrastive word pairs, and phrases with speakers with AOS (Square et al., 1985, 1986; Square-Storer & Hayden, 1989). Generalization to untrained items was not evident, but anecdotal reports indicated generalized use of trained phrases beyond the treatment setting. Freed and colleagues (1997) trained an individual with severe AOS and aphasia in the production of 30 functional words and phrases. Results were similar to those reported by Square and colleagues in that the participant successfully learned the trained items, but generalization was not evident to untrained items. Stimulus generalization in the form of use of trained productions in novel situations was reported anecdotally. Bose and colleagues (2001) examined the impact of the type of sentence construction on the effects of PROMPT. Specifically they measured the precision of production of short sentences grouped by imperatives, active declaratives, and interrogatives in an individual with moderate AOS and aphasia. Findings indicated positive results for imperatives and active declaratives, but

not for interrogatives. No generalization to untrained items was observed; maintenance effects were positive for gains made with imperatives and active declaratives. It is of importance to note that the positive results reported by Freed and colleagues and Square and colleagues represent supporting data from independent research groups, which is an important component in the demonstration of treatment efficacy (Chambless & Hollon, 1998).

Sound-Production Treatment

Sound-Production Treatment (SPT; Wambaugh, 2004; Wambaugh & Nessler, 2004) has been evaluated more extensively than other treatments for AOS. SPT was designed to facilitate improved production of specific sounds targeted for treatment. Sounds selected for treatment are those that are produced in error on a relatively consistent basis at some level of production. The level of production at which sound-production difficulty may be evidenced and at which treatment is directed includes syllables, monosyllabic words, multisyllabic words, phrases, and sentences. SPT combines modeling, repetition, minimal-pair contrast, integral stimulation, articulatory placement cueing, and feedback in a response-contingent hierarchy. The original SPT hierarchy is shown in Appendix 36.6. Modifications to the original hierarchy have been made based upon research findings and the desire to incorporate principles of motor learning. The most recent version of SPT is shown in Appendix 36.7. As seen in Appendix 36.7, the minimal-contrast item is introduced only upon incorrect production of the target item. Additional repetitions are elicited upon a correct response in order to maximize repeated practice, and a reduced-feedback schedule is used with those additional repetitions. In addition, the silent-juncture step was eliminated. As noted previously, the SPT hierarchy (both versions) is response contingent. Steps of the hierarchy are used only as needed. In addition, the steps of the hierarchy are not reversed upon a correct response.

Research with SPT has shown that when eight to 10 exemplars of the target sound are trained to criterion, response generalization to untrained exemplars of the target sound may be expected to occur at levels of accuracy that approximate trained items (Wambaugh, 2004; Wambaugh & Nessler, 2004; Wambaugh et al., 1998, 1999). Generalization to untrained sounds that are unrelated (i.e., are not cognates or closely related in manner of production) is likely to be minimal. Partial generalization has been observed for sounds that demonstrate similar manner of production with similar types of errors (Wambaugh & Cort, 1998). Stimulus generalization has not been evaluated extensively; consequently, predictions cannot be made concerning these effects with SPT. However, positive stimulus generalization to longer and more complex production conditions has been observed for some speakers (Wambaugh, 2004; Wambaugh & Nessler, 2004; Wambaugh et al., 1998b).

SPT has been modified with successful results for application to multiple sound targets (Wambaugh & Nessler, 2004), sentences containing numerous target words/sounds (Wambaugh et al., 1998b), and words elicited through sentence completion (Wambaugh & Nessler, 2004). Although much remains to be clarified about the outcomes associated with SPT, it can be expected that SPT will result in improved production of targeted sounds for speakers with AOS.

Treatment for AOS and Aphasia

Virtually all of the participants described in the AOS treatment literature presented with some type and degree of aphasia (Wambaugh et al., 2006a). Unfortunately, the descriptions of the accompanying aphasia and its impact on verbal expression have usually not been provided in sufficient detail to allow inferences about its effect on treatment outcomes. Most treatments for AOS, with a few exceptions (such as those focused on AAC), have provided relatively superficial attention to the accompanying aphasia. The consideration of aphasia has most often been reflected in the selection of treatment stimuli. That is, in the selection of items for treatment, the following factors, which impact language production as well as speech production, have sometimes been taken into account: frequency of occurrence, length of stimuli, functionality, and patient preference. It is our impression that treatments for AOS have generally been designed to work around the constraints of the patient's language disorder in order to focus on the motor-speech deficit.

One treatment for aphasia that has been specifically modified to accommodate the presence of AOS and that has incorporated treatment techniques considered to facilitate speech production in AOS is Response Elaboration Training (RET; Kearns, 1985). RET was developed to promote increased production of content and length of utterances through the use of modeling and forward-chaining applied to patient-initiated verbalizations. Wambaugh and Martinez (2000) modified RET by incorporating additional modeling, integral stimulation, and repeated practice of utterances to make the treatment more amenable for application with persons with significant AOS. Wambaugh and Martinez reported positive changes in production of verbal content upon application of modified RET in three speakers with chronic AOS and aphasia. The effects of modified RET on speech-production accuracy have not been examined. Although it is likely that changes in speech production in AOS will necessitate significant amounts of repeated practice, modifications to existing aphasia treatments, such as RET, may allow clinicians to target both speech and language deficits simultaneously in the future.

Treatment Summary

Persons with aphasia may also have neuromotor speech disorders such as AOS and dysarthria. The presentation of such disorders will be unique for each individual, as will the communication disruption resulting from the combination of aphasia and AOS/dysarthria. Significant evidence exists indicating that persons with aphasia and neuromotor speech disorders can benefit from treatment directed toward their speech disruption.

KEY POINTS

1. Thanks to the advent of new, mainly noninvasive, technologies, we have learned a great deal about the brain regions that subserve speech production. Areas such as M1, which were thought to be purely motor, appear to play a role in higher level cognitive functions relating to movement, not simply in the execution of movement.

2. Several cortical regions, such as the left IFG, have been shown to play a role in both language and speech behaviors. This may explain why speech and language deficits frequently co-occur after damage to the left hemisphere.

3. Speech production and speech perception, once believed to be separate processes, appear to be tightly linked in the brain.

4. In light of what we have learned about the role that different brain regions play in speech production, we can understand how damage to different brain regions could produce similar deficits. For example, based on what we know about their function, we can understand why damage to the left IFG or the left IPL could result in problems in producing longer words.

5. Apraxia of speech (AOS) and unilateral upper motor neuron dysarthria may occur with aphasia and may exacerbate its effects, particularly in terms of verbal expression. Other forms of dysarthria may be present with aphasia, but rarely will they be the result of the same neurologic event that caused the aphasia.

6. Clinicians must understand the impact of both the language and motor aspects of verbal-production disorders associated with brain damage to the language-dominant hemisphere.

7. Clinicians should be aware of the treatment recommendations and options described in the AOS Treatment Guidelines (Wambaugh et al., 2006a, 2006b).

8. Clinicians should base treatment decisions on balanced consideration of the best available evidence, clinical experience, theoretical rationale, and patient needs and preferences.

ACTIVITIES FOR REFLECTION AND DISCUSSION

1. It appears that Broca's area plays a role in multiple aspects of speech and language behavior. Discuss how it might be possible for a brain region to have such diverse functions and yet still be efficient.

2. Describe how our view of the relationship between speech perception and speech production has changed. Discuss whether what we know about this relationship would change your approach to evaluation and/or treatment of motor-speech disorders.

3. Develop at least two explanations for why, after decades of study, there is still no universal agreement on the location of the lesion that produces apraxia of speech.

4. Review the characteristics that are considered *necessary* for a diagnosis of AOS and those that are *consistent with* a diagnosis of AOS, but that *should not be used* for differential diagnosis. Revisit the early descriptions of AOS (e.g., Darley et al., 1975) and discuss how the diagnostic descriptors have changed.

5. Describe the speech characteristics of a patient with AOS (real or fictitious). Discuss the possible advantages and disadvantages of an articulatory-kinematic approach versus a rate/rhythm control approach for treating this patient.

6. Review the various ways in which speech may be sampled when assessing AOS. Discuss patient-specific considerations that should be taken into account when selecting methods for sampling.

References

Academy of Neurologic Communication Disorders and Sciences (ANCDS)(2007). www.ancds.org. Retrieved 11/23/07

Alario, F. X., Chainay, H., Lehéricy, S., & Cohen, L. (2006). The role of the Supplementary Motor Area (SMA) in word production. *Brain Research, 1076*, 129–143.

Alexander, M. P., Naeser, M. A., & Palumbo, C. (1990). Broca's area aphasia. *Neurology, 41*, 353–362.

Amiez, C., Koastopoulos, P., Champod, A.-S., & Petrides, M. (2006). Local morphology predicts functional organization of the dorsal premotor region in the human brain. *Journal of Neuroscience, 26*, 2724–2731.

Amunts, K., Schleicher, A., Bürgel, U., Mohlberg, H., Uylings, H.B., & Zilles, K. (1999). Broca's region revisited: cytoarchitecture and intersubject variability. *Journal of Comparative Neurophysiology, 412*, 319–341.

Amunts, K., Schleicher, A., Ditterich, A., & Zilles, K. (2003). Broca's region: Cytarchitectonic asymmetry and developmental changes. *The Journal of Comparative Neurology, 465*, 72–89.

Amunts, K., Weiss, P. H., Mohlber, H., Pieperhoff, P., Eickhoff, S., Gurd, J. M., et al. (2004). Analysis of neural mechanisms underlying verbal fluency in cytoarchitectonically defined sterotaxic space— The roles of Brodmann areas 44 and 45. *NeuroImage, 22*, 42–56.

Anwander, A., Tittgemeyer, von Cramon, D. Y., Friederici, A., & Knösche, T. R. (2006). Connectivity-based parcellation of Broca's

area. *Cerebral Cortex* [Epub ahead of print]. Articulate Instruments (2006). www.articulateinstruments.com

Asanuma, H. & Rosen, I. (1972). Topographical organization of cortical efferent zones projecting to distal forelimb muscles in the monkey. *Experimental Brain Research, 14*, 243–256.

Assmus, A., Marshall, J. C., Ritzl, A., Noth, J., Zilles, K., & Fink. G. R. (2003). Left inferior parietal cortex integrates time and space during collision judgments. *NeuroImage, 20*(Suppl. 1), S82–S88.

Aten, J. L. (1986). Aphasia and severe apraxia of speech: Charting the treatment course. In R. Marshall (Ed.), *Case studies in aphasia rehabilitation* (pp. 119–132). Austin, TX: Pro-Ed.

Augustine, J. (1996). Circuitry and functional aspects of the insular lobe in primates including humans. *Brain Research Reviews, 22*, 229–244.

Bailey, S. (1983). Blissymbols and aphasia therapy: A case study. In C. Code & D. Muller (Eds.), *Aphasia Therapy* (pp. 178–186). London: Edward Arnold.

Barinaga, M. (1995). Remapping the motor cortex. *Science, 268*, 1696–1698.

Binkofski, F., & Buccino, G. (2004). Motor functions of the Broca's region. *Brain and Language, 89*, 362–369.

Blumstein, S. E. (2001). Deficits in speech production and speech perception in aphasia. In R. Berndt (Ed.), *Handbook of neuropsychology* (Vol. 3, 2nd ed.). The Netherlands: Elsevier.

Bohland, J. W., & Guenther, F. H. (2006). An fMRI investigation of syllable sequence production. *NeuroImage, 32*, 821–841.

Bose. A., & Square, P. A. (2001). PROMPT treatment method and apraxia of speech. *ASHA Division 2 Newsletter, 11*(4), 5–8.

Bose, A., Square, P. A., Schlosser, R., & van Lieshout, P. (2001). Effects of PROMPT therapy on speech motor function in a person with aphasia. *Aphasiology, 15*(8), 767–785.

Brendel, B., Ziegler, W., & Deger, K. (2000). The synchronization paradigm in the treatment of apraxia of speech. *Journal of Neurolinguistics, 13*, 241–327.

Broca, P. (1861). Remarques sur le siége de la faculté du langage articulé, suivies d'une observation d'aphémie. *Bulletin de la Société Anatomique, 6*, 330–357.

Brodmann, K. (2006). Brodmann's localisation in the cerebral cortex (L. J. Gary, Trans.). New York: Springer. (Original work published 1909)

Buckingham, H. W. (1979). Explanation in apraxia with consequences for the concept of apraxia of speech. *Brain and Language, 8*, 202–226.

Buckingham, H.W., & Yule, G. (1987). Phonemic false evaluation: Theoretical and clinical aspects. *Clinical Linguistics and Phonetics, 1*, 113–125.

Burton, M. W., Small, S. L., & Blumstein, S. E. (2000). The role of segmentation in phonological processing: An fMRI investigation. *Journal of Cognitive Neuroscience, 12*, 679–690.

Catani, J., Jones, D. K., & ffytche, D. H. (2005). Perisylvian language networks of the human brain. *Annals of Neurology, 57*, 8–16.

Chambless, D. L., & Hollon, S. D. (1998). Defining empirically supported therapies. *Journal of Consulting and Clinical Psychology, 66*, 7–18.

Chee, M. W .L., Soon, C. S., Lee, H. L., & Pallier, C. (2004). Left insula activation: A marker for language attainment in bilinguals. *Proceedings of the National Academy of Sciences, 101*, 15265–15270.

Cheney, P. D., & Fetz, E. E. (1985). Comparable patterns of muscle facilitation evoked by individual corticomotoneuronal (CM) cells and by single intracortical microstimuli in primates: Evidence for functional groups of CM cells. *Journal of Neurophysiology, 53*, 786–804.

Chumpelik, D. (1984). The PROMPT system of therapy. *Seminars in Speech and Language, 5*, 139–156.

Classen, J., Liepert, J., Wise, S., Hallett, M., & Cohen, L. (1998). Rapid plasticity of human cortical movement representation induced by practice. *Journal of Neurophysiology, 79*, 1117–1123.

Code, C., & Gaunt, C. (1986). Treating severe speech and limb apraxia in a case of aphasia. *British Journal of Disorders of Communication, 21*(1), 11–20.

Croot, K. (2002). Diagnosis of AOS: Definition and criteria. *Seminars in Speech and Language, 23*(4), 267–279.

Croot, K., van Heyst, J., Deacon, B., & Law, S. (June, 2006). *Reduction of acquired stutter in a man with apraxia of speech*. Paper presented at the annual Clinical Aphasiology Conference, Gent, Belgium.

Crosson, B., Sadek, J. R., Maron, L., Gokcay, D., Mohr, C. M., Auerbach, E. J., et al. (2001). Relative shift in activity from medial to lateral frontal cortex during internally versus externally guided word generation. *Journal of Cognitive Neuroscience, 13*, 272–283.

Darley, F. L., Aronson, A. E., & Brown, J. R. (1975). *Motor speech disorders*. Philadelphia, PA: W. B. Saunders.

de Pellegrino, G., Fadiga, L., Fogassi, L., Gallese, V., & Rizzolatti, G. (1992). Understanding motor events: A neurophysiological study. *Experimental Brain Research, 91*, 176–180.

Deal, J. L., & Florance, C. L. (1978). Modification of the eight-step continuum for treatment of apraxia of speech in adults. *Journal of Speech and Hearing Disorders, 43*, 89–95.

Devlin, J. T., Matthews, P. M., & Rushworth, M. F. S. (2003). Semantic processing in the left inferior prefrontal cortex: A combined functional magnetic resonance imaging and transcranial magnetic stimulation study. *Journal of Cognitive Neuroscience, 15*, 71–84.

Dowden, P. A., Marshall, R. C., & Tompkins, C. A. (1981). Amer-Ind sign as a communicative facilitator for aphasic and apraxic patients. In R. H. Brookshire (Ed.), *Clinical aphasiology: Conference proceedings* (pp. 133–140). Minneapolis, BRK.

Dronkers, N. F., Redfern, B., & Shapiro, J. K. (1993). Neuroanatomic correlates of production deficits in severe Broca's aphasia. *Journal of Clinical and Experimental Neuropsychology, 15*, 59–60.

Dronkers, N.F. (1996). A new brain region for coordinating speech articulation. *Nature, 384*, 159–161.

Duffy, J. R. (2005). *Motor speech disorders. Substrates, differential diagnosis, and management* (2nd ed.). St. Louis, MO: Elsevier Mosby.

Duffy, J. R., & Folger, W. N. (1996). Dysarthria associated with unilateral central nervous system lesion: A retrospective study. *Journal of Medical Speech-Language Pathology, 4*, 57–70.

Duffy, J. R., & Yorkston, K. M. (2003). Medical intervention for spasmodic dysphonia and some related conditions: A systematic review. *Journal of Medical Speech-Language Pathology, 11*(4), ix–ivii.

Dupont, S., Bouilleret, V., Hasboun, D., Semah, F., & Baulac, M. (2003). Functional anatomy of insula: New insights from imaging. *Surgical and Radiologic Anatomy, 25*, 113–119.

Dworkin, J. P., & Abkarian, G. G. (1996). Treatment of phonation in a patient with apraxia and dysarthria secondary to severe closed head injury. *Journal of Medical Speech-Language Pathology, 2*, 105–115.

Dworkin, J. P., Abkarian, G. G., & Johns, D. F. (1988). Apraxia of speech: The effectiveness of a treatment regime. *Journal of Speech and Hearing Disorders, 53*, 280–294.

Ehrsson, H., Fagergren, A., & Forssberg, H. (2001). Differential fronto-parietal activation depending on force used in a precision grip task: An fmri study. *Journal of Neurophysiology, 85*, 2613–2623, 2001.

Eickhoff, S. B., Amunts, K., Mohlberg, H., & Zilles, K. (2006). The human parietal operculum. II. Sterotaxic maps and correlation with functional imaging results. *Cerebral Cortex, 16*, 268–279.

Eickhoff, S. B., Schleicher, A., Zilles, K., & Amunts, K. (2006). The human parietal operculum. I. Cytoarchitectonic mapping of subdivisions. *Cerebral Cortex, 16*, 1–14.

Fadiga, L., Fogassi, G., Pavesi, G., & Rizzolatti, G. (1995). Motor facilitation during action observation: A magnetic stimulation study. *Journal of Neurophysiology, 73*, 2608–2611.

Fawcus, M., & Fawcus, R. (1990). Information transfer in four cases of severe articulatory dyspraxia. *Aphasiology, 4*(2), 207–212.

Florance, C. L., & Deal, J. L. (1977). A treatment protocol for nonverbal stroke patients. In R. H. Brookshire (Ed.), *Clinical aphasiology: Conference proceedings* (pp. 59–67). Minneapolis: BRK.

Freed, D. B., Marshall, R. C., & Frazier, K. E. (1997). Long-term effectiveness of PROMPT treatment in a severely apractic-aphasic speaker. *Aphasiology, 11*(4/5), 365–372.

Freud, S. (1953). *On aphasia: A critical study*. Stengel, E. (trans.). New York. International Universities Press. (Original work published 1891).

Friederici, A. (2002). Toward a neural basis of auditory sentence processing. *Trends in Cognitive Sciences, 6*, 78–84.

Geyer, S., Schleicher, & Zilles, K. (1999). Areas 3a, 3b, and 1 of human somatosensory cortex. 1. Microstructural organization and interindividual variability. *NeuroImage, 10*, 63–83.

Geyer, S., Schormann, T., Mohlberg, H., Zilles, K. (2000). Areas 3a, 3b, and 1 of human primary somatosensory cortex. Part 2. Spatial normalization to standard anatomical space. *NeuroImage, 11*, 684–696.

Ghez, C., & Krakauer, J. (2000). The organization of movement. In E. R. Kandel, J. H. Schwartz, & T. M. Jessell (Eds.), *Principles of neural science* (4th ed., pp. 653–673). New York: McGraw-Hill.

Ghosh, S., & Porter, R. (1988). Morphology of pyramidal neurones in monkey motor cortex and the synaptic actions of their intracortical axon collaterals. *Journal of Physiology, 400*, 593–615.

Graziano, M. S. A., Taylor, C. S. R., & Moore, T. (2002). Complex movements evoked by microstimulation of the precentral cortex. *Neuron, 34*, 841–851.

Greenlee, J. D. W., Oya, H., Kawasaki, H., Volkov, I. O., Kaufman, O. P., Kovach, C., et al. (2004). A functional connection between inferior frontal gyrus and orofacial motor cortex in human. *Journal of Neurophysiology, 92*, 1153–1164.

Guenther, F. H., Ghosh, S. S., & Tourville, J. A. (2006). Neural modeling and imaging of the cortical interactions underlying syllable production. *Brain and Language, 96*, 280–301.

Gunji, A., Hoshiyama, M., & Kakigi, R. (2001). Auditory response following vocalization: A magnetoencephalographic study. *Clinical Neurophysiology, 112*, 514–520.

Halsband, U., Forssberg, H. J. (1990). Premotor cortex and conditional motor learning in man. *Brain, 113*, 207–222.

Hanson, E. K., & Yorkston, K. M. (2004). Speech supplementation techniques for dysarthria: A systematic review. *Journal of Medical Speech-Language Pathology, 12*(2) xi–xxix.

Hayden, D. (1999). *PROMPT level 11 certification workshop manual*. Santa Fe, NM: PROMPT Institute.

Hayden, D. (2004). A tactually-grounded treatment approach to speech production disorders (pp. 255–297). In I. J. Stockman (Ed.) *Movement and Action Links to Intelligent Behavior, From Theory to Practice*. San Diego: Elsevier Academic Press.

Hickok, G., & Poeppel, D. (2004). Dorsal and ventral streams: A framework for understanding aspects of the functional anatomy of language. *Cognition, 92,* 67–99.

Hillis, A. E., Work, M., Barker, P. B., Jacobs, M. A., Breese, E. L., & Maurer, K. (2004). Re-examining the brain regions crucial for orchestrating speech articulation. *Brain, 127,* 1479–1487.

Holtzapple, P., & Marshall, N. (1977). The application of multi-phonemic articulation therapy with apraxic patients. In R. H. Brookshire (Ed.), *Clinical aphasiology: Conference proceedings* (pp. 46–58). Minneapolis: BRK.

Howard, S., & Varley, R. (1995). Using electropalatography to treat severe acquired apraxia of speech. *European Journal of Disorders of Communication, 30*(2), 246–255.

Huang, C. S., Sirisko, M. A., Hiraba, H., Murray, G. M., & Sessle, B. J. (1988). Organization of the primate face motor cortex as revealed by intracortical microstimulation and electrophysiological identification of afferent inputs and corticobulbar projections. *Journal of Neurophysiology, 59,* 796–818.

Huang, C. S., Hiraba, H., & Sessle, C. J. (1989). Input-output relationships of the primary face motor cortex in the monkey (Macaca fascicularis). *Journal of Neurophysiology, 61,* 350–362.

Huntley, G. W. & Jones, E. G. (1991). Relationship of intrinsic connections to forelimb movement representations in monkey motor cortex: a correlative anatomic and physiological study. *Journal of Neurophysiology, 66,* 390–419.

Indefrey, P., & Levelt, W. J. M. (2004). The spatial and temporal signatures of word production components. *Cognition, 92,* 101–144.

Jackson, J. H. (1931). *Selected writings of John Hughlings Jackson.* London: Hodder and Stoughton.

Kahn, H., Stannard, T., & Skinner, J. (1998). The use of words versus nonwords in the treatment of apraxia of speech: A case study. *ASHA Division 2 Perspectives, 8*(3), 5–9.

Katz, W. F., Bharadwaj, S. V., & Carstens, B. (1999). Electromagnetic articulography treatment for an adult with Broca's aphasia and apraxia of speech. *Journal of Speech, Language, and Hearing Research, 42*(6), 1355–1366.

Kayelemetrics (2007). Multispeech Model 3700. www.kayelemtrics. com. Retrieval date 11/23/07.

Kearns, K. P. (1985). Response elaboration training for patient initiated utterances (pp. 196–204). In R.H.Brookshire (Ed.), Clinical Aphasiology. Minneapolis, MN: BRK Publishers.

Keith, R. L., & Aronson, A. E. (1975). Singing as therapy for apraxia of speech and aphasia: Report of a case. *Brain and Language, 2,* 483–488.

Kent, R. D., Weismer, G., Kent, J. F., & Rosenbek, J. C. (1989). Toward phonetic intelligibility testing in dysarthria. *Journal of Speech and Hearing Disorders, 54,* 482–499.

Kimura, D., & Watson, N. (1989). The relation between oral movement control and speech. *Brain and Language, 37,* 565–590.

Knock, T. R., Ballard, K. J., Robin, D. A., & Schmidt, R. A. (2000). Influence of order of stimulus presentation on speech motor learning: A principled approach to treatment for apraxia of speech. *Aphasiology, 14*(5/6), 653–668.

Krainik, A., Duffau, H., Capelle, L., Cornu, P., Boch, A. L., Mangin, J. F., et al. (2004). Role of the healthy hemisphere in recovery after resection of the supplementary motor area. *Neurology, 62,* 1323–1332.

Krainik, A., Lehericy, S., Duffau, H., Capelle, L., Chainay, H., Cornu, P., et al. (2003). Postoperative speech disorder after medial frontal surgery. *Neurology, 60,* 587–594.

Kremer, S., Chassagnon, S., Hoffman, D., Benabid, A. L., Kahane, P. (2001). The cingulate hidden hand. *Journal of Neurology, Neurosurgery, and Psychiatry, 70,* 264–268.

Kurowski, K., Hazen, E., & Blumstein, S. E. (2003). The nature of speech production impairments in anterior aphasics: An acoustic analysis of voicing in fricative consonants. *Brain and Language, 84,* 353–371.

Lane, V. W., & Samples, J. M. (1981). Facilitating communiction skills in adult apraxics: Application of blissymbols in a group setting. *Journal of Communication Disorders, 14,* 157–167.

LaPointe, L. L. (1984). Sequential treatment of split lists: A case report. In J. Rosenbek, M. McNeil, & A. Aronson (Eds.), *Apraxia of speech: Physiology, acoustics, linguistics, management* (pp. 277–286). San Diego: College Hill.

Lasker, J. P., & Bedrosian, J.L. (2001). Promoting acceptance of augmentative and alternative communication by adults with acquired communication disorders. *AAC: Augmentative & Alternative Communication, 17*(3), 141–153.

Lehéricy, S., Ducros, M., Krainik, A., Francois, C., Van de Moortele, P.- F., Ugurbil, K., et al. (2004). 3-D diffusion tensor axonal tracking shows distinct SMA and pre-SMA projections to the human striatum. *Cerebral Cortex, 14,* 1302–1309.

Levelt, W. J. M. (2001). Spoken word production: A theory of lexical access. *Proceedings of the National Academy of Sciences, 98,* 13464–13471.

Liberman, A. M., & Mattingly, I. G. (1985). The motor theory of speech perception revised. *Cognition, 21,* 1–36.

Liepmann, H. (1913). Motor aphasia, anarthria, and apraxia. Transactions of the 17th International Congress of Medicine (Section XI, Part II), 97–106.

LoCasto, P. C., Krebs-Noble, D., Gullapalli, R. P., & Burton, M. W. (2004). An fMRI investigation of speech and tone segmentation. *Journal of Cognitive Neuroscience, 16,* 1612–1624.

LogoMetrix (2007). www.logometrix.org. Retrieval date 11/23/07.

Lustig, A. P., & Tompkins, C. A. (2002). A written comprehension strategy for a speaker with aphasia and apraxia of speech: Treatment outcomes and social validity. *Aphasiology, 16*(4/5/6), 507–521.

Makuuchi, M. (2005). Is Broca's area crucial for imitation? *Cerebral Cortex, 15,* 563–570.

Marcuse, E. K., Shiffman, R. N., Homer, C. J., Lannon, C. M., Harbaugh, N., Hodgson, E. S., et al. (2004). Classifying recommendations for clinical practice guidelines. American Academy of Pediatrics Policy Statement. *Pediatrics, 114*(3), 874–877.

Marshall, J. C., & Fink, G. R. (2003). Cerebral localization, then and now. *NeuroImage, 20,* 2–7.

Marshall, R. C., Gandour, J., & Windsor, J. (1988). Selective impairment of phonation: A case study. *Brain and Language, 35,* 313–339.

Mauszycki, S. C. (2006). *Variability of sound production in apraxia of speech and aphasia: Perceptual analyses.* Unpublished doctoral dissertation.

Mauszycki, S. C., & Wambaugh, J. L. (2006). *The effects of rate control treatment on consonant production accuracy in apraxia of speech.* Manuscript in preparation.

Mauszycki, S. C., & Wambaugh, J. L. (in press). The effects of rate control treatment on consonant production accuracy in mild apraxia of speech. *Aphasiology.*

McHenry, M., & Wilson, R. (1994). The challenge of unintelligible speech following traumatic brain injury. *Brain Injury, 8*(4), 363–375.

McNeil, M. R., Robin, D. A., & Schmidt, R. A. (1997). Apraxia of speech: Definition, differentiation, and treatment. In M. R.

McNeil (Ed.), *Clinical management of sensorimotor speech disorders* (pp. 311–344). New York: Thieme.

Mines, M., Hanson, B., & Shoup, J. (1978). Frequency of occurrence of phoneme in conversational English. *Language and Speech, 21*, 221–241.

Mohr, J. P., Pessin, M. S., Finkelstein, S., Funkenstein, H. H., Duncan, G. W., Davis, K. R. (1978). Broca aphasia: pathologic and clinical. *Neurology, 28*, 311–324.

MRC Pscyholinguistic Database (2007).www.psy.uwa.edu.au/mrcdatabase/uwa_mrc.htm. Retrieval date 11/23/07.

Naeser, M. A., & Hayward, R. W. (1978). Lesion localization in aphasia with cranial computed tomography and the Boston Diagnostic Aphasia Exam. *Neurology, 28*, 545–551.

Naselaris, T., Merchant, H., Amirikian, B., & Georgopoulos, A. P. (2006). Large-scale organization of preferred directions in the motor cortex II: Analysis of local distributions. *Journal of Neurophysiology.* [E-pub ahead of print, September 13, 2006]. http://jn.physiology.org/cgi/content/short/00488.2006vi.

Nishitani, N., Schürmann, M., Amunts, K., & Hari, R. (2005). Broca's region: From action to language. *Physiology, 20*, 60–69.

Nolte, J. (1993). *The human brain. An introduction to its functional anatomy* (3rd ed.). Baltimore: Mosby Year Book.

Odell, K. H. (2002). Considerations in target selection in apraxia of speech treatment. *Seminars in Speech and Language, 23*(4), 309–323.

Paninski, L., Fellows, M. R., Hatsopoulos, N. G., & Donoghue, J. P. (2004). Spatiotemporal tuning of motor cortical neurons for hand position and velocity. *Journal of Neurophysiology, 91*, 515–532.

Paus, T., Tomaiuolo, F., Otaky, N., MacDonald, D., Petrides, M., Atlas, J., et al. (1996). Human cingulate and paracingulate sulci: Pattern, variability, asymmetry, and probabilistic map. *Cerebral Cortex, 6*, 207–214.

Pell, M. D. (2006). Cerebral mechanisms for understanding emotional prosody in speech. *Brain and Language, 96*, 221–234.

Penfield, W., & Roberts, L. (1959). Speech and brain mechanisms. Princeton, NJ: Princeton University Press.

Picard, N., & Strick, P. L. (1996). Motor areas of the medial wall: A review of their location and functional activation. *Cerebral Cortex, 6*, 342–353.

Picard, N., & Strick, P. L. (2001). Imaging the premotor areas. *Neurobiology, 11*, 663–672.

Poeppel, D., & Hickok, G. (2004). Towards a new functional anatomy of language. *Cognition, 92*, 1–12.

Purves, D., Augustine, G., & Fitzpatrick, D. (2001). *Neuroscience* (2nd ed.). Sunderland, MA: Sinaur.

Rabidoux, P., Florance, C., & McCauslin, L. (1980). The use of a Handi Voice in the treatment of a severely apractic nonverbal patient. In R. H. Brookshire (Ed.), *Clinical Aphasiology Conference Proceedings* (pp. 294–301). Minneapolis, BRK.

Raymer, A. M., Haley, M. A., & Kendall, D. L. (2002). Overgeneralization in treatment for severe apraxia of speech: A case study. *Journal of Medical Speech-Language Pathology, 10*(4), 313–317.

Raymer, A. M., & Thompson, C. K. (1991). Effects of verbal plus gestural treatment in a patient with aphasia and severe apraxia of speech. In T. E. Prescott (Ed.), *Clinical Aphasiology* (Vol. 20, pp. 285–298). Austin, TX: Pro-Ed.

Rizzolatti, G., & Arbib, M. A. (1998). Language within our grasp. *Trends in Neurosciences, 21*, 188–194.

Rizzolatti, G., Fadiga, L., Gallese, V., & Fogassi, L. (1996). Premotor cortex and the recognition of motor actions. *Cognitive Brain Research, 3*, 131–141.

Rose, M., & Douglas, J. (2006). A comparison of verbal and gestural treatments for a word production deficit resulting from acquired apraxia of speech. *Aphasiology, 20*(12), 1186–1209.

Rosenbek, J. C., Lemme, M. L., Ahern, M. B., et al. (1973). A treatment for apraxia of speech in adults. *J Speech Hear Disord, 38*, 462–472.

Rosenbek, J. C., Collins, M., Wertz, R. T. (1976). Intersystemic reorganization for apraxia of speech. In R. H. Brookshire (Ed.), *Clinical aphasiology: Conference proceedings* (pp. 255–260). Minneapolis, BRK.

Rubow, R. T., Rosenbek, J. C., Collins, M. J., & Longstreth, D. (1982). Vibrotactile stimulation for intersystemic reorganization in the treatment of apraxia of speech. *Archives of Physical Medicine Rehabilitation, 63*, 150–153.

Rushworth, M. F., Behrens, T. E., Johansen-Berg, H. (2006). Connection patterns distinguish 3 regions of human parietal cortex. *Cerebral Cortex, 16*, 1418–1430.

Rushworth, M. F. S., Johansen-Berg. H., Göbel, S., & Devlin, J. T. (2003). The left parietal and premotor cortices: Motor attention and selection. *NeuroImage, 20*(Suppl 1), S89–S100.

Saarinen, T., Laaksonen, H., Parviainen, T., & Salmelin. R. (2006). Motor cortex dynamics of speech and non-speech mouth movements. *Cerebral Cortex, 16*, 212–222.

Sanes, J. N., & Donoghue, J. P. (2000). Plasticity and primary motor cortex. *Annual Review of Neuroscience, 23*, 393–415.

Sanes, J. N., Donoghue, J. P., Thangaraj, V., Edelman, R. R., & Warach, S. (1995). Shared neural substrates controlling hand movements in human motor cortex. *Science, 268*, 1775–1777.

Schluter, N. D., Rushworth, M. F. S., Passingham, R. E., & Mills, K. R. (1998). Temporary interference in human lateral premotor cortex suggests dominance for the selection of movements: A study using transcranial magnetic stimulation. *Brain, 121*, 785–799.

Schmidt, R. A., & Lee, T. D. (1999). *Motor control and learning. A behavioral emphasis.* (3rd ed.). Champaign, IL: Human Kinetics.

Schubotz, R. I., & von Cramon, D. (2003). Functional-anatomical concepts of human premotor cortex: Evidence from fMRI and PET studies. *NeuroImage, 20*, S120–S131.

Schulz, G. M., Varga, M., Jeffires, K., Ludlow, C. L., & Braun, A. R. (2005). Functional neuroanatomy of human vocalization: An $H_2{}^{15}0$ PET study. *Cerebral Cortex, 15*, 1835–1847.

Schütz-Bosbach, S., Mancini, B., Aglioti, S. M., & Haggard, P. (2006). Self and other in the human motor system. *Current Biology, 16*, 1830–1834.

Scott, S. K., & Wise, R. J. S. (2004). The functional neuroanatomy of prelexical processing in speech perception. *Cognition, 92*, 13–45.

Shuster, L. I. & Wambaugh, J.L. (2000). Perceptual and acoustic analyses of speech sound errors in apraxia of speech accompanied by aphasia. *Aphasiology, 14*, 635–651.

Shuster, L. I., & Lemieux, S. K. (2005). An fMRI investigation of covertly and overtly produced mono- and multisyllabic words. *Brain and Language, 93*, 20–31.

Simmons, N. N. (1978). Finger counting as an intersystemic reorganizer in apraxia of speech. In R. H. Brookshire (Ed.), *Clinical aphasiology: Conference proceedings* (pp. 174–179). Minneapolis, BRK.

Simmons, N. N. (1980). Choice of stimulus modes in treating apraxia of speech: A case study. In R. H. Brookshire (Ed.), *Clinical aphasiology: Conference proceedings* (pp. 302–307). Minneapolis, BRK.

Simonyan, K., & Jürgens, U. (2005). Afferent cortical connections of the motor cortical larynx area in the rhesus monkey. *Neuroscience, 130,* 133–149.

Skelly, M. (1979). *Amer-Ind gestural code based on universal American Indian hand talk.* New York: Elsevier.

Skelly, M., Schinsky, L., Smith, R. W., & Fust, R. S. (1974). American Indian Sign (AMERIND) as a facilitator of verbalization for the oral verbal apraxic. *Journal of Speech and Hearing Disorders, 39,* 445–456.

Southwood, H. (1987). The use of prolonged speech in the treatment of apraxia of speech. In R. H. Brookshire (Ed.), *Clinical Aphasiology Conference Proceedings* (pp. 277–287). Minneapolis, BRK.

Spencer, K. A., Yorkston, K. M., & Duffy, J. R. (2003). Behavioral management of respiratory/phonatory dysfunction from dysarthria: A flowchart for guidance in clinical decision-making. *Journal of Medical Speech-Language Pathology, 11*(2), xxxix–ixi.

Square, P .A., Chumpelik, D. A., & Adams, S. (1985). Efficacy of the PROMPT system for the treatment of acquired apraxia of speech. In R.H. Brookshire (Ed.), *Clinical Aphasiology Conference Proceedings* (pp. 319–320). Minneapolis, BRK.

Square, P. A., Chumpelik, D. A., Morningstar, D., & Adams, S. (1986). Efficacy of the PROMPT system for the treatment of acquired apraxia of speech: A follow-up investigation. In R. H. Brookshire (Ed.), *Clinical Aphasiology Conference Proceedings* (pp. 221–226). Minneapolis, BRK.

Square, P. A., & Martin, R. E. (1994). The nature and treatment of neuromotor speech disorders in aphasia. In R. H. Chapey (Ed.), *Language intervention strategies in adult aphasia* (3rd ed., pp. 467–499). Baltimore, MD: Williams & Wilkins.

Square, P. A., Roy, E. A., & Martin, R. E. (1997). Apraxia of speech: Another form of praxis disruption. In L. J. G. Rothi and K. M. Heilman (Eds), *Apraxia: The neuropsychology of action* (pp. 173–206). East Sussex: Psychology Press.

Square, P. A., Martin, R. E., & Bose, A. (2001). Nature and treatment of neuromotor speech disorders in aphasia. In R. H. Chapey (Ed.), *Language intervention strategies in adult aphasia* (4th ed., pp. 847–884).

Square-Storer, P. A. & Apeldoorn, S. (1991). An acoustic study of apraxia of speech in patients with different lesion loci. In C.A. Moore, K. M. Yorkston and D. R. Beukelman (Eds), *Dysarthria and apraxia of speech: Perspectives on management* (pp. 217–286). Baltimore: Paul H. Brookes Publishing.

Square-Storer, P. A., & Hayden, D. C. (1989). PROMPT treatment. In P. Square-Storer (Ed.), *Acquired apraxia of speech in aphasic adults* (pp. 190–219). Hove and London: Lawrence Erlbaum.

Talairach, J., & Tournoux, P. (1988). *Co-planar stereotaxic atlas of the human brain.* New York: Thieme Medical.

Tjaden, K. (2000). Exploration of a treatment technique for prosodic disturbance following stroke. *Clinical Linguistics and Phonetics, 14*(8), 619–641.

Tomaiuolo, F., MacDonald, J. D., Caramanos, Z., Posner, G., Chiavaras, M., Evans, A. C., et al. (1999). Morphology, mor-

phometry and probability mapping of the pars opercularis of the inferior frontal gyrus: An in vivo MRI analysis. *European Journal of Neuroscience, 11,* 3033–3046.

Uylings, H. B., Jacobsen, A. M., Zilles, K., & Amunts, K. (2006). Left-right asymmetry in volume and number of neurons in adult Broca's area. *Cortex, 42,* 652–658.

Van Riper, C. (1939). Speech correction: Principles and methods. Engelwood Cliffs, NJ: Prentice Hall.

Vorobiev, V., Govoni, P., Rizzolatti, G., Matelli, M., & Luppino, G. (1998). Parcellation of human mesial area 6: Cytoarchitectonic evidence for three separate areas. *European Journal of Neuroscience, 10,* 2199–2203.

Wambaugh, J. L., Doyle, P. J., Kalinyak, M. M., & West, J. E. (1996). A minimal contrast treatment for apraxia of speech. *Clinical Aphasiology,* 97–108.

Wambaugh, J. L., & Martinez, A. L. (2000). Effects of rate and rhythm control treatment on consonant production accuracy in apraxia of speech. *Aphasiology, 14*(8), 851–871.

Wambaugh, J. L. (2002). A summary of treatments for apraxia of speech and review of replicated approaches. *Seminars in Speech and Language, 23*(4), 293–308.

Wambaugh, J. L. (2004). Stimulus generalization effects of sound production treatment for apraxia of speech. *Journal of Medical Speech-Language Pathology, 12*(2), 77–97.

Wambaugh, J. L. (2006). Treatment guidelines for apraxia of speech: Lessons for future research. *Journal of Medical Speech-Language Pathology, 14*(4), 317–321.

Wambaugh, J. L., & Cort, R. C. (1998, January). *Treatment for AOS: Perceptual and VOT changes in sound production.* Poster session presented at the biennial Motor Speech Conference, Tuscon, AZ.

Wambaugh, J. L., Duffy, J. R., McNeil, M. R., Robin, D. A., & Rogers, M. (2006a). Treatment guidelines for acquired apraxia of speech: A synthesis and evaluation of the evidence. *Journal of Medical Speech Language Pathology, 14*(2), xv–xxxiii.

Wambaugh, J. L., Duffy, J. R., McNeil, M. R., Robin, D. A., & Rogers, M. (2006b). Treatment guidelines for acquired apraxia of speech: Treatment descriptions and recommendations. *Journal of Medical Speech Language Pathology, 14*(2), xxxv–ixvii.

Wambaugh, J. L., Kalinyak-Fliszar, M. M., West, J. E., & Doyle, P. J. (1998a). Effects of treatment for sound errors in apraxia of speech and aphasia. *Journal of Speech, Language, Hearing Research, 41,* 725–743.

Wambaugh, J. L., Martinez, A. L., McNeil, M. R., & Rogers, M. A. (1999). Sound production treatment for apraxia of speech: Overgeneralization and maintenance effects. *Aphasiology, 13*(9–11), 821–837.

Wambaugh, J. L., & Martinez, A. L. (2000). Effects of modified response elaboration training with apraxic and aphasic speakers. *Aphasiology, 5/6,* 603–617.

Wambaugh, J. L., & Nessler, C. (2004). Modification of Sound Production Treatment for aphasia: Generalization effects. *Aphasiology, 18*(5/6/7), 407–427.

Wambaugh, J., Nessler, C., Bennett, J., & Mauszycki, S. C. (2004). Variability in apraxia of speech: A perceptual and VOT analysis. *Journal of Medical Speech Language Pathology, 12*(4), 221–227.

Wambaugh, J. L., West, J. E., & Doyle, P. J. (1998b). Treatment for apraxia of speech: Effects of targeting sound groups. *Aphasiology, 12,* 731–743.

Warren, D. W., Allen, G., & King, H. A. (1984). Physiologic and perceptual effects of induced anterior open bite. *Folia Phoniatrica, 36,* 164–173.

Watkins, K., & Paus, T. (2004). Modulation of motor excitability during speech perception: The role of Broca's area. *Journal of Cognitive Neuroscience, 16,* 978–987.

Wernicke, C. (1874). Der aphasische symptomenkomplex. Breslau, Germany: Cohn & Weigert.

Wernicke, C. (1885). Die neueren arbeiten uber aphasie. Forschritte der Medizin, 3, 824–830.

Wertz, R. T., LaPointe, L. L., & Rosenbek, J. C. (1984). *Apraxia of speech in adults: The disorder and its management.* Orlando, FL: Grune & Stratton.

Wertz, R. T., LaPointe, L. L., & Rosenbek, J. C. (1984). *Apraxia of speech in adults: The disorder and its management.* Orlando, FL: Grune & Stratton. Square-Storer, P.A. (1989). *Acquired apraxia of speech in aphasic adults.* London: Taylor & Francis.

Wilson, S. M., Saygin, A. P., Sereno, M. I., & Iacoboni, M. (2004). Listening to speech activates motor areas involved in speech production. *Nature Neuroscience, 7,* 701–702.

Wise, R. J. S., Scott, S. K., Blank, S. C., Mummery, C. J., Murphy, K., & Warburton, E. A. (2001). Separate neural subsystems within "Wernicke's area." *Brain, 124,* 83–95.

Yorkston, K. M., & Beukelman, D. R. (1981). *Assessment of intelligibility of dysarthric speech.* Austin, TX: Pro-ed.

Yorkston, K. M., & Waugh, P .F. (1989). Use of augmentative communication devices with apractic individuals. In P. Square-Storer (Ed.), *Acquired apraxia of speech in aphasic adults* (pp. 267–283). Hove and London: Lawrence Erlbaum.

Yorkston, K. M., Spencer, K., Duffy, J., Beukelman, D., Gopher, L. A., et al. (2001). Evidence-based practice guidelines for dysarthria: Management of velopharyngeal function. *Journal of Medical Speech-Language Pathology, 9*(4), 257–273.

Yorkston, K. M., Spencer, K., Duffy J. R. (2003). Behavioral management of respiratory/phonatory dysfunction from dysarthria: A systematic review of the evidence. *Journal of Medical Speech-Language Pathology, 11*(2), xiii–xxxviii.

Yorkston, K. M., Hakel, M., Beukelman, D. R., & Fager, S. (2006). Evidence for effectiveness of treatment of loudness, rate or prosody in dysarthria: A systematic review. *Journal of Medical Speech-Language Pathology.* Manuscript submitted for publication.

APPENDIX 36.1
Consonant-Production Probe

Syllable Initial Stops

<u>d</u>	<u>t</u>	<u>b</u>	<u>p</u>	<u>g</u>	<u>k</u>
deer	tear	beer	peer	gore	core
dip	tip	bop	pop	gap	cap
die	tie	buy	pie	gay	Kay
dot	tot	bit	pit	got	cot
dame	tame	ban	pan	game	came

Syllable Final Stops

<u>d</u>	<u>t</u>	<u>b</u>	<u>p</u>	<u>g</u>	<u>k</u>
pad	pat	pub	pup	pug	puck
god	got	gab	gap	gag	gawk
sad	sat	sob	sap	sag	sack
tad	tat	tab	tap	tag	tack
ride	right	rib	rip	rig	Rick

Syllable Initial Fricatives

<u>s</u>	<u>z</u>	<u>f</u>	<u>v</u>	<u>sh</u>	<u>th</u>
sin	zen	fin	vine	shine	thin
same	zoom	fame	voom	shame	thumb
sore	czar	fear	veer	shore	Thor
sit	zit	fit	vet	sheet	thought
sauce	Zeus	face	vase	shoes	thaws

Syllable Final Fricatives

<u>s</u>	<u>z</u>	<u>f</u>	<u>v</u>	<u>sh</u>	<u>th</u>
bus	buzz	buff	pave	bush	bath
sauce	saws	safe	save	sash	Seth
face	faze	fife	five	fish	faith
race	raise	roof	rave	rash	wrath
kiss	keys	cuff	cove	cash	Keith

Syllable Initial Affricate/Nasals/Glides/Liquids

<u>ch</u>	<u>j</u>	<u>m</u>	<u>n</u>	<u>r</u>	<u>w</u>	<u>l</u>
choke	joke	mine	nine	wren	win	line
chain	Jane	met	net	right	wit	light
chill	Jill	mail	nail	rail	wail	liar
choice	juice	mice	nice	rash	wish	lash
cheat	jet	mock	knock	rack	wick	lack

Syllable Final Affricates/Nasal/Liquids

<u>ch</u>	<u>j</u>	<u>m</u>	<u>n</u>	<u>r</u>	<u>l</u>
fetch	judge	fame	fan	fire	file
batch	budge	bum	bun	bear	bale
latch	ledge	lime	line	wire	while
witch	wedge	some	sun	sore	soil
notch	nudge	numb	nun	near	kneel

Blends

<u>s-blends</u>	<u>l-blends</u>	<u>r-blends</u>
ski	clown	crown
star	black	break
sled	flag	freeze
swing	sled	trip
small	glass	grass

(From Wambaugh, et al., 1998a)

APPENDIX 36.2
Example of Lists of Balanced Multisyllabic Words

Bi-Syllabic Words by Initial Phoneme

h	f	m	s	d	r	n
hazel	focus	minus	sausage	deca[l]	raisin	notice
hyphen	faucet	mason	siphon	diesel	rebate	nylon
humus	famous	mobile	siren	demon	rotate	nation
haven	feline	motive	sinus	donut	regal	native

Tri-Syllabic Words by Initial Phoneme

h	f	m	s	d	r	n
hesitate	feminine	magazine	sanitize	dedicate	radical	nominate
habitat	physical	marathon	sedative	deficit	relative	navigate
homicide	fabulous	monotone	silicone	dominate	renovate	negative
halogen	pheromone	medicate	salivate	decorate	ridicule	nicotine

Bi-Syllabic Words by Final Phoneme

z	d	m	s	l	k	p
rabies	nomad	forum	bogus	vocal	basic	tulip
topaz	Cupid	Salem	recess	rival	lilac	julep
series	lucid	totem	Venus	legal	cubic	gallop
pisces	moped	serum	cautious	naval	Kodak	bebop

Tri-Syllabic Words by Final Phoneme

z	d	m	s	l	k	p
memorize	latitude	catacomb	nemesis	chemical	bailiwick	teletype
paralyze	renegade	maximum	paradise	topical	tomahawk	leadership
televise	marinade	synonym	Genesis	parallel	Similac	lollipop
maximize	solitude	minimum	populous	monorail	Tillamook	handicap

(From Mauszycki, S. C. (2006). Variability of sound production in apraxia of speech and aphasia: Perceptual analyses. Unpublished doctoral dissertation.)

APPENDIX 36.3
Examples of Sentence-Completion Items

/s/

1. (see) Before I can read the newspaper, I need to put on my glasses because I can't _____.
2. (set) A track-and-field runner always gets ready when he or she hears the phrase: "On your marks, get _____."
3. (seal) In order for a passport to be legal, the immigration department has to stamp a _____.
4. (Sue) My best friend's name is Susan but I call her by the nicknames of Susie or _____.
5. (sigh) Everybody knows when my father is extremely tired and ready to go to sleep because he tends to yawn and _____.

/p/

1. (pie) Julie usually makes desserts when she has company. Last Saturday, her parents came and she baked a delicious apple _____.
2. (pail) The little boy wanted to build a sandcastle, so his mom bought him a shovel and a _____.
3. (pet) We have a goldfish, a hamster, and a dog in my house. I'm responsible for the hamster because she is my _____.
4. (pat) Every time I get home, my dog wants me to play with him and give him a friendly _____.
5. (pier) I tied my boat up at the dock or the _____.

/v/

1. (vee) The little boy learned today to write words such as violin, van, and vase, which are words that begin with the letter _____.
2. (veil) A bride bought her wedding gown, shoes, and accessories. But later she realized that she did not buy a _____.
3. (view) If you live on the mountain and look over the city, you have a beautiful _____.
4. (vet) My dog has been very sick for the past two days. I need to take her to the _____.
5. (veal) Instead of making my beef stew with beef, I prefer to use the meat of a calf, which is better known as _____.

/k/

1. (key) I was frustrated because I locked myself out. Fortunately, I remembered that I was carrying an extra _____.

2. (cut) My hair is too long. I need to go to my hairdresser and get a new hair _____.
3. (cot) Grandpa came to visit. Mom said to my brother: "Grandpa can sleep in your bed and you can unfold the _____."
4. (coo) When I went to New York, I visited Central Park. I loved to feed the pigeons and hear their _____.
5. (car) I've been riding the bus for many years. I finally saved enough money to buy a good _____.

/ʃ/

1. (shoe) The little boy is almost ready to go outside and play. He'll be ready once he ties his left _____.
2. (shot) The flu can be deadly in older people. That's why older people have been encouraged to have a flu _____.
3. (shut) The little boy was so tired that when his mom finished reading the story, his eyes were already _____.
4. (share) At the beginning of the school semester, the teacher did not have enough books for all the children so she said: "We'll have to _____."
5. (she) We saw a beautiful dog at the pet shop. We wanted to get a "he" so we asked: "Is it a he or a _____?"

/dʒ/

1. (jail) A man committed a crime and was caught. He was sentenced to 15 years in _____.
2. (Jew) My friend believes in Judaism, so everyone considers him a _____.
3. (jaw) The boxer threw a punch near his opponent's mouth and broke his _____.
4. (jar) The little boy was so hungry that he couldn't wait for his lunch and grabbed some cookies from the cookie _____.
5. (gee) The little girl learned in class today that the words girl, game, goat, and guitar begin with the letter _____.

/l/

1. (light) I was reading a book and all of the sudden the room became dark. I told my husband to turn on the _____.

2. (late) Tim is never on time. He usually gets to school ten to fifteen minutes _____.
3. (lit) Julie doesn't like to live in a dark house. When she was looking for a home, she made sure that it was well-_____.
4. (low) Ted wants to apply for medical school but he needs to retake the test because he scored too _____.
   (lie) I tried to believe what they said but it was very hard for me because they always _____.

/m/

1. (mitt) Tim was ready to play baseball. He brought a ball and a bat, but then he realized that he forgot to bring his baseball _____.
2. (me) Julie's mom told her to call home as soon as possible. So when Julie was leaving, mom said: "Don't forget to call _____."
3. (mate) Ted is always dating but never seems to find the right person. He's still searching for the perfect _____.
4. (mow) The big kids share the yard work with their dad. The grass is tall and dad asked: "Who is going to _____?"
5. (moo) I would like to live on a farm. I love to hear the horses neigh, the ducks quack, the pigs oink, and the cows _____.

/n/

1. (knit) I know how to cross-stitch, sew, and crochet, but I don't know how to _____.
2. (know) The teacher asked a question about what the children were studying in class. A kid raised his hand and said "I _____."
3. (night) The mom put her son in his bed, covered him with a blanket, gave him a kiss, and said: "Good _____!"
4. (need) The Boy Scouts were knocking on every door, asking for donations for families in _____.
5. (knee) The boy was running and tripped over a rock. He was crying because he scraped his left _____.

(From Wambaugh, J. L., & Nessler, C. 2004)

APPENDIX 36.4
Metronome and Hand-tapping Treatment

Level One:- Clinician Model, Unison Production, Beginning Patient Production

A. S/T[a]
B. Metronome setting: 93 bpm
C. Treatment steps:
   1. CM[b] - 1 production
   2. Patient taps along (no verbal production), while clinician produces word - 5 productions
   3. UPT[c]- 3 productions
   4. PPT[d] - 1 production
D. Target-item presentation: Clinician presents experimental words (treatment items only) in random order. Clinician presents as many items per session as possible.
E. Feedback: Clinician provides positive or negative feedback about tapping, production of correct number of syllables, and/or production of syllables on beat, *but not about sound accuracy*
F. Scoring: "+" or "−" for PPT step ("+" = correct use of tapping with production of correct number of syllables on the beat)

Criterion: 95% accuracy for entire treatment session in two consecutive sessions

Level Two:- Faded Clinician Model, Repeated Patient Production

A. S/T
B. Metronome setting: 93 bpm
C. Treatment steps:
   1. CM - 1 production
   2. PPT - 3 productions
   a) If any errors in tapping to the beat or in producing the correct number of syllables: CM (1 production) plus UPT (3 productions); if errors remain: clinician presents next target word
   b) If correct, clinician begins treatment steps with next word
D. Target item presentation: same as Level 1
E. Feedback: same as Level 1
F. Scoring: "+" or "−" for first production of PPT step

Criterion: 95% accuracy for entire treatment session in two consecutive sessions

Level Three:- No Clinician Model, Repeated Patient Production

A. S/T
B. Metronome setting: 93 bpm
C. Treatment steps:
   1. Clinician says word with normal rate and prosody (no metronome or tapping)

2. PPT - 3 productions
   a) If any errors in tapping to the beat or in producing correct number of syllables: CM (1 production) plus PPT (3 productions); if errors remain: CM (1 production) plus UPT (3 productions); if errors remain: clinician presents next target word
   b) If correct, clinician begins treatment steps with next word
D. Target item presentation: same as Level 1
E. Feedback: same as Level 1
F. Scoring: "+" or "−" for first production of PPT step

Criterion: 95% accuracy for entire treatment session in two consecutive sessions

Level Four:- Increased Rate of Production

A. Metronome setting: 100 to 110 bpm
B. Treatment steps: same as Level 3
C. Target item presentation: same as Level 1
D. Feedback: same as Level 1
E. Scoring: "+" or "−" for first production of PPT step

Criterion: 95% accuracy for entire treatment session in two consecutive sessions and no decrease in accuracy of trained items on probes

Level Five:- Syncopated Production

A. Clinician explains concept of syncopation: The target word will be produced in two beats, with the first syllable on downbeat of hand tap, the second syllable on the upbeat, and the third syllable on the downbeat of second hand tap.
B. S/T
C. Metronome setting: 100 bpm
D. Treatment steps: apply syncopation sequentially at each of preceding levels, beginning with Level 1

Abbreviations

[a]**Schematic/tapping review (S/T)**: Clinician explains/reviews schematic of stress pattern for words under treatment; clinician and patient practice tapping with the schematic (_ _ ↓).
[b]**Clinician model (CM)**: Clinician produces word with metronome (one syllable per beat), while tapping
[c]**Unison production and tapping (UPT)**: Clinician and patient simultaneously produce target word, while tapping
[d]**Patient production and tapping (PPT)**: Patient produces target word, while tapping; clinician provides no model or assistance

(From Wambaugh, J. L., & Martinez, A. L. (2000).

APPENDIX 36.5
Eight-Step Continuum

Step 1. Integral Stimulation. The target utterance is produced simultaneously by the client and clinician simultaneously with auditory and visual stimulation. "Watch me, listen to me" plus simultaneous production.

Step 2. Integral Stimulation and Delayed Production. The clinician provides a model of the utterance, then asks the client to produce the utterance while the clinician produces the utterance without sound. That is, the auditory model is eliminated during simultaneous production.

Step 3. Integral Stimulation and Delayed Production with No Visual Cue. The clinician provides a model while instructing the client to watch and listen. The client is asked to repeat the utterance. "I'll say it first, then you say it after me."

Step 4. Integral Stimulation and Successive Productions. The clinician provides a verbal model and the client is asked to produce the target several times without any cues.

Step 5. Written Stimuli and Simultaneous Production. The client reads the target utterance aloud with written stimulus present.

Step 6. Written Stimuli and Delayed Production. The clinician provides the written utterance, then the client is asked to produce the utterance after the written stimulus is removed.

Step 7. Appropriate Utterance Elicited by Question. The clinician asks a question that is appropriate for eliciting the target utterance.

Step 8. Appropriate Response in Role-Playing Situation. The clinician and others assume roles to elicit the target utterance in a contextually appropriate situation.

(From Rosenbek, J. C., .)

APPENDIX 36.6
Original Sound-Production Treatment Hierarchy

Step 1—Modeling/Imitation: The therapist produces the minimal contrast pair* and instructs the speaker to repeat the pair (e.g., "say pie ... buy"). If the speaker cannot repeat the paired words together, each member of the pair is presented separately. If the target sound and contrasting sound are correct, feedback about accuracy is provided, another production of the target word is elicited, and the next pair is presented. If either sound is incorrect, feedback about accuracy is provided and this step is reattempted. If either sound is incorrect upon second attempt, feedback is provided and Step 2 is attempted.

Step 2—Modeling plus Written Letter Cue/Imitation: The therapist points to printed letters representing the target sound and contrasting sound while modeling production of the minimal-pair items. The speaker is asked to repeat each item. If both sounds are correct, feedback is provided and the next pair is presented. If either sound is incorrect, feedback is provided and Step 3 is attempted.

Step 3—Integral Stimulation: If only the target sound or both sounds are incorrect in Step 2, then the target sound *only* is focused upon at this step. If only the contrasting sound is incorrect, then that sound is focused upon. Using the single item (i.e., nonpaired item), the therapist instructs the speaker to "watch me, listen to me, and say it with me". If correct, then feedback is provided, another production is elicited, and the next pair is presented. If the contrasting sound is incorrect, feedback is provided and the next pair is presented. If the target sound is incorrect, the therapist provides feedback and moves to Step 4.

Step 4—Modeling with Silent Juncture/Imitation: The clinician models the target word using a silent juncture, separating the sound from the rest of the word (e.g., "Say the word like this, p . . . ie). The speaker is instructed to repeat the word. If correct, feedback is provided and the next pair is presented. If incorrect, feedback is provided and the clinician moves to Step 5.

Step 5—Articulatory Placement and Modeling: The therapist provides verbal articulatory placement instructions specific to the speaker's perceived error, models the sound in isolation, and asks the speaker to repeat the sound. If correct or incorrect, feedback is provided and the clinician moves to the next pair of contrasts at Step 1.

*__Modifications to the Minimal-Pair Presentation:__

A. 80% to 100% correct production at Step 1 in a single trial (10 items), use hierarchy exactly as above.
B. 50% to 79% correct production at Step 1 in a single trial, use single items in alternate trials instead of contrast pairs at every trial (i.e., use only the target item without the minimal-contrast item).

C. 0% to 49% correct production at Step 1 in a single trial, use two single-item trials alternately with one minimal-pair trial.

__Notes__:

- 10 exemplars of the target sound presented in random order constitute one trial
- As many productions as possible should be attempted per session (attempt to complete a minimum of seven 10-item trials)
- Continue treatment until at least 80% of trained items are produced correctly in PROBES (not during application of treatment) in two of three consecutive sessions

(From Wambaugh et al., 1998a)

APPENDIX 36.7
Modified Sound-Production Treatment

1) Clinician produces the target item and requests a repetition
   a) if correct, the clinician provides positive feedback concerning accuracy, requests five additional repetitions,* and moves to the next target item
   b) if incorrect, the clinician gives feedback and says: "Now, let's try a different word" and models the *minimal contrast word*
      • if correct, the clinician says: "Now, let's go back to the other word" & goes to Step 2 with the target word
      • if incorrect, the clinician gives feedback, and attempts production of the contrast word with integral stimulation for a maximum of 3 trials; the clinician then moves to Step 2 with the target word
2) The clinician shows the letter representing the target sound, models the *target item*, and requests a repetition
   a) if correct, the clinician provides feedback, requests five additional repetitions,* and moves to the next item
   b) if incorrect, the clinician goes to Step 3

3) The clinician requests production of the target item using integral stimulation: "watch me, listen to me, and say it with me," for a maximum of three trials
   a) if correct, the clinician provides feedback, requests five additional repetitions,* and moves to the next item
   b) if incorrect, the clinician moves to Step 4
4) The clinician provides articulatory placement cues appropriate to the participant's error and requests production of the target item using integral stimulation; if correct, request additional repetitions (five times*)
   a) if correct, the clinician provides feedback, requests five additional repetitions,* and moves to the next item
   b) if incorrect, the clinician provides feedback and moves to the next item

*Feedback is provided on approximately 60% of attempts.
(From Wambaugh, J. L., & Nessler, C. (2004). Modification of Sound Production Treatment for aphasia: Generalization effects. *Aphasiology, 18*(5/6/7), 407–427.)

APPENDIX 36.8
Modified Response Elaboration Training

Treatment Steps

Step 1. The clinician presents a picture and elicits a response (e.g., "Tell me about this picture.", What does this remind you of?", "Tell me what's happening.")

A. If the response is correct,* the clinician moves to Step 2.

B. If there is no or an incorrect response, the clinician models two response options (e.g., "You could say something like . . . noun phrase [NP] or verb phrase [VP].") If the response is correct, the clinician moves to Step 2.

C. If there is no or an incorrect response, the clinician models a one-word response and requests a repetition (e.g., "Say noun." or "Say verb.") If the response is correct, the clinician moves to Step 2.

D. If there is no or an incorrect response, the clinician uses integral stimulation, with a maximum of four attempts, to elicit the noun or verb production. If the response is correct, the clinician moves to Step 2. In the event of an incorrect or no response, the next item is presented.

Step 2. The clinician models and reinforces the participant's production from Step 1 (e.g., "Shoe. Great. That's a shoe.")

Step 3. The clinician requests an elaboration of the response from Step 1 (e.g., "What's happening with the shoe?")

A. If the response is correct, the clinician moves to Step 4.

B. If there is no or an incorrect response, the clinician models two response options (e.g., "You could say something like . . . noun phrase [NP] or verb phrase [VP].") and requests a response. If the response is correct, the clinician moves to Step 4.

C. If there is no or an incorrect response, the clinician models a one-word response and requests a repetition (e.g., "Say noun." or "Say verb.") If the response is correct, the clinician moves to Step 4.

D. If there is no or an incorrect response, the clinician uses integral stimulation, with a maximum of four attempts, to elicit

the noun or verb production. If the response is correct, the clinician moves to Step 4. In the event of an incorrect or no response, the next item is presented.

Step 4. The clinician reinforces the production from Step 3 and models a phrase/sentence that combines the participant's productions from Steps 1 and 3 (e.g., "Right, tie. Tie shoe.")

Step 5. The clinician models the combined production again and requests a repetition.

A. If the response is correct, the clinician requests three more productions, using integral stimulation as needed. The clinician moves to Step 6.

B. If there is an incorrect or no response, the clinician attempts to elicit four productions of the target, using integral stimulation. The clinician moves to Step 6.

Step 6. The clinician removes the picture, waits for at least 5 seconds, returns the picture, and requests that the participant again describe the picture.

A. If the entire† elaborated response is produced, the clinician reinforces the production and moves to the next item.

B. If a partial elaborated response is produced, the clinician reinforces the production, models the entire elaboration, and requests a production with integral stimulation. The clinician then moves to the next item.

C. If no response, the clinician reinforces the production, models the entire elaboration, and requests a production with integral stimulation. The clinician then moves to the next item.

D. If an alternate correct response is produced, the clinician reinforces the production and moves to the next item.

*Any appropriate, intelligible noun, pronoun, verb, adjective, adverb, or preposition; not perseverative, stereotypic, or reiterative.
†Omission of functors is not considered incorrect.
(From Wambaugh, J. L., & Martinez, A. L. (2000).)

Author Index

Aaronson, D., 802
AARP Public Policy Institute, 206
Aarsland, D., 993
Abe, K., 50, 551
Abernathy, C. D., 22
Abidi, R., 259
Abikof, H., 914, 924
Abkarian, G. G., 1024, 1025
Abo, M., 191
Abrams, W., 13
Abramson, R. K., 256
Abrous, D. N., 13
Absher, J. R., 535
Abutalebi, J., 250, 251
Abu-Zeid, H. A. H., 787
Academy of Neurologic Communication
    Disorders and Sciences (ANCDS), 14, 177,
    437, 438, 1018, 1019
Ackles, P., 967
ADA. See Americans with Disabilities Act
Adamovich, B. L. B., 88, 904, 968
Adams, H. P., 30, 34, 572
Adams, J. E., 856
Adams, J. H., 881, 892
Adams, M. R., 428
Adams, R., 967
Adams, S., 1027
Adger, D., 738
Adolfsson, R., 193
Adolphs, R., 37, 774, 976
Adrian, J. A., 413, 832, 862
Afford, R. J., 566
Aftonomos, L. B., 586, 587, 761, 832, 853,
    864, 868
Agan, J., 329
Agency for Health Care Research and Quality,
    254
Ager, C., 52
Aging Eye, 334
Aglioti, S., 251, 259, 1014
Agran, M., 892, 914
Agranowitz, A., 376, 383
Agrell, B., 94
Aguado, G., 109
AHCPR, 880, 902
Ahern, M. B., 1018, 1021
Ahlsen, E., 519, 520
Ahlskog, J. E., 551
Aichert, I., 113
Alajouanine, M. S., 568
Alarcon, N., 89, 295, 524, 545, 546, 550,
    557, 820
Alario, F. X., 1012

Alazraki, N. P., 50
Albers, G. W., 45
Albert, M., 253, 259, 297, 437, 438,
    758, 760, 772, 773, 786, 826, 830,
    837, 840, 965
Albert, M. A., 507, 518
Albert, M. L., 56, 75, 92, 96, 102, 108, 191,
    192, 195, 197, 198, 415, 416, 451, 515, 575,
    582, 583, 585
Albert, N., 384
Alderman, N., 904, 905, 926, 927
Alexander, D., 583
Alexander, M. P., 21, 27, 32, 33, 35, 49,
    96, 108, 552, 566, 567, 569, 583, 611, 667,
    881, 885, 893, 894, 919, 967, 1014
Alibali, M. W., 919, 920
Ali-Cherif, A., 11, 566
Aliminosa, D., 600
Al-Khawaja, I., 70
Allamano, N., 257
Allan, E., 326
Allan, K., 365
Allchin, J., 106
Allen, C. C., 967
Allen, G., 1011
Allen, K. E., 229, 230, 233
Allen, M., 102
Allport, A., 585
Allport, D. A., 95, 610
Aloia, M., 992
Alperovitch, A., 993
Alpress, F., 229
Altarriba, J., 252, 265
Altenmuller, E., 757
Altieri, M., 48
Altman, I. M., 885
Alvarez, P., 708, 715
Alves, W. M., 192
Alvord, E. C., 880
Alzheimer's Association, 349, 991
Alzheimer's Disease and Related Disorders
    Association, 176
American Academy of Audiology, 335
American Academy of Family Physicians,
    336
American Academy of Neurology, 861
American Association of University Women,
    176, 177
American Heart Association, 10, 52
American Medical Association, 210
American Medical Association (AMA), 213
American Psychiatric Association, 988,
    992

American Speech-Language-Hearing
    Association (ASHA), 15, 166, 176,
    177, 178, 212, 219, 220, 222, 246,
    306, 319, 321, 350, 356, 386, 457, 815, 891,
    988, 1003
American Stroke Association, 382
American Telemedicine Association, 180
Americans with Disabilities Act (ADA), 306
Amiez, C., 1013
Amirikian, B., 1011
Amitrano, A., 619
Ammons, J., 50
Amunts, K., 1013, 1014, 1015
Anastasi, A., 77
ANCDS. See Academy of Neurologic
    Communication Disorders and Sciences
Andersen, G., 975
Andersen, K., 993
Anderson, J. R., 902
Anderson, K., 52
Anderson, N., 207
Anderson, N. B., 217
Anderson, P. E., 207
Anderson, S. W., 20, 894, 905, 910, 926
Andersson, S., 307, 308
Andrews, M., 206
Andrews, R. J., 188
Andriaanse, H. P., 238
Angelini, F. J., 233
Annegers, J. F., 880
Ansaldo, A., 114, 979
Ansell, B. J., 423, 424
Anthony, J. C., 995
Antiplatelet Trialists Collaboration, 46
Antonello, R. M., 251
Antonucci, S. M., 612
Anwander, A., 1013
Apeldoorn, S., 1015
Aphasia Hope Foundaion, 382
Appelros, P., 964
Appicciafuoco, A., 411
Applebaum, J. S., 587
Arabatzi, M., 741, 747
Aram, D. M., 165
Aran, D. M., 34
Arbib, M. A., 621, 1013, 1014
Archer, C. R., 35
Archibald, T. M., 968
Ardila, A., 171, 186, 192, 246, 255, 256,
    257
Arguin, M., 769
Arima, K., 552
Arkin, S. M., 1002

Armstrong, E., 70, 80, 101, 106, 107, 109, 110, 115, 116, 118, 119, 120, 295, 301, 302, 307, 309, 342, 524
Armstrong, J., 342
Armstrong, L., 256, 996
Armus, S. R., 426
Arne, L., 34
Aronson, A. E., 65, 90, 205, 865, 1011, 1026
Aronson, M., 376, 377, 379, 756
Arrigoni, G., 568
Arruda, J. E., 967
Arseni, C., 35
Asante, M. K., 246
Asanuma, H., 1011
Ash, S., 89, 548, 549, 554
ASHA. *See* American Speech-Language-Hearing Association
Ashayery, H., 259
Ashbaugh, J., 215, 217
Ashcraft, M., 919
Ashman, A. F., 899
Ashtry, F., 56, 57
Asking, M., 378
Asplund, K., 11, 193
Assel, M. A., 910
Asslid, R., 47
Assmus, A., 1015
Astrom, M., 193
Aten, J. L., 110, 377, 382, 386, 387, 389, 391, 392, 1022, 1024
Atkins-Mair, D. L., 53
Audet, T., 964, 967
Auerbach, S., 508
Augustine, G., 1010, 1013
Augustine, J., 1015
Augustine, L., 432
Aureille, E., 966
Aurelia, J., 492
Auriacombe, S., 993
Ausman, J. I., 259
Austermann, S., 361, 588
Austin, J., 115
Australian Association of Speech and Hearing, 246
Ausubel, D., 477
Auther, L. L., 117
Avent, J., 83, 90, 117, 120, 126, 180, 302, 338, 339, 361, 376, 377, 382, 386, 391, 588
Avery, J., 14
Avrutin, S., 424
Ayala, J., 414
Azouvi, P., 547
Azuma, T., 995, 999

Babbage, C., 853
Babcock, P., 418, 776
Bach, D., 1000
Bach, M., 1000
Bachman, D. L., 56, 80, 94, 507, 922
Bach-Y-Rita, P., 188
Backus, O., 377, 379, 756
Baddeley, A. D., 95, 97, 601, 714, 726, 904, 920, 922, 988, 989, 991, 998
Badecker, W., 102, 103, 611
Baer, D. M., 392, 393, 394, 520, 929, 1001
Baguley, I. J., 895

Bahrami, A., 56
Bahrick, H. P., 249, 714
Bahrick, L. E., 249
Bailey, J., 617, 999
Bailey, K. G. D., 648
Bailey, P., 413, 610, 617
Bailey, S., 71, 124, 1026
Bain, B., 1001
Bain, H., 49
Baines, K. A., 80, 119, 579
Bainton, D., 756
Bak, T., 575
Bakas, T., 364
Baker, E., 102, 105, 418, 586, 864
Baker, M., 550
Baker, R., 78, 249, 253, 256
Baker, S., 902, 918
Baker, T., 785
Bakke, B. L., 716
Baldo, J., 764
Ball, M., 119
Ballard, K. J., 92, 173, 425, 597, 601, 643, 718, 745, 746, 748, 778, 1022
Baly, A., 999
Bambauer, D. E., 51
Bambauer, K. Z., 51
Bandera, R., 991
Bandur, D. L., 756, 757, 761, 770, 775
Bandura, A., 488
Bang, O. Y., 569, 573
Banja, S., 328
Banker, B. Q., 544
Bannerman, D. J., 930, 931
Barat, M., 34
Barbarotto, R., 616
Baressi, B., 7, 71
Bargh, J. A., 910, 912
Barinaga, M., 1011
Barker, L. M., 180
Barker, P. B., 767, 964, 1014
Barker-Collo, S. L., 78
Barkley, R. A., 914, 926
Barnes, M., 893
Barnes, R., 565
Barnes, S., 336
Barnett, H. J., 46
Baron, C. R., 180, 973
Baron, J. C., 50, 188, 406
Barona, A., 124, 994
Barr, A., 865
Barresi, B., 108, 174, 196, 255, 256, 578, 581, 582, 607, 657, 741, 768, 771, 773, 817, 830, 970, 974
Barrett, A. M., 659
Barrett, H. M., 256
Barrette, J., 305, 363
Barry, C., 673
Barry, P., 297
Barsalou, L. W., 919
Bartels-Tobin, L. R., 85, 971
Barth, J. T., 888
Bartha, M., 894
Barthel, G., 712
Bartlett, C. L., 81, 123, 572
Bartolomeo, P., 964, 965
Barton, M., 413, 417

Basford, J. R., 52
Basili, A., 484, 502, 611, 696, 971
Basilico, D., 648
Bassett, S. S., 995
Basso, A., 81, 96, 123, 124, 125, 186, 188, 189, 192, 193, 198, 437, 565, 566, 567, 568, 572, 575, 705, 710, 711, 719, 756, 763
Bastiaanse, R., 103, 113, 174, 620, 737, 738, 741
Bates, B., 52
Bates, D. G., 78
Bates, E., 64, 74, 79, 113, 114, 249, 253, 257, 265, 705
Battle, D. E., 246, 248
Bauer, P. J., 937
Bauer, R. M., 65, 91, 719, 976
Baum, C., 299
Baum, S. R., 86, 418, 424, 427, 977, 978
Baumeister, R. F., 891, 902, 910
Baumgaertner, A., 965, 972, 973, 974, 975, 978
Bautz-Holter, E., 291, 360
Bava, A., 251
Bawden, K., 295, 338
Bayard, K., 220
Bayles, K. A., 87, 88, 256, 437, 988, 991, 993, 994, 995, 996, 997, 999, 1000, 1002, 1003
Baylis, G. C., 524
Baynes, K., 519
Bays, C., 337, 360
Beach, T. G., 551
Beach, W. A., 554
Bear, D., 415, 975, 976
Beard, L. C., 174
Beattie, A., 894
Beatty, P. W., 973
Beauchamp, B. G., 767
Beaulieu, M-D., 229
Bechera, A., 926
Beck, A. T., 994
Becker, R., 975
Beckers, K., 885
Bedenbaugh, P. H., 692
Bedrosian, J. L., 1026
Beecham, R., 260, 262
Beeke, S., 118, 299
Beekman, L., 426, 509
Beeman, M., 973
Beeson, P., 64, 82, 96, 102, 196, 197, 381, 382, 389, 390, 419, 597, 598, 599, 602, 612, 619, 654, 657, 658, 659, 663, 665, 666, 667, 668, 669, 670, 671, 673, 674, 769, 775, 782, 783, 785, 814, 1001
Begley, C. E., 217
Behrens, S. J., 977
Behrens, T. E., 1015
Behrmann, M., 599, 617, 622, 671
Beis, J. M., 965
Béland, R., 260
Belanger, L., 337
Belanger, S. A., 92
Belin, P., 190, 191, 264, 757
Bell, A., 293, 301
Bell, B. D., 102, 613
Bell, K. L., 993
Bell, S., 212

Bellaire, K. J., 584
Belleville, S., 905, 997
Belleza, T., 886
Bellugi, V., 20
Belz, P., 930
Benabid, A. L., 1012
Benaim, C., 94
Bench, C. J., 967
Bender, D. B., 535
Benedet, M. J., 735, 741
Bengston, V. L., 856
Benke, T., 968
Bennett, D. A., 988
Bennett, J., 1019
Benoit, N., 554
Benowitz, L. I., 971, 976
Benson, A. L., 410
Benson, D. F., 28, 186, 192, 327, 437, 507, 609,
    767, 782, 861, 893, 896, 905, 927
Benson, F., 105, 895
Benton, A. I., 910
Benton, A. L., 21, 73, 74, 75, 76, 106, 110, 123,
    255, 410, 571, 578, 777, 881, 905, 995
Ben-Yishay, Y., 920
Beretta, A., 104
Berg, E. A., 97, 98
Berg, M., 68, 69, 119, 120, 126
Bergeman, C. S., 206
Berger, S. A., 249
Bergeron, H., 352
Bergner, M., 81
Bergstralh, E. J., 43
Berk, L. E., 899, 914, 924
Berko, J., 111, 424, 777
Berko, R., 13
Berman, M., 205, 492
Berndt, R. S., 37, 102, 103, 104, 109, 110, 188,
    410, 413, 422, 425, 571, 572, 597, 600, 601,
    602, 610, 611, 612, 613, 614, 619, 632, 634,
    639, 640, 641, 643, 644, 645, 646, 647, 648,
    655, 664, 696, 704, 735, 736, 743, 767, 768,
    775, 776, 777
Bernholtz, N. D., 745
Bernstein-Ellis, E., 114, 118, 169, 180, 290,
    295, 302, 304, 376, 377, 380, 381, 382, 390,
    391, 392, 394
Berrios, G. E., 544, 992
Berry, T., 586, 864
Bertelson, P., 536
Berthier, M., 123
Best, W., 110, 197, 580, 618, 620, 624, 726,
    775, 776
Bester, S., 68
Beth, R. E., 991
Bettinardi, V., 37
Bettoni, C., 249
Beukelman, D., 93, 107, 295, 297, 306, 454,
    457, 458, 492, 601, 815, 817, 819, 820, 821,
    822, 825, 827, 828, 886, 1018, 1020
Beveridge, M. A., 762
Bevington, L. J., 381
Bezdudnaya, T., 533
Bharadwaj, S. V., 1022
Bhat, S., 259
Bhatnagar, S. C., 566
Bhogal, S. K., 714, 757

Bianchetti, A., 997
Biber, C., 423
Bick, K., 989
Biddle, K. R., 893
Biedermann, B., 565, 582
Biemiller, A., 891, 912
Bienias, J. L., 988
Biggers, A., 12
Bigler, E., 327
Bihrle, A. M., 969, 972
Biller, J., 30, 319, 357, 572
Billups, J. J., 229
Binetti, G., 997
Binkofski, F., 1013, 1014
Bioulac, B., 34
Birch, H. G., 409
Bird, F., 931
Bird, H., 110, 111, 190, 735
Bishop, D. S., 94
Bishop, D. V. M., 75
Bishop, R., 319
Bisiach, E., 410, 777
Bissett, J., 340
Bizzi, E., 715
Bjork, R. A., 715
Bjorklund, D. F., 910
Black, C., 713
Black, F. W., 997
Black, M., 126, 174, 638, 758, 759, 777
Black, S. E., 179, 236, 290, 363, 517, 547,
    565, 779
Blackman, N., 377, 379, 750, 756
Blackstone, S., 68, 69, 119, 120, 126
Blackwell, B., 56
Blair, J. R., 75
Blair, M., 548
Blake, M. L., 85, 86, 969, 970, 971, 973,
    975
Blanc, M., 250, 253
Blank, K., 437
Blank, S. C., 190, 1016
Blanken, G., 109, 568
Blishen, B. R., 786
Bliss, L. S., 893
Bloise, C. G. R., 174, 965, 975
Blomert, L., 80, 119, 297, 513
Blonder, L. X., 86, 712, 976
Bloom, D., 380
Bloom, L., 9, 382, 383, 478, 479, 480
Bloom, P., 106
Bloom, R. L., 109, 971, 976
Blum, A., 971
Blumer, D., 895
Blumstein, S. E., 102, 113, 415, 418, 423, 740,
    837, 1014, 1017
Boada, R., 781
Boake, C., 885
Boatman, D., 507, 508, 514, 609
Bobaljik, D. B., 736, 747
Bock, J., 641, 642
Bock, R. D., 404
Boczko, F., 999, 1000
Boden, M., 477
Bodrova, E., 899
Boen, J. R., 880
Boeve, B. F., 547, 548, 551, 554

Bogen, J., 697
Bogousslavsky, J., 50, 572
Bohland, J. W., 1009, 1014, 1015
Bohmer, F., 1000
Bois, M., 253
Boiten, J., 190
Bolduc, M., 337
Boles, L., 69, 89, 108, 118, 295, 303, 304, 306,
    308, 452, 779
Boling, E., 826
Boll, T. J., 888
Boller, F., 102, 411, 413, 424, 431, 514, 515,
    765, 967, 991, 993
Bollinger, R. L., 180, 386, 432, 433, 810
Bolt, E., 910
Bolter, J. D., 853
Bolwinick, J., 485
Bombard, T., 69, 108, 118
Bonaffini, N., 48
Bond, M., 886, 894
Bondar, J., 895
Bondi, M., 991
Bonita, R., 42
Bookheimer, S., 251
Boone, D., 376, 411, 431
Boone, J. R., 611
Boone, R. R., 14
Booth, S., 118, 294, 295
Borenstein, P., 376, 378, 379, 382, 384
Borgwaldt, S., 252
Borkowski, J. G., 96, 915, 994, 995
Borod, J. C., 193, 971, 975, 976
Borthwick, S. E., 256, 996
Bos, M., 252
Bosch, L., 250
Boschen, K., 364
Bose, A., 425, 647, 745, 778, 1022, 1023,
    1028
Boser, K. I., 645
Boser, K. K., 761
Bosje, M., 174, 620
Boston, B. O., 219
Bottenberg, D., 109, 174, 427
Bouchard, R., 28
Bouchard-Lamothe, D., 292, 366
Boucher, V., 427
Bouilleret, V., 1015
Boulay, N., 419, 618
Bourbon, T., 967
Bourgeois, M. S., 87, 168, 171, 179, 295, 302,
    361, 745, 998, 999, 1001, 1003
Bourhis, R., 293
Bouvier, G., 26
Bowden, J., 999
Bowen, A., 964
Bowen, D., 991
Bowen, S. E., 233
Bower, G. H., 714
Bowers, D., 964, 971, 976, 977
Bowers, L., 75, 100
Boyajian, A. E., 930
Boyeson, M. G., 56
Boyle, M., 69, 337, 419, 426, 450, 499, 500,
    519, 520, 619, 622
Boynton, W., 880
Braak, E., 989, 993

Braak, H., 989, 993
Braber, N., 103, 776
Bracchi, M., 705
Bracy, O. L., 858, 860
Bradburn, N., 297
Bradley, W. G., 48
Brady, C. B., 991
Bragoni, M., 56, 57
Brammer, M. J., 757
Brandt, J. P., 21
Branker, B., 544
Brashers-Krug, T., 715
Brassard, C., 70, 290, 294, 323, 337, 351, 419, 618, 760
Brassell, E. G., 70, 71, 124, 125, 192, 578
Braswell, D., 100
Braun, A., 768, 1009
Braunling-McMorrow, D., 924
Braverman, K. M., 484, 502
Brawley, E., 322, 334, 335
Brazzeli, M., 894
Brecher, A., 109, 180, 420, 597, 612, 832, 852
Breedin, S., 776
Breen, K., 106, 418, 998
Breese, E. L., 412, 614, 616, 782, 1014
Breier, J. I., 190
Brendel, B., 1024, 1025
Brennan, A., 363
Brennan, D. M., 180
Brenneise-Sarshad, R., 174, 427
Brenner, T., 895
Brentnall, S., 916
Bresnan, J., 639, 736
Bressi, S., 37, 991
Brianti, R., 894
Brickencamp, R., 98
Bricker, A. L., 420
Brickman, A. M., 992
Briggs, P., 231
Brigstocke, G., 319
Brindely, P., 376, 377
Brindley, P., 757
Brislin, R. W., 246
Broadbent, N. J., 989
Broca, P., 20, 21, 26, 1011, 1013
Broderick, J., 42, 43
Brodie, J., 361
Brodin, J., 865
Brodmann, K., 1010
Broida, H., 756
Bronson, M. B., 910
Brooks, B. M., 922, 923
Brooks, D. N., 894
Brooks, J. L., 966
Brooks, R. L., 968
Brookshire, R. H., 3, 4, 5, 56, 67, 70, 71, 75, 85, 87, 88, 101, 102, 107, 108, 109, 110, 120, 124, 127, 165, 167, 169, 171, 174, 258, 297, 377, 380, 384, 386, 387, 406, 408, 413, 415, 416, 421, 424, 425, 426, 427, 428, 429, 430, 431, 432, 433, 436, 457, 508, 514, 515, 516, 669, 765, 779, 780, 806, 810, 887, 965, 969, 971, 972, 974
Brothers, L., 895
Brotherton, F. A., 924

Broussolle, E., 554, 555
Brown, A. L., 899, 904
Brown, B. B., 779
Brown, C. M., 103
Brown, C. S., 861
Brown, F., 930
Brown, G., 894, 994
Brown, J. A., 53
Brown, J. E., 230, 232
Brown, J. R., 65, 891, 1011
Brown, J. W., 7, 110, 430, 573, 705, 977
Brown, K., 177
Brown, L., 98, 100, 819
Brown, N. A., 205, 221
Brown, R. D., 43
Brown, R. S., 217
Brown, V. J., 534
Brown, V. L., 75
Brownell, H. H., 86, 101, 410, 583, 740, 772, 969, 970, 971, 972, 973, 975
Brownell, J., 221
Brownell, M. T., 914
Brubaker, S. H., 855
Bruce, C., 178, 306, 620, 763, 775
Brumfitt, S. M., 80, 94, 292, 293, 307, 308, 319, 362
Bruner, J., 476, 477, 896
Brunet, P., 554
Brunner, R. J., 34, 49
Bruno, J., 833
Brush, J. A., 997, 999
Brust, J. C., 30, 566, 572
Bruun, B., 566
Bryan, K. L., 85, 178, 638
Bryant, B. R., 75, 578, 657
Bryden, J., 894
Bryer, A., 517
Brysbaert, M., 249
Bub, D., 89, 103, 109, 111, 112, 545, 546, 549, 550, 551, 552, 610, 611, 668, 698, 769, 964, 967, 995
Buccino, G., 1013, 1014
Buchel, C., 37
Buchman, A. S., 609
Buchtel, H. A., 609
Buck, R., 771, 976
Buckingham, H. W., 1015, 1016
Buckle, L., 895, 905
Buckner, R. L., 190, 894, 991
Bucks, R., 98
Budka, H., 552
Buiza, J. J., 413, 832, 862
Bulgren, J. A., 919
Bunch, W. H., 80
Bundesen, C., 964
Bunn, E. M., 37
Buonaguro, A., 123, 193, 891
Buonomano, D. V., 689, 701, 728
Burani, C., 613
Burbaum, L. J., 769
Burchardt, T., 328
Burchert, F., 741
Burger, L. K., 598
Burgess, C., 973
Burgess, P., 892, 904, 905

Burgio, F., 96, 179, 763
Burk, F., 252, 265
Burke, J. E., 96
Burke, W. H., 928
Burkhardt, P., 740
Burns, M., 91, 98
Burns, R. B., 246
Burr, J. A., 247
Burris, G. A., 376, 377, 379
Burton, M. W., 639, 775, 1013, 1014
Buschke, H., 894
Bushell, C., 740
Bushnell, D. L., 50
Busk, P. L., 196
Butfield, E., 492
Butler, I., 206, 894
Butt, P., 98
Butters, N., 258, 894, 989, 991
Butterworth, B., 536, 632
Button, J., 293
Buxant, P., 361
Buxbaum, L. J., 964, 965
Buzolich, M., 67
Buzzard, M., 977
Bylsma, F. W., 992
Byng, S., 10, 66, 77, 81, 82, 115, 126, 127, 174, 192, 259, 290, 292, 294, 301, 305, 307, 308, 309, 310, 328, 349, 350, 355, 356, 357, 360, 379, 453, 484, 509, 598, 600, 618, 638, 647, 648, 745, 758, 759, 768, 777, 857, 858, 862
Byrne, M. E., 171

Cabeza, R., 894
Cai, Y., 910
Cain, R., 762
Cairns, A. Y., 361
Cairns, D., 638, 642
Calabrese, D. B., 904
Calautti, C., 406
Calderon, J., 992
Caldognetto, E. M., 977
Caligiuri, M. P., 377
Calkins, M., 334
Callaghan, S., 804
Caltagirone, C., 11, 568
Calvanio, R., 966
Calvert, G. A., 757
Calvin, J., 421
Camp, C., 333, 996, 997, 999, 1003
Campanella, D. J., 414
Campbell, C. R., 102, 108
Campbell, D. T., 164, 169, 172, 194
Campbell, T. F., 76, 178, 516
Campione, J. C., 899, 904
Campsie, L., 894
Canadian Cooperative Study Group, 46
Canadian Institutes of Health Research, 176
Cancelliere, A. E. B., 976
Caneman, G., 965
Cannito, M. D., 425, 426
Cannito, M. P., 102, 426, 509, 747, 765
Canter, G., 102, 416, 419, 420, 421, 422, 423, 424, 426, 451, 509, 567, 578, 582, 765, 774, 783, 974
Cantor, N., 80

Cao, Y., 191, 757
Capasso, R., 103, 619
Caperton, C. J., 319
Capitani, E., 188, 192, 568, 610, 613, 616, 705, 756
Caplan, B., 965
Caplan, D., 9, 81, 82, 103, 104, 108, 109, 111, 112, 423, 425, 609, 623, 648, 735, 736, 765, 969
Caplan, L. R., 967
Capo, M., 915, 940
Capon, A., 189
Cappa, S. F., 35, 37, 50, 111, 124, 250, 251, 427, 566, 610, 612, 757, 968
Cappelletti, J. Y., 610
Caramazza, A., 37, 75, 89, 102, 103, 109, 252, 410, 413, 421, 423, 597, 598, 599, 600, 601, 607, 609, 610, 611, 612, 614, 615, 617, 619, 633, 634, 636, 640, 641, 646, 656, 657, 665, 666, 668, 671, 672, 696, 736, 758
Carbone, G., 610
Cardebat, D., 50, 190
Cardell, E. A., 668
Cardol, M., 291, 294, 296, 300, 304, 305
Carew, T. J., 716
Carey, P., 423, 764
CARF. See Commission on Accreditation of Rehabilitation Facilities
Carino, B. V., 246
Carlan, M., 725
Carlomagno, S., 264, 361, 411, 520, 600
Carlson, G. S., 583, 586, 761, 832, 864
Carlson, J. I., 928
Carlsson, M., 357
Carmines, E. G., 76
Carney, N., 895, 902, 918, 921
Caroselli, J., 319
Carpenter, E., 206
Carpenter, P. A., 190
Carpenter, S., 552
Carper, J. M., 193
Carr, E. G., 902, 923, 928, 930, 931
Carr, T., 302, 414, 509, 600
Carroll, E., 644, 736
Carroll, V., 406, 407, 408, 411, 416, 421, 430, 433
Carstens, B., 1022
Carter, G., 998
Carter, J., 124
Carter, P., 124
Casadio, P., 361, 520
Caselli, R. J., 547, 551
Casey, P. F., 508
Casper, M. L., 11
Castelein, P., 360, 361, 366, 367
Castellani, R. J., 550
Castro-Caldas, A., 33
Cataldo, M. D., 926
Catani, J., 1009, 1015
Catani, M., 697
Catsman-Berrevoets, C. E., 56
Cattani, B., 257
Cattelani, R., 894, 895
Cavanaugh, J., 533
Cavus, I., 54

Cazden, C. B., 486
Cazzato, G., 251
Ceccaldi, M., 9, 555
Cegla, B., 584
Celery, K., 519
Cenkovich, F., 52
Cenoz, J., 250
Centers for Disease Control and Prevention, 10, 11, 12, 15, 880, 881
Central Brain Tumor Registry of the United States, 12
Cercy, S. P., 992
Cermak, L., 516, 738
Cesaro, P., 50
Chadwick, O., 894
Chainay, H., 1012
Chambers, N., 304
Chambless, D. L., 1028
Champod, A.-S., 1013
Champoux, R., 756
Chan, K. L., 975
Chan, S. W.-C., 251, 257
Chang, A., 760
Chang, E. C., 73
Chang, F., 637
Chang, S., 782, 783
Channon, S., 895
Chapey, R., 3, 64, 65, 66, 67, 69, 70, 74, 77, 79, 80, 81, 82, 84, 85, 95, 96, 97, 105, 114, 125, 126, 127, 128, 129, 159, 160, 203, 279, 452, 469, 470, 472, 473, 475, 478, 484, 485, 487, 502, 523, 761, 781, 854
Chapman, S., 118, 554, 555, 766, 780, 781, 891, 893, 1001, 1003
Charbel, F., 259
Chargualaf, J., 782
Chartrand, T. L., 912
Charuvastra, A., 550
Chary, P., 260
Chase, K. N., 965
Chassagnon, S., 1012
Chastain, R., 124, 994
Chatterjee, A., 103, 111, 648
Chaudhary, P., 569, 611
Chavada, S., 965
Chee, M. W. L., 251, 1015
Cheek, W. R., 35
Chelune, G. J., 764
Chen, H. C., 252
Chen, S., 257
Chenery, H. J., 418, 668
Cheney, P. D., 1011
Cheng, L. L., 253, 254
Chengappa, S., 259
Chenven, H., 376, 382, 391
Cherney, L. R., 70, 86, 107, 186, 190, 191, 192, 197, 665, 774, 965, 966, 974
Cherrie, C., 246
Cherry, B. J., 967
Chertkow, H., 9, 610, 698, 995
Chester, S. L., 114, 853
Cheung, S. W., 692
Chial, M. R., 164
Chialant, D., 607, 610, 611

Chiat, S., 422, 620, 638, 641, 642, 643, 668, 764, 784
Chiavari, L., 610
CHIEF. See Craig Hospital Inventory of Environmental Factors
Chieffi, S., 411
Childers, J. B., 714
Childs, K. E., 905
Chiou, H. H., 73, 78
Chissom, B. S., 658
Chitiri, H.-F., 249
Chitsaz, A., 56
Chobor, K. L., 977
Choi, D., 10
Choi, H., 206
Choi, N. W., 787
Chokron, S., 964, 965
Cholewa, J., 611
Chomsky, N., 14, 479, 485, 706, 736, 738, 747
Choy, J., 740
Christensen, A. L., 74
Christensen, B., 256
Christiansen, J. A., 111, 112, 424, 735
Christinaz, D., 861
Christman, M. A., 432
Chrotowski, J., 56
Chubon, R. A., 298
Chui, D., 51
Chui, H. C., 964, 992
Chujo, T., 173
Chuma, T., 54
Chumpelik, D., 174, 1022, 1027
Chung, A., 782
Churchill, C., 239
Chytas, P., 205
Ciarocco, N. J., 891
Cicciarelli, A. W., 188
Cicero, B. A., 976
Cicerone, K., 860, 892, 895, 902, 918, 920, 966
Cicone, M., 976
Cifu, D., 290
Cifu, D. X., 229, 230, 239, 242
Cimino, C. R., 971, 972, 976
Cimino-Knight, A. M., 691, 697
Cioe, J., 689
Cipolotti, L., 568, 609
Clare, L., 998
Clarfield, A. M., 87
Clark, A. E., 417
Clark, D. G., 89, 95, 550, 551, 554
Clark, D. O., 357
Clark, E., 71, 124
Clark, H., 66, 69, 82, 88, 97, 109, 124, 126, 217, 293, 481
Clark, M. S., 52
Clark, N., 519
Clark, R. E., 989
Clarkberg, M., 206
Clarke, S., 905, 968
Classen, J., 1011
Clausen, N. S., 668, 669, 670, 785
Clayton, M. C., 659
Clearman, R., 304
Cleary, S., 997, 1002
Clemens, C., 205

Clemmons, D., 896
Cline, H., 13
Clinical Aphasiology Conference, 177
Cloninger, C. J., 902
Cloutier, R., 352
Coad, M. L., 886
Coates, R., 27, 49, 186
Cochran, R. M., 582
Cochrane, R., 391, 392, 497
Cockburn, J., 92, 97, 904
Code, C., 94, 101, 102, 115, 121, 124, 192, 193, 203, 264, 292, 297, 309, 323, 337, 342, 362, 513, 524, 893, 1026
Coelho, C., 14, 69, 70, 88, 89, 92, 109, 110, 127, 403, 419, 450, 452, 470, 499, 500, 519, 520, 583, 619, 622, 771, 772, 830, 856, 893
Cohan, M., 87
Cohen, E., 245
Cohen, G., 701
Cohen, J. A., 35, 171
Cohen, L., 54, 554, 555, 1011, 1012
Cohen, M. P., 56
Cohen, N. J., 96
Cohen, R. M., 967
Cohen, S. B., 174, 880
Cohen-Schneider, R., 306, 381
Cohn, R., 212
Coker, S. B., 56
Colby, K. M., 861
Cole, L., 246
Cole, M., 544
Coleman, M., 306, 763
Coles, R., 308, 388
Cole-Virtue, J., 102
Colheart, M., 657, 660
Collard, M., 49
Collard, S., 967
Collin, C. F., 70
Collins, D., 229
Collins, M., 566, 567, 568, 569, 574, 575, 577, 578, 580, 581, 582, 584, 803, 829, 866, 880, 888, 1026
Colombo, A., 566, 574, 600
Colombo, L., 613
Colombo, N., 894
Colombo, P., 11
Colonna, A., 568
Colosimo, C., 35
Colsher, P. L., 978
Coltheart, M., 77, 78, 82, 83, 259, 578, 597, 598, 600, 607, 612, 613, 656, 660, 663, 893
Comfort, A., 206
Commission on Accreditation of Rehabilitation Facilities (CARF), 240, 242
Conforta, A. B., 54
Confraria, A., 33
Conley, A., 419, 619
Conlon, C. P., 108, 174, 520, 583
Connell, P. J., 172, 393
Connis, D., 319
Connor, D. J., 992
Connor, L. T., 507
Connors, C. K., 98
Consolini, T., 7
Conway, R. N. F., 899

Conway, T. W., 721, 722
Cook, D. A., 240
Cook, J. C., 376, 756
Cook, R. G., 896
Cook, T. D., 194
Cooper, J., 895
Cooper, L., 488
Cooper, W. E., 978
Coopersmith, H., 975
Cope, D. N., 237, 238, 880, 886, 939
Copeland, M., 376, 757
Copper, B., 206, 207
Corbeil, R. R., 1000
Corbetta, M., 190, 437, 966
Corbin, J., 178, 390
Corbin, M. A., 376
Corbin, M. L., 383
Corder, L. S., 13
Cordes, A. K., 76, 77
Corey-Bloom, J., 992
Corlew, M. M., 410
Cormier, L. S., 220, 221
Cormier, W. H., 220, 221
Cornelissen, K., 191, 414
Cornelius, B., 56
Cornell, S., 30, 572
Cornell, T., 740
Cornman, C. B., 229
Correia, L., 421, 427, 779
Corrigan, J., 297
Corrington, K., 714
Corsi, L., 930
Cort, R. C., 1028
Corwin, M., 565
Coslett, H. B., 97, 105, 108, 539, 609, 656, 659, 769, 964, 965, 966, 976, 977
Costa, A., 250, 252, 607
Costa, L. D., 894
Costeff, D. N., 895
Côté, J., 352
Côté, L., 990, 991
Cotman, C. W., 991
Cotton, J., 488
Coull, J. T., 967
Court, J. H., 818, 819
Courville, J., 881, 884
Cox, C. L., 533
Cox, D., 361, 418, 565, 645, 710, 777, 778, 864, 991
Coyle, J. T., 991
Crabtree, J. W., 533
Craenhals, A., 552
Crago, M. B., 246
Craig, A. H., 94
Craig, H., 64, 480
Craig Hospital Research Department, 364
Craik, F., 714, 716, 894, 967
Cramazza, A., 75
Cramer, S. C., 53
Cranberg, M. D., 894
Crandell, C., 335
Crary, M. A., 71, 81, 259
Crawford, A. B., 195, 437, 524, 762
Crawford, J. R., 895
Crépeau, F., 905

Crerar, M. A., 197, 762, 832, 860, 865
Crimmins, D. B., 931, 932
Crinion, J., 50, 51, 251
Crisostomo, E. A., 56
Crisp, J., 119, 178, 295
Crittsinger, B. A., 376
Crockford, C., 120
Croft, S., 257
Cronbach, L. J., 77
Croot, K., 1017, 1019
Cropley, A., 96, 472
Crosky, C. S., 428
Crosson, B., 108, 123, 530, 531, 533, 535, 536, 537, 538, 539, 611, 615, 674, 704, 1012
Croteau, C., 14, 70, 323
Crow, E., 70, 71
Crowe, S., 894
Cruice, M., 121, 122, 179, 291, 295, 296, 308, 351, 355, 356, 362
Cruickshank, M., 206, 207
Crum, R. M., 995
Cubelli, R., 7, 830
Cudworth, C., 672, 784
Cuerva, A. G., 56
Cuetos, F., 109, 613
Culbertson, W., 71
Culham, J., 609
Culioli, A., 260
Cullen, N. K., 894
Cullinan, W. L., 861
Cullum, C. M., 327
Cummings, J. L., 86, 91, 94, 975, 992
Cunningham, R., 74, 110, 308, 361, 363, 578, 580
Curl, R. M., 896
Curtis, C., 319
Curtis, G., 764
Curtis, S., 56, 382
Curtiss, S., 112, 416, 423
Cushner, K., 246
Cutler, A., 249, 427, 515
Czvik, P., 517

Dabul, B., 92, 93, 380, 756
Dagenbach, D., 535
D'Agostino, R. B., 256
Daigle, T., 977
Dalen, J. E., 46
D'Alessandro, P., 547
Damasio, A., 7, 8, 9, 21, 28, 29, 34, 35, 37, 566, 567, 611, 612, 774, 775, 894, 899, 901, 905, 922, 926, 927, 964
Damasio, D., 37
Damasio, H., 9, 20, 21, 22, 23, 24, 26, 27, 28, 29, 30, 32, 34, 35, 37, 38, 572, 611, 735, 774, 775, 894, 901, 905, 926, 964, 976, 977
Damico, H., 300
Damico, J. S., 74, 119, 120, 121, 128, 129, 178, 293, 294, 295, 296, 297, 298, 299, 300, 301, 302, 307, 360, 361, 394, 523, 816
D'Amour, D., 229, 240
Danault, S., 260
Daniele, A., 35
Daniels, S., 196, 611
Daniloff, J. K., 101, 102, 108, 427, 768

Daniloff, R., 101, 427
Danly, M., 978
Danys, I., 43
Dapretto, M., 251
Darley, F. L., 3, 65, 71, 90, 92, 93, 123, 124, 125, 166, 167, 174, 207, 208, 377, 403, 409, 410, 411, 418, 421, 425, 426, 429, 433, 437, 457, 509, 524, 544, 549, 757, 803, 855, 860, 869, 891, 1011, 1017, 1030
Darley, R., 390
Dartigues, J. F., 993
Daselaar, S. M., 989
David, R. M., 77, 78, 125, 750, 756
Davidoff, M., 859, 866
Davidson, B., 69, 298, 350, 351, 382
Davidson, R. A., 966, 967
Davidson, W., 548, 549, 611
Davies, C., 580
Davies, K. G., 613
Davies, P., 991
Davies, R., 551, 552, 783
Davis, A., 293, 301, 509, 520, 618
Davis, C., 109, 229, 242, 519, 611
Davis, D. G., 990
Davis, G., 385
Davis, G. A., 70, 82, 85, 88, 107, 114, 116, 117, 124, 125, 174, 196, 377, 378, 380, 381, 384, 385, 386, 391, 403, 426, 482, 497, 566, 567, 586, 587, 777, 830, 859
Davis, J. N., 55, 56
Davis, K. L., 996
Davis, K. R., 26, 1014
Davis, P. N., 246
Davison, A. N., 991
Davolt, S., 211
Daw, J., 217
Dawson, D. V., 56, 965
Day, A. L., 26
Day, E. A., 714
Dayus, B., 921
De Bastiani, P., 673
de Bleser, R., 73, 109, 252, 256, 567, 568, 611, 737, 741
de Bot, K., 248, 250
de Brabander, J. M., 990
De Deyn, P. P., 256, 536
De Gelder, B., 536
de Groot, A. M. B., 250, 252, 253
de Groot, I., 296
de Haan, R., 296, 323, 922
De Jong, B., 291
de Luca, G., 260, 264
de Partz, M. P., 600, 664
de Pellegrino G., 1013
De Renzi, E., 192, 566, 568, 574, 575, 578, 775, 861
de Riesthal, M., 123, 125, 192
De Ruyter, F., 757
de Ruyter, F., 437, 524, 814
De Tanti, A., 257
de Vos, R. A. I., 993
de Witt, D., 967
De Witte, L., 536, 537
Deacon, B., 1019

Deal, J. L., 81, 168, 259, 756, 865, 968, 1022, 1027
Deal, L. A., 756, 968
Dean, E. C., 197, 832, 854, 860, 865
Dean, M. P., 638
Deaudon, C., 698
Decaix, C., 965
Deci, E. L., 891, 931
Deco, G., 691, 701
DeCoste, D., 830
DeDe, G., 418, 620
Defer, G., 50
Defoor-Hill, L., 394
Degaonkar, M., 964
Deger, K., 1024, 1025
DeGiovani, R., 292
deGreiff, A., 967
Dehaene, S., 251
Dehlin, O., 94
Deiner, H.-C., 967
Dejerine, J., 29
DeKosky, S. T., 976
Del Grosso Destreri, N., 783
Del Pesce, M., 967
Del Pozo, F., 205
Del Tredici, K., 993
Delacoste, C., 785
Delcey, M., 80
DeLeon, J., 597, 995
Deleval, J., 572
D'Elia, L. F., 98
Delis, D. C., 98, 971, 995
Dell, G. S., 598, 603, 636, 637, 641, 699, 700, 774
Della Sala, S., 566, 991
Deloche, G., 105, 110, 264, 421, 617, 859, 864
DeLong, E. R., 187, 571, 572
DeLong, M. R., 991
Demain, C., 376, 757
Dember, W., 477
Demery, J. A., 91, 719
Demeurisse, G., 189
Demonet, J. F., 757
Demos, G., 90, 471
Dempster, F. N., 713
den Ouden, D. B., 113
Denburg, N. L., 71
Denckla, M. B., 96, 909
Denes, G., 609, 972, 977
Dening, T. R., 992
Denman, A., 115
Dennis, F., 361
Dennis, M., 893, 905
Denzin, N. K., 178
DeRenzi, E., 11, 75, 91, 411, 547, 861, 964
Derman, S., 380
D'Erme, P., 568, 964
DeRosa, E. A., 52
Deser, T., 109, 110
Desimone, R., 534, 535
Deslauriers, L., 252, 264, 265
Desmarais, G., 905
Desrochers, A., 79, 85, 256
Detterman, D. K., 896, 902

Dettinger, E., 206
Deutsch, G., 967
Devault, S. M., 376
Devitt, E. W., 859
Devlieger, P. J., 248
Devlin, J., 1013
Dewaele, J. M., 245
Di Piero, V., 48, 50
Di Pietro, M., 180, 620, 862
Diamond, P. T., 192
Dichgans, J., 757
Dick, F., 103
Dick, J. P., 547
Dick, M. B., 991
Dick, W., 229
Dickey, M. W., 740
Dickson, D. W., 550
Didic, M., 555
Diener, E., 12, 304
Diener, H., 46
Diener, R., 298
Dietz, A., 823, 825
Diggs, C., 484, 502, 971
Dijkstra, T., 245, 249, 250, 252
Diller, L., 180, 905, 920
Diner, E., 66
DiPellegrino, G., 964
Dippel, D. W. J., 71, 420
Dipper, L. T., 638
Dirkx, T., 866
DiSimoni, F., 71, 90, 92, 174, 429, 803
Disimoni, R., 390
Ditterich, A., 1013
Djundja, D., 712
Dodd, D., 919, 920
Dodd, M. L., 53
Doesborgh, S. J. C., 71, 420, 761
Dogil, G., 113
Dollaghan, C. A., 76, 129, 178, 194
Dolphin, M. K., 377
Donabedian, A., 164
Donaldson, N., 319
Donaldson, R., 583
Donati, F., 558
Donnellan, A. M., 931
Donnelly, R. E., 893
Donoghue, J. P., 1011
Donovan, J. J., 713
Donovan, N. J., 178
Doolittle, G. C., 205
Dordain, M., 864
Dore, J., 115, 480, 481
Dores, P. A., 931
Dorland's Illustrated Medical Dictionary, 42
Doss, S., 931
Doucet, N., 256
Douglas, J. M., 92, 102, 110, 119, 122, 413, 621, 771, 886, 996
Douglass, E., 377, 379
Dowden, P., 815, 1026
Dowling, S. M., 967
Downes, J., 921
Dowswell, G., 327
Doyel, A. W., 107, 118
Doyle, D., 892

Doyle, P. J., 81, 92, 103, 108, 116, 122, 128, 171, 173, 178, 197, 291, 294, 295, 296, 298, 357, 508, 553, 710, 745, 1022, 1023
Doyon, J., 989
Drachman, D. A., 991
Dressler, R. A., 855
Drew, R., 450, 519, 618, 620, 815
Dribbon, M., 833
Dromerick, A. W., 569
Dronkers, N. F., 92, 168, 192, 259, 260, 549, 550, 551, 554, 556, 574, 865, 995, 1015
Druback, D. A., 53
Druks, J., 75, 578, 621, 644, 736, 741
Drummond, S., 93
Dubois, J., 260
Dubois, M. F., 992
duBoulay, G. H. D., 994
Ducanis, A. J., 232, 233
Ducarne, B., 554
Duchan, J., 66, 126, 179, 236, 279, 290, 292, 293, 303, 307, 309, 328, 349, 350, 355, 360, 362, 363, 496, 497, 509, 517, 565, 588, 779
Duffy, F. D., 379, 411
Duffy, J. R., 65, 89, 92, 93, 102, 127, 196, 205, 403, 406, 411, 452, 470, 543, 544, 545, 547, 549, 550, 551, 554, 555, 556, 771, 865, 969, 971, 1011, 1014, 1015, 1017, 1018, 1020, 1026, 1029
Duffy, R. J., 92, 118, 325, 771, 772, 830, 893, 971, 976
Dugbartey, A. T., 96
Dumond, D. L., 428
Duncan, D. M., 249
Duncan, G. W., 26, 35
Duncan, J., 964, 965
Duncan, P., 319
Duncan, P. W., 52, 56
Dunkle, R. E., 95
Dunlap, G., 902, 905, 930
Dunn, E. S., 75
Dunn, H., 377, 379
Dunn, L. M., 75
Dupont, S., 1015
Durand, V. M., 931, 932
Durgunoglu, A. Y., 250
Dusatko, D., 520, 777
Dutta, A., 717
Duvernoy, H., 22
Dvonch, V. M., 80
Dwivedi, V. D., 978
Dworetsky, B., 415
Dworkin, J. P., 1024, 1025
Dwyer, C., 968
Dyer, W. M., 205
Dywan, J., 905

Eales, C., 308, 388
Earp, J., 323
Easterbrook, A., 779
Easton, J. D., 51
Eastwood, C., 935
Eastwood, M. R., 52
Eayrs, C. B., 726, 727
Ebbinghaus, H., 713
Ebert, A. D., 536

Eccarius, M., 826, 828
Eccles, J. C., 406
Eccles, M., 14
Echiverri, H. C., 56
Eckert, T. L., 930
ECSTC, 51
Edelman, G. M., 578, 580
Edelman, R. R., 1011
Edmonds, L., 173, 179, 260, 263, 265, 723, 724
Edmundson, A., 178, 306, 453, 484, 618, 763
Edwards, D., 299
Edwards, J., 248
Edwards, S., 111, 112, 113, 741, 747
Edwards-Schaefer, P., 343
Egan, J., 307, 391, 763
Egelko, S., 327
Egnor, H., 670
Egolf, D. B., 114, 853
Ehlhardt, L., 763, 940
Ehrlich, J. S., 893
Ehrsson, H., 1013
Eickhoff, S., 1015
Eischeid, T., 828
Eisenberg, A., 249
Eisenberg, H. M., 893, 967
Eisenson, J., 73, 376, 377, 379, 382, 394, 409, 521, 578, 756, 767, 855, 859, 860, 869, 968
Elbard, H., 68
Elbert, T., 712
Elias, M. F., 256
Elias, P. K., 256
Elias, S., 13
Elliott, R., 90
Ellis, A., 77, 102, 110, 197, 413, 597, 609, 610, 611, 613, 617, 618, 657, 666, 695, 782, 783, 832, 860, 865
Ellis, G., 382, 387
Ellis, N., 246
Ellis-Hill, C., 337
Ellmo, W. J., 904
Ellsworth, T. A., 619, 620, 642, 643, 644
Elman, R., 66, 84, 114, 115, 118, 129, 169, 174, 175, 180, 279, 290, 295, 302, 304, 307, 308, 309, 310, 362, 376, 377, 379, 381, 382, 389, 390, 391, 392, 394, 524
Elman, S., 309, 524
Elmslie, H., 904
Emanuelli, S., 361, 520
Emery, P., 518
Emmons, R., 298
Emre, M., 993
Emslie, H., 905, 921
Enderby, P., 70, 71, 93, 195, 198, 451, 756, 761, 832, 857, 864, 866
Engel, P. A., 552
Engelborghs, S., 536
Engell, B., 122, 300, 355
Englert, C. S., 499
English, A. C., 95, 470
English, H. B., 95, 470
English, L., 517
Engvik, H., 571, 572
Erbaugh, J., 994
Erickson, J. G., 248
Erickson, R. J., 507

Eriksson, P. S., 13
Erlich, J., 297
Ernest-Baron, C., 102, 427
Eslinger, P., 21, 34, 566, 905
Estes, W. K., 714
Estrada, P., 257
European Carotid Trialists' Collaborative Group, 46
Evans, A. C., 251
Evans, D. A., 988
Evans, D. H., 47
Evans, J. J., 727, 904, 905, 916, 921, 922, 998
Evans, K. L., 423
Evans, P., 899
Evans, R., 126, 319, 338, 339, 488
Ewart, C., 211
Ewert, J., 894
Ewing, S., 377, 379, 382, 391, 394
Ezekowitz, M. D., 51

Fabbro, F., 251, 259, 260
Faber, M., 110
Fadiga, L., 1013, 1014
Fagan, S. C., 124
Fager, S., 1018
Fagergren, A., 1013
Faglioni, P., 192, 566, 568, 756
Fahey, K. B., 117
Faich, G., 880
Fair, J., 173
Falanga, A., 609
Falconer, J. A., 233
Falk, G. D., 905
Family Caregiver Alliance, 206
Family Caregivers Online, 336
Farabola, M., 193, 565, 566, 567, 572, 575
Farah, M. J., 91, 609, 610, 693, 964
Farber, J. F., 995
Farina, E., 610
Faroqi-Shah, Y., 736, 746
Farrier, L., 170
Farrow, C. E., 967
Farrow, V., 580
Fassbender, L. L., 931
Fassbinder, W., 972
Fastenau, P. S., 71
Faust, M., 102
Fawcett, J. T., 246
Fawcus, M., 376, 377, 382, 389, 391, 522, 1026
Fawcus, R., 522, 1026
Faxio, F., 610
Fazio, F., 37
FDA. See Food and Drug Administration
Fedio, P., 966, 991
Feeney, D., 56, 188, 880
Feeney, J., 880, 892
Feeney, T. J., 96, 173, 879, 880, 891, 892, 895, 896, 897, 898, 899, 900, 902, 903, 904, 905, 906, 910, 912, 913, 915, 923, 927, 928, 929, 930, 931, 933, 935, 936, 937, 939, 940
Feher, E., 416
Feigin, V. L., 11
Feinstein, A., 88
Feldman, E., 255

Feldman, L., 978
Fellows, M. R., 1011
Felmingham, K., 895
Fenaughty, A., 205
Fenstad, J. E., 854
Fergus, S. L., 360
Ferguson, A., 117, 178, 301, 307, 779
Ferketic, M., 80, 123, 178, 255, 298, 319, 356
Fernandez, B., 190
Ferrada-Videla, M., 229
Ferrand, L., 252, 264
Ferrari, C., 75
Ferrari, P., 192, 566
Ferraro, K., 343
Ferraro, V., 648
Ferreira, C. T., 610
Ferreira, F., 648
Ferreres, A. R., 257
Ferreri, T., 536
Ferris, S. H., 995
Ferro, J. M., 187, 189, 192, 567, 572, 575
Ferroni, A., 547
Fetz, E. E., 1011
Feuerstein, R., 904
Fey, M., 117, 482, 902
ffytche, D. H., 1009, 1015
Fickas, S., 763, 940
Fidopiastis, C. M., 923
Field, M. J., 205
Fields, W. S., 46
Fife, D., 880
Filley, C. M., 894
Fillingham, J. K., 432, 718, 726, 727
The FIM System, 80
Findley, L. J., 554
Fink, G. R., 190, 565, 1015, 1016
Fink, R. B., 103, 180, 414, 420, 597, 619, 640,
    643, 647, 648, 726, 745, 762, 832, 852, 862
Finkelstein, S., 26, 969
Finlayson, A., 68
Fischer, R. S., 32, 33, 667
Fischette, M. R., 33
Fischler, I., 106
Fishbourne, R. P., 658
Fisher, M., 48
Fisher, R. S., 217
Fishman, J. A., 249
Fitch-West, J., 71
Fitz-Gibbon, C. T., 869
Fitzpatrick, D., 1010, 1013
Fitzpatrick, P. M., 108, 174, 581, 771, 830
FitzpatrickDeSalme, E. J., 893
Fitzsimons, G. M., 910
Fivush, R., 937
Flack, J. M., 11, 12
Flaherty, D., 76
Flavell, J., 891, 892, 899, 915, 919, 920
Fleet, W. S., 965
Flege, J. E., 249
Fleiss, J. L., 168
Fleming, P. D., 552
Fletcher, J. M., 894
Fletcher, R., 323, 768
Flexer, C., 335
Flick, C. L., 239

Florance, C., 115, 116, 1022, 1026, 1027
Flores, D. K., 191
Flower, W., 15, 222
Flowers, C. R., 179, 417, 423, 424, 971, 977
Flynn, C. D., 53
Flynn, M., 965
Fodor, I. G., 427
Fogassi, G., 1014
Fogassi, L., 1013, 1014
Foldi, N. S., 116, 426, 972
Folstein, M. F., 98, 994, 995, 1002
Folstein, M. R., 975
Folstein, S. E., 995, 1002
Food and Drug Administration (FDA), 49, 51
Forbes, M., 125, 264, 570, 572
Ford, A. B., 43
Ford, J., 382
Forde, E., 567, 693, 720
Fordyce, D. J., 891
Foreman, M. D., 995
Foresti, A., 7
Forssberg, H., 1013
Forster, S., 377
Fortier-Blanc, J., 205
Foss, J. W., 996
Fossett, T. R. D., 549
Fougeyrollas, P., 66, 281, 351, 352, 353, 354,
    357, 359, 364, 365
Foundas, A. L., 611, 612, 613, 616
Fowler, C. G., 91
Fowler, R., 930
Fox, H. B., 217
Fox, L., 295, 304, 338, 817, 824
Fox, P. T., 967
Fraansen, M., 620
Frackowiak, R. S., 37, 50, 547, 554, 967
Frady, M., 13
Fragassi, N. A., 609
Fralish, K., 924
Frame, S., 293, 779
Franchi, D., 967
Francis, D., 519, 609, 618
Francis, G., 999
Francis, W. N., 613
Francois, L. K., 195
Frank, A., 297
Frank, C., 89, 94
Frank, E. M., 256, 524
Frank, R., 22, 30, 37
Franklin, L. R., 781
Franklin, S., 110, 111, 173, 413, 599, 609, 610,
    611, 617, 619, 620, 643, 718, 735
Franklin, T. C., 74, 76
Frankoski, R. F., 46
Franssen, E., 995
Franssen, M., 174
Franz, S. I., 756
Fraser, C., 54
Fraser, R. T., 896
Frattali, C. M., 14, 79, 80, 119, 120, 121, 128,
    129, 130, 164, 178, 255, 290, 291, 295, 297,
    298, 319, 356, 376, 377, 437, 487, 550, 551,
    555, 579, 768
Frayne, S. M., 246
Frazier, C. H., 756

Frazier, K. E., 171, 1028
Fredman, M., 260, 264
Freed, D. B., 93, 110, 125, 171, 173, 174, 179,
    417, 418, 519, 776, 1028
Freedman, M., 32
Freedman-Stern, R. F., 107, 785
Freeman, S., 221
Freemann, R., 771
Freese, P., 300
French, S., 305
Frenck-Mestre, C., 249
Freud, S., 1015
Frick, T., 826
Friden, T. P., 756, 803
Fridlund, B., 307, 308
Fridman, E. A., 54
Fridriksson, J., 110, 511
Friederici, A., 416, 423, 424, 509, 689, 706,
    783, 1013, 1014
Friedland, J., 379, 380, 381, 382, 384
Friedland, R. P., 995
Friedman, H. M., 411
Friedman, M. H., 379
Friedman, O., 101
Friedman, R. B., 413, 597, 609, 663, 667,
    767, 769
Friedmann, N., 103, 738, 740, 741
Fried-Oken, M., 824
Friedrich, F. A., 534
Friedrich, F. J., 696, 964
Fristoe, M., 768
Friston, K., 37
Frith, C. D., 37, 967
Fromhoff, F. A., 937
Fromkin, V., 740
Fromm, D., 34, 80, 178, 192, 297, 437, 524,
    572, 579, 757, 814
Fruhwald, T., 1000
Fucetola, R., 193, 437
Fuchs, L. S., 918
Fuchs, S., 895
Fuh, J. L., 550
Fuhrer, M., 304
Fukui, T., 552, 554, 555
Fuld, P. A., 894
Fuller, K., 866
Functional Communication Measure, 80
Funfgeld, M., 378
Funkenstein, H. H., 26
Funnell, E., 585, 610, 611, 674
Fust, R. S., 384
Fuster, J. M., 534
Fytche, D. H., 697

Gabriel, C., 172
Gabrieli, J. D., 96
Gaddie, A., 172, 496, 520, 573
Gaddie-Cariola, A., 394
Gadler, H. P., 865
Gage, F. H., 13
Gagnon, D. A., 699, 774
Gailey, G., 291, 306, 497
Gaines, K., 11
Gainotti, G., 11, 35, 37, 411, 568, 610, 964
Gajar, A., 924

Galaburda, A. M., 27, 30
Galasko, D., 992
Galens, J., 246
Gallagher, A. J., 423
Gallagher, D., 994
Gallagher, R., 111, 112, 424, 735
Gallagher, T., 80, 114, 213, 481
Gallese, V., 1013, 1014
Galt, J. R., 50
Galynker, I., 52
Gandek, B., 357
Gandour, J., 251, 1027
Ganguley, B., 566
Gannaway, R., 293, 779
Garcia, L., 79, 85, 256, 279, 305, 349, 351,
    360, 363, 427
García-Albea, J. E., 252
Gardner, B., 413, 428, 864
Gardner, H., 102, 410, 415, 416, 417, 420,
    515, 567, 570, 576, 586, 774, 864, 969,
    971, 972, 976
Gardner, R., 864
Garrett, K., 67, 71, 173, 295, 297, 306, 377,
    382, 387, 392, 393, 522, 584, 817, 818, 819,
    820, 821, 824, 826, 827, 828
Garrett, M. F., 597, 634, 635, 636, 637, 641,
    646, 769
Garron, D. C., 609
Gasper, S. M., 716
Gass, S. M., 250
Gatehouse, C., 775
Gates, G. A., 91
Gathercole, S., 720
Gaudreau, J., 419, 618
Gaunt, C., 1026
Gaviria, M., 259
Gazdar, G., 736
Geffner, D., 213
Gehlbach, S. H., 81
Geigenbaum, E. A., 865
Geigenberger, A., 977
Gelfer, C. E., 35
Genereux, S., 306
Genesee, F., 260
Gennarelli, T. A., 881
Gentile, A., 253
Gentry, B., 246
George, K. P., 123, 191
George, P., 757
Georgeadis, A. C., 180
Georges, J. B., 584
Georgopoulos, A. P., 91, 1011
Gerard, R., 219
Gerber, S., 118, 119
Gerberich, S. G., 880
Gerdau, R., 13
German, D. J., 75, 105, 578
Germani, M. J., 770
Gernsbacher, M. A., 757
Gerratt, B. R., 102, 420
Gersh, F., 21
Gershaw, N. J., 923
Gersten, J. W., 52
Gersten, R., 902, 918
Gerstenberger, D., 94, 333

Gerstman, L. J., 110, 430, 573, 971, 977
Geschwind, N., 9, 21, 28, 29, 33, 507, 690, 767,
    857, 891
Geyer, S., 1014
Ghaemi, M., 50, 190
Ghez, C., 1010
Ghidella, C., 305, 307, 763
Ghosh, S., 1011, 1014, 1015
Giangreco, M. F., 902
Giap, B. T., 894
Gibbon, B., 229, 240, 242
Gibbs, L., 81
Gierut, J., 746
Gilbert, B., 997
Gilbert, E., 999
Gilbert, T. P., 384
Giles, H., 207, 293, 301
Gilhooly, K. J., 613
Gill, H. S., 204
Gillilan, L. A., 44
Gillispie, M., 1002
Gillum, R. F., 11
Gilpin, S., 10, 115, 290, 328, 355
Ginsberg, G. M., 90
Gioia, G., 98, 904
Giordani, B., 888
Girling, D. M., 544
Giroire, J. M., 34
Giusiano, B., 610
Giustolisi, L., 35, 611
Gjengedal, E., 334
Glasberg, J. J., 52
Glaser, R., 409, 411
Glass, T., 319
Gleason, J. B., 416, 745
Gleick, J., 701
Glenberg, A. M., 714
Glenn, C. G., 696
Glennen, S., 830
Glickstein, J. K., 1002
Glindemann, R., 520, 757
Glisky, E. L., 863, 922
Glomset, J. A., 44
Gloning, K., 192, 193
Glosser, G., 96, 109, 110, 114, 427, 663,
    771, 830
Gluck, M. A., 894
Glucroft, B., 557
Glueckauf, R., 119, 122
Glykas, M., 205
Göbel, S., 1015
Gobin, P., 570
Goda, A. J., 108, 128, 508
Godduhn, J., 377
Godfrey, C. M., 377, 379
Goedert, M., 990
Goertzen, C. D., 53
Goettl, B. P., 714
Goff, D. C., 12
Goffin, J., 50
Goffman, E., 327
Goffman, I., 291, 307, 308
Goggin, J. P., 249, 257
Gold, B. T., 574
Gold, M., 56, 537, 540, 711

Goldberg, D., 214
Goldberg, E., 98
Goldberg, G., 52, 539
Goldberg, M. S., 43
Goldberg, S. A., 854, 858, 865
Goldblum, M. C., 259
Goldenberg, G., 124, 189, 190, 508, 537
Goldenberg, M., 975
Goldfader, P. R., 35
Goldman, J., 990, 991
Goldman, P. S., 910
Goldman-Rakic, P. S., 534, 700
Goldrick, M., 598, 607, 611, 774, 775
Goldsmith, T., 973
Goldstein, A. P., 923
Goldstein, B., 246
Goldstein, F. C., 880, 892
Goldstein, H., 171, 173, 178, 431, 745, 757
Goldstein, J., 409
Goldstein, K., 6, 94, 105, 421, 492, 811, 860
Goldstein, L. B., 55
Goleman, D., 229, 232
Golin, A. K., 232, 233
Gollnick, D., 246
Golper, L. A., 229, 232
Golper, L. C., 80, 84, 363, 366, 417, 518
Gomez-Tortosa, E., 259
Gomis, M., 11
Gonatas, N., 549
Gontkovsky, S., 319
Gonzales, J., 56
Gonzalez, M., 413, 832, 862
Gonzalez-Rothi, L. J., 450, 530, 535, 536, 597,
    599, 600, 602, 607, 648, 674, 689, 704, 718,
    721, 722, 776
Goodale, M. A., 609
Goodenough, C., 758
Goodglass, H., 3, 4, 7, 8, 9, 21, 27, 35, 71, 72,
    74, 75, 79, 96, 102, 105, 109, 110, 111, 112,
    113, 125, 192, 196, 255, 256, 389, 411, 413,
    415, 416, 418, 423, 424, 427, 457, 492, 507,
    508, 566, 567, 574, 578, 601, 607, 632, 644,
    657, 666, 698, 724, 735, 736, 738, 741, 745,
    764, 765, 767, 768, 771, 774, 776, 777, 782,
    783, 817, 857, 970, 974, 995
Goodman, J. S., 718
Goodman, P., 14, 77, 480
Goodman, R. A., 75, 597, 656, 666
Goodman-Schulman, R., 600, 657
Goodwin, C., 101, 178, 291, 293, 294, 301
Goplerud, E., 212
Goral, M., 245, 249, 252
Gordon, B., 547, 609, 610, 611, 698, 738
Gordon, E., 376, 380
Gordon, H., 259, 837
Gordon, J. K., 81
Goren, A. R., 90
Gorno-Tempini, M., 37, 549, 550, 551, 554,
    555, 556
Görtler, M., 536
Gottlieb, S. H., 11, 12
Gouaze, A., 26
Goulding, P. J., 547
Goulet, P., 612, 969, 973
Govoni, P., 1012

Gowan, J., 296, 471
Grabow, J. D., 880
Grabowski, T. J., 22, 37, 611, 774, 775
Grade, C., 56
Graetz, P., 256, 424
Graff-Radford, N., 21, 35, 550, 552, 978
Grafman, J., 550, 893, 894, 896, 899, 901, 919, 922, 967
Graham, D. I., 881, 892
Graham, K. S., 557, 611
Graham, L. F., 421, 578
Graham, M., 302, 382, 386, 387, 598
Graham, S., 861, 914
Grainger, J., 252
Grand, M., 51
Granger, C. V., 80, 297
Granier, J. P., 92
Grant, D., 97, 98, 488
Grant, I., 74
Grantham, R. B., 248
Grasby, P. M., 967
Graser, J. M., 904
Grassi, M. P., 193
Grassly, J., 620
Gray, J. A. M., 14
Gray, L., 380, 509
Grayson, E., 617
Graziano, M. S. A., 1011
Green, D. W., 250
Green, E., 411, 413, 424, 431, 758, 765
Green, G., 511
Green, J., 550, 552
Greenbaum, S., 769
Greene, R. L., 714
Greener, J., 195, 198, 451
Greenhalgh, T., 297
Greenhouse, J. B., 192, 195, 572
Greenlee, J. D. W., 1010
Greenlee, R., 56
Greenwald, M. L., 425, 607, 608, 609, 612, 614, 615, 620, 622, 641, 655, 659
Greenwood, A., 620
Greenwood, R. J., 96, 885
Grendel, M., 249
Grenier, L. H., 992
Gresham, F. M., 902, 924
Gresham, G. E., 52
Grey, J. E., 217
Grice, H. P., 117
Griffin, P., 583
Griffin, S., 124
Griffin, Z. M., 637, 641
Grilc, B., 1000
Grill, J. J., 76
Grimshaw, J., 14
Grinspin, D. R., 238
Grip, J. C., 197, 665, 774
Grober, E., 75, 705
Grodzinsky, Y., 103, 634, 736, 738, 740, 741
Grogan, S., 765
Groher, M., 893
Grol, R., 14
Gronwall, D. M. A., 98, 725, 880, 888
Grosjean, F., 246, 248, 249, 250, 252, 265
Gross, M., 967

Grossi, D., 609
Grossman, M., 89, 424, 548, 549, 554
Grossman, R. G., 881, 886, 891, 893
Grosswasser, Z., 895
Grubeck-Loebenstein, B., 13
Gruen, A., 484, 502
Grujic, Z., 552
Gudykunst, W. B., 246
Guenther, F. H., 1009, 1014, 1015
Guerrini, C., 725
Guilford, J. P., 9, 64, 95, 96, 97, 471, 472, 473, 474, 475, 476, 478, 483, 484, 485, 487, 492
Gullapalli, R. P., 1013
Gunji, A., 1009
Gupta, A., 94
Gupta, S., 50, 56
Gurd, J. M., 1013
Gurland, G. B., 118, 119
Guyard, H., 854, 865
Gybels, J., 50
Gyoubu, T., 544

Haaland, K. Y., 76
Haan, M. N., 222
Haarbauer-Krupa, J., 619, 880, 891, 918, 919
Haarmann, H. J., 111, 112
Haas, D., 539
Haas, G., 508
Haas, J., 880
Haberman, S., 424
Habib, M., 11, 566
Hachinski, V. C., 992, 994
Hack, N., 738
Hada, J., 537
Haden, C. A., 937
Haendiges, A. N., 102, 110, 634, 639, 641, 643, 648, 736, 767, 775, 776
Hageman, C. F., 415, 429, 430
Hagen, C., 756, 886, 891, 893
Hagenlocker, D., 993
Haggard, P., 1014
Hagiwara, H., 740
Hagoort, P., 103
Haine, R. A., 937
Haire, A., 340
Hake, H., 488
Hakel, M., 1018
Hakuta, K., 248, 249
Haley, K., 297, 299
Haley, M. A., 672, 784, 1022
Haley, W., 323
Halkar, R. K., 50
Hall, K. M., 80, 880, 886, 894
Hall, L. K., 249
Halle, J. W., 896
Halle, M., 747
Hallett, M., 922, 1011
Halliday, M., 109, 515
Halligan, P. W., 92, 96, 965
Hallowell, B., 3, 4, 5, 203, 205, 208, 210, 211, 212, 213, 214, 215, 216, 217, 218, 219, 220, 811, 856, 902
Hallowell, E. M., 926
Halm, M., 340
Halper, A. S., 85, 966

Halpern, H., 413, 416, 421, 422, 891
Halsband, U., 251, 1013
Hamburg, D. A., 856
Hamby, S., 969
Hamers, J., 250, 253
Hamilton, M., 994
Hammill, D. D., 75, 98
Hammons, J., 94
Hamrin, E., 357
Hamsher, K., 21, 255
Han, B., 323
Hand, L., 893
Hand, P. J., 48
Handlesman, J. A., 230
Hanks, R. A., 89
Hanley, J. R., 673, 783
Hanlon, R. E., 110, 430, 569, 573, 583
Hanna, G., 101
Hanna, J. E., 425, 735
Hanna, J. S., 664
Hanna, P. R., 664
Hanratty, K., 698
Hansen, A. M., 174
Hansen, L. A., 992
Hanson, B., 1019
Hanson, E. K., 1018
Hanson, J., 246
Hanson, W. R., 49, 50, 52, 187, 188, 416, 508, 756
Hanton, G., 894
Happe, F., 971
Harchik, A. E., 930, 931
Hardt, E. J., 246
Hardy, J. C., 428
Hardy, R. J., 46
Harford, C., 104
Hari, R., 1014
Harley, B., 250
Harley, T. A., 595, 637, 641, 699
Harlock, W., 27, 49, 186
Harlow, H., 477
Harrington, G., 519
Harris, E. H., 1018, 1021
Harris, J. L., 521
Harris, K. R., 914
Harris, L., 319, 357
Harris, M., 488
Harris, P. J., 902
Harris, R. J., 248
Harris, V. M., 587
Harrison, R. P., 482
Harruff, R. C., 880
Harskamp, F. V., 56
Hart, E. J., 894
Hart, J., 37, 609, 610, 611, 698
Hart, K., 304
Hart, R. P., 554, 555, 895
Hart, S., 87
Hartley, L. L., 88, 120, 893
Hartman, E. C., 207, 208
Hartman, J., 572
Hartshorne, N. J., 880
Hartsuiker, R. J., 636, 641, 650
Harvey, P. D., 89
Harvey, R. L., 52

Harward, H. N., 893, 897
Hasan, R., 109, 515
Hasboun, D., 1015
Haselkorn, J., 319
Hashimoto, N., 621
Haslam, C., 922
Hatfield, M. F., 599
Hatsopoulos, N. G., 1011
Hauck, K., 904
Hauk, O., 420
Havighurst, R., 298
Haviland, S. E., 481
Hawes, A., 572
Hayden, D., 1022, 1027, 1028
Hayden, M. E., 905
Hayes, R. B., 14
Hayes, S., 565
Haynes, R. B., 14, 51, 166
Hayward, R. W., 27, 28, 49, 1014
Hazen, E., 1017
Hazenberg, G. J., 544
He, J., 12
Head, H., 4, 69
Health Advocate, 218
Healton, E. B., 30, 572
Heath, P. D., 544
Heaton, R., 74, 106, 764, 818
Heaton, S., 922
Hebb, D. O., 701
Hebert, L. E., 988
Hebert, R., 967, 992
Hécaen, H., 260
Hechtman, L., 914, 924
Hedber-Borenstein, E., 378
Hedberg, N., 109, 427
Heeringa, H. M., 80, 579
Heeschen, C., 118, 738
Heidler, J., 189, 508, 524, 597, 767, 782,
    783, 964
Heidler-Gary, J., 611
Heikkila, V. M., 229
Heilman, K. M., 35, 91, 92, 93, 533, 534, 539,
    609, 610, 611, 616, 621, 648, 656, 691, 696,
    697, 719, 721, 722, 724, 776, 891, 964, 965,
    966, 967, 971, 975, 976, 977
Heindel, W. C., 989, 991
Heinrich, J. J., 508
Heiss, W. D., 50, 190, 191, 192, 565
Held, J. P., 43
Hellblom, A., 571, 572
Hellerstein, J., 220
Hellige, J. B., 967
Hellings, C., 70
Helm, N., 191, 384, 431, 582, 768, 773, 837
Helm-Estabrooks, N., 21, 56, 71, 72, 73, 76,
    88, 92, 93, 98, 108, 111, 125, 174, 187, 197,
    297, 409, 437, 451, 508, 518, 558, 565, 570,
    572, 575, 577, 578, 581, 582, 583, 585, 586,
    659, 744, 745, 756, 763, 768, 771, 773, 777,
    778, 786, 817, 818, 819, 826, 830, 840, 904
Helmick, J. W., 414
Hemsley, G., 94, 193, 323, 337
Hemyari, P., 880
Henderson, J., 88, 904
Henderson, L. W., 74, 256

Henderson, V. L., 786
Hendler, J., 893
Hendrick, D. L., 432
Hendricks, R., 319
Hengst, J. A., 115, 293, 294, 301, 779
Henley, S., 192
Hennes, H. J., 229
Henri, B. P., 205, 210, 211, 212, 213, 214, 215,
    216, 217, 218, 219, 220, 902
Henry, K., 918
Henry, M., 597, 598, 599, 602, 654, 667
Henson, H., 508
Henson, R. A., 544
Herbert, R., 197, 580, 620, 726, 776, 967
Heredia, R. R., 265
Herholz, K., 191
Heritage, J., 178
Hermann, B. P., 613
Hermann, M., 94, 124, 193, 337, 362, 378
Hernandez, A. E., 74, 79, 251, 253
Hernandez, D., 256
Heron, J., 178
Heron, M. P., 11
Herrin, J. S., 233
Herrmann, D., 868
Herrmann, M., 94, 290, 362, 536, 568, 569, 771
Hersh, D., 291, 381, 382, 391
Hersh, N. A., 921
Herskovits, E., 964
Herweyer, S., 999
Herzog, H., 966
Hesketh, A., 300, 769
Hichwa, R. D., 37, 611, 775
Hickey, E., 110, 295, 303, 517, 999
Hickin, J., 197, 580, 620, 624, 726, 776
Hickman, C. S., 205
Hickok, G., 424, 1015, 1016
Hickson, L., 69, 89, 179, 221, 256, 291, 294,
    296, 298, 350, 351, 355, 356, 362, 363, 831
Hickson, M., 513
Hier, D. B., 11, 597, 993
Highley, A. P., 118
Hijdra, A., 50
Hilari, K., 121, 192, 294, 295, 298, 300, 351,
    356, 357, 358
Hildebrandt, N., 103, 104, 736, 765
Hillary, F. G., 716
Hiller, M. D., 217
Hillis, A., 37, 64, 77, 82, 89, 102, 108, 124, 126,
    189, 406, 412, 508, 520, 524, 538, 548, 567,
    595, 597, 598, 599, 600, 601, 603, 607, 608,
    609, 610, 611, 612, 614, 615, 616, 617, 619,
    620, 621, 622, 623, 634, 636, 640, 641, 654,
    657, 660, 661, 665, 668, 669, 671, 672, 674,
    719, 736, 767, 782, 783, 784, 964, 971,
    1014, 1016
Hillis Trupe, A. E., 600, 668, 669
Hillman, T. C., 50
Hiltbronner, B., 32
Hilton, N., 921
Hilton, R., 617
Hinckley, J. J., 66, 69, 70, 85, 114, 118, 123,
    179, 180, 260, 262, 263, 265, 295, 297, 302,
    304, 329, 338, 414, 509, 600, 971
Hindenlang, J., 126, 179, 295, 304, 308, 517

Hinnach, S. E., 106
Hinton, G. E., 692, 693
Hintzman, D. L., 714
Hiraba, H., 1011
Hird, K., 250
Hirsch, B. D., 221
Hirsch, F. M., 197, 356, 597, 668
Hirsch, J., 251
Hirsch, K. W., 102, 110, 613
Hirst, W., 768, 972
Hitch, G., 989
Ho, K., 205, 584
Hochhalter, A. K., 716
Hodges, J. R., 89, 546, 548, 552, 557, 598, 610,
    611, 991, 992, 998
Hodges, R. E., 664
Hodgson, C., 432, 718
Hoen, B., 294, 295, 306
Hoen, R., 378, 379
Hoepfner, R., 96, 97, 471, 472, 473, 474, 476,
    483, 484, 485, 492
Hoerster, L., 999
Hoffman, D., 1012
Hoffman, E., 319
Hoffman, P., 499, 500
Hoffman, R. E., 54
Hofstede, B. T. M., 113, 114
Hofstetter, R. C., 992
Hogan, A., 362
Hogh, P., 229
Hohenstein, J., 249
Hohl, B., 558
Holbrook, M., 80, 323
Holcomb, H. J., 967
Holland, A. L., 34, 66, 69, 70, 80, 82, 89, 102,
    114, 116, 117, 118, 119, 122, 123, 124, 125,
    127, 128, 178, 180, 187, 192, 247, 253, 255,
    257, 260, 264, 290, 292, 295, 297, 298, 300,
    301, 302, 308, 319, 356, 361, 376, 377, 381,
    382, 384, 386, 389, 390, 391, 392, 394, 406,
    409, 419, 432, 433, 437, 452, 455, 457, 486,
    497, 508, 510, 511, 517, 524, 552, 570, 571,
    572, 576, 578, 579, 580, 588, 600, 619, 659,
    775, 779, 814, 840, 842, 843, 844, 846, 887,
    893, 924, 991, 1001
Holley, S., 220
Hollingsworth, A. L., 691, 697
Hollinshead, W., 880
Hollon, S. D., 1028
Holm, V. A., 229
Holman, B. L., 50
Holmes, D., 923
Holmes, T., 999
Holt, B. L., 429
Holtzapple, P., 71, 421, 578, 1023
Holub, R. J., 716
Holzemer, W. L., 219
Holzer, W. L., 219
Homan, R. W., 978
Homma, A., 549
Honig, L. S., 991
Hood, B. S., 967
Hoodin, R. B., 583
Hoops, H., 121, 409, 411, 416, 423
Hopcutt, B., 300
Hopkins, H. K., 886

Hopper, T., 95, 295, 302, 303, 306, 361, 363, 517, 588, 779, 988, 997, 999, 1002
Hori, T., 26
Horn, L. C., 991
Horn, S., 337
Hornak, J., 927
Horner, J., 75, 187, 411, 429, 433, 571, 572, 578, 583, 657, 965
Horner, R. H., 392, 393, 394, 902
Hornseth, J., 488
Horowitz, D. M., 856
Horton, G., 923
Horton, S., 299
Hoshiyama, M., 1009
Hotz, G., 88, 904
Hough, M. S., 102, 425, 426, 427, 509, 765, 780, 969, 970
Houghton, G., 674
Houghton, P., 119
Houle, S., 894
Housman, K. A., 240
Houston, M., 12, 256
Hovda, D. A., 56
Howard, D., 67, 73, 75, 100, 102, 105, 110, 197, 410, 416, 420, 457, 580, 599, 610, 611, 613, 614, 615, 620, 624, 632, 718, 726, 735, 773, 775, 776, 869
Howard, S., 1022, 1023
Howe, T., 294, 295, 305, 306, 350, 363, 382, 831
Howieson, D. B., 71
Howland, J., 102
Hoyert, D. L., 11
Hoyt, P., 509
Huang, C. S., 1011
Hubbard, D. J., 433
Hubbard-Wiley, P., 246
Huber, M., 383
Huber, W., 73, 78, 256, 300, 355, 425, 437, 520, 565, 648, 757
Huberman, A., 390
Hubley, A. M., 74
Huck, S. W., 169
Hudson, J. A., 937
Hudson, L., 552
Hufeisen, B., 250
Hugdahl, K., 535
Hughes, C., 892
Hughes, D. L., 392, 393, 394
Hughy, J., 485
Hula, W. D., 178, 357
Humphrey, G. K., 609
Humphreys, G. W., 252, 264, 519, 567, 598, 609, 617, 693, 720, 893, 964, 967
Hunkin, N. M., 726, 727, 922, 998
Hunt, J., 424
Hunt, M. I., 388
Hunter, M., 78
Huntley, G. W., 1011
Huntley, R. A., 102, 540, 776
Hurford, J. R., 250
Hurwitz, B., 297
Husain, M., 965
Hutchinson, A., 14
Hutchinson, T. J., 76

Huth, C., 173, 306
Hutter, B., 300
Hütter, B.-O., 355
Huvelle, R., 49
Hux, K., 119, 814, 823, 825, 828
Hyde, M. K., 745
Hyde, M. R., 21, 416, 745
Hyltenstam, K., 249, 250
Hynan, L. S., 1001

Iacoboni, M., 697, 975, 1011
Iavarone, A., 600
ICF. *See* International Classification of Functioning, Disability and Health
Ide, J., 716
IDEA: Federal Register, 880, 881
Idrissi, A., 260
Ielasi, W., 427
Ignativicius, D. D., 240
Ikoma, K., 54
Ilinsky, I. A., 21, 35
Imao, G., 544
Imbornone, E., 610
Indefrey, P., 1014
Ingham, D., 756
Inglehart, J. K., 217
Ingles, J. L., 895, 902, 920
Ingram, J. C. L., 418
Ingstad, B., 326
Insalaco, D., 343, 665
Inskip, W. M., 376, 377, 379
International Classification of Functioning, Disability and Health (ICF), 10, 64, 65, 66, 80, 82, 85, 91, 114, 120, 126, 127, 128, 164, 210, 295, 350, 351, 376, 831
Inzaghi, M. G., 257
Iorio, L., 609
Ireland, C., 295, 306, 328, 333
Ireland, S., 290
Irvin, L. K., 902
Irvine, D., 535
Irwin, W., 120, 437, 524
Isaac, J. T. R., 533
Isaacs, E., 220
Isquith, P. K., 904
Itkonen, T., 930
Ittelson, W., 323
Ivancic, M. T., 926
Iverson, V. S., 902
Ivnik, R. J., 74, 256
Iwata, B. A., 905
Izard, C. E., 893, 922

Jack, C. R., 549
Jack, C. R., Jr., 547
Jackson, C. A., 50, 416, 423, 508
Jackson, H. H., 4, 484, 837, 851
Jackson, J. H., 1011
Jackson, S., 78, 102, 108, 123, 167, 770
Jacobs, B. J., 196, 425, 597, 599, 620, 636, 643, 646, 648, 726, 745, 746, 778, 815
Jacobs, D. M., 79, 993
Jacobs, H. E., 891, 894, 895, 896, 928
Jacobs, J. R., 971
Jacobs, M. A., 1014

Jacobsen, A. M., 1013
Jacobson, R., 56, 250, 632
Jacques, P., 975
Jagaroo, V., 824
Jake, J., 250
James, T. W., 609
James, W., 902
Jane, J. A., 888
Janer, K. W., 967
Janghorbani, M., 56
Jansen Steur, E. N. H., 993
Jarecki, J. M., 426, 765
Jarvis, S., 249
Jarvis-Selinger, S., 205
Jefferson, A. L., 992
Jefferson, G., 117
Jeffires, K., 1009
Jehkonen, M., 965
Jenike, M., 327
Jenkins, D., 884, 894
Jenkins, H., 838
Jenkins, J. J., 6, 81, 102, 377, 382, 404, 405, 411, 412, 420, 477, 756, 803, 855
Jenkins, W. M., 450, 603
Jennett, B., 886
Jennings, E., 470
Jennings, F., 765
Jennings, R., 967
Jensen, G., 488
Jessell, T. M., 603
Jessner, U., 250
Jezewski, M., 326
Jimenez-Pabon, E., 6, 81, 377, 382, 404, 756, 838, 855
Jin, K., 13
Jinks, A. F. G., 419
Joanette, Y., 86, 114, 292, 379, 612, 969, 970, 971, 973, 978, 979
Johannsen-Horbach, H., 180, 378, 379, 380, 568, 584, 771, 831, 832
Johansen-Berg, H., 1015
Johns, D. F., 1024, 1025
Johnsen, S., 819
Johnson, A., 290, 485, 757, 902
Johnson, A. F., 123, 191
Johnson, C., 211
Johnson, D. A., 924
Johnson, J. P., 102, 411, 415, 516
Johnson, L., 764
Johnson, N., 552
Johnson, S. C., 51
Johnson, S. K., 100
Johnson, W., 166
Johnson, Z., 921
Johnston, A., 172
Johnston, J. M., 382
Johnston, R. A., 701
Johnston, S. S., 923
Joint Commission on Accreditation of Healthcare Organizations (JCAHO), 166, 212, 240, 242
Joint Committee for Stroke Facilities, 45, 46
Jokel, R., 557
Jones, D., 102, 382, 391, 420, 697, 1009, 1015
Jones, E. G., 1011

Jones, E. V., 639
Jones, J. A., 53
Jones, K. J., 110, 325, 417, 423, 764, 776
Jones, L., 7, 8, 404, 416, 578
Jones, R. S., 726, 727
Jones, T., 50
Jong, C. N., 894
Jonker, C., 989
Jonkers, R., 737
Jorgensen, H. S., 11, 124, 186
Josephs, K. A., 549, 550, 551, 552, 553, 554,
    555, 556
Judge, K. S., 999
Junqué, C., 260, 264
Juola, J. F., 412
Jürgens, U., 1014
Just, M. A., 190

Kadon, N., 54
Kaga, K., 618
Kagan, A., 70, 115, 179, 236, 279, 290, 291,
    292, 294, 295, 296, 297, 299, 300, 303, 304,
    305, 306, 310, 328, 342, 343, 352, 356, 362,
    363, 364, 366, 381, 388, 497, 508, 517, 565,
    588, 779
Kahan, T., 571, 572
Kahana, B., 327
Kahana, E., 327
Kahana, M., 327
Kahane, P., 1012
Kahn, H. J., 616, 1023
Kahn, R., 337
Kahneman, D., 12, 66
Kahrs, J., 757
Kakigi, R., 1009
Kalinyak-Fliszar, M., 197, 710, 1022
Kalisky, Z., 894
Kalra, L., 319
Kandel, E. R., 603
Kane, A., 672, 767, 784
Kang, S.-M., 247
Kaori, M., 173
Kaplan, E., 7, 21, 71, 79, 109, 196, 255, 256,
    389, 413, 427, 451, 452, 457, 492, 507, 508,
    566, 567, 574, 578, 601, 607, 657, 724, 741,
    771, 774, 817, 830, 857, 904, 905, 970, 974,
    995
Kaplan, G. A., 222
Kaplan, J., 969, 971, 972, 975, 976
Kaplan, L. R., 30, 572
Kaplan, R. F., 967
Kaplan, R. M., 639
Kapur, N., 544, 921
Kapur, S., 894
Karbe, H., 50, 190, 191, 549, 565
Karcher, L., 425, 643, 764
Karlsson, G. M., 964
Karnath, H. O., 92
Karow, C. M., 418, 776, 975, 976
Karpf, C., 861
Kartsounis, L. D., 554, 673
Kaschak, M. P., 757
Kashima, H., 90
Kaszniak, A. W., 87, 88, 523, 991, 993
Katsuki-Nakamura, J., 426, 515

Katsumata, A., 566, 570
Katz, B., 415, 853
Katz, D. I., 881, 884, 885, 893
Katz, J. M., 570
Katz, R., 203, 213, 216
Katz, R. B., 671
Katz, R. C., 180, 196, 207, 208, 210, 257, 665,
    762, 852, 853, 854, 855, 856, 857, 858, 859,
    860, 861, 862, 863, 865, 866
Katz, S., 43
Katz, W. F., 1022
Katzman, R., 989
Kaufer, D. I., 86
Kaufman, A. S., 75
Kaufman, M., 515
Kaufman, N. L., 75
Kauschke, C., 737
Kavale, K., 902, 920
Kawabata, K., 50, 565
Kawahigashi, J. N., 856
Kawamura, M., 552
Kay, B., 206
Kay, G. C., 764
Kay, J., 75, 77, 78, 82, 102, 103, 108, 109, 111,
    453, 484, 578, 611, 612, 618, 656, 657, 666
Kay, T., 887
Kayser, H., 254, 256
Kazis, A., 256
Kean, M., 297, 513, 646
Kearns, K. P., 163, 168, 170, 171, 172, 173,
    174, 175, 179, 180, 197, 214, 295, 350, 362,
    363, 376, 377, 382, 385, 388, 391, 392, 393,
    394, 419, 433, 469, 496, 497, 517, 520, 583,
    585, 599, 747, 858, 1024, 1029
Keefe, J. S., 89
Keenan, E. L., 52
Keenan, J. A., 492
Keenan, J. S., 70, 71, 124, 125, 192, 578, 855
Keeton, R. J., 764
Keidel, M., 967
Keil, K., 523
Keith, R., 71, 390
Keith, R. L., 174, 803, 855, 1026
Keith, R. W., 87, 98
Kellar, L. A., 765
Keller, C., 94, 333
Keller, R., 967
Kelly, B., 969
Kelly, R. J., 91
Kelly-Hayes, M., 43, 325
Kelso, D., 866
Kemeny, S., 768
Kemmerer, D., 109, 639, 737
Kempler, D., 50, 74, 79, 416, 420, 423, 508,
    544, 552, 972
Ken, L., 89
Kendall, D., 414, 711, 720, 721, 722, 724, 1022
Kendall, P., 164
Kenin, M., 188, 576
Kennedy, C. H., 902, 930
Kennedy, M., 14, 73, 78, 129, 894, 918
Kennedy, P., 544
Kennedy, S. H., 976
Kent, J. C., 93
Kent, J. F., 1020

Kent, R. D., 93, 165, 166, 173, 553, 978, 1020
Kenyon, L. C., 549
Kerlinger, F. N., 163
Kern, L., 905
Kerns, K. A., 922
Kerr, P., 205
Kerschensteiner, M., 425
Kertesz, A., 7, 11, 27, 28, 32, 49, 71, 72, 79, 81,
    88, 89, 123, 124, 125, 186, 187, 188, 189,
    192, 193, 196, 256, 437, 507, 548, 549, 550,
    551, 552, 554, 556, 565, 566, 567, 568, 570,
    572, 574, 575, 576, 578, 580, 610, 611, 657,
    666, 668, 705, 720, 724, 741, 756, 787, 817,
    818, 819, 857, 976
Kessels, F., 190
Kessels, R. P. C., 922
Kessler, J., 50, 190, 191, 565
Ketonen, L., 48
Ketterson, T. U., 178
Keyserlingk, A. G., 565, 567, 573
Khaw, K., 12
Khazei, A., 205
Kiernan, R. J., 98
Kilborn, K., 249
Kilgard, M. P., 450, 727
Killackey, J., 738
Kim, E. S., 997
Kim, H., 256
Kim, J., 764
Kim, K. H., 251
Kim, M., 103, 735, 737, 745
Kim, Y., 411, 514
Kimbarow, M. L., 69
Kimelman, M., 214, 310
Kimelman, M. D. Z., 81, 102, 174, 427,
    436, 515
Kimura, D., 11, 1015
Kimura, M., 534
Kincade, M., 966
Kincaid, J. P., 658
King, H. A., 1011
King, J. M., 557, 820
King, N., 757
King, P. S., 429
King, R. B., 95
Kingston, D., 293, 779
Kinsella, G., 97, 99, 325, 379, 894
Kinsella, K., 206, 988
Kiosseoglu, G., 256
Kiran, S., 127, 173, 179, 197, 256, 258, 260,
    263, 264, 265, 266, 422, 425, 595, 600, 618,
    621, 622, 623, 708, 710, 720, 723, 724, 745,
    746, 778
Kirchner, D., 114, 115, 116, 117, 118, 119,
    120, 480
Kirkevold, M., 334
Kirshner, H., 507, 508
Kirsner, K., 250
Kirwin, M. M., 76
Kisley, C. A., 380
Kiss, K., 737
Kitselman, K., 520, 777, 968
Klatzky, R. L., 95
Kleczewska, M. K., 586, 832, 864
Klees, B., 319

Klein, B., 423, 764
Klein, D., 251
Klein, J. A., 53
Klein, K., 509, 567, 582
Klein, L., 119
Klein, P., 923
Kleinman, J., 611
Klima, E. S., 20
Klippi, A., 118, 293
Klonoff, P. S., 894
Knibb, J. A., 89, 546, 550, 552, 553, 556
Knight, J. A., 85
Knight, R. T., 865
Knighton, K., 841
Knock, T. R., 718, 1022, 1023
Knopman, D. S., 27, 49, 50, 189, 508
Knösche, T. R., 1013
Knowlton, B., 708, 894
Knox, A. W., 412
Kobayashi, K., 544
Koch, A., 523
Koch, U., 568
Kodras, J., 295
Koegel, L. K., 902
Koegel, R. L., 902
Koehl, M., 13
Koelman, T. W., 52
Koenig, H. G., 94
Koenig-Bruhin, M., 558
Koetsier, J. C., 52
Koff, E., 573, 976
Kohen, F. P., 180, 617, 619
Kohn, S., 111, 418, 422, 609, 611, 616,
    735, 865
Kohnert, K., 74, 79, 252, 253, 256, 259,
    260, 264
Kokmen, E., 549
Kolb, B., 689
Kolk, H., 111, 112, 113, 114, 125, 423, 637,
    641, 648, 650, 706, 738
Koller, J. J., 696
Konorski, J., 28
Kooistra, C. A., 964
Koopman, H., 736
Kordus, R. N., 718
Kornhuber, H. H., 34, 49
Korpelainen, J., 229
Kosinski, M., 357
Koski, L., 967
Koskiniemi, M., 894
Koss, E., 995
Kosslyn, S. M., 976
Koster, C., 297, 513
Kotten, A., 854
Koudstaal, S. R., 46
Koul, R., 565, 587
Kovach, T., 220
Kozniewska, H., 28
Kraat, A., 301, 815
Kraemer, H. C., 861
Kragh-Sorensen, P., 993
Krainen, G. H., 856
Krainik, A., 1012
Krakauer, J., 1010
Kramer, J. H., 992

Kramer, L., 977
Kraus, J. F., 880
Krause, B. J., 251
Krause, N., 323
Kravetz,, S., 102
Krchnavek, B., 904
Krebs-Noble, D., 1013
Krefft, T. A., 550, 552
Kregel, J., 896
Kremer, S., 1012
Kremin, H., 613, 864
Kretschmann, C. M., 43
Kreutzer, J. S., 885, 887, 896
Kricos, P., 335, 342
Kroenke, K., 364
Kroll, J. F., 250
Kronick, D., 856
Kubat-Silman, A. K., 535
Kubik, S., 22
Kubos, K. L., 975
Kucera, H., 613
Kudo, T., 421
Kufera, J., 893
Kuhl, D. E., 49, 50
Kulke, F., 109
Kuller, L. H., 11
Kumar, R., 565, 567
Kung, H., 11
Kurachi, M., 544
Kurland, L. T., 880
Kurowski, K., 1017
Kurtz, P. F., 926
Kurtzke, J. F., 787
Kushner, M., 544
Kusunoki, T., 73
Kvigne, K., 334
Kwakkel, G., 52

Laake, K., 291, 360
Laaksonen, H., 1011
Laasko, M., 118, 124, 414
Labar, D. R., 569
Labarthe, D. R., 12
Labov, W., 114, 785
Labovitz, G., 212
Ladavas, E., 967
Lafaury, P. J., 253
Lafond, D., 292, 379
Laganaro, K. M., 260, 261
Laganaro, M., 123, 180, 620, 862
Lahey, M., 9, 66, 68, 69, 70, 74, 81, 82, 100,
    114, 478, 479, 480
Lai, Q., 713
Lai, S. J., 567
Laiacona, M., 102, 192, 193, 257, 610, 613,
    616, 705
Laihinen, A., 251
Laine, M., 73, 257, 414, 619, 657, 726, 774
Laird, L., 425, 647, 745, 778
Lallanranta, T., 229
Lalor, E., 250
Lambert, J. D., 206
Lambon Ralph, M. A., 432, 607, 610, 718, 776
Lambrecht, K. J., 413
Lamping, D. L., 357

Landis, L., 102, 420
Landrum, P. K., 237, 240
Landry, S. H., 910
Lane, M., 229, 595
Lane, V. W., 1026
Lang, A. E., 993
Lang, M., 110, 410, 777
Langdon, H. W., 247, 253, 254
Langdon, N. A., 928
Lange, K. L., 422, 704
Langenbahn, D. M., 180, 905
Langer, E. J., 856
Langmore, S. E., 783
Lankhorse, G. J., 52
Lanzoni, S., 738
LaPointe, L. L., 65, 75, 85, 121, 123, 125, 166,
    292, 294, 295, 308, 377, 411, 414, 421, 429,
    433, 507, 508, 515, 567, 578, 657, 660, 810,
    814, 853, 855, 858, 1022, 1023
LaPointe, S., 636
Larfeuil, C., 101
Larkins, B., 351
Larkins, B. M., 89
Laroche, C., 305, 360, 363
Larrabee, G. J., 98
Larsen, C., 15, 222
Larsen, J. P., 993
Larsen, R., 298, 910
Larson, D., 49, 189
Larson, S. C., 75
Laska, A., 125, 571, 572
Lasker, J., 67, 71, 295, 306, 817, 818, 819, 822,
    824, 826, 828, 1026
Lasky, E. Z., 102, 415, 416, 516
Laterre, E. C., 552
Lau, W. K., 27, 189, 610
Laughlin, S. A., 21
Lauritzen, L., 975
Law, P., 484, 502
Law, S., 257, 1019
Law, W., 56
Laws, E. R., 880
Lawton, M., 327, 363, 364
Lazerson, A., 476, 477
Lazorthes, G., 26
le Grand, H., 419, 620, 726
le Grand, H. R., 599
Le Moal, M., 13
Leander, W. J., 231
Leavitt, J., 991
LeBlanc, J. E., 905
LeBlanc, K., 305, 352, 363
Leblanc, Y., 205
Lecours, A. R., 9, 124, 566, 767, 964
LeDorze, G., 14, 70, 101, 253, 258, 290, 294,
    306, 323, 337, 351, 419, 611, 618, 620, 760
LeDoux, J. E., 893, 972
Lee, A., 205
Lee, H. L., 251, 1015
Lee, J., 293, 739, 741
Lee, K.-M., 251
Lee, L., 75
Lee, M., 409, 738, 741
Lee, R. G., 50
Lee, T. D., 1023

Leek, E. C., 610
Leff, B., 205
Lefkowitz, N., 380, 509
Lefrancois, G., 477
Legatt, A. D., 30, 572
Leger, A., 191, 757
Legg, C., 517
Lehéricy, S., 1012
Lehman, M. T., 966, 969, 972, 973
Lehman-Blake, M. T., 551, 555, 970, 972, 973
Lehmann, T. S., 714
Lehner, L., 111, 418
Lehoux, P., 205
Lehtonen, M., 257
Leicester, J., 576
Leigh, W. A., 217
Leiguarda, R., 56
Leith, W., 14
Leiwo, M., 299, 300, 302
Lekka, G., 256
Lemak, N. A., 46
Lemhöfer, K., 245, 252
Lemieux, S. K., 1009, 1015
Lemme, M., 109, 168, 174, 175, 427, 1018, 1021
Lennon, T., 13
Lenzi, G. L., 50, 975
Leon, S. A., 979
Leonard, A., 572
Leonard, C. L., 86, 418, 557, 969
Leonard, L. B., 426, 482
Leonard, L. L., 116, 117
Leonardi-Bee, J., 46
Leong, D. J., 899
Lepper, M. R., 858
LeRhun, E., 89
Leri, J., 756
Leslie, J., 92
Lesniewicz, K., 969, 970, 971
Lesser, R., 78, 82, 83, 117, 120, 299, 423, 424, 578, 612, 656, 657, 666
Letenneur, I., 993
Leung, M. T., 257
Levander, M., 965
Leve, A. R., 43
Levelt, W., 636, 637, 642, 647, 774, 1014
Levey, S., 249
Levin, B. E., 255
Levin, H. S., 880, 881, 886, 891, 892, 894, 895
Levin, J., 206
Levin, W., 206
Levine, B. A., 738
Levine, D. N., 966, 969
Levine, H. L., 21, 573
Levine, J. A., 51
Levita, E., 123, 188, 192, 193, 565, 570, 571, 572, 575, 576, 577, 580, 582, 891
Levkoff, S., 206
Levy, E. S., 245
Lewis, D. L., 415
Lewis, J., 217, 427
Lewis, M., 304, 308
Lewis, R., 967
Lezak, M. D., 71, 82, 87, 95, 97, 887, 894, 909
Lhermitte, F., 537

Lhermitte, R., 260, 632
Li, E. C., 70, 107, 419, 422, 520, 776, 777, 780, 781
Li, L., 422, 425
Li, P., 252, 257, 265
Li, Y., 343
Liao, K. K., 550
Libben, G., 73, 255, 258
Liberman, A. M., 1010
Lichtenberg, P. A., 256
Lichtheim, L., 691, 700
Liddle, P. F., 37
Lieberman, R., 213, 411, 429
Lieberman, R. J., 213, 411
Lieberthal, T., 599, 617, 622
Liepert, J., 1011
Liepmann, H., 28, 1015
Light, J., 816, 820
Lightfoot, E., 343
Liles, B. J., 893
Liles, B. Z., 109, 110, 118, 415, 893, 971
Limburg, M., 50, 323
Lin, K. N., 550
Lincoln, N., 80, 94, 119, 193, 580
Lincoln, Y. S., 178
Lindamood, P. C., 721
Lindamood, P. D., 721
Lindeboom, J., 544
Lindeman, E., 319
Lindfors, J. W., 486, 487
Lindquist, K., 930
Lindsay, J., 118, 290, 360, 391, 618
Linebarger, M. C., 646, 648, 704, 740, 865
Linebaugh, C., 110, 111, 115, 122, 412, 418, 599, 769, 970, 972
Linebaugh, G. W., 413
Linell, S., 376, 378
Ling, A. R., 566
Lipsey, J. R., 975
Lissauer, H., 609
Litvan, I., 550
Liu, H., 265
Livingston, M. G., 894
Lloyd, J. J., 49
Lloyd, K., 924
Lloyd, L. L., 584, 768
Lo, A., 966
LoCasto, P. C., 1013
Lock, S., 109, 178, 303
Lockhart, R. S., 714, 716
Lodder, J., 190
Logan, C. G., 37
Logie, R., 613, 991
LogoMetrix, 1022
Logue, P. E., 995
Lojek-Osiejuk, E., 969, 971
Lolk, A., 993
Lomas, J., 68, 80, 115, 119, 120, 188, 297, 299, 356, 388, 389, 392, 457, 570, 578, 580
Lombardi, F., 894
Lommel, M., 428
London, R., 756
Long, B., 310
Longan, D., 205
Longman, D. J. A., 714

Longoni, F., 966, 968
Longstreth, D., 1026
Loomis, M. E., 231
Lorch, M. P., 195, 422, 735, 976
Lorenze, E. J., 52
Lorge, I., 421
Lorimer, W., 231
Loring, D. W., 71
Losanno, N., 361, 520
Lott, C., 229
Lott, P., 108
Lott, S. L., 769
Lott, S. N., 413, 597
Lovati, L., 260
Love, R., 14, 100, 416, 488, 767, 965
Love, T., 75, 740
Lovegreen, L., 327
Loverme, S. R., Jr., 35, 49
Loverso, F., 108, 389, 392, 429, 516, 583, 667, 745, 858, 860, 861, 866, 867
Lovett, M., 893
Lowell, S., 419, 619, 622, 1001
LPAA Project Group, 10, 279, 290, 291, 292, 310, 369, 376, 377, 588
Lu, L. H., 776
Lu, S., 79
Lubinski, R., 115, 306, 319, 325, 334, 343, 344, 363, 470, 472, 484, 485, 486, 502, 1001
Lucariello, J. M., 937
Lucas, E., 114, 480
Lucas, R. W., 860
Lucchelli, F., 775
Lucius-Hoene, G., 771
Ludlow, C. L., 189, 777, 1009
Ludy, C., 92, 764
Luecke, J., 205
Lum, T., 343
Luppino, G., 1012
Luria, A., 193, 632, 858, 899, 909
Luring, B., 557
Lustig, A. P., 1027
Lustig, C., 991
Luterman, D. M., 83, 308, 361, 362, 377, 379, 382
Lutsep, H., 46, 53
Lux, W. E., 569
Luzzatti, C., 102, 192, 256, 257, 544, 547, 568, 737
Lynch, E. W., 246
Lynch, W. J., 124, 857
Lyon, J., 108, 114, 118, 122, 123, 279, 290, 291, 294, 295, 297, 299, 303, 304, 306, 308, 310, 328, 337, 360, 361, 376, 377, 379, 499, 507, 517, 585, 786, 826, 944

Maas, E., 745
Macciocchi, S. N., 192
MacDonald, J., 902
MacDonald, S., 98, 904
Mace, F. C., 930
MacGinitie, W. H., 75
Mack, J., 423, 514
MacKay, I. R. A., 249
Mackay, R., 328, 349, 362

MacKenzie, A., 760
MacKenzie, I. R. A., 552
Mackey, W. F., 245
Mackisack, E. L., 966, 969, 970, 972
MacLennan, D. L., 56, 101, 174
MacMillan, P. J., 895
MacPhail, J., 999
MacWhinney, B., 249, 250, 257
Madden, M., 121
Madureira, S., 192
Mager, U., 584
Magito-McLaughlin, D., 902, 928
Magloire, J., 251, 657
Magni, E., 997
Magnusson, M., 865
Mahendra, N., 78, 251, 999, 1002
Maher, L. M., 92, 103, 111, 196, 414, 450, 608, 611, 616, 619, 648, 659, 660, 712, 726
Maiberger, R., 975
Majesky, S., 109
Makely, M., 53
Makenzie, C., 382, 384, 391
Makhlouf, M. S., 550
Makoni, S., 248, 250
Makris, N., 697
Makuuchi, M., 1014
Malec, J. F., 895
Malin, J. P., 56
Malone, D. M., 242
Malone, R. L., 379
Maly, J., 537
Mammucari, A., 192, 976
Mampaey, E., 256
Manaster, H., 380
Mancini, B., 1014
Mandell, A. M., 552
Maneta, A., 618
Manion, J., 231
Manjaly, Z. M., 410
Manly, J. J., 993
Manly, T., 966
Mann, D. M. A., 546, 548, 552
Mann, L., 902, 920
Mann, W., 335
Manning, L., 965
Manochiopinig, S., 118, 119
Mansur, L. L., 79, 255
Manton, K. G., 13
Manuel-Dupont, S., 255
Maraganore, D. M., 551
Marantz, A., 736, 738, 747
Marckmann, G., 757
Marcuse, E. K., 1021
Marder, K., 993
Margolin, D. I., 657, 673, 782
Marguardt, T. P., 768, 772
Mariage, T. V., 499
Mariën, P., 256, 536
Marin, G., 247
Marin, O. S. M., 633, 639, 655, 696, 704
Marini, A., 86
Mark, V. W., 188, 571, 572, 574, 575, 964
Markel, N. N., 853
Markesbery, W. R., 990, 992
Marks, N., 206

Markson, E., 207
Markwardt, F. C., 75
Marquardsen, J., 11, 43
Marquardt, T. P., 255, 376, 377, 379, 382, 391, 975
Marsh, E. B., 609
Marshall, J., 77, 96, 101, 102, 103, 257, 295, 301, 422, 423, 597, 618, 620, 638, 641, 642, 643, 647, 648, 660, 663, 668, 764, 777, 784, 965, 1015, 1016
Marshall, M. M., 894
Marshall, N., 1023
Marshall, R. C., 98, 110, 123, 125, 171, 179, 180, 188, 192, 236, 302, 376, 377, 382, 389, 413, 417, 418, 429, 430, 437, 451, 507, 515, 516, 517, 519, 520, 521, 522, 524, 569, 572, 581, 776, 975, 976, 1026, 1027, 1028
Martelli, M. F., 895
Marthas, M. S., 232, 233
Martin, A., 37, 966, 991
Martin, A. D., 73, 77, 407, 484, 517, 519, 620, 837
Martin, A. W., 80, 579
Martin, C., 775
Martin, D., 246, 254, 991
Martin, E. M., 259
Martin, G., 902
Martin, J. E., 892, 914, 918
Martin, N., 414, 595, 617, 619, 622, 641, 647, 699, 720, 726, 745, 762, 774, 778
Martin, R. C., 103, 416, 634, 757
Martin, R. E., 1009, 1015, 1026
Martin, W. R. W., 50
Martinage, D. P., 894
Martinez, A., 197, 205, 520, 1019, 1022, 1024, 1025, 1029
Marty, S., 265
Martyn, P., 376, 757
Maruszewski, M., 417
Marwitz, J. H., 885
Marx, M., 477
Masand, P., 569
Masayk, T. J., 47
Mashima, P. A., 205
Masih, A. K., 565
Maslow, A., 342
Massaro, M., 168, 171, 173, 174, 175, 419
Massey, E. W., 965
Masson, V., 854
Masters, S. E., 716
Masterson, J., 75, 259, 578, 741
Masterson, R. J., 549
Masullo, C., 11
Matarrese, M., 37
Matchar, D. B., 55
Mateer, C. A., 88, 89, 764, 920, 922
Matejka, J., 897
Matelli, M., 1012
Matsuo, Y., 54
Matthews, B. A. J., 855, 858
Matthews, C. G., 74
Matthews, C. T., 429
Matthews, P. M., 1013
Mattingly, I. G., 1010
Mattson, P., 902, 920

Matyas, T. A., 413, 621
Mauer, B. A., 71
Mauner, G., 740
Maurer, K., 1014
Mauro, B. C., 930
Mauszycki, S. C., 1019, 1024, 1025
Mavroudakis, N., 572
Max, J. E., 895
Maxim, J., 118, 178, 299
Maxwell, R. E., 880
Mayberg, M. R., 46, 51
Mayer, J., 106, 113
Mayer, N. H., 893
Mayo, N. E., 43
Mazaux, J. M., 34, 73
Mazoyer, B. M., 37
Mazziotta, J., 251
Mazzocchi, F., 28, 49, 566
McAfee, J., 83, 90, 129
McAllister, B. L., 992, 994
McAlonan, K., 533
McBride, K. E., 756
McBurney, D. H., 552
McCabe, A., 893, 937
McCabe, P., 124, 125, 186, 187, 192, 193, 549, 565, 568, 570, 572, 575, 576, 580, 611
McCaffrey, R., 124, 246
McCall, D., 106, 361, 418, 565, 586, 645, 710, 761, 777, 778, 864
McCallum, A. F., 195
McCarthy, G., 37
McCarthy, R. A., 37, 610, 696, 967
McCauley, R. J., 76, 100
McCauslin, L., 1026
McCleary, C., 768
McClelland, J. L., 598, 692, 693, 694, 695, 700, 701, 705, 708, 709, 715, 776
McCloskey, M., 600, 709
McColl, M., 379, 380, 381, 382, 384
McConnell, F., 488
McCooey, R., 115, 351
McCormick, G., 339
McCormick, L., 479
McCullagh, E., 319
McCullagh, S., 88
McDearmon, J. R., 411, 417
McDermott, F. B., 187, 571, 572
McDicken, W. N., 47
McDonald, S., 86, 88, 119, 521, 893, 895, 969
McDowell, I., 357, 360
McFarling, D., 35
McGarry, K., 781
McGilly, K., 899
McGlone, J., 11, 192
McGlynn, E. A., 860
McGrath, J., 927
McHenry, M., 1024, 1025
McHugh, P. B., 994, 995, 1002
McHugh, P. R., 975, 995
McHugh, R. E., 419, 519
McKeel, D. W., 550
McKeith, I. G., 992
McKelvey, M., 823, 824, 825
McKenna, K., 295, 305, 763, 964
McKenna, P., 567

McKinlay, W. W., 894
McKitrick, L. A., 997
McKoon, G., 969
McLaurin, D., 212
McLean, A., Jr., 237
McNamara, P., 738
McNaughton, B. L., 708
McNeil, M. R., 73, 75, 81, 92, 102, 103, 108, 173, 174, 178, 213, 264, 357, 409, 411, 427, 429, 430, 436, 515, 516, 543, 544, 549, 550, 553, 554, 557, 578, 583, 599, 816, 858, 1017, 1018, 1022, 1023
McPherson, J. R., 242
McPherson, S. E., 992
McQuade, D., 928
McReynolds, L. V., 168, 170, 172, 173, 392, 393, 858
McRoberts, H. A., 786
McWreath, J. M., 356
Meador, D., 249
Meadows, M. E., 967
Mechanic, D., 222
Mechelli, A., 251
Medford, I., 967
Megens, J., 50
Mehler, J., 249
Mehler, M. F., 544
Mehrabian, A., 853
Meichenbaum, D., 891, 892, 912, 914, 915, 918, 924
Meikle, M., 756
Meinzer, M., 712, 726
Meline, T., 77
Mellancamp, P., 207
Melton, A. W., 714
Melvold, J., 111
MEND. *See* Miami Emergency Neurologic Deficit
Mendelsohn, D., 893
Mendelson, M., 994
Mendez, M. F., 550
Menefee, L., 893, 905
Menn, L., 111, 113, 257, 640, 736
Mentis, M., 893
Merbitz, C. T., 197, 665, 774
Merchant, H., 1011
Mercier, L., 967
Merck Institute of Aging and Health, 13
Merens, T. A., 56
Merians, A. S., 718
Mertz, T., 192
Merzenich, M. M., 450, 603, 689, 701, 727, 728
Mesaros, R. A., 931
Messerli, P., 124, 192
Messick, C., 214
Messick, S., 76, 129
Messmer, C. L., 923
Mesulam, M. M., 13, 89, 544, 545, 546, 547, 548, 549, 550, 551, 552, 553, 554, 893, 895, 899, 901, 964, 965, 976, 977, 978
Metoki, H., 12
Metter, E. J., 42, 49, 50, 52, 171, 187, 416, 508
Metz, D. E., 166, 169
Meyer, A. S., 636
Meyer, E., 251

Meyer, J. S., 50
Meyers, C. A., 891
Meyers, J., 98
Meyers, K., 98
Meyers-Briggs, I., 231
Miami Emergency Neurologic Deficit (MEND), 71
Miceli, G., 11, 103, 111, 192, 422, 611, 619, 671, 696, 705
Michael, J., 928
Michallet, B., 323, 338, 339
Michel, M.-C., 245
Michelow, D., 969, 972
Miklossy, J., 50
Mikolic, J. M., 178, 357
Milan, M. A., 924
Milberg, W., 418
Milders, M., 895
Miles, M., 390
Miller, B. L., 550
Miller, D., 597, 609
Miller, G., 95
Miller, J. W., 550
Miller, M., 103
Miller, M. D., 914
Miller, N., 73, 249, 256, 265
Miller, P., 891, 892, 915, 919, 920
Miller, R. G., 319, 997
Miller, S., 891, 892, 915, 919, 920
Miller, W. R., 994
Miller-Loncar, C. L., 910
Millis, S. R., 89
Mills, C. K., 756
Mills, K. R., 1013
Mills, R., 110, 412, 413, 858, 859, 860, 861
Milman, L., 251
Milner, A. D., 92, 609
Milner, B., 251
Milo, T. J., 50
Milroy, L., 117, 178, 293
Milton, I., 999
Milton, S. B., 391, 392, 497, 582
Minamimoto, T., 534
Mines, M., 1019
Mingazzini, G., 544
Minifie, F., 214, 221
Miozzo, A., 37, 612
Miozzo, M., 251, 252, 610, 611
Miravalles, G., 257
Mirenda, P. L., 931
Mitchell, D., 229
Mitchum, C. C., 109, 425, 597, 600, 601, 602, 613, 614, 619, 632, 634, 639, 641, 643, 644, 645, 647, 648, 664, 704, 736, 767, 775, 776
Mithaug, D. E., 914
Miura, K., 190
Mizuno, M., 90
Mlcoch, A. G., 42, 50, 56
Moberg, P., 535, 611
Mock, J., 994
Mogentale, C., 725
Mogil, S., 380, 509
Mohlberg, H., 1014, 1015
Mohr, J. P., 26, 35, 576, 597, 1014
Mohs, R. C., 996

Moir, L., 387
Molrine, C. J., 79, 256
Moncrief, E., 828
Monetta, L., 86
Monfils, M. H., 53
Monheit, M. A., 964
Moniz, D., 931
Monroe, P., 49
Monsalve, A., 613
Monsch, A., 258
Montagna, C. G., 830
Monteleone, D., 964
Montgomery, E. B., 995
Montgomery, M. W., 893
Montrul, S., 249
Moonis, M., 48
Moore, M., 218
Moore, P., 229
Moore, S., 220
Moore, T., 1011
Moore, W. H., 413
Moore, W. S., 51
Moorhouse, B., 996
Moos, R., 323
Moossy, J., 552
The Moran Company, 218
Moran, J., 534
Moraschini, S., 188, 566
Moreines, J., 516
Moretti, J. L., 50
Moretti, R., 251, 259
Morgan, A., 56, 187, 508, 558, 565, 570, 572, 578, 585, 586, 778, 786, 817
Morgan, D., 336
Morgan, F., 488
Morganlander, J. C., 55
Moriarty, L., 607
Moritz, T., 56
Morley, G. K., 56
Morningstar, D., 1027
Moro, A., 111
Morris, E. K., 902
Morris, J., 413, 610, 617, 618, 619, 643
Morris, J. C., 544, 550
Morris, J. D., 535
Morris, J. N., 996
Morris, M., 608
Morris, R. G., 757
Morrison, E., 470, 523, 854
Morrison, M. H., 856
Morrow, L., 110, 964
Mortensen, H., 229
Mortimer, J. A., 992
Mortley, J., 761, 832, 864
Morton, J., 599, 620, 718, 726
Morton, V. M., 894
Moscovitch, M., 894
Moses, J., 971
Moskowitz, M. A., 246
Moss, A., 173
Moss, B., 307, 308
Moss, H. E., 765
Moss, S., 600, 659
Moulard, G., 859
Mounin, G., 632

Mourant, R. R., 923
Moya, K. L., 969
Moyer, S. B., 657, 769
MRC Psycholinguistic Database, 1019
Muir Gray, J. A., 166
Müller, D., 193, 292, 297, 308, 310, 362, 379
Muller, R. A., 50
Muma, J., 9, 64, 65, 475, 476, 480, 482, 485
Mummery, C. J., 551, 1016
Mungas, D., 246, 992
Munoz, D. G., 548, 552
Munoz, M., 255, 302, 361
Muraski, A., 756
Murdoch, B., 86, 88, 90, 566
Murison, R., 291, 296, 355
Murphy, H. H., 713
Murphy, J., 14, 207
Murphy, K., 1016
Murphy, S. L., 11
Murray, G. M., 1011
Murray, L. L., 65, 66, 67, 69, 70, 74, 77, 80, 81,
    82, 85, 88, 95, 96, 97, 102, 105, 106, 108,
    109, 110, 114, 116, 118, 124, 125, 126, 127,
    128, 425, 557, 643, 648, 763, 764, 775
Murray, L. S., 881
Murray, R. C., 550, 555, 922
Murray, S., 305
Murray, S. J., 763
Murray, V., 571, 572
Murtha, S., 698
Musen, G., 894
Musso, M., 191
Musson, N. D., 180, 386
Mutchler, J. E., 247
Myers, A. S., 774
Myers, C. E., 894
Myers, J. L., 643, 745, 762
Myers, J. S., 380
Myers, M. K. S., 205
Myers, P. S., 85, 86, 860, 963, 965, 966, 968,
    969, 970, 971, 972, 973, 974, 975, 979
Myerson, R., 421, 758
Myers-Scotton, C., 250

Na, D. L., 256
Nadeau, S. E., 108, 126, 127, 530, 531, 532,
    533, 534, 535, 536, 537, 538, 539, 607, 611,
    674, 689, 691, 694, 697, 700, 704, 706, 707,
    711, 723, 724
Naeser, M. A., 21, 27, 28, 32, 34, 49, 54, 124,
    189, 190, 251, 257, 406, 424, 508, 565, 566,
    573, 574, 575, 582, 586, 588, 778, 1014
Naesser, M., 193
Nagarajan, S. S., 692
Nagaratnam, N., 565, 573
Nagaratnam, S., 565
Nagy, V. T., 858, 859, 861, 862, 863
Nahemow, L., 363, 364
Naigles, L., 249
Nakamura, J., 544
Nakano, I., 552
Nakayama, H., 11, 186
Nakles, K., 171
Naremore, R., 480
Naselaris, T., 1011

Nash Koury, L., 1001
Nation, J. E., 165, 410
National Academy on an Aging Society, 13
National Aphasia Association, 211, 241, 290,
    343, 381
National Center for Evidence-Based Practice in
    Communication Disorders, 15
National Center for Health Statistics, 210
National Center for Injury Prevention and
    Control, 349
National Committee on Quality Assurance
    (NCQA), 212, 218
National Faculty Center, 78
National Head Injury Foundation, 340
National Institute for Deafness and Other
    Communication Disorders (NIDCD), 11,
    176, 177, 246
National Institute of Neurological Disorders
    and Stroke Study Group, 51
National Institute on Aging, 991
National Institute on Disability and
    Rehabilitation Research, 326
National Institutes of Health (NIH), 11, 246,
    896, 940
National Joint Committee for the
    Communicative Needs of Persons with
    Severe Disabilities, 281
National Stroke Association, 241, 349, 382
National Stroke Foundation, 340
Naujokat, C., 565
N-CEP registry of clinical practice guidelines
    and systematic reviews, 129
Neary, D., 49, 546, 547, 548, 552, 553, 557
Neault, M. J., 360
Nebel, K., 967
Nebes, R. D., 991
Needham, P., 916
Neils, J., 74
Neils-Strunjas, J., 74, 85
Neiman, M. R., 92
Neisser, U., 9, 64, 95, 470
Nelson, E. M., 248
Nelson, H., 75
Nelson, K., 937
Nelson, M., 340
Nelson, N. A., 787
Nelson, N. W., 102, 111
Nelson, T. R., 584
Nemoto, T., 90
Nespor, M., 427
Nespoulous, J.-L., 611, 969
Nessler, C., 1019, 1023, 1028, 1029
Nestor, P. J., 551, 554, 556
Netsu, R., 768, 772
Neugarten, B., 298
Neuman-Stritzel, T., 293, 779
Neustadt, G. K., 1002
New Jersey Speech and Hearing Association,
    369
Newacheck, P. W., 217
Newbery, J., 307
Newcombe, F., 75, 423, 663, 881
Newell, C., 357, 360
Newhart, M., 595, 611, 964
Newhoff, M., 116, 380, 381, 426

Newmark, D., 220
Newton, A., 924
Newton, M., 336, 484, 502
Ng, K., 887, 975
Niccum, N., 28, 49, 189, 508
Nicholas, L. E., 56, 75, 101, 102, 107, 108, 109,
    110, 120, 169, 171, 172, 173, 174, 258, 297,
    386, 415, 416, 421, 424, 425, 426, 427, 431,
    457, 515, 748, 765, 778, 779, 780, 974
Nicholas, L. S., 432
Nicholas, M., 88, 173, 187, 361, 508, 565, 570,
    571, 572, 576, 577, 578, 585, 586, 817, 976
Nicholson, D. E., 718
Nickel, D., 411
Nickels, L., 81, 102, 105, 110, 174, 410, 416,
    420, 519, 565, 607, 611, 613, 618, 620, 638,
    647, 664, 769, 770, 775, 777, 782, 784
Nicklay, C. K., 509, 567, 582
NIDCD. *See* National Institute for Deafness
    and Other Communication Disorders
Nielsen, N. P., 253
Nielson, J. M., 376, 383
Nielson, K. A., 991
Nieman, H., 967
Niemann, K., 565
NIH. *See* National Institutes of Health
NIH Stroke Scale, 71
Niles, S., 1002
Nilipour, R., 257, 259, 260
Nimmo-Smith, I., 966
Nippold, M., 110, 417, 781, 902
Nishitani, N., 1014
Nkase-Thompson, R., 70
Nobbs, H., 52
Nobre, A., 37
Nocentini, U., 422
Noe, E., 993
Noel, G., 49
Noel, M., 337
Noell, J. W., 902
Noll, D. C., 191
Noll, J. D., 419, 423, 768, 776
Noll, S., 290
Nolte, J., 1015, 1016
Noots-Villers, P., 360, 366
Nordahl, S., 967
Noreau, L., 297, 357, 364
Norris, D., 249
Norris, J., 499, 500
North American Symptomatic Carotid
    Endarterectomy Trial Collaborators, 49
North, B., 413
North Carolina State Board of Education, 884
Northcutt, S., 295
Northen, B., 547
Northouse, L. L., 231, 232
Northouse, P. G., 231, 232
Norton-Ford, J., 164
Noth, J., 1015
Nourjah, P., 880
Nussbaum, M., 328
Nyberg, L., 894
Nybo, T., 894
Nydevik, I., 964
Nye, C., 195

Ober, B. A., 995
Oberlander, J. B., 217
Obler, L. K., 75, 113, 192, 245, 253, 257, 259, 260, 507, 640, 736, 971, 976, 993
O'Boyle, R., 337
Ochipa, C., 92, 610, 611, 619, 622, 659
Ochs, E., 480
O'Connor, M., 257
Oddy, M., 884
Odekar, A., 811
Odell, K. H., 80, 436, 866, 965, 1023
O'Donnell, V. M., 886
Odor, J. P., 854
Oelschlaeger, M., 121, 293, 294, 295
Oesch-Serra, C., 249
O'Fallon, W. M., 43
O'Flaherty, C. A., 122, 886
Ogar, J., 92, 309
Ogasawara, K., 205
Ogden, J. A., 965
Ogletree, B. T., 815
Ogrezeanu, V., 123, 124, 125
Oh, S., 89
O'Halloran, C., 513
O'Halloran, R., 119, 120
O'Hanlon, A. M., 996
Ohmoto, T., 566, 570
Ohyama, M., 190
Ojemann, G. A., 37
Oke, A., 967
Okuda, B., 50, 565, 567
Oldendorf, W. H., 48
O'Lear, J., 939
Oleyar, K. S., 173
Olgar, J., 524
Olness, G. S., 107
Olsen, R. S., 413
Olsen, T. S., 11, 125, 186
Olsen, W. O., 409, 411
Olson, A., 964
Olson, E., 323
Olswang, L., 295, 517, 524, 1001
Olver, J. H., 887
Ono, M., 22
Ono, Y., 566, 567, 570
Onslow, M., 205
Oomen, C., 125
Opie, M., 257
Oradei, D. M., 377, 379
Orchard-Lisle, V., 599, 610, 614, 620, 718
O'Reilly, R. C., 701, 708, 728
Orgogozo, J. M., 73
Orjada, S., 665
Orpwood, L., 422
Orr, A., 334
Orsulic-Jeras, S., 999
Osborne, F., 197, 580, 620, 624, 726, 776
Osgood, W., 477
Osiejek, E., 387, 391
Osnes, P. P., 394
Oster, E., 75
Ostrove, J. M., 971
O'Sullivan, T., 124
Otsuki, M., 549
Ottenbacher, K. J., 80, 886

Otto, F., 205
Overmier, J. B., 716
Overton Venet, M., 260, 261
Owens, R., 113
Oxbury, S., 611
Oxenham, D., 307, 363, 391, 763
Ozolins, U., 254

Pace, G. M., 926
Pachalska, M., 376, 382, 383, 389
Packard, D., 295, 338
Packard, J., 251
Packard, M., 179, 180, 295, 297, 304, 328
Padakannaya, P., 259
Padovani, A., 975
Paivio, A., 610
Pajak, T. F., 43
Palinscar, A. S., 899, 904
Pallier, C., 250, 1015
Palmer, S., 319, 914
Palmore, E., 207
Paltan-Ortiz, J., 552
Palumbo, C., 27, 124, 566, 573, 575, 589, 1014
Pan, H. C., 567
Panaccio, J., 996
Pandya, D. N., 30
Pang, D., 881
Paniagua, F. A., 248
Paninski, L., 1011
Pansari, K., 94
Panzeri, M., 536
Paolucci, S., 52, 125, 188
Papagno, C., 568
Papanicolaou, A. C., 967
Pappenheim, M., 28
Paquier, P. F., 96
Paradign Health Corporation Publications, 23
Paradis, J., 427
Paradis, M., 73, 78, 245, 249, 250, 251, 254, 255, 257, 258, 259, 260, 265, 509
Pardo, J., 565
Pardo, J. V., 967
Parent, A., 43, 537
Parisi, D., 423, 424
Park, G. H., 103, 768
Park, H. S., 260, 264
Park, J.-H., 713
Park, N. W., 895, 902, 920
Parker, D. H., 658
Parker, L. S., 892
Parkerson, G. R., 81
Parkin, A. J., 726, 922
Parkison, R. C., 861
Parr, S., 10, 115, 174, 290, 291, 294, 296, 306, 307, 308, 310, 328, 355, 360, 362, 363, 367, 379, 391, 588
Parrent, A. G., 775
Parris, B., 783
Parris, D., 418, 620
Parrish, T. B., 551
Parviainen, T., 1011
Pascual-Leone, A., 54, 922
Pashek, G. V., 81, 102, 187, 415, 425, 427, 508, 511, 515, 516, 570, 571, 572, 576, 621, 765
Pasquarello, M., 340

Pasquier, F., 89
Passingham, R. E., 1013
Pate, D. S., 646, 704
Paterson, B., 89
Patronas, N., 550
Patterson, J., 64, 94, 106, 111, 126, 600
Patterson, J. P., 104, 106
Patterson, K., 75, 77, 100, 546, 552, 557, 597, 598, 599, 600, 610, 611, 615, 620, 660, 663, 692, 694, 718, 726, 776, 991
Patterson, M., 411
Patterson, R., 126, 297
Patton, M., 229
Paul, A., 379
Paul, D. R., 122, 236, 298, 300
Paul, R. H., 992
Paul-Brown, D., 319
Paule, L., 764
Paulman, R. G., 905
Paus, T., 1009, 1010, 1011, 1012
Pavesi, G., 1014
Pavlenko, A., 249
Pawlik, G., 190, 565
Payne, J., 119, 120, 126, 297, 298, 880
Payne-Johnson, J. C., 79
PDP Research Group, 700
Peach, R. K., 92, 423, 565, 570, 575, 580, 581, 642, 646
Pear, J., 902
Pearce, S., 119, 521, 893
Pearson, D. M., 422, 735
Pease, D. M., 110
Peasin, M. S., 967
Pedersen, P. M., 11, 92, 125, 413
Pederson, P. M., 186, 188, 192, 193
Peelle, L., 492
Peizer, E. R., 179
Pell, M. D., 977, 1016
Pelletier, R., 978
Pellijeff, A., 895
Penfield, W., 1011
Penman, R., 378, 381, 382, 391
Penn, C., 70, 114, 117, 118, 119, 120, 247, 253, 260, 262, 292, 297, 360, 361, 382, 391, 971, 974
Pennington, B. F., 910
Pennypacker, H. S., 382
Perani, D., 37, 190, 250, 251, 610, 964
Perera, K., 779
Perez, A., 613
Perkins, J., 217, 539, 779
Perkins, L., 117, 118, 119, 178, 293, 294, 295, 299
Perkins, S. M., 364
Perlesz, A., 894
Perry, M., 206
Perry, R. J., 992
Pertheram, B., 308
Pessin, M. S., 26
Pet, R., 94
Peters, D. P., 865
Peters, J., 241, 382
Peters, L. J., 865
Peters, S., 673, 783
Peters, T., 212

Petersen, R. C., 89, 545, 546, 547, 548, 550, 551
Petersen, S. E., 37, 190, 535, 967
Peterson, C., 477, 937
Peterson, L. R., 725
Peterson, M. J., 725
Petheram, B., 307, 761, 762, 860
Petheram, D., 832
Petrides, M., 894, 967, 1013
Petrone, P., 966
Petrosino, L., 213
Petrov, V., 26
Pettit, S., 192
Pfalzgraf, B., 382
Phelps, E., 714
Phelps, M. E., 49, 50
Philbrick, K. L., 549
Philip, I., 13
Philippa, H., 762
Phillips, D., 123, 179, 188, 192, 429, 519, 572
Phillips, J. M., 534
Phillips, S. J., 43
Piasetsky, E. B., 920
Picard, N., 1011, 1012, 1013
Piccirilli, M., 547
Pichora-Fuller, M. K., 335
Pick, A., 632
Pickard, L., 68
Pickersgill, M. J., 193
Pieniadz, J. M., 573
Pierce, K., 815
Pierce, R. S., 79, 102, 256, 424, 425, 426, 427, 509, 765, 770, 780
Piercy, M., 568
Pieres, E., 488
Pietron, H., 415
Pigatt, T., 256
Pillon, B., 264
Pimentel, J., 377, 392, 393
Pimentel, P. A., 85
Pinango, M., 740
Pinault, D., 533
Pincus, D., 971
Pindzola, R. H., 102, 776
Pineda, D. A., 79
Pinker, S., 471, 639
Pitres, A., 35
Pizzamiglio, L., 192, 411, 423, 424
Plante, E., 64, 251, 769, 782
Plaut, D., 598, 603, 623, 674, 692, 694, 695, 698, 700, 701, 705, 710, 723
Plautz, E. J., 53
Pleger, B., 56
Plog, F., 78
Plue, L. D., 364
Plum, F., 44
Plunkett, K., 701
Podolsky, L., 381
Podraza, B. L., 418
Poeck, K., 73, 256, 415, 425, 437, 544, 547, 567, 568, 757
Poeppel, D., 1015, 1016
Pogue, J., 895
Poizner, H., 20
Polk, M., 27, 189, 549, 610

Polkey, C. E., 663
Pollatsek, A., 657
Pollock, A., 973
Pollock, J. -Y., 737, 741, 747
Polster, M. R., 609, 610
Poncet, M., 9, 11, 555, 566, 610
Ponsford, J., 97, 887
Pontón, M. O., 246
Ponzio, J., 292, 379
Poole, E., 7, 787, 817, 818
Poot, R., 253
Poppe, P., 33
Porch, B. E., 71, 72, 73, 120, 123, 174, 196, 385, 386, 409, 410, 430, 508, 574, 578, 768, 771, 800, 803, 804, 817, 855, 858, 861, 865
Porter, G., 73
Porter, I. L., 380
Porter, R., 1011
Porteus, S. D., 98
Posner, J. B., 44
Posner, M. E., 964
Posner, M. I., 534, 905, 907, 964
Post, J., 14
Post, M., 319
Postma, A., 125
Potechin, G., 179, 295, 350, 363, 496, 517
Potechin Scher, G., 173, 174
Potter, H. H., 969, 971, 972
Potter, R. E., 411, 417
Poulsen, K., 338
Poulsen, S., 295
Pound, C., 290, 291, 292, 300, 301, 302, 308, 309, 310, 328, 360, 362, 378, 379, 381, 382, 391, 588, 618, 674
Povlishock, J. T., 881, 893
Powell, G., 71, 124
Powell, J. H., 885
Power, A. E., 708
Power, E., 101, 102
Prather, P., 704, 740
Pratt, K. H., 557
Pratt, S. R., 544, 557, 816
Premack, D., 864
Prescott, T. E., 73, 75, 103, 174, 175, 409, 429, 516, 578, 745, 857, 858, 860, 863, 866
Press, D. Z., 993
Pressley, M., 902, 915, 918
Price, C., 37, 50, 51, 190, 757
Price, D. L., 28, 991
Price, T. R., 975
Priest, J. D., 880
Prigatano, G. P., 885, 891, 894
Pring, T., 257, 422, 618, 620, 623, 638, 641, 642, 643, 668, 764, 784
Prins, R. S., 188, 570, 576, 756
Prinz, P., 116
Prior, M., 259
Prizmic, Z., 910
Proctor, P. W., 717
Propst, M. A., 56
Proshansky, H., 323
Provinciali, L., 967
Prutting, C., 114, 115, 116, 117, 118, 119, 120, 409, 480, 481, 893
Puente, A. E., 246, 255

Pullum, J., 736
Pulvermüller, F., 197, 361, 407, 414, 420, 450, 520, 712, 726
Purdy, M., 96, 124, 125, 126, 179, 295, 304, 308, 517, 523
Purell, C., 726
Purtillo, R. B., 217
Purves, D., 1010, 1011, 1013, 1014
Puskaric, N. J., 102
Putnam, R., 323
Puts-Zwartes, R. A., 380
Pyle, W. H., 713
Pynte, J., 249
Pyypponen, V., 291

Qu, L., 206
Quadagno, J., 206
Quadfasel, F., 8
Quadfaset, F., 33
Quatember, R., 192
Quayhagen, M., 1000
Quillen, D. A., 91
Quiniou, R., 854
Quinlan, P. T., 598
Quirk, K., 921

Raaijmakers, J. G., 989
Raaschou, H. O., 11, 186
Rabidoux, P., 1026
Rackley, A., 1001
Radanovic, M., 79, 255
Radonjic, V., 376, 377, 382, 383, 384, 388, 391
Radosevich, D. J., 713
Rafal, R. D., 534, 964
Raichle, M. E., 44, 50, 190, 967
Raison-Van Ruymbeke, A. M., 552
Rajan, I., 13
Rakuscek, N., 376, 377, 382, 383, 384, 388, 391
Ralph, M., 610, 769
Ramage, A., 95, 673
Ramasubbu, R., 976
Ramsberger, G., 96, 111, 125, 297, 299, 522, 570, 578, 583, 586, 745, 772, 774, 778, 817
Rand Corporation, 321
Randall, V. R., 217
Rao, K., 975
Rao, P. L., 771, 772
Rao, P. R., 583
Rapcsak, S. Z., 125, 597, 654, 657, 663, 666, 667, 668, 671, 673, 674, 769, 783, 965, 967
Raphal, R. D., 964, 965
Rapp, B., 557, 558, 597, 598, 600, 601, 607, 610, 611, 654, 666, 672, 674, 774, 775, 784
Rappaport, M., 886
Raskin, S. A., 763, 764
Raskins, P., 764
Ratcliff, R., 969
Ratey, J. J., 926
Rath, J. F., 180, 905
Rattok, J., 920
Rau, M. T., 417, 518
Ravaud, J. F., 80
Ravel, M., 544
Raven, J., 98, 568, 787, 818, 819, 866
Raybeck, D., 868

Raymer, A. M., 56, 75, 76, 77, 92, 100, 108, 109, 180, 419, 535, 536, 537, 583, 597, 599, 602, 607, 608, 609, 610, 611, 612, 613, 614, 615, 616, 617, 619, 620, 621, 622, 623, 642, 643, 644, 672, 698, 717, 718, 721, 723, 726, 784, 1022, 1023, 1024, 1026
Rayner, H., 295
Rayner, K., 657
Razzano, C., 192
Recanzone, G., 603
Records, N. L., 102, 298, 300, 413
Rectem, D., 552
Redfern, B., 1015
Redford, B., 56
Redinger, R. A., 377, 379, 380
Reed, B. R., 992
Reed, G. M., 350
Reed, V. A., 118
Reese, E., 937
Reeve, C. E., 902, 910
Reggia, J. A., 613, 664
Regli, F., 50
Rehak, A., 969, 971, 976
Reich, P. A., 636, 699
Reichle, J., 902, 923, 931
Reichle, T., 771
Reichman, S., 645, 648
Reid, R., 914
Reif, L., 978
Reinmuth, O. M., 34, 552
Reinvang, I., 571, 572
Reisberg, B., 994, 995
Reisi, A., 56
Rekate, H. L., 34
Relkin, N. R., 251
Remy, P., 264
Rende, B., 297, 299, 522, 523
Renvall, K., 414, 619
Repo, M., 383, 389
Resnick, L. B., 918
Retchin, S. M., 217
Reuterskiöld, C., 421
Revell, T., 205
Rewega, M. A., 197, 295, 361, 597, 668, 671, 779
Rey, G. J., 73, 255, 256, 578
Reyes, B. A., 249
Reynolds, C., 124, 994
Rheingold, H., 853, 859
Rice, B., 379, 381, 384
Rich, S. A., 996
Richard, F., 89
Richardson, M. E., 609, 612
Richardson, W. L., 166
Richardson, W. S., 14, 166
Richter, R. W., 566
Ricker, J. H., 89, 894
Riddoch, J., 259
Riddoch, M. J., 598, 609, 617, 967
Riege, W. H., 50, 52, 187
Rifat, S. L., 52
Rigrodsky, S., 420, 431, 470, 488, 523, 837, 854
Riis, J. O., 975
Rijnders, P., 323
Riley, G. A., 922

Riley, K. P., 992
Riley, L., 860
Rilling, E., 770
Rimel, R. W., 888
Ringel, R., 214, 221
Rintala, D., 304
Ripich, D. N., 87, 993, 1002
Rising, K., 669
Risley, T. R., 929
Rispens, J., 741
Risser, A. H., 70, 71, 76, 77, 78, 79, 85
Ritgert, B. A., 614
Ritterman, S., 780, 781
Ritzl, A., 1015
Rivas-Vasquez, R., 255
Rivers, D. L., 965
Rivlin, L., 323
Rizzo, A. A., 922
Rizzo, M., 21, 964
Rizzolatti, G., 1012, 1013, 1014
Roach, A., 612
Roberts, J. A., 174, 420
Roberts, L., 1011
Roberts, M. M., 746
Roberts, P. M., 245, 252, 253, 254, 256, 257, 258, 260, 261, 264, 265, 266
Robertson, I., 97, 98, 860, 868, 892, 966
Robertson, L. C., 966
Robey, R. R., 14, 125, 129, 164, 180, 186, 193, 195, 196, 197, 437, 524, 576, 657, 674, 762, 769, 814, 852, 861
Robin, D. A., 92, 553, 718, 964, 977, 1017, 1018, 1022
Robinson, A. J., 81
Robinson, D. L., 535
Robinson, J., 931
Robinson, R. G., 95, 193, 327, 967, 975
Robinson, T. R., 914
Robson, J., 620, 668, 764, 784
Rocca, A., 48
Rochette, A., 967
Rochon, E., 112, 425, 557, 645, 646, 647, 648, 743, 745, 778
Rock, A., 880
Rockstroh, B., 712
Rodesch, G., 572
Rodgers, J. A., 1000
Rodin, J., 856
Rodriguez, A., 619, 621, 623
Rodriguez, J., 192
Rodriguez, R., 124
Rodríguez-Campello, A., 11
Rodríguez-Forwells, A., 252
Rodriquez, L. S. M., 229
Rodwin, M. A., 217
Roediger, H. L., 250
Roelofs, A., 636, 774
Rogers, C., 220, 221
Rogers, M., 89, 295, 303, 306, 524, 545, 546, 550, 557, 558, 559, 820, 1017, 1018, 1019, 1022
Rogers, R. L., 658
Rogers-Warren, A. K., 392, 393, 487
Rogoff, B., 899
Rolland, J., 307, 308, 325

Rolls, E. T., 691, 701, 708, 709, 715, 901, 927
Rolnick, M., 121, 409, 411, 416
Román, G. C., 992
Roman, M., 971, 972
Romani, C., 610, 671
Rombouts, S. A., 989
Romero, M., 79
Rondeau, G., 110
Roquer, J., 11
Rorden, C., 965
Rosamond, W. D., 43
Rosazza, C., 610
Rose, D. E., 409, 411
Rose, D. F., 34
Rose, M., 92, 101, 102, 108, 110, 413, 621, 771, 1022
Rose, S. B., 609, 610
Rose, T., 295, 307, 382
Roselli, M., 79, 171
Rosen, A. K., 246
Rosen, H. J., 190, 191
Rosen, I., 1011
Rosen, T. J., 704
Rosen, W. G., 996
Rosenbaum, G., 994
Rosenbek, J., 93, 125, 127, 165, 166, 167, 168, 178, 433, 508, 567, 582, 583, 689, 721, 722, 854, 855, 857, 860, 978, 979, 1018, 1020, 1021, 1022, 1023, 1026, 1027
Rosenberg, C. R., 715
Rosenberg, R. N., 554
Rosenberg, W., 14, 166
Rosenberger, P. B., 576
Rosenfeld, N., 117, 482
Rosenthal, R., 976
Rosenthal, T., 470, 477
Rosin, P., 229, 230, 242
Ross, E. D., 977, 978
Ross, G., 259, 896
Ross, J. S., 47
Ross, K., 79, 81, 82, 108, 121, 122, 123, 300, 319, 321, 350, 360, 361, 362
Ross, R., 44, 308
Ross, T., 256
Rosselli, M., 255
Rosser, M. N., 547, 554
Rossi, B., 968
Rossor, M. N., 568
Ross-Swain, D., 98, 904
Roth, C. R., 212
Roth, H. L., 691, 696, 697, 698
Roth, P. A., 1000
Roth, R. M., 904
Roth, V. M., 180, 361, 520, 865
Rothi, L. J., 35, 76, 77, 91, 92, 100, 102, 108, 109, 126, 127, 414, 540, 607, 608, 609, 610, 611, 612, 614, 616, 617, 619, 621, 623, 656, 659, 674, 689, 721, 723
Roueche, J. R., 891
Rouselle, M., 859
Rowe, J., 337
Rowley, D., 192
Roy, E. A., 1015
Roy, P., 192, 294

Royal College of Speech and Language Therapists: Clinical Guidelines, 129
Royen, E. A., 50
Rozzini, L., 997
Rüb, U., 993
Rubens, A. B., 28, 29, 49, 50, 125, 189, 192, 508, 668
Rubin, A. J., 30
Rubin, M. J., 572
Rubin, N. P., 89, 546
Rubow, R. T., 1026
Ruderman, J., 52
Rudorf, E. H., 664
Ruff, M., 376
Ruff, R. M., 75, 880, 888, 967
Ruggieri, P. M., 47
Rule, A., 895
Rumelhart, D. E., 692, 693, 700, 701
Rummans, T. A., 549
Rushakoff, G. E., 860
Rushworth, M. F. S., 1013, 1015
Russo, M., 206
Rutter, M., 894
Ryalls, R., 978
Ryan, R. M., 891, 931
Ryff, C., 66, 298, 300

Saarinen, T., 1011
Sabe, L., 56
Sacchett, C., 108
Sacco, R. L., 11, 46
Sachett, C., 301
Sackett, D. L., 14, 51, 129, 166
Sacks, H., 117
Saddy, J. D., 972
Saerens, J., 256
Saffell, D., 180, 617, 619
Saffran, E. M., 102, 103, 111, 112, 422, 609, 610, 632, 633, 636, 637, 639, 640, 641, 644, 646, 647, 648, 655, 659, 696, 699, 704, 735, 740, 743, 745, 762, 769, 774
Safilios-Rothchild, C., 326
Safran, A., 891
Sag, I., 736
Sage, K., 432, 607, 718, 769
Sahs, A. L., 208
Saint-Cyr, J. A., 993
Saito, A., 246
Sakai, F., 50
Sakurai, Y., 552, 555
Salamon, G., 11, 26, 566
Salamoura, A., 249
Saletta, P., 257
Salmelin, R., 1011
Salmon, D. J., 992
Salmon, D. P., 894, 989, 991, 992, 995
Salmon, S., 747
Salmon, S. J., 412
Salter, K., 70
Saltz, E., 476
Salvatore, A., 415, 515, 516, 578, 579, 582, 584
Salverezza, F., 56
Sample, D. M., 597
Samples, J. M., 1026
Sampson, E. E., 232, 233

Sampson, H., 98
Sanchez-Casas, R., 252
Sanderson, C., 80
Sandin, K., 290
Sandler, H. m., 169
Sandok, B. A., 46, 52
Sands, E., 71, 123, 124, 192, 492, 575, 756, 840
Sandson, J., 96, 550, 614, 641, 776
Sandy, T. J., 992
Sanes, J. N., 1011
SantaCruz, K., 993
Santo Pietro, M. J., 420, 431, 999, 1000
Santora, T. A., 880
Sarno, J., 123, 575
Sarno, M., 119, 120, 123, 319, 379, 492, 840
Sarno, M. R., 570, 571, 572, 576
Sarno, M. T., 188, 192, 193, 219, 241, 290, 291, 292, 297, 304, 307, 310, 311, 377, 382, 394, 403, 433, 438, 565, 570, 571, 572, 575, 576, 577, 579, 580, 582, 756, 760, 891, 893, 968
Sarwar, M., 891
Sasanuma, S., 257, 260, 261, 264, 572
Sato, M., 549
Saur, D., 50, 191
Saurwein-Teissl, M., 13
Saxe, J. G., 349
Saygin, A. P., 1011
Scaff, M., 255
Scanlon, D., 902
Scannell, G., 658
Scarpa, M., 11, 566, 574
Schacter, D. L., 893, 894, 920, 922, 989, 996
Scharp, V. L., 163, 519
Scharre, D. W., 609
Schartz, M., 914
Schatz, J., 190
Scheerer, M., 6
Schegloff, E. A., 117, 118, 363
Scheibel, R. S., 895
Scheifelbusch, R. L., 229
Schell, L. M., 101
Schelper, R. L., 21, 35
Scheltens, P. H., 544, 991
Schempp, B., 584
Schendel, L., 422
Schepers, V., 319
Scher, G. P., 393, 394, 520
Scherr, P. A., 988
Scherzer, B. P., 905
Schiavetti, N., 164, 166, 169, 172
Schieffelin, B., 480
Schienberg, S., 117
Schiff, H. B., 27
Schinco, K. A., 880
Schinsky, L., 384, 583
Schlacter, D. L., 863
Schlaghecken, F., 37
Schlanger, B. B., 376, 377, 378, 379, 977
Schlanger, P. H., 376, 377, 378, 379, 771, 977
Schlaug, G., 44, 49
Schleicher, A., 1013, 1014, 1015
Schlenk, C., 648
Schlenk, K.-J., 648
Schlesinger, R., 206, 207
Schloss, C. N., 924

Schloss, P. J., 924
Schlosser, R., 297, 300, 360, 366, 1022, 1023
Schluter, N. D., 1013
Schmalzl, L., 782, 784
Schmeichel, B. J., 902, 910
Schmel'kov, V. N., 52
Schmidt, N. D., 237, 240, 241, 902
Schmidt, R. A., 553, 715, 717, 718, 1017, 1022, 1023
Schmitt, F. A., 990, 995
Schmitter-Edgecombe, M., 901, 910
Schneider, P., 899
Schneider, S. L., 422, 557, 597, 636, 642, 643, 704
Schneider, S. S., 746
Schneider, W., 535, 915
Schneiderman, E. I., 972
Schnider, A., 123, 180, 609, 620, 862
Schoenle, P. W., 416
Schokker, J., 297, 513
Scholes, R., 977
Scholte op Reimer, W., 323
Schonitzer, D., 13
Schonle, P. W., 757, 783
Schormann, T., 1014
Schreiner, C. E., 692
Schreiner, R., 101
Schreuder, R., 250
Schubitowski, Y. D., 859
Schubotz, R. I., 1011, 1012, 1013, 1015
Schuell, H., 6, 7, 71, 72, 79, 81, 102, 127, 256, 382, 403, 404, 405, 406, 407, 408, 409, 411, 412, 414, 415, 416, 420, 421, 430, 432, 433, 450, 451, 452, 458, 459, 470, 485, 487, 492, 508, 578, 756, 803, 811, 838, 840, 855, 857, 859
Schuloff, C., 427
Schulte, E., 430, 431
Schulteis, M., 922, 923
Schulte-Monting, J., 575
Schultz, D. A., 376
Schultz, M., 125, 293, 779
Schultz, M. C., 14, 164, 193, 195, 437, 762, 769
Schultz, R., 94, 524
Schulz, G. M., 1009
Schulz, R., 167, 856
Schum, R. L., 255, 256
Schumacher, J. G., 172, 173, 174
Schumaker, J. B., 919
Schürmann, M., 1014
Schütz-Bosbach, S., 1014
Schwanenflugel, P., 106
Schwartz, A. H., 855
Schwartz, H., 769, 964
Schwartz, J., 220, 603
Schwartz, L., 895
Schwartz, M., 81, 101, 102, 103, 109, 112, 180, 422, 539, 549, 597, 600, 609, 612, 632, 633, 636, 639, 640, 643, 646, 647, 655, 699, 704, 735, 740, 743, 745, 762, 774, 776, 777, 778, 832, 852, 862, 865, 893
Schwartz, N., 66
Schwartz, R. L., 76, 539
Schwartz-Crowley, R., 484, 502
Schwarz, I. E., 781, 902

Schwarz, N., 12
Schweinhart, L. J., 910
Schwenkries, P., 56
Scofield, J., 425, 647, 745, 778
Scolaro, C., 56
Scott, A. G., 163
Scott, C., 453, 484, 618, 768, 857, 858, 862
Scott, G., 881, 892
Scott, R., 205
Scott, S. K., 1015, 1016
Scott, W., 477
Scott-Findlay, S., 89
Scotti, G., 568
Scottish Intercollegiate Guideline Network, 319
Scovel, T., 250
Screen, M. R., 217
Seacat, G., 376
Searle, J., 108, 115, 480, 481
Sebastián-Galles, N., 250
Seddoh, S., 113
Seel, R., 885
Seeman, T., 337
Seemiuller, E., 34
Sefer, J. W., 377, 404, 756
Segal, A. Z., 570
Segal, O., 724
Segalowitz, S. J., 905
Segarra, J. M., 28, 33
Segui, J., 249
Seibert, G. B., 978
Seibold, M. S., 971
Seidenberg, M., 598, 610, 692, 694, 695, 701, 705
Seiger, A., 964
Seitz, R. J., 251
Sejinowski, T. J., 715
Seki, K., 660
Seliger, H. W., 249, 250
Seligman, M., 856, 994
Selinger, M., 745, 857, 858, 860, 863, 866
Selinker, L., 249, 250
Sellers, C., 343
Selnes, O. A., 27, 28, 29, 49, 50, 189, 508, 547, 567
Semah, F., 1015
Semel, E., 101
Semenza, C., 37, 536, 609, 977
Semple, J. M., 87
Semple, W. E., 967
Sen, A., 328
Seoane, J., 205
Sereno, M. I., 1011
Serio, C., 885
Seron, X., 264, 421, 552, 617, 859, 863
Sessle, B. J., 1011
Shadden, B., 70, 106, 107, 290, 329, 360, 362, 365, 367, 371, 379
Shadmehr, R., 715
Shafer, S. Q., 566
Shaffer, D., 894
Shah, A. P., 978
Shallice, T., 35, 37, 598, 610, 611, 667, 693, 696, 892, 893, 967
Shammi, P., 893

Shankle, W. R., 991
Shanks, J. E., 91
Shankweiler, D., 192
Shankwilder, D., 123
Shapira, J. S., 550
Shapiro, B. E., 978
Shapiro, D. C., 718
Shapiro, J. K., 1015
Shapiro, K., 103, 611, 612
Shapiro, L. P., 173, 197, 422, 425, 597, 704, 708, 735, 738, 745, 746, 777, 778
Sharwood Smith, M. A., 249
Shatin, L., 376, 756
Shaw, R., 404
Shaw, R. E., 377
Shea, C. H., 713
Sheard, C., 118
Shebilske, W. L., 714
Sheehan, V. M., 383
Sheeran, P., 80, 94, 319, 362
Sheets, A., 246
Sheinker, A., 923
Sheinker, J., 923
Sheldon, J. B., 930
Shelton, J., 103, 361, 418, 565, 610, 645, 710, 777, 778, 864
SHEP Cooperative Research Group, 43
Sheppard, A., 11, 566, 705
Sherbenou, R., 100, 819
Sheremata, W. A., 28
Sherman, C., 381
Sherman, D., 51, 421
Sherman, E. M. S., 77
Sherman, J. A., 930, 931
Sherman, J. C., 423
Sherman, S. M., 533
Sherman, W., 13
Sherr, R. L., 180, 905
Sherratt, S. M., 971, 974
Sherron, P., 896
Shetty, H., 94, 570
Shewan, C. M., 72, 74, 75, 102, 167, 168, 416, 420, 424, 437, 578, 756, 757, 761, 765, 770, 786, 787, 788
Shewell, C., 718
Shibuya, H., 964
Shiel, A., 922, 998
Shiffrin, D., 178, 293
Shill, M., 125
Shimamura, A. P., 894, 991
Shindler, A. G., 993
Shindo, M., 618
Shinn, R., 214
Shinton, R., 12
Shiota, J., 552
Shipley, J. G., 83, 90, 129
Shisler, R. J., 96, 111, 524
Shlonsky, A., 81
Shobe, A., 554
Shoben, E., 106
Shoup, J., 1019
Shrier, R., 415, 418
Shrout, P. E., 168
Shubert, T., 13
Shubitowski, Y., 168, 431, 859

Shulman, G., 966
Shulz, R., 123
Shum, D., 922
Shumway, E., 306
Shuren, J., 719
Shuster, L., 125, 1009, 1015, 1016
Sicks, J. D., 43
Sicotte, C., 205
Sidman, M., 576, 922
Sidtis, J. J., 977, 978
Siegel, G. M., 102, 392, 420, 423, 457
Siegenthaler, B. M., 409
Siegert, R., 126
Siegler, R. S., 919, 920
Sieroff, E., 965
Sigma Xi Research Society, 177
Signer, M., 220
Signoret, J. -L., 264
Siirtola, M., 570, 572, 576
Siirtola, T., 570, 572, 576
Silberman, E. K., 975
Silbershatz, H., 256
Silkes, J., 853
Silliman, R., 323
Silvast, M., 301
Silverberg, R., 259
Silveri, M., 11, 35, 37, 178, 411, 422, 610, 611, 671, 964
Silverman, F. H., 163, 165, 166, 168, 177, 583, 856
Silverman, M., 492, 575, 756, 840
Simmons, N. N., 168, 179, 290, 293, 301, 303, 382, 385, 388, 392, 394, 497, 519, 583, 1026, 1027
Simmons, R., 206
Simmons-Mackie, N., 79, 115, 119, 120, 125, 127, 128, 129, 178, 179, 236, 279, 290, 292, 293, 294, 295, 296, 297, 298, 299, 300, 301, 302, 303, 304, 305, 306, 307, 309, 310, 342, 350, 356, 360, 361, 363, 366, 394, 453, 499, 517, 523, 524, 565, 588, 779, 816
Simon, D., 180, 905
Simonyan, K., 1014
Simpson, G. B., 973
Simpson, T., 971, 972
Sims, E., 585
Sims, N., 991
Sin, G., 597, 609
Singer, B., 66
Singer, S., 13
Singh, S., 307
Singley, M. K., 902
Sinner, C. A., 195, 437, 762
Sinyor, D., 52, 975
Sipilae, H., 251
Sirigu, A., 893
Sirisko, M. A., 1011
Sisterhen, C., 50, 583
Sittner, M., 522
Sivan, A. B., 98, 255, 256, 578
Sjardin, H., 253
Ska, B., 969
Skelly, M., 108, 384, 409, 428, 583, 771, 772, 1026
Skenes, L., 76

Skidmore, R., 47
Skilbeck, C. E., 77, 80, 125, 860
Skinner, B. F., 855, 858, 910, 926
Skinner, J., 616, 1023
Sklar, M., 71, 578
Skoloda, T. E., 233
Slama, H., 92
Slifer, K. J., 926
Sliwinski, M., 75
Slobin, D., 478, 479, 642
Smaldino, J., 335
Small, S., 15, 180, 190, 191, 192, 549, 1014
Smart, M., 305, 763
Smith, A., 382, 391, 406, 756
Smith, B., 488, 966
Smith, D. C., 861
Smith, D. S., 52
Smith, F., 476, 477, 487
Smith, G., 215, 217, 619
Smith, G. E., 256
Smith, K., 110, 773, 826
Smith, K. C., 410, 777
Smith, K. E., 910
Smith, K. L., 611
Smith, K. R., 35
Smith, L., 180, 249, 298
Smith, P., 56, 382
Smith, R., 583
Smith, R. D., 858
Smith, R. W., 384
Smith, S., 249, 294, 991
Smith, S. C., 192, 357
Smith, S. W., 914
Smith, V. O. G., 568
Smith-Knapp, K., 297
Smithpeter, J. V., 413
Smolensky, P., 692, 693
Sniezek, J. E., 880
Snodgrass, J., 105, 252, 613
Snow, C., 902, 918
Snow, C. E., 188, 756
Snow, E., 570, 576
Snow, P. A., 122
Snow, P. C., 886
Snow, W. G., 894
Snowden, J. S., 49, 87, 546, 547, 548, 552, 557
Snowdon, D. A., 992
Snyder, L. S., 126
Soardi, S., 37, 612
Sobecks, J., 197, 425, 708, 746, 778
Sobel, L., 49
Sobel, P., 420, 597, 832
Sohlberg, M. M., 14, 88, 89, 100, 763, 764, 920, 921, 940, 968
Sokol, S., 600
Solomon, G. E., 569
Solomon, J., 740
Soma, Y., 549
Sommers, B., 206
Sommers, R., 411
Sonderman, J. C., 406, 432
Sonies, B. C., 555
Sonty, S. P., 551
Soon, C. S., 251, 1015
Sooy, D., 15, 222

Sorgato, P., 11, 566
Sorin-Peters, R., 295, 304, 308, 365
Sosin, D. M., 880
Sotnick, P., 326
Soubrouillard, C., 9
Southwood, H., 1024, 1025
Southwood, M. H., 648
Sparks, R., 191, 384, 391, 411, 511, 513, 514, 837, 838, 840, 842, 843, 844, 846
Sparks, S., 236
Spatt, J., 124, 189, 190, 508
Specht, K., 966
Speechley, M., 714, 757
Speedie, L., 696, 977
Spellacy, F. J., 71
Spencer, K. A., 94, 108, 128, 508, 1018
Sperry, R. W., 976
Spicher, C., 361
Spikman, J. M., 97
Spinelli, C., 520, 777
Spinnler, H., 567, 568, 894, 991
Sportiche, D., 736
Spradley, J., 296, 297
Spradlin, J., 392, 457, 896
Sprafkin, R. P., 923
Spreen, O., 70, 71, 73, 75, 76, 77, 78, 79, 85, 95, 97, 106, 123, 124, 256, 421, 571, 578, 995
Spriestersbach, D. C., 166
Springer, L., 103, 252, 265, 387, 389, 520, 648, 757
Square, P., 179, 236, 290, 363, 517, 565, 779, 1009, 1015, 1017, 1018, 1019, 1021, 1022, 1023, 1026, 1027, 1028
Square-Storer, P. A., 1015, 1023, 1028
Squire, L. R., 95, 536, 708, 715, 893, 894, 922, 989
Squires, E. J., 726, 922
Srinivasan, M., 508
St. Michel, G., 282, 352, 364
Staats, A., 477, 488
Stablum, F., 725
Stach, C., 196
Stadie, N., 252, 264, 770
Stallard, E., 13
Staltari, C., 387
Stampp, M. S., 996
Stanczak, L., 623
Stanley, J. C., 164, 169, 172
Stanley, J. M., 233
Stannard, T., 616, 1023
Stapleton, J. H., 567
Stark, A. J., 667
Starkstein, S., 327
Starkstein, S. E., 56, 95, 193
Starr, L. B., 975
Statlender, S., 423
Staub, C. P., 880
Steel, G., 996
Steele, R. D., 583, 586, 587, 761, 832, 853, 864, 868
Stegall, M. H., 217
Stegmayr, B., 11
Stein, M., 437, 524, 757, 814
Stein, S., 972

Steinmetz, H., 251
Steinmetz, J., 994
Stemberger, J. P., 699
Stemmer, B., 114, 968
Stenger, A., 217
Stepien, L., 28
Steriade, M., 537
Stern, C., 704
Stern, G., 756
Stern, R., 80, 94, 95, 297
Stern, S., 337
Stern, Y., 993
Sternberg, R. J., 896, 902
Steven, D. A., 775
Stevens, A. B., 996
Stewart, D. G., 229, 230, 239, 242
Stewart, J. D., 609
Stewart, N., 336
Stiassny-Eder, D., 573, 575
Stickgold, R., 715
Stiegler, L., 309, 524
Stierwalt, J. A. G., 88
Stimley, M. A., 419, 776
Stoddard, L. T., 576, 922
Stoicheff, M. L., 110, 428, 432, 858
Stoioff, M., 409
Stokes, T., 392, 394, 520, 1001
Stone, S. P., 96
Stout, C. E., 432, 810
Strait, M., 415, 515
Strasser, D. C., 233, 242
Straughan, P. T., 976
Straus, S., 14, 166
Strauss, A., 178, 390
Strauss, E., 73, 77, 78, 95, 97, 106, 123, 124, 256
Strick, P. L., 1011, 1012, 1013
Stringer, A. Y., 91, 979
Stringfellow, A., 971, 975
Stroke Scales, 71
Stuart, S., 822
Stude, P., 967
Studer-Eichenberger, F., 558
Sturm, J., 319
Sturm, W., 966, 967, 968
Stuss, D. T., 893, 895, 896, 905, 927, 967
Subirana, A., 193
Sue, L. I., 551
Sugai, G., 902
Suger, G., 34, 49
Sugishita, M., 73, 660
Sugita, K., 552
Sugita, M., 50, 565
Sugiu, K., 566, 570
Sullivan, D. M., 619
Sullivan, K. J., 718
Summala, H., 229
Sundance, P., 237, 238
Sundt, T. M., 46
Sung, J. M., 248
Sutcliffe, A., 763
Sutcliffe, L. M., 80, 94
Sutton, M. A., 716
Svec, W. R., 598
Sveen, U., 291, 308, 360

Swank, P. R., 910
Sweeper, S., 922
Sweet, A. P., 902, 918
Sweet, R. D., 35
Swinburn, K., 73, 190, 757
Swindell, C. S., 34, 81, 94, 119, 125, 192, 511, 570, 572
Swinnen, S. P., 718
Swinney, D., 427, 515, 740
Swisher, L., 76, 188, 576, 968
Syder, D., 71
Symington, C., 894
Szekeres, S. F., 174, 619, 879, 880, 887, 891, 892, 910, 912, 913, 918, 919, 933, 939
Szilda, G., 26

Tabouret-Kelly, A., 260
Tachibana, H., 50, 565
Tailby, R., 922
Tainturier, M. -J., 654, 666
Ta'ir, J., 696
Tait, M. E., 597, 746
Takeuchi, N., 54
Talairach, J., 1012
Talbot, P. R., 49
Tallberg, I. M., 256
Talley, J. L., 764
Tallis, R. C., 964
Tamiya, T., 566, 570
Tan, E. W. L., 251
Tan, L. L., 196
Tanaka, H., 50, 565
Tanaka, Y., 618
Tannen, D., 292, 293
Tanner, D., 71, 94, 333
Taquemori, L., 79
Tate, R. L., 881
Tatemichi, T. K., 96, 539
Tatum, W. O., 56
Taveras, J., 35
Taylor, A. E., 609, 993
Taylor, C., 207, 1011
Taylor, D., 51, 293, 887
Taylor, H. G., 894
Taylor, J. R., 554
Taylor, M. L., 454, 457
Taylor, M. T., 407
Taylor, W., 126
Taylor-Sarno, M., 260
Teasdale, G., 886
Teasdale, J. D., 935
Teasell, R., 70, 714, 757
Tegenthoff, M., 56
Tegner, R., 965, 966
Tempo, P. M., 246
ter Keurs, M., 103
Teraes, M., 251
Terr, A., 376
Terrace, H. S., 922
Terrell, S., 248
Teskey, G. C., 53
Testa, H. J., 49
Tetnowski, J. A., 74, 76
Tetreault, S., 323
Thal, L. F., 992

Thal, L. J., 992
Tham, K., 966
Thangaraj, V., 1011
Thelander, M., 294, 378
Theodoros, D. G., 88
Theurkauf, J., 21
Thiel, A., 50, 190, 191, 757
Thiel, T., 251
Thistlethwaite, N., 516
Thoene, A., 920
Thom, T., 42, 43
Thomas, B. E., 188, 571
Thomas, C., 757
Thomas, C. A., 770
Thomas, K., 778, 864
Thomas, L., 535
Thomas, L. L., 924
Thomas, T. N., 12
Thommessen, B., 291, 360
Thompson, C., 111, 112, 214, 295, 298, 301, 319
Thompson, C. K., 103, 114, 124, 127, 128, 171, 172, 173, 178, 191, 196, 197, 255, 356, 377, 392, 419, 422, 425, 435, 450, 519, 550, 557, 559, 578, 579, 582, 583, 584, 595, 597, 599, 600, 601, 618, 620, 621, 622, 623, 636, 641, 642, 643, 644, 646, 648, 704, 708, 710, 723, 725, 726, 728, 735, 736, 737, 738, 740, 741, 742, 743, 745, 746, 747, 748, 777, 778, 924, 1001, 1026
Thompson, J. L., 118, 781
Thompson, J. M., 885, 895
Thompson, L., 994
Thomsen, I. V., 891, 894
Thornburg, L., 778, 864
Thorndike, E. L., 421
Thráinsson, H., 736, 747
Threats, T., 79, 121, 350, 351, 356, 366
Thron, A., 565
Throwalls, A., 964
Thulborn, K. R., 190
Thurman, D. J., 880
Thurstone, L. L., 74, 75
Thurstone, T. G., 74, 75
Tidy, J. A., 726
Tikofsky, R. S., 50, 409
Timberlake, W., 8
Timko, M. L., 965
Tipper, S., 967
Tiraboschi, P., 992
Tison, F., 993
Tissot, A., 124, 192
Tissot, R. J., 632
Tittgemeyer, M., 1013
Tjaden, K., 1024, 1025
Tobin, S., 298
Todd-Pokropek, A., 192
Todis, B., 923, 940
Toffolo, D., 115
Toffolo, R., 513
Togher, L., 893
Tomaiuolo, F., 1013
Tomasello, M., 714
Tombaugh, T. N., 74
Tomblin, J., 300

Tomlinson, B. E., 989
Tomoeda, C. K., 88, 256, 988, 993, 994, 995, 996, 999, 1000, 1002
Tompkins, C. A., 78, 86, 94, 95, 96, 102, 123, 125, 126, 163, 165, 166, 167, 168, 170, 171, 173, 174, 175, 178, 188, 417, 419, 426, 429, 507, 519, 520, 781, 965, 966, 969, 970, 971, 972, 973, 974, 975, 977, 978, 1026, 1027
Tonkonogy, J., 27
Tonkovich, J. D., 257, 376, 392, 583, 856
Toole, J. F., 43
Toppin, C. J., 102
Toraldo, A., 257
Torrance, E., 100, 472, 484, 488
Torre, P., 251
Torrence, E., 96
Toshiko, W., 173
Toth, J. P., 967
Tournoux, P., 1012
Tourville, J. A., 1014
Toussaint, L., 56
Tower, C. D., 79
Trabucchi, M., 997
Trahan, D. E., 98
Tranel, D., 20, 21, 30, 31, 37, 39, 109, 572, 611, 612, 737, 774, 775, 894, 901, 905, 910, 922, 926, 967, 976, 977
Trappl, R., 192
Traub, M., 894
Traynor, C., 93
Treadgold, L. G., 921
Treisman, A., 106
Trentini, P., 830
Treves, A., 691, 701, 708, 709, 715
Trimble, M. R., 91
Trojanowski, J. Q., 549
Trooskin, S. Z., 880
Troske, K., 220
Trosset, M. W., 991, 995
Trost-Cardmone, J. E., 609
Trouard, T. P., 251
Trout, A. L., 914
Trupe, E. H., 549, 971
Truscott, B. L., 43
Tsantali, S., 256
Tseng, C. H., 436
Tsolaki, M., 256
Tsuji, S., 549
Tsvetkova, L. S., 376
Tuchman, L. I., 230
Tucker, D. M., 967, 975, 977
Tucker, F., 437
Tucker, G., 90
Tuffash, E., 654
Tuffiash, E., 89, 612
Tulving, E., 894, 989
Tuomainen, J., 657, 774
Tupper, A., 192
Tureen, L., 377, 379, 756
Turing, A. M., 853
Turkheimer, F., 190
Turkka, J., 229
Turkstra, L., 14, 88, 885, 893, 904, 905, 928, 934, 968
Turnblom, M., 380

Turnbull, A., 323
Turnbull, H. R., 323
Turner, J., 610, 617
Turner, R. S., 549
Turner, S., 179
Tyler, L. K., 605, 608
Tyrrell, P. J., 547, 554
Tzeng, O., 257

Uhden, L. D., 781
Ukita, H., 551
Ukita, N., 50
Ulatowska, H. K., 79, 107, 116, 118, 766, 780, 781, 785
Ullman, M. T., 725
Ulrich, S. R., 406
Umiltà, C., 725
Underhill, B., 212
Ungerleider, L. G., 989
Unwin, H., 56
Uomoto, J. M., 170
Urayse, D., 971, 974
Urbanczyk, B., 937
Urbani, F., 77
Urrea, D., 417
Urrutia, J., 557
Uryase, D., 118
U.S. Department of Health and Human Services, 52
U.S. Department of Transportation, 880
U.S. Department of Veteran's Affairs, 176, 215, 233, 856
U.S. General Acccounting Office, 13
U.S. Government Accountability Office, 218, 220
Uylings, H. B. M., 990, 1013

Vagges, K., 977
Vago, R. M., 249
Vaid, J., 260
Vail, S., 597, 671
Valenstein, E., 964, 976
Valentino, D. A., 967
Valk, J., 544
Vallar, G., 50, 92, 964
Valle, R., 247
Van Amerongen, N. M., 264
van de Sandt-Koenderman, M. W. M. E., 264, 420, 761, 762, 815, 856, 861, 864
Van Demark, A. A., 428
van den Bos, G., 296, 323
Van den Broek, M. D., 921
Van den Eijnden, E., 252
Van den Heuvel, E., 326, 340
Van der Flier, W. M., 991
van der Gaag, A., 180, 382, 390, 391, 395
Van der Linden, M., 997
Van der Werf, Y. D., 534
Van Eekhout, P., 554, 757
van Harskamp, F., 125, 126, 127, 264, 377
Van Hell, J. G., 249, 252
van Heutgen, C. M., 76
Van Heuven, W., 250, 252
van Heyst, J., 1019
Van Horn, G., 572

Van Lancker, D., 420, 509, 567, 582, 972, 977, 978
Van Lancker-Sidtis, D., 252, 977
van Lieshout, P., 1022
van Loon, J., 50
Van Mourik, M., 761
Van Pelt, D., 404
van Praag, H., 13
Van Riper, C., 1021
van Vendendaal, H., 238
Van Wijnendaele, I., 249
Van Zagten, M., 190
van Zomeren, A. H., 97
van Zonneveld, R., 738
VanBiervliet, A., 343
VanDam, A., 56
Vandenberghe, R. R., 89
Vanderwart, M., 613
Vanderwoort, M., 105
VanGrunsven, M. F., 648
Vanhalle, C., 997
Vanier, M., 566, 735
Varga, M., 1009
Vargha-Khadem, F., 663, 709
Varian, T., 212
Varley, R., 1022, 1023
Varney, N., 21, 81, 101, 105, 893, 905
Vasilakakos, M., 254
Vass, K., 552
Vasterling, J. J., 611
Vaughn, G. R., 855, 865
Velkoff, V., 206, 988
Vellet, S., 910
Velozo, C. A., 178
Veltman, D. J., 989
Vendrell, J., 260
Vendrell, P., 260
Vendrell-Brucet, J., 260
Ventry, I. M., 164, 166, 169, 172
Verbeeten, B., 50
Verderber, R. F., 361
Verfaellie, M., 96, 965, 967, 971
Vervaet, A., 256
Vestergaard, K., 975
Veteran's Administration Cooperative Study Group on Antihypertensive Agents, 43
Vickery, C., 319
Vigliocco, G., 636, 769
Vignolo, L. A., 28, 35, 49, 91, 186, 192, 411, 492, 566, 567, 578, 609, 756, 861
Vikingstad, E. M., 191
Villa, G., 11, 568, 611, 671, 696
Villarreal, R. P., 257
Villarroel, V., 205
Vincent, C., 357
Vinter, K., 125, 413
Vinz, B., 536
Virata, T., 761
Visch-Brink, E. G., 125, 126, 127, 264, 377
Visser-Meily, A., 319
Vital, C., 34
Vitevitch, M. S., 695
Voeller, K. S., 724
Vogel, D., 102, 124, 426, 747
Vogel, S., 765

Vohn, R., 966
Vohs, K. D., 891
Volk, J., 669
Vollmer, T. R., 905
Volpe, A. D., 780, 781
Von Arbin, M., 571, 572
von Cramon, D. Y., 1011, 1012, 1013, 1015
von Monakow, C., 698
Vorano, L., 260
Vorobiev, V., 1012
Vrtunski, B., 411
Vygotsky, L. S., 899, 904, 910, 924

Wachterman, M., 206
Wacker, D. P., 902, 923, 931
Waddington, M. M., 26
Wade, D. T., 70, 97, 927
Wade, J., 761, 762, 832
Wafters, W. C., 35
Wagenaar, E., 188, 570, 576
Wagenaar, R. C., 52
Wagner, E., 81, 323
Wahner, H. W., 547
Wahrborg, P., 94, 308, 327, 376, 378
Waite, J. S., 377, 379
Waksman, D. D., 923
Waksman, S., 923
Wales, R., 969
Walker, H. M., 902, 923
Walker, J. A., 534, 964, 967
Walker, J. P., 977, 978
Walker, K. A., 967
Walker, M. P., 715
Walker, W., 884
Walker-Batson, D., 56, 382, 383, 389, 391, 524
Wallace, G., 75, 221, 246, 253, 257, 421, 451, 509, 567, 582, 610, 765, 774
Wallace, R. B., 222
Wallace, S., 814
Waller, A., 361
Waller, M., 425, 426, 509
Wallesch, C., 34, 49, 94, 180, 193, 290, 378, 536, 568, 575, 584, 771, 831, 832
Walshaw, D., 119, 178, 295
Walters, G., 613
Walters, R., 488
Waltz, A. G., 56
Wambaugh, J. L., 92, 197, 419, 520, 553, 619, 710, 776, 1009, 1016, 1017, 1018, 1019, 1020, 1021, 1022, 1023, 1024, 1025, 1026, 1027, 1028, 1029
Wang, L., 102, 768, 771
Wang, S. J., 550
Wang, W., 250
Wapner, W., 567, 570, 576, 969, 970, 971, 972, 976
Warach, S., 1011
Warburton, E., 190, 757, 1016
Ward, A., 926
Ward, C., 291, 363
Ward, C. D., 110, 361
Ward, C. H., 994
Warden, M. R., 76
Ward-Lonergan, J., 108, 187, 361, 508, 565, 572, 585, 817

Ward-Longergan, J., 817
Ware, J. E., 357
Warren, D. W., 1011
Warren, R. G., 128
Warren, R. L., 165, 172, 173, 175, 177, 395
Warren, S., 487
Warren, S. F., 392, 393
Warrington, E. K., 35, 37, 106, 418, 422, 547, 567, 568, 609, 610, 611, 693, 696, 991
Wasterlain, C. G., 49
Watamori, T., 260, 261, 264
Watanabe, I., 54
Waterman, R., 212
Waters, G., 103, 418, 620, 623, 765, 969
Watkins, K., 1009, 1010, 1011
Watkins, L. B., 102, 411
Watkins, R., 899
Watson, M. G., 894
Watson, N., 1015
Watson, P., 916
Watson, R. T., 92, 964, 965, 977
Watt, J., 771
Waugh, P. F., 1026
Wearing, D., 96
Webb, W. G., 100, 416, 767
Weber, C., 778, 864
Weber, L. S., 899
Webster, J., 67, 619, 643
Webster Ross, G., 259
Webster's New Collegiate Dictionary, 128, 483
Wechsler, D., 75, 97, 98
Weddell, R., 894
Weekes, B., 782
Weekes, B. S., 257
Weeks, D. L., 718
Ween, J. E., 96
Weese, G. D., 534
Wegner, M. L., 515
Wehman, P., 894, 896, 902
Wehmeyer, M., 892, 914
Wei, J. Y., 206
Weidner, W. E., 102, 409, 411, 415, 416, 419, 516
Weigl, E., 418
Weikart, D. P., 910
Weiler, M. D., 967
Weiller, C., 190, 538, 610
Weinand, M., 53
Weinberger, M., 319, 357
Weiner, D. A., 507
Weiner, M. F., 554, 1001
Weiner, M. W., 992
Weingartner, H., 975
Weinrich, M., 361, 419, 565, 583, 586, 645, 710, 761, 777, 778, 832, 864
Weinstein, S., 409
Weintraub, S., 89, 102, 256, 415, 515, 545, 546, 548, 549, 551, 552, 578, 724, 977
Weisenburg, T., 756
Weismer, G., 1020
Weismer, J. F., 93
Weiss, D., 437, 756
Weiss, S. J., 584
Weissling, K., 814, 823, 825
Wekstein, D. R., 990

Welch, K. M., 191, 757
Welch, L. W., 74
Wells, A., 126, 297
Wells, C. R., 569
Wells, J., 868
Welsh, M. C., 910
Weltens, B., 249
Wender, D., 260, 264
Wenig, B., 930
Weniger, D., 77, 256
Wenz, C., 378
Wepman, J., 6, 7, 8, 15, 125, 376, 383, 403, 404, 406, 407, 408, 416, 417, 421, 429, 451, 452, 485, 487, 492, 495, 496, 497, 518, 519, 520, 523, 578, 756, 968
Werdner, W., 776
Werhahn, K. J., 54
Wernicke, C., 20, 21, 27, 1016
Wersinger, J., 377
Wertman, E., 696
Wertz, R. T., 79, 81, 82, 85, 108, 117, 120, 121, 122, 123, 124, 125, 166, 167, 168, 169, 170, 171, 174, 180, 192, 196, 204, 236, 259, 319, 350, 360, 361, 362, 377, 382, 385, 391, 392, 395, 409, 420, 430, 431, 433, 437, 508, 524, 567, 574, 586, 665, 756, 757, 761, 762, 803, 832, 853, 855, 856, 858, 859, 860, 861, 862, 864, 865, 866, 1018, 1021, 1022, 1023, 1025, 1026
Wertz, R. W., 968
Wertz, T., 300
Werven, G. W., 205, 865
Wesolowski, M. D., 928
Wessinger, M., 535
West, J. E., 710, 1022
West, J. F., 515
West, M. D., 896
Westbury, C., 89, 545, 546, 549, 550, 551, 552
Westby, C., 296, 297, 899
Wester, K., 535
Wester, P. O., 11
Westernoff, F., 246
Weston, R., 206
Weylman, S. T., 969, 971, 972, 976
Whatmough, C., 698
Wheeler, K. M., 858
Whelton, P. K., 12
Whisnant, J. P., 43, 46
Whitaker, H. A., 837
White, L., 259
White, R. M., 919, 920
Whiteaker, A., 34
Whitehead, V., 698
Whitehouse, P., 410
Whiteneck, G., 351, 357
White-Thompson, M., 618
Whitney, C., 768
Whitney, J. L., 171, 173, 431, 757
Whitten, P., 205
Whitworth, A., 67, 68, 82, 100, 179, 253, 297, 299
WHO. *See* World Health Organization
WHOQOL Group, 356, 357
WHOQOL: Measuring quality of life, 121, 122

WHOQOL-BREF. *See* World Health Organization Quality of LIfe
Whurr, R., 71, 195, 198, 451
Whyte, E. M., 94
Whyte, J., 89
Wichter, M. D., 609
Wicks, L. B., 217
Wiebers, D. O., 43
Wiederholt, J. L., 75, 578, 657
Wiegers, J., 762
Wiener, D., 260
Wiener, J., 902
Wiener, M., 109, 427, 771, 830
Wiese, H., 967
Wiggins, R., 294
Wiggins, R. D., 192
Wiig, E., 88, 101
Wiig, E. W., 253
Wilcox, J., 293, 301, 377, 378, 385, 391, 426, 586, 587
Wilcox, M., 830
Wilcox, M. H., 385
Wilcox, M. J., 116, 174, 482, 499, 509, 520, 587, 777, 859
Wilkes-Gibbs, D., 293
Wilkins, A. M., 967
Wilkins, D., 764
Wilkinson, G. S., 75
Wilkinson, K. M., 824
Wilkinson, M., 893
Wilkinson, R., 118, 178, 299
Willer, B., 886
Williams, A., 207
Williams, J., 340
Williams, J. N., 249
Williams, J. P., 918
Williams, L., 319
Williams, L. S., 121, 357, 364
Williams, M., 75, 98, 100
Williams, P., 339
Williams, P. L., 43
Williams, S. E., 411, 419, 422, 776, 780, 781
Williamson, D. H., 892
Williamson, P. A., 967
Willich, S. N., 11
Willison, J., 75
Willmes, K., 73, 256, 300, 355, 437, 520, 757, 967
Willows, D. M., 249
Wilshire, C. E., 105, 108, 109
Wilson, B. A., 92, 96, 97, 98, 600, 623, 904, 905, 916, 920, 921, 922, 994, 998
Wilson, J., 995
Wilson, L., 205
Wilson, R., 91, 1024, 1025
Wilson, S. M., 1011
Wilssens, I., 536
Wimmer, A., 537
Winckel, J., 306
Windsor, J., 1027
Wineburgh, L., 15
Wingfield, A., 4, 8, 21, 764
Winhuisen, L., 54
Winkel, G., 323
Winner, E., 774, 971, 972

Winograd, T., 509
Winsler, A., 899
Winstein, C. J., 718
Winter, J., 998
Wipplinger, M., 414
Wirz, S., 118, 119
Wise, R. J., 50, 190, 757, 1015, 1016
Wise, S., 1011
Wisotzek, I. E., 924
Wityk, R., 767
Wohl, C., 178, 255, 298, 319, 356
Wolf, M. M., 929
Wolf, P. A., 256
Wolfe, G. R., 858, 860, 866
Wolfeck, B. B., 423
Wollack, J. A., 965
Wolters, E. C., 544
Wong, A. B., 964
Wong, K., 740
Wong, P. C. M., 642, 646
Wong, Y., 966
Wood, D., 896, 926
Wood, R. E., 718
Wood, V., 70
Woodcock, J. P., 47
Woodruff, W. W., 965
Woolf, C., 290, 360, 391
Woolf, S. H., 14
Woolfolk, E., 75
Work, M., 1014, 1016
World Health Organization (WHO), 4, 9–10,
    42, 164, 195, 281, 291, 295, 296, 305, 328,
    350, 351, 385, 831, 885, 1003
World Health Organization Quality of Life
    (WHOQOL-BREF), 122
Worrall, L. E., 14, 69, 79, 89, 119, 120, 121,
    123, 128, 179, 221, 256, 290, 291, 292, 294,
    295, 296, 298, 300, 305, 307, 343, 350, 351,
    355, 356, 362, 363, 382, 391, 513, 763, 831
Worsley, J., 294, 378
Wotton, G., 295, 306, 333
Wozniak, M. A., 641
Wright, D., 544
Wright, H. H., 96, 426
Wright, J., 80
Wright, M., 360
Wrisberg, C. A., 717, 718
Wu, G. Y., 13
Wulfeck, B., 114, 257, 705
Wunderlich, A., 977, 978

Wurtz, R. H., 533
Wykle, M., 1002
Wylie, T., 967
Wyller, T., 11, 291, 360

Xu, J., 768
Xu, X. J., 190, 191
Xuereb, J., 546, 552

Yajima, M., 660
Yalom, I. D., 377
Yamada, T., 21
Yamaguchi, F., 50
Yamamoto, M., 50
Yamanouchi, H., 552
Yamasaki, Y., 259
Yanagihara, T., 50, 547, 551
Yang, B. J., 567
Yang, F., 567
Yang, T. C., 567
Yarbrough, S. C., 928
Yardley, A., 477
Yarnell, P., 49
Yasuda, K., 567, 921, 922
Yates, A. J., 552
Yedor, K., 393, 394, 496, 520, 585
Yelnik, A., 80
Yesavage, J. A., 80, 94
Yiu, E., 256, 343, 363
Ylvisaker, M., 14, 88, 96, 173, 174, 879, 880,
    881, 885, 887, 891, 892, 893, 894, 895, 896,
    897, 898, 899, 900, 902, 903, 904, 905, 906,
    910, 912, 913, 915, 918, 919, 921, 923, 924,
    925, 926, 927, 928, 929, 930, 931, 933, 934,
    935, 936, 937, 939, 940
Yoder, C. Y., 868
Yokoyama, K., 967
Yong, M., 246
Yorkston, K., 93, 170, 174, 297, 437, 454, 457,
    458, 492, 601, 815, 894, 1018, 1020, 1026
Yoshihata, H., 173
Youakim, M., 535
Youmans, G., 302, 361
Young, A., 77
Young, A. W., 695
Young, L., 517
Young, M., 304
Young, N. A., 53
Young, P. H., 881
Young, R., 246, 323

Young-Charles, H., 392
Youse, K., 89
Yule, G., 1016
Yunis, C., 11, 12

Zafonte, R. D., 894
Zahn, R., 565, 574, 575
Zahn, T. P., 967
Zaidel, D. W., 697
Zaidel, E., 697, 976
Zalagens, M. R., 893
Zanetti, O., 997, 998
Zangwill, O., 492
Zanobia, M. E., 193
Zanobio, M. E., 705
Zarcone, J. R., 905
Zasler, N. D., 887, 895
Zatorre, R. J., 251
Zatz, L. M., 49
Zawacki, T., 91
Zeches, J., 170
Zechner, K., 865
Zeller, R. A., 76
Zemva, N., 128, 323
Zencius, A. H., 928
Zettin, M., 37, 977
Zhao, C., 13
Ziegler, W., 113, 977, 978, 1024, 1025
Zientz, J., 1001, 1002
Zilbovicius, M., 264
Zilhka, E., 994
Zilles, K., 1013, 1014, 1015
Zillmer, E., 98
Zimmerman, B., 470, 477
Zingeser, L., 109, 422, 611, 612, 613, 735
Ziol, E., 1002
Ziolko, M., 338
Zipoli, R. P., 129
Zivin, J., 10, 51
Zoghaib, C., 68
Zola, S., 989
Zola-Morgan, S., 708, 715
Zonca, G., 257
Zorthian, A., 519
Zorzi, M., 610, 674
Zou, D. J., 13
Zraik, R. I., 14
Zurif, E., 704, 738, 740, 864
Zurif, E. B., 421, 423, 427, 515, 586, 633, 758
Zwahlen, J., 558

Subject Index

In this index, page numbers followed by the letter "*f*" designate figures; page numbers followed by the letter "*t*" designate tables; (see also) cross-references designate related topics or more detailed subtopic breakdowns.

AAC. *See* Augmentative or Alternative Communication Systems
Aachen Aphasia Test, 73, 78, 256, 558
Abstract attitude, 6
Abstraction, 476–477
Abstractness, 421
ACESA. *See* Assessment of Communication Effectiveness in Severe Aphasia
Acetylcholine, 990–991
Acetylcholinesterase, 990
Acoustic treatment, 335
Acoustic-articulatory motor pattern associator network, 694–695
ACS. *See* Activity Card Sort
ACT. *See* Anagram and Copy Treatment
Action for Dysphasic Adults, 388
Action Naming Test, 741
Activation theory, 973, 975
Activities and participation, 10
Activities of daily living (ADL), 52, 55, 206
    Alzheimer's disease and, 997
    primary progressive aphasia and, 546
Activity Card Sort (ACS), 299
Activity limitations, 10
AD. *See* Alzheimer's disease
ADA. *See* Americans with Disabilities Act
Adaptation, 294
ADAS. *See* Alzheimer's Disease Assessment Scale
ADHD. *See* Attention deficit hyperactivity disorder
ADL. *See* Activities of daily living
Administrative tasks, 209–212
ADP. *See* Aphasia Diagnostic Profiles
Advocacy, 214, 309–310
    context-based treatment and, 524
    treatments based on, 382–384
Advocacy reports, 382–384
Adynamic aphasia, 711
Age
    aphasia and, 192, 206, 550
    bilingualism and, 250
    global aphasia and, 572
    primary progressive aphasia and, 550
    prognosis formulation and, 192
Ageism, 206–207
Aging
    communication and, 13
    ecological model of, 363–364, 364*f*
    financial aspects of, 207
    language intervention and, 206
    successful, 207

Agnosia, 65
    visual, 609
Agrammatism, 633–634
    assessment of, 741–744
    computer-aided communication and, 762
    defining, 735–736
    morphologic, 704
    spontaneous language profile for, 745*t*
    theoretic underpinnings of, 736–741
    treatment of, 741–750
Agraphia, 9, 667, 667*t*
    deep, 661–671, 663*f*
    phonologic, 662*f*, 667–671
    surface, 661*f*, 670–671
    treatment for, 663–666
AI. *See* Artificial intelligence
Akinetic mutism, 37–38, 39*f*, 56
Alexia, 9
    assessment of, 656–657
    deep, 661–666, 663*f*
    phonologic, 661–663, 662*f*
    profiles of, 656*t*
    pure, 656–660
    surface, 660–661, 661*f*
    treatment for, 657–661, 663–666
    unspecified, 665–666
ALFA. *See* Assessment of Language-Related Functional Activities
Allographics conversion process, 666, 783
    impairment of, 672–674, 673*f*
    treatment of, 673–674
Allographs, 666
ALS. *See* Amyotrophic lateral sclerosis
Alternative meanings, 972–973, 975
Alzheimer's disease (AD), 20, 87, 543, 545, 552, 894, 988, 994
    activities of daily living and, 997
    behavioral treatment for, 996–1003
    caregiver training and, 1001–1002
    cognitive stimulation and, 1000–1001
    communication ability and, 993
    conceptual information and, 991
    development of, 989–991, 990*f*
    functional maintenance therapy and, 1002
    generalization and, 1001
    group therapy for, 999–1000
    hippocampus and, 989–990, 990*f*
    memory and, 991
    Montessori activities and, 999
    multicomponent treatment programs for, 999–1000
    naming and, 991

neurochemical deficiencies in, 990–991
    recognition memory and, 998–999
    sensory stimulation and, 999
    spaced-retrieval training for, 996–997, 1002
    spared-memory processes and, 997–998
    verbal fluency and, 991
Alzheimer's Disease Assessment Scale (ADAS), 996
Alzheimer's Quick Test, 88
Ambient noise, 335
American Sign Language (ASL), 20
American-Indian Code, 583, 772
Americans with Disabilities Act (ADA), 215, 280–281, 306
Amitriptyline (Elavil), 55*t*
Amnesia, 922
Amnesic aphasia. *See* Anomic aphasia
Amphetamine, 55*t*, 56
Amsterdam-Nijmegen Everyday Language Test, 80, 522, 571
Amygdala, 26
Amyotrophic lateral sclerosis (ALS), 552, 555
Anagram and Copy Treatment (ACT), 197, 668–670, 670*f*
Aneurysm, 47
Angiography, 47
Anomia, 776
    compensations and, 518–520
    computer-assisted therapy for, 862
    direct approaches for, 519–520
    indirect approaches to, 518–519
    noun, 708
    traumatic brain injury and, 891
    verb, 708
    Wernicke's aphasia and, 518–520
Anomic aphasia, 8, 35, 37, 38*f*, 307, 570, 720–721, 817
Anticoagulation, 46
Antiplatelet agents, 46, 51. *See also* Aspirin
Anxiolytics, 55
AOS. *See* Apraxia of speech
Apathy syndrome, 52
Aphasia
    AAC relation with, 815–817
    acquiring, 3–4
    adynamic, 711
    age and, 192, 206, 550
    anomic, 8, 35, 37, 38*f*, 307, 570, 720–721, 817
    atypical, 36*f*, 37*f*
    bilingual, 252–260, 261*t*–263*t*, 263–267
    bilingual/multilingual, 178–179, 245

Aphasia (*continued*)

brain anatomy and, 21–24, 26

Broca's, 8, 20–21, 25*f*, 27*f*, 259, 309–310, 410, 419, 537, 567, 569, 570–571, 704–706, 735, 817, 827, 855

  canonical sentence computation and, 738

  neuroanatomy of, 26–27, 27*f*

  sentence deficits and, 632–634

characteristics of, 125

childhood, 3–4

classification of, 81, 405–406, 547–548, 817

conceptual frameworks for

  body structure and function, activity, and participation, 9–10

  concrete-abstract, 6

  information processing, 9

  microgenetic view of, 7

  multidimensional, 7–9

  problem solving, 9

  propositional language, 4, 6

  psycholinguistic, 9

  thought process, 6

  unidimensional, 6–7

conduction, 8, 28–30, 29*f*, 570, 690–691, 697–698, 706

context and therapy for, 716

crossed, 33, 35*f*

culture and, 326–327

declarative memory and, 709–710

defining, 3–4, 20, 65, 403–404

determining presence of, 84–90

disability and, 349–350

drawing and, 108

environment and, 830–831

epidemiology of, 10–13

etiologies of, 10–13, 547*t*, 569–570

fluent, 7–8, 187–188

future trends in, 15

gender and, 206

gerontology and, 206–207

gesture and, 101–102

global, 8, 30–31, 30*f*, 31*f*, 32*f*, 187, 259, 840

  affect and, 569

  age and, 572

  assessment and, 577

  behavioral treatment targets and, 577–578

  cognition and, 568

  communication and, 568–569

  comprehension and, 567

  demographics of, 566

  depression and, 569

  etiology of, 569–570

  evolution of, 570–572, 572*t*

  expression and, 567–568

  formal tests and, 578–579, 578*t*

  goal revisions and, 576–577

  hemiplegia and, 572–573

  incidence of, 566

  informal tests and, 578*t*, 579–580

  intervention and, 575–578

  language and, 567–568

  lesion site and, 566–567, 575

  Melodic Intonation Therapy and, 840

neuroimaging of, 573–574

prognosis for, 565, 572–576

recovery from, 570–575

treatment of, 565, 576, 580–588, 581*t*

historical overview of, 20–21, 756–757

incidence of, 10–11

information processing and, 816

infrequency of, 891

interdisciplinary approaches to, 13

with intermittent auditory imperception, 406

interpersonal relationships and, 381

interpreting strategies and, 648

irreversible, 406

language intervention in, rationale for, 15

lexical-semantic impairment in, 696–698

life areas framework of, 295–296, 296*f*

life changes from, 13–14

life consequences of, 365

nature of, 404–405

nonfluent, 8, 57, 187–188, 735

optic, 609

PDP model and, 696–698

with persisting dysfluency, 405

perspective of subject in, 296

phonologic impairment in, 696–698, 718–721

prevention of, 12

primary progressive, 8–9, 37, 85, 89, 543–544, 820–821

  age and, 550

  character of, 549–550

  classification of, 547–548

  clinical presentation of, 548–549

  deficits accompanying, 550–551

  defining, 543–544

  demographics of, 545*t*, 550

  diagnostic criteria for, 546–547

  epidemiology of, 545*t*

  histologic pathology of, 551–553

  historical perspective of, 544–546

  management of, 556–559

  neuroimaging of, 551

  PPAOS and, 554–555

procedural memory and, 709–710

progressive, 8–9, 37

progressive nonfluent, 548, 552, 556

referring to people with, 4, 5*t*

resource allocation models and, 436–437

risk factors for, 11

with scattered findings, 405

Scheull's model of, 404–405

with sensorimotor involvement, 405–406

sentence-level deficits in, 632–634

severity classification of, 81–82, 187, 188, 296, 407, 818

simple, 405

social model of, 292

societal awareness of, 342–343

sources of symptoms in, 637–641

stages of, 324*t*–325*t*

stroke and, 10–12

structure and therapy for, 716

subcortical, 530, 537–540, 538*f*

as symbolic processing weakness, 816–817

symptoms of, 403–404

systems analysis approach to, 800–803

tests for

  comprehensive, 71–74

  observational, 68–70, 74, 76

  psychometric considerations for, 76–77

  screening, 70–71, 71*t*

  specific language functions and, 74, 75*t*–76*t*

thalamic, 530–537

transcortical motor, 8, 32, 34*f*, 840

transcortical sensory, 8, 9, 31–32, 33*f*, 611, 840

traumatic brain injury and, 891

type evolution of, 187

verbal retention span and, 416

with visual involvement, 405

Wernicke's, 7–8, 9, 21, 27–28, 28*f*, 191, 259, 567, 569, 570–571, 697–698, 705–706, 764, 817, 840

  assessment of, 510–511, 512*t*–513*t*, 513

  causes of, 507

  characteristics of, 507–508, 508*t*

  Melodic Intonation Therapy and, 840

  neuroanatomy of, 27–28, 28*f*

  prognosis and, 508

  rapid discharge and, 509

  sentence deficits and, 632

  speech patterns in, 517

  therapeutic window for, 509

  treatment of, 514–521

word retrieval and, 774–777

Aphasia Bill of Rights, 241

Aphasia Center Lifelink, 389

Aphasia centers, 343, 389

Aphasia Diagnostic Profiles (ADP), 71, 72, 578

Aphasia family groups, 339–340

The Aphasia Handbook (Sarno & Peters), 382

Aphasia Language Performance Scales, 70, 578

Aphasia Needs Assessment, 820

Aphasia quotient (AQ), 573, 587, 818

Aphasia Tutor, 867

Aphasic Depression Rating Scale, 94

Aphasiologist(s)

  administrative tasks of, 209–211

  advocacy by, 214

  assessment by, 208

  client selection for, 207–208

  consultation by, 208

  counseling by, 209

  education and, 211

  ethical decision-making and, 213

  excellence in, 220–221

  fundraising and, 213

  intervention by, 208

  marketing and, 211–212

  patient communication with, 307–308

  quality assurance and, 212

  referral from, 209

  research by, 213–214

  roles of, 207–214

Apolipoprotein E, 991

Apomorphine, 55*t*

Apprenticeship learning model, 899, 900*t*, 922

Apraxia Battery for Adults, 92

Apraxia, constructional, 964, 971
Apraxia, ideomotor, 550
Apraxia of limbs, 92–93, 550
Apraxia of speech (AOS), 65, 92, 309–310, 543,
  552. *See also* Primary progressive
  apraxia of speech
  AAC and, 1021, 1026–1027
  articulatory-kinematic approaches to,
    1021–1024
  assessment of, 1019–1021
  considerations in treatment of, 1018–1019,
    1018*t*
  cueing for, 1022
  defining, 1017
  eight-step task continuum for, 1027
  feedback and, 1022
  inferior frontal gyrus and, 1014
  insula and, 1015–1016
  intersystemic facilitation/reorganization
    approaches to, 1026
  rate/rhythm control approach to,
    1024–1026
  severity of, 1018, 1018*t*
  singing and, 1026
  therapy approaches for, 1021–1029
Aprosodia, 975
APT. *See* Attention Processing Training
AQ. *See* Aphasia quotient
Argument Structure Complexity Hypothesis,
  738
Arizona Battery for Communication Disorders
  in Dementia, 88, 256, 994–996, 995*t*,
  1000
Arousal
  hyper, 966
  impairment in, 539
  right hemisphere damage and, 966–967
Arteriogram, 46
Arteriovenous malformation (AVM), 28, 29*f*, 47
Artificial intelligence (AI), 865
ASHA CQL. *See* Communication Quality of
  Life Scale
ASHA FACS. *See* ASHA Functional
  Assessment of Communications
  Skills for Adults
ASHA Functional Assessment of
  Communications Skills for Adults
  (ASHA FACS), 120, 123, 178, 356,
  386, 579, 886*t*
ASL. *See* American Sign Language
Aspirin, 46, 51
Assessment. *See also* specific measures
  AAC and, 817–821
  of agrammatism, 741–744
  alexia and, 656–657
  aphasiologists and, 208
  apraxia of speech and, 1019–1021
  attention and, 97
  attention deficits and, 967–968
  bilingualism/multilingualism and, 254–255
  biographical information and, 511
  of clinical performance on tasks, 454
  cognition and, 97–98, 98*t*, 100, 483–484,
    818–819
  comprehension and, 613–614

of content production, 108–109
context-based treatment and, 510–511,
  512*t*–513*t*, 513
defining, 66–67
dementia and, 994–996, 994*t*
depression and, 80, 94, 95, 569, 975–976,
  994
error patterns and, 614, 614*t*
executive functions and, 100
of functional communication, 119–121,
  119*t*
further development in, 128–129
gesture and, 101–102
global aphasia and, 577
goals of, 67, 67*t*
  aphasia presence and, 84–90
  cognitive ability analysis and, 95–98, 100
  complicating conditions and, 90–95
  intervention goals, 126–128
  language content comprehension,
    100–102
  language content production and,
    105–111
  language form comprehension and,
    102–105, 104*t*
  pragmatics, 113–121
  production of language form and,
    111–113
  quality of life, 121–123
  therapy prognosis determination,
    123–126
in-house translation for, 257–258
interview for, 511, 513
lexical model and, 612–614, 613*t*, 614*t*
memory and, 97–98
observation and, 510–511
para-standardized testing for, 511,
  512*t*–513*t*
participation measures for, 299–300
of pragmatics, 118–119, 119*t*
process of, 67–74, 76–84
psychosocial adjustment and, 362
quality of life and, 300
real-life behavior, 178
of recovery, 906
social model and, 295–300, 297*t*–298*t*
social-validity, 178
Thematic Language Stimulation and,
  453–456
thinking and, 98, 100
traumatic brain injury and, 903–906, 904*t*,
  909
of treatments, 174
Wernicke's aphasia and, 510–511,
  512*t*–513*t*, 513
Assessment of Communication Effectiveness in
  Severe Aphasia (ACESA), 74, 580
Assessment of Intelligibility of Dysarthric
  Speech, 93, 1020
Assessment of Language-Related Functional
  Activities (ALFA), 80, 579
Atherosclerosis, 44
Atrial fibrillation, 44, 46
Attention, 763–764
  assessing, 97

impairment of, 539, 965
information processing and, 476
neglect and, 965
right hemisphere damage and, 966–968
selective, 967
sustained, 967
Attention deficit hyperactivity disorder
  (ADHD), 725, 914, 924
Attention deficits, 966–968
  communication and, 967
  treatment of, 967–968
Attention Processing Training (APT), 764
Attentional networks, 967–968
Attentional systems, 534
Attrition, language, 249
Atypical aphasia, 36*f*, 37*f*
Auditory association cortex, 691
Auditory comprehension, 764–766
  computerized treatment and, 861, 867
  Melodic Intonation Therapy and, 839
  speech rate and, 415
  treatment based on, 581–582, 581*t*
Auditory Comprehension Test for Sentences,
  781
Auditory cortex. *See* Primary auditory cortex
Auditory deficit
  imperception and, 406, 430
  information capacity deficit and, 429
  noise buildup, 429
  pattern of, 429–430
  retention deficit in, 429
  slow rise time, 429
Auditory imperception, 406, 430
Auditory perception, 406, 430, 764
Auditory perceptual clarity, 409
Auditory processing, 764–766
Auditory stimulation, 411
Auditory system, 406
Augmentative communication devices,
  864–865, 868, 869
Augmentative or Alternative Communication
  Systems (AAC), 71, 558, 762, 861,
  864–865, 869
  aphasia relation with, 815–817
  apraxia of speech and, 1021, 1026–1027
  assessment for, 817–821
  augmented input/comprehension and, 821
  communication books and, 821–824
  computer-based treatment and, 831–832,
    852–853, 868
  drawing in, 826–827, 828*f*
  environment and, 830–831
  future trends in, 833
  generalization of, 832–833
  gesture and, 828–830
  interventions in, 821–832
  multifaceted interventions with, 815–816
  overview of, 814–815
  technology and, 824–826, 825*f*
  written choice communication and,
    827–828, 828*f*
Augmented comprehension, 821
Augmented input, 821
AUSWEGE, 865
Auto-associator network, 692–693, 700, 703

Automatic language, 454
Automatic serial naming, 106
Automatic speech, 773
Automatic-closure naming, 106
Autonomy, developing, 910, 912, 914–915
AVM. *See* Arteriovenous malformation
Axonal injury, 884*f*

Back to the Drawing Board (BDB), 585–586
BASA. *See* Boston Assessment of Severe Aphasia
Basal ganglia, 21, 25*f*, 26, 34, 989, 991, 1010, 1014
    insula and, 1015
    motor-speech disorders and, 1009
    neglect and, 964
BDAE. *See* Boston Diagnostic Aphasia Examination
BDB. *See* Back to the Drawing Board
Beck Depression Inventory, 994
Bedside tests, 70, 71*t*
Behavior management
    antecedent-focused, 928–931, 928*t*, 929*t*
    communication alternatives and, 931, 932*t*–933*t*, 933–934
    consequence-based, 926–927, 927*t*, 931
    positive, 928–931, 933–934
    social skills training and, 931
Behavior modification, 858
Behavior Rating Inventory of Executive Function, 904
Behavioral Assessment of the Dysexecutive Syndrome, 904
Behavioral disorders
    arousal, 539
    attention, 539
    concept formation, 540
    frontal systems dysfunction, 539–540
    nonlinguistic, 539–540
    treatment and, 577–578
Behavioral impairment, 894–895
    importance of, 923
    rehabilitation for, 923–926
Behavioral rehabilitation, 894–903, 897*t*, 898*t*, 923–926
Behavioral tests, 484
Bias, 76, 169
Bifemelane, 195
Bilingual aphasia
    culture and, 252–253
    future trends for, 265–266
    impairment types in, 258–259
    interpreters and, 254
    intervention issues for, 260, 264–265
    language choice and treatment of, 265
    level of bilingualism and, 253–254
    multi-language testing and, 254–255
    patterns in, 258
    recovery and, 258–260
    test-retest reliability and, 258
    tests for, 255–257
    treatment and, 260, 261*t*–263*t*, 264–265
Bilingual Aphasia Test (BAT), 255
Bilingualism
    age and, 250
    defining, 248–250
    level of, 253–254

localization and, 250–252
    types of, 250
Biographical information, assessment and, 511
BIRCO-39 Scales, 885
Blissymbols, 264, 584–585
Blocked practice, 1023
Body structure and function, 10
BOSS. *See* Burden of Stroke Scale
Boston Assessment of Severe Aphasia (BASA), 73–74, 107, 187, 570–571, 578–579, 586, 772, 817
Boston Classification System, 817–818
Boston Diagnostic Aphasia Examination (BDAE), 7, 71, 72, 73, 79, 82, 85, 196, 255, 256–257, 259, 389, 567, 578, 582, 657, 666, 741, 817, 970, 971*f*, 995
Boston Naming Test, 71, 74, 79, 256, 578, 582, 721, 781
Bradykinesia, 992
Brain. *See also* Traumatic brain injury
    auto-associator networks in, 700, 703
    bilingualism and, 250–252
    blood supply to, 43–44
    imaging of, 47–51
    infection in, 46
    information in, 690
    injury to, 85, 88–89
    knowledge storage and, 689–691
    motor-speech disorders and, 1009–1016
    PDP model emulating, 700–701
    recurrent connections in, 700
    structure of, 689–690
    systems analysis model of, 800–803, 802*f*
    tumors in, 46
    two-way connections in, 700
    vascular supply of, 26
Brain damage
    aphasia and, 3
    knowledge and, 690–691
Brain plasticity, 52, 188, 689, 1011
Brain-behavior relationships, 858
Brainvox, 22
Brief orthographic exposure, 659–660
Brief Test of Head Injury, 88, 904
Broca's aphasia, 8, 20–21, 25*f*, 259, 309–310, 410, 419, 537, 567, 569, 570–571, 704, 705, 706, 735, 817, 827, 855
    canonical sentence computation and, 738
    neuroanatomy of, 26–27, 27*f*
    sentence deficits and, 632–634
Broca's area, 21, 25*f*, 190, 566, 691, 697*f*, 1016
Brodmann's regions, 22*f*, 23
Bromocriptine, 55*t*, 56–57, 195
Brown-Peterson paradigm, 725
Brubaker on Disk, 868
Burden of Stroke Scale (BOSS), 178

CA. *See* Conversation Analysis
CADL. *See* Communicative Activities of Daily Living
CADL-2. *See* Communication Activities of Daily Living-2
CAI. *See* Computer-assisted instruction
Calcarine fissure (CF), 24

Canonical sentence computation, 737–738
Capability profile, 817–820
Capitation, 216
Captain's Log, 868
Carbamazepine (Tegretol), 55*t*
CARM. *See* Complex Aphasia Rehabilitation Model
Carotid artery, 26, 46, 47, 51
Carotid endarterectomy (CEA), 46, 47, 51
CART. *See* Copy and Recall Treatment
Case rate arrangements, 215
Case-managers, 234
CAT. *See* Comprehensive Aphasia Test; Computer-aided therapy
Category naming, 105
CBD. *See* Corticobasal degeneration
CBF. *See* Cerebral blood flow
CBM. *See* Cognitive behavior modification
CC. *See* Corpus callosum
CEA. *See* Carotid endarterectomy
Central nervous system (CNS), degenerative disease of, 543
Cerebellum, 530, 989, 991
    motor-speech disorders and, 1009
Cerebral artery, 26
    global aphasia and, 566–567, 569
Cerebral blood flow (CBF), 49, 775
Cerebral cortex, 24, 55, 530
    insula and, 1015
    motor-speech disorders and, 1010, 1010*f*
Cerebral dominance, 9
Cerebral edema, 188, 883*f*
Cerebral infarcts, 690
Cerebral tumors, 20
Cerebrovascular accident (CVA), 10, 42, 279, 352, 569. *See also* Stroke
Cerebrovascular disease, 20, 990*t*
    dementia and, 992
CETI. *See* Communication Effectiveness Index
CF. *See* Calcarine fissure
Chaotic order, 701
CHART. *See* Craig Hospital Assessment and Reporting Technique
Chart Links, 856
Childhood aphasia, 3–4
Cholesterol, 11
Choline acetyltransferase, 990
Cholinergic system, 990–991
Choroidal artery, 26
Circle of Willis, 26, 44
CIT. *See* Constraint Induced Therapy
Civil rights, 206–207
CJD. *See* Creutzfeldt-Jakob disease
Classification. *See also* International Classification of Functioning, Disability and Health; International Classification of Impairments, Disabilities and Handicaps
    of aphasia, 81, 405–406, 547–548, 817
    Boston System for, 817–818
    of dementia, 994*t*, 995
    of primary progressive aphasia, 547–548
    of primary progressive apraxia of speech, 554–555
    of severity, 81–82, 187, 188, 296, 407, 818

Clinical accountability, 391–392

Clinical decision making, incomplete evidence and, 937, 939

Clinical investigation, 172–173, 392

Clinical meaningfulness, 177

Clinical significance, 164–165, 177–178

Clonidine, 55, 55*t*

Closed head injury (CHI), 881, 882*f*

CNS. *See* Central nervous system

Cochrane systematic review, 195

Code switching, 482

Code-Müller Protocols, 362

Code-switching, 250

Cognition, 9, 501
  analysis of, 95–98, 100
  aspects of, 955
  assessment of, 97–98, 98*t*, 100, 483–484, 818–819
  cognitive therapy and, 488–490
  communication and, 350, 993
  computerized treatment and, 860, 868
  defining, 470–471, 478, 919–920
  developmental, 898–899
  functional rehabilitation approaches to, 915
  global aphasia and, 568
  impairment of, 543, 920
  increasing flexibility of, 522–524
  language and, 763–764, 781
  mental operations and, 95–96
  models of, 598
  primary progressive aphasia and, 550
  rehabilitation for, 894–903, 907*t*–908*t*
  retraining, 920–921
  structure of intellect model and, 96–97, 471

Cognitive approach
  accountability and, 485–487
  future trends in, 502–503
  integration in, 491–492
  intervention and, 484–487
  Life Participation Approach to Aphasia and, 496–497, 497*t*, 498*t*, 499–502
  rationale for, 484–485
  response elaboration training and, 496–497
  tasks for, 492
  therapy objectives of, 487–492
  therapy plan for, 493*t*–495*t*
  therapy principles of, 488
  traumatic brain injury and, 919–923
  virtual reality and, 922–923
  Wepman thought process therapy and, 495–496

Cognitive behavior modification (CBM), 914

Cognitive Linguistic Quick Test (CQLT), 763, 818

Cognitive neuropsychological approaches, 264
  basic assumptions of, 597–598
  clinical applications and, 612–616
  definitions for, 595–596
  future trends in, 649
  generalization and, 621–623
  goal of, 596
  lexical processing model in, 607–612
  limitations of, 600–602, 623
  treatment focusing with, 598–600
  treatment methods and, 617–621

Cognitive neuropsychology, 607

Cognitive semantic therapy, 485, 502–503

Cognitive stimulation, 1000–1001

Cohesion analysis, 109–110

Collaborative referencing, 779

Collateral sprouting, 188

Combined cues, 419

Communication. *See also* Augmentative or Alternative Communication Systems
  aging and, 13
  Alzheimer-type dementia and, 993
  attention deficits and, 967
  barriers to, 232–233
  behavior management and, 931, 932*t*–933*t*, 933–934
  behavioral impairment and, 894–895
  cognition and, 350, 993
  as collaboration, 293
  compensatory, 786
  culture and, 246–248, 247*t*
  dementia and, 993
  drawing for, 108, 585–586, 826–827, 828*f*
  dyadic nature of, 321
  environment and, 114, 329, 330*t*–332*t*, 332, 334–336
  functional, 119–121, 119*t*
    assessment of, 119–121, 119*t*
    baseline, 453–454
    global aphasia and, 579, 580
    quality of life and, 129–130
    Thematic Language Stimulation and, 452–454
  gestural, 771–772
  gestural-verbal, 771–772
  global aphasia and, 568–569
  group, 230–231
  intent in, 115–117
  levels of, 361
  memory impairment and, 894
  natural interaction in, 293–294
  non-aphasic deficits in, 407, 891–895, 892*t*
  non-speech aids for, 583–587
  partner behaviors and, 179
  partner-dependent, 818, 818*t*
  partner-independent, 818, 818*t*
  partners for, 114–115, 337–341, 363, 896, 937
  patient-therapist, 307–308
  patterns of, 233
  pragmatics and, 113–121
  as problem solving/decision making task, 469
  psychosocial impairment and, 894–895
  right hemisphere damage and, 85–86, 963–964
  social approach view of, 293, 300–302
  strategies for, 569
  system of, 758*f*
  team interventions and, 230–231
  team processes and, 233
  traumatic brain injury and, 888, 891–895, 892*t*
  written choice, 827–828, 829*f*

Communication Activities of Daily Living-2 (CADL-2), 119–121, 119*t*, 178, 579

Communication boards, 584

Communication books, 821–824
  content of, 821–822
  goals of, 822
  instruction in using, 824
  organization of, 822–824

Communication Effectiveness Index (CETI), 68*t*, 80, 120, 356, 457, 580, 587

Communication Effectiveness Survey, 886*t*

Communication Environment Inventory, 329, 330*t*–332*t*

Communication intervention
  psychosocial intervention and, 291–292
  self-actualization skills and, 342

Communication Profile, 120

Communication Quality of Life Scale (ASHA CQL), 122

Communication-impaired environment, 329, 332

Communication-related quality of life (CRQOL), 121

Communicative Activities of Daily Living (CADL), 80, 81–82, 386, 390, 457

Communicative confidence
  counseling for, 308
  empowerment and, 308–309
  increasing, 307–309

Communicative Profiling System (CPS), 120, 296

Community Integration Questionnaire, 886*t*

Compensatory communication, 786

Compensatory strategies, 915–916, 917*t*–918*t*, 918–919

Compensatory-strategy training, 301–302

Complementarity principle, 249

Complementizer phrase (CP), 736–737, 737*f*, 741, 747

Complex Aphasia Rehabilitation Model (CARM), 389

Complicating conditions
  apraxia, 92
  auditory and visual agnosia, 91
  auditory and visual sensitivity, 91
  case history and, 90
  dysarthria, 93
  hemiparesis, 93
  identification of, 90–95
  interviews for, 90
  limb apraxia, 92–93
  medical conditions, 93–94
  motoric impairments, 92
  post-stroke psychobehavioral disorders, 94
  rating scales for, 94–95
  right hemisphere function, 91–92

Comprehension
  assessing, 100–102
  auditory, 764–766
  connected language and, 101
  context-based treatment of, 514–517
  form words and, 102–103
  gesture and, 101–102
  impairments of, 617–618
  influential variables in, 102
  lexical model and, 613–614
  morphology and, 102–103

Comprehension (*continued*)
POSSE strategy for, 499
prosodic, 977–978
reading, 455, 654–656, 768–770, 862–863,
867–868
receptive vocabulary and, 100–102
restitutive treatments for, 617
sentence, 633–634, 636–637, 637*f*
substitutive treatments for, 617–618
syntactic constructions and, 103–105, 104*t*
taking responsibility for, 517
treatments for, 618
visual, 768
word, 607
Comprehensive Aphasia Test (CAT), 73
Comprehensive aphasia tests, 71–74
Comprehensive Apraxia Test, 92
Computed tomography (CT), 33, 46, 48, 49,
189–190, 555, 566, 573–574, 575
Computer aided visual communication (C-
ViC), 583, 586, 761–762, 778, 864
Computer Based Microword protocol, 197
Computer Reading Treatment, 196
Computer-aided therapy (CAT), 180, 413, 565,
862
AAC and, 831–832
generalization and, 832
limitations of, 832
Computer-Assisted Anomia Rehabilitation,
862
Computer-assisted instruction (CAI), 865
Computerized aphasia treatment
administrative functions and, 856–857
artificial intelligence applications in, 865
auditory comprehension and, 861, 867
behavioral modification and, 858
brain-behavior relationships and, 858
cognitive problems and, 868
commercial products for, 867–868
definitions for, 852–853
drill and practice in, 859
educational models and, 858–859
efficacy of, 855, 860–867
emotional factors in, 856
feedback and, 858
future trends in, 868–869
generalization and, 855–856
independence and, 856
limitations of, 853–854
modality considerations in, 857
models for, 858–859
patient candidacy for, 860
prognosis and, 855, 860
reading comprehension and, 862–863,
867–868
recreational programs and, 857
simulations in, 859, 865
stimulation and, 859
structure of, 857–858
tasks in, 859
telemedicine and, 865
traditional treatments compared with,
866–867
treatment supplementing, 855
tutorials in, 859

verbal output and, 861–862, 867
writing and, 863–864, 868
Computerized Patient Records System, 856
Computer-only treatment (COT), 852, 862
Concept formation, 476
impairment of, 540
Concept manipulation, 703
rehabilitation for, 725
sentence production and, 704
Concept representation
distributed, 692–693, 693*f*, 703
PDP model and, 692–693, 697*f*
thalamic aphasia and, 537
Condensed practice, 712–714, 713*f*
Conditional Statements, 868
Conduction aphasia, 8, 28–30, 29*f*, 570,
690–691, 697–698, 706
Confidence interval, 171
Confrontation naming, 106
Connected language, 101, 110*t*
Connected utterances, 435
Connectionist models, 691–692, 715, 721*f*
Consequential bias, 76
Constraint Induced Therapy (CIT), 197, 712,
713, 726
Construct validity, 76
Constructional apraxia, 964, 971
Content production, 105–111
analysis of, 112–113
cohesion analysis of, 109–110
error analysis of, 109
form words and, 111
morphology and, 111
neurolinguistic assessment of, 108–109
neuropsychological assessment of, 108–109
phonology and, 113
syntactic constructions and, 111–112,
112*t*
variables influencing, 110–111
Content validity, 76
Content-oriented activities, 231
Context
aphasia therapy and, 716
dependence on, 901
establishing, 514, 515*t*
rehabilitation sensitive to, 898–899, 901
skill, 715
stimulation approach and, 425–427
structural, 716
Context-based treatment
assessment for, 510–511, 512*t*–513*t*, 513
caregiver training and, 517
cognitive flexibility and, 522–524
comprehension and, 517
confidence development in, 521–524
future trends in, 524
information exchange and, 517–520
linguistic variables in, 515–517
measurement in, 522
naturalistic quality of, 509
outcomes and, 510
perseveration and, 518–520
rationale for, 508–510
research and, 524
self-correction and, 520

temporal variables in, 515–516
treatment phase of, 514–521
Contextual photographs, 823–824, 838*f*
Contextual priming, 414, 619
Continuous quality improvement (CQI), 233
Contrast medium, 47
Contrastive stress drills, 1026
Contrecoup injury, 884*f*
Controlled Oral Word Association Test, 74,
721, 995
Contusion, 884*f*
Convergent semantic tests, 483
Convergent thinking, 96, 501–502
cognitive therapy and, 488–491
in structure of intellect model, 472
Conversation
intervention and, 300–301
Language-Oriented Treatment and,
779–781
scaffolded, 302–303
supported, 302–303
Conversation Analysis (CA), 299
Conversation therapy, 301
Conversational coaching, 302, 361, 588, 779
Conversational partners, 363
Conversational prompting, 582
Conversational verbal tasks, 435
Copular constructions, 638
Copy and Recall Treatment (CART), 197,
669–670, 672
Corpus callosum (CC), 23, 24, 690
Cortical reorganization, 189
Cortical rim, 25*f*
Corticobasal degeneration (CBD), 545, 548,
550–551, 552, 555
COT. *See* Computer-only treatment
Coumadin, 51. *See also* Warfarin
Counseling, 308
Coup injury, 884*f*
CP. *See* Complementizer phrase
CPS. *See* Communicative Profiling System
CQI. *See* Continuous quality improvement
CQLT. *See* Cognitive Linguistic Quick Test
Craig Hospital Assessment and Reporting
Technique (CHART), 357–358, 364
Creutzfeldt-Jakob disease (CJD), 552
Criterion-related validity, 76
Crossed aphasia, 33, 35*f*
Cross-modality cueing, 660
Cross-training, 230
CRQOL. *See* Communication-related quality
of life
CT. *See* Computed tomography
Cueing, 264
algorithms for, 861
apraxia of speech therapy with, 1022
combined, 419
cross-modality, 660
functional, 410
hierarchy for, 111*t*, 669*t*, 776–777, 777*f*
Language-Oriented Treatment and, 760
Melodic Intonation Therapy and, 843
neglect and, 966
perceptual, 410
personalized, 519

phonemic, 620, 696
phonologic hierarchy for, 618–620
rhythmic, 1025
self, 418, 861, 966
semantic, 418, 419, 776
sentence production and, 420
stimulation approach and, 417–420
verbal, 843
visual, 334–335
Cultural milieu, 326–327
Culturally and linguistically diverse (CLD), 245–248, 253–254, 266
Culture
bilingual aphasia and, 252–253
communication and, 246–248, 247t
data collection and, 78, 248
diversity of, 245–248
CVA. *See* Cerebrovascular accident
C-ViC. *See* Computer aided visual communication
Cyclophosphamide, 570
Cytoarchitectonic fields, 21–24, 22f, 26

DA. *See* Dopamine
Dartmouth COOP Charts, 355
Data collection, 67–74, 76–81
direct observations for, 69–70
ethnocultural considerations in, 78–79
predictive considerations in, 78
psychometrics and, 76–77
reliability in, 77
reported observations for, 68–69
screening tests for, 70–71, 71t
standardization and, 77–78
Deafness, 20
Deblocking function, 418
Decision making, 474
Declarative memory, 535–536, 708–710, 715, 989
aphasia and, 709–710
Decontextualized cognitive retraining, 920–921
Deep agraphia, 661–663, 663f, 667–668
treating, 668–671
treatment of, 663–666
Deep alexia, 661–663, 663f
treatment of, 663–666
Deep dysgraphia, 668
Defective utterances, 517
Degenerative central nervous system disease, 543
Dementia, 85, 333, 545
assessment of, 994–996, 994t
caregiver training and, 1001–1002
causes of, 87t
cerebrovascular disease and, 992
cognitive stimulation and, 1000–1001
communication ability and, 993
course of, 86–87
depression and, 994
etiologies of, 989, 990t
functional maintenance therapy for, 1002
future trends in, 1003
generalization and, 1001
Lewy body disease and, 992
measurement issues in, 1003

memory and, 988–989, 993
multicomponent treatment programs for, 999–1000
neuropsychological tests sensitive to, 994–996, 994t
Parkinson's disease and, 992–993
pragmatics and, 995
progressive, 49
pseudo, 994
screening tests for, 994–995, 994t
semantic, 547, 548, 552, 556
semantic dysfunction and, 611
semantic skills and, 995
sensory stimulation and, 999
severity scales for, 994t, 995
site of lesion in, 87
spaced-retrieval training for, 1002
stages of, 87–88
syndrome of, 988
vascular, 992
volunteers in treatment for, 1002–1003
Dementia with Lewy bodies (DLB), 992
Depression, 85, 327, 335
assessment and, 80, 94, 95, 569, 975–976, 994
dementia and, 994
global aphasia and, 569
identifying symptoms of, 95
post-stroke, 94
recovery and, 52, 975–976
right hemisphere damage and, 975–976
stroke recovery and, 52, 975–976
Desipramine, 55t
Dextran, 195
Diabetes, 11, 46
Diagnosis-related group system (DRG), 215
Diagnostic and Statistical Manual of Mental Disorders, 4th Edition (DSM-IV), 988, 989, 992
Dialects, 249–250
Diaschisis, 188
Diazepam, 55t
Dietitians, 235
Difficulty
level of, 780
order of, 428
Diffusion tensor imaging (DTI), 1009
Dilantin, 55t. *See also* Phenytoin
Direct language treatment groups, 384–385
Direction following, 434
Disability, 10
adaptation v., 294
aphasia and, 349–350
measures of severity of, 885, 886t
Disability Creation Process (DCP), 352–353, 352f, 355, 360
operational definitions of, 353–354
Disability models. *See also* Disability Creation Process; International Classification of Functioning, Disability and Health; International Classification of Impairments, Disabilities and Handicaps
aphasia and, 355–358, 360–366
applying, 354–355

environmental factors in, 354
life activities/roles in, 353
overview of, 350–354
personal factors in, 353–354, 360–362
Disability Rating Scale, 886t
Disconnection syndromes, 690–691
Discounted fee-for-service arrangements, 215
Discourse, 779–781
narrative, 970
Discourse Comprehension Test, 101
Discourse impairment, 893–894
alternative meanings and, 972–973, 975
compensation strategies and, 919
evaluation of, 973–974
informative content production and, 971–972
macrostructure deficits, 969–970
selection/integration deficits, 970–971
treatment of, 974–975
Discourse patterns, treatment on, 748
Discourse schemas, 919
Discourse skills, 117–118
Discourse structures, 480t, 481–483
Discriminability, 411–412
Disinhibition hypothesis, 927t
Distributed practice, 712–714, 713f
Distributed representation, 692–693, 693f, 703
DIVA model, 1015
Divergent semantic tests, 483
Divergent thinking, 96
cognitive therapy and, 490–491
in structure of intellect model, 472
DLB. *See* Dementia with Lewy bodies
DNR. *See* Do-not-resuscitate orders
Do-not-resuscitate orders (DNR), 213
Dopamine (DA), 55, 56, 57
Drawing, communication with, 108, 585–586, 826–827, 828f
DRG. *See* Diagnosis-related group system
Drill and practice, 859
DSM-IV. *See* Diagnostic and Statistical Manual of Mental Disorders, 4th Edition
DTI. *See* Diffusion tensor imaging
Duke-UNC Health Profile, 81
DynaVox, 868
Dysarthria, 20, 36f, 65, 93, 550, 554
unilateral upper motor neuron, 1017
Dysarthria Examination Battery, 93
Dysgraphia
computer-based treatment and, 862
deep, 668
surface, 862
Dyslexia, 767, 769–770
computer-based treatment and, 862
surface, 862
Dysphagia, 550

EBP. *See* Evidence-based practice
Echocardiography, 47
Echolalia, 33
Ecological model of aging, 363–364, 364f
ECP. *See* Everyday communication partner
ECS. *See* Electrical cortical stimulation
Educational models, computerized treatment and, 858–859

EEG. *See* Electroencephalography
Effect size, 171
Efficacy research, 164
Elavil, 55*t*. *See also* Amitriptyline
Electrical cortical stimulation (ECS), 53–54
Electrocardiogram, 47
Electroencephalography (EEG), 551, 555
Electrolarynx, 1027
Electromagnetic articulography (EMA), 1022
Electronic scheduling devices, 868
Electropalatography (EPG), 1022–1023
EMA. *See* Electromagnetic articulography
Embolism, 44, 538, 992
    transient ischemic attacks and, 46
Emotional support, 338
Endarterectomy, 46, 47, 51
Entorhinal cortex, 989
Environment, 296
    AAC and, 830–831
    aphasia-friendly, 830–831
    communication, 114, 330*t*–332*t*
    communication-impaired, 329, 332
    communication-promoting, 334–336
    cultural, 326–327
    defining, 321, 322*f*, 362–363
    external, 321–322
    handicap and, 354
    ICF and, 10
    IFC and, 831
    importance of, 366
    improvement of, 362–364
    internal, 327–328
    Life Participation Approach to Aphasia and,
        281
    participation measures and, 300
    partners in, 364–366
    physical, 322
    social, 322–323, 325–326
Environmental intervention, 329
    acoustic treatment in, 335
    aphasia family groups and, 339–340
    applications of, 368*t*–369*t*, 369
    concerns in, 333*t*
    environmental factors and, 362–364
    furniture arrangement and, 335–336
    lighting and, 334–335
    philosophy of, 328–329
    props in, 336
    respite and, 340
    safety issues and, 336
    self-actualization skills and, 341–342
    self-efficacy skills and, 341–342
    self-help groups and, 339–340
    skills improvement in, 333–334
    societal awareness and, 342–343
    staff inservice and, 340–341
    stimulation and, 337–338
    stroke education and, 338–339
    visual cues in, 334–335
    wellness programs and, 340
Environmental partner, 364–366
Environmental press, 364, 364*f*
Environmental props, 336
EPG. *See* Electropalatography
Episodic memory, 991

Error analysis, 109
Error patterns, assessment and, 614, 614*t*
Errorless learning, 726–728, 902, 922, 998
Ethics, 213, 221
Ethnocentrism, 232–233
Ethnographic interviews, 296
Evaluation systémique des objectifs prioritaires
        en réadaptation (Systemic Evaluation
        of Priority Goals in Rehabilitation)
        (ESOPE), 366, 367*f*
Evaluative thinking, 96, 781
    cognitive therapy and, 490–491
    in structure of intellect model, 472
Everyday communication partner (ECP), 896,
        912, 926
Everyday Communicative Needs Assessment,
        120, 121*t*
Everyday Language Test, 513
Evidence-based practice (EBP), 14–15, 81, 129,
        166, 172, 175, 194, 258, 319
Evidential bias, 76
Evolution, global aphasia and, 570–572, 572*t*
Examining for Aphasia–Third Edition, 578
Executive-function abilities, 96, 550
    ADHD and, 914
    assessing, 100
    defining, 909–910, 910*t*
    functional rehabilitation approaches to, 915
    impairment of, 891–892
    rehabilitation of, 894–903, 907*t*–908*t*
    scripts for, 910, 911*t*, 912, 914–915
    structured event complexes and, 901
    teaching and, 912, 913*f*
Explicit memory, 726
Extension studies, 174
External memory aids, 921
External validity, 164
Extralinguistic deficits
    alternative meanings and, 972–973, 975
    discourse and, 969–975
    emotional content and, 975–977
    evaluation of, 973–974
    facial expression deficits and, 976
    informative content production and,
        971–972
    integration and, 970–971
    macrostructure, 969–970
    prosodic processing and, 977–979
    selection and, 970–971
    treatment of, 974–975

Facial expression deficits, 976
Family, 323, 339, 340
    counseling and support groups for, 379–382
    generalization and, 833
    Melodic Intonation Therapy and, 851
Family Interaction Analysis, 115, 116*t*
FAS Verbal Fluency Test, 995
FAST. *See* Functional Assessment Staging Scale
FCP. *See* Functional Communication Profile
FDG. *See* Fluorodeoxyglucose
Feedback
    apraxia of speech therapy with, 1022
    computerized treatment and, 858
    in-treatment, 717–718

Language-Oriented Treatment and, 760
    stimulation approach and, 431–432
Feedback loops, 801
Figurative language, 781
FIM. *See* Functional Independence Measure
5-HT. *See* Serotonin
Flat affect, 975–976
Fluent aphasias, 7–8, 187–188
Fluorodeoxyglucose (FDG), 50
Fluoxitine, 55*t*
FMT. *See* Functional maintenance therapy
Form words, 102–103
    production of, 111
Frenchay Activities Index, 80
Frenchay Dysarthria Assessment, 93
Frontal systems, dysfunction of, 539–540
Frontolimbic damage, 891, 892–893, 892*t*, 899
Frontotemporal lobar degeneration (FTLD),
        548, 552, 556
FTLD. *See* Frontotemporal lobar degeneration
Functional Assessment Measure, 80, 886*t*
Functional Assessment of Communicative
        Skills for Adults, 80
Functional Assessment of Verbal Reasoning and
        Executive Strategies, 904
Functional Assessment Staging Scale (FAST),
        995
Functional Auditory Comprehension Task, 578
Functional communication
    assessment of, 119–121, 119*t*
    baseline, 453–454
    global aphasia and, 579, 580
    quality of life and, 129–130
    Thematic Language Stimulation and,
        452–454
Functional Communication Measure, 80
Functional Communication Profile (FCP), 120,
        123, 571, 577, 579, 757
Functional cues, 410
Functional Drawing Training, 586
Functional Independence Measure (FIM), 80
Functional Life Scale, 123
Functional Linguistic Communication
        Inventory, 88, 996
Functional magnetic resonance imaging
        (fMRI), 21, 50–51, 54, 190–192, 251,
        573–574, 575, 603, 757, 967, 968,
        1009, 1012, 1013, 1015, 1016
Functional maintenance therapy (FMT), 1002
Functional outcome, 178
Functional rehabilitation, 319
Functional representation, 636, 639–640
Functional-level impairments, 639–640
Functional-to-positional level, treatment of,
        643–646
Furniture arrangement, 335–336

GABA. *See* Gamma-aminobutyric-acid
Galveston Orientation and Amnesia Test
        (GOAT), 886*t*
Games, context and, 521, 521*t*
Gamma-aminobutyric-acid (GABA), 55, 532,
        535
GDS. *See* Geriatric Depression Scale; Global
        Deterioration Scale

Gender
  language intervention and, 206
  primary progressive aphasia and, 550
  salary/status and, 220
Generality, 163, 171, 178
Generalization, 476–477
  AAC and, 832–833
  Alzheimer's disease and, 1001
  complexity and, 746
  comprehension and, 648
  computer-based treatment and, 832,
    855–856, 861
  constraint induced therapy and, 726
  family and, 833
  gesture and, 830
  intervention promoting, 833
  lack of, 644
  lexical impairment and, 621–623
  mechanisms of, 710–712, 711t
  neglect and, 966
  PDP model and, 710–712
  planning for, 832–833
  semantic therapy and, 723
  across tasks, 622
  tense-agreement forms and, 748
  traumatic brain injury and, 902
  of treatment effects, 647–648
  untrained stimuli and, 622–623
Generalization planning, 393–394
Geriatric Depression Scale (GDS), 80, 94
Gerontology, aphasia and, 206–207
Gestural communication, 771–772
Gestural programs, 583–584
Gestural-verbal communication, 771–772
Gesture, 101–102, 771–772
  AAC and, 828–830
  content production with, 108
  generalization of, 830
  speech production enhancement with, 1026
  substitutive word-retrieval treatment and,
    621
  training for, 829–830
Glasgow Coma Scale (GCS), 886t, 888
Glasgow Outcome Scale, 885, 886t
Global aphasia, 8, 30–31, 30f, 31f, 32f, 187,
    259, 578t, 581–588
  affect and, 569
  age and, 572
  assessment and, 577
  behavioral treatment targets and, 577–578
  cognition and, 568
  communication and, 568–569
  comprehension and, 567
  demographics of, 566
  depression and, 569
  etiology of, 569–570
  evolution of, 570–572, 572t
  expression and, 567–568
  formal tests and, 578–579, 578t
  goal revisions and, 576–577
  hemiplegia and, 572–573
  incidence of, 566
  informal tests and, 578t, 579–580
  intervention and, 575–578
  language and, 567–568, 574–575

lesion site and, 566–567, 575
  Melodic Intonation Therapy and, 840
  neuroimaging of, 573–574
  prognosis for, 565, 575–576
  recovery from, 570–575
  treatment of, 565, 576, 580
    functional approaches to, 581t, 583–588
    impairment-based, 581–583, 581t
    social approaches to, 581t, 588
Global Deterioration Scale (GDS), 995
Goal Attainment Scaling, 366
Goal-attainment scales, 300
Grammar, 479
  class of, 775
  naming and, 775
  rehabilitation strategies for, 724–726
  stimulation approach and, 423–425
  Wernicke's aphasia and, 507–508
  working memory and, 724–725
Grammatical expression, 707
Grammatical morphology, 740–741,
    749f
  articles in, 706–707
  auxiliary verbs in, 706–707
  PDP model and, 702, 706–707
  prepositions in, 707
  pronouns in, 707
  treatment of, 747–748
Graphemes, 655, 664t
Grapheme-to-phoneme conversion, 769
Grapheme-to-sound conversion, 767
Graphemic buffer, 666
  impairment of, 671–672, 672f, 783
  treatment for, 671–672
Graphemic input lexicon, 654
Graphemic lexicon, 767
Graphemic output buffer, 666
Graphemic output lexicon, 666
Graphic expression, 782–786
Graphomotor access, 783
Gray Oral Reading Tests, 578, 657
Group therapy, 302
  Alzheimer's disease and, 999–1000
  clinical accountability and, 391–392
  family counseling and, 379–382
  family support groups and, 379–382
  future trends in, 394–395
  generalization planning and, 393–394
  guiding principles of, 392–394
  history of, 376–377
  multipurpose, 388–391
  psychosocial groups for, 377–379
  traumatic brain injury rehabilitation and,
    934
Group treatment approaches, 179–180, 231
Gus Multimedia Speech System, 587
Gyri, 21–24, 24f, 26
  left posterior inferior frontal, 1013–1014
  motor-speech disorders and, 1009
  superior temporal, 1016

Haldol, 55t. See also Halperidol
Halperidol (Haldol), 55t
Hamilton Rating Scale, 994
Hand tapping, 844, 847, 1024, 1024t

Handicap, 10
  environmental factors in, 354
  life activities and roles and, 353
  personal factors in, 353–354
Handicap Creation Process, 66
HCFA Outcomes and Assessment Information
    Set (OASIS), 166
Head injury. See Closed head injury;
    Penetrating head injury; Traumatic
    brain injury
Health Environmental Factors Model, 831
Health Insurance Portability and
    Accountability Act (HIPAA), 215
Health-maintenance organization (HMO), 216
Heart disease, 11
Hebbian learning, 701, 708, 727
Helm Elicited Language Program for Syntax
    Stimulation (HELPSS), 744–745,
    777–779
HELPSS. See Helm Elicited Language
    Program for Syntax Stimulation
Hematoma, 46
Hemiparesis, 52, 93, 573
Hemiplegia, 52, 56, 565
  global aphasia and, 572–573
Hemorrhagic stroke, 45
Heparin, 51
Heschl's gyrus, 530
99mTc Hexamethylpropylene amine oxide
    (HMPAO), 49
High-overall-prediction method (HOAP),
    803–804
HIPAA. See Health Insurance Portability and
    Accountability Act
Hippocampus, 26, 709, 989
  Alzheimer's disease and, 989–990, 990f
  damage to, 893, 899, 922
HMO. See Health-maintenance organization
HMPAO. See 99mTc hexamethylpropylene
    amine oxide
HOAP. See High-overall-prediction method
Holistic treatment approach, 389. See also
    Complex Aphasia Rehabilitation
    Model
Home health settings, language intervention in,
    205
Hospitals
  language intervention in, 203–204
  rehabilitation, 218
How the Mind Works (Pinker), 471
Human rights issues, 280–281
Huntington's disease, 87
Hyperarousal, 966
Hypertension, 11, 46
Hypothesis formation, 67–68, 81–82
Hypothesis testing, 67–68, 82–84

ICF. See International Classification of
    Functioning, Disability and Health
ICIDH. See International Classification of
    Impairments, Disabilities and Handicaps
IDEA. See Individuals with Disabilities
    Education Act
Idebenone, 195
Ideomotor apraxia, 550

Ideomotor praxis, 92
IFCI. *See* Inpatient Functional Communication Interview
Imagery and gesture therapy, 642
Imitation of contrasts, 1023
Immediate social milieu, 322–323, 325–326
IMP. *See* N-isopropyl-p-iodoamphetamine
Impairment
    adaptation v., 294
    bilingual aphasia and, 258–259
Implicit memory, 726–727, 922, 989
    traumatic brain injury and, 902
Implied meaning, 426
Indirect language treatment groups, 384–385
Individuals with Disabilities Education Act (IDEA), 215, 230, 880, 881
Infantilization and Oppositionality hypothesis, 927*t*
Inference, 969, 970
Inferotemporal cortex, 534
Inflection phrase (IP), 736
Information exchange
    brain and, 690
    improving, 517–520
Information load, 416
Information processing, 9, 474–476
    aphasia and, 816
    memory and, 475–476
Initiation hypothesis, 927*t*
Inpatient Functional Communication Interview (IFCI), 120, 513, 522
Institutional Review Board, 175
Insula, 1015–1016
Integration deficits, 970–971
Intelligence, defining, 471
Intelligent CAI (ICAI), 865
Interaction competence scale, 522, 523*t*
Interdisciplinary teams, 230, 231
Interlanguage, 250
Internal consistency, 77, 163
    task, 803
Internal environment, 327–328
Internal validity, 164, 170
International Classification of Functioning, Disability and Health (ICF), 10, 65–66, 66*f*, 84, 114, 120, 126, 164, 295, 360, 363, 376, 885
    activity and, 79–80
    environment and, 831
    intervention and, 350–352, 351*f*
    societal participation and, 80–81
International Classification of Impairments, Disabilities and Handicaps (ICIDH), 9–10, 351, 351*f*, 352
International Quality fo Life Assessment Project, 855
Interpreters, 254
Interpreting strategies, 648
Interprofessional Perception Scale, 233
Interrater reliability, 77
Intersystemic reorganization/facilitation, 1026
Intervention
    ICF framework and, 350–352, 351*f*
    personal factors and, 360–362

Intervention outcomes, 320*f*. *See also* Treatment outcomes
Intonation, 113, 837
IP. *See* Inflection phrase
Irreversible aphasia syndrome, 406
Ischemic penumbra, 51
Ischemic strokes, 44–45, 530, 887
    dementia and, 992
    imaging of, 48
    subcortical aphasia and, 538
Isolated speech areas, 32–33

Johns Hopkins University Dyslexia and Dysgraphia Battery, 656, 678–686
Judgement, 472, 781. *See also* Evaluative thinking

Key-word technique, 1022
Knowledge
    brain damage and, 690–691
    brain structures and, 689–691
    managerial units of, 919
    nondeclarative, 690
    PDP model and, 692
    word sequence, 725–726

Language. *See also* Bilingualism; Parallel distributed processing model of language
    attrition of, 249
    choice of, 265
    cognition and, 763–764, 781
    components of, 64–65, 65*f*
    comprehension of, 100–105, 104*t*, 197
    concrete, 6
    connected, 101, 106–108, 110*t*
    content of, 100–102, 105–111, 478–479
    defining, 478–483
    figurative, 781
    form of, 102–105, 104*t*, 479–480
    functional links between, 252
    human experience and, 14
    influential variables in, 102
    learning, 692
    mechanism of, 404–405
    Melodic Intonation Therapy and, 839
    morphology of, 102–103
    naming and, 105–106
    neurophysiology of, 404
    nonpropositional, 837
    paraphrasic, 7–8
    processing of, 82
    propositional aspects of, 4, 6
    psycholinguistic approaches to, 9
    Scheull's model of, 404–405
    structure-of-intellect model and, 478, 478*f*
    use of, 480–483
    verbal, 839
    verbal fluency and, 105–106
Language Activities of Daily Living, 858, 867
Language intervention
    aging and, 206
    constraint-induced, 414, 712
    content of, 758
    delivery contexts for, 203–206
    economics of, 215–220

    future trends is, 221–222
    generalization planning and, 394–395
    legislative issues affecting, 214–215
    managed care and, 217–220
Language Master, 855
Language Modalities Test for Aphasia, 7, 578
Language performance, studies of, 196
Language, Speech and Hearing centers, language intervention in, 204
Language-Oriented Treatment (LOT), 756
    auditory comprehension and, 764–766
    auditory perception and, 764
    auditory processing and, 764–766
    automatic speech and, 773
    branching and, 760
    compensatory communication and, 786
    computers in, 761–763
    content and, 758–759
    conversation/discourse and, 779–781
    criterion response and, 760
    cueing and, 760
    data recording and, 760
    demographics of, 786–787, 787*t*
    difficulty levels and, 759–760, 765*f*
    efficacy study of, 786–790, 787*t*, 788*t*, 789*f*, 790*f*
    evolution of, 757–761
    feedback and, 760
    future trends for, 790
    gestural/gestural-verbal communication and, 771–772
    gestures and, 771–772
    graphic expression and, 782–786
    graphomotor access, 783
    guiding principles of, 761
    methodology of, 759–760
    oral expression and, 772–782
    oral reading and, 774
    oral spelling and, 774
    patient-clinician relationship in, 760–761
    philosophy of, 757–758
    phonologic-articulatory production and, 773
    rationale for, 757–758
    repetition and, 773–774
    social signals and, 771
    speech acts and, 772
    visual comprehension, 768
    visual perception, 768
    visual processing and, 766–771
    word orthography and, 783–785
    word retrieval and, 774–777
Lateral premotor areas, 1012–1013
LaTrobe Communication Questionnaire, 886*t*
Learning, 476–478
    apprenticeship model of, 899, 900*t*, 922
    errorless, 726–728, 902, 922, 998
    Hebbian, 701, 708, 727
    mechanisms of, 715
    motor, 1023
    problem solving and, 477–478
    scaffolding and, 922
    self-determined, 892
    Structure-of-Intellect Model and, 476
    traumatic brain injury and, 902
Left posterior inferior frontal gyrus, 1013–1014

Letter-to-sound conversion, 655
impaired, 661–663, 661f
strengthening, 663–665, 664t
Lewy bodies, 87, 545, 990t, 992
Parkinson's disease and, 993
Lexical agraphia. *See* Surface agraphia
Lexical phonologic output, 611–612
tasks involving, 615–616
Lexical phonologic recognition, 615
Lexical processing, 596–597, 596f
assessment and, 612–614, 613t, 614t
clinical applications of, 612–616
comprehension impairments and, 617–618
error patterns and, 614, 614t
gesture and, 621
model of, 607–612, 608f
naming impairments and, 618–621
orthographics mechanisms and, 620–621
phonologic output and, 611–612
phonologic recognition and, 609–610
recovery and, 616–617
stage-specific analysis and, 614–616
treatment and, 617–621
visual recognition and, 608–609
Lexical semantic route, 655
Lexical stimuli, 612–613
Lexical treatment, 663–666
pure alexia and, 657–660
surface alexia and, 660–661
Lexical-semantic access
PDP model and, 691–692
thalamic aphasia and, 536
Lexical-Semantic Activation Inhibition
Treatment (L-SAIT), 557
Lexical-semantic impairment, rehabilitation
strategies for, 718–721
Lexical-semantic memory, 709
Life activities
disability models and, 353
disrupted, 355–358, 360
handicap and, 353
inventory of, 299t
Life expectancy, 206
PPAOS and, 555
primary progressive aphasia and, 550
Life Participation Approach to Aphasia
(LPAA), 10, 84, 369, 376, 377
cognitive intervention and, 496–497, 497t,
498t, 499–502
core values of, 281–282
defining, 279
focus of, 280t
origins of, 280–281
Life Satisfaction Questionnaire, 357
Life-H scale, 357–358, 359f, 360
Lifelink, 389
Limbic system, 893. *See also* Frontolimbic
damage
insula and, 1015
Lindamood Phoneme Sequencing Program,
721
Lingraphica, 586–587
LingraphiCARE America, 868
Linguistic visuoperceptual clarity, 411
Linguistic-Specific Approach (LST), 778

Linguistic-specific treatment, 196
Listening drills, 857
Long-term care centers, language intervention
in, 204
Loose training approaches, 394–395
LOT. *See* Language-Oriented Treatment
Lotus Notes, 856
LPAA. *See* Life Participation Approach to
Aphasia
LST. *See* Linguistic-Specific Approach

Macrostructure deficits, 969–970
Magnetic resonance imaging (MRI), 21, 22, 33,
34, 46, 47–49, 551, 555, 566, 569,
1013. *See also* Diffusion tensor
imaging; Functional magnetic
resonance imaging
Magnetic resonance perfusion, 603
Magnetoencephalography (MEG), 1009
Maintenance groups, 387
Managed care, 216–220
accreditation of, 218
consequences of, 217–219
positive impacts of, 219–220
Managed-care organizations (MCO), 212, 214,
216–219
Managerial knowledge units, 919
MAP kinase, 716
Mapping Therapy, 745, 762, 777–778
Mapping-deficit hypothesis, 646—647
Massed practice, 713
MAST. *See* Mississippi Aphasia Screening Test
Mayo-Portland Adaptability Inventory, 885
MCO. *See* Managed-care organizations
MDS. *See* Minimum Data Set
Meaningfulness, 420–421
Measure of Cognitive-Linguistic Abilities, 904
Measure of the Quality of the Environment
(MQE), 364, 365f
Medial premotor areas, 1012
Medicaid, 214–215, 218
Medical chart, 510
Medical social workers, 234
Medicare, 214–215, 218, 232, 865. *See also*
Diagnosis-related group system;
Prospective-payment system
MEG. *See* Magnetoencephalography
Melodic intonation, 840–842, 842f
Melodic Intonation Therapy (MIT), 191, 264,
384, 391, 427, 772
candidacy for, 839–840
cueing in, 843
examination for, 838
family and, 851
hand tapping and, 844, 847
linguistic content and, 842
objectives of, 837–838
phonologic patterns for, 843t
principles of, 838–839
repetition and, 838, 843
session scoring for, 844
techniques in, 843–844
therapeutic hierarchy of, 838, 843–848,
845t, 847t, 848t, 849t–850t, 851
therapies concurrent with, 848, 851

Memory, 95–96, 500–501, 763–764. *See also*
Knowledge
aids for, 921–922
Alzheimer's disease and, 991, 997–999
aphasia and, 709–710
assessing, 97–98
cognitive therapy and, 488–491
declarative, 535–536, 708–710, 715, 989
dementia and, 988–989
episodic, 991
explicit, 726
impairment of, 894, 921
implicit, 726–727, 902, 922, 989
information processing and, 475–476
lexical-semantic, 709
nondeclarative, 536, 989
PDP model and, 708–710
POSSE strategy for, 499
procedural, 708–710, 715, 902
recognition, 998–999
retrieval of, 894
semantic, 483, 991
spared, 997–998
in structure of intellect model, 471–472
thalamic aphasia and, 536
traumatic brain injury and, 894, 902, 921
working, 724–725, 989, 991
MEND. *See* Miami Emergency Neurologic
Deficit Prehospital Checklist
Mental deficits, 4
Message exchange task, 522, 522t
Message length, 416–417
Message redundancy, 416–417
Message representation, 636, 638–639
Message-level impairment, 638–639, 641–642
Message-to-functional level, treatment of,
642–643
Metalinguistic dialogue, 453
Metaphor, traumatic brain injury rehabilitation
and, 934–936
Methylphenidate (Ritalin), 55t, 569
Metronomic pacing, 1024–1025, 1024t
Meyers-Briggs Inventory, 231
Miami Emergency Neurologic Deficit
Prehospital Checklist (MEND), 71
Microworld Project, 865
Midbrain, 55, 530, 531f
arousal impairment and, 539
Midbrain reticular formation (MRF), 531f,
532–533
Mini-Mental State Examination (MMSE), 995,
1002
Minimum Data Set (MDS), 218
Minnesota Test for Differential Diagnosis of
Aphasia (MTDDA), 9, 71–72, 79,
256–257, 508t, 578
Mississippi Aphasia Screening Test (MAST), 70
MIT. *See* Melodic Intonation Therapy
MMSE. *See* Mini-Mental State Examination
MOR. *See* Multiple oral reading
Morphologic agrammatism, 704
Morphology, 102–103
comprehension and, 424
grammatical, 740–741, 747–748, 749f
production of, 111

Motivation, traumatic brain injury rehabilitation and, 934–936
Motor cortex. *See* Primary motor cortex
Motor impairment, 4
Motor learning, 1023
Motor neuron disease, 552
Motor-speech disorders, 1016
    defining features of, 1017
    insula and, 1015–1016
    left posterior inferior frontal gyrus and, 1013–1014
    management of, 1017–1029
    neuroanatomy of, 1009–1016
    parietal lobe and, 1014–1015
    premotor areas and, 1012–1013
    primary motor cortex and, 1010–1011
    superior temporal gyrus and, 1016
MRF. *See* Midbrain reticular formation
MRI. *See* Magnetic resonance imaging
MS. *See* Multiple sclerosis
MTDDA. *See* Minnesota Test for Differential Diagnosis of Aphasia
MultiCue, 856, 861
Multidimensional scoring, 802–803
Multidisciplinary teams, 230
Multilingual Aphasia Examination, 73, 255–256, 578
Multimedia Microworld, 762
Multimodal Communication Screening Task for Persons with Aphasia, 71
Multi-Modal Communication Screening Task for Persons with Aphasia, 819
Multiple oral reading (MOR), 657–659, 659*t*, 665
Multiple sclerosis (MS), 46
Multipurpose therapy groups, 388–391
Multi-skilling, 230
Multi-Speech, 1020
Muscimol, 535
Mutism, akinetic, 37–38, 39*f*, 56
Myocardial infarction, 44

Naming, 83*f*
    accuracy in, 419
    Alzheimer's disease and, 991
    automatic serial, 106
    automatic-closure, 106
    category, 105
    confrontation, 106
    deficits of, 422
    grammatical class and, 775
    impairments of, 618–621
    pathways for, 696–698
    recognition, 106
    repetition, 106
    therapies for, 643–644, 719, 727
National Outcomes Measurement System (NOMS), 173, 321
National support groups, 241
NE. *See* Norephinephrine
Needs profile, 820
Negative rhetoric, 307
Negative symptom complex, 52
Neglect, 964–966
    attention and, 965

basal ganglia and, 964
evaluation of, 965–966
generalization and, 966
lesion sites in, 964
self-cueing and, 966
symptoms of, 964–965
thalamus and, 964
treatment of, 966
Nelson Reading Skills Test, 101
Neocortex, 990
NeueWEGE, 865
Neural networks, 689–691
    attractors in, 701
    auto-associator networks in, 692–693, 700, 703
    emergent behavior of, 700
    pattern associator, 705
    reorganization of, 728
Neuritic plaques, 990, 990*f*
Neurobehavioral Functioning Inventory, 885
Neurofibrillary tangles, 990, 990*f*
Neurogenesis, 689
Neurogenic disorders, 13. *See also* Aphasia
Neurologic diseases, 543
Neurologic impairment, 52, 165*t*
Neurologic incidents, 3–4
Neurological deficit, 85
Neurology, restorative, 52–57
Neurophysiological studies
    post-rehabilitation, 191–192
    recovery-phase, 190–191
Neuroplasticity, 52. *See also* Brain plasticity
Neurosensory Center Comprehensive Examination for Aphasia, 73, 123, 571, 578
N-isopropyl-p-iodoamphetamine (IMP), 49
Noise
    ambient, 335
    buildup of, 429
    control of, 335
NOMS. *See* National Outcomes Measurement System
Noncanonical sentence computation, 738–740
Non-contextual photographs, 823, 838*f*
Nondeclarative knowledge, 690
Nondeclarative memory, 536, 989
Nonfluent aphasias, 8, 57, 187–188, 735
Nonlinguistic visuoperceptual clarity, 409–411
Nonpropositional language, 837
Non-speech communication aids, 583–587
Nontraditional treatment approaches, evaluating, 179–180
Norephinephrine (NE), 55, 56
Normal comparison data, 174–175
Northwestern Assessment of Verb Inflection, 743, 744*t*
Northwestern Assessment of Verbs and Sentences, 742, 742*f*, 743*t*, 744*f*
Nortriptyline (Pamelor), 55*t*
Noun phrases (NPs), 735, 778
Nouns, assigning, 640
NP-movement, 739–740, 740*f*, 746
NPs. *See* Noun phrases
NR. *See* Reticular nucleus
Nucleus basalis of Meynert, 991

Nurses, 234
Nursing facilities, language intervention in, 204

OASIS. *See* HCFA Outcomes and Assessment Information Set
Object and Action Naming Battery, 578
Object-Action Naming Test, 721
Observation
    assessment and, 510–511
    direct, 69–70
    nonstandard, 74, 76
    reported, 68–69
    structured, 70
    unstructured, 69–70
Occipital cortex, 690
Occipital lobe, 32
Occupational therapy (OT), 235–236
OIL. *See* Orthographic input lexicon
OOL. *See* Orthographic output lexicon
Optic aphasia, 609
Oral expression, 772–782
    automatic speech and, 773
    phonologic-articulatory production and, 773
    repetition and, 773–774
    word retrieval and, 774–777
Oral reading, 197, 578, 657–659, 659*t*, 665, 774
Oral Reading for Language in Aphasia (ORLA), 197, 665
Oral reading treatments, 197, 665. *See also* Multiple oral reading; Oral Reading for Language in Aphasia
Oral spelling, 774
ORLA. *See* Oral Reading for Language in Aphasia
Orthographic input lexicon (OIL), 654, 767
Orthographic output lexicon (OOL), 666, 782, 784
Orthographic word-retrieval treatments, 620–621
Orthography-to-phonology conversion (OPC), 767
OT. *See* Occupational therapy
Outcome-oriented rehabilitation, 240
Outcomes and Assessment Information Set. *See* HCFA Outcomes and Assessment Information Set
Outcomes research, 164

PACE therapy. *See* Promoting Aphasic Communicative Effectiveness
Paced Auditory Serial Addition Test (PASAT), 725
Pacing board, 1024–1025
PALPA. *See* Psycholinguistic Assessments of Language Processing in Aphasia
Pamelor, 55*t*. *See also* Nortriptyline
Parallel distributed processing model of language (PDP model), 691*f*
    acoustic-articulatory motor pathway in, 694–695
    aphasia and, 696–698
    articulatory domain in, 692
    auditory domain in, 691–692
    brain emulation by, 700–701

chaotic order and, 701
concept manipulation and, 703–704, 725
concepts representations in, 692–693, 697*f*
generalization and, 710–712
grammar and, 702–708
grammatical morphology and, 702, 706–707
heuristic value of, 701
knowledge in, 692
lexicons and, 695–696
memory and, 708–710
naming therapy and, 719
phonologic sequence therapy and, 719–721, 722*t*
phonologic/semantic/lexical-semantic processing and, 691–692
phrase structure rules and, 702, 705–706
properties of, 699*t*
rationale for, 698–701
reading model of, 694–695, 694*f*
rehabilitation strategies and, 718–728
semantic therapy and, 721, 723–724, 724*t*
semantic/conceptual domain in, 692
sentence organization and, 702–704
syntax and, 702–706
working memory and, 724–725
Paraphrasias, 7–8
Para-standardized testing, 511, 512*t*–513*t*
Parietal cortex, 697*f*
Parietal lobe, 23, 1010
motor-speech disorders and, 1014–1015
Parkinson's disease (PD), 56, 87, 545, 990*t*
dementia and, 992–993
Lewy bodies and, 993
Parkinson's disease with dementia (PDD), 993
Participation, 298
activities and, 10, 298–299
environment and, 300
goal-attainment scales for, 300
ICF and, 80–81
increasing, 304–305
measures of, 299–300
social intervention and, 298–300
societal, 80–81
Partner training, 303–304, 306, 588, 779–780
PAS. *See* Predicate-argument structures
PASAT. *See* Paced Auditory Serial Addition Test
Pathways: Moving Beyond Stroke and Aphasia (Ewing & Pfalzgraf), 382
Patient Competency Rating Scale, 885
Pattern associator networks, 705
PCAD. *See* Personal Communication Assistant for Dysphasic People
PD. *See* Parkinson's disease
PDD. *See* Parkinson's disease with dementia
PDP model. *See* Parallel distributed processing model of language
Penetrating head injury, 881, 882*f*
Per diem arrangements, 215
Perception
auditory, 406, 430, 764
information processing and, 476
visual, 456, 768
Perceptual cues, 410

Perisylvian region, 691, 697, 697*f*
Perseveration, 456, 518
Personal Communication Assistant for Dysphasic People (PCAD), 762
Personal identity, 365
Personal Wellness Inventory, 123
Personalized cueing, 519
PGC. *See* Phoneme-to-grapheme conversion
Pharmacists, 234–235
Phenobarbitol, 55*t*
Phenytoin (Dilantin), 55, 55*t*
Phoneme occurrences, 687
Phoneme-to-grapheme conversion (PGC), 666, 782, 784
cueing hierarchy for, 669*t*
Phonemic cues, 620, 696
Phonetic derivation, 1022, 1023
Phonetic placement, 1022, 1023
Phonologic agraphia, 662*f*, 667–668
treating, 668–671
Phonologic alexia, 661–663, 662*f*
Phonologic buffer, 655
Phonologic cueing hierarchy, 618–620
Phonologic dysgraphia, 783
Phonologic impairment, 696–698, 718–721
Phonologic input lexicon, 695
Phonologic loop, 989
Phonologic output
impairment of, 665
lexical, 611–612, 615–616
lexicon of, 654
PDP model and, 691–692
Phonologic output lexicon, 654
Phonologic paraphasic errors, 696
Phonologic processing, 691–692, 721*f*
Phonologic recognition, 609–610
Phonologic sequence therapy, 719–721, 722*t*
Phonologic treatment, 565, 601, 618*t*, 619–620
Phonological buffer, 655
Phonological reading route, 655
Phonology, production of, 113
Phrase structure building, 738
Physical therapy (PT), 235–236
PICA. *See* Porch Index of Communicative Ability
Pick's disease, 20, 37, 87, 548, 552, 555
Picture description tasks, 106–107, 107*t*
Piracetam, 195
PNFA. *See* Progressive nonfluent aphasia
Point-to tasks, 433–434
Pons, 55
Porch Index of Communicative Ability (PICA), 56, 71, 72–73, 73*t*, 81, 123, 187, 385, 386, 410, 415, 428, 429, 508*t*, 522, 574, 578, 585, 757, 800, 802, 817, 855, 861, 863, 865, 867
future trends of, 811
patient selection and, 803–804
patient-clinician team and, 809–810
response reinforcement and, 811
stimulus selection and, 805–807, 806*t*
task shifting and, 810–811
treatment format and, 807–809
treatment plan design and, 803–809

treatment priorities and, 810
treatment task selection and, 804–805, 805*f*
Positional level, 636, 637
impairment of, 640–641
Positron emission tomography (PET), 21, 48, 49–50, 54, 190, 251, 551, 565, 603, 757, 775, 968, 1009
POSSE strategy, 499
Post-stroke depression (PSD), 52, 94, 975–976
PPA. *See* Primary progressive aphasia
PPAOS. *See* Primary progressive apraxia of speech
PPO. *See* Preferred provider organization
PPS. *See* Prospective-payment system
Practical significance, 164
Practice effect, 838
Pragmatic Protocol, 115
Pragmatics, 113–121
assessment of, 118–119, 119*t*
communication and, 113–121
communicative intent, 115–117
dementia and, 995
discourse skills, 117–118
speech acts, 115–117
structure-of-intellect model and, 480–481
training for, 923–924
Prazosin, 55, 55*t*
Predicate-argument structures (PAS), 643
Predictability, 426
Preferred provider organization (PPO), 216
Prefrontal cortex, 989
Premotor areas, 1009
lateral, 1012–1013
medial, 1012
neuroanatomy of, 1011–1013
Preparatory training, 583–584
Prestimulation, stimulation approach and, 417–420
Presynaptic marker proteins, 990
Preventive care, 219
Pribedil, 195
Primary auditory cortex, 1016
Primary motor cortex, 1010*f*
neuroanatomy of, 1009–1011
plasticity of, 1011
Primary physicians, 233–234
Primary progressive aphasia (PPA), 8–9, 37, 85, 89, 820–821
activities of daily living and, 546
age and, 550
character of, 549–550
classification of, 547–548
clinical presentation of, 548–549
cognition and, 550
deficits accompanying, 550–551
defining, 543–544
demographics of, 545*t*, 550
diagnostic criteria for, 546–547
epidemiology of, 545*t*
histologic pathology of, 551–553
historical perspective of, 544–546
management of, 556–559
neuroimaging of, 551
PPAOS and, 554–555

Primary progressive apraxia of speech
        (PPAOS), 543
    classification of, 554–555
    clinical presentation of, 555
    deficits accompanying, 555
    defining, 553
    demographics of, 555
    diagnostic criteria for, 554
    histologic pathology of, 556
    historical perspective on, 553–554
    management of, 556–559
    neuroimaging of, 555–556
    primary progressive aphasia and,
        554–555
Priming, contextual, 414, 619
Problem solving, 9, 474
    learning and, 477–478
    spelling as, 671
Problem-focused treatment, 521
Procedural memory, 708–710, 715
    aphasia and, 709–710
    traumatic brain injury and, 902
Procedural reliability, 163, 169
Process-oriented activities, 231
Professional ethnocentrism, 232–233
Professional integrity, 219
Profile of the Communication Environment of
        the Adult Aphasic, 115
Prognosis formulation
    age and, 192
    aphasia characteristics and, 125
    assessment goals and, 123–126
    biographical variables for, 123–124
    computerized treatment and, 855, 860
    gender and, 192–193
    global aphasia and, 565, 572–575
    handedness and, 193
    limitations to, 575–576
    medical variables for, 124
    neuropsychological variables for, 124–125
    personality/social variables for, 125–126
    psychosocial factors in, 193
    stimulability and, 125
    Wernicke's aphasia and, 508
Programmed Assistance to Learning, 855
Progressive aphasia, 8–9, 37
Progressive degenerative diseases, 37
Progressive dementia, 49
Progressive nonfluent aphasia (PNFA), 548,
        552, 556
Progressive supranuclear palsy, 87, 545
Promoting Aphasic Communicative
        Effectiveness (PACE), 264, 385–386,
        391, 520, 587–588, 830
PROMPT. See Prompts for Restructuring Oral
        and Muscular Phonetic Targets
Prompts
    conversational, 582
    stimulation approach and, 417–420
    surface, 1025
Prompts for Restructuring Oral and Muscular
        Phonetic Targets (PROMPT),
        1022–1023, 1027–1028
Propositional language, 837
Propranolol, 55t

Prosodic processing deficits, 977–979
    comprehension and, 977–978
    evaluation of, 978–979
    production and, 978
    treatment for, 979
Prosody patterns, 840–841, 841f, 846
Prospective-payment system (PPS), 215, 218
Prosthetic communities, 306
PSD. See Post-stroke depression
Pseudodementia, 994
PSSCogReHab, 868
Psychiatric disorders, 89–90
Psycholinguistic approaches to language, 9
Psycholinguistic Assessments of Language
        Processing in Aphasia (PALPA), 78,
        83f, 103, 578, 656–657, 666
Psychologists, 235
Psychometrics, 76–77
Psychosocial adjustment, assessing, 362
Psychosocial group therapy, 377–379
Psychosocial impairment
    importance of, 923
    rehabilitation for, 894–903, 923–926
Psychosocial rehabilitation, 291–292, 377–379,
        894–903, 897t, 898t, 923–926
Psychosocial support, 308, 377
PT. See Physical therapy
Pure alexia, 656–660
Putamen, 34, 530, 531f
    global aphasia and, 567
Pyramids and Palm Trees test, 100

QOL. See Quality of life
Qualitative research approach, 178
Quality assurance, 212, 218
Quality of life (QOL), 121–123, 296
    assessment and, 121–123, 300
    family-reported, 122
    functional communication and, 129–130
    measures of, 121, 122, 356–358, 358f, 359f,
        855

Radiography, 48. See also Computed
        tomography
Radiopharmaceuticals, 49
Rancho Los Amigos Levels of Cognitive
        Functioning, 886t, 887
Random practice, 1023
Randomized controlled clinical trial (RCT),
        194
Rate control, 1024–1026, 1024t
Rating Scale of Attentional Behavior, 99f
Rating scales, 94–95
Raven's Colored Progressive Matrices (RCPM),
        568, 570, 866
Raven's Progressive Matrices, 818
rCBF. See Regional cerebral blood flow
RCT. See Randomized controlled clinical trial
Reactive plasticity, 689
Reading. See also Alexia
    compensation in, 658f
    comprehension mechanism for,
        654–656
    comprehension of, 455, 768–770, 862–863,
        867–868

computer-based treatment and, 862–863,
        867–868
    dyslexia and, 769–770
    impairments of, 656–657
    oral, 197, 578, 657–659, 659t, 665, 774
    PDP model and, 694–695, 694f
    representations and, 694
    semantic system and, 654–656, 655f, 658f
    tasks for, 436, 455, 619
    treatment of, 769
Reading Comprehension Adults, 867
Reading Comprehension Battery for Aphasia,
        578
Real-life behavior assessment, 178
Receptive vocabulary, 100–101
Reciprocal scaffolding, 588
Recognition level, mechanisms of, 608–610
Recognition memory, 998–999
Recognition naming, 106
Recognition/understanding, 95
Recovery
    aphasia severity and, 187, 188
    assessment of, 906
    bilingual aphasia and, 258–260
    collaboration in, 936–937
    depression and, 52, 975–976
    global aphasia and, 570–575
    lesion site/size and, 189–190
    lexical processing and, 616–617
    neural mechanisms of, 188–189, 748–750,
        749f
    neuroanatomical factors in, 189–190
    neurophysiologic studies of, 190–191
    pattern of, 187–188
    personal factors in, 192–193
    phonologic routes and, 698
    priorities in, 236–237, 237t
    settings of, 237–239, 238t
    spontaneous, 186, 190, 769
    stroke and, 52–57, 975–976
    time course of, 186–187
    traumatic brain injury and, 887–888,
        936–937, 938t–939t
Recovery-compensation continuum, 389
Recreation therapy, 235
Recurrent connections, 700–701
Reduced Syntax Therapy (REST), 648
Regenerative sprouting, 188
Regional cerebral blood flow (rCBF), 49
Rehabilitation
    behavioral disorders and, 539–540
    cognition and, 894–903, 907t–908t, 915
    cognitive neuroscience and, 899, 901–902
    community and, 240–241
    of concept manipulation, 725
    context-sensitive, 898–899, 901
    culture and, 326–327
    developmental cognitive psychology and,
        898–899
    everyday routine-based, 896–903, 898t, 903t
    executive-function abilities, 894–903,
        907t–908t, 915
    functional, 319
    goals on, 237
    grammar and, 724–726

group therapy and, 934
inpatient, 218
interprofessional strategies for, 366–367
national support groups and, 241
neurophysiologic studies following, 191–192
neuropsychology and, 899, 901–902
outcome-oriented, 240
processes enabling, 689
psychosocial/behavioral, 291–292, 377–379, 894–903, 897t, 898t, 923–926
scaffolding and, 896
of semantic impairment, 721, 723–724, 724t
settings of, 239–240
stroke and, 52
training model for, 899, 900t
traumatic brain injury and, 895–899, 897t, 898t, 900t, 901–903, 903t, 923–926, 934–936
Vygotskyan apprenticeship model for, 899, 900t, 922
Rehabilitation Act, 215
Rehabilitation centers, language intervention in, 204
Reimbursement schemes, 215–216
Life Participation Approach to Aphasia and, 281
Reliability, 77, 164
bilingualism and, 258
data collection and, 77
defining, 163
interrater, 77
procedural, 163, 169
research evaluation and, 168
test-retest, 258
Reminiscence therapy, 521
Repetition, 454
Language-Oriented Treatment and, 773–774
Melodic Intonation Therapy and, 838, 843
naming, 106
oral expression and, 773–774
stimulus, 414–415
tasks, 434
Replication studies, 174
Representations
concept, 537, 692–693, 693f, 697f, 703
distributed, 692–693, 693f, 703
functional, 636, 639–640
impairments involving, 637–641
message, 636, 638–639
PDP model and, 692–693, 697f
positional level, 636, 637, 640–641
reading and, 694
semantic, 610
stress, 427–428
thalamic aphasia and, 537
translating between, 637
visual object tasks for, 614–615
word, 703–704
Request-Response-Evaluation (RRE), 300
Research
aphasiologists and, 213–214
clinical processes and, 165–166
consultation assistance for, 176–177

context-based treatment and, 524
efficacy, 164
evaluating, 166–172, 194
extending, 174
funding, 176–177
initiating, 175–176
interdisciplinary collaboration and, 240
managed care and, 219–220
meta-analyses of, 195
normal comparison data and, 174–175
outcomes, 164, 173, 193–195, 196t
primary studies, 196
process of, 163–164
qualitative, 178
replicating, 174
systematic reviews of, 195
Thematic Language Stimulation, 457–459, 458f
treatment assessment, 174
treatment evaluation, 164, 173, 193–195, 196t
Research and Human Rights Committee, 175
Resource allocation models, 436–437
Resource-utilization group (RUG), 218
Respite programs, 340
Response(s)
characteristics of, 431
criterion, 760
Language-Oriented Treatment and, 760
mode of, 430
patterns of, 803, 803t
reinforcement of, 811
stimulation approach and, 430–431
switching, 434
temporal relationship in, 430
Response Elaboration Training (RET), 197, 393–394, 419, 520–521, 1029
cognitive intervention and, 496–497
REST. See Reduced Syntax Therapy
Restorative neurology, 52–57
RET. See Response Elaboration Training
Retelling, 435
Reticular nucleus (NR), 532–533
Revised Interprofessional Attitude Scale (RIPS), 233
Revised Token Test, 103, 578
Rey Complex Figure Test, 98
RH attentional networks, 967–968
RHD. See Right hemisphere damage
Rheumatic heart disease, 46
Rhythm control, 1024–1026
Rhythmic cues, 1025
Right hemisphere damage (RHD), 85–86, 85t
arousal and, 966–967
attention deficits and, 966–968
attention/perception disorders and, 86
cognitive deficit and, 86
communication disorders and, 85–86, 963–964
depression and, 975–976
discourse deficits in, 969–975
emotional content and, 975–977
extralinguistic deficits in, 968–979
facial expression deficits and, 976
future directions in, 979–980

linguistic defects in, 968
neglect and, 964–966
nonlinguistic deficits associated with, 964–968
prosodic processing and, 977–979
sustained attention and, 967
RIPS. See Revised Interprofessional Attitude Scale
Ritalin, 55t. See also Methylphenidate
Rivermead Behavioral Memory Test (RBMT), 97, 904
Role release, 230
Role/code switching, 482–483
Ross Information Processing Assessment, 904
RRE. See Request-Response-Evaluation
RUG. See Resource-utilization group
Ryff Psychological Well-Being scale, 355

SADQ. See Stroke Aphasia Depression Questionnaire
SAQOL. See Stroke and Aphasia Quality of Life Scale
SCA. See Supported Conversation for Adults with Aphasia
Scaffolded conversations, 302–303, 588
Scaffolding. See also Support systems
learning and, 922
reciprocal, 588
rehabilitation and, 896
Scales of Cognitive Ability for Traumatic Brain Injury, 88, 903
Schizophrenia, 20
Schuell-Wepman-Darley Multimodal-stimulation (SWDM), 195, 196
Science
clinical decision making and, 165–166
clinicians' use of, 166
diagnostic process and, 167t
principles of, 164–165, 165t
Screening instruments, 70–71, 71t
SCT. See Semantic cueing treatment
SD. See Semantic dementia
Segmental phonology, 113
Selection deficits, 970–971
Selective attention, 967
Selective engagement, 704, 707
Self-actualization, 341–342
Self-advocacy, 308–309, 937, 938t–939t
Self-coaching, 924–926, 925t, 926t
Self-correction, 520, 668
Self-cueing, 418, 861
neglect and, 966
Self-determined learning, 892
Self-efficacy, 341–342
Self-esteem, 362
Self-help groups, 308
environmental intervention and, 339–340
Self-initiated verbal tasks, 435
Self-regulation
defining, 909–910
impairment of, 891–892
scripts for, 910, 911t, 912, 914–915
Self-talk, 912, 914
Semantic awareness tests, 483
Semantic complexity, 422

Semantic comprehension training, 618–619
Semantic cueing treatment (SCT), 619
Semantic cues, 418, 419, 776
Semantic dementia (SD), 547, 548, 552, 556
Semantic evaluation tests, 483
Semantic feature analysis (SFA), 419, 519–520
Semantic memory
    Alzheimer's disease and, 991
    tests of, 483
Semantic system
    dementia and, 995
    impairment of, 610–611, 665, 668, 721,
        723–725, 724t
    PDP model and, 691–692
    reading and, 654–656, 655f, 658f
    representations and, 610
    tasks involving, 615
    treatment of, 618–619, 618t, 642, 668
Semantic word category, 421–423
Semantically reversible sentences, 634
Semantic-feature matrix training, 619
Sensory deficits, 4
Sensory stimulation, 406, 999
Sentence comprehension, 633–634, 636–637,
        637f
Sentence Comprehension Test, 742
Sentence computation, 737–740
Sentence construction, 454
Sentence formulation, 777–779
Sentence hierarchy, 777
Sentence processing
    aphasic, 638
    normal, 634, 636–637
Sentence Processing Resource Pack, 103
Sentence production, 424, 634, 635f, 636
    concept modification and, 704
    cueing and, 420
    interpreting strategies and, 648
Sentence Production Priming Test, 742
Sentence recognition, 416
Sentence structure, non-canonical, 645–646, 647f
Sentence verification, 434
Sentence-level deficits, 632–634
Sentence/phrase completion, 435
Sequencing deficits, 416
Serotonin (5-HT), 55
Setting events, 928–930, 929t, 930t
Severity classification, 81–82, 187, 188, 296,
        407, 818
SF-36 Health Survey, 855
SFA. See Semantic feature analysis
Shewan Spontaneous Language Analysis
        (SSLA), 74
Shortened PICA (SPICA), 390
Sickness Impact Profile, 80–81
Simulations, computerized, 859, 865
Sinemet, 56
Singing, apraxia of speech and, 1026
Single photon emission computed tomography
        (SPECT), 48, 49–50, 190, 551, 555
Single-subject experimental designs, 172–173
Skill contexts, 715
Sklar Aphasia Scale, 578
SLP. See Speech-language pathology
SMA. See Supplementary motor area

SOAP note, 83–84, 84f
Social action, 309–310
Social approach to intervention, 565
    activities/participation and, 298–299
    assessment and, 295–300, 297t–298t
    caveats of, 309
    effectiveness of, 295
    elements of, 291
    enhancing communication in, 300–302
    future of, 310
    goals of, 295
    integrating, 291–292
    medical approach v., 291
    participation measurement in, 299–300
    principles of, 292–295
    rationale for, 290
Social interaction scripts, 924–926
Social isolation, 335
Social model
    defining, 292
    intervention within, 300–310
Social network theory, 68, 120, 298f
Social networks, 68, 69f
Social Services Subsidy, 215
Social signals, 771
Social skills training (SST), 923–924, 931
Socialization, 337
Social-validity assessments, 178
Sociolinguistic treatment groups, 384–385
Somatic marker theory, 899, 901, 927t
Somatoparaphrenia, 964
Somatosensory cortex, 530, 728
Somatosensory error map, 1015
Sound-Production Treatment (SPT),
        1028–1029
Sound-to-letter conversion
    impaired, 667–668
    overreliance on, 670–671
    strengthening, 668
Spaced-retrieval training (SRT), 996–997, 1002
Spacing effect, 714–716
SPARCC. See Supporting Partners of People
        with Aphasia in Relationships and
        Conversation
Specific event complexes, 919
SPECT. See Single photon emission computed
        tomography
Spectroscopy, 603
Speech acts, 115–117, 772
Speech areas, 32–33, 566. See also Broca's area;
        Wernicke's area
Speech production, 197
    gestures enhancing, 1026
Speech rate, auditory comprehension and, 415
Speech-language pathology (SLP), 236, 241,
        254, 309, 319, 333, 369, 380
    phases of, 393
Speech-language treatment groups
    advocacy reports and, 382–384
    direct, 384–385
    indirect, 385
    maintenance, 387–388
    overview of, 382
    sociolinguistic, 385–387
    transition, 387

Spelling
    impairments of, 666–668
    lexical treatments for, 668–670
    mechanisms of, 666
    oral, 774
    problem-solving approach to, 671
SPICA. See Shortened PICA
Spiroperidol, 55t
Splenium, 24, 690
Spontaneous recovery, 186, 190, 769
Spouse intervention groups, 380–381
Sprechgesang, 842, 846, 847
SPT. See Sound-Production Treatment
SRT. See Spaced-retrieval training
SSLA. See Shewan Spontaneous Language
        Analysis
SS-QOL. See Stroke-Specific Quality of Life
        Scale
SST. See Social skills training
Standard error, 171
Standardization, 77–78
Stenosis, 44, 47
Stereotypes, 246–248, 567–568
Stimulation approach, 404, 410
    abstractness and, 421
    auditory ability tasks in, 433–434
    auditory deficit and, 429–430
    auditory delivery and, 411
    auditory perceptual clarity in, 409
    client selection for, 407
    combined sensory modalities in, 412–414
    compatibility of, 433
    computerized treatment and, 859
    consequences/feedback and, 431–432
    context and, 425–427
    cues and, 417–420
    defining, 406, 470
    discriminability in, 411–412
    efficacy of, 437
    frequency and, 420–421
    future trends in, 437–439
    general principles of, 408
    grammar and, 423–425
    length/redundancy and, 416–417
    linguistic visuoperceptual clarity in, 411
    meaningfulness and, 420–421
    nonlinguistic visuoperceptual clarity in,
        409–411
    order of difficulty and, 428
    parts of speech in, 421–423
    philosophical underpinnings of, 407–408
    physical factors and, 428–429
    prestimulation and, 417–420
    prompts and, 417–420
    psychological factors and, 428–429
    rate/pause and, 415–416
    rationale of, 406
    reading/writing tasks in, 436
    repetition in, 414–415
    response characteristics and, 430–431
    response considerations in, 430–431
    response mode and, 430
    semantic word category and, 421–423
    sequence of, 432–433
    starting, 432–433

stress and, 427–428
structure of stimulation in, 409–421
success criteria in, 433
syntax and, 423–425
temporal relationship and, 430–431
Thematic Language Stimulation and, 450
verbal and auditory tasks in, 434–435
Stimulus properties, 716–717
Stimulus repetition, 414–415
Stimulus-recognition processes, 608
Story Retelling test. *See* Arizona Battery for
Communication Disorders in
Dementia
Strategic behavior, 915–916, 918–919
Strategy and device trials, 820
Stress, 113
Stress patterning, 1024*t*
Stress representation, 427–428
Stroke, 20
    acute therapy for, 51
    aphasia and, 10–12
    chronic therapy for, 51–52
    cultural factors in, 11
    definition of, 10, 42
    depression and, 52, 94, 975–976
    diagnosis of, 44*t*, 46–47
    diagnostic studies for, 47–51
    environmental intervention and, 338–339
    epidemiology of, 42–43
    ethnic factors in, 11
    etiology of, 43–44
    global aphasia and, 569
    hemorrhagic, 45
    ischemic, 44–45, 48, 530, 538, 887, 992
    neurologic findings in, 45*t*
    pharmaceuticals and recovery form, 54–56
    prevention of, 12, 12*t*, 43
    racial factors in, 11
    recovery from, 52–57, 975–976
    rehabilitation after, 52
    risk factors for, 11, 43, 43*t*
    stages of, 323, 324*t*–325*t*, 325, 338–339
    thalamic gating function and, 533–534
    transient ischemic attacks and, 45–46
    treatment of, 51–52
Stroke and Aphasia Quality of Life Scale
    (SAQOL), 121, 358*f*
Stroke Aphasia Depression Questionnaire
    (SADQ), 80, 94
Stroke clubs, 387
Stroke education, 338–339
Stroke-like syndromes, 46
Stroke-Specific Quality of Life Scale
    (SS-QOL), 121, 357
Structural context, 716
Structured event complexes, 901
Structure-of-Intellect Model, 9, 64, 96–97,
    469, 470*f*
    cognition in, 96–97, 471
    cognitive stimulation approach and, 485
    composite abilities in, 473–474
    content in, 472–473
    convergent thinking in, 472
    divergent thinking in, 472
    evaluative thinking in, 472

information processing and, 474–476, 475*f*
language model in, 478, 478*f*
learning in, 476
memory in, 471–472
mental operations in, 471–472
pragmatics and, 480–481
products of, 97, 473
Subcortical aphasia, 530. *See also* Thalamic aphasia
    behavioral disorders related to, 539–540
    nonthalamic, 537–539, 538*f*
Subject-verb-object constructions (SVO),
    735, 738
Sulci, 21–24, 22*f*, 24*f*, 26
    intraparietal, 1015
Supervision Rating Scale, 885
Supplementary motor area (SMA), 1011–1012
Support systems
    cognitive/behavioral impairment and,
        896–897, 897*t*
    family, 379–382
    partner training for, 306
    prosthetic communities for, 306
    providing, 305–307
    resources for, 306–307
Supported Conversation for Adults with
    Aphasia (SCA), 179, 363, 588, 779
Supported conversations, 302–303
Supporting Partners of People with Aphasia in
    Relationships and Conversation
    (SPPARC), 178
Suppression theory, 973, 975
Suprasegmental phonology, 113
Surface agraphia, 661*f*, 670–671
    treatment of, 671
Surface alexia, 660–661, 661*f*
Surface dysgraphia, 862
Surface dyslexia, 862
Surface prompts, 1025
Sustained attention, 967
SVO. *See* Subject-verb-object constructions
SWDM. *See* Schuell-Wepman-Darley
    Multimodal-stimulation
Sylvian fissure (SF), 23, 530, 569
Symptom awareness, 456
Syntactic constructions, 103–105, 104*t*,
    111–112, 112*t*
Syntactic deficits, treatment of, 744–747
Syntactic stimulation, 196
Syntax
    complexity of, 426
    disorders of, 704–705
    PDP model and, 702–706
    phrase structure rules and, 702, 705–706
    sentence organization and, 702–704
    stimulation approach and, 423–425
    thalamic aphasia and, 536–537
    treatment and, 196–197
Systems analysis approach, 800–802
    internal consistency of tasks and, 803
    multidimensional scoring and, 802–803
    treatment plan design and, 803–809

Task orientation, 456
Tasks for Assessing Motor Speech Planning or
    Programmin Capacity, 92

Tauopathy, 552
Team interventions, 229, 366–367
    documentation and, 240
    evaluations and, 240
    group barriers in, 232–233
    group communication for, 230–231
    leadership for, 232
    models of, 230
    team development for, 231–232
    team members for, 233–236
    treatments and, 240
    weak links in, 233
Tegretol, 55*t*. *See also* Carbamazepine
Tele-Communicology, 865
Telehealth, language intervention in, 205–206
Telemedicine, 865
Temporal lobe, 23
Test of Adolescent and Adult Word Finding,
    105
Test of Problem Solving, 484
Test-retest reliability, 258
Test-retest stability, 77
Thalamic aphasia, 530–537
    concept representation and, 537
    lexical-semantic access and, 536
    memory and, 536
    syntax and, 536–537
Thalamic gating mechanism, 531*f*
    disorders of, 535–537
    operation of, 532–533
    purpose of, 534–535
    stroke and, 533–534
Thalamus, 21, 55, 1010
    behavioral disorders related to, 539–540
    functioning of, 530, 531*f*
    motor-speech disorders and, 1009
    neglect and, 964
    tumors of, 35
Thematic content, 451–452
Thematic Language Stimulation (TLS)
    assessment for, 453–456
    behavioral considerations in, 455–456
    clinical performance on tasks and, 454
    cognitive considerations in, 455–456
    concept of, 450–451
    definition of, 451
    formal testing and, 454–455
    functional communication and, 452–454
    future trends in, 459
    goal definition in, 457
    metalinguistic dialogue and, 453
    Organization and delivery for, 451–452
    patient involvement in, 455–456
    research with, 457–459, 458*f*
    results of, 457–458, 457*f*
    stimulation approach and, 450
    stimulation delivery in, 452
    thematic content in, 451–452
    treatment delivery in, 456–457
    visual perception and, 456
Thematic mapping
    impairment of, 647
    therapies for, 647
Therapeutic set, 514
Therapeutic window, 509

Therapist Helper, 857
Thinking
  assessing, 98, 100
  convergent, 96, 472, 488–491, 501–502
  creative, 484
  divergent, 96, 472, 490–491
  evaluative, 96, 472, 490–491, 781
  structure of intellect model and, 472
  types of, 96
Third-party payers, 215
Thought process therapy, 495–496
Thrombolytic therapy, 49
Thrombosis, 44, 538, 992
  transient ischemic attacks and, 46
Thurstone Word Fluency Test, 74
TIA. *See* Transient ischemic attacks
Tissue plasminogen activator (t-PA), 51, 57
TLS. *See* Thematic Language Stimulation
TMA. *See* Transcortical motor aphasia
TMS. *See* Transcranial magnetic stimulation
Token economies, 931
Token Test, 71, 415, 430, 571, 578, 861. *See also*
    Revised Token Test
Torrance Test of Creative Thinking, 484
Total quality improvement (TQI), 233
Total quality management (TQM), 212
t-PA. *See* Tissue plasminogen activator
TQI. *See* Total quality improvement
TQM. *See* Total quality management
Traffic Sign Tutor, 868
Transactional success, 522
Transcortical motor aphasia (TMA), 8, 32, 34*f*,
    840
Transcortical sensory aphasia (TSA), 8, 9,
    31–32, 33*f*, 611, 840
Transcranial magnetic stimulation (TMS), 54,
    190, 565, 582, 1009, 1013, 1016
Transdisciplinary teams, 230
Transfer, 476–477. *See also* Generalization
  traumatic brain injury and, 902
Transient ischemic attacks (TIA), 45–46
Transition groups, 387
Traumatic brain injury (TBI), 88–89
  anomia and, 891
  aphasia and, 891
  assessment of, 903–906, 904*t*, 909
  attention deficits and, 968
  behavioral impairment from, 894–895
  behavioral/psychosocial rehabilitation for,
    923–926
  cognitive interventions for, 919–923
  collaboration in recovery from, 936–937
  communication and, 888, 891–895, 892*t*
  compensatory strategies and, 915–916,
    917*t*–918*t*, 918–919
  context dependence and, 901
  disability following, 884–885, 886*t*,
    887–888, 891–895, 892*t*
  economic support and, 902–903
  epidemiology of, 880–881
  errorless learning and, 902
  executive dysfunction and, 901
  factors in, 888, 889*f*
  frontolimbic, 891, 892–893, 892*t*
  future trends for, 939–940

generalization and, 902
group therapy and, 934
long-term communication-related outcome
    and, 888, 891–895
measures of, 885, 886*t*
memory aids for, 921
memory impairment from, 894, 902
motivation and rehabilitation from,
    934–936
non-aphasic communication disorders with,
    891–895, 892*t*
outcome prediction and, 885, 886*t*, 887
pathophysiology of, 881, 882*f*, 883*f*, 884,
    884*f*
primary impact damage in, 881, 882*f*, 884*f*
processing capacity and, 901–902
psychosocial impairment from, 894–895
recovery from, 887–888, 936–937,
    938*t*–939*t*
rehabilitation from, 895–899, 897*t*, 898*t*,
    900*t*, 901–903, 903*t*, 923–926,
    934–936
risk factors for, 880–881
secondary damage in, 881, 883*f*, 884
self-advocacy and recovery from, 937,
    938*t*–939*t*
service settings and, 888
Trazodone, 55*t*
Treatment effectiveness, 164
  bilingualism and, 260, 261*t*–263*t*, 264–265
  generalization of, 647–648
  interpreting, 646–649
  investigating, 172–173
Treatment format, 807–809
Treatment interactions, 170
Treatment methods. *See also* Specific
    approaches
  assessing, 174
  auditory comprehension and, 581–582, 581*t*
  bilingual aphasia and, 264
  feedback and, 717–718
  functional approaches to, 581*t*, 583–588
  history of, 756–757
  impairment-based, 581–583, 581*t*
  lexical-semantic impairment and, 718–721
  PDP model and, 718–728
  phonologic impairment and, 718–721
  PICA and, 803–811
  priorities in, 810
  semantic impairment and, 721, 723–724,
    724*t*
  social approaches to, 581*t*, 588
  time distribution in, 712–716
  verbal expression and, 581*t*, 582–583
Treatment of underlying forms (TUF), 736,
    745
Treatment of underlying forms for grammatical
    morphology or functional categories
    (TUF$_{FUNCAT}$), 747–748, 748–749
Treatment of underlying forms for Syntax
    (TUF$_{Syntax}$), 745, 748
Treatment outcomes
  context-based treatment and, 510
  language comprehension and, 197
  measurement of, 164

meta-analyses of, 195
overall language performance and, 196
primary studies on, 196
reading/writing and, 197
research on, 164, 173, 193–195, 196*t*
speech production/fluency and, 197
syntax and, 196–197
systematic reviews of, 195
time distribution and, 712–716
types of, 320–321, 320*f*
word retrieval and, 197
Tree Pruning Hypothesis, 738, 740–741, 741*f*
TSA. *See* Transcortical sensory aphasia
TUF. *See* Treatment of underlying forms
TUF$_{FUNCAT}$. *See* Treatment of underlying forms
    for grammatical morphology or
    functional categories
TUF$_{Syntax}$. *See* Treatment of underlying forms
    for Syntax
Turn-taking rules, 482–483
Tutorials, computerized, 859

Ultrasound, 47. *See also* Echocardiography
Unilateral upper motor neuron dysarthria
    (UUMN dysarthria), 1017
University clinics, language intervention in,
    204–205
UUMN dysarthria. *See* Unilateral upper motor
    neuron dysarthria

VaD. *See* Vascular dementia
VADS. *See* Visual Analogue Dysphoric Scale
    (VADS)
Validity, 164
  construct, 76
  content, 76
  criterion-related, 76
  defining, 163–164
  external, 164
  internal, 164, 170
  research evaluation and, 168–169, 170
  social, 178
  treatment interactions and, 170
VAMS. *See* Visual Analogue Mood Scale
    (VAMS)
Variable practice, 1023
Vascular dementia (VaD), 992, 994
VASES. *See* Visual Analogue Self-Esteem Scale
    (VASES)
VAT. *See* Visual Action Therapy
VBM. *See* Voxel-based morphometry
VCIU. *See* Voluntary Control of Involuntary
    Utterances
Verb and Sentence Test, 103, 741
Verb difficulty, 639
Verb generation, 704
Verb morphology, 644–645, 645*t*
Verb phrase (VP), 737, 737*f*
Verb production, 641–646
Verbal association, 435
Verbal cueing, 843
Verbal expression, 582–583
Verbal fluency, 105–106, 991, 995
Verbal output, computerized treatment and,
    861–862, 867

Verbal Picture Naming Plus, 867
Verbal retention span, 416
Verb-retrieval impairment, 638
Verb-retrieval therapy, 642
    non-canonical sentence structures and,
        645–646, 647f
    verb morphology and, 644–645
    word form and, 643–644
Veterans Affairs Department, 215, 233, 856
Veterans Health Administration, 215
Vibrotactile stimulation, 1026
Vigilance, 967
Virtual reality (VR), 922–923
Visual Action Therapy (VAT), 581, 583,
    771–772, 830
Visual agnosia, 609
Visual Analogue Dysphoric Scale (VADS), 80,
    94
Visual Analogue Mood Scale (VAMS), 80, 94
Visual Analogue Self-Esteem Scale (VASES),
    80, 94–95, 362
Visual comprehension, 768
Visual Confrontation Naming, 856, 867
Visual cortex, 24, 530
Visual cues, 334–335
Visual input lexicon, 654
Visual object recognition, 608–609
Visual object representation tasks, 614–615
Visual output lexicon, 666
Visual perception, 456, 768
Visual processing, 766–771
Visual Retrieval Language System, 389
Visual scene display, 824, 824f, 825f
Vocabulary
    receptive, 100–101
    written, 654

Vocal stress, 427–428
Voice recognition software, 763
Voluntary Control of Involuntary Utterances
    (VCIU), 582
Voxel-based morphometry (VBM), 551
VP. *See* Verb phrase
VR. *See* Virtual reality

WAB. *See* Western Aphasia Battery
WAB Aphasia Quotient, 390
Warfarin, 51
Wechsler Memory Scale, 97
Wellness, 207, 340
Wepman thought process therapy, 495–496
Wernicke-Lichtheim information processing
    model, 691–692
Wernicke's aphasia, 7–8, 9, 21, 191, 259, 567,
    569, 570–571, 697–698, 705–706,
    764, 817
    assessment of, 510–511, 512t–513t, 513
    causes of, 507
    characteristics of, 507–508, 508t
    Melodic Intonation Therapy and, 840
    neuroanatomy of, 27–28, 28f
    prognosis and, 508
    rapid discharge and, 509
    sentence deficits and, 632
    speech patterns in, 517
    therapeutic window for, 509
    treatment of, 514–521
Wernicke's area, 21, 189–190, 507–508, 566,
    573, 575, 697f, 1016
Western Aphasia Battery (WAB), 7, 71, 72, 79,
    81, 85, 187, 256, 259, 386, 390,
    570–571, 573, 587, 657, 666, 741,
    781, 817–818, 863

"Wh-" questions, 435
What Is Aphasia? (Ewing & Pfalzgraf), 382, 499,
    501
Wh-movement, 739, 739f, 746
WHOQOL Instrument, 122, 123,
    356–357
Wisconsin Card Sorting Test, 97, 764, 818
Women, ageism and, 207
Word availability, 703–704
Word comprehension, impairment of, 607
Word form, 643–644
Word frequency, 420–421
Word generation, 1012
Word Intelligibility Test, 1020
Word level, 416
Word orthography, 783–785
Word processing software, 868
Word representations, 703–704
Word retrieval, 197, 421, 774–777
    impairment of, 607
    restitutive treatments for, 618–620,
        618t
    substitutive treatments for, 620–621
Word sequence knowledge, 725–726
Word-exchange errors, 636
Word-intelligibility test, 93, 93t
Word-meaning deafness, 609
Working memory, 724–725, 989, 991
Working Memory Hypothesis, 927t
Writing tasks, 436, 455
    computer-based treatment and, 863–864,
        868
Written choice communication, 827–828,
    829f

Yes/no questions, 434